D0242736

# The Lothian Joint Formulary for Adults

## Abbreviated drug list

First and second choice drugs
from the
Lothian Joint Formulary
for hospitals
and general practice
(www.ljf.scot.nhs.uk)

September 2009
(review date March 2010)

# Contents

| Chapter | Page |
|---|---|

Introduction 1

1: Gastro-intestinal system 2

2: Cardiovascular system 3

3: Respiratory system 5

4: Central nervous system 6

5: Infections 9

6: Endocrine system 12

7: Obstetrics, gynaecology
and urinary-tract disorders 14

8: Malignant disease and immunosuppression 16

9: Nutrition and blood 17

10: Musculoskeletal and joint diseases 18

11: Eyes 19

12: Ear, nose and oropharynx 20

13: Skin 21

14: Vaccines and immunoglobulins *not included*

15: Anaesthesia 25

16: Appendices- *these are available on the website
(www.ljf.scot.nhs.uk) and contain additional information
including palliative care and prescribing in pregnancy*

# Introduction

This abbreviated drug list only includes the names of those drugs suggested as first or second choice in the Lothian Joint Formulary. Drugs recommended as first choice are shaded in grey. Users should refer to the full document and the BNF for further detail and more specific information.

The most up to date version of the Lothian Joint Formulary is maintained in electronic form at **www.ljf.scot.nhs.uk**

For enquiries contact:
prescribing@nhslothian.scot.nhs.uk
Tel:    0131 537 8516

## Key

Drug name shaded grey:         recommended first choice drug

A+B    :         A and B to be administered together

A±B    :         A to be given with or without B

---

### Non-formulary drugs

When patients require a non-formulary drug, because formulary drugs have proven to be ineffective or not tolerated, please communicate the reasons for this when patients transfer from hospital to general practice and vice versa.

---

## 1: GASTRO-INTESTINAL SYSTEM

### 1.1 Antacids and alginates
co-magaldrox 195/220
compound alginic acid preps

### 1.2
**(a) antispasmodics**
mebeverine

**(b) motility stimulants**
metoclopramide
domperidone

### 1.3 Drugs for dyspepsia and GORD

*Antacids:*
co-magaldrox

*Alginates:*
compound alginic acid preps

*$H_2$-receptor antagonists:*
ranitidine

*Proton pump inhibitors:*
lansoprazole
omeprazole

**Drugs for the treatment of peptic ulcers**

**(a) ulcers associated with Helicobacter pylori**

*First choice (for 1 week only):*
lansoprazole (*or* omeprazole)
+ amoxicillin
+ clarithromycin

*Second choice (for eradication failure) (for 1 week only):*
Lansoprazole (*or* omeprazole)
+ amoxicillin
+ metronidazole

*(patients allergic to penicillin may receive tetracycline instead of amoxicillin in one of the above regimens)*

**(b) NSAID-associated ulcers and dyspepsia**
lansoprazole
omeprazole

### 1.4 Antidiarrhoeal drugs

oral rehydration therapy *for acute diarrhoea*
loperamide
codeine phosphate

### 1.5 Drugs for inflammatory bowel disease

**(a) acute exacerbation of ulcerative proctitis or distal inflammatory bowel disease**

*Local treatment:*
mesalazine suppositories
mesalazine foam enema

*Systemic treatment:*
prednisolone
oral mesalazine

**(b) maintenance of remission of colonic inflammatory bowel disease**
Pentasa® (mesalazine m/r)
Asacol® MR (mesalazine m/r)

**(c) steroid-sparing treatment for inflammatory bowel disease**
azathioprine

### 1.6 Laxatives

**(a) acute constipation**
senna
glycerol
bisacodyl

**(b) chronic constipation**
ispaghula husk
senna

**(c) faecal loading of rectum**
sodium citrate enema
phosphate enema

### 1.7 Ano-rectal preparations
Anusol-HC®

### 1.9.4 Pancreatic exocrine insufficiency
Creon®

# 2: CARDIOVASCULAR SYSTEM

**2.1.1 Cardiac glycosides**
digoxin

**2.2.1 Thiazide diuretics**
bendroflumethiazide

**2.2.2 Loop diuretics**
furosemide

**2.2.3 Potassium-sparing diuretics and aldosterone antagonists**
spironolactone
amiloride

**2.2.4 Potassium-sparing diuretics with other diuretics**
co-amilofruse

**2.3.3 Drugs for arrhythmias**

*To be initiated on specialist advice*

*Class 1 (membrane stabilising drugs):*
lidocaine
flecainide

*Class 2 (beta-blockers):*
atenolol

*Class 3 anti-arrhythmic agents:*
amiodarone
sotalol

*Class 4 (calcium-channel blockers):*
verapamil

*Other anti-arrhythmics:*
adenosine
atropine
digoxin

**2.4 Beta-adrenoceptor blocking drugs**
atenolol
bisoprolol

**2.5.4 Alpha-adrenoceptor blocking drugs**
doxazosin

**2.5.5.1 Angiotensin-converting enzyme inhibitors**

*Hypertension:*
lisinopril

*Heart failure and prophylaxis of cardiovascular events:*
lisinopril
ramipril

**2.5.5.2 Angiotensin-II receptor antagonists**

*Heart failure or hypertension:*
candesartan

*Diabetic nephropathy in type 2 diabetes mellitus:*
irbesartan

**2.6.1 Nitrates**

glyceryl trinitrate
isosorbide mononitrate

**2.6.2 Calcium-channel blockers**
*Hypertension:*
amlodipine

*Angina:*
(a) patients not receiving beta-blocker
diltiazem
verapamil

(b) patients receiving beta-blocker
amlodipine

*Supraventricular arrhythmias:*
verapamil

**2.7 Sympathomimetics**

*Sympathomimetics:*
adrenaline

*Inotropic sympathomimetics:*
dobutamine
dopamine

*Vasoconstrictor sympathomimetics:*
noradrenaline acid tartrate

### 2.8.1  Parenteral anticoagulants

*Prophylaxis of DVT:*
> enoxaparin
>
>> unfractionated heparin
>> *where immediate effect is*
>> *needed or reversibility is*
>> *appropriate or in patients*
>> *with CrCl < 30 ml/min*

*Unstable angina non ST and ST*
*segment elevation myocardial*
*infarction:*
> fondaparinux

*Treatment of DVT and PE:*
> enoxaparin
>
>> unfractionated heparin
>> *where immediate effect is*
>> *needed or reversibility is*
>> *appropriate or in patients*
>> *with CrCL < 30 ml/min*

### 2.8.2  Oral anticoagulants
warfarin

*Prophylaxis of venous*
*thromboembolism in orthopaedics*
> rivaroxaban

### 2.9  Antiplatelet drugs

*Secondary prevention in cerebro-*
*vascular disease, cardiovascular*
*disease and peripheral vascular*
*disease:*
> aspirin

*Acute coronary syndrome*
*Non ST elevation myocardial*
*infarction:*
>> aspirin + clopidogrel *for up*
>> *to 3 months then stop*
>> *clopidogrel*

*ST elevation myocardial infarction:*
> aspirin + clopidogrel *for 1*
> *month*

*Prevention of coronary artery stent*
*occlusion:*
>> aspirin + clopidogrel *for 3*
>> *months (bare metal stents)*
>> *or 12 months (drug-eluting*
>> *stents) then stop*
>> *clopidogrel*

*Secondary prevention in*
*cerebrovascular disease*
> aspirin + dipyrimadole m/r

### 2.10  Fibrinolytic drugs

*Acute myocardial infarction:*
> tenecteplase

*Acute ischaemic stroke:*
> alteplase

### 2.11  Antifibrinolytic drugs and haemostatics

> tranexamic acid *for*
> *menorrhagia*

### 2.12  Lipid-regulating drugs

> simvastatin
> atorvastatin

## 3: RESPIRATORY SYSTEM

### 3.1.1 Beta$_2$-agonist bronchodilators

**(a)** short-acting beta$_2$-agonist bronchodilators

> salbutamol
> terbutaline

**(b)** long-acting beta$_2$-agonist bronchodilators

> salmeterol
> formoterol

### 3.1.2 Anticholinergic bronchodilators

*Mild symptoms of COPD:*
> ipratropium bromide

*Moderate-severe symptoms of COPD:*
> tiotropium

### 3.1.3 Theophylline preparations

*Oral:*
> theophylline
> (Uniphyllin Continus®)

*Injection (hospital only):*
> aminophylline

### 3.2 Corticosteroids

**(a)** inhaled corticosteroids
> beclometasone (Clenil Modulite®)
> budesonide
> fluticasone

**(b)** other corticosteroids
*Oral:*
> prednisolone

*Intravenous injection:*
> hydrocortisone

**(c)** combination products
> Seretide®
> Symbicort®

### 3.3.1 Cromoglicate

> sodium cromoglicate

### 3.3.2 Leukotriene receptor antagonists

> montelukast

### 3.4.1 Antihistamines

> chlorphenamine
> cetirizine
> loratadine

### 3.4.3 Allergic emergencies

> adrenaline
> chlorphenamine
> hydrocortisone

### 3.7 Mucolytics

> dornase alfa *for cystic fibrosis*

> nebulised saline *for bronchiectasis*

## 4: CENTRAL NERVOUS SYSTEM

**4.1.1 Hypnotics**
no treatment
temazepam

**4.1.2 Drugs used in the treatment of anxiety**
**(a) acute anxiety state**
diazepam

**(b) anxiety disorders**
*Generalised anxiety disorder, panic disorder, social anxiety disorder, post traumatic stress disorder:*
non-pharmacological therapy
paroxetine

*Obsessive-compulsive disorder:*
non-pharmacological therapy
fluoxetine

**4.2.1 Antipsychotic drugs**
**(a) treatment of acute psychoses**
chlorpromazine
risperidone
olanzapine

**(b) rapid control of agitation and aggression**
haloperidol + lorazepam
olanzapine

**(c) antipsychotics for older patients**
amisulpride
quetiapine

**(c) treatment resistant psychoses**
clozapine

**(f) antipsychotic depot injections**
flupentixol decanoate
zuclopenthixol decanoate

**4.2.3 Mood stabilisers in the treatment of mania**

*Maintenance treatment of bipolar disorder with mood stabilisers:*
lithium (Priadel®)
sodium valproate

**4.3 Antidepressant drugs**

**1. Drug treatment of major depression**

*Newly diagnosed depression:*
fluoxetine
citalopram

*Recurrence of depression:*
previously successful antidepressant

**2. Antidepressants for treatment of anxiety disorders**

see 4.1.2 (b)

**4.4 CNS stimulants**

**(a) narcolepsy:**
modafinil

**(b) attention deficit hyperactivity disorder (ADHD):**
methylphenidate

**4.5 Drugs used in the treatment of obesity**

diet and lifestyle changes
orlistat

**4.6 Drugs used in nausea and vertigo**
**(a) drug treatment of nausea and vomiting**
*Gastric stasis:*
metoclopramide
domperidone

*Migraine:*
metoclopramide
domperidone

*Motion sickness:*
cyclizine

*Opioid-induced (not palliative care)*
cyclizine
prochlorperazine

**(b)** **drug treatment of labyrinthine vertigo**
cinnarizine
prochlorperazine

## 4.7 Analgesics

Dysmenorrhoea, see 7.0 (a).
Musculoskeletal and joint pain (including gout) see 10.1.
Migraine, see 4.7.4.
Peri-operative analgesics, see 15.1.4.2.

*Step 1: mild pain*
ibuprofen
paracetamol
diclofenac sodium

*Step 2: mild to moderate pain*
co-codamol 8/500 ± NSAID (ibuprofen or diclofenac sodium)

co-codamol 30/500 ± NSAID (ibuprofen or diclofenac sodium)

*Step 3: moderate to severe pain*
morphine + paracetamol ± NSAID (ibuprofen or diclofenac sodium)

### 4.7.3 Adjuvant analgesics for chronic pain
amitriptyline

**Neuropathic pain**
amitriptyline
gabapentin

### 4.7.4 Antimigraine drugs

### 4.7.4.1 Treatment of the acute migraine attack

**(a)** **Step 1**
aspirin
ibuprofen
paracetamol

**(b)** **Step 2**
sumatriptan
almotriptan

### 4.7.4.2 Migraine prophylaxis

propranolol
sodium valproate

### 4.7.4.3 Drug treatment of cluster headache

**(a)** **acute attacks**
sumatriptan subcutaneous
sumatriptan nasal

**(b)** **prophylaxis**
verapamil

### 4.8.1 Control of epilepsy

carbamazepine
sodium valproate
lamotrigine

### 4.8.2 Treatment of prolonged seizures and status epilepticus

*Step 1 (in community):*
diazepam rectal solution
midazolam buccal

*Step 2 (in hospital):*
lorazepam injection
diazepam injection (emulsion)
midazolam buccal

*Step 3 (in hospital):*
phenobarbital injection
phenytoin injection

*Step 4:* admit to ITU

| 4.9 | Drugs used in parkinsonism and related disorders |
|---|---|

**4.9.1 Dopaminergic drugs used in parkinsonism**

(a) **dopamine-agonists**
ropinirole
pramipexole

(b) **levodopa**
co-beneldopa (Madopar®)
co-careldopa (Sinemet®)

**4.9.2 Antimuscarinic drugs used in parkinsonism**
orphenadrine

**4.9.3 Drugs used in intractable hiccups, essential tremor and related disorders**

(a) **intractable hiccups**
chlorpromazine

(b) **essential tremor or tremors associated with anxiety or thyrotoxicosis**
propranolol

**4.10 Drugs used in substance dependence**

(a) **acute opioid withdrawal symptoms**
lofexidine
symptomatic relief

(b) **opioid maintenance prescribing**
methadone
dihydrocodeine

(d) **opioid detoxification**
buprenorphine
lofexidine
dihydrocodeine

(e) **opioid relapse prevention**
naltrexone

(f) **acute benzodiazepine withdrawal symptoms**
diazepam
carbamazepine

(g) **benzodiazepine prescribing**
diazepam

(i) **alcohol dependence**

*Outpatients and general practice:*
chlordiazepoxide

*In-patients:*
diazepam
chlordiazepoxide

**Maintenance of abstinence**
disulfiram
acamprosate

**Vitamin supplementation**
*Prophylaxis of Wernicke-Korsakoff syndrome:*
thiamine (vitamin B$_1$)
parenteral vitamins B & C
(Pabrinex®)

*Treatment of patients with Wernicke-Korsakoff syndrome (hospital in-patients):*
parenteral vitamins B & C
(Pabrinex®)

(j) **cigarette smoking**

*Step 1:* smoking cessation support based on assessment of patient's motivation to quit

*Step 2:* continuous therapy (patch*) (plus cessation support)* intermittent thrapy (lozenges/gum) *(plus cessation support)*

*Step 3:* bupropion *(plus cessation support)*

**4.11 Drugs for dementia**

*For hospital initiation and treatment under shared care protocol:*
donepezil
galantamine
rivastigmine

## 5: INFECTIONS

This section advises on 1st and 2nd choice anti-infective agents for the treatment of common infections in general practice and hospital. Hospital doctors should refer to departmental antibiotic guidelines for advice regarding treatment of severe infections, and specific treatments within specialised units (including prophylaxis for surgical, medical and dental procedures).

### (a) Gastro-intestinal

*Threadworms:*
mebendazole

*Giardiasis:*
metronidazole

*Campylobacter enteritis, shigellosis or salmonellosis:*
no antibiotic treatment

*Acute cholecystitis:*
no antibiotic treatment
co-amoxiclav

*Travellers' diarrhoea:*
rehydration
trimethoprim
ciprofloxacin

*Colstridium difficile diarrhea:*
stop the offending antibiotic
and start metronidazole

### (b) Respiratory

*Upper respiratory tract infection:*
no antibiotic treatment

*Lower respiratory tract infection (including bronchitis) in otherwise healthy individuals:*
no antibiotic treatment

*Lower respiratory tract infection with pre-existing lung disease and/or other complicating factors:*
amoxicillin
doxycycline

*Community acquired pneumonia:*
amoxicillin
clarithromycin

### (c) Urinary tract
**Women**
*Cystitis and uncomplicated UTI:*
trimethoprim
nitrofurantoin

*Pyelonephritis and complicated UTI:*
co-amoxiclav
ciprofloxacin

**Men**
*Urinary tract infection:*
trimethoprim
ciprofloxacin

*Tender epididymis/epidiymitis:*
ofloxacin

*Orchitis:*
ciprofloxacin

*Acute prostatitis:*
trimethoprim
ciprofloxacin

### (d) Genital system
*Thrush (vaginal candidiasis):*
clotrimazole pessaries
fluconazole (oral)

*Bacterial vaginosis:*
metronidazole orally or
vaginal gel
clindamycin vaginal cream

*Chlamydia:*
azithromycin

*Trichomoniasis:*
metronidazole

*Non-specific urethritis:*
azithromycin
doxycycline

*Uncomplicated gonorrhoea:*
cefixime (oral)

*Pelvic inflammatory disease:*
metronidazole + ofloxacin

*Genital herpes:*
aciclovir

*Bartholins gland infection:*
co-amoxiclav

*Genital warts:*
podophyllotoxin (topical)
liquid nitrogen (topical)

**(e)  Wound and skin infection**

*Cellulitis:*
flucloxacillin

*Surgical wounds, abscesses,*
*mastitis, wound infection:*
flucloxacillin
co-amoxiclav

*Animal and human bites:*
co-amoxiclav
doxycycline + metronidazole

*Episiotomy infection:*
co-amoxiclav
erythromycin + metronidazole

*Impetigo:*
flucloxacillin

*Fungal nail infections (if treatment*
*required):*
terbinafine
itraconazole

*Athlete's foot*
clotrimazole 1% cream
terbinafine 1% cream

**(f)  Diabetic ulcers**

*Deep ulcer*
ciprofloxacin +
clindamycin

flucloxacillin
+ metronidazole
+ ciprofloxacin

**(g)  MRSA**

*Soft tissue infections (choice of*
*treatment depends upon the extent*
*of infection):*
Mild:  silver sulfadiazine 1% cream

Moderate:  doxycycline

Severe/extensive: doxycycline
+ rifampicin

*Chest infections (MRSA):*
doxycycline (add
rifampicin for severe
illness)

*Urinary tract infection (MRSA):*
doxycycline
trimethoprim

*Decontamination (MRSA):*
no treatment

**(h)  ENT**

*Tonsillitis/pharyngitis:*
no antibiotic treatment
penicillin V

*Sinusitis:*
no antibiotic treatment
amoxicillin
clarithromycin

*Otitis externa* (see 12.1.1):
Ear toilet
Otomize® ear spray
Locorten-Vioform® drops
clotrimazole 1% solution

*Otitis media:*
no antibiotic treatment
amoxicillin

*Oral thrush:*
nystatin

**(i)  Dental infections**

*Acute gingivitis*
mechanical cleansing (if
possible)
+ chlorhexidine mouthwash

*Acute ulcerative gingivitis*
Metronidazole + mechanical
cleansing of teeth and gums
when inflammation has settled

*Dental abscess:*
drainage + amoxicillin

**(j) Eyes**

*Bacterial conjunctivitis:*
no treatment
chloramphenicol eye
drops/ointment

*Chlamydia conjunctivitis:*
azithromycin (oral)

*Herpes simplex corneal infection:*
aciclovir eye ointment

*Ophthalmic zoster:*
aciclovir (oral)

*Blepharitis:*
fusidic acid eye drops

*Corneal ulcers:*
Refer to hospital

*Corneal abrasions:*
chloramphenicol eye oint

**(k) Central nervous system**

*Meningitis, initial "blind"
treatment (pre-hospital):*
benzylpenicillin

*Hospital in-patient treatment:*
see hospital guidelines

**(m) Varicella zoster
(chickenpox)**

no treatment
aciclovir dispersible

**(n) Herpes zoster (shingles)**

aciclovir dispersible

## 6: ENDOCRINE SYSTEM

### 6.1.1 Insulins

Insulin should be initiated on specialist advice only. Choice depends on the particular needs of the individual patient, taking into account lifestyle, age, preference and capabilities. Type of insulin, device and needle size should be specified. Care should be taken to write the brand name in full.

### 6.1.2 Antidiabetes drugs

(a) **biguanides**
metformin

(b) **sulphonylureas**
gliclazide
glipizide

(c) **other antidiabetes drugs**
(i) **glitazones**
**(thiazoldinediones)**
pioglitazone

### 6.1.4 Treatment of hypoglycaemia

*Choice of treatment depends on the clinical situation and includes:*
glucose *(oral)*
glucagon *injection*
glucose *iv infusion 20%*

### 6.1.6 Diagnostic and monitoring agents for diabetes mellitus

(a) **capillary blood glucose monitoring**

Accu-Chek® Aviva
Accu-Chek® Compact Plus
FreeStyle® Lite
Optium Xceed® (for use with Optium® Plus test strips or MediSense® Optium® β-Ketone test strips)
Glucomen® LX
One Touch® Ultra 2®/Ultra Smart®/Ultra Easy®

(b) **capillary blood ketone monitoring**
Medisense ® Optium β-ketone test strips

(c) **urine testing for glucose**
Diastix®

(d) **urine testing for ketones**
Ketostix®

### 6.2 Thyroid and antithyroid drugs, and parathyroid disease

### 6.2.1 Hypothyroidism
levothyroxine

### 6.2.2 Hyperthyroidism
(a) **antithyroid drugs**
*To be initiated on specialist advice*
carbimazole

(b) **beta-blockers**
propranolol

### 6.2.3 Hypoparathyroidism
alfacalcidol

### 6.3 Corticosteroids
(a) **replacement therapy**
hydrocortisone
fludrocortisone

(b) **pharmacological therapy**
prednisolone
dexamethasone
hydrocortisone
methylprednisolone

### 6.4.1 HRT for menopausal symptoms

(a) **women who have not had a hysterectomy**
*Sequential combined (oral):*
Elleste-Duet®
Femoston®
Prempak C®

*Sequential combined (transdermal):*
Evorel® Sequi
FemSeven Sequi®

*Continuous combined (oral):*
Kliovance®
Premique® Low Dose

*Continuous combined (transdermal)*
Evorel® Conti

**(b)     women who have had a
          hysterectomy**

*Unopposed oestrogens (oral):*
          Elleste-Solo®
          Premarin®

*Unopposed oestrogens
          (transdermal):*
          Evorel®

## 6.4.2 Male sex hormones

          testosterone *injection*
                    (Sustanon®)
          testosterone *gel*

## 6.5     Pituitary hormones and anti-oestrogens

### 6.5.1     Anterior pituitary hormones
*Corticotrophins for testing:*
          tetracosactide

### 6.5.2     Posterior pituitary hormones and antagonists

**(a)     diabetes insipidus**
          desmopressin *nasal spray*
          desmopressin *tablets*

**(b)     antidiuretic hormone
          antagonists**
          demeclocycline

**(c)     oesophageal varices**
          terlipressin *(hospital use only)*

## 6.6     Drugs affecting bone metabolism
*(for bisphosphonates used in
malignant disease, see 8.4)*

**(a)     prevention of
          postmenopausal
          osteoporosis**

*Early menopause (< 45 years old):*
          HRT (see 6.4.1)

          combined oral
                    contraception (see 7.3)

*Institutionalised or housebound
older patients:*
          Calcichew-D₃ Forte®
          Calfovit D₃®

**(b)     treatment of
          postmenopausal
          osteoporosis**

          alendronate +
          Calcichew-D₃ Forte®

**(c)     corticosteroid-induced
          osteoporosis (treatment
          and prevention)**

          alendronate +
          Calcichew-D₃ Forte®

**(d)     male osteoporosis**

*Specialist referral should be
considered*
          alendronate +
          Calcichew-D₃ Forte®

## 6.7     Other endocrine drugs

### 6.7.1     Dopamine-receptor agonists

*Treatment of hyperprolactinaemia:*

          quinagolide
          bromocriptine
          cabergoline

### 6.7.4     Acromegaly

          octreotide
          lanreotide

# 7: OBSTETRICS, GYNAECOLOGY & URINARY-TRACT DISORDERS

## 7.0 Treatment of disorders occurring in obstetrics and gynaecology

**(a) dysmenorrhoea**
paracetamol
ibuprofen
naproxen

**(b) menorrhagia**
*Contraception required:*
combined oral
contraceptive (see 7.3)

*Contraception not required:*
tranexamic acid
naproxen

**(c) frequent irregular periods**
*Contraception required:*
combined oral
contraceptive (see 7.3)

*Contraception not required:*
norethisterone
medroxyprogesterone
acetate

**(d) endometriosis**
combined oral
contraceptive (see 7.3)
medroxyprogesterone
acetate
nafarelin *(on specialist advice)*

**(e) lichen sclerosus**
clobetasol propionate 0.05% ointment (Dermovate®)
diflucortolone valerate 0.3% ointment (Nerisone Forte®)

**(f) infertility**
*To be initiated and prescribed on specialist advice:*
clomifene citrate
chorionic gonadotrophin
follitropin alfa and beta
tamoxifen

**(h) premenstrual tension**
no drug treatment
fluoxetine

**(i) galactorrhoea**
no treatment

**(j) polycystic ovarian syndrome**
*Oligomenorrhoea:*
combined oral
contraceptive (see 7.3)
medroxyprogesterone
acetate
*Hirsutism:*
co-cyprindiol 2000/35
Marvelon®

## 7.1.1 Oxytocics
*Prevention and treatment of post-partum haemorrhage:*
Syntometrine®

## 7.2.1 Preparations for vaginal atrophy
Ovestin®
Vagifem®

## 7.3 Contraceptives

### 7.3.1 Combined oral
**(a) contraceptives**
Ovranette®
Katya 30/75®
Marvelon®

**(b) transdermal**
Evra®

**Emergency contraception**
Levonelle®-1500

## 7.3.2 Progestogen-only contraceptives
Micronor®
Norgeston®
Cerazette®

**Long-acting progestogen-only methods**

**(a) injectable progestogen-only methods**
medroxyprogesterone
acetate (Depo-Provera®)

**(b) contraceptive implants**
etonogestrel (Implanon®)

**(c) hormone releasing intra-uterine systems**
Mirena®

**7.3.4    Contraceptive devices**

**(a)    intra-uterine devices**

TT380 Slimline
Nova-T® 380
Mirena®

**(b)    diaphragms**

Reflexions®
Ortho®

**7.3.3    Spermicidal contraceptives**

Gygel®

**7.4    Drugs for genito-urinary disorders**

**7.4.1    Drugs for symptoms caused by benign prostatic obstruction**

**(a)    alpha-blockers**

alfuzosin
tamsulosin m/r
doxazosin

**(c)    5α-reductase inhibitors**

finasteride
dutasteride

**7.4.2    Drugs for urinary frequency, enuresis and incontinence**

**(a)    Urinary frequency due to bladder instability**

oxybutynin hydrochloride
solifenacin

**(b)    Stress urinary incontinence in women**
pelvic floor muscle exercises

duloxetine on specialist advice + pelvic floor muscle exercises

**7.4.3    Drugs used in dysuria**

*Alkalinisation of urine:*
potassium citrate

*Acidification of urine:*
ascorbic acid

**7.4.4    Catheter maintenance solutions**
*Dissolution of encrustation in lumen of the catheter:*
Solution G (Uro-Tainer® Twin Suby G)

*Dissolution of blood clots following urological surgery:*
sodium chloride 0.9% (Uro-Tainer Sodium Chloride®)

*Bladder infection:*
Catheter maintenance solutions are not recommended

**7.4.5    Drugs for erectile failure (impotence)**

sildenafil tablets (Viagra®)
tadalafil tablets
alprostadil injection
(Caverject® Dual Chamber)

## 8: MALIGNANT DISEASE and IMMUNOSUPPRESSION

### 8.2 Drugs affecting the immune response

#### 8.2.1 Antiproliferative immunosuppressants
azathioprine
mycophenolate mofetil (MMF)

#### 8.2.2 Corticosteroids and other immunosuppressants

**(a) corticosteroids**
dexamethasone
prednisolone

**(b) other immunosuppressants**
tacrolimus
ciclosporin

### 8.3 Sex hormones and hormone antagonists in malignant disease
*(on specialist advice)*

#### 8.3.2 Progestogens
medroxyprogesterone acetate
megestrol acetate

#### 8.3.4 Hormone antagonists

##### 8.3.4.1 Breast cancer

**(a) neo-adjuvant therapy of postmenopausal breast cancer** *(given for at least 3 months prior to surgery or radiotherapy)*
letrozole
tamoxifen

**(b) extended adjuvant therapy** *(given for 3 years after completion of 5 years of tamoxifen only)*

*Postmenopausal breast cancer:*
letrozole

**(c) metastatic breast cancer** *(continued until the disease progresses)*

*No prior adjuvant tamoxifen:*
letrozole
tamoxifen

*Prior adjuvant tamoxifen:*
letrozole
exemestane

##### 8.3.4.2 Prostate cancer and gonadorelin analogues

*Anti-androgen:*
bicalutamide
flutamide

*Gonadorelin analogue:*
triptorelin
goserelin
leuprorelin acetate

##### 8.3.4.3 Somatostatin analogues

*Short-acting:*
octreotide

*Long-acting:*
lanreotide
octreotide depot (Sandostatin LAR®)

### 8.4 Bisphosphonates used in malignant disease

*(for bisphosphonates used in osteoporosis, see 6.6)*

*Hypercalcaemia of malignancy:*
disodium pamidronate

*Prevention of skeletal related events in patients with breast cancer on the advice of an oncologist/ haematologist:*
ibandronic acid
zoledronic acid

*Prevention of skeletal related events in patients with multiple myeloma on the advice of an oncologist/ haematologist:*
zoledronic acid
disodium pamidronate

# 9: NUTRITION and BLOOD

## 9.1.1 Iron-deficiency anaemias

### 9.1.1.1 oral iron
ferrous sulphate
ferrous fumarate

### 9.1.1.2 parenteral iron
iron dextran (CosmoFer®)
iron sucrose (Venofer®)

## 9.1.2 Drugs used in megaloblastic anaemias

**(a) vitamin B$_{12}$ deficiency**
hydroxocobalamin

**(b) folate deficiency**
folic acid

## 9.1.3 Drugs for renal anaemia
epoetin
darbepoetin alfa

## 9.1.6 Drugs used in neutropenia
*Hospital use only*
filgrastim
lenograstim

## 9.2 Fluids and electrolytes

### 9.2.1.1 Oral potassium
Sando-K® effervescent tabs
Kay-Cee-L® syrup

**Potassium removal**
calcium polystyrene
sulphonate

### 9.2.1.2 Oral sodium and water
*Sodium depletion (e.g. salt-losing bowel, renal disease):*
sodium chloride m/r

*Oral rehydration therapy:*
Electrolade®

### 9.2.1.3 Oral bicarbonate
*Chronic acidotic states:*
sodium bicarbonate

*Hyperchloraemic acidosis:*
potassium bicarbonate

## 9.4 Oral nutritional supplements

*Milk style:*
Clinutren® 1.5 200ml
Fortisip® Bottle 200ml

*Fruit juice style:*
Clinutren® Fruit 200ml
Fortijuce® Bottle 200ml

*Yoghurt style:*
Fortifresh® 200ml

*Milk style with fibre:*
Clinutren® 1.5 Fibre 200ml
Fortisip® Multi Fibre 200ml

### 9.5.1.1 Calcium supplements
Calcichew®
Sandocal®

## 9.6 Vitamins
## 9.6.2 Vitamin B group
see 4.10 (g)

## 9.6.3 Vitamin C
ascorbic acid

## 9.6.4 Vitamin D
alfacalcidol

**Calcium and vitamin D supplements for osteoporosis** (see 6.6)
Calcichew-D$_3$ Forte®
Calfovit D$_3$®

## 9.6.6 Vitamin K
*Malabsorption syndromes (water-soluble preparation required):*
menadiol sodium phosphate

*Fat soluble formula (not malabsorption):*
phytomenadione

## 10: MUSCULOSKELETAL and JOINT DISEASES

### 10.1 Drugs used in rheumatic diseases and gout

#### 10.1.1 NSAIDs
ibuprofen
diclofenac sodium

*Patients at high risk of serious gastro-intestinal adverse events:*
NSAID (see 10.1.1)
+ lansoprazole *(or* omeprazole) (see 1.3)

#### 10.1.2.1 Systemic corticosteroids

*Oral:*
prednisolone

*Intravenous injection:*
methylprednisolone sodium succinate (Solu-Medrone®)

*Intramuscular depot injection:*
methylprednisolone acetate (Depo-Medrone®)

#### 10.1.2.2 Local corticosteroid injections

*Soft tissue injection:*
hydrocortisone acetate

*Intra-articular injection (only to be administered by appropriately trained staff):*

methylprednisolone acetate (Depo-Medrone®)

triamcinolone acetonide (Adcortyl® Intra-articular or Kenalog® Intra-articular)

#### 10.1.3 Conventional disease-modifying antirheumatic drugs
sulfasalazine e/c

*Initiated in consultation with a specialist (second choices):*
methotrexate
leflunomide
sodium aurothiomalate
penicillamine
azathioprine
hydroxychloroquine
prednisolone

*Initiated in consultation with a specialist (third choices):*
ciclosporin (Neoral®)
cyclophosphamide

*Tumour necrosis factor (TNF) antagonists (cytokine inhibitors):*
etanercept

#### 10.1.4 Drugs for treatment of gout

**(a)    acute attacks of gout**
indometacin
diclofenac sodium
colchicine

**(b)    prophylaxis of gout**
allopurinol

### 10.2 Drugs used in neuromuscular disorders

#### 10.2.1 Drugs used in myasthenia gravis
pyridostigmine bromide
neostigmine

#### 10.2.2 Skeletal muscle relaxants
baclofen
dantrolene sodium
diazepam

#### 10.2.3 Drugs used in acute exacerbations of multiple sclerosis

methylprednisolone sodium succinate injection

dexamethasone tablets

# 11: EYES

## 11.3 Anti-infective eye preparations

See 5 (j)

## 11.4 Corticosteroids and anti-inflammatory preps

**(a)** corticosteroids

betamethasone 0.1% eye drops/ointment

Maxidex® eye drops

**(b)** NSAIDs

ketorolac 0.5% eye drops

## 11.4.2 Other anti-inflammatory preparations

sodium cromoglicate 2% eye drops *for prophylaxis*

Otrivine-Antistin® eye drops *for acute treatment*

## 11.5 Mydriatics and cycloplegics

**(a)** therapeutic uses

*Antimuscarinics:*
atropine 1% eye drops/ointment
cyclopentolate 1% eye drops

*Sympathomimetic:*
phenylephrine 2.5% eye drops

**(b)** diagnostic uses

*Antimuscarinic:*
tropicamide 0.5% or 1% eye drops

## 11.6 Treatment of glaucoma

**(a)** prostaglandin analogues

travoprost eye drops

**(b)** beta-blockers

timolol 0.25% eye drops

**(c)** carbonic anhydrase inhibitors

dorzolamide 2% eye drops

acetazolamide (systemic)

**(d)** alpha$_2$-agonists

brimonidine 0.2% eye drops

**(e)** miotics

pilocarpine 1%, 2% or 4% eye drops

## 11.7 Local anaesthetics

oxybuprocaine 0.4% eye drops
tetracaine 1% eye drops

## 11.8.1 Preparations for tear deficiency

*Eye drops:*
hypromellose 0.3%

polyvinyl alcohol (Liquifilm Tears®)

carbomers

*Eye ointment:*
Lacri-Lube®

## 11.8.2 Ocular diagnostic stains

fluorescein 1% or 2% eye drops

fluorescein ophthalmic strips

## 12: EAR, NOSE and OROPHARYNX

### 12.1.1 Treatment of otitis externa

*If eardrum not perforated:*
Otomize® ear spray

*If perforated eardrum suspected:*
Locorten-Vioform® ear drops

*If suspected fungal infection:*
clotrimazole 1% solution

### 12.1.3 Removal of ear wax

almond oil ear drops

sodium bicarbonate 5% ear drops

### 12.2.1 Drugs used in chronic rhinosinusitus (including nasal polyps)

beclometasone dipropionate *nasal spray*

mometasone furoate *nasal spray*

### 12.2.2 Topical nasal decongestants

sodium chloride 0.9% *nasal drops*

ephedrine *nasal drops*

### 12.2.3 Anti-infective nasal preparations

Naseptin® cream

### 12.3.1 Drugs for oral ulceration and inflammation

*Aphthous ulcers:*

Difflam® *oral rinse* ± chlorhexidine gluconate

hydrocortisone sodium succinate *lozenge*

triamcinolone in adhesive basis *oral paste*

### 12.3.2 Oral thrush

nystatin

### 12.3.4 Mouthwashes, gargles and dentifrices

chlorhexidine gluconate *mouthwash*

hydrogen peroxide *mouthwash BP for Vincent's infection*

### 12.3.5 Treatment of dry mouth

Biotene Oralbalance®
AS Saliva Orthana®

## 13: SKIN

### 13.2.1 Emollients (moisturisers)
*Ointment base*
> white soft paraffin 50%/
> liquid paraffin 50%
> Epaderm® ointment
> emulsifying ointment BP

*Cream base*
> aqueous cream BP
> Diprobase® cream
> Aveeno® cream

*Soap substitutes*
> aqueous cream BP
> emulsifying ointment
> Dermol® 500 lotion
> Diprobase® cream
> Epaderm® ointment

### 13.2.1.1 Emollient bath additives

*Emollient bath/shower products
without antiseptic:*
> Oilatum® shower emollient/
> emollient bath additive
> Balneum® bath oil
> E45® emollient bath oil

*Emollient bath/shower products
with antiseptic:*
> Oilatum® Plus bath additive
> Emulsiderm® liquid
> emulsion
> Dermol®

### 13.2.2 Barrier preparations
> zinc & castor oil ointment
> Conotrane® cream

### 13.3 (a) topical antipruritics
> calamine cream or lotion
> crotamiton cream
> 1% menthol in aqueous
> cream

#### (b) topical local anaesthetics
> Emla® cream

#### (c) chronic urticaria
> cetirizine
> loratadine

### 13.4 Topical corticosteroids

*Mild corticosteroid:*
> hydrocortisone 0.5%, 1%,
> 2.5%

*Moderately potent corticosteroid:*
> clobetasone butyrate 0.05%
> (Eumovate®)

> betamethasone valerate
> 0.025% (Betnovate-RD®)

> fluocinolone acetonide
> 0.00625% (Synalar 1 in
> 4 Dilution®)

*Potent corticosteroid:*
> betamethasone valerate
> 0.1%

> fluocinolone acetonide
> 0.025% (Synalar®)

*Very potent corticosteroid:*
> clobetasol propionate
> 0.05%

### 13.5.1 Preparations for atopic eczema

*First step:*
> emollients ± antiseptic (see
> 13.2.1)
> topical corticosteroid
> (see 13.4)

*Second step:*
> ichthammol 1% with zinc
> oxide 15% in yellow soft
> paraffin

### 13.5.2 Preparations for psoriasis

*Vitamin D and analogues*
calcitriol
calcipotriol

*Other topical preparations for
psorasis used in
combinatiuon:*
coal tar
dithranol
emollients (see 13.2.1)
mild/moderate topical
corticosteroids *for face/
flexures* (see 13.4)
salicylic acid containing
preparations *for scaling*

### 13.6 Acne and rosacea
### (a) acne

*Topical treatment:*
benzoyl peroxide
antibiotics
retinoids (adapalene,
isotretinoin or tretinoin)

*Systemic treatment:*
oxytetracycline
erythromycin
lymecycline
(an option in women is
co-cyprindiol)

*Under specialist supervision only:*
isotretinoin (oral)

### (b) rosacea

azelaic acid gel
oxytetracycline (oral)
metronidazole topical
lymecycline

### 13.7 Preparations for warts
and calluses
salicylic acid
formaldehyde

### 13.8.1 Sunscreening
preparations

Delph® lotion (SPF 30)
Sunsense® Ultra Lotion
(SPF 60)
Uvistat® cream (SPF 30 or
50)
E45 Sun® (SPF 50)

### 13.8.1.1 Actinic keratosis
### (a) small non tender
keratoses
no treatment
diclofenac gel 3%
(Solaraze®)

### (a) extensive thicker
keratoses
cryotherapy
fluorouracil (Efudix®)

### 13.8.2 Camouflagers
Dermablend®

### 13.9 Shampoos and some other
scalp preparations
coconut oil containing
shampoos
Polytar® liquid
ketoconazole shampoo
T/Gel® shampoo

### 13.10.1 Anti-infective skin
preparations
*(see also chapter 5)*

*Antiseptics*
silver sulfadiazine cream
*for Gram -ve organisms*

silver nitrate solution 0.5%
w/v *for exudative leg
eczema or ulcers*

eosin solution 2% w/v *for
flexures*

potassium permanganate
*for infected eczema of
hands and feet*

*Topical antibiotics*
fusidic acid topical *for
Gram +ve organisms*

metronidazole topical *for
anaerobes*

### 13.10.2 Antifungal preparations
*(see also chapter 5)*
clotrimazole cream
terbinafine cream

### 13.10.4 Parasiticidal preparations
*(a) scabies:*
    permethrin

*(b) head lice:*
    dimeticone (Hedrin®)
    malathion
    phenothrin

*(c) pubic lice:*
    malathion
    permethrin

### 13.11 Disinfectants & cleansers
*(a) cleansers:*
    sodium chloride 0.9%

*(b) disinfectants:*
    chlorhexidine
    povidone-iodine

### 13.12 Antiperspirants
    aluminium chloride
    hexahydrate

### 13.13.1 Wound management products

**(a) alginate dressings**
    Activheal® Alginate
    Sorbsan®

**(b)(i) foam dressings**
*with adhesive border*
    Allevyn® Adhesive
    Tegaderm®Foam Adhesive
*without adhesive border*
    Tegaderm® Foam
    Allevyn®

**(b)(ii) soft silicone foam dressings**
*without border*
    Mepilex®
*with border*
    Mepilex Border®

**(c) hydrogel dressings**
*hydrogels*
    Activheal® Hydrogel
    Purilon® Gel
*sheet hydrogels*
    ActiformCool®

**(d)(i) hydrocolloid dressings**
*standard dressings*
    DuoDERM® Signal®
    Comfeel® Plus
*thin dressings*
    DuoDERM® Extra Thin
    Comfeel® Plus Transparent

**(d)(ii) hydrocolloid fibre dressings**
    Aquacel® *ribbon or sheet*

**(e) vapour-permeable films and membranes**
    Tegaderm®
*With absorbent pad:*
    Tegaderm® Plus Pad

**(f) Low adherence dressings and wound contact materials**
*Silicone coated knitted viscose primary dressings*
    N-A Ultra®
*Silicone dressings*
    Mepitel®

**(g) Odour management dressings**
*Activated charcoal non-absorbent dressing*
    Actisorb® Silver 220
*Activated charcoal absorbent dressing*
    CarboFLEX®

**(i) Surgical absorbent dressings**
*High absorbency*
    Eclypse®
    Mesorb®
*Low absorbency*
    Relcase®

**(k) Antimicrobial**
**(k)(i) Silver based dressings**
*Absorbent/fibrous*
    Aquacel® Ag
    Acticoat® Absorbent
*Silver releasing sheet*
    Acticoat® / Acticoat® 7
*Silver ointment*
    Flamazine® (silver sulfadiazine 1%w/w)
*Silver foam*
    Allevyn® Ag (without adhesive border)
    Mepilex® Ag

**(k)(ii)   Honey Based Products**

*Honey Ointment*
> Activon® Tube

*Absorbent Honey Dressing*
> Algivon®

*Tulle dressing*
> Activon Tulle®

*Low adherent dressing*
> Actilite®

**(k)(iii)   Iodine Based Products**

*Absorbent (0.9% cadexomer iodine)*
> Iodosorb® ointment
> Iodoflex® Paste

*Non-absorbent(povidone iodine)*
> Inadine®

**(l)     Protease Modulating Products**
> Promogran® Prisma®

**(m)   Scar Management Products**

*Flat sheet*
> Dermatix®

*Gel spray*
> Kelo-cote®

**(n)   Skin Protectors**

*Unbroken skin*
> Cavilon Durable Barrier Cream

*Broken skin*
> Cavilon No-sting Barrier Film

**(o)     Specialist Products for Plastic Surgery** (Only for use on advice from plastic surgery outpatients)
> Urgotul®
> Urgotul® SS0
> Urgotul® Duo
> Urgotul® Duo (with silver)

**13.13.2 Bandages**
**(b)     light-weight conforming** *bandages*
> K-Band®
> Acti-Wrap®

**(c)     tubular bandages**
*elasticated viscose bandage*
> Comfigrip®

*elasticated viscose stockinette*
> Comfifast®

*non-elasticated viscose bandage* stockinette

**(d)     Light support bandages**
> K-Lite®
> Soffcrepe®

**(e)     Light compression bandages (single)**
> K-Plus®

**(f)     Short stretch compression bandages (single)**
> Actico® (cohesive)
> Actiban®

**(g)     High compression bandages** (single not mutilayer)
> Setopress®

**(h)     Cohesive bandages (light compression)** (single)
> Profore® #4
> Ultra Four® #4
> Co-plus®

**(i)     Light compression multi-layer kits**
> Ultra Four® RC
> Profore® Lite

**(j)     High compression multi-layer kits**
*2 layer system*
> Coban®

*4 layer system*
> Ultra Four® 4 Layer System
> Profore® 4 Layer System

**(k)     Orthopaedic wadding**
> Soffban® (synthetic)
> Soffban® (natural)

**(l)     Medicated bandages**
> Steripaste®
> Ichthopaste®

**13.13.3 Adhesive tapes**
*Permeable Non-woven*
> Clinipore®

*Permeable Aperture Non-woven*
> Mefix®

*Permeable Aperture Woven (synthetic)*
> Hapla Band®

*Impermeable plastic*
> Sleek®

# 15: ANAESTHESIA

## 15.1 General anaesthesia

### 15.1.1 Intravenous anaesthetics
*Specialist training required*
> propofol
> thiopental
> etomidate emulsion

### 15.1.2 Inhalational anaesthetics
*Specialist training required*
> isoflurane
> ± nitrous oxide

> sevoflurane
> ± nitrous oxide

### Inhalational analgesia
*Specialist training required*
> nitrous oxide

### 15.1.3 Antimuscarinic drugs
> atropine sulphate
> glycopyrronium bromide

### 15.1.4.1 Anxiolytics and sedative techniques
*Pre-operative sedation:*
> diazepam
> temazepam
> lorazepam

*Intravenous sedation (specialist training required):*
> midazolam

### 15.1.4.2 Peri-operative analgesics
*Step 1:  mild pain*
> ibuprofen
> paracetamol
> diclofenac sodium

*Step 2:  mild to moderate pain*
> co-codamol 30/500 ±
> NSAID (ibuprofen or
> diclofenac sodium)

dihydrocodeine (short-term)
*Step 3:  moderate to severe pain*
> morphine + paracetamol
> ± NSAID (ibuprofen or
> diclofenac sodium)

### 15.1.4.3 Opioid analgesics used in anaesthesia
> morphine
> diamorphine

### 15.1.5 Neuromuscular blocking agents

*Specialist training required*
> atracurium besilate
> vecuronium bromide

*Rapid sequence induction*
> suxamethonium chloride
> rocuronium bromide

### 15.1.6 Anticholinesterases used in anaesthesia
> neostigmine metilsulfate

### 15.1.7 Antagonists for central and respiratory depression
*Opioid-induced respiratory depression:*
> naloxone

*Reversal of benzodiazepine-induced respiratory depression in anaesthesia:*
> flumazenil

### 15.1.8.1 Drugs for malignant hyperthermia due to anaesthesia
> dantrolene sodium

## 15.2 Local anaesthesia
*Skin surface application:*
> Emla® cream
> tetracaine gel (Ametop®)

*Skin infiltration:*
> lidocaine ± adrenaline
> bupivacaine ± adrenaline

*Biers block:*
> prilocaine 0.5%

*Digital nerve block:*
> lidocaine
> bupivacaine
*Intra-articular:*
> bupivacaine
> lidocaine

# British National Formulary

**BNF 58**

**September 2009**

**bnf.org**

Published jointly by
**BMJ Group**
Tavistock Square, London WC1H 9JP, UK
and
**RPS Publishing**
RPS Publishing is the wholly-owned publishing organisation of the Royal Pharmaceutical Society of Great Britain
1 Lambeth High Street, London, SE1 7JN, UK

Copyright © BMJ Group and RPS Publishing 2009

ISBN: 978 0 85369 848 7

ISSN: 0260-535X

Printed by GGP Media GmbH, Pössneck, Germany

A catalogue record for this book is available from the British Library.

Paper copies may be obtained through any bookseller or direct from:

Pharmaceutical Press
c/o Macmillan Distribution (MDL)
Brunel Rd
Houndmills
Basingstoke
RG21 6XS
UK
Tel: +44 (0) 1256 302 699
Fax: +44 (0) 1256 812 521
E-mail: direct@macmillan.co.uk
www.pharmpress.com
RPS Publishing also supplies the BNF in digital formats suitable for standalone use or for small networks, for use over an intranet and for use on a personal digital assistant (PDA).

## Distribution of BNFs
The UK health departments distribute BNFs to NHS hospitals, doctors, dental surgeons, and community pharmacies. In England, BNFs are mailed individually to NHS general practitioners and community pharmacies; contact the DH Publication Orderline for extra copies or changes relating to mailed BNFs.
Tel: 0300 123 1002
In Wales, telephone the Business Services Centre
Tel: 01495 332 000
For further information on the supply of copies of the BNF to NHS organisations, see http://tinyurl.com/2uebpp.

The BNF is designed as a digest for rapid reference and it may not always include all the information necessary for prescribing and dispensing. Also, less detail is given on areas such as obstetrics, malignant disease, and anaesthesia since it is expected that those undertaking treatment will have specialist knowledge and access to specialist literature. *BNF for Children* should be consulted for detailed information on the use of medicines in children. The BNF should be interpreted in the light of professional knowledge and supplemented as necessary by specialised publications and by reference to the product literature. Information is also available from medicines information services (see inside front cover).

# Preface

# Contents

The BNF is a joint publication of the British Medical Association and the Royal Pharmaceutical Society of Great Britain. It is published biannually under the authority of a Joint Formulary Committee which comprises representatives of the two professional bodies and of the UK Health Departments. The Dental Advisory Group oversees the preparation of advice on the drug management of dental and oral conditions; the Group includes representatives of the British Dental Association. The Nurse Prescribers' Advisory Group advises on the content relevant to nurses.

The BNF aims to provide prescribers, pharmacists and other healthcare professionals with sound up-to-date information about the use of medicines.

The BNF includes key information on the selection, prescribing, dispensing and administration of medicines. Medicines generally prescribed in the UK are covered and those considered less suitable for prescribing are clearly identified. Little or no information is included on medicines promoted for purchase by the public.

Information on drugs is drawn from the manufacturers' product literature, medical and pharmaceutical literature, UK health departments, regulatory authorities, and professional bodies. Advice is constructed from clinical literature and reflects, as far as possible, an evaluation of the evidence from diverse sources. The BNF also takes account of authoritative national guidelines and emerging safety concerns. In addition, the editorial team receives advice on all therapeutic areas from expert clinicians; this ensures that the BNF's recommendations are relevant to practice.

The BNF is designed as a digest for rapid reference and it may not always include all the information necessary for prescribing and dispensing. Also, less detail is given on areas such as obstetrics, malignant disease, and anaesthesia since it is expected that those undertaking treatment will have specialist knowledge and access to specialist literature. *BNF for Children* should be consulted for detailed information on the use of medicines in children. The BNF should be interpreted in the light of professional knowledge and supplemented as necessary by specialised publications and by reference to the product literature. Information is also available from medicines information services (see inside front cover).

It is **vital** to use the most recent edition of the BNF for making clinical decisions. The more important changes for this edition are listed on p. xi.

The BNF on the internet (bnf.org) includes additional information of relevance to healthcare professionals dealing with medicines. Other digital versions of the BNF—including intranet and personal digital assistant (PDA) versions—are produced in parallel with the paper version.

The BNF welcomes comments from healthcare professionals. Comments and constructive criticism should be sent to:
British National Formulary,
Royal Pharmaceutical Society of Great Britain,
1 Lambeth High Street, London SE1 7JN.
editor@bnf.org

Preface                                            iii
Acknowledgements                                   iv
How to use the BNF                                 ix
Changes for this edition                           xi
Significant changes                                xi
Dose changes                                       xi
Classification changes                             xii
Deleted preparations                               xii
New preparations included in this edition          xiii
Late additions                                     xiii
Name changes                                       xiv
Guidance on prescribing                            1
General guidance                                   1
Prescription writing                               4
Emergency supply of medicines                      6
Controlled Drugs and drug dependence               7
Adverse reactions to drugs                         11
Prescribing for children                           13

For detailed advice on medicines used for children consult *BNF for Children*

Prescribing in palliative care                     15
Prescribing for the elderly                        19
Prescribing in dental practice                     21
Drugs and sport                                    26
Emergency treatment of poisoning                   27
Notes on drugs and Preparations
1:  Gastro-intestinal system                       37
2:  Cardiovascular system                          72
3:  Respiratory system                             150
4:  Central nervous system                         185
5:  Infections                                     288
6:  Endocrine system                               372
7:  Obstetrics, gynaecology, and
    urinary-tract disorders                        434
8:  Malignant disease and immunosuppression        465
9:  Nutrition and blood                            512
10: Musculoskeletal and joint diseases             559
11: Eye                                            590
12: Ear, nose, and oropharynx                      608
13: Skin                                           624
14: Immunological products and vaccines            669
15: Anaesthesia                                    697
Appendixes and indices
Appendix 1:  Interactions                          720
Appendix 2:  Liver disease                         804
Appendix 3:  Renal impairment                      815
Appendix 4:  Pregnancy                             831
Appendix 5:  Breast-feeding                        852
Appendix 6:  Intravenous additives                 867
Appendix 7:  Borderline substances                 880
Appendix 8:  Wound management products
             and elasticated garments              911
Appendix 9:  Cautionary and advisory labels
             for dispensed medicines               932
Dental Practitioners' Formulary                    947
Nurse Prescribers' Formulary                       950
Non-medical prescribing                            954
Index of manufacturers                             955
Index                                              971

# Acknowledgements

The Joint Formulary Committee is grateful to individuals and organisations that have provided advice and information to the BNF.

The principal contributors for this edition were:

U.J. Adderley, I.H. Ahmed-Jushuf, K.W. Ah-See, S.P. Allison, M.N. Badminton, T.P. Baglin, P.R.J. Barnes, D.N. Bateman, S.L. Bloom, D. Bowsher, E.M. Brown, R.J. Buckley, I.F. Burgess, D.J. Burn, J.J. Coleman, R. Dinwiddie, P.N. Durrington, D.A.C. Elliman, M.D. Feher, B.G. Gazzard, A.M. Geretti, A.H. Ghodse, N.J.L. Gittoes, P.J. Goadsby, J. Guillebaud, D.J. Hatch, B.G. Higgins, S.H.D. Jackson, A. Jones, J.R. Kirwan, P.G. Kopelman, A.J. Krentz, T.H. Lee, D.N.J. Lockwood, M.G. Lucas, L. Luzzatto, A. MacDonald, A.G. Marson, P.D. Mason, K.E.L. McColl, G.M. Mead, E. Miller, J.M. Neuberger, D.J. Nutt, L.P. Ormerod, W.J. Penny, A.B. Provan, M.M. Ramsay, D.J. Rowbotham, J.W. Sander, J.A.T. Sandoe, M. Schacter, G.J. Shortland, D.B. Silk, S.C.E. Sporton, M.A. Stroud, J.P. Thompson, D.A. Warrell, R.P. Walt, A.D. Weeks, A. Wilcock, C.E. Willoughby, M.M Yaqoob.

M.J. Kendall, senior medical adviser for BNF Publications, has also provided valuable assistance.

Expert advice on the management of oral and dental conditions was kindly provided by M. Addy, P. Coulthard, A. Crighton, M.A.O. Lewis, J.G. Meechan, N.D. Robb, R.A. Seymour, R. Welbury, and J.M. Zakrzewska. S. Kaur provided valuable advice on dental prescribing policy.

Members of the British Association of Dermatologists Therapy Guidelines Subcommittee, H.K. Bell, L.C. Fuller, J. Hughes, S. Hulley, J. Lear, N.J. Levell, A.J. McDonagh, S. Punjabi, M.J. Tidman, P.D. Yesudian, and M.F.M. Mustapa (Secretariat) have provided valuable advice.

Members of the Advisory Committee on Malaria Prevention, B.A. Bannister, R.H. Behrens, P.L. Chiodini, F. Genasi, L. Goodyer, D. Hill, R. Jecock, G. Kassianos, D.G. Lalloo, G. Lea, G. Pasvol, M. Powell, D.V. Shingadia, D.A. Warrell, C.J.M. Whitty, and C. Lucas (Secretariat) have also provided valuable advice.

The Joint British Societies' Coronary Risk Prediction Charts have been reproduced with the kind permission of P.N. Durrington who has also provided the BNF with access to the computer program for assessing coronary and stroke risk.

R. Suvarna and colleagues at the MHRA have provided valuable assistance.

Correspondents in the pharmaceutical industry have provided information on new products and commented on products in the BNF. NHS Prescription Services has supplied the prices of products in the BNF.

Numerous doctors, pharmacists, nurses and others have sent comments and suggestions.

The BNF has valuable access to the *Martindale* data banks by courtesy of S. Sweetman and staff.

J.E. Macintyre and staff provided valuable technical assistance.

C. Adetola, N. Bansal, A. Breewood, K.L. d'Almeida, M. Davis, C. Fischetti, S. Foad, E.H. Glover, D.T.H. Griffiths, T. Hamp, A. Harvey, J. Humphreys, J.M. James, E. Laughton, A. McLaughlin, A. Melen, H.M.N. Neill, O. Ojeleye, A. Parkin, R.G. Taljaard, and E.J. Tong provided considerable assistance during the production of this edition of the BNF.

Xpage have provided technical assistance with the editorial database and typesetting software.

# BNF Staff

**Managing Editor: Knowledge Creation**
John Martin *BPharm, PhD, MRPharmS*

**Assistant Editors**
Leigh Anne Claase *BSc, PhD, MRPharmS*
Bryony Jordan *BSc, DipPharmPract, MRPharmS*
Colin R. Macfarlane *BPharm, MSc, MRPharmS*
Allison F. Patterson *BPharm, MRPharmS*
Rachel S. M. Ryan *BPharm, MRPharmS*
Shama M. S. Wagle *BPharm, DipPharmPract, MRPharmS*

**Staff Editors**
Onatefe Akporobaro-Iwudibia *MPharm, MRPharmS*
Sejal Amin *BPharm, MSc, MRPharmS*
Angela K. Bennett *MPharm, DipPharmPract, MRPharmS*
Susan E. Clarke *BPharm, DipClinPharm, MRPharmS*
Julia A. Dickin *MPharm, MRPharmS*
Belén Granell Villen *BSc, PGDipClinPharm, MRPharmS*
Manjula Halai *BScChem, MPharm, MRPharmS*
Emma E. Harris *MPharm, DipPharmPract, MRPharmS*
Amy E. Harvey *MPharm, PGDipCommPharm, MRPharmS*
Paul S. Maycock *MPharm, DipPharmPract, MRPharmS*
Elizabeth Nix *DipPharm(NZ), MRPharmS*
Rupal M. Patel *BSc, MRPharmS*
Sanjay Patel *BPharm, MRPharmS*
Claire L. Preston *BPharm, MRPharmS*
Shaistah J. Qureshi *MPharm, MRPharmS*
Vinaya K. Sharma *BPharm, MSc, PGDipPIM, MRPharmS*

**Editorial Assistant**
Jennifer L. Palmer *RegPharmTech*

**Senior BNF Administrator**
Heidi Homar *BA*

**Administrative Assistant**
Cristina Lopez-Bueno *BA*

**Managing Editor: Digital Development and Delivery**
Cornelia Schnelle *MPhil*

**Digital Development Editor**
Philip D. Lee *BSc, PhD*

**Digital Development Assistants**
Robert C. Buckingham *BSc*
Michelle Cartwright
Zephyr M.Wastell

**Terminologist**
Sarah Peck *BSc*

**Head of Publishing Services**
John Wilson

**BNF Publishing Director**
Duncan S. T. Enright *MA, PGCE, MInstP, FIDM*

**Managing Director, RPS Publishing**
Robert Bolick *BA, MA*

# Joint Formulary Committee 2008–2009

**Chair**
Derek G. Waller
*BSc, MB, BS, DM, FRCP*

**Deputy Chair**
Alison Blenkinsopp
*PhD, BPharm, FRPharmS*

**Committee Members**
Jeffrey K. Aronson
*MA, MB ChB, DPhil, FRCP, FBPharmacolS, FFPM*
Anthony J. Avery
*BMedSci, MB ChB, DM, FRCGP*
Beth Hird
*BPharm, MSc, MRPharmS, SP, IP*
W. Moira Kinnear
*BSc, MSc, MRPharmS*
Donal O'Donoghue
*MRCP, FRCP*
Gul Root
*BSc(Pharm), MRPharmS, DMS*
Rafe Suvarna
*MBBS, BSc, FFPM, DAvMed, DipIMC*
Carwen Wynne Howells
*BPharm, FRPharmS*

**Executive Secretary**
Heidi Homar
*BA*

# Dental Advisory Group 2008–2009

**Chair**
David Wray
*MD, BDS, MB ChB, FDSRCPS, FDSRCS Ed, F MedSci*

**Committee Members**
Christine Arnold
*BDS, DDPHRCS, MCDH*

Barry Cockcroft
*BDS, FDSRCS (Eng)*

Duncan S.T. Enright
*MA, PGCE, MInstP, FIDM*

Amy E. Harvey
*MPharm, PGDipCommPharm, MRPharmS*

Martin J. Kendall
*OBE, MD, FRCP, FFPM*

Lesley P. Longman
*BSc, BDS, FDSRCS Ed, PhD*

John Martin
*BPharm, PhD, MRPharmS*

Michelle Moffat
*BDS, MFDS RCS Ed, M Paed Dent RCPS, FDS (Paed Dent) RCS Ed*

Richard J. Oliver
*BDS, BSc, PhD, FDSRCPS, FDS (OS) RCPS*

Rachel S.M. Ryan
*BPharm, MRPharmS*

**Secretary**
Arianne J. Matlin
*MA, MSc, PhD*

**Executive Secretary**
Heidi Homar
*BA*

> **Advice on dental practice**
> The **British Dental Association** has contributed to the advice on medicines for dental practice through its representatives on the Dental Advisory Group.

# Nurses Prescribers' Advisory Group 2008–2009

**Chair**
Nicky A. Cullum
*PhD, RGN*

**Committee Members**
Una J. Adderley
*MSc, BA, RGN, DN*

Rebecca F. Cheatle
*BSc, RGN*

Michele L. Cossey
*BPharm, MSc, MRPharmS*

Molly Courtenay
*PhD, MSc, Cert Ed, BSc, RGN*

Duncan S.T. Enright
*MA, PGCE, MInstP, FIDM*

Penny M. Franklin
*RN, RCN, RSCPHN(HV), MA, PGCE*

Margaret F. Helliwell
*MB, BS, BSc, MFPHM, FRCP (Edin)*

Bryony Jordan
*BSc, DipPharmPract, MRPharmS*

Martin J. Kendall
*OBE, MD, FRCP, FFPM*

Fiona Lynch
*BSc, MSc, RGN, RSCN*

John Martin
*BPharm, PhD, MRPharmS*

Paul S. Maycock
*MPharm, DipPharmPract, MRPharmS*

Maureen P. Morgan
*RN, RHV, MBA*

Elizabeth J. Plastow
*RMN, RGN, RSCPHN(HV), MSc, PGDipEd*

Paul G.H. Robinson
Gul Root
*BSc, MRPharmS, DMS*

Jill M. Shearer
*BSc, RGN, RM*

Rabina Tindale
*RGN, RSCN, BSc, DipAEN, PGCE*

Vicky Vidler
*MA, RGN, RSCN*

**Executive Secretary**
Heidi Homar
*BA*

# How the BNF is constructed

The BNF is unique in bringing together authoritative, independent guidance on best practice with clinically validated drug information, enabling healthcare professionals to select safe and effective medicines for individual patients.

Information in the BNF has been validated against emerging evidence, best-practice guidelines, and advice from a network of clinical experts.

Hundreds of changes are made between editions, and the most clinically significant changes are listed at the front of each edition (pp. xi–xiii).

## Joint Formulary Committee

The Joint Formulary Committee (JFC) is responsible for the content of the BNF. The JFC includes doctors appointed by the BMJ Publishing Group, pharmacists appointed by the Royal Pharmaceutical Society of Great Britain, and representatives from the Medicines and Healthcare products Regulatory Agency (MHRA) and the UK health departments. The JFC decides on matters of policy and reviews amendments to the BNF in the light of new evidence and expert advice. The Committee meets quarterly and each member also receives proofs of all BNF chapters for review before publication.

## Editorial team

BNF staff editors are pharmacists with a sound understanding of how drugs are used in clinical practice. Each staff editor is responsible for editing, maintaining, and updating specific chapters of the BNF. During the publication cycle the staff editors review information in the BNF against a variety of sources (see below).

Amendments to the text are drafted when the editors are satisfied that any new information is reliable and relevant. The draft amendments are passed to expert advisers for comment and then presented to the Joint Formulary Committee for consideration. Additionally, for each edition, sections are chosen from every chapter for thorough review. These planned reviews aim to verify all the information in the selected sections and to draft any amendments to reflect the current best practice.

Staff editors prepare the text for publication and undertake a number of checks on the knowledge at various stages of the production.

## Expert advisers

The BNF uses about 60 expert clinical advisers (including doctors, pharmacists, nurses, and dentists) throughout the UK to help with the production of each edition. The role of these expert advisers is to review existing text and to comment on amendments drafted by the staff editors. These clinical experts help to ensure that the BNF remains reliable by:

- commenting on the relevance of the text in the context of best clinical practice in the UK;

- checking draft amendments for appropriate interpretation of any new evidence;

- providing expert opinion in areas of controversy or when reliable evidence is lacking;

- advising on areas where the BNF diverges from summaries of product characteristics;

- providing independent advice on drug interactions, prescribing in hepatic impairment, renal impairment, pregnancy, breast-feeding, children, the elderly, palliative care, and the emergency treatment of poisoning.

In addition to consulting with regular advisers, the BNF calls on other clinical specialists for specific developments when particular expertise is required.

The BNF also works closely with a number of expert bodies that produce clinical guidelines. Drafts or prepublication copies of guidelines are routinely received for comment and for assimilation into the BNF.

## Sources of BNF information

The BNF uses a variety of sources for its information; the main ones are shown below.

**Summaries of product characteristics** The BNF receives summaries of product characteristics (SPCs) of all new products as well as revised SPCs for existing products. The SPCs are the principal source of product information and are carefully processed, despite the ever-increasing volume of information being issued by the pharmaceutical industry. Such processing involves:

- verifying the approved names of all relevant ingredients including 'non-active' ingredients (the BNF is committed to using approved names and descriptions as laid down by the Medicines Act);

- comparing the indications, cautions, contra-indications, and side-effects with similar existing drugs. Where these are different from the expected pattern, justification is sought for their inclusion or exclusion;

- seeking independent data on the use of drugs in pregnancy and breast-feeding;

- incorporating the information into the BNF using established criteria for the presentation and inclusion of the data;

- checking interpretation of the information by two staff editors before submitting to a senior editor; changes relating to doses receive an extra check;

- identifying potential clinical problems or omissions and seeking further information from manufacturers or from expert advisers;

- careful validation of any areas of divergence of the BNF from the SPC before discussion by the Committee (in the light of supporting evidence);

- constructing, with the help of expert advisers, a comment on the role of the drug in the context of similar drugs.

Much of this processing is applicable to the following sources as well.

**Expert advisers** The role of expert clinical advisers in providing the appropriate clinical context for all BNF information is discussed above.

**Literature** Staff editors monitor core medical and pharmaceutical journals. Research papers and reviews relating to drug therapy are carefully processed. When a difference between the advice in the BNF and the paper is noted, the new information is assessed for reliability and relevance to UK clinical practice. If necessary, new text is drafted and discussed with expert advisers and the Joint Formulary Committee. The BNF enjoys a close working relationship with a number of national information providers.

**Systematic reviews** The BNF has access to various databases of systematic reviews (including the Cochrane Library and various web-based resources). These are used for answering specific queries, for reviewing existing text and for constructing new text. Staff editors receive training in critical appraisal, literature evaluation, and search strategies. Reviews published in Clinical Evidence are used to validate BNF advice.

**Consensus guidelines** The advice in the BNF is checked against consensus guidelines produced by expert bodies. A number of bodies make drafts or pre-publication copies of the guidelines available to the BNF; it is therefore possible to ensure that a consistent message is disseminated. The BNF routinely processes guidelines from the National Institute for Health and Clinical Excellence (NICE), the Scottish Medicines Consortium (SMC), and the Scottish Intercollegiate Guidelines Network (SIGN).

**Reference sources** Textbooks and reference sources are used to provide background information for the review of existing text or for the construction of new text. The BNF team works closely with the editorial team that produces *Martindale: The Complete Drug Reference*. The BNF has access to *Martindale* information resources and each team keeps the other informed of significant developments and shifts in the trends of drug usage.

**Statutory information** The BNF routinely processes relevant information from various Government bodies including Statutory Instruments and regulations affecting the Prescription only Medicines Order. Official compendia such as the British Pharmacopoeia and its addenda are processed routinely to ensure that the BNF complies with the relevant sections of the Medicines Act. The BNF itself is named as an official compendium in the Medicines Act.

The BNF maintains close links with the Home Office (in relation to controlled drug regulations) and the Medicines and Healthcare products Regulatory Agency (including the British Pharmacopoeia Commission). Safety warnings issued by the Commission on Human Medicines (CHM) and guidelines on drug use issued by the UK health departments are processed as a matter of routine.

Relevant professional statements issued by the Royal Pharmaceutical Society of Great Britain are included in the BNF as are guidelines from bodies such as the Royal College of General Practitioners.

The BNF reflects information from the Drug Tariff, the Scottish Drug Tariff, and the Northern Ireland Drug Tariff.

**Pricing information** The Prescription Pricing Division provides information on prices of medicinal products and appliances in the BNF. The BNF also receives and processes price lists from product suppliers.

**Comments from readers** Readers of the BNF are invited to send in comments. Numerous letters and emails are received during the preparation of each edition. Such feedback helps to ensure that the BNF provides practical and clinically relevant information. Many changes in the presentation and scope of the BNF have resulted from comments sent in by users.

**Comments from industry** Each manufacturer is provided with a complimentary copy of the BNF and invited to comment on it. Close scrutiny of the BNF by the manufacturers provides an additional check and allows them an opportunity to raise issues about the BNF's presentation of the role of various drugs; this is yet another check on the balance of the BNF's advice. All comments are looked at with care and, where necessary, additional information and expert advice are sought.

**Virtual user groups** The BNF has set up virtual user groups across various healthcare professions (e.g. doctors, pharmacists, nurses, dentists). The aim of these groups will be to provide feedback to the editors and publishers to ensure that BNF publications continue to serve the needs of its users.

**Market research** Market research is conducted at regular intervals to gather feedback on specific areas of development, such as drug interactions or changes to the way information is presented in digital formats.

> The BNF is an independent professional publication that is kept up-to-date and addresses the day-to-day prescribing information needs of healthcare professionals. Use of this resource throughout the health service helps to ensure that medicines are used safely, effectively, and appropriately.

# How to use the BNF

## Notes on conditions, drugs and preparations

The main text consists of classified notes on clinical conditions, drugs and preparations. These notes are divided into 15 chapters, each of which is related to a particular system of the body or to an aspect of medical care. Each chapter is then divided into sections which begin with appropriate *notes for prescribers*. These notes are intended to provide information to doctors, dental surgeons, pharmacists, nurses, and other healthcare professionals to facilitate the selection of suitable treatment. Guidance on dental and oral conditions is identified by means of a relevant heading (e.g. Dental and Orofacial pain) in the appropriate sections of the BNF. The notes are followed by details of relevant drugs and preparations. Preparations which can be prescribed by dental surgeons using NHS form FP10D (GP14 in Scotland, WP10D in Wales) are identified within the BNF by means of a note headed Dental Prescribing on NHS.

> For information available since publication of this edition see bnf.org

## Guidance on prescribing

This part includes information on prescription writing, controlled drugs and dependence, prescribing for children and the elderly, and prescribing in palliative care. Advice is given on the reporting of adverse reactions.

---

###  DRUG NAME

**Indications** details of uses and indications

**Cautions** details of precautions required (with cross-references to appropriate Appendixes) and also any monitoring required
Counselling Verbal explanation to the patient of specific details of the drug treatment (e.g. posture when taking a medicine)

**Contra-indications** details of any contra-indications to use of drug

**Side-effects** details of common and more serious side-effects

**Dose**
- Dose and frequency of administration (max. dose); CHILD and ELDERLY details of dose for specific age group
- By alternative route, dose and frequency

¹**Approved Name** (Non-proprietary) PoM
Pharmaceutical form, colour, coating, active ingredient and amount in dosage form, net price, pack size = basic NHS price. Label: (as in Appendix 9)
1.Exceptions to the prescribing status are indicated by a note or footnote.

**Proprietary Name** (Manufacturer) PoM NHS
Pharmaceutical form, sugar-free, active ingredient mg/mL, net price, pack size = basic NHS price. Label: (as in Appendix 9)
Excipients include clinically important excipients or electrolytes
Note Specific notes about the product e.g. handling

## Preparations

Preparations usually follow immediately after the drug which is their main ingredient.

Preparations are included under a non-proprietary title, if they are marketed under such a title, if they are not otherwise prescribable under the NHS, or if they may be prepared extemporaneously.

If proprietary preparations are of a distinctive colour this is stated.

In the case of compound preparations the indications, cautions, contra-indications, side-effects, and interactions of all constituents should be taken into account for prescribing.

## Drugs

Drugs appear under pharmacopoeial or other non-proprietary titles. When there is an *appropriate current monograph* (Medicines Act 1968, Section 65) preference is given to a name at the head of that monograph; otherwise a British Approved Name (BAN), if available, is used (see also Name changes).

The symbol ◢ is used to denote those preparations that are considered by the Joint Formulary Committee to be less suitable for prescribing. Although such preparations may not be considered as drugs of first choice, their use may be justifiable in certain circumstances.

### Prescription-only medicines PoM

This symbol has been placed against those preparations that are available only on a prescription issued by an appropriate practitioner. For more detailed information see *Medicines, Ethics and Practice*, No. 33, London, Pharmaceutical Press, 2009 (and subsequent editions as available).

The symbol CD indicates that the preparation is subject to the prescription requirements of the Misuse of Drugs Act. For regulations governing prescriptions for such preparations see p. 7.

### Preparations not available for NHS prescription NHS

This symbol has been placed against those preparations included in the BNF that are not prescribable under the NHS. Those prescribable only for specific disorders have a footnote specifying the condition(s) for which the preparation remains available. Some preparations which are not *prescribable* by brand name under the NHS may nevertheless be *dispensed* using the brand name providing that the prescription shows an appropriate non-proprietary name.

### Prices

Prices have been calculated from the basic cost used in pricing NHS prescriptions dispensed in May 2009, see also Prices in the BNF p. x for details.

The BNF also includes advice on medical emergencies and other medical problems in dental practice, together with a review of the oral side-effects of drugs.

An index of conditions relevant to dental surgeons is included.

## Emergency treatment of poisoning

This chapter provides information on the management of acute poisoning when first seen in the home, although aspects of hospital-based treatment are mentioned.

## Appendixes and indexes

The appendixes include information on interactions, liver disease, renal impairment, pregnancy, breast-feeding, intravenous additives, borderline substances, wound management products, and cautionary and advisory labels for dispensed medicines. They are designed for use in association with the main body of the text.

The Dental Practitioners' List and the Nurse Prescribers' List are also included in this section. The indexes consist of the Index of Manufacturers and the Main Index.

## Patient packs

Directive 92/27/EEC specifies the requirements for the labelling of medicines and outlines the format and content of patient information leaflets to be supplied with every medicine; the directive also requires the use of Recommended International Non-proprietary Names for drugs (see p. xiv).

All medicines have approved labelling and patient information leaflets; anyone who supplies a medicine is responsible for providing the relevant information to the patient (see also Appendix 9).

Many medicines are available in manufacturers' original packs complete with patient information leaflets. Where patient packs are available, the BNF shows the number of dose units in the packs. In particular clinical circumstances, where patient packs need to be split or medicines are provided in bulk dispensing packs, manufacturers will provide additional supplies of patient information leaflets on request.

During the revision of each edition of the BNF careful note is taken of the information that appears on the patient information leaflets. Where it is considered appropriate to alert a prescriber to some specific limitation appearing on the patient information leaflet (for example, in relation to pregnancy) this advice now appears in the BNF.

The patient information leaflet also includes details of all inactive ingredients in the medicine. A list of common E numbers and the inactive ingredients to which they correspond is now therefore included in the BNF (see inside back cover).

## PACT and SPA

PACT (Prescribing Analyses and Cost) and SPA (Scottish Prescribing Analysis) provide prescribers with information about their prescribing.

The *PACT Standard Report*, or in Scotland SPA *Level 1 Report*, is sent to all general practitioners on a quarterly basis. The PACT Standard Report contains an analysis of the practitioner's prescribing and the practice prescribing over the last 3 months, and gives comparisons with the local Primary Care Trust equivalent practice and with a national equivalent. The report also contains details of the practice prescribing for a specific topic; a different topic is chosen each quarter.

The *PACT Catalogue*, or in Scotland SPA *Level 2 Report*, provides a full inventory of the prescriptions issued by a prescriber. The PACT catalogue is available on request for periods between 1 and 24 months. To allow the prescriber to target specific areas of prescribing, a Catalogue may be requested to cover individual preparations, BNF sections, or combinations of BNF chapters.

PACT is also available electronically (www.nhsbsa.nhs.uk). This system gives users on-line access through NHSnet to the 3 years' prescribing data held on the NHS Prescription Services' database; tools for analysing the data are also provided.

## Prices in the BNF

Basic **net prices** are given in the BNF to provide an indication of relative cost. Where there is a choice of suitable preparations for a particular disease or condition the relative cost may be used in making a selection. Cost-effective prescribing must, however, take into account other factors (such as dose frequency and duration of treatment) that affect the total cost. The use of more expensive drugs is justified if it will result in better treatment of the patient or a reduction of the length of an illness or the time spent in hospital.

Prices have generally been calculated from the net cost used in pricing NHS prescriptions dispensed in May 2009. Unless an original pack is available these prices are based on the largest pack size of the preparation in use in community pharmacies. The price for an extemporaneously prepared preparation has been omitted where the net cost of the ingredients used to make it would give a misleadingly low impression of the final price. In Appendix 8 prices stated are per dressing or bandage.

The unit of 20 is still sometimes used as a basis for comparison, but where suitable original packs or patient packs are available these are priced instead.

Gross prices vary as follows:

1. Costs to the NHS are greater than the net prices quoted and include professional fees and overhead allowances;

2. Private prescription charges are calculated on a separate basis;

3. Over-the-counter sales are at retail price, as opposed to basic net price, and include VAT.

BNF prices are not, therefore, suitable for quoting to patients seeking private prescriptions or contemplating over-the-counter purchases.

A fuller explanation of costs to the NHS may be obtained from the Drug Tariff. Separate drug tariffs are applicable to England and Wales, Scotland, and Northern Ireland; prices in the different tariffs may vary.

# Changes for this edition

## Significant changes

The BNF is revised twice yearly and numerous changes are made between issues. All copies of BNF No. 57 (March 2009) should therefore be withdrawn and replaced by BNF No. 58 (September 2009). Significant changes have been made in the following sections for BNF No. 58:

Salicylate poisoning, Emergency treatment of poisoning

Paracetamol poisoning, Emergency treatment of poisoning

Ethylene glycol and methanol poisoning, Emergency treatment of poisoning

Infliximab for acute exacerbations of ulcerative colitis [NICE guidance], section 1.5

Management of arrhythmias [updated advice on atrial flutter, paroxysmal supraventricular tachycardia and ventricular tachycardia], section 2.3.1

Use of beta-adrenoceptor blocking drugs in patients with COPD, section 2.4

Rivaroxaban [NICE guidance], section 2.8.2

Corticosteroids [updated advice], section 3.2

Over-the-counter cough and cold medicines [MHRA/CHM advice], section 3.9.1 and section 12.2.2

Tricyclic and related antidepressant drugs [section updated and reorganised], section 4.3.1

*Clostridium difficile* infection, section 5.1, Table 1

Peritonitis, section 5.1, Table 1

Hospital-acquired pneumonia, section 5.1, Table 1

Antibacterial prophylaxis for endoscopic retrograde cholangiopancreatography, percutaneous endoscopic gastronomy or jejunostomy, section 5.1, Table 2

Oseltamivir and zanamivir [prophylaxis and treatment of influenza in pregnancy and breast-feeding], section 5.3.4

Oseltamivir, zanamivir, and amantadine for the prophylaxis and treatment of influenza [updated NICE guidance], section 5.3.4

Intravenous quinine to treat benign malaria in patients unable to take oral therapy, section 5.4.1

Measurement of HbA$_{1c}$ [update on units to express HbA$_{1c}$], section 6.1.1

Diabetes and surgery, section 6.1.1

Use of insulin detemir and insulin glargine for type 2 diabetes [NICE guidance updated], section 6.1.1.2

Use of a thiazolidinedione for type 2 diabetes [NICE guidance updated], section 6.1.2.3

Use of sitagliptin and vildagliptin for type 2 diabetes [NICE guidance], section 6.1.2.3

Use of exenatide for type 2 diabetes [NICE guidance], section 6.1.2.3

Nocturnal enuresis [updated advice], section 7.4.2

Administration of vinca alkaloids [NPSA advice], section 8.1.4

Drugs unsafe for use in acute porphyrias, section 9.8.2

Management of rheumatoid arthritis, section 10.1

Management of osteoarthritis, section 10.1

Cytokine modulators [section reorganised], section 10.1.3

Topical oral pain relief products containing salicylates [CHM advice], section 12.3.1

Efalizumab [suspension of marketing authorisation], section 13.5.3

Isotretinoin [pregnancy prevention], section 13.6.2

Immunoglobulins [section reorganised and updated], section 14.5

Adjustment of drug dosages in renal impairment [updated advice and terminology], appendix 3

Enteral feeds and nutritional supplements for adults [new tables], appendix 7

Wound management products [table to aid choice of dressing, and all sections reorganised], appendix 8

Changes to Dental Practitioners' Fomulary, p. 948

## Dose changes

Changes in dose statements introduced into BNF No. 58:

Abacavir, p. 341

Aciclovir [varicella and herpes zoster], p. 349

Alprostadil, p. 437

Atracurium [surgery or intubation], p. 709

Atomoxetine, p. 221

Atropine sulphate [organophosphorous insecticide poisoning, text], p. 36

Atropine sulphate [control of muscarinic side-effects of edrophonium], p. 703

*Axsain*®, p. 589

*Binocrit*®, p. 519

Chloroquine [prophylaxis of malaria], p. 362

Ciprofloxacin, p. 329

*Concerta*® XL, p. 222

Cyanocobalamin [by mouth], p. 516

*Daktarin*® oral gel, p. 619

Dantrolene [malignant hyperthermia], p. 713

Darunavir, p. 344

Dasatinib [accelerated and blast phase chronic myeloid leukaemia, acute lymphoblastic leukaemia], p. 488

Dexamethasone injection, p. 570

Dexamfetamine [refractory ADHD], p. 221

Diamorphine [myocardial infarction], p. 239

Diazepam [status epilepticus], p. 266

Diazepam [premedication], p. 705

Efavirenz, p. 347

*Efexor*® XL [depression], p. 220

*EMLA*®, p. 715

*Equasym XL*®, p. 222

Estramustine phosphate, p. 471

European viper venom antiserum [text], p. 36

Fentanyl injection, p. 708

*Flixotide®* [by dry powder inhalation], p. 168

Folic acid [megaloblastic anaemia], p. 517

*Galphenol®*, p. 183

Glycopyrronium bromide [control of muscarinic side-effects of neostigmine], p. 703

*Grazax®*, p. 175

Halothane, p. 702

Hydrocortisone, p. 152

Hydroxyzine hydrochloride, p. 173

Levetiracetam, p. 259

*Medikinet XL®*, p. 222

Methylphenidate [ADHD], p. 222

Metronidazole [extra-intestinal amoebiasis], p. 366

Midazolam [status epilepticus], p. 267

Mirtazapine, p. 218

Nortriptyline [nocturnal enuresis], p. 212

*Otrivine-Antistin®*, p. 595

Oxytocin [induction of labour], p. 436

Palifermin, p. 469

Pancuronium [intubation], p. 710

Parecoxib, p. 707

Pizotifen [paediatric dose], p. 251

Prednisolone [inflammatory bowel disease], p. 57

Promethazine hydrochloride, p. 190

*Pulmicort®* [by aerosol inhalation], p. 168

Ranitidine [prophylaxis of stress ulceration], p. 46

Risperidone [psychoses], p. 203

Salbutamol [by inhalation of aerosol or nebulised solution], p. 152

Sevoflurane [induction of anaesthesia], p. 702

Sodium cromoglicate [by aerosol inhalation], p. 170

Terbutaline [by inhalation of aerosol or nebulised solution], p. 152

*Timentin®*, p. 302

*Ursofalk®* [primary biliary cirrhosis], p. 70

*Varilrix®*, p. 689

*Varivax®*, p. 689

Vecuronium, p. 711

*Welldorm®* elixir, p. 189

*Zacin®*, p. 589

Zanamivir, p. 355

*Zelapar®*, p. 275

Zidovudine, p. 343

## Classification changes

Classification changes have been made in the following sections for BNF No. 58:

**Section** 1.6.5 Bowel cleansing preparations [title change]

**Section 14.5.1** Normal immunoglobulin [new sub-section]

**Section 14.5.2** Disease-specific immunoglobulins [new sub-section]

**Section 14.5.3** Anti-D (RhO) immunoglobulin [new sub-section]

## Deleted preparations

Preparations listed below have been discontinued during the compilation of BNF No. 58, or are still available but are not considered suitable for inclusion by the Joint Formulary Committee (see footnote)

*Aquasept®*

*Beclazone Easi-Breathe®*

*Bonefos®* concentrate

*Burinex A®*

*Cabaser®*

*Carisoma®*

*Cedocard Retard®*

*Drogenil®*

*Effico®¹*

*Endoxana®*

*Estracombi®*

*Euglucon®*

*Feldene®* injection

*Flagyl®* intravenous infusion

*Full Marks®* lotion and mousse

Gentian mixture, Alkaline, BP¹

*Halycitrol®*

*Hibisol®*

*Hycosan®*

*IONSYS®*

*Kapake®* effervescent tablets

*Maxolon®* paediatric liquid and syrup

*Metatone®¹*

*Mitoxana®*

*Motilium®* suspension

*Neo-Cortef®*

*Nystan®* tablets

Paraldehyde injection

*Paraplatin®*

*Prioderm®* lotion

Procaine

*Rapolyte®*

*Seconal Sodium®*

*Ster-Zac Bath Concentrate®*

*Tri-Adcortyl Otic®*

*Vibramycin®* capsules

*Vioform-Hydrocortisone®*

1. Not considered suitable for inclusion by the Joint Formulary Committee

## New preparations included in this edition

Preparations included in the relevant sections of BNF No. 58:

*Abraxane*®, p. 491

*Avamys*®, p. 614

*Azarga*®, p. 601

*Berinert*®, p. 178

*Bramitob*®, p. 312

*Denzapine*® suspension, p. 202

*Diafalk*®, p. 66

*Effentora*®, p. 240

*Efient*®, p. 137

*Extavia*®, p. 501

*Firmagon*®, p. 510

*Flamascard*®, p. 135

*Foraven XL*®, p. 220

*Intanza*®, p. 681

*Ixiaro*®, p. 681

*Kuvan*®, p. 540

Levofolinic acid, p. 469

*LMX 4*®, p. 715

*Nevanac*®, p. 606

*Nicorette*® *Invisi* patches, p. 281

*NuvaRing*®, p. 447

*Periogard*® oromucosal solution, p. 621

*Qlaira*®, p. 449

*Ranexa*®, p. 121

*Sandocal*® +D 600, p. 551

*Sevikar*®, p. 109

*Siklos*®, p. 522

*Stelara*®, p. 646

*Targinact*®, p. 244

*Tifaxin XL*®, p. 220

*Valdoxan*®, p. 218

*Venaxx XL*®, p. 220

*Venlalic* ® *XL*, p. 220

*Vidaza*®, p. 476

*Virgan*®, p. 593

*Xerotin*®, p. 622

*Xomolix*®, p. 227

*Zeridame*® SR, p. 246

# Late additions

**Vantas**® (Orion) ▼ [PoM]

Implant, histrelin (as acetate) 50 mg, net price 1 pack (containing implantation device and implant) = £990.00

BNF section 8.3.4.2. For palliative treatment of advanced prostate cancer

**Zarzio**® (Sandoz) ▼ [PoM]

Injection, prefilled syringe, filgrastim, net price 30 million-units (300 micrograms)/0.5 mL = £59.00; 48 million-units (480 micrograms)/0.5 mL = £94.00

**Note** Biosimilar medicine, p. 1

BNF section 9.1.6. (Specialist use only) reduction in duration of neutropenia and incidence of febrile neutropenia in cytotoxic chemotherapy for malignancy (except chronic myeloid leukaemia and myelodysplastic syndromes); reduction in duration of neutropenia in myeloablative therapy followed by bone-marrow transplantation; mobilisation of peripheral blood progenitor cells for harvesting and subsequent autologous or allogeneic infusion; severe congenital neutropenia, cyclic neutropenia, or idiopathic neutropenia and history of severe or recurrent infections (distinguish carefully from other haematological disorders, consult product literature); persistent neutropenia in advanced HIV infection

# Name changes

European Law requires use of the Recommended International Non-proprietary Name (rINN) for medicinal substances. In most cases the British Approved Name (BAN) and rINN were identical. Where the two differed, the BAN was modified to accord with the rINN.

The following list shows those substances for which the former BAN has been modified to accord with the rINN. Former BANs have been retained as synonyms in the BNF.

**Adrenaline and noradrenaline** Adrenaline and noradrenaline are the terms used in the titles of monographs in the European Pharmacopoeia and are thus the official names in the member states. For these substances, BP 2009 shows the European Pharmacopoeia names and the rINNs at the head of the monographs; the BNF has adopted a similar style.

| Former BAN | New BAN |
|---|---|
| adrenaline | *see above* |
| amethocaine | tetracaine |
| aminacrine | aminoacridine |
| amoxycillin | amoxicillin |
| amphetamine | amfetamine |
| amylobarbitone sodium | amobarbital sodium |
| beclomethasone | beclometasone |
| bendrofluazide | bendroflumethiazide |
| benzhexol | trihexyphenidyl |
| benzphetamine | benzfetamine |
| busulphan | busulfan |
| butobarbitone | butobarbital |
| carticaine | articaine |
| cephalexin | cefalexin |
| cephradine | cefradine |
| chloral betaine | cloral betaine |
| chlorbutol | chlorobutanol |
| chlormethiazole | clomethiazole |
| chlorpheniramine | chlorphenamine |
| chlorthalidone | chlortalidone |
| cholecalciferol | colecalciferol |
| cholestyramine | colestyramine |
| clomiphene | clomifene |
| colistin sulphomethate sodium | colistimethate sodium |
| corticotrophin | corticotropin |
| cyclosporin | ciclosporin |
| cysteamine | mercaptamine |
| danthron | dantron |
| dexamphetamine | dexamfetamine |
| dibromopropamidine | dibrompropamidine |
| dicyclomine | dicycloverine |
| dienoestrol | dienestrol |
| dimethicone(s) | dimeticone |
| dimethyl sulphoxide | dimethyl sulfoxide |
| dothiepin | dosulepin |
| doxycycline hydrochloride (hemihydrate hemiethanolate) | doxycycline hyclate |
| eformoterol | formoterol |

| Former BAN | New BAN |
|---|---|
| ethamsylate | etamsylate |
| ethinyloestradiol | ethinylestradiol |
| ethynodiol | etynodiol |
| flumethasone | flumetasone |
| flupenthixol | flupentixol |
| flurandrenolone | fludroxycortide |
| frusemide | furosemide |
| guaiphenesin | guaifenesin |
| hexachlorophane | hexachlorophene |
| hexamine hippurate | methenamine hippurate |
| hydroxyurea | hydroxycarbamide |
| indomethacin | indometacin |
| lignocaine | lidocaine |
| methotrimeprazine | levomepromazine |
| methyl cysteine | mecysteine |
| methylene blue | methylthioninium chloride |
| methicillin | meticillin |
| mitozantrone | mitoxantrone |
| nicoumalone | acenocoumarol |
| noradrenaline | *see above* |
| oestradiol | estradiol |
| oestriol | estriol |
| oestrone | estrone |
| oxpentifylline | pentoxifylline |
| phenobarbitone | phenobarbital |
| pipothiazine | pipotiazine |
| polyhexanide | polihexanide |
| pramoxine | pramocaine |
| procaine penicillin | procaine benzylpenicillin |
| prothionamide | protionamide |
| quinalbarbitone | secobarbital |
| riboflavine | riboflavin |
| salcatonin | calcitonin (salmon) |
| sodium calciumedetate | sodium calcium edetate |
| sodium cromoglycate | sodium cromoglicate |
| sodium ironedetate | sodium feredetate |
| sodium picosulphate | sodium picosulfate |
| sorbitan monostearate | sorbitan stearate |
| stibocaptate | sodium stibocaptate |
| stilboestrol | diethylstilbestrol |
| sulphacetamide | sulfacetamide |
| sulphadiazine | sulfadiazine |
| sulphamethoxazole | sulfamethoxazole |
| sulphapyridine | sulfapyridine |
| sulphasalazine | sulfasalazine |
| sulphathiazole | sulfathiazole |
| sulphinpyrazone | sulfinpyrazone |
| tetracosactrin | tetracosactide |
| thiabendazole | tiabendazole |
| thioguanine | tioguanine |
| thiopentone | thiopental |
| thymoxamine | moxisylyte |
| thyroxine sodium | levothyroxine sodium |
| tribavirin | ribavirin |
| trimeprazine | alimemazine |
| urofollitrophin | urofollitropin |

# Guidance on prescribing
## General guidance

Medicines should be prescribed only when they are necessary, and in all cases the benefit of administering the medicine should be considered in relation to the risk involved. This is particularly important during pregnancy, when the risk to both mother and fetus must be considered (for further details see Prescribing in Pregnancy, Appendix 4).

It is important to discuss treatment options carefully with the patient to ensure that the patient is content to take the medicine as prescribed (see also Taking Medicines to Best Effect, below). In particular, the patient should be helped to distinguish the adverse effects of prescribed drugs from the effects of the medical disorder. When the beneficial effects of the medicine are likely to be delayed, the patient should be advised of this.

**Taking medicines to best effect**  Difficulties in adherence to drug treatment occur regardless of age. Factors contributing to poor compliance with prescribed medicines include:

- prescription not collected or not dispensed;
- purpose of medicine not clear;
- perceived lack of efficacy;
- real or perceived adverse-effects;
- patients' perception of the risk and severity of side-effects may differ from that of the prescriber;
- instructions for administration not clear;
- physical difficulty in taking medicines (e.g. swallowing the medicine, handling small tablets, or opening medicine containers);
- unattractive formulation (e.g. unpleasant taste);
- complicated regimen.

The prescriber and the patient should agree on the health outcomes that the patient desires and on the strategy for achieving them ('concordance'). The prescriber should be sensitive to religious, cultural, and personal beliefs that can affect a patient's acceptance of medicines.

Taking the time to explain to the patient (and relatives) the rationale and the potential adverse effects of treatment may improve adherence. Reinforcement and elaboration of the physician's instructions by the pharmacist also helps. Advising the patient of the possibility of alternative treatments may encourage the patient to seek advice rather than merely abandon unacceptable treatment.

Simplifying the drug regimen may help; the need for frequent administration may reduce adherence, although there appears to be little difference in adherence between once-daily and twice-daily administration. Combination products reduce the number of drugs taken but at the expense of the ability to titrate individual doses.

**Biosimilar medicines**  A biosimilar medicine is a new biological product that is similar to a medicine that has already been authorised to be marketed (the biological reference medicine) in the European Union. The active substance of a biosimilar medicine is similar, but not identical, to the biological reference medicine. Biological products are different from standard chemical products in terms of their complexity and although theoretically there should be no important differences between the biosimilar and the biological reference medicine in

terms of safety or efficacy, when prescribing biological products, it is good practice to use the brand name. This will ensure that substitution of a biosimilar medicine does not occur when the medicine is dispensed.

Biosimilar medicines have black triangle status (▼) at the time of initial marketing. It is important to report suspected adverse reactions to biosimilar medicines using the Yellow Card Scheme (p. 11). For biosimilar medicines, adverse reaction reports should clearly state the brand name of the suspected medicine.

**Complementary and alternative medicine**  An increasing amount of information on complementary and alternative medicine is becoming available. The scope of the BNF is restricted to the discussion of conventional medicines but reference is made to complementary treatments if they affect conventional therapy (e.g. interactions with St John's wort—see Appendix 1). Further information on herbal medicines is available at www.mhra.gov.uk.

**Abbreviation of titles**  In general, titles of drugs and preparations should be written *in full*. Unofficial abbreviations should not be used as they may be misinterpreted.

**Non-proprietary titles**  Where non-proprietary ('generic') titles are given, they should be used in prescribing. This will enable any suitable product to be dispensed, thereby saving delay to the patient and sometimes expense to the health service. The only exception is where there is a demonstrable difference in clinical effect between each manufacturer's version of the formulation, making it important that the patient should always receive the same brand; in such cases, the brand name or the manufacturer should be stated. Non-proprietary titles should **not** be invented for the purposes of prescribing generically since this can lead to confusion, particularly in the case of compound and modified-release preparations.

Titles used as headings for monographs may be used freely in the United Kingdom but in other countries may be subject to restriction.

Many of the non-proprietary titles used in this book are titles of monographs in the European Pharmacopoeia, British Pharmacopoeia, or British Pharmaceutical Codex 1973. In such cases the preparations must comply with the standard (if any) in the appropriate publication, as required by the Medicines Act (Section 65).

**Proprietary titles**  Names followed by the symbol® are or have been used as proprietary names in the United Kingdom. These names may in general be applied only to products supplied by the owners of the trade marks.

**Marketing authorisation and BNF advice**  In general the *doses, indications, cautions, contra-indications,* and *side-effects* in the BNF reflect those in the manufacturers' data sheets or Summaries of Product Characteristics (SPCs) which, in turn, reflect those in the corresponding marketing authorisations (formerly known as Product Licences). The BNF does not generally include proprietary medicines that are not supported by a valid Summary of Product Characteristics or when the marketing

General guidance

authorisation holder has not been able to supply essential information. When a preparation is available from more than one manufacturer, the BNF reflects advice that is the most clinically relevant regardless of any variation in the marketing authorisations. Unlicensed products can be obtained from 'special-order' manufacturers or specialist importing companies, see p. 969.

Where an unlicensed drug is included in the BNF, this is indicated in square brackets after the entry. When the BNF suggests a use (or route) that is outside the licensed indication of a product ('off-label' use), this too is indicated. Unlicensed use of medicines becomes necessary if the clinical need cannot be met by licensed medicines; such use should be supported by appropriate evidence and experience.

The doses stated in the BNF are intended for general guidance and represent, unless otherwise stated, the usual range of doses that are generally regarded as being suitable for adults.

> Prescribing medicines outside the recommendations of their marketing authorisation alters (and probably increases) the prescriber's professional responsibility and potential liability. The prescriber should be able to justify and feel competent in using such medicines.

**Oral syringes** An **oral syringe** is supplied when oral liquid medicines are prescribed in doses other than multiples of 5 mL. The oral syringe is marked in 0.5-mL divisions from 1 to 5 mL to measure doses of less than 5 mL (other sizes of oral syringe may also be available). It is provided with an adaptor and an instruction leaflet. The *5-mL spoon* is used for doses of 5 mL (or multiples thereof).

> To avoid inadvertent intravenous administration of oral liquid medicines, only an appropriate **oral** or **enteral syringe** should be used to measure an oral liquid medicine (if a medicine spoon or graduated measure cannot be used); these syringes should **not** be compatible with intravenous or other parenteral devices. Oral or enteral syringes should be clearly labelled 'Oral' or 'Enteral' in a large font size; it is the healthcare practitioner's responsibility to label the syringe with this information if the manufacturer has not done so.

**Strengths and quantities** The strength or quantity to be contained in capsules, lozenges, tablets, etc. should be stated by the prescriber.

If a pharmacist receives an incomplete prescription for a systemically administered preparation and considers it would not be appropriate for the patient to return to the doctor, the following procedures will apply[1]:

(a) an attempt must always be made to contact the prescriber to ascertain the intention;

(b) if the attempt is successful the pharmacist must, where practicable, subsequently arrange for details of quantity, strength where applicable, and dosage to be inserted by the prescriber on the incomplete form;

(c) where, although the prescriber has been contacted, it has not proved possible to obtain the written intention regarding an incomplete prescription, the pharmacist may endorse the form 'p.c.' (prescriber contacted) and add

details of the quantity and strength where applicable of the preparation supplied, and of the dose indicated. The endorsement should be initialled and dated by the pharmacist;

(d) where the prescriber cannot be contacted and the pharmacist has sufficient information to make a professional judgement the preparation may be dispensed. If the quantity is missing the pharmacist may supply sufficient to complete up to 5 days' treatment; except that where a combination pack (i.e. a proprietary pack containing more than one medicinal product) or oral contraceptive is prescribed by name only, the smallest pack shall be dispensed. In all cases the prescription must be endorsed 'p.n.c.' (prescriber not contacted), the quantity, the dose, and the strength (where applicable) of the preparation supplied must be indicated, and the endorsement must be initialled and dated;

(e) if the pharmacist has any doubt about exercising discretion, an incomplete prescription must be referred back to the prescriber.

**Excipients** Branded oral liquid preparations that do not contain *fructose, glucose,* or *sucrose* are described as 'sugar-free' in the BNF. Preparations containing hydrogenated glucose syrup, mannitol, maltitol, sorbitol, or xylitol are also marked 'sugar-free' since there is evidence that they do not cause dental caries. Patients receiving medicines containing cariogenic sugars should be advised of appropriate dental hygiene measures to prevent caries. Sugar-free preparations should be used whenever possible.

Where information on the presence of *aspartame, gluten, sulphites, tartrazine, arachis (peanut) oil* or *sesame oil* is available, this is indicated in the BNF against the relevant preparation.

Information is provided on *selected excipients* in skin preparations (section 13.1.3), in vaccines (section 14.1), and on *selected preservatives* and *excipients* in eye drops and injections. Pressurised metered aerosols containing *chlorofluorocarbons* (CFCs) have also been identified throughout the BNF (see section 3.1.1.1).

The presence of *benzyl alcohol* and *polyoxyl castor oil* (polyethoxylated castor oil) in injections is indicated in the BNF. Benzyl alcohol has been associated with a fatal toxic syndrome in preterm neonates, and therefore, parenteral preparations containing the preservative should not be used in neonates. Polyoxyl castor oils, used as vehicles in intravenous injections, have been associated with severe anaphylactoid reactions.

The presence of *propylene glycol* in oral or parenteral medicines is indicated in the BNF; it can cause adverse effects if its elimination is impaired, e.g. in renal failure, in neonates and young children, and in slow metabolisers of the substance. It may interact with disulfiram and metronidazole.

The *lactose* content in most medicines is too small to cause problems in most lactose intolerant patients. However, in severe lactose intolerance, the lactose content should be determined before prescribing. The amount of lactose varies according to manufacturer, product, formulation, and strength.

> In the absence of information on excipients in the BNF and in the product literature (available at www.emc.medicines.org.uk), contact the manufacturer (see Index of Manufacturers) if it is essential to check details.

**Extemporaneous preparation** A product should be dispensed extemporaneously only when no product with a marketing authorisation is available.

---

1. These recommendations are acceptable for **prescription-only medicines** (PoM). For items marked CD see also Controlled Drugs and Drug Dependence, p. 7.

The BP direction that a preparation must be *freshly prepared* indicates that it must be made not more than 24 hours before it is issued for use. The direction that a preparation should be *recently prepared* indicates that deterioration is likely if the preparation is stored for longer than about 4 weeks at 15–25° C.

The term **water** used without qualification means either potable water freshly drawn direct from the public supply and suitable for drinking or freshly boiled and cooled purified water. The latter should be used if the public supply is from a local storage tank or if the potable water is unsuitable for a particular preparation (Water for injections, section 9.2.2).

**Drugs and driving** Prescribers should advise patients if treatment is likely to affect their ability to drive motor vehicles. This applies especially to drugs with sedative effects; patients should be warned that these effects are increased by alcohol. General information about a patient's fitness to drive is available from the Driver and Vehicle Licensing Agency at www.dvla.gov.uk (see also Appendix 9).

**Patents** In the BNF, certain drugs have been included notwithstanding the existence of actual or potential patent rights. In so far as such substances are protected by Letters Patent, their inclusion in this Formulary neither conveys, nor implies, licence to manufacture.

**Health and safety** When handling chemical or biological materials particular attention should be given to the possibility of allergy, fire, explosion, radiation, or poisoning. Substances such as corticosteroids, some antimicrobials, phenothiazines, and many cytotoxics, are irritant or very potent and should be handled with caution. Contact with the skin and inhalation of dust should be avoided.

**Safety in the home** Patients must be warned to keep all medicines out of the reach of children. All solid dose and all oral and external liquid preparations must be dispensed in a reclosable *child-resistant container* unless:

- the medicine is in an original pack or patient pack such as to make this inadvisable;
- the patient will have difficulty in opening a child-resistant container;
- a specific request is made that the product shall not be dispensed in a child-resistant container;
- no suitable child-resistant container exists for a particular liquid preparation.

All patients should be advised to dispose of *unwanted medicines* by returning them to a supplier for destruction.

**Name of medicine** The name of the medicine should appear on the label unless the prescriber indicates otherwise.

(a) The strength is also stated on the label in the case of tablets, capsules, and similar preparations that are available in different strengths.

(b) If it is the wish of the prescriber that a description such as 'The Sedative Tablets' should appear on the label, the prescriber should write the desired description on the prescription form.

(c) The arrangement will extend to approved names, proprietary names or titles given in the BP, BPC, BNF, DPF, or NPF.

(d) The name written on the label is that used by the prescriber on the prescription.

(e) When a prescription is written other than on an NHS prescription form the name of the prescribed preparation will be stated on the label of the dispensed medicine unless the prescriber indicates otherwise.

(f) The Council of the Royal Pharmaceutical Society advises that the labels of dispensed medicines should indicate the total quantity of the product dispensed in the container to which the label refers. This requirement applies equally to solid, liquid, internal, and external preparations. If a product is dispensed in more than one container, the reference should be to the amount in each container.

---

Non-proprietary names of **compound preparations** which appear in the BNF are those that have been compiled by the British Pharmacopoeia Commission or another recognised body; whenever possible they reflect the names of the active ingredients.

Prescribers should avoid creating their own compound names for the purposes of generic prescribing; such names do not have an approved definition and can be misinterpreted.

Special care should be taken to avoid errors when prescribing compound preparations; in particular the hyphen in the prefix 'co-' should be retained.

Special care should also be taken to avoid creating generic names for **modified-release** preparations where the use of these names could lead to confusion between formulations with different lengths of action.

---

**Security and validity of prescriptions** The Councils of the British Medical Association and the Royal Pharmaceutical Society have issued a joint statement on the security and validity of prescriptions.

In particular, prescription forms should:

- not be left unattended at reception desks;
- not be left in a car where they may be visible; and
- when not in use, be kept in a locked drawer within the surgery and at home.

Where there is any doubt about the authenticity of a prescription, the pharmacist should contact the prescriber. If this is done by telephone, the number should be obtained from the directory rather than relying on the information on the prescription form, which may be false.

**Patient group direction (PGD)** In most cases, the most appropriate clinical care will be provided on an individual basis by a prescriber to a specific individual patient. However, a Patient Group Direction for supply and administration of medicines by other healthcare professionals can be used where it would benefit patient care without compromising safety.

A Patient Group Direction is a written direction relating to the supply and administration (or administration only) of a licensed prescription-only medicine by certain classes of healthcare professionals; the Direction is signed by a doctor (or dentist) and a pharmacist. Further information on Patient Group Directions is available in Health Service Circular HSC 2000/026 (England), HDL (2001) 7 (Scotland), and WHC (2000) 116 (Wales) and at www.portal.nelm.nhs.uk/PGD.

**NICE and Scottish Medicines Consortium** Advice issued by the National Institute for Health and Clinical Excellence (NICE) is included in the BNF when relevant. The BNF also includes advice issued by the Scottish Medicines Consortium (SMC) when a medicine is restricted or not recommended for use within NHS Scotland. If advice within a NICE Single Technology Appraisal differs from SMC advice, the Scottish Executive expects NHS Boards within NHS Scotland to comply with the SMC advice. Details of the advice together with updates can be obtained from www.nice.org.uk and from www.scottishmedicines.org.uk.

General guidance

# Prescription writing

> **Shared care**
> In its guidelines on responsibility for prescribing (circular EL (91) 127) between hospitals and general practitioners, the Department of Health has advised that legal responsibility for prescribing lies with the doctor who signs the prescription.

Prescriptions[1] should be written legibly in ink or otherwise so as to be indelible[2], should be dated, should state the full name and address of the patient, and should be signed in ink by the prescriber[3]. The age and the date of birth of the patient should preferably be stated, and it is a legal requirement in the case of prescription-only medicines to state the age for children under 12 years.

The following should be noted:

(a) The unnecessary use of decimal points should be avoided, e.g. 3 mg, not 3.0 mg.

Quantities of 1 gram or more should be written as 1 g etc.

Quantities less than 1 gram should be written in milligrams, e.g. 500 mg, not 0.5 g.

Quantities less than 1 mg should be written in micrograms, e.g. 100 micrograms, not 0.1 mg.

When decimals are unavoidable a zero should be written in front of the decimal point where there is no other figure, e.g. 0.5 mL, not .5 mL.

Use of the decimal point is acceptable to express a range, e.g. 0.5 to 1 g.

(b) 'Micrograms' and 'nanograms' should **not** be abbreviated. Similarly 'units' should **not** be abbreviated.

(c) The term 'millilitre' (ml or mL)[4] is used in medicine and pharmacy, and cubic centimetre, c.c., or cm³ should not be used.

(d) Dose and dose frequency should be stated; in the case of preparations to be taken 'as required' a **minimum dose interval** should be specified.

When doses other than multiples of 5 mL are prescribed for *oral liquid preparations* the dose-volume will be provided by means of an **oral syringe**, see p. 2 (except for preparations intended to be measured with a pipette).

Suitable quantities:

Elixirs, Linctuses, and Paediatric Mixtures (5-mL dose), 50, 100, or 150 mL

Adult Mixtures (10-mL dose), 200 or 300 mL

Ear Drops, Eye drops, and Nasal Drops, 10 mL (or the manufacturer's pack)

Eye Lotions, Gargles, and Mouthwashes, 200 mL

(e) For suitable quantities of dermatological preparations, see section 13.1.2.

(f) The names of drugs and preparations should be written clearly and **not** abbreviated, using approved titles **only** (see also advice in box on p. 3 to **avoid** creating generic titles for modified-release preparations).

(g) The quantity to be supplied may be stated by indicating the number of days of treatment required in the box provided on NHS forms. In most cases the exact amount will be supplied. This does not apply to items directed to be used as required—if the dose and frequency are not given then the quantity to be supplied needs to be stated.

When several items are ordered on one form the box can be marked with the number of days of treatment provided the quantity is added for any item for which the amount cannot be calculated.

(h) Although directions should preferably be in **English without abbreviation**, it is recognised that some Latin abbreviations are used (for details see Inside Back Cover).

(i) Medical and dental practitioners may prescribe unlicensed medicines (i.e. those without marketing authorisation) or withdrawn medicines. The prescriber should inform the patient or the patient's carer that the product does not have a marketing authorisation.

**Prescribing by dental surgeons**    Until new prescribing arrangements are in place for NHS prescriptions, dental surgeons should use form FP10D (GP14 in Scotland, WP10D in Wales) to prescribe only those items listed in the Dental Practitioners' Formulary.

| Pharmacy Stamp | Age 1yr 3mths | Title, Forename, Surname & Address Master Peter Patient |
|---|---|---|
| | D.o.B 2/4/2007 | Flat 1 50 Stanhope Street Newtown TE22 1ST |
| *Please don't stamp over age box* Number of days' treatment N.B. Ensure dose is stated | 5 | |
| Endorsements | | Amoxicillin oral suspension 125mg/5ml sugar-free 125mg three times daily Supply 100ml [No more items on this prescription] |

Signature of Prescriber    Good    Date 02/07/08

For dispenser No. of Prescns. on form

Anyborough Health Authority
Dr D O Good    345543
7 High Street
Anytown KB1 CD2
Tel: 0111 222 333

**NHS**                                    FP10NC0105

---

1. These recommendations are acceptable for **prescription-only medicines** ([PoM]). For items marked [CD] see also Controlled Drugs and Drug Dependence, p. 7.
2. It is permissible to issue carbon copies of NHS prescriptions as long as they are signed in ink.
3. Computer-generated facsimile signatures do not meet the legal requirement.
4. The use of capital 'L' in mL is a printing convention throughout the BNF; both 'mL' and 'ml' are recognised SI abbreviations.

The Act and Regulations do not set any limitations upon the number and variety of substances which the dental surgeon may administer to patients in the surgery or may order by private prescription—provided the relevant legal requirements are observed the dental surgeon may use or order whatever is required for the clinical situation. There is no statutory requirement for the dental surgeon to communicate with a patient's medical practitioner when prescribing for dental use. There are, however, occasions when this would be in the patient's interest and such communication is to be encouraged. For legal requirements relating to prescriptions for Controlled Drugs, see p. 7.

## Computer-issued prescriptions

For computer-issued prescriptions the following advice, based on the recommendations of the Joint GP Information Technology Committee, should also be noted:

1. The computer must print out the date, the patient's surname, one forename, other initials, and address, and may also print out the patient's title and date of birth. The age of children under 12 years and of adults over 60 years must be printed in the box available; the age of children under 5 years should be printed in years and months. A facility may also exist to print out the age of patients between 12 and 60 years.

2. The doctor's name must be printed at the bottom of the prescription form; this will be the name of the doctor responsible for the prescription (who will normally sign it). The doctor's surgery address, reference number, and Primary Care Trust (PCT[1]) are also necessary. In addition, the surgery telephone number should be printed.

3. When prescriptions are to be signed by general practitioner registrars, assistants, locums, or deputising doctors, the name of the doctor printed at the bottom of the form must still be that of the responsible principal.

4. Names of medicines must come from a dictionary held in the computer memory, to provide a check on the spelling and to ensure that the name is written in full. The computer can be programmed to recognise both the non-proprietary and the proprietary name of a particular drug and to print out the preferred choice, but should not print out both names. For medicines not in the dictionary, separate checks are required—the user must be warned that no check was possible and the entire prescription must be entered in the lexicon.

5. The dictionary may contain information on the usual doses, formulations, and pack sizes to produce standard predetermined prescriptions for common preparations, and to provide a check on the validity of an individual prescription on entry.

6. The prescription must be printed in English without abbreviation; information may be entered or stored in abbreviated form. The dose must be in numbers, the frequency in words, and the quantity in numbers in brackets, thus: 40 mg four times daily (112). It must also be possible to prescribe by indicating the length of treatment required, see (h) above.

7. The BNF recommendations should be followed as in (a), (b), (c), (d), and (e) above.

8. Checks may be incorporated to ensure that all the information required for dispensing a particular drug has been filled in. For instructions such as 'as directed' and 'when required', the maximum daily dose should normally be specified.

9. Numbers and codes used in the system for organising and retrieving data must never appear on the form.

10. Supplementary warnings or advice should be written in full, should not interfere with the clarity of the prescription itself, and should be in line with any warnings or advice in the BNF; numerical codes should not be used.

11. A mechanism (such as printing a series of non-specific characters) should be incorporated to cancel out unused space, or wording such as 'no more items on this prescription' may be added after the last item. Otherwise the doctor should delete the space manually.

12. To avoid forgery the computer may print on the form the number of items to be dispensed (somewhere separate from the box for the pharmacist). The number of items per form need be limited only by the ability of the printer to produce clear and well-demarcated instructions with sufficient space for each item and a spacer line before each fresh item.

13. Handwritten alterations should only be made in exceptional circumstances—it is preferable to print out a new prescription. Any alterations must be made in the doctor's own handwriting and countersigned; computer records should be updated to fully reflect any alteration. Prescriptions for drugs used for contraceptive purposes (but which are not promoted as contraceptives) may need to be marked in handwriting with the symbol ♀ (or endorsed in another way to indicate that the item is prescribed for contraceptive purposes).

14. Prescriptions for controlled drugs can be printed from the computer, but the prescriber's signature must be handwritten[2].

15. The strip of paper on the side of the FP10SS[3] may be used for various purposes but care should be taken to avoid including confidential information. It may be advisable for the patient's name to appear at the top, but this should be preceded by 'confidential'.

16. In rural dispensing practices prescription requests (or details of medicines dispensed) will normally be entered in one surgery. The prescriptions (or dispensed medicines) may then need to be delivered to another surgery or location; if possible the computer should hold up to 10 alternatives.

17. Prescription forms that are reprinted or issued as a duplicate should be labelled clearly as such.

2. See Controlled Drugs and Drug Dependence p. 7; the prescriber may use a date stamp.
3. GP10SS in Scotland, WP10SS in Wales.

# Emergency supply of medicines

*Emergency supply of medicines*

## Emergency supply requested by member of the public

Pharmacists are sometimes called upon by members of the public to make an emergency supply of medicines. The Prescription Only Medicines (Human Use) Order 1997 allows exemptions from the Prescription Only requirements for emergency supply to be made by a person lawfully conducting a retail pharmacy business provided:

(a) that the pharmacist has interviewed the person requesting the prescription-only medicine and is satisfied:

  (i) that there is immediate need for the prescription-only medicine and that it is impracticable in the circumstances to obtain a prescription without undue delay;

  (ii) that treatment with the prescription-only medicine has on a previous occasion been prescribed for the person requesting it;

  (iii) as to the dose that it would be appropriate for the person to take;

(b) that no greater quantity shall be supplied than will provide 5 days' treatment of phenobarbital, phenobarbital sodium, or Controlled Drugs in Schedules 4 or 5[1], or 30 days' treatment for other prescription-only medicines, except when the prescription-only medicine is:

  (i) insulin, an ointment or cream, or a preparation for the relief of asthma in an aerosol dispenser when the smallest pack can be supplied;

  (ii) an oral contraceptive when a full cycle may be supplied;

  (iii) an antibiotic in liquid form for oral administration when the smallest quantity that will provide a full course of treatment can be supplied;

(c) that an entry shall be made by the pharmacist in the prescription book stating:

  (i) the date of supply;

  (ii) the name, quantity and, where appropriate, the pharmaceutical form and strength;

  (iii) the name and address of the patient;

  (iv) the nature of the emergency;

(d) that the container or package must be labelled to show:

  (i) the date of supply;

  (ii) the name, quantity and, where appropriate, the pharmaceutical form and strength;

  (iii) the name of the patient;

  (iv) the name and address of the pharmacy;

  (v) the words 'Emergency supply';

  (vi) the words 'Keep out of the reach of children' (or similar warning);

(e) that the prescription-only medicine is not a substance specifically excluded from the emergency supply provision, and does not contain a Controlled Drug specified in Schedules 1, 2, or 3 to the Misuse of Drugs Regulations 2001 except for phenobarbital or phenobarbital sodium for the treatment of epilepsy: for details see *Medicines, Ethics and Practice*, No. 33, London, Pharmaceutical Press, 2009 (and subsequent editions as available)[1].

## Emergency supply requested by prescriber

Emergency supply of a prescription-only medicine may also be made at the request of a doctor, a dentist, a supplementary prescriber, a community practitioner nurse prescriber, a nurse, pharmacist, or optometrist independent prescriber, or a doctor or dentist from the European Economic Area or Switzerland, provided:

(a) that the pharmacist is satisfied that the prescriber by reason of some emergency is unable to furnish a prescription immediately;

(b) that the prescriber has undertaken to furnish a prescription within 72 hours;

(c) that the medicine is supplied in accordance with the directions of the prescriber requesting it;

(d) that the medicine is not a Controlled Drug specified in Schedules 1, 2, or 3 to the Misuse of Drugs Regulations 2001 except for phenobarbital or phenobarbital sodium for the treatment of epilepsy: for details see *Medicines, Ethics and Practice*, No. 33, London, Pharmaceutical Press, 2009 (and subsequent editions as available)[1];

(e) that an entry shall be made in the prescription book stating:

  (i) the date of supply;

  (ii) the name, quantity and, where appropriate, the pharmaceutical form and strength;

  (iii) the name and address of the practitioner requesting the emergency supply;

  (iv) the name and address of the patient;

  (v) the date on the prescription;

  (vi) when the prescription is received the entry should be amended to include the date on which it is received.

## Royal Pharmaceutical Society's guidelines

1. The pharmacist should consider the medical consequences of *not* supplying a medicine in an emergency.

2. If the pharmacist is unable to make an emergency supply of a medicine the pharmacist should advise the patient how to obtain essential medical care.

For conditions that apply to supplies made at the request of a patient see *Medicines, Ethics and Practice*, No. 33, London Pharmaceutical Press, 2009 (and subsequent editions).

---

1. Doctors or dentists from the European Economic Area and Switzerland, or their patients, cannot request an emergency supply of Controlled Drugs, or drugs that do not have a UK marketing authorisation.

# Controlled Drugs and drug dependence

The Misuse of Drugs Act, 1971 prohibits certain activities in relation to 'Controlled Drugs', in particular their manufacture, supply, and possession. The penalties applicable to offences involving the different drugs are graded broadly according to the *harmfulness attributable to a drug when it is misused* and for this purpose the drugs are defined in the following three classes:

**Class A** includes: alfentanil, cocaine, diamorphine (heroin), dipipanone, lysergide (LSD), methadone, methylenedioxymethamfetamine (MDMA, 'ecstasy'), morphine, opium, pethidine, phencyclidine, remifentanil, and class B substances when prepared for injection

**Class B** includes: oral amphetamines, barbiturates, cannabis, cannabis resin, codeine, ethylmorphine, glutethimide, pentazocine, phenmetrazine, and pholcodine

**Class C** includes: certain drugs related to the amphetamines such as benzfetamine and chlorphentermine, buprenorphine, diethylpropion, mazindol, meprobamate, pemoline, pipradrol, most benzodiazepines, zolpidem, androgenic and anabolic steroids, clenbuterol, chorionic gonadotrophin (HCG), non-human chorionic gonadotrophin, somatotropin, somatrem, and somatropin

The Misuse of Drugs Regulations 2001 define the classes of person who are authorised to supply and possess controlled drugs while acting in their professional capacities and lay down the conditions under which these activities may be carried out. In the regulations drugs are divided into five schedules each specifying the requirements governing such activities as import, export, production, supply, possession, prescribing, and record keeping which apply to them.

**Schedule 1** includes drugs such as cannabis and lysergide which are not used medicinally. Possession and supply are prohibited except in accordance with Home Office authority.

**Schedule 2** includes drugs such as diamorphine (heroin), morphine, remifentanil, pethidine, secobarbital, glutethimide, amfetamine, and cocaine and are subject to the full controlled drug requirements relating to prescriptions, safe custody (except for secobarbital), the need to keep registers, etc. (unless exempted in Schedule 5).

**Schedule 3** includes the barbiturates (except secobarbital, now Schedule 2), buprenorphine, diethylpropion, mazindol, meprobamate, midazolam, pentazocine, phentermine, and temazepam. They are subject to the special prescription requirements (except for temazepam) but not to the safe custody requirements (except for buprenorphine, diethylpropion, and temazepam) nor to the need to keep registers (although there are requirements for the retention of invoices for 2 years).

**Schedule 4** includes in Part I benzodiazepines (except temazepam and midazolam, which are in Schedule 3) and zolpidem, which are subject to minimal control. Part II includes androgenic and anabolic steroids, clenbuterol, chorionic gonadotrophin (HCG), non-human chorionic gonadotrophin, somatotropin, somatrem, and somatropin. Controlled drug prescription requirements do not apply and Schedule 4 Controlled Drugs are not subject to safe custody requirements.

**Schedule 5** includes those preparations which, because of their strength, are exempt from virtually all Controlled Drug requirements other than retention of invoices for two years.

**Prescriptions** Preparations in Schedules 2 and 3 of the Misuse of Drugs Regulations 2001 (and subsequent amendments) are identified throughout the BNF by the symbol ⌖ (Controlled Drug). The principal legal requirements relating to medical prescriptions are listed below (see also Department of Health Guidance, p. 8).

---

**Prescription requirements**

Prescriptions for Controlled Drugs that are subject to prescription requirements[1] must be indelible,[2] and must be *signed* by the prescriber, *be dated*, and specify the prescriber's *address*. The prescription must always state:

- the name and address of the patient;
- in the case of a preparation, the form[3] and where appropriate the strength[4] of the preparation;
- either the total quantity (in both words and figures) of the preparation[5], or the number (in both words and figures) of dosage units, as appropriate, to be supplied; in any other case, the total quantity (in both words and figures) of the Controlled Drug to be supplied;
- the dose;[6]
- the words 'for dental treatment only' if issued by a dentist.

---

A pharmacist is **not** allowed to dispense a Controlled Drug unless all the information required by law is given on the prescription. In the case of a prescription for a Controlled Drug in Schedule 2 or 3, a pharmacist can amend the prescription if it specifies the total quantity only in words or in figures or if it contains minor typographical errors, provided that such amendments are indelible and clearly attributable to the pharmacist. Failure to comply with the regulations concerning the writing of prescriptions will result in inconvenience to patients and delay in supplying the necessary medicine. A prescription for a Controlled Drug in Schedules 2, 3, or 4 is valid for 28 days from the date stated thereon[7].

---

1. All preparations in Schedules 2 and 3, except temazepam.
2. A machine-written prescription is acceptable. The prescriber's signature must be handwritten.
3. The dosage form (e.g. tablets) must be included on a Controlled Drugs prescription irrespective of whether it is implicit in the proprietary name (e.g. *MST Continus*) or whether only one form is available.
4. When more than one strength of a preparation exists the strength required must be specified.
5. The Home Office has advised that quantities of liquid preparations, such as methadone oral solution, should be written in millilitres.
6. The instruction 'one as directed' constitutes a dose but 'as directed' does not.
7. The prescriber may forward-date the prescription; the start date may also be specified in the body of the prescription.

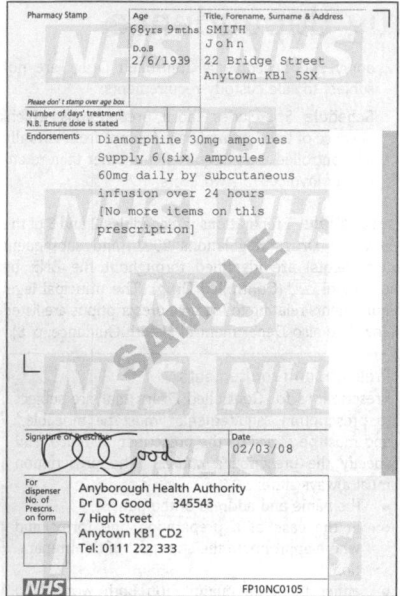

| Pharmacy Stamp | Age 68yrs 9mths | Title, Forename, Surname & Address |
| | D.O.B. 2/6/1939 | SMITH John |
| | | 22 Bridge Street Anytown KB1 5SX |

Please don't stamp over age box
Number of days' treatment
N.B. Ensure dose is stated

Endorsements
Diamorphine 30mg ampoules
Supply 6(six) ampoules
60mg daily by subcutaneous
infusion over 24 hours
[No more items on this
prescription]

Signature of prescriber    O O Good    Date 02/03/08

For dispenser No. of Prescrs. on form
Anyborough Health Authority
Dr D O Good    345543
7 High Street
Anytown KB1 CD2
Tel: 0111 222 333

NHS    FP10NC0105

**Instalments and 'repeats'** A prescription may order a Controlled Drug to be dispensed by instalments; the amount of instalments and the intervals to be observed must be specified.[1] Prescriptions ordering 'repeats' on the same form are **not** permitted for Controlled Drugs in Schedules 2 or 3.

**Private prescriptions** Private prescriptions for Controlled Drugs in Schedules 2 and 3 must be written on specially designated forms provided by Primary Care Trusts in England, Health Boards in Scotland, Local Health Boards in Wales, or the Northern Ireland Central Services Agency; in addition, prescriptions must specify the *prescriber's identification number*. Prescriptions to be supplied by a pharmacist in hospital are exempt from the requirements for private prescriptions.

**Department of Health guidance** Guidance (June 2006) issued by the Department of Health in England on prescribing and dispensing of Controlled Drugs requires:

- in general, prescriptions for Controlled Drugs in Schedules 2, 3, and 4 to be limited to a supply of up to 30 days' treatment; exceptionally, to cover a justifiable clinical need and after consideration of any risk, a prescription can be issued for a longer

period, but the reasons for the decision should be recorded on the patient's notes;

- the patient's identifier to be shown on NHS and private prescriptions for Controlled Drugs in Schedules 2 and 3.

Further information is available at www.dh.gov.uk/controlleddrugs. For a sample prescription, see above.

**Dependence and misuse** The most serious drugs of addiction are **cocaine**, **diamorphine** (heroin), **morphine**, and the **synthetic opioids**. For arrangements for prescribing of diamorphine, dipipanone, or cocaine for addicts, see p. 10.

Despite marked reduction in the prescribing of **amphetamines**, there is concern that abuse of illicit amfetamine and related compounds is widespread.

**Benzodiazepines** are commonly misused. The misuse of **barbiturates** is now uncommon, in line with declining medicinal use and consequent availability.

**Cannabis** (Indian hemp) has no approved medicinal use and cannot be prescribed by doctors. Its use is illegal but widespread. Cannabis is a mild hallucinogen seldom accompanied by a desire to increase the dose; withdrawal symptoms are unusual. **Lysergide** (lysergic acid diethylamide, LSD) is a much more potent hallucinogen; its use can lead to severe psychotic states which can be life-threatening.

There are concerns at an increase in the availability and misuse of other drugs with variously combined hallucinogenic, anaesthetic, or sedative properties. These include ketamine and gamma-hydroxybutyrate (sodium oxybate, GHB).

**Prescribing drugs likely to cause dependence or misuse** The prescriber has three main responsibilities:

- To avoid creating dependence by introducing drugs to patients without sufficient reason. In this context, the proper use of the morphine-like drugs is well understood. The dangers of other Controlled Drugs are less clear because recognition of dependence is not easy and its effects, and those of withdrawal, are less obvious.

- To see that the patient does not gradually increase the dose of a drug, given for good medical reasons, to the point where dependence becomes more likely. This tendency is seen especially with hypnotics and anxiolytics (for CSM advice see section 4.1). The prescriber should keep a close eye on the amount prescribed to prevent patients from accumulating stocks. A minimal amount should be prescribed in the first instance, or when seeing a new patient for the first time.

- To avoid being used as an unwitting source of supply for addicts. Methods include visiting more than one doctor, fabricating stories, and forging prescriptions.

Patients under temporary care should be given only small supplies of drugs unless they present an unequivocal letter from their own doctor. Doctors should also remember that their own patients may be attempting to collect prescriptions from other prescribers, especially in hospitals. It is sensible to reduce dosages steadily or to issue weekly or even daily prescriptions for small amounts if it is apparent that dependence is occurring.

1. A total of 14 days' treatment by instalment of any drug listed in Schedule 2 of the Misuse of Drugs Regulations, buprenorphine, and diazepam may be prescribed in England. In *England*, forms FP10(MDA) (blue) and FP10H(MDA) (blue) should be used. In *Scotland*, forms GP10 (peach), HBP (blue), or HBPA (pink) should be used. In *Wales* a total of 14 days' treatment by instalment of any drug listed in Schedules 2–5 of the Misuse of Drugs Regulations may be prescribed. In Wales, form WP10(MDA) or form WP10HP(AD) should be used.

The stealing and misuse of prescription forms could be minimised by the following precautions:

- do not leave unattended if called away from the consulting room or at reception desks; do not leave in a car where they may be visible; when not in use, keep in a locked drawer within the surgery and at home;
- draw a diagonal line across the blank part of the form under the prescription;
- write the quantity in words and figures when prescribing drugs prone to abuse; this is obligatory for controlled drugs (see Prescriptions, above);
- alterations are best avoided but if any are made they should be clear and unambiguous; add initials against altered items;
- if prescriptions are left for collection they should be left in a safe place in a sealed envelope.

**Travelling abroad** Prescribed drugs listed in Schedule 4 Part II (CD Anab) and Schedule 5 of the Misuse of Drugs Regulations 2001 are not subject to export or import licensing. However, patients intending to travel abroad for more than 3 months carrying any amount of drugs listed in Schedules 2, 3, or 4 Part I (CD Benz) will require a personal export/import licence. Further details can be obtained at www.drugs.homeoffice.gov.uk/drugs-laws/licensing/personal, or from the Home Office by contacting licensing_enquiry.aadu@homeoffice.gsi.gov.uk (in cases of emergency, telephone 0207 035 0484).

Applications must be supported by a covering letter from the prescriber and should give details of:

- the patient's name and address;
- the quantities of drugs to be carried;
- the strength and form in which the drugs will be dispensed;
- the country or countries of destination;
- the dates of travel to and from the United Kingdom.

Applications for licences should be sent to the Home Office, Drugs Licensing, Peel Building, 2 Marsham Street, London, SW1P 4DF. Alternatively, completed application forms can be emailed to licensing_enquiry.aadu@homeoffice.gsi.gov.uk with a scanned copy of the covering letter from the prescriber. A minimum of two weeks should be allowed for processing the application.

Patients travelling for less than 3 months do not require a personal export/import licence for carrying Controlled Drugs, but are advised to carry a letter from the prescribing doctor. Those travelling for more than 3 months are advised to make arrangements to have their medication prescribed by a practitioner in the country they are visiting.

Doctors who want to take Controlled Drugs abroad while accompanying patients may similarly be issued with licences. Licences are not normally issued to doctors who want to take Controlled Drugs abroad solely in case a family emergency should arise.

Personal export/import licences do not have any legal status outside the UK and are issued only to comply with the Misuse of Drugs Act and to facilitate passage through UK Customs and Excise control. For clearance in the country to be visited it is necessary to approach that country's consulate in the UK.

# Notification of drug misusers

Doctors should report cases of drug misuse to their regional or national drug misuse database or centre—see below for contact telephone numbers. The National Drugs Treatment Monitoring System (NDTMS) was introduced in England in April 2001; regional (NDTMS) centres replace the Regional Drug Misuse Databases. A similar system has been introduced in Wales.

Notification to regional (NDTMS) or national centre should be made when a patient starts treatment for drug misuse. All types of problem drug misuse should be reported including opioid, benzodiazepine, and CNS stimulant.

The regional (NDTMS) or national centres are now the only national and local source of epidemiological data on people presenting with problem drug misuse; they provide valuable information to those working with drug misusers and those planning services for them. The databases cannot, however be used as a check on multiple prescribing for drug addicts because the data are anonymised.

Enquiries about the regional (NDTMS) or national centres (including information on how to submit data) can be made to one of the centres listed below:

ENGLAND

*Eastern*
Tel: (01223) 767 904
Fax: (01223) 330 345

*South East*
Tel: (01865) 334 734
Fax: (01865) 334 964

*London*
Tel: (020) 7972 1986
Fax: (020) 7972 1998

*North West*
Tel: (0151) 231 4533
Fax: (0151) 231 4515

*North East*
Tel: (0191) 334 0372
Fax: (0191) 334 0391

*Yorkshire and the Humber*
Tel: (0113) 341 2923
Fax: (0113) 341 3082

*South Western*
Tel: (0117) 970 6474 ext 311
Fax: (0117) 970 7021

*East Midlands*
Tel: (0115) 971 2745
Fax: (0115) 971 2404

*West Midlands*
Tel: (0121) 415 8556
Fax: (0121) 414 8197

SCOTLAND
Tel: (0131) 551 8715
Fax: (0131) 551 1392

WALES
Tel: (029) 2050 3343
Fax: (029) 2050 2330

In **Northern Ireland**, the Misuse of Drugs (Notification of and Supply to Addicts) (Northern Ireland) Regulations 1973 require doctors to send particulars of persons whom they consider to be addicted to certain controlled drugs to the Chief Medical Officer of the Department of Health and Social Services. The Northern Ireland contacts are:

Medical contact:

Dr Ian McMaster
C3 Castle Buildings
Belfast, BT4 3FQ
Tel: (028) 9052 2421
Fax: (028) 9052 0718
ian.mcmaster@dhsspsni.gov.uk

Administrative contact:

Public Health Information & Research Branch
Annex 2
Castle Building
Belfast, BT4 3SQ
Tel: (028) 9052 2520

Public Health Information & Research Branch also maintains the Northern Ireland Drug Misuse Database (NIDMD) which collects detailed information on those presenting for treatment, on drugs misused and injecting behaviour; participation is not a statutory requirement.

## Prescribing of diamorphine (heroin), dipipanone, and cocaine for addicts

The Misuse of Drugs (Supply to Addicts) Regulations 1997 require that only medical practitioners who hold a special licence issued by the Home Secretary may prescribe, administer, or supply diamorphine, dipipanone (*Diconal®*), or cocaine in the treatment of drug addiction; other practitioners must refer any addict who requires these drugs to a treatment centre. Whenever possible the addict will be introduced by a member of staff from the treatment centre to a pharmacist whose agreement has been obtained and whose pharmacy is conveniently sited for the patient. Prescriptions for weekly supplies will be sent to the pharmacy by post and will be dispensed on a daily basis as indicated by the doctor. If any alterations of the arrangements are requested by the addict, the portion of the prescription affected must be represcribed and not merely altered.

General practitioners and other doctors do not require a special licence for prescribing diamorphine, dipipanone, and cocaine for patients (including addicts) for *relieving pain* from organic disease or injury.

For guidance on prescription writing, see p. 7.

# Adverse reactions to drugs

Any drug may produce unwanted or unexpected adverse reactions. Rapid detection and recording of adverse reactions is of vital importance so that unrecognised hazards are identified promptly and appropriate regulatory action is taken to ensure that medicines are used safely. Doctors, dentists, coroners, pharmacists, and nurses (see also self-reporting below) are urged to report suspected adverse reactions directly to the Medicines and Healthcare products Regulatory Agency (MHRA) through the Yellow Card Scheme using the electronic form at www.yellowcard.gov.uk. Alternatively, prepaid Yellow Cards for reporting are available from the address below and are also bound in this book (inside back cover).

Medicines and Healthcare products Regulatory Agency
CHM
Freepost
London SW8 5BR
Tel: 0800 731 6789

Suspected adverse reactions to *any* therapeutic agent should be reported, including drugs *(self-medication* as well as those *prescribed)*, blood products, vaccines, radiographic contrast media, complementary and herbal products.

A 24-hour Freefone service is available to all parts of the UK for advice and information on suspected adverse drug reactions; contact the National Yellow Card Information Service at the MHRA on 0800 731 6789. Outside office hours a telephone-answering machine will take messages.

The following Yellow Card Centres may *follow up* reports:

Yellow Card Centre
Northwest
70 Pembroke Place
Liverpool L69 3GF
Tel: (0151) 794 8206

Yellow Card Centre Wales
Freepost
Cardiff CF4 1ZZ
Tel: (029) 2074 4181
(direct line)

Yellow Card Centre
Northern & Yorkshire
Wolfson Unit
Claremont Place
Newcastle upon
Tyne NE2 4HH
Tel: (0191) 260 6181
(direct line)

Yellow Card Centre West
Midlands
Freepost SW2991
Birmingham B18 7BR
Tel: (0121) 507 5672

Yellow Card Centre
Scotland
CARDS, Royal Infirmary
of Edinburgh
Freepost RRAR-RUXE-
GJGX
Edinburgh EH16 4SA
Tel: (0131) 242 2919

The MHRA's database facilitates the monitoring of adverse drug reactions.

More detailed information on reporting and a list of products currently under intensive monitoring can be found on the MHRA website: www.mhra.gov.uk.

> *Drug Safety Update* is a monthly newsletter from the MHRA and the Commission on Human Medicines (CHM); it is available at www.mhra.gov.uk/mhra/drugsafetyupdate.

**Self-reporting** Patients, parents, and carers can also report suspected adverse reactions to the MHRA. Reports can be submitted directly to the MHRA through the Yellow Card Scheme using the electronic form at www.yellowcard.gov.uk or by telephone on 0808 100 3352. Alternatively, patient Yellow Cards are available from pharmacies.

**Prescription-event monitoring** In addition to the MHRA's Yellow Card Scheme, an independent scheme monitors the safety of new medicines using a different approach. The Drug Safety Research Unit identifies patients who have been prescribed selected new medicines and collects data on clinical events in these patients. The data are submitted on a voluntary basis by general practitioners on green forms. More information about the scheme and the Unit's educational material is available from www.dsru.org.

**Newer drugs and vaccines** Only limited information is available from clinical trials on the safety of new medicines. Further understanding about the safety of medicines depends on the availability of information from routine clinical practice.

The black triangle symbol (▼) identifies newly licensed medicines that are monitored intensively by the MHRA. Such medicines include new active substances, biosimilar medicines, medicines that have been licensed for administration by a new route or drug delivery system, or for significant new indications which may alter the established risks and benefits of that drug, or that contain a new combination of active substances. There is no standard time for which products retain a black triangle; safety data are usually reviewed after 2 years.

Spontaneous reporting is particularly valuable for recognising possible new hazards rapidly. For medicines showing the black triangle symbol, the MHRA asks that **all** suspected reactions (including those considered not to be serious) are reported through the Yellow Card Scheme. An adverse reaction should be reported even if it is not certain that the drug has caused it, or if the reaction is well recognised, or if other drugs have been given at the same time.

**Established drugs and vaccines** Doctors, dentists, coroners, pharmacists and nurses are asked to report *all* serious suspected reactions, including those that are fatal, life-threatening, disabling, incapacitating, or which result in or prolong hospitalisation; they should be reported even if the effect is well recognised. Examples include anaphylaxis, blood disorders, endocrine disturbances, effects on fertility, haemorrhage from any site, renal impairment, jaundice, ophthalmic disorders, severe CNS effects, severe skin reactions, reactions in pregnant women, and any drug interactions. Reports of serious adverse reactions are required to enable comparison with other drugs of a similar class. Reports of overdoses (deliberate or accidental) can complicate the assessment of adverse drug reactions, but provide important information on the potential toxicity of drugs.

For established drugs there is no need to report well-known, relatively minor side-effects, such as dry mouth with tricyclic antidepressants or constipation with opioids.

**Adverse reactions to medical devices** Suspected adverse reactions to medical devices including dental or surgical materials, intra-uterine devices, and contact lens fluids should be reported. Information on reporting these can be found at: www.mhra.gov.uk.

**Side-effects in the BNF** The BNF includes clinically relevant side-effects for most drugs; an exhaustive list is not included for drugs that are used by specialists (e.g. cytotoxic drugs and drugs used in anaesthesia). Where causality has not been established, side-effects in the manufacturers' literature may be omitted from the BNF.

Recognising that hypersensitivity reactions can occur with virtually all medicines, this effect is not generally listed, unless the drug carries an increased risk of such reactions. The BNF also omits effects that are likely to have little clinical consequence (e.g. transient increase in liver enzymes).

Side-effects are generally listed in order of frequency and arranged broadly by body systems. Occasionally a rare side-effect might be listed first if it is considered to be particularly important because of its seriousness.

In the product literature the frequency of side-effects is generally described as follows:

| | |
|---|---|
| Very common | greater than 1 in 10 |
| Common | 1 in 100 to 1 in 10 |
| Uncommon ['less commonly' in BNF] | 1 in 1000 to 1 in 100 |
| Rare | 1 in 10 000 to 1 in 1000 |
| Very rare | less than 1 in 10 000 |

## Special problems

**Delayed drug effects** Some reactions (e.g. cancers, chloroquine retinopathy, and retroperitoneal fibrosis) may become manifest months or years after exposure. Any suspicion of such an association should be reported directly to the MHRA through the Yellow Card Scheme.

**The elderly** Particular vigilance is required to identify adverse reactions in the elderly.

**Congenital abnormalities** When an infant is born with a congenital abnormality or there is a malformed aborted fetus doctors are asked to consider whether this might be an adverse reaction to a drug and to report all drugs (including self-medication) taken during pregnancy.

**Children** Particular vigilance is required to identify and report adverse reactions in children, including those resulting from the unlicensed use of medicines; **all** suspected reactions should be reported directly to the MHRA through the Yellow Card Scheme.

## Prevention of adverse reactions

Adverse reactions may be prevented as follows:

- never use any drug unless there is a good indication. If the patient is pregnant do not use a drug unless the need for it is imperative;

- allergy and idiosyncrasy are important causes of adverse drug reactions. Ask if the patient had previous reactions;

- ask if the patient is already taking other drugs *including self-medication drugs, health supplements, complementary and alternative therapies*; interactions may occur;

- age and hepatic or renal disease may alter the metabolism or excretion of drugs, so that much smaller doses may be needed. Genetic factors may also be responsible for variations in metabolism, notably of isoniazid and the tricyclic antidepressants;

- prescribe as few drugs as possible and give very clear instructions to the elderly or any patient likely to misunderstand complicated instructions;

- whenever possible use a familiar drug; with a new drug, be particularly alert for adverse reactions or unexpected events;

- warn the patient if serious adverse reactions are liable to occur.

## Oral side-effects of drugs

Drug-induced disorders of the mouth may be due to a local action on the mouth or to a systemic effect manifested by oral changes. In the latter case urgent referral to the patient's medical practitioner may be necessary.

### Oral mucosa

Medicaments left in contact with or applied directly to the oral mucosa can lead to inflammation or ulceration; the possibility of allergy should also be borne in mind.

**Aspirin** tablets allowed to dissolve in the sulcus for the treatment of toothache can lead to a white patch followed by ulceration.

Flavouring agents, particularly **essential oils**, may sensitise the skin, but mucosal swelling is not usually prominent.

The oral mucosa is particularly vulnerable to ulceration in patients treated with cytotoxic drugs, e.g. **methotrexate**. Other drugs capable of causing oral ulceration include **captopril** (and other ACE inhibitors), **gold**, **nicorandil, NSAIDs, pancreatin, penicillamine, proguanil**, and **protease inhibitors**.

*Erythema multiforme* (including Stevens-Johnson syndrome) may follow the use of a wide range of drugs including **antibacterials, antiretrovirals, sulphonamide derivatives**, and **anticonvulsants**; the oral mucosa may be extensively ulcerated, with characteristic target lesions on the skin. Oral lesions of *toxic epidermal necrolysis* (Lyell's syndrome) have been reported with a similar range of drugs.

*Lichenoid eruptions* are associated with **ACE inhibitors, NSAIDs, methyldopa, chloroquine, oral antidiabetics, thiazide diuretics**, and **gold**.

*Candidiasis* can complicate treatment with **antibacterials** and **immunosuppressants** and is an occasional side-effect of **corticosteroid inhalers**, see also p. 166.

### Teeth and Jaw

*Brown staining* of the teeth frequently follows the use of **chlorhexidine** mouthwash, spray or gel, but can readily be removed by polishing. **Iron** salts in liquid form can stain the enamel black. Superficial staining has been reported rarely with **co-amoxiclav** suspension.

*Intrinsic staining* of the teeth is most commonly caused by **tetracyclines**. They will affect the teeth if given at any time from about the fourth month *in utero* until the age of twelve years; they are contra-indicated during pregnancy, in breast-feeding women, and in children under 12 years. All tetracyclines can cause permanent, unsightly staining in children, the colour varying from yellow to grey.

Excessive ingestion of **fluoride** leads to *dental fluorosis* with mottling of the enamel and areas of hypoplasia or pitting; fluoride supplements occasionally cause mild mottling (white patches) if the dose is too large for the child's age (taking into account the fluoride content of the local drinking water and of toothpaste).

*Osteonecrosis of the jaw* has been reported in patients receiving a bisphosphonate by the intravenous route and, rarely, in those taking a biphosphonate orally. If possible, dental surgical procedures should be avoided during and after bisphosphonate treatment, see also p. 422.

### Periodontium

*Gingival overgrowth* (gingival hyperplasia) is a side-effect of **phenytoin** and sometimes of **ciclosporin** or of **nifedipine** (and some other calcium-channel blockers).

*Thrombocytopenia* may be drug related and may cause bleeding at the gingival margins, which may be spontaneous or may follow mild trauma (such as toothbrushing).

### Salivary glands

The most common effect that drugs have on the salivary glands is to *reduce flow* (xerostomia). Patients with a persistently dry mouth may have poor oral hygiene; they are at an increased risk of dental caries and oral infections (particularly candidiasis). Many drugs have been implicated in xerostomia, particularly **antimuscarinics** (anticholinergics), **antidepressants** (including tricyclic antidepressants, and selective serotonin re-uptake inhibitors), **alpha-blockers**, **antihistamines**, **antipsychotics**, **baclofen**, **bupropion**, **clonidine**, 5HT$_1$ agonists, **opioids**, **sibutramine**, and **tizanidine**. Excessive use of **diuretics** can also result in xerostomia.

Some drugs (e.g. clozapine, neostigmine) can *increase saliva production* but this is rarely a problem unless the patient has associated difficulty in swallowing.

Pain in the salivary glands has been reported with some **antihypertensives** (e.g. clonidine, methyldopa) and with **vinca alkaloids**.

Swelling of the salivary glands can occur with **iodides**, **antithyroid drugs**, **phenothiazines**, **ritodrine**, and **sulphonamides**.

### Taste

There can be *decreased* taste acuity or *alteration* in taste sensation. Drugs implicated include **amiodarone**, **calcitonin**, **captopril** (and other ACE inhibitors), **carbimazole**, **clarithromycin**, **gold**, **griseofulvin**, **lithium salts**, **metformin**, **metronidazole**, **penicillamine**, **phenindione**, **propafenone**, **protease inhibitors**, **terbinafine**, and **zopiclone**.

## Defective medicines

During the manufacture or distribution of a medicine an error or accident may occur whereby the finished product does not conform to its specification. While such a defect may impair the therapeutic effect of the product and could adversely affect the health of a patient, it should **not** be confused with an Adverse Drug Reaction where the product conforms to its specification.

The Defective Medicines Report Centre assists with the investigation of problems arising from licensed medicinal products thought to be defective and co-ordinates any necessary protective action. Reports on suspect defective medicinal products should include the brand or the non-proprietary name, the name of the manufacturer or supplier, the strength and dosage form of the product, the product licence number, the batch number or numbers of the product, the nature of the defect, and an account of any action already taken in consequence. The Centre can be contacted at:

The Defective Medicines Report Centre
Medicines and Healthcare products Regulatory Agency
17–157 Market Towers
1 Nine Elms Lane
London SW8 5NQ
(020) 7084 2574 (weekdays 9.00 am–5.00 pm)
or (020) 7210 3000 (urgent calls outside office hours)
info@mhra.gsi.gov.uk

# Prescribing for children

For detailed advice on medicines used for children, consult *BNF for Children*

Children, and particularly neonates, differ from adults in their response to drugs. Special care is needed in the neonatal period (first 30 days of life) and doses should always be calculated with care. At this age, the risk of toxicity is increased by reduced drug clearance and differing target organ sensitivity.

Whenever possible, intramuscular injections should be **avoided** in children because they are painful.

Where possible, medicines for children should be prescribed within the terms of the marketing authorisation (product licence). However, many children may require medicines not specifically licensed for paediatric use.

Although medicines cannot be promoted outside the limits of the licence, the Medicines Act does not prohibit the use of unlicensed medicines. It is recognised that the informed use of unlicensed medicines or of licensed medicines for unlicensed applications ('off-label' use) is often necessary in paediatric practice.

**Adverse drug reactions in children** The reporting of all suspected adverse drug reactions in children is **strongly encouraged** through the Yellow Card Scheme (see p. 11) even if the intensive monitoring symbol (▼) has been removed, because experience in children may still be limited.

The identification and reporting of adverse reactions to drugs in children is particularly important because:

- the action of the drug and its pharmacokinetics in children (especially in the very young) may be different from that in adults;
- drugs are not extensively tested in children;
- many drugs are not specifically licensed for use in children and are used 'off-label';
- suitable formulations may not be available to allow precise dosing in children;
- the nature and course of illnesses and adverse drug reactions may differ between adults and children.

**Prescription writing** Prescriptions should be written according to the guidelines in Prescription Writing (p. 4) Inclusion of age is a legal requirement in the case of prescription-only medicines for children under 12 years of age, but it is preferable to state the age for **all** prescriptions for children.

It is particularly important to state the strengths of capsules or tablets. Although liquid preparations are particularly suitable for children, they may contain sugar which encourages dental decay. Sugar-free medicines are preferred for long-term treatment.

Many children are able to swallow tablets or capsules and may prefer a solid dose form; involving the child and parents in choosing the formulation is helpful.

When a prescription for a liquid oral preparation is written and the dose ordered is smaller than 5 mL an **oral syringe** will be supplied (for details, see p. 2). Parents should be advised not to add any medicines to the infant's feed, since the drug may interact with the milk or other liquid in it; moreover the ingested dosage may be reduced if the child does not drink all the contents.

Parents must be warned to keep **all** medicines out of reach of children, see Safety in the Home, p. 3.

## Rare paediatric conditions

Information on substances such as *biotin* and *sodium benzoate* used in rare metabolic conditions is included in *BNF for Children*; further information can be obtained from:

Alder Hey Children's Hospital
Drug Information Centre
Liverpool  L12 2AP
Tel: (0151) 252 5381

Great Ormond Street Hospital for Children
Pharmacy
Great Ormond St
London  WC1N 3JH
Tel: (020) 7405 9200

## Dosage in children

Children's doses in the BNF are stated in the individual drug entries as far as possible, except where paediatric use is not recommended, information is not available, or there are special hazards.

Doses are generally based on body-weight (in kilograms) or the following age ranges:

first month (neonate)

up to 1 year (infant)

1–5 years

6–12 years

Unless the age is specified, the term 'child' in the BNF includes persons aged 12 years and younger.

**Dose calculation** Many children's doses are standardised by **weight** (and therefore require multiplying by the body-weight in kilograms to determine the child's dose); occasionally, the doses have been standardised by **body surface area** (in $m^2$). These methods should be used rather than attempting to calculate a child's dose on the basis of doses used in adults.

For most drugs the adult maximum dose should not be exceeded. For example if the dose is stated as 8 mg/kg (max. 300 mg), a child weighing 10 kg should receive 80 mg but a child weighing 40 kg should receive 300 mg (rather than 320 mg).

Young children may require a higher dose per kilogram than adults because of their higher metabolic rates. Other problems need to be considered. For example, calculation by body-weight in the overweight child may result in much higher doses being administered than necessary; in such cases, dose should be calculated from an ideal weight, related to height and age (see inside back cover).

**Body surface area (BSA) estimates** are often preferable to body-weight for calculation of paediatric doses since many physiological phenomena correlate better with body surface area. Body surface area can be estimated from weight. For more information, refer to *BNF for Children*.

Where the dose for children is not stated, prescribers should consult *BNF for Children* or seek advice from a medicines information centre.

**Dose frequency** Antibacterials are generally given at regular intervals throughout the day. Some flexibility should be allowed in children to avoid waking them during the night. For example, the night-time dose may be given at the child's bedtime.

Where new or potentially toxic drugs are used, the manufacturers' recommended doses should be carefully followed.

# Prescribing in palliative care

Palliative care is the active total care of patients whose disease is not responsive to curative treatment. Control of pain, of other symptoms, and of psychological, social and spiritual problems, is paramount to provide the best quality of life for patients and their families. Careful assessment of symptoms and needs of the patient should be undertaken by a multidisciplinary team.

Specialist palliative care is available in most areas as day hospice care, home-care teams (often known as Macmillan teams), in-patient hospice care, and hospital teams. Many acute hospitals and teaching centres now have consultative, hospital-based teams.

Hospice care of terminally ill patients has shown the importance of symptom control and psychosocial support of the patient and family. Families should be included in the care of the patient if they wish.

Many patients wish to remain at home with their families. Although some families may at first be afraid of caring for the patient at home, support can be provided by community nursing services, social services, voluntary agencies and hospices together with the general practitioner. The family may be reassured by the knowledge that the patient will be admitted to a hospital or hospice if the family cannot cope.

**Drug treatment**   The number of drugs should be as few as possible, for even the taking of medicine may be an effort. Oral medication is usually satisfactory unless there is severe nausea and vomiting, dysphagia, weakness, or coma, when parenteral medication may be necessary.

## Pain

Analgesics are more effective in preventing pain than in the relief of established pain; it is important that they are given regularly.

**Paracetamol** (p. 234) or a **NSAID** (section 10.1.1) given regularly will often make the use of opioid analgesics unnecessary. A NSAID may also control the pain of *bone secondaries*; if necessary, flurbiprofen or indometacin can be given rectally. Radiotherapy, bisphosphonates (section 6.6.2), and radioactive isotopes of **strontium** (*Metastron®* available from GE Healthcare) may also be useful for pain due to bone metastases.

An opioid analgesic (section 4.7.2) such as **codeine** (p. 239), alone or in combination with a non-opioid analgesic at adequate dosage, may be helpful in the control of moderate pain if non-opioid analgesics alone are not sufficient. Alternatively, **tramadol** (p. 245) can be considered for moderate pain. If these preparations do not control the pain, **morphine** (p. 242) is the most useful opioid analgesic. Alternatives to morphine, including **hydromorphone** (p. 241), **methadone** (p. 241), **oxycodone** (p. 243), and transdermal **fentanyl** (see p. 16 and p. 240) are best initiated by those with experience in palliative care. Initiation of an opioid analgesic should not be delayed by concern over a theoretical likelihood of psychological dependence (addiction).

### Equivalent single doses of opioid analgesics

These equivalences are intended **only** as an approximate guide; patients should be carefully monitored after **any** change in medication and dose titration may be required

| Analgesic | Dose |
|---|---|
| Morphine salts (oral) | 10 mg |
| Diamorphine hydrochloride (intramuscular) | 3 mg |
| Hydromorphone hydrochloride | 1.3 mg |
| Oxycodone (oral) | 5 mg |

**Oral route**   Morphine (p. 242) is given *by mouth* as an oral solution or as standard ('immediate release') tablets regularly every 4 hours, the initial dose depending largely on the patient's previous treatment. A dose of 5–10 mg is enough to replace a weaker analgesic (such as paracetamol), but 10–20 mg or more is required to replace a strong one (comparable to morphine itself). If the first dose of morphine is no more effective than the previous analgesic, the next dose should be increased by 30–50%, the aim being to choose the lowest dose that prevents pain. The dose should be adjusted with careful assessment of the pain, and the use of adjuvant analgesics (such as NSAIDs) should also be considered. Although morphine in a dose of 5–20 mg is usually adequate there should be no hesitation in increasing it stepwise according to response to 100 mg or occasionally up to 500 mg or higher if necessary. It may be possible to omit the overnight dose if double the usual dose is given at bedtime.

If pain occurs between regular doses of morphine ('breakthrough pain'), an additional dose ('rescue dose') should be given. An additional dose should also be given 30 minutes before an activity that causes pain (e.g. wound dressing). Fentanyl lozenges are also licensed for breakthrough pain.

When the pain is controlled and the patient's 24-hour morphine requirement is established, the daily dose can be given as a *modified-release preparation* in a single dose or in two divided doses.

Preparations suitable for twice-daily administration include *Morphgesic® SR* tablets (p. 243), *MST Continus®* tablets or suspension (p. 243), and *Zomorph®* capsules (p. 243). *MXL®* capsules (p. 243) allow administration of the total daily morphine requirement as a single dose.

The starting dose of modified-release morphine preparations designed for twice daily administration is usually 10–20 mg every 12 hours if no other analgesic (or only paracetamol) has been taken previously, but to replace a weaker opioid analgesic (such as co-codamol) the starting dose is usually 20–30 mg every 12 hours. Increments should be made to the dose, not to the frequency of administration, which should remain at every 12 hours.

The effective dose of modified-release preparations can alternatively be determined by giving the oral solution of morphine every 4 hours in increasing doses until the pain has been controlled, and then transferring the patient to the same total 24-hour dose of morphine given as the modified-release preparation (divided into two portions for 12-hourly administration). The first dose of the modified-release preparation is given 4 hours after the last dose of the oral solution.[1]

Morphine, as oral solution or standard formulation tablets, should be prescribed for breakthrough pain; the dose should be about one-sixth of the total daily dose of oral morphine repeated every 4 hours if necessary (review pain management if analgesic required more frequently).

**Oxycodone** (p. 243) can be used in patients who require an opioid but cannot tolerate morphine. If the patient is already receiving an opioid, oxycodone should be started at a dose equivalent to the current analgesic (see Equivalent Single Doses of Opioid Analgesics table, p. 15).

**Levomepromazine** (methotrimeprazine, p. 197) is licensed to treat pain in palliative care, and may be of benefit in some patients. It should be reserved for use in conjunction with strong opioid analgesics in distressed patients with severe pain unresponsive to other measures.

**Parenteral route**  If the patient becomes unable to swallow, the equivalent intramuscular dose of morphine is half the oral solution dose; in the case of the modified-release tablets it is half the total 24-hour dose (which is then divided into 6 portions to be given every 4 hours). **Diamorphine** (p. 239) is preferred for injection because, being more soluble, it can be given in a smaller volume. The equivalent intramuscular (or subcutaneous) dose is approximately a third of the oral dose of morphine. *Subcutaneous infusion* of diamorphine via continuous infusion device can be useful (for details, see p. 17).

If the patient can resume taking medicines by mouth, then oral morphine may be substituted for subcutaneous infusion of diamorphine. See table of approximate equivalent doses of morphine and diamorphine, p. 19.

**Rectal route**  Morphine (p. 243) is also available for *rectal administration* as suppositories; alternatively **oxycodone** (p. 243) suppositories can be obtained on special order.

**Transdermal route**  Transdermal preparations of fentanyl and buprenorphine are available (section 4.7.2); they are not suitable for acute pain or in patients whose analgesic requirements are changing rapidly because the long time to steady state prevents rapid titration of the dose. Prescribers should ensure that they are familiar with the correct use of transdermal preparations (see under Fentanyl, p. 240) because inappropriate use has caused fatalities.

The following 24-hour doses of morphine **by mouth** are considered to be approximately equivalent to the fentanyl patches shown:

Morphine salt 45 mg daily ≡ fentanyl '12' patch

Morphine salt 90 mg daily ≡ fentanyl '25' patch

Morphine salt 180 mg daily ≡ fentanyl '50' patch

Morphine salt 270 mg daily ≡ fentanyl '75' patch

Morphine salt 360 mg daily ≡ fentanyl '100' patch

Morphine (as oral solution or standard formulation tablets) is given for breakthrough pain.

**Gastro-intestinal pain**  The pain of *bowel colic* may be reduced by loperamide 2–4 mg 4 times daily. *Hyoscine*

*hydrobromide* (section 4.6) may also be helpful, given sublingually at a dose of 300 micrograms 3 times daily as *Kwells®* tablets. For the dose by subcutaneous infusion, see p. 18).

Gastric distension pain due to pressure on the stomach may be helped by a preparation incorporating an antacid with an antiflatulent (section 1.1.1) and a prokinetic such as domperidone 10 mg 3 times daily before meals.

**Muscle spasm**  The pain of muscle spasm can be helped by a muscle relaxant such as diazepam 5–10 mg daily or baclofen 5–10 mg 3 times daily.

**Neuropathic pain**  Patients with neuropathic pain (section 4.7.3) may benefit from a trial of a tricyclic antidepressant for several weeks. An anticonvulsant may be added or substituted if pain persists; gabapentin and pregabalin (both section 4.8.1) are licensed for neuropathic pain.

Pain due to nerve compression may be reduced by a corticosteroid such as dexamethasone 8 mg daily, which reduces oedema around the tumour, thus reducing compression.

**Nerve blocks** can be considered when pain is localised to a specific area. **Transcutaneous electrical nerve stimulation** (TENS) may also help.

---

## Miscellaneous conditions

> Unlicensed indications or routes
> Several recommendations in this section involve unlicensed indications or routes.

**Anorexia**  Anorexia may be helped by prednisolone 15–30 mg daily or dexamethasone 2–4 mg daily.

**Capillary bleeding**  Capillary bleeding can be treated with tranexamic acid (section 2.11) by mouth; treatment is usually discontinued one week after the bleeding has stopped, or, if necessary, it can be continued at a reduced dose. Alternatively, gauze soaked in tranexamic acid 100 mg/mL or adrenaline (epinephrine) solution 1 mg/mL (1 in 1000) can be applied to the affected area.

**Constipation**  Constipation is a very common cause of distress and is almost invariable after administration of an opioid analgesic. It should be prevented if possible by the regular administration of laxatives; a faecal softener with a peristaltic stimulant (e.g. co-danthramer) or lactulose solution with a senna preparation should be used (section 1.6.2 and section 1.6.3). Methylnaltrexone (section 1.6.6) is licensed for the treatment of opioid-induced constipation.

**Convulsions**  Patients with cerebral tumours or uraemia may be susceptible to convulsions. Prophylactic treatment with phenytoin or carbamazepine (section 4.8.1) should be considered. When oral medication is no longer possible, diazepam as suppositories 10–20 mg every 4 to 8 hours, or phenobarbital by injection 50–200 mg twice daily is continued as prophylaxis. For the use of midazolam by subcutaneous infusion using a continuous infusion device, see below.

**Dry mouth**  Dry mouth may be relieved by good mouth care and measures such as the sucking of ice or pineapple chunks or the use of artificial saliva (section 12.3.5); dry mouth associated with candidiasis can be treated by oral preparations of nystatin or miconazole

---

1. Studies have indicated that administration of the last dose of the *oral solution* with the first dose of the *modified-release tablets* is not necessary.

(section 12.3.2); alternatively, fluconazole can be given by mouth (section 5.2). Dry mouth may be caused by certain medications including opioids, antimuscarinic drugs (e.g. hyoscine), antidepressants and some antiemetics; if possible, an alternative preparation should be considered.

**Dysphagia** A corticosteroid such as dexamethasone 8 mg daily may help, temporarily, if there is an obstruction due to tumour. See also Dry Mouth, p. 16.

**Dyspnoea** Breathlessness at rest may be relieved by regular oral morphine in carefully titrated doses, starting at 5 mg every 4 hours. Diazepam 5–10 mg daily may be helpful for dyspnoea associated with anxiety. A corticosteroid, such as dexamethasone 4–8 mg daily, may also be helpful if there is bronchospasm or partial obstruction.

**Excessive respiratory secretion** Excessive respiratory secretion (death rattle) may be reduced by subcutaneous injection of hyoscine hydrobromide 400–600 micrograms every 4 to 8 hours; however, care must be taken to avoid the discomfort of dry mouth. Alternatively glycopyrronium can be given by subcutaneous or intramuscular injection in a dose of 200 micrograms every 4 hours. For the dose by subcutaneous infusion using a continuous infusion device, see p. 18.

**Fungating tumours** Fungating tumours can be treated by regular dressing and antibacterial drugs; systemic treatment with metronidazole (section 5.1.11) is often required but topical metronidazole (section 13.10.1.2) is also used.

**Hiccup** Hiccup due to gastric distension may be helped by a preparation incorporating an antacid with an antiflatulent (section 1.1.1). If this fails, metoclopramide 10 mg every 6 to 8 hours by mouth or by subcutaneous or intramuscular injection can be added; if this also fails, baclofen 5 mg twice daily, or nifedipine 10 mg three times daily, or chlorpromazine 10–25 mg every 6 to 8 hours can be tried.

**Hypercalcaemia** see section 9.5.1.2

**Insomnia** Patients with advanced cancer may not sleep because of discomfort , cramps, night sweats, joint stiffness, or fear. There should be appropriate treatment of these problems before hypnotics are used. Benzodiazepines, such as temazepam (section 4.1.1), may be useful.

**Intractable cough** Intractable cough may be relieved by moist inhalations or by regular administration of oral morphine in an initial dose of 5 mg every 4 hours. Methadone linctus should be avoided because it has a long duration of action and tends to accumulate.

**Nausea and vomiting** Nausea and vomiting are common in patients with advanced cancer. Ideally, the cause should be determined before treatment with an antiemetic (section 4.6) is started.

Nausea and vomiting may occur with opioid therapy particularly in the initial stages but can be prevented by giving an antiemetic such as haloperidol or metoclopramide. An antiemetic is usually necessary only for the first 4 or 5 days and therefore combined preparations containing an opioid with an antiemetic are not recommended because they lead to unnecessary antiemetic therapy (and associated side-effects when used long-term).

Metoclopramide has a prokinetic action and is used in a dose of 10 mg 3 times daily by mouth for nausea and vomiting associated with gastritis, gastric stasis, and functional bowel obstruction. Drugs with antimuscarinic effects antagonise prokinetic drugs and, if possible, should not be used concurrently.

Haloperidol is used by mouth in an initial dose of 1.5 mg once or twice daily (can be increased if necessary to 5–10 mg daily in divided doses) for most metabolic causes of vomiting (e.g. hypercalcaemia, renal failure).

Cyclizine is given in a dose of 50 mg up to 3 times daily by mouth. It is used for nausea and vomiting due to mechanical bowel obstruction, raised intracranial pressure, and motion sickness.

Antiemetic therapy should be reviewed every 24 hours; it may be necessary to substitute the antiemetic or to add another one.

Levomepromazine (methotrimeprazine) can be used if first-line antiemetics are inadequate; it is given by mouth in a dose of 6–50 mg daily (6-mg tablets available from 'special-order' manufacturers or specialist importing companies, see p. 969) in 1–2 divided doses. For the dose by subcutaneous infusion, see p. 18. Dexamethasone 8–16 mg daily by mouth can be used as an adjunct.

For the administration of antiemetics by subcutaneous infusion using a continuous infusion device, see below.

For the treatment of nausea and vomiting associated with cancer chemotherapy, see section 8.1.

**Pruritus** Pruritus, even when associated with obstructive jaundice, often responds to simple measures such as application of emollients (section 13.2.1). In the case of obstructive jaundice, further measures include administration of colestyramine (section 1.9.2).

**Raised intracranial pressure** Headache due to raised intracranial pressure often responds to a high dose of a corticosteroid, such as dexamethasone 16 mg daily for 4 to 5 days, subsequently reduced to 4–6 mg daily if possible; dexamethasone should be given before 6 p.m. to reduce the risk of insomnia.

**Restlessness and confusion** Restlessness and confusion may require treatment with haloperidol 1–3 mg by mouth every 8 hours. Levomepromazine (methotrimeprazine) is also used occasionally for restlessness. For the dose by subcutaneous infusion using a continuous infusion device, see p. 18.

# Continuous infusion devices

Although drugs can usually be administered *by mouth* to control the symptoms of advanced cancer, the parenteral route may sometimes be necessary. Repeated administration of *intramuscular injections* can be difficult in a cachectic patient. This has led to the use of portable continuous infusion devices, such as syringe drivers, to give a *continuous subcutaneous infusion*, which can provide good control of symptoms with little discomfort or inconvenience to the patient.

> **Syringe driver rate settings**
> Staff using syringe drivers should be **adequately trained** and different rate settings should be **clearly identified** and **differentiated**; incorrect use of syringe drivers is a common cause of medication errors.

Indications for the **parenteral route** are:

- the patient is unable to take medicines by mouth owing to *nausea and vomiting, dysphagia, severe weakness,* or *coma;*

- there is *malignant bowel obstruction* in patients for whom further surgery is inappropriate (avoiding the need for an intravenous infusion or for insertion of a nasogastric tube);

- occasionally when the patient *does not wish* to take regular medication by mouth.

## Bowel colic and excessive respiratory secretions

Hyoscine hydrobromide effectively reduces respiratory secretions and is sedative (but occasionally causes paradoxical agitation); it is given in a *subcutaneous infusion dose* of 0.6–2.4 mg/24 hours.

Hyoscine butylbromide is effective in bowel colic, is less sedative than hyoscine hydrobromide, but is not always adequate for the control of respiratory secretions; it is given in a *subcutaneous infusion dose* of 20–60 mg/24 hours (**important:** this dose of *hyoscine butylbromide* must not be confused with the much lower dose of *hyoscine hydrobromide,* above).

Glycopyrronium 0.6–1.2 mg/24 hours by subcutaneous infusion may also be used.

## Convulsions

If a patient has previously been receiving an antiepileptic drug *or* has a primary or secondary cerebral tumour *or* is at risk of convulsion (e.g. owing to uraemia) antiepileptic medication should *not* be stopped. Midazolam is the benzodiazepine antiepileptic of choice for *continuous subcutaneous infusion,* and it is given initially in a dose of 20–40 mg/24 hours.

## Nausea and vomiting

Haloperidol is given in a *subcutaneous infusion dose* of 2.5–10 mg/24 hours.

Levomepromazine (methotrimeprazine) is given in a *subcutaneous infusion dose* of 5–25 mg/24 hours but sedation can limit the dose.

Cyclizine is particularly likely to precipitate if mixed with diamorphine or other drugs (see under Mixing and Compatibility, below); it is given in a *subcutaneous infusion dose* of 150 mg/24 hours.

Metoclopramide can cause skin reactions; it is given in a *subcutaneous infusion dose* of 30–100 mg/24 hours.

Octreotide (section 8.3.4.3), which stimulates water and electrolyte absorption and inhibits water secretion in the small bowel, can be used by subcutaneous infusion in a dose of 300–600 micrograms/24 hours to reduce intestinal secretions and vomiting.

## Pain control

Diamorphine is the preferred opioid since its high solubility permits a large dose to be given in a small volume (see under Mixing and Compatibility, below). The table on p. 19 shows approximate equivalent doses of morphine and diamorphine.

## Restlessness and confusion

Haloperidol has little sedative effect; it is given in a *subcutaneous infusion dose* of 5–15 mg/24 hours.

Levomepromazine (methotrimeprazine) has a sedative effect; it is given in a *subcutaneous infusion dose* of 12.5–200 mg/24 hours.

Midazolam is a sedative and an antiepileptic that may be used in addition to an antipsychotic drug in a very restless patient; it is given in a *subcutaneous infusion dose* of 20–100 mg/24 hours.

## Mixing and compatibility

The general principle that injections should be given into separate sites (and should not be mixed) does not apply to the use of syringe drivers in palliative care. Provided that there is evidence of compatibility, selected injections can be mixed in syringe drivers. Not all types of medication can be used in a subcutaneous infusion. In particular, chlorpromazine, prochlorperazine, and diazepam are **contra-indicated** as they cause skin reactions at the injection site; to a lesser extent cyclizine and levomepromazine (methotrimeprazine) also sometimes cause local irritation.

In theory injections dissolved in water for injections are more likely to be associated with pain (possibly owing to their hypotonicity). The use of physiological saline (sodium chloride 0.9%) however increases the likelihood of precipitation when more than one drug is used; moreover subcutaneous infusion rates are so slow (0.1–0.3 mL/hour) that pain is not usually a problem when water is used as a diluent.

Diamorphine can be given by subcutaneous infusion in a strength of up to 250 mg/mL; up to a strength of 40 mg/mL either *water for injections* or *physiological saline* (sodium chloride 0.9%) is a suitable diluent—above that strength only *water for injections* is used (to avoid precipitation).

The following can be mixed with *diamorphine*:

| | |
|---|---|
| Cyclizine[1] | Hyoscine hydrobromide |
| Dexamethasone[2] | Levomepromazine |
| Haloperidol[3] | Metoclopramide[4] |
| Hyoscine butylbromide | Midazolam |

Subcutaneous infusion solution should be monitored regularly both to check for precipitation (and discoloration) and to ensure that the infusion is running at the correct rate.

## Problems encountered with syringe drivers

The following are problems that may be encountered with syringe drivers and the action that should be taken:

- if the subcutaneous infusion runs *too quickly* check the rate setting and the calculation;

- if the subcutaneous infusion runs *too slowly* check the start button, the battery, the syringe driver, the cannula, and make sure that the injection site is not inflamed;

- if there is an *injection site reaction* make sure that the site does not need to be changed—firmness or swelling at the site of injection is not in itself an indication for change, but pain or obvious inflammation is.

---

1. Cyclizine may precipitate at concentrations above 10 mg/mL *or* in the presence of sodium chloride 0.9% *or* as the concentration of diamorphine relative to cyclizine increases; mixtures of diamorphine and cyclizine are also likely to precipitate after 24 hours.
2. Special care is needed to avoid precipitation of dexamethasone when preparing it.
3. Mixtures of haloperidol and diamorphine are likely to precipitate after 24 hours if haloperidol concentration is above 2 mg/mL.
4. Under some conditions infusions containing metoclopramide become discoloured; such solutions should be discarded.

## Equivalent doses of morphine sulphate and diamorphine hydrochloride

These equivalences are *approximate only* and should be adjusted according to response

| MORPHINE | | PARENTERAL DIAMORPHINE | |
|---|---|---|---|
| Morphine sulphate oral solution or standard tablets | Morphine sulphate by subcutaneous infusion | Diamorphine hydrochloride by intramuscular injection | Diamorphine hydrochloride by subcutaneous infusion |
| **every 4 hours** | **every 24 hours** | **every 4 hours** | **every 24 hours** |
| 5 mg | 15 mg | 1.25–2.5 mg | 10 mg |
| 10 mg | 30 mg | 2.5–5 mg | 20 mg |
| 15 mg | 45 mg | 5 mg | 30 mg |
| 20 mg | 60 mg | 7.5 mg | 40 mg |
| 30 mg | 90 mg | 10 mg | 60 mg |
| 40 mg | 120 mg | 12.5 mg | 80 mg |
| 60 mg | 180 mg | 20 mg | 120 mg |
| 80 mg | 240 mg | 27.5 mg | 160 mg |
| 100 mg | 300 mg | 35 mg | 200 mg |
| 130 mg | 390 mg | 42.5 mg | 260 mg |
| 160 mg | 480 mg | 55 mg | 320 mg |
| 200 mg | 600 mg | 65 mg | 400 mg |

If breakthrough pain occurs give a subcutaneous (preferable) or intramuscular injection equivalent to one-sixth of the total 24-hour subcutaneous infusion dose. It is kinder to give an intermittent bolus injection *subcutaneously*—absorption is smoother so that the risk of adverse effects at peak absorption is avoided (an even better method is to use a subcutaneous butterfly needle).

To minimise the risk of infection no individual subcutaneous infusion solution should be used for longer than 24 hours.

# Prescribing for the elderly

Old people, especially the very old, require special care and consideration from prescribers. *Medicines for Older People*, a component document of the National Service Framework for Older People,[1] describes how to maximise the benefits of medicines and how to avoid excessive, inappropriate, or inadequate consumption of medicines by older people.

**Appropriate prescribing** Elderly patients often receive multiple drugs for their multiple diseases. This greatly increases the risk of drug interactions as well as adverse reactions, and may affect compliance (see Taking medicines to best effect under General guidance). The balance of benefit and harm of some medicines may be altered in the elderly. Therefore, elderly patients' medicines should be reviewed regularly and medicines which are not of benefit should be stopped.

Non-pharmacological measures may be more appropriate for symptoms such as headache, sleeplessness, and lightheadedness when associated with social stress as in widowhood, loneliness, and family dispersal.

In some cases prophylactic drugs are inappropriate if they are likely to complicate existing treatment or introduce unnecessary side-effects, especially in elderly patients with poor prognosis or with poor overall health. However, elderly patients should not be denied medi-

cines which may help them, such as anticoagulants or antiplatelet drugs for atrial fibrillation, antihypertensives, statins, and drugs for osteoporosis.

**Form of medicine** Frail elderly patients may have difficulty swallowing tablets; if left in the mouth, ulceration may develop. They should always be encouraged to take their tablets or capsules with enough fluid, and whilst in an upright position to avoid the possibility of oesophageal ulceration. It can be helpful to discuss with the patient the possibility of taking the drug as a liquid if available.

**Manifestations of ageing** In the very old, manifestations of normal ageing may be mistaken for disease and lead to inappropriate prescribing. In addition, age-related muscle weakness and difficulty in maintaining balance should not be confused with neurological disease. Disorders such as lightheadedness not associated with postural or postprandial hypotension are unlikely to be helped by drugs.

**Sensitivity** The nervous system of elderly patients is more sensitive to many commonly used drugs, such as opioid analgesics, benzodiazepines, antipsychotics, and antiparkinsonian drugs, all of which must be used with caution. Similarly, other organs may also be more susceptible to the effects of drugs such as antihypertensives and NSAIDs.

1. Department of Health. National Service Framework for Older People. London: Department of Health, March 2001.

## Pharmacokinetics

Pharmacokinetic changes can markedly increase the tissue concentration of a drug in the elderly, especially in debilitated patients.

The most important effect of age is reduced renal clearance. Many aged patients thus *excrete drugs slowly*, and are *highly susceptible to nephrotoxic drugs*. Acute illness can lead to rapid reduction in renal clearance, especially if accompanied by dehydration. Hence, a patient stabilised on a drug with a narrow margin between the therapeutic and the toxic dose (e.g. digoxin) can rapidly develop adverse effects in the aftermath of a myocardial infarction or a respiratory-tract infection. The hepatic metabolism of lipid soluble drugs is reduced in elderly patients because there is a reduction in liver volume. This is important for drugs with a narrow therapeutic window.

## Adverse reactions

Adverse reactions often present in the elderly in a vague and non-specific fashion. *Confusion* is often the presenting symptom (caused by almost any of the commonly used drugs). Other common manifestations are *constipation* (with antimuscarinics and many tranquillisers) and postural *hypotension* and *falls* (with diuretics and many psychotropics).

**Hypnotics** Many hypnotics with long half-lives have serious hangover effects, including drowsiness, unsteady gait, slurred speech, and confusion. Hypnotics with short half-lives should be used but they too can present problems (section 4.1.1). Short courses of hypnotics are occasionally useful for helping a patient through an acute illness or some other crisis but every effort must be made to avoid dependence. Benzodiazepines impair balance, which can result in falls.

**Diuretics** Diuretics are overprescribed in old age and should **not** be used on a long-term basis to treat simple gravitational oedema which will usually respond to increased movement, raising the legs, and support stockings. A few days of diuretic treatment may speed the clearing of the oedema but it should rarely need continued drug therapy.

**NSAIDs** Bleeding associated with aspirin and other NSAIDs is more common in the elderly who are more likely to have a fatal or serious outcome. NSAIDs are also a special hazard in patients with cardiac disease or renal impairment which may again place older patients at particular risk.

Owing to the *increased susceptibility of the elderly* to the *side-effects of NSAIDs* the following recommendations are made:

- for *osteoarthritis, soft-tissue lesions*, and *back pain*, first try measures such as weight reduction (if obese), warmth, exercise, and use of a walking stick;
- for *osteoarthritis, soft-tissue lesions, back pain*, and *pain in rheumatoid arthritis*, paracetamol should be used first and can often provide adequate pain relief;
- alternatively, a low-dose NSAID (e.g. ibuprofen up to 1.2 g daily) may be given;
- for pain relief when either drug is inadequate, paracetamol in a full dose plus a low-dose NSAID may be given;

- if necessary, the NSAID dose can be increased or an opioid analgesic given with paracetamol;
- do not give two NSAIDs at the same time.

For advice on prophylaxis of NSAID-induced peptic ulcers if continued NSAID treatment is necessary, see section 1.3.

**Other drugs** Other drugs which commonly cause adverse reactions are *antiparkinsonian drugs, antihypertensives, psychotropics*, and *digoxin*. The usual maintenance dose of digoxin in very old patients is 125 micrograms daily (62.5 micrograms in those with renal disease); lower doses are often inadequate but toxicity is common in those given 250 micrograms daily.

Drug-induced blood disorders are much more common in the elderly. Therefore drugs with a tendency to cause bone marrow depression (e.g. *co-trimoxazole, mianserin*) should be avoided unless there is no acceptable alternative.

The elderly generally require a lower maintenance dose of *warfarin* than younger adults; once again, the outcome of bleeding tends to be more serious.

## Guidelines

Always consider whether a drug is indicated at all.

**Limit range** It is a sensible policy to prescribe from a limited range of drugs and to be thoroughly familiar with their effects in the elderly.

**Reduce dose** Dosage should generally be substantially lower than for younger patients and it is common to start with about 50% of the adult dose. Some drugs (e.g. long-acting antidiabetic drugs such as glibenclamide and chlorpropamide) should be avoided altogether.

**Review regularly** Review repeat prescriptions regularly. In many patients it may be possible to stop some drugs, provided that clinical progress is monitored. It may be necessary to reduce the dose of some drugs as renal function declines.

**Simplify regimens** Elderly patients benefit from simple treatment regimens. Only drugs with a clear indication should be prescribed and whenever possible given once or twice daily. In particular, regimens which call for a confusing array of dosage intervals should be avoided.

**Explain clearly** Write full instructions on every prescription (*including* repeat prescriptions) so that containers can be properly labelled with full directions. Avoid imprecisions like 'as directed'. Child-resistant containers may be unsuitable.

**Repeats and disposal** Instruct patients what to do when drugs run out, and also how to dispose of any that are no longer necessary. Try to prescribe matching quantities.

If these guidelines are followed most elderly people will cope adequately with their own medicines. If not then it is essential to enrol the help of a third party, usually a relative or a friend.

# Prescribing in dental practice

The following is a list of topics of particular relevance to dental surgeons.

> Advice on the drug management of dental and oral conditions has been integrated into the BNF. For ease of access, guidance on such conditions is usually identified by means of a relevant heading (e.g. Dental and Orofacial Pain) in the appropriate sections of the BNF.

### General guidance
Prescribing by dental surgeons, p. 4
Oral side-effects of drugs, p. 12
Medical emergencies in dental practice, below
Medical problems in dental practice, p. 23

### Drug management of dental and oral conditions
Dental and orofacial pain, p. 232
   Neuropathic pain, p. 246
   Non-opioid analgesics, p. 233
   Opioid analgesics, p. 238
   Non-steroidal anti-inflammatory drugs, p. 561
Oral infections
   Bacterial infections, p. 289
     Phenoxymethylpenicillin, p. 296
     Broad-spectrum penicillins (amoxicillin and ampicillin), p. 298
     Cephalosporins (cefalexin and cefradine), p. 303
     Tetracyclines, p. 308
     Macrolides (erythromycin and azithromycin) , p. 313
     Clindamycin, p. 315
     Metronidazole, p. 327
     Fusidic acid p. 658
   Fungal infections, p. 618
     Local treatment, p. 618
     Systemic treatment, p. 332
   Viral infections
     Herpetic gingivostomatitis, local treatment, p. 620
     Herpetic gingivostomatitis, systemic treatment, p. 348 and p. 620
     Herpes labialis, p. 661
Anaesthetics, anxiolytics and hypnotics
   Anaesthesia, sedation, and resuscitation in dental practice, p. 698
   Hypnotics, p. 186
   Peri-operative anxiolytics, p. 704
   Local anaesthesia, p. 714
**Oral ulceration and inflammation, p. 616**
**Mouthwashes, gargles and dentifrices, p. 620**
**Dry mouth, p. 621**
**Minerals**
   Fluorides, p. 545
**Aromatic inhalations, p. 182**
**Nasal decongestants, p. 615**

**Dental Practitioners' Formulary, p. 947**

**Changes to Dental Practitioners' Formulary, p. 948**

## Medical emergencies in dental practice

This section provides guidelines on the management of the more common medical emergencies which may arise in dental practice. Dental surgeons and their staff should be familiar with standard resuscitation procedures, but in all circumstances it is advisable to summon medical assistance as soon as possible. For an **algorithm** of the procedure for **cardiopulmonary resuscitation**, see inside back cover.

> **The drugs referred to in this section include:**
> Adrenaline Injection (Epinephrine Injection), adrenaline 1 in 1000, (adrenaline 1 mg/mL as acid tartrate), 1-mL amps
> Aspirin Dispersible Tablets 300 mg
> Glucagon Injection, glucagon (as hydrochloride), 1-unit vial (with solvent)
> Glucose (for administration by mouth)
> Glyceryl Trinitrate Spray
> Midazolam Injection, midazolam (as hydrochloride) 2 mg/mL, 5-mL amps, or 5 mg/mL, 2-mL amps
> Oxygen
> Salbutamol Aerosol Inhalation, salbutamol 100 micrograms/metered inhalation

### Adrenal insufficiency

Adrenal insufficiency may follow prolonged therapy with corticosteroids and can persist for years after stopping. A patient with adrenal insufficiency may become hypotensive under the stress of a dental visit (important: see also p. 395 for details of corticosteroid cover before dental surgical procedures under general anaesthesia).

**Management**

- Lay the patient flat
- Give **oxygen** (see section 3.6)
- Transfer patient urgently to hospital

### Anaphylaxis

A severe allergic reaction may follow oral or parenteral administration of a drug. Anaphylactic reactions in dentistry may follow the administration of a drug or contact with substances such as latex in surgical gloves. In general, the more rapid the onset of the reaction the more profound it tends to be. Symptoms may develop within minutes and rapid treatment is essential.

Anaphylactic reactions may also be associated with *additives* and *excipients* in foods and medicines (see Excipients, p. 2). Refined arachis (peanut) oil, which may be present in some medicinal products, is unlikely to cause an allergic reaction—nevertheless it is wise to check the full formula of preparations which may contain allergenic fats or oils (including those for topical application, particularly if they are intended for use in the mouth or for application to the nasal mucosa).

*Prescribing in dental practice*

**Symptoms and signs**

- Paraesthesia, flushing, and swelling of face
- Generalised itching, especially of hands and feet
- Bronchospasm and laryngospasm (with wheezing and difficulty in breathing)
- Rapid weak pulse together with fall in blood pressure and pallor; finally cardiac arrest

**Management**

First-line treatment includes securing the airway, restoration of blood pressure (laying the patient flat and raising the feet, or in the recovery position if unconscious or nauseous and at risk of vomiting), and administration of **adrenaline** (epinephrine) injection. This is given **intramuscularly** in a dose of 500 micrograms (0.5 mL adrenaline injection 1 in 1000); a preparation delivering a dose of 300 micrograms (0.3 mL adrenaline injection 1 in 1000) is available for immediate *self-administration*. The dose is repeated if necessary at 5-minute intervals according to blood pressure, pulse, and respiratory function. **Oxygen** administration is also of primary importance (see section 3.6). Arrangements should be made to transfer the patient to hospital urgently.

> For further details on the management of anaphylaxis including details of paediatric doses of adrenaline, see p. 176

## Asthma

Patients with asthma may have an attack while at the dental surgery. Most attacks will respond to 2 puffs of the patient's short-acting beta$_2$ agonist inhaler such as **salbutamol** 100 micrograms/puff; further puffs are required if the patient does not respond rapidly. If the patient is unable to use the inhaler effectively, further puffs should be given through a large-volume spacer device (or, if not available, through a plastic or paper cup with a hole in the bottom for the inhaler mouthpiece). If the response remains unsatisfactory, or if further deterioration occurs, then the patient should be transferred urgently to hospital. Whilst awaiting transfer, **oxygen** (section 3.6) should be given with salbutamol 5 mg or terbutaline 10 mg by nebuliser; if a nebuliser is unavailable, then 4–10 puffs of salbutamol 100 micrograms/metered inhalation should be given (preferably by a large-volume spacer), and repeated every 10–20 minutes if necessary. If asthma is part of a more generalised anaphylactic reaction, an intramuscular injection of **adrenaline** (as detailed under Anaphylaxis above) should be given.

For a table describing the management of acute asthma, see p. 152

Patients with severe chronic asthma or whose asthma has deteriorated previously during a dental procedure may require an increase in their prophylactic medication before a dental procedure. This should be discussed with the patient's medical practitioner and may include increasing the dose of inhaled or oral corticosteroid.

## Cardiac emergencies

If there is a history of *angina* the patient will probably carry **glyceryl trinitrate** spray or tablets (or isosorbide dinitrate tablets) and should be allowed to use them. Hospital admission is not necessary if symptoms are mild and resolve rapidly with the patient's own medication. See also Coronary Artery Disease on p. 24.

*Arrhythmias* may lead to a sudden reduction in cardiac output with loss of consciousness. Medical assistance should be summoned. For advice on pacemaker interference, see also Pacemakers, p. 24.

The pain of *myocardial infarction* is similar to that of angina but generally more severe and more prolonged. For general advice see also Coronary Artery Disease on p. 24

**Symptoms and signs of myocardial infarction**

- Progressive onset of severe, crushing pain across front of chest; pain may radiate towards the shoulder and down arm, or into neck and jaw
- Skin becomes pale and clammy
- Nausea and vomiting are common
- Pulse may be weak and blood pressure may fall
- Breathlessness

**Initial management of myocardial infarction**

Call immediately for medical assistance and an ambulance, as appropriate.

Allow the patient to rest in the position that feels most comfortable; in the presence of breathlessness this is likely to be sitting position, whereas the syncopal patient should be laid flat; often an intermediate position (dictated by the patient) will be most appropriate. **Oxygen** may be administered (see section 3.6).

Sublingual glyceryl trinitrate may relieve pain. Intramuscular injection of drugs should be avoided because absorption may be too slow (particularly when cardiac output is reduced) and pain relief is inadequate. Intramuscular injection also increases the risk of local bleeding into the muscle if the patient is given a thrombolytic drug.

Reassure the patient as much as possible to relieve further anxiety. If available, aspirin in a single dose of 300 mg should be given. A note (to say that aspirin has been given) should be sent with the patient to the hospital. For further details on the initial management of myocardial infarction, see p. 137.

If the patient collapses and loses consciousness attempt standard resuscitation measures. For an **algorithm** of the procedure for **cardiopulmonary resuscitation**, see inside back cover.

## Epileptic seizures

Patients with epilepsy must continue with their normal dosage of anticonvulsant drugs when attending for dental treatment. It is not uncommon for epileptic patients not to volunteer the information that they are epileptic but there should be little difficulty in recognising a tonic-clonic (grand mal) seizure.

**Symptoms and signs**

- There may be a brief warning (but variable)
- Sudden loss of consciousness, the patient becomes rigid, falls, may give a cry, and becomes cyanotic (tonic phase)
- After 30 seconds, there are jerking movements of the limbs; the tongue may be bitten (clonic phase)
- There may be frothing from mouth and urinary incontinence
- The seizure typically lasts a few minutes; the patient may then become flaccid but remain unconscious. After a variable time the patient regains consciousness but may remain confused for a while

## Management

During a convulsion try to ensure that the patient is not at risk from injury but make no attempt to put anything in the mouth or between the teeth (in mistaken belief that this will protect the tongue). Give **oxygen** (section 3.6) to support respiration if necessary.

Do not attempt to restrain convulsive movements.

After convulsive movements have subsided place the patient in the coma (recovery) position and check the airway.

After the convulsion the patient may be confused ('post-ictal confusion') and may need reassurance and sympathy. The patient should not be sent home until fully recovered. Seek medical attention or transfer the patient to hospital if it was the first episode of epilepsy, or if the convulsion was atypical, prolonged (or repeated), or if injury occurred.

Medication should only be given if convulsive seizures are prolonged (convulsive movements lasting 5 minutes or longer) or repeated rapidly.

**Midazolam** injection solution can be given by the buccal route [unlicensed use] in a single dose of 10 mg. For further details on the management of status epilepticus, including details of paediatric doses of midazolam, see p. 267.

Partial seizures similarly need very little active management (in an automatism only a minimum amount of restraint should be applied to prevent injury). Again, the patient should be observed until post-ictal confusion has completely resolved.

## Hypoglycaemia

Insulin-treated diabetic patients attending for dental treatment under local anaesthesia should inject insulin and eat meals as normal. If food is omitted the blood glucose will fall to an abnormally low level (hypoglycaemia). Patients can often recognise the symptoms themselves and this state responds to sugar in water or a few lumps of sugar. Children may not have such prominent changes but may appear unduly lethargic.

### Symptoms and signs

- Shaking and trembling
- Sweating
- 'Pins and needles' in lips and tongue
- Hunger
- Palpitation
- Headache (occasionally)
- Double vision
- Difficulty in concentration
- Slurring of speech
- Confusion
- Change of behaviour; truculence
- Convulsions
- Unconsciousness

### Management

Initially glucose 10–20 g is given by mouth either in liquid form or as granulated sugar or sugar lumps. Approximately 10 g of glucose is available from 2 teaspoons sugar, 3 sugar lumps, *GlucoGel®* (formerly known as *Hypostop® Gel*; glucose 10 g/25 g tube, available from BBI Healthcare), *Dextrogel®* (glucose 10 g/25 g tube, available from M & A Pharmachem), and non-diet

versions of *Lucozade® Energy Original* 55 mL, *Coca-Cola®* 100 mL, *Ribena® Blackcurrant* 18 mL (to be diluted). If necessary this may be repeated in 10–15 minutes.

If glucose cannot be given by mouth, if it is ineffective, or if the hypoglycaemia causes unconsciousness, **glucagon** 1 mg (1 unit) should be given by intramuscular (or subcutaneous) injection; a child under 8 years or of body-weight under 25 kg should be given 500 micrograms. Once the patient regains consciousness oral glucose should be administered as above. If glucagon is ineffective or contra-indicated, the patient should be transferred urgently to hospital. The patient must also be admitted to hospital if hypoglycaemia is caused by an oral antidiabetic drug.

## Syncope

Insufficient blood supply to the brain results in loss of consciousness. The commonest cause is a vasovagal attack or simple faint (syncope) due to emotional stress.

### Symptoms and signs

- Patient feels faint
- Low blood pressure
- Pallor and sweating
- Yawning and slow pulse
- Nausea and vomiting
- Dilated pupils
- Muscular twitching

### Management

- Lay the patient as flat as is reasonably comfortable and, in the absence of associated breathlessness, raise the legs to improve cerebral circulation
- Loosen any tight clothing around the neck
- Once consciousness is regained, give sugar in water or a cup of sweet tea

### Other possible causes

Postural hypotension can be a consequence of rising abruptly or of standing upright for too long; antihypertensive drugs predispose to this. When rising, susceptible patients should take their time. Management is as for a vasovagal attack.

Under stressful circumstances, some patients hyperventilate. This gives rise to feelings of faintness but does not usually result in syncope. In most cases reassurance is all that is necessary; rebreathing from cupped hands or a bag may be helpful but calls for careful supervision.

Adrenal insufficiency or arrhythmias are other possible causes of syncope, see p. 21 and p. 24.

## Medical problems in dental practice

Individuals presenting at the dental surgery may also suffer from an unrelated medical condition; this may require modification to the management of their dental condition. If the patient has systemic disease or is taking other medication, the matter may need to be discussed with the patient's general practitioner or hospital consultant.

For advice on adrenal insufficiency, anaphylaxis, asthma, cardiac emergencies, epileptic seizures, hypoglycaemia and syncope see under Medical Emergencies in Dental Practice.

## Allergy

Patients should be asked about any history of allergy; those with a history of atopic allergy (asthma, eczema, hay fever, etc.) are at special risk. Those with a history of a severe allergy or of anaphylactic reactions are at high risk—it is essential to confirm that they are not allergic to any medication, or to any dental materials or equipment (including latex gloves). See also Anaphylaxis on p. 21.

## Arrhythmias

Patients, especially those who suffer from heart failure or who have sustained a myocardial infarction, may have irregular cardiac rhythm. Atrial fibrillation is a common arrhythmia even in patients with normal hearts and is of little concern except that dental surgeons should be aware that such patients may be receiving anticoagulant therapy. The patient's medical practitioner should be asked whether any special precautions are necessary. Premedication (e.g. with temazepam) may be useful in some instances for very anxious patients.

See also Cardiac emergencies, p. 22 and Dental Anaesthesia, p. 714.

## Cardiac prostheses

For an account of the risk of infective endocarditis in patients with prosthetic heart valves, see Infective Endocarditis, below. For advice on patients receiving anticoagulants, see Thromboembolic disease, below.

## Coronary artery disease

Patients are vulnerable for at least 4 weeks following a myocardial infarction or following any sudden increase in the symptoms of angina. It would be advisable to check with the patient's medical practitioner before commencing treatment. See also Cardiac Emergencies on p. 22.

Treatment with low-dose aspirin (75 mg daily), clopidogrel, or dipyridamole should not be stopped routinely nor should the dose be altered before dental procedures.

A Working Party of the British Society for Antimicrobial Chemotherapy has not recommended antibiotic prophylaxis for patients following coronary artery bypass surgery.

## Cyanotic heart disease

Patients with cyanotic heart disease are at risk in the dental chair, particularly if they have pulmonary hypertension. In such patients a syncopal reaction increases the shunt away from the lungs, causing more hypoxia which worsens the syncopal reaction—a vicious circle that may prove fatal. The advice of the cardiologist should be sought on any patient with congenital cyanotic heart disease. Treatment in hospital is more appropriate for some patients with this condition.

## Hypertension

Patients with hypertension are likely to be receiving antihypertensive drugs such as those described in section 2.5. Their blood pressure may fall dangerously low under general anaesthesia, see also under Dental Anaesthesia on p. 714.

## Immunosuppression and indwelling intraperitoneal catheters

See Table 2, section 5.1

## Infective endocarditis

While almost any dental procedure can cause bacteraemia, there is no clear association with the development of infective endocarditis. Routine daily activities such as tooth brushing also produce a bacteraemia and may present a greater risk of infective endocarditis than a single dental procedure.

Antibacterial prophylaxis and chlorhexidine mouthwash are **not** recommended for the prevention of endocarditis in patients undergoing dental procedures. Such prophylaxis may expose patients to the adverse effects of antimicrobials when the evidence of benefit has not been proven.

**Reduction of oral bacteraemia**  Patients at risk of endocarditis[1] should be advised to maintain the highest possible standards of oral hygiene in order to reduce the:

- need for dental extractions or other surgery;
- chances of severe bacteraemia if dental surgery is needed;
- possibility of 'spontaneous' bacteraemia.

**Postoperative care**  Patients at risk of endocarditis[1] should be warned to report to the doctor or dental surgeon any unexplained illness that develops after dental treatment. Any infection in patients at risk of endocarditis[1] should be investigated promptly and treated appropriately to reduce the risk of endocarditis.

**Patients on anticoagulant therapy**  For general advice on dental surgery in patients receiving oral anticoagulant therapy see Thromboembolic Disease, below.

## Joint prostheses

See Table 2, section 5.1

## Liver disease

Liver disease may alter the response to drugs and drug prescribing should be kept to a minimum in patients with severe liver disease. Problems are likely mainly in patients with *jaundice*, *ascites*, or evidence of *encephalopathy*.

For a table of drugs to be avoided or used with caution in liver disease see Appendix 2.

## Pacemakers

Pacemakers prevent asystole or severe bradycardia. Some ultrasonic scalers, electronic apex locators, electro-analgesic devices, and electrocautery devices interfere with the normal function of pacemakers (including shielded pacemakers) and should not be used. The

---

1. Patients at risk of endocarditis include those with valve replacement, acquired valvular heart disease with stenosis or regurgitation, structural congenital heart disease (including surgically corrected or palliated structural conditions, but excluding isolated atrial septal defect, fully repaired ventricular septal defect, fully repaired patent ductus arteriosus, and closure devices considered to be endothelialised), hypertrophic cardiomyopathy, or a previous episode of infective endocarditis.

manufacturer's literature should be consulted whenever possible. If severe bradycardia occurs in a patient fitted with a pacemaker, electrical equipment should be switched off and the patient placed supine with the legs elevated. If the patient loses consciousness and the pulse remains slow or is absent, cardiopulmonary resuscitation (see inside back cover) may be needed. Call immediately for medical assistance and an ambulance, as appropriate.

A Working Party of the British Society for Antimicrobial Chemotherapy does not recommend antibacterial prophylaxis for patients with pacemakers.

## Pregnancy

Drugs taken during pregnancy can be harmful to the fetus and should be prescribed only if the expected benefit to the mother is thought to be greater than the risk to the fetus; all drugs should be avoided if possible during the first trimester.

Appendix 4 includes information on drug treatment during pregnancy.

## Breast-feeding

Some drugs taken by the mother whilst breast-feeding can be transferred to the breast milk, and may affect the infant.

Appendix 5 includes information on drug treatment during breast-feeding.

## Renal impairment

The use of drugs in patients with reduced renal function can give rise to many problems. Many of these problems can be avoided by reducing the dose or by using alternative drugs.

Special care is required in renal transplantation and immunosuppressed patients; if necessary such patients should be referred to specialists.

For a table of drugs to be avoided or used with caution in renal impairment see Appendix 3.

## Thromboembolic disease

Patients receiving **heparin** or oral anticoagulants such as **warfarin, acenocoumarol** (nicoumalone), **phenindione, dabigatran etexilate**, or **rivaroxaban** may be liable to excessive bleeding after extraction of teeth or other dental surgery. Often dental surgery can be delayed until the anticoagulant therapy has been completed.

For a patient requiring long-term therapy with warfarin, the patient's medical practitioner should be consulted and the International Normalised Ratio (INR) should be assessed 72 hours before the dental procedure. This allows sufficient time for dose modification if necessary. In those with an unstable INR (including those who require weekly monitoring of their INR, or those who have had some INR measurements greater than 4.0 in the last 2 months), the INR should be assessed within 24 hours of the dental procedure. Patients requiring minor dental procedures (including extractions) who have an INR below 4.0 may continue warfarin without dose adjustment. There is no need to check the INR for a patient requiring a non-invasive dental procedure.

If possible, a single extraction should be done first; if this goes well further teeth may be extracted at subsequent visits (two or three at a time). Measures should be taken to minimise bleeding during and after the procedure. This includes the use of sutures and a haemostatic such as oxidised cellulose, collagen sponge or resorbable gelatin sponge. Scaling and root planing should initially be restricted to a limited area to assess the potential for bleeding.

For a patient on long-term warfarin, the advice of the clinician responsible for the patient's anticoagulation should be sought if:

- the INR is unstable, or if the INR is greater than 4.0;
- the patient has thrombocytopenia, haemophilia, or other disorders of haemostasis, or suffers from liver impairment, alcoholism, or renal failure;
- the patient is receiving antiplatelet drugs, cytotoxic drugs or radiotherapy.

Intramuscular injections are *contra-indicated* in patients on anticoagulant therapy, and in those with any disorder of haemostasis.

A local anaesthetic containing a vasoconstrictor should be given by infiltration, or by intraligamentary or mental nerve injection if possible. If regional nerve blocks cannot be avoided the local anaesthetic should be given cautiously using an aspirating syringe.

Drugs which have potentially serious interactions with anticoagulants include aspirin and other NSAIDs, carbamazepine, imidazole and triazole antifungals (including miconazole), erythromycin, clarithromycin, and metronidazole; for details of these and other interactions with anticoagulants, see Appendix 1 (dabigatran etexilate, heparin, phenindione, rivaroxaban, and coumarins). Although studies have failed to demonstrate an interaction, common experience in anticoagulant clinics is that the INR can be altered following a course of an oral broad-spectrum antibiotic, such as ampicillin or amoxicillin.

Information on the treatment of patients who take anticoagulants is available at www.npsa.nhs.uk/patientsafety/alerts-and-directives/alerts/anticoagulant

Prescribing in dental practice

# Drugs and sport

UK Sport advises that athletes are personally responsible should a prohibited substance be detected in their body. An advice card listing examples of permitted and prohibited substances is available from:

Drug-Free Sport
UK Sport
40 Bernard Street
London  WC1N 1ST
Tel: 0800 528 0004
drug-free@uksport.gov.uk
www.uksport.gov.uk

A similar card detailing classes of drugs and doping methods prohibited in football is available from the Football Association.

> **General Medical Council's advice**
> Doctors who prescribe or collude in the provision of drugs or treatment with the intention of improperly enhancing an individual's performance in sport contravene the GMC's guidance, and such actions would usually raise a question of a doctor's continued registration. This does not preclude the provision of any care or treatment where the doctor's intention is to protect or improve the patient's health.

**Drugs and sport**

# Emergency treatment of poisoning

These notes provide only an overview of the treatment of poisoning, and it is strongly recommended that either TOXBASE or the UK National Poisons Information Service (see below) be consulted when there is doubt about the degree of risk or about management.

**Hospital admission** Patients who have features of poisoning should generally be admitted to hospital. Patients who have taken poisons with delayed action should also be admitted, even if they appear well. Delayed-action poisons include aspirin, iron, paracetamol, tricyclic antidepressants, and co-phenotrope (diphenoxylate with atropine, *Lomotil®*); the effects of modified-release preparations are also delayed. A note of all relevant information, including what treatment has been given, should accompany the patient to hospital.

## Further information and advice

TOXBASE, the primary clinical toxicology database of the National Poisons Information Service, is available on the internet to registered users at www.toxbase.org. It provides information about routine diagnosis, treatment, and management of patients exposed to drugs, household products, and industrial and agricultural chemicals.

> Specialist information and advice on the treatment of poisoning is available day and night from the UK National Poisons Information Service on the following number:
> Tel: 0844 892 0111

Advice on laboratory analytical services can be obtained from TOXBASE or from the National Poisons Information Service.

Help with identifying capsules or tablets may be available from a regional medicines information centre (see inside front cover).

## General care

It is often impossible to establish with certainty the identity of the poison and the size of the dose. Fortunately this is not usually important because only a few poisons (such as opioids, paracetamol, and iron) have specific antidotes; few patients require active removal of the poison. In most patients, treatment is directed at managing symptoms as they arise. Nevertheless, knowledge of the type and timing of poisoning can help in anticipating the course of events. All relevant information should be sought from the poisoned individual and from carers or parents. However, such information should be interpreted with care because it may not be complete or entirely reliable. Sometimes symptoms arise from other illnesses and patients should be assessed carefully. Accidents may involve domestic and industrial products (the contents of which are not generally known). The National Poisons Information Service should be consulted when there is doubt about any aspect of suspected poisoning.

## Respiration

Respiration is often impaired in unconscious patients. An obstructed airway requires immediate attention. In the absence of trauma, the airway should be opened with simple measures such as chin lift or jaw thrust. An oropharyngeal or nasopharyngeal airway may be useful in patients with reduced consciousness to prevent obstruction, provided ventilation is adequate. Intubation and ventilation should be considered in patients whose airway cannot be protected or who have respiratory acidosis because of inadequate ventilation; such patients should be monitored in a critical care area.

Most poisons that impair consciousness also depress respiration. Assisted ventilation (either mouth-to-mouth or using a bag-valve-mask device) may be needed. Oxygen is not a substitute for adequate ventilation, although it should be given in the highest concentration possible in poisoning with carbon monoxide and irritant gases.

Respiratory stimulants do not help and should be **avoided**.

## Blood pressure

Hypotension is common in severe poisoning with central nervous system depressants. A systolic blood pressure of less than 70 mmHg may lead to irreversible brain damage or renal tubular necrosis. Hypotension should be corrected initially by tilting down the head of the bed and administration of either sodium chloride intravenous infusion or a colloidal infusion. Vasoconstrictor sympathomimetics (section 2.7.2) are rarely required and their use may be discussed with the National Poisons Information Service.

Fluid depletion without hypotension is common after prolonged coma and after aspirin poisoning due to vomiting, sweating, and hyperpnoea.

Hypertension, often transient, occurs less frequently than hypotension in poisoning; it may be associated with sympathomimetic drugs such as amphetamines, phencyclidine, and cocaine.

## Heart

Cardiac conduction defects and arrhythmias can occur in acute poisoning, notably with tricyclic antidepressants, some antipsychotics, and some antihistamines. Arrhythmias often respond to correction of underlying hypoxia, acidosis, or other biochemical abnormalities. Ventricular arrhythmias that cause serious hypotension require treatment. If the QT interval is prolonged, specialist advice should be sought because the use of some anti-arrhythmic drugs may be inappropriate. Supraventricular arrhythmias are seldom life-threatening and drug treatment is best withheld until the patient reaches hospital.

## Body temperature

Hypothermia may develop in patients of any age who have been deeply unconscious for some hours, particularly following overdose with barbiturates or phenothiazines. It may be missed unless core temperature is measured using a low-reading rectal thermometer or by some other means. Hypothermia is best treated by wrapping the patient (e.g. in a 'space blanket') to conserve body heat.

Hyperthermia can develop in patients taking CNS stimulants; children and the elderly are also at risk when taking therapeutic doses of drugs with antimuscarinic properties. Hyperthermia is initially managed by removing all unnecessary clothing and using a fan. Sponging with tepid water will promote evaporation; iced water should **not** be used. Advice should be sought from the National Poisons Information Service on the management of severe hyperthermia resulting from conditions such as the serotonin syndrome.

Both hypothermia and hyperthermia require **urgent** hospitalisation for assessment and supportive treatment.

## Convulsions

Single short-lived convulsions do not require treatment. If convulsions are protracted or recur frequently, lorazepam 4 mg or diazepam (preferably as emulsion) 10 mg should be given by slow intravenous injection into a large vein (section 4.8.2). Benzodiazepines should not be given by the intramuscular route for convulsions. If the intravenous route is not readily available, diazepam can be administered as a rectal solution or midazolam [unlicensed use] can be given by the buccal route (section 4.8.2).

## Removal and elimination

### Prevention of absorption

Given by mouth, **activated charcoal** can bind many poisons in the gastro-intestinal system, thereby *reducing their absorption*. The **sooner** it is given the **more effective** it is, but it may still be effective up to 1 hour after ingestion of the poison—longer in the case of modified-release preparations or of drugs with antimuscarinic (anticholinergic) properties. It is relatively safe and is particularly useful for the prevention of absorption of poisons that are toxic in small amounts, such as antidepressants.

For the use of charcoal in active elimination techniques, see below.

### Active elimination techniques

Repeated doses of **activated charcoal** by mouth *enhance the elimination* of some drugs after they have been absorbed; repeated doses are given after overdosage with:

| | |
|---|---|
| Carbamazepine | Quinine |
| Dapsone | Theophylline |
| Phenobarbital | |

The usual dose of activated charcoal in adults and children over 12 years of age is 50 g initially then 50 g every 4 hours. Vomiting should be treated (e.g. with an antiemetic drug) since it may reduce the efficacy of charcoal treatment. In cases of intolerance, the dose may be reduced and the frequency increased (e.g. 25 g every 2 hours *or* 12.5 g every hour) but this may compromise efficacy.

In children under 12 years of age, activated charcoal is given in a dose of 1 g/kg (max. 50 g) every 4 hours; the dose may be reduced and the frequency increased if not tolerated.

Other techniques intended to enhance the elimination of poisons after absorption are only practicable in hospital and are only suitable for a small number of severely poisoned patients. Moreover, they only apply to a limited number of poisons. Examples include:

- haemodialysis for salicylates, phenobarbital, methyl alcohol (methanol), ethylene glycol, and lithium;
- alkalinisation of the urine for salicylates.

## Removal from the gastro-intestinal tract

Gastric lavage is rarely required; for substances that cannot be removed effectively by other means (e.g. iron), it should be considered only if a life-threatening amount has been ingested within the previous hour. It should be carried out only if the airway can be protected adequately. Gastric lavage is contra-indicated if a corrosive substance or a petroleum distillate has been ingested, but it may occasionally be considered in patients who have ingested drugs that are not adsorbed by charcoal, such as iron or lithium. Induction of *emesis* (e.g. with ipecacuanha) is **not** recommended because there is no evidence that it affects absorption and it may increase the risk of aspiration.

*Whole bowel irrigation* (by means of a bowel cleansing preparation) has been used in poisoning with certain modified-release or enteric-coated formulations, in severe poisoning with iron and lithium salts, and if illicit drugs are carried in the gastro-intestinal tract ('body-packing'). However, it is not clear that the procedure improves outcome and advice should be sought from the National Poisons Information Service.

## CHARCOAL, ACTIVATED

**Indications** reduction of absorption of poisons in the gastro-intestinal system; see also active elimination techniques, above

**Cautions** drowsy or comatose patient (risk of aspiration); reduced gastro-intestinal motility (risk of obstruction); **not** for poisoning with petroleum distillates, corrosive substances, alcohols, malathion, and metal salts including iron and lithium salts

**Side-effects** black stools

**Dose**

- Reduction of absorption, ADULT and CHILD over 12 years, 50 g; CHILD under 12 years, 1 g/kg (max. 50 g)
- Active elimination, see notes above
Note Activated charcoal doses in BNF may differ from those in product literature. Suspension or reconstituted powder may be mixed with soft drinks (e.g. caffeine-free diet cola) or fruit juices to mask the taste

**Actidose-Aqua® Advance** (Cambridge)
Oral suspension, activated charcoal 1.04 g/5 mL, net price 50-g pack (240 mL) = £8.69

**Carbomix®** (Beacon)
Powder, activated charcoal, net price 25-g pack = £8.50, 50-g pack = £11.90

**Charcodote®** (TEVA UK)
Oral suspension, activated charcoal 1 g/5 mL, net price 50-g pack = £11.88

## Specific drugs

### Alcohol

Acute intoxication with alcohol (ethanol) is common in adults but also occurs in children. The features include ataxia, dysarthria, nystagmus, and drowsiness, which may progress to coma, with hypotension and acidosis. Aspiration of vomit is a special hazard and hypoglycaemia may occur in children and some adults. Patients are managed supportively, with particular attention to maintaining a clear airway and measures to reduce the risk of aspiration of gastric contents. The blood glucose is measured and glucose given if indicated.

> The **National Poisons Information Service** (Tel: 0844 892 0111) will provide specialist advice on all aspects of poisoning day and night

### Analgesics (non-opioid)

**Aspirin** The main features of salicylate poisoning are hyperventilation, tinnitus, deafness, vasodilatation, and sweating. Coma is uncommon but indicates very severe poisoning. The associated acid-base disturbances are complex.

Treatment must be in hospital, where plasma salicylate, pH, and electrolytes can be measured; absorption of aspirin may be slow and the plasma-salicylate concentration may continue to rise for several hours, requiring repeated measurement. Plasma-salicylate concentration may not correlate with clinical severity in the young and the elderly, and clinical and biochemical assessment is necessary. Generally, the clinical severity of poisoning is low below a plasma-salicylate concentration of 500 mg/litre (3.6 mmol/litre), unless there is evidence of metabolic acidosis. Activated charcoal can be given within 1 hour of ingesting more than 125 mg/kg of aspirin. Fluid losses should be replaced and intravenous sodium bicarbonate may be given (ensuring plasma-potassium concentration is within the reference range) to enhance urinary salicylate excretion (optimum urinary pH 7.5–8.5).

Plasma-potassium concentration should be corrected before giving sodium bicarbonate as hypokalaemia may complicate alkalinisation of the urine.

Haemodialysis is the treatment of choice for severe salicylate poisoning and should be considered when the plasma-salicylate concentration exceeds 700 mg/litre (5.1 mmol/litre) or in the presence of severe metabolic acidosis.

**NSAIDs** Mefenamic acid has important consequences in overdosage because it can cause convulsions, which if prolonged or recurrent require treatment, see p. 28.

Overdosage with ibuprofen may cause nausea, vomiting, epigastric pain, and tinnitus, but more serious toxicity is very uncommon. Activated charcoal followed by symptomatic measures are indicated if more than 400 mg/kg has been ingested within the preceding hour.

**Paracetamol** Single or repeated doses totalling as little as 10–15 g (20–30 tablets) or 150 mg/kg of paracetamol taken within 24 hours may cause severe hepatocellular necrosis and, much less frequently, renal tubular necrosis. Patients at *high-risk* of liver damage, including those taking enzyme-inducing drugs or who are malnourished (see below), may develop liver toxicity with as little as 75 mg/kg of paracetamol (equivalent to approx. 5 g (10 tablets) in a 70-kg patient) taken within 24 hours. Nausea and vomiting, the only early features of poisoning, usually settle within 24 hours. Persistence beyond this time, often associated with the onset of right subcostal pain and tenderness, usually indicates development of hepatic necrosis. Liver damage is maximal 3–4 days after ingestion and may lead to encephalopathy, haemorrhage, hypoglycaemia, cerebral oedema, and death.

Therefore, despite a lack of significant early symptoms, patients who have taken an overdose of paracetamol should be transferred to hospital urgently.

Administration of activated charcoal should be considered if paracetamol in excess of 150 mg/kg or 12 g, **whichever is the smaller** (or in excess of 75 mg/kg for those considered to be at *high risk*, see below), is thought to have been ingested within the previous hour.

**Acetylcysteine** protects the liver if infused within 24 hours of ingesting paracetamol. It is most effective if given within 8 hours of ingestion, after which effectiveness declines sharply; if more than 24 hours have elapsed advice should be sought either from the National Poisons Information Service or from a liver unit on the management of serious liver damage. Giving acetylcysteine by mouth [unlicensed route] is an alternative if intravenous access is not possible—contact the National Poisons Information service for advice. In remote areas, **methionine** by mouth is an alternative only if acetylcysteine cannot be given promptly. Once the patient reaches hospital the need to continue treatment with the antidote will be assessed from the plasma-paracetamol concentration (related to the time from ingestion).

Patients at risk of liver damage and therefore requiring treatment can be identified from a single measurement of the plasma-paracetamol concentration, related to the time from ingestion, provided this time interval is not less than 4 hours; earlier samples may be misleading. The concentration is plotted on a paracetamol treatment graph, with a reference line ('normal treatment line') joining plots of 200 mg/litre (1.32 mmol/litre) at 4 hours and 6.25 mg/litre (0.04 mmol/litre) at 24 hours (see p. 30). Those whose plasma-paracetamol concentration is above the *normal treatment line* are treated with acetylcysteine by intravenous infusion (or, if acetylcysteine is not available, with methionine by mouth, provided the overdose has been taken **within 10–12 hours** *and* the patient is not vomiting).

Patients at *high-risk* of liver damage include those:

- taking liver enzyme-inducing drugs (e.g. carbamazepine, phenobarbital, phenytoin, primidone, rifampicin, alcohol, and St John's wort);
- who are malnourished (e.g. in anorexia, cystic fibrosis, in alcoholism, or those who are HIV-positive);
- who have not eaten for a few days.

These patients can develop toxicity at **lower** plasma-paracetamol concentration and should be treated if the concentration is above the *high-risk treatment line* (which joins plots that are at 50% of the plasma-paracetamol concentrations of the normal treatment line).

The prognostic accuracy of plasma-paracetamol concentration taken after 15 hours is uncertain, but a

Emergency treatment of poisoning

Patients whose plasma-paracetamol concentrations are above the **normal treatment line** should be treated with acetylcysteine by intravenous infusion (or, if acetylcysteine cannot be used, with methionine by mouth, provided the overdose has been taken **within 10–12 hours** and the patient is not vomiting).

Patients at *high-risk* of liver damage include those:

- taking liver enzyme-inducing drugs (e.g. carbamazepine, phenobarbital, phenytoin, primidone, rifampicin, alcohol, St John's wort);
- who are malnourished (e.g. in anorexia, cystic fibrosis, in alcoholism, or those who are HIV-positive);
- who have not eaten for a few days.

These patients should be treated if their plasma-paracetamol concentration is above the **high-risk treatment line.**

The prognostic accuracy after 15 hours is uncertain but a plasma-paracetamol concentration above the relevant treatment line should be regarded as carrying a serious risk of liver damage.

Graph reproduced courtesy of University of Wales College of Medicine Therapeutics and Toxicology Centre

concentration above the relevant treatment line should be regarded as carrying a serious risk of liver damage.

The plasma-paracetamol concentration may be difficult to interpret when paracetamol has been ingested over several hours. If there is doubt about timing or the need for treatment then the patient should be treated with an antidote.

## ACETYLCYSTEINE

**Indications** paracetamol overdosage, see notes above

**Cautions** asthma (see side-effects below but do not delay acetylcysteine treatment)

**Side-effects** hypersensitivity-like reactions managed by reducing infusion rate or suspending until reaction settled—contact the National Poisons Information Service if reaction severe (rash also managed by giving antihistamine; acute asthma managed by giving nebulised short-acting beta$_2$ agonist)

**Dose**

- By intravenous infusion, ADULT and CHILD, initially 150 mg/kg (max. 16.5 g) over 15 minutes, then 50 mg/kg (max. 5.5 g) over 4 hours then 100 mg/kg (max. 11 g) over 16 hours

  Administration Dilute requisite dose in glucose intravenous infusion 5% as follows: ADULT and CHILD over 12 years, initially 200 mL given over 15 minutes, then 500 mL over 4 hours, then 1 litre over 16 hours; CHILD under 12 years, body-weight over 20 kg, initially 100 mL given over 15 minutes, then 250 mL over 4 hours, then 500 mL over 16 hours; CHILD body-weight under 20 kg, initially 3 mL/kg given over 15 minutes, then 7 mL/kg over 4 hours, then 14 mL/kg over 16 hours

  Note Manufacturer also recommends other infusion fluids, but glucose 5% is preferable

**Acetylcysteine** (Non-proprietary) [PoM]
Injection, acetylcysteine 200 mg/mL, net price 10-mL amp = £2.50

**Parvolex®** (UCB Pharma) [PoM]
Injection, acetylcysteine 200 mg/mL, net price 10-mL amp = £2.25

## ▌ METHIONINE

**Indications** paracetamol overdosage, see notes above

**Cautions** hepatic impairment (Appendix 2)

**Side-effects** nausea, vomiting, drowsiness, irritability

**Dose**

- ADULT and CHILD over 6 years initially 2.5 g, followed by 3 further doses of 2.5 g every 4 hours, CHILD under 6 years initially 1 g, followed by 3 further doses of 1 g every 4 hours

**Methionine** (Pharma Nord)
Tablets, f/c, methionine 500 mg, net price 20-tab pack = £9.95

**Methionine** (UCB Pharma)
Tablets, DL-methionine 250 mg, net price 200-tab pack = £87.76

◀ **With paracetamol (co-methiamol)**
Section 4.7.1

## Analgesics (opioid)

Opioids (narcotic analgesics) cause coma, respiratory depression, and pinpoint pupils. The specific antidote **naloxone** is indicated if there is coma or bradypnoea. Since naloxone has a shorter duration of action than many opioids, close monitoring and repeated injections are necessary according to the respiratory rate and depth of coma. When repeated administration of naloxone is required, it can be given by continuous intravenous infusion instead and the rate of infusion adjusted according to vital signs. The effects of some opioids, such as buprenorphine, are only partially reversed by naloxone. Dextropropoxyphene and methadone have very long durations of action; patients may need to be monitored for long periods following large overdoses.

Naloxone reverses the opioid effects of dextropropoxyphene; the long duration of action of dextropropoxyphene calls for prolonged monitoring and further doses of naloxone may be required. Norpropoxyphene, a metabolite of dextropropoxyphene, also has cardiotoxic effects which may require treatment with **sodium**

**bicarbonate**, or **magnesium sulphate**, or both; arrhythmias may occur for up to 12 hours.

> The **National Poisons Information Service** (Tel: 0844 892 0111) will provide specialist advice on all aspects of poisoning day and night

## ▌ NALOXONE HYDROCHLORIDE

**Indications** overdosage with opioids; reversal of opioid-induced respiratory depression and reversal of neonatal respiratory depression resulting from opioid administration to mother during labour (section 15.1.7)

**Cautions** physical dependence on opioids; cardiac irritability; naloxone is short-acting, see notes above

**Dose**

- By intravenous injection, 0.4–2 mg; if no response repeat at intervals of 2–3 minutes to a max. of 10 mg (then review diagnosis); further doses may be required if respiratory function deteriorates; CHILD 10 micrograms/kg; if no response give subsequent dose of 100 micrograms/kg (then review diagnosis); further doses may be required if respiratory function deteriorates

- By subcutaneous *or* intramuscular injection, ADULT and CHILD dose as for intravenous injection but use only if intravenous route not feasible (onset of action slower)

- By continuous intravenous infusion using an infusion pump, 4 mg diluted in 20 mL intravenous infusion solution [unlicensed concentration] at a rate adjusted according to response (initial rate may be set at 60% of initial intravenous injection dose (see above) and infused over 1 hour)

  Important Doses used in acute opioid overdosage may not be appropriate for the management of opioid-induced respiratory depression and sedation in those receiving palliative care and in chronic opioid use; see also section 15.1.7 for management of postoperative respiratory depression

[1]**Naloxone** (Non-proprietary) [PoM]
Injection, naloxone hydrochloride 400 micrograms/mL, net price 1-mL amp = £4.50; 1 mg/mL, 2-mL prefilled syringe = £8.36

[1]**Minijet® Naloxone** (UCB Pharma) [PoM]
Injection, naloxone hydrochloride 400 micrograms/mL, net price 1-mL disposable syringe = £19.90, 2-mL disposable syringe = £12.96, 5-mL disposable syringe = £12.68

## Antidepressants

**Tricyclic and related antidepressants** Tricyclic and related antidepressants cause dry mouth, coma of varying degree, hypotension, hypothermia, hyperreflexia, extensor plantar responses, convulsions, respiratory failure, cardiac conduction defects, and arrhythmias. Dilated pupils and urinary retention also occur. Metabolic acidosis may complicate severe poisoning; delirium with confusion, agitation, and visual and auditory hallucinations are common during recovery.

Assessment in hospital is strongly advised in case of poisoning by *tricyclic and related antidepressants* but

---

1. [PoM] restriction does not apply where administration is for saving life in emergency

symptomatic treatment can be given before transfer. Supportive measures to ensure a clear airway and adequate ventilation during transfer are mandatory. Intravenous lorazepam or intravenous diazepam (preferably in emulsion form) may be required to treat convulsions. Activated charcoal given within 1 hour of the overdose reduces absorption of the drug. Although arrhythmias are worrying, some will respond to correction of hypoxia and acidosis. The use of anti-arrhythmic drugs is best avoided, but intravenous infusion of sodium bicarbonate can arrest arrhythmias or prevent them in those with an extended QRS duration. Diazepam given by mouth is usually adequate to sedate delirious patients but large doses may be required.

### Selective serotonin re-uptake inhibitors (SSRIs)

Symptoms of poisoning by selective serotonin re-uptake inhibitors include nausea, vomiting, agitation, tremor, nystagmus, drowsiness, and sinus tachycardia; convulsions may occur. Rarely, severe poisoning results in the serotonin syndrome, with marked neuropsychiatric effects, neuromuscular hyperactivity, and autonomic instability; hyperthermia, rhabdomyolysis, renal failure, and coagulopathies may develop.

Management of SSRI poisoning is supportive. Activated charcoal given within 1 hour of the overdose reduces absorption of the drug. Convulsions can be treated with lorazepam, diazepam, or buccal midazolam [unlicensed use] (see p. 28). Contact the National Poisons Information Service for the management of hyperthermia or the serotonin syndrome.

## Antimalarials

Overdosage with quinine, chloroquine, or hydroxychloroquine is extremely hazardous and difficult to treat. Urgent advice from the National Poisons Information Service is essential. Life-threatening features include arrhythmias (which can have a very rapid onset) and convulsions (which can be intractable).

## Beta-blockers

Therapeutic overdosages with beta-blockers may cause lightheadedness, dizziness, and possibly syncope as a result of bradycardia and hypotension; heart failure may be precipitated or exacerbated. These complications are most likely in patients with conduction system disorders or impaired myocardial function. Bradycardia is the most common arrhythmia caused by beta-blockers, but sotalol may induce ventricular tachyarrhythmias (sometimes of the torsade de pointes type). The effects of massive overdosage can vary from one beta-blocker to another; propranolol overdosage in particular may cause coma and convulsions.

*Acute massive overdosage* must be managed in hospital and expert advice should be obtained. Maintenance of a clear airway and adequate ventilation is mandatory. An intravenous injection of atropine is required to treat bradycardia and hypotension (3 mg for an adult, 40 micrograms/kg (max. 3 mg) for a child). Cardiogenic shock unresponsive to atropine is probably best treated with an intravenous injection of glucagon 2–10 mg (CHILD 50–150 micrograms/kg, max. 10 mg) [unlicensed indication and dose] in glucose 5% (with precautions to protect the airway in case of vomiting) followed by an intravenous infusion of 50 micrograms/kg/hour. If glucagon is not available, intravenous isoprenaline (available from 'special-order' manufacturers or specialist importing companies, see p. 969) is an alternative. A cardiac pacemaker can be used to increase the heart rate.

## Calcium-channel blockers

Features of calcium-channel blocker poisoning include nausea, vomiting, dizziness, agitation, confusion, and coma in severe poisoning. Metabolic acidosis and hyperglycaemia may occur. Verapamil and diltiazem have a profound cardiac depressant effect causing hypotension and arrhythmias, including complete heart block and asystole. The dihydropyridine calcium-channel blockers cause severe hypotension secondary to profound peripheral vasodilatation.

Activated charcoal should be considered if the patient presents within 1 hour of overdosage with a calcium-channel blocker; repeated doses of activated charcoal are considered if a modified-release preparation is involved. In patients with significant features of poisoning, calcium chloride or calcium gluconate (section 9.5.1.1) is given by injection; atropine is given to correct symptomatic bradycardia. In severe cases, an insulin and glucose infusion may be required in the management of hypotension and myocardial failure. For the management of hypotension, the choice of inotropic sympathomimetic depends on whether hypotension is secondary to vasodilatation or to myocardial depression—advice should be sought from the National Poisons Information Service.

## Hypnotics and anxiolytics

**Benzodiazepines** Benzodiazepines taken alone cause drowsiness, ataxia, dysarthria, and occasionally minor and short-lived depression of consciousness. Activated charcoal can be given within 1 hour of ingesting a significant quantity of benzodiazepine, provided the patient is awake and the airway is protected. Benzodiazepines potentiate the effects of other central nervous system depressants taken concomitantly. Use of the benzodiazepine antagonist flumazenil can be hazardous, particularly in mixed overdoses involving tricyclic antidepressants or in benzodiazepine-dependent patients. Flumazenil should be used on **expert advice** only.

## Iron salts

Iron poisoning in childhood is usually accidental. The symptoms are nausea, vomiting, abdominal pain, diarrhoea, haematemesis, and rectal bleeding. Hypotension and hepatocellular necrosis can occur later. Coma, shock, and metabolic acidosis indicate severe poisoning.

Advice should be sought from the National Poisons Information Service if a significant quantity of iron has been ingested within the previous hour.

Mortality is reduced by intensive and specific therapy with **desferrioxamine**, which chelates iron. The serum-iron concentration is measured as an emergency and intravenous desferrioxamine given to chelate absorbed iron in excess of the expected iron binding capacity. In **severe toxicity** intravenous desferrioxamine should be given *immediately* without waiting for the result of the serum-iron measurement.

## ◢ DESFERRIOXAMINE MESILATE
### (Deferoxamine Mesilate)

**Indications** iron poisoning; chronic iron overload (section 9.1.3)
**Cautions** section 9.1.3
**Side-effects** section 9.1.3
**Dose**
- By continuous intravenous infusion, ADULT and CHILD up to 15 mg/kg/hour, reduced after 4–6 hours; max. 80 mg/kg in 24 hours (in severe cases, higher doses on advice from the National Poisons Information Service)

◢ **Preparations**
Section 9.1.3

## Lithium

Most cases of lithium intoxication occur as a complication of long-term therapy and are caused by reduced excretion of the drug due to a variety of factors including dehydration, deterioration of renal function, infections, and co-administration of diuretics or NSAIDs (or other drugs that interact). Acute deliberate overdoses may also occur with delayed onset of symptoms (12 hours or more) owing to slow entry of lithium into the tissues and continuing absorption from modified-release formulations.

The early clinical features are non-specific and may include apathy and restlessness which could be confused with mental changes arising from the patient's depressive illness. Vomiting, diarrhoea, ataxia, weakness, dysarthria, muscle twitching, and tremor may follow. Severe poisoning is associated with convulsions, coma, renal failure, electrolyte imbalance, dehydration, and hypotension.

Therapeutic lithium concentrations are within the range of 0.4–1.0 mmol/litre; concentrations in excess of 2.0 mmol/litre are usually associated with serious toxicity and such cases may need treatment with haemodialysis if neurological symptoms or renal failure are present. In acute overdosage much higher serum-lithium concentrations may be present without features of toxicity and all that is usually necessary is to take measures to increase urine output (e.g. by increasing fluid intake but avoiding diuretics). Otherwise, treatment is supportive with special regard to electrolyte balance, renal function, and control of convulsions. The stomach should be emptied by gastric lavage if it can be performed within 1 hour of ingesting significant quantities of lithium. Whole-bowel irrigation should be considered for significant ingestion, but advice should be sought from the National Poisons Information Service, p. 27.

## Phenothiazines and related drugs

Phenothiazines cause less depression of consciousness and respiration than other sedatives. Hypotension, hypothermia, sinus tachycardia, and arrhythmias may complicate poisoning. Dystonic reactions can occur with therapeutic doses (particularly with prochlorperazine and trifluoperazine), and convulsions may occur in severe cases. Arrhythmias may respond to correction of hypoxia, acidosis, and other biochemical abnormalities, but specialist advice should be sought if arrhythmias result from a prolonged QT interval; the use of some anti-arrhythmic drugs can worsen such arrhythmias. Dystonic reactions are rapidly abolished by injection

of drugs such as procyclidine (section 4.9.2) or diazepam (section 4.8.2, emulsion preferred).

## Atypical antipsychotic drugs

Features of poisoning by atypical antipsychotic drugs (section 4.2.1) include drowsiness, convulsions, extrapyramidal symptoms, hypotension, and ECG abnormalities (including prolongation of the QT interval). Management is supportive. Activated charcoal can be given within 1 hour of ingesting a significant quantity of an atypical antipsychotic drug.

## Stimulants

**Amphetamines** These cause wakefulness, excessive activity, paranoia, hallucinations, and hypertension followed by exhaustion, convulsions, hyperthermia, and coma. The early stages can be controlled by diazepam or lorazepam; advice should be sought from the National Poisons Information Service (p. 27) on the management of hypertension. Later, tepid sponging, anticonvulsants, and artificial respiration may be needed.

**Cocaine** Cocaine stimulates the central nervous system, causing agitation, dilated pupils, tachycardia, hypertension, hallucinations, hyperthermia, hypertonia, and hyperreflexia; cardiac effects include chest pain, myocardial infarction, and arrhythmias.

Initial treatment of cocaine poisoning involves intravenous administration of diazepam to control agitation and cooling measures for hyperthermia (see Body temperature, p. 27); hypertension and cardiac effects require specific treatment and expert advice should be sought.

**Ecstasy** Ecstasy (methylenedioxymethamfetamine, MDMA) may cause severe reactions, even at doses that were previously tolerated. The most serious effects are delirium, coma, convulsions, ventricular arrhythmias, hyperthermia, rhabdomyolysis, acute renal failure, acute hepatitis, disseminated intravascular coagulation, adult respiratory distress syndrome, hyperreflexia, hypotension and intracerebral haemorrhage; hyponatraemia has also been associated with ecstasy use.

Treatment of methylenedioxymethamfetamine poisoning is supportive, with diazepam to control severe agitation or persistent convulsions and close monitoring including ECG. Self-induced water intoxication should be considered in patients with ecstasy poisoning.

'Liquid ecstasy' is a term used for sodium oxybate (gamma-hydroxybutyrate, GHB), which is a sedative.

> The **National Poisons Information Service** (Tel: 0844 892 0111) will provide specialist advice on all aspects of poisoning day and night

## Theophylline

Theophylline and related formulations and toxicity can therefore be delayed. They cause vomiting (which may be severe and intractable), agitation, restlessness, dilated pupils, sinus tachycardia, and hyperglycaemia. More serious effects are haematemesis, convulsions, and supraventricular and ventricular arrhythmias. Severe hypokalaemia may develop rapidly.

Repeated doses of activated charcoal can be used to eliminate theophylline even if more than 1 hour has elapsed after ingestion and especially if a modified-release preparation has been taken (see also under Active Elimination Techniques, p. 28). Ondansetron (section 4.6) may be effective for severe vomiting that is resistant to other antiemetics [unlicensed indication]. Hypokalaemia is corrected by intravenous infusion of potassium chloride and may be so severe as to require 60 mmol/hour (high doses require ECG monitoring). Convulsions should be controlled by intravenous administration of lorazepam or diazepam (emulsion preferred). Sedation with diazepam may be necessary in agitated patients.

Provided the patient does **not** suffer from asthma, a short-acting beta-blocker (section 2.4) can be administered intravenously to reverse severe tachycardia, hypokalaemia, and hyperglycaemia.

## Other poisons

Consult either the National Poisons Information Service day and night or TOXBASE, see p. 27.

## Cyanides

Oxygen should be administered to patients with cyanide poisoning. The choice of antidote depends on the severity of poisoning, certainty of diagnosis, and the cause. Dicobalt edetate is the antidote of choice when there is a strong clinical suspicion of severe cyanide poisoning. Dicobalt edetate itself is toxic, associated with anaphylactic reactions, and is potentially fatal if administered in the absence of cyanide poisoning. A regimen of sodium nitrite followed by sodium thiosulphate is an alternative if dicobalt edetate is not available.

Hydroxocobalamin can be considered for victims of smoke inhalation who show signs of significant cyanide poisoning. The usual dose is 5 g (70 mg/kg in children) by intravenous infusion (given once or twice according to severity). *Cyanokit®* provides hydroxocobalamin 2.5 g/bottle (no other preparation of hydroxocobalamin is suitable)—contact the National Poisons Information Service for advice.

## ■ DICOBALT EDETATE

**Indications** severe poisoning with cyanides

**Cautions** owing to toxicity to be used only for definite cyanide poisoning when patient tending to lose, or has lost, consciousness; **not** to be used as a precautionary measure

**Side-effects** hypotension, tachycardia, and vomiting; anaphylactic reactions including facial and laryngeal oedema and cardiac abnormalities

**Dose**

• By intravenous injection, ADULT 300 mg over 1 minute (5 minutes if condition less serious) followed immediately by 50 mL of glucose intravenous infusion 50%; if response inadequate a second dose of both may be given, but risk of cobalt toxicity; CHILD consult the National Poisons Information Service

¹**Dicobalt Edetate** (Cambridge) ᴘᴏᴹ
Injection, dicobalt edetate 15 mg/mL, net price 20-mL (300-mg) amp = £13.75

## ■ SODIUM NITRITE

**Indications** poisoning with cyanides (used in conjunction with sodium thiosulphate)

**Side-effects** flushing and headache due to vasodilatation

**Dose**

• By intravenous injection over 5–20 minutes (as sodium nitrite injection 30 mg/mL), 300 mg; CHILD 4–10 mg/kg (max. 300 mg)

¹**Sodium Nitrite** ᴘᴏᴹ
Injection, sodium nitrite 3% (30 mg/mL) in water for injections
Available from 'special-order' manufacturers or specialist importing companies, see p. 969

## ■ SODIUM THIOSULPHATE

**Indications** in conjunction with sodium nitrite for cyanide poisoning

**Dose**

• By intravenous injection over 10 minutes (as sodium thiosulphate injection 500 mg/mL), 12.5 g; dose may be repeated in severe cyanide poisoning if dicobalt edetate not available; CHILD 400 mg/kg (max. 12.5 g); dose may be repeated in severe cyanide poisoning if dicobalt edetate not available

¹**Sodium Thiosulphate** ᴘᴏᴹ
Injection, sodium thiosulphate 50% (500 mg/mL) in water for injections
Available from 'special-order' manufacturers or specialist importing companies, see p. 969

## Ethylene glycol and methanol

**Fomepizole** (available from 'special-order' manufacturers or specialist importing companies, see p. 969) is the treatment of choice for ethylene glycol and methanol (methyl alcohol) poisoning. If necessary, **ethanol** (by mouth or by intravenous infusion) can be used, but with caution. Advice on the treatment of ethylene glycol and methanol poisoning should be obtained from the National Poisons Information Service. It is important to start antidote treatment promptly in cases of suspected poisoning with these agents.

## Heavy metals

Heavy metal antidotes include dimercaprol and sodium calcium edetate. Other antidotes include succimer (DMSA) and unithiol (DMPS) [both unlicensed]; they may be useful in certain cases of heavy metal poisoning but the advice of the National Poisons Information Service should be sought.

## ■ DIMERCAPROL
(BAL)

**Indications** poisoning by antimony, arsenic, bismuth, gold, mercury

**Cautions** hypertension, renal impairment (discontinue or use with extreme caution if impairment develops during treatment; elderly, pregnancy and breast-feeding; **interactions:** Appendix 1 (dimercaprol)

**Contra-indications** not indicated for iron, cadmium, or selenium poisoning; severe hepatic impairment (unless due to arsenic poisoning)

---

1. ᴘᴏᴹ restriction does not apply where administration is for saving life in emergency

**Side-effects** hypertension, tachycardia, malaise, nausea, vomiting, salivation, lacrimation, sweating, burning sensation (mouth, throat, and eyes), feeling of constriction of throat and chest, headache, muscle spasm, abdominal pain, tingling of extremities; pyrexia in children; local pain and abscess at injection site

**Dose**

- By intramuscular injection, ADULT and CHILD 2.5–3 mg/kg every 4 hours for 2 days, 2–4 times on the third day, then 1–2 times daily for 10 days or until recovery

**Dimercaprol** (Sovereign) ᴾᵒᴹ
Injection, dimercaprol 50 mg/mL. Net price 2-mL amp = £42.73
Note Contains arachis (peanut) oil as solvent

---

## SODIUM CALCIUM EDETATE
(Sodium Calciumedetate)

**Indications** lead poisoning

**Cautions** renal impairment

**Side-effects** nausea, diarrhoea, abdominal pain, pain at site of injection, thrombophlebitis if given too rapidly, renal damage particularly in overdosage; hypotension, lacrimation, myalgia, nasal congestion, sneezing, malaise, thirst, fever, chills, headache, and zinc depletion also reported

**Dose**

- By intravenous infusion, ADULT and CHILD 40 mg/kg twice daily for up to 5 days; if necessary, a second course can be given at least 7 days after the first course, a third course can be given at least 7 days after the second course

**Ledclair®** (Durbin) ᴾᵒᴹ
Injection, sodium calcium edetate 200 mg/mL, net price 5-mL amp = £7.29

---

## Noxious gases

**Carbon monoxide** Carbon monoxide poisoning is usually due to inhalation of smoke, car exhaust, or fumes caused by blocked flues or incomplete combustion of fuel gases in confined spaces.

Immediate treatment of carbon monoxide poisoning is essential. The person should be moved to fresh air, the airway cleared, and high-flow **oxygen** 100% administered through a tight-fitting mask with an inflated face seal. Artificial respiration should be given as necessary and continued until adequate spontaneous breathing starts, or stopped only after persistent and efficient treatment of cardiac arrest has failed. The patient should be admitted to hospital because complications may arise after a delay of hours or days. Cerebral oedema may occur in severe poisoning and is treated with an intravenous infusion of mannitol (section 2.2.5). Referral for hyperbaric oxygen treatment should be discussed with the National Poisons Information Service if the victim is or has been unconscious, or has psychiatric or neurological features other than a headache, or has myocardial ischaemia or an arrhythmia, or has a blood carboxyhaemoglobin concentration of more than 20%, or is pregnant.

**Sulphur dioxide, chlorine, phosgene, ammonia**
All of these gases can cause upper respiratory tract and conjunctival irritation. Pulmonary oedema, with severe breathlessness and cyanosis may develop suddenly up to 36 hours after exposure. Death may occur. Patients are kept under observation and those who develop pulmonary oedema are given oxygen. Assisted ventilation may be necessary in the most serious cases.

---

## CS Spray

CS spray, which is used for riot control, irritates the eyes (hence 'tear gas') and the respiratory tract; symptoms normally settle spontaneously within 15 minutes. If symptoms persist, the patient should be removed to a well-ventilated area, and the exposed skin washed with soap and water after removal of contaminated clothing. Contact lenses should be removed and rigid ones washed (soft ones should be discarded). Eye symptoms should be treated by irrigating the eyes with physiological saline (or water if saline is not available) and advice sought from an ophthalmologist. Patients with features of severe poisoning, particularly respiratory complications, should be admitted to hospital for symptomatic treatment.

---

## Nerve agents

Treatment of nerve agent poisoning is similar to organophosphorus insecticide poisoning (see below), but advice must be sought from the National Poisons Information Service. The risk of cross-contamination is significant; adequate decontamination and protective clothing for healthcare personnel are essential. In emergencies involving the release of nerve agents, kits ('NAAS pods') containing **pralidoxime** can be obtained through the Ambulance Service from the National Blood Service (or the Welsh Blood Service in South Wales or designated hospital pharmacies in Northern Ireland and Scotland—see TOXBASE for list of designated centres).

> The **National Poisons Information Service** (Tel: 0844 892 0111) will provide specialist advice on all aspects of poisoning day and night

---

## Pesticides

**Organophosphorus insecticides** Organophosphorus insecticides are usually supplied as powders or dissolved in organic solvents. All are absorbed through the bronchi and intact skin as well as through the gut and inhibit cholinesterase activity, thereby prolonging and intensifying the effects of acetylcholine. Toxicity between different compounds varies considerably, and onset may be delayed after skin exposure.

Anxiety, restlessness, dizziness, headache, miosis, nausea, hypersalivation, vomiting, abdominal colic, diarrhoea, bradycardia, and sweating are common features of organophosphorus poisoning. Muscle weakness and fasciculation may develop and progress to generalised flaccid paralysis, including the ocular and respiratory muscles. Convulsions, coma, pulmonary oedema with copious bronchial secretions, hypoxia, and arrhythmias occur in severe cases. Hyperglycaemia and glycosuria without ketonuria may also be present.

Further absorption of the organophosphorus insecticide should be prevented by moving the patient to fresh air, removing soiled clothing, and washing contaminated skin. In severe poisoning it is vital to ensure a clear airway, frequent removal of bronchial secretions, and adequate ventilation and oxygenation; gastric lavage may be considered provided that the airway is protected. **Atropine** will reverse the muscarinic effects of acetylcholine and is given by intravenous injection in a dose of 2 mg (20 micrograms/kg (max. 2 mg) in a child) as atropine sulphate every 5 to 10 minutes (according to the severity of poisoning) until the skin becomes flushed and dry, the pupils dilate, and bradycardia is abolished.

**Pralidoxime chloride**, a cholinesterase reactivator, is used as an adjunct to atropine in moderate or severe poisoning. It improves muscle tone within 30 minutes of administration. Pralidoxime chloride is continued until the patient has not required atropine for 12 hours. Pralidoxime chloride can be obtained from designated centres, the names of which are held by the National Poisons Information Service (see p. 27).

### ■ PRALIDOXIME CHLORIDE

**Indications** adjunct to atropine in the treatment of poisoning by organophosphorus insecticide or nerve agent

**Cautions** renal impairment, myasthenia gravis

**Contra-indications** poisoning with carbamates or with organophosphorus compounds without anti-cholinesterase activity

**Side-effects** drowsiness, dizziness, disturbances of vision, nausea, tachycardia, headache, hyperventilation, and muscular weakness

**Dose**

- By intravenous infusion, ADULT and CHILD initially 30 mg/kg over 20 minutes, followed by 8 mg/kg/hour; usual max. 12 g in 24 hours

**Note** The loading dose may be administered by intravenous injection (diluted to a concentration of 50 mg/mL with water for injections) over at least 5 minutes if pulmonary oedema is present or if it is not practical to administer an intravenous infusion; pralidoxime chloride doses in BNF may differ from those in product literature

**¹Pralidoxime chloride** PoM

Injection, powder for reconstitution, pralidoxime chloride 1 g/vial

Available as *Protopam*® (from designated centres for organophosphorus insecticide poisoning or from the National Blood Service (or Welsh Ambulance Services for Mid West and South East Wales)—see TOXBASE for list of designated centres)

1. PoM restriction does not apply where administration is for saving life in emergency

## Snake bites and animal stings

**Snake bites** Envenoming from snake bite is uncommon in the UK. Many exotic snakes are kept, some illegally, but the only indigenous venomous snake is the adder (*Vipera berus*). The bite may cause local and systemic effects. Local effects include pain, swelling, bruising, and tender enlargement of regional lymph nodes. Systemic effects include early anaphylactic symptoms (transient hypotension with syncope, angioedema, urticaria, abdominal colic, diarrhoea, and vomiting), with later persistent or recurrent hypotension, ECG abnormalities, spontaneous systemic bleeding, coagulopathy, adult respiratory distress syndrome, and acute renal failure. Fatal envenoming is rare but the

potential for severe envenoming must not be underestimated.

Early anaphylactic symptoms should be treated with **adrenaline (epinephrine)** (section 3.4.3). Indications for antivenom treatment include systemic envenoming, especially hypotension (see above), ECG abnormalities, vomiting, haemostatic abnormalities, and marked local envenoming such that after bites on the hand or foot, swelling extends beyond the wrist or ankle within 4 hours of the bite. For both **adults** and **children**, the contents of one vial (10 mL) of **European viper venom antiserum** (available from Movianto) is given *by intravenous injection* over 10–15 minutes or *by intravenous infusion* over 30 minutes after diluting in sodium chloride intravenous infusion 0.9% (use 5 mL diluent/kg bodyweight). The dose can be repeated in 1–2 hours if symptoms of **systemic envenoming** persist. For patients who present with clinical features of severe envenoming (e.g. shock, ECG abnormalities, or local swelling that has advanced from the foot to above the knee or from the hand to above the elbow within 2 hours of the bite), an initial dose of 2 vials (20 mL) of the antiserum is recommended. Adrenaline (epinephrine) injection must be immediately to hand for treatment of anaphylactic reactions to the antivenom (for the management of anaphylaxis, see section 3.4.3).

Antivenom is available for bites by certain foreign snakes and spiders, stings by scorpions and fish. For information on identification, management, and for supply in an emergency, telephone the National Poisons Information Service (Tel: 0844 892 0111)

**Insect stings** Stings from ants, wasps, hornets, and bees cause local pain and swelling but seldom cause severe direct toxicity unless many stings are inflicted at the same time. If the sting is in the mouth or on the tongue local swelling may threaten the upper airway. The stings from these insects are usually treated by cleaning the area with a topical antiseptic. Bee stings should be removed as quickly as possible. Anaphylactic reactions require immediate treatment with intramuscular **adrenaline (epinephrine)**; self-administered intramuscular adrenaline (e.g. *EpiPen*®) is the best first-aid treatment for patients with severe hypersensitivity. An inhaled bronchodilator should be used for asthmatic reactions. For the management of anaphylaxis, see section 3.4.3. A short course of an oral **antihistamine** or a **topical corticosteroid** may help to reduce inflammation and relieve itching. A vaccine containing extracts of bee and wasp venom can be used to reduce the risk of anaphylaxis and systemic reactions in patients with systemic hypersensitivity to bee or wasp stings (section 3.4.2).

**Marine stings** The severe pain of weeverfish (*Trachinus vipera*) and Portuguese man-o'-war stings can be relieved by immersing the stung area immediately in uncomfortably hot, but not scalding, water (not more than 45°C). People stung by jellyfish and Portuguese man-o'-war around the UK coast should be removed from the sea as soon as possible. Adherent tentacles should be lifted off carefully (wearing gloves or using tweezers) or washed off with seawater. Alcoholic solutions, including suntan lotions, should **not** be applied because they can cause further discharge of stinging hairs. Ice packs will reduce pain and a slurry of baking soda (sodium bicarbonate), but not vinegar, may be useful for treating stings from UK species.

# 1 Gastro-intestinal system

**1.1 Dyspepsia and gastro-oesophageal reflux disease** 37

1.1.1 Antacids and simeticone 38

1.1.2 Compound alginates and proprietary indigestion preparations 40

**1.2 Antispasmodics and other drugs altering gut motility** 41

**1.3 Antisecretory drugs and mucosal protectants** 43

1.3.1 H₂-receptor antagonists 45

1.3.2 Selective antimuscarinics 47

1.3.3 Chelates and complexes 47

1.3.4 Prostaglandin analogues 47

1.3.5 Proton pump inhibitors 48

**1.4 Acute diarrhoea** 50

1.4.1 Adsorbents and bulk-forming drugs 51

1.4.2 Antimotility drugs 51

**1.5 Chronic bowel disorders** 52

1.5.1 Aminosalicylates 54

1.5.2 Corticosteroids 56

1.5.3 Drugs affecting the immune response 57

1.5.4 Food allergy 58

**1.6 Laxatives** 59

1.6.1 Bulk-forming laxatives 59

1.6.2 Stimulant laxatives 60

1.6.3 Faecal softeners 62

1.6.4 Osmotic laxatives 63

1.6.5 Bowel cleansing preparations 65

1.6.6 Peripheral opioid-receptor antagonists 66

**1.7 Local preparations for anal and rectal disorders** 67

1.7.1 Soothing haemorrhoidal preparations 67

1.7.2 Compound haemorrhoidal preparations with corticosteroids 67

1.7.3 Rectal sclerosants 68

1.7.4 Management of anal fissures 68

**1.8 Stoma care** 68

**1.9 Drugs affecting intestinal secretions** 69

1.9.1 Drugs affecting biliary composition and flow 69

1.9.2 Bile acid sequestrants 70

1.9.3 Aprotinin 70

1.9.4 Pancreatin 70

This chapter also includes advice on the drug management of the following:
*Clostridium difficile* infection, p. 53
constipation, p. 59
Crohn's disease, p. 52
diverticular disease. p. 53
food allergy, p. 58
*Helicobacter pylori* infection, p. 43
irritable bowel syndrome, p. 53
NSAID-associated ulcers, p. 44
ulcerative colitis, p. 52

## 1.1 Dyspepsia and gastro-oesophageal reflux disease

1.1.1 Antacids and simeticone

1.1.2 Compound alginates and proprietary indigestion preparations

### Dyspepsia

Dyspepsia covers pain, fullness, early satiety, bloating, and nausea. It can occur with gastric and duodenal ulceration (section 1.3) and gastric cancer but most commonly it is of uncertain origin.

Urgent endoscopic investigation is required if dyspepsia is accompanied by 'alarm features' (e.g. bleeding, dysphagia, recurrent vomiting, or weight loss). Urgent investigation should also be considered for patients over 55 years with unexplained, recent-onset dyspepsia that has not responded to treatment.

Patients with dyspepsia should be advised about lifestyle changes (see Gastro-oesophageal reflux disease, below). Some medications may cause dyspepsia—these should be stopped, if possible. Antacids may provide some symptomatic relief.

If symptoms persist in *uninvestigated dyspepsia*, treatment involves a **proton pump inhibitor** (section 1.3.5) for 4 weeks. A proton pump inhibitor can be used intermittently to control symptoms long-term. Patients with uninvestigated dyspepsia, who do not respond to an initial trial with a proton pump inhibitor, should be tested for *Helicobacter pylori* and given eradication therapy (section 1.3) if *H. pylori* is present. Alternatively, particularly in populations where *H. pylori* infection is more likely, the 'test and treat' strategy for *H. pylori* can be used before a trial with a proton pump inhibitor.

If *H. pylori* is present in patients with *functional (investigated, non-ulcer) dyspepsia*, eradication therapy should be provided. If symptoms persist, treatment with either a **proton pump inhibitor** (section 1.3.5) or a **histamine H₂-receptor antagonist** (section 1.3.1) can be given for 4 weeks. These antisecretory drugs can be used intermittently to control symptoms long term. However, most patients with functional dyspepsia do not benefit symptomatically from *H. pylori* eradication therapy or antisecretory drugs.

## Gastro-oesophageal reflux disease

Gastro-oesophageal reflux disease (including non-erosive gastro-oesophageal reflux and erosive oesophagitis) is associated with heartburn, acid regurgitation, and sometimes, difficulty in swallowing (dysphagia); oesophageal inflammation (oesophagitis), ulceration, and stricture formation may occur and there is an association with asthma.

The management of gastro-oesophageal reflux disease includes drug treatment, lifestyle changes and, in some cases, surgery. Initial treatment is guided by the severity of symptoms and treatment is then adjusted according to response. The extent of healing depends on the severity of the disease, the treatment chosen, and the duration of therapy.

Patients with gastro-oesophageal reflux disease should be advised about lifestyle changes (avoidance of excess alcohol and of aggravating foods such as fats); other measures include weight reduction, smoking cessation, and raising the head of the bed.

For *mild symptoms* of gastro-oesophageal reflux disease, initial management may include the use of **antacids** and **alginates**. Alginate-containing antacids can form a 'raft' that floats on the surface of the stomach contents to reduce reflux and protect the oesophageal mucosa. **Histamine H₂-receptor antagonists** (section 1.3.1) may relieve symptoms and permit reduction in antacid consumption. However, **proton pump inhibitors** (section 1.3.5) provide more effective relief of symptoms than H₂-receptor antagonists. When symptoms abate, treatment is titrated down to a level which maintains remission (e.g. by giving treatment intermittently).

For *severe symptoms* of gastro-oesophageal reflux disease or for patients with a proven or severe pathology (e.g. *oesophagitis, oesophageal ulceration, oesophagopharyngeal reflux, Barrett's oesophagus*), initial management involves the use of a **proton pump inhibitor** (section 1.3.5); patients need to be reassessed if symptoms persist despite treatment for 4–6 weeks with a proton pump inhibitor. When symptoms abate, treatment is titrated down to a level which maintains remission (e.g. by reducing the dose of the proton pump inhibitor or by giving it intermittently, or by substituting treatment with a histamine H₂-receptor antagonist). However, for endoscopically confirmed *erosive, ulcerative,* or *stricturing* disease, or *Barrett's oesophagus*, treatment with a proton pump inhibitor usually needs to be maintained at the minimum effective dose.

A prokinetic drug such as **metoclopramide** (section 4.6) may improve gastro-oesophageal sphincter function and accelerate gastric emptying.

**Children**  Gastro-oesophageal reflux disease is common in infancy but most symptoms resolve without treatment between 12 and 18 months of age. In infants, mild or moderate reflux without complications can be managed initially by changing the frequency and volume of feed; a feed thickener or thickened formula feed can be used (with advice of a dietitian—see Appendix 7 for suitable products). If necessary, a suitable alginate-containing preparation can be used instead of thickened feeds. For older children, life-style changes similar to those for adults (see above) may be helpful followed if necessary by treatment with an alginate-containing preparation.

Children who do not respond to these measures or who have problems such as respiratory disorders or suspected oesophagitis need to be referred to hospital; an H₂-receptor antagonist (section 1.3.1) may be needed to reduce acid secretion. If the oesophagitis is resistant to H₂-receptor blockade, the proton pump inhibitor omeprazole (section 1.3.5) can be tried.

## 1.1.1  Antacids and simeticone

Antacids (usually containing aluminium or magnesium compounds) can often relieve symptoms in *ulcer dyspepsia* and in *non-erosive gastro-oesophageal reflux* (see also section 1.1); they are also sometimes used in functional (non-ulcer) dyspepsia but the evidence of benefit is uncertain. Antacids are best given when symptoms occur or are expected, usually between meals and at bedtime, 4 or more times daily; additional doses may be required up to once an hour. Conventional doses e.g. 10 mL 3 or 4 times daily of liquid magnesium–aluminium antacids promote ulcer healing, but less well than antisecretory drugs (section 1.3); proof of a relationship between healing and neutralising capacity is lacking. Liquid preparations are more effective than tablet preparations.

**Aluminium-** and **magnesium-containing** antacids (e.g. aluminium hydroxide, and magnesium carbonate, hydroxide and trisilicate), being relatively insoluble in water, are long-acting if retained in the stomach. They are suitable for most antacid purposes. Magnesium-containing antacids tend to be laxative whereas aluminium-containing antacids may be constipating; antacids containing both magnesium and aluminium may reduce these colonic side-effects. Aluminium accumulation does not appear to be a risk if renal function is normal (see also Appendix 3).

The acid-neutralising capacity of preparations that contain more than one antacid may be the same as simpler preparations. Complexes such as **hydrotalcite** confer no special advantage.

**Sodium bicarbonate** should no longer be prescribed alone for the relief of dyspepsia but is present as an ingredient in many indigestion remedies. However, it retains a place in the management of urinary-tract disorders (section 7.4.3) and acidosis (section 9.2.1.3 and section 9.2.2). Sodium bicarbonate should be avoided in patients on salt-restricted diets.

**Bismuth-containing** antacids (unless chelates) are not recommended because absorbed bismuth can be neurotoxic, causing encephalopathy; they tend to be constipating. **Calcium-containing** antacids (section 1.1.2) can induce rebound acid secretion: with modest doses the clinical significance is doubtful, but prolonged high doses also cause hypercalcaemia and alkalosis, and can precipitate the milk-alkali syndrome.

**Simeticone** (activated dimeticone) is added to an antacid as an antifoaming agent to relieve flatulence. These preparations may be useful for the relief of hiccup in palliative care. **Alginates**, added as protectants, may be useful in gastro-oesophageal reflux disease (section 1.1 and section 1.1.2). The amount of additional ingredient or antacid in individual preparations varies widely, as does their sodium content, so that preparations may not be freely interchangeable.

See also section 1.3 for drugs used in the treatment of peptic ulceration.

**Interactions** Antacids should preferably not be taken at the same time as other drugs since they may impair absorption. Antacids may also damage enteric coatings designed to prevent dissolution in the stomach. See also **Appendix 1** (antacids, calcium salts).

> **Low Na⁺**
> The words 'low Na⁺' added after some preparations indicate a sodium content of less than 1 mmol per tablet or 10-mL dose.

## Aluminium- and magnesium-containing antacids

### ◼ ALUMINIUM HYDROXIDE

**Indications** dyspepsia; hyperphosphataemia (section 9.5.2.2)

**Cautions** see notes above; renal impairment (Appendix 3); **interactions:** Appendix 1 (antacids)

**Contra-indications** hypophosphataemia; neonates and infants

**Side-effects** see notes above

◂Aluminium-only preparations

**Aluminium Hydroxide** (Non-proprietary)
Tablets, dried aluminium hydroxide 500 mg. Net price 20 = 28p
Dose 1–2 tablets chewed 4 times daily and at bedtime or as required

**Alu-Cap®** (3M)
Capsules, green/red, dried aluminium hydroxide 475 mg (low Na⁺). Net price 120-cap pack = £3.75
Dose antacid, 1 capsule 4 times daily and at bedtime; CHILD not recommended for antacid therapy

◂Co-magaldrox
Co-magaldrox is a mixture of aluminium hydroxide and magnesium hydroxide; the proportions are expressed in the form x/y where x and y are the strengths in milligrams per unit dose of magnesium hydroxide and aluminium hydroxide respectively

**Maalox®** (Sanofi-Aventis)
Suspension, sugar-free, co-magaldrox 195/220 (magnesium hydroxide 195 mg, dried aluminium hydroxide 220 mg/5 mL (low Na⁺)). Net price 500 mL = £2.79
Dose ADULT and CHILD over 14 years, 10–20 mL 20–60 minutes after meals and at bedtime or when required

**Mucogel®** (Chemidex)
Suspension, sugar-free, co-magaldrox 195/220 (magnesium hydroxide 195 mg, dried aluminium

hydroxide 220 mg/5 mL (low Na⁺)). Net price 500 mL = £1.71
Dose ADULT and CHILD over 12 years, 10–20 mL 3 times daily, 20–60 minutes after meals, and at bedtime or when required

### ◼ MAGNESIUM CARBONATE

**Indications** dyspepsia

**Cautions** renal impairment (Appendix 3); see also notes above; **interactions:** Appendix 1 (antacids)

**Contra-indications** hypophosphataemia

**Side-effects** diarrhoea; belching due to liberated carbon dioxide

**Aromatic Magnesium Carbonate Mixture, BP**
(**Aromatic Magnesium Carbonate Oral Suspension**)
Oral suspension, light magnesium carbonate 3%, sodium bicarbonate 5%, in a suitable vehicle containing aromatic cardamom tincture. Contains about 6 mmol Na⁺/10 mL. Net price 200 mL = 66p
Dose 10 mL 3 times daily in water

For **preparations** also containing aluminium, see above and section 1.1.2.

### ◼ MAGNESIUM TRISILICATE

**Indications** dyspepsia

**Cautions** see under Magnesium Carbonate

**Contra-indications** see under Magnesium Carbonate

**Side-effects** diarrhoea, belching due to liberated carbon dioxide; silica-based renal stones reported on long-term treatment

**Magnesium Trisilicate Tablets, Compound, BP**
Tablets, magnesium trisilicate 250 mg, dried aluminium hydroxide 120 mg
Dose 1–2 tablets chewed when required

**Magnesium Trisilicate Mixture, BP**
(**Magnesium Trisilicate Oral Suspension**)
Oral suspension, 5% each of magnesium trisilicate, light magnesium carbonate, and sodium bicarbonate in a suitable vehicle with a peppermint flavour. Contains about 6 mmol Na⁺/10 mL
Dose 10–20 mL in water 3 times daily or as required; CHILD 5–12 years, 5–10 mL in water 3 times daily or as required

For **preparations** also containing aluminium, see above and section 1.1.2.

## Aluminium-magnesium complexes

### ◼ HYDROTALCITE
Aluminium magnesium carbonate hydroxide hydrate

**Indications** dyspepsia

**Cautions** see notes above; **interactions:** Appendix 1 (antacids)

**Side-effects** see notes above

**Hydrotalcite** (Peckforton)
Suspension, hydrotalcite 500 mg/5 mL (low Na⁺). Net price 500-mL pack = £1.96
Dose 10 mL between meals and at bedtime; CHILD 6–12 years 5 mL between meals and at bedtime
Note The brand name *Altacite®* ⃞ is used for hydrotalcite suspension; for *Altacite Plus®* suspension, see below

**Gastro-intestinal system**

**1**

## Antacid preparations containing simeticone

### Altacite Plus® (Peckforton)

Suspension, sugar-free, co-simalcite 125/500 (simeticone 125 mg, hydrotalcite 500 mg)/5 mL (low Na⁺). Net price 500 mL = £1.96

Dose 10 mL between meals and at bedtime when required; CHILD 8–12 years 5 mL between meals and at bedtime when required

### Asilone® (Thornton & Ross)

Suspension, sugar-free, dried aluminium hydroxide 420 mg, simeticone 135 mg, light magnesium oxide 70 mg/5 mL (low Na⁺). Net price 500 mL = £1.95

Dose ADULT and CHILD over 12 years, 5–10 mL after meals and at bedtime or when required up to 4 times daily

### Maalox Plus® (Sanofi-Aventis)

Suspension, sugar-free, dried aluminium hydroxide 220 mg, simeticone 25 mg, magnesium hydroxide 195 mg/5 mL (low Na⁺). Net price 500 mL = £2.79

Dose 5–10 mL 4 times daily (after meals and at bedtime) or when required; CHILD under 5 years 5 mL 3 times daily, over 5 years appropriate proportion of adult dose

## Simeticone alone

**Simeticone** (activated dimeticone) is an antifoaming agent. It is licensed for infantile colic but evidence of benefit is uncertain.

### Dentinox® (DDD)

Colic drops (= emulsion), simeticone 21 mg/2.5-mL dose. Net price 100 mL = £1.73

Dose colic or wind pains, NEONATE and INFANT 2.5 mL with or after each feed (max. 6 doses in 24 hours); may be added to bottle feed

Note The brand name *Dentinox®* is also used for other preparations including teething gel

### Infacol® (Forest) ◣

Liquid, sugar-free, simeticone 40 mg/mL (low Na⁺). Net price 50 mL = £2.26. Counselling, use of dropper

Dose colic or wind pains, NEONATE and INFANT 0.5–1 mL before feeds

<table>
<tr><td>1.1.2</td><td>Compound alginates and proprietary indigestion preparations</td></tr>
</table>

Alginate taken in combination with an antacid increases the viscosity of stomach contents and can protect the oesophageal mucosa from acid reflux. Some alginate-containing preparations form a viscous gel ('raft') that floats on the surface of the stomach contents, thereby reducing symptoms of reflux.

Antacids may damage enteric coatings designed to prevent dissolution in the stomach. For **interactions**, see Appendix 1 (antacids, calcium salts).

## Alginate raft-forming oral suspensions

The following preparations contain sodium alginate, sodium bicarbonate, and calcium carbonate in a suitable flavoured vehicle, and conform to the specification for Alginate Raft-forming Oral Suspension, BP.

### Acidex® (Pinewood)

Liquid, sugar-free, sodium alginate 250 mg, sodium bicarbonate 133.5 mg, calcium carbonate 80 mg/5 mL. Contains about 3 mmol Na⁺/5 mL. Net price 500 mL (aniseed- or peppermint-flavour) = £2.30

Dose 10–20 mL after meals and at bedtime; CHILD 6–12 years 5–10 mL after meals and at bedtime

### Peptac® (IVAX)

Suspension, sugar-free, sodium bicarbonate 133.5 mg, sodium alginate 250 mg, calcium carbonate 80 mg/5 mL. Contains 3.1 mmol Na⁺/5 mL. Net price 500 mL (aniseed- or peppermint-flavoured) = £2.16

Dose 10–20 mL after meals and at bedtime; CHILD 6–12 years 5–10 mL after meals and at bedtime

## Other compound alginate preparations

### Gastrocote® (Actavis)

Tablets, alginic acid 200 mg, dried aluminium hydroxide 80 mg, magnesium trisilicate 40 mg, sodium bicarbonate 70 mg. Contains about 1 mmol Na⁺/tablet. Net price 100-tab pack = £3.51

Cautions diabetes mellitus (high sugar content)

Dose ADULT and CHILD over 6 years, 1–2 tablets chewed 4 times daily (after meals and at bedtime)

Liquid, sugar-free, peach-coloured, dried aluminium hydroxide 80 mg, magnesium trisilicate 40 mg, sodium alginate 220 mg, sodium bicarbonate 70 mg/5 mL. Contains 2.13 mmol Na⁺/5 mL. Net price 500 mL = £2.67

Dose ADULT and CHILD over 6 years, 5–15 mL 4 times daily (after meals and at bedtime)

### Gaviscon® Advance (R&C)

Tablets, sugar-free, sodium alginate 500 mg, potassium bicarbonate 100 mg. Contains 2.25 mmol Na⁺, 1 mmol K⁺/tablet. Net price 60-tab pack (peppermint-flavoured) = £3.13

Excipients include aspartame (section 9.4.1)

Dose ADULT and CHILD over 12 years, 1–2 tablets to be chewed after meals and at bedtime; CHILD 6–12 years, 1 tablet to be chewed after meals and at bedtime (under medical advice only)

Suspension, sugar-free, aniseed- or peppermint flavour, sodium alginate 500 mg, potassium bicarbonate 100 mg/5 mL. Contains 2.3 mmol Na⁺, 1 mmol K⁺/5 mL, net price 250 mL = £2.61, 500 mL = £5.21

Dose ADULT and CHILD over 12 years, 5–10 mL after meals and at bedtime; CHILD 2–12 years, 2.5–5 mL after meals and at bedtime (under medical advice only)

### Gaviscon Infant® (R&C)

Oral powder, sugar-free, sodium alginate 225 mg, magnesium alginate 87.5 mg, with colloidal silica and mannitol/dose (half dual-sachet). Contains 0.92 mmol Na⁺/dose. Net price 15 dual-sachets (30 doses) = £2.46

Dose INFANT body-weight under 4.5 kg, 1 'dose' (half dual-sachet) mixed with feeds (or water in breast-fed infants) when required (max. 6 times in 24 hours); body-weight over 4.5 kg, 2 'doses' (1 dual-sachet) mixed with feeds (or water in breast-fed infants) when required (max. 6 times in 24 hours); CHILD 2 'doses' (1 dual-sachet) in water after each meal (max. 6 times in 24 hours)

Note Not to be used in preterm neonates, or where excessive water loss likely (e.g. fever, diarrhoea, vomiting, high room temperature), or if intestinal obstruction. Not to be used with other preparations containing thickening agents

Important Each half of the dual-sachet is identified as 'one dose'. To avoid errors prescribe as 'dual-sachet' with directions in terms of 'dose'

### Rennie® Duo (Roche Consumer Health)

Suspension, sugar-free, calcium carbonate 600 mg, magnesium carbonate 70 mg, sodium alginate

150 mg/5 mL. Contains 2.6 mmol Na⁺/5 mL. Net
price 500 mL (mint flavour) = £2.67
**Dose** ADULT and CHILD over 12 years, 10 mL after meals and at
bedtime; an additional 10 mL may be taken between doses for
heartburn if necessary, max. 80 mL daily
**Excipients** include propylene glycol

**Topal®** (Fabre)
Tablets, alginic acid 200 mg, dried aluminium hydroxide 30 mg, light magnesium carbonate 40 mg with
lactose 220 mg, sucrose 880 mg, sodium bicarbonate
40 mg (low Na⁺). Net price 42-tab pack = £1.67
**Cautions** diabetes mellitus (high sugar content)
**Dose** ADULT and CHILD over 12 years, 1–3 tablets chewed 4 times
daily (after meals and at bedtime)

## 1.2 Antispasmodics and other drugs altering gut motility

Drugs in this section include antimuscarinic compounds
and drugs believed to be direct relaxants of intestinal
smooth muscle. The smooth muscle relaxant properties
of antimuscarinic and other antispasmodic drugs may
be useful in *irritable bowel syndrome* and in *diverticular
disease*.

The dopamine-receptor antagonists metoclopramide
and domperidone (section 4.6) stimulate transit in the
gut.

### Antimuscarinics

Antimuscarinics (formerly termed 'anticholinergics')
reduce intestinal motility. They are used for the management of *irritable bowel syndrome* and *diverticular disease*.
However, their value has not been established and
response varies. Other indications for antimuscarinic
drugs include arrhythmias (section 2.3.1), asthma and
airways disease (section 3.1.2), motion sickness (section
4.6), parkinsonism (section 4.9.2), urinary incontinence
(section 7.4.2), mydriasis and cycloplegia (section 11.5),
premedication (section 15.1.3) and as an antidote to
organophosphorus poisoning (p. 36).

Antimuscarinics that are used for gastro-intestinal
smooth muscle spasm include the tertiary amines **atropine sulphate** and **dicycloverine hydrochloride**
(dicyclomine hydrochloride) and the quaternary
ammonium compounds **propantheline bromide** and
**hyoscine butylbromide**. The quaternary ammonium
compounds are less lipid soluble than atropine and are
less likely to cross the blood–brain barrier; they are also
less well absorbed from the gastro-intestinal tract.

Dicycloverine hydrochloride has a much less marked
antimuscarinic action than atropine and may also have
some direct action on smooth muscle. Hyoscine butylbromide is advocated as a gastro-intestinal antispasmodic, but it is poorly absorbed; the injection is useful
in endoscopy and radiology. Atropine and the belladonna alkaloids are outmoded treatments, any clinical
virtues being outweighed by atropinic side-effects.

**Cautions** Antimuscarinics should be used with caution
in Down's syndrome, in children and in the elderly; they
should also be used with caution in gastro-oesophageal

reflux disease, diarrhoea, ulcerative colitis, acute myocardial infarction, hypertension, conditions characterised by tachycardia (including hyperthyroidism, cardiac insufficiency, cardiac surgery), pyrexia, pregnancy
(Appendix 4), and in individuals susceptible to angle-
closure glaucoma. **Interactions:** Appendix 1 (antimuscarinics).

**Contra-indications** Antimuscarinics are contra-indicated in myasthenia gravis (but may be used to decrease
muscarinic side-effects of anticholinesterases—section
10.2.1), paralytic ileus, pyloric stenosis and prostatic
enlargement.

**Side-effects** Side-effects of antimuscarinics include
constipation, transient bradycardia (followed by tachycardia, palpitation and arrhythmias), reduced bronchial
secretions, urinary urgency and retention, dilatation of
the pupils with loss of accommodation, photophobia,
dry mouth, flushing and dryness of the skin. Side-effects
that occur occasionally include confusion (particularly
in the elderly), nausea, vomiting, and giddiness; very
rarely, angle-closure glaucoma may occur.

### ■ ATROPINE SULPHATE

**Indications** symptomatic relief of gastro-intestinal
disorders characterised by smooth muscle spasm;
mydriasis and cycloplegia (section 11.5); premedi-
cation (section 15.1.3); see also notes above
**Cautions** see notes above; also breast-feeding
(Appendix 5)
**Contra-indications** see notes above
**Side-effects** see notes above
**Dose**
● 0.6–1.2 mg at night

**Atropine** (Non-proprietary) PoM ◢
Tablets, atropine sulphate 600 micrograms. Net price
28-tab pack = £13.43
Available from CP

### ■ DICYCLOVERINE HYDROCHLORIDE
(Dicyclomine hydrochloride)

**Indications** symptomatic relief of gastro-intestinal
disorders characterised by smooth muscle spasm
**Cautions** see notes above
**Contra-indications** see notes above; also infants
under 6 months; breast-feeding (Appendix 5)
**Side-effects** see notes above
**Dose**
● 10–20 mg 3 times daily; INFANT 6–24 months 5–10 mg
3–4 times daily, 15 minutes before feeds; CHILD 2–12
years 10 mg 3 times daily

**Merbentyl®** (Sanofi-Aventis) PoM
Tablets, dicycloverine hydrochloride 10 mg, net price
100-tab pack = £4.84; 20 mg (*Merbentyl 20®*), 84-tab
pack = £8.14

Syrup, dicycloverine hydrochloride 10 mg/5 mL, net
price 120 mL = £1.77
**Note** Dicycloverine hydrochloride can be sold to the public
provided that max. single dose is 10 mg and max. daily dose
is 60 mg

**◀Compound preparations**

**Kolanticon®** (Peckforton)

Gel, sugar-free, dicycloverine hydrochloride 2.5 mg, dried aluminium hydroxide 200 mg, light magnesium oxide 100 mg, simeticone 20 mg/5 mL, net price 200 mL = £2.21, 500 mL = £2.79

Dose ADULT and CHILD over 12 years, 10–20 mL every 4 hours when required

## ■ HYOSCINE BUTYLBROMIDE

**Indications** symptomatic relief of gastro-intestinal or genito-urinary disorders characterised by smooth muscle spasm; bowel colic and excessive respiratory secretions (see Prescribing in Palliative Care, p. 18)

**Cautions** see notes above; also breast-feeding (Appendix 5)

**Contra-indications** see notes above

**Side-effects** see notes above

**Dose**

- By mouth (but poorly absorbed, see notes above), smooth muscle spasm, 20 mg 4 times daily; CHILD 6–12 years, 10 mg 3 times daily

  Irritable bowel syndrome, 10 mg 3 times daily, increased if required up to 20 mg 4 times daily

- By intramuscular or slow intravenous injection, acute spasm and spasm in diagnostic procedures, 20 mg repeated after 30 minutes if necessary (may be repeated more frequently in endoscopy), max. 100 mg daily; CHILD 2–18 years see BNF for Children

**Buscopan®** (Boehringer Ingelheim) [PoM]

Tablets, coated, hyoscine butylbromide 10 mg, net price 56-tab pack = £2.25

Note Hyoscine butylbromide tablets can be sold to the public, provided single dose does not exceed 20 mg, daily dose does not exceed 80 mg, and pack does not contain a total of more than 240 mg

Injection, hyoscine butylbromide 20 mg/mL, net price 1-mL amp = 22p

## ■ PROPANTHELINE BROMIDE

**Indications** symptomatic relief of gastro-intestinal disorders characterised by smooth muscle spasm; urinary frequency (section 7.4.2); gustatory sweating (section 6.1.5)

**Cautions** see notes above; also hepatic and renal impairment; breast-feeding (Appendix 5)

**Contra-indications** see notes above

**Side-effects** see notes above

**Dose**

- ADULT and CHILD over 12 years, 15 mg 3 times daily at least 1 hour before meals and 30 mg at night, max. 120 mg daily

**Pro-Banthine®** (Concord) [PoM]

Tablets, pink, s/c, propantheline bromide 15 mg, net price 112-tab pack = £18.38. Label: 23

## Other antispasmodics

**Alverine**, **mebeverine**, and **peppermint oil** are believed to be direct relaxants of intestinal smooth muscle and may relieve pain in *irritable bowel syndrome* and *diverticular disease*. They have no serious adverse effects but, like all antispasmodics, should be avoided in paralytic ileus. Peppermint oil occasionally causes heartburn.

## ■ ALVERINE CITRATE

**Indications** adjunct in gastro-intestinal disorders characterised by smooth muscle spasm; dysmenorrhoea

**Cautions** pregnancy; breast-feeding (Appendix 5)

**Contra-indications** paralytic ileus

**Side-effects** nausea; headache, dizziness; pruritus, rash; hepatitis also reported

**Dose**

- ADULT and CHILD over 12 years, 60–120 mg 1–3 times daily

**Spasmonal®** (Norgine)

Capsules, alverine citrate 60 mg (blue/grey), net price 100-cap pack = £11.48; 120 mg (*Spasmonal® Forte*, blue/grey), 60-cap pack = £13.26

## ■ MEBEVERINE HYDROCHLORIDE

**Indications** adjunct in gastro-intestinal disorders characterised by smooth muscle spasm

**Cautions** pregnancy (Appendix 4); avoid in acute porphyria (section 9.8.2.)

**Contra-indications** paralytic ileus

**Side-effects** rarely allergic reactions (including rash, urticaria, angioedema)

**Dose**

- ADULT and CHILD over 10 years 135–150 mg 3 times daily preferably 20 minutes before meals; CHILD under 10 years see BNF for Children

[1]**Mebeverine Hydrochloride** (Non-proprietary) [PoM]

Tablets, mebeverine hydrochloride 135 mg, net price 100-tab pack = £9.43

Oral suspension, mebeverine hydrochloride (as mebeverine embonate) 50 mg/5 mL, net price 300 mL = £107.00

1. Mebeverine hydrochloride can be sold to the public for symptomatic relief of irritable bowel syndrome provided that max. single dose is 135 mg and max. daily dose is 405 mg; for uses other than symptomatic relief of irritable bowel syndrome provided that max. single dose is 100 mg and max. daily dose is 300 mg

**Colofac®** (Solvay) [PoM]

Tablets, s/c, mebeverine hydrochloride 135 mg, net price 100-tab pack = £7.52

**◀Modified release**

**Colofac® MR** (Solvay) [PoM]

Capsules, m/r, mebeverine hydrochloride 200 mg, net price 60-cap pack = £6.67. Label: 25

Dose irritable bowel syndrome, 1 capsule twice daily preferably 20 minutes before meals; CHILD 12–18 years see BNF for Children

**◀Compound preparations**

[1]**Fybogel® Mebeverine** (R&C) [PoM]

Granules, buff, effervescent, ispaghula husk 3.5 g, mebeverine hydrochloride 135 mg/sachet. Contains 2.5 mmol K⁺/sachet, net price 10 sachets = £2.50. Label: 13, 22, counselling, see below

Excipients include aspartame (section 9.4.1)

Dose irritable bowel syndrome, ADULT and CHILD over 12 years, 1 sachet in water, morning and evening 30 minutes before food; an additional sachet may also be taken before the midday meal if necessary

**Counselling** Preparations that swell in contact with liquid should always be carefully swallowed with water and should not be taken immediately before going to bed

1. 10-sachet pack can be sold to the public

### ▌ PEPPERMINT OIL

**Indications** relief of abdominal colic and distension, particularly in irritable bowel syndrome

**Cautions** sensitivity to menthol

**Side-effects** heartburn, perianal irritation; rarely, allergic reactions (including rash, headache, bradycardia, muscle tremor, ataxia)

**Local irritation** Capsules should not be broken or chewed because peppermint oil may irritate mouth or oesophagus

**Dose**

● See preparations

**Colpermin®** (McNeil)

Capsules, m/r, e/c, light blue/dark blue, blue band, peppermint oil 0.2 mL. Net price 100-cap pack = £12.05. Label: 5, 22, 25
Excipients include arachis (peanut) oil

**Dose** ADULT and CHILD over 15 years, 1–2 capsules, swallowed whole with water, 3 times daily for up to 3 months if necessary

**Mintec®** (Shire)

Capsules, e/c, green/ivory, peppermint oil 0.2 mL. Net price 84-cap pack = £7.04. Label: 5, 22, 25

**Dose** ADULT over 18 years, 1–2 capsules swallowed whole with water, 3 times daily before meals for up to 2–3 months if necessary

## Motility stimulants

**Metoclopramide** and **domperidone** (section 4.6) are dopamine receptor antagonists which stimulate gastric emptying and small intestinal transit, and enhance the strength of oesophageal sphincter contraction. They are used in some patients with *functional dyspepsia* that has not responded to a proton pump inhibitor or a $H_2$-receptor antagonist. Metoclopramide is also used to speed the transit of barium during intestinal follow-through examination, and as accessory treatment for *gastro-oesophageal reflux disease*. For the management of gastroparesis in patients with diabetes, see section 6.1.5. Metoclopramide and domperidone are useful in non-specific and in cytotoxic-induced nausea and vomiting. Metoclopramide and occasionally domperidone can cause acute dystonic reactions, particularly in young women and children—for further details of this and other side-effects, see section 4.6.

### ▌1.3 Antisecretory drugs and mucosal protectants

| | |
|---|---|
| **1.3.1** | **H2-receptor antagonists** |
| **1.3.2** | **Selective antimuscarinics** |
| **1.3.3** | **Chelates and complexes** |
| **1.3.4** | **Prostaglandin analogues** |
| **1.3.5** | **Proton pump inhibitors** |

Peptic ulceration commonly involves the stomach, duodenum, and lower oesophagus; after gastric surgery it involves the gastro-enterostomy stoma.

Healing can be promoted by general measures, stopping smoking and taking antacids and by antisecretory drug treatment, but relapse is common when treatment ceases. Nearly all duodenal ulcers and most gastric ulcers not associated with NSAIDs are caused by *Helicobacter pylori*.

The management of *H. pylori* infection and of NSAID-associated ulcers is discussed below.

## *Helicobacter pylori* infection

Eradication of *Helicobacter pylori* reduces recurrence of gastric and duodenal ulcers and the risk of rebleeding. The presence of *H. pylori* should be confirmed before starting eradication treatment. Acid inhibition combined with antibacterial treatment is highly effective in the eradication of *H. pylori*; reinfection is rare. Antibiotic-associated colitis is an uncommon risk.

For initial treatment, a one-week triple-therapy regimen that comprises a proton pump inhibitor, clarithromycin, and *either* amoxicillin *or* metronidazole can be used. However, if a patient has been treated with metronidazole for other infections, a regimen containing a proton pump inhibitor, amoxicillin and clarithromycin is preferred for initial therapy. If a patient has been treated with a macrolide for other infections, a regimen containing a proton pump inhibitor, amoxicillin and metronidazole is preferred for initial therapy. These regimens eradicate *H. pylori* in about 85% of cases. There is usually no need to continue antisecretory treatment (with a proton pump inhibitor or $H_2$-receptor antagonist), however, if the ulcer is large, or complicated by haemorrhage or perforation, then antisecretory treatment is continued for a further 3 weeks. Treatment failure usually indicates antibacterial resistance or poor compliance. Resistance to amoxicillin is rare. However, resistance to clarithromycin and metronidazole is common and can develop during treatment.

Two-week triple-therapy regimens offer the possibility of higher eradication rates compared to one-week regimens, but adverse effects are common and poor compliance is likely to offset any possible gain.

Two-week dual-therapy regimens using a proton pump inhibitor and a single antibacterial are licensed, but produce low rates of *H. pylori* eradication and are **not** recommended.

Tinidazole is also used occasionally for *H. pylori* eradication as an alternative to metronidazole; tinidazole should be combined with antisecretory drugs and other antibacterials.

A two-week regimen comprising a proton pump inhibitor (e.g. omeprazole 20 mg twice daily) *plus* tripotassium dicitratobismuthate 120 mg four times daily, *plus* tetracycline 500 mg four times daily, *plus* metronidazole 400 mg three times daily can be used for eradication failure. Alternatively, the patient can be referred for endoscopy and treatment based on the results of culture and sensitivity testing.

For the role of *H. pylori* eradication therapy in patients starting or taking a NSAID, see NSAID-associated Ulcers, p. 44. For *H. pylori* eradication in patients with dyspepsia, see also section 1.1.

**1**

**Gastro-intestinal system**

## Recommended regimens for *Helicobacter pylori* eradication in adults

| Acid suppressant | Antibacterial | | | Price for 7-day course |
|---|---|---|---|---|
| | Amoxicillin | Clarithromycin | Metronidazole | |
| Esomeprazole 20 mg twice daily | 1 g twice daily | 500 mg twice daily | – | £17.89 |
| | – | 250 mg twice daily | 400 mg twice daily | £13.34 |
| Lansoprazole 30 mg twice daily | 1 g twice daily | 500 mg twice daily | – | £10.19 |
| | 1 g twice daily | – | 400 mg twice daily | £4.40 |
| | – | 250 mg twice daily | 400 mg twice daily | £5.64 |
| Omeprazole 20 mg twice daily | 1 g twice daily | 500 mg twice daily | – | £9.50 |
| | 500 mg 3 times daily | – | 400 mg 3 times daily | £3.61 |
| | – | 250 mg twice daily | 400 mg twice daily | £4.95 |
| Pantoprazole 40 mg twice daily | 1 g twice daily | 500 mg twice daily | – | £18.93 |
| | – | 250 mg twice daily | 400 mg twice daily | £14.38 |
| Rabeprazole 20 mg twice daily | 1 g twice daily | 500 mg twice daily | – | £17.41 |
| | – | 250 mg twice daily | 400 mg twice daily | £12.86 |

## Test for *Helicobacter pylori*

[13]C-Urea breath test kits are available for the diagnosis of gastro-duodenal infection with *Helicobacter pylori*. The test involves collection of breath samples before and after ingestion of an oral solution of [13]C-urea; the samples are sent for analysis by an appropriate laboratory. The test should not be performed within 4 weeks of treatment with an antibacterial or within 2 weeks of treatment with an antisecretory drug. A specific [13]C-urea breath test kit for children is available (*Helicobacter Test INFAI for children of the age 3–11®*). However, the appropriateness of testing for *H.pylori* infection in children has not been established.

**diabact UBT®** (MDE) [PoM]
Tablets, [13]C-urea 50 mg, net price 1 kit (including 1 tablet, 4 breath-sample containers, straws) = £19.95 (analysis included), 10-kit pack (hosp. only) = £74.50 (analysis not included)

**Helicobacter Test INFAI®** (Infai) [PoM]
Oral powder, [13]C-urea 75 mg, net price 1 kit (including 4 breath-sample containers, straws) = £19.20 (spectrometric analysis included), 1 kit (including 2 breath bags) = £14.20 (spectroscopic analysis not included), 50-test set = £855.00 (spectrometric analysis included); 45 mg (*Helicobacter Test INFAI for children of the age 3–11®*), 1 kit (including 4 breath-sample containers, straws) = £19.20 (spectrometric analysis included)

**Pylobactell®** (Torbet) [PoM]
Soluble tablets, [13]C-urea 100 mg, net price 1 kit (including 6 breath-sample containers, 30-mL mixing and administration vial, straws) = £20.75 (analysis included)

## NSAID-associated ulcers

Gastro-intestinal bleeding and ulceration can occur with NSAID use (section 10.1.1). The risk of serious upper gastro-intestinal side-effects varies between individual NSAIDs (see CSM advice, p. 562). Whenever possible, the NSAID should be **withdrawn** if an ulcer occurs.

Patients at high risk of developing gastro-intestinal complications include those aged over 65 years, those with a history of peptic ulcer disease or serious gastro-intestinal complication, those taking other medicines that increase the risk of gastro-intestinal side-effects, or those with serious co-morbidity. In those at risk of ulceration, a proton pump inhibitor can be considered for protection against gastric and duodenal ulcers associated with non-selective NSAIDs; a $H_2$-receptor antagonist such as ranitidine given at twice the usual dose or misoprostol are alternatives. Colic and diarrhoea may limit the dose of misoprostol.

NSAID use and *H. pylori* infection are independent risk factors for gastro-intestinal bleeding and ulceration. In patients already taking a NSAID, eradication of *H. pylori* is unlikely to reduce the risk of NSAID-induced bleeding or ulceration. However, in patients with dyspepsia or a history of gastric or duodenal ulcer, who are *H. pylori* positive, and who are about to start long-term treatment with a non-selective NSAID, eradication of *H. pylori* may reduce the overall risk of ulceration.

If the *NSAID can be discontinued* in a patient who has developed an ulcer, a proton pump inhibitor usually produces the most rapid healing, but the ulcer can be treated with a $H_2$-receptor antagonist or misoprostol.

If *treatment with a non-selective NSAID needs to continue*, the following options are suitable:

- Treat ulcer with a proton pump inhibitor and on healing continue the proton pump inhibitor (dose not normally reduced because asymptomatic ulcer recurrence may occur);

- Treat ulcer with a proton pump inhibitor and on healing switch to misoprostol for maintenance therapy (colic and diarrhoea may limit the dose of misoprostol);

- Treat ulcer with a proton pump inhibitor and switch non-selective NSAID to a cyclo-oxygenase-2 selective inhibitor, but see NSAIDs and Cardiovascular Events, p. 561; on healing, continuation of the proton pump inhibitor in patients with a history of upper gastro-intestinal bleeding may provide further protection against recurrence.

If *treatment with a cyclo-oxygenase-2 selective inhibitor needs to continue,* treat ulcer with a proton pump inhibitor; on healing continuation of the proton pump inhibitor in patients with a history of upper gastro-intestinal bleeding may provide further protection against recurrence.

## 1.3.1 H$_2$-receptor antagonists

Histamine **H$_2$-receptor antagonists** heal *gastric and duodenal ulcers* by reducing gastric acid output as a result of histamine H$_2$-receptor blockade; they are also used to relieve symptoms of *gastro-oesophageal reflux disease* (section 1.1). H$_2$-receptor antagonists should not normally be used for *Zollinger-Ellison syndrome* because proton pump inhibitors (section 1.3.5) are more effective.

Maintenance treatment with low doses for the prevention of peptic ulcer disease has largely been replaced in *Helicobacter pylori* positive patients by eradication regimens (section 1.3).

H$_2$-receptor antagonists are used for the treatment of *functional dyspepsia* (section 1.1). H$_2$-receptor antagonists may be used for the treatment of *uninvestigated dyspepsia* in patients without alarm features.

H$_2$-receptor antagonist therapy can promote healing of *NSAID-associated ulcers* (particularly duodenal) (section 1.3).

Treatment with a H$_2$-receptor antagonist has not been shown to be beneficial in haematemesis and melaena, but prophylactic use reduces the frequency of bleeding from *gastroduodenal erosions in hepatic coma,* and possibly in other conditions requiring intensive care. H$_2$-receptor antagonists also reduce the risk of *acid aspiration* in obstetric patients at delivery (Mendelson's syndrome).

**Cautions** H$_2$-receptor antagonists should be used with caution in renal impairment (Appendix 3), pregnancy (Appendix 4), and in breast-feeding (Appendix 5). H$_2$-receptor antagonists might mask symptoms of gastric cancer; particular care is required in those whose symptoms change and in those who are middle-aged or older.

**Side-effects** Side-effects of the H$_2$-receptor antagonists include diarrhoea and other gastro-intestinal disturbances, altered liver function tests (rarely liver damage), headache, dizziness, rash, and tiredness. Rare side-effects include acute pancreatitis, bradycardia, AV block, confusion, depression, and hallucinations particularly in the elderly or the very ill, hypersensitivity reactions (including fever, arthralgia, myalgia, anaphylaxis), blood disorders (including agranulocytosis, leucopenia, pancytopenia, thrombocytopenia), and skin reactions (including erythema multiforme and toxic epidermal necrolysis). There have been occasional reports of gynaecomastia and impotence.

**Interactions** Cimetidine retards oxidative hepatic drug metabolism by binding to microsomal cytochrome P450. It should be avoided in patients stabilised on warfarin, phenytoin, and theophylline (or aminophylline), but other interactions (see **Appendix 1**) may be of less clinical relevance. Famotidine, nizatidine, and ranitidine do not share the drug metabolism inhibitory properties of cimetidine.

## CIMETIDINE

**Indications** benign gastric and duodenal ulceration, stomal ulcer, reflux oesophagitis, Zollinger–Ellison syndrome, other conditions where gastric acid reduction is beneficial (see notes above and section 1.9.4)

**Cautions** see notes above; also hepatic impairment (Appendix 2); **interactions**: Appendix 1 (histamine H$_2$-antagonists) and notes above

**Side-effects** see notes above; also alopecia; very rarely tachycardia, galactorrhoea, interstitial nephritis

**Dose**

• 400 mg twice daily (with breakfast and at night) *or* 800 mg at night (benign gastric and duodenal ulceration) for at least 4 weeks (6 weeks in gastric ulceration, 8 weeks in NSAID-associated ulceration); when necessary the dose may be increased to 400 mg 4 times daily; INFANT under 1 year 20 mg/kg daily in divided doses has been used; CHILD 1–12 years, 25–30 mg/kg daily in divided doses; max. 400 mg 4 times daily

   Maintenance, 400 mg at night *or* 400 mg morning and night

• Reflux oesophagitis, 400 mg 4 times daily for 4–8 weeks

• Prophylaxis of stress ulceration, 200–400 mg every 4–6 hours

• Gastric acid reduction (prophylaxis of acid aspiration; do not use syrup), obstetrics 400 mg at start of labour, then up to 400 mg every 4 hours if required (max. 2.4 g daily); surgical procedures 400 mg 90–120 minutes before induction of general anaesthesia

• Short-bowel syndrome, 400 mg twice daily (with breakfast and at bedtime) adjusted according to response

• To reduce degradation of pancreatic enzyme supplements, 0.8–1.6 g daily in 4 divided doses 1–1½ hours before meals

**¹Cimetidine** (Non-proprietary) ⟮PoM⟯

   Tablets, cimetidine 200 mg, net price 60-tab pack = £1.96; 400 mg, 60-tab pack = £2.30; 800 mg, 30-tab pack = £1.99

   Oral solution, cimetidine 200 mg/5 mL, net price 300 mL = £14.24
   Excipients may include propylene glycol (see Excipients, p. 2)

1. Cimetidine can be sold to the public for adults and children over 16 years (provided packs do not contain more than 2 weeks' supply) for the short-term symptomatic relief of heartburn, dyspepsia, and hyperacidity (max. single dose 200 mg, max. daily dose 800 mg), and for the prophylactic management of nocturnal heartburn (single night-time dose 100 mg)

**Tagamet®** (Chemidex) ⟮PoM⟯

   Tablets, all green, f/c, cimetidine 200 mg, net price 120-tab pack = £19.58; 400 mg, 60-tab pack = £22.62; 800 mg, 30-tab pack = £22.62

   Syrup, orange, cimetidine 200 mg/5 mL. Net price 600 mL = £28.49
   Excipients include propylene glycol 10%, (see Excipients, p. 2)

## ■ FAMOTIDINE

**Indications** see under Dose

**Cautions** see notes above; **interactions:** Appendix 1 (histamine H$_2$-antagonists) and notes above

**Side-effects** see notes above; also *very rarely* anorexia, cholestatic jaundice, interstitial pneumonia, anxiety, paraesthesia, insomnia, decreased libido, dry mouth, and taste disturbances

**Dose**

- Benign gastric and duodenal ulceration, treatment, 40 mg at night for 4–8 weeks; maintenance (duodenal ulceration), 20 mg at night
- Reflux oesophagitis, 20–40 mg twice daily for 6–12 weeks; maintenance, 20 mg twice daily
- CHILD not recommended

**¹Famotidine** (Non-proprietary) ⓅoM
Tablets, famotidine 20 mg, net price 28-tab pack = £3.56; 40 mg, 28-tab pack = £4.40
1. Famotidine can be sold to the public for adults and children over 16 years (provided packs do not contain more than 2 weeks' supply) for the short-term symptomatic relief of heartburn, dyspepsia, and hyperacidity, and for the prevention of these symptoms when associated with consumption of food or drink including when they cause sleep disturbance (max. single dose 10 mg, max. daily dose 20 mg)

**Pepcid®** (MSD) ⓅoM
Tablets, f/c, famotidine 20 mg (beige), net price 28-tab pack = £13.37; 40 mg (brown), 28-tab pack = £25.40

## ■ NIZATIDINE

**Indications** see under Dose

**Cautions** see notes above; also avoid rapid intravenous injection (risk of arrhythmias and postural hypotension); hepatic impairment (Appendix 2); **interactions:** Appendix 1 (histamine H$_2$-antagonists) and notes above

**Side-effects** see notes above; also sweating; rarely hyperuricaemia

**Dose**

- By mouth, benign gastric, duodenal or NSAID-associated ulceration, treatment, 300 mg in the evening *or* 150 mg twice daily for 4–8 weeks; maintenance, 150 mg at night
Gastro-oesophageal reflux disease, 150–300 mg twice daily for up to 12 weeks
- By intravenous infusion, for short-term use in peptic ulcer as alternative to oral route (for hospital inpatients), by intermittent intravenous infusion over 15 minutes, 100 mg 3 times daily, *or* by continuous intravenous infusion, 10 mg/hour; max. 480 mg daily
- CHILD not recommended

**¹Nizatidine** (Non-proprietary) ⓅoM
Capsules, nizatidine 150 mg, net price 30-cap pack = £3.60; 300 mg, 30-cap pack = £5.52
1. Nizatidine can be sold to the public for the prevention and treatment of symptoms of food-related heartburn and meal-induced indigestion in adults and children over 16 years; max. single dose 75 mg, max. daily dose 150 mg for max. 14 days

**Axid®** (Flynn) ⓅoM
Capsules, nizatidine 150 mg (pale yellow/dark yellow), net price 28-cap pack (hosp. only) = £6.87, 30-

cap pack = £7.97; 300 mg (pale yellow/brown), 30-cap pack = £15.80

Injection, nizatidine 25 mg/mL. For dilution and use as an intravenous infusion. Net price 4-mL amp = £1.14

## ■ RANITIDINE

**Indications** see under Dose, other conditions where reduction of gastric acidity is beneficial (see notes above and section 1.9.4)

**Cautions** see notes above; also acute porphyria; **interactions:** Appendix 1 (histamine H$_2$-antagonists) and notes above

**Side-effects** see notes above; also *rarely* tachycardia, agitation, visual disturbances, alopecia, vasculitis; *very rarely* interstitial nephritis

**Dose**

- By mouth, benign gastric and duodenal ulceration, chronic episodic dyspepsia, ADULT and CHILD over 12 years, 150 mg twice daily *or* 300 mg at night for 4–8 weeks in benign gastric and duodenal ulceration, up to 6 weeks in chronic episodic dyspepsia, and up to 8 weeks in NSAID-associated ulceration (in duodenal ulcer 300 mg can be given twice daily for 4 weeks to achieve a higher healing rate); CHILD 3–12 years, (benign gastric and duodenal ulceration) 2–4 mg/kg (max. 150 mg) twice daily for 4–8 weeks
Prophylaxis of NSAID-associated gastric or duodenal ulcer [unlicensed dose], ADULT and CHILD over 12 years, 300 mg twice daily
Gastro-oesophageal reflux disease, ADULT and CHILD over 12 years, 150 mg twice daily *or* 300 mg at night for up to 8 weeks or if necessary 12 weeks (moderate to severe, 600 mg daily in 2–4 divided doses for up to 12 weeks); long-term treatment of healed gastro-oesophageal reflux disease, 150 mg twice daily; CHILD 3–12 years, 2.5–5 mg/kg (max. 300 mg) twice daily
Gastric acid reduction (prophylaxis of acid aspiration) in obstetrics, ADULT and CHILD over 12 years, by mouth, 150 mg at onset of labour, then every 6 hours; surgical procedures, by intramuscular *or* slow intravenous injection, 50 mg 45–60 minutes before induction of anaesthesia (intravenous injection diluted to 20 mL and given over at least 2 minutes), or by mouth, 150 mg 2 hours before induction of anaesthesia and also when possible on the preceding evening
- By intramuscular injection, 50 mg every 6–8 hours
- By slow intravenous injection, ADULT and CHILD over 12 years, 50 mg diluted to 20 mL and given over at least 2 minutes; may be repeated every 6–8 hours
- Prophylaxis of stress ulceration [unlicensed dose], ADULT and CHILD over 12 years, by slow intravenous injection over at least 2 minutes, 50 mg diluted to 20 mL every 8 hours (may be changed to 150 mg twice daily by mouth when oral feeding commences)

**Ranitidine** (Non-proprietary) ⓅoM
Tablets, ranitidine (as hydrochloride) 150 mg, net price 60-tab pack = £1.18; 300 mg, 30-tab pack = £1.28
Brands include *Ranitic®*

Effervescent tablets, ranitidine (as hydrochloride) 150 mg, net price 60-tab pack = £10.77; 300 mg, 30-tab pack = £11.27. Label: 13
Excipients may include sodium (check with supplier)

Oral solution, ranitidine (as hydrochloride) 75 mg/
5 mL, net price 100 mL = £7.44, 300 mL = £21.43
Excipients may include alcohol (check with supplier)

**Note** Ranitidine can be sold to the public for adults and
children over 16 years (provided packs do not contain more
than 2 weeks' supply) for the short-term symptomatic relief of
heartburn, dyspepsia, and hyperacidity, and for the prevention
of these symptoms when associated with consumption of food
or drink (max. single dose 75 mg, max. daily dose 300 mg)

Injection, ranitidine (as hydrochloride) 25 mg/mL,
net price 2-mL amp = £1.07

**Zantac®** (GSK) PoM
Tablets, f/c, ranitidine (as hydrochloride) 150 mg, net
price 60-tab pack = £1.30; 300 mg, 30-tab pack =
£1.30

Effervescent tablets, pale yellow, ranitidine (as
hydrochloride) 150 mg (contains 14.3 mmol Na⁺/
tablet), net price 60-tab pack = £24.93; 300 mg (contains 20.8 mmol Na⁺/tablet), 30-tab pack = £24.52.
Label: 13
Excipients include aspartame (section 9.4.1)

Syrup, sugar-free, ranitidine (as hydrochloride)
75 mg/5 mL, net price 300 mL = £20.76
Excipients include alcohol 8%

Injection, ranitidine (as hydrochloride) 25 mg/mL,
net price 2-mL amp = 57p

## 1.3.2 Selective antimuscarinics

**Pirenzepine** is a selective antimuscarinic drug which
was used for the treatment of gastric and duodenal
ulcers. It has been discontinued.

## 1.3.3 Chelates and complexes

**Tripotassium dicitratobismuthate** is a bismuth chelate
effective in healing gastric and duodenal ulcers. For the
role of tripotassium dicitratobismuthate in a *Helicobacter
pylori* eradication regimen for those who have not
responded to first-line regimens, see section 1.3.

The bismuth content of tripotassium dicitratobismuthate is low but absorption has been reported; encephalopathy (described with older high-dose bismuth preparations) has not been reported.

**Sucralfate** may act by protecting the mucosa from acid-
pepsin attack in gastric and duodenal ulcers. It is a
complex of aluminium hydroxide and sulphated sucrose
but has minimal antacid properties. It should be used
with caution in patients under intensive care (**important:** reports of bezoar formation, see CSM advice
below)

### TRIPOTASSIUM DICITRATOBISMUTHATE

**Indications** benign gastric and duodenal ulceration;
see also *Helicobacter pylori* infection, section 1.3

**Cautions** see notes above; **interactions:** Appendix 1
(tripotassium dicitratobismuthate)

**Contra-indications** renal impairment (avoid if severe);
pregnancy (Appendix 4)

**Side-effects** may darken tongue and blacken faeces;
*less commonly* nausea, vomiting, diarrhoea, constipation, rash, and pruritus reported

**De-Noltab®** (Astellas)
Tablets, f/c, tripotassium dicitratobismuthate 120 mg.
Contains 2 mmol K⁺/tablet. Net price 112-tab pack =
£7.27. Counselling, see below
Dose 2 tablets twice daily *or* 1 tablet 4 times daily; taken for 28
days followed by further 28 days if necessary; maintenance not
indicated but course may be repeated after interval of 1 month;
CHILD not recommended

Counselling To be swallowed with half a glass of water; twice-
daily dosage to be taken 30 minutes before breakfast and main
evening meal; four-times-daily dosage to be taken as follows: one
dose 30 minutes before breakfast, midday meal and main evening
meal, and one dose 2 hours after main evening meal; milk should
not be drunk by itself during treatment but small quantities may
be taken in tea or coffee or on cereal; antacids, fruit, or fruit juice
should not be taken half an hour before or after a dose; may
darken tongue and blacken faeces

### SUCRALFATE

**Indications** see under Dose

**Cautions** renal impairment (Appendix 3); pregnancy
and breast-feeding; administration of sucralfate and
enteral feeds should be separated by 1 hour; **interactions:** Appendix 1 (sucralfate)

Bezoar formation Following reports of bezoar formation
associated with sucralfate, the CSM has advised caution in
seriously ill patients, especially those receiving concomitant
enteral feeds or those with predisposing conditions such as
delayed gastric emptying

**Side-effects** constipation; *less frequently* diarrhoea,
nausea, indigestion, flatulence, gastric discomfort,
back pain, dizziness, headache, drowsiness, bezoar
formation (see above), dry mouth and rash

**Dose**

- Benign gastric and duodenal ulceration and chronic
gastritis, ADULT and CHILD over 15 years, 2 g twice daily
(on rising and at bedtime) *or* 1 g 4 times daily 1 hour
before meals and at bedtime, taken for 4–6 weeks or in
resistant cases up to 12 weeks; max. 8 g daily

- Prophylaxis of stress ulceration, ADULT and CHILD over
15 years, 1 g 6 times daily; max. 8 g daily

- CHILD under 15 years see *BNF for Children*

**Antepsin®** (Chugai) PoM
Tablets, scored, sucralfate 1 g, net price 50-tab pack =
£5.53. Label: 5
Note Crushed tablets may be dispersed in water

Suspension, sucralfate, 1 g/5 mL, net price 250 mL
(aniseed- and caramel-flavoured) = £5.53. Label: 5

## 1.3.4 Prostaglandin analogues

**Misoprostol**, a synthetic prostaglandin analogue has
antisecretory and protective properties, promoting healing of *gastric and duodenal ulcers*. It can prevent NSAID-
associated ulcers, its use being most appropriate for the
frail or very elderly from whom NSAIDs cannot be
withdrawn.

For comment on the use of misoprostol to induce abortion or labour [unlicensed indications], see section 7.1.1.

### MISOPROSTOL

**Indications** see notes above and under Dose

**Cautions** conditions where hypotension might precipitate severe complications (e.g. cerebrovascular disease, cardiovascular disease)

**1 Gastro-intestinal system**

**Contra-indications** pregnancy or planning pregnancy (Appendix 4), (increases uterine tone)—**important:** women of childbearing age, see also below, and breast-feeding (Appendix 5)

Women of childbearing age Manufacturer advises that misoprostol should not be used in women of childbearing age unless the patient requires non-steroidal anti-inflammatory (NSAID) therapy and is at high risk of complications from NSAID-induced ulceration. In such patients it is advised that misoprostol should only be used if the patient takes *effective contraceptive measures* and has been advised of the *risks of taking misoprostol if pregnant.*

**Side-effects** diarrhoea (may occasionally be severe and require withdrawal, reduced by giving single doses not exceeding 200 micrograms and by avoiding magnesium-containing antacids); also reported: abdominal pain, dyspepsia, flatulence, nausea and vomiting, abnormal vaginal bleeding (including intermenstrual bleeding, menorrhagia, and postmenopausal bleeding), rashes, dizziness

**Dose**

- Benign gastric and duodenal ulceration and NSAID-associated ulceration, ADULT over 18 years, 800 micrograms daily (in 2–4 divided doses) with breakfast (or main meals) and at bedtime; treatment should be continued for at least 4 weeks and may be continued for up to 8 weeks if required
- Prophylaxis of NSAID-induced gastric and duodenal ulcer, ADULT over 18 years, 200 micrograms 2–4 times daily taken with the NSAID

**Cytotec®** (Pharmacia) ▱⒫⒪⒨
Tablets, scored, misoprostol 200 micrograms, net price 60-tab pack = £10.03. Label: 21

◢With diclofenac or naproxen
Section 10.1.1

## 1.3.5 Proton pump inhibitors

Proton pump inhibitors inhibit gastric acid secretion by blocking the hydrogen-potassium adenosine triphosphatase enzyme system (the 'proton pump') of the gastric parietal cell. Proton pump inhibitors are effective short-term treatments for *gastric* and *duodenal ulcers*; they are also used in combination with antibacterials for the eradication of *Helicobacter pylori* (see p. 43 for specific regimens). Following endoscopic treatment of severe peptic ulcer bleeding, an intravenous, high-dose proton pump inhibitor reduces the risk of rebleeding and the need for surgery [unlicensed use]. Proton pump inhibitors can be used for the treatment of *dyspepsia* and *gastro-oesophageal reflux disease* (section 1.1).

Proton pump inhibitors are also used for the prevention and treatment of NSAID-associated ulcers (see p. 44). In patients who need to continue NSAID treatment after an ulcer has healed, the dose of proton pump inhibitor should normally not be reduced because asymptomatic ulcer deterioration may occur.

A proton pump inhibitor can be used to control excessive secretion of gastric acid in *Zollinger–Ellison syndrome*; high doses are often required.

**Cautions** Proton pump inhibitors should be used with caution in patients with liver disease (Appendix 2), in pregnancy (Appendix 4) and in breast-feeding (Appendix 5). Proton pump inhibitors may mask the symptoms of gastric cancer; particular care is required in those

presenting with 'alarm features' (see p. 37), in such cases gastric malignancy should be ruled out before treatment.

**Side-effects** Side-effects of the proton pump inhibitors include gastro-intestinal disturbances (including nausea, vomiting, abdominal pain, flatulence, diarrhoea, constipation), and headache. Less frequent side-effects include dry mouth, peripheral oedema, dizziness, sleep disturbances, fatigue, paraesthesia, arthralgia, myalgia, rash, and pruritus. Other side-effects reported rarely or very rarely include taste disturbance, stomatitis, hepatitis, jaundice, hypersensitivity reactions (including anaphylaxis, bronchospasm), fever, depression, hallucinations, confusion, gynaecomastia, interstitial nephritis, hyponatraemia, blood disorders (including leucopenia, leucocytosis, pancytopenia, thrombocytopenia), visual disturbances, sweating, photosensitivity, alopecia, Stevens-Johnson syndrome, and toxic epidermal necrolysis. By decreasing gastric acidity, proton pump inhibitors may increase the risk of gastro-intestinal infections (including *Clostridium difficile* infection).

### ▉ ESOMEPRAZOLE

**Indications** see under Dose

**Cautions** see notes above; renal impairment (Appendix 3); **interactions:** Appendix 1 (proton pump inhibitors)

**Side-effects** see notes above

**Dose**

- By mouth duodenal ulcer associated with *Helicobacter pylori*, see eradication regimens on p. 43
 NSAID-associated gastric ulcer, ADULT over 18 years, 20 mg once daily for 4–8 weeks; prophylaxis in patients with an increased risk of gastroduodenal complications who require continued NSAID treatment, 20 mg daily
 Gastro-oesophageal reflux disease, ADULT and CHILD over 12 years, 40 mg once daily for 4 weeks, continued for further 4 weeks if not fully healed or symptoms persist; maintenance 20 mg daily; symptomatic treatment in the absence of oesophagitis, 20 mg daily for up to 4 weeks, then in ADULTS over 18 years 20 mg daily when required
 Zollinger–Ellison syndrome, ADULT over 18 years, initially 40 mg twice daily, adjusted according to response; usual range 80–160 mg daily (above 80 mg in 2 divided doses)
 Counselling Do not chew or crush tablets, swallow whole *or* disperse in water
- By intravenous injection over at least 3 minutes *or* by intravenous infusion, ADULT over 18 years, gastro-oesophageal reflux disease, 40 mg once daily; symptomatic reflux disease without oesophagitis, treatment of NSAID-associated gastric ulcer, prevention of NSAID-associated gastric or duodenal ulcer, 20 mg daily; continue until oral administration possible

**Nexium®** (AstraZeneca) ▱⒫⒪⒨
Tablets, f/c, esomeprazole (as magnesium trihydrate) 20 mg (light pink), net price 28-tab pack = £18.50 (also 7-tab pack, hosp. only); 40 mg (pink), 28-tab pack = £25.19 (also 7-tab pack, hosp. only). Counselling, administration

Injection, powder for reconstitution, esomeprazole (as sodium salt), net price 40-mg vial = £5.21

# LANSOPRAZOLE

**Indications** see under Dose

**Cautions** see notes above; **interactions:** Appendix 1 (proton pump inhibitors)

**Side-effects** see notes above; also glossitis, pancreatitis, anorexia, restlessness, tremor, impotence, petechiae, and purpura; *very rarely* colitis, raised serum cholesterol or triglycerides

**Dose**

* Benign gastric ulcer, 30 mg daily in the morning for 8 weeks
* Duodenal ulcer, 30 mg daily in the morning for 4 weeks; maintenance 15 mg daily
* NSAID-associated duodenal or gastric ulcer, 30 mg once daily for 4 weeks, continued for further 4 weeks if not fully healed; prophylaxis, 15–30 mg once daily
* Eradication of *Helicobacter pylori* associated with duodenal ulcer or ulcer-like dyspepsia, see eradication regimens on p. 43
* Zollinger-Ellison syndrome (and other hypersecretory conditions), initially 60 mg once daily adjusted according to response; daily doses of 120 mg or more given in two divided doses
* Gastro-oesophageal reflux disease, 30 mg daily in the morning for 4 weeks, continued for further 4 weeks if not fully healed; maintenance 15–30 mg daily
* Acid-related dyspepsia, 15–30 mg daily in the morning for 2–4 weeks
* CHILD under 18 years see *BNF for Children*

Note Lansoprazole doses in BNF may differ from those in product literature

**Lansoprazole** (Non-proprietary) [PoM]
Capsules, enclosing e/c granules, lansoprazole 15 mg, net price 28-cap pack = £1.80; 30 mg, 28-cap pack = £3.09. Label: 5, 22, 25
Dental prescribing on NHS Lansoprazole capsules may be prescribed

**Zoton®** (Wyeth) [PoM]
FasTab® (= orodispersible tablet), lansoprazole 15 mg, net price 28-tab pack = £2.99; 30 mg, 14-tab pack = £2.74, 28-tab pack = £5.50. Label: 5, 22, counselling, administration
Excipients include aspartame (section 9.4.1)
Counselling Tablets should be placed on the tongue, allowed to disperse and swallowed, or may be swallowed whole with a glass of water. Alternatively, tablets can be dispersed in a small amount of water and administered by an oral syringe or nasogastric tube

# OMEPRAZOLE

**Indications** see under Dose

**Cautions** see notes above; **interactions:** Appendix 1 (proton pump inhibitors)

**Side-effects** see notes above; also agitation and impotence

**Dose**

* By mouth, benign gastric and duodenal ulcers, 20 mg once daily for 4 weeks in duodenal ulceration or 8 weeks in gastric ulceration; in severe or recurrent cases increase to 40 mg daily; maintenance for recurrent duodenal ulcer, 20 mg once daily; prevention of relapse in duodenal ulcer, 10 mg daily increasing to 20 mg once daily if symptoms return

NSAID-associated duodenal or gastric ulcer and gastroduodenal erosions, 20 mg once daily for 4 weeks,

continued for further 4 weeks if not fully healed; prophylaxis in patients with a history of NSAID-associated duodenal or gastric ulcers, gastroduodenal lesions, or dyspeptic symptoms who require continued NSAID treatment, 20 mg once daily

Duodenal or benign gastric ulcer associated with *Helicobacter pylori*, see eradication regimens on p. 43

Zollinger–Ellison syndrome, initially 60 mg once daily; usual range 20–120 mg daily (above 80 mg in 2 divided doses)

Gastric acid reduction during general anaesthesia (prophylaxis of acid aspiration), 40 mg on the preceding evening then 40 mg 2–6 hours before surgery

Gastro-oesophageal reflux disease, 20 mg once daily for 4 weeks, continued for further 4–8 weeks if not fully healed; 40 mg once daily has been given for 8 weeks in gastro-oesophageal reflux disease refractory to other treatment; maintenance 20 mg once daily

Acid reflux disease (long-term management), 10 mg daily increasing to 20 mg once daily if symptoms return

Acid-related dyspepsia, 10–20 mg once daily for 2–4 weeks according to response

Severe ulcerating reflux oesophagitis, CHILD over 1 year, body-weight 10–20 kg, 10 mg once daily increased if necessary to 20 mg once daily for 4–12 weeks; body-weight over 20 kg, 20 mg once daily increased if necessary to 40 mg once daily for 4–12 weeks; to be initiated by hospital paediatrician

* By intravenous injection over 5 minutes *or* by intravenous infusion over 20–30 minutes, prophylaxis of acid aspiration, 40 mg completed 1 hour before surgery

Benign gastric ulcer, duodenal ulcer and gastro-oesophageal reflux, 40 mg once daily until oral administration possible

* Severe peptic ulcer bleeding [unlicensed indication], initial intravenous infusion of 80 mg over 40–60 minutes, then by continuous intravenous infusion, 8 mg/hour for 72 hours (then change to oral therapy)

Counselling Swallow whole, *or* disperse *MUPS®* tablets in water, *or* mix capsule contents or *MUPS®* tablets with fruit juice or yoghurt. Preparations consisting of an e/c tablet within a capsule should **not** be opened

**Omeprazole** (Non-proprietary) [PoM]
Capsules, enclosing e/c granules, omeprazole 10 mg, net price 28-cap pack = £1.82; 20 mg, 28-cap pack = £1.71; 40 mg, 7-cap pack = £2.03, 28-cap pack = £58.00. Counselling, administration
Note Some preparations consist of an e/c tablet within a capsule; brands include *Mepradec®*
Dental prescribing on NHS Gastro-resistant omeprazole capsules may be prescribed

[1]Tablets, e/c, omeprazole 10 mg, net price 28-tab pack = £5.21; 20 mg, 28-tab pack = £4.70; 40 mg, 7-tab pack = £4.47. Label: 25

Intravenous infusion, powder for reconstitution, omeprazole (as sodium salt), net price 40-mg vial = £5.14

1. Omeprazole 10 mg tablets can be sold to the public for the short-term relief of reflux-like symptoms (e.g. heartburn) in adults over 18 years, max. daily dose 20 mg for max. 4 weeks, and a pack size of 28 tablets

**Losec®** (AstraZeneca) [PoM]
MUPS® (multiple-unit pellet system = dispersible tablets), f/c, omeprazole 10 mg (light pink), net price

**1 Gastro-intestinal system**

28-tab pack = £7.75; 20 mg (pink), 28-tab pack = £11.60; 40 mg (red-brown), 7-tab pack = £5.80. Counselling, administration

Capsules, enclosing e/c granules, omeprazole 10 mg (pink), net price 28-cap pack = £7.75; 20 mg (pink/brown), 28-cap pack = £11.60; 40 mg (brown), 7-cap pack = £5.80. Counselling, administration

Intravenous infusion, powder for reconstitution, omeprazole (as sodium salt), net price 40-mg vial = £5.41

Injection, powder for reconstitution, omeprazole (as sodium salt), net price 40-mg vial (with solvent) = £5.41

## ■ PANTOPRAZOLE

**Indications** see under Dose

**Cautions** see notes above; also renal impairment (Appendix 3); **interactions:** Appendix 1 (proton pump inhibitors)

**Side-effects** see notes above; also raised serum cholesterol or triglycerides

**Dose**
- By mouth, benign gastric ulcer, ADULT over 18 years, 40 mg daily in the morning for 4 weeks, continued for further 4 weeks if not fully healed

  Gastro-oesophageal reflux disease, ADULT and CHILD over 12 years, 20–40 mg daily in the morning for 4 weeks, continued for further 4 weeks if not fully healed; maintenance 20 mg daily, increased to 40 mg daily if symptoms return

  Duodenal ulcer, ADULT over 18 years, 40 mg daily in the morning for 2 weeks, continued for further 2 weeks if not fully healed

  Duodenal ulcer associated with *Helicobacter pylori*, see eradication regimens on p. 43

  Prophylaxis of NSAID-associated gastric or duodenal ulcer in patients with an increased risk of gastroduodenal complications who require continued NSAID treatment, ADULT over 18 years, 20 mg daily

  Zollinger–Ellison syndrome (and other hypersecretory conditions), ADULT over 18 years, initially 80 mg once daily adjusted according to response (ELDERLY max. 40 mg daily); daily doses above 80 mg given in 2 divided doses

- By intravenous injection over at least 2 minutes *or* by intravenous infusion, ADULT over 18 years, duodenal ulcer, gastric ulcer, and gastro-oesophageal reflux, 40 mg daily until oral administration can be resumed

  Zollinger–Ellison syndrome (and other hypersecretory conditions), ADULT over 18 years, initially 80 mg (160 mg if rapid acid control required) then 80 mg once daily adjusted according to response; daily doses above 80 mg given in 2 divided doses

**Pantoprazole** (Non-proprietary) ℗oM
Tablets, e/c, pantoprazole 20 mg, net price 28-tab pack = £11.83; 40 mg, 28-tab pack = £20.57. Label: 25

**Protium®** (Nycomed) ℗oM
Tablets, yellow, e/c, pantoprazole (as sodium sesquihydrate) 20 mg, net price 28-tab pack = £11.83; 40 mg, 28-tab pack = £20.57. Label: 25

Injection, powder for reconstitution, pantoprazole (as sodium salt), net price 40-mg vial = £5.11

## ■ RABEPRAZOLE SODIUM

**Indications** see under Dose

**Cautions** see notes above; **interactions:** Appendix 1 (proton pump inhibitors)

**Side-effects** see notes above; also cough, influenza-like syndrome, and rhinitis; *less commonly* chest pain and nervousness; *rarely* anorexia and weight gain

**Dose**
- Benign gastric ulcer, 20 mg daily in the morning for 6 weeks, continued for further 6 weeks if not fully healed
- Duodenal ulcer, 20 mg daily in the morning for 4 weeks, continued for further 4 weeks if not fully healed
- Gastro-oesophageal reflux disease, 20 mg once daily for 4–8 weeks; maintenance 10–20 mg daily; symptomatic treatment in the absence of oesophagitis, 10 mg daily for up to 4 weeks, then 10 mg daily when required
- Duodenal and benign gastric ulcer associated with *Helicobacter pylori*, see eradication regimens on p. 43
- Zollinger–Ellison syndrome, initially 60 mg once daily adjusted according to response (max. 120 mg daily); doses above 100 mg daily given in 2 divided doses
- CHILD not recommended

**Pariet®** (Janssen-Cilag, Eisai) ℗oM
Tablets, e/c, rabeprazole sodium 10 mg (pink), net price 28-tab pack = £11.56; 20 mg (yellow), 28-tab pack = £17.54. Label: 25

## 1.4 Acute diarrhoea

### 1.4.1 Adsorbents and bulk-forming drugs
### 1.4.2 Antimotility drugs

The priority in acute diarrhoea, as in gastro-enteritis, is the prevention or reversal of fluid and electrolyte depletion. This is particularly important in infants and in frail and elderly patients. For details of oral rehydration preparations, see section 9.2.1.2. Severe depletion of fluid and electrolytes requires immediate admission to hospital and urgent replacement.

**Antimotility drugs** (section 1.4.2) relieve symptoms of acute diarrhoea. They are used in the management of uncomplicated acute diarrhoea in adults; fluid and electrolyte replacement may be necessary in case of dehydration. However, antimotility drugs are **not** recommended for acute diarrhoea in young children.

Antispasmodics (section 1.2) are occasionally of value in treating abdominal cramp associated with diarrhoea but they should **not** be used for primary treatment. Antispasmodics and antiemetics should be **avoided** in young children with gastro-enteritis because they are rarely effective and have troublesome side-effects.

Antibacterial drugs are generally unnecessary in simple gastro-enteritis because the complaint usually resolves quickly without them, and infective diarrhoeas in the UK often have a viral cause. Systemic bacterial infection does, however, need appropriate systemic treatment; for drugs used in campylobacter enteritis, shigellosis, and salmonellosis, see Table 1, section 5.1. **Ciprofloxacin** is occasionally used for prophylaxis against travellers' diarrhoea, but routine use is **not** recommended. Lactobacillus preparations have not been shown to be effective.

Colestyramine (cholestyramine, section 1.9.2), binds unabsorbed bile salts and provides symptomatic relief of diarrhoea following ileal disease or resection.

## 1.4.1 Adsorbents and bulk-forming drugs

Adsorbents such as kaolin are **not** recommended for *acute diarrhoeas*. Bulk-forming drugs, such as ispaghula, methylcellulose, and sterculia (section 1.6.1) are useful in controlling diarrhoea associated with diverticular disease.

### ▍ KAOLIN, LIGHT

**Indications** diarrhoea but see notes above
**Cautions** interactions: Appendix 1 (kaolin)

**Kaolin Mixture, BP**
(Kaolin Oral Suspension)
Oral suspension, light kaolin or light kaolin (natural) 20%, light magnesium carbonate 5%, sodium bicarbonate 5% in a suitable vehicle with a peppermint flavour.
**Dose** 10–20 mL every 4 hours

## 1.4.2 Antimotility drugs

Antimotility drugs have a role in the management of uncomplicated *acute diarrhoea* in adults but not in young children; see also section 1.4. However, in severe cases, fluid and electrolyte replacement (section 9.2.1.2) are of primary importance.

For comments on the role of antimotility drugs in *chronic bowel disorders* see section 1.5. For their role in *stoma care* see section 1.8.

Loperamide can be used for faecal incontinence [unlicensed indication] after the underlying cause of incontinence has been addressed.

### ▍ CODEINE PHOSPHATE

**Indications** see notes above; cough suppression (section 3.9.1); pain (section 4.7.2)
**Cautions** see section 4.7.2; tolerance and dependence may occur with prolonged use; **interactions:** Appendix 1 (opioid analgesics)
**Contra-indications** see section 4.7.2; also conditions where inhibition of peristalsis should be avoided, where abdominal distension develops, or in acute diarrhoeal conditions such as acute ulcerative colitis or antibiotic-associated colitis
**Side-effects** see section 4.7.2
**Dose**
● See preparations

**Codeine Phosphate** (Non-proprietary) ℞
Tablets, codeine phosphate 15 mg, net price 28 = £1.08; 30 mg, 28 = £1.24; 60 mg, 28 = £1.73. Label: 2
**Dose** ADULT and CHILD over 12 years, acute diarrhoea, 30 mg 3–4 times daily (range 15–60 mg)
**Note** As for schedule 2 controlled drugs, travellers needing to take codeine phosphate tablets abroad may require a doctor's letter explaining why codeine is necessary.

### ▍ CO-PHENOTROPE

A mixture of diphenoxylate hydrochloride and atropine sulphate in the mass proportions 100 parts to 1 part respectively

**Indications** adjunct to rehydration in acute diarrhoea (but see notes above); control of faecal consistency after colostomy or ileostomy (section 1.8)
**Cautions** see under Codeine Phosphate (section 4.7.2); also young children are particularly susceptible to **overdosage** and symptoms may be delayed and observation is needed for at least 48 hours after ingestion; presence of subclinical doses of atropine may give rise to atropine side-effects in susceptible individuals or in overdosage (section 1.2); **interactions:** Appendix 1 (antimuscarinics, opioid analgesics)
**Contra-indications** see under Antimuscarinics (section 1.2) and Codeine Phosphate (section 4.7.2); also jaundice
**Side-effects** see under Antimuscarinics (section 1.2) and Codeine Phosphate (section 4.7.2); also fever
**Dose**
● See preparations

**Co-phenotrope** (Non-proprietary) ℞
Tablets, co-phenotrope 2.5/0.025 (diphenoxylate hydrochloride 2.5 mg, atropine sulphate 25 micrograms), net price 100 = £8.95
Brands include *Lomotil*®
**Dose** initially 4 tablets, followed by 2 tablets every 6 hours until diarrhoea controlled; CHILD under 4 years see *BNF for Children*, 4–9 years 1 tablet 3 times daily, 9–12 years 1 tablet 4 times daily, 12–16 years 2 tablets 3 times daily, but see also notes above
**Note** Co-phenotrope 2.5/0.025 can be sold to the public for adults and children over 16 years (provided packs do not contain more than 20 tablets) as an adjunct to rehydration in acute diarrhoea (max. daily dose 10 tablets)

### ▍ LOPERAMIDE HYDROCHLORIDE

**Indications** symptomatic treatment of acute diarrhoea; adjunct to rehydration in acute diarrhoea in adults and children over 4 years (but see notes above); chronic diarrhoea in adults only
**Cautions** see notes above; also liver disease; pregnancy (Appendix 4); **interactions:** Appendix 1 (loperamide)
**Contra-indications** conditions where inhibition of peristalsis should be avoided, where abdominal distension develops, or in conditions such as active ulcerative colitis or antibiotic-associated colitis
**Side-effects** abdominal cramps, dizziness, drowsiness, and skin reactions including urticaria; paralytic ileus and abdominal bloating also reported
**Dose**
● Acute diarrhoea, 4 mg initially followed by 2 mg after each loose stool for up to 5 days; usual dose 6–8 mg daily; max. 16 mg daily; CHILD under 4 years not recommended; 4–8 years, 1 mg 3–4 times daily for up to 3 *days only*; 8–12 years, 2 mg 4 times daily for up to 5 days
● Chronic diarrhoea in adults, initially, 4–8 mg daily in divided doses, subsequently adjusted according to response and given in 2 divided doses for maintenance; max. 16 mg daily; CHILD under 18 years see *BNF for Children*
● Faecal incontinence [unlicensed indication], initially 500 micrograms daily, adjusted according to response; max. 16 mg daily in divided doses

**Loperamide** (Non-proprietary) PoM

Capsules, loperamide hydrochloride 2 mg, net price 30-cap pack = £1.06

Tablets, loperamide hydrochloride 2 mg, net price 30-tab pack = £2.15
Brands include *Norimode*®

Note Loperamide can be sold to the public, for adults and children over 12 years, provided it is licensed and labelled for the treatment of acute diarrhoea

**Imodium**® (Janssen-Cilag) PoM

Capsules, green/grey, loperamide hydrochloride 2 mg. Net price 30-cap pack = £1.09

Syrup, sugar free, red, loperamide hydrochloride 1 mg/5 mL. Net price 100 mL = 94p

◀Compound preparations

**Imodium**® **Plus** (McNeil)

Caplets (= tablets), loperamide hydrochloride 2 mg, simeticone 125 mg, net price 6-tab pack = £2.27, 12-tab pack = £3.56

Dose acute diarrhoea with abdominal colic, initially 2 caplets (CHILD 12–18 years 1 caplet) then 1 caplet after each loose stool; max. 4 caplets daily for up to 2 days; CHILD under 12 years not recommended

### MORPHINE

**Indications** see notes above; cough in terminal disease (section 3.9.1); pain (section 4.7.2)

**Cautions** see notes above and under Morphine Salts (section 4.7.2)

**Contra-indications** see notes above and under Morphine Salts (section 4.7.2)

**Side-effects** see notes above and under Morphine Salts (section 4.7.2); sedation and the risk of dependence are greater

**Dose**

• See preparation

**Kaolin and Morphine Mixture, BP** ▱
(Kaolin and Morphine Oral Suspension)

Oral suspension, light kaolin or light kaolin (natural) 20%, sodium bicarbonate 5%, with chloroform and morphine tincture 4% in a suitable vehicle. Contains anhydrous morphine 550–800 micrograms/10 mL.

Dose ADULT and CHILD over 12 years, 10 mL every 6 hours in water

## 1.5 Chronic bowel disorders

Once tumours are ruled out individual symptoms of chronic bowel disorders need specific treatment including dietary manipulation as well as drug treatment and the maintenance of a liberal fluid intake.

## Inflammatory bowel disease

Chronic inflammatory bowel diseases include *ulcerative colitis* and *Crohn's disease*. Effective management requires drug therapy, attention to nutrition, and in severe or chronic active disease, surgery.

**Aminosalicylates** (balsalazide, mesalazine, olsalazine, and sulfasalazine), **corticosteroids** (hydrocortisone, beclometasone, budesonide, and prednisolone), and **drugs that affect the immune response** form the basis of drug treatment.

**Treatment of acute ulcerative colitis and Crohn's disease** Acute mild to moderate disease affecting the rectum (proctitis) or the recto-sigmoid (distal colitis) is treated initially with local application of an aminosalicylate (section 1.5.1); alternatively, a local corticosteroid can be used but it is less effective. A combination of a local aminosalicylate and a local corticosteroid can be used for proctitis that does not respond to a local aminosalicylate alone. Foam preparations and suppositories are especially useful when patients have difficulty retaining liquid enemas.

Diffuse inflammatory bowel disease or disease that does not respond to local therapy requires oral treatment. Mild disease affecting the upper colon can be treated with an oral aminosalicylate alone; a combination of a local and an oral aminosalicylate can be used in proctitis or distal colitis. Refractory or moderate inflammatory bowel disease usually requires adjunctive use of an oral corticosteroid such as **prednisolone** (section 1.5.2) for 4–8 weeks. Modified-release **budesonide** is licensed for Crohn's disease affecting the ileum and the ascending colon; it causes fewer systemic side-effects than oral prednisolone but may be less effective. **Beclometasone dipropionate** by mouth is licensed as an adjunct to mesalazine for mild to moderate ulcerative colitis, but it is not known whether it is as effective as other corticosteroids.

Severe inflammatory bowel disease calls for hospital admission and treatment with an intravenous corticosteroid (such as hydrocortisone or methylprednisolone, section 6.3.2); other therapy may include intravenous fluid and electrolyte replacement, and possibly parenteral nutrition. Specialist supervision is required for patients who fail to respond adequately to these measures. Patients with severe ulcerative colitis that has not responded to intravenous corticosteroids, may benefit from a short course of intravenous **ciclosporin** [unlicensed indication] (section 1.5.3). Patients with unresponsive or chronically active Crohn's disease may benefit from **azathioprine** (section 1.5.3), **mercaptopurine** (section 1.5.3), or once-weekly **methotrexate** (section 1.5.3) [all unlicensed indications].

**Infliximab** (section 1.5.3) is licensed for the management of severe active Crohn's disease and severe ulcerative colitis in patients whose condition has not responded adequately to treatment with a corticosteroid and a conventional immunosuppressant or who are intolerant of them.

NICE guidance
**Infliximab for Crohn's disease (April 2002)**
Infliximab is recommended for the treatment of severe active Crohn's disease (with or without fistulae) when treatment with immunomodulating drugs and corticosteroids has failed or is not tolerated and when surgery is inappropriate. Treatment may be repeated if the condition responded to the initial course but relapsed subsequently. Infliximab should be prescribed only by a gastroenterologist.

NICE guidance
**Infliximab for subacute manifestations of ulcerative colitis (April 2008)**
Infliximab is **not** recommended for the treatment of subacute manifestations of moderate to severe active ulcerative colitis that would normally be managed in an outpatient setting.

> **NICE guidance**
> **Infliximab for acute exacerbations of ulcerative colitis (December 2008)**
> Infliximab is recommended as an option for the treatment of acute exacerbations of severe ulcerative colitis when treatment with ciclosporin is contra-indicated or inappropriate.

**Adalimumab** (section 1.5.3) is licensed for the treatment of severe active Crohn's disease in patients whose condition has not responded adequately to treatment with a corticosteroid and a conventional immunosuppressant, or who are intolerant of them. For inducing remission, adalimumab should be used in combination with a corticosteroid, but it may be given alone if a corticosteroid is inappropriate or is not tolerated. Adalimumab may also be used for Crohn's disease in patients who have relapsed while taking infliximab or who cannot tolerate infliximab because of hypersensitivity reactions.

**Maintenance of remission of acute ulcerative colitis and Crohn's disease** Smoking cessation (section 4.10) reduces the risk of relapse in Crohn's disease and should be encouraged. **Aminosalicylates** are of great value in the maintenance of remission of ulcerative colitis. They are of less value in the maintenance of remission of Crohn's disease; an oral formulation of mesalazine is licensed for the long-term management of ileal disease. Corticosteroids are **not** suitable for maintenance treatment because of their side-effects. In resistant or frequently relapsing cases either **azathioprine** (section 1.5.3) [unlicensed indication] or **mercaptopurine** (section 1.5.3) [unlicensed indication], given under close supervision may be helpful. Methotrexate (section 1.5.3) is tried in Crohn's disease if azathioprine or mercaptopurine cannot be used [unlicensed indication]. Maintenance therapy with infliximab should be considered for patients with Crohn's disease or ulcerative colitis who respond to the initial induction course of infliximab; fixed-interval dosing is superior to intermittent dosing. **Adalimumab** is licensed for maintenance therapy in Crohn's disease.

**Fistulating Crohn's disease** Treatment may not be necessary for simple, asymptomatic perianal fistulas. **Metronidazole** (section 5.1.11) or **ciprofloxacin** (section 5.1.12) can improve symptoms of fistulating Crohn's disease but complete healing occurs rarely [unlicensed indication]. Metronidazole by mouth is used at a dose of 10–20 mg/kg daily in divided doses (usual dose 400–500 mg 3 times daily); it is usually given for 1 month but no longer than 3 months because of concerns about peripheral neuropathy. Ciprofloxacin by mouth is given at a dose of 500 mg twice daily. Other antibacterials should be given if specifically indicated (e.g. sepsis associated with fistulas and perianal disease) and for managing bacterial overgrowth in the small bowel. Fistulas may also require surgical exploration and local drainage.

Either **azathioprine** or **mercaptopurine** is used as a second-line treatment for fistulating Crohn's disease and continued for maintenance [unlicensed indication]. **Infliximab** is used for fistulating Crohn's disease refractory to conventional treatments; fixed-interval dosing is superior to intermittent dosing. Maintenance therapy with infliximab should be considered for patients who

respond to the initial induction course of infliximab. **Adalimumab** can be used if there is intolerance to infliximab [unlicensed indication].

**Adjunctive treatment of inflammatory bowel disease** Due attention should be paid to diet; high-fibre or low-residue diets should be used as appropriate. Irritable bowel syndrome during remission of ulcerative colitis calls for avoidance of a high-fibre diet and possible treatment with an antispasmodic (section 1.2).

Antimotility drugs such as codeine and loperamide, and antispasmodic drugs may precipitate paralytic ileus and megacolon in active ulcerative colitis; treatment of the inflammation is more logical. Laxatives may be required in proctitis. Diarrhoea resulting from the loss of bile-salt absorption (e.g. in terminal ileal disease or bowel resection) may improve with **colestyramine** (section 1.9.2), which binds bile salts.

## *Clostridium difficile* infection

Antibiotic-associated colitis is caused by colonisation of the colon with *Clostridium difficile*, which may follow antibiotic therapy. It is usually of acute onset, but may become chronic; it is a particular hazard of ampicillin, amoxicillin, co-amoxiclav, third-generation cephalosporins, clindamycin, and quinolones, but few antibiotics are free of this side-effect. Oral **metronidazole** (see section 5.1.11) or oral **vancomycin** (see section 5.1.7) are used as specific treatment; vancomycin may be preferred for very sick patients. Metronidazole can be given by intravenous infusion if oral treatment is inappropriate.

## Diverticular disease

Diverticular disease is treated with a high-fibre diet, **bran supplements**, and **bulk-forming drugs** (section 1.6.1). **Antispasmodics** may provide symptomatic relief when colic is a problem (section 1.2). **Antibacterials** are used only when the diverticula in the intestinal wall become infected (specialist referral). Antimotility drugs which slow intestinal motility, e.g. codeine, diphenoxylate, and loperamide could possibly exacerbate the symptoms of diverticular disease and are contra-indicated.

## Irritable bowel syndrome

Irritable bowel syndrome can present with pain, constipation, or diarrhoea. In some patients there may be important psychological aggravating factors which respond to reassurance and possibly specific treatment e.g. with an antidepressant.

The **fibre** intake of patients with irritable bowel syndrome should be reviewed. If an increase in dietary fibre is required, soluble fibre (e.g. ispaghula husk, sterculia, or oats) is recommended; insoluble fibre (e.g. bran) may exacerbate symptoms and its use should be discouraged. A **laxative** (section 1.6) can be used to treat constipation. An osmotic laxative, such as a macrogol, is preferred; lactulose may cause bloating. **Loperamide** (section 1.4.2) may relieve diarrhoea and **antispasmodic drugs** (section 1.2) may relieve pain. Opioids with a central action, such as codeine, are better avoided because of the risk of dependence.

**1**

**Gastro-intestinal system**

A **tricyclic antidepressant** (section 4.3.1) can be used for abdominal pain or discomfort [unlicensed indication] in patients who have not responded to laxatives, loperamide, or antispasmodics. Low doses of a tricyclic antidepressant are used (e.g. amitriptyline, initially 5–10 mg each night, increased if necessary in steps of 10 mg at intervals of at least 2 weeks to max. 30 mg each night). A **selective serotonin reuptake inhibitor** (section 4.3.3) may be considered in those who do not respond to a tricyclic antidepressant [unlicensed indication].

## Malabsorption syndromes

Individual conditions need specific management and also general nutritional consideration. Coeliac disease (gluten enteropathy) usually needs a gluten-free diet and pancreatic insufficiency needs pancreatin supplements (section 1.9.4)

For further information on foods for special diets (ACBS), see Appendix 7.

## 1.5.1 Aminosalicylates

**Sulfasalazine** is a combination of 5-aminosalicylic acid ('5-ASA') and sulfapyridine; sulfapyridine acts only as a carrier to the colonic site of action but still causes side-effects. In the newer aminosalicylates, **mesalazine** (5-aminosalicylic acid), **balsalazide** (a prodrug of 5-aminosalicylic acid) and **olsalazine** (a dimer of 5-aminosalicylic acid which cleaves in the lower bowel), the sulphonamide-related side-effects of sulfasalazine are avoided, but 5-aminosalicylic acid alone can still cause side-effects including blood disorders (see recommendation below) and lupus-like syndrome also seen with sulfasalazine.

**Cautions** Renal function should be monitored before starting an oral aminosalicylate, at 3 months of treatment, and then annually during treatment (more frequently in renal impairment). Aminosalicylates should be used with caution in renal impairment (Appendix 3), during pregnancy (Appendix 4) and breast-feeding (Appendix 5); blood disorders can occur (see recommendation below).

> **Blood disorders**
> Patients receiving aminosalicylates should be advised to report any unexplained bleeding, bruising, purpura, sore throat, fever or malaise that occurs during treatment. A blood count should be performed and the drug stopped immediately if there is suspicion of a blood dyscrasia.

**Contra-indications** Aminosalicylates should be avoided in salicylate hypersensitivity.

**Side-effects** Side-effects of the aminosalicylates include diarrhoea, nausea, vomiting, abdominal pain, exacerbation of symptoms of colitis, headache, hypersensitivity reactions (including rash and urticaria); side-effects that occur rarely include acute pancreatitis, hepatitis, myocarditis, pericarditis, lung disorders (including eosinophilia and fibrosing alveolitis), peripheral neuropathy, blood disorders (including agranulocytosis, aplastic anaemia, leucopenia, methaemoglobin-

aemia, neutropenia, and thrombocytopenia—see also recommendation above), renal dysfunction (interstitial nephritis, nephrotic syndrome), myalgia, arthralgia, skin reactions (including lupus erythematosus-like syndrome, Stevens-Johnson syndrome), alopecia.

### ■ BALSALAZIDE SODIUM

**Indications** treatment of mild to moderate ulcerative colitis and maintenance of remission

**Cautions** see notes above; also history of asthma; **interactions:** Appendix 1 (aminosalicylates)
    **Blood disorders** See recommendation above

**Contra-indications** see notes above; also severe hepatic impairment

**Side-effects** see notes above; also cholelithiasis

**Dose**
- Acute attack, 2.25 g 3 times daily until remission occurs or for up to max. 12 weeks
- Maintenance, 1.5 g twice daily, adjusted according to response (max. 6 g daily)
- CHILD under 18 years see *BNF for Children*

**Colazide®** (Almirall) ▣PoM▣
    Capsules, beige, balsalazide sodium 750 mg. Net price 130-cap pack = £39.00. Label: 21, 25, counselling, blood disorder symptoms (see recommendation above)

### ■ MESALAZINE

**Indications** treatment of mild to moderate ulcerative colitis and maintenance of remission; see also under preparations

**Cautions** see notes above; elderly; **interactions:** Appendix 1 (aminosalicylates)
    **Blood disorders** See recommendation above

**Contra-indications** see notes above; also severe hepatic impairment (Appendix 2)

**Side-effects** see notes above

**Dose**
- See under preparations, below
    **Note** The delivery characteristics of oral mesalazine preparations may vary; these preparations should not be considered interchangeable

**Asacol®** (Procter & Gamble Pharm.) ▣PoM▣
    Foam enema, mesalazine 1 g/metered application, net price 14-application canister with disposable applicators and plastic bags = £27.26. Counselling, blood disorder symptoms (see recommendation above)
    Excipients include disodium edetate, hydroxybenzoates (parabens), polysorbate 20, sodium metabisulphite
    **Dose** acute attack affecting the rectosigmoid region, 1 metered application (mesalazine 1 g) into the rectum daily for 4–6 weeks; acute attack affecting the descending colon, 2 metered applications (mesalazine 2 g) once daily for 4–6 weeks; CHILD 12–18 years, see *BNF for Children*

    Suppositories, mesalazine 250 mg, net price 20-suppos pack = £4.92; 500 mg, 10-suppos pack = £4.92. Counselling, blood disorder symptoms (see recommendation above)
    **Dose** acute attack or maintenance, by rectum 0.75–1.5 g daily in divided doses, with last dose at bedtime; CHILD 12–18 years, see *BNF for Children*

**Asacol® MR** (Procter & Gamble Pharm.) ▣PoM▣
    Tablets, red, e/c, mesalazine 400 mg, net price 90-tab pack = £30.00, 120-tab pack = £40.00. Label: 5, 25,

counselling, blood disorder symptoms (see recommendation above)

**Dose** ulcerative colitis, acute attack, 2.4 g daily in divided doses; maintenance of remission of ulcerative colitis and Crohn's ileo-colitis, 1.2–2.4 g daily in divided doses; CHILD 12–18 years, see *BNF for Children*

Tablets, red-brown, e/c, mesalazine 800 mg, net price 180-tab pack = £119.99. Label: 5, 25, counselling, blood disorder symptoms (see recommendation above)

**Dose** ADULT over 18 years, ulcerative colitis, acute attack, 2.4–4.8 g daily in divided doses; maintenance of remission of ulcerative colitis and Crohn's ileo-colitis, up to 2.4 g daily in divided doses

**Note** Preparations that lower stool pH (e.g. lactulose) may prevent release of mesalazine

**Ipocol®** (Sandoz) PoM
Tablets, e/c, mesalazine 400 mg, net price 120-tab pack = £41.62. Label: 5, 25, counselling, blood disorder symptoms (see recommendation above)

**Dose** acute attack, 2.4 g daily in divided doses; maintenance, 1.2–2.4 g daily in divided doses; CHILD 12–18 years, see *BNF for Children*

**Note** Preparations that lower stool pH (e.g. lactulose) may prevent release of mesalazine

**Mesren® MR** (IVAX) PoM
Tablets, red-brown, e/c, mesalazine 400 mg, net price 90-tab pack = £19.50, 120-tab pack = £26.00. Label: 5, 25, counselling, blood disorder symptoms (see recommendation above)

**Dose** ADULT and CHILD over 12 years, acute attack, 2.4 g daily in divided doses; maintenance, 1.2–2.4 g daily in divided doses

**Mezavant® XL** (Shire) PoM
Tablets, m/r, red-brown, e/c, mesalazine 1.2 g, net price 60-tab pack = £62.44. Label: 21, 25, counselling, blood disorder symptoms (see recommendations above)

**Dose** ADULT over 18 years, acute attack, 2.4 g once daily, increase if necessary to 4.8 g once daily (review treatment at 8 weeks); maintenance, 2.4 g once daily

**Pentasa®** (Ferring) PoM
Tablets, m/r, scored, mesalazine 500 mg (grey), net price 100-tab pack = £24.21. Counselling, administration, see dose, blood disorder symptoms (see recommendation above)

**Dose** ADULT and CHILD over 15 years, acute attack, up to 4 g daily in 2–3 divided doses; maintenance, 1.5 g daily in 2–3 divided doses; tablets may be dispersed in water, but should not be chewed; CHILD 5–15 years see *BNF for Children*

Granules, m/r, pale brown, mesalazine 1 g/sachet, net price 50-sachet pack = £28.82; 2 g/sachet, 60-sachet pack = £72.05. Counselling, administration, see dose, blood disorder symptoms (see recommendation above)

**Dose** ADULT and CHILD over 12 years, acute attack, up to 4 g daily in 2–4 divided doses; maintenance, 2 g once daily; granules should be placed on tongue and washed down with water or orange juice without chewing; CHILD 5–12 years see *BNF for Children*

Retention enema, mesalazine 1 g in 100-mL pack. Net price 7 enemas = £17.73. Counselling, blood disorder symptoms (see recommendation above)

**Dose** by rectum ADULT and CHILD over 12 years, 1 enema at bedtime

Suppositories, mesalazine 1 g. Net price 28-suppos pack = £40.01. Counselling, blood disorder symptoms (see recommendation above)

**Dose** by rectum ulcerative proctitis, ADULT and CHILD over 15 years, acute attack, 1 g daily for 2–4 weeks; maintenance, 1 g daily; CHILD 12–15 years see *BNF for Children*

**Salofalk®** (Dr Falk) PoM
Tablets, e/c, yellow, mesalazine 250 mg. Net price 100-tab pack = £16.50. Label: 5, 25, counselling, blood disorder symptoms (see recommendation above)

**Dose** ADULT and CHILD over 15 years, acute attack, 1.5 g daily in 3 divided doses; maintenance, 0.75–1.5 g daily in divided doses; CHILD 12–15 years see *BNF for Children*

Granules, m/r, grey, e/c, vanilla-flavoured, mesalazine 500 mg/sachet, net price 100-sachet pack = £29.30; 1 g/sachet, 50-sachet pack = £29.30; 1.5 g/sachet, 60-sachet pack = £49.80. Label: 25, counselling, administration, see dose, blood disorder symptoms (see recommendation above)

Excipients include aspartame (section 9.4.1)

**Dose** ADULT and CHILD over 15 years, acute attack, 1.5–3 g once daily (preferably in the morning) or 0.5–1 g 3 times daily; maintenance, 500 mg 3 times daily; CHILD 6–15 years, body-weight under 40 kg see *BNF for Children*, body-weight over 40 kg, adult dose; granules should be placed on tongue and washed down with water without chewing

**Note** Preparations that lower stool pH (e.g. lactulose) may prevent release of mesalazine

Suppositories, mesalazine 500 mg. Net price 30-suppos pack = £15.10. Counselling, blood disorder symptoms (see recommendation above)

**Dose** ADULT and CHILD over 15 years, acute attack, by rectum, 0.5–1 g 2–3 times daily adjusted according to response; CHILD 12–15 years see *BNF for Children*

Enema, mesalazine 2 g in 59-mL pack. Net price 7 enemas = £30.50. Counselling, blood disorder symptoms (see recommendation above)

**Dose** acute attack *or* maintenance, by rectum, 2 g daily at bedtime; CHILD 12–18 years see *BNF for Children*

Rectal foam, mesalazine 1 g/metered application, net price 14-application canister with disposable applicators and plastic bags = £30.75. Counselling, blood disorder symptoms (see recommendation above)

Excipients include cetostearyl alcohol, disodium edetate, polysorbate 60, propylene glycol, sodium metabisulphite

**Dose** mild ulcerative colitis affecting sigmoid colon and rectum, ADULT and CHILD over 12 years, 2 metered applications (mesalazine 2 g) into the rectum at bedtime increased if necessary to 2 metered applications (mesalazine 2 g) twice daily

## ▌ OLSALAZINE SODIUM

**Indications** treatment of mild ulcerative colitis and maintenance of remission

**Cautions** see notes above; **interactions:** Appendix 1 (aminosalicylates)
**Blood disorders** See recommendation above

**Contra-indications** see notes above

**Side-effects** see notes above; watery diarrhoea common; also reported, tachycardia, palpitation, pyrexia, blurred vision, and photosensitivity

**Dose**
- ADULT and CHILD over 12 years, acute attack, 1 g daily in divided doses after meals increased if necessary over 1 week to max. 3 g daily (max. single dose 1 g); maintenance, 500 mg twice daily after meals
- CHILD under 12 years see *BNF for Children*

**Dipentum®** (UCB Pharma) PoM
Capsules, brown, olsalazine sodium 250 mg. Net price 112-cap pack = £19.77. Label: 21, counselling, blood disorder symptoms (see recommendation above)

Tablets, yellow, scored, olsalazine sodium 500 mg. Net price 60-tab pack = £21.18. Label: 21, counselling, blood disorder symptoms (see recommendation above)

**1**

**Gastro-intestinal system**

## SULFASALAZINE
(Sulphasalazine)

**Indications** treatment of mild to moderate and severe ulcerative colitis and maintenance of remission; active Crohn's disease; rheumatoid arthritis (section 10.1.3)

**Cautions** see notes above; also history of allergy; hepatic impairment; G6PD deficiency (section 9.1.5); slow acetylator status; risk of haematological and hepatic toxicity (differential white cell, red cell, and platelet counts initially and at monthly intervals for first 3 months; liver function tests at monthly intervals for first 3 months); upper gastro-intestinal side-effects common over 4 g daily; acute porphyria (section 9.8.2); **interactions:** Appendix 1 (aminosalicylates) **Blood disorders** See recommendation above

**Contra-indications** see notes above; also sulphonamide hypersensitivity; child under 2 years of age

**Side-effects** see notes above; also loss of appetite; fever; blood disorders (including Heinz body anaemia, megaloblastic anaemia); hypersensitivity reactions (including exfoliative dermatitis, epidermal necrolysis, pruritus, photosensitisation, anaphylaxis, serum sickness); ocular complications (including periorbital oedema); stomatitis, parotitis; ataxia, aseptic meningitis, vertigo, tinnitus, insomnia, depression, hallucinations; kidney reactions (including proteinuria, crystalluria, haematuria); oligospermia; urine may be coloured orange; some soft contact lenses may be stained

**Dose**
- By mouth, acute attack 1–2 g 4 times daily (but see **cautions**) until remission occurs (if necessary corticosteroids may also be given), reducing to a maintenance dose of 500 mg 4 times daily; CHILD 2–12 years see *BNF for Children*
- By rectum, in suppositories, alone or in conjunction with oral treatment 0.5–1 g morning and night after a bowel movement; CHILD 5–12 years see *BNF for Children*

**Sulfasalazine** (Non-proprietary) [PoM]
Tablets, sulfasalazine 500 mg. Net price 112 = £9.11. Label: 14, counselling, blood disorder symptoms (see recommendation above), contact lenses may be stained

Tablets, e/c, sulfasalazine 500 mg. Net price 112-tab pack = £16.15. Label: 5, 14, 25, counselling, blood disorder symptoms (see recommendation above), contact lenses may be stained
Brands include *Sulazine EC*®

**Salazopyrin**® (Pharmacia) [PoM]
Tablets, yellow, scored, sulfasalazine 500 mg. Net price 112-tab pack = £6.97. Label: 14, counselling, blood disorder symptoms (see recommendation above), contact lenses may be stained

EN-Tabs® (= tablets e/c), yellow, f/c, sulfasalazine 500 mg. Net price 112-tab pack = £8.43. Label: 5, 14, 25, counselling, blood disorder symptoms (see recommendation above), contact lenses may be stained

Suspension, yellow, sulfasalazine 250 mg/5 mL. Net price 500 mL = £18.84. Label: 14, counselling, blood disorder symptoms (see recommendation above), contact lenses may be stained

Suppositories, yellow, sulfasalazine 500 mg. Net price 10 = £3.30. Label: 14, counselling, blood dis-

order symptoms (see recommendation above), contact lenses may be stained

## 1.5.2 Corticosteroids

For the role of corticosteroids in acute ulcerative colitis and Crohn's disease, see Inflammatory Bowel Disease, p. 52.

## BECLOMETASONE DIPROPIONATE

**Indications** adjunct to aminosalicylates in acute mild to moderate ulcerative colitis; asthma (section 3.2); allergic and vasomotor rhinitis (section 12.2.1); oral ulceration [unlicensed indication] (section 12.3.1)

**Cautions** section 6.3.2; **interactions:** Appendix 1 (corticosteroids)

**Contra-indications** section 6.3.2

**Side-effects** section 6.3.2; also nausea, constipation, headache, and drowsiness

**Dose**
- 5 mg in the morning; max. duration of treatment 4 weeks; CHILD safety and efficacy not established

**Clipper**® (Chiesi) [PoM]
Tablets, m/r, ivory, beclometasone dipropionate 5 mg, net price 30-tab pack = £57.66. Label: 25

## BUDESONIDE

**Indications** see preparations

**Cautions** section 6.3.2; **interactions:** Appendix 1 (corticosteroids)

**Contra-indications** section 6.3.2

**Side-effects** section 6.3.2

**Dose**
- See preparations

**Budenofalk**® (Dr Falk) [PoM]
Capsules, pink, enclosing e/c pellets, budesonide 3 mg, net price 100-cap pack = £76.50. Label: 5, 10, steroid card, 22, 25
**Dose** mild to moderate Crohn's disease affecting ileum or ascending colon, chronic diarrhoea due to collagenous colitis, ADULT over 18 years, 3 mg 3 times daily for up to 8 weeks; reduce dose for the last 2 weeks of treatment (see also section 6.3.2); CHILD 12–18 years see *BNF for Children*

Rectal foam, budesonide 2 mg/metered application, net price 14-application canister with disposable applicators and plastic bags = £58.22
**Excipients** include cetyl alcohol, disodium edetate, propylene glycol, sorbic acid
**Dose** ulcerative colitis affecting sigmoid colon and rectum, by rectum, ADULT over 18 years, 1 metered application (budesonide 2 mg) once daily for up to 8 weeks

**Entocort**® (AstraZeneca) [PoM]
CR Capsules, grey/pink, enclosing e/c, m/r granules, budesonide 3 mg, net price 100-cap pack = £99.00. Label: 5, 10, steroid card, 25
**Note** Dispense in original container (contains desiccant)
**Dose** mild to moderate Crohn's disease affecting the ileum or ascending colon, 9 mg once daily in the morning for up to 8 weeks; reduce dose for the last 2–4 weeks of treatment (see also section 6.3.2); CHILD 12–18 years see *BNF for Children*

Enema, budesonide 2 mg/100 mL when dispersible tablet reconstituted in isotonic saline vehicle, net price pack of 7 dispersible tablets and bottles of vehicle = £33.00

**Dose** ulcerative colitis involving rectal and recto-sigmoid disease, by rectum, 1 enema at bedtime for 4 weeks; CHILD 12–18 years see *BNF for Children*

## HYDROCORTISONE

**Indications** ulcerative colitis, proctitis, proctosigmoiditis

**Cautions** section 6.3.2; systemic absorption may occur; prolonged use should be avoided

**Contra-indications** intestinal obstruction, bowel perforation, recent intestinal anastomoses, extensive fistulas; untreated infection

**Side-effects** section 6.3.2; also local irritation

**Dose**

- By rectum see preparations

**Colifoam®** (Meda) PoM

Foam in aerosol pack, hydrocortisone acetate 10%, net price 14-application canister with applicator = £8.21

Excipients include cetyl alcohol, hydroxybenzoates (parabens), propylene glycol

**Dose** initially 1 metered application (125 mg hydrocortisone acetate) inserted into the rectum once or twice daily for 2–3 weeks, then once on alternate days; CHILD 2–18 years see *BNF for Children*

## PREDNISOLONE

**Indications** ulcerative colitis, and Crohn's disease; other indications, see section 6.3.2, see also preparations

**Cautions** section 6.3.2; systemic absorption may occur with rectal preparations; prolonged use should be avoided

**Contra-indications** section 6.3.2; intestinal obstruction, bowel perforation, recent intestinal anastomoses, extensive fistulas; untreated infection

**Side-effects** section 6.3.2

**Dose**

- By mouth, initially 20–40 mg daily (up to 60 mg daily in some cases), preferably taken in the morning after breakfast; continued until remission occurs, followed by reducing doses
- By rectum, see preparations

◢Oral preparations
Section 6.3.2

◢Rectal preparations

**Predenema®** (Forest) PoM

Retention enema, prednisolone 20 mg (as sodium metasulphobenzoate) in 100-mL single-dose disposable pack. Net price 1 (standard tube) = 71p, 1 (long tube) = £1.21

**Dose** ulcerative colitis, by rectum, ADULT and CHILD over 12 years, initially 20 mg at bedtime for 2–4 weeks, continued if good response

**Predfoam®** (Forest) PoM

Foam in aerosol pack, prednisolone 20 mg (as metasulphobenzoate sodium)/metered application, net price 14-application canister with disposable applicators = £6.32

Excipients include cetostearyl alcohol, disodium edetate, polysorbate 20, sorbic acid

**Dose** proctitis and distal ulcerative colitis, 1 metered application (20 mg prednisolone) inserted into the rectum once or twice daily

for 2 weeks, continued for further 2 weeks if good response; CHILD not recommended

**Predsol®** (UCB Pharma) PoM

Retention enema, prednisolone 20 mg (as sodium phosphate) in 100-mL single-dose disposable packs fitted with a nozzle. Net price 7 = £6.00

**Dose** rectal and rectosigmoidal ulcerative colitis and Crohn's disease, by rectum, initially 20 mg at bedtime for 2–4 weeks, continued if good response; CHILD not recommended

Suppositories, prednisolone 5 mg (as sodium phosphate). Net price 10 = £1.35

**Dose** ADULT and CHILD proctitis and rectal complications of Crohn's disease, by rectum, 5 mg inserted night and morning after a bowel movement

## 1.5.3 Drugs affecting the immune response

For the role of **azathioprine**, **ciclosporin**, **mercaptopurine**, and **methotrexate** in the treatment of inflammatory bowel disease, see p. 52.

## AZATHIOPRINE

**Indications** see under Inflammatory Bowel Disease, p. 52; autoimmune conditions and prophylaxis of transplant rejection (section 8.2.1); rheumatoid arthritis (section 10.1.3)

**Cautions** section 8.2.1

**Contra-indications** section 8.2.1

**Side-effects** section 8.2.1

**Dose**

- Severe acute Crohn's disease, maintenance of remission of Crohn's disease or ulcerative colitis [unlicensed indications], ADULT over 18 years, by mouth, 2–2.5 mg/kg daily; some patients may respond to lower doses

◢Preparations
Section 8.2.1

## CICLOSPORIN
(Cyclosporin)

**Indications** severe acute ulcerative colitis refractory to corticosteroid treatment [unlicensed indication]; transplantation and graft-versus-host disease, nephrotic syndrome (section 8.2.2); rheumatoid arthritis (section 10.1.3); atopic dermatitis and psoriasis (section 13.5.3)

**Cautions** section 8.2.2

**Contra-indications** section 8.2.2

**Side-effects** section 8.2.2

**Dose**

- By continuous intravenous infusion, ADULT over 18 years, 2 mg/kg daily over 24 hours; dose adjusted according to blood-ciclosporin concentration and response

◢Preparations
Section 8.2.2

1

Gastro-intestinal system

## MERCAPTOPURINE

**Indications** see under Inflammatory Bowel disease, p. 52; acute leukaemias and chronic myeloid leukaemia (section 8.1.3)

**Cautions** section 8.1.3

**Contra-indications** section 8.1.3

**Side-effects** section 8.1.3

**Dose**

- Severe acute Crohn's disease, maintenance of remission of Crohn's disease or ulcerative colitis [unlicensed indications], ADULT over 18 years, by mouth, 1–1.5 mg/kg daily; some patients may respond to lower doses

◢Preparations
Section 8.1.3

## METHOTREXATE

**Indications** see under Inflammatory Bowel Disease, p. 52; malignant disease (section 8.1.3); rheumatoid arthritis (section 10.1.3); psoriasis (section 13.5.3)

**Cautions** section 10.1.3

**Contra-indications** section 10.1.3

**Side-effects** section 10.1.3

**Dose**

- By intramuscular injection, severe Crohn's disease [unlicensed indication], ADULT over 18 years, induction of remission, 25 mg once weekly; maintenance, 15 mg once weekly
- By mouth, maintenance of remission of severe Crohn's disease [unlicensed indication], ADULT over 18 years, 10–25 mg once weekly

> **Important**
> Note that the above dose is a **weekly** dose. To avoid error with low-dose methotrexate, it is recommended that:
> - the patient is carefully advised of the **dose** and **frequency** and the reason for taking methotrexate and any other prescribed medicine (e.g. folic acid);
> - only one strength of methotrexate tablet (usually 2.5 mg) is prescribed and dispensed;
> - the prescription and the dispensing label clearly show the dose and frequency of methotrexate administration;
> - the patient is warned to report immediately the onset of any feature of blood disorders (e.g. sore throat, bruising, and mouth ulcers), liver toxicity (e.g. nausea, vomiting, abdominal discomfort, and dark urine), and respiratory effects (e.g. shortness of breath).

◢Preparations
Section 10.1.3

## Cytokine modulators

**Infliximab** and **adalimumab** are monoclonal antibodies which inhibit the pro-inflammatory cytokine, tumour necrosis factor alpha. They should be used under specialist supervision. Adequate resuscitation facilities must be available when infliximab is used.

## ADALIMUMAB

**Indications** see under Inflammatory Bowel Disease, p. 53; ankylosing spondylitis, psoriatic arthritis, rheumatoid arthritis, juvenile idiopathic arthritis, (section 10.1.3); psoriasis (section 13.5.3)

**Cautions** section 10.1.3

**Contra-indications** section 10.1.3

**Side-effects** section 10.1.3

**Dose**

- By subcutaneous injection, severe active Crohn's disease, ADULT over 18 years, initially 80 mg, then 40 mg 2 weeks after initial dose or accelerated regimen, initially 160 mg in 4 divided doses over 1–2 days, then 80 mg 2 weeks after initial dose; maintenance, 40 mg on alternate weeks, increased if necessary to 40 mg weekly; review treatment if no response within 12 weeks of initial dose

◢Preparations
Section 10.1.3

## INFLIXIMAB

**Indications** see under Inflammatory Bowel Disease, p. 52; ankylosing spondylitis, rheumatoid arthritis (section 10.1.3); psoriasis (section 13.5.3)

**Cautions** see section 10.1.3; also history of dysplasia or colon carcinoma

**Hypersensitivity reactions** Risk of delayed hypersensitivity if drug-free interval exceeds 16 weeks

**Contra-indications** see section 10.1.3

**Side-effects** see section 10.1.3; also hepatosplenic T-cell lymphoma

**Dose**

- By intravenous infusion, severe active Crohn's disease, ADULT over 18 years, initially 5 mg/kg, then 5 mg/kg 2 weeks after initial dose; then if the condition has responded, maintenance either 5 mg/kg 6 weeks after initial dose, then 5 mg/kg every 8 weeks or further dose of 5 mg/kg if signs and symptoms recur; CHILD 6–18 years, initially 5 mg/kg, then 5 mg/kg 2 weeks and 6 weeks after initial dose, then 5 mg/kg every 8 weeks; interval between maintenance doses adjusted according to response; discontinue if no response within 10 weeks of initial dose

Fistulating Crohn's disease, ADULT over 18 years, initially 5 mg/kg, then 5 mg/kg 2 weeks and 6 weeks after initial dose, then if condition has responded, consult product literature for guidance on further doses; CHILD under 18 years, see *BNF for Children*

Severe active ulcerative colitis, ADULT over 18 years, initially 5 mg/kg, then 5 mg/kg 2 weeks and 6 weeks after initial dose, then 5 mg/kg every 8 weeks; discontinue if no response 14 weeks after initial dose

◢Preparations
Section 10.1.3

## 1.5.4 Food allergy

Allergy with classical symptoms of vomiting, colic and diarrhoea caused by specific foods such as shellfish should be managed by strict avoidance. The condition should be distinguished from symptoms of occasional food intolerance in those with irritable bowel syndrome. **Sodium cromoglicate** (sodium cromoglycate) may be helpful as an adjunct to dietary avoidance.

## SODIUM CROMOGLICATE
(Sodium cromoglycate)

**Indications** food allergy (in conjunction with dietary restriction); asthma (section 3.3); allergic conjunctivitis (section 11.4.2); allergic rhinitis (section 12.2.1)

**Side-effects** occasional nausea, rashes, and joint pain

**Dose**

- 200 mg 4 times daily before meals; may be increased if necessary after 2–3 weeks to a max. of 40 mg/kg daily and then reduced according to response; CHILD 2–14 years 100 mg 4 times daily before meals; may be increased if necessary after 2–3 weeks to a max. of 40 mg/kg daily and then reduced according to response

  **Counselling** Capsules may be swallowed whole or the contents dissolved in hot water and diluted with cold water before taking

**Nalcrom®** (Sanofi-Aventis) [PoM]

Capsules, sodium cromoglicate 100 mg. Net price 100-cap pack = £59.75. Label: 22, counselling, see dose above

## 1.6 Laxatives

|       |                                   |
|-------|-----------------------------------|
| 1.6.1 | **Bulk-forming laxatives**        |
| 1.6.2 | **Stimulant laxatives**           |
| 1.6.3 | **Faecal softeners**              |
| 1.6.4 | **Osmotic laxatives**             |
| 1.6.5 | **Bowel cleansing preparations**  |
| 1.6.6 | **Peripheral opioid-receptor antagonists** |

Before prescribing laxatives it is important to be sure that the patient *is* constipated and that the constipation is *not* secondary to an underlying undiagnosed complaint.

It is also important for those who complain of constipation to understand that bowel habit can vary considerably in frequency without doing harm. Some people tend to consider themselves constipated if they do not have a bowel movement each day. A useful definition of constipation is the passage of hard stools less frequently than the patient's own normal pattern and this can be explained to the patient.

Misconceptions about bowel habits have led to excessive laxative use. Abuse may lead to hypokalaemia.

Thus, laxatives should generally be **avoided** except where straining will exacerbate a condition (such as angina) or increase the risk of rectal bleeding as in haemorrhoids. Laxatives are also of value in *drug-induced constipation*, for the expulsion of *parasites* after anthelmintic treatment, and to clear the alimentary tract before *surgery and radiological procedures*. Prolonged treatment of constipation is sometimes necessary.

For the role of laxatives in the treatment of irritable bowel syndrome, see p. 53.

**Children** Laxatives should be prescribed by a healthcare professional experienced in the management of constipation in children. Delays of greater than 3 days between stools may increase the likelihood of pain on passing hard stools leading to anal fissure, anal spasm

and eventually to a learned response to avoid defaecation.

If increased fluid and fibre intake is insufficient, an osmotic laxative containing macrogols or lactulose (section 1.6.4) can be used. If there is evidence of minor faecal retention, the addition of a stimulant laxative (section 1.6.2) may overcome withholding but may lead to colic or, in the presence of faecal impaction in the rectum, an increase of faecal overflow.

In children with faecal impaction, an oral preparation containing macrogols is used to clear faecal mass and to establish and maintain soft well-formed stools. Rectal administration of laxatives may be effective but this route is frequently distressing for the child and may lead to persistent withholding. If the impacted mass is not expelled following treatment with macrogols, referral to hospital may be necessary. Enemas may be administered under heavy sedation in hospital or alternatively, a bowel cleansing preparation (section 1.6.5) may be tried. In severe cases or where the child is afraid, a manual evacuation under anaesthetic may be appropriate.

Long-term regular use of laxatives is essential to maintain well-formed stools and prevent recurrence of faecal impaction; intermittent use may provoke relapses.

> For children with chronic constipation, it may be necessary to exceed the licensed doses of some laxatives. Parents and carers of children should be advised to adjust the dose of laxative in order to establish a regular pattern of bowel movements in which stools are soft, well-formed, and passed without discomfort.

**Pregnancy** If dietary and lifestyle changes fail to control constipation in pregnancy, moderate doses of poorly absorbed laxatives may be used. A bulk-forming laxative should be tried first. An osmotic laxative, such as lactulose, can also be used. Bisacodyl or senna may be suitable, if a stimulant effect is necessary.

> The laxatives that follow have been divided into 5 main groups (sections 1.6.1–1.6.5). This simple classification disguises the fact that some laxatives have a complex action.

## 1.6.1 Bulk-forming laxatives

Bulk-forming laxatives relieve constipation by increasing faecal mass which stimulates peristalsis; patients should be advised that the full effect may take some days to develop.

Bulk-forming laxatives are of particular value in those with small hard stools, but should not be required unless fibre cannot be increased in the diet. A balanced diet, including adequate fluid intake and fibre is of value in preventing constipation.

Bulk-forming laxatives are useful in the management of patients with *colostomy, ileostomy, haemorrhoids, anal fissure, chronic diarrhoea associated with diverticular disease, irritable bowel syndrome,* and as adjuncts in *ulcerative colitis* (section 1.5). Adequate fluid intake must be

Gastro-intestinal system

**1**

maintained to avoid intestinal obstruction. Unprocessed wheat **bran**, taken with food or fruit juice, is a most effective bulk-forming preparation. Finely ground bran, though more palatable, has poorer water-retaining properties, but can be taken as bran bread or biscuits in appropriately increased quantities. Oat bran is also used.

**Methylcellulose**, **ispaghula**, and **sterculia** are useful in patients who cannot tolerate bran. Methylcellulose also acts as a faecal softener.

## ISPAGHULA HUSK

**Indications** see notes above

**Cautions** adequate fluid intake should be maintained to avoid intestinal obstruction—it may be necessary to supervise elderly or debilitated patients or those with intestinal narrowing or decreased motility

**Contra-indications** difficulty in swallowing, intestinal obstruction, colonic atony, faecal impaction

**Side-effects** flatulence, abdominal distension, gastro-intestinal obstruction or impaction; hypersensitivity reported

**Dose**

* See preparations below

**Counselling** Preparations that swell in contact with liquid should always be carefully swallowed with water and should not be taken immediately before going to bed

**Fibrelief®** (Manx)

Granules, sugar- and gluten-free, ispaghula husk 3.5 g/sachet (natural or orange flavour), net price 10 sachets = £1.23, 30 sachets = £2.07. Label: 13, counselling, see above

Excipients include aspartame (section 9.4.1)

**Dose** ADULT and CHILD over 12 years, 1–6 sachets daily in water in 1–3 divided doses

**Fybogel®** (R&C)

Granules, buff, effervescent, sugar- and gluten-free, ispaghula husk 3.5 g/sachet (low Na⁺), net price 30 sachets (plain, lemon, or orange flavour) = £1.84. Label: 13, counselling, see above

Excipients include aspartame 16 mg/sachet (see section 9.4.1)

**Dose** 1 sachet or 2 level 5-mL spoonfuls in water twice daily preferably after meals; CHILD (but see section 1.6) 2–12 years ⅓–1 level 5-mL spoonful in water, twice daily preferably after meals (CHILD 2–6 years on specialist practitioner's advice only)

**Isogel®** (Potters)

Granules, brown, sugar- and gluten-free, ispaghula husk 90%. Net price 200 g = £2.67. Label: 13, counselling, see above

**Dose** constipation, 2 level 5-mL spoonfuls in water once or twice daily, preferably at mealtimes; CHILD (but see section 1.6) 2–12 years, 1 level 5-mL spoonful in water once or twice daily, preferably at mealtimes

Diarrhoea (section 1.4.1), 1 level 5-mL spoonful 3 times daily

**Note** May be difficult to obtain

**Ispagel Orange®** (LPC)

Granules, beige, effervescent, sugar- and gluten-free, ispaghula husk 3.5 g/sachet, net price 30 sachets = £2.10. Label: 13, counselling, see above

Excipients include aspartame (section 9.4.1)

**Dose** 1 sachet in water 1–3 times daily; CHILD (but see section 1.6) 2–12 years see BNF for Children

**Regulan®** (Procter & Gamble)

Powder, beige, sugar- and gluten-free, ispaghula husk 3.4 g/5.85-g sachet (orange or lemon/lime flavour).

Net price 30 sachets = £2.44. Label: 13, counselling, see above

Excipients include aspartame (section 9.4.1)

**Dose** 1 sachet in 150 mL water 1–3 times daily; CHILD (but see section 1.6) 2–6 years, see BNF for Children; 6–12 years 2.5–5 mL in water 1–3 times daily

## METHYLCELLULOSE

**Indications** see notes above; adjunct in obesity (but see section 4.5.1)

**Cautions** see under Ispaghula Husk

**Contra-indications** see under Ispaghula Husk; also infective bowel disease

**Side-effects** see under Ispaghula Husk

**Dose**

* See preparations below

**Counselling** Preparations that swell in contact with liquid should always be carefully swallowed with water and should not be taken immediately before going to bed

**Celevac®** (Amdipharm)

Tablets, pink, scored, methylcellulose '450' 500 mg, net price 112-tab pack = £3.22. Counselling, see above and dose

**Dose** constipation and diarrhoea, 3–6 tablets twice daily; in constipation the dose should be taken with at least 300 mL liquid; in diarrhoea, ileostomy, and colostomy control, avoid liquid intake for 30 minutes before and after dose; CHILD 7–12 years see BNF for Children

Adjunct in obesity (but see section 4.5.1), 3 tablets with at least 300 mL warm liquid 30 minutes before food or when hungry

## STERCULIA

**Indications** see notes above

**Cautions** see under Ispaghula Husk

**Contra-indications** see under Ispaghula Husk

**Side-effects** see under Ispaghula Husk

**Dose**

* See under preparations below

**Counselling** Preparations that swell in contact with liquid should always be carefully swallowed with water and should not be taken immediately before going to bed

**Normacol®** (Norgine)

Granules, coated, gluten-free, sterculia 62%. Net price 500 g = £5.94; 60 × 7-g sachets = £4.99. Label: 25, 27, counselling, see above

**Dose** 1–2 heaped 5-mL spoonfuls, or the contents of 1–2 sachets, washed down without chewing with plenty of liquid once or twice daily after meals; CHILD (but see section 1.6) 6–12 years half adult dose

**Normacol Plus®** (Norgine)

Granules, brown, coated, gluten-free, sterculia 62%, frangula (standardised) 8%. Net price 500 g = £6.34; 60 × 7 g sachets = £5.34. Label: 25, 27, counselling, see above

**Dose** constipation and after haemorrhoidectomy, 1–2 heaped 5-mL spoonfuls or the contents of 1–2 sachets washed down without chewing with plenty of liquid once or twice daily after meals; CHILD 6–12 years see BNF for Children

## 1.6.2 Stimulant laxatives

Stimulant laxatives include **bisacodyl**, **sodium picosulfate**, and members of the **anthraquinone** group, **senna** and **dantron** (danthron). The indications for dantron are limited (see below) by its potential carcinogenicity (based on *rodent* carcinogenicity studies) and evidence of genotoxicity. Powerful stimulants such as **cascara** (an anthraquinone) and **castor oil** are obsolete. **Docusate sodium** probably acts both as a stimulant and as a softening agent.

Stimulant laxatives increase intestinal motility and often cause abdominal cramp; they should be avoided in intestinal obstruction. Excessive use of stimulant laxatives can cause diarrhoea and related effects such as hypokalaemia; however, prolonged use may be justifiable in some circumstances (see section 1.6 for the use of stimulant laxatives in children).

**Glycerol** suppositories act as a rectal stimulant by virtue of the mildly irritant action of glycerol.

The **parasympathomimetics** bethanechol, distigmine, neostigmine, and pyridostigmine (see section 7.4.1 and section 10.2.1) enhance parasympathetic activity in the gut and increase intestinal motility. They are rarely used for their gastro-intestinal effects. Organic obstruction of the gut must first be excluded and they should not be used shortly after bowel anastomosis.

## ■ BISACODYL

**Indications** see under Dose

**Cautions** see notes above; pregnancy, see p. 59

**Contra-indications** see notes above, acute surgical abdominal conditions, acute inflammatory bowel disease, severe dehydration

**Side-effects** see notes above; nausea and vomiting; colitis also reported; *suppositories*, local irritation

**Dose**

- Constipation, by mouth, 5–10 mg at night; CHILD (but see section 1.6) 4–18 years see *BNF for Children*

  By rectum in suppositories, 10 mg in the morning; CHILD (but see section 1.6) 2–18 years see *BNF for Children*

- Before radiological procedures and surgery, by mouth, 10–20 mg the night before procedure and by rectum in suppositories, 10 mg the following morning; CHILD 4–10 years by mouth, 5 mg the night before procedure and by rectum in suppositories, 5 mg the following morning; over 10 years, adult dose

**Note** tablets act in 10–12 hours; suppositories act in 20–60 minutes

**Bisacodyl** (Non-proprietary)

Tablets, e/c, bisacodyl 5 mg. Net price 100 = £3.27. Label: 5, 25

Suppositories, bisacodyl 10 mg. Net price 12 = 89p

Paediatric suppositories, bisacodyl 5 mg. Net price 5 = 94p

**Note** The brand name *Dulcolax*® ᴹˢ (Boehringer Ingelheim) is used for bisacodyl tablets, net price 10-tab pack = 74p; suppositories (10 mg), 10 = £1.57; paediatric suppositories (5 mg), 5 = 94p

The brand names *Dulcolax*® *Liquid* and *Dulcolax*® *Perles* are used for sodium picosulfate preparations

## ■ DANTRON
(Danthron)

**Indications** only for constipation in terminally ill patients of all ages

**Cautions** see notes above; *rodent* studies indicate potential carcinogenic risk; avoid prolonged contact with skin (as in incontinent patients or infants wearing

nappies)—risk of irritation and excoriation; pregnancy (Appendix 4) and breast-feeding (Appendix 5)

**Contra-indications** See notes above

**Side-effects** see notes above; urine may be coloured red

**Dose**

- See under preparations

### ◀With poloxamer '188' (as co-danthramer)

**Note** Co-danthramer suspension 5 mL = one co-danthramer capsule, **but** strong co-danthramer suspension 5 mL = two strong co-danthramer capsules

**Co-danthramer** (Non-proprietary) ᴾᵒᴹ

Capsules, co-danthramer 25/200 (dantron 25 mg, poloxamer '188' 200 mg). Net price 60-cap pack = £12.86. Label: 14, (urine red)

**Dose** 1–2 capsules at bedtime; CHILD 1 capsule at bedtime (restricted indications, see notes above)

Strong capsules, co-danthramer 37.5/500 (dantron 37.5 mg, poloxamer '188' 500 mg). Net price 60-cap pack = £15.55. Label: 14, (urine red)

**Dose** ADULT and CHILD over 12 years, 1–2 capsules at bedtime (restricted indications, see notes above)

Suspension, co-danthramer 25/200 in 5 mL (dantron 25 mg, poloxamer '188' 200 mg/5 mL). Net price 300 mL = £11.27, 1 litre = £37.57. Label: 14, (urine red)

**Dose** 5–10 mL at night; CHILD 2.5–5 mL (restricted indications, see notes above)

Brands include *Codalax*® ᴹˢ, *Danlax*®

Strong suspension, co-danthramer 75/1000 in 5 mL (dantron 75 mg, poloxamer '188' 1 g/5 mL). Net price 300 mL = £30.13. Label: 14, (urine red)

**Dose** ADULT and CHILD over 12 years, 5 mL at night (restricted indications, see notes above)

Brands include *Codalax Forte*® ᴹˢ

### ◀With docusate sodium (as co-danthrusate)

**Co-danthrusate** (Non-proprietary) ᴾᵒᴹ

Capsules, co-danthrusate 50/60 (dantron 50 mg, docusate sodium 60 mg). Net price 63-cap pack = £14.50. Label: 14, (urine red)

**Dose** 1–3 capsules at night; CHILD 6–12 years 1 capsule at night (restricted indications, see notes above)

Brands include *Normax*® ᴹˢ

Suspension, yellow, co-danthrusate 50/60 (dantron 50 mg, docusate sodium 60 mg/5 mL). Net price 200 mL = £8.75. Label: 14, (urine red)

**Dose** 5–15 mL at night; CHILD 6–12 years 5 mL at night (restricted indications, see notes above)

Brands include *Normax*®

## ■ DOCUSATE SODIUM
(Dioctyl sodium sulphosuccinate)

**Indications** constipation, adjunct in abdominal radiological procedures

**Cautions** see notes above; do not give with liquid paraffin; rectal preparations not indicated if haemorrhoids or anal fissure; pregnancy (Appendix 4); breast-feeding (Appendix 5)

**Contra-indications** see notes above

**Side-effects** see notes above

**Dose**

- By mouth, chronic constipation, up to 500 mg daily in divided doses; CHILD (but see section 1.6) 6 months–2 years 12.5 mg 3 times daily, 2–12 years

**Gastro-intestinal system** 1

12.5–25 mg 3 times daily (use paediatric oral solution only)

Note Oral preparations act within 1–2 days

With barium meal, ADULT and CHILD over 12 years, 400 mg

**Dioctyl®** (UCB Pharma)

Capsules, yellow/white, docusate sodium 100 mg, net price 30-cap pack = £1.92, 100-cap pack = £6.40

**Docusol®** (Typharm)

Adult oral solution, sugar-free, docusate sodium 50 mg/5 mL, net price 300 mL = £5.49

Paediatric oral solution, sugar-free, docusate sodium 12.5 mg/5 mL, net price 300 mL = £5.29

◢**Rectal preparations**

**Norgalax Micro-enema®** (Norgine)

Enema, docusate sodium 120 mg in 10-g single-dose disposable packs. Net price 10-g unit = 57p

Dose ADULT and CHILD (but see section 1.6) over 12 years, 10-g unit

## GLYCEROL
(Glycerin)

**Indications** constipation

**Dose**
● See below

**Glycerol Suppositories, BP**
(Glycerin Suppositories)

Suppositories, gelatin 140 mg, glycerol 700 mg, purified water to 1 g, net price 12 = £1.04 (1 g), £1.02 (2 g), £1.47 (4 g)

Dose 1 suppository moistened with water before use, when required. The usual sizes are for INFANT under 1 year, small (1-g mould), CHILD 1–12 years medium (2-g mould), ADULT and CHILD over 12 years, large (4-g mould)

## SENNA

**Indications** constipation

**Cautions** see notes above; pregnancy, see p. 59

**Contra-indications** see notes above

**Side-effects** see notes above

**Dose**
● See under preparations

Note Acts in 8–12 hours

**Senna** (Non-proprietary)

Tablets, total sennosides (calculated as sennoside B) 7.5 mg. Net price 60 = £1.89

Dose 2–4 tablets, usually at night; initial dose should be low then gradually increased; CHILD (but see section 1.6) 6–12 years, half adult dose in the morning (on doctor's advice only)

Note Lower dose on packs on sale to the public

Brands include Senokot® ᴺᴴˢ

**Manevac®** (Galen)

Granules, coated, senna fruit 12.4%, ispaghula 54.2%, net price 400 g = £7.45. Label: 25, 27, counselling, see Ispaghula Husk

Dose 1–2 level 5-mL spoonfuls with water or warm drink after supper and, if necessary, before breakfast or every 6 hours in resistant cases for 1–3 days; CHILD (but see section 1.6) 5–12 years 1 level 5-mL spoonful daily

Counselling Preparations that swell in contact with liquid should always be carefully swallowed with water and should not be taken immediately before going to bed

**Senokot®** (R&C)

Tablets ᴺᴴˢ, see above

Syrup, sugar-free, brown, total sennosides (calculated as sennoside B) 7.5 mg/5 mL, net price 500 mL = £2.69

Dose 10–20 mL, usually at bedtime; CHILD (but see section 1.6) 1 month–2 years see BNF for Children, 2–6 years 2.5–5 mL in the morning, 6–12 years 5–10 mL at night or in the morning

Note Lower dose on packs on sale to the public

## SODIUM PICOSULFATE
(Sodium picosulphate)

**Indications** constipation; bowel evacuation before abdominal radiological and endoscopic procedures on the colon, and surgery (section 1.6.5); acts within 6–12 hours

**Cautions** see notes above; active inflammatory bowel disease (avoid if fulminant); pregnancy, see p. 59; breast-feeding (Appendix 5)

**Contra-indications** see notes above; severe dehydration

**Side-effects** see notes above

**Dose**
● 5–10 mg at night; CHILD (but see section 1.6) 1 month–4 years 250 micrograms/kg (max. 5 mg) at night; 4–10 years 2.5–5 mg at night; over 10 years, adult dose

**Sodium Picosulfate** (Non-proprietary)

Elixir, sodium picosulfate 5 mg/5 mL, net price 100 mL = £1.85

Note The brand name Dulcolax® Liquid (Boehringer Ingelheim) is used for sodium picosulfate elixir 5 mg/5 mL

**Dulcolax®** (Boehringer Ingelheim)

Perles® (= capsules), sodium picosulfate 2.5 mg, net price 20-cap pack = £1.93, 50-cap pack = £2.73

Note The brand name Dulcolax® is also used for bisacodyl tablets and suppositories

◢**Bowel cleansing preparations**

Section 1.6.5

## Other stimulant laxatives

Unstandardised preparations of cascara, frangula, rhubarb, and senna should be **avoided** as their laxative action is unpredictable. Aloes, colocynth, and jalap should be **avoided** as they have a drastic purgative action.

## 1.6.3 Faecal softeners

Liquid paraffin, the traditional lubricant, has disadvantages (see below). Bulk laxatives (section 1.6.1) and non-ionic surfactant 'wetting' agents e.g. docusate sodium (section 1.6.2) also have softening properties. Such drugs are useful for oral administration in the management of haemorrhoids and anal fissure; glycerol (section 1.6.2) is useful for rectal use.

Enemas containing **arachis oil** (ground-nut oil, peanut oil) lubricate and soften impacted faeces and promote a bowel movement.

## ARACHIS OIL

**Indications** see notes above

**Dose**
● See below

**Arachis Oil Enema** (Non-proprietary)
Enema, arachis (peanut) oil in 130-mL single-dose disposable packs. Net price 130 mL = £7.98

Dose to soften impacted faeces, 130 mL; the enema should be warmed before use; CHILD (but see section 1.6) under 3 years not recommended; over 3 years reduce adult dose in proportion to body-weight (medical supervision only), see *BNF for Children*

## LIQUID PARAFFIN

**Indications** constipation

**Cautions** avoid prolonged use; contra-indicated in children under 3 years

**Side-effects** anal seepage of paraffin and consequent anal irritation after prolonged use, granulomatous reactions caused by absorption of small quantities of liquid paraffin (especially from the emulsion), lipoid pneumonia, and interference with the absorption of fat-soluble vitamins

**Dose**
• See under preparation

**Liquid Paraffin Oral Emulsion, BP**
Oral emulsion, liquid paraffin 5 mL, vanillin 5 mg, chloroform 0.025 mL, benzoic acid solution 0.2 mL, methylcellulose-20 200 mg, saccharin sodium 500 micrograms, water to 10 mL

Dose ADULT over 18 years, 10–30 mL at night when required
Counselling Should not be taken immediately before going to bed

## 1.6.4 Osmotic laxatives

Osmotic laxatives increase the amount of water in the large bowel, either by drawing fluid from the body into the bowel or by retaining the fluid they were administered with.

**Lactulose** is a semi-synthetic disaccharide which is not absorbed from the gastro-intestinal tract. It produces an osmotic diarrhoea of low faecal pH, and discourages the proliferation of ammonia-producing organisms. It is therefore useful in the treatment of *hepatic encephalopathy*.

**Macrogols** are inert polymers of ethylene glycol which sequester fluid in the bowel; giving fluid with macrogols may reduce the dehydrating effect sometimes seen with osmotic laxatives.

Saline purgatives such as **magnesium hydroxide** are commonly abused but are satisfactory for occasional use; adequate fluid intake should be maintained. **Magnesium salts** are useful where rapid bowel evacuation is required. **Sodium salts** should be avoided as they may give rise to sodium and water retention in susceptible individuals. **Phosphate enemas** are useful in bowel clearance before radiology, endoscopy, and surgery.

## LACTULOSE

**Indications** constipation (may take up to 48 hours to act), hepatic encephalopathy (portal systemic encephalopathy)

**Cautions** lactose intolerance; **interactions:** Appendix 1 (lactulose)

**Contra-indications** galactosaemia, intestinal obstruction

**Side-effects** flatulence, cramps, and abdominal discomfort

**Dose**
• See under preparations below

**Lactulose** (Non-proprietary)
Solution, lactulose 3.1–3.7 g/5 mL with other ketoses. Net price 300-mL pack = £2.64, 500-mL pack = £2.95

Dose constipation, initially 15 mL twice daily, adjusted according to patient's needs; CHILD (adjusted according to response but see section 1.6) under 1 year 2.5 mL twice daily, 1–5 years 5 mL twice daily, 5–10 years 10 mL twice daily

Hepatic encephalopathy, 30–50 mL 3 times daily, subsequently adjusted to produce 2–3 soft stools daily; CHILD 12–18 years see *BNF for Children*
Brands include *Duphalac®* , *Lactugal®* , *Regulose®*

## MACROGOLS
(Polyethylene glycols)

**Indications** see preparations below

**Cautions** pregnancy (Appendix 4); breast-feeding (Appendix 5); discontinue if symptoms of fluid and electrolyte disturbance; see also preparations below

**Contra-indications** intestinal perforation or obstruction, paralytic ileus, severe inflammatory conditions of the intestinal tract (such as Crohn's disease, ulcerative colitis, and toxic megacolon), see also preparations below

**Side-effects** abdominal distension and pain, nausea

**Dose**
• See preparations below

**Macrogol Oral Powder, Compound** (Non-proprietary)
Oral powder, macrogol '3350' (polyethylene glycol '3350') 13.125 g, sodium bicarbonate 178.5 mg, sodium chloride 350.7 mg, potassium chloride 46.6 mg/sachet, net price 20-sachet pack = £4.45, 30-sachet pack = £6.68. Label: 13

Cautions patients with cardiovascular impairment should not take more than 2 sachets in any 1 hour

Dose chronic constipation, ADULT and CHILD over 12 years, 1–3 sachets daily in divided doses usually for up to 2 weeks; contents of each sachet dissolved in half a glass (approx. 125 mL) of water; maintenance, 1–2 sachets daily

Faecal impaction, ADULT and CHILD over 12 years, 8 sachets daily dissolved in 1 litre of water and drunk within 6 hours, usually for max. 3 days

After reconstitution the solution should be kept in a refrigerator and discarded if unused after 6 hours

**Laxido®** (Galen)
Oral powder, orange-flavoured, macrogol '3350' (polyethylene glycol '3350') 13.125 g, sodium bicarbonate 178.5 mg, sodium chloride 350.7 mg, potassium chloride 46.6 mg/sachet, net price 20-sachet pack = £3.56, 30-sachet pack = £5.34. Label: 13

Note Also available in natural flavour (sugar-free)

Cautions patients with cardiovascular impairment should not take more than 2 sachets in any 1 hour

Dose chronic constipation, ADULT and CHILD over 12 years, 1–3 sachets daily in divided doses usually for up to 2 weeks; contents of each sachet dissolved in half a glass (approx. 125 mL) of water; maintenance, 1–2 sachets daily

Faecal impaction, ADULT and CHILD over 12 years, 8 sachets daily dissolved in 1 litre of water and drunk within 6 hours, usually for max. 3 days

After reconstitution the solution should be kept in a refrigerator and discarded if unused after 6 hours

**Movicol®** (Norgine)
Oral powder, macrogol '3350' (polyethylene glycol '3350') 13.125 g, sodium bicarbonate 178.5 mg, sodium chloride 350.7 mg, potassium chloride 46.6 mg/sachet, net price 20-sachet pack (lime and lemon flavour) = £4.45, 30-sachet pack (lime- and lemon- or

**1**
Gastro-intestinal system

chocolate- or plain-flavoured) = £6.68, 50–sachet pack (lime- and lemon- or plain-flavoured) = £11.13. Label: 13

Note Amount of potassium chloride varies according to flavour of *Movicol*® as follows: plain-flavour (sugar-free) = 50.2 mg/sachet; lime and lemon flavour = 46.6 mg/sachet; chocolate flavour = 31.7 mg/sachet. 1 sachet when reconstituted with 125 mL water provides K⁺ 5.4 mmol/litre

Cautions patients with cardiovascular impairment should not take more than 2 sachets in any 1 hour

Dose chronic constipation, ADULT and CHILD over 12 years, 1–3 sachets daily in divided doses usually for up to 2 weeks; contents of each sachet dissolved in half a glass (approx. 125 mL) of water; maintenance, 1–2 sachets daily

Faecal impaction, ADULT and CHILD over 12 years, 8 sachets daily dissolved in 1 litre of water and drunk within 6 hours, usually for max. 3 days

After reconstitution the solution should be kept in a refrigerator and discarded if unused after 6 hours

### Movicol®-Half (Norgine)
Oral powder, sugar-free, macrogol '3350' (polyethylene glycol '3350') 6.563 g, sodium bicarbonate 89.3 mg, sodium chloride 175.4 mg, potassium chloride 23.3 mg/sachet, net price 20-sachet pack (lime and lemon flavour) = £2.67, 30-sachet pack = £4.01. Label: 13

Cautions patients with cardiovascular impairment should not take more than 4 sachets in any 1 hour

Dose chronic constipation, ADULT and CHILD over 12 years, 2–6 sachets daily in divided doses usually for up to 2 weeks; content of each sachet dissolved in quarter of a glass (approx. 60–65 mL) of water; maintenance, 2–4 sachets daily

Faecal impaction, ADULT and CHILD over 12 years, 16 sachets daily dissolved in 1 litre of water and drunk within 6 hours, usually for max. 3 days

After reconstitution the solution should be kept in a refrigerator and discarded if unused after 6 hours

### Movicol® Paediatric Plain (Norgine) ▣PoM
Oral powder, sugar-free, macrogol '3350' (polyethylene glycol '3350') 6.563 g, sodium bicarbonate 89.3 mg, sodium chloride 175.4 mg, potassium chloride 25.1 mg/sachet, net price 30-sachet pack = £4.45. Label: 13

Cautions with high doses, impaired gag reflex, reflux oesophagitis, impaired consciousness

Contra-indications cardiovascular impairment; renal impairment

Dose chronic constipation and recurrence of faecal impaction, CHILD 2–6 years 1 sachet daily; 7–11 years 2 sachets daily; adjust according to response, max. 4 sachets daily

Faecal impaction, CHILD (taken in divided doses over 12 hours each day until impaction resolves or for max. 7 days) 5–11 years 4 sachets on first day then increased in steps of 2 sachets daily to 12 sachets daily; content of each sachet dissolved in quarter of a glass (approx. 60–65 mL) of water

After reconstitution the solution should be kept in a refrigerator and discarded if unused after 24 hours

---

## ▮ MAGNESIUM SALTS

Indications see under preparations below

Cautions renal impairment (Appendix 3; risk of magnesium accumulation); hepatic impairment (see Appendix 2); elderly and debilitated; see also notes above; interactions: Appendix 1 (antacids)

Contra-indications acute gastro-intestinal conditions

Side-effects colic

Dose
● See preparations

### ◀Magnesium hydroxide
### Magnesium Hydroxide Mixture, BP
Aqueous suspension containing about 8% hydrated magnesium oxide. Do not store in cold place

Dose constipation, 30–45 mL with water at bedtime when required; CHILD 3–12 years, 5–10 mL with water at bedtime when required

### ◀Magnesium hydroxide with liquid paraffin
### Liquid Paraffin and Magnesium Hydroxide Oral Emulsion, BP ▭
Oral emulsion, 25% liquid paraffin in aqueous suspension containing 6% hydrated magnesium oxide

Dose constipation, 5–20 mL when required

Note Liquid paraffin and magnesium hydroxide preparations on sale to the public include: *Milpar*® ▣

### ◀Magnesium sulphate
### Magnesium Sulphate
Label: 13, 23

Dose rapid bowel evacuation (acts in 2–4 hours) 5–10 g in a glass of water preferably before breakfast

Note Magnesium sulphate is on sale to the public as Epsom Salts

### ◀Bowel cleansing preparations
Section 1.6.5

---

## ▮ PHOSPHATES (RECTAL)

Indications rectal use in constipation; bowel evacuation before abdominal radiological procedures, endoscopy, and surgery

Cautions elderly and debilitated; with enema, electrolyte disturbances, renal impairment, congestive heart failure, ascites, uncontrolled hypertension, maintain adequate hydration

Contra-indications acute gastro-intestinal conditions (including gastro-intestinal obstruction, inflammatory bowel disease, and conditions associated with increased colonic absorption)

Side-effects local irritation; with enema, electrolyte disturbances

Dose
● See under preparations

### Carbalax® (Forest)
Suppositories, sodium acid phosphate (anhydrous) 1.3 g, sodium bicarbonate 1.08 g, net price 12 = £2.01

Dose constipation, ADULT and CHILD over 12 years, 1 suppository, inserted 30 minutes before evacuation required; moisten with water before use

### Fleet® Ready-to-use Enema (De Witt)
Enema, sodium acid phosphate 21.4 g, sodium phosphate 9.4 g/118 mL, net price 133-mL pack (delivers 118 mL dose) with standard tube = 57p

Dose ADULT and CHILD (but see section 1.6) over 12 years, 118 mL; CHILD 3–12 years, on doctor's advice only (under 3 years not recommended)

### Phosphates Enema BP Formula B
Enema, sodium dihydrogen phosphate dihydrate 12.8 g, disodium phosphate dodecahydrate 10.24 g, purified water, freshly boiled and cooled, to 128 mL. Net price 128 mL with standard tube = £2.98, with long rectal tube = £3.98

Dose 128 mL; CHILD (but see section 1.6) over 3 years, reduced according to body weight see *BNF for Children*

## ■ SODIUM CITRATE (RECTAL)

**Indications** rectal use in constipation

**Cautions** elderly and debilitated; see also notes above

**Contra-indications** acute gastro-intestinal conditions

**Dose**

- See under preparations

### Micolette Micro-enema® (Pinewood)

Enema, sodium citrate 450 mg, sodium lauryl sulphoacetate 45 mg, glycerol 625 mg, together with potassium sorbate and sorbitol in a viscous solution, in 5-mL single-dose disposable packs with nozzle. Net price 5 mL = 38p

Dose ADULT and CHILD over 3 years, 5–10 mL (but see section 1.6)

### Micralax Micro-enema® (UCB Pharma)

Enema, sodium citrate 450 mg, sodium alkylsulphoacetate 45 mg, sorbic acid 5 mg, together with glycerol and sorbitol in a viscous solution in 5-mL single-dose disposable packs with nozzle. Net price 5 mL = 41p

Dose ADULT and CHILD over 3 years, 5 mL (but see section 1.6)

### Relaxit Micro-enema® (Crawford)

Enema, sodium citrate 450 mg, sodium lauryl sulphate 75 mg, sorbic acid 5 mg, together with glycerol and sorbitol in a viscous solution in 5-mL single-dose disposable packs with nozzle. Net price 5 mL = 32p

Dose ADULT and CHILD (but see section 1.6) 5 mL (insert only half nozzle length in child under 3 years)

## 1.6.5 Bowel cleansing preparations

Bowel cleansing preparations are used before colonic surgery, colonoscopy, or radiological examination to ensure the bowel is free of solid contents. They are **not** treatments for constipation.

**Cautions** Bowel cleansing preparations should be used with caution in patients with fluid and electrolyte disturbances. Adequate hydration should be maintained during treatment. Bowel cleansing preparations should also be used with caution in children, in the elderly, in those who are debilitated, in renal impairment (Appendix 3), or during pregnancy and breast-feeding.

**Contra-indications** Bowel cleansing preparations are contra-indicated in patients with gastro-intestinal obstruction or perforation, gastric retention, or toxic megacolon.

**Side-effects** Side-effects of bowel cleansing preparations include nausea, vomiting, abdominal pain (usually transient—reduced by taking more slowly), and abdominal distention. Less frequent side-effects include headache, dizziness, dehydration, and electrolyte disturbances.

## ■ MACROGOLS

**Indications** see notes above

**Cautions** see notes above; also heart failure; acute inflammatory bowel disease; impaired gag reflex, impaired consciousness or possibility of regurgitation or aspiration

**Contra-indications** see notes above; also gastro-intestinal ulceration

**Side-effects** see notes above; also fatigue, sleep disturbances, and anal discomfort

**Dose**

- See preparations

### Klean-Prep® (Norgine)

Oral powder, sugar-free, macrogol '3350' (polyethylene glycol '3350') 59 g, anhydrous sodium sulphate 5.685 g, sodium bicarbonate 1.685 g, sodium chloride 1.465 g, potassium chloride 743 mg/sachet, net price 4 sachets = £8.23. Label: 10, patient information leaflet, 13, counselling

Excipients include aspartame (section 9.4.1)

Four sachets when reconstituted with water to 4 litres provides an iso-osmotic solution for bowel cleansing before surgery, colonoscopy or radiological procedures

Dose a glass (approx. 250 mL) of reconstituted solution every 10–15 minutes, or by nasogastric tube 20–30 mL/minute, until 4 litres have been consumed or watery stools are free of solid matter; CHILD not recommended

The solution from all 4 sachets should be drunk within 4–6 hours (250 mL drunk rapidly every 10–15 minutes); flavouring such as clear fruit cordials may be added if required; to facilitate gastric emptying domperidone or metoclopramide may be given 30 minutes before starting.

Alternatively the administration may be divided into two, e.g. taking the solutions from 2 sachets on the evening before examination and the remaining 2 on the morning of the examination

After reconstitution the solution should be kept in a refrigerator and discarded if unused after 24 hours

Note 1 sachet when reconstituted with 1 litre of water provides $Na^+$ 125 mmol, $K^+$ 10 mmol

### Moviprep® (Norgine)

Oral powder, lemon-flavoured, *Sachet A* (containing macrogol '3350' (polyethylene glycol '3350') 100 g, anhydrous sodium sulphate 7.5 g, sodium chloride 2.691 g, potassium chloride 1.015 g) and *Sachet B* (containing ascorbic acid 4.7 g, sodium ascorbate 5.9 g), net price 4-sachet pack (2 each of sachet A and B) = £9.87. Label: 10, patient information leaflet, 13, counselling, see below

Excipients include aspartame (section 9.4.1)

Contra-indications G6PD deficiency

Dose bowel evacuation for surgery, colonoscopy or radiological examination, ADULT over 18 years, 2 litres of reconstituted solution on the evening before procedure *or* 1 litre of reconstituted solution on the evening before procedure and 1 litre of reconstituted solution early on the morning of procedure; treatment should be completed at least 1 hour before colonoscopy

Counselling One pair of sachets (A and B) should be reconstituted in 1 litre of water (providing absorbable $Na^+$ 56.2 mmol, $K^+$ 14.2 mmol/litre) and taken over 1–2 hours. Solid food should not be taken during treatment. 1 litre of other clear fluid should also be taken during treatment

## ■ MAGNESIUM CITRATE

Reconstitution of a sachet containing 11.57 g magnesium carbonate and 17.79 g anhydrous citric acid produces a solution containing magnesium citrate

**Indications** see preparations

**Cautions** see notes above

**Contra-indications** see notes above

**Side-effects** see notes above

**Dose**

- See preparations

### Citramag® (Sanochemia)

Oral powder, sugar-free, effervescent, magnesium carbonate 11.57 g, anhydrous citric acid 17.79 g/sachet, net price 10-sachet pack (lemon and lime flavour) = £17.20. Label: 10, patient information leaflet, 13, counselling, see below

**Dose** bowel evacuation for surgery, colonoscopy or radiological examination, on day before procedure, 1 sachet at 8 a.m. and 1 sachet between 2 and 4 p.m.; CHILD 5–10 years one-third adult dose; over 10 years and frail ELDERLY one-half adult dose

**Counselling** The patient information leaflet advises that hot water (200 mL) is needed to make the solution and provides guidance on the timing and procedure for reconstitution; it also mentions need for high fluid, low residue diet beforehand (according to hospital advice), and explains that only clear fluids can be taken after *Citramag®* until procedure completed

### PHOSPHATES (ORAL)

**Indications** see preparations

**Cautions** see notes above; also cardiac disease (avoid in congestive cardiac failure)

**Contra-indications** see notes above; also acute inflammatory bowel disease; ascites; congestive cardiac failure

**Side-effects** see notes above; also chest pain and asthenia

**Dose**

• See preparations

**Diafalk®** (Dr Falk)

Tablets, monobasic sodium phosphate monohydrate 1.102 g, disodium phosphate 398 mg. Contains 13.6 mmol $Na^+$/tablet. Net price 32-tab pack = £7.20. Label: 10, patient information leaflet, counselling, see below

**Dose** bowel evacuation before diagnostic procedure, ADULT over 18 years, 4 tablets every 15 minutes until a total of 20 tablets have been consumed on the evening before procedure, then on the next day (starting 3–5 hours before procedure) 4 tablets every 15 minutes until a total of 12 tablets have been consumed; do not repeat course within 7 days

**Counselling** On the day before procedure, a light, low-fibre breakfast may be consumed in the morning, clear liquid diet recommended after 12 noon. Each dose of 4 tablets to be taken with 250 mL clear liquid. Copious intake of water or other clear liquids recommended during treatment

**Fleet Phospho-soda®** (De Witt)

Oral solution, sugar-free, sodium dihydrogen phosphate dihydrate 24.4 g, disodium phosphate dodeca-hydrate 10.8 g/45 mL. Contains about 217 mmol $Na^+$/45 mL. Net price 2 × 45-mL bottles = £4.79. Label: 10, patient information leaflet, counselling

**Dose** bowel evacuation before colonic surgery, colonoscopy or radiological examination, ADULT and CHILD over 15 years, 45 mL diluted with half a glass (120 mL) of cold water, followed by one full glass (240 mL) of cold water

Timing of doses is dependent on the time of the procedure

For morning procedure, first dose should be taken at 7 a.m. and second at 7 p.m. on day before the procedure

For afternoon procedure, first dose should be taken at 7 p.m. on day before and second dose at 7 a.m. on day of the procedure

Solid food must not be taken during dosing period; clear liquids or water should be substituted for meals

Acts within half to 6 hours of first dose

### SODIUM PICOSULFATE WITH MAGNESIUM CITRATE

**Indications** see preparations

**Cautions** see notes above; also inflammatory bowel disease; recent gastro-intestinal surgery; cardiac disease (avoid in congestive cardiac failure)

**Contra-indications** see notes above; also gastro-intestinal ulceration; ascites; congestive cardiac failure

**Side-effects** see notes above; also anal discomfort, sleep disturbances, fatigue, and rash

**Dose**

• See preparations

**CitraFleet®** (De Witt)

Oral powder, sodium picosulfate 10 mg/sachet, with magnesium citrate. Contains 86 mmol $Mg^{2+}$ and 5 mmol $K^+$/sachet. Net price 2-sachet pack (lemon-flavoured) = £3.25. Label: 10, patient information leaflet, 13, counselling, see below

**Dose** bowel evacuation on day before radiological examination, endoscopy, or surgery, ADULT over 18 years, 1 sachet before 8 a.m. then 1 sachet 6–8 hours later

Acts within 3 hours of first dose

**Counselling** One sachet should be reconstituted with 150 mL (approx. half a glass) of cold water; patients should be warned that heat is generated during reconstitution and that the solution should be allowed to cool before drinking. Low residue diet recommended on the day before procedure and copious intake of water or other clear fluids recommended during treatment

**Picolax®** (Ferring)

Oral powder, sugar-free, sodium picosulfate 10 mg/sachet, with magnesium citrate. Contains 87 mmol $Mg^{2+}$ and 5 mmol $K^+$/sachet. Net price 2-sachet pack = £3.39. Label: 10, patient information leaflet, 13, counselling, see below

**Dose** bowel evacuation on day before radiological procedure, endoscopy, or surgery, ADULT and CHILD over 9 years, 1 sachet before 8 a.m. then 1 sachet 6–8 hours later; CHILD 1–2 years, quarter sachet before 8 a.m. then quarter sachet 6–8 hours later; 2–4 years, half sachet before 8 a.m. then half sachet 6–8 hours later; 4–9 years, 1 sachet before 8 a.m. then half sachet 6–8 hours later

Acts within 3 hours of first dose

**Counselling** One sachet should be reconstituted with 150 mL (approx. half a glass) of cold water; patients should be warned that heat is generated during reconstitution and that the solution should be allowed to cool before drinking. Low residue diet recommended on the day before procedure and copious intake of water or other clear fluids recommended during treatment

## 1.6.6 Peripheral opioid-receptor antagonists

**Methylnaltrexone** is a peripherally acting opioid-receptor antagonist that is licensed for the treatment of opioid-induced constipation in patients receiving palliative care, when response to other laxatives is inadequate; it should be used as an adjunct to existing laxative therapy. Methylnaltrexone does not alter the central analgesic effect of opioids. For the prevention of opioid-induced constipation in palliative care, see p. 16.

### METHYLNALTREXONE BROMIDE

**Indications** opioid-induced constipation in terminally ill patients, when response to other laxatives is inadequate

**Cautions** diverticular disease; faecal impaction; patients with colostomy or peritoneal catheter; renal impairment (Appendix 3); pregnancy (Appendix 4); breast-feeding (Appendix 5)

**Contra-indications** gastro-intestinal obstruction; acute surgical abdominal conditions; severe hepatic impairment (Appendix 2)

**Side-effects** abdominal pain, nausea, diarrhoea, flatulence; dizziness; injection site reactions

**Dose**

• By subcutaneous injection, ADULT over 18 years, body-weight under 38 kg, 150 micrograms/kg on alternate days; body-weight 38–62 kg, 8 mg on alternate days; body-weight 62–114 kg, 12 mg on alternate days; body-weight over 114 kg, 150 micrograms/kg on alternate days; may be given less frequently depending on response; 2 consecutive doses may be given 24 hours apart if no response to treatment on the preceding day; rotate sites of injection; max. duration of treatment 4 months

**Note** May act within 30–60 minutes

**Relistor®** (Wyeth) ▼ PoM

Injection, methylnaltrexone bromide 20 mg/mL, net price 0.6-mL vial = £21.05, 7-vial pack (with syringes and needles) = £147.35

## 1.7    Local preparations for anal and rectal disorders

| | |
|---|---|
| 1.7.1 | **Soothing haemorrhoidal preparations** |
| 1.7.2 | **Compound haemorrhoidal preparations with corticosteroids** |
| 1.7.3 | **Rectal sclerosants** |
| 1.7.4 | **Management of anal fissures** |

Anal and perianal pruritus, soreness, and excoriation are best treated by application of bland ointments and suppositories (section 1.7.1). These conditions occur commonly in patients suffering from haemorrhoids, fistulas, and proctitis. Cleansing with attention to any minor faecal soiling, adjustment of the diet to avoid hard stools, the use of bulk-forming materials such as bran (section 1.6.1) and a high residue diet are helpful. In proctitis these measures may supplement treatment with corticosteroids or sulfasalazine (see section 1.5).

When necessary topical preparations containing **local anaesthetics** (section 1.7.1) or **corticosteroids** (section 1.7.2) are used provided perianal thrush has been excluded. Perianal thrush is best treated with **nystatin** by mouth and by local application (see section 5.2, section 7.2.2, and section 13.10.2).

For the management of *anal fissures*, see section 1.7.4.

## 1.7.1    Soothing haemorrhoidal preparations

Soothing preparations containing mild astringents such as bismuth subgallate, zinc oxide, and hamamelis may give symptomatic relief in haemorrhoids. Many proprietary preparations also contain lubricants, vasoconstrictors, or mild antiseptics.

**Local anaesthetics** are used to relieve pain associated with *haemorrhoids* and *pruritus ani* but good evidence is lacking. Lidocaine (lignocaine) ointment (section 15.2) is used before emptying the bowel to relieve pain associated with *anal fissure*. Alternative local anaesthetics

include tetracaine (amethocaine), cinchocaine (dibucaine), and pramocaine (pramoxine), but they are more irritant. Local anaesthetic ointments can be absorbed through the rectal mucosa therefore excessive application should be **avoided**, particularly in infants and children. Preparations containing local anaesthetics should be used for short periods only (no longer than a few days) since they may cause sensitisation of the anal skin.

## 1.7.2    Compound haemorrhoidal preparations with corticosteroids

Corticosteroids are often combined with local anaesthetics and soothing agents in preparations for haemorrhoids. They are suitable for occasional short-term use after exclusion of infections, such as herpes simplex; prolonged use can cause atrophy of the anal skin. See section 13.4 for general comments on topical corticosteroids and section 1.7.1 for comment on local anaesthetics.

**Children** Haemorrhoids in children are rare. Treatment is usually symptomatic and the use of a locally applied cream is appropriate for short periods; however, local anaesthetics can cause stinging initially and this may aggravate the child's fear of defaecation.

**Anugesic-HC®** (Pfizer) PoM

Cream, benzyl benzoate 1.2%, bismuth oxide 0.875%, hydrocortisone acetate 0.5%, Peru balsam 1.85%, pramocaine hydrochloride 1%, zinc oxide 12.35%. Net price 30 g (with rectal nozzle) = £3.71

**Dose** apply night and morning and after a bowel movement; do not use for longer than 7 days; CHILD not recommended

Suppositories, buff, benzyl benzoate 33 mg, bismuth oxide 24 mg, bismuth subgallate 59 mg, hydrocortisone acetate 5 mg, Peru balsam 49 mg, pramocaine hydrochloride 27 mg, zinc oxide 296 mg, net price 12 = £2.69

**Dose** insert 1 suppository night and morning and after a bowel movement; do not use for longer than 7 days; CHILD not recommended

**Anusol-HC®** (McNeil) PoM

Ointment, benzyl benzoate 1.25%, bismuth oxide 0.875%, bismuth subgallate 2.25%, hydrocortisone acetate 0.25%, Peru balsam 1.875%, zinc oxide 10.75%. Net price 30 g (with rectal nozzle) = £3.50

**Dose** apply night and morning and after a bowel movement; do not use for longer than 7 days; CHILD not recommended

**Note** A proprietary brand (*Anusol Plus HC®* ointment) is on sale to the public

Suppositories, benzyl benzoate 33 mg, bismuth oxide 24 mg, bismuth subgallate 59 mg, hydrocortisone acetate 10 mg, Peru balsam 49 mg, zinc oxide 296 mg. Net price 12 = £2.46

**Dose** insert 1 suppository night and morning and after a bowel movement; do not use for longer than 7 days; CHILD not recommended

**Note** A proprietary brand (*Anusol Plus HC®* suppositories) is on sale to the public

**Perinal®** (Dermal)

Spray application, hydrocortisone 0.2%, lidocaine hydrochloride 1%. Net price 30-mL pack = £6.21

**Dose** ADULT and CHILD over 14 years, spray once over the affected area up to 3 times daily; do not use for longer than 7 days without medical advice; CHILD under 14 years on medical advice only

1

Gastro-intestinal system

**Proctofoam HC®** (Meda) PoM
Foam in aerosol pack, hydrocortisone acetate 1%, pramocaine hydrochloride 1%. Net price 21.2-g pack (approx. 40 applications) with applicator = £5.06
Dose haemorrhoids and proctitis, 1 applicatorful (4–6 mg hydrocortisone acetate, 4–6 mg pramocaine hydrochloride) by rectum 2–3 times daily and after each bowel movement (max. 4 times daily); do not use for longer than 7 days; CHILD not recommended

**Proctosedyl®** (Aventis Pharma) PoM
Ointment, cinchocaine (dibucaine) hydrochloride 0.5%, hydrocortisone 0.5%. Net price 30 g = £10.34 (with cannula)
Dose apply morning and night and after a bowel movement, externally or by rectum; do not use for longer than 7 days

Suppositories, cinchocaine (dibucaine) hydrochloride 5 mg, hydrocortisone 5 mg. Net price 12 = £4.66
Dose insert 1 suppository night and morning and after a bowel movement; do not use for longer than 7 days

**Scheriproct®** (Valeant) PoM
Ointment, cinchocaine (dibucaine) hydrochloride 0.5%, prednisolone hexanoate 0.19%. Net price 30 g = £3.00
Dose apply twice daily for 5–7 days (3–4 times daily on 1st day if necessary), then once daily for a few days after symptoms have cleared

Suppositories, cinchocaine (dibucaine) hydrochloride 1 mg, prednisolone hexanoate 1.3 mg. Net price 12 = £1.41
Dose insert 1 suppository daily after a bowel movement, for 5–7 days (in severe cases initially 2–3 times daily)

**Ultraproct®** (Meadow) PoM
Ointment, cinchocaine (dibucaine) hydrochloride 0.5%, fluocortolone caproate 0.095%, fluocortolone pivalate 0.092%, net price 30 g (with rectal nozzle) = £4.57
Dose apply twice daily for 5–7 days (3–4 times daily on 1st day if necessary), then once daily for a few days after symptoms have cleared

Suppositories, cinchocaine (dibucaine) hydrochloride 1 mg, fluocortolone caproate 630 micrograms, fluocortolone pivalate 610 micrograms, net price 12 = £2.15
Dose insert 1 suppository daily after a bowel movement, for 5–7 days (in severe cases initially 2–3 times daily) then 1 suppository every other day for 1 week

**Uniroid-HC®** (Chemidex) PoM
Ointment, cinchocaine (dibucaine) hydrochloride 0.5%, hydrocortisone 0.5%. Net price 30 g (with applicator) = £4.23
Dose ADULT and CHILD over 12 years, apply twice daily and after a bowel movement, externally or by rectum; do not use for longer than 7 days; CHILD under 12 years on medical advice only

Suppositories, cinchocaine (dibucaine) hydrochloride 5 mg, hydrocortisone 5 mg. Net price 12 = £1.91
Dose ADULT and CHILD over 12 years, insert 1 suppository twice daily and after a bowel movement; do not use for longer than 7 days

**Xyloproct®** (AstraZeneca) PoM
Ointment (water-miscible), aluminium acetate 3.5%, hydrocortisone acetate 0.275%, lidocaine 5%, zinc oxide 18%, net price 20 g (with applicator) = £2.26
Dose apply several times daily; short-term use only

## 1.7.3 Rectal sclerosants

Oily phenol injection is used to inject haemorrhoids particularly when unprolapsed.

### PHENOL

**Indications** see notes above
**Side-effects** irritation, tissue necrosis

**Oily Phenol Injection, BP** PoM
phenol 5% in a suitable fixed oil. Net price 5-mL amp = £5.00
Dose 2–3 mL into the submucosal layer at the base of the pile; several injections may be given at different sites, max. total injected 10 mL at any one time
Available from UCB Pharma

## 1.7.4 Management of anal fissures

The management of *anal fissures* requires stool softening by increasing dietary fibre in the form of bran or by using a bulk-forming laxative. Short-term use of local anaesthetic preparations may help (section 1.7.1). If these measures are inadequate, the patient should be referred for specialist treatment in hospital. The use of a topical nitrate (e.g. glyceryl trinitrate 0.4% ointment) may be considered. Before considering surgery, topical diltiazem 2% may be used twice daily [unlicensed indication] in patients with chronic anal fissures unresponsive to topical nitrates.

The *Scottish Medicines Consortium* (p. 3) has advised (January 2008) that glyceryl trinitrate 0.4% ointment (*Rectogesic®*) is **not** recommended for use within NHS Scotland for the relief of pain associated with chronic anal fissure.

### GLYCERYL TRINITRATE

**Indications** anal fissure; angina, left ventricular failure (section 2.6.1); extravasation (section 10.3)
**Cautions** section 2.6.1
**Contra-indications** section 2.6.1
**Side-effects** section 2.6.1; also diarrhoea, burning, itching, and rectal bleeding
**Dose**
• See preparations

**Rectogesic®** (Strakan) ▼ PoM
Rectal ointment, glyceryl trinitrate 0.4%, net price 30 g = £34.80
Excipients include lanolin, propylene glycol
Dose ADULT over 18 years, apply 2.5 cm of ointment to anal canal every 12 hours until pain stops; max. duration of use 8 weeks
Note 2.5 cm of ointment contains glyceryl trinitrate 1.5 mg; discard tube 8 weeks after first opening

## 1.8 Stoma care

Prescribing for patients with stoma calls for special care. The following is a brief account of some of the main points to be borne in mind.

*Enteric-coated* and *modified-release* preparations are **unsuitable**, particularly in patients with an ileostomy, as there may not be sufficient release of the active ingredient.

**Laxatives** Enemas and washouts should **not** be prescribed for patients with an ileostomy as they may cause rapid and severe loss of water and electrolytes.

Colostomy patients may suffer from constipation and whenever possible should be treated by increasing fluid intake or dietary fibre. **Bulk-forming drugs** (section 1.6.1) should be tried. If they are insufficient, as small a dose as possible of senna (section 1.6.2) should be used.

**Antidiarrhoeals** Drugs such as **loperamide, codeine phosphate**, or **co-phenotrope** (diphenoxylate with atropine) are effective. Bulk-forming drugs (section 1.6.1) may be tried but it is often difficult to adjust the dose appropriately.

**Antibacterials** should **not** be given for an episode of acute diarrhoea.

**Antacids** The tendency to diarrhoea from magnesium salts or constipation from aluminium salts may be increased in these patients.

**Diuretics** Diuretics should be used with caution in patients with an ileostomy as they may become excessively dehydrated and potassium depletion may easily occur. It is usually advisable to use a **potassium-sparing** diuretic (see section 2.2.3).

**Digoxin** Patients with a stoma are particularly susceptible to hypokalaemia if on digoxin therapy and potassium supplements or a potassium-sparing diuretic may be advisable (for comment see section 9.2.1.1).

**Potassium supplements** Liquid formulations are preferred to modified-release formulations (see above).

**Analgesics** Opioid analgesics (see section 4.7.2) may cause troublesome constipation in colostomy patients. When a non-opioid analgesic is required **paracetamol** is usually suitable but anti-inflammatory analgesics may cause gastric irritation and bleeding.

**Iron preparations** Iron preparations may cause loose stools and sore skin in these patients. If this is troublesome and if iron is definitely indicated an intramuscular iron preparation (see section 9.1.1.2) should be used. Modified-release preparations should be **avoided** for the reasons given above.

**Care of stoma** Patients are usually given advice about the use of *cleansing agents*, *protective creams*, *lotions*, *deodorants*, or *sealants* whilst in hospital, either by the surgeon or by stoma care nurses. Voluntary organisations offer help and support to patients with stoma.

## 1.9   Drugs affecting intestinal secretions

**1.9.1 Drugs affecting biliary composition and flow**

**1.9.2 Bile acid sequestrants**

**1.9.3 Aprotinin**

**1.9.4 Pancreatin**

## 1.9.1   Drugs affecting biliary composition and flow

The use of laparoscopic cholecystectomy and of endoscopic biliary techniques has limited the place of the bile acid **ursodeoxycholic acid** in gallstone disease. Ursodeoxycholic acid is suitable for patients with unimpaired gall bladder function, small or medium-sized radiolucent stones, and whose mild symptoms are not amenable to other treatment; it should be used cautiously in those with liver disease (but see below). Patients should be given dietary advice (including avoidance of excessive cholesterol and calories) and they require radiological monitoring. Long-term prophylaxis may be needed after complete dissolution of the gallstones has been confirmed because they may recur in up to 25% of patients within one year of stopping treatment.

Ursodeoxycholic acid is also used in primary biliary cirrhosis; liver tests improve in most patients but the effect on overall survival is uncertain. Ursodeoxycholic acid has also been tried in primary sclerosing cholangitis [unlicensed indication].

### URSODEOXYCHOLIC ACID

**Indications** see under Dose and under preparations

**Cautions** see notes above; **interactions**: Appendix 1 (ursodeoxycholic acid)

**Contra-indications** radio-opaque stones, pregnancy (Appendix 4), non-functioning gall bladder, inflammatory diseases and other conditions of the small intestine, colon and liver which interfere with enterohepatic circulation of bile salts

**Side-effects** nausea, vomiting, diarrhoea; gallstone calcification; pruritus

**Dose**

- Dissolution of gallstones, 8–12 mg/kg daily as a single dose at bedtime *or* in two divided doses, for up to 2 years; treatment is continued for 3–4 months after stones dissolve

- Primary biliary cirrhosis, see under *Ursofalk®*

**Ursodeoxycholic Acid** (Non-proprietary) ⓅⓄⓂ
Tablets, ursodeoxycholic acid 150 mg, net price 60-tab pack = £18.51. Label: 21
Capsules, ursodeoxycholic acid 250 mg, net price 60-cap pack = £35.11. Label: 21

**Destolit®** (Norgine) ⓅⓄⓂ
Tablets, scored, ursodeoxycholic acid 150 mg, net price 60-tab pack = £17.67. Label: 21

**Urdox®** (CP) ⓅⓄⓂ
Tablets, f/c, ursodeoxycholic acid 300 mg, net price 60-tab pack = £26.50. Label: 21

**1** Gastro-intestinal system

**Ursofalk®** (Dr Falk) ▢PoM

Capsules, ursodeoxycholic acid 250 mg, net price 60-cap pack = £30.75, 100-cap pack = £32.50. Label: 21

Suspension, sugar-free, ursodeoxycholic acid 250 mg/5 mL, net price 250 mL = £27.50. Label: 21

Dose primary biliary cirrhosis, 10–15 mg/kg daily as a single daily dose or in 2–4 divided doses

Dissolution of gallstones, see Dose, above

**Ursogal®** (Galen) ▢PoM

Tablets, scored, ursodeoxycholic acid 150 mg, net price 60-tab pack = £17.05. Label: 21

Capsules, ursodeoxycholic acid 250 mg, net price 60-cap pack = £30.50. Label: 21

## Other preparations for biliary disorders

A **terpene** mixture (*Rowachol®*) raises biliary cholesterol solubility. It is not considered to be a useful adjunct.

**Rowachol®** (Rowa) ▢PoM ◢

Capsules, green, e/c, borneol 5 mg, camphene 5 mg, cineole 2 mg, menthol 32 mg, menthone 6 mg, pinene 17 mg in olive oil. Net price 50-cap pack = £7.35. Label: 22

Dose 1–2 capsules 3 times daily before food (but see notes above)

Interactions: Appendix 1 (*Rowachol®*)

## 1.9.2 Bile acid sequestrants

**Colestyramine** (cholestyramine) is an anion-exchange resin that is not absorbed from the gastro-intestinal tract. It relieves diarrhoea and pruritus by forming an insoluble complex with bile acids in the intestine. Colestyramine can interfere with the absorption of a number of drugs. Colestyramine is also used in hypercholesterolaemia (section 2.12).

### COLESTYRAMINE
(Cholestyramine)

**Indications** pruritus associated with partial biliary obstruction and primary biliary cirrhosis; diarrhoea associated with Crohn's disease, ileal resection, vagotomy, diabetic vagal neuropathy, and radiation; hypercholesterolaemia (section 2.12)

**Cautions** see section 2.12

**Contra-indications** see section 2.12

**Side-effects** see section 2.12

**Dose**

- Pruritus, 4–8 g daily in a suitable liquid; CHILD 1–18 years see *BNF for Children*

- Diarrhoea, initially 4 g daily increased by 4 g at weekly intervals to 12–24 g daily in a suitable liquid in 1–4 divided doses, then adjusted as required; max. 36 g daily; CHILD 1–18 years see *BNF for Children*

Counselling Other drugs should be taken at least 1 hour before or 4–6 hours after colestyramine to reduce possible interference with absorption

Note The contents of each sachet should be mixed with at least 150 mL of water or other suitable liquid such as fruit juice, skimmed milk, thin soups, and pulpy fruits with a high moisture content

◢**Preparations**

Section 2.12

## 1.9.3 Aprotinin

Aprotinin is no longer used for the treatment of acute pancreatitis.

## 1.9.4 Pancreatin

Supplements of pancreatin are given by mouth to compensate for reduced or absent exocrine secretion in cystic fibrosis, and following pancreatectomy, gastrectomy, or chronic pancreatitis. They assist the digestion of starch, fat, and protein. Pancreatin may also be necessary if a tumour (e.g. pancreatic cancer) obstructs outflow from the pancreas.

Pancreatin is inactivated by gastric acid therefore pancreatin preparations are best taken with food (or immediately before or after food). Gastric acid secretion may be reduced by giving cimetidine or ranitidine an hour beforehand (section 1.3). Concurrent use of antacids also reduces gastric acidity. Enteric-coated preparations deliver a higher enzyme concentration in the duodenum (provided the capsule contents are swallowed whole without chewing). Higher-strength preparations are also available (**important:** see CSM advice below).

Since pancreatin is also inactivated by heat, excessive heat should be avoided if preparations are mixed with liquids or food; the resulting mixtures should not be kept for more than one hour.

Dosage is adjusted according to size, number, and consistency of stools, so that the patient thrives; extra allowance will be needed if snacks are taken between meals.

Pancreatin can irritate the perioral skin and buccal mucosa if retained in the mouth, and excessive doses can cause perianal irritation. The most frequent side-effects are gastro-intestinal, including nausea, vomiting, and abdominal discomfort; hyperuricaemia and hyperuricosuria have been associated with very high doses. Hypersensitivity reactions occur occasionally and may affect those handling the powder.

### PANCREATIN

**Indications** see above

**Cautions** see above and (for higher-strength preparations) see below

**Side-effects** see above and (for higher-strength preparations) see below

**Dose**

- See preparations

**Creon® 10 000** (Solvay)

Capsules, brown/clear, enclosing buff-coloured e/c granules of pancreatin (pork), providing: protease 600 units, lipase 10 000 units, amylase 8000 units. Net price 100-cap pack = £14.00. Counselling, see dose

Dose ADULT and CHILD initially 1–2 capsules with each meal either taken whole or contents mixed with fluid or soft food (then swallowed immediately without chewing)

**Creon® Micro** (Solvay)

Gastro-resistant granules, brown, pancreatin (pork), providing: protease 200 units, lipase 5000 units, amylase 3600 units per 100 mg, net price 20 g = £31.50 Counselling, see dose

Dose ADULT and CHILD initially 100 mg with each meal either taken whole or mixed with acidic fluid or soft food (then swallowed immediately without chewing)

**Nutrizym 10®** (Merck)

Capsules, red/yellow, enclosing e/c minitablets of pancreatin (pork), providing minimum of: protease 500 units, lipase 10 000 units, amylase 9000 units. Net price 100 = £14.47. Counselling, see dose

Dose ADULT and CHILD 1–2 capsules with meals and 1 capsule with snacks, swallowed whole or contents taken with water or mixed with soft food (then swallowed immediately without chewing); higher doses may be required according to response

**Pancrex®** (Paines & Byrne)

Granules, pancreatin (pork), providing minimum of: protease 300 units, lipase 5000 units, amylase 4000 units/g. Net price 300 g = £20.39. Label: 25, counselling, see dose

Dose ADULT and CHILD 5–10 g just before meals washed down or mixed with a little milk or water

**Pancrex V®** (Paines & Byrne)

Capsules, pancreatin (pork), providing minimum of: protease 430 units, lipase 8000 units, amylase 9000 units. Net price 300-cap pack = £15.80. Counselling, see dose

Dose ADULT and CHILD over 1 year 2–6 capsules with each meal, swallowed whole or sprinkled on food; INFANT up to 1 year contents of 1–2 capsules mixed with feeds

Capsules '125', pancreatin (pork), providing minimum of: protease 160 units, lipase 2950 units, amylase 3300 units, net price 300-cap pack = £9.72. Counselling, see dose

Dose NEONATE contents of 1–2 capsules mixed with feeds

Tablets, e/c, pancreatin (pork), providing minimum of: protease 110 units, lipase 1900 units, amylase 1700 units. Net price 300-tab pack = £4.51. Label: 5, 25, counselling, see dose

Dose ADULT and CHILD 5–15 tablets before each meal

Tablets forte, e/c, pancreatin (pork), providing minimum of: protease 330 units, lipase 5600 units, amylase 5000 units. Net price 300-tab pack = £13.74. Label: 5, 25, counselling, see dose

Dose ADULT and CHILD 6–10 tablets before each meal

Powder, pancreatin (pork), providing minimum of: protease 1400 units, lipase 25 000 units, amylase 30 000 units/g. Net price 300 g = £24.28. Counselling, see dose

Dose ADULT and CHILD over 1 month, 0.5–2 g before each meal, washed down or mixed with liquid; NEONATE 250–500 mg with each feed

◀ **Higher-strength preparations**

The **CSM** has advised of data associating the high-strength pancreatin preparations *Nutrizym 22®* and *Pancreatin HL®* with the development of large bowel strictures (fibrosing colonopathy) in children with cystic fibrosis aged between 2 and 13 years. No association was found with *Creon® 25 000*. The following was recommended:

- *Pancrease HL®*, *Nutrizym 22®*, *Panzytrat® 25 000* [now discontinued] should not be used in children aged 15 years or less with cystic fibrosis;

- the total dose of pancreatic enzyme supplements used in patients with cystic fibrosis should not usually exceed 10 000 units of lipase per kg body-weight daily;

- if a patient on any pancreatin preparation develops new abdominal symptoms (or any change in existing abdominal symptoms) the patient should be reviewed to exclude the possibility of colonic damage.

Possible risk factors are gender (boys at greater risk than girls), more severe cystic fibrosis, and concomitant use of laxatives. The peak age for developing fibrosing colonopathy is between 2 and 8 years.

**Counselling** It is important to ensure adequate hydration at all times in patients receiving higher-strength pancreatin preparations.

**Creon® 25 000** (Solvay) [PoM]

Capsules, orange/clear, enclosing brown-coloured e/c pellets of pancreatin (pork), providing: protease (total) 1000 units, lipase 25 000 units, amylase 18 000 units, net price 100-cap pack = £28.25. Counselling, see above and under dose

Dose ADULT and CHILD initially 1 capsule with meals either taken whole or contents mixed with fluid or soft food (then swallowed immediately without chewing)

**Creon® 40 000** (Solvay) [PoM]

Capsules, brown/clear, enclosing brown-coloured e/c granules of pancreatin (pork), providing: protease (total) 1600 units, lipase 40 000 units, amylase 25 000 units, net price 100-cap pack = £60.00. Counselling, see above and under dose

Dose ADULT and CHILD 1–2 capsules with meals either taken whole or contents mixed with fluid or soft food (then swallowed immediately without chewing)

**Nutrizym 22®** (Merck) [PoM]

Capsules, red/yellow, enclosing e/c minitablets of pancreatin (pork), providing minimum of: protease 1100 units, lipase 22 000 units, amylase 19 800 units. Net price 100-cap pack = £33.33. Counselling, see above and under dose

Dose ADULT and CHILD over 15 years, 1–2 capsules with meals and 1 capsule with snacks, swallowed whole or contents taken with water or mixed with soft food (then swallowed immediately without chewing)

**Pancrease HL®** (Janssen-Cilag) [PoM]

Capsules, enclosing light brown e/c minitablets of pancreatin (pork), providing minimum of: protease 1250 units, lipase 25 000 units, amylase 22 500 units. Net price 100 = £32.34. Counselling, see above and under dose

Dose ADULT and CHILD over 15 years, 1–2 capsules during each meal and 1 capsule with snacks swallowed whole or contents mixed with slightly acidic liquid or soft food (then swallowed immediately without chewing)

**1**

**Gastro-intestinal system**

# 2 Cardiovascular system

**2.1 Positive inotropic drugs**    72
2.1.1 Cardiac glycosides    72
2.1.2 Phosphodiesterase inhibitors    74

**2.2 Diuretics**    **74**
2.2.1 Thiazides and related diuretics    75
2.2.2 Loop diuretics    76
2.2.3 Potassium-sparing diuretics and aldosterone antagonists    78
2.2.4 Potassium-sparing diuretics with other diuretics    79
2.2.5 Osmotic diuretics    80
2.2.6 Mercurial diuretics    80
2.2.7 Carbonic anhydrase inhibitors    80
2.2.8 Diuretics with potassium    80

**2.3 Anti-arrhythmic drugs**    **81**
2.3.1 Management of arrhythmias    81
2.3.2 Drugs for arrhythmias    82

**2.4 Beta-adrenoceptor blocking drugs**    **86**

**2.5 Hypertension and heart failure**    **93**
2.5.1 Vasodilator antihypertensive drugs    95
2.5.2 Centrally acting antihypertensive drugs    98
2.5.3 Adrenergic neurone blocking drugs    99
2.5.4 Alpha-adrenoceptor blocking drugs    99
2.5.5 Drugs affecting the renin-angiotensin system    101
2.5.5.1 Angiotensin-converting enzyme inhibitors    102
2.5.5.2 Angiotensin-II receptor antagonists    107
2.5.5.3 Renin inhibitors    110

**2.6 Nitrates, calcium-channel blockers, and other antianginal drugs**    **110**
2.6.1 Nitrates    111
2.6.2 Calcium-channel blockers    114
2.6.3 Other antianginal drugs    120
2.6.4 Peripheral vasodilators and related drugs    121

**2.7 Sympathomimetics**    **123**
2.7.1 Inotropic sympathomimetics    123
2.7.2 Vasoconstrictor sympathomimetics    124

2.7.3 Cardiopulmonary resuscitation    125

**2.8 Anticoagulants and protamine**    **125**
2.8.1 Parenteral anticoagulants    125
2.8.2 Oral anticoagulants    130
2.8.3 Protamine sulphate    133

**2.9 Antiplatelet drugs**    **133**

**2.10 Myocardial infarction and fibrinolysis**    **137**
2.10.1 Management of myocardial infarction    137
2.10.2 Fibrinolytic drugs    138

**2.11 Antifibrinolytic drugs and haemostatics**    **140**

**2.12 Lipid-regulating drugs**    **142**

**2.13 Local sclerosants**    **149**

This chapter also includes advice on the drug management of the following:
angina, p. 110
arrhythmias, p. 81
cardiovascular disease risk, p. 93 and p. 142
heart failure, p. 101
hypertension, p. 93
myocardial infarction, p. 137
phaeochromocytoma, p. 101

## 2.1 Positive inotropic drugs

2.1.1 Cardiac glycosides
2.1.2 Phosphodiesterase inhibitors

Positive inotropic drugs increase the force of contraction of the myocardium; for sympathomimetics with inotropic activity see section 2.7.1.

## 2.1.1 Cardiac glycosides

Cardiac glycosides increase the force of myocardial contraction and reduce conductivity within the atrioventricular (AV) node. Digoxin is the most commonly used cardiac glycoside.

Cardiac glycosides are most useful for controlling ventricular response in persistent atrial fibrillation and atrial flutter (section 2.3.1). For reference to the role of digoxin in heart failure, see section 2.5.5.

For management of atrial fibrillation the maintenance dose of the cardiac glycoside can usually be determined by the ventricular rate at rest, which should not be allowed to fall below 60 beats per minute except in special circumstances, e.g. with the concomitant administration of a beta-blocker.

Digoxin is now rarely used for rapid control of heart rate (see section 2.3 for the management of supraventricular arrhythmias). Even with intravenous administration, response may take many hours; persistence of tachycardia is therefore not an indication for exceeding the recommended dose. The intramuscular route is **not** recommended.

In patients with heart failure who are in sinus rhythm a loading dose is not required, and a satisfactory plasma-digoxin concentration can be achieved over a period of about a week.

Digoxin has a long half-life and maintenance doses need to be given only once daily (although higher doses may be divided to avoid nausea). **Digitoxin** also has a long half-life and maintenance doses need to be given only once daily or on alternate days. Renal function is the most important determinant of digoxin dosage, whereas elimination of digitoxin depends on metabolism by the liver.

Unwanted effects depend both on the concentration of the cardiac glycoside in the plasma and on the sensitivity of the conducting system or of the myocardium, which is often increased in heart disease. It can sometimes be difficult to distinguish between toxic effects and clinical deterioration because symptoms of both are similar. The plasma concentration alone cannot indicate toxicity reliably, but the likelihood of toxicity increases progressively through the range 1.5 to 3 micrograms/litre for digoxin. Cardiac glycosides should be used with special care in the elderly, who may be particularly susceptible to digitalis toxicity.

Regular monitoring of plasma-digoxin concentration during maintenance treatment is not necessary unless problems are suspected. Hypokalaemia predisposes the patient to digitalis toxicity; it is managed by giving a potassium-sparing diuretic or, if necessary, potassium supplementation.

Toxicity can often be managed by discontinuing digoxin; serious manifestations require urgent specialist management. **Digoxin-specific antibody fragments** are available for reversal of life-threatening overdosage (see below).

## ■ DIGOXIN

**Indications** heart failure (see also section 2.5.5), supraventricular arrhythmias (particularly atrial fibrillation and atrial flutter; see also section 2.3.2)

**Cautions** recent myocardial infarction; sick sinus syndrome; thyroid disease; reduce dose in the elderly; severe respiratory disease; hypokalaemia, hypomagnesaemia, hypercalcaemia, and hypoxia (risk of digitalis toxicity); monitor serum electrolytes and renal function; avoid rapid intravenous administration (risk of hypertension and reduced coronary flow); renal impairment (Appendix 3); pregnancy (Appendix 4); **interactions:** Appendix 1 (cardiac glycosides)

**Contra-indications** intermittent complete heart block, second degree AV block; supraventricular arrhythmias associated with accessory conducting pathways e.g. Wolff-Parkinson-White syndrome; ventricular tachycardia or fibrillation; hypertrophic cardiomyopathy (unless concomitant atrial fibrillation and heart failure—but use with caution); myocarditis; constrictive pericarditis (unless to control atrial fibrillation or improve systolic dysfunction—but use with caution)

**Side-effects** see notes above; also nausea, vomiting, diarrhoea; arrhythmias, conduction disturbances; dizziness; blurred or yellow vision; rash, eosinophilia; *less commonly* depression; *very rarely* anorexia, intestinal ischaemia and necrosis, psychosis, apathy, confusion, headache, fatigue, weakness, gynaecomastia on long-term use, and thrombocytopenia

**Dose**

- Rapid digitalisation, for atrial fibrillation or flutter, by mouth, 0.75–1.5 mg over 24 hours in divided doses
- Maintenance, for atrial fibrillation or flutter, by mouth, according to renal function and initial loading dose; usual range 125–250 micrograms daily
- Heart failure (for patients in sinus rhythm), by mouth, 62.5–125 micrograms once daily
- Emergency loading dose, for atrial fibrillation or flutter, by intravenous infusion (but rarely necessary), 0.75–1 mg over at least 2 hours (see also Cautions) then maintenance dose by mouth on the following day

**Note** The above doses may need to be reduced if digoxin (or another cardiac glycoside) has been given in the preceding 2 weeks. Digoxin doses in the BNF may differ from those in product literature. For plasma concentration monitoring, blood should ideally be taken at least 6 hours after a dose

**Digoxin** (Non-proprietary) ▣
Tablets, digoxin 62.5 micrograms, net price 28 = £1.63; 125 micrograms, 28 = £1.29; 250 micrograms, 28 = £1.29

Injection, digoxin 250 micrograms/mL, net price 2-mL amp = 70p
Available from Antigen

Paediatric injection, digoxin 100 micrograms/mL
Available from 'special-order' manufacturers or specialist importing companies, see p. 969

**Lanoxin**® (GSK) ▣
Tablets, digoxin 125 micrograms, net price 20 = 32p; 250 micrograms (scored), 20 = 32p

Injection, digoxin 250 micrograms/mL, net price 2-mL amp = 66p

**Lanoxin-PG**® (GSK) ▣
Tablets, blue, digoxin 62.5 micrograms, net price 20 = 32p

Elixir, yellow, digoxin 50 micrograms/mL. Do not dilute, measure with pipette. Net price 60 mL = £5.35.
Counselling, use of pipette

## ■ DIGITOXIN

**Indications** heart failure, supraventricular arrhythmias (particularly atrial fibrillation)

**Cautions** see under Digoxin

**Contra-indications** see under Digoxin

**Side-effects** see under Digoxin

**Dose**

- Maintenance, 100 micrograms daily *or* on alternate days; may be increased to 200 micrograms daily if necessary

**Digitoxin** (Non-proprietary) ▣
Tablets, digitoxin 100 micrograms, net price 28 = £4.11

## Digoxin-specific antibody

**Digoxin-specific antibody fragments** are indicated for the treatment of known or strongly suspected digoxin or digitoxin overdosage when measures beyond the withdrawal of the cardiac glycoside and correction of any electrolyte abnormalities are felt to be necessary (see also notes above).

**Digibind®** (GSK) [PoM]
Injection, powder for preparation of infusion, digoxin-specific antibody fragments (F(ab)) 38 mg, net price per vial = £93.97 (hosp. and poisons centres only)
**Dose** consult product literature

### 2.1.2 Phosphodiesterase inhibitors

**Enoximone** and **milrinone** are selective phosphodiesterase inhibitors which exert most of their effect on the myocardium. Sustained haemodynamic benefit has been observed after administration, but there is no evidence of any beneficial effect on survival.

### ■ ENOXIMONE

**Indications** congestive heart failure where cardiac output reduced and filling pressures increased
**Cautions** heart failure associated with hypertrophic cardiomyopathy, stenotic or obstructive valvular disease or other outlet obstruction; monitor blood pressure, heart rate, ECG, central venous pressure, fluid and electrolyte status, renal function, platelet count, hepatic enzymes; avoid extravasation; hepatic impairment (Appendix 2); renal impairment (Appendix 3); pregnancy (Appendix 4); breast-feeding (Appendix 5); **interactions:** Appendix 1 (phosphodiesterase inhibitors)
**Side-effects** ectopic beats; less frequently ventricular tachycardia or supraventricular arrhythmias (more likely in patients with pre-existing arrhythmias); hypotension; also headache, insomnia, nausea and vomiting, diarrhoea; occasionally, chills, oliguria, fever, urinary retention; upper and lower limb pain

**Dose**
- By slow intravenous injection (rate not exceeding 12.5 mg/minute), diluted before use, initially 0.5–1 mg/kg, then 500 micrograms/kg every 30 minutes until satisfactory response or total of 3 mg/kg given; maintenance, initial dose of up to 3 mg/kg may be repeated every 3–6 hours as required
- By intravenous infusion, initially 90 micrograms/kg/minute over 10–30 minutes, followed by continuous or intermittent infusion of 5–20 micrograms/kg/minute
Total dose over 24 hours should not usually exceed 24 mg/kg

**Perfan®** (INCA-Pharm) [PoM]
Injection, enoximone 5 mg/mL. For dilution before use. Net price 20-mL amp = £15.02
**Excipients** include alcohol, propylene glycol
**Note** Plastic apparatus should be used; crystal formation if glass used

### ■ MILRINONE

**Indications** short-term treatment of severe congestive heart failure unresponsive to conventional maintenance therapy (not immediately after myocardial infarction); acute heart failure, including low output states following heart surgery
**Cautions** see under Enoximone; also correct hypokalaemia; renal impairment (Appendix 3); pregnancy (Appendix 4); breast-feeding (Appendix 5); **interactions:** Appendix 1 (phosphodiesterase inhibitors)
**Side-effects** ectopic beats, ventricular tachycardia, supraventricular arrhythmias (more likely in patients with pre-existing arrhythmias), hypotension; headache; *less commonly* ventricular fibrillation, chest pain, tremor, hypokalaemia, thrombocytopenia; *very rarely* bronchospasm, anaphylaxis, and rash

**Dose**
- By intravenous injection over 10 minutes, either undiluted or diluted before use, 50 micrograms/kg followed by intravenous infusion at a rate of 375–750 nanograms/kg/minute, usually for up to 12 hours following surgery or for 48–72 hours in congestive heart failure; max. daily dose 1.13 mg/kg

**Primacor®** (Sanofi-Aventis) [PoM]
Injection, milrinone (as lactate) 1 mg/mL, net price 10-mL amp = £16.61

### 2.2 Diuretics

2.2.1  Thiazides and related diuretics
2.2.2  Loop diuretics
2.2.3  Potassium-sparing diuretics and aldosterone antagonists
2.2.4  Potassium-sparing diuretics with other diuretics
2.2.5  Osmotic diuretics
2.2.6  Mercurial diuretics
2.2.7  Carbonic anhydrase inhibitors
2.2.8  Diuretics with potassium

**Thiazides** (section 2.2.1) are used to relieve oedema due to chronic heart failure (section 2.5.5) and, in lower doses, to reduce blood pressure.

**Loop diuretics** (section 2.2.2) are used in pulmonary oedema due to left ventricular failure and in patients with chronic heart failure (section 2.5.5).

**Combination diuretic therapy** may be effective in patients with oedema resistant to treatment with one diuretic. Vigorous diuresis, particularly with loop diuretics, may induce acute hypotension; rapid reduction of plasma volume should be avoided.

**Elderly** Lower initial doses of diuretics should be used in the elderly because they are particularly susceptible to the side-effects. The dose should then be adjusted according to renal function. Diuretics should not be used continuously on a long-term basis to treat simple gravitational oedema (which will usually respond to increased movement, raising the legs, and support stockings).

**Potassium loss** Hypokalaemia may occur with both thiazide and loop diuretics. The risk of hypokalaemia depends on the duration of action as well as the potency and is thus greater with thiazides than with an equipotent dose of a loop diuretic.

Hypokalaemia is dangerous in severe cardiovascular disease and in patients also being treated with cardiac glycosides. Often the use of potassium-sparing diuretics (section 2.2.3) avoids the need to take potassium supplements.

In hepatic failure, hypokalaemia caused by diuretics can precipitate encephalopathy, particularly in alcoholic cirrhosis; diuretics may also increase the risk of hypomagnesaemia in alcoholic cirrhosis, leading to arrhythmias. Spironolactone, a potassium-sparing diuretic (section 2.2.3), is chosen for oedema arising from cirrhosis of the liver.

Potassium supplements or potassium-sparing diuretics are seldom necessary when thiazides are used in the routine treatment of hypertension (see also section 9.2.1.1).

## 2.2.1 Thiazides and related diuretics

Thiazides and related compounds are moderately potent diuretics; they inhibit sodium reabsorption at the beginning of the distal convoluted tubule. They act within 1 to 2 hours of oral administration and most have a duration of action of 12 to 24 hours; they are usually administered early in the day so that the diuresis does not interfere with sleep.

In the management of *hypertension* a low dose of a thiazide, e.g. bendroflumethiazide (bendrofluazide) 2.5 mg daily, produces a maximal or near-maximal blood pressure lowering effect, with very little biochemical disturbance. Higher doses cause more marked changes in plasma potassium, sodium, uric acid, glucose, and lipids, with little advantage in blood pressure control. For reference to the use of thiazides in chronic heart failure see section 2.5.5.

**Bendroflumethiazide** (bendrofluazide) is widely used for mild or moderate heart failure and for hypertension—alone in the treatment of mild hypertension or with other drugs in more severe hypertension.

**Chlortalidone** (chlorthalidone), a thiazide-related compound, has a longer duration of action than the thiazides and may be given on alternate days to control oedema. It is also useful if acute retention is liable to be precipitated by a more rapid diuresis or if patients dislike the altered pattern of micturition caused by other diuretics.

Other thiazide diuretics (including benzthiazide, clopamide, cyclopenthiazide, hydrochlorothiazide, and hydroflumethiazide) do not offer any significant advantage over bendroflumethiazide or chlortalidone.

**Metolazone** is particularly effective when combined with a loop diuretic (even in renal failure); profound diuresis can occur and the patient should therefore be monitored carefully.

**Xipamide** and **indapamide** are chemically related to chlortalidone. Indapamide is claimed to lower blood pressure with less metabolic disturbance, particularly less aggravation of diabetes mellitus.

**Cautions** See also section 2.2. Thiazides and related diuretics can exacerbate diabetes, gout, and systemic lupus erythematosus. Electrolytes should be monitored, particularly with high doses, long-term use, or in renal impairment. Thiazides and related diuretics should also be used with caution in nephrotic syndrome, hyperaldosteronism, malnourishment, hepatic impairment (avoid if severe; Appendix 2), renal impairment (Appendix 3), pregnancy (Appendix 4), and breast-feeding (Appendix 5); **interactions**: Appendix 1 (diuretics)

**Contra-indications** Thiazides and related diuretics should be avoided in refractory hypokalaemia, hyponatraemia and hypercalcaemia, symptomatic hyperuricaemia, and Addison's disease.

**Side-effects** Side-effects of thiazides and related diuretics include mild gastro-intestinal disturbances, postural hypotension, altered plasma-lipid concentrations, metabolic and electrolyte disturbances including hypokalaemia (see also notes above), hyponatraemia, hypomagnesaemia, hypercalcaemia, hyperglycaemia, hypochloraemic alkalosis, hyperuricaemia, and gout. Less common side-effects include blood disorders such as agranulocytosis, leucopenia, and thrombocytopenia, and impotence. Pancreatitis, intrahepatic cholestasis, cardiac arrhythmias, headache, dizziness, paraesthesia, visual disturbances, and hypersensitivity reactions (including pneumonitis, pulmonary oedema, photosensitivity, and severe skin reactions) have also been reported.

### BENDROFLUMETHIAZIDE
#### (Bendrofluazide)

**Indications** oedema, hypertension (see also notes above)

**Cautions** see notes above

**Contra-indications** see notes above

**Side-effects** see notes above

**Dose**
- Oedema, initially 5–10 mg daily in the morning *or* on alternate days; maintenance 5–10 mg 1–3 times weekly
- Hypertension, 2.5 mg daily in the morning; higher doses rarely necessary (see notes above)

**Bendroflumethiazide** (Non-proprietary) PoM
Tablets, bendroflumethiazide 2.5 mg, net price 28 = 81p; 5 mg, 28 = 85p
Brands include *Aprinox*®, *Neo-NaClex*®

### CHLORTALIDONE
#### (Chlorthalidone)

**Indications** ascites due to cirrhosis in stable patients (under close supervision), oedema due to nephrotic syndrome, hypertension (see also notes above), mild to moderate chronic heart failure; diabetes insipidus (see section 6.5.2)

**Cautions** see notes above

**Contra-indications** see notes above

**Side-effects** see notes above; also *rarely* jaundice and allergic interstitial nephritis

**Dose**

- Oedema, up to 50 mg daily
- Hypertension, 25 mg daily in the morning, increased to 50 mg daily if necessary (but see notes above)
- Heart failure, 25–50 mg daily in the morning, increased if necessary to 100–200 mg daily (reduce to lowest effective dose for maintenance)

**Hygroton®** (Alliance) [PoM]
Tablets, yellow, scored, chlortalidone 50 mg, net price 28-tab pack = £1.52

### ■ CYCLOPENTHIAZIDE

**Indications** oedema, hypertension (see also notes above); heart failure

**Cautions** see notes above

**Contra-indications** see notes above

**Side-effects** see notes above; also *rarely* depression

**Dose**

- Heart failure, 250–500 micrograms daily in the morning increased if necessary to 1 mg daily (reduce to lowest effective dose for maintenance)
- Hypertension, initially 250 micrograms daily in the morning, increased if necessary to 500 micrograms daily (but see notes above)
- Oedema, up to 500 micrograms daily for a short period

**Navidrex®** (Goldshield) [PoM]
Tablets, scored, cyclopenthiazide 500 micrograms, net price 28-tab pack = £1.27
Excipients include gluten

### ■ INDAPAMIDE

**Indications** essential hypertension

**Cautions** see notes above; also acute porphyria (section 9.8.2)

**Contra-indications** see notes above; also hypersensitivity to sulphonamides

**Side-effects** see notes above; also palpitation, diuresis with doses above 2.5 mg daily

**Dose**

- 2.5 mg daily in the morning

**Indapamide** (Non-proprietary) [PoM]
Tablets, s/c, indapamide 2.5 mg, net price 28-tab pack = £1.27, 56-tab pack = £1.88

**Natrilix®** (Servier) [PoM]
Tablets, f/c, indapamide 2.5 mg. Net price 30-tab pack = £4.32, 60-tab pack = £8.64

**◢ Modified release**

**Ethibide XL®** (Genus) [PoM]
Tablets, m/r, indapamide 1.5 mg, net price 30-tab pack = £4.05. Label: 25
Dose hypertension, 1 tablet daily, preferably in the morning

**Natrilix SR®** (Servier) [PoM]
Tablets, m/r, indapamide 1.5 mg, net price 30-tab pack = £4.32. Label: 25
Dose hypertension, 1 tablet daily, preferably in the morning

### ■ METOLAZONE

**Indications** oedema, hypertension (see also notes above)

**Cautions** see notes above; also acute porphyria (section 9.8.2)

**Contra-indications** see notes above

**Side-effects** see notes above; also chills, chest pain

**Dose**

- Oedema, 5–10 mg daily in the morning, increased if necessary to 20 mg daily in resistant oedema, max. 80 mg daily
- Hypertension, initially 5 mg daily in the morning; maintenance 5 mg on alternate days

**Metenix 5®** (Sanofi-Aventis) [PoM]
Tablets, blue, metolazone 5 mg, net price 100-tab pack = £18.20

### ■ XIPAMIDE

**Indications** oedema, hypertension (see also notes above)

**Cautions** see notes above; also acute porphyria (section 9.8.2)

**Contra-indications** see notes above

**Side-effects** see notes above

**Dose**

- Oedema, initially 40 mg daily in the morning, increased to 80 mg in resistant cases; maintenance 20 mg in the morning
- Hypertension, 20 mg daily in the morning

**Diurexan®** (Viatris) [PoM]
Tablets, scored, xipamide 20 mg, net price 140-tab pack = £19.46

## 2.2.2 Loop diuretics

Loop diuretics are used in pulmonary oedema due to left ventricular failure; intravenous administration produces relief of breathlessness and reduces pre-load sooner than would be expected from the time of onset of diuresis. Loop diuretics are also used in patients with chronic heart failure. Diuretic-resistant oedema (except lymphoedema and oedema due to peripheral venous stasis or calcium-channel blockers) can be treated with a loop diuretic combined with a thiazide or related diuretic (e.g. bendroflumethiazide 5–10 mg daily or metolazone 5–20 mg daily).

If necessary, a loop diuretic can be added to antihypertensive treatment to achieve better control of blood pressure in those with resistant hypertension, or in patients with impaired renal function or heart failure.

Loop diuretics inhibit reabsorption from the ascending limb of the loop of Henlé in the renal tubule and are powerful diuretics. Hypokalaemia may develop, and care is needed to avoid hypotension. If there is an enlarged prostate, urinary retention may occur; this is less likely if small doses and less potent diuretics are used initially.

**Furosemide** (frusemide) and **bumetanide** are similar in activity; both act within 1 hour of oral administration and diuresis is complete within 6 hours so that, if necessary, they can be given twice in one day without interfering with sleep. Following intravenous administration they have a peak effect within 30 minutes. The diuresis associated with these drugs is dose related. In patients with impaired renal function very large doses may occasionally be needed; in such doses both drugs can cause deafness and bumetanide can cause myalgia.

**Torasemide** has properties similar to those of furosemide and bumetanide, and is indicated for oedema and for hypertension.

---

## FUROSEMIDE
### (Frusemide)

**Indications** oedema (see notes above); resistant hypertension (see notes above)

**Cautions** section 2.2; also monitor electrolytes; hypotension; prostatic enlargement; impaired micturition; gout; diabetes; intravenous administration rate should not usually exceed 4 mg/minute, however single doses of up to 80 mg may be administered more rapidly; a lower infusion rate may be considered in those with renal impairment; hepatorenal syndrome; hepatic impairment (Appendix 2); renal impairment (Appendix 3); pregnancy (Appendix 4); breast-feeding (Appendix 5); **interactions:** Appendix 1 (diuretics)

**Contra-indications** hypovolaemia, dehydration, severe hypokalaemia, severe hyponatraemia; comatose or precomatose states associated with liver cirrhosis; renal failure due to nephrotoxic or hepatotoxic drugs, anuria

**Side-effects** mild gastro-intestinal disturbances; hypotension; hyperglycaemia (less common than with thiazides); hyperuricaemia and gout; electrolyte disturbances including hyponatraemia, hypokalaemia (see also section 2.2), hypocalcaemia, and hypomagnesaemia, metabolic alkalosis; *rarely* paraethesia, blood disorders (including thrombocytopenia, leucopenia, agranulocytosis, aplastic anaemia, haemolytic anaemia), bone marrow depression (withdraw treatment), tinnitus and deafness (usually with large parenteral doses and rapid administration, in renal impairment, or in hypoproteinaemia), and hypersensitivity reactions (including rashes, photosensitivity, eosinophilia, exfoliative dermatitis, purpura, and anaphylaxis), pancreatitis, intrahepatic cholestasis; temporary increase in plasma cholesterol and triglyceride concentration also reported

**Dose**
- By mouth, oedema, initially 40 mg in the morning; maintenance 20–40 mg daily; CHILD 1–3 mg/kg daily, max. 40 mg daily

  Resistant oedema, 80–120 mg daily

  Resistant hypertension, 40–80 mg daily
- By intramuscular injection *or* slow intravenous injection (rate of administration, see Cautions above), initially 20–50 mg, increased if necessary in steps of 20 mg not less than every 2 hours; doses greater than 50 mg by intravenous infusion only; max. 1.5 g daily; CHILD 0.5–1.5 mg/kg daily, max. 20 mg daily

**Furosemide** (Non-proprietary) ▣PoM
Tablets, furosemide 20 mg, net price 28 = 81p; 40 mg, 28 = 85p; 500 mg, 28 = £3.66
Brands include *Froop®*, *Rusyde®*

Oral solution, sugar-free, furosemide, net price 20 mg/5 mL, 150 mL = £12.46; 40 mg/5 mL, 150 mL = £15.99; 50 mg/5 mL, 150 mL = £17.39
Brands include *Frusol®* (contains alcohol 10%)

Injection, furosemide 10 mg/mL, net price 2-mL amp = 55p, 5-mL amp = 66p, 25-mL amp = £2.50

**Lasix®** (Sanofi-Aventis) ▣PoM
Injection, furosemide 10 mg/mL, net price 2-mL amp = 75p
Note Large-volume furosemide injections also available; brands include *Minijet®*

---

## BUMETANIDE

**Indications** oedema (see notes above)

**Cautions** see under Furosemide; hepatic impairment (Appendix 2); pregnancy (Appendix 4); breast-feeding (Appendix 5)

**Contra-indications** see under Furosemide

**Side-effects** see under Furosemide; also headache, dizziness, fatigue, gynaecomastia, myalgia

**Dose**
- By mouth, 1 mg in the morning, repeated after 6–8 hours if necessary; severe cases, 5 mg daily increased by 5 mg every 12–24 hours according to response; ELDERLY, 500 micrograms daily may be sufficient
- By intravenous injection, 1–2 mg, repeated after 20 minutes if necessary; ELDERLY, 500 micrograms daily may be sufficient
- By intravenous infusion, 2–5 mg over 30–60 minutes; ELDERLY, 500 micrograms daily may be sufficient
- By intramuscular injection, 1 mg initially then adjusted according to response; ELDERLY, 500 micrograms daily may be sufficient

**Bumetanide** (Non-proprietary) ▣PoM
Tablets, bumetanide 1 mg, net price 28-tab pack = £1.25; 5 mg, 28-tab pack = £2.48

Oral liquid, bumetanide 1 mg/5 mL, net price 150 mL = £128.00

Injection, bumetanide 500 micrograms/mL, net price 4-mL amp = £1.79

**Burinex®** (LEO) ▣PoM
Tablets, scored, bumetanide 1 mg, net price 28-tab pack = £1.52; 5 mg, 28 = £9.67

---

## TORASEMIDE

**Indications** oedema (see notes above), hypertension

**Cautions** see under Furosemide; hepatic impairment (Appendix 2); renal impairment (Appendix 3); pregnancy (Appendix 4)

**Contra-indications** see under Furosemide

**Side-effects** see under Furosemide; also dry mouth; rarely limb paraesthesia

**Dose**
- Oedema, 5 mg once daily, preferably in the morning, increased if required to 20 mg once daily; usual max. 40 mg daily
- Hypertension, 2.5 mg daily, increased if necessary to 5 mg once daily

**Torasemide** (Non-proprietary) ▣PoM
Tablets, torasemide 5 mg, net price 28-tab pack = £5.64; 10 mg, 28-tab pack = £8.10

**Torem®** (Roche) ▣PoM
Tablets, torasemide 2.5 mg, net price 28-tab pack = £3.43; 5 mg (scored), 28-tab pack = £4.97; 10 mg (scored), 28-tab pack = £8.14

**2**

**Cardiovascular system**

Cardiovascular system

2

### 2.2.3 Potassium-sparing diuretics and aldosterone antagonists

Amiloride and triamterene on their own are weak diuretics. They cause retention of potassium and are therefore given with thiazide or loop diuretics as a more effective alternative to potassium supplements. See section 2.2.4 for compound preparations with thiazides or loop diuretics.

Potassium supplements must **not** be given with potassium-sparing diuretics. Administration of a potassium-sparing diuretic to a patient receiving an ACE inhibitor or an angiotensin-II receptor antagonist can also cause severe hyperkalaemia.

### AMILORIDE HYDROCHLORIDE

**Indications** oedema; potassium conservation when used as an adjunct to thiazide or loop diuretics for hypertension, congestive heart failure, or hepatic cirrhosis with ascites

**Cautions** monitor electrolytes; diabetes mellitus; elderly; renal impairment (manufacturers advise avoid if severe; Appendix 3); pregnancy (Appendix 4); breast-feeding (Appendix 5); **interactions**: Appendix 1 (diuretics)

**Contra-indications** hyperkalaemia; anuria; Addison's disease

**Side-effects** include gastro-intestinal disturbances, dry mouth, rashes, confusion, postural hypotension, hyperkalaemia, hyponatraemia

**Dose**

* Used alone, initially 10 mg daily *or* 5 mg twice daily, adjusted according to response; max. 20 mg daily
* With other diuretics, congestive heart failure and hypertension, initially 5–10 mg daily; cirrhosis with ascites, initially 5 mg daily

**Amiloride** (Non-proprietary) [PoM]
Tablets, amiloride hydrochloride 5 mg, net price 28-tab pack = 97p
Oral solution, sugar-free, amiloride hydrochloride 5 mg/5 mL, net price 150 mL = £39.73
Brands include *Amilamont®* (Excipients include propylene glycol, see Excipients, p. 2)

◢Compound preparations with thiazide or loop diuretics
Section 2.2.4

### TRIAMTERENE

**Indications** oedema, potassium conservation with thiazide and loop diuretics

**Cautions** see under Amiloride Hydrochloride; may cause blue fluorescence of urine

**Contra-indications** see under Amiloride Hydrochloride

**Side-effects** include gastro-intestinal disturbances, dry mouth, rashes; slight decrease in blood pressure, hyperkalaemia, hyponatraemia; photosensitivity and blood disorders also reported; triamterene found in kidney stones

**Dose**

* Initially 150–250 mg daily, reducing to alternate days after 1 week; taken in divided doses after breakfast and lunch; lower initial dose when given with other diuretics
**Counselling** Urine may look slightly blue in some lights

**Dytac®** (Goldshield) [PoM]
Capsules, maroon, triamterene 50 mg, net price 30-cap pack = £17.35 Label: 14, (see above), 21

◢Compound preparations with thiazides or loop diuretics
Section 2.2.4

### Aldosterone antagonists

**Spironolactone** potentiates thiazide or loop diuretics by antagonising aldosterone; it is a potassium-sparing diuretic. Spironolactone is of value in the treatment of oedema and ascites caused by cirrhosis of the liver; furosemide (section 2.2.2) can be used as an adjunct. Low doses of spironolactone are beneficial in severe heart failure, see section 2.5.5.

Spironolactone is also used in primary hyperaldosteronism (Conn's syndrome). It is given before surgery or if surgery is not appropriate, in the lowest effective dose for maintenance.

**Eplerenone** is licensed for use as an adjunct in left ventricular dysfunction with evidence of heart failure after a myocardial infarction (see also section 2.5.5 and section 2.10.1).

Potassium supplements must **not** be given with aldosterone antagonists.

### EPLERENONE

**Indications** adjunct in stable patients with left ventricular dysfunction with evidence of heart failure, following myocardial infarction (start therapy within 3–14 days of event)

**Cautions** measure plasma-potassium concentration before treatment, during initiation, and when dose changed; elderly; hepatic impairment (Appendix 2); renal impairment (avoid if eGFR less than 50 mL/minute/1.73 m²; Appendix 3); pregnancy; breast-feeding (Appendix 5); **interactions**: Appendix 1 (diuretics)

**Contra-indications** hyperkalaemia; concomitant use of potassium-sparing diuretics or potassium supplements

**Side-effects** diarrhoea, nausea; hypotension; dizziness; hyperkalaemia; rash; *less commonly* flatulence, vomiting, atrial fibrillation, postural hypotension, arterial thrombosis, dyslipidaemia, pharyngitis, headache, insomnia, gynaecomastia, pyelonephritis, hyponatraemia, dehydration, eosinophilia, asthenia, malaise, back pain, leg cramps, impaired renal function, azotaemia, sweating and pruritus

**Dose**

* Initially 25 mg once daily, increased within 4 weeks to 50 mg once daily; CHILD not recommended

**Inspra®** (Pfizer) ▼ [PoM]
Tablets, yellow, f/c, eplerenone 25 mg, net price 28-tab pack = £42.72; 50 mg, 28-tab pack = £42.72

## ■ SPIRONOLACTONE

**Indications** oedema and ascites in cirrhosis of the liver, malignant ascites, nephrotic syndrome, congestive heart failure (section 2.5.5); primary hyperaldosteronism

**Cautions** potential metabolic products carcinogenic in *rodents*; elderly; monitor electrolytes (discontinue if hyperkalaemia); acute porphyria (section 9.8.2); hepatic impairment; renal impairment (manufacturers advise avoid if severe; Appendix 3); pregnancy (Appendix 4); breast-feeding (Appendix 5); **interactions**: Appendix 1 (diuretics)

**Contra-indications** hyperkalaemia, hyponatraemia; Addison's disease

**Side-effects** gastro-intestinal disturbances; impotence, gynaecomastia; menstrual irregularities; lethargy, headache, confusion; rashes; hyperkalaemia (discontinue); hyponatraemia; hepatotoxicity, osteomalacia, and blood disorders reported

**Dose**
- 100–200 mg daily, increased to 400 mg if required; CHILD initially 3 mg/kg daily in divided doses
- Heart failure, see section 2.5.5

**Spironolactone** (Non-proprietary) ℗ₒₘ
Tablets, spironolactone 25 mg, net price 28 = £1.79; 50 mg, 28 = £2.49; 100 mg, 28 = £3.38. Label: 21
Oral suspensions, spironolactone 5 mg/5 mL, 10 mg/5 mL, 25 mg/5 mL, 50 mg/5 mL, and 100 mg/5 mL. Label: 21
Available from 'special-order' manufacturers or specialist importing companies, see p. 969

**Aldactone®** (Pharmacia) ℗ₒₘ
Tablets, f/c, spironolactone 25 mg (buff), net price 100-tab pack = £8.89; 50 mg (off-white), 100-tab pack = £17.78; 100 mg (buff), 28-tab pack = £9.96. Label: 21

**■ With thiazides or loop diuretics**
Section 2.2.4

## 2.2.4 Potassium-sparing diuretics with other diuretics

Although it is preferable to prescribe thiazides (section 2.2.1) and potassium-sparing diuretics (section 2.2.3) separately, the use of fixed combinations may be justified if compliance is a problem. Potassium-sparing diuretics are not usually necessary in the routine treatment of hypertension, unless hypokalaemia develops. For **interactions**, see Appendix 1 (diuretics).

**■ Amiloride with thiazides**
**Co-amilozide** (Non-proprietary) ℗ₒₘ
Tablets, co-amilozide 2.5/25 (amiloride hydrochloride 2.5 mg, hydrochlorothiazide 25 mg), net price 28-tab pack = £2.43
Brands include *Moduret 25®*
Dose hypertension, initially 1 tablet daily, increased if necessary to max. 2 tablets daily
Congestive heart failure, initially 1 tablet daily, increased if necessary to max. 4 tablets daily
Oedema and ascites in cirrhosis of the liver, initially 2 tablets daily, increased if necessary to max. 4 tablets daily; reduce for maintenance if possible

Tablets, co-amilozide 5/50 (amiloride hydrochloride 5 mg, hydrochlorothiazide 50 mg), net price 28 = £1.06
Brands include *Amil-Co®*, *Moduretic®*
Dose hypertension, initially ½ tablet daily, increased if necessary to max. 1 tablet daily
Congestive heart failure, initially ½ tablet daily, increased if necessary to max. 2 tablets daily
Oedema and ascites in cirrhosis of the liver, initially 1 tablet daily, increased if necessary to max. 2 tablets daily; reduce for maintenance if possible

**Navispare®** (Goldshield) ℗ₒₘ
Tablets, f/c, orange, amiloride hydrochloride 2.5 mg, cyclopenthiazide 250 micrograms, net price 28-tab pack = £2.70
Excipients include gluten
Dose hypertension, 1–2 tablets in the morning

**■ Amiloride with loop diuretics**
**Co-amilofruse** (Non-proprietary) ℗ₒₘ
Tablets, co-amilofruse 2.5/20 (amiloride hydrochloride 2.5 mg, furosemide 20 mg), net price 28-tab pack = £1.24, 56-tab pack = £1.61
Brands include *Frumil LS®*
Dose oedema, 1 tablet in the morning

Tablets, co-amilofruse 5/40 (amiloride hydrochloride 5 mg, furosemide 40 mg), net price 28-tab pack = £1.30, 56-tab pack = £1.64
Brands include *Frumil®*
Dose oedema, 1–2 tablets in the morning

Tablets, co-amilofruse 10/80 (amiloride hydrochloride 10 mg, furosemide 80 mg), net price 28-tab pack = £9.33
Dose oedema, 1 tablet in the morning

**Amiloride with bumetanide** (Non-proprietary) ℗ₒₘ
Tablets, amiloride hydrochloride 5 mg, bumetanide 1 mg, net price 28-tab pack = £29.60
Dose oedema, 1–2 tablets daily

**■ Triamterene with thiazides**
**Counselling** Urine may look slightly blue in some lights

**Co-triamterzide** (Non-proprietary) ℗ₒₘ
Tablets, co-triamterzide 50/25 (triamterene 50 mg, hydrochlorothiazide 25 mg), net price 30-tab pack = 95p. Label: 14, (see above), 21
Dose hypertension, 1 tablet daily after breakfast, increased if necessary, max. 4 daily
Oedema, 2 tablets daily (1 after breakfast and 1 after midday meal) increased to 3 daily if necessary (2 after breakfast and 1 after midday meal); usual maintenance in oedema, 1 daily or 2 on alternate days; max. 4 daily
Brands include *Triam-Co®*

**Dyazide®** (Goldshield) ℗ₒₘ
Tablets, peach, scored, co-triamterzide 50/25 (triamterene 50 mg, hydrochlorothiazide 25 mg), net price 30-tab pack = 95p. Label: 14, (see above), 21
Dose hypertension, 1 tablet daily after breakfast, increased if necessary, max. 4 daily
Oedema, 2 tablets daily (1 after breakfast and 1 after midday meal) increased to 3 daily if necessary (2 after breakfast and 1 after midday meal); usual maintenance in oedema, 1 daily or 2 on alternate days; max. 4 daily

**Dytide®** (Goldshield) ℗ₒₘ
Capsules, clear/maroon, triamterene 50 mg, benzthiazide 25 mg, net price 30-cap pack = £17.35. Label: 14, (see above), 21
Dose oedema, initially 3 capsules daily (2 after breakfast and 1 after midday meal) for 1 week then 1 or 2 on alternate days

**2**

**Cardiovascular system**

**Kalspare®** (DHP Healthcare) PoM ⬛

Tablets, orange, f/c, scored, triamterene 50 mg, chlortalidone 50 mg, net price 28-tab pack = £3.05. Label: 14, (see above), 21
Dose hypertension, oedema, 1–2 tablets in the morning

◢**Triamterene with loop diuretics**
Counselling Urine may look slightly blue in some lights

**Frusene®** (Orion) PoM

Tablets, yellow, scored, triamterene 50 mg, furosemide 40 mg, net price 56-tab pack = £4.41. Label: 14, (see above), 21
Dose oedema, ½–2 tablets daily in the morning

◢**Spironolactone with thiazides**
**Co-flumactone** (Non-proprietary) PoM ⬛

Tablets, co-flumactone 25/25 (hydroflumethiazide 25 mg, spironolactone 25 mg), net price 100-tab pack = £20.23
Brands include *Aldactide 25®*
Dose congestive heart failure, initially 4 tablets daily; range 1–8 tablets daily (but not recommended because spironolactone generally given in lower dose)

Tablets, co-flumactone 50/50 (hydroflumethiazide 50 mg, spironolactone 50 mg), net price 28-tab pack = £10.70
Brands include *Aldactide 50®*
Dose congestive heart failure, initially 2 tablets daily; range 1–4 tablets daily (but not recommended because spironolactone generally given in lower dose)

◢**Spironolactone with loop diuretics**
**Lasilactone®** (Sanofi-Aventis) PoM

Capsules, blue/white, spironolactone 50 mg, furosemide 20 mg, net price 28-cap pack = £7.97
Dose resistant oedema, 1–4 capsules daily

## 2.2.5 Osmotic diuretics

Mannitol is an osmotic diuretic that can be used to treat cerebral oedema and raised intra-ocular pressure.

### ▎ MANNITOL

**Indications** see notes above; glaucoma (section 11.6)
**Cautions** extravasation causes inflammation and thrombophlebitis; monitor fluid and electrolyte balance, serum osmolality, and, pulmonary and renal function; assess cardiac function before and during treatment; renal impairment (Appendix 3); pregnancy (Appendix 4); breast-feeding (Appendix 5); **interactions**: Appendix 1 (mannitol)
**Contra-indications** severe cardiac failure; severe pulmonary oedema; intracranial bleeding (except during craniotomy); anuria; severe dehydration
**Side-effects** *less commonly* hypotension, thrombophlebitis, fluid and electrolyte imbalance; *rarely* dry mouth, thirst, nausea, vomiting, oedema, raised intracranial pressure, arrhythmia, hypertension, pulmonary oedema, chest pain, headache, convulsions, dizziness, chills, fever, urinary retention, focal osmotic nephrosis, dehydration, cramp, blurred vision, rhinitis, skin necrosis, and hypersensitivity reactions (including urticaria and anaphylaxis); *very rarely* congestive heart failure and acute renal failure

**Dose**
- Cerebral oedema and raised intra-ocular pressure, by intravenous infusion over 30–60 minutes, 0.25–2 g/kg repeated if necessary 1–2 times after 4–8 hours
Note For mannitol 20%, an in-line filter is recommended (15-micron filters have been used)

**Mannitol** (Baxter) PoM

Intravenous infusion, mannitol 10%, net price 500-mL *Viaflex®* bag = £1.87, 500-mL *Viaflo®* bag = £2.15; 20%, net price 250-mL *Viaflex®* bag = £2.70, 250-mL *Viaflo®* bag = £3.10, 500-mL *Viaflex®* bag = £2.72, 500-mL *Viaflo®* bag = £3.12

## 2.2.6 Mercurial diuretics

Mercurial diuretics are effective but are now almost never used because of their nephrotoxicity.

## 2.2.7 Carbonic anhydrase inhibitors

The carbonic anhydrase inhibitor **acetazolamide** is a weak diuretic and is little used for its diuretic effect. It is used for prophylaxis against mountain sickness [unlicensed indication] but is not a substitute for acclimatisation.

Acetazolamide and eye drops of dorzolamide and brinzolamide inhibit the formation of aqueous humour and are used in glaucoma (section 11.6).

## 2.2.8 Diuretics with potassium

Many patients on diuretics do not need potassium supplements (section 9.2.1.1). For many of those who do, the amount of potassium in combined preparations may not be enough, and for this reason their use is to be discouraged.

Diuretics with potassium and potassium-sparing diuretics should **not** usually be given together.
Counselling Modified-release potassium tablets should be swallowed whole with plenty of fluid during meals while sitting or standing

**Centyl K®** (LEO) PoM ⬛

Tablets, green, s/c, bendroflumethiazide 2.5 mg, potassium 7.7 mmol for modified release, net price 56-tab pack = £7.50. Label: 25, 27, counselling, see above

**Diumide-K Continus®** (Teofarma) PoM ⬛

Tablets, white/orange, f/c, furosemide 40 mg, potassium 8 mmol for modified release, net price 30-tab pack = £3.00. Label: 25, 27, counselling, see above

**Neo-NaClex-K®** (Goldshield) PoM ⬛

Tablets, pink/white, f/c, bendroflumethiazide 2.5 mg, potassium 8.4 mmol for modified release, net price 100 tab-pack = £8.99. Label: 25, 27, counselling, see above
Note May be difficult to obtain

Cardiovascular system

2

## 2.3 Anti-arrhythmic drugs

### 2.3.1 Management of arrhythmias
### 2.3.2 Drugs for arrhythmias

## 2.3.1 Management of arrhythmias

Management of an arrhythmia requires precise diagnosis of the type of arrhythmia, and electrocardiography is essential; underlying causes such as heart failure require appropriate treatment.

**Ectopic beats** If ectopic beats are spontaneous and the patient has a normal heart, treatment is rarely required and reassurance to the patient will often suffice. If they are particularly troublesome, beta-blockers are sometimes effective and may be safer than other suppressant drugs.

**Atrial fibrillation** Atrial fibrillation can be managed by either controlling the ventricular rate or by attempting to restore and maintain sinus rhythm. All patients with atrial fibrillation should be assessed for their risk of stroke and thromboembolism, and thromboprophylaxis given if necessary (see below).

Ventricular rate can be controlled with a beta-blocker (section 2.4), or diltiazem [unlicensed indication], or verapamil. If rate control is inadequate during normal activities, digoxin can be added; in those who require additional rate control during exercise, a combination of diltiazem or verapamil with digoxin should be used, but care is required if ventricular function is diminished. Digoxin is usually only effective for controlling ventricular rate at rest, therefore digoxin monotherapy should only be used in predominantly sedentary patients; digoxin is also used if atrial fibrillation is accompanied by congestive heart failure.

Sinus rhythm can be restored by electrical cardioversion, or pharmacological cardioversion with an intravenous anti-arrhythmic drug e.g. flecainide or amiodarone. If necessary, sotalol or amiodarone can be started 4 weeks before electrical cardioversion to increase success of the procedure. If drug treatment is required to maintain sinus rhythm, a beta-blocker is used. If a standard beta-blocker is not appropriate or is ineffective, an oral anti-arrhythmic drug such as sotalol (section 2.4), flecainide, propafenone, or amiodarone, is required.

In symptomatic paroxysmal atrial fibrillation, ventricular rhythm is controlled with a beta-blocker. Alternatively, if symptoms persist or a beta-blocker is not appropriate, an oral anti-arrhythmic drug such as sotalol, flecainide, propafenone, or amiodarone can be given (see also Paroxysmal Supraventricular Tachycardia below, and Supraventricular Arrhythmias).

All haemodynamically unstable patients with acute-onset atrial fibrillation should undergo electrical cardioversion. Intravenous amiodarone, or alternatively flecainide, can be used in non-life-threatening cases where electrical cardioversion is delayed. If urgent ventricular rate control is required, a beta-blocker, verapamil, or amiodarone can be given intravenously.

All patients with atrial fibrillation should be assessed for their risk of stroke and the need for thromboprophylaxis. Anticoagulants (section 2.8) are indicated for those with a history of ischaemic stroke, transient ischaemic attacks, or thromboembolic events, and those with valve disease, heart failure, or impaired left ventricular function; anticoagulants should be considered for those with cardiovascular disease, diabetes, hypertension, or thyrotoxicosis, and in the elderly. Anticoagulants are also indicated during cardioversion procedures. Aspirin (section 2.9) is less effective than warfarin at preventing emboli, but may be appropriate if there are no other risk factors for stroke, or if warfarin is contra-indicated.

**Atrial flutter** Like atrial fibrilliation, treatment options for atrial flutter involve either controlling the ventricular rate or attempting to restore and maintain sinus rhythm. However, atrial flutter generally responds less well to drug treatment than atrial fibrillation.

Control of the ventricular rate is usually an interim measure pending restoration of sinus rhythm. Ventricular rate can be controlled by administration of a beta-blocker (section 2.4), diltiazem [unlicensed indication], or verapamil (section 2.6.2); an intravenous beta-blocker or verapamil is preferred for rapid control. Digoxin (section 2.1.1) can be added if rate control remains inadequate, and may be particularly useful in those with heart failure.

Conversion to sinus rhythm can be achieved by electrical cardioversion (by cardiac pacing or direct current), pharmacological cardioversion, or catheter ablation. If the duration of atrial flutter is unknown, or it has lasted for over 48 hours, cardioversion should not be attempted until the patient has been fully anticoagulated (see section 2.8.2). Alternatively, anticoagulation can be commenced and a left atrial thrombus should be ruled out immediately before cardioversion.

Direct current cardioversion is usually the treatment of choice when rapid conversion to sinus rhythm is necessary (e.g. when atrial flutter is associated with haemodynamic compromise); catheter ablation is preferred for the treatment of recurrent atrial flutter. There is a limited role for anti-arrhythmic drugs as their use is not always successful. Flecainide or propafenone can slow atrial flutter resulting in 1:1 conduction to the ventricles and should therefore be prescribed in conjunction with a ventricular rate controlling drug such as a beta-blocker, diltiazem [unlicensed indication] or verapamil. Amiodarone can be used when other drug treatments are contra-indicated or ineffective.

All patients should be assessed for their risk of stroke and the need for thromboprophylaxis; the choice of anticoagulant is based on the same criteria as for atrial fibrillation (see notes above).

**Paroxysmal supraventricular tachycardia** This will often terminate spontaneously or with reflex vagal stimulation such as a Valsalva manoeuvre, immersing the face in ice-cold water, or carotid sinus massage; such manoeuvres should be performed with ECG monitoring.

If the effects of reflex vagal stimulation are transient or ineffective, or if the arrhythmia is causing severe symptoms, intravenous adenosine (section 2.3.2) should be given. If adenosine is ineffective or contra-indicated, intravenous verapamil (section 2.6.2) is an alternative, but it should be avoided in patients recently treated with beta-blockers (see p. 119).

Failure to terminate paroxysmal supraventricular tachycardia with reflex vagal stimulation or drug treatment may suggest an arrhythmia of atrial origin, such as focal atrial tachycardia or atrial flutter.

Treatment with direct current cardioversion is needed in haemodynamically unstable patients or when the above measures have failed to restore sinus rhythm (and an alternative diagnosis has not been found).

Recurrent episodes of paroxysmal supraventricular tachycardia can be treated by catheter ablation, or prevented with drugs such as diltiazem, verapamil, beta-blockers including sotalol (section 2.4), flecainide or propafenone (section 2.3.2).

**Arrhythmias after myocardial infarction**   In patients with a paroxysmal tachycardia or rapid irregularity of the pulse it is best not to administer an anti-arrhythmic until an ECG record has been obtained. Bradycardia, particularly if complicated by hypotension, should be treated with 500 micrograms of atropine sulphate given intravenously; the dose may be repeated every 3–5 minutes if necessary up to a maximum total dose of 3 mg. If there is a risk of asystole, or if the patient is unstable and has failed to respond to atropine, adrenaline should be given by intravenous infusion in a dose of 2–10 micrograms/minute, adjusted according to response.

For further advice, refer to the most recent recommendations of the Resuscitation Council (UK) available at www.resus.org.uk.

**Ventricular tachycardia**   Pulseless ventricular tachycardia or ventricular fibrillation should be treated with immediate defibrillation (see Cardiopulmonary Resuscitation, section 2.7.3).

Patients with unstable sustained ventricular tachycardia, who continue to deteriorate with signs of hypotension or reduced cardiac output, should receive direct current cardioversion to restore sinus rhythm. If this fails, intravenous amiodarone (section 2.3.2) should be administered and direct current cardioversion repeated.

Patients with sustained ventricular tachycardia who are haemodynamically stable can be treated with intravenous anti-arrhythmic drugs. Amiodarone is the preferred drug. Sotalol (section 2.4), flecainide, propafenone (section 2.3.2), and, although less effective, lidocaine (lignocaine) (section 2.3.2) have all been used. If sinus rhythm is not restored, direct current cardioversion or pacing should be considered. Catheter ablation is an alternative if cessation of the arrhythmia is not urgent. Non-sustained ventricular tachycardia can be treated with a beta-blocker (section 2.4).

All patients presenting with ventricular tachycardia should be referred to a specialist. Following restoration of sinus rhythm, patients who remain at high risk of cardiac arrest will require maintenance therapy. Most patients will be treated with an implantable cardioverter defibrillator. Beta-blockers or sotalol (in place of a standard beta-blocker), or amiodarone (in combination with a standard beta-blocker), can be used in addition to the device in some patients; alternatively, they can be used alone when use of an implantable cardioverter defibrillator is not appropriate.

*Torsade de pointes* is a form of ventricular tachycardia associated with a long QT syndrome (usually drug-induced, but other factors including hypokalaemia,

severe bradycardia, and genetic predisposition are also implicated). Episodes are usually self-limiting, but are frequently recurrent and can cause impairment or loss of consciousness. If not controlled, the arrhythmia can progress to ventricular fibrillation and sometimes death. Intravenous infusion of magnesium sulphate (section 9.5.1.3) is usually effective. A beta-blocker (but not sotalol) and atrial (or ventricular) pacing can be considered. Anti-arrhythmics can further prolong the QT interval, thus worsening the condition.

## 2.3.2 Drugs for arrhythmias

Anti-arrhythmic drugs can be classified clinically into those that act on supraventricular arrhythmias (e.g. verapamil), those that act on both supraventricular and ventricular arrhythmias (e.g. disopyramide), and those that act on ventricular arrhythmias (e.g. lidocaine (lignocaine)).

They can also be classified according to their effects on the electrical behaviour of myocardial cells during activity:

> Class I: membrane stabilising drugs (e.g. lidocaine, flecainide)
>
> Class II: beta-blockers
>
> Class III: amiodarone and sotalol (also Class II)
>
> Class IV: calcium-channel blockers (includes verapamil but not dihydropyridines)

This latter classification (the Vaughan Williams classification) is of less clinical significance.

**Cautions**   The negative inotropic effects of anti-arrhythmic drugs tend to be additive. Therefore special care should be taken if two or more are used, especially if myocardial function is impaired. Most or all drugs that are effective in countering arrhythmias can also provoke them in some circumstances; moreover, hypokalaemia enhances the arrhythmogenic (pro-arrhythmic) effect of many drugs.

### Supraventricular arrhythmias

**Adenosine** is usually the treatment of choice for terminating paroxysmal supraventricular tachycardia. As it has a very short duration of action (half-life only about 8 to 10 seconds, but prolonged in those taking dipyridamole), most side-effects are short lived. Unlike verapamil, adenosine can be used after a beta-blocker. Verapamil may be preferable to adenosine in asthma.

Oral administration of a **cardiac glycoside** (such as digoxin, section 2.1.1) slows the ventricular response in cases of atrial fibrillation and atrial flutter. However, intravenous infusion of digoxin is rarely effective for rapid control of ventricular rate. Cardiac glycosides are contra-indicated in supraventricular arrhythmias associated with accessory conducting pathways (e.g. Wolff-Parkinson-White syndrome).

**Verapamil** (section 2.6.2) is usually effective for supraventricular tachycardias. An initial intravenous dose (**important**: serious beta-blocker interaction hazard, see p. 119) may be followed by oral treatment; hypotension may occur with large doses. It should not be used for tachyarrhythmias where the QRS complex is wide (i.e. broad complex) unless a supraventricular origin has been established beyond reasonable doubt. It is also contra-indicated in atrial fibrillation or atrial flutter associated with accessory conducting pathways (e.g. Wolff-Parkinson-White syndrome). It should not be used in children with arrhythmias without specialist advice; some supraventricular arrhythmias in childhood can be accelerated by verapamil with dangerous consequences.

Intravenous administration of a **beta-blocker** (section 2.4) such as esmolol or propranolol, can achieve rapid control of the ventricular rate.

Drugs for both supraventricular and ventricular arrhythmias include **amiodarone**, **beta-blockers** (see p. 87), **disopyramide**, **flecainide**, **procainamide** (available from 'special-order' manufacturers or specialist importing companies, see p. 969), and **propafenone**, see below under Supraventricular and Ventricular Arrhythmias.

---

### ▌ADENOSINE

**Indications**   rapid reversion to sinus rhythm of paroxysmal supraventricular tachycardias, including those associated with accessory conducting pathways (e.g. Wolff-Parkinson-White syndrome); aid to diagnosis of broad or narrow complex supraventricular tachycardias

**Cautions**   atrial fibrillation or flutter with accessory pathway (conduction down anomalous pathway may increase); heart transplant (see below); **interactions**: Appendix 1 (adenosine)

**Contra-indications**   second- or third-degree AV block and sick sinus syndrome (unless pacemaker fitted); prolonged QT syndrome; severe hypotension; decompensated heart failure; chronic obstructive lung disease

**Side-effects**   include transient facial flush, chest pain, dyspnoea, bronchospasm, choking sensation, nausea, light-headedness; severe bradycardia reported (requiring temporary pacing); ECG may show transient rhythm disturbances

**Dose**

- By rapid intravenous injection into central or large peripheral vein, 6 mg over 2 seconds with cardiac monitoring; if necessary followed by 12 mg after 1–2 minutes, and then by 12 mg after a further 1–2 minutes; increments should not be given if high level AV block develops at any particular dose

  **Important** Patients with a **heart transplant** are very sensitive to effects of adenosine and should receive initial dose of 3 mg over 2 seconds, followed if necessary by 6 mg after 1–2 minutes, and then by 12 mg after a further 1–2 minutes.

  Also, if essential to give with dipyridamole reduce initial dose to 0.5–1 mg

  **Note** Adenosine doses in the BNF may differ from those in product literature

**Adenocor®** (Sanofi-Aventis) [PoM]

Injection, adenosine 3 mg/mL in physiological saline, net price 2-mL vial = £4.45 (hosp. only)

**Note** Intravenous infusion of adenosine (*Adenoscan®*, Sanofi Winthrop) may be used in conjunction with radionuclide myocardial perfusion imaging in patients who cannot exercise adequately or for whom exercise is inappropriate—consult product literature

## Supraventricular and ventricular arrhythmias

**Amiodarone** is used in the treatment of arrhythmias particularly when other drugs are ineffective or contra-indicated. It may be used for paroxysmal supraventricular, nodal and ventricular tachycardias, atrial fibrillation and flutter, and ventricular fibrillation. It may also be used for tachyarrhythmias associated with Wolff-Parkinson-White syndrome. It should be initiated only under hospital or specialist supervision. Amiodarone may be given by intravenous infusion as well as by mouth, and has the advantage of causing little or no myocardial depression. Unlike oral amiodarone, intravenous amiodarone may act relatively rapidly.

Intravenous injection of amiodarone may be used in cardiopulmonary resuscitation for ventricular fibrillation or pulseless tachycardia unresponsive to other interventions (section 2.7.3).

Amiodarone has a very long half-life (extending to several weeks) and only needs to be given once daily (but high doses may cause nausea unless divided). Many weeks or months may be required to achieve steady-state plasma-amiodarone concentration; this is particularly important when drug interactions are likely (see also Appendix 1).

Most patients taking amiodarone develop corneal microdeposits (reversible on withdrawal of treatment); these rarely interfere with vision, but drivers may be dazzled by headlights at night. However, if vision is impaired or if optic neuritis or optic neuropathy occur, amiodarone must be stopped to prevent blindness and expert advice sought. Because of the possibility of phototoxic reactions, patients should be advised to shield the skin from light during treatment and for several months after discontinuing amiodarone; a wide-spectrum sunscreen (section 13.8.1) to protect against both long-wave ultraviolet and visible light should be used.

Amiodarone contains iodine and can cause disorders of thyroid function; both hypothyroidism and hyperthyroidism may occur. Clinical assessment alone is unreliable, and laboratory tests should be performed before treatment and every 6 months. Thyroxine (T4) may be raised in the absence of hyperthyroidism; therefore tri-iodothyronine (T3), T4, and thyroid-stimulating hormone (thyrotrophin, TSH) should all be measured. A raised T3 and T4 with a very low or undetectable TSH concentration suggests the development of thyrotoxicosis. The thyrotoxicosis may be very refractory, and amiodarone should usually be withdrawn at least temporarily to help achieve control; treatment with carbimazole may be required. Hypothyroidism can be treated with replacement therapy without withdrawing amiodarone if it is essential; careful supervision is required.

Pneumonitis should always be suspected if new or progressive shortness of breath or cough develops in a patient taking amiodarone. Fresh neurological symptoms should raise the possibility of peripheral neuropathy.

Amiodarone is also associated with hepatotoxicity and treatment should be discontinued if severe liver function abnormalities or clinical signs of liver disease develop.

**Beta-blockers** act as anti-arrhythmic drugs principally by attenuating the effects of the sympathetic system on automaticity and conductivity within the heart, for details see section 2.4. For special reference to the role of **sotalol** in ventricular arrhythmias, see p. 88.

**Disopyramide** may be given by intravenous injection to control arrhythmias after myocardial infarction (including those not responding to lidocaine (lignocaine)), but it impairs cardiac contractility. Oral administration of disopyramide is useful but it has an antimuscarinic effect which limits its use in patients susceptible to angle-closure glaucoma or prostatic hypertrophy.

**Flecainide** belongs to the same general class as lidocaine and may be of value for serious symptomatic ventricular arrhythmias. It may also be indicated for junctional re-entry tachycardias and for paroxysmal atrial fibrillation. However, it can precipitate serious arrhythmias in a small minority of patients (including those with otherwise normal hearts).

**Propafenone** is used for the prophylaxis and treatment of ventricular arrhythmias and also for some supraventricular arrhythmias. It has complex mechanisms of action, including weak beta-blocking activity (therefore caution is needed in obstructive airways disease—contra-indicated if severe).

Drugs for supraventricular arrhythmias include **adenosine**, **cardiac glycosides**, and **verapamil**; see above under Supraventricular Arrhythmias. Drugs for ventricular arrhythmias include **lidocaine**; see under Ventricular Arrhythmias, p. 86.

Mexiletine and procainamide are both available from 'special-order' manufacturers or specialist importing companies, see p. 969. Mexiletine can be used for life-threatening ventricular arrhythmias; procainamide is given by intravenous injection to control ventricular arrhythmias.

## ▌ AMIODARONE HYDROCHLORIDE

**Indications** see notes above (should be initiated in hospital or under specialist supervision)

**Cautions** liver-function and thyroid-function tests required before treatment and then every 6 months (see notes above for tests of thyroid function); hypokalaemia (measure serum-potassium concentration before treatment); chest x-ray required before treatment; heart failure; elderly; severe bradycardia and conduction disturbances in excessive dosage; intravenous use may cause moderate and transient fall in blood pressure (circulatory collapse precipitated by rapid administration or overdosage) or severe hepatocellular toxicity (monitor transaminases closely); give by central venous catheter **only**, infusion via peripheral veins may cause pain and inflammation; ECG monitoring and resuscitation facilities must be available during intravenous use; acute porphyria (section 9.8.2); **interactions:** Appendix 1 (amiodarone)

**Contra-indications** (except in cardiac arrest) sinus bradycardia, sino-atrial heart block; unless pacemaker fitted avoid in severe conduction disturbances or sinus node disease; thyroid dysfunction; iodine sensitivity; avoid *intravenous use* in severe respiratory failure, circulatory collapse, or severe arterial hypotension; avoid bolus injection in congestive heart failure or cardiomyopathy; pregnancy (Appendix 4); breast-feeding (Appendix 5)

**Side-effects** nausea, vomiting, taste disturbances, raised serum transaminases (may require dose reduction or withdrawal if accompanied by acute liver

disorders), jaundice; bradycardia (see Cautions); pulmonary toxicity (including pneumonitis and fibrosis); tremor, sleep disorders; hypothyroidism, hyperthyroidism; reversible corneal microdeposits (sometimes with night glare); phototoxicity, persistent slate-grey skin discoloration (see also notes above), injection-site reactions; *less commonly* onset or worsening of arrhythmia, conduction disturbances (see Cautions); peripheral neuropathy and myopathy (usually reversible on withdrawal); *very rarely* chronic liver disease including cirrhosis, sinus arrest, bronchospasm (in patients with severe respiratory failure), ataxia, benign intracranial hypertension, headache, vertigo, epididymo-orchitis, impotence, haemolytic or aplastic anaemia, thrombocytopenia, rash (including exfoliative dermatitis), hypersensitivity including vasculitis, alopecia, impaired vision due to optic neuritis or optic neuropathy (including blindness), anaphylaxis on rapid injection, also hypotension, respiratory distress syndrome, sweating, and hot flushes

**Dose**

• By mouth, 200 mg 3 times daily for 1 week reduced to 200 mg twice daily for a further week; maintenance, usually 200 mg daily or the minimum required to control the arrhythmia

• By intravenous infusion via central venous catheter, initially 5 mg/kg over 20–120 minutes with ECG monitoring; subsequent infusion given if necessary according to response up to max. 1.2 g in 24 hours

• Ventricular fibrillation or pulseless ventricular tachycardia refractory to defibrillation, section 2.7.3

**Amiodarone** (Non-proprietary) PoM

Tablets, amiodarone hydrochloride 100 mg, net price 28-tab pack = £1.36; 200 mg, 28-tab pack = £1.41. Label: 11

Injection, amiodarone hydrochloride 30 mg/mL, net price 10-mL prefilled syringe = £20.90
Excipients may include benzyl alcohol (avoid in neonates unless no safer alternative available, see Excipients, p. 2)

Sterile concentrate, amiodarone hydrochloride 50 mg/mL, net price 3-mL amp = £1.33, 6-mL amp = £2.86. For dilution and use as an infusion
Excipients may include benzyl alcohol (avoid in neonates unless no safer alternative available, see Excipients, p. 2)

**Cordarone X**® (Sanofi-Aventis) PoM

Tablets, scored, amiodarone hydrochloride 100 mg, net price 28-tab pack = £4.28; 200 mg, 28-tab pack = £6.99. Label: 11

Sterile concentrate, amiodarone hydrochloride 50 mg/mL, net price 3-mL amp = £1.33. For dilution and use as an infusion
Excipients include benzyl alcohol (avoid in neonates unless no safer alternative available, see Excipients, p. 2)

## ▌ DISOPYRAMIDE

**Indications** ventricular arrhythmias, especially after myocardial infarction; supraventricular arrhythmias

**Cautions** monitor for hypotension, hypoglycaemia, ventricular tachycardia, ventricular fibrillation or torsade de pointes (discontinue if occur); atrial flutter or atrial tachycardia with partial block, bundle branch block, heart failure (avoid if severe); prostatic enlargement; susceptibility to angle-closure glaucoma; hepatic impairment (Appendix 2); renal impairment (Appendix 3); pregnancy (Appendix 4); breast-feeding

(Appendix 5); **interactions:** Appendix 1 (disopyramide)

**Contra-indications** second- and third-degree heart block and sinus node dysfunction (unless pacemaker fitted); cardiogenic shock; severe uncompensated heart failure

**Side-effects** ventricular tachycardia, ventricular fibrillation or torsade de pointes (usually associated with prolongation of QRS complex or QT interval—see Cautions above), myocardial depression, hypotension, AV block; antimuscarinic effects include dry mouth, blurred vision, urinary retention, and very rarely angle-closure glaucoma; gastro-intestinal irritation; psychosis, cholestatic jaundice, hypoglycaemia also reported (see Cautions above)

**Dose**

- By mouth, 300–800 mg daily in divided doses
- By slow intravenous injection, 2 mg/kg over at least 5 minutes to a max. of 150 mg, with ECG monitoring, followed immediately *either* by 200 mg by mouth, then 200 mg every 8 hours for 24 hours *or* 400 micrograms/kg/hour by intravenous infusion; max. 300 mg in first hour and 800 mg daily

**Disopyramide** (Non-proprietary) ℗ℴ𝕄
Capsules, disopyramide (as phosphate) 100 mg, net price 84 = £21.92; 150 mg, 84 = £28.66

**Rythmodan®** (Sanofi-Aventis) ℗ℴ𝕄
Capsules, disopyramide 100 mg (green/beige), net price 84-cap pack = £14.14; 150 mg, 84-cap pack = £18.76

Injection, disopyramide (as phosphate) 10 mg/mL, net price 5-mL amp = £2.61

◢**Modified release**
**Rythmodan Retard®** (Sanofi-Aventis) ℗ℴ𝕄
Tablets, m/r, scored, f/c, disopyramide (as phosphate) 250 mg, net price 56-tab pack = £27.72. Label: 25
Dose 250–375 mg every 12 hours

---

## FLECAINIDE ACETATE

**Indications** *Capsules, tablets, and injection:* AV nodal reciprocating tachycardia, arrhythmias associated with accessory conducting pathways (e.g. Wolff-Parkinson-White syndrome), disabling symptoms of paroxysmal atrial fibrillation in patients without left ventricular dysfunction (arrhythmias of recent onset will respond more readily)
*Immediate-release tablets only:* symptomatic sustained ventricular tachycardia, disabling symptoms of premature ventricular contractions or non-sustained ventricular tachycardia in patients resistant to or intolerant of other therapy
*Injection only:* ventricular tachyarrhythmias resistant to other treatment

**Cautions** patients with pacemakers (especially those who may be pacemaker dependent because stimulation threshold may rise appreciably); atrial fibrillation following heart surgery; elderly (accumulation may occur); ECG monitoring and resuscitation facilities must be available during intravenous use; hepatic impairment (Appendix 2); renal impairment (Appendix 3); pregnancy (Appendix 4); breast-feeding (Appendix 5); **interactions:** Appendix 1 (flecainide)

**Contra-indications** heart failure; abnormal left ventricular function; history of myocardial infarction

and either asymptomatic ventricular ectopics or asymptomatic non-sustained ventricular tachycardia; long-standing atrial fibrillation where conversion to sinus rhythm not attempted; haemodynamically significant valvular heart disease; avoid in sinus node dysfunction, atrial conduction defects, second-degree or greater AV block, bundle branch block or distal block unless pacing rescue available

**Side-effects** oedema, pro-arrhythmic effects; dyspnoea; dizziness, asthenia, fatigue, fever; visual disturbances; *rarely* pneumonitis, hallucinations, depression, confusion, amnesia, dyskinesia, convulsions, peripheral neuropathy; *also reported* gastro-intestinal disturbances, anorexia, hepatic dysfunction, flushing, syncope, drowsiness, tremor, vertigo, headache, anxiety, insomnia, ataxia, paraesthesia, anaemia, leucopenia, thrombocytopenia, corneal deposits, tinnitus, increased antinuclear antibodies, hypersensitivity reactions (including rash, urticaria, and photosensitivity), increased sweating

**Dose**

- By mouth (initiated under direction of hospital consultant), ventricular arrhythmias, initially 100 mg twice daily (max. 400 mg daily usually reserved for rapid control or in heavily built patients), reduced after 3–5 days to the lowest dose that controls arrhythmia
Supraventricular arrhythmias, 50 mg twice daily, increased if required to max. 300 mg daily
- By slow intravenous injection (in hospital), 2 mg/kg over 10–30 minutes, max. 150 mg, with ECG monitoring; followed if required by infusion at a rate of 1.5 mg/kg/hour for 1 hour, subsequently reduced to 100–250 micrograms/kg/hour for up to 24 hours; max. cumulative dose in first 24 hours, 600 mg; transfer to *oral* treatment, as above

**Flecainide** (Non-proprietary) ℗ℴ𝕄
Tablets, flecainide acetate 50 mg, net price 60-tab pack = £9.07; 100 mg, 60-tab pack = £13.59

**Tambocor®** (3M) ℗ℴ𝕄
Tablets, flecainide acetate 50 mg, net price 60-tab pack = £13.25; 100 mg (scored), 60-tab pack = £19.00

Injection, flecainide acetate 10 mg/mL, net price 15-mL amp = £4.40

◢**Modified release**
**Tambocor® XL** (Meda) ℗ℴ𝕄
Capsules, m/r, grey/pink, flecainide acetate 200 mg, net price 30-cap pack = £14.77. Label: 25
Dose supraventricular arrhythmias, 200 mg once daily
Note Not to be used to control arrhythmias in acute situations; patients stabilised on 200 mg daily immediate-release flecainide may be transferred to *Tambocor® XL*

---

## PROPAFENONE HYDROCHLORIDE

**Indications** ventricular arrhythmias; paroxysmal supraventricular tachyarrhythmias which include paroxysmal atrial flutter or fibrillation and paroxysmal re-entrant tachycardias involving the AV node or accessory pathway, where standard therapy ineffective or contra-indicated

**Cautions** heart failure; elderly; pacemaker patients; great caution in obstructive airways disease owing to beta-blocking activity (contra-indicated if severe); hepatic impairment (Appendix 2); renal impairment; pregnancy (Appendix 4); breast-feeding (Appendix 5); **interactions:** Appendix 1 (propafenone)

**2**

**Cardiovascular system**

**Contra-indications** uncontrolled congestive heart failure, cardiogenic shock (except arrhythmia induced), severe bradycardia, electrolyte disturbances, severe obstructive pulmonary disease, marked hypotension; myasthenia gravis; unless adequately paced avoid in sinus node dysfunction, atrial conduction defects, second degree or greater AV block, bundle branch block or distal block

**Side-effects** antimuscarinic effects including constipation, blurred vision, and dry mouth; dizziness, nausea and vomiting, fatigue, bitter taste, diarrhoea, headache, and allergic skin reactions reported; postural hypotension, particularly in elderly; bradycardia, sino-atrial, atrioventricular, or intraventricular blocks; arrhythmogenic (pro-arrhythmic) effect; rarely hypersensitivity reactions (cholestasis, blood disorders, lupus syndrome), seizures; myoclonus also reported

**Dose**
- Body-weight 70 kg and over, initially 150 mg 3 times daily after food under direct hospital supervision with ECG monitoring and blood pressure control (if QRS interval prolonged by more than 20%, reduce dose or discontinue until ECG returns to normal limits); may be increased at intervals of at least 3 days to 300 mg twice daily and, if necessary, to max. 300 mg 3 times daily; body-weight under 70 kg, reduce dose; ELDERLY may respond to lower doses

**Arythmol®** (Abbott) ▣PoM
Tablets, f/c, propafenone hydrochloride 150 mg, net price 90-tab pack = £7.37; 300 mg, 60-tab pack = £9.34. Label: 21, 25

## Ventricular arrhythmias

**Lidocaine** (lignocaine) is relatively safe when used by slow intravenous injection. Although it has been used in suppression of ventricular tachycardia and reducing the risk of ventricular fibrillation following myocardial infarction, it has not been shown to reduce mortality when used prophylactically in this condition. In patients with cardiac or hepatic failure doses may need to be reduced to avoid convulsions, depression of the central nervous system, or depression of the cardiovascular system.

**Moracizine** is available from 'special-order' manufacturers or specialist importing companies (see p. 969) for the prophylaxis and treatment of serious and life-threatening ventricular arrhythmias for patients already stabilised on moracizine.

Drugs for both supraventricular and ventricular arrhythmias include **amiodarone, beta-blockers, disopyramide, flecainide, procainamide** (available from 'special-order' manufacturers or specialist importing companies, see p. 969), and **propafenone**, see above under Supraventricular and Ventricular Arrhythmias.

**Mexiletine** is available from 'special-order' manufacturers or specialist importing companies (see p. 969) for treatment of life-threatening ventricular arrhythmias.

### ▌ LIDOCAINE HYDROCHLORIDE
(Lignocaine hydrochloride)

**Indications** ventricular arrhythmias, especially after myocardial infarction

**Cautions** lower doses in congestive cardiac failure and following cardiac surgery; monitor ECG and have resuscitation facilities available; elderly; hepatic impairment (Appendix 2); renal impairment (Appendix 3); pregnancy (Appendix 4); **interactions:** Appendix 1 (lidocaine)

**Contra-indications** sino-atrial disorders, all grades of atrioventricular block, severe myocardial depression; acute porphyria (section 9.8.2)

**Side-effects** dizziness, paraesthesia, or drowsiness (particularly if injection too rapid); other CNS effects include confusion, respiratory depression and convulsions; hypotension and bradycardia (may lead to cardiac arrest); *rarely* hypersensitivity reactions including anaphylaxis

**Dose**
- By intravenous injection, in patients without gross circulatory impairment, 100 mg as a bolus over a few minutes (50 mg in lighter patients or those whose circulation is severely impaired), followed immediately by infusion of 4 mg/minute for 30 minutes, 2 mg/minute for 2 hours, then 1 mg/minute; reduce concentration further if infusion continued beyond 24 hours (ECG monitoring and specialist advice for infusion)

**Note** Following *intravenous injection* lidocaine has a short duration of action (lasting for 15–20 minutes). If an *intravenous infusion* is not immediately available the initial *intravenous injection* of 50–100 mg can be repeated if necessary once or twice at intervals of not less than 10 minutes

**Lidocaine** (Non-proprietary) ▣PoM
Injection 2%, lidocaine hydrochloride 20 mg/mL, net price 2-mL amp = 27p; 5-mL amp = 28p; 10-mL amp = 60p; 20-mL amp = 61p
*Available from Braun*

Infusion, lidocaine hydrochloride 0.1% (1 mg/mL) and 0.2% (2 mg/mL) in glucose intravenous infusion 5%. 500-mL containers
*Available from Baxter*

**Minijet® Lignocaine** (UCB Pharma) ▣PoM
Injection, lidocaine hydrochloride 1% (10 mg/mL), net price 10-mL disposable syringe = £5.34; 2% (20 mg/mL), 5-mL disposable syringe = £5.20

## 2.4 Beta-adrenoceptor blocking drugs

Beta-adrenoceptor blocking drugs (beta-blockers) block the beta-adrenoceptors in the heart, peripheral vasculature, bronchi, pancreas, and liver.

Many beta-blockers are now available and in general they are all equally effective. There are, however, differences between them which may affect choice in treating particular diseases or individual patients.

Intrinsic sympathomimetic activity (ISA, partial agonist activity) represents the capacity of beta-blockers to stimulate as well as to block adrenergic receptors. **Oxprenolol, pindolol, acebutolol,** and **celiprolol** have intrinsic sympathomimetic activity; they tend to cause less bradycardia than the other beta-blockers and may also cause less coldness of the extremities.

Some beta-blockers are lipid soluble and some are water soluble. **Atenolol, celiprolol, nadolol,** and **sotalol** are the most water-soluble; they are less likely to enter the brain, and may therefore cause less sleep disturbance and nightmares. Water-soluble beta-blockers are excreted by the kidneys and dosage reduction is often necessary in renal impairment.

Beta-blockers with a relatively short duration of action have to be given two or three times daily. Many of these are, however, available in modified-release formulations so that administration once daily is adequate for hypertension. For angina twice-daily treatment may sometimes be needed even with a modified-release formulation. Some beta-blockers such as atenolol, bisoprolol, carvedilol, celiprolol, and nadolol have an intrinsically longer duration of action and need to be given only once daily.

Beta-blockers slow the heart and can depress the myocardium; they are contra-indicated in patients with second- or third-degree heart block. Beta-blockers should also be avoided in patients with worsening unstable heart failure; care is required when initiating a beta-blocker in those with stable heart failure (see also section 2.5.5). **Sotalol** may prolong the QT interval, and it occasionally causes life-threatening ventricular arrhythmias (**important:** particular care is required to avoid hypokalaemia in patients taking sotalol).

**Labetalol, celiprolol, carvedilol,** and **nebivolol** are beta-blockers that have, in addition, an arteriolar vasodilating action, by diverse mechanisms, and thus lower peripheral resistance. There is no evidence that these drugs have important advantages over other beta-blockers in the treatment of hypertension.

Beta-blockers can precipitate asthma and this effect can be dangerous. Beta-blockers should be **avoided** in patients with a history of asthma or bronchospasm; if there is no alternative, a cardioselective beta-blocker can be used with extreme caution under specialist supervision. Patients with well-controlled chronic obstructive pulmonary disease (without significant reversible airways obstruction) can be treated with a beta-blocker for a co-existing condition if necessary; in such circumstances, a cardioselective beta-blocker should be initiated at a low dose by a specialist, and the patient monitored for adverse effects. **Atenolol, bisoprolol, metoprolol, nebivolol,** and (to a lesser extent) **acebutolol,** have less effect on the beta$_2$ (bronchial) receptors and are, therefore, relatively *cardioselective*, but they are **not** *cardiospecific*. They have a lesser effect on airways resistance but are **not** free of this side-effect.

Beta-blockers are also associated with fatigue, coldness of the extremities (may be less common with those with ISA, see above), and sleep disturbances with nightmares (may be less common with the water-soluble beta-blockers, see above).

Beta-blockers are not contra-indicated in diabetes; however, they can lead to a small deterioration of glucose tolerance and interfere with metabolic and autonomic responses to hypoglycaemia. Cardioselective beta-blockers (see above) may be preferable and beta-blockers should be avoided altogether in those with frequent episodes of hypoglycaemia. Beta blockers, especially when combined with a thiazide diuretic, should be avoided for the routine treatment of uncomplicated hypertension in patients with diabetes or in those at high risk of developing diabetes.

**Hypertension** The mode of action of beta-blockers in hypertension is not understood, but they reduce cardiac output, alter baroceptor reflex sensitivity, and block peripheral adrenoceptors. Some beta-blockers depress plasma renin secretion. It is possible that a central effect may also partly explain their mode of action.

Beta-blockers are effective for reducing blood pressure but other antihypertensives (section 2.5) are usually more effective for reducing the incidence of stroke, myocardial infarction, and cardiovascular mortality, especially in the elderly. Other antihypertensives are therefore preferred for routine initial treatment of uncomplicated hypertension.

In general, the dose of a beta-blocker does not have to be high; for example, atenolol is given in a dose of 25–50 mg daily and it is rarely necessary to increase the dose to 100 mg.

Beta-blockers can be used to control the pulse rate in patients with *phaeochromocytoma* (section 2.5.4). However, they should never be used alone as beta-blockade without concurrent alpha-blockade may lead to a hypertensive crisis. For this reason phenoxybenzamine should always be used together with the beta-blocker.

**Angina** By reducing cardiac work beta-blockers improve exercise tolerance and relieve symptoms in patients with *angina* (for further details on the management of stable and unstable angina see section 2.6). As with hypertension there is no good evidence of the superiority of any one drug, although occasionally a patient will respond better to one beta-blocker than to another. There is some evidence that sudden withdrawal may cause an exacerbation of angina and therefore gradual reduction of dose is preferable when beta-blockers are to be stopped. There is a risk of precipitating heart failure when beta-blockers and verapamil are used together in established ischaemic heart disease (**important:** see p. 119).

**Myocardial infarction** For advice on the management of ST-segment-elevation myocardial infarction see section 2.10.1; for advice on the management of non-ST-segment-elevation myocardial infarction see section 2.6. Several studies have shown that some beta-blockers can reduce the recurrence rate of *myocardial infarction.* However, uncontrolled heart failure, hypotension, bradyarrhythmias, and obstructive airways disease render beta-blockers unsuitable in some patients following a myocardial infarction. **Atenolol** and **metoprolol** may reduce early mortality after intravenous and subsequent oral administration in the acute phase, while **acebutolol, metoprolol, propranolol,** and **timolol** have protective value when started in the early convalescent phase. The evidence relating to other beta-blockers is less convincing; some have not been tested in trials of secondary prevention. Sudden cessation of a beta-blocker can cause a rebound worsening of myocardial ischaemia.

**Arrhythmias** Beta-blockers act as *anti-arrhythmic drugs* principally by attenuating the effects of the sympathetic system on automaticity and conductivity within the heart. They can be used in conjunction with digoxin to control the ventricular response in atrial fibrillation, especially in patients with thyrotoxicosis. Beta-blockers are also useful in the management of supraventricular tachycardias, and are used to control those following myocardial infarction (see above).

**2**

**Cardiovascular system**

**Esmolol** is a relatively cardioselective beta-blocker with a very short duration of action, used intravenously for the short-term treatment of supraventricular arrhythmias, sinus tachycardia, or hypertension, particularly in the peri-operative period. It may also be used in other situations, such as acute myocardial infarction, where sustained beta blockade might be hazardous.

**Sotalol**, a non-cardioselective beta-blocker with additional class III anti-arrhythmic activity, is used for prophylaxis in paroxysmal supraventricular arrhythmias. It also suppresses ventricular ectopic beats and non-sustained ventricular tachycardia. It has been shown to be more effective than lidocaine (lignocaine) in the termination of spontaneous sustained ventricular tachycardia due to coronary disease or cardiomyopathy. However, it may induce torsade de pointes in susceptible patients.

**Heart failure**   Beta-blockers may produce benefit in heart failure by blocking sympathetic activity. **Bisoprolol** and **carvedilol** reduce mortality in any grade of stable heart failure; **nebivolol** is licensed for stable mild to moderate heart failure in patients over 70 years. Treatment should be initiated by those experienced in the management of heart failure (section 2.5.5).

**Thyrotoxicosis**   Beta-blockers are used in pre-operative preparation for thyroidectomy. Administration of propranolol can reverse clinical symptoms of *thyrotoxicosis* within 4 days. Routine tests of increased thyroid function remain unaltered. The thyroid gland is rendered less vascular thus making surgery easier (section 6.2.2).

**Other uses**   Beta-blockers have been used to alleviate some symptoms of *anxiety*, probably patients with palpitation, tremor, and tachycardia respond best (see also section 4.1.2 and section 4.9.3). Beta-blockers are also used in the *prophylaxis of migraine* (section 4.7.4.2). Betaxolol, carteolol, levobunolol, metipranolol and timolol are used topically in *glaucoma* (section 11.6).

## ▶ PROPRANOLOL HYDROCHLORIDE

**Indications**   see under Dose

**Cautions**   see notes above; also avoid abrupt withdrawal especially in ischaemic heart disease; first-degree AV block; portal hypertension (risk of deterioration in liver function); diabetes; history of obstructive airways disease (introduce cautiously and monitor lung function—see also Bronchospasm below); myasthenia gravis; symptoms of hypoglycaemia and thyrotoxicosis may be masked (also see notes above); psoriasis; history of hypersensitivity—may increase sensitivity to allergens and result in more serious hypersensitivity response, also may reduce response to adrenaline (epinephrine) (see also section 3.4.3); reduce dose of oral propranolol in hepatic impairment; renal impairment (Appendix 3); pregnancy (Appendix 4); breast-feeding (Appendix 5); **interactions**: Appendix 1 (beta-blockers), **important**: verapamil interaction, see also p. 119

**Contra-indications**   asthma (but see Bronchospasm below), uncontrolled heart failure, Prinzmetal's angina, marked bradycardia, hypotension, sick sinus syndrome, second- or third- degree AV block, cardiogenic shock, metabolic acidosis, severe per-

ipheral arterial disease; phaeochromocytoma (apart from specific use with alpha-blockers, see also notes above)

**Bronchospasm**   The CSM advised that beta-blockers, including those considered to be cardioselective, should not be given to patients with a history of asthma or bronchospasm. However, in rare situations when there is no alternative, a cardioselective beta-blocker can be given to these patients with extreme caution and under specialist supervision.

**Side-effects**   see notes above; also gastro-intestinal disturbances; bradycardia, heart failure, hypotension, conduction disorders, peripheral vasoconstriction (including exacerbation of intermittent claudication and Raynaud's phenomenon); bronchospasm (see above), dyspnoea; headache, fatigue, sleep disturbances, paraesthesia, dizziness, vertigo, psychoses; sexual dysfunction; purpura, thrombocytopenia; visual disturbances; exacerbation of psoriasis, alopecia; *rarely* rashes and dry eyes (reversible on withdrawal); **overdosage**: see Emergency Treatment of Poisoning, p. 32

**Dose**

● By mouth, hypertension, initially 80 mg twice daily, increased at weekly intervals as required; maintenance 160–320 mg daily

Prophylaxis of variceal bleeding in portal hypertension, initially 40 mg twice daily, increased to 80 mg twice daily according to heart rate; max. 160 mg twice daily

Phaeochromocytoma (only with an alpha-blocker), 60 mg daily for 3 days before surgery *or* 30 mg daily in patients unsuitable for surgery

Angina, initially 40 mg 2–3 times daily; maintenance 120–240 mg daily

Arrhythmias, hypertrophic cardiomyopathy, anxiety tachycardia, and thyrotoxicosis (adjunct), 10–40 mg 3–4 times daily

Anxiety with symptoms such as palpitation, sweating, tremor, 40 mg once daily, increased to 40 mg 3 times daily if necessary

Prophylaxis after myocardial infarction, 40 mg 4 times daily for 2–3 days, then 80 mg twice daily, beginning 5 to 21 days after infarction

Migraine prophylaxis and essential tremor, initially 40 mg 2–3 times daily; maintenance 80–160 mg daily

● By intravenous injection, arrhythmias and thyrotoxic crisis, 1 mg over 1 minute; if necessary repeat at 2-minute intervals; max. total dose 10 mg (5 mg in anaesthesia)

**Note** Excessive bradycardia can be countered with intravenous injection of atropine sulphate 0.6–2.4 mg in divided doses of 600 micrograms; for **overdosage** see Emergency Treatment of Poisoning, p. 32

**Propranolol** (Non-proprietary) ▣ℙₒₘ

Tablets, propranolol hydrochloride 10 mg, net price 28 = 90p; 40 mg, 28 = 95p; 80 mg, 56 = £1.65; 160 mg, 56 = £3.05. Label: 8
Brands include *Angilol*®

Oral solution, propranolol hydrochloride 5 mg/5 mL, net price 150 mL = £12.50; 10 mg/5 mL, 150 mL = £16.45; 50 mg/5 mL, 150 mL = £19.98. Label: 8
Brands include *Syprol*®

**Inderal**® (AstraZeneca) ▣ℙₒₘ

Injection, propranolol hydrochloride 1 mg/mL, net price 1-mL amp = 21p

◢**Modified release**

**Note** Modified-release preparations can be used for once daily administration

**Half-Inderal LA®** (AstraZeneca) [PoM]

Capsules, m/r, lavender/pink, propranolol hydrochloride 80 mg, net price 28-cap pack = £5.40. Label: 8, 25

**Note** Modified-release capsules containing propranolol hydrochloride 80 mg also available; brands include *Bedranol SR®*, *Half Beta Prograne®*

**Inderal-LA®** (AstraZeneca) [PoM]

Capsules, m/r, lavender/pink, propranolol hydrochloride 160 mg, net price 28-cap pack = £1.91. Label: 8, 25

**Note** Modified-release capsules containing propranolol hydrochloride 160 mg also available; brands include *Bedranol SR®*, *Beta Prograne®*, *Slo-Pro®*

## ACEBUTOLOL

**Indications** see under Dose

**Cautions** see under Propranolol Hydrochloride; renal impairment (Appendix 3)

**Contra-indications** see under Propranolol Hydrochloride

**Side-effects** see under Propranolol Hydrochloride

**Dose**

• Hypertension, initially 400 mg once daily *or* 200 mg twice daily, increased after 2 weeks to 400 mg twice daily if necessary

• Angina, initially 400 mg once daily *or* 200 mg twice daily; 300 mg 3 times daily in severe angina; up to 1.2 g daily has been used

• Arrhythmias, 0.4–1.2 g daily in 2–3 divided doses

**Sectral®** (Sanofi-Aventis) [PoM]

Capsules, acebutolol (as hydrochloride) 100 mg (buff/white), net price 84-cap pack = £14.97; 200 mg (buff/pink), 56-cap pack = £19.18. Label: 8

Tablets, f/c, acebutolol 400 mg (as hydrochloride), net price 28-tab pack = £18.62. Label: 8

## ATENOLOL

**Indications** see under Dose

**Cautions** see under Propranolol Hydrochloride; renal impairment (Appendix 3)

**Contra-indications** see under Propranolol Hydrochloride

**Side-effects** see under Propranolol Hydrochloride

**Dose**

• By mouth, hypertension, 25–50 mg daily (higher doses rarely necessary)

Angina, 100 mg daily in 1 or 2 doses

Arrhythmias, 50–100 mg daily

• By intravenous injection, arrhythmias, 2.5 mg at a rate of 1 mg/minute, repeated at 5-minute intervals to a max. of 10 mg

**Note** Excessive bradycardia can be countered with intravenous injection of atropine sulphate 0.6–2.4 mg in divided doses of 600 micrograms; for **overdosage** see Emergency Treatment of Poisoning, p. 32

• By intravenous infusion, arrhythmias, 150 micrograms/kg over 20 minutes, repeated every 12 hours if required

Early intervention within 12 hours of myocardial infarction (section 2.10.1), by intravenous injection over 5 minutes, 5 mg, then by mouth, 50 mg after 15 minutes, 50 mg after 12 hours, then 100 mg daily

**Atenolol** (Non-proprietary) [PoM]

Tablets, atenolol 25 mg, net price 28-tab pack = 82p; 50 mg, 28-tab pack = 86p; 100 mg, 28-tab pack = 86p. Label: 8

Brands include *Atenix®*

**Tenormin®** (AstraZeneca) [PoM]

'25' tablets, f/c, atenolol 25 mg, net price 28-tab pack = £1.16. Label: 8

LS tablets, orange, f/c, scored, atenolol 50 mg, net price 28-tab pack = £2.04. Label: 8

Tablets, orange, f/c, scored, atenolol 100 mg, net price 28-tab pack = £3.46. Label: 8

Syrup, sugar-free, atenolol 25 mg/5 mL, net price 300 mL = £8.55. Label: 8

Injection, atenolol 500 micrograms/mL, net price 10-mL amp = 96p (hosp. only)

◢**With diuretic**

**Co-tenidone** (Non-proprietary) [PoM]

Tablets, co-tenidone 50/12.5 (atenolol 50 mg, chlortalidone 12.5 mg), net price 28-tab pack = £1.15; co-tenidone 100/25 (atenolol 100 mg, chlortalidone 25 mg), 28-tab pack = £1.25. Label: 8

**Dose** hypertension, 1 tablet daily (but see also under Dose above)

**Kalten®** (BPC 100) [PoM]

Capsules, red/ivory, atenolol 50 mg, co-amilozide 2.5/25 (anhydrous amiloride hydrochloride 2.5 mg, hydrochlorothiazide 25 mg), net price 28-cap pack = £10.01. Label: 8

**Dose** hypertension, 1 capsule daily

**Tenoret 50®** (AstraZeneca) [PoM]

Tablets, brown, f/c, co-tenidone 50/12.5 (atenolol 50 mg, chlortalidone 12.5 mg), net price 28-tab pack = £1.15. Label: 8

**Dose** hypertension, 1 tablet daily

**Tenoretic®** (AstraZeneca) [PoM]

Tablets, brown, f/c, co-tenidone 100/25 (atenolol 100 mg, chlortalidone 25 mg), net price 28-tab pack = £1.25. Label: 8

**Dose** hypertension, 1 tablet daily (but see also under Dose above)

◢**With calcium-channel blocker**

**Note** Only indicated when calcium-channel blocker or beta-blocker alone proves inadequate. For cautions, contra-indications, and side-effects of nifedipine see section 2.6.2

**Beta-Adalat®** (Bayer) [PoM]

Capsules, reddish-brown, atenolol 50 mg, nifedipine 20 mg (m/r), net price 28-cap pack = £10.00. Label: 8, 25

**Dose** hypertension, 1 capsule daily, increased if necessary to twice daily; elderly, 1 daily

Angina, 1 capsule twice daily

**Tenif®** (AstraZeneca) [PoM]

Capsules, reddish-brown, atenolol 50 mg, nifedipine 20 mg (m/r), net price 28-cap pack = £10.63. Label: 8, 25

**Dose** hypertension, 1 capsule daily, increased if necessary to twice daily; elderly, 1 daily

Angina, 1 capsule twice daily

**2**

**Cardiovascular system**

## ◼ BISOPROLOL FUMARATE

**Indications**  see under Dose

**Cautions**  see under Propranolol Hydrochloride; ensure heart failure not worsening before increasing dose; hepatic impairment (Appendix 2); renal impairment (Appendix 3)

**Contra-indications**  see under Propranolol Hydrochloride; also acute or decompensated heart failure requiring intravenous inotropes; sino-atrial block

**Side-effects**  see under Propranolol Hydrochloride

**Dose**

- Hypertension and angina, usually 10 mg once daily (5 mg may be adequate in some patients); max. 20 mg daily

- Adjunct in stable moderate to severe heart failure (section 2.5.5), initially 1.25 mg once daily (in the morning) for 1 week then, if well tolerated, increased to 2.5 mg once daily for 1 week, then 3.75 mg once daily for 1 week, then 5 mg once daily for 4 weeks, then 7.5 mg once daily for 4 weeks, then 10 mg once daily; max. 10 mg daily

**Bisoprolol Fumarate** (Non-proprietary) ⒫ⓄⓂ

Tablets, bisoprolol fumarate 5 mg, net price 28-tab pack = £1.23; 10 mg, 28-tab pack = £1.31. Label: 8

**Cardicor®** (Merck) ⒫ⓄⓂ

Tablets, f/c, bisoprolol fumarate 1.25 mg, net price 28-tab pack = £5.90; 2.5 mg (scored), 28-tab pack = £3.90; 3.75 mg (scored, white-yellow), 28-tab pack = £5.90; 5 mg (scored, light yellow), 28-tab pack = £5.90; 7.5 mg (scored, yellow), 28-tab pack = £5.90; 10 mg (scored, orange), 28-tab pack = £5.90. Label: 8

**Emcor®** (Merck) ⒫ⓄⓂ

LS Tablets, yellow, f/c, scored, bisoprolol fumarate 5 mg, net price 28-tab pack = £11.30. Label: 8

Tablets, orange, f/c, scored, bisoprolol fumarate 10 mg, net price 28-tab pack = £12.68. Label: 8

## ◼ CARVEDILOL

**Indications**  hypertension; angina; adjunct to diuretics, digoxin, or ACE inhibitors in symptomatic chronic heart failure

**Cautions**  see under Propranolol Hydrochloride; monitor renal function during dose titration in patients with heart failure who also have renal impairment, low blood pressure, ischaemic heart disease, or diffuse vascular disease

**Contra-indications**  see under Propranolol Hydrochloride; acute or decompensated heart failure requiring intravenous inotropes; hepatic impairment

**Side-effects**  postural hypotension, dizziness, headache, fatigue, gastro-intestinal disturbances, bradycardia; occasionally diminished peripheral circulation, peripheral oedema and painful extremities, dry mouth, dry eyes, eye irritation or disturbed vision, impotence, disturbances of micturition, influenza-like symptoms; rarely angina, AV block, exacerbation of intermittent claudication or Raynaud's phenomenon; allergic skin reactions, exacerbation of psoriasis, nasal stuffiness, wheezing, depressed mood, sleep disturbances, paraesthesia, heart failure, changes in liver enzymes, thrombocytopenia, leucopenia also reported

**Dose**

- Hypertension, initially 12.5 mg once daily, increased after 2 days to usual dose of 25 mg once daily; if necessary may be further increased at intervals of at least 2 weeks to max. 50 mg daily in single or divided doses; ELDERLY initial dose of 12.5 mg daily may provide satisfactory control

- Angina, initially 12.5 mg twice daily, increased after 2 days to 25 mg twice daily

- Adjunct in heart failure (section 2.5.5) initially 3.125 mg twice daily (with food), dose increased at intervals of at least 2 weeks to 6.25 mg twice daily, then to 12.5 mg twice daily, then to 25 mg twice daily; increase to highest dose tolerated, max. 25 mg twice daily in patients with severe heart failure or body-weight less than 85 kg and 50 mg twice daily in patients over 85 kg

**Carvedilol** (Non-proprietary) ⒫ⓄⓂ

Tablets, carvedilol 3.125 mg, net price 28-tab pack = £5.73; 6.25 mg, 28-tab pack = £6.09; 12.5 mg, 28-tab pack = £1.54; 25 mg, 28-tab pack = £2.17. Label: 8

**Eucardic®** (Roche) ⒫ⓄⓂ

Tablets, scored, carvedilol 3.125 mg (pink), net price 28-tab pack = £7.27; 6.25 mg (yellow), 28-tab pack = £8.08; 12.5 mg (peach), 28-tab pack = £8.99; 25 mg, 28-tab pack = £11.22. Label: 8

## ◼ CELIPROLOL HYDROCHLORIDE

**Indications**  mild to moderate hypertension

**Cautions**  see under Propranolol Hydrochloride; renal impairment (avoid if eGFR less than 15 mL/minute/1.73 m²; Appendix 3)

**Contra-indications**  see under Propranolol Hydrochloride

**Side-effects**  headache, dizziness, fatigue, nausea and somnolence; also bradycardia, bronchospasm; depression and pneumonitis reported rarely

**Dose**

- 200 mg once daily in the morning, increased to 400 mg once daily if necessary

**Celiprolol** (Non-proprietary) ⒫ⓄⓂ

Tablets, celiprolol hydrochloride 200 mg, net price 28-tab pack = £5.74; 400 mg, 28-tab pack = £38.58. Label: 8, 22

**Celectol®** (Winthrop) ⒫ⓄⓂ

Tablets, f/c, scored, celiprolol hydrochloride 200 mg (yellow), net price 28-tab pack = £19.83; 400 mg, 28-tab pack = £39.65. Label: 8, 22

## ◼ ESMOLOL HYDROCHLORIDE

**Indications**  short-term treatment of supraventricular arrhythmias (including atrial fibrillation, atrial flutter, sinus tachycardia); tachycardia and hypertension in peri-operative period

**Cautions**  see under Propranolol Hydrochloride; renal impairment

**Contra-indications**  see under Propranolol Hydrochloride

**Side-effects**  see under Propranolol Hydrochloride; also on infusion venous irritation and thrombophlebitis

**Dose**

- By intravenous infusion, usually within range 50–200 micrograms/kg/minute (consult product literature for details of dose titration and doses during peri-operative period)

**Brevibloc®** (Baxter) [PoM]

Injection, esmolol hydrochloride 10 mg/mL, net price 10-mL vial = £7.79, 250-mL infusion bag = £89.69

---

## LABETALOL HYDROCHLORIDE

**Indications** hypertension (including hypertension in pregnancy, hypertension with angina, and hypertension following acute myocardial infarction); hypertensive crisis (but see section 2.5); controlled hypotension in anaesthesia

**Cautions** see under Propranolol Hydrochloride; interferes with laboratory tests for catecholamines; liver damage (see below); renal impairment (Appendix 3)
**Liver damage** Severe hepatocellular damage reported after both short-term and long-term treatment. Appropriate laboratory tests needed at first symptom of liver dysfunction and if laboratory evidence of damage (or if jaundice) labetalol should be stopped and not restarted

**Contra-indications** see under Propranolol Hydrochloride

**Side-effects** postural hypotension (avoid upright position during and for 3 hours after intravenous administration), tiredness, weakness, headache, rashes, scalp tingling, difficulty in micturition, epigastric pain, nausea, vomiting; liver damage (see above); rarely lichenoid rash

**Dose**

- By mouth, initially 100 mg (50 mg in elderly) twice daily with food, increased at intervals of 14 days to usual dose of 200 mg twice daily; up to 800 mg daily in 2 divided doses (3–4 divided doses if higher); max. 2.4 g daily
- By intravenous injection, 50 mg over at least 1 minute, repeated after 5 minutes if necessary; max. total dose 200 mg
  **Note** Excessive bradycardia can be countered with intravenous injection of atropine sulphate 0.6–2.4 mg in divided doses of 600 micrograms; for **overdosage** see Emergency Treatment of Poisoning, p. 32
- By intravenous infusion, 2 mg/minute until satisfactory response then discontinue; usual total dose 50–200 mg, (**not** recommended for phaeochromocytoma, see under Phaeochromocytoma, section 2.5.4)

  Hypertension of pregnancy, 20 mg/hour, doubled every 30 minutes; usual max. 160 mg/hour
  Hypertension following myocardial infarction, 15 mg/hour, gradually increased to max. 120 mg/hour

**Labetalol Hydrochloride** (Non-proprietary) [PoM]

Tablets, f/c, labetalol hydrochloride 100 mg, net price, 56 = £9.46; 200 mg, 56 = £14.64; 400 mg, 56 = £20.87. Label: 8, 21

**Trandate®** (UCB Pharma) [PoM]

Tablets, all orange, f/c, labetalol hydrochloride 50 mg, net price 56-tab pack = £3.64; 100 mg, 56-tab pack = £4.01; 200 mg, 56-tab pack = £6.51; 400 mg, 56-tab pack = £9.05. Label: 8, 21

Injection, labetalol hydrochloride 5 mg/mL, net price 20-mL amp = £2.04

---

## METOPROLOL TARTRATE

**Indications** see under Dose
**Cautions** see under Propranolol Hydrochloride; hepatic impairment (Appendix 2)
**Contra-indications** see under Propranolol Hydrochloride
**Side-effects** see under Propranolol Hydrochloride
**Dose**

- By mouth, hypertension, initially 100 mg daily, increased if necessary to 200 mg daily in 1–2 divided doses; max. 400 mg daily (but high doses rarely necessary)
  Angina, 50–100 mg 2–3 times daily
  Arrhythmias, usually 50 mg 2–3 times daily; up to 300 mg daily in divided doses if necessary
  Migraine prophylaxis, 100–200 mg daily in divided doses
  Hyperthyroidism (adjunct), 50 mg 4 times daily
- By intravenous injection, arrhythmias, up to 5 mg at rate 1–2 mg/minute, repeated after 5 minutes if necessary, total dose 10–15 mg
  **Note** Excessive bradycardia can be countered with intravenous injection of atropine sulphate 0.6–2.4 mg in divided doses of 600 micrograms; for **overdosage** see Emergency Treatment of Poisoning, p. 32

  In surgery, by slow intravenous injection 2–4 mg at induction or to control arrhythmias developing during anaesthesia; 2-mg doses may be repeated to a max. of 10 mg

  Early intervention within 12 hours of infarction, by intravenous injection 5 mg every 2 minutes to a max. of 15 mg, followed after 15 minutes by 50 mg by mouth every 6 hours for 48 hours; maintenance 200 mg daily in divided doses

**Metoprolol Tartrate** (Non-proprietary) [PoM]

Tablets, metoprolol tartrate 50 mg, net price 28 = £1.28, 56 = £1.55; 100 mg, 28 = £1.81, 56 = £2.11. Label: 8

**Betaloc®** (AstraZeneca) [PoM]

Injection, metoprolol tartrate 1 mg/mL, net price 5-mL amp = 42p

**Lopresor®** (Novartis) [PoM]

Tablets, f/c, scored, metoprolol tartrate 50 mg (pink), net price 56-tab pack = £2.57; 100 mg (blue), 56-tab pack = £6.68. Label: 8

◀ **Modified release**

**Betaloc-SA®** (AstraZeneca) [PoM]

Durules® (= tablets, m/r), metoprolol tartrate 200 mg, net price 28-tab pack = £4.56. Label: 8, 25
**Dose** hypertension, angina, 200 mg daily in the morning, increased to 400 mg daily if necessary; migraine prophylaxis, 200 mg daily

**Lopresor SR®** (Novartis) [PoM]

Tablets, m/r, yellow, f/c, metoprolol tartrate 200 mg, net price 28-tab pack = £9.80. Label: 8, 25
**Dose** hypertension, 200 mg daily; angina, 200–400 mg daily; migraine prophylaxis, 200 mg daily

---

## NADOLOL

**Indications** see under Dose
**Cautions** see under Propranolol Hydrochloride; hepatic impairment; renal impairment (Appendix 3)
**Contra-indications** see under Propranolol Hydrochloride

**2**

**Cardiovascular system**

**Side-effects** see under Propranolol Hydrochloride

**Dose**

- Hypertension, initially 80 mg once daily, increased in increments of up to 80 mg at weekly intervals if required; max. 240 mg daily (higher doses rarely necessary)
- Angina, initially 40 mg once daily, increased at weekly intervals if required; usual max. 160 mg daily (rarely up to 240 mg may be required)
- Arrhythmias, initially 40 mg once daily, increased at weekly intervals up to 160 mg if required; reduce to 40 mg if bradycardia occurs
- Migraine prophylaxis, initially 40 mg once daily, increased in 40 mg increments at weekly intervals according to response; usual maintenance dose 80–160 mg once daily
- Thyrotoxicosis (adjunct), 80–160 mg once daily

**Corgard®** (Sanofi-Synthelabo) (PoM)
Tablets, blue, scored, nadolol 80 mg, net price 28-tab pack = £5.00. Label: 8

---

## NEBIVOLOL

**Indications** essential hypertension; adjunct in stable mild to moderate heart failure in patients over 70 years

**Cautions** see under Propranolol Hydrochloride; renal impairment (Appendix 3)

**Contra-indications** see under Propranolol Hydrochloride; also acute or decompensated heart failure requiring intravenous inotropes; hepatic impairment (Appendix 2)

**Side-effects** see under Propranolol Hydrochloride; also oedema and depression

**Dose**

- Hypertension, 5 mg daily; ELDERLY initially 2.5 mg daily, increased if necessary to 5 mg daily
- Adjunct in heart failure (section 2.5.5), initially 1.25 mg once daily, then if tolerated increased at intervals of 1–2 weeks to 2.5 mg once daily, then to 5 mg once daily, then to max. 10 mg once daily

**Nebivolol** (Non-proprietary) (PoM)
Tablets, nebivolol (as hydrochloride) 5 mg, net price 28-tab pack = £9.23. Label: 8

**Nebilet®** (Menarini) (PoM)
Tablets, scored, nebivolol (as hydrochloride) 5 mg, net price 28-tab pack = £9.23. Label: 8
Note Also available as *Hypoloc®*

---

## OXPRENOLOL HYDROCHLORIDE

**Indications** see under Dose

**Cautions** see under Propranolol Hydrochloride; reduce dose in hepatic impairment

**Contra-indications** see under Propranolol Hydrochloride

**Side-effects** see under Propranolol Hydrochloride

**Dose**

- Hypertension, 80–160 mg daily in 2–3 divided doses, increased as required; max. 320 mg daily
- Angina, 80–160 mg daily in 2–3 divided doses; max. 320 mg daily
- Arrhythmias, 40–240 mg daily in 2–3 divided doses; max. 240 mg daily
- Anxiety symptoms (short-term use), 40–80 mg daily in 1–2 divided doses

**Oxprenolol** (Non-proprietary) (PoM)
Tablets, coated, oxprenolol hydrochloride 20 mg, net price 56 = £1.86; 40 mg, 56 = £3.73; 80 mg, 56 = £6.20; 160 mg, 20 = £2.36. Label: 8

**Trasicor®** (Amdipharm) (PoM)
Tablets, f/c, oxprenolol hydrochloride 20 mg (contain gluten), net price 56-tab pack = £1.86; 40 mg (contain gluten), 56-tab pack = £3.73; 80 mg (yellow), 56-tab pack = £6.20. Label: 8

◢Modified release

**Slow-Trasicor®** (Amdipharm) (PoM)
Tablets, m/r, f/c, oxprenolol hydrochloride 160 mg, net price 28-tab pack = £6.63. Label: 8, 25
Dose hypertension, angina, initially 160 mg once daily; if necessary may be increased to max. 320 mg daily

◢With diuretic

**Trasidrex®** (Goldshield) (PoM)
Tablets, red, s/c, co-prenozide 160/0.25 (oxprenolol hydrochloride 160 mg (m/r), cyclopenthiazide 250 micrograms), net price 28-tab pack = £10.66. Label: 8, 25
Dose hypertension, 1 tablet daily, increased if necessary to 2 daily as a single dose

---

## PINDOLOL

**Indications** see under Dose

**Cautions** see under Propranolol Hydrochloride

**Contra-indications** see under Propranolol Hydrochloride; severe renal impairment (Appendix 3)

**Side-effects** see under Propranolol Hydrochloride

**Dose**

- Hypertension, initially 5 mg 2–3 times daily *or* 15 mg once daily, increased as required at weekly intervals; usual maintenance 15–30 mg daily; max. 45 mg daily
- Angina, 2.5–5 mg up to 3 times daily

**Pindolol** (Non-proprietary) (PoM)
Tablets, pindolol 5 mg, net price 100-tab pack = £7.81. Label: 8

**Visken®** (Amdipharm) (PoM)
Tablets, scored, pindolol 5 mg, net price 56-tab pack = £5.85; 15 mg, 28-tab pack = £8.79. Label: 8

◢With diuretic

**Viskaldix®** (Amdipharm) (PoM)
Tablets, scored, pindolol 10 mg, clopamide 5 mg, net price 28-tab pack = £6.70. Label: 8
Dose hypertension, 1 tablet daily in the morning, increased if necessary to 2 daily; max. 3 daily

---

## SOTALOL HYDROCHLORIDE

**Indications** *Tablets and injection:* life-threatening arrhythmias including ventricular tachyarrhythmias, symptomatic non-sustained ventricular tachyarrhythmias
*Tablets only:* prophylaxis of paroxysmal atrial tachycardia or fibrillation, paroxysmal AV re-entrant tachycardias (both nodal and involving accessory pathways), paroxysmal supraventricular tachycardia

after cardiac surgery, maintenance of sinus rhythm following cardioversion of atrial fibrillation or flutter

*Injection only:* electrophysiological study of inducible ventricular and supraventricular arrhythmias; temporary substitution for tablets

**CSM advice.** The use of sotalol should be limited to the treatment of ventricular arrhythmias or prophylaxis of supraventricular arrhythmias (see above). It should no longer be used for angina, hypertension, thyrotoxicosis or for secondary prevention after myocardial infarction; when stopping sotalol for these indications, the dose should be reduced gradually

**Cautions** see under Propranolol Hydrochloride; renal impairment (avoid if eGFR less than 10 mL/minute/1.73 m²; Appendix 3); correct hypokalaemia, hypomagnesaemia, or other electrolyte disturbances; severe or prolonged diarrhoea; **interactions:** Appendix 1 (beta-blockers), **important:** verapamil interaction see also p. 119

**Contra-indications** see under Propranolol Hydrochloride; congenital or acquired long QT syndrome; torsade de pointes; renal failure

**Side-effects** see under Propranolol Hydrochloride; arrhythmogenic (pro-arrhythmic) effect (torsade de pointes—increased risk in women)

**Dose**
● By mouth with ECG monitoring and measurement of corrected QT interval, arrhythmias, initially 80 mg daily in 1–2 divided doses increased gradually at intervals of 2–3 days to usual dose of 160–320 mg daily in 2 divided doses; higher doses of 480–640 mg daily for life-threatening ventricular arrhythmias under specialist supervision
● By intravenous injection over 10 minutes, acute arrhythmias, 20–120 mg with ECG monitoring, repeated if necessary with 6-hour intervals between injections

Diagnostic use, see product literature

**Note** Excessive bradycardia can be countered with intravenous injection of atropine sulphate 0.6–2.4 mg in divided doses of 600 micrograms; for **overdosage** see Emergency Treatment of Poisoning, p. 32

**Sotalol** (Non-proprietary) PoM
Tablets, sotalol hydrochloride 40 mg, net price 56 = £1.29; 80 mg, 56 = £1.91; 160 mg, 28 = £2.12. Label: 8

**Beta-Cardone®** (UCB Pharma) PoM
Tablets, scored, sotalol hydrochloride 40 mg (green), net price 56-tab pack = £1.29; 80 mg (pink), 56-tab pack = £1.91; 200 mg, 28-tab pack = £2.40. Label: 8

**Sotacor®** (Bristol-Myers Squibb) PoM
Tablets, scored, sotalol hydrochloride 80 mg, net price 28-tab pack = £3.12; 160 mg, 28-tab pack = £6.16. Label: 8
Injection, sotalol hydrochloride 10 mg/mL, net price 4-mL amp = £1.57

---

▌ **TIMOLOL MALEATE**

**Indications** see under Dose; glaucoma (section 11.6)

**Cautions** see under Propranolol Hydrochloride; hepatic impairment (Appendix 2); renal impairment (Appendix 3)

**Contra-indications** see under Propranolol Hydrochloride

**Side-effects** see under Propranolol Hydrochloride

**Dose**
● Hypertension, initially 10 mg daily in 1–2 divided doses; gradually increased if necessary to max. 60 mg daily; usual maintenance dose 10–30 mg daily (doses above 30 mg daily given in divided doses)
● Angina, initially 5 mg twice daily increased if necessary by 10 mg daily every 3–4 days; max. 30 mg twice daily
● Prophylaxis after myocardial infarction, initially 5 mg twice daily, increased after 2 days to 10 mg twice daily if tolerated
● Migraine prophylaxis, 10–20 mg daily in 1–2 divided doses

**Betim®** (Valeant) PoM
Tablets, scored, timolol maleate 10 mg, net price 30-tab pack = £2.08. Label: 8

◢**With diuretic**
**Prestim®** (Valeant) PoM
Tablets, scored, timolol maleate 10 mg, bendroflumethiazide 2.5 mg, net price 30-tab pack = £3.49. Label: 8
**Dose** hypertension, 1–2 tablets daily; max. 4 daily

---

## 2.5 Hypertension and heart failure

**2.5.1** Vasodilator antihypertensive drugs
**2.5.2** Centrally acting antihypertensive drugs
**2.5.3** Adrenergic neurone blocking drugs
**2.5.4** Alpha-adrenoceptor blocking drugs
**2.5.5** Drugs affecting the renin-angiotensin system

Lowering raised blood pressure decreases the risk of stroke, coronary events, heart failure, and renal impairment. Advice on antihypertensive therapy in this section takes into account the recommendations of the Joint British Societies (JBS2: British Societies' guidelines on prevention of cardiovascular disease in clinical practice. *Heart* 2005; **91** (Suppl V): v1–v52).

Possible causes of hypertension (e.g. renal disease, endocrine causes), contributory factors, risk factors, and the presence of any complications of hypertension, such as left ventricular hypertrophy, should be established. Patients should be given advice on lifestyle changes to reduce blood pressure or cardiovascular risk; these include smoking cessation, weight reduction, reduction of excessive intake of alcohol, reduction of dietary salt, reduction of total and saturated fat, increasing exercise, and increasing fruit and vegetable intake.

**Thresholds and targets for treatment** The following thresholds for treatment[1] are recommended:

● Accelerated (malignant) hypertension (with papilloedema or fundal haemorrhages and exudates) *or* acute cardiovascular complications, admit for **immediate treatment**;

---

1. Thresholds and targets for treatment based on blood pressure measured in clinic may not apply to ambulatory or home blood-pressure monitoring, which usually give lower values.

**2**

**Cardiovascular system**

- Where the initial blood pressure is systolic ≥ 220 mmHg *or* diastolic ≥ 120 mmHg, **treat immediately**;

- Where the initial blood pressure is systolic 180–219 mmHg *or* diastolic 110–119 mmHg, confirm over 1–2 weeks then **treat** if these values are sustained;

- Where the initial blood pressure is systolic 160–179 mmHg *or* diastolic 100–109 mmHg, *and* the patient has cardiovascular complications, target-organ damage (e.g. left ventricular hypertrophy, renal impairment) or diabetes mellitus (type 1 or 2), confirm over 3–4 weeks then **treat** if these values are sustained;

- Where the initial blood pressure is systolic 160–179 mmHg *or* diastolic 100–109 mmHg, but the patient has *no* cardiovascular complications, no target-organ damage, or no diabetes, advise lifestyle changes, reassess weekly initially and **treat** if these values are sustained on repeat measurements over 4–12 weeks;

- Where the initial blood pressure is systolic 140–159 mmHg *or* diastolic 90–99 mmHg *and* the patient has cardiovascular complications, target-organ damage or diabetes, confirm within 12 weeks and **treat** if these values are sustained;

- Where the initial blood pressure is systolic 140–159 mmHg *or* diastolic 90–99 mmHg and *no* cardiovascular complications, no target-organ damage, or no diabetes, advise lifestyle changes and **reassess** monthly; **treat** persistent mild hypertension if the 10-year cardiovascular disease risk is 20% or more.[1]

A target systolic blood pressure < 140 mmHg *and* diastolic blood pressure < 90 mmHg is suggested. A lower target systolic blood pressure < 130 mmHg *and* diastolic blood pressure < 80 mmHg should be considered for those with established atherosclerotic cardiovascular disease, diabetes, or chronic renal failure. In some individuals it may not be possible to reduce blood pressure below the suggested targets despite the use of appropriate therapy.

**Drug treatment of hypertension** Response to drug treatment for hypertension may be affected by the patient's age and ethnic background. An **ACE inhibitor** (section 2.5.5.1) or an **angiotensin-II receptor antagonist** (section 2.5.5.2) may be the most appropriate initial drug in younger Caucasians; however a **beta-blocker** may be considered if an ACE inhibitor or an angiotensin-II receptor antagonist is not tolerated or is contra-indicated (see also Hypertension in Pregnancy, p. 95). Afro-Caribbean patients and those aged over 55 years respond less well to ACE inhibitors and angiotensin-II receptor antagonists, therefore a **thiazide** (section 2.2.1) or a **calcium-channel blocker** (section 2.6.2) may be chosen for initial treatment.

Beta-blockers, especially when combined with a thiazide diuretic, should be avoided for the routine treatment of uncomplicated hypertension in patients with diabetes or in those at high risk of developing diabetes.

1. Cardiovascular disease risk may be determined from the chart issued by the Joint British Societies (*Heart* 2005; **91** (Suppl V): v1–v52)—see inside back cover. The Joint British Societies' 'Cardiac Risk Assessor' computer programme may also be used to determine cardiovascular disease risk.

A single antihypertensive drug is often not adequate and other antihypertensive drugs are usually added in a step-wise manner until control is achieved. Unless it is necessary to lower the blood pressure urgently, an interval of at least 4 weeks should be allowed to determine response.

Where two antihypertensive drugs are needed, an ACE inhibitor *or* an angiotensin-II receptor antagonist may be combined with *either* a thiazide *or* a calcium-channel blocker.

If control is inadequate with 2 drugs, a thiazide *and* a calcium-channel blocker may be added. The addition of an **alpha-blocker** (section 2.5.4), **spironolactone**, another diuretic, or a beta-blocker should be considered in resistant hypertension. In patients with *primary hyperaldosteronism*, spironolactone (section 2.2.3) is effective.

**Other measures to reduce cardiovascular risk**
Aspirin (section 2.9) in a dose of 75 mg daily reduces the risk of cardiovascular events and myocardial infarction. Unduly high blood pressure must be controlled before aspirin is given. Unless contra-indicated, aspirin is recommended for all patients with established cardiovascular disease or those with a 10-year cardiovascular disease risk[1] of 20% or more and aged over 50 years. Aspirin is also of benefit in those with diabetes (see also section 2.9).

Lipid-regulating drugs can also be of benefit in cardiovascular disease or in those who are at high risk of developing cardiovascular disease (section 2.12).

**Hypertension in the elderly** Benefit from antihypertensive therapy is evident up to at least 80 years of age, but it is probably inappropriate to apply a strict age limit when deciding on drug therapy. Patients who reach 80 years of age while taking antihypertensive drugs should continue treatment, provided that it continues to be of benefit and does not cause significant side-effects. The thresholds for treatment are diastolic pressure averaging ≥ 90 mmHg *or* systolic pressure averaging ≥ 160 mmHg over 3 to 6 months' observation (despite appropriate lifestyle interventions). Treatment with a low dose of a thiazide or a dihydropyridine calcium-channel blocker is effective. An ACE inhibitor (or an angiotensin-II receptor antagonist) (section 2.5.5) can be added if necessary.

**Isolated systolic hypertension** Isolated systolic hypertension (systolic pressure ≥ 160 mmHg, diastolic pressure < 90 mmHg) is associated with an increased cardiovascular disease risk, particularly in those aged over 60 years. Systolic blood pressure averaging 160 mmHg or higher over 3 to 6 months (despite appropriate lifestyle interventions) should be lowered in those over 60 years, even if diastolic hypertension is absent. Treatment with a low dose of a thiazide or a dihydropyridine calcium-channel blocker is effective. An ACE inhibitor (or an angiotensin-II receptor antagonist) (section 2.5.5) can be added if necessary. Patients with severe postural hypotension should not receive blood pressure lowering drugs.

Isolated systolic hypertension in younger patients is uncommon but treatment may be indicated in those with a threshold systolic pressure of 160 mmHg (or less if at increased risk of cardiovascular disease, see above).

**Hypertension in diabetes** For patients with diabetes, the aim should be to maintain systolic pressure

< 130 mmHg and diastolic pressure < 80 mmHg. However, in some individuals, it may not be possible to achieve this level of control despite appropriate therapy. Most patients require a combination of antihypertensive drugs.

Hypertension is common in type 2 diabetes and antihypertensive treatment prevents macrovascular and microvascular complications. In type 1 diabetes, hypertension usually indicates the presence of diabetic nephropathy. An ACE inhibitor (or an angiotensin-II receptor antagonist) may have a specific role in the management of diabetic nephropathy (section 6.1.5); in patients with type 2 diabetes, an ACE inhibitor (or an angiotensin-II receptor antagonist) can delay progression of microalbuminuria to nephropathy.

**Hypertension in renal disease** The threshold for antihypertensive treatment in patients with renal impairment or persistent proteinuria is a systolic blood pressure ≥ 140 mmHg *or* a diastolic blood pressure ≥ 90 mmHg. Optimal blood pressure is a systolic blood pressure < 130 mmHg and a diastolic pressure < 80 mmHg, or lower if proteinuria exceeds 1 g in 24 hours. An ACE inhibitor (or an angiotensin-II receptor antagonist) should be considered for patients with proteinuria; however, ACE inhibitors should be used with caution in renal impairment, see section 2.5.5.1. Thiazide diuretics may be ineffective and high doses of loop diuretics may be required. A dihydropyridine calcium channel blocker can be added.

**Hypertension in pregnancy** High blood pressure in pregnancy may usually be due to pre-existing essential hypertension or to pre-eclampsia. **Methyldopa** (section 2.5.2) is safe in pregnancy. Beta-blockers are effective and safe in the third trimester. Modified-release preparations of **nifedipine** [unlicensed] are also used for hypertension in pregnancy. Intravenous administration of **labetalol** (section 2.4) can be used to control hypertensive crises; alternatively, **hydralazine** (section 2.5.1) may be used by the intravenous route. For use of **magnesium sulphate** in pre-eclampsia and eclampsia, see section 9.5.1.3.

**Accelerated or very severe hypertension** Accelerated (or malignant) hypertension or very severe hypertension (e.g. diastolic blood pressure > 140 mmHg) requires urgent treatment in hospital, but it is not an indication for parenteral antihypertensive therapy. Normally treatment should be by mouth with a beta-blocker (atenolol or labetalol) or a long-acting calcium-channel blocker (e.g. amlodipine or modified-release nifedipine). Within the first 24 hours the diastolic blood pressure should be reduced to 100–110 mmHg. Over the next 2 or 3 days blood pressure should be further reduced using a calcium-channel blocker, diuretic, ACE inhibitor, beta-blocker, or vasodilator, alone or in combination. Rapid reduction in blood pressure can reduce organ perfusion leading to cerebral infarction and blindness, deterioration in renal function, and myocardial ischaemia. **Sodium nitroprusside** [unlicensed] by intravenous infusion is the drug of choice on the rare occasions when parenteral treatment is necessary.

For advice on short-term management of hypertensive episodes in phaeochromocytoma, see under Phaeochromocytoma, section 2.5.4.

## 2.5.1 Vasodilator antihypertensive drugs

Vasodilators have a potent hypotensive effect, especially when used in combination with a beta-blocker and a thiazide. **Important:** for a warning on the hazards of a very rapid fall in blood pressure, see Accelerated or Very Severe Hypertension, above.

**Diazoxide** has been used by intravenous injection in hypertensive emergencies.

**Hydralazine** is given by mouth as an adjunct to other antihypertensives for the treatment of resistant hypertension but is rarely used; when used alone it causes tachycardia and fluid retention. The incidence of side-effects is lower if the dose is kept below 100 mg daily, but systemic lupus erythematosus should be suspected if there is unexplained weight loss, arthritis, or any other unexplained ill health.

**Sodium nitroprusside** [unlicensed] is given by intravenous infusion to control severe hypertensive crises on the rare occasions when parenteral treatment is necessary.

**Minoxidil** should be reserved for the treatment of severe hypertension resistant to other drugs. Vasodilatation is accompanied by increased cardiac output and tachycardia and the patients develop fluid retention. For this reason the addition of a beta-blocker and a diuretic (usually furosemide, in high dosage) are mandatory. Hypertrichosis is troublesome and renders this drug unsuitable for women.

Prazosin, doxazosin, and terazosin (section 2.5.4) have alpha-blocking and vasodilator properties.

**Ambrisentan, bosentan, epoprostenol** (section 2.8.1), **iloprost, sildenafil,** and **sitaxentan** are licensed for the treatment of some types of pulmonary hypertension and should be used under specialist supervision. Bosentan is also licensed to reduce the number of new digital ulcers in patients with systemic sclerosis and ongoing digital ulcer disease.

The *Scottish Medicines Consortium* (p. 3) has advised (November 2005) that iloprost (*Ventavis®*) is accepted for restricted use within NHS Scotland in patients in whom bosentan is ineffective or not tolerated, and should only be prescribed by specialists in the Scottish Pulmonary Vascular Unit.

The *Scottish Medicines Consortium* (p. 3) has advised (October 2008) that ambrisentan (*Volibris®*) should be prescribed only by specialists in the Scottish Pulmonary Vascular Unit or other similar specialists.

### ◢ AMBRISENTAN

**Indications** pulmonary arterial hypertension

**Cautions** not to be initiated in significant anaemia; monitor haemoglobin concentration or haematocrit after 1 month and 3 months of starting treatment, and periodically thereafter (reduce dose or discontinue treatment if significant decrease in haemoglobin concentration or haematocrit observed); monitor liver function before treatment, and monthly thereafter—discontinue if liver enzymes raised significantly or if symptoms of liver impairment develop; hepatic impairment (avoid if severe; Appendix 2); renal impairment (Appendix 3)

**2 Cardiovascular system**

**Contra-indications** pregnancy (Appendix 4); breast-feeding (Appendix 5)

**Side-effects** abdominal pain, constipation; palpitation, flushing, peripheral oedema; upper respiratory-tract disorders; headache; anaemia; *less commonly* hypersensitivity reactions (including angioedema and rash)

**Dose**

- ADULT over 18 years, 5 mg once daily, increased if necessary to 10 mg once daily

**Volibris®** (GSK) ▼ PoM

Tablets, f/c, ambrisentan 5 mg (pale pink), net price 30-tab pack = £1651.07; 10 mg (dark pink), 30-tab pack = £1651.07

---

### ▌ BOSENTAN

**Indications** pulmonary arterial hypertension; systemic sclerosis with ongoing digital ulcer disease (to reduce number of new digital ulcers)

**Cautions** not to be initiated if systemic systolic blood pressure is below 85 mmHg; monitor haemoglobin before and during treatment (monthly for first 4 months, then 3-monthly); avoid abrupt withdrawal; monitor liver function before treatment, at monthly intervals during treatment, and 2 weeks after dose increase (reduce dose or suspend treatment if liver enzymes raised significantly)—discontinue if symptoms of liver impairment; hepatic impairment (Appendix 2); **interactions**: Appendix 1 (bosentan)

**Contra-indications** acute porphyria (section 9.8.2) pregnancy (Appendix 4); breast-feeding (Appendix 5)

**Side-effects** gastro-intestinal disturbances, dry mouth, rectal haemorrhage, hepatic impairment (see Cautions, above); flushing, hypotension, palpitation, oedema, chest pain; dyspnoea; headache, dizziness, fatigue; back pain and pain in extremities; anaemia; hypersensitivity reactions (including rash, pruritus, and anaphylaxis)

**Dose**

- Pulmonary arterial hypertension, initially 62.5 mg twice daily increased after 4 weeks to 125 mg twice daily; max. 250 mg twice daily; CHILD under 12 years see *BNF for Children*
- Systemic sclerosis with ongoing digital ulcer disease, initially 62.5 mg twice daily increased after 4 weeks to 125 mg twice daily

**Tracleer®** (Actelion) ▼ PoM

Tablets, f/c, orange, bosentan (as monohydrate) 62.5 mg, net price 56-tab pack = £1493.07; 125 mg, 56-tab pack = £1493.07

---

### ▌ DIAZOXIDE

**Indications** hypertensive emergency including severe hypertension associated with renal disease (but see section 2.5); hypoglycaemia (section 6.1.4)

**Cautions** ischaemic heart disease; renal impairment (Appendix 3); pregnancy and labour (Appendix 4); **interactions**: Appendix 1 (diazoxide)

**Side-effects** tachycardia, hypotension, hyperglycaemia, sodium and water retention; *rarely* cardiomegaly, hyperosmolar non-ketotic coma, leucopenia, thrombocytopenia, and hirsuitism

**Dose**

- By rapid intravenous injection (less than 30 seconds), 1–3 mg/kg to max. single dose of 150 mg (see below); may be repeated after 5–15 minutes if required

**Note** Single doses of 300 mg have been associated with angina and with myocardial and cerebral infarction

**Eudemine®** (Goldshield) PoM ◢

Injection, diazoxide 15 mg/mL, net price 20-mL amp = £30.00

Tablets, see section 6.1.4

---

### ▌ HYDRALAZINE HYDROCHLORIDE

**Indications** moderate to severe hypertension (adjunct); heart failure (with long-acting nitrate, but see section 2.5.5); hypertensive crisis (including during pregnancy) (but see section 2.5)

**Cautions** hepatic impairment (Appendix 2); renal impairment (Appendix 3); coronary artery disease (may provoke angina, avoid after myocardial infarction until stabilised), cerebrovascular disease; occasionally blood pressure reduction too rapid even with low parenteral doses; pregnancy (Appendix 4); breast-feeding (Appendix 5); manufacturer advises test for antinuclear factor and for proteinuria every 6 months and check acetylator status before increasing dose above 100 mg daily, but evidence of clinical value unsatisfactory; **interactions**: Appendix 1 (hydralazine)

**Contra-indications** idiopathic systemic lupus erythematosus, severe tachycardia, high output heart failure, myocardial insufficiency due to mechanical obstruction, cor pulmonale, dissecting aortic aneurysm; acute porphyria (section 9.8.2)

**Side-effects** tachycardia, palpitation, flushing, hypotension, fluid retention, gastro-intestinal disturbances; headache, dizziness; systemic lupus erythematosus-like syndrome after long-term therapy with over 100 mg daily (or less in women and in slow acetylator individuals) (see also notes above); rarely rashes, fever, peripheral neuritis, polyneuritis, paraesthesia, arthralgia, myalgia, increased lacrimation, nasal congestion, dyspnoea, agitation, anxiety, anorexia; blood disorders (including leucopenia, thrombocytopenia, haemolytic anaemia), abnormal liver function, jaundice, raised plasma creatinine, proteinuria and haematuria reported

**Dose**

- By mouth, hypertension, 25 mg twice daily, increased to usual max. 50 mg twice daily (see notes above)

  Heart failure (initiated in hospital) 25 mg 3–4 times daily, increased every 2 days if necessary; usual maintenance dose 50–75 mg 4 times daily

- By slow intravenous injection, hypertension with renal complications and hypertensive crisis, 5–10 mg diluted with 10 mL sodium chloride 0.9%; may be repeated after 20–30 minutes (see Cautions)
- By intravenous infusion, hypertension with renal complications and hypertensive crisis, initially 200–300 micrograms/minute; maintenance usually 50–150 micrograms/minute

**Hydralazine** (Non-proprietary) PoM

Tablets, hydralazine hydrochloride 25 mg, net price 56 = £12.40; 50 mg, 56 = £19.20

**Apresoline®** (Amdipharm) [PoM]
Tablets, yellow, s/c, hydralazine hydrochloride 25 mg,
net price 84-tab pack = £3.38
Excipients include gluten

Injection, powder for reconstitution, hydralazine
hydrochloride, net price 20-mg amp = £2.19

## ILOPROST

**Indications** idiopathic or familial pulmonary arterial
hypertension

**Cautions** unstable pulmonary hypertension with
advanced right heart failure; hypotension (do not
initiate if systolic blood pressure below 85 mmHg);
acute pulmonary infection; chronic obstructive
pulmonary disease; severe asthma; hepatic impairment (Appendix 2); **interactions:** Appendix 1 (iloprost)

**Contra-indications** unstable angina; within 6 months
of myocardial infarction; decompensated cardiac
failure (unless under close medical supervision);
severe arrhythmias; congenital or acquired heart-
valve defects; within 3 months of cerebrovascular
events; pulmonary veno-occlusive disease; conditions
which increase risk of bleeding; pregnancy (Appendix
4); breast-feeding (Appendix 5)

**Side-effects** vasodilatation, hypotension, syncope,
cough, headache, throat or jaw pain; nausea, vomiting, diarrhoea, chest pain, dyspnoea, bronchospasm,
and wheezing also reported

**Dose**

• By inhalation of nebulised solution, initial dose
2.5 micrograms increased to 5 micrograms for second dose, if tolerated maintain at 5 micrograms 6–9
times daily according to response; reduce to
2.5 micrograms 6–9 times daily if higher dose not
tolerated; CHILD 8–18 years see *BNF for Children*

**Ventavis®** (Schering Health) ▼ [PoM]
Nebuliser solution, iloprost (as trometamol)
10 micrograms/mL, net price 30 × 1-mL (10 microgram) unit-dose vials = £407.94, 168 × 1-mL =
£2284.49. For use with *Prodose®* [NHS] or *Venta-Neb®*
[NHS] nebuliser

## MINOXIDIL

**Indications** severe hypertension, in addition to a
diuretic and a beta-blocker

**Cautions** see notes above; angina; after myocardial
infarction (until stabilised); lower doses in dialysis
patients; acute porphyria (section 9.8.2); renal
impairment (Appendix 3); pregnancy (Appendix 4);
**interactions:** Appendix 1 (vasodilator antihypertensives)

**Contra-indications** phaeochromocytoma

**Side-effects** sodium and water retention; weight gain,
peripheral oedema, tachycardia, hypertrichosis;
reversible rise in creatinine and blood urea nitrogen;
occasionally, gastro-intestinal disturbances, breast
tenderness, rashes

**Dose**

• Initially 5 mg (ELDERLY, 2.5 mg) daily, in 1–2 divided
doses, increased in steps of 5–10 mg at intervals of at
least 3 days; max. 100 mg daily (seldom necessary to
exceed 50 mg daily)

**Loniten®** (Pharmacia) [PoM]
Tablets, scored, minoxidil 2.5 mg, net price 60-tab
pack = £8.88; 5 mg, 60-tab pack = £15.83; 10 mg, 60-
tab pack = £30.68

## SILDENAFIL

**Indications** pulmonary arterial hypertension; erectile
dysfunction (section 7.4.5)

**Cautions** hypotension (avoid if systolic blood pressure
below 90 mmHg); intravascular volume depletion; left
ventricular outflow obstruction; cardiovascular disease; autonomic dysfunction; pulmonary veno-
occlusive disease; anatomical deformation of the
penis, predisposition to priapism; bleeding disorders
or active peptic ulceration; consider gradual withdrawal; hepatic impairment (avoid if severe; Appendix
2); renal impairment (Appendix 3); pregnancy
(Appendix 4); breast-feeding (Appendix 5); **interactions:** Appendix 1 (sildenafil)

**Contra-indications** recent history of stroke or myocardial infarction, history of non-arteritic anterior
ischaemic optic neuropathy; hereditary degenerative
retinal disorders; avoid concomitant use of nitrates

**Side-effects** gastro-intestinal disturbances, dry
mouth; flushing, oedema; bronchitis, cough; headache, migraine, night sweats, paraesthesia, insomnia,
anxiety, tremor, vertigo; fever, influenza-like symptoms; anaemia; back and limb pain, myalgia; visual
disturbances, retinal haemorrhage, photophobia,
painful red eyes; nasal congestion, epistaxis; cellulitis,
alopecia; *less commonly* gynaecomastia, priapism; *also
reported* rash, retinal vascular occlusion and non-
arteritic anterior ischaemic optic neuropathy (discontinue if sudden visual impairment), and sudden
hearing loss (advise patient to seek medical help)

**Dose**

• 20 mg 3 times daily; CHILD under 18 years see *BNF for
Children*

**Revatio®** (Pfizer) ▼ [PoM]
Tablets, f/c, sildenafil (as citrate), 20 mg, net price 90-
tab pack = £373.50

**Viagra®** (Pfizer) [PoM] [NHS]
Section 7.4.5 (erectile dysfunction)

## SITAXENTAN SODIUM

**Indications** pulmonary arterial hypertension

**Cautions** test liver function before treatment and
monitor monthly during treatment (discontinue
treatment if liver enzymes significantly raised); measure haemoglobin concentration before treatment,
after 1–3 months, then every 3 months; pregnancy
(Appendix 4); **interactions:** Appendix 1 (sitaxentan)

**Contra-indications** hepatic impairment; breast-feeding (Appendix 5)

**Side-effects** gastro-intestinal disturbances; peripheral
oedema, flushing; headache, insomnia, fatigue, dizziness; decreased haemoglobin, prolonged prothrombin
time, increased INR; muscle cramp; nasal congestion,
epistaxis

**Dose**

• ADULT over 18 years 100 mg once daily

**Cardiovascular system** *(vertical sidebar)*

**2** *(vertical sidebar marker)*

**Thelin®** (Encysive) ▼ [PoM]

Tablets, f/c, yellow-orange, sitaxentan sodium 100 mg, net price 28-tab pack = £1540.00

**Note** All orders of Thelin should be based on a prescription from a specialist in Pulmonary Arterial Hypertension, who has received appropriate training as part of the Programmed Access to Sitaxentan Sodium (PASS) scheme. Orders should be placed with Polarspeed at 01525 217211

---

## ◼ SODIUM NITROPRUSSIDE

**Indications** hypertensive crisis (but see section 2.5); controlled hypotension in anaesthesia; acute or chronic heart failure

**Cautions** hypothyroidism, hyponatraemia, ischaemic heart disease, impaired cerebral circulation, elderly; hypothermia; monitor blood pressure and blood-cyanide concentration and if treatment exceeds 3 days, also blood-thiocyanate concentration; avoid sudden withdrawal—terminate infusion over 15–30 minutes; hepatic impairment (Appendix 2); renal impairment (Appendix 3); pregnancy (Appendix 4); breast-feeding (Appendix 5); **interactions:** Appendix 1 (sodium nitroprusside)

**Contra-indications** severe vitamin $B_{12}$ deficiency; Leber's optic atrophy; compensatory hypertension

**Side-effects** associated with over rapid reduction in blood pressure (reduce infusion rate): headache, dizziness, nausea, retching, abdominal pain, perspiration, palpitation, anxiety, retrosternal discomfort; occasionally reduced platelet count, acute transient phlebitis

**Cyanide** Side-effects caused by excessive plasma concentration of the cyanide metabolite include tachycardia, sweating, hyperventilation, arrhythmias, marked metabolic acidosis (discontinue and give antidote, see p. 34)

**Dose**

- Hypertensive crisis, by intravenous infusion, initially 0.5–1.5 micrograms/kg/minute, then increased in steps of 500 nanograms/kg/minute every 5 minutes within range 0.5–8 micrograms/kg/minute (lower doses if already receiving other antihypertensives); stop if response unsatisfactory with max. dose in 10 minutes

  **Note** Lower initial dose of 300 nanograms/kg/minute has been used

- Maintenance of blood pressure at 30–40% lower than pretreatment diastolic blood pressure, 20–400 micrograms/minute (lower doses for patients being treated with other antihypertensives)

- Controlled hypotension in surgery, by intravenous infusion, max. 1.5 micrograms/kg/minute

- Heart failure, by intravenous infusion, initially 10–15 micrograms/minute, increased every 5–10 minutes as necessary; usual range 10–200 micrograms/minute normally for max. 3 days

**Sodium Nitroprusside** (Non-proprietary) [PoM]

Intravenous infusion, powder for reconstitution, sodium nitroprusside 10 mg/mL

Available from 'special-order' manufacturers or specialist importing companies, see p. 969

---

## 2.5.2 Centrally acting antihypertensive drugs

**Methyldopa** is a centrally acting antihypertensive; it may be used for the management of hypertension in pregnancy. Side-effects are minimised if the daily dose is kept below 1 g.

**Clonidine** has the disadvantage that sudden withdrawal may cause a hypertensive crisis.

**Moxonidine**, a centrally acting drug, is licensed for mild to moderate essential hypertension. It may have a role when thiazides, calcium-channel blockers, ACE inhibitors, and beta-blockers are not appropriate or have failed to control blood pressure.

---

## ◼ CLONIDINE HYDROCHLORIDE

**Indications** hypertension; migraine (section 4.7.4.2); menopausal flushing (section 6.4.1.1)

**Cautions** must be withdrawn gradually to avoid hypertensive crisis; Raynaud's syndrome or other occlusive peripheral vascular disease; history of depression; avoid in acute porphyria (section 9.8.2); pregnancy (Appendix 4); breast-feeding (Appendix 5); **interactions:** Appendix 1 (clonidine)

**Driving** Drowsiness may affect performance of skilled tasks (e.g. driving); effects of alcohol may be enhanced

**Side-effects** dry mouth, sedation, depression, fluid retention, bradycardia, Raynaud's phenomenon, headache, dizziness, euphoria, nocturnal unrest, rash, nausea, constipation, rarely impotence

**Dose**

- By mouth, 50–100 micrograms 3 times daily, increased every second or third day; usual max. dose 1.2 mg daily

- By slow intravenous injection, 150–300 micrograms; max. 750 micrograms in 24 hours

**Catapres®** (Boehringer Ingelheim) [PoM] ▱

Tablets, scored, clonidine hydrochloride 100 micrograms, net price 100-tab pack = £5.32; 300 micrograms, 100-tab pack = £12.39. Label: 3, 8

Injection, clonidine hydrochloride 150 micrograms/mL, net price 1-mL amp = 28p

**Dixarit®** [PoM] ▱

Section 4.7.4.2

---

## ◼ METHYLDOPA

**Indications** hypertension

**Cautions** monitor blood counts and liver-function before treatment and at intervals during first 6–12 weeks or if unexplained fever occurs; history of depression; positive direct Coombs' test in up to 20% of patients (may affect blood cross-matching); interference with laboratory tests; hepatic impairment (avoid in active liver disease; Appendix 2); renal impairment (Appendix 3); **interactions:** Appendix 1 (methyldopa)

**Driving** Drowsiness may affect performance of skilled tasks (e.g. driving); effects of alcohol may be enhanced

**Contra-indications** depression, active liver disease, phaeochromocytoma; acute porphyria (section 9.8.2)

**Side-effects** gastro-intestinal disturbances, dry mouth, stomatitis, sialadenitis; bradycardia, exacerbation of angina, postural hypotension, oedema; sedation, headache, dizziness, asthenia, myalgia, arthralgia, paraesthesia, nightmares, mild psychosis, depression, impaired mental acuity, parkinsonism, Bell's palsy; hepatitis, jaundice; pancreatitis; haemolytic anaemia; bone-marrow depression, leucopenia, thrombocytopenia, eosinophilia; hypersensitivity reactions including lupus erythematosus-like syndrome, drug fever, myocarditis, pericarditis; rashes (including toxic epidermal necrolysis); nasal congestion, failure of ejaculation, impotence, decreased libido, gynaecomastia, hyperprolactinaemia, amenorrhoea

**Dose**

- Initially 250 mg 2–3 times daily, increased gradually at intervals of at least 2 days, max. 3 g daily; ELDERLY initially 125 mg twice daily, increased gradually, max. 2 g daily

**Methyldopa** (Non-proprietary) PoM

Tablets, coated, methyldopa (anhydrous) 125 mg, net price 56-tab pack = £14.32; 250 mg, 56-tab pack = £6.80; 500 mg, 56-tab pack = £10.17. Label: 3, 8

**Aldomet**® (MSD) PoM

Tablets, all yellow, f/c, methyldopa (anhydrous) 250 mg, net price 60 = £1.88; 500 mg, 30 = £1.90. Label: 3, 8

### MOXONIDINE

**Indications** mild to moderate essential hypertension

**Cautions** avoid abrupt withdrawal (if concomitant treatment with beta-blocker has to be stopped, discontinue beta-blocker first, then moxonidine after a few days); susceptibility to angle-closure glaucoma; renal impairment (avoid if eGFR less than 30 mL/minute/1.73 m²; Appendix 3); **interactions:** see Appendix 1 (moxonidine)

**Contra-indications** history of angioedema; conduction disorders (sick sinus syndrome, sino-atrial block, second- or third-degree AV block); bradycardia; life-threatening arrhythmia; severe heart failure; severe coronary artery disease, unstable angina; severe liver disease; also on theoretical grounds: Raynaud's syndrome, intermittent claudication, epilepsy, depression, Parkinson's disease; pregnancy (Appendix 4); breast-feeding (Appendix 5)

**Side-effects** dry mouth; headache, fatigue, dizziness, nausea, sleep disturbance (rarely sedation), asthenia, vasodilatation; *rarely* skin reactions; *very rarely* angle-closure glaucoma

**Dose**

- 200 micrograms once daily in the morning, increased if necessary after 3 weeks to 400 micrograms daily in 1–2 divided doses; max. 600 micrograms daily in 2 divided doses (max. single dose 400 micrograms)

**Moxonidine** (Non-proprietary) PoM

Tablets, f/c, moxonidine 200 micrograms, net price 28-tab pack = £5.12; 300 micrograms, net price 28-tab pack = £8.10; 400 micrograms, net price 28-tab pack = £5.89. Label: 3

**Physiotens**® (Solvay) PoM

Tablets, f/c, moxonidine 200 micrograms (pink), net price 28-tab pack = £9.72; 300 micrograms (red), 28-tab pack = £11.49; 400 micrograms (red), 28-tab pack = £13.26. Label: 3

### 2.5.3 Adrenergic neurone blocking drugs

Adrenergic neurone blocking drugs prevent the release of noradrenaline from postganglionic adrenergic neu-

rones. These drugs do not control supine blood pressure and may cause postural hypotension. For this reason they have largely fallen from use, but may be necessary with other therapy in resistant hypertension.

**Guanethidine**, which also depletes the nerve endings of noradrenaline, is licensed for rapid control of blood pressure.

### GUANETHIDINE MONOSULPHATE

**Indications** hypertensive crisis (but see section 2.5)

**Cautions** coronary or cerebral arteriosclerosis, asthma, history of peptic ulceration; renal impairment (avoid if eGFR less than 40 mL/minute/1.73 m²; Appendix 3); pregnancy (Appendix 4); **interactions:** Appendix 1 (adrenergic neurone blockers)

**Contra-indications** phaeochromocytoma, heart failure

**Side-effects** postural hypotension, failure of ejaculation, fluid retention, nasal congestion, headache, diarrhoea, drowsiness

**Dose**

- By intramuscular injection, 10–20 mg, repeated after 3 hours if required

**Ismelin**® (Amdipharm) PoM 

Injection, guanethidine monosulphate 10 mg/mL, net price 1-mL amp = £1.56

### 2.5.4 Alpha-adrenoceptor blocking drugs

**Prazosin** has post-synaptic alpha-blocking and vasodilator properties and rarely causes tachycardia. It may, however, reduce blood pressure rapidly after the first dose and should be introduced with caution. **Doxazosin**, **indoramin**, and **terazosin** have properties similar to those of prazosin.

Alpha-blockers can be used with other antihypertensive drugs in the treatment of resistant hypertension (section 2.5).

**Prostatic hyperplasia** Alfuzosin, doxazosin, indoramin, prazosin, tamsulosin, and terazosin are indicated for benign prostatic hyperplasia (section 7.4.1).

### DOXAZOSIN

**Indications** hypertension (see notes above); benign prostatic hyperplasia (section 7.4.1)

**Cautions** care with initial dose (postural hypotension); cataract surgery (risk of intra-operative floppy iris syndrome); susceptibility to heart failure; hepatic impairment (Appendix 2); pregnancy (Appendix 4); breast-feeding (Appendix 5); **interactions:** Appendix 1 (alpha-blockers)

**Driving** May affect performance of skilled tasks e.g. driving

**Side-effects** gastro-intestinal disturbances; oedema, hypotension, postural hypotension; dyspnoea, rhinitis, coughing; asthenia, fatigue, vertigo, dizziness, headache, paraesthesia, sleep disturbance, anxiety, depression; respiratory-tract infection, urinary-tract infection, influenza-like symptoms; back pain, myalgia; *less commonly* weight changes, flushing, syncope, tremor, agitation, micturition disturbance, impotence,

**2**

**Cardiovascular system**

epistaxis, arthralgia, tinnitus, hypersensitivity reactions (including pruritus, purpura, rash), alopecia; *very rarely* cholestasis, hepatitis, jaundice, bronchospasm, gynaecomastia, priapism, abnormal ejaculation, leucopenia, thrombocytopenia, blurred vision

**Dose**

- Hypertension, 1 mg daily, increased after 1–2 weeks to 2 mg once daily, and thereafter to 4 mg once daily, if necessary; max. 16 mg daily

**Doxazosin** (Non-proprietary) (PoM)

Tablets, doxazosin (as mesilate) 1 mg, net price 28-tab pack = 93p; 2 mg, 28-tab pack = £1.00; 4 mg, 28-tab pack = £1.48. Counselling, initial dose, driving
Brands include *Doxadura*®

**Cardura**® (Pfizer) (PoM)

Tablets, doxazosin (as mesilate) 1 mg, net price 28-tab pack = £10.56; 2 mg, 28-tab pack = £14.08. Counselling, initial dose, driving

◢Modified-release

**Doxazosin** (Non-proprietary) (PoM)

Tablets, m/r, doxazosin (as mesilate) 4 mg, net price 28-tab pack = £6.33. Label: 25, counselling, initial dose, driving
Dose hypertension, benign prostatic hyperplasia, 4 mg once daily, increased to 8 mg once daily after 4 weeks if necessary
Brands include *Doxadura*® XL, *Slocinx*® XL

**Cardura**® **XL** (Pfizer) (PoM)

Tablets, m/r, doxazosin (as mesilate) 4 mg, net price 28-tab pack = £5.70; 8 mg, 28-tab pack = £9.98. Label: 25, counselling, driving, initial dose
Dose hypertension, benign prostatic hyperplasia, 4 mg once daily, increased to 8 mg once daily after 4 weeks if necessary

## INDORAMIN

**Indications** hypertension (see notes above); benign prostatic hyperplasia (section 7.4.1)

**Cautions** avoid alcohol (enhances rate and extent of absorption); control incipient heart failure before initiating indoramin; elderly; Parkinson's disease; epilepsy (convulsions in *animal* studies); history of depression; cataract surgery (risk of floppy iris syndrome); hepatic impairment; renal impairment; **interactions:** Appendix 1 (alpha-blockers)
Driving Drowsiness may affect performance of skilled tasks (e.g. driving); effects of alcohol may be enhanced

**Contra-indications** established heart failure

**Side-effects** see section 7.4.1; drowsiness, sedation; *less commonly* dry mouth, hypotension, syncope, nasal congestion, dizziness, depression, fatigue, headache, weight gain, failure of ejaculation; *rarely* hypersensitivity reactions (including rash and puritus); diarrhoea, nausea, palpitation, urinary frequency and incontinence, and priapism also reported

**Dose**

- Hypertension, initially 25 mg twice daily, increased by 25–50 mg daily at intervals of 2 weeks; max. daily dose 200 mg in 2–3 divided doses

**Baratol**® (Amdipharm) (PoM)

Tablets, blue, f/c, indoramin (as hydrochloride) 25 mg, net price 84-tab pack = £9.00. Label: 2

**Doralese**® (PoM)

Section 7.4.1 (prostatic hyperplasia)

## PRAZOSIN

**Indications** hypertension (see notes above); congestive heart failure (but see section 2.5.5); Raynaud's syndrome (see also section 2.6.4); benign prostatic hyperplasia (section 7.4.1)

**Cautions** first dose may cause collapse due to hypotension (therefore should be taken on retiring to bed); elderly; cataract surgery (risk of intraoperative floppy iris syndrome); hepatic impairment (Appendix 2); renal impairment (Appendix 3); pregnancy (Appendix 4); breast-feeding (Appendix 5); **interactions:** Appendix 1 (alpha-blockers)
Driving May affect performance of skilled tasks e.g. driving

**Contra-indications** not recommended for congestive heart failure due to mechanical obstruction (e.g. aortic stenosis)

**Side-effects** see section 7.4.1; also gastro-intestinal disturbances; postural hypotension, oedema, palpitation; dyspnoea, nasal congestion; drowsiness, headache, depression, nervousness, vertigo; urinary frequency; weakness; blurred vision; *less commonly* tachycardia, insomnia, paraesthesia, sweating, impotence, arthralgia, eye disorders, tinnitus, epistaxis, allergic reactions including rash, pruritus, and urticaria; *rarely* pancreatitis, flushing, vasculitis, bradycardia, hallucinations, worsening of narcolepsy, gynaecomastia, priapism, urinary incontinence, and alopecia

**Dose**

- Hypertension (see notes above), 500 micrograms 2–3 times daily for 3–7 days, the initial dose on retiring to bed at night (to avoid collapse, see Cautions); increased to 1 mg 2–3 times daily for a further 3–7 days; further increased if necessary to max. 20 mg daily in divided doses

- Congestive heart failure (but see section 2.5.5), 500 micrograms 2–4 times daily (initial dose at bedtime, see above), increasing to 4 mg daily in divided doses; maintenance 4–20 mg daily in divided doses (but rarely used)

- Raynaud's syndrome (but efficacy not established, see section 2.6.4), initially 500 micrograms twice daily (initial dose at bedtime, see above) increased, if necessary, after 3–7 days to usual maintenance 1–2 mg twice daily

**Prazosin** (Non-proprietary) (PoM)

Tablets, prazosin (as hydrochloride) 500 micrograms, net price 56-tab pack = £2.51; 1 mg, 56-tab pack = £3.23; 2 mg, 56-tab pack = £4.39; 5 mg, 56-tab pack = £8.75. Counselling, initial dose, driving

**Hypovase**® (Pfizer) (PoM)

Tablets, prazosin (as hydrochloride) 500 micrograms, net price 60-tab pack = £2.69; 1 mg, scored, 60-tab pack = £3.46. Counselling, initial dose, driving

## TERAZOSIN

**Indications** mild to moderate hypertension (see notes above); benign prostatic hyperplasia (section 7.4.1)

**Cautions** first dose may cause collapse due to hypotension (within 30–90 minutes, therefore should be taken on retiring to bed) (may also occur with rapid dose increase); pregnancy (Appendix 4); **interactions:** Appendix 1 (alpha-blockers)
Driving May affect performance of skilled tasks e.g. driving

**Side-effects** see section 7.4.1; also drowsiness, dizziness, lack of energy, peripheral oedema; urinary frequency and priapism reported

**Dose**

- Hypertension, 1 mg at bedtime (compliance with bedtime dose important, see Cautions); dose doubled after 7 days if necessary; usual maintenance dose 2–10 mg once daily; more than 20 mg daily rarely improves efficacy

**Terazosin** (Non-proprietary) [PoM]

Tablets, terazosin (as hydrochloride) 2 mg, net price 28-tab pack = £2.34; 5 mg, 28-tab pack = £2.78; 10 mg, 28-tab pack = £7.06. Counselling, initial dose, driving

**Hytrin®** (Amdipharm) [PoM]

Tablets, terazosin (as hydrochloride) 2 mg (yellow), net price 28-tab pack = £2.29; 5 mg (tan), 28-tab pack = £4.29; 10 mg (blue), 28-tab pack = £8.57; starter pack (for hypertension) of 7 × 1-mg tabs with 21 × 2-mg tabs = £13.00. Counselling, initial dose, driving

## Phaeochromocytoma

Long-term management of phaeochromocytoma involves surgery. Alpha-blockers are used in the short-term management of hypertensive episodes in phaeochromocytoma. Once alpha blockade is established, tachycardia can be controlled by the cautious addition of a beta-blocker (section 2.4); a cardioselective beta-blocker is preferred.

**Phenoxybenzamine**, a powerful alpha-blocker, is effective in the management of phaeochromocytoma but it has many side-effects. **Phentolamine** is a short-acting alpha-blocker used mainly during surgery of phaeochromocytoma; its use for the diagnosis of phaeochromocytoma has been superseded by measurement of catecholamines in blood and urine.

**Metirosine** (available from 'special-order' manufacturers or specialist importing companies, see p. 969) inhibits the enzyme tyrosine hydroxylase, and hence the synthesis of catecholamines. It is rarely used in the pre-operative management of phaeochromocytoma, and long term in patients unsuitable for surgery; an alpha-adrenoceptor blocking drug may also be required. Metirosine should **not** be used to treat essential hypertension.

## ▊ PHENOXYBENZAMINE HYDROCHLORIDE

**Indications** hypertensive episodes in phaeochromocytoma

**Cautions** elderly; congestive heart failure; severe heart disease (see also Contra-indications); cerebrovascular disease (avoid if history of cerebrovascular accident); renal impairment; carcinogenic in *animals*; avoid in acute porphyria (section 9.8.2); avoid infusion in hypovolaemia; avoid extravasation (irritant to tissues); pregnancy (Appendix 4); breast-feeding (Appendix 5)

**Contra-indications** history of cerebrovascular accident; during recovery period after myocardial infarction (usually 3–4 weeks)

**Side-effects** postural hypotension with dizziness and marked compensatory tachycardia, lassitude, nasal congestion, miosis, inhibition of ejaculation; rarely gastro-intestinal disturbances; decreased sweating

and dry mouth after intravenous infusion; idiosyncratic profound hypotension within few minutes of starting infusion

**Dose**

- See under preparations

**Phenoxybenzamine** (Goldshield) [PoM]

Injection concentrate, phenoxybenzamine hydrochloride 50 mg/mL. To be diluted before use, net price 2-mL amp = £57.14 (hosp. only)

Dose by *intravenous infusion* (preferably through large vein), adjunct in severe shock (but rarely used) and phaeochromocytoma, 1 mg/kg daily over at least 2 hours; do not repeat within 24 hours (intensive care facilities needed)

Caution Owing to risk of contact sensitisation healthcare professionals should avoid contamination of hands

**Dibenyline®** (Goldshield) [PoM]

Capsules, red/white, phenoxybenzamine hydrochloride 10 mg, net price 30-cap pack = £10.84

Dose phaeochromocytoma, 10 mg daily, increased by 10 mg daily; usual dose 1–2 mg/kg daily in 2 divided doses

Note May be difficult to obtain

## ▊ PHENTOLAMINE MESILATE

**Indications** hypertensive episodes due to phaeochromocytoma e.g. during surgery; diagnosis of phaeochromocytoma

**Cautions** monitor blood pressure (avoid in hypotension), heart rate; renal impairment; gastritis, peptic ulcer; elderly; pregnancy (Appendix 4) and breast-feeding (Appendix 5); **interactions:** Appendix 1 (alpha-blockers)

**Contra-indications** hypotension; history of myocardial infarction; coronary insufficiency, angina, or other evidence of coronary artery disease

**Side-effects** postural hypotension, tachycardia, dizziness, flushing; nausea and vomiting, diarrhoea, nasal congestion; also acute or prolonged hypotension, angina, chest pain, arrhythmias

**Dose**

- Hypertensive episodes, by intravenous injection, 2–5 mg repeated if necessary
- Diagnosis of phaeochromocytoma, consult product literature

**Rogitine®** (Alliance) [PoM]

Injection, phentolamine mesilate 10 mg/mL, net price 1-mL amp = £1.53

Excipients include sulphites

## 2.5.5 Drugs affecting the renin-angiotensin system

2.5.5.1  Angiotensin-converting enzyme inhibitors

2.5.5.2  Angiotensin-II receptor antagonists

2.5.5.3  Renin inhibitors

## Heart failure

Drug treatment of heart failure due to left ventricular systolic dysfunction is covered below; optimal management of heart failure with preserved left ventricular function is not established.

**2** Cardiovascular system

The treatment of chronic heart failure aims to relieve symptoms, improve exercise tolerance, reduce the incidence of acute exacerbations, and reduce mortality. An **ACE inhibitor**, titrated to a 'target dose' (or the maximum tolerated dose if lower), and a **beta-blocker** is recommended to achieve these aims. A **diuretic** is also necessary in most patients to reduce symptoms of fluid overload.

An ACE inhibitor (section 2.5.5.1) is generally advised for patients with asymptomatic left ventricular dysfunction or symptomatic heart failure. An **angiotensin-II receptor antagonist** (section 2.5.5.2) may be a useful alternative for patients who, because of side-effects such as cough, cannot tolerate ACE inhibitors; a relatively high dose of the angiotensin-II receptor antagonist may be required to produce benefit.

The beta-blockers bisoprolol and carvedilol (section 2.4) are of value in any grade of stable heart failure and left-ventricular systolic dysfunction; nebivolol (section 2.4) is licensed for stable mild to moderate heart failure in patients over 70 years. Beta-blocker treatment should be started by those experienced in the management of heart failure, at a very low dose and titrated very slowly over a period of weeks or months. Symptoms may deteriorate initially, calling for adjustment of concomitant therapy.

Patients with fluid overload should also receive either a loop or a thiazide diuretic (with salt or fluid restriction where appropriate). A **thiazide diuretic** (section 2.2.1) may be of benefit in patients with mild heart failure and good renal function; however, thiazide diuretics are ineffective in patients with poor renal function (eGFR less than 30 mL/minute/1.73 m², see Appendix 3) and a **loop diuretic** (section 2.2.2) is preferred. If diuresis with a single diuretic is insufficient, a combination of a loop diuretic and a thiazide diuretic may be tried; addition of metolazone (section 2.2.1) may also be considered but the resulting diuresis may be profound and care is needed to avoid potentially dangerous electrolyte disturbances.

The aldosterone antagonist **spironolactone** (section 2.2.3) can be considered for patients with moderate to severe heart failure who are already taking an ACE inhibitor and a beta-blocker; low doses of spironolactone (usually 25 mg daily) reduce symptoms and mortality in these patients. If spironolactone cannot be used, eplerenone (section 2.2.3) may be considered for the management of heart failure after an acute myocardial infarction with evidence of left ventricular dysfunction. Close monitoring of serum creatinine and potassium is necessary with any change in treatment or in the patient's condition.

**Digoxin** (section 2.1.1) improves symptoms of heart failure and exercise tolerance and reduces hospitalisation due to acute exacerbations but it does not reduce mortality. Digoxin is reserved for patients with atrial fibrillation and also for selected patients in sinus rhythm who remain symptomatic despite treatment with an ACE inhibitor, a beta-blocker, and a diuretic.

Patients who cannot tolerate an ACE inhibitor or an angiotensin-II receptor antagonist, or in whom they are contra-indicated, may be given **isosorbide dinitrate** (section 2.6.1) with **hydralazine** (section 2.5.1), but this combination may be poorly tolerated. In African-American patients, the combination of isosorbide dinitrate and hydralazine may be considered in addition to standard therapy if necessary.

## 2.5.5.1 Angiotensin-converting enzyme inhibitors

Angiotensin-converting enzyme inhibitors (ACE inhibitors) inhibit the conversion of angiotensin I to angiotensin II. They have many uses and are generally well tolerated. The main indications of ACE inhibitors are shown below.

**Heart failure** ACE inhibitors are used in all grades of heart failure, usually combined with a beta-blocker (section 2.5.5). Potassium supplements and potassium-sparing diuretics should be discontinued before introducing an ACE inhibitor because of the risk of hyperkalaemia. However, a low dose of spironolactone may be beneficial in severe heart failure (section 2.5.5) and can be used with an ACE inhibitor provided serum potassium is monitored carefully. Profound first-dose hypotension may occur when ACE inhibitors are introduced to patients with heart failure who are already taking a high dose of a loop diuretic (e.g. furosemide 80 mg daily or more). Temporary withdrawal of the loop diuretic reduces the risk, but may cause severe rebound pulmonary oedema. Therefore, for patients on high doses of loop diuretics, the ACE inhibitor may need to be initiated under specialist supervision, see below. An ACE inhibitor can be initiated in the community in patients who are receiving a low dose of a diuretic or who are not otherwise at risk of serious hypotension; nevertheless, care is required and a very low dose of the ACE inhibitor is given initially.

**Hypertension** An ACE inhibitor may be the most appropriate initial drug for hypertension in younger Caucasian patients; Afro-Caribbean patients, those aged over 55 years, and those with primary aldosteronism respond less well (see section 2.5). ACE inhibitors are particularly indicated for hypertension in patients with type 1 diabetes with nephropathy (see also section 6.1.5). They may reduce blood pressure very rapidly in some patients particularly in those receiving diuretic therapy (see Cautions, below); the first dose should preferably be given at bedtime.

**Diabetic nephropathy** For comment on the role of ACE inhibitors in the management of diabetic nephropathy, see section 6.1.5.

**Prophylaxis of cardiovascular events** ACE inhibitors are used in the early and long-term management of patients who have had a myocardial infarction, see section 2.10.1. ACE inhibitors may also have a role in preventing cardiovascular events.

**Initiation under specialist supervision** ACE inhibitors should be initiated under specialist supervision and with careful clinical monitoring in those with severe heart failure or in those:

- receiving multiple or high-dose diuretic therapy (e.g. more than 80 mg of furosemide daily or its equivalent);
- with hypovolaemia;
- with hyponatraemia (plasma-sodium concentration below 130 mmol/litre);
- with hypotension (systolic blood pressure below 90 mmHg);
- with unstable heart failure;
- receiving high-dose vasodilator therapy;
- known renovascular disease.

**Renal effects** Renal function and electrolytes should be checked before starting ACE inhibitors (or increasing the dose) and monitored during treatment (more frequently if features mentioned below present); hyperkalaemia and other side-effects of ACE inhibitors are more common in those with impaired renal function and the dose may need to be reduced (Appendix 3). Although ACE inhibitors now have a specialised role in some forms of renal disease, including chronic kidney disease, they also occasionally cause impairment of renal function which may progress and become severe in other circumstances (at particular risk are the elderly). A specialist should be involved if renal function is significantly reduced as a result of treatment with an ACE inhibitor.

Concomitant treatment with NSAIDs increases the risk of renal damage, and potassium-sparing diuretics (or potassium-containing salt substitutes) increase the risk of hyperkalaemia.

In patients with severe bilateral renal artery stenosis (or severe stenosis of the artery supplying a single functioning kidney), ACE inhibitors reduce or abolish glomerular filtration and are likely to cause severe and progressive renal failure. They are therefore not recommended in patients known to have these forms of critical renovascular disease.

ACE inhibitor treatment is unlikely to have an adverse effect on overall renal function in patients with severe unilateral renal artery stenosis and a normal contralateral kidney, but glomerular filtration is likely to be reduced (or even abolished) in the affected kidney and the long-term consequences are unknown.

ACE inhibitors are therefore best avoided in patients with known or suspected renovascular disease, unless the blood pressure cannot be controlled by other drugs. If ACE inhibitors are used, they should be initiated only under specialist supervision and renal function should be monitored regularly.

ACE inhibitors should also be used with particular caution in patients who may have undiagnosed and clinically silent renovascular disease. This includes patients with peripheral vascular disease or those with severe generalised atherosclerosis.

**Cautions** ACE inhibitors need to be initiated with care in patients receiving diuretics (**important**: see Concomitant diuretics, below); first doses can cause hypotension especially in patients taking high doses of diuretics, on a low-sodium diet, on dialysis, dehydrated or with heart failure (see above). They should also be used with caution in peripheral vascular disease or generalised atherosclerosis owing to risk of clinically silent renovascular disease; for use in known renovascular disease, see Renal Effects above. The risk of agranulocytosis is possibly increased in collagen vascular disease (blood counts recommended). ACE inhibitors should be used with care in patients with severe or symptomatic aortic stenosis (risk of hypotension) and in hypertrophic cardiomyopathy. They should also be used with care (or avoided) in those with a history of idiopathic or hereditary angioedema. If jaundice or marked elevations of hepatic enzymes occur during treatment then the ACE inhibitor should be discontinued—risk of hepatic necrosis (see also Appendix 2; hepatic impairment). ACE inhibitors should be used with caution in breast-feeding (Appendix 5). **Interactions:** Appendix 1 (ACE inhibitors).

**Anaphylactoid reactions** To prevent anaphylactoid reactions, ACE inhibitors should be avoided during dialysis with high-flux polyacrylonitrile membranes and during low-density lipoprotein apheresis with dextran sulphate; they should also be withheld before desensitisation with wasp or bee venom.

**Concomitant diuretics** ACE inhibitors can cause a very rapid fall in blood pressure in volume-depleted patients; treatment should therefore be initiated with very low doses. If the dose of diuretic is greater than 80 mg furosemide or equivalent, the ACE inhibitor should be initiated under close supervision and in some patients the diuretic dose may need to be reduced or the diuretic discontinued at least 24 hours beforehand (may not be possible in heart failure—risk of pulmonary oedema). If high-dose diuretic therapy cannot be stopped, close observation is recommended after administration of the first dose of ACE inhibitor, for at least 2 hours or until the blood pressure has stabilised.

**Contra-indications** ACE inhibitors are contra-indicated in patients with hypersensitivity to ACE inhibitors (including angioedema). ACE inhibitors should not be used in pregnancy (Appendix 4).

**Side-effects** ACE inhibitors can cause profound hypotension (see Cautions) and renal impairment (see Renal effects above), and a persistent dry cough. They can also cause angioedema (onset may be delayed; higher incidence reported in Afro-Caribbean patients), rash (which may be associated with pruritus and urticaria), pancreatitis, and upper respiratory-tract symptoms such as sinusitis, rhinitis, and sore throat. Gastro-intestinal effects reported with ACE inhibitors include nausea, vomiting, dyspepsia, diarrhoea, constipation, and abdominal pain. Altered liver function tests, cholestatic jaundice, hepatitis, fulminant hepatic necrosis, and hepatic failure have been reported—discontinue if marked elevation of hepatic enzymes or jaundice. Hyperkalaemia, hypoglycaemia, and blood disorders including thrombocytopenia, leucopenia, neutropenia, and haemolytic anaemia have also been reported. Other reported side-effects include headache, dizziness, fatigue, malaise, taste disturbance, paraesthesia, bronchospasm, fever, serositis, vasculitis, myalgia, arthralgia, positive antinuclear antibody, raised erythrocyte sedimentation rate, eosinophilia, leucocytosis, and photosensitivity.

**Combination products** Products incorporating an ACE inhibitor with a thiazide diuretic or a calcium-channel blocker are available for the management of hypertension. Use of these combination products should be reserved for patients whose blood pressure has not responded adequately to a single antihypertensive drug and who have been stabilised on the individual components of the combination in the same proportions.

---

### ▌ CAPTOPRIL

**Indications** mild to moderate essential hypertension alone or with thiazide therapy and severe hypertension resistant to other treatment; congestive heart failure with left ventricular dysfunction (adjunct—see section 2.5.5); following myocardial infarction, see dose; diabetic nephropathy (microalbuminuria greater than 30 mg/day) in type 1 diabetes

**Cautions** see notes above

**Contra-indications** see notes above

**Side-effects** see notes above; tachycardia, serum sickness, weight loss, stomatitis, maculopapular rash, photosensitivity, flushing and acidosis

**Dose**

- Hypertension, used alone, initially 12.5 mg twice daily; if used in addition to diuretic (see notes above), or in elderly, initially 6.25 mg twice daily (first dose at bedtime); usual maintenance dose 25 mg twice daily; max. 50 mg twice daily (rarely 3 times daily in severe hypertension)

- Heart failure (adjunct), initially 6.25–12.5 mg 2–3 times daily under close medical supervision (see notes above), increased gradually at intervals of at least 2 weeks up to max. 150 mg daily in divided doses if tolerated

- Prophylaxis after infarction in clinically stable patients with asymptomatic or symptomatic left ventricular dysfunction (radionuclide ventriculography or echo-cardiography undertaken before initiation), initially 6.25 mg, starting as early as 3 days after infarction, then increased over several weeks to 150 mg daily (if tolerated) in divided doses

- Diabetic nephropathy, 75–100 mg daily in divided doses; if further blood pressure reduction required, other antihypertensives may be used in conjunction with captopril; in severe renal impairment, initially 12.5 mg twice daily (if concomitant diuretic therapy required, loop diuretic rather than thiazide should be chosen)

**Captopril** (Non-proprietary) ▣ᴾᵒᴹ
Tablets, captopril 12.5 mg, net price 56-tab pack = £1.53; 25 mg, 56-tab pack = £1.73; 50 mg, 56-tab pack = £2.48
Brands include *Ecopace®*, *Kaplon®*, *Tensopril®*

**Capoten®** (Squibb) ᴾᵒᴹ
Tablets, captopril 12.5 mg (scored), net price 56-tab pack = £9.44; 25 mg, 56-tab pack = £10.75; 50 mg (scored), 56-tab pack = £18.33 (also available as *Acepril®*)

◀**With diuretic**
**Note** For mild to moderate hypertension in patients stabilised on the individual components in the same proportions. For cautions, contra-indications, and side-effects of thiazides, see section 2.2.1

**Co-zidocapt** (Non-proprietary) ᴾᵒᴹ
Tablets, co-zidocapt 12.5/25 (hydrochlorothiazide 12.5 mg, captopril 25 mg), net price 28-tab pack = £14.10
Brands include *Capto-co®*

Tablets, co-zidocapt 25/50 (hydrochlorothiazide 25 mg, captopril 50 mg), net price 28-tab pack = £14.00
Brands include *Capto-co®*

**Capozide®** (Squibb) ᴾᵒᴹ
LS tablets, scored, co-zidocapt 12.5/25 (hydro-chlorothiazide 12.5 mg, captopril 25 mg), net price 28-tab pack = £10.05

Tablets, scored, co-zidocapt 25/50 (hydrochloro-thiazide 25 mg, captopril 50 mg), net price 28-tab pack = £7.16 (also available as *Acezide®*)

## ■ CILAZAPRIL

**Indications** essential hypertension; congestive heart failure (adjunct—see section 2.5.5)

**Cautions** see notes above

**Contra-indications** see notes above; ascites

**Side-effects** see notes above; dyspnoea and bronchitis

**Dose**

- Hypertension, initially 1 mg once daily (reduced to 500 micrograms daily if used in addition to diuretic (see notes above), in the elderly, and in renal impairment), then adjusted according to response; usual maintenance dose 2.5–5 mg once daily; max. 5 mg daily

- Heart failure (adjunct), initially 500 micrograms once daily under close medical supervision (see notes above), increased gradually to 1–2.5 mg once daily if tolerated; max. 5 mg once daily

**Vascace®** (Roche) ᴾᵒᴹ
Tablets, f/c, cilazapril 500 micrograms (white), net price 30-tab pack = £3.76; 1 mg (yellow), 30-tab pack = £6.19; 2.5 mg (pink), 28-tab pack = £7.34; 5 mg (brown), 28-tab pack = £12.76

## ■ ENALAPRIL MALEATE

**Indications** hypertension; symptomatic heart failure (adjunct—see section 2.5.5); prevention of symptomatic heart failure in patients with asymptomatic left ventricular dysfunction

**Cautions** see notes above

**Contra-indications** see notes above

**Side-effects** see notes above; also dyspnoea; depression, asthenia; blurred vision; *less commonly* dry mouth, peptic ulcer, anorexia, ileus; arrhythmias, palpitation, flushing; confusion, nervousness, drowsiness, insomnia, vertigo; impotence; muscle cramps; tinnitus; alopecia, sweating; hyponatraemia; *rarely* stomatitis, glossitis, Raynaud's syndrome, pulmonary infiltrates, allergic alveolitis, dream abnormalities, gynaecomastia, Stevens-Johnson syndrome, toxic epidermal necrolysis, exfoliative dermatitis, pemphigus; *very rarely* gastro-intestinal angioedema

**Dose**

- Hypertension, used alone, initially 5 mg once daily; if used in addition to diuretic (see notes above), or in renal impairment, lower initial doses may be required; usual maintenance dose 20 mg once daily; max. 40 mg once daily

- Heart failure (adjunct), asymptomatic left ventricular dysfunction, initially 2.5 mg once daily under close medical supervision (see notes above), increased gradually over 2–4 weeks to 10–20 mg twice daily if tolerated

**Enalapril Maleate** (Non-proprietary) ᴾᵒᴹ
Tablets, enalapril maleate 2.5 mg, net price 28-tab pack = £1.28; 5 mg, 28-tab pack = £1.03; 10 mg, 28-tab pack = £1.10; 20 mg, 28-tab pack = £1.21
Brands include *Ednyt®*

**Innovace®** (MSD) ᴾᵒᴹ
Tablets, enalapril maleate 2.5 mg, net price 28-tab pack = £5.35; 5 mg (scored), 28-tab pack = £7.51; 10 mg (red), 28-tab pack = £10.53; 20 mg (peach), 28-tab pack = £12.51

*(sidebar)* **2** | **Cardiovascular system**

◀**With diuretic**

Note For mild to moderate hypertension in patients stabilised on the individual components in the same proportions. For cautions, contra-indications, and side-effects of thiazides, see section 2.2.1

**Innozide®** (MSD) [PoM]

Tablets, yellow, scored, enalapril maleate 20 mg, hydrochlorothiazide 12.5 mg, net price 28-tab pack = £12.82

Note Non-proprietary tablets containing enalapril maleate (20 mg) and hydrochlorothiazide (12.5 mg) are available

## FOSINOPRIL SODIUM

**Indications** hypertension; congestive heart failure (adjunct—see section 2.5.5)

**Cautions** see notes above

**Contra-indications** see notes above

**Side-effects** see notes above; chest pain; musculoskeletal pain

**Dose**

- Hypertension, initially 10 mg daily, increased if necessary after 4 weeks; usual dose range 10–40 mg (doses over 40 mg not shown to increase efficacy); if used in addition to diuretic see notes above

- Heart failure (adjunct), initially 10 mg once daily under close medical supervision (see notes above), increased gradually to 40 mg once daily if tolerated

**Fosinopril sodium** (Non-proprietary) [PoM]

Tablets, fosinopril sodium 10 mg, net price 28-tab pack = £2.32; 20 mg, 28-tab pack = £2.65

**Staril®** (Squibb) [PoM]

Tablets, fosinopril sodium 10 mg, net price 28-tab pack = £10.76; 20 mg, 28-tab pack = £11.62

## IMIDAPRIL HYDROCHLORIDE

**Indications** essential hypertension

**Cautions** see notes above

**Contra-indications** see notes above

**Side-effects** see notes above; dry mouth, glossitis, ileus; bronchitis, dyspnoea; sleep disturbances, depression, confusion, blurred vision, tinnitus, impotence

**Dose**

- Initially 5 mg daily before food; if used in addition to diuretic (see notes above), in elderly, in patients with heart failure, angina or cerebrovascular disease, or in renal or hepatic impairment, initially 2.5 mg daily; if necessary increase dose at intervals of at least 3 weeks; usual maintenance dose 10 mg once daily; max. 20 mg daily (elderly, 10 mg daily)

**Tanatril®** (Chiesi) [PoM]

Tablets, scored, imidapril hydrochloride 5 mg, net price 28-tab pack = £6.52; 10 mg, 28-tab pack = £7.36; 20 mg, 28-tab pack = £8.84

## LISINOPRIL

**Indications** hypertension (but see notes above); symptomatic heart failure (adjunct—see section 2.5.5); short-term treatment following myocardial infarction in haemodynamically stable patients; renal complications of diabetes mellitus

**Cautions** see notes above

**Contra-indications** see notes above

**Side-effects** see notes above; also *less commonly* tachycardia, palpitation, cerebrovascular accident, myocardial infarction, Raynaud's syndrome, confusion, mood changes, vertigo, sleep disturbances, asthenia, impotence; *rarely* dry mouth, gynaecomastia, alopecia, psoriasis; *very rarely* allergic alveolitis, pulmonary infiltrates, profuse sweating, pemphigus, Stevens-Johnson syndrome, and toxic epidermal necrolysis

**Dose**

- Hypertension, initially 10 mg once daily; if used in addition to diuretic (see notes above) or in cardiac decompensation or in volume depletion, initially 2.5–5 mg once daily; usual maintenance dose 20 mg once daily; max. 80 mg once daily

- Heart failure (adjunct), initially 2.5 mg once daily under close medical supervision (see notes above); increased in steps no greater than 10 mg at intervals of at least 2 weeks up to max. 35 mg once daily if tolerated

- Prophylaxis after myocardial infarction, systolic blood pressure over 120 mmHg, 5 mg within 24 hours, followed by further 5 mg 24 hours later, then 10 mg after a further 24 hours, and continuing with 10 mg once daily for 6 weeks (or continued if heart failure); systolic blood pressure 100–120 mmHg, initially 2.5 mg once daily, increased to maintenance dose of 5 mg once daily

  Note Should not be started after myocardial infarction if systolic blood pressure less than 100 mmHg; temporarily reduce maintenance dose to 5 mg and if necessary 2.5 mg daily if systolic blood pressure 100 mmHg or less during treatment; withdraw if prolonged hypotension occurs (systolic blood pressure less than 90 mmHg for more than 1 hour)

- Renal complications of diabetes mellitus, initially 2.5–5 mg once daily adjusted according to response; usual dose range 10–20 mg once daily

**Lisinopril** (Non-proprietary) [PoM]

Tablets, lisinopril (as dihydrate) 2.5 mg, net price 28-tab pack = 89p; 5 mg, 28-tab pack = 97p; 10 mg, 28-tab pack = £1.05; 20 mg, 28-tab pack = £1.29

**Carace®** (Bristol-Myers Squibb) [PoM]

Tablets, scored, lisinopril 5 mg, net price 28-tab pack = £8.18; 10 mg (yellow), 28-tab pack = £10.10; 20 mg (orange), 28-tab pack = £11.43

**Zestril®** (AstraZeneca) [PoM]

Tablets, lisinopril (as dihydrate) 2.5 mg, net price 28-tab pack = £1.78; 5 mg (pink), 28-tab pack = £1.31; 10 mg (pink), 28-tab pack = £2.05; 20 mg (pink), 28-tab pack = £2.17

◀**With diuretic**

Note For mild to moderate hypertension in patients stabilised on the individual components in the same proportions. For cautions, contra-indications, and side-effects of thiazides, see section 2.2.1

**Carace Plus®** (Bristol-Myers Squibb) [PoM]

Carace 10 Plus tablets, blue, lisinopril 10 mg, hydrochlorothiazide 12.5 mg, net price 28-tab pack = £10.10

Carace 20 Plus tablets, yellow, scored, lisinopril 20 mg, hydrochlorothiazide 12.5 mg, net price 28-tab pack = £11.43

**2**

**Cardiovascular system**

**Lisicostad®** (Genus) [PoM]

Lisicostad 10/12.5 mg tablets, scored, lisinopril (as dihydrate) 10 mg, hydrochlorothiazide 12.5 mg, net price 28-tab pack = £10.99

Lisicostad 20/12.5 mg tablets, scored, lisinopril (as dihydrate) 20 mg, hydrochlorothiazide 12.5 mg, net price 28-tab pack = £11.99

**Zestoretic®** (AstraZeneca) [PoM]

Zestoretic 10 tablets, peach, lisinopril (as dihydrate) 10 mg, hydrochlorothiazide 12.5 mg, net price 28-tab pack = £13.01

Zestoretic 20 tablets, lisinopril (as dihydrate) 20 mg, hydrochlorothiazide 12.5 mg, net price 28-tab pack = £14.72

## MOEXIPRIL HYDROCHLORIDE

**Indications**  essential hypertension

**Cautions**  see notes above

**Contra-indications**  see notes above

**Side-effects**  see notes above; arrhythmias, angina, chest pain, syncope, cerebrovascular accident, myocardial infarction; appetite and weight changes; dry mouth, photosensitivity, flushing, nervousness, mood changes, anxiety, drowsiness, sleep disturbance, tinnitus, influenza-like syndrome, sweating and dyspnoea

**Dose**

- Used alone, initially 7.5 mg once daily; if used in addition to diuretic (see notes above), with nifedipine, in elderly, in renal or hepatic impairment, initially 3.75 mg once daily; usual range 15–30 mg once daily; doses above 30 mg daily not shown to increase efficacy

**Perdix®** (UCB Pharma) [PoM]

Tablets, f/c, pink, scored, moexipril hydrochloride 7.5 mg, net price 28-tab pack = £6.04; 15 mg, 28-tab pack = £6.96

## PERINDOPRIL ERBUMINE

**Indications**  hypertension (but see notes above); symptomatic heart failure (adjunct—see section 2.5.5); prophylaxis of cardiac events following myocardial infarction or revascularisation in stable coronary artery disease

**Cautions**  see notes above

**Contra-indications**  see notes above

**Side-effects**  see notes above; asthenia, mood and sleep disturbances

**Dose**

- Hypertension, initially 4 mg once daily in the morning for 1 month, subsequently adjusted according to response; if used in addition to diuretic (see notes above), in elderly, in renal impairment, in cardiac decompensation, or in volume depletion, initially 2 mg once daily; max. 8 mg daily
- Heart failure (adjunct), initially 2 mg once daily in the morning under close medical supervision (see notes above), increased after at least 2 weeks to max. 4 mg once daily if tolerated
- Following myocardial infarction or revascularisation, initially 4 mg once daily in the morning increased after 2 weeks to 8 mg once daily if tolerated; ELDERLY 2 mg once daily for 1 week, then 4 mg once daily for 1 week, thereafter increased to 8 mg once daily if tolerated

**Perindopril** (Non-proprietary) [PoM]

Tablets, perindopril erbumine (= *tert*-butylamine) 2 mg, net price 30-tab pack = £3.46; 4 mg, 30-tab pack = £3.43; 8 mg, 30-tab pack = £3.52. Label: 22

◢**Perindopril arginine**

**Coversyl® Arginine** (Servier) [PoM]

Tablets, f/c, perindopril arginine 2.5 mg (white), net price 30-tab pack = £9.09; 5 mg (light green, scored), 30-tab pack = £10.22; 10 mg (green), 30-tab pack = £11.36. Label: 22

Dose  Hypertension, initially 5 mg once daily in the morning for 1 month, subsequently adjusted according to response; if used in addition to diuretic (see notes above), in elderly, in renal impairment, in cardiac decompensation, or in volume depletion, initially 2.5 mg once daily; max. 10 mg daily

Heart failure (adjunct), initially 2.5 mg once daily in the morning under close medical supervision (see notes above), increased after 2 weeks to max. 5 mg once daily if tolerated

Following myocardial infarction or revascularisation, initially 5 mg once daily in the morning increased after 2 weeks to 10 mg once daily if tolerated; ELDERLY 2.5 mg once daily for 1 week, then 5 mg once daily for 1 week, thereafter increased to 10 mg once daily if tolerated

◢**Perindopril arginine with diuretic**

Note  For hypertension not adequately controlled by perindopril alone. For cautions, contra-indications, and side-effects of indapamide, see section 2.2.1

**Coversyl® Arginine Plus** (Servier) [PoM]

Tablets, f/c, perindopril arginine 5 mg, indapamide 1.25 mg, net price 30-tab pack = £13.04. Label: 22

## QUINAPRIL

**Indications**  essential hypertension; congestive heart failure (adjunct—see section 2.5.5)

**Cautions**  see notes above

**Contra-indications**  see notes above

**Side-effects**  see notes above; asthenia, chest pain, oedema, flatulence, nervousness, depression, insomnia, blurred vision, impotence, and back pain

**Dose**

- Hypertension, initially 10 mg once daily; with a diuretic (see notes above), in elderly, or in renal impairment initially 2.5 mg daily; usual maintenance dose 20–40 mg daily in single or 2 divided doses; up to 80 mg daily has been given
- Heart failure (adjunct), initial dose 2.5 mg daily under close medical supervision (see notes above), increased gradually to 10–20 mg daily in 1–2 divided doses if tolerated; max. 40 mg daily

**Quinapril** (Non-proprietary) [PoM]

Tablets, quinapril (as hydrochloride) 5 mg, net price 28-tab pack = £1.81; 10 mg, 28-tab pack = £2.10; 20 mg, 28-tab pack = £2.50; 40 mg, 28-tab pack = £3.01

Brands include *Quinil®*

**Accupro®** (Pfizer) [PoM]

Tablets, f/c, quinapril (as hydrochloride) 5 mg (brown), net price 28-tab pack = £8.60; 10 mg (brown), 28-tab pack = £8.60; 20 mg (brown), 28-tab pack = £10.79; 40 mg (red-brown), 28-tab pack = £9.75

**2  Cardiovascular system**

◀**With diuretic**

Note For hypertension in patients stabilised on the individual components in the same proportions. For cautions, contra-indications, and side-effects of thiazides, see section 2.2.1

**Accuretic®** (Pfizer) (PoM)

Tablets, pink, f/c, scored, quinapril (as hydrochloride) 10 mg, hydrochlorothiazide 12.5 mg, net price 28-tab pack = £11.75

## ▌ RAMIPRIL

**Indications** mild to moderate hypertension; congestive heart failure (adjunct—see section 2.5.5); following myocardial infarction in patients with clinical evidence of heart failure; susceptible patients over 55 years, prevention of myocardial infarction, stroke, cardiovascular death or need of revascularisation procedures (consult product literature)

**Cautions** see notes above

**Contra-indications** see notes above

**Side-effects** see notes above; arrhythmias, angina, chest pain, syncope, cerebrovascular accident, myocardial infarction, loss of appetite, stomatitis, dry mouth, skin reactions including erythema multiforme and pemphigoid exanthema; precipitation or exacerbation of Raynaud's syndrome; conjunctivitis, onycholysis, confusion, nervousness, depression, anxiety, impotence, decreased libido, alopecia, bronchitis and muscle cramps

**Dose**

● Hypertension, initially 1.25 mg once daily, increased at intervals of 1–2 weeks; usual range 2.5–5 mg once daily; max. 10 mg once daily; if used in addition to diuretic see notes above

● Heart failure (adjunct), initially 1.25 mg once daily under close medical supervision (see notes above), increased gradually at intervals of 1–2 weeks to max. 10 mg daily if tolerated (daily doses of 2.5 mg or more may be taken in 1–2 divided doses)

● Prophylaxis after myocardial infarction (started in hospital 3 to 10 days after infarction), initially 2.5 mg twice daily, increased after 2 days to 5 mg twice daily; maintenance 2.5–5 mg twice daily
Note If initial 2.5-mg dose not tolerated, give 1.25 mg twice daily for 2 days before increasing to 2.5 mg twice daily, then 5 mg twice daily

● Prophylaxis of cardiovascular events or stroke, initially 2.5 mg once daily, increased after 1 week to 5 mg once daily, then increased after a further 3 weeks to 10 mg once daily

**Ramipril** (Non-proprietary) (PoM)

Capsules, ramipril 1.25 mg, net price 28-cap pack = £1.07; 2.5 mg, 28-cap pack = £1.17; 5 mg, 28-cap pack = £1.31; 10 mg, 28-cap pack = £1.49

Tablets, ramipril 1.25 mg, net price 28-tab pack = £1.85; 2.5 mg, 28-tab pack = £1.58; 5 mg, 28-tab pack = £1.88; 10 mg, 28-tab pack = £2.30

**Tritace®** (Aventis Pharma) (PoM)

Tablets, scored, ramipril 1.25 mg (white), net price 28-tab pack = £5.09; 2.5 mg (yellow), 28-tab pack = £7.22; 5 mg (red), 28-tab pack = £10.05; 10 mg (white), 28-tab pack = £13.68

Titration pack, tablets, 35-day starter pack of ramipril 7 × 2.5 mg with 21 × 5 mg and 7 × 10 mg, net price = £13.00

◀**With calcium-channel blocker**

Note For hypertension in patients stabilised on the individual components in the same proportions. For cautions, contra-indications, and side-effects of felodipine, see section 2.6.2

**Triapin®** (Aventis Pharma) (PoM)

Triapin® tablets, f/c, brown, ramipril 5 mg, felodipine 5 mg (m/r), net price 28-tab pack = £16.13. Label: 25

Triapin mite® tablets, f/c, orange, ramipril 2.5 mg, felodipine 2.5 mg (m/r), net price 28-tab pack = £24.55. Label: 25

## ▌ TRANDOLAPRIL

**Indications** mild to moderate hypertension; following myocardial infarction in patients with left ventricular dysfunction

**Cautions** see notes above

**Contra-indications** see notes above

**Side-effects** see notes above; also ileus, dry mouth; tachycardia, palpitation, arrhythmias, angina, transient ischaemic attacks, cerebral haemorrhage, myocardial infarction, syncope; dyspnoea, bronchitis; asthenia, nervousness, sleep disturbances; hot flushes; alopecia, sweating, skin reactions including Stevens-Johnson syndrome, toxic epidermal necrolysis, and psoriasis-like efflorescence

**Dose**

● Hypertension, initially 500 micrograms once daily, increased at intervals of 2–4 weeks; usual range 1–2 mg once daily; max. 4 mg daily; if used in addition to diuretic see notes above

● Prophylaxis after myocardial infarction (starting as early as 3 days after infarction), initially 500 micrograms once daily, gradually increased to max. 4 mg once daily
Note If symptomatic hypotension develops during titration, do not increase dose further; if possible, reduce dose of any adjunctive treatment and if this is not effective or feasible, reduce dose of trandolapril

**Trandolapril** (Non-proprietary) (PoM)

Capsules, trandolapril 500 micrograms, net price 14-cap pack = £1.39; 1 mg, 28-cap pack = £6.77; 2 mg, 28-cap pack = £6.77; 4 mg, 28-cap pack = £11.45

**Gopten®** (Abbott) (PoM)

Capsules, trandolapril 500 micrograms (red/yellow), net price 14-cap pack = £1.35; 1 mg (red/orange), 28-cap pack = £6.59; 2 mg (red/red), 28-cap pack = £6.59; 4 mg (red/maroon), 28-cap pack = £11.19

◀**With calcium-channel blocker**

Note For hypertension in patients stabilised on the individual components in the same proportions. For cautions, contra-indications, and side-effects of verapamil, see section 2.6.2

**Tarka®** (Abbott) ▼ (PoM) ◢

Capsules, pink, trandolapril 2 mg, verapamil hydrochloride 180 mg (m/r), net price 28 cap-pack = £10.29. Label: 25

### ▌ 2.5.5.2  Angiotensin-II receptor antagonists

Candesartan, eprosartan, irbesartan, losartan, olmesartan, telmisartan, and valsartan are angiotensin-II receptor antagonists with many properties similar to those of the ACE inhibitors. However, unlike ACE inhibitors, they do not inhibit the breakdown of bradykinin

**2**

**Cardiovascular system**

and other kinins, and thus are unlikely to cause the persistent dry cough which commonly complicates ACE inhibitor therapy. They are therefore a useful alternative for patients who have to discontinue an ACE inhibitor because of persistent cough.

An angiotensin-II receptor antagonist may be used as an alternative to an ACE inhibitor in the management of heart failure (section 2.5.5) or diabetic nephropathy (section 6.1.5).

**Cautions** Angiotensin-II receptor antagonists should be used with caution in renal artery stenosis (see also Renal Effects under ACE Inhibitors, section 2.5.5.1). Monitoring of plasma-potassium concentration is advised, particularly in the elderly and in patients with renal impairment; lower initial doses may be appropriate in these patients. Angiotensin-II receptor antagonists should be used with caution in aortic or mitral valve stenosis and in hypertrophic cardiomyopathy. Those with primary aldosteronism, and Afro-Caribbean patients (particularly those with left ventricular hypertrophy), may not benefit from an angiotensin-II receptor antagonist. **Interactions:** Appendix 1 (angiotensin-II receptor antagonists).

**Contra-indications** Angiotensin-II receptor antagonists, like the ACE inhibitors, should also be avoided in pregnancy (Appendix 4) and breast-feeding (Appendix 5).

**Side-effects** Side-effects are usually mild. Symptomatic hypotension including dizziness may occur, particularly in patients with intravascular volume depletion (e.g. those taking high-dose diuretics). Hyperkalaemia occurs occasionally; angioedema has also been reported with some angiotensin-II receptor antagonists.

## ▌CANDESARTAN CILEXETIL

**Indications** hypertension; heart failure with impaired left ventricular systolic function in conjunction with an ACE inhibitor, or when ACE inhibitors are not tolerated (see also section 2.5.5)

**Cautions** see notes above; hepatic impairment (Appendix 2); renal impairment (Appendix 3)

**Contra-indications** see notes above; also cholestasis

**Side-effects** see notes above; also vertigo, headache; *very rarely* nausea, hepatitis, blood disorders, hyponatraemia, back pain, arthralgia, myalgia, rash, urticaria, pruritus

**Dose**

- Hypertension, initially 8 mg (hepatic impairment 2 mg, renal impairment or intravascular volume depletion 4 mg) once daily, increased if necessary at intervals of 4 weeks to max. 32 mg once daily; usual maintenance dose 8 mg once daily
- Heart failure, initially 4 mg once daily, increased at intervals of at least 2 weeks to 'target' dose of 32 mg once daily or to max. tolerated dose

**Amias®** (Takeda) ℗ℴ𝕄
Tablets, candesartan cilexetil 2 mg (white), net price 7-tab pack = £2.99; 4 mg (white, scored), 7-tab pack = £3.24, 28-tab pack = £8.15; 8 mg (pink, scored), 28-tab pack = £9.89; 16 mg (pink, scored), 28-tab pack = £12.72; 32 mg (pink, scored), 28-tab pack = £16.13

## ▌EPROSARTAN

**Indications** hypertension (see also notes above)

**Cautions** see notes above; also hepatic impairment (Appendix 2); renal impairment (Appendix 3)

**Contra-indications** see notes above

**Side-effects** see notes above; also flatulence, hypertriglyceridaemia, arthralgia, rhinitis; *rarely* headache, asthenia, anaemia, hypersensitivity reactions (including rash, pruritus, urticaria); *very rarely* nausea

**Dose**

- 600 mg once daily (elderly over 75 years, mild to moderate hepatic impairment, renal impairment, initially 300 mg once daily); if necessary increased after 2–3 weeks to 800 mg once daily

**Teveten®** (Solvay) ℗ℴ𝕄
Tablets, f/c, eprosartan (as mesilate) 300 mg (white), net price 28-tab pack = £10.00; 400 mg (pink), 56-tab pack = £15.77; 600 mg (white), 28-tab pack = £14.31. Label: 21

## ▌IRBESARTAN

**Indications** hypertension; renal disease in hypertensive type 2 diabetes mellitus (see also notes above)

**Cautions** see notes above

**Contra-indications** see notes above

**Side-effects** see notes above; also nausea, vomiting; fatigue; musculoskeletal pain; *less commonly* diarrhoea, dyspepsia, flushing, tachycardia, chest pain, cough, and sexual dysfunction; *rarely* rash, urticaria; *very rarely* headache, myalgia, arthralgia, tinnitus, taste disturbance, hepatitis, renal dysfunction, and cutaneous vasculitis

**Dose**

- Hypertension, initially 150 mg once daily, increased if necessary to 300 mg once daily (in haemodialysis or in ELDERLY over 75 years, initial dose of 75 mg once daily may be used); CHILD not recommended
- Renal disease in hypertensive type 2 diabetes mellitus, initially 150 mg once daily, increased to 300 mg once daily if tolerated (in haemodialysis or in ELDERLY over 75 years, consider initial dose of 75 mg once daily); CHILD not recommended

**Aprovel®** (Bristol-Myers Squibb, Sanofi-Synthelabo) ℗ℴ𝕄
Tablets, f/c, irbesartan 75 mg, net price 28-tab pack = £9.89; 150 mg, 28-tab pack = £12.08; 300 mg, 28-tab pack = £16.25

◀**With diuretic**
Note For hypertension not adequately controlled with irbesartan alone. For cautions, contra-indications, and side-effects of thiazides, see section 2.2.1

**CoAprovel®** (Bristol-Myers Squibb, Sanofi-Synthelabo) ℗ℴ𝕄
Tablets, f/c, irbesartan 150 mg, hydrochlorothiazide 12.5 mg (peach), net price 28-tab pack = £12.08; irbesartan 300 mg, hydrochlorothiazide 12.5 mg (peach), 28-tab pack = £16.25; irbesartan 300 mg, hydrochlorothiazide 25 mg (pink), 28-tab pack = £16.25

## ▌LOSARTAN POTASSIUM

**Indications** hypertension (including reduction of stroke risk in hypertension with left ventricular hypertrophy); chronic heart failre when ACE inhibitors are unsuitable or contra-indicated; diabetic nephropathy in type 2 diabetes mellitus (see also notes above)

**Cautions** see notes above; severe heart failure; hepatic impairment (avoid if severe; Appendix 2);

**Contra-indications** see notes above

**Side-effects** see notes above; asthenia, fatigue, vertigo; *less commonly* gastro-intestinal disturbance, angina, palpitation, dyspnoea, headache, urticaria, pruritus, rash; *rarely* atrial fibrillation, cerebrovascular accident, syncope, paraesthesia; hepatitis, anaphylaxis, cough, anaemia (in severe renal disease or following renal transplantation), thrombocytopenia, arthralgia, myalgia, and vasculitis (including Henoch-Schönlein purpura) also reported

**Dose**

• Hypertension, diabetic nephropathy in type 2 diabetes mellitus, usually 50 mg once daily (intravascular volume depletion, initially 25 mg once daily); if necessary increased after several weeks to 100 mg once daily; ELDERLY over 75 years initially 25 mg daily

• Chronic heart failure, 12.5 mg once daily, increased at weekly intervals to 50 mg once daily if tolerated

**Cozaar®** (MSD) ▼ PoM

Tablets, f/c, losartan potassium 12.5 mg (blue), net price 28-tab pack = £8.09; 25 mg (white), net price 28-tab pack = £16.18; 50 mg (white, scored), 28-tab pack = £12.80; 100 mg (white), 28-tab pack = £16.18

◢**With diuretic**

Note For hypertension not adequately controlled with losartan alone. For cautions, contra-indications, and side-effects of thiazides, see section 2.2.1

**Cozaar-Comp®** (MSD) PoM

Tablets 50/12.5, yellow, f/c, losartan potassium 50 mg, hydrochlorothiazide 12.5 mg, net price 28-tab pack = £12.80

Tablets 100/12.5, white, f/c, losartan potassium 100 mg, hydrochlorothiazide 12.5 mg, net price 28-tab pack = £16.18

Tablets 100/25, yellow, f/c, losartan potassium 100 mg, hydrochlorothiazide 25 mg, net price 28-tab pack = £16.18

## ▌ OLMESARTAN MEDOXOMIL

**Indications** hypertension (see also notes above)

**Cautions** see notes above; hepatic impairment (avoid in severe impairment; Appendix 2); renal impairment (avoid if eGFR less than 20 mL/minute/1.73 m²; Appendix 3)

**Contra-indications** see notes above; biliary obstruction

**Side-effects** see notes above; also gastro-intestinal disturbances; chest pain, peripheral oedema, hypertriglyceridaemia; fatigue; influenza-like symptoms; cough, pharyngitis, rhinitis; urinary-tract infection; haematuria, hyperuricaemia; arthritis, musculoskeletal pain; *less commonly* angina, vertigo, rash; *very rarely* headache, thrombocytopenia, myalgia, pruritus, urticaria

**Dose**

• Initially 10 mg once daily; if necessary increased to 20 mg once daily; max. 40 mg daily

**Olmetec®** (Sankyo) PoM

Tablets, f/c, olmesartan medoxomil 10 mg, net price 28-tab pack = £10.95; 20 mg, 28-tab pack = £12.95; 40 mg, 28-tab pack = £17.50

◢**With calcium-channel blocker**

Note For hypertension in patients stabilised on the individual components in the same proportions. For cautions, contra-indications, and side-effects of amlodipine, see section 2.6.2

**Sevikar®** (Daiichi Sankyo) ▼ PoM

Tablets 20/5, white, f/c, olmesartan medoxomil 20 mg, amlodipine (as besilate) 5 mg, net price 28-tab pack = £16.95

Tablets 40/5, ivory, f/c, olmesartan medoxomil 40 mg, amlodipine (as besilate) 5 mg, net price 28-tab pack = £16.95

Tablets 40/10, brownish-red, f/c, olmesartan medoxomil 40 mg, amlodipine (as besilate) 10 mg, net price 28-tab pack = £16.95

◢**With diuretic**

Note For hypertension not adequately controlled with olmesartan alone. For cautions, contra-indications, and side-effects of thiazides, see section 2.2.1

**Olmetec Plus®** (Sankyo) ▼ PoM

Tablets, f/c, olmesartan medoxomil 20 mg, hydrochlorothiazide 12.5 mg (red-yellow), net price 28-tab pack = £12.95; olmesartan medoxomil 20 mg, hydrochlorothiazide 25 mg (pink), 28-tab pack = £12.95

## ▌ TELMISARTAN

**Indications** hypertension (see also notes above)

**Cautions** see notes above; hepatic impairment (Appendix 2; avoid in severe impairment); renal impairment (Appendix 3)

**Contra-indications** see notes above; biliary obstruction

**Side-effects** see notes above; also gastro-intestinal disturbances; chest pain; influenza-like symptoms including pharyngitis and sinusitis; urinary-tract infection; arthralgia, myalgia, back pain, leg cramps; eczema; *less commonly* dry mouth, flatulence, anxiety, vertigo, tendinitis-like symptoms, abnormal vision, increased sweating; *rarely* bradycardia, tachycardia, dyspnoea, insomnia, depression, blood disorders, increase in uric acid, eosinophilia, rash, and pruritus; syncope and asthenia also reported

**Dose**

• Usually 40 mg once daily (but 20 mg may be sufficient), increased if necessary after at least 4 weeks, to max. 80 mg once daily

**Micardis®** (Boehringer Ingelheim) PoM

Tablets, telmisartan 20 mg, net price 28-tab pack = £8.00; 40 mg, 28-tab pack = £12.50; 80 mg, 28-tab pack = £17.00

◢**With diuretic**

Note For patients with hypertension not adequately controlled by telmisartan alone. For cautions, contra-indications, and side-effects of thiazides, see section 2.2.1

**Micardis Plus®** (Boehringer Ingelheim) PoM

Tablets 40/12.5, red/white, telmisartan 40 mg, hydrochlorothiazide 12.5 mg, net price 28-tab pack = £12.50

Tablets 80/12.5, red/white, telmisartan 80 mg, hydrochlorothiazide 12.5 mg, net price 28-tab pack = £17.00

Tablets 80/25, yellow/white, telmisartan 80 mg, hydrochlorothiazide 25 mg, net price 28-tab pack = £17.00

## ■ VALSARTAN

**Indications** hypertension; heart failure when ACE inhibitors cannot be used, or in conjunction with an ACE inhibitor when a beta-blocker cannot be used (see also section 2.5.5); myocardial infarction with left ventricular failure or left ventricular systolic dysfunction (adjunct—see section 2.5.5 and section 2.10.1)

**Cautions** see notes above; hepatic impairment (avoid if severe; Appendix 2); renal impairment (Appendix 3)

**Contra-indications** see notes above, biliary cirrhosis, cholestasis

**Side-effects** see notes above; renal impairment; *less commonly* gastro-intestinal disturbance, syncope, fatigue, cough, headache, acute renal failure; neutropenia, thrombocytopenia, myalgia, and hypersensitivity reactions (including rash, pruritus, vasculitis, and serum sickness) also reported

**Dose**

- Hypertension, usually 80 mg once daily (initially 40 mg once daily in intravascular volume depletion); if necessary increased at intervals of 4 weeks up to max. 320 mg daily
- Heart failure, initially 40 mg twice daily increased at intervals of at least 2 weeks up to max. 160 mg twice daily
- Myocardial infarction, initially 20 mg twice daily increased over several weeks to 160 mg twice daily if tolerated

**Diovan®** (Novartis) PoM
Capsules, valsartan 40 mg (grey), net price 28-cap pack = £13.97; 80 mg (grey/pink), 28-cap pack = £13.97; 160 mg (dark grey/pink), 28-cap pack = £18.41

Tablets, f/c, valsartan 40 mg (yellow, scored), net price 7-tab pack = £3.49; 320 mg (dark grey-violet), 28-tab pack = £20.23

**◄With diuretic**
Note For hypertension not adequately controlled by valsartan alone. For cautions, contra-indications, and side-effects of thiazides, see section 2.2.1

**Co-Diovan®** (Novartis) ▼ PoM
Tablets 80/12.5, orange, f/c, valsartan 80 mg, hydrochlorothiazide 12.5 mg, net price 28-tab pack = £13.97

Tablets 160/12.5, red, f/c, valsartan 160 mg, hydrochlorothiazide 12.5 mg, net price 28-tab pack = £18.41

Tablets 160/25, brown-orange, f/c, valsartan 160 mg, hydrochlorothiazide 25 mg, net price 28-tab pack = £18.41

## 2.5.5.3 Renin inhibitors

Renin inhibitors inhibit renin directly; renin converts angiotensinogen to angiotensin I. **Aliskiren** is licensed for the treatment of hypertension, either alone or in combination with other antihypertensives.

## ■ ALISKIREN

**Indications** essential hypertension

**Cautions** patients taking concomitant diuretics, on a low-sodium diet, or who are dehydrated (first doses may cause hypotension—initiate with care); renal artery stenosis; patients at risk of renal impairment; renal impairment (Appendix 3); monitor plasma-potassium concentration and renal function in renal impairment, diabetes mellitus, and heart failure; **interactions**: Appendix 1 (aliskiren)

**Contra-indications** pregnancy (Appendix 4); breast-feeding (Appendix 5)

**Side-effects** diarrhoea; *less commonly* rash; *rarely* angioedema; acute renal failure (reversible on discontinuation of treatment), anaemia, and hyperkalaemia also reported

**Dose**

- ADULT over 18 years, 150 mg once daily, increased if necessary to 300 mg once daily

**Rasilez®** (Novartis) ▼ PoM
Tablets, f/c, aliskiren (as hemifumarate) 150 mg (pink), net price 28-tab pack = £19.80; 300 mg (red), net price 28-tab pack = £23.80. Label: 21

## 2.6 Nitrates, calcium-channel blockers, and other antianginal drugs

2.6.1  **Nitrates**

2.6.2  **Calcium-channel blockers**

2.6.3  **Other antianginal drugs**

2.6.4  **Peripheral vasodilators and related drugs**

Nitrates, calcium-channel blockers, and potassium-channel activators have vasodilating effects. Vasodilators can act in heart failure by arteriolar dilatation which reduces both peripheral vascular resistance and left ventricular pressure during systole resulting in improved cardiac output. They can also cause venous dilatation which results in dilatation of capacitance vessels, increase of venous pooling, and diminution of venous return to the heart (decreasing left ventricular end-diastolic pressure).

## Angina

It is important to distinguish unstable angina from stable angina. *Stable angina* usually results from atherosclerotic plaques in the coronary arteries and is often precipitated by exertion and relieved by rest. *Unstable angina* is usually due to plaque rupture and is often characterised by new onset severe angina or sudden worsening of previously stable angina. Treatment of stable and unstable angina involves management of acute anginal pain, and long-term management to prevent angina attacks and to reduce the risk of cardiovascular events.

**Stable angina** Acute attacks of stable angina should be managed with sublingual **glyceryl trinitrate**; sublingual glyceryl trinitrate can also be taken before performing activities that are known to bring on an attack. If attacks occur more than twice a week, regular drug therapy is required and should be introduced in a stepwise manner according to response.

**2 Cardiovascular system**

Patients with mild or moderate stable angina should be given a **beta-blocker** (section 2.4). In those with left-ventricular dysfunction, beta-blocker treatment should be started at a very low dose and titrated very slowly over a period of weeks or months (section 2.5.5).

For those patients in whom beta-blockers are not tolerated or are contra-indicated, a long-acting **nitrate** (section 2.6.1) or a rate-limiting **calcium-channel blocker** (diltiazem or verapamil, section 2.6.2) can be used; in patients with left-ventricular dysfunction, diltiazem and verapamil are contra-indicated because heart failure may be precipitated (**important**: see p. 114); however, a long-acting dihydropyridine calcium-channel blocker, such as amlodipine or felodipine, is suitable. Nicorandil or ivabradine (section 2.6.3) are alternatives.

When a single drug fails to control symptoms, combination treatment can be used. A calcium-channel blocker can be added to a beta-blocker, although combining verapamil with a beta-blocker should be avoided (see p. 119); combinations including diltiazem and a beta-blocker should be used with caution. Long-acting nitrates can also be used with a beta-blocker or a calcium-channel blocker, if appropriate. Combinations that include nicorandil or ranolazine (section 2.6.3) can also be considered.

Patients should be referred to a specialist if a combination of two drugs fails to control symptoms. Revascularisation procedures may be appropriate.

**Unstable angina** Unstable angina and non-ST-segment elevation myocardial infarction (NSTEMI) are managed similarly. The aims of management are to provide supportive care and pain relief during the acute attack and to prevent further cardiac events and death. For advice on the management of patients with acute ST-segment elevation myocardial infarction (STEMI), see section 2.10.1.

**Initial management  Oxygen** (section 3.6) should be administered if there is evidence of hypoxia, pulmonary oedema, or continuing myocardial ischaemia; hyperoxia should be avoided and particular care is required in patients with chronic obstructive airways disease.

**Nitrates** (section 2.6.1) are used to relieve ischaemic pain. If sublingual glyceryl trinitrate is not effective, intravenous or buccal glyceryl trinitrate or intravenous isosorbide dinitrate is given. If pain continues, **diamorphine** or **morphine** (section 4.7.2) can be given by slow intravenous injection; an antiemetic such as metoclopramide should also be given (section 4.6).

**Aspirin** (chewed or dispersed in water) is given for its antiplatelet effect in a dose of 300 mg (section 2.9). If aspirin is given before arrival at hospital, a note saying that it has been given should be sent with the patient. **Clopidogrel** in a dose of 300 mg (section 2.9) and a **low molecular weight heparin** or **fondaparinux** (section 2.8.1) should also be given.

Patients without contra-indications should receive **beta-blockers** (section 2.4) which should be continued indefinitely. In patients without left-ventricular dysfunction and in whom beta-blockers are inappropriate, **diltiazem** or **verapamil** can be given (section 2.6.2).

The glycoprotein IIb/IIIa inhibitors **eptifibatide** and **tirofiban** (section 2.9) are recommended (with aspirin and heparin) for unstable angina or for non-ST-segment elevation myocardial infarction in patients at a high risk of either myocardial infarction or death.

Abciximab, eptifibatide, or tirofiban can also be used with aspirin and heparin in patients undergoing percutaneous coronary intervention, to reduce the immediate risk of vascular occlusion.

Revascularisation procedures are often appropriate for patients with unstable angina.

**Long-term management** The need for long-term angina treatment or for coronary angiography should be assessed. Most patients will require standard angina treatment (see Stable angina) to prevent recurrence of symptoms.

**Prevention of cardiovascular events** Patients with stable and unstable angina should be given advice and treatments to reduce their cardiovascular risk. The importance of life-style changes, especially stopping smoking, should be emphasised. Patients should take **aspirin** indefinitely in a dose of 75 mg daily. A combination of aspirin and clopidogrel is given for up to 12 months in patients with non-ST-segment elevation acute coronary syndromes (section 2.9). An **ACE inhibitor** (section 2.5.5.1) and a **statin** (section 2.12) should also be given.

## 2.6.1 Nitrates

Nitrates have a useful role in *angina* (for details on the management of stable angina, see section 2.6). Although they are potent coronary vasodilators, their principal benefit follows from a reduction in venous return which reduces left ventricular work. Unwanted effects such as flushing, headache, and postural hypotension may limit therapy, especially when angina is severe or when patients are unusually sensitive to the effects of nitrates.

*Sublingual* **glyceryl trinitrate** is one of the most effective drugs for providing rapid symptomatic relief of angina, but its effect lasts only for 20 to 30 minutes; the 300-microgram tablet is often appropriate when glyceryl trinitrate is first used. The *aerosol spray* provides an alternative method of rapid relief of symptoms for those who find difficulty in dissolving sublingual preparations. Duration of action may be prolonged by *modified-release* and *transdermal* preparations (but tolerance may develop, see below).

**Isosorbide dinitrate** is active *sublingually* and is a more stable preparation for those who only require nitrates infrequently. It is also effective by mouth for prophylaxis; although the effect is slower in onset, it may persist for several hours. Duration of action of up to 12 hours is claimed for *modified-release* preparations. The activity of isosorbide dinitrate may depend on the production of active metabolites, the most important of which is isosorbide mononitrate. **Isosorbide mononitrate** itself is also licensed for angina prophylaxis; modified-release formulations (for once daily administration) are available.

Glyceryl trinitrate or isosorbide dinitrate may be tried by *intravenous injection* when the sublingual form is ineffective in patients with chest pain due to myocardial infarction or severe ischaemia. Intravenous injections are also useful in the treatment of congestive heart failure.

**Tolerance** Many patients on long-acting or transdermal nitrates rapidly develop tolerance (with reduced therapeutic effects). Reduction of blood-nitrate concentrations to low levels for 4 to 8 hours each day usually maintains effectiveness in such patients. If tolerance is suspected during the use of transdermal patches they should be left off for several consecutive hours in each 24 hours; in the case of modified-release tablets of isosorbide dinitrate (and conventional formulations of isosorbide mononitrate), the second of the two daily doses should be given after about 8 hours rather than after 12 hours. Conventional formulations of isosorbide mononitrate should not usually be given more than twice daily unless small doses are used; modified-release formulations of isosorbide mononitrate should only be given once daily, and used in this way do not produce tolerance.

## ◼ GLYCERYL TRINITRATE

**Indications** prophylaxis and treatment of angina; congestive heart failure; anal fissure (section 1.7.4); extravasation (section 10.3)

**Cautions** hypothyroidism, malnutrition, hypothermia; recent history of myocardial infarction; hypoxaemia or other ventilation and perfusion abnormalities; susceptibility to angle-closure glaucoma; metal-containing transdermal systems should be removed before cardioversion or diathermy; avoid abrupt withdrawal; tolerance (see notes above); severe hepatic impairment; severe renal impairment; pregnancy (Appendix 4); breast-feeding (Appendix 5); **interactions:** Appendix 1 (nitrates)

**Contra-indications** hypersensitivity to nitrates; hypotensive conditions and hypovolaemia; hypertrophic cardiomyopathy, aortic stenosis, cardiac tamponade, constrictive pericarditis, mitral stenosis; toxic pulmonary oedema; head trauma, cerebral haemorrhage; marked anaemia

**Side-effects** postural hypotension, tachycardia (but paradoxical bradycardia also reported); throbbing headache, dizziness; *less commonly* nausea, vomiting, heartburn; flushing; temporary hypoxaemia; rash; application site reactions with transdermal patches; *very rarely* angle-closure glaucoma
Injection Specific side-effects following injection (particularly if given too rapidly) include severe hypotension, diaphoresis, apprehension, restlessness, muscle twitching, retrosternal discomfort, palpitation, abdominal pain, syncope; prolonged administration has been associated with methaemoglobinaemia

**Dose**
- Sublingually, 0.3–1 mg, repeated as required
- By intravenous infusion, 10–200 micrograms/minute
- By transdermal application, see under preparations

### ◼ Short-acting tablets and sprays
**Glyceryl Trinitrate** (Non-proprietary)
Sublingual tablets, glyceryl trinitrate 300 micrograms, net price 100 = £2.71; 500 micrograms, 100 = £2.70; 600 micrograms, 100 = £11.33. Label: 16
Note Glyceryl trinitrate tablets should be supplied in glass containers of not more than 100 tablets, closed with a foil-lined cap, and containing no cotton wool wadding; they should be discarded after 8 weeks in use

Aerosol spray, glyceryl trinitrate 400 micrograms/metered dose, net price 200-dose unit = £3.13
Dose treatment or prophylaxis of angina, spray 1–2 doses under tongue and then close mouth

**Coro-Nitro Pump Spray®** (Ayrton Saunders)
Aerosol spray, glyceryl trinitrate 400 micrograms/metered dose, net price 200-dose unit = £3.13
Dose treatment or prophylaxis of angina, spray 1–2 doses under tongue and then close mouth

**Glytrin Spray®** (Sanofi-Synthelabo)
Aerosol spray, glyceryl trinitrate 400 micrograms/metered dose, net price 200-dose unit = £3.35
Dose treatment or prophylaxis of angina, spray 1–2 doses under tongue and then close mouth
Cautions flammable

**GTN 300 mcg** (Martindale)
Sublingual tablets, glyceryl trinitrate 300 micrograms, net price 100 = £2.71. Label: 16

**Nitrolingual Pumpspray®** (Merck)
Aerosol spray, glyceryl trinitrate 400 micrograms/metered dose, net price 200-dose unit = £3.51
Dose treatment or prophylaxis of angina, spray 1–2 doses under tongue and then close mouth

**Nitromin®** (Egis)
Aerosol spray, glyceryl trinitrate 400 micrograms/metered dose, net price 180-dose unit = £2.63, 200-dose unit = £2.71
Dose treatment or prophylaxis of angina, spray 1–2 doses under tongue and then close mouth

### ◼ Longer-acting tablets
**Suscard®** (Forest)
Buccal tablets, m/r, glyceryl trinitrate 2 mg, net price 100-tab pack = £12.70; 3 mg, 100-tab pack = £18.33; 5 mg, 100-tab pack = £24.96. Counselling, see below
Dose treatment of angina, 2 mg as required, increased to 3 mg if necessary; prophylaxis 2–3 mg 3 times daily; 5 mg in severe angina
Unstable angina (adjunct), up to 5 mg with ECG monitoring
Congestive heart failure, 5 mg 3 times daily, increased to 10 mg 3 times daily in severe cases
Acute heart failure, 5 mg repeated until symptoms abate
Counselling Tablets have rapid onset of effect; they are placed between upper lip and gum, and left to dissolve; vary site to reduce risk of dental caries

### ◼ Parenteral preparations
Note Glass or polyethylene apparatus is preferable; loss of potency will occur if PVC is used

**Glyceryl Trinitrate** (Non-proprietary) [PoM]
Injection, glyceryl trinitrate 5 mg/mL. To be diluted before use. Net price 5-mL amp = £6.49; 10-mL amp = £12.98
Excipients may include ethanol, propylene glycol (see Excipients, p. 2)

**Nitrocine®** (UCB Pharma) [PoM]
Injection, glyceryl trinitrate 1 mg/mL. To be diluted before use or given undiluted with syringe pump. Net price 10-mL amp = £5.88; 50-mL bottle = £13.77
Excipients include propylene glycol (see Excipients, p. 2)

**Nitronal®** (Merck) [PoM]
Injection, glyceryl trinitrate 1 mg/mL. To be diluted before use or given undiluted with syringe pump. Net price 5-mL vial = £1.84; 50-mL vial = £15.06

### ◼ Transdermal preparations
**Deponit®** (UCB Pharma)
Patches, self-adhesive, transparent, glyceryl trinitrate, '5' patch (releasing approx. 5 mg/24 hours when in contact with skin), net price 28 = £12.77; '10' patch (releasing approx.10 mg/24 hours), 28 = £14.06
Dose prophylaxis of angina, apply one '5' or one '10' patch to lateral chest wall, upper arm, thigh, abdomen, or shoulder; increase to two '10' patches every 24 hours if necessary; replace every 24 hours, siting replacement patch on different area; see also notes above (Tolerance)

**Minitran®** (3M)

Patches, self-adhesive, transparent, glyceryl trinitrate, '5' patch (releasing approx. 5 mg/24 hours when in contact with skin), net price 30 = £11.62; '10' patch (releasing approx. 10 mg/24 hours), 30 = £12.87; '15' patch (releasing approx. 15 mg/24 hours), 30 = £14.19

**Dose** prophylaxis of angina, apply one '5' patch to chest or upper arm; replace every 24 hours, siting replacement patch on different area; adjust dose according to response; see also notes above (Tolerance)

Maintenance of venous patency ('5' patch only), consult product literature

**Nitro-Dur®** (Schering-Plough)

Patches, self-adhesive, buff, glyceryl trinitrate, '0.2 mg/h' patch (releasing approx. 5 mg/24 hours when in contact with skin), net price 28 = £10.80; '0.4 mg/h' patch (releasing approx. 10 mg/24 hours), 28 = £11.95; '0.6 mg/h' patch (releasing approx.15 mg/24 hours), 28 = £13.15

**Dose** prophylaxis of angina, apply one '0.2 mg/h' patch to chest or outer upper arm; replace every 24 hours, siting replacement patch on different area; adjust dose according to response; see also notes above (Tolerance)

**Percutol®** (TEVA UK)

Ointment, glyceryl trinitrate 2%, net price 60 g = £9.55. Counselling, see administration below

**Excipients** include wool fat

**Dose** prophylaxis of angina, usual dose 1–2 inches of ointment measured on to *Applirule®*, and applied (usually to chest, arm, or thigh) without rubbing in and secured with surgical tape, every 3–4 hours as required; to determine dose, ½ inch on first day then increased by ½ inch/day until headache occurs, then reduced by ½ inch

**Note** Approx. 800 micrograms/hour absorbed from 1 inch of ointment

**Transiderm-Nitro®** (Novartis)

Patches, self-adhesive, pink, glyceryl trinitrate, '5' patch (releasing approx. 5 mg/24 hours when in contact with skin), net price 28 = £21.31; '10' patch (releasing approx. 10 mg/24 hours), 28 = £23.43

**Dose** prophylaxis of angina, apply one '5' or one '10' patch to lateral chest wall; replace every 24 hours, siting replacement patch on different area; max. two '10' patches daily; see also notes above (Tolerance)

Prophylaxis of phlebitis and extravasation ('5' patch only), consult product literature

**Trintek®** (Goldshield)

Patches, self-adhesive, glyceryl trinitrate, '5' patch (releasing approx. 5 mg/24 hours when in contact with skin), net price 30 = £11.84; '10' patch (releasing approx. 10 mg/24 hours), net price 30 = £13.10; '15' patch (releasing approx. 15 mg/24 hours), net price 30 = £14.42

**Dose** prophylaxis of angina, apply one '5' patch to lateral chest wall; replace every 24 hours, siting replacement patch on different area; adjust dose according to response, max one '15' patch daily; see also notes above (Tolerance)

## ISOSORBIDE DINITRATE

**Indications** prophylaxis and treatment of angina; left ventricular failure

**Cautions** see under Glyceryl Trinitrate

**Contra-indications** see under Glyceryl Trinitrate

**Side-effects** see under Glyceryl Trinitrate

**Dose**

- By mouth, daily in divided doses, angina 30–120 mg, left ventricular failure 40–160 mg, up to 240 mg if required

- By intravenous infusion, 2–10 mg/hour; higher doses up to 20 mg/hour may be required

◢ **Short-acting tablets and sprays**

**Isosorbide Dinitrate** (Non-proprietary)

Tablets, isosorbide dinitrate 10 mg, net price 56-tab pack = £9.53; 20 mg, 56-tab pack = £11.67

**Angitak®** (LPC)

Aerosol spray, isosorbide dinitrate 1.25 mg/metered dose, net price 200-dose unit = £3.95

**Dose** treatment or prophylaxis of angina, spray 1–3 doses under tongue whilst holding breath; allow 30 second interval between each dose

◢ **Modified-release preparations**

**Isoket Retard®** (UCB Pharma)

Retard-20 tablets, m/r, scored, isosorbide dinitrate 20 mg, net price 56-tab pack = £2.58. Label: 25

Retard-40 tablets, m/r, scored, isosorbide dinitrate 40 mg, net price 56-tab pack = £6.36. Label: 25

**Dose** prophylaxis of angina, 40 mg daily in 1–2 divided doses, increased if necessary to 60–80 mg daily in 2–3 divided doses

◢ **Parenteral preparations**

**Isoket®** (UCB Pharma) PoM

Injection 0.05%, isosorbide dinitrate 500 micrograms/mL. To be diluted before use or given undiluted with syringe pump. Net price 50-mL bottle = £7.15

Injection 0.1%, isosorbide dinitrate 1 mg/mL. To be diluted before use. Net price 10-mL amp = £2.69; 50-mL bottle = £13.36; 100-mL bottle = £25.98

**Note** Glass or polyethylene infusion apparatus is preferable; loss of potency if PVC used

## ISOSORBIDE MONONITRATE

**Indications** prophylaxis of angina; adjunct in congestive heart failure

**Cautions** see under Glyceryl Trinitrate

**Contra-indications** see under Glyceryl Trinitrate

**Side-effects** see under Glyceryl Trinitrate

**Dose**

- Initially 20 mg 2–3 times daily or 40 mg twice daily (10 mg twice daily in those who have not previously received nitrates); up to 120 mg daily in divided doses if required

**Isosorbide Mononitrate** (Non-proprietary)

Tablets, isosorbide mononitrate 10 mg, net price 56 = £1.02; 20 mg, 56 = £1.04; 40 mg, 56 = £1.46. Label: 25

Brands include *Angeze®*

**Elantan®** (UCB Pharma)

Elantan 10 tablets, scored, isosorbide mononitrate 10 mg, net price 56-tab pack = £1.32; 84-tab pack = £4.97. Label: 25

Elantan 20 tablets, scored, isosorbide mononitrate 20 mg, net price 56-tab pack = £1.73; 84-tab pack = £6.13. Label: 25

Elantan 40 tablets, scored, isosorbide mononitrate 40 mg, net price 56-tab pack = £2.81; 84-tab pack = £10.56. Label: 25

**Ismo®** (Riemser)

Ismo 10 tablets, isosorbide mononitrate 10 mg, net price 60-tab pack = £3.31. Label: 25

Ismo 20 tablets, scored, isosorbide mononitrate 20 mg, net price 60-tab pack = £4.85. Label: 25

**2**

**Cardiovascular system**

◀ **Modified release**

**Chemydur® 60XL** (Sovereign) PoM

Tablets, m/r, scored, ivory, isosorbide mononitrate 60 mg, net price 28-tab pack = £5.76. Label: 25

**Dose** prophylaxis of angina, 1 tablet in the morning (half a tablet for 2–4 days to minimise possibility of headache), increased if necessary to 2 tablets

**Elantan LA®** (UCB Pharma)

Elantan LA 25 capsules, m/r, brown/white, enclosing white micropellets, isosorbide mononitrate 25 mg, net price 28-cap pack = £2.64. Label: 25

**Dose** prophylaxis of angina, 1 capsule in the morning, increased if necessary to 2 capsules

Elantan LA 50 capsules, m/r, brown/pink, enclosing white micropellets, isosorbide mononitrate 50 mg, net price 28-cap pack = £3.69. Label: 25

**Dose** prophylaxis of angina, 1 capsule daily in the morning, increased if necessary to 2 capsules

**Imdur®** (AstraZeneca)

Durules® (= tablets m/r), yellow, f/c, scored, isosorbide mononitrate 60 mg, net price 28-tab pack = £10.71. Label: 25

**Dose** prophylaxis of angina, 1 tablet in the morning (half a tablet if headache occurs), increased to 2 tablets in the morning if required

**Isib 60XL®** (Ranbaxy)

Tablets, m/r, scored, yellow, isosorbide mononitrate 60 mg, net price 28-tab pack = £8.15. Label: 25

**Dose** prophylaxis of angina, 1 tablet in the morning (half a tablet for 2–4 days if headache occurs), increased if necessary to 2 tablets

**Note** Also available as Cibral 60XL®, Xismox 60XL®

**Ismo Retard®** (Riemser)

Tablets, m/r, s/c, isosorbide mononitrate 40 mg, net price 30-tab pack = £10.71. Label: 25

**Dose** prophylaxis of angina, 1 tablet daily in morning

**Isodur®** (Galen)

Isodur 25XL capsules, m/r, brown/white, isosorbide mononitrate 25 mg, net price 28-cap pack = £5.50. Label: 25

Isodur 50XL capsules, m/r, brown/pink, isosorbide mononitrate 50 mg, net price 28-cap pack = £6.50. Label: 25

**Dose** prophylaxis of angina, 25–50 mg daily in the morning, increased if necessary to 50–100 mg once daily

**Isotard®** (ProStrakan)

Isotard 25XL tablets, m/r, ivory, isosorbide mononitrate 25 mg, net price 28-tab pack = £5.95. Label: 25

Isotard 40XL tablets, m/r, ivory, isosorbide mononitrate 40 mg, net price 28-tab pack = £6.78. Label: 25

Isotard 50XL tablets, m/r, ivory, isosorbide mononitrate 50 mg, net price 28-tab pack = £6.78. Label: 25

Isotard 60XL tablets, m/r, ivory, isosorbide mononitrate 60 mg, net price 28-tab pack = £5.75. Label: 25

**Dose** prophylaxis of angina, 25–60 mg daily in the morning (if headache occurs with 60-mg tablet, half a 60-mg tablet may be given for 2–4 days), increased if necessary to 50–120 mg daily

**Modisal LA®** (UCB Pharma)

Modisal LA25 capsules, m/r, brown/white, isosorbide mononitrate 25 mg, net price 28-cap pack = £6.22. Label: 25

Modisal LA50 capsules, m/r, brown/peach, isosorbide mononitrate 50 mg, net price 28-cap pack = £10.03. Label: 25

**Dose** prophylaxis of angina, 25–50 mg daily in the morning, increased if necessary to 100 mg once daily

**Modisal XL®** (Sandoz)

Tablets, m/r, ivory, isosorbide mononitrate 60 mg, net price 28-tab pack = £10.36. Label: 25

**Dose** prophylaxis of angina, 1 tablet daily in the morning (half a tablet for first 2–4 days to minimise possibility of headache), increased if necessary to 2 tablets once daily

**Monomax®** (Chiesi)

Monomax® SR, capsules, m/r, isosorbide mononitrate 40 mg, net price 28-cap pack = £8.31; 60 mg, 28-cap pack = £9.03. Label: 25

**Dose** prophylaxis of angina, 40–60 mg daily in the morning, increased if necessary to 120 mg daily

**Note** Also available as Angeze SR®

Monomax® XL tablets, m/r, isosorbide mononitrate 60 mg, net price 28-tab pack = £5.75. Label: 25

**Dose** prophylaxis of angina, 1 tablet in the morning (half a tablet for first 2–4 days to minimise possibility of headache), increased if necessary to 2 tablets

**Monomil XL®** (IVAX) PoM

Tablets, m/r, isosorbide mononitrate 60 mg, net price 28-tab pack = £4.32. Label: 25

**Dose** prophylaxis of angina, 1 tablet daily in the morning (half a tablet daily for first 2–4 days to minimise possibility of headache), increased if necessary to 2 tablets once daily

**Monosorb XL 60®** (Dexcel) PoM

Tablets, m/r, f/c, isosorbide mononitrate 60 mg, net price 28-tab pack = £16.66. Label: 25

**Dose** prophylaxis of angina, 1 tablet daily in the morning (half a tablet for first 2–4 days to minimise possibility of headache), increased if necessary to 2 tablets

**Note** Also available as Monigen® XL, Trangina® XL

**Zemon®** (Neolab)

Zemon 40XL tablets, m/r, ivory, isosorbide mononitrate 40 mg, net price 28-tab pack = £14.25. Label: 25

Zemon 60XL tablets, scored, m/r, ivory, isosorbide mononitrate 60 mg, net price 28-tab pack = £11.14. Label: 25

**Dose** prophylaxis of angina, 40–60 mg daily in the morning (half a 60-mg tablet may be given for 2–4 days to minimise possibility of headache), increased if necessary to 80–120 mg once daily

## 2.6.2 Calcium-channel blockers

Calcium-channel blockers (less correctly called 'calcium-antagonists') interfere with the inward displacement of calcium ions through the slow channels of active cell membranes. They influence the myocardial cells, the cells within the specialised conducting system of the heart, and the cells of vascular smooth muscle. Thus, myocardial contractility may be reduced, the formation and propagation of electrical impulses within the heart may be depressed, and coronary or systemic vascular tone may be diminished.

Calcium-channel blockers differ in their predilection for the various possible sites of action and, therefore, their therapeutic effects are disparate, with much greater variation than those of beta-blockers. There are important differences between verapamil, diltiazem, and the dihydropyridine calcium-channel blockers (amlodipine, felodipine, isradipine, lacidipine, lercanidipine, nicardipine, nifedipine, and nimodipine). Verapamil and diltiazem should usually be **avoided** in heart failure because they may further depress cardiac function and cause clinically significant deterioration.

**2 Cardiovascular system**

**Verapamil** is used for the treatment of angina (section 2.6), hypertension (section 2.5), and arrhythmias (section 2.3.2). It is a highly negatively inotropic calcium channel-blocker and it reduces cardiac output, slows the heart rate, and may impair atrioventricular conduction. It may precipitate heart failure, exacerbate conduction disorders, and cause hypotension at high doses and should **not** be used with beta-blockers (see p. 119). Constipation is the most common side-effect.

**Nifedipine** relaxes vascular smooth muscle and dilates coronary and peripheral arteries. It has more influence on vessels and less on the myocardium than does verapamil, and unlike verapamil has no anti-arrhythmic activity. It rarely precipitates heart failure because any negative inotropic effect is offset by a reduction in left ventricular work. Short-acting formulations of nifedipine are not recommended for angina or long-term management of hypertension; their use may be associated with large variations in blood pressure and reflex tachycardia. **Nicardipine** has similar effects to those of nifedipine and may produce less reduction of myocardial contractility. **Amlodipine** and **felodipine** also resemble nifedipine and nicardipine in their effects and do not reduce myocardial contractility and they do not produce clinical deterioration in heart failure. They have a longer duration of action and can be given once daily. Nifedipine, nicardipine, amlodipine, and felodipine are used for the treatment of angina (section 2.6) or hypertension. All are valuable in forms of angina associated with coronary vasospasm. Side-effects associated with vasodilatation such as flushing and headache (which become less obtrusive after a few days), and ankle swelling (which may respond only partially to diuretics) are common.

**Isradipine, lacidipine,** and **lercanidipine** have similar effects to those of nifedipine and nicardipine; they are indicated for hypertension only.

**Nimodipine** is related to nifedipine but the smooth muscle relaxant effect preferentially acts on cerebral arteries. Its use is confined to prevention and treatment of vascular spasm following aneurysmal subarachnoid haemorrhage.

**Diltiazem** is effective in most forms of angina (section 2.6); the longer-acting formulation is also used for hypertension. It may be used in patients for whom beta-blockers are contra-indicated or ineffective. It has a less negative inotropic effect than verapamil and significant myocardial depression occurs rarely. Nevertheless because of the risk of bradycardia it should be used with caution in association with beta-blockers.

**Unstable angina** Calcium-channel blockers do not reduce the risk of myocardial infarction in unstable angina. The use of diltiazem or verapamil should be reserved for patients resistant to treatment with beta-blockers.

**Withdrawal** There is some evidence that sudden withdrawal of calcium-channel blockers may be associated with an exacerbation of angina.

---

### ■ AMLODIPINE

**Indications** hypertension, prophylaxis of angina

**Cautions** hepatic impairment (Appendix 2); pregnancy (Appendix 4); **interactions:** Appendix 1 (calcium-channel blockers)

**Contra-indications** cardiogenic shock, unstable angina, significant aortic stenosis; acute porphyria (section 9.8.2); breast-feeding (Appendix 5)

**Side-effects** abdominal pain, nausea; palpitation, flushing, oedema; headache, dizziness, sleep disturbances, fatigue; *less commonly* gastro-intestinal disturbances, dry mouth, taste disturbances, hypotension, syncope, chest pain, dyspnoea, rhinitis, mood changes, asthenia, tremor, paraesthesia, urinary disturbances, impotence, gynaecomastia, weight changes, myalgia, muscle cramps, back pain, arthralgia, visual disturbances, tinnitus, pruritus, rashes (including isolated reports of erythema multiforme), sweating, alopecia, purpura, and skin discolouration; *very rarely* gastritis, pancreatitis, hepatitis, jaundice, cholestasis, gingival hyperplasia, myocardial infarction, arrhythmias, tachycardia, vasculitis, coughing, peripheral neuropathy, hyperglycaemia, thrombocytopenia, angioedema, and urticaria

**Dose**

- Hypertension or angina, initially 5 mg once daily; max. 10 mg once daily

**Note** Tablets from various suppliers may contain different salts (e.g. amlodipine besilate, amlodipine maleate, and amlodipine mesilate) but the strength is expressed in terms of amlodipine (base); tablets containing different salts are considered interchangeable

**Amlodipine** (Non-proprietary) ▣Pom▣
Tablets, amlodipine (as maleate or as mesilate) 5 mg, net price 28-tab pack = £1.08; 10 mg, 28-tab pack = £1.24
Brands include *Amlostin*®

**Istin**® (Pfizer) ▣Pom▣
Tablets, amlodipine (as besilate) 5 mg, net price 28-tab pack = £11.08; 10 mg, 28-tab pack = £16.55

**◢With valsartan**
**Note** For hypertension in patients stabilised on the individual components in the same proportions. For cautions, contra-indications, and side-effects of valsartan, see section 2.5.5.2

**Exforge**® (Novartis) ▼ ▣Pom▣
Tablets 5/80, f/c, dark yellow, amlodipine 5 mg, valsartan 80 mg, net price 28-tab pack = £13.97
Tablets 5/160, f/c, dark yellow, amlodipine 5 mg, valsartan 160 mg, net price 28-tab pack = £18.41
Tablets 10/160, f/c, light yellow, amlodipine 10 mg, valsartan 160 mg, net price 28-tab pack = £18.41

---

### ■ DILTIAZEM HYDROCHLORIDE

**Indications** prophylaxis and treatment of angina; hypertension

**Cautions** reduce dose in hepatic and renal impairment; heart failure or significantly impaired left ventricular function, bradycardia (avoid if severe), first degree AV block, or prolonged PR interval; **interactions:** Appendix 1 (calcium-channel blockers)

**Contra-indications** severe bradycardia, left ventricular failure with pulmonary congestion, second- or third-degree AV block (unless pacemaker fitted), sick sinus syndrome; acute porphyria (but see section 9.8.2); pregnancy; breast-feeding (Appendix 5)

**Side-effects** bradycardia, sino-atrial block, AV block, palpitation, dizziness, hypotension, malaise, asthenia, headache, hot flushes, gastro-intestinal disturbances, oedema (notably of ankles); rarely rashes (including erythema multiforme and exfoliative dermatitis), photosensitivity; hepatitis, gynaecomastia, gum

**2**

**Cardiovascular system**

hyperplasia, extrapyramidal symptoms, depression reported

**Dose**

- Angina, 60 mg 3 times daily (elderly initially twice daily); increased if necessary to 360 mg daily
- Longer-acting formulations, see under preparations below

◀**Standard formulations**

Note These formulations are licensed as generics and there is no requirement for brand name dispensing. Although their means of formulation has called for the strict designation 'modified-release' their duration of action corresponds to that of tablets requiring administration 3 times daily

**Diltiazem** (Non-proprietary) ⒫ⓄⓂ

Tablets, m/r (but see note above), diltiazem hydrochloride 60 mg, net price 84 = £3.34. Label: 25
Brands include Optil®

**Tildiem®** (Sanofi-Synthelabo) ⒫ⓄⓂ

Tablets, m/r (but see note above), off-white, diltiazem hydrochloride 60 mg, net price 90-tab pack = £7.96. Label: 25

◀**Longer-acting formulations**

Note Different versions of modified-release preparations may not have the same clinical effect. To avoid confusion between these different formulations of diltiazem, prescribers should specify the brand to be dispensed

**Adizem-SR®** (Napp) ⒫ⓄⓂ

Capsules, m/r, diltiazem hydrochloride 90 mg (white), net price 56-cap pack = £8.62; 120 mg (brown/white), 56-cap pack = £9.59; 180 mg (brown/white), 56-cap pack = £14.36. Label: 25

Tablets, m/r, f/c, scored, diltiazem hydrochloride 120 mg, net price 56-tab pack = £14.72. Label: 25
Dose mild to moderate hypertension, usually 120 mg twice daily (dose form not appropriate for initial dose titration)
Angina, initially 90 mg twice daily (elderly, dose form not appropriate for initial dose titration); increased to 180 mg twice daily if required

**Adizem-XL®** (Napp) ⒫ⓄⓂ

Capsules, m/r, diltiazem hydrochloride 120 mg (pink/blue), net price 28-cap pack = £9.28; 180 mg (dark pink/blue), 28-cap pack = £10.53; 200 mg (brown), 28-cap pack = £6.40; 240 mg (red/blue), 28-cap pack = £11.69; 300 mg (maroon/blue), 28-cap pack = £9.28. Label: 25
Dose angina and mild to moderate hypertension, initially 240 mg once daily, increased if necessary to 300 mg once daily; in elderly and in hepatic or renal impairment, initially 120 mg daily

**Angitil SR®** (Chiesi) ⒫ⓄⓂ

Capsules, m/r, diltiazem hydrochloride 90 mg (white), net price 56-cap pack = £7.55; 120 mg (brown), 56-cap pack = £8.39; 180 mg (brown), 56-cap pack = £13.53. Label: 25
Dose angina and mild to moderate hypertension, initially 90 mg twice daily; increased if necessary to 120 mg or 180 mg twice daily

**Angitil XL®** (Chiesi) ⒫ⓄⓂ

Capsules, m/r, diltiazem hydrochloride 240 mg (white), net price 28-cap pack = £9.07; 300 mg (yellow), 28-cap pack = £8.24. Label: 25
Dose angina and mild to moderate hypertension, initially 240 mg once daily (elderly and in hepatic and renal impairment, dose form not appropriate for initial dose titration); increased if necessary to 300 mg once daily

**Calcicard CR®** (IVAX) ⒫ⓄⓂ

Tablets, m/r, both f/c, diltiazem hydrochloride 90 mg, net price 56-tab pack = £6.33; 120 mg, 56-tab pack = £7.04. Label: 25
Dose mild to moderate hypertension, initially 90 mg or 120 mg twice daily; up to 360 mg daily may be required: ELDERLY and in hepatic and renal impairment, initially 120 mg once daily; up to 240 mg daily may be required
Angina, initially 90 mg or 120 mg twice daily; up to 480 mg daily in divided doses may be required; ELDERLY and in hepatic and renal impairment, dose form not appropriate for initial dose titration; up to 240 mg daily may be required

**Dilcardia SR®** (Generics) ⒫ⓄⓂ

Capsules, m/r, diltiazem hydrochloride 60 mg (pink/white), net price 56-cap pack = £8.31; 90 mg (pink/yellow), 56-cap pack = £10.33; 120 mg (pink/orange), 56-cap pack = £11.49. Label: 25
Dose angina and mild to moderate hypertension, initially 90 mg twice daily; increased if necessary to 180 mg twice daily; ELDERLY and in hepatic or renal impairment, initially 60 mg twice daily, max. 90 mg twice daily

**Dilzem SR®** (Cephalon) ⒫ⓄⓂ

Capsules, m/r, all beige, diltiazem hydrochloride 60 mg, net price 56-cap pack = £6.15; 90 mg, 56-cap pack = £11.51; 120 mg, 56-cap pack = £13.14. Label: 25
Dose angina and mild to moderate hypertension, initially 90 mg twice daily (elderly 60 mg twice daily); up to 180 mg twice daily may be required

**Dilzem XL®** (Cephalon) ⒫ⓄⓂ

Capsules, m/r, diltiazem hydrochloride 120 mg, net price 28-cap pack = £7.93; 180 mg, 28-cap pack = £11.77; 240 mg, 28-cap pack = £11.24. Label: 25
Dose angina and mild to moderate hypertension, initially 180 mg once daily (elderly and in hepatic and renal impairment, 120 mg once daily); if necessary may be increased to 360 mg once daily

**Slozem®** (Merck) ⒫ⓄⓂ

Capsules, m/r, diltiazem hydrochloride 120 mg (pink/clear), net price 28-cap pack = £7.00; 180 mg (pink/clear), 28-cap pack = £7.80; 240 mg (red/clear), 28-cap pack = £8.20; 300 mg (red/white), 28-cap pack = £8.50. Label: 25
Dose angina and mild to moderate hypertension, initially 240 mg once daily (elderly and in hepatic and renal impairment, 120 mg once daily); if necessary may be increased to 360 mg once daily

**Tildiem LA®** (Sanofi-Synthelabo) ⒫ⓄⓂ

Capsules, m/r, diltiazem hydrochloride 200 mg (pink/grey, containing white pellets), net price 28-cap pack = £6.40; 300 mg (white/yellow, containing white pellets), 28-cap pack = £7.22. Label: 25
Dose angina and mild to moderate hypertension, initially 200 mg once daily before or with food, increased if necessary to 300–400 mg daily, max. 500 mg daily; ELDERLY and in hepatic or renal impairment, initially 200 mg daily, increased if necessary to 300 mg daily

**Tildiem Retard®** (Sanofi-Synthelabo) ⒫ⓄⓂ

Tablets, m/r, diltiazem hydrochloride 90 mg, net price 56-tab pack = £7.27; 120 mg, 56-tab pack = £7.15. Label: 25
Counselling Tablet membrane may pass through gastro-intestinal tract unchanged, but being porous has no effect on efficacy
Dose mild to moderate hypertension, initially 90 mg or 120 mg twice daily; increased if necessary to 360 mg daily in divided doses; ELDERLY and in hepatic or renal impairment, initially 120 mg once daily; increased if necessary to 120 mg twice daily
Angina, initially 90 mg or 120 mg twice daily; increased if necessary to 480 mg daily in divided doses; ELDERLY and in hepatic or renal impairment, dose form not appropriate for initial titration; up to 120 mg twice daily may be required

**Viazem XL®** (Genus) [PoM]
Capsules, m/r, diltiazem hydrochloride 120 mg (lavender), net price 28-cap pack = £6.60; 180 mg (white/blue-green), 28-cap pack = £7.36; 240 mg (blue-green/lavender), 28-cap pack = £7.74; 300 mg (white/lavender), 28-cap pack = £8.03; 360 mg (blue-green), 28-cap pack = £14.13. Label: 25
Dose angina and mild to moderate hypertension, initially 180 mg once daily, adjusted according to response to 240 mg once daily; max. 360 mg once daily; ELDERLY and in hepatic or renal impairment, initially 120 mg once daily, adjusted according to response

**Zemtard®** (Galen) [PoM]
Zemtard 120XL capsules, m/r, brown/orange, diltiazem hydrochloride 120 mg, net price 28-cap pack = £6.10. Label: 25

Zemtard 180XL capsules, m/r, grey/pink, diltiazem hydrochloride 180 mg, net price 28-cap pack = £6.20 Label: 25

Zemtard 240XL capsules, m/r, blue, diltiazem hydrochloride 240 mg, net price 28-cap pack = £6.30. Label: 25

Zemtard 300XL capsules, m/r, white/blue, diltiazem hydrochloride 300 mg, net price 28-cap pack = £6.70. Label: 25
Dose angina and mild to moderate hypertension, 180–300 mg once daily, increased if necessary to 360 mg once daily in hypertension and to 480 mg once daily in angina; ELDERLY and in hepatic or renal impairment, initially 120 mg once daily

## FELODIPINE

**Indications** hypertension, prophylaxis of angina
**Cautions** withdraw if ischaemic pain occurs or existing pain worsens shortly after initiating treatment or if cardiogenic shock develops; severe left ventricular dysfunction; avoid grapefruit juice (may affect metabolism); reduce dose in hepatic impairment; breast-feeding (Appendix 5); **interactions:** Appendix 1 (calcium-channel blockers)
**Contra-indications** unstable angina, uncontrolled heart failure; significant aortic stenosis; within 1 month of myocardial infarction; acute porphyria (section 9.8.2); pregnancy (Appendix 4)
**Side-effects** flushing, headache, palpitation, dizziness, fatigue, gravitational oedema; rarely rash, pruritus, cutaneous vasculitis, gum hyperplasia, urinary frequency, impotence, fever
**Dose**
- Hypertension, initially 5 mg (elderly 2.5 mg) daily in the morning; usual maintenance 5–10 mg once daily; doses above 20 mg daily rarely needed
- Angina, initially 5 mg daily in the morning, increased if necessary to 10 mg once daily

**Felodipine** (Non-proprietary) [PoM]
Tablets, m/r, felodipine 2.5 mg, net price 28-tab pack = £6.44; 5 mg, 28-tab pack = £4.30; 10 mg, 28-tab pack = £5.78, 30-tab pack = £12.87. Label: 25
Brands include *Cardioplen XL®*, *Felogen XL®*, *Felotens XL®*, *Keloc SR®*, *Neofel XL®*, *Parmid XL®*, *Vascalpha®*

**Plendil®** (AstraZeneca) [PoM]
Tablets, m/r, f/c, felodipine 2.5 mg (yellow), net price 28-tab pack = £6.44; 5 mg (pink), 28-tab pack = £4.30; 10 mg (brown), 28-tab pack = £5.78. Label: 25

## ISRADIPINE

**Indications** hypertension
**Cautions** sick sinus syndrome (if pacemaker not fitted); avoid grapefruit juice (may affect metabolism); poor cardiac reserve; reduce dose in hepatic or renal impairment; pregnancy (Appendix 4); **interactions:** Appendix 1 (calcium-channel blockers)
**Contra-indications** cardiogenic shock; symptomatic or tight aortic stenosis; during or within 1 month of myocardial infarction; unstable angina; acute porphyria (section 9.8.2); breast-feeding (Appendix 5)
**Side-effects** abdominal discomfort; tachycardia, palpitation, flushing, peripheral oedema; dyspnoea; headache, fatigue, dizziness; polyuria; rash; *less commonly* hypotension, weight gain; *very rarely* vomiting, nausea, gum hyperplasia, anorexia, drowsiness, arrhythmia, bradycardia, heart failure, cough, depression, paraesthesia, anxiety, erectile dysfunction, blood disorders (such as thrombocytopenia, leucopenia, anaemia), arthralgia, visual disturbance, hypersensitivity reactions; hepatitis and gynaecomastia also reported
**Dose**
- 2.5 mg twice daily, increased if necessary after 3–4 weeks to 5 mg twice daily (exceptionally up to 10 mg twice daily); ELDERLY (or in hepatic or renal impairment) 1.25 mg twice daily, increased if necessary after 3–4 weeks according to response, maintenance dose of 2.5 mg or 5 mg once daily may be sufficient

**Prescal®** (Novartis) [PoM]
Tablets, yellow, scored, isradipine 2.5 mg, net price 56-tab pack = £16.54

## LACIDIPINE

**Indications** hypertension
**Cautions** cardiac conduction abnormalities; poor cardiac reserve; avoid grapefruit juice (may affect metabolism); hepatic impairment (Appendix 2); **interactions:** Appendix 1 (calcium-channel blockers)
**Contra-indications** cardiogenic shock, unstable angina, aortic stenosis; avoid within 1 month of myocardial infarction; acute porphyria (section 9.8.2); pregnancy (Appendix 4); breast-feeding (Appendix 5)
**Side-effects** flushing, palpitation, oedema; headache, dizziness; *rarely* gastro-intestinal disturbances, gum hyperplasia, aggravation of angina, mood disturbances, asthenia, polyuria, muscle cramps, skin rash (including pruritus and erythema)
**Dose**
- Initially 2 mg as a single daily dose, preferably in the morning; increased after 3–4 weeks to 4 mg daily, then if necessary to 6 mg daily

**Motens®** (Boehringer Ingelheim) [PoM]
Tablets, both f/c, lacidipine 2 mg, net price 28-tab pack = £4.50; 4 mg (scored), 28-tab pack = £7.00

## LERCANIDIPINE HYDROCHLORIDE

**Indications** mild to moderate hypertension
**Cautions** left ventricular dysfunction; sick sinus syndrome (if pacemaker not fitted); avoid grapefruit juice (may affect metabolism); hepatic impairment (Appendix 2); **interactions:** Appendix 1 (calcium-channel blockers)

**2**
**Cardiovascular system**

**Contra-indications** aortic stenosis; unstable angina, uncontrolled heart failure; within 1 month of myocardial infarction; renal impairment (avoid if eGFR less than 30 mL/minute/1.73 m²); acute porphyria (section 9.8.2); pregnancy (Appendix 4); breast-feeding

**Side-effects** flushing, peripheral oedema, palpitation, tachycardia, headache, dizziness, asthenia; also gastro-intestinal disturbances, hypotension, drowsiness, myalgia, polyuria, rash

**Dose**

• Initially 10 mg once daily; increased, if necessary, after at least 2 weeks to 20 mg daily

**Zanidip®** (Recordati) ℞
Tablets, f/c, lercanidipine hydrochloride 10 mg (yellow), net price 28-tab pack = £5.70; 20 mg (pink), 28-tab pack = £10.82. Label: 22

## NICARDIPINE HYDROCHLORIDE

**Indications** prophylaxis of angina; mild to moderate hypertension

**Cautions** withdraw if ischaemic pain occurs or existing pain worsens within 30 minutes of initiating treatment or increasing dose; congestive heart failure or significantly impaired left ventricular function; elderly; avoid grapefruit juice (may affect metabolism); hepatic impairment (Appendix 2); renal impairment (Appendix 3); pregnancy (Appendix 4); **interactions:** Appendix 1 (calcium-channel blockers)

**Contra-indications** cardiogenic shock; advanced aortic stenosis; unstable or acute attacks of angina; avoid within 1 month of myocardial infarction; acute porphyria (section 9.8.2); breast-feeding (Appendix 5)

**Side-effects** dizziness, headache, peripheral oedema, flushing, palpitation, nausea; also gastro-intestinal disturbances, drowsiness, insomnia, tinnitus, hypotension, rashes, dyspnoea, paraesthesia, frequency of micturition; thrombocytopenia, depression and impotence reported

**Dose**

• Initially 20 mg 3 times daily, increased, after at least three days, to 30 mg 3 times daily (usual range 60–120 mg daily)

**Nicardipine** (Non-proprietary) ℞
Capsules, nicardipine hydrochloride 20 mg, net price 56-cap pack = £3.00; 30 mg, 56-cap pack = £4.49

**Cardene®** (Astellas) ℞
Capsules, nicardipine hydrochloride 20 mg (blue/white), net price 56-cap pack = £8.57; 30 mg (blue/pale blue), 56-cap pack = £9.95

◢Modified release
**Cardene SR®** (Astellas) ℞
Capsules, m/r, nicardipine hydrochloride 30 mg, net price 56-cap pack = £10.21; 45 mg (blue), 56-cap pack = £14.86. Label: 25
Dose mild to moderate hypertension, initially 30 mg twice daily; usual effective dose 45 mg twice daily (range 30–60 mg twice daily)

## NIFEDIPINE

**Indications** prophylaxis of angina; hypertension; Raynaud's phenomenon

**Cautions** see notes above; also withdraw if ischaemic pain occurs or existing pain worsens shortly after

initiating treatment; poor cardiac reserve; heart failure or significantly impaired left ventricular function (heart failure deterioration observed); severe hypotension; elderly; diabetes mellitus; hepatic impairment (Appendix 2); may inhibit labour; pregnancy (Appendix 4); breast-feeding (Appendix 5); avoid grapefruit juice (may affect metabolism); **interactions:** Appendix 1 (calcium-channel blockers)

**Contra-indications** cardiogenic shock; advanced aortic stenosis; within 1 month of myocardial infarction; unstable or acute attacks of angina; acute porphyria (section 9.8.2)

**Side-effects** gastro-intestinal disturbance; hypotension, oedema, vasodilatation, palpitation; headache, dizziness, lethargy, asthenia; *less commonly* tachycardia, syncope, chills, nasal congestion, dyspnoea, anxiety, sleep disturbance, vertigo, migraine, paraesthesia, tremor, polyuria, dysuria, nocturia, erectile dysfunction, epistaxis, myalgia, joint swelling, visual disturbance, sweating, hypersensitivity reactions (including angioedema, jaundice, pruritus, urticaria, and rash); *rarely* anorexia, gum hyperplasia, mood disturbances, hyperglycaemia, male infertility, purpura, and photosensitivity reactions; also reported dysphagia, intestinal obstruction, intestinal ulcer, bezoar formation (with some modified-release preparations), gynaecomastia, agranulocytosis, and anaphylaxis

**Dose**

• See preparations below

**Nifedipine** (Non-proprietary) ℞
Capsules, nifedipine 5 mg, net price 84-cap pack = £2.89; 10 mg, 84-cap pack = £3.90
Dose angina prophylaxis (but not recommended, see notes above) and Raynaud's phenomenon, initially 5 mg 3 times daily, adjusted according to response to 20 mg 3 times daily
Hypertension, not recommended therefore no dose stated

**Adalat®** (Bayer) ℞
Capsules, orange, nifedipine 5 mg, net price 90-cap pack = £5.84; 10 mg, 90-cap pack = £7.44
Dose angina prophylaxis (but not recommended, see notes above) and Raynaud's phenomenon, initially 5 mg 3 times daily, adjusted according to response to max. 20 mg 3 times daily
Hypertension, not recommended therefore no dose stated

◢Modified release
Note Different versions of modified-release preparations may not have the same clinical effect. To avoid confusion between these different formulations of nifedipine, prescribers should specify the brand to be dispensed. Modified-release formulations may not be suitable for dose titration in hepatic disease

**Adalat® LA** (Bayer) ℞
LA 20 tablets, m/r, f/c, pink, nifedipine 20 mg, net price 28-tab pack = £5.06. Label: 25
LA 30 tablets, m/r, f/c, pink, nifedipine 30 mg, net price 28-tab pack = £7.13. Label: 25
LA 60 tablets, m/r, f/c, pink, nifedipine 60 mg, net price 28-tab pack = £9.31. Label: 25
Counselling Tablet membrane may pass through gastro-intestinal tract unchanged, but being porous has no effect on efficacy
Dose hypertension, 20–30 mg once daily, increased if necessary to max. 90 mg once daily
Angina prophylaxis, 30 mg once daily, increased if necessary to max. 90 mg once daily
Cautions dose form not appropriate for use in hepatic impairment or where there is a history of oesophageal or gastro-intestinal obstruction, decreased lumen diameter of the gastro-intestinal tract, or inflammatory bowel disease (including Crohn's disease)

**Adalat® Retard** (Bayer) PoM

Retard 10 tablets, m/r, f/c, grey-pink, nifedipine 10 mg, net price 56-tab pack = £7.48. Label: 25

Retard 20 tablets, m/r, f/c, grey-pink, nifedipine 20 mg, net price 56-tab pack = £8.98. Label: 25

Dose hypertension and angina prophylaxis, 10 mg twice daily, adjusted according to response to 40 mg twice daily

**Adipine® MR** (Chiesi) PoM

Tablets, m/r, nifedipine 10 mg (apricot), net price 56-tab pack = £5.73; 20 mg (pink), 56-tab pack = £7.14. Label: 21, 25

Dose hypertension and angina prophylaxis, 20 mg twice daily after food (initial titration 10 mg twice daily); max. 40 mg twice daily

**Adipine® XL** (Chiesi) PoM

Tablets, m/r, red, nifedipine 30 mg, net price 28-tab pack = £5.66; 60 mg, 28-tab pack = £8.50. Label: 25

Dose hypertension and angina prophylaxis, 30 mg once daily, increased if necessary; max. 90 mg once daily

**Coracten SR®** (UCB Pharma) PoM

Capsules, m/r, nifedipine 10 mg (grey/pink, enclosing yellow pellets), net price 60-cap pack = £3.90; 20 mg (pink/brown, enclosing yellow pellets), 60-cap pack = £5.41. Label: 25

Dose hypertension and angina prophylaxis, initially 10 mg twice daily, increased if necessary to max. 40 mg twice daily

**Coracten XL®** (UCB Pharma) PoM

Capsules, m/r, nifedipine 30 mg (brown), net price 28-cap pack = £4.89; 60 mg (orange), 28-cap pack = £7.34. Label: 25

Dose hypertension and angina prophylaxis, 30 mg once daily, increased if necessary; max. 90 mg once daily

**Fortipine LA 40®** (Goldshield) PoM

Tablets, m/r, red, nifedipine 40 mg, net price 30-tab pack = £9.60. Label: 21, 25

Dose hypertension and angina prophylaxis, 40 mg once daily, increased if necessary to 80 mg daily in 1–2 divided doses

**Hypolar® Retard 20** (Sandoz) PoM

Tablets, m/r, red, f/c, nifedipine 20 mg, net price 56-tab pack = £5.75. Label: 25

Dose hypertension and angina prophylaxis, 20 mg twice daily, increased if necessary to 40 mg twice daily

**Nifedipress® MR** (Dexcel) PoM

Tablets, m/r, pink, nifedipine 10 mg, net price 56-tab pack = £2.02; 20 mg, 56-tab pack = £2.02. Label: 25

Dose hypertension and angina prophylaxis, initially 10 mg twice daily adjusted according to response to 40 mg twice daily

Note Also available as Calchan® MR, Kentipine® MR

**Tensipine MR®** (Genus) PoM

Tablets, m/r, pink-grey, nifedipine 10 mg, net price 56-tab pack = £4.30; 20 mg, 56-tab pack = £5.49. Label: 21, 25

Dose hypertension and angina prophylaxis, initially 10 mg twice daily adjusted according to response to 40 mg twice daily

**Valni XL®** (Winthrop) PoM

Tablets, m/r, red, nifedipine 30 mg, net price 28-tab pack = £7.29; 60 mg, 28-tab pack = £9.31. Label: 25

Dose severe hypertension and prophylaxis of angina, 30 mg once daily, increased if necessary to max. 90 mg once daily

Cautions dose form not appropriate for use in hepatic impairment, or where there is a history of oesophageal or gastro-intestinal obstruction, decreased lumen diameter of the gastro-intestinal tract, inflammatory bowel disease, or ileostomy after proctocolectomy

◢**With atenolol**

Section 2.4

◢ **NIMODIPINE**

**Indications** prevention and treatment of ischaemic neurological deficits following aneurysmal subarachnoid haemorrhage

**Cautions** cerebral oedema or severely raised intracranial pressure; hypotension; avoid concomitant administration of nimodipine tablets and infusion, other calcium-channel blockers, or beta-blockers; concomitant nephrotoxic drugs; avoid grapefruit juice (may affect metabolism); hepatic impairment (Appendix 2); renal impairment (Appendix 3); pregnancy (Appendix 4); **interactions:** Appendix 1 (calcium-channel blockers, alcohol (infusion only))

**Contra-indications** within 1 month of myocardial infarction; unstable angina; acute porphyria (section 9.8.2)

**Side-effects** hypotension, variation in heart-rate, flushing, headache, gastro-intestinal disorders, nausea, sweating and feeling of warmth; thrombocytopenia and ileus reported

**Dose**

- Prevention, by mouth, 60 mg every 4 hours, starting within 4 days of aneurysmal subarachnoid haemorrhage and continued for 21 days

- Treatment, by intravenous infusion via central catheter, initially 1 mg/hour (up to 500 micrograms/hour if body-weight less than 70 kg or if blood pressure unstable), increased after 2 hours to 2 mg/hour if no severe fall in blood pressure; continue for at least 5 days (max. 14 days); if surgical intervention during treatment, continue for at least 5 days after surgery; max. total duration of nimodipine use 21 days

**Nimotop®** (Bayer) PoM

Tablets, yellow, f/c, nimodipine 30 mg, net price 100-tab pack = £37.33

Intravenous infusion, nimodipine 200 micrograms/mL; also contains ethanol 20% and macrogol '400' 17%. Net price 50-mL vial (with polyethylene infusion catheter) = £7.47

Note Polyethylene, polypropylene, or glass apparatus should be used; PVC should be avoided

◢ **VERAPAMIL HYDROCHLORIDE**

**Indications** see under Dose and preparations

**Cautions** first-degree AV block; acute phase of myocardial infarction (avoid if bradycardia, hypotension, left ventricular failure); patients taking beta-blockers (**important:** see below); hepatic impairment (Appendix 2); children, specialist advice only (section 2.3.2); pregnancy (Appendix 4) and breast-feeding (Appendix 5); avoid grapefruit juice (may affect metabolism); **interactions:** Appendix 1 (calcium-channel blockers)
Verapamil and beta-blockers **Verapamil** injection should not be given to patients recently treated with beta-blockers because of the risk of hypotension and asystole. The suggestion that when verapamil injection has been given first, an interval of 30 minutes before giving a beta-blocker is sufficient has not been confirmed.
It may also be hazardous to give verapamil and a beta-blocker together by mouth (should only be contemplated if myocardial function well preserved).

**Contra-indications** hypotension, bradycardia, second- and third-degree AV block, sick sinus syndrome, cardiogenic shock, sino-atrial block; history of heart failure or significantly impaired left ventricular function, even if controlled by therapy; atrial flutter or

**2**

**Cardiovascular system**

fibrillation associated with accessory conducting pathways (e.g. Wolff-Parkinson-White syndrome); acute porphyria (section 9.8.2)

**Side-effects** constipation; less commonly nausea, vomiting, flushing, headache, dizziness, fatigue, ankle oedema; rarely allergic reactions (erythema, pruritus, urticaria, angioedema, Stevens-Johnson syndrome); myalgia, arthralgia, paraesthesia, erythromelalgia; increased prolactin concentration; rarely gynaecomastia and gingival hyperplasia after long-term treatment; after intravenous administration or high doses, hypotension, heart failure, bradycardia, heart block, and asystole

**Dose**

- By mouth, supraventricular arrhythmias (but see also Contra-indications), 40–120 mg 3 times daily
  Angina, 80–120 mg 3 times daily
  Hypertension, 240–480 mg daily in 2–3 divided doses
- By slow intravenous injection over 2 minutes (3 minutes in elderly), supraventricular arrhythmias (but see also Contra-indications), 5–10 mg (preferably with ECG monitoring); in paroxysmal tachyarrhythmias a further 5 mg after 5–10 minutes if required

**Verapamil** (Non-proprietary) [PoM]

Tablets, coated, verapamil hydrochloride 40 mg, net price 84-tab pack = £1.55; 80 mg, 84-tab pack = £1.73; 120 mg, 28-tab pack = £1.44; 160 mg, 56-tab pack = £22.42

Oral solution, verapamil hydrochloride 40 mg/5 mL, net price 150 mL = £36.90
Brands include *Zolvera*®

**Cordilox**® (Dexcel) [PoM]

Tablets, yellow, f/c, verapamil hydrochloride 40 mg, net price 84-tab pack = £1.50; 80 mg, 84-tab pack = £2.05; 120 mg, 28-tab pack = £1.15; 160 mg, 56-tab pack = £2.80

Injection, verapamil hydrochloride 2.5 mg/mL, net price 2-mL amp = £1.11

**Securon**® (Abbott) [PoM]

Injection, verapamil hydrochloride 2.5 mg/mL, net price 2-mL amp = £1.08

◀**Modified release**

**Half Securon SR**® (Abbott) [PoM]

Tablets, m/r, f/c, verapamil hydrochloride 120 mg, net price 28-tab pack = £7.86. Label: 25
Dose see *Securon SR*®

**Securon SR**® (Abbott) [PoM]

Tablets, m/r, pale green, f/c, scored, verapamil hydrochloride 240 mg, net price 28-tab pack = £5.66. Label: 25
Dose hypertension, 240 mg daily (new patients initially 120 mg), increased if necessary to max. 480 mg daily (doses above 240 mg daily as 2 divided doses)
Angina, 240 mg twice daily (may sometimes be reduced to once daily)
Prophylaxis after myocardial infarction where beta-blockers not appropriate (started at least 1 week after infarction), 360 mg daily in divided doses, given as 240 mg in the morning and 120 mg in the evening *or* 120 mg 3 times daily

**Univer**® (Cephalon) [PoM]

Capsules, m/r, verapamil hydrochloride 120 mg (yellow/dark blue), net price 28-cap pack = £4.96;

180 mg (yellow), 56-cap pack = £11.98; 240 mg (yellow/dark blue), 28-cap pack = £8.08. Label: 25
Dose hypertension, 240 mg daily, max. 480 mg daily (new patients, initial dose 120 mg); angina, 360 mg daily, max. 480 mg daily

**Verapress MR**® (Dexcel) [PoM]

Tablets, m/r, pale green, f/c, verapamil hydrochloride 240 mg, net price 28-tab pack = £6.04. Label: 25
Dose hypertension, 1 tablet daily, increased to twice daily if necessary; angina, 1 tablet twice daily (may sometimes be reduced to once daily)
Note Also available as *Cordilox*® *MR*

**Vertab**® **SR 240** (Chiesi) [PoM]

Tablets, m/r, pale green, f/c, scored, verapamil hydrochloride 240 mg, net price 28-tab pack = £8.29. Label: 25
Dose mild to moderate hypertension, 240 mg daily, increased to twice daily if necessary; angina, 240 mg twice daily (may sometimes be reduced to once daily)

## 2.6.3  Other antianginal drugs

**Nicorandil**, a potassium-channel activator with a nitrate component, has both arterial and venous vasodilating properties and is licensed for the prevention and long-term treatment of angina (section 2.6). Nicorandil has similar efficacy to other antianginal drugs in controlling symptoms; it may produce additional symptomatic benefit in combination with other antianginal drugs [unlicensed indication].

**Ivabradine** lowers the heart rate by its action on the sinus node. It is licensed for the treatment of angina in patients in normal sinus rhythm when beta-blockers are contra-indicated or not tolerated.

**Ranolazine** is licensed as adjunctive therapy in patients who are inadequately controlled or intolerant of first-line antianginal drugs.

### ■ IVABRADINE

**Indications** treatment of angina in patients in normal sinus rhythm (see notes above)

**Cautions** mild heart failure including asymptomatic left ventricular dysfunction; monitor for atrial fibrillation or other arrhythmias (treatment ineffective); hypotension (avoid if severe); retinitis pigmentosa; elderly; hepatic impairment (avoid if severe; Appendix 2); renal impairment (Appendix 3); **interactions**: Appendix 1 (ivabradine)

**Contra-indications** severe bradycardia (not to be initiated if heart rate below 60 beats per minute); cardiogenic shock; acute myocardial infarction; immediately after cerebrovascular accident; sicksinus syndrome; sino-atrial block; moderate to severe heart failure; patients with pacemaker; unstable angina; second- and third-degree heart block; congenital QT syndrome; pregnancy (Appendix 4); breastfeeding (Appendix 5)

**Side-effects** bradycardia, first-degree heart block, ventricular extrasystoles; headache, dizziness; visual disturbances including phosphenes and blurred vision; *less commonly* nausea, constipation, diarrhoea, palpitations, supraventricular extrasystoles, dyspnoea, vertigo, muscle cramps, eosinophilia, hyperuricaemia, and raised plasma-creatinine concentration

**Dose**

- Initially 5 mg twice daily, increased if necessary after 3–4 weeks to 7.5 mg twice daily (if not tolerated reduce dose to 2.5–5 mg twice daily); ELDERLY initially 2.5 mg twice daily
  **Note** Ventricular rate at rest should not be allowed to fall below 50 beats per minute

**Procoralan®** (Servier) ▼ [PoM]
Tablets, pink, f/c, ivabradine (as hydrochloride) 5 mg (scored), net price 56-tab pack = £39.00; 7.5 mg, 56-tab pack = £39.00

## NICORANDIL

**Indications**  prophylaxis and treatment of angina

**Cautions**  hypovolaemia; low systolic blood pressure; acute pulmonary oedema; acute myocardial infarction with acute left ventricular failure and low filling pressures; pregnancy (Appendix 4); **interactions:** Appendix 1 (nicorandil)
**Driving** Patients should be warned not to drive or operate machinery until it is established that their performance is unimpaired

**Contra-indications**  cardiogenic shock; left ventricular failure with low filling pressures; hypotension; breast-feeding

**Side-effects**  headache (especially on initiation, usually transitory); cutaneous vasodilatation with flushing; nausea, vomiting, dizziness, weakness also reported; *rarely* oral ulceration, myalgia, and rash; at high dosage, reduction in blood pressure and/or increase in heart rate; angioedema, hepatic dysfunction, and anal ulceration also reported

**Dose**

- Initially 10 mg twice daily (if susceptible to headache 5 mg twice daily); usual dose 10–20 mg twice daily; up to 30 mg twice daily may be used

**Ikorel®** (Rhône-Poulenc Rorer) [PoM]
Tablets, scored, nicorandil 10 mg, net price 60-tab pack = £8.18; 20 mg, 60-tab pack = £15.54

## RANOLAZINE

**Indications**  as adjunctive therapy in the treatment of stable angina in patients inadequately controlled or intolerant of first-line antianginal therapies

**Cautions**  moderate to severe congestive heart failure; QT interval prolongation; elderly; body-weight less than 60 kg; hepatic impairment (avoid if moderate or severe;Appendix 2); renal impairment (avoid if eGFR less than 30 mL/minute/1.73 m²; Appendix 3); pregnancy (Appendix 4); **interactions:** Appendix 1 (ranolazine)

**Contra-indications**  breast-feeding

**Side-effects**  constipation, nausea, vomiting; dizziness, headache, asthenia; *less commonly* abdominal pain, weight loss, dry mouth, dyspepsia, flatulence; hot flush, hypotension, syncope, prolonged QT interval, peripheral oedema; dyspnoea, cough, epistaxis; lethargy, hypoaesthesia, drowsiness, tremor, anxiety, insomnia, anorexia; dysuria, haematuria, chromaturia; dehydration; pain in extremities, muscle cramp, joint swelling; visual disturbance; tinnitus; pruritus, sweating; *rarely* pancreatitis, erosive duodenitis; cold extremities; throat tightness; amnesia, loss of consciousness, disorientation; erectile dysfunction;

parosmia, impaired hearing; allergic dermatitis, urticaria, rash

**Dose**

- ADULT over 18 years, initially 375 mg twice daily, increased after 2–4 weeks to 500 mg twice daily and then adjusted according to response to max. 750 mg twice daily (reduce dose to 375–500 mg twice daily if not tolerated)

**Ranexa®** (Menarini) ▼ [PoM]
Tablets, m/r, ranolazine 375 mg (blue), net price 60-tab pack = £48.98; 500 mg (orange), 60-tab pack = £48.98; 750 mg (green), 60-tab pack = £48.98.
Label: 25, patient alert card

## 2.6.4 Peripheral vasodilators and related drugs

Peripheral vascular disease can be either occlusive (e.g. *intermittent claudication*) in which occlusion of the peripheral arteries is caused by atherosclerosis, or vasospastic (e.g. *Raynaud's syndrome*).

Peripheral arterial occlusive disease is associated with an increased risk of cardiovascular events; this risk is reduced by measures such as smoking cessation (section 4.10), effective control of blood pressure (section 2.5), regulating blood lipids (section 2.12), optimising glycaemic control in diabetes (section 6.1), taking aspirin in a dose of 75 mg daily (section 2.9), and possibly weight reduction in obesity (section 4.5). Exercise training, treatment with cilostazol or naftidrofuryl (see below), and possibly statin therapy can improve symptoms of intermittent claudication.

**Cilostazol** is licensed for use in intermittent claudication to improve walking distance in patients without peripheral tissue necrosis who do not have pain at rest. Patients receiving cilostazol should be assessed for improvement after 3 months. The *Scottish Medicines Consortium* (p. 3) has advised (October 2005) that cilostazol is not recommended for the treatment of intermittent claudication within NHS Scotland.

**Naftidrofuryl** can alleviate symptoms of intermittent claudication and improve pain-free walking distance in moderate disease. Patients taking naftidrofuryl should be assessed for improvement after 3–6 months.

Inositol nicotinate, pentoxifylline (oxpentifylline), and cinnarizine are not established as being effective for the treatment of intermittent claudication.

Management of *Raynaud's syndrome* includes avoidance of exposure to cold and stopping smoking. More severe symptoms may require vasodilator treatment, which is most often successful in primary Raynaud's syndrome. **Nifedipine** (section 2.6.2) is useful for reducing the frequency and severity of vasospastic attacks. Alternatively, **naftidrofuryl** may produce symptomatic improvement; **inositol nicotinate** (a nicotinic acid derivative) may also be considered. Cinnarizine, pentoxifylline, prazosin, and moxisylyte (thymoxamine) are not established as being effective for the treatment of Raynaud's syndrome.

Vasodilator therapy is not established as being effective for *chilblains* (section 13.13).

2

Cardiovascular system

2 Cardiovascular system

## CILOSTAZOL

**Indications** intermittent claudication in patients without rest pain and no peripheral tissue necrosis

**Cautions** atrial or ventricular ectopy, atrial fibrillation, atrial flutter; diabetes mellitus (higher risk of intra-ocular bleeding); concomitant drugs that increase risk of bleeding; hepatic impairment (Appendix 2); **inter-actions:** Appendix 1 (cilostazol)

**Contra-indications** predisposition to bleeding (e.g. active peptic ulcer, haemorrhagic stroke in previous 6 months, surgery in previous 3 months, proliferative diabetic retinopathy, poorly controlled hypertension); history of ventricular tachycardia, of ventricular fibrillation and of multifocal ventricular ectopics; prolongation of QT interval, congestive heart failure; renal impairment (if eGFR less than 25 mL/minute/ 1.73 m²); pregnancy (Appendix 4); breast-feeding (Appendix 5)

**Side-effects** gastro-intestinal disturbances; tachy-cardia, palpitation, angina, arrhythmia, chest pain, oedema; rhinitis; dizziness, headache; asthenia; rash, pruritus, ecchymosis; *less commonly* gastritis, conges-tive heart failure, postural hypotension, dyspnoea, pneumonia, cough, insomnia, abnormal dreams, anxiety, hyperglycaemia, diabetes mellitus, anaemia, haemorrhage, myalgia, hypersensitivity reactions (including Stevens-Johnson syndrome and toxic epi-dermal necrolysis in rare cases); *rarely* anorexia, hypertension, paresis, increased urinary frequency, bleeding disorders, renal impairment, conjunctivitis, tinnitus, and jaundice

**Dose**

● 100 mg twice daily (30 minutes before or 2 hours after food)

**Pletal®** (Otsuka) (PoM)
Tablets, cilostazol 50 mg, net price 56-tab pack = £35.31; 100 mg, 56-tab pack = £35.31

## INOSITOL NICOTINATE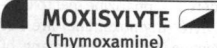

**Indications** peripheral vascular disease; hyperlipid-aemia (section 2.12)

**Cautions** cerebrovascular insufficiency, unstable angina

**Contra-indications** recent myocardial infarction, acute phase of a cerebrovascular accident; pregnancy (Appendix 4)

**Side-effects** nausea, vomiting, hypotension, flushing, syncope, oedema, headache, dizziness, paraesthesia, rash

**Dose**

● 3 g daily in 2–3 divided doses; max. 4 g daily

**Hexopal®** (Genus)
Tablets, scored, inositol nicotinate 500 mg, net price 20 = £4.10
Tablets forte, scored, inositol nicotinate 750 mg, net price 112-tab pack = £34.02

## MOXISYLYTE
(Thymoxamine)

**Indications** primary Raynaud's syndrome (short-term treatment)

**Cautions** diabetes mellitus

**Contra-indications** active liver disease; pregnancy (Appendix 4)

**Side-effects** nausea, diarrhoea, flushing, headache, dizziness; hepatic reactions including cholestatic jaundice and hepatitis reported to CSM

**Dose**

● Initially 40 mg 4 times daily, increased to 80 mg 4 times daily if poor initial response; discontinue after 2 weeks if no response

**Opilon®** (Concord) (PoM)
Tablets, yellow, f/c, moxisylyte 40 mg (as hydro-chloride), net price 112-tab pack = £95.98. Label: 21

## NAFTIDROFURYL OXALATE

**Indications** see under Dose

**Side-effects** nausea, epigastric pain, rash, hepatitis, hepatic failure

**Dose**

● Peripheral vascular disease (see notes above), 100–200 mg 3 times daily

● Cerebral vascular disease, 100 mg 3 times daily

**Naftidrofuryl** (Non-proprietary) (PoM)
Capsules, naftidrofuryl oxalate 100 mg, net price 84-cap pack = £5.24. Label: 25, 27

**Praxilene®** (Merck) (PoM)
Capsules, pink, naftidrofuryl oxalate 100 mg, net price 84-cap pack = £8.26. Label: 25, 27

## PENTOXIFYLLINE
(Oxpentifylline)

**Indications** peripheral vascular disease; venous leg ulcers [unlicensed indication] (Appendix A8.2.5)

**Cautions** hypotension, coronary artery disease; renal impairment (Appendix 3), severe hepatic impairment; avoid in acute porphyria (section 9.8.2); **interactions:** Appendix 1 (pentoxifylline)

**Contra-indications** cerebral haemorrhage, extensive retinal haemorrhage, acute myocardial infarction; pregnancy and breast-feeding

**Side-effects** gastro-intestinal disturbances, dizziness, agitation, sleep disturbances, headache; *rarely* flush-ing, tachycardia, angina, hypotension, thrombocyto-penia, intrahepatic cholestasis, hypersensitivity reac-tions including rash, pruritus and bronchospasm

**Dose**

● 400 mg 2–3 times daily

**Trental®** (Aventis Pharma) (PoM)
Tablets, m/r, pink, s/c, pentoxifylline 400 mg, net price 90-tab pack = £19.68. Label: 21, 25

## Other preparations used in peripheral vascular disease

Rutosides (oxerutins, *Paroven®*) are not vasodilators and are not generally regarded as effective preparations as capillary sealants or for the treatment of cramps; side-effects include headache, flushing, rashes, mild gastro-intestinal disturbances.

**Paroven®** (Novartis Consumer Health) ◢
Capsules, yellow, oxerutins 250 mg, net price 120-cap pack = £13.05
**Dose** relief of symptoms of oedema associated with chronic venous insufficiency, 500 mg twice daily

# 2.7 Sympathomimetics

### 2.7.1 Inotropic sympathomimetics
### 2.7.2 Vasoconstrictor sympathomimetics
### 2.7.3 Cardiopulmonary resuscitation

The properties of sympathomimetics vary according to whether they act on alpha or on beta adrenergic receptors. Adrenaline (epinephrine) (section 2.7.3) acts on both alpha and beta receptors and increases both heart rate and contractility (beta$_1$ effects); it can cause peripheral vasodilation (a beta$_2$ effect) or vasoconstriction (an alpha effect).

## 2.7.1 Inotropic sympathomimetics

The cardiac stimulants **dobutamine** and **dopamine** act on beta$_1$ receptors in cardiac muscle, and increase contractility with little effect on rate.

**Dopexamine** acts on beta$_2$ receptors in cardiac muscle to produce its positive inotropic effect; and on peripheral dopamine receptors to increase renal perfusion; it is reported not to induce vasoconstriction.

**Isoprenaline** injection is available from 'special-order' manufacturers or specialist importing companies, see p. 969.

**Shock** Shock is a medical emergency associated with a high mortality. The underlying causes of shock such as haemorrhage, sepsis, or myocardial insufficiency should be corrected. The profound hypotension of shock must be treated promptly to prevent tissue hypoxia and organ failure. Volume replacement is essential to correct the hypovolaemia associated with haemorrhage and sepsis but may be detrimental in cardiogenic shock. Depending on haemodynamic status, cardiac output may be improved by the use of sympathomimetic inotropes such as adrenaline (epinephrine), dobutamine or dopamine (see notes above). In septic shock, when fluid replacement and inotropic support fail to maintain blood pressure, the vasoconstrictor noradrenaline (norepinephrine) (section 2.7.2) may be considered. In cardiogenic shock peripheral resistance is frequently high and to raise it further may worsen myocardial performance and exacerbate tissue ischaemia.

The use of sympathomimetic inotropes and vasoconstrictors should preferably be confined to the intensive care setting and undertaken with invasive haemodynamic monitoring.

For advice on the management of anaphylactic shock, see section 3.4.3.

## DOBUTAMINE

**Indications** inotropic support in infarction, cardiac surgery, cardiomyopathies, septic shock, and cardiogenic shock

**Cautions** hyperthyroidism; pregnancy (Appendix 4); **interactions:** Appendix 1 (sympathomimetics)

**Side-effects** tachycardia and marked increase in systolic blood pressure indicate overdosage; phlebitis; *rarely* thrombocytopenia

**Dose**
• By intravenous infusion, 2.5–10 micrograms/kg/minute, adjusted according to response

**Dobutamine** (Non-proprietary) ▣PoM
Strong sterile solution, dobutamine (as hydrochloride) 12.5 mg/mL. For dilution and use as an intravenous infusion. Net price 20-mL amp = £5.20

## DOPAMINE HYDROCHLORIDE

**Indications** cardiogenic shock in infarction or cardiac surgery

**Cautions** correct hypovolaemia; low dose in shock due to acute myocardial infarction—see notes above; hyperthyroidism; pregnancy (Appendix 4); **interactions:** Appendix 1 (sympathomimetics)

**Contra-indications** tachyarrhythmia, phaeochromocytoma

**Side-effects** nausea and vomiting, peripheral vasoconstriction, hypotension, hypertension, tachycardia

**Dose**
• By intravenous infusion, 2–5 micrograms/kg/minute initially (see notes above)

**Dopamine** (Non-proprietary) ▣PoM
Sterile concentrate, dopamine hydrochloride 40 mg/mL, net price 5-mL amp = £3.88; 160 mg/mL, 5-mL amp = £14.75. For dilution and use as an intravenous infusion

Intravenous infusion, dopamine hydrochloride 1.6 mg/mL in glucose 5% intravenous infusion, net price 250-mL container (400 mg) = £11.69; 3.2 mg/mL, 250-mL container (800 mg) = £22.93 (both hosp. only)

**Select-A-Jet® Dopamine** (UCB Pharma) ▣PoM
Strong sterile solution, dopamine hydrochloride 40 mg/mL, net price 5-mL vial = £5.51; 10-mL vial = £8.86. For dilution and use as an intravenous infusion

## DOPEXAMINE HYDROCHLORIDE

**Indications** inotropic support and vasodilator in exacerbations of chronic heart failure and in heart failure associated with cardiac surgery

**Cautions** myocardial infarction, recent angina, hypokalaemia, hyperglycaemia; correct hypovolaemia before starting and during treatment, monitor blood pressure, pulse, plasma potassium, and blood glucose; hyperthyroidism; avoid abrupt withdrawal; pregnancy; **interactions:** Appendix 1 (sympathomimetics)

**Contra-indications** left ventricular outlet obstruction such as hypertrophic cardiomyopathy or aortic stenosis; phaeochromocytoma, thrombocytopenia

**Side-effects** nausea, vomiting; tachycardia, bradycardia, arrhythmias, angina, myocardial infarction; tremor, headache; dyspnoea; reversible thrombocytopenia; sweating

**Dose**
• By intravenous infusion into central or large peripheral vein, 500 nanograms/kg/minute, may be

2

Cardiovascular system

increased to 1 microgram/kg/minute and further increased up to 6 micrograms/kg/minute in increments of 0.5–1 microgram/kg/minute at intervals of not less than 15 minutes

**Dopacard®** (Cephalon) PoM
Strong sterile solution, dopexamine hydrochloride 10 mg/mL (1%). For dilution and use as an intravenous infusion. Net price 5-mL amp = £20.18
Note Contact with metal in infusion apparatus should be minimised

## 2.7.2 Vasoconstrictor sympathomimetics

Vasoconstrictor sympathomimetics raise blood pressure transiently by acting on alpha-adrenergic receptors to constrict peripheral vessels. They are sometimes used as an emergency method of elevating blood pressure where other measures have failed (see also section 2.7.1).

The danger of vasoconstrictors is that although they raise blood pressure they also reduce perfusion of vital organs such as the kidney.

Spinal and epidural anaesthesia may result in sympathetic block with resultant hypotension. Management may include intravenous fluids (which are usually given prophylactically), oxygen (section 3.6), elevation of the legs, and injection of a pressor drug such as ephedrine. As well as constricting peripheral vessels **ephedrine** also accelerates the heart rate (by acting on beta receptors). Use is made of this dual action of ephedrine to manage associated bradycardia (although intravenous injection of atropine sulphate 400 to 600 micrograms may also be required if bradycardia persists).

### ▌ EPHEDRINE HYDROCHLORIDE

**Indications**  see under Dose
**Cautions**  hyperthyroidism, diabetes mellitus, ischaemic heart disease, hypertension, susceptibility to angle-closure glaucoma, elderly, pregnancy (Appendix 4); may cause acute urine retention in prostatic hypertrophy; **Interactions:** Appendix 1 (sympathomimetics)
**Contra-indications**  breast-feeding (Appendix 5)
**Side-effects**  nausea, vomiting, anorexia; tachycardia (sometimes bradycardia), arrhythmias, anginal pain, vasoconstriction with hypertension, vasodilation with hypotension, dizziness and flushing; dyspnoea; headache, anxiety, restlessness, confusion, psychoses, insomnia, tremor; difficulty in micturition, urine retention; sweating, hypersalivation; changes in blood-glucose concentration; *very rarely* angle-closure glaucoma
**Dose**
● Reversal of hypotension from spinal or epidural anaesthesia, by slow intravenous injection of a solution containing ephedrine hydrochloride 3 mg/mL, 3–6 mg (max. 9 mg) repeated every 3–4 minutes according to response to max. 30 mg

**Ephedrine Hydrochloride** (Non-proprietary) PoM
Injection, ephedrine hydrochloride 3 mg/mL, net price 10-mL amp = £2.83; 30 mg/mL, net price 1-mL amp = £1.70

### ▌ METARAMINOL

**Indications**  acute hypotension (see notes above); priapism (section 7.4.5) [unlicensed indication]
**Cautions**  see under Noradrenaline Acid Tartrate; longer duration of action than noradrenaline (norepinephrine), see below; cirrhosis; pregnancy (Appendix 4); breast-feeding (Appendix 5)
**Hypertensive response** Metaraminol has a longer duration of action than noradrenaline, and an excessive vasopressor response may cause a prolonged rise in blood pressure
**Contra-indications**  see under Noradrenaline Acid Tartrate
**Side-effects**  see under Noradrenaline Acid Tartrate; tachycardia; fatal ventricular arrhythmia reported in Laennec's cirrhosis
**Dose**
● By intravenous infusion, 15–100 mg, adjusted according to response
● In emergency, by intravenous injection, 0.5–5 mg then by intravenous infusion, 15–100 mg, adjusted according to response

**Metaraminol** (Non-proprietary) PoM
Injection, metaraminol 10 mg (as tartrate)/mL
Available from 'special-order' manufacturers or specialist importing companies, see p. 969

### ▌ NORADRENALINE ACID TARTRATE/ NOREPINEPHRINE BITARTRATE

**Indications**  see under dose
**Cautions**  coronary, mesenteric, or peripheral vascular thrombosis; following myocardial infarction, Prinzmetal's variant angina, hyperthyroidism, diabetes mellitus; hypoxia or hypercapnia; uncorrected hypovolaemia; elderly; extravasation at injection site may cause necrosis; **interactions:** Appendix 1 (sympathomimetics)
**Contra-indications**  hypertension (monitor blood pressure and rate of flow frequently); pregnancy (Appendix 4)
**Side-effects**  hypertension, headache, bradycardia, arrhythmias, peripheral ischaemia
**Dose**
● Acute hypotension, by intravenous infusion, via central venous catheter, of a solution containing noradrenaline acid tartrate 80 micrograms/mL (equivalent to noradrenaline base 40 micrograms/mL) at an initial rate of 0.16–0.33 mL/minute, adjusted according to response
● Cardiac arrest, by rapid intravenous *or* intracardiac injection, 0.5–0.75 mL of a solution containing noradrenaline acid tartrate 200 micrograms/mL (equivalent to noradrenaline base 100 micrograms/mL)

**Noradrenaline/Norepinephrine** (Non-proprietary) PoM
Injection, noradrenaline acid tartrate 2 mg/mL (equivalent to noradrenaline base 1 mg/mL). For dilution before use. Net price 2-mL amp = £1.01, 4-mL amp = £1.50, 20-mL amp = £6.35

### ▌ PHENYLEPHRINE HYDROCHLORIDE

**Indications**  acute hypotension (see notes above); priapism (section 7.4.5) [unlicensed indication]

**Cautions** see under Noradrenaline Acid Tartrate; longer duration of action than noradrenaline (norepinephrine), see below; coronary disease
**Hypertensive response** Phenylephrine has a longer duration of action than noradrenaline, and an excessive vasopressor response may cause a prolonged rise in blood pressure

**Contra-indications** see under Noradrenaline Acid Tartrate; severe hyperthyroidism; pregnancy (Appendix 4)

**Side-effects** see under Noradrenaline Acid Tartrate; tachycardia or reflex bradycardia

**Dose**

- By subcutaneous or intramuscular injection, 2–5 mg, followed if necessary by further doses of 1–10 mg
- By slow intravenous injection of a 1 mg/mL solution, 100–500 micrograms repeated as necessary after at least 15 minutes
- By intravenous infusion, initial rate up to 180 micrograms/minute reduced to 30–60 micrograms/minute according to response

**Phenylephrine** (Sovereign) [PoM]
Injection, phenylephrine hydrochloride 10 mg/mL (1%), net price 1-mL amp = £5.50

## 2.7.3 Cardiopulmonary resuscitation

The algorithm for cardiopulmonary resuscitation (see inside back cover) reflects the most recent recommendations of the Resuscitation Council (UK). These guidelines are available at www.resus.org.uk.

Cardiac arrest can be associated with ventricular fibrillation, pulseless ventricular tachycardia, asystole, and electromechanical dissociation (pulseless electrical activity). **Adrenaline (epinephrine)** 1 in 10 000 (100 micrograms/mL) is recommended in a dose of 1 mg (10 mL) by intravenous injection repeated every 3–5 minutes if necessary. Administration through a central line is preferred, however if adrenaline is injected through a peripheral line, it must be flushed with at least 20 mL Sodium Chloride 0.9% injection to aid entry into the central circulation. Intravenous injection of **amiodarone** 300 mg or 5 mg/kg (from a prefilled syringe or diluted in 20 mL Glucose 5%) should be considered after adrenaline to treat ventricular fibrillation or pulseless ventricular tachycardia in cardiac arrest refractory to defibrillation. An additional dose of amiodarone 150 mg (or 2.5 mg/kg) can be given by intravenous injection if necessary, followed by an intravenous infusion of amiodarone 900 mg over 24 hours. **Lidocaine**, in a dose of 1 mg/kg, is an alternative if amiodarone is not available; a total dose of 3 mg/kg should not be exceeded during the first hour. **Atropine** 3 mg by intravenous injection (section 15.1.3) as a single dose is also used in non-shockable cardiopulmonary resuscitation to block vagal activity.

During cardiopulmonary arrest if intravenous access cannot be obtained, the intraosseous route can be considered; if circulatory access cannot be obtained at all, the endotracheal route can be considered for some drugs.

For the management of acute anaphylaxis see section 3.4.3.

### ADRENALINE/EPINEPHRINE

**Indications** see notes above

**Cautions** heart disease, hypertension, arrhythmias, cerebrovascular disease, phaeochromocytoma; diabetes mellitus, hyperthyroidism; susceptibility to angle-closure glaucoma; elderly; **interactions:** Appendix 1 (sympathomimetics)

**Side-effects** nausea, vomiting; tachycardia, arrhythmias, palpitation, cold extremities, hypertension (risk of cerebral haemorrhage); dyspnoea, pulmonary oedema (on excessive dosage or extreme sensitivity); anxiety, tremor, restlessness, headache, weakness, dizziness; hyperglycaemia; urinary retention; sweating; tissue necrosis at injection site and angle-closure glaucoma also reported

**Dose**

- See notes above

**Adrenaline/Epinephrine 1 in 10 000, Dilute** (Non-proprietary) [PoM]
Injection, adrenaline (as acid tartrate) 100 micrograms/mL. 10-mL amp.
Brands include *Minijet® Adrenaline*

## 2.8 Anticoagulants and protamine

**2.8.1 Parenteral anticoagulants**
**2.8.2 Oral anticoagulants**
**2.8.3 Protamine sulphate**

The main use of anticoagulants is to prevent thrombus formation or extension of an existing thrombus in the slower-moving venous side of the circulation, where the thrombus consists of a fibrin web enmeshed with platelets and red cells. They are therefore widely used in the prevention and treatment of deep-vein thrombosis in the legs.

Anticoagulants are of less use in preventing thrombus formation in arteries, for in faster-flowing vessels thrombi are composed mainly of platelets with little fibrin. They are used to prevent thrombi forming on prosthetic heart valves.

## 2.8.1 Parenteral anticoagulants

### Heparin

**Heparin** initiates anticoagulation rapidly but has a short duration of action. It is often referred to as 'standard' or 'unfractionated heparin' to distinguish it from the **low molecular weight heparins** (see p. 127), which have a longer duration of action. Although a low molecular weight heparin is generally preferred for routine use, heparin can be used in those at high risk of bleeding because its effect can be terminated rapidly by stopping the infusion.

**Treatment** For the initial treatment of deep-vein thrombosis and pulmonary embolism a low molecular weight heparin is used; alternatively, heparin is given as an intravenous loading dose, followed by continuous

*2 Cardiovascular system*

intravenous infusion (using an infusion pump) or by intermittent subcutaneous injection. Intermittent intravenous injection of heparin is no longer recommended. An oral anticoagulant (usually warfarin, section 2.8.2) is started at the same time as the heparin (the heparin needs to be continued for at least 5 days and until the INR has been in the therapeutic range for 2 consecutive days). Laboratory monitoring, preferably on a daily basis, is essential; determination of the activated partial thromboplastin time (APTT) is the most widely used measure. A low molecular weight heparin or, in some circumstances, heparin is also used in regimens for the management of myocardial infarction (section 2.10.1) and unstable angina (section 2.6).

**Prophylaxis** In patients undergoing general surgery, a low molecular weight heparin is effective for the prevention of postoperative deep-vein thrombosis and pulmonary embolism in 'high-risk' patients (i.e. those with obesity, malignant disease, history of deep-vein thrombosis or pulmonary embolism, patients over 40 years, or those with an established thrombophilic disorder or who are undergoing major or complicated surgery). Subcutaneous injection of low-dose heparin is an alternative; this regimen does not require laboratory monitoring.

To combat the increased risk in major orthopaedic surgery an adjusted dose regimen of heparin (with monitoring), low molecular weight heparin (p. 127) or fondaparinux (p. 130) can be used—a low molecular weight heparin is probably more effective.

**Pregnancy** Heparins are used for the management of venous thromboembolism in pregnancy because they do not cross the placenta. Low molecular weight heparins are preferred because they have a lower risk of osteoporosis and of heparin-induced thrombocytopenia. Low molecular weight heparins are eliminated more rapidly in pregnancy, requiring alteration of the dosage regimen for drugs such as dalteparin, enoxaparin, and tinzaparin. Treatment should be stopped at the onset of labour and advice sought from a specialist on continuing therapy after birth.

**Extracorporeal circuits** Heparin is also used in the maintenance of extracorporeal circuits in cardiopulmonary bypass and haemodialysis.

**Haemorrhage** If haemorrhage occurs it is usually sufficient to withdraw heparin, but if rapid reversal of the effects of heparin is required, protamine sulphate (section 2.8.3) is a specific antidote (but only partially reverses the effects of low molecular weight heparins).

### ■ HEPARIN

**Indications** see under Dose

**Cautions** see notes above; also elderly; concomitant use of drugs that increase risk of bleeding; hepatic impairment (Appendix 2); renal impairment (Appendix 3); pregnancy (Appendix 4); **interactions:** Appendix 1 (heparin)

**Heparin-induced thrombocytopenia** Clinically important heparin-induced thrombocytopenia is immune-mediated and does not usually develop until after 5–10 days; it can be complicated by thrombosis. Platelet counts should be measured just before treatment with heparin or low molecular weight heparins, and regular monitoring of platelet counts is recommended if given for longer than 4 days. Signs of heparin-induced thrombocytopenia include a 50% reduction of platelet count, thrombosis, or skin allergy. If heparin-induced thrombocytopenia is strongly suspected or confirmed, heparin should be **stopped** and an alternative anticoagulant, such as lepirudin or danaparoid, should be given. Ensure platelet counts return to normal range in those who require warfarin

**Hyperkalaemia** Inhibition of aldosterone secretion by heparin (including low molecular weight heparins) can result in hyperkalaemia; patients with diabetes mellitus, chronic renal failure, acidosis, raised plasma potassium or those taking potassium-sparing drugs seem to be more susceptible. The risk appears to increase with duration of therapy and the CSM has recommended that plasma-potassium concentration should be measured in patients at risk of hyperkalaemia before starting heparin and monitored regularly thereafter, particularly if heparin is to be continued for longer than 7 days

**Contra-indications** haemophilia and other haemorrhagic disorders, thrombocytopenia (including history of heparin-induced thrombocytopenia), recent cerebral haemorrhage, severe hypertension; severe liver disease (including oesophageal varices), peptic ulcer; after major trauma or recent surgery to eye or nervous system; acute bacterial endocarditis; spinal or epidural anaesthesia with treatment doses of heparin; hypersensitivity to heparin or to low molecular weight heparins

**Side-effects** haemorrhage (see notes above), thrombocytopenia (see Cautions), *rarely* rebound hyperlipidaemia following heparin withdrawal, priapism, hyperkalaemia (see Cautions), osteoporosis (risk lower with low molecular weight heparins), alopecia on prolonged use, injection-site reactions, skin necrosis, and hypersensitivity reactions (including urticaria, angioedema, and anaphylaxis)

**Dose**
- Treatment of deep-vein thrombosis, pulmonary embolism, unstable angina, and acute peripheral arterial occlusion, by intravenous injection, loading dose of 5000 units *or* 75 units/kg (10 000 units in severe pulmonary embolism), followed by continuous intravenous infusion of 18 units/kg/hour *or* treatment of deep-vein thrombosis, by subcutaneous injection of 15 000 units every 12 hours (laboratory monitoring essential—preferably on a daily basis, and dose adjusted accordingly); CHILD under 18 years *see* BNF for Children

- Prophylaxis in orthopaedic surgery, see notes above

- Prophylaxis in general and gynaecological surgery (see notes above), by subcutaneous injection, 5000 units 2 hours before surgery, then every 8–12 hours for 7–10 days or until patient is ambulant (monitoring not needed); during pregnancy (with monitoring), 5000–10 000 units every 12 hours (**important:** prevention of prosthetic heart-valve thrombosis in pregnancy calls for **specialist management**)

- Haemodialysis by intravenous injection initially 1000–5000 units, followed by continuous intravenous infusion of 250–1000 units/hour

- Myocardial infarction, see section 2.10.1

- Prevention of clotting in extracorporeal circuits, consult product literature

Doses above reflect the guidelines of the British Society for Haematology; for doses of the low molecular weight heparins, see p. 127

**Heparin Sodium** (Non-proprietary) [PoM]
Injection, heparin sodium 1000 units/mL, net price 1-mL amp = 37p, 5-mL amp = 93p, 5-mL vial = 92p, 10-mL amp = £1.60, 20-mL amp = £2.63; 5000 units/mL,

1-mL amp = 72p, 5-mL amp = £1.87, 5-mL vial = £2.09; 25 000 units/mL, 0.2-mL amp = 92p, 1-mL amp = £1.90, 5-mL vial = £3.68
**Excipients** may include benzyl alcohol (avoid in neonates, see Excipients, p. 2)

**Heparin Calcium** (Non-proprietary) PoM
Injection, heparin calcium 25 000 units/mL, net price 0.2-mL amp = 73p

## Low molecular weight heparins

Low molecular weight heparins (**bemiparin, dalteparin, enoxaparin,** and **tinzaparin**) are usually preferred over unfractionated heparin in the *prevention* of venous thromboembolism because they are as effective and they have a lower risk of heparin-induced thrombocytopenia. Also, the standard prophylactic regimen does not require monitoring. In orthopaedic practice low molecular weight heparins are probably more effective than unfractionated heparin; fondaparinux (p. 130) can also be used. The duration of action of low molecular weight heparins is longer than that of unfractionated heparin and *once-daily subcutaneous* administration is possible for some indications, making them convenient to use.

Low molecular weight heparins are also used in the *treatment* of deep-vein thrombosis, pulmonary embolism, myocardial infarction (section 2.10.1), unstable coronary artery disease (section 2.6) and for the prevention of clotting in extracorporeal circuits.

Dalteparin is also licensed for the extended treatment and prophylaxis of venous thromboembolism in patients with solid tumours; treatment is recommended for a duration of 6 months.

Routine monitoring of anti-Factor Xa activity is not usually required during treatment with low molecular weight heparins, but may be necessary in patients at increased risk of bleeding (e.g. in renal impairment and those who are underweight or overweight).

**Haemorrhage** See under Heparin.

**Pregnancy** See under Heparin.

### ■ BEMIPARIN SODIUM

**Indications** see notes above and under preparations
**Cautions** see under Heparin and notes above
**Contra-indications** see under Heparin; breast-feeding (Appendix 5)
**Side-effects** see under Heparin
**Dose**
● See under preparations below

**Zibor®** (Amdipharm) ▼ PoM
Injection, bemiparin sodium 12 500 units/mL, net price 2500-unit (0.2-mL) prefilled syringe = £1.86; 17 500 units/mL, 3500-unit (0.2-mL) prefilled syringe = £2.75
**Dose** prophylaxis of deep-vein thrombosis, by subcutaneous injection, moderate risk, 2500 units 2 hours before or 6 hours after surgery then 2500 units every 24 hours for 7–10 days; high risk, 3500 units 2 hours before or 6 hours after surgery then 3500 units every 24 hours for 7–10 days
Prevention of clotting in extracorporeal circuits, consult product literature

Injection, bemiparin sodium 25 000 units/mL, net price 0.2-mL (5000-unit) prefilled syringe = £4.22, 0.3-

mL (7500-unit) prefilled syringe = £5.34, 0.4-mL (10 000-unit) prefilled syringe = £8.44
**Dose** treatment of deep-vein thrombosis (with or without pulmonary embolism), by subcutaneous injection, 115 units/kg every 24 hours for 5–9 days (and until adequate oral anticoagulation established)

### ■ DALTEPARIN SODIUM

**Indications** see notes above and under preparations
**Cautions** see under Heparin and notes above
**Contra-indications** see under Heparin
**Side-effects** see under Heparin
**Dose**
● See under preparations below

**Fragmin®** (Pharmacia) PoM
Injection (single-dose syringe), dalteparin sodium 12 500 units/mL, net price 2500-unit (0.2-mL) syringe = £1.86; 25 000 units/mL, 5000-unit (0.2-mL) syringe = £2.82, 7500-unit (0.3-mL) syringe = £4.23, 10 000-unit (0.4-mL) syringe = £5.65, 12 500-unit (0.5-mL) syringe = £7.06, 15 000-unit (0.6-mL) syringe = £8.47, 18 000-unit (0.72-mL) syringe = £10.16
**Dose** prophylaxis of deep-vein thrombosis, in surgical patients, by subcutaneous injection, moderate risk, 2500 units 1–2 hours before surgery then 2500 units every 24 hours for 5–7 days or longer; high risk, 2500 units 1–2 hours before surgery, then 2500 units 8–12 hours later (or 5000 units on the evening before surgery, then 5000 units on the following evening), then 5000 units every 24 hours for 5–7 days or longer (5 weeks in hip replacement)
Prophylaxis of deep-vein thrombosis in medical patients, by subcutaneous injection, 5000 units every 24 hours
Treatment of deep-vein thrombosis and of pulmonary embolism, by subcutaneous injection, as a single daily dose, ADULT body-weight under 46 kg, 7500 units daily; body-weight 46–56 kg, 10 000 units daily; body-weight 57–68 kg, 12 500 units daily; body-weight 69–82 kg, 15 000 units daily; body-weight 83 kg and over, 18 000 units daily, with oral anticoagulant treatment until prothrombin complex concentration in therapeutic range (usually for at least 5 days); monitoring of anti-Factor Xa not usually required; for patients at increased risk of haemorrhage, see below
Treatment of venous thromboembolism in pregnancy [unlicensed indication], by subcutaneous injection, early pregnancy body-weight under 50 kg, 5000 units twice daily; body-weight 50–70 kg, 6000 units twice daily; body-weight 70–90 kg, 8000 units twice daily; body-weight over 90 kg, 10 000 units twice daily
Extended treatment and prophylaxis of venous thromboembolism in patients with solid tumours, by subcutaneous injection, ADULT body-weight over 40 kg, 200 units/kg (max. 18 000 units) as a single daily dose for 30 days, followed by 150 units/kg (max. 18 000 units) as a single daily dose for a further 5 months; interrupt treatment or reduce dose in chemotherapy-induced thrombocytopenia—consult product literature

Injection, dalteparin sodium 2500 units/mL (for subcutaneous or intravenous use), net price 4-mL (10 000-unit) amp = £5.12; 10 000-units/mL (for subcutaneous or intravenous use), 1-mL (10 000-unit) amp = £5.12; 25 000 units/mL (for subcutaneous use only), 4-mL (100 000-unit) vial = £48.66
**Excipients** include benzyl alcohol (in 100 000-unit/4 mL multidose vial) (avoid in neonates, see Excipients, p. 2)
**Dose** treatment of deep-vein thrombosis and of pulmonary embolism, by subcutaneous injection, 200 units/kg (max. 18 000 units) as a single daily dose (or 100 units/kg twice daily if increased risk of haemorrhage) with oral anticoagulant treatment until prothrombin complex concentration in therapeutic range (usually for at least 5 days)
**Note** For monitoring, blood should be taken 3–4 hours after a dose (recommended plasma concentration of anti-Factor Xa 0.5–1 unit/mL); monitoring not required for once-daily treatment regimen and not generally necessary for twice-daily regimen
Unstable coronary artery disease, by subcutaneous injection, 120 units/kg every 12 hours (max. 10 000 units twice daily) for 5–8 days
Prevention of clotting in extracorporeal circuits, consult product literature

Injection (graduated syringe), dalteparin sodium 10 000 units/mL, net price 1-mL (10 000-unit) syringe = £5.65

**Dose** unstable coronary artery disease (including non-ST-segment-elevation myocardial infarction), by subcutaneous injection, 120 units/kg every 12 hours (max. 10 000 units twice daily) for up to 8 days; beyond 8 days (if awaiting angiography or revascularisation) women body-weight less than 80 kg and men less than 70 kg, 5000 units every 12 hours, women body-weight greater than 80 kg and men greater than 70 kg, 7500 units every 12 hours, until day of procedure (max. 45 days)

## ENOXAPARIN SODIUM

**Indications** see notes above and under preparations

**Cautions** see under Heparin and notes above; low body-weight (increased risk of bleeding)

**Contra-indications** see under Heparin; breast-feeding (Appendix 5)

**Side-effects** see under Heparin

**Dose**

- See under preparation below

**Clexane®** (Rhône-Poulenc Rorer) (PoM)

Injection, enoxaparin sodium 100 mg/mL, net price 20-mg (0.2-mL, 2000-units) syringe = £3.03, 40-mg (0.4-mL, 4000-units) syringe = £4.04, 60-mg (0.6-mL, 6000-units) syringe = £4.57, 80-mg (0.8-mL, 8000-units) syringe = £5.19, 100-mg (1-mL, 10 000-units) syringe = £6.43; 300 mg (3-mL, 30 000-units) vial (*Clexane® Multidose*) = £21.33; 150 mg/mL (*Clexane® Forte*), 120-mg (0.8-mL, 12 000-units) syringe = £9.77, 150-mg (1-mL, 15 000-units) syringe = £11.10

**Excipients** include benzyl alcohol (in 300 mg multidose vials) (avoid in neonates, see Excipients, p. 2)

**Dose** prophylaxis of deep-vein thrombosis especially in surgical patients, by subcutaneous injection, *moderate risk*, 20 mg (2000 units) approx. 2 hours before surgery then 20 mg (2000 units) every 24 hours for 7–10 days; *high risk* (e.g. orthopaedic surgery), 40 mg (4000 units) 12 hours before surgery then 40 mg (4000 units) every 24 hours for 7–10 days

Prophylaxis of deep-vein thrombosis in medical patients, by subcutaneous injection, 40 mg (4000 units) every 24 hours for at least 6 days and continued until patient ambulant (max. 14 days)

Treatment of deep-vein thrombosis or pulmonary embolism, by subcutaneous injection, 1.5 mg/kg (150 units/kg) every 24 hours, usually for at least 5 days (and until adequate oral anticoagulation established)

Treatment of acute ST-segment elevation myocardial infarction, ADULT under 75 years, by intravenous injection, 30 mg (3000 units) followed by subcutaneous injection, 1 mg/kg (100 units/kg), then by subcutaneous injection, 1 mg/kg every 12 hours for up to 8 days (max. 100 mg (10 000 units) for first two subcutaneous doses only); ELDERLY over 75 years, by subcutaneous injection *only*, 750 micrograms/kg (75 units/kg) every 12 hours (max. 75 mg (7500 units) for first two doses only); patients undergoing percutaneous coronary intervention, additional dose, by intravenous injection, 300 micrograms/kg (30 units/kg) at time of procedure if last subcutaneous dose given more than 8 hours previously

**Note** When administered in conjunction with a thrombolytic, enoxaparin should be given between 15 minutes before and 30 minutes after the start of thrombolytic therapy

Unstable angina and non-ST-segment-elevation myocardial infarction, by subcutaneous injection, 1 mg/kg (100 units/kg) every 12 hours usually for 2–8 days (minimum 2 days)

Prevention of clotting in extracorporeal circuits, consult product literature

Treatment of venous thromboembolism in pregnancy [unlicensed indication], by subcutaneous injection, early pregnancy body-weight under 50 kg, 40 mg (4000 units) twice daily; body-weight 50–70 kg, 60 mg (6000 units) twice daily; body-weight 70–90 kg, 80 mg (8000 units) twice daily; body-weight over 90 kg, 100 mg (10 000 units) twice daily

## TINZAPARIN SODIUM

**Indications** see notes above and under preparations

**Cautions** see under Heparin and notes above; elderly with renal impairment (avoid if age over 90 years with renal impairment)

**Contra-indications** see under Heparin; breast-feeding (Appendix 5)

**Side-effects** see under Heparin

**Dose**

- See under preparations below

**Innohep®** (LEO) (PoM)

Injection, tinzaparin sodium 10 000 units/mL, net price 2500-unit (0.25-mL) syringe = £1.98, 3500-unit (0.35-mL) syringe = £2.77, 4500-unit (0.45-mL) syringe = £3.56, 20 000-unit (2-mL) vial = £10.56

**Excipients** include benzyl alcohol (in vial) (avoid in neonates, see Excipients, p. 2)

**Dose** prophylaxis of deep-vein thrombosis, by subcutaneous injection, general surgery, 3500 units 2 hours before surgery, then 3500 units every 24 hours for 7–10 days; orthopaedic surgery, 50 units/kg 2 hours before surgery, then 50 units/kg every 24 hours for 7–10 days *or* 4500 units 12 hours before surgery, then 4500 units every 24 hours for 7–10 days

Prevention of clotting in extracorporeal circuits, consult product literature

Injection, tinzaparin sodium 20 000 units/mL, net price 0.5-mL (10 000-unit) syringe = £8.63, 0.7-mL (14 000-unit) syringe = £12.08, 0.9-mL (18 000-unit) syringe = £15.53, 2-mL (40 000-unit) vial = £34.20

**Excipients** include benzyl alcohol (in vial) (avoid in neonates, see Excipients, p. 2), sulphites (in 20 000 units/mL vial and syringe)

**Dose** treatment of deep-vein thrombosis and of pulmonary embolism, by subcutaneous injection, 175 units/kg once daily for at least 6 days (and until adequate oral anticoagulation established)

Treatment of venous thromboembolism in pregnancy [unlicensed indication], by subcutaneous injection, 175 units/kg once daily (based on early pregnancy body-weight)

**Note** Treatment regimens do not require anticoagulation monitoring

# Heparinoids

**Danaparoid** is a heparinoid used for prophylaxis of deep-vein thrombosis in patients undergoing general or orthopaedic surgery. Providing there is no evidence of cross-reactivity, it also has a role in patients who develop thrombocytopenia in association with heparin.

## DANAPAROID SODIUM

**Indications** prevention of deep-vein thrombosis in general or orthopaedic surgery; thromboembolic disease in patients with history of heparin-induced thrombocytopenia

**Cautions** recent bleeding or risk of bleeding; concomitant use of drugs that increase risk of bleeding; antibodies to heparins (risk of antibody-induced thrombocytopenia); body-weight over 90 kg (monitor anti factor Xa activity); hepatic impairment (Appendix 2); renal impairment (Appendix 3); pregnancy (Appendix 4); breast-feeding (Appendix 5)

**Contra-indications** haemophilia and other haemorrhagic disorders, thrombocytopenia (unless patient has heparin-induced thrombocytopenia), recent cerebral haemorrhage, severe hypertension, active peptic ulcer (unless this is the reason for operation), diabetic retinopathy, acute bacterial endocarditis, spinal or epidural anaesthesia with treatment doses of danaparoid

**Side-effects** bleeding; hypersensitivity reactions (including rash)

**Dose**

- Prevention of deep-vein thrombosis, by subcutaneous injection, 750 units twice daily for 7–10 days; initiate treatment before operation (with last preoperative dose 1–4 hours before surgery)
- Thromboembolic disease in patients with history of heparin-induced thrombocytopenia, by intravenous injection, 2500 units (1250 units if body-weight under 55 kg, 3750 units if over 90 kg), followed by intravenous infusion of 400 units/hour for 2 hours, *then* 300 units/hour for 2 hours, *then* 200 units/hour for 5 days

**Orgaran®** (Organon) [PoM]
Injection, danaparoid sodium 1250 units/mL, net price 0.6-mL amp (750 units) = £27.19

## Hirudins

**Lepirudin**, a recombinant hirudin, is licensed for anticoagulation in patients with Type II (immune) heparin-induced thrombocytopenia who require parenteral antithrombotic treatment. The dose of lepirudin is adjusted according to activated partial thromboplastin time (APTT). **Bivalirudin**, a hirudin analogue, is a thrombin inhibitor which is licensed for acute coronary syndromes in patients planned for urgent or early intervention in combination with aspirin and clopidogrel, and as an anticoagulant for patients undergoing percutaneous coronary intervention. The *Scottish Medicines Consortium* (p. 3) has advised (November 2008) that bivalirudin is accepted for restricted use for patients with acute coronary syndromes planned for urgent or early intervention who would have been considered for treatment with unfractionated heparin combined with a glycoprotein IIb/IIIa inhibitor.

### ■ BIVALIRUDIN

**Indications** acute coronary syndromes in patients planned for urgent or early intervention; anticoagulation for patients undergoing percutaneous coronary intervention (PCI)

**Cautions** exposure to lepirudin (theoretical risk from lepirudin antibodies); brachytherapy procedures; concomitant use of drugs that increase risk of bleeding; renal impairment (avoid if eGFR less than 30 mL/minute/1.73 m²; Appendix 3); pregnancy (Appendix 4); breast-feeding (Appendix 5)

**Contra-indications** severe hypertension; subacute bacterial endocarditis; active bleeding; bleeding disorders

**Side-effects** bleeding (discontinue); *less commonly* nausea, vomiting, tachycardia, bradycardia, hypotension, angina, dyspnoea, allergic reactions (including isolated reports of anaphylaxis), headache, thrombocytopenia, anaemia, back and chest pain, and injection-site reactions; *very rarely* thrombosis

**Dose**

- Acute coronary syndromes (in addition to aspirin and clopidogrel), initially by intravenous injection, 100 micrograms/kg then by intravenous infusion 250 micrograms/kg/hour (for up to 72 hours in

medically managed patients); patients proceeding to percutaneous coronary intervention or coronary artery bypass surgery *without* cardiopulmonary bypass, additional bolus dose by intravenous injection 500 micrograms/kg, then by intravenous infusion 1.75 mg/kg/hour for duration of procedure; following percutaneous coronary intervention, reduce infusion rate to 250 micrograms/kg/hour for 4–12 hours as necessary; patients proceeding to coronary artery bypass surgery *with* cardiopulmonary bypass, discontinue intravenous infusion 1 hour before procedure and treat with unfractionated heparin

- Anticoagulation in patients undergoing percutaneous coronary intervention, initially by intravenous injection, 750 micrograms/kg then by intravenous infusion 1.75 mg/kg/hour for up to 4 hours after procedure

**Angiox®** (The Medicines Company) ▼ [PoM]
Injection, powder for reconstitution, bivalirudin, net price 250-mg vial = £310.00

### ■ LEPIRUDIN

**Indications** thromboembolic disease requiring parenteral anticoagulation in patients with heparin-induced thrombocytopenia type II

**Cautions** hepatic impairment (Appendix 2); renal impairment (Appendix 3); recent bleeding or risk of bleeding including recent puncture of large vessels, organ biopsy, recent major surgery, stroke, bleeding disorders, severe hypertension, bacterial endocarditis; concomitant use of drugs that increase risk of bleeding; determine activated partial thromboplastin time 4 hours after start of treatment (or after infusion rate altered) and at least once daily thereafter

**Contra-indications** pregnancy and breast-feeding

**Side-effects** bleeding; reduced haemoglobin concentration without obvious source of bleeding; fever, hypersensitivity reactions (including rash); injection-site reactions

**Dose**

- Initially by slow intravenous injection (of 5 mg/mL solution), 400 micrograms/kg followed by continuous intravenous infusion of 150 micrograms/kg/hour (max. 16.5 mg/hour), adjusted according to activated partial thromboplastin time, for 2–10 days (longer if necessary)

**Refludan®** (Celgene) [PoM]
Injection, powder for reconstitution, lepirudin, net price 50-mg vial = £57.00

## Heparin flushes

The use of heparin flushes should be kept to a minimum. For maintaining patency of peripheral venous catheters, sodium chloride injection 0.9% is as effective as heparin flushes. The role of heparin flushes in maintaining patency of arterial and central venous catheters is unclear.

**Heparin Sodium** (Non-proprietary) [PoM]
Solution, heparin sodium 10 units/mL, net price 5-mL amp = 25p; 100 units/mL, 2-mL amp = 28p
Dose to maintain patency of catheters, cannulas, etc. 10–200 units flushed through every 4–8 hours. Not for therapeutic use
Excipients may include benzyl alcohol (avoid in neonates, see Excipients, p. 2)

2

Cardiovascular system

**Sidebar:** 2 Cardiovascular system

## Epoprostenol

**Epoprostenol** (prostacyclin) can be given to inhibit platelet aggregation during renal dialysis either alone or with heparin. It is also licensed for the treatment of primary pulmonary hypertension resistant to other treatment, usually with oral anticoagulation. Since its half-life is only about 3 minutes it must be given by continuous intravenous infusion. It is a potent vasodilator and therefore its side-effects include flushing, headache, and hypotension.

### ■ EPOPROSTENOL

**Indications** see notes above

**Cautions** anticoagulant monitoring required when given with heparin; haemorrhagic diathesis; dose titration for pulmonary hypertension should be in hospital (risk of pulmonary oedema); concomitant use of drugs that increase risk of bleeding; pregnancy (Appendix 4)

**Contra-indications** severe left ventricular dysfunction

**Side-effects** see notes above; also bradycardia, tachycardia, pallor, sweating with higher doses; gastro-intestinal disturbances; lassitude, anxiety, agitation; dry mouth, jaw pain, chest pain; also reported, hyperglycaemia and injection-site reactions

**Dose**

● See product literature

**Flolan**® (GSK) [PoM]

Infusion, powder for reconstitution, epoprostenol (as sodium salt), net price 500-microgram vial (with diluent) = £62.05; 1.5-mg vial (▼) (with diluent) = £125.00

## Fondaparinux

**Fondaparinux sodium** is a synthetic pentasaccharide that inhibits activated factor X.

### ■ FONDAPARINUX SODIUM

**Indications** prophylaxis of venous thromboembolism in medical patients immobilised because of acute illness, and patients undergoing major orthopaedic surgery of the legs or abdominal surgery; treatment of deep-vein thrombosis and of pulmonary embolism; treatment of unstable angina or non-ST-segment elevation myocardial infarction; treatment of ST-segment elevation myocardial infarction

**Cautions** bleeding disorders; active gastro-intestinal ulcer disease; recent intracranial haemorrhage; brain, spinal, or ophthalmic surgery; spinal or epidural anaesthesia (risk of spinal haematoma—avoid if using treatment doses); risk of catheter thrombus during percutaneous coronary intervention; low bodyweight; elderly patients; concomitant use of drugs that increase risk of bleeding; hepatic impairment (Appendix 2); renal impairment (Appendix 3); pregnancy (Appendix 4); breast-feeding (Appendix 5)

**Contra-indications** active bleeding; bacterial endocarditis

**Side-effects** bleeding, purpura, anaemia; *less commonly* gastro-intestinal disturbances, oedema, hepatic impairment, chest pain, dyspnoea, thrombocytopenia, thrombocythaemia, rash, pruritus; *rarely* hypotension, flushing, cough, vertigo, dizziness, anxiety, drowsi-

ness, confusion, headache, hypokalaemia, hyperbilirubinaemia, injection-site reactions; also reported atrial fibrillation, tachycardia, and pyrexia

**Dose**

● See under preparation below

**Arixtra**® (GSK) ▼ [PoM]

Injection, fondaparinux sodium 5 mg/mL, net price 0.3-mL (1.5-mg) prefilled syringe = £6.41

Dose prophylaxis of venous thromboembolism after surgery, by subcutaneous injection, 2.5 mg 6 hours after surgery then 2.5 mg once daily for 5–9 days (longer after hip surgery); CHILD under 17 years not recommended

Prophylaxis of venous thromboembolism in medical patients, by subcutaneous injection, 2.5 mg once daily usually for 6–14 days; CHILD under 17 years not recommended

Injection, fondaparinux sodium 5 mg/mL, net price 0.5-mL (2.5-mg) prefilled syringe = £6.41

Dose prophylaxis of venous thromboembolism after surgery, by subcutaneous injection, 2.5 mg 6 hours after surgery then 2.5 mg once daily for 5–9 days (longer after hip surgery); CHILD under 17 years not recommended

Prophylaxis of venous thromboembolism in medical patients, by subcutaneous injection, 2.5 mg once daily usually for 6–14 days; CHILD under 17 years not recommended

Unstable angina and non-ST-segment elevation myocardial infarction, by subcutaneous injection, 2.5 mg once daily for up to 8 days (or until hospital discharge if sooner); CHILD under 17 years not recommended

ST-segment elevation myocardial infarction, initially by intravenous injection or infusion, 2.5 mg for first day, thereafter by subcutaneous injection 2.5 mg once daily for up to 8 days (or until hospital discharge if sooner); CHILD under 17 years not recommended

Injection, fondaparinux sodium 12.5 mg/mL, net price 0.4-mL (5-mg) prefilled syringe = £11.89, 0.6-mL (7.5-mg) prefilled syringe = £11.89, 0.8-mL (10-mg) prefilled syringe = £11.89

Dose treatment of deep-vein thrombosis and of pulmonary embolism, by subcutaneous injection, ADULT body-weight under 50 kg, 5 mg every 24 hours; body-weight 50–100 kg, 7.5 mg every 24 hours; body-weight over 100 kg, 10 mg every 24 hours; usually for at least 5 days (and until adequate oral anticoagulation established); CHILD under 17 years not recommended

## 2.8.2 Oral anticoagulants

### Coumarins and phenindione

The oral anticoagulants, **warfarin**, **acenocoumarol** (nicoumalone) and **phenindione**, antagonise the effects of vitamin K, and take at least 48 to 72 hours for the anticoagulant effect to develop fully; if an immediate effect is required, heparin must be given concomitantly.

**Uses** The main indication for these oral anticoagulants is *deep-vein thrombosis*. Patients with *pulmonary embolism* should also be treated, as should those with *atrial fibrillation who are at risk of embolisation* (see also section 2.3.1), and those with *mechanical prosthetic heart valves* (to prevent emboli developing on the valves); an antiplatelet drug may also be useful in these patients but this combination increases the risk of bleeding.

Warfarin is the drug of choice; acenocoumarol (nicoumalone) and phenindione are seldom required.

These oral anticoagulants should not be used in cerebral artery thrombosis or peripheral artery occlusion as first-line therapy; aspirin (section 2.9) is more appropriate for reduction of risk in transient ischaemic attacks. Heparin or a low molecular weight heparin (section 2.8.1) is usually preferred for the prophylaxis of venous thromboembolism in patients undergoing surgery; alternatively, warfarin can be continued in selected patients currently taking long-term warfarin and who are at high risk of thromboembolism (seek expert advice).

**Dose** Whenever possible, the base-line prothrombin time should be determined but the initial dose should not be delayed whilst awaiting the result.

For patients who require rapid anticoagulation the usual adult induction dose of warfarin is 10 mg[1] on the first day; subsequent doses depend upon the prothrombin time, reported as INR (international normalised ratio). For patients who do not require rapid anticoagulation, a lower loading dose can be used over 3–4 weeks. The daily maintenance dose of warfarin is usually 3–9 mg (taken at the **same time** each day). The following indications and target INRs[2] take into account recommendations of the British Society for Haematology[3]:

- INR 2.5 for treatment of deep-vein thrombosis and pulmonary embolism (including those associated with antiphospholipid syndrome or for recurrence in patients no longer receiving warfarin), for atrial fibrillation, cardioversion (higher target values, such as an INR of 3, can be used for up to 4 weeks before the procedure to avoid cancellations due to low INR; anticoagulation should continue for at least 4 weeks following the procedure), dilated cardiomyopathy, mural thrombus, symptomatic inherited thrombophilia, coronary artery thrombosis (if anticoagulated), and paroxysmal nocturnal haemoglobinuria;

- INR 3.5 for recurrent deep-vein thrombosis and pulmonary embolism (in patients currently receiving warfarin with INR above 2);

- For mechanical prosthetic heart valves, the recommended target INR depends on the type and location of the valve. Generally, a target INR of 3 is recommended for mechanical aortic valves, and 3.5 for mechanical mitral valves.

**Monitoring** It is essential that the INR be determined daily or on alternate days in early days of treatment, *then* at longer intervals (depending on response[4]) *then* up to every 12 weeks.

**Haemorrhage** The main adverse effect of all oral anticoagulants is haemorrhage. Checking the INR and omitting doses when appropriate is essential; if the anticoagulant is stopped but not reversed, the INR should be measured 2–3 days later to ensure that it is falling. The following recommendations (which take into

1. First dose reduced if base-line prothrombin time prolonged, if liver-function tests abnormal, or if patient in cardiac failure, on parenteral feeding, less than average body weight, elderly, or receiving other drugs known to potentiate oral anticoagulants.
2. An INR which is within 0.5 units of the target value is generally satisfactory; larger deviations require dosage adjustment. Target values (rather than ranges) are now recommended.
3. Guidelines on Oral Anticoagulation (warfarin): third edition—2005 update. *Br J Haematol* 2005; **132**: 277–285.
4. Change in patient's clinical condition, particularly associated with liver disease, intercurrent illness, or drug administration, necessitates more frequent testing. See also interactions, Appendix 1 (warfarin). Major changes in diet (especially involving salads and vegetables) and in alcohol consumption may also affect warfarin control.

account the recommendations of the British Society for Haematology[3]) are based on the result of the INR and whether there is major or minor bleeding; the recommendations apply to patients taking warfarin:

- Major bleeding—stop warfarin; give phytomenadione (vitamin $K_1$) 5–10 mg by slow intravenous injection; give dried prothrombin complex (factors II, VII, IX, and X—section 2.11), 30–50 units/kg *or* fresh frozen plasma 15 mL/kg (if dried prothrombin complex not available)

- INR > 8.0, no bleeding or minor bleeding—stop warfarin, restart when INR < 5.0; if there are other risk factors for bleeding give phytomenadione (vitamin $K_1$) 500 micrograms by slow intravenous injection or 5 mg by mouth (for partial reversal of anticoagulation give smaller oral doses of phytomenadione e.g. 0.5–2.5 mg using the intravenous preparation orally); repeat dose of phytomenadione if INR still too high after 24 hours

- INR 6.0–8.0, no bleeding or minor bleeding—stop warfarin, restart when INR < 5.0

- INR < 6.0 but more than 0.5 units above target value—reduce dose or stop warfarin, restart when INR < 5.0

- Unexpected bleeding at therapeutic levels—always investigate possibility of underlying cause e.g. unsuspected renal or gastro-intestinal tract pathology

**Pregnancy** Warfarin, acenocoumarol, and phenindione are teratogenic and should not be given in the first trimester of pregnancy. Women of child-bearing age should be warned of this danger since stopping warfarin before the sixth week of gestation may largely avoid the risk of fetal abnormality. These oral anticoagulants cross the placenta with risk of placental or fetal haemorrhage, especially during the last few weeks of pregnancy and at delivery. Therefore, if at all possible, they should be avoided in pregnancy, especially in the first and third trimesters. Difficult decisions may have to be made, particularly in women with prosthetic heart valves, atrial fibrillation, or with a history of recurrent venous thrombosis or pulmonary embolism.

**Treatment booklets** Anticoagulant treatment booklets should be issued to patients, and are available for distribution to local healthcare professionals from Health Authorities and from:

3M Security Printing and
Systems Limited
Gorse Street
Chadderton
Oldham
OL9 9QH
0845 610 1112
nhsforms@spsl.uk.com

These booklets include advice for patients on anticoagulant treatment, an alert card to be carried by the patient at all times, and a section for recording of INR results and dosage information. Electronic copies and further advice are also available at www.npsa.nhs.uk/nrls/alerts-and-directives/alerts/anticoagulant.

## WARFARIN SODIUM

**Indications** prophylaxis of embolisation in rheumatic heart disease and atrial fibrillation; prophylaxis after insertion of prosthetic heart valve; prophylaxis and treatment of venous thrombosis and pulmonary embolism; transient ischaemic attacks

**Cautions** see notes above; also recent surgery; concomitant use of drugs that increase risk of bleeding; bacterial endocarditis (increased risk of bleeding; use only if warfarin otherwise indicated); hepatic impairment (Appendix 2); renal impairment (avoid if severe); breast-feeding; (Appendix 5); avoid cranberry juice; **interactions:** Appendix 1 (coumarins)

**Contra-indications** peptic ulcer, severe hypertension; pregnancy (see notes above and Appendix 4)

**Side-effects** haemorrhage—see notes above; other side-effects reported include hypersensitivity, rash, alopecia, diarrhoea, unexplained drop in haematocrit, 'purple toes', skin necrosis, jaundice, hepatic dysfunction; also nausea, vomiting, and pancreatitis

**Dose**

● See notes above

**Warfarin** (Non-proprietary) [PoM]
Tablets, warfarin sodium 500 micrograms (white), net price 28-tab pack = £1.17; 1 mg (brown), 28-tab pack = £1.05; 3 mg (blue), 28-tab pack = £1.15; 5 mg (pink), 28-tab pack = £1.21. Label: 10, anticoagulant card
Brands include *Marevan*®

### ▌ACENOCOUMAROL
(Nicoumalone)

**Indications** see under Warfarin Sodium
**Cautions** see under Warfarin Sodium
**Contra-indications** see under Warfarin Sodium
**Side-effects** see under Warfarin Sodium
**Dose**

● 4 mg on first day, 4–8 mg on second day; maintenance dose usually 1–8 mg daily adjusted according to response

**Sinthrome**® (Alliance) [PoM]
Tablets, acenocoumarol 1 mg, net price 100-tab pack = £4.27. Label: 10, anticoagulant card

### ▌PHENINDIONE

**Indications** prophylaxis of embolisation in rheumatic heart disease and atrial fibrillation; prophylaxis after insertion of prosthetic heart valve; prophylaxis and treatment of venous thrombosis and pulmonary embolism

**Cautions** see under Warfarin Sodium; **interactions:** Appendix 1 (phenindione)

**Contra-indications** see under Warfarin Sodium; breast-feeding (Appendix 5)

**Side-effects** see under Warfarin Sodium; also hypersensitivity reactions including rashes, exfoliative dermatitis, exanthema, fever, leucopenia, agranulocytosis, eosinophilia, diarrhoea, renal and hepatic damage; urine coloured pink or orange

**Dose**

● 200 mg on day 1; 100 mg on day 2; maintenance dose usually 50–150 mg daily

**Phenindione** (Non-proprietary) [PoM]
Tablets, phenindione 10 mg, net price 28-tab pack = £14.75; 25 mg, 28-tab pack = £17.96; 50 mg, 28-tab pack = £21.22. Label: 10, anticoagulant card, 14, (urine pink or orange)

## Dabigatran etexilate

**Dabigatran etexilate**, a direct thrombin inhibitor, is given orally for prophylaxis of venous thromboembolism in adults after total hip replacement or total knee replacement surgery. Dabigatran etexilate has a rapid onset of action and does not require therapeutic monitoring. The most common side-effect is haemorrhage and patients should be monitored for signs of bleeding or anaemia; treatment should be stopped if severe bleeding occurs.

> **NICE guidance**
> **Dabigatran etexilate for the prevention of venous thromboembolism after hip or knee replacement surgery in adults (September 2008)**
> Dabigatran etexilate is an option for the prophylaxis of venous thromboembolism in adults after total hip replacement or total knee replacement surgery.

### ▌DABIGATRAN ETEXILATE

**Indications** see notes above

**Cautions** see notes above; also elderly; body-weight less than 50 kg; recent surgery; anaesthesia with postoperative indwelling epidural catheter (risk of paralysis—give initial dose at least 2 hours after catheter removal and monitor neurological signs); bacterial endocarditis (increased risk of bleeding); bleeding disorders; active gastro-intestinal ulceration; concomitant use of drugs that increase risk of bleeding; renal impairment (avoid if eGFR less than 30 mL/minute/1.73 m²; Appendix 3); **interactions:** Appendix 1 (dabigatran etexilate)

**Contra-indications** active bleeding; impaired haemostasis; severe hepatic impairment (Appendix 2); pregnancy (Appendix 4); breast-feeding (Appendix 5)

**Side-effects** haemorrhage—see notes above; *less commonly* hepatobiliary disorders

**Dose**

● Prophylaxis of venous thromboembolism following total knee replacement surgery, ADULT over 18 years, 110 mg (ELDERLY over 75 years, 75 mg) 1–4 hours after surgery, *then* 220 mg (ELDERLY over 75 years, 150 mg) once daily for 9 days

● Prophylaxis of venous thromboembolism following total hip replacement surgery, ADULT over 18 years, 110 mg (ELDERLY over 75 years, 75 mg) 1–4 hours after surgery, *then* 220 mg (ELDERLY over 75 years, 150 mg) once daily for 27–34 days

**Pradaxa**® (Boehringer Ingelheim) ▼ [PoM]
Capsules, blue/ivory, dabigatran etexilate (as mesilate) 75 mg, net price 10-cap pack = £21.00, 60-cap pack = £126.00; 110 mg 10-cap pack = £21.00, 60-cap pack = £126.00 (all hosp. only). Label: 25

## Rivaroxaban

**Rivaroxaban**, a direct inhibitor of activated factor X, is given orally for prophylaxis of venous thromboembolism in adults after hip or knee replacement surgery. Rivaroxaban does not require therapeutic monitoring. The common side-effects are nausea and haemorrhage and patients should be monitored for signs of bleeding or anaemia; treatment should be stopped if severe bleeding occurs.

### NICE guidance
**Rivaroxaban for the prevention of venous thromboembolism after total hip or total knee replacement in adults (April 2009)**
Rivaroxaban is an option for the prophylaxis of venous thromboembolism in adults after total hip replacement or total knee replacement surgery.

## RIVAROXABAN

**Indications** see notes above

**Cautions** see notes above; also bleeding disorders; concomitant use of drugs that increase risk of bleeding; severe hypertension; active or recent gastrointestinal ulceration; vascular retinopathy; anaesthesia with postoperative indwelling epidural catheter (risk of paralysis—monitor neurological signs and wait at least 18 hours after rivaroxaban dose before removing catheter and do not give next dose until at least 6 hours after catheter removal); recent surgery; hepatic impairment (Appendix 2); renal impairment (avoid if eGFR less than 15 mL/minute/1.73 m²; Appendix 3); **interactions:** (Appendix 1)

**Contra-indications** active bleeding; pregnancy (Appendix 4); breast-feeding (Appendix 5)

**Side-effects** nausea; haemorrhage (see notes above); *less commonly* constipation, diarrhoea, dyspepsia, dry mouth, vomiting, hypotension, oedema, tachycardia, thrombocythaemia, syncope, dizziness, headache, renal impairment, pain in extremities, pruritus, and rash; jaundice also reported

**Dose**
● Prophylaxis of venous thromboembolism following knee replacement surgery, ADULT over 18 years, 10 mg once daily for 2 weeks starting 6–10 hours after surgery
● Prophylaxis of venous thromboembolism following hip replacement surgery, ADULT over 18 years, 10 mg once daily for 5 weeks starting 6–10 hours after surgery

**Xarelto®** (Bayer) ▼ [PoM]
Tablets, red, f/c, rivaroxaban 10 mg, net price 10-tab pack = £45.00, 30-tab pack = £135.00, 100-tab pack = £450.00

## 2.8.3 Protamine sulphate

**Protamine sulphate** is used to treat overdosage of heparin, and low molecular weight heparins. The long half-life of low molecular weight heparins should be taken into consideration when determining the dose of protamine sulphate; the effects of low molecular weight heparins can persist for up to 24 hours after administration. Excessive doses of protamine sulphate can have an anticoagulant effect.

## PROTAMINE SULPHATE
(Protamine Sulfate)

**Indications** see above

**Cautions** see above; also monitor activated partial thromboplastin time or other appropriate blood clotting parameters; increased risk of allergic reaction to protamine (including previous treatment with protamine or protamine insulin, allergy to fish, men who are infertile or who have had a vasectomy)

**Side-effects** nausea, vomiting, lassitude, flushing, hypotension, hypertension, bradycardia, dyspnoea, rebound bleeding, back pain; hypersensitivity reactions (including angioedema, anaphylaxis) and pulmonary oedema reported

**Dose**
● Overdosage with intravenous injection of heparin, by intravenous injection (rate not exceeding 5 mg/minute), 1 mg neutralises 80–100 units heparin when given within 15 minutes of heparin; if longer than 15 minutes since heparin, less protamine required (consult product literature for details) as heparin rapidly excreted; max. 50 mg
● Overdosage with intravenous infusion of heparin, by intravenous injection (rate not exceeding 5 mg/minute), 25–50 mg once heparin infusion stopped
● Overdosage with subcutaneous injection of heparin, 1 mg neutralises 100 units heparin; give 25–50 mg by intravenous injection (rate not exceeding 5 mg/minute) then any remaining dose given by intravenous infusion over 8–16 hours; max. total dose 50 mg
● Overdosage with subcutaneous injection of low molecular weight heparin, by intermittent intravenous injection (rate not exceeding 5 mg/minute) or by continuous intravenous infusion, 1 mg neutralises approx. 100 units low molecular weight heparin (consult product literature of low molecular weight heparin for details); max. 50 mg

**Protamine Sulphate** (Non-proprietary) [PoM]
Injection, protamine sulphate 10 mg /mL, net price 5-mL amp = £1.43, 10-mL amp = £4.15

## 2.9 Antiplatelet drugs

Antiplatelet drugs decrease platelet aggregation and may inhibit thrombus formation in the arterial circulation, where anticoagulants have little effect.

A single dose of **aspirin** 300 mg is given as soon as possible after an ischaemic event, preferably dispersed in water or chewed. The initial dose is followed by long-term treatment of aspirin 75 mg daily in order to prevent further cardiovascular disease events.

Long-term use of aspirin, in a dose of 75 mg daily, is also of benefit for all patients with established cardiovascular disease, for patients with a 10-year cardiovascular disease risk[1] of 20% or more and aged over 50 years, for patients with diabetes aged over 50 years or who have

---

1. Cardiovascular disease risk may be determined from the chart issued by the Joint British Societies (*Heart* 2005; **91** (Suppl V): v1–v52)—see inside back cover. The Joint British Societies' 'Cardiac Risk Assessor' computer programme may also be used to determine cardiovascular disease risk.

**2 Cardiovascular system**

had diabetes for more than 10 years, and for patients with diabetes who are receiving antihypertensive treatment. Unduly high blood pressure must be controlled before aspirin is given.

Aspirin in a dose of 75 mg daily is also given following coronary bypass surgery. For details on the use of aspirin in atrial fibrillation see section 2.3.1, for stable angina see section 2.6 and for intermittent claudication see section 2.6.4.

If the patient is at a high risk of gastro-intestinal bleeding, a proton pump inhibitor (section 1.3.5) can be added.

**Clopidogrel** is licensed for the prevention of ischaemic events in patients with a history of symptomatic ischaemic disease. Clopidogrel, in combination with low-dose aspirin, is also licensed for acute coronary syndrome without ST-segment elevation (section 2.6); in these circumstances the combination is usually given for 12 months (there is no evidence of benefit beyond 12 months). Clopidogrel, in combination with low-dose aspirin, is also licensed for acute myocardial infarction with ST-segment elevation (section 2.10.1); the combination should be continued for at least 4 weeks. Use of clopidogrel with aspirin increases the risk of bleeding. Clopidogrel monotherapy is an alternative when aspirin is contra-indicated, for example in those with aspirin hypersensitivity, or when aspirin is not tolerated despite the addition of a proton pump inhibitor.

The *Scottish Medicines Consortium* (p. 3) has advised (February 2004) that clopidogrel be accepted for restricted use for the treatment of confirmed acute coronary syndrome (without ST-segment elevation), in combination with aspirin. The *Scottish Medicines Consortium* has also advised (July 2007) that clopidogrel be accepted for restricted use for patients with ST-segment elevation acute myocardial infarction in combination with aspirin; treatment with clopidogrel is restricted to 4 weeks only. Clopidogrel should be initiated in hospital inpatients **only**.

---

**NICE guidance**
**Clopidogrel in the treatment of non-ST-segment elevation acute coronary syndrome (July 2004)**
Clopidogrel in combination with low-dose aspirin is recommended for the management of non-ST-segment elevation acute coronary syndrome in those at moderate to high risk of myocardial infarction or of death.
Clopidogrel in combination with low-dose aspirin may be used for up to 12 months after the last event of non-ST-segment elevation acute coronary syndrome.

---

**Dipyridamole** is used by mouth as an adjunct to oral anticoagulation for prophylaxis of thromboembolism associated with prosthetic heart valves. Modified-release preparations are licensed for secondary prevention of ischaemic stroke and transient ischaemic attacks.

A combination of modified-release dipyridamole and low-dose aspirin is used after an ischaemic stroke or transient ischaemic attack, and may reduce the risk of recurrent stroke and other cardiovascular events compared to aspirin alone (see also NICE guidance below).

---

**NICE guidance**
**Clopidogrel and modified-release dipyridamole in the prevention of occlusive vascular events (May 2005)**
The combination of modified-release dipyridamole and aspirin is recommended to prevent occlusive vascular events in those who have had a transient ischaemic attack or an ischaemic stroke; this combination should be used for 2 years after the last event. Long-term treatment with low-dose aspirin is continued after this period.
Clopidogrel monotherapy may be used for those who cannot tolerate low-dose aspirin and have had an occlusive vascular event or have symptomatic peripheral arterial disease.

---

**Prasugrel**, in combination with aspirin, is licensed for the prevention of atherothrombotic events in patients with acute coronary syndrome undergoing percutaneous coronary intervention; the combination is usually given for up to 12 months.

**Glycoprotein IIb/IIIa inhibitors**  Glycoprotein IIb/IIIa inhibitors prevent platelet aggregation by blocking the binding of fibrinogen to receptors on platelets. **Abciximab** is a monoclonal antibody which binds to glycoprotein IIb/IIIa receptors and to other related sites; it is licensed as an adjunct to heparin and aspirin for the prevention of ischaemic complications in high-risk patients undergoing percutaneous transluminal coronary intervention. Abciximab should be used once only (to avoid additional risk of thrombocytopenia). **Eptifibatide** and **tirofiban** also inhibit glycoprotein IIb/IIIa receptors; they are licensed for use with heparin and aspirin to prevent early myocardial infarction in patients with unstable angina (section 2.6) or non-ST-segment-elevation myocardial infarction. Abciximab, eptifibatide and tirofiban should be used by specialists only.

For use of epoprostenol, see section 2.8.1.

---

**NICE guidance**
**Glycoprotein IIb/IIIa inhibitors for acute coronary syndromes (September 2002)**
A glycoprotein IIb/IIIa inhibitor (abciximab, eptifibatide, and tirofiban) should be considered for the management of unstable angina or non-ST-segment-elevation myocardial infarction.
A glycoprotein IIb/IIIa inhibitor is recommended for patients at high risk of myocardial infarction or death when early percutaneous coronary intervention is desirable but does not occur immediately; either eptifibatide or tirofiban is recommended in addition to other appropriate drug treatment.
A glycoprotein IIb/IIIa inhibitor is recommended as an adjunct to percutaneous coronary intervention:
- when early percutaneous coronary intervention is indicated but it is delayed;
- in patients with diabetes;
- if the procedure is complex.
Note Only abciximab is licensed as an adjunct to percutaneous coronary intervention

---

## ▌ ABCIXIMAB

**Indications**  prevention of ischaemic cardiac complications in patients undergoing percutaneous coronary intervention; short-term prevention of myocardial infarction in patients with unstable angina not responding to conventional treatment and who are scheduled for percutaneous coronary intervention (use under specialist supervision)

**Cautions** measure baseline prothrombin time, activated clotting time, activated partial thromboplastin time, platelet count, haemoglobin and haematocrit; monitor haemoglobin and haematocrit 12 hours and 24 hours after start of treatment and platelet count 2–4 hours and 24 hours after start of treatment; concomitant use of drugs that increase risk of bleeding; discontinue if uncontrollable serious bleeding occurs or emergency cardiac surgery needed; consult product literature for details of procedures to minimise bleeding; elderly; hepatic impairment (Appendix 2); renal impairment (Appendix 3); pregnancy (Appendix 4)

**Contra-indications** active internal bleeding; major surgery, intracranial or intraspinal surgery or trauma within last 2 months; stroke within last 2 years; intracranial neoplasm, arteriovenous malformation or aneurysm, severe hypertension, haemorrhagic diathesis, thrombocytopenia, vasculitis, hypertensive retinopathy; breast-feeding (Appendix 5)

**Side-effects** bleeding manifestations; nausea, vomiting, hypotension, bradycardia, chest pain, back pain, headache, fever, puncture site pain, thrombocytopenia; *rarely* cardiac tamponade, adult respiratory distress, hypersensitivity reactions

**Dose**

- ADULT initially by intravenous injection over 1 minute, 250 micrograms/kg, then by intravenous infusion, 125 nanograms/kg/minute (max. 10 micrograms/minute); for prevention of ischaemic complications start 10–60 minutes before percutaneous coronary intervention and continue infusion for 12 hours; for unstable angina start up to 24 hours before possible percutaneous coronary intervention and continue infusion for 12 hours after intervention

**ReoPro®** (Lilly) [PoM]
Injection, abciximab 2 mg/mL, net price 5-mL vial = £250.24

▌ **ASPIRIN (antiplatelet)**
(Acetylsalicylic Acid)

**Indications** prophylaxis of cerebrovascular disease or myocardial infarction (see section 2.10.1 and notes above)

**Cautions** asthma; uncontrolled hypertension; previous peptic ulceration (but manufacturers may advise avoidance of low-dose aspirin in history of peptic ulceration); concomitant use of drugs that increase risk of bleeding; G6PD deficiency (section 9.1.5); hepatic impairment (avoid if severe; Appendix 2); renal impairment (avoid if severe; Appendix 3); pregnancy (Appendix 4); **interactions:** Appendix 1 (aspirin)

**Contra-indications** use other than as an antiplatelet in children and adolescents under 16 years (Reye's syndrome, section 4.7.1); active peptic ulceration; haemophilia and other bleeding disorders; breast-feeding (Appendix 5)

Hypersensitivity Aspirin and other NSAIDs are **contra-indicated** in history of hypersensitivity to aspirin or any other NSAID—which includes those in whom attacks of asthma, angioedema, urticaria, or rhinitis have been precipitated by aspirin or any other NSAID

**Side-effects** bronchospasm; gastro-intestinal irritation, gastro-intestinal haemorrhage (occasionally major), also other haemorrhage (e.g. subconjunctival)

**Dose**

- See notes above

[1]**Aspirin** (Non-proprietary) [PoM]
Dispersible tablets, aspirin 75 mg, net price 28 = 82p; 300 mg, see section 4.7.1. Label: 13, 21, 32

Tablets, e/c, aspirin 75 mg, net price 28-tab pack = 94p; 56-tab pack = £1.07; 300 mg, see section 4.7.1. Label: 5, 25, 32
Brands include *Micropirin®*

**Angettes 75®** (Bristol-Myers Squibb)
Tablets, aspirin 75 mg, net price 28-tab pack = 84p. Label: 32

**Caprin®** (Pinewood) [PoM]
Tablets, e/c, pink, aspirin 75 mg, net price 28-tab pack = £1.55, 56-tab pack = £3.08, 100-tab pack = £5.24; 300 mg, see section 4.7.1. Label: 5, 25, 32

**Nu-Seals® Aspirin** (Alliance) [PoM]
Tablets, e/c, aspirin 75 mg, net price 56-tab pack = £3.12; 300 mg, see section 4.7.1. Label: 5, 25, 32
Note Tablets may be chewed at diagnosis for rapid absorption

◢**Modified release**
Note Modified release aspirin should **not** be used in acute situations when a rapid onset of action is required

**Flamasacard®** (Abbey) [PoM]
Capsules, m/r, white/red, aspirin 162.5 mg, net price 30-cap pack = £2.70. Label: 25, 32
Dose secondary prophylaxis following a coronary or cerebrovascular ischaemic event, 1 capsule once daily

▌ **CLOPIDOGREL**

**Indications** prevention of atherosclerotic events in peripheral arterial disease, or within 35 days of myocardial infarction, or within 6 months of ischaemic stroke; prevention of artherosclerotic events in acute coronary syndrome without ST-segment elevation (given with aspirin—see notes above) and in acute myocardial infarction with ST-segment elevation (given with aspirin—see notes above)

**Cautions** patients at risk of increased bleeding from trauma, surgery or other pathological conditions; concomitant use of drugs that increase risk of bleeding; discontinue 7 days before elective surgery if antiplatelet effect not desirable; liver impairment (Appendix 2); renal impairment (Appendix 3); pregnancy (Appendix 4); **interactions:** Appendix 1 (clopidogrel)

**Contra-indications** active bleeding, breast-feeding (Appendix 5)

**Side-effects** dyspepsia, abdominal pain, diarrhoea; bleeding disorders (including gastro-intestinal and intracranial); *less commonly* nausea, vomiting, gastritis, flatulence, constipation, gastric and duodenal ulcers, headache, dizziness, paraesthesia, leucopenia, decreased platelets (very rarely severe thrombocytopenia), eosinophilia, rash, and pruritus; *rarely* vertigo; *very rarely* colitis, pancreatitis, hepatitis, acute liver

---

1. Aspirin tablets 75 mg may be sold to the public in packs of up to 100 tablets; for details relating to other strengths see section 4.7.1 and *Medicines, Ethics and Practice*, No. 33, London, Pharmaceutical Press, 2009 (and subsequent editions as available)

**Cardiovascular system** (sidebar)

**2** (sidebar)

failure, vasculitis, confusion, hallucinations, taste disturbance, stomatitis, bronchospasm, interstitial pneumonitis, blood disorders (including thrombocytopenic purpura, agranulocytosis and pancytopenia), and hypersensitivity-like reactions (including fever, glomerulonephritis, arthralgia, Stevens-Johnson syndrome, toxic epidermal necrolysis, lichen planus)

**Dose**

- Prevention of artherosclerotic events in peripheral arterial disease or after myocardial infarction or ischaemic stroke, 75 mg once daily
- Acute coronary syndrome (without ST-segment elevation), initially 300 mg then 75 mg daily (with aspirin—see notes above)
- Acute myocardial infarction (with ST-segment elevation), initially 300 mg then 75 mg daily (with aspirin—see notes above); initial dose omitted if patient over 75 years

**Plavix®** (Bristol-Myers Squibb, Sanofi-Synthelabo) PoM
Tablets, pink, f/c, clopidogrel (as hydrogen sulphate) 75 mg, net price 30-tab pack = £36.35; 300 mg, 30-tab pack = £145.42

## DIPYRIDAMOLE

**Indications** see notes above and under Dose

**Cautions** rapidly worsening angina, aortic stenosis, recent myocardial infarction, left ventricular outflow obstruction, heart failure; may exacerbate migraine; hypotension; myasthenia gravis (risk of exacerbation); coagulation disorders; concomitant use of drugs that increase risk of bleeding; breast-feeding (Appendix 5); interactions: Appendix 1 (dipyridamole)

**Side-effects** gastro-intestinal effects, dizziness, myalgia, throbbing headache, hypotension, hot flushes and tachycardia; worsening symptoms of coronary heart disease; hypersensitivity reactions such as rash, urticaria, severe bronchospasm and angioedema; increased bleeding during or after surgery; thrombocytopenia reported

**Dose**

- By mouth, 300–600 mg daily in 3–4 divided doses Modified-release preparations, see under preparation below
- By intravenous Injection, diagnostic only, consult product literature

**Dipyridamole** (Non-proprietary) PoM
Tablets, coated, dipyridamole 25 mg, net price 84 = £3.53; 100 mg, 84 = £3.19. Label: 22

Oral suspension, dipyridamole 50 mg/5 mL, net price 150 mL = £37.38

**Persantin®** (Boehringer Ingelheim) PoM
Tablets, s/c, dipyridamole 25 mg (orange), net price 84-tab pack = £1.49; 100 mg, 84-tab pack = £4.16. Label: 22

Injection, dipyridamole 5 mg/mL, net price 2-mL amp = 12p

◢ **Modified release**

**Persantin® Retard** (Boehringer Ingelheim) PoM
Capsules, m/r, red/orange containing yellow pellets, dipyridamole 200 mg, net price 60-cap pack = £7.50. Label: 21, 25
**Dose** secondary prevention of ischaemic stroke and transient ischaemic attacks (used alone or with aspirin), adjunct to oral anticoagulation for prophylaxis of thromboembolism associated

with prosthetic heart valves, 200 mg twice daily preferably with food
**Note** Dispense in original container (pack contains a desiccant) and discard any capsules remaining 6 weeks after opening

◢ **With aspirin**

For cautions, contra-indications and side-effects of aspirin, see under Aspirin, above

**Asasantin® Retard** (Boehringer Ingelheim) PoM
Capsules, red/ivory, aspirin 25 mg, dipyridamole 200 mg (m/r), net price 60-cap pack = £7.79. Label: 21, 25
**Dose** secondary prevention of ischaemic stroke and transient ischaemic attacks, 1 capsule twice daily
**Note** Dispense in original container (pack contains a desiccant) and discard any capsules remaining 6 weeks after opening

## EPTIFIBATIDE

**Indications** prevention of early myocardial infarction in patients with unstable angina or non-ST-segment-elevation myocardial infarction and with last episode of chest pain within 24 hours (use under specialist supervision)

**Cautions** risk of bleeding, concomitant drugs that increase risk of bleeding—discontinue immediately if uncontrolled serious bleeding; measure baseline prothrombin time, activated partial thromboplastin time, platelet count, haemoglobin, haematocrit and serum creatinine; monitor haemoglobin, haematocrit and platelets within 6 hours after start of treatment then at least once daily; discontinue if thrombolytic therapy, intra-aortic balloon pump or emergency cardiac surgery necessary; hepatic impairment (Appendix 2); renal impairment (avoid if eGFR less than 30 mL/minute/1.73 m²; Appendix 3); pregnancy (Appendix 4); breast-feeding (Appendix 5)

**Contra-indications** abnormal bleeding within 30 days, major surgery or severe trauma within 6 weeks, stroke within last 30 days or any history of haemorrhagic stroke, intracranial disease (aneurysm, neoplasm or arteriovenous malformation), severe hypertension, haemorrhagic diathesis, increased prothrombin time or INR, thrombocytopenia, significant hepatic impairment; breast-feeding

**Side-effects** bleeding manifestations; *very rarely* anaphylaxis and rash

**Dose**

- Initially by intravenous injection, 180 micrograms/kg, then by intravenous infusion, 2 micrograms/kg/minute for up to 72 hours (up to 96 hours if percutaneous coronary intervention during treatment)

**Integrilin®** (GSK) PoM
Injection, eptifibatide 2 mg/mL, net price 10-mL (20-mg) vial = £13.89

Infusion, eptifibatide 750 micrograms/mL, net price 100-mL (75-mg) vial = £43.65

## PRASUGREL

**Indications** in combination with aspirin for the prevention of atherothrombotic events in patients with acute coronary syndrome undergoing percutaneous coronary intervention

**Cautions** patients at increased risk of bleeding (e.g. from recent trauma, surgery, gastro-intestinal bleeding, or active peptic ulcer disease); concomitant use of drugs that increase risk of bleeding; discontinue at least 7 days before elective surgery if antiplatelet effect not desirable; elderly; body-weight less than 60 kg; hepatic impairment (avoid if severe; Appendix 2); renal impairment (Appendix 3); pregnancy (Appendix 4); breast-feeding (Appendix 5); **interactions**: Appendix 1 (prasugrel)

**Contra-indications**  active bleeding; history of stroke or transient ischaemic attack

**Side-effects**  haemorrhage (including gastro-intestinal and intracranial), haematoma; haematuria; anaemia; rash

**Dose**

- ADULT over 18 years, (with aspirin—see notes above) initially 60 mg as a single dose then body-weight over 60 kg, 10 mg once daily *or* body-weight under 60 kg or ELDERLY over 75 years, 5 mg once daily

**Efient®** (Lilly) ▼ [PoM]
Tablets, f/c, prasugrel (as hydrochloride) 5 mg (yellow), net price 28-tab pack = £47.56; 10 mg (beige), 28-tab pack = £47.56

---

### ▌ TIROFIBAN

**Indications**  prevention of early myocardial infarction in patients with unstable angina or non-ST-segment-elevation myocardial infarction and with last episode of chest pain within 12 hours (use under specialist supervision)

**Cautions**  major surgery or severe trauma within 3 months (avoid if within 6 weeks); traumatic or protracted cardiopulmonary resuscitation, organ biopsy or lithotripsy within last 2 weeks; risk of bleeding including active peptic ulcer within 3 months; acute pericarditis, aortic dissection, haemorrhagic retinopathy, vasculitis, haematuria, faecal occult blood; severe heart failure, cardiogenic shock, anaemia; puncture of non-compressible vessel within 24 hours; concomitant drugs that increase risk of bleeding (including within 48 hours of thrombolytic administration); monitor platelet count, haemoglobin and haematocrit before treatment, 2–6 hours after start of treatment and then at least once daily; discontinue if thrombolytic therapy, intra-aortic balloon pump or emergency cardiac surgery necessary; discontinue immediately if serious bleeding uncontrolled by pressure occurs; hepatic impairment (avoid if severe; Appendix 2); renal impairment (Appendix 3); pregnancy (Appendix 4); **interactions**: Appendix 1 (tirofiban)

**Contra-indications**  abnormal bleeding within 30 days, stroke within 30 days or any history of haemorrhagic stroke, intracranial disease (aneurysm, neoplasm or arteriovenous malformation), severe hypertension, haemorrhagic diathesis, increased prothrombin time or INR, thrombocytopenia; breast-feeding (Appendix 5)

**Side-effects**  bleeding manifestations; reversible thrombocytopenia

**Dose**

- By intravenous infusion, initially 400 nanograms/kg/minute for 30 minutes, then 100 nanograms/kg/minute for at least 48 hours (continue during and for 12–24 hours after percutaneous coronary intervention); max. duration of treatment 108 hours

**Aggrastat®** (MSD) [PoM]
Concentrate for intravenous infusion, tirofiban (as hydrochloride) 250 micrograms/mL. For dilution before use, net price 50-mL (12.5-mg) vial = £146.11

Intravenous infusion, tirofiban (as hydrochloride) 50 micrograms/mL, net price 250-mL *Intravia®* bag = £160.72

---

## ▌2.10  Myocardial infarction and fibrinolysis

### 2.10.1  Management of myocardial infarction
### 2.10.2  Fibrinolytic drugs

---

## ▌2.10.1  Management of myocardial infarction

> Local guidelines for the management of myocardial infarction should be followed where they exist

Myocardial infarction is part of the spectrum of acute coronary syndromes which includes unstable angina, and myocardial infarction with or without ST-segment elevation.

These notes give an overview of the initial and long-term management of myocardial infarction with ST-segment elevation. For advice on the management of non-ST-segment elevation myocardial infarction and unstable angina, see section 2.6. The aims of management of ST-segment elevation myocardial infarction are to provide supportive care and pain relief, to promote reperfusion and to reduce mortality. Oxygen, nitrates, and diamorphine or morphine can provide initial support and pain relief; aspirin and percutaneous coronary intervention or thrombolytics promote reperfusion; long-term use of aspirin, beta-blockers, ACE inhibitors, and statins help to reduce mortality further.

**Initial management**  **Oxygen** (section 3.6) should be administered if there is evidence of hypoxia, pulmonary oedema, or continuing myocardial ischaemia; hyperoxia should be avoided and particular care is required in patients with chronic obstructive airways disease.

The pain (and anxiety) of myocardial infarction is managed with slow intravenous injection of **diamorphine** or **morphine** (section 4.7.2); an antiemetic such as metoclopramide (or, if left ventricular function is not compromised, cyclizine) by intravenous injection should also be given (section 4.6).

**Aspirin** (chewed or dispersed in water) is given for its antiplatelet effect (section 2.9); a dose of 300 mg is suitable. If aspirin is given before arrival at hospital, a note saying that it has been given should be sent with the patient. **Clopidogrel**, in a dose of 300 mg, should also be given (section 2.9).

Patency of the occluded artery can be restored by percutaneous coronary intervention or by giving a **thrombolytic drug** (section 2.10.2), unless contra-indicated. Percutaneous coronary intervention is the preferred method and patients should receive a **glycopro-**

tein IIb/IIIa inhibitor (section 2.9) to reduce the risk of immediate vascular occlusion. In patients who cannot be offered percutaneous coronary intervention within 90 minutes of diagnosis, a thrombolytic drug should be administered. A **low molecular weight heparin** or **fondaparinux** (section 2.8.1) should also be given to all patients; anticoagulant treatment should be continued for up to 8 days, or until percutaneous coronary intervention, or hospital discharge.

**Heparin [unfractionated]** can be considered for use in myocardial infarction if there is a high risk of systemic or pulmonary embolism. It should also be considered as initial therapy during the first 48 hours in patients treated with thrombolytics (consult thrombolytic product literature and local protocols (where they exist) for details of heparin dosage).

**Nitrates** (section 2.6.1) are used to relieve ischaemic pain. If sublingual glyceryl trinitrate is not effective, intravenous glyceryl trinitrate or isosorbide dinitrate is given.

Early administration of some **beta-blockers** (section 2.4) has been shown to be of benefit and should be given to patients without contra-indications.

**ACE inhibitors** (section 2.5.5.1), and angiotensin-II receptor antagonists (section 2.5.5.2) if an ACE inhibitor cannot be used, are also of benefit to patients who have no contra-indications; in hypertensive and normotensive patients treatment with an ACE inhibitor, or an angiotensin-II receptor antagonist, can be started within 24 hours of the myocardial infarction and continued for at least 5–6 weeks (see below for long-term treatment).

All patients should be closely monitored for hyperglycaemia; those with diabetes or raised blood-glucose concentration should receive **insulin**.

**Long-term management**   Long-term management involves the use of several drugs which should ideally be started before the patient is discharged from hospital.

**Aspirin** (section 2.9) should be given to all patients, unless contra-indicated, at a dose of 75 mg daily. The addition of **clopidogrel** (section 2.9) has been shown to reduce morbidity and mortality. For those intolerant of clopidogrel, and who are at low risk of bleeding, the combination of **warfarin** (section 2.8.2) and aspirin should be considered. In those intolerant of both aspirin and clopidogrel, warfarin alone can be used. Warfarin should be continued for those who are already being treated for another indication, such as atrial fibrillation, with the addition of aspirin if there is a low risk of bleeding. The combination of aspirin with clopidogrel or warfarin increases the risk of bleeding.

**Beta-blockers** (section 2.4) should be given to all patients in whom they are not contra-indicated. Acebutolol, metoprolol, propranolol, and timolol are suitable; for patients with left ventricular dysfunction, carvedilol, bisoprolol, or long-acting metoprolol may be appropriate (section 2.5.5).

**Diltiazem** [unlicensed] or **verapamil** (section 2.6.2) can be considered if a beta-blocker cannot be used; however, they are contra-indicated in those with left ventricular dysfunction. Other calcium-channel blockers have no place in routine long-term management after a myocardial infarction.

An **ACE inhibitor** (section 2.5.5.1) should be considered for all patients, especially those with evidence of left

ventricular dysfunction. If an ACE inhibitor cannot be used, an angiotensin-II receptor antagonist may be used for patients with heart failure. A relatively high dose of either the ACE inhibitor or angiotensin-II receptor antagonist may be required to produce benefit.

**Nitrates** (section 2.6.1) are used for patients with angina.

**Eplerenone** (section 2.2.3) is licensed for use following a myocardial infarction in those with left ventricular dysfunction and evidence of heart failure.

For the role of **statins** in preventing recurrent cardiovascular events, see section 2.12.

## 2.10.2 Fibrinolytic drugs

Fibrinolytic drugs act as thrombolytics by activating plasminogen to form plasmin, which degrades fibrin and so breaks up thrombi.

The value of thrombolytic drugs for the treatment of *myocardial infarction* has been established (section 2.10.1). **Streptokinase** and **alteplase** have been shown to reduce mortality. **Reteplase** and **tenecteplase** are also licensed for acute myocardial infarction. Thrombolytic drugs are indicated for any patient with acute myocardial infarction for whom the benefit is likely to outweigh the risk of treatment. Trials have shown that the benefit is greatest in those with ECG changes that include ST segment elevation (especially in those with anterior infarction) and in patients with bundle branch block. Patients should not be denied thrombolytic treatment on account of age alone because mortality in the elderly is high and the reduction in mortality is the same as in younger patients.

Alteplase, reteplase and streptokinase need to be given within 12 hours of symptom onset, ideally within 1 hour; use after 12 hours requires specialist advice. Tenecteplase should be given as early as possible and usually within 6 hours of symptom onset.

Alteplase, streptokinase, and **urokinase** can be used for other thromboembolic disorders such as deep-vein thrombosis and pulmonary embolism. Alteplase is also used for acute ischaemic stroke. Treatment must be started promptly.

Urokinase is also licensed to restore the patency of occluded intravenous catheters and cannulas blocked with fibrin clots.

> **NICE guidance**
> **Alteplase for the treatment of acute ischaemic stroke (June 2007)**
> Alteplase, used in accordance with the licence for *Actilyse®*, is recommended for the treatment of acute ischaemic stroke.

**Cautions**   Thrombolytic drugs should be used with caution if there is a risk of bleeding including that from venepuncture or invasive procedures. They should also be used with caution in external chest compression, pregnancy (Appendix 4), elderly, hypertension, conditions in which thrombolysis might give rise to embolic complications such as enlarged left atrium with atrial fibrillation (risk of dissolution of clot and subsequent embolisation), and recent or concurrent use of drugs that increase the risk of bleeding.

**Contra-indications**  Thrombolytic drugs are contra-indicated in recent haemorrhage, trauma, or surgery (including dental extraction), coagulation defects, bleeding diatheses, aortic dissection, aneurysm, coma, history of cerebrovascular disease especially recent events or with any residual disability, recent symptoms of possible peptic ulceration, heavy vaginal bleeding, severe hypertension, active pulmonary disease with cavitation, acute pancreatitis, pericarditis, bacterial endocarditis, severe liver disease, and oesophageal varices; also in the case of streptokinase, previous allergic reactions to either streptokinase or anistreplase (no longer available).

Prolonged persistence of antibodies to streptokinase and anistreplase (no longer available) can reduce the effectiveness of subsequent treatment; therefore, streptokinase should not be used again beyond 4 days of first administration of either streptokinase or anistreplase.

**Side-effects**  Side-effects of thrombolytics are mainly nausea and vomiting and bleeding. When thrombolytics are used in myocardial infarction, reperfusion arrhythmias and recurrent ischaemia and angina may occur. Reperfusion may also cause cerebral and pulmonary oedema. Hypotension can also occur and can usually be controlled by elevating the patient's legs, or by reducing the rate of infusion or stopping it temporarily. Back pain, fever, and convulsions have been reported. Bleeding is usually limited to the site of injection, but intracerebral haemorrhage or bleeding from other sites can occur. Serious bleeding calls for discontinuation of the thrombolytic and may require administration of coagulation factors and antifibrinolytic drugs (e.g. tranexamic acid). Rarely further embolism may occur (either due to clots that break away from the original thrombus or to cholesterol crystal emboli). Thrombolytics can cause allergic reactions (including rash, flushing and uveitis) and anaphylaxis has been reported (for details of management see Allergic Emergencies, section 3.4.3). Guillain-Barré syndrome has been reported rarely after streptokinase treatment.

### ALTEPLASE
(rt-PA, tissue-type plasminogen activator)

**Indications**  acute myocardial infarction (see notes above and section 2.10.1); pulmonary embolism; acute ischaemic stroke (treatment under specialist neurology physician **only**)

**Cautions**  see notes above; *in acute stroke*, monitor for intracranial haemorrhage, monitor blood pressure (antihypertensive recommended if systolic above 180 mmHg or diastolic above 105 mmHg)

**Contra-indications**  see notes above; *in acute stroke*, convulsion accompanying stroke, severe stroke, history of stroke in patients with diabetes, stroke in last 3 months, hypoglycaemia, hyperglycaemia

**Side-effects**  see notes above; also risk of cerebral bleeding increased in acute stroke

**Dose**

● Myocardial infarction, accelerated regimen (initiated within 6 hours of symptom onset), 15 mg by intravenous injection, followed by intravenous infusion of 50 mg over 30 minutes, then 35 mg over 60

minutes (total dose 100 mg over 90 minutes); in patients less than 65 kg, 15 mg by intravenous injection, followed by intravenous infusion of 0.75 mg/kg over 30 minutes, then 0.5 mg/kg over 60 minutes (max. total dose 100 mg over 90 minutes)

● Myocardial infarction, initiated within 6–12 hours of symptom onset, 10 mg by intravenous injection, followed by intravenous infusion of 50 mg over 60 minutes, then 4 infusions each of 10 mg over 30 minutes (total dose 100 mg over 3 hours; max. 1.5 mg/kg in patients less than 65 kg)

● Pulmonary embolism, 10 mg by intravenous injection over 1–2 minutes, followed by intravenous infusion of 90 mg over 2 hours; max. 1.5 mg/kg in patients less than 65 kg

● Acute stroke (treatment **must** begin within 3 hours of symptom onset), by intravenous administration over 60 minutes, 900 micrograms/kg (max. 90 mg); initial 10% of dose by intravenous injection, remainder by intravenous infusion; ELDERLY over 80 years not recommended

**Actilyse®** (Boehringer Ingelheim) PoM
Injection, powder for reconstitution, alteplase 10 mg (5.8 million units)/vial, net price per vial (with diluent) = £120.00; 20 mg (11.6 million units)/vial (with diluent and transfer device) = £180.00; 50 mg (29 million-units)/vial (with diluent, transfer device, and infusion bag) = £300.00

### RETEPLASE

**Indications**  acute myocardial infarction (see notes above and section 2.10.1)

**Cautions**  see notes above; breast-feeding (Appendix 5)

**Contra-indications**  see notes above

**Side-effects**  see notes above

**Dose**

● By intravenous injection (initiated within 12 hours of symptom onset), 10 units over not more than 2 minutes, followed after 30 minutes by a further 10 units

**Rapilysin®** (Actavis) PoM
Injection, powder for reconstitution, reteplase 10 units/vial, net price pack of 2 vials (with 2 prefilled syringes of diluent and transfer device) = £640.13

### STREPTOKINASE

**Indications**  acute myocardial infarction (see notes above and section 2.10.1); deep-vein thrombosis, pulmonary embolism, acute arterial thromboembolism, and central retinal venous or arterial thrombosis

**Cautions**  see notes above

**Contra-indications**  see notes above

**Side-effects**  see notes above

**Dose**

● Myocardial infarction (initiated within 12 hours of symptom onset), by intravenous infusion, 1.5 million units over 60 minutes

● Deep-vein thrombosis, pulmonary embolism, acute arterial thromboembolism, central retinal venous or arterial thrombosis, by intravenous infusion, 250 000 units over 30 minutes, then 100 000 units every hour for up to 12–72 hours according to condition with monitoring of clotting parameters (consult product literature)

**Streptase®** (CSL Behring) PoM
Injection, powder for reconstitution, streptokinase, net price 250 000-unit vial = £15.91; 750 000-unit vial = £41.72; 1.5 million-unit vial = £83.44 (hosp. only)

### TENECTEPLASE

**Indications** acute myocardial infarction (see notes above and section 2.10.1)

**Cautions** see notes above; breast-feeding (Appendix 5)

**Contra-indications** see notes above

**Side-effects** see notes above

**Dose**
- By intravenous injection over 10 seconds (initiated within 6 hours of symptom onset), 30–50 mg according to body-weight—consult product literature; max. 50 mg

**Metalyse®** (Boehringer Ingelheim) PoM
Injection, powder for reconstitution, tenecteplase, net price 40-mg (8000-unit) vial = £502.25; 50-mg (10 000-unit) vial = £502.25 (both with prefilled syringe of water for injection)

### UROKINASE

**Indications** thromboembolic occlusive vascular disease including deep-vein thrombosis, pulmonary embolism, and peripheral vascular occlusion; occluded intravenous catheters and cannulas blocked by fibrin clots

**Cautions** see notes above

**Contra-indications** see notes above

**Side-effects** see notes above

**Dose**
- Deep-vein thrombosis, by intravenous infusion, initially 4400 units/kg in 15 mL sodium chloride 0.9% over 10 minutes, followed by 4400 units/kg/hour for 12–24 hours
- Pulmonary embolism, by intravenous infusion, initially 4400 units/kg in 15 mL sodium chloride 0.9% over 10 minutes, followed by 4400 units/kg/hour for 12 hours *or* by injection into pulmonary artery, initially 15 000 units/kg, subsequent doses adjusted according to response; max. 3 doses in 24 hours
- Peripheral vascular occlusion, consult product literature
- Occluded catheters and cannulas, by injection directly into catheter or cannula, 5000–25 000 units in 2 mL sodium chloride 0.9%; leave for up to 4 hours then aspirate the lysate

**Syner-KINASE®** (Syner-Med) PoM
Injection, powder for reconstitution, urokinase, net price 25 000 unit vial = £45.95; 100 000 unit vial = £112.95
Note 10 000-unit vial, 50 000-unit vial, and 250 000-unit vial also available from 'special-order' manufacturers or specialist importing companies, see p. 969

## 2.11 Antifibrinolytic drugs and haemostatics

Fibrin dissolution can be impaired by the administration of **tranexamic acid**, which inhibits fibrinolysis. It can be used to prevent bleeding or to treat bleeding associated with excessive fibrinolysis (e.g. in prostatectomy, bladder surgery, in dental extraction in patients with haemophilia, in conisation of the cervix, and in traumatic hyphaema) and in the management of menorrhagia. Tranexamic acid may also be used in hereditary angioedema, epistaxis, and in thrombolytic overdose.

**Desmopressin** (section 6.5.2) is used in the management of mild to moderate haemophilia and von Willebrand's disease. It is also used for fibrinolytic response testing.

**Etamsylate** (ethamsylate) reduces capillary bleeding in the presence of a normal number of platelets. It does not act by fibrin stabilisation, but probably by correcting abnormal adhesion.

### ETAMSYLATE
(Ethamsylate)

**Indications** blood loss in menorrhagia

**Contra-indications** acute porphyria (see section 9.8.2)

**Side-effects** nausea, headache, rashes

**Dose**
- 500 mg 4 times daily during menstruation

**Dicynene®** (Sanofi-Synthelabo) PoM
Tablets, scored, etamsylate 500 mg, net price 100–tab pack = £8.44

### TRANEXAMIC ACID

**Indications** see notes above

**Cautions** renal impairment (Appendix 3); massive haematuria (avoid if risk of ureteric obstruction); not for use in disseminated intravascular coagulation; irregular menstrual bleeding (establish cause before initiating therapy); pregnancy (Appendix 4); regular liver function tests in long-term treatment of hereditary angioedema

**Contra-indications** thromboembolic disease

**Side-effects** nausea, vomiting, diarrhoea (reduce dose); *rarely* disturbances in colour vision (discontinue), thromboembolic events, allergic skin reactions; giddiness and hypotension on rapid intravenous injection

**Dose**
- By mouth, local fibrinolysis, 1–1.5 g (*or* 15–25 mg/kg) 2–3 times daily
  Menorrhagia (initiated when menstruation has started), 1 g 3 times daily for up to 4 days; max. 4 g daily
  Hereditary angioedema, 1–1.5 g 2–3 times daily
  Epistaxis, 1 g 3 times daily for 7 days
- By slow intravenous injection, local fibrinolysis, 0.5–1 g 3 times daily
- By continuous intravenous infusion, local fibrinolysis, following initial treatment by intravenous injection, 25–50 mg/kg over 24 hours

**Tranexamic acid** (Non-proprietary) ⒫Ⓞⓜ
Tablets, tranexamic acid 500 mg, net price 60-tab pack = £6.90

**Cyklokapron®** (Meda) ⒫Ⓞⓜ
Tablets, f/c, scored, tranexamic acid 500 mg, net price 60-tab pack = £14.30

**Cyklokapron®** (Pfizer) ⒫Ⓞⓜ
Injection, tranexamic acid 100 mg/mL, net price 5-mL amp = £1.55

## Blood products

### ▌ ANTITHROMBIN III CONCENTRATE
Dried antithrombin III is prepared from human plasma

**Indications** congenital deficiency of antithrombin III
**Side-effects** nausea, flushing, headache, dizziness; *rarely* allergic reactions and fever
Available from BPL (Dried Antithrombin III)
**Note** Preparation of recombinant human antithrombin (antithrombin alfa) available from LEO (*ATryn*® ▼) indicated for the prophylaxis of venous thromboembolism in surgery in patients with congenital antithrombin deficiency

### ▌ DRIED PROTHROMBIN COMPLEX
(Human Prothrombin Complex)
Dried prothrombin complex is prepared from human plasma by a suitable fractionation technique, and contains factor IX, together with variable amounts of factors II, VII, and X

**Indications** treatment and peri-operative prophylaxis of haemorrhage in patients with congenital deficiency of factors II, VII, IX, or X if purified specific coagulation factors not available; treatment and peri-operative prophylaxis of haemorrhage in patients with acquired deficiency of factors II, VII, IX, or X (e.g. during warfarin treatment—see section 2.8.2)
**Cautions** risk of thrombosis; disseminated intravascular coagulation; history of myocardial infarction or coronary heart disease; hepatic disease; postoperative use
**Contra-indications** angina; recent myocardial infarction (except in life-threatening haemorrhage following overdosage of oral anticoagulants, and before induction of fibrinolytic therapy); history of heparin-induced thrombocytopenia
**Side-effects** thrombotic events (including disseminated intravascular coagulation); *very rarely* pyrexia, antibody formation, hypersensitivity reactions (including anaphylaxis); nephrotic syndrome also reported
Available from CSL Behring (*Beriplex® P/N*▼)

### ▌ DROTRECOGIN ALFA (ACTIVATED)
Recombinant activated protein C

**Indications** adjunctive treatment of severe sepsis with multiple organ failure—start treatment within 24 hours (and no later than 48 hours) after onset of organ failure
**Cautions** increased risk of bleeding, concomitant use of drugs that increase risk of bleeding; pregnancy (Appendix 4); breast-feeding (Appendix 5); **interactions**: Appendix 1 (drotrecogin alfa)

**Contra-indications** internal bleeding; intracranial neoplasm or cerebral herniation; chronic severe hepatic disease; thrombocytopenia; not recommended for use in children under 18 years or in single organ failure
**Side-effects** bleeding; headache; ecchymosis; pain
Available from Lilly (*Xigris®*)

> **NICE guidance**
> **Drotrecogin alfa (activated) for severe sepsis (September 2004)**
> Drotrecogin alfa (activated) should be considered for adults with severe sepsis that has resulted in the failure of two or more major organs and who are receiving optimum intensive care support. Drotrecogin alfa (activated) should be initiated and supervised only by a specialist consultant with intensive care skills and experience in the care of patients with sepsis.

### ▌ FACTOR VIIa (RECOMBINANT)
Eptacog alfa (activated)

**Indications** treatment and prophylaxis of haemorrhage in patients with haemophilia A or B with inhibitors to factors VIII or IX, acquired haemophilia, factor VII deficiency, or Glanzmann's thrombasthenia
**Cautions** risk of thrombosis or disseminated intravascular coagulation
**Side-effects** *very rarely* nausea, thrombotic events (including myocardial infarction and cerebrovascular accident), coagulation disorders, fever, pain, and allergic reactions including rash
Available from Novo Nordisk (*NovoSeven®* ▼)

### ▌ FACTOR VIII FRACTION, DRIED
(Human Antihaemophilic Fraction, Dried)
Dried factor VIII fraction is prepared from human plasma by a suitable fractionation technique

**Indications** treatment and prophylaxis of haemorrhage in congenital factor VIII deficiency (haemophilia A), acquired factor VIII deficiency, von Willebrand's disease
**Cautions** monitor for development of factor VIII inhibitors; intravascular haemolysis after large or frequently repeated doses in patients with blood groups A, B, or AB—less likely with high potency concentrates
**Side-effects** gastro-intestinal disturbances, taste disturbances; flushing, palpitation; dyspnoea, coughing; headache, dizziness, paraesthesia, drowsiness; blurred vision; antibody formation; hypersensitivity reactions including hypotension, angioedema, chills, fever, urticaria, and anaphylaxis

Available from Biotest UK (*Haemoctin®* ▼), CSL Behring (*Haemate® P*), BPL (*Optivate®*, High Purity Factor VIII and von Willebrand factor concentrate; *8Y®*), Grifols (*Alphanate®*; *Fanhdi®*), Octapharma (*Octanate®* ▼)
**Note** Preparation of recombinant human antihaemophilic factor VIII (octocog alfa) available from CSL Behring (*Helixate® NexGen*), Baxter (*Advate®*), Bayer (*Kogenate® Bayer*); preparation of recombinant human antihaemophilic factor VIII (moroctocog alfa) available from Wyeth (*ReFacto AF®* ▼); octocog alfa and moroctocog alfa are not indicated for use in von Willebrand's disease

Cardiovascular system

2

### FACTOR VIII INHIBITOR BYPASSING FRACTION

Preparations with factor VIII inhibitor bypassing activity are prepared from human plasma

**Indications** treatment and prophylaxis of haemorrhage in patients with congenital factor VIII deficiency (haemophilia A) and factor VIII inhibitors; treatment of haemorrhage in non-haemophiliac patients with acquired factor VIII inhibitors
**Contra-indications** disseminated intravascular coagulation
**Side-effects** paraesthesia; pyrexia; allergic reactions including hypotension, flushing, urticaria, rash, and anaphylaxis
Available from Baxter (*FEIBA®*)

### FACTOR IX FRACTION, DRIED

Dried factor IX fraction is prepared from human plasma by a suitable fractionation technique; it may also contain clotting factors II, VII, and X

**Indications** treatment and prophylaxis of haemorrhage in congenital factor IX deficiency (haemophilia B)
**Cautions** risk of thrombosis—principally with former low purity products
**Contra-indications** disseminated intravascular coagulation
**Side-effects** gastro-intestinal disturbances; headache, dizziness; allergic reactions, including chills, fever
Available from CSL Behring (*Mononine®*), BPL (*Replenine®-VF*, Dried Factor IX Fraction), Grifols (*AlphaNine®*)
**Note** Preparation of recombinant coagulation factor IX (nonacog alfa) available from Wyeth (*BeneFIX®*)

### FACTOR XIII FRACTION, DRIED
(Human Fibrin-stabilising Factor, Dried)

**Indications** congenital factor XIII deficiency
**Side-effects** rarely, allergic reactions and fever
Available from CSL Behring (*Fibrogammin® P*)

### FRESH FROZEN PLASMA

Fresh frozen plasma is prepared from the supernatant liquid obtained by centrifugation of one donation of whole blood

**Indications** to replace coagulation factors or other plasma proteins where their concentration or functional activity is critically reduced, e.g. to reverse warfarin effect
**Cautions** need for compatibility
**Contra-indications** circulatory overload; avoid use as a volume expander
**Side-effects** allergic reactions including chills, fever, bronchospasm; adult respiratory distress syndrome
Available from Regional Blood Transfusion Services and BPL
**Note** A preparation of solvent/detergent treated human plasma (frozen) from pooled donors is available from Octapharma (*Octaplas®*)

### PROTEIN C CONCENTRATE

Protein C is prepared from human plasma

**Indications** congenital protein C deficiency
**Cautions** hypersensitivity to heparin

**Side-effects** fever, arrhythmia, bleeding and thrombosis reported; *rarely* allergic reactions
Available from Baxter (*Ceprotin®*)

## 2.12 Lipid-regulating drugs

Preventative measures should be taken in individuals with a high risk of developing cardiovascular disease (primary prevention) and to prevent recurrence of events in those with established cardiovascular disease (secondary prevention).

Individuals at high risk include those who already have atherosclerotic disease, those with diabetes mellitus aged over 40 years, and those with familial hypercholesterolaemia. The risk also increases with age; those over 75 years are at particularly high risk, especially if they smoke or have hypertension.

Preventative measures are also required for other individuals who may be at high risk of developing atherosclerotic cardiovascular disease; those with a 10-year risk of cardiovascular disease[1] of 20% or more stand to benefit most from drug treatment. The risk is assessed on the basis of lipid concentration as well as smoking status, blood pressure, gender, and age; other risk factors, such as premature menopause, ethnicity, obesity, triglyceride concentration, chronic kidney disease, impaired glucose tolerance, and a family history of premature cardiovascular disease, should also be taken into account when assessing risk in individual patients.

Lowering the concentration of low-density lipoprotein (LDL) cholesterol and raising high-density lipoprotein (HDL) cholesterol slows the progression of atherosclerosis and may even induce regression. All patients at high risk of cardiovascular disease should be advised to make lifestyle modifications that include beneficial changes to diet, exercise, weight management, alcohol consumption, and smoking cessation. Lipid-regulating drug treatment must be combined with advice on diet and lifestyle measures, lowering of raised blood pressure (section 2.5), the use of low-dose aspirin (section 2.9), and management of diabetes (section 6.1).

The prescribing of drug therapy in homozygous familial hypercholesterolaemia should be undertaken in a specialist centre.

A **statin** (see p. 143) reduces the risk of cardiovascular disease events, irrespective of serum cholesterol concentration, and is the drug of first choice for primary and secondary prevention of cardiovascular disease. If statins are contra-indicated or not tolerated, a **fibrate** (p. 147) or a **bile acid sequestrant** (p. 145) may be considered for *primary* or *secondary* prevention; **nicotinic acid** (p. 148) is also an option for *secondary* prevention. Fibrates, bile acid sequestrants, or nicotinic acid should not be used in combination with a statin for *primary* prevention of cardiovascular disease. In secondary prevention of cardiovascular events, consider adjusting doses of lipid-regulating drugs if a total

---

1. Cardiovascular disease risk may be determined from the chart issued by the Joint British Societies (*Heart* 2005; **91** (Suppl V): v1–v52)—see inside back cover. The Joint British Societies' 'Cardiac Risk Assessor' computer programme may also be used to determine cardiovascular disease risk.

cholesterol concentration of less than 4 mmol/litre *or* a LDL-cholesterol concentration of less than 2 mmol/litre is not achieved with initial treatment.

A statin is also the drug of first choice for treating hypercholesterolaemia and moderate hypertriglyceridaemia. Severe hyperlipidaemia not adequately controlled with a maximal dose of a statin may require the use of an additional lipid-regulating drug such as **ezetimibe** or **colestyramine**; such treatment should generally be supervised by a specialist.

A number of conditions, some familial, are characterised by very high LDL-cholesterol concentration, high triglyceride concentration, or both. A **fibrate** is added to statin therapy if triglycerides remain high even after the LDL-cholesterol concentration has been reduced adequately; **nicotinic acid** may also be used to further lower triglyceride or LDL-cholesterol concentration.

Combination of a statin with a fibrate or with nicotinic acid carries an increased risk of side-effects (including rhabdomyolysis—see CSM advice below) and should be used under specialist supervision; monitoring of liver function and creatine kinase should also be considered. The concomitant administration of gemfibrozil with a statin increases the risk of rhabdomyolysis considerably—this combination should **not** be used.

Patients with hypothyroidism should receive adequate thyroid replacement therapy before assessing the requirement for lipid-regulating treatment because correcting hypothyroidism itself may resolve the lipid abnormality. Untreated hypothyroidism increases the risk of myositis with lipid-regulating drugs.

---

**CSM advice (muscle effects)**
The CSM has advised that rhabdomyolysis associated with lipid-regulating drugs such as the fibrates and statins appears to be rare (approx. 1 case in every 100 000 treatment years) but may be increased in those with renal impairment and possibly in those with hypothyroidism (see also notes above). Concomitant treatment with drugs that increase plasma-statin concentration increase the risk of muscle toxicity; concomitant treatment with a fibrate and a statin may also be associated with an increased risk of serious muscle toxicity.

---

## Statins

The statins (**atorvastatin**, **fluvastatin**, **pravastatin**, **rosuvastatin**, and **simvastatin**) competitively inhibit 3-hydroxy-3-methylglutaryl coenzyme A (HMG CoA) reductase, an enzyme involved in cholesterol synthesis, especially in the liver. Statins are more effective than other lipid-regulating drugs at lowering LDL-cholesterol concentration but they are less effective than the fibrates in reducing triglyceride concentration. However, statins reduce cardiovascular disease events and total mortality irrespective of the initial cholesterol concentration.

Statins should be considered for all patients, including the elderly, with symptomatic cardiovascular disease such as those with coronary heart disease (including history of angina or acute myocardial infarction), occlusive arterial disease (including peripheral vascular disease, non-haemorrhagic stroke, or transient ischaemic attacks).

In patients with diabetes mellitus, the risk of developing cardiovascular disease depends on the duration and complications of diabetes, age, and concomitant risk factors. Statin therapy should be considered for *all* patients over 40 years with diabetes mellitus (type 1 and 2). In younger patients with diabetes, treatment with a statin should be considered if there is target-organ damage, poor glycaemic control (HbA$_{1c}$ greater than 9%), low HDL-cholesterol and raised triglyceride concentration, hypertension, or a family history of premature cardiovascular disease.

Statins are also used for the prevention of cardiovascular disease events in asymptomatic individuals who are at increased risk (see p. 142). Statin treatment should also be considered if the total cholesterol concentration to HDL-cholesterol ratio exceeds 6.

**Cautions** Statins should be used with caution in those with a history of liver disease or with a high alcohol intake (use should be avoided in active liver disease). Hypothyroidism should be managed adequately before starting treatment with a statin (see above). There is little information available on a rational approach to liver-function monitoring; however, a NICE guideline[1] suggests that liver enzymes should be measured before treatment, and repeated within 3 months and at 12 months of starting treatment, unless indicated at other times by signs or symptoms suggestive of hepatotoxicity. Those with serum transaminases that are raised, but less than 3 times the upper limit of the reference range, should **not** be routinely excluded from statin therapy. Those with serum transaminases of more than 3 times the upper limit of the reference range should discontinue statin therapy. Statins should be used with caution in those with risk factors for myopathy or rhabdomyolysis; patients should be advised to report unexplained muscle pain (see Muscle Effects below). Statins should be avoided in acute porphyria (section 9.8.2) but rosuvastatin is thought to be safe. **Interactions:** Appendix 1 (statins).

**Contra-indications** Statins are contra-indicated in active liver disease (or persistently abnormal liver function tests), in pregnancy (adequate contraception required during treatment and for 1 month afterwards) and during breast-feeding (see Appendix 4 and Appendix 5).

**Side-effects** The statins can cause various muscular side-effects, including myositis, which can lead to rhabdomyolysis. Muscular effects are rare but often significant (see below and CSM advice (Muscle Effects) above). Statins can cause gastro-intestinal disturbances, and very rarely pancreatitis. They can also cause altered liver function tests, and rarely hepatitis and jaundice; hepatic failure has been reported very rarely. Other side-effects include sleep disturbance, headache, dizziness, depression, paraesthesia, asthenia, peripheral neuropathy, amnesia, fatigue, sexual dysfunction, thrombocytopenia, arthralgia, visual disturbance, alopecia and hypersensitivity reactions (including rash, pruritus, urticaria, and very rarely lupus erythematosus-like reactions). In very rare cases, statins can cause interstitial lung disease; if patients develop symptoms such as

---

1. NICE clinical guideline 67 (May 2008). Lipid Modification—Cardiovascular risk assessment and the modification of blood lipids for the primary and secondary prevention of cardiovascular disease

dyspnoea, cough, and weight loss, they should seek medical attention.

**Muscle effects** Myalgia, myositis, and myopathy have been reported with the statins; if myopathy is suspected and creatine kinase is markedly elevated (more than 5 times upper limit of normal), or muscular symptoms are severe, treatment should be discontinued; in patients at high risk of muscle effects, a statin should not be started if creatine kinase is elevated. Patients at high risk of myopathy include those with a personal or family history of muscular disorders, previous history of muscular toxicity or liver disease, and the elderly (see also CSM advice p. 143). There is also an increased incidence of myopathy if a statin is given at a high dose or given with a fibrate, with lipid-lowering doses of nicotinic acid, or with immunosuppressants such as ciclosporin; close monitoring of liver function and, if symptomatic, of creatine kinase is required in patients receiving these drugs. Rhabdomyolysis with acute renal impairment secondary to myoglobinuria has also been reported.

**Counselling** Advise patient to report promptly unexplained muscle pain, tenderness, or weakness.

## ATORVASTATIN

**Indications** primary hypercholesterolaemia, heterozygous familial hypercholesterolaemia, homozygous familial hypercholesterolaemia or combined (mixed) hyperlipidaemia in patients who have not responded adequately to diet and other appropriate measures; prevention of cardiovascular events in patients with type 2 diabetes and at least one additional risk factor for cardiovascular disease

**Cautions** see notes above; also haemorrhagic stroke

**Contra-indications** see notes above

**Side-effects** see notes above; also chest pain; back pain; *less commonly* anorexia, malaise, weight gain, hypoglycaemia, hyperglycaemia, tinnitus; *rarely* cholestatic jaundice, peripheral oedema; *very rarely* taste disturbances, gynaecomastia, hearing loss, Stevens-Johnson Syndrome, and toxic epidermal necrolysis

**Dose**

- Primary hypercholesterolaemia and combined hyperlipidaemia, usually 10 mg once daily; if necessary, may be increased at intervals of at least 4 weeks to max. 80 mg once daily; CHILD 10–17 years usually 10 mg once daily (limited experience with doses above 20 mg daily)
- Familial hypercholesterolaemia, initially 10 mg daily, increased at intervals of at least 4 weeks to 40 mg once daily; if necessary, further increased to max. 80 mg once daily (or 40 mg once daily combined with anion-exchange resin in heterozygous familial hypercholesterolaemia); CHILD 10–17 years initially 10 mg daily, increased if necessary after at least 4 weeks to 20 mg once daily (limited experience with higher doses)
- Prevention of cardiovascular events in type 2 diabetes, 10 mg once daily

Note Max. 10 mg daily with concomitant ciclosporin; max. 20 mg daily (or temporarily discontinue atorvastatin) with concomitant clarithromycin; max. 40 mg daily (or temporarily discontinue atorvastatin) with concomitant itraconazole

**Lipitor®** (Pfizer) ℞

Tablets, all f/c, atorvastatin (as calcium trihydrate) 10 mg, net price 28-tab pack = £18.03; 20 mg, 28-tab pack = £24.64; 40 mg 28-tab pack = £24.64; 80 mg, 28-tab pack = £28.21. Counselling, muscle effects, see notes above

## FLUVASTATIN

Note The *Scottish Medicines Consortium* (p. 3) has advised (February 2004) that fluvastatin is accepted for restricted use for the secondary prevention of coronary events after percutaneous coronary angioplasty; if the patient has previously been receiving another statin, then there is no need to change the statin

**Indications** adjunct to diet in primary hypercholesterolaemia or combined (mixed) hyperlipidaemia (types IIa and IIb); adjunct to diet to slow progression of coronary atherosclerosis in primary hypercholesterolaemia and concomitant coronary heart disease; prevention of coronary events after percutaneous coronary intervention

**Cautions** see notes above

**Contra-indications** see notes above

**Side-effects** see notes above; also *very rarely* vasculitis

**Dose**

- Hypercholesterolaemia or combined hyperlipidaemia, initially 20–40 mg daily in the evening, adjusted at intervals of at least 4 weeks; up to 80 mg daily may be required; CHILD under 18 years, not recommended
- Prevention of progression of coronary atherosclerosis, 40 mg daily in the evening
- Following percutaneous coronary intervention, 80 mg daily

**Lescol®** (Novartis) ℞

Capsules, fluvastatin (as sodium salt) 20 mg (brown/yellow), net price 28-cap pack = £15.26; 40 mg (brown/orange), 28-cap pack = £15.26, 56-cap pack = £30.53. Counselling, muscle effects, see notes above

◀**Modified release**

**Lescol® XL** (Novartis) ℞

Tablets, m/r, yellow, fluvastatin (as sodium salt) 80 mg, net price 28-tab pack = £19.20. Label: 25, counselling, muscle effects, see notes above

Dose 80 mg once daily (dose form not appropriate for initial dose titration in hypercholesterolaemia or combined hyperlipidaemia)

## PRAVASTATIN SODIUM

**Indications** adjunct to diet for primary hypercholesterolaemia or combined (mixed) hyperlipidaemias in patients who have not responded adequately to dietary control; adjunct to diet to prevent cardiovascular events in patients with hypercholesterolaemia; prevention of cardiovascular events in patients with previous myocardial infarction or unstable angina; reduction of hyperlipidaemia in patients receiving immunosuppressive therapy following solid-organ transplantation

**Cautions** see notes above; renal impairment (Appendix 3)

**Contra-indications** see notes above

**Side-effects** see notes above; *less commonly* abnormal urination (including dysuria, nocturia and frequency); *very rarely* fulminant hepatic necrosis

**Dose**

- Hypercholesterolaemia or combined hyperlipidaemias, 10–40 mg once daily at night, adjusted at intervals of at least 4 weeks
- Familial hypercholesterolaemia, CHILD 8–14 years 10–20 mg once daily at night, 14–18 years 10–40 mg once daily at night

*(sidebar)* 2 Cardiovascular system

- Prevention of cardiovascular events, 40 mg once daily at night
- Post-transplantation hyperlipidaemia, initially 20 mg once daily at night, increased if necessary (under close medical supervision) to max. 40 mg once daily at night

**Pravastatin** (Non-proprietary) [PoM]
Tablets, pravastatin sodium 10 mg, net price 28-tab pack = £1.71; 20 mg, 28-tab pack = £2.13; 40 mg, 28-tab pack = £2.78. Counselling, muscle effects, see notes above

**Lipostat®** (Squibb) [PoM]
Tablets, all yellow, pravastatin sodium 10 mg, net price 28-tab pack = £14.46; 20 mg, 28-tab pack = £26.53; 40 mg, 28-tab pack = £26.53. Counselling, muscle effects, see notes above

### ■ ROSUVASTATIN

**Indications**  primary hypercholesterolaemia (type IIa including heterozygous familial hypercholesterolaemia), mixed dyslipidaemia (type IIb), or homozygous familial hypercholesterolaemia in patients who have not responded adequately to diet and other appropriate measures

**Cautions**  see notes above; patients of Asian origin (see under Dose); max. dose 20 mg in patients with risk factors for myopathy or rhabdomyolysis (including personal or family history of muscular disorders or toxicity); renal impairment (avoid if eGFR less than 30 mL/minute/1.73 m²; Appendix 3)

**Contra-indications**  see notes above

**Side-effects**  see notes above; also proteinuria; *very rarely* haematuria

**Dose**
- Initially 5–10 mg once daily increased if necessary at intervals of at least 4 weeks to 20 mg once daily, increased after further 4 weeks to 40 mg daily only in severe hypercholesterolaemia with high cardiovascular risk and under specialist supervision; ELDERLY initially 5 mg once daily; patient of ASIAN origin, initially 5 mg once daily increased if necessary to max. 20 mg daily

Note Initially 5 mg once daily with concomitant fibrate increased if necessary to max. 20 mg daily

**Crestor®** (AstraZeneca) [PoM]
Tablets, f/c, rosuvastatin (as calcium salt) 5 mg (yellow), net price 28-tab pack = £18.03; 10 mg (pink), 28-tab pack = £18.03; 20 mg (pink), 28-tab pack = £26.02; 40 mg (pink), 28-tab pack = £29.69. Counselling, muscle effects, see notes above

### ■ SIMVASTATIN

**Indications**  primary hypercholesterolaemia, homozygous familial hypercholesterolaemia or combined (mixed) hyperlipidaemia in patients who have not responded adequately to diet and other appropriate measures; prevention of cardiovascular events in patients with atherosclerotic cardiovascular disease or diabetes mellitus

**Cautions**  see notes above; renal impairment (Appendix 3)

**Contra-indications**  see notes above

**Side-effects**  see notes above; also *rarely* anaemia

**Dose**
- Primary hypercholesterolaemia, combined hyperlipidaemia, 10–20 mg daily at night, adjusted at intervals of at least 4 weeks; usual range 10–80 mg once daily at night
- Homozygous familial hypercholesterolaemia, 40 mg daily at night *or* 80 mg daily in 3 divided doses (with largest dose at night)
- Prevention of cardiovascular events, initially 20–40 mg once daily at night, adjusted at intervals of at least 4 weeks; max. 80 mg once daily at night

Note Max. 10 mg daily with concomitant ciclosporin, danazol, or fibrate (except fenofibrate). Max. 20 mg daily with concomitant amiodarone or verapamil. Max. 40 mg daily with diltiazem

**¹Simvastatin** (Non-proprietary) [PoM]
Tablets, simvastatin 10 mg, net price 28-tab pack = 84p; 20 mg, 28-tab pack = 94p; 40 mg, 28-tab pack = £1.32; 80 mg, 28-tab pack = £2.87. Counselling, muscle effects, see notes above
Brands include *Simvador®*

**¹Zocor®** (MSD) [PoM]
Tablets, all f/c, simvastatin 10 mg (peach), net price 28-tab pack = £18.03; 20 mg (tan), 28-tab pack = £29.69; 40 mg (red), 28-tab pack = £29.69; 80 mg (red), 28-tab pack = £29.69. Counselling, muscle effects, see notes above

**◢With ezetimibe**
Note For homozygous familial hypercholesterolaemia, primary hypercholesterolaemia, and mixed hyperlipidaemia in patients stabilised on the individual components in the same proportions, or for patients not adequately controlled by statin alone. For cautions, contra-indications, and side-effects of ezetimibe, see Ezetimibe

**Inegy®** (MSD, Schering-Plough) ▼ [PoM]
Tablets, simvastatin 20 mg, ezetimibe 10 mg, net price 28-tab pack = £33.42; simvastatin 40 mg, ezetimibe 10 mg, 28-tab pack = £38.98; simvastatin 80 mg, ezetimibe 10 mg, 28-tab pack = £41.21. Counselling, muscle effects, see notes above

## Bile acid sequestrants

**Colesevelam**, **colestipol**, and **colestyramine** (cholestyramine) are bile acid sequestrants used in the management of hypercholesterolaemia. They act by binding bile acids, preventing their reabsorption; this promotes hepatic conversion of cholesterol into bile acids; the resultant increased LDL-receptor activity of liver cells increases the clearance of LDL-cholesterol from the plasma. Bile acid sequestrants effectively reduce LDL-cholesterol but can aggravate hypertriglyceridaemia.

**Cautions**  Bile acid sequestrants interfere with the absorption of fat-soluble vitamins; supplements of vitamins A, D, and K may be required when treatment is prolonged. **Interactions**: Appendix 1 (bile acid sequestrants)

---

1. Simvastatin 10 mg tablets can be sold to the public to reduce risk of first coronary event in individuals at moderate risk of coronary heart disease (approx. 10–15% risk of major event in 10 years), max. daily dose 10 mg and pack size of 28 tablets; treatment should form part of a programme to reduce risk of coronary heart disease; a proprietary brand *Zocor Heart-Pro®* is on sale to the public

**2**

Cardiovascular system

**Side-effects** As bile acid sequestrants are not absorbed, gastro-intestinal side-effects predominate. Constipation is common, but diarrhoea has occurred, as have nausea, vomiting, and gastro-intestinal discomfort. Hypertriglyceridaemia may be aggravated. An increased bleeding tendency has been reported due to hypoprothrombinaemia associated with vitamin K deficiency.

**Counselling** Other drugs should be taken at least 1 hour before or 4–6 hours after bile acid sequestrants to reduce possible interference with absorption. Colesevelam and a statin can be taken at the same time.

## COLESEVELAM HYDROCHLORIDE

**Indications** primary hypercholesterolaemia as an adjunct to dietary measures, either alone or with a statin

**Cautions** see notes above; also gastro-intestinal motility disorders, major gastro-intestinal surgery, inflammatory bowel disease, hepatic impairment; pregnancy (Appendix 4); breast-feeding (Appendix 5)

**Contra-indications** bowel or biliary obstruction

**Side-effects** see notes above; also headache; myalgia

**Dose**
- Monotherapy, 3.75 g daily in 1–2 divided doses; max. 4.375 g daily
- Combination therapy with statin, 2.5–3.75 g daily in 1–2 divided doses

**Cholestagel®** (Genzyme) ▼ PoM
Tablets, f/c, colesevelam hydrochloride 625 mg, net price 180-cap pack = £89.05. Label: 21, counselling, avoid other drugs at same time (see notes above)

## COLESTYRAMINE
(Cholestyramine)

**Indications** hyperlipidaemias, particularly type IIa, in patients who have not responded adequately to diet and other appropriate measures; primary prevention of coronary heart disease in men aged 35–59 years with primary hypercholesterolaemia who have not responded to diet and other appropriate measures; pruritus associated with partial biliary obstruction and primary biliary cirrhosis (section 1.9.2); diarrhoeal disorders (section 1.9.2)

**Cautions** see notes above; pregnancy (Appendix 4); breast-feeding (Appendix 5); **interactions**: Appendix 1 (colestyramine)

**Contra-indications** complete biliary obstruction (not likely to be effective)

**Side-effects** see notes above; intestinal obstruction reported rarely and hyperchloraemic acidosis reported on prolonged use

**Dose**
- Lipid reduction, initially 4 g daily increased by 4 g at weekly intervals to 12–24 g daily in 1–4 divided doses, then adjusted as required; max. 36 g daily
- Pruritus, see section 1.9.2
- Diarrhoeal disorders, see section 1.9.2
- CHILD 6–12 years, see *BNF for Children*

**Note** The contents of each sachet should be mixed with at least 150 mL of water or other suitable liquid such as fruit juice, skimmed milk, thin soups, and pulpy fruits with a high moisture content

**Colestyramine** (Non-proprietary) PoM
Powder, sugar-free, colestyramine (anhydrous) 4 g/sachet, net price 50-sachet pack = £17.59. Label: 13, counselling, avoid other drugs at same time (see notes above)
Excipients may include aspartame (section 9.4.1)

**Questran®** (Bristol-Myers Squibb) PoM
Powder, colestyramine (anhydrous) 4 g/sachet, net price 50-sachet pack = £10.97. Label: 13, counselling, avoid other drugs at same time (see notes above)
Excipients include sucrose 3.79 g/sachet

**Questran Light®** (Bristol-Myers Squibb) PoM
Powder, sugar-free, colestyramine (anhydrous) 4 g/sachet, net price 50-sachet pack = £16.47. Label: 13, counselling, avoid other drugs at same time (see notes above)
Excipients include aspartame (section 9.4.1)

## COLESTIPOL HYDROCHLORIDE

**Indications** hyperlipidaemias, particularly type IIa, in patients who have not responded adequately to diet and other appropriate measures

**Cautions** see notes above; pregnancy (Appendix 4); breast-feeding (Appendix 5); **interactions**: Appendix 1 (colestipol)

**Side-effects** see notes above

**Dose**
- Initially 5 g 1–2 times daily in liquid increased if necessary in 5-g increments at intervals of 1 month to max. 30 g daily (in 1–2 divided doses)

**Note** The contents of each sachet should be mixed with at least 100 mL of water or other suitable liquid such as fruit juice, skimmed milk, thin soups, yoghurt, and pulpy fruits with a high moisture content

**Colestid®** (Pharmacia) PoM
Granules, yellow, colestipol hydrochloride 5 g/sachet, net price 30 sachets = £15.05. Label: 13, counselling, avoid other drugs at same time (see notes above)

Colestid Orange, granules, yellow/orange, colestipol hydrochloride 5 g/sachet, with aspartame, net price 30 sachets = £15.05. Label: 13, counselling, avoid other drugs at same time (see notes above)

## Ezetimibe

**Ezetimibe** inhibits the intestinal absorption of cholesterol. It is licensed as an adjunct to dietary manipulation in patients with primary hypercholesterolaemia in combination with a statin or alone (if a statin is inappropriate), in patients with homozygous familial hypercholesterolaemia in combination with a statin, and in patients with homozygous familial sitosterolaemia (phytosterolaemia). If ezetimibe is used in combination with a statin, there is an increased risk of rhabdomyolysis (see also CSM advice on p. 143).

> **NICE guidance**
> **Ezetimibe for the treatment of primary hypercholesterolaemia (November 2007)**
> Ezetimibe, used in accordance with the licensed indications for *Ezetrol®*, is an option for the treatment of adults with primary hypercholesterolaemia.

## ◼ EZETIMIBE

**Indications** adjunct to dietary measures and statin treatment in primary hypercholesterolaemia and homozygous familial hypercholesterolaemia (ezetimibe alone in primary hypercholesterolaemia if statin inappropriate or not tolerated); adjunct to dietary measures in homozygous sitosterolaemia

**Cautions** hepatic impairment (avoid if moderate or severe; Appendix 2); pregnancy (Appendix 4); breast-feeding (Appendix 5); **interactions:** Appendix 1 (ezetimibe)

**Side-effects** gastro-intestinal disturbances; headache, fatigue; myalgia; *rarely* arthralgia, hypersensitivity reactions (including rash, angioedema, and anaphylaxis), hepatitis; *very rarely* pancreatitis, cholelithiasis, cholecystitis, thrombocytopenia, raised creatine kinase, myopathy, and rhabdomyolysis

**Dose**
- ADULT and CHILD over 10 years, 10 mg once daily

**Ezetrol®** (MSD, Schering-Plough) ▼ PoM
Tablets, ezetimibe 10 mg, net price 28-tab pack = £26.31

◢**With simvastatin**
See under Simvastatin

---

## Fibrates

**Bezafibrate, ciprofibrate, fenofibrate,** and **gemfibrozil** act mainly by decreasing serum triglycerides; they have variable effects on LDL-cholesterol. Although a fibrate can reduce the risk of coronary heart disease events in those with low HDL-cholesterol or with raised triglycerides, a statin should be used first. Fibrates are first-line therapy only in those whose serum-triglyceride concentration is greater than 10 mmol/litre or in those who cannot tolerate a statin. In type 2 diabetes a fibrate can be added to a statin for those with a serum-triglyceride concentration exceeding 2.3 mmol/litre, despite 6 months of treatment with a statin and optimal glycaemic control.

Fibrates can cause a myositis-like syndrome, especially if renal function is impaired. Also, combination of a fibrate with a statin increases the risk of muscle effects (especially rhabdomyolysis) and should be used with caution (see CSM advice on p. 143) and monitoring of liver function and creatinine kinase should be considered; gemfibrozil and statins should **not** be used concomitantly.

## ◼ BEZAFIBRATE

**Indications** hyperlipidaemias of types IIa, IIb, III, IV, and V in patients who have not responded adequately to diet and other appropriate measures; also see notes above

**Cautions** correct hypothyroidism before initiating treatment (see p. 143); hepatic impairment (avoid if severe; Appendix 2); renal impairment (avoid if eGFR less than 15 mL/minute/1.73 m²; Appendix 3; see also under Myotoxicity below); **interactions:** Appendix 1 (fibrates)

**Myotoxicity** Special care needed in patients with renal disease, as progressive increases in serum creatinine concentration or failure to follow dosage guidelines may result in myotoxicity (rhabdomyolysis); discontinue if myotoxicity suspected or creatine kinase concentration increases significantly

**Contra-indications** hypoalbuminaemia, primary biliary cirrhosis, gall bladder disease, nephrotic syndrome, pregnancy (Appendix 4); breast-feeding (Appendix 5)

**Side-effects** gastro-intestinal disturbances, anorexia; *less commonly* cholestasis, weight gain, dizziness, headache, fatigue, drowsiness, renal impairment, raised serum creatinine (unrelated to renal impairment), erectile dysfunction, myotoxicity (with myasthenia or myalgia)—special risk in renal impairment (see Cautions), urticaria, pruritus, photosensitivity reactions; *very rarely* gallstones, hypoglycaemia, anaemia, leucopenia, thrombocytopenia, increased platelet count, alopecia, Stevens-Johnson syndrome, and toxic epidermal necrolysis

**Dose**
- See preparations below

**Bezafibrate** (Non-proprietary) PoM
Tablets, bezafibrate 200 mg, net price 100-tab pack = £10.25. Label: 21
**Dose** 200 mg 3 times daily; CHILD over 10 years, see *BNF for Children*

**Bezalip®** (Roche) PoM
Tablets, f/c, bezafibrate 200 mg, net price 100-tab pack = £8.79. Label: 21
**Dose** 200 mg 3 times daily; CHILD over 10 years, see *BNF for Children*

◢**Modified release**
**Bezafibrate** (Non-proprietary) PoM
Tablets, m/r, bezafibrate 400 mg, net price 28-tab pack = £7.68. Label: 21, 25
**Dose** 400 mg once daily (dose form not appropriate in patients with renal impairment)
Brands include *Fibrazate® XL, Zimbacol® XL*

**Bezalip® Mono** (Roche) PoM
Tablets, m/r, f/c, bezafibrate 400 mg, net price 30-tab pack = £7.77. Label: 21, 25
**Dose** 400 mg once daily (dose form not appropriate in patients with renal impairment)

## ◼ CIPROFIBRATE

**Indications** hyperlipidaemias of types IIa, IIb, III, and IV in patients who have not responded adequately to diet; also see notes above

**Cautions** see under Bezafibrate; renal impairment (avoid if severe; Appendix 3)

**Contra-indications** see under Bezafibrate

**Side-effects** see under Bezafibrate

**Dose**
- 100 mg daily

**Modalim®** (Winthrop) PoM
Tablets, scored, ciprofibrate 100 mg. Net price 28-tab pack = £17.66

## ◼ FENOFIBRATE

**Indications** hyperlipidaemias of types IIa, IIb, III, IV, and V in patients who have not responded adequately to diet and other appropriate measures; also see notes above

**Cautions** see under Bezafibrate; liver function tests recommended every 3 months for first year (discontinue treatment if significantly raised); renal impairment (avoid if eGFR less than 15 mL/minute/1.73 m²; Appendix 3)

2

Cardiovascular system

**Contra-indications** gall bladder disease; photosensitivity to ketoprofen; severe hepatic impairment (Appendix 2); pregnancy (Appendix 4); breast-feeding (Appendix 5)

**Side-effects** see under Bezafibrate; also *very rarely* hepatitis, pancreatitis, and interstitial pneumopathies

**Dose**

- See preparations below

**Fenofibrate** (Non-proprietary) [PoM]

Capsules, fenofibrate (micronised) 200 mg, net price 28-cap pack = £14.23. Label: 21

Dose 1 capsule daily (dose form not appropriate for children or in renal impairment)

Capsules, fenofibrate (micronised) 267 mg, net price 28-cap pack = £21.75. Label: 21

Dose severe hyperlipidaemia, 1 capsule daily (dose form not appropriate for children or in renal impairment)

**Lipantil®** (Solvay) [PoM]

Lipantil® Micro 67 capsules, yellow, fenofibrate (micronised) 67 mg, net price 90-cap pack = £23.30. Label: 21

Dose initially 3 capsules daily in divided doses; usual range 2–4 capsules daily; CHILD 4–15 years 1 capsule/20 kg daily

Lipantil® Micro 200 capsules, orange, fenofibrate (micronised) 200 mg, net price 28-cap pack = £17.95. Label: 21

Dose initially 1 capsule daily (dose form not appropriate for children or in renal impairment)

Lipantil® Micro 267 capsules, orange/cream, fenofibrate (micronised) 267 mg, net price 28-cap pack = £21.75. Label: 21

Dose severe hyperlipidaemia, 1 capsule daily (dose form not appropriate for children or in renal impairment)

**Supralip® 160** (Solvay) [PoM]

Tablets, f/c, fenofibrate (micronised) 160 mg, net price 28-tab pack = £7.50. Label: 21

Dose 160 mg daily (dose form not appropriate for children or in renal impairment)

## ▉ GEMFIBROZIL

**Indications** hyperlipidaemias of types IIa, IIb, III, IV and V in patients who have not responded adequately to diet and other appropriate measures; primary prevention of cardiovascular disease in men with hyperlipidaemias that have not responded to diet and other appropriate measures; also see notes above

**Cautions** lipid profile, blood counts, and liver-function tests before initiating long-term treatment; preferably avoid use with statins (high risk of rhabdomyolysis); correct hypothyroidism before initiating treatment (see p. 143); elderly; renal impairment (avoid if eGFR less than 30 mL/minute/1.73 m²; Appendix 3); **interactions:** Appendix 1 (fibrates)

**Contra-indications** alcoholism, biliary-tract disease including gallstones; photosensitivity to fibrates; hepatic impairment (Appendix 2); pregnancy (Appendix 4); breast-feeding (Appendix 5)

**Side-effects** gastro-intestinal disturbances; headache, fatigue, vertigo; eczema, rash; *less commonly* atrial fibrillation; *rarely* pancreatitis, appendicitis, disturbances in liver function including hepatitis and cholestatic jaundice, dizziness, paraesthesia, sexual dysfunction, thrombocytopenia, anaemia, leucopenia, eosinophilia, bone-marrow suppression, myalgia, myopathy, myasthenia, myositis accompanied by increase in creatine kinase (discontinue if raised sig-

nificantly), blurred vision, exfoliative dermatitis, alopecia, and photosensitivity)

**Dose**

- 1.2 g daily, usually in 2 divided doses; range 0.9–1.2 g daily; CHILD not recommended

**Gemfibrozil** (Non-proprietary) [PoM]

Capsules, gemfibrozil 300 mg, net price 112-cap pack = £46.70. Label: 22

Tablets, gemfibrozil 600 mg, net price 30-tab pack = £12.28, 56-tab pack = £33.34. Label: 22

**Lopid®** (Pfizer) [PoM]

'300' capsules, white/maroon, gemfibrozil 300 mg, net price 112-cap pack = £35.57. Label: 22

'600' tablets, f/c, gemfibrozil 600 mg, net price 56-tab pack = £35.57. Label: 22

## Nicotinic acid group

The value of **nicotinic acid** is limited by its side-effects, especially vasodilatation. In doses of 1.5 to 3 g daily it lowers both cholesterol and triglyceride concentrations by inhibiting synthesis; it also increases HDL-cholesterol. Nicotinic acid is licensed for use with a statin if the statin alone cannot adequately control dyslipidaemia (raised LDL-cholesterol, triglyceridaemia, and low HDL-cholesterol); it can be used alone if the patient is intolerant of statins (for advice on treatment of dyslipidaemia, including use of combination treatment, see p. 142).

Acipimox seems to have fewer side-effects than nicotinic acid but may be less effective in its lipid-modulating capabilities.

## ▉ ACIPIMOX

**Indications** hyperlipidaemias of types IIb and IV in patients who have not responded adequately to diet and other appropriate measures

**Cautions** renal impairment (avoid if eGFR less than 30 mL/minute/1.73 m²; Appendix 3)

**Contra-indications** peptic ulcer; pregnancy (Appendix 4); breast-feeding (Appendix 5)

**Side-effects** vasodilatation, flushing, itching, rashes, urticaria, erythema; heartburn, epigastric pain, nausea, diarrhoea, headache, malaise, dry eyes; rarely angioedema, bronchospasm, anaphylaxis

**Dose**

- Usually 500–750 mg daily in divided doses

**Olbetam®** (Pharmacia) [PoM]

Capsules, brown/pink, acipimox 250 mg, net price 90-cap pack = £46.33. Label: 21

## ▉ NICOTINIC ACID

**Indications** adjunct to statin in dyslipidaemia or used alone if statin not tolerated (see also p. 142)

**Cautions** unstable angina, acute myocardial infarction, diabetes mellitus, gout, history of peptic ulceration; hepatic impairment (Appendix 2); renal impairment; pregnancy (Appendix 4); **interactions:** Appendix 1 (nicotinic acid)

**Contra-indications** arterial bleeding; active peptic ulcer disease; breast-feeding

**Side-effects** diarrhoea, nausea, vomiting, abdominal pain, dyspepsia, flushing; pruritus, rash; *less commonly* tachycardia, palpitation, shortness of breath, peripheral oedema, headache, dizziness, increase in uric acid, hypophosphataemia, prolonged prothrombin time, and reduced platelet count; *rarely* hypotension, syncope, rhinitis, insomnia, reduced glucose tolerance, myalgia, myopathy, and myasthenia; *very rarely* anorexia, rhabdomyolysis

**Note** Prostaglandin-mediated symptoms (such as flushing) can be reduced by low initial doses taken with meals or, if patient taking aspirin, aspirin dose should be taken 30 minutes before nicotinic acid

**Dose**
- See under preparation

◢**Modified release**
**Niaspan®** (Abbott) PoM

Tablets, m/r, nicotinic acid 500 mg, net price 56-tab pack = £18.98; 750 mg, 56-tab pack = £28.88; 1 g, 56-tab pack = £38.23; 21-day starter pack of 7 × 375-mg tab with 7 × 500-mg tab and 7 × 750-mg tab = £15.40. Label: 21, 25

**Dose** 375 mg once daily at night (after a low-fat snack) for 1 week, then 500 mg once daily at night for 1 week, then 750 mg once daily at night for 1 week, then 1 g once daily at night for 4 weeks, increased if necessary in steps of 500 mg at intervals of at least 4 weeks to max. 2 g daily; usual maintenance dose 1–2 g once daily at night

## Omega-3 fatty acid compounds

The omega-3 fatty acid compounds comprise omega-3-acid ethyl esters (*Omacor®*) and omega-3-marine triglycerides (*Maxepa®*). Omega-3 fatty acid compounds may be used to reduce triglycerides, as an alternative to a fibrate and in addition to a statin, in patients with combined (mixed) hyperlipidaemia not adequately controlled with a statin alone. A triglyceride concentration exceeding 10 mmol/litre is associated with acute pancreatitis and lowering the concentration reduces this risk. The fat content of omega-3 fatty acid compounds (including excipients in the preparations) should be taken into consideration when treating hypertriglyceridaemia. There is little clinical trial evidence that the triglyceride lowering effect decreases the risk of cardiovascular disease.

The *Scottish Medicines Consortium* (p. 3) has advised (November 2002) that omega-3-acid ethyl esters (*Omacor®*) is **not** recommended for use within NHS Scotland for the treatment of hypertriglyceridaemia.

### ▋ OMEGA-3-ACID ETHYL ESTERS

**Indications** adjunct to diet and statin in type IIb or III hypertriglyceridaemia; adjunct to diet in type IV hypertriglyceridaemia; adjunct in secondary prevention in those who have had a myocardial infarction in the preceding 3 months

**Cautions** haemorrhagic disorders, anticoagulant treatment (bleeding time increased); hepatic impairment (Appendix 2); pregnancy (Appendix 4)

**Contra-indications** breast-feeding (Appendix 5)

**Side-effects** gastro-intestinal disturbances; *less commonly* taste disturbances, dizziness, and hypersensitivity reactions; *rarely* hepatic disorders, headache, hyperglycaemia, acne, and rash; *very rarely* hypotension, nasal dryness, urticaria, and increased white cell count

**Dose**
- See under preparation below

**Omacor®** (Solvay)

Capsules, 1 g of omega-3-acid ethyl esters 90 containing eicosapentaenoic acid 460 mg and decosahexaenoic acid 380 mg, net price 28-cap pack = £14.24, 100-cap pack = £50.84. Label: 21

**Dose** hypertriglyceridaemia, initially 2 capsules daily with food, increased if necessary to 4 capsules daily

Secondary prevention after myocardial infarction, 1 capsule daily with food

### ▋ OMEGA-3-MARINE TRIGLYCERIDES

**Indications** adjunct in the reduction of plasma triglycerides in severe hypertriglyceridaemia

**Cautions** haemorrhagic disorders, anticoagulant treatment; aspirin-sensitive asthma; type 2 diabetes

**Side-effects** occasional nausea and belching

**Dose**
- See under preparations below

**Maxepa®** (Seven Seas)

Capsules, 1 g (approx. 1.1 mL) concentrated fish oils containing eicosapentaenoic acid 170 mg, docosahexaenoic acid 115 mg. Vitamin A content less than 100 units/g, vitamin D content less than 10 units/g, net price 200-cap pack = £27.28. Label: 21

**Dose** 5 capsules twice daily with food

Liquid, golden-coloured, concentrated fish oils containing eicosapentaenoic acid 170 mg, docosahexaenoic acid 115 mg/g (1.1 mL). Vitamin A content less than 100 units/g, vitamin D content less than 10 units/g, net price 150 mL = £20.46. Label: 21

**Dose** 5 mL twice daily with food

## **2.13** Local sclerosants

Ethanolamine oleate and sodium tetradecyl sulphate are used in sclerotherapy of varicose veins, and phenol is used in haemorrhoids (section 1.7.3).

### ▋ ETHANOLAMINE OLEATE
(Monoethanolamine Oleate)

**Indications** sclerotherapy of varicose veins

**Cautions** extravasation may cause necrosis of tissues

**Contra-indications** inability to walk, acute phlebitis, oral contraceptive use, obese legs

**Side-effects** allergic reactions (including anaphylaxis)

**Ethanolamine Oleate** (UCB Pharma) PoM

Injection, ethanolamine oleate 5%, net price 2-mL amp = £3.19, 5-mL amp = £2.28

**Dose** by slow injection into empty isolated segment of vein, 2–5 mL divided between 3–4 sites; repeated at weekly intervals

### ▋ SODIUM TETRADECYL SULPHATE

**Indications** sclerotherapy of varicose veins

**Cautions** see under Ethanolamine Oleate

**Contra-indications** see under Ethanolamine Oleate

**Side-effects** see under Ethanolamine Oleate

**Fibro-Vein®** (STD Pharmaceutical) PoM

Injection, sodium tetradecyl sulphate 0.2%, net price 5-mL amp = £5.51; 0.5%, 2-mL amp = £2.87; 1%, 2-mL amp = £3.31; 3%, 2-mL amp = £4.07, 5-mL vial = £10.25

**Dose** by slow injection into empty isolated segment of vein, 0.1–1 mL according to site and condition being treated (consult product literature)

**2 Cardiovascular system**

# 3 Respiratory system

**3.1 Bronchodilators** 150
**3.1.1** Adrenoceptor agonists 154
**3.1.1.1** Selective beta₂ agonists 154
**3.1.1.2** Other adrenoceptor agonists 158
**3.1.2** Antimuscarinic bronchodilators 159
**3.1.3** Theophylline 160
**3.1.4** Compound bronchodilator preparations 161
**3.1.5** Peak flow meters, inhaler devices and nebulisers 161
**3.2 Corticosteroids** 165
**3.3 Cromoglicate and related therapy and leukotriene receptor antagonists** 169
**3.3.1** Cromoglicate and related therapy 169
**3.3.2** Leukotriene receptor antagonists 170
**3.4 Antihistamines, hyposensitisation, and allergic emergencies** 171
**3.4.1** Antihistamines 171
**3.4.2** Allergen Immunotherapy 174
**3.4.3** Allergic emergencies 175
**3.5 Respiratory stimulants and pulmonary surfactants** 178
**3.5.1** Respiratory stimulants 178
**3.5.2** Pulmonary surfactants 179
**3.6 Oxygen** 179
**3.7 Mucolytics** 181
**3.8 Aromatic inhalations** 182
**3.9 Cough preparations** 182
**3.9.1** Cough suppressants 182
**3.9.2** Expectorant and demulcent cough preparations 184
**3.10 Systemic nasal decongestants** 184

This chapter also includes advice on the drug management of the following:
acute severe asthma, p. 153
anaphylaxis, p. 176
angioedema, p. 178
chronic asthma, p. 151
chronic obstructive pulmonary disease, p. 153
croup, p. 154

## 3.1 Bronchodilators

**3.1.1** Adrenoceptor agonists
**3.1.2** Antimuscarinic bronchodilators
**3.1.3** Theophylline
**3.1.4** Compound bronchodilator preparations
**3.1.5** Peak flow meters, inhaler devices and nebulisers

### Asthma

Drugs used in the management of asthma include beta₂ agonists (section 3.1.1), antimuscarinic bronchodilators (section 3.1.2), theophylline (section 3.1.3), corticosteroids (section 3.2), cromoglicate and nedocromil (section 3.3.1), leukotriene receptor antagonists (section 3.3.2), and, in specialist centres, omalizumab (section 3.4.2).

For tables outlining the management of chronic and acute asthma, see p. 151 and p. 152. For advice on the management of medical emergencies in dental practice, see p. 22.

### Administration of drugs for asthma

**Inhalation** This route delivers the drug directly to the airways; the dose required is smaller than when given by mouth and side-effects are reduced. See also Inhaler devices, section 3.1.5.

*Solutions for nebulisation* are available for use in severe acute asthma. They are administered over 5–10 minutes from a nebuliser, usually driven by oxygen in hospital. See also Nebulisers, section 3.1.5.

**Oral** The oral route is used when administration by inhalation is not possible. Systemic side-effects occur more frequently when a drug is given orally rather than by inhalation. Drugs given by mouth for the treatment of asthma include beta₂ agonists, corticosteroids, theophylline, and leukotriene receptor antagonists.

**Parenteral** Drugs such as beta₂ agonists, corticosteroids, and aminophylline can be given by injection in acute severe asthma when administration by nebulisation is inadequate or inappropriate. If the patient is being treated in the community, urgent transfer to hospital should be arranged.

### Pregnancy and breast-feeding

It is particularly important that asthma should be well controlled during pregnancy; when this is achieved asthma has no important effects on pregnancy, labour, or on the fetus. Drugs for asthma should preferably be administered by inhalation to minimise exposure of the

# Management of chronic asthma

Start at **step most appropriate** to initial severity; before initiating a new drug consider whether diagnosis is correct, check compliance and inhaler technique, and eliminate trigger factors for acute exacerbations

## Adult and Child over 5 years

### Step 1: occasional relief bronchodilator
Inhaled short-acting beta$_2$ agonist as required (up to once daily)
**Note** Move to step 2 if needed more than twice a week, or if night-time symptoms more than once a week, or if exacerbation in the last 2 years

### Step 2: regular inhaled preventer therapy
Inhaled short-acting beta$_2$ agonist as required
*plus*
Regular standard-dose[1] inhaled corticosteroid (alternatives[2] are considerably less effective)

### Step 3: inhaled corticosteroid + long-acting inhaled beta$_2$ agonist
Inhaled short-acting beta$_2$ agonist as required
*plus*
Regular standard-dose[1] inhaled corticosteroid
*plus*
Regular inhaled long-acting beta$_2$ agonist (salmeterol *or* formoterol)
*If asthma not controlled*
Increase dose of inhaled corticosteroid to upper end of standard dose range[1]
*and*
*Either* stop long-acting beta$_2$ agonist if of no benefit
*Or* continue long-acting beta$_2$ agonist if of some benefit
*If asthma still not controlled and long-acting beta$_2$ agonist stopped, add one of*

    Leukotriene receptor antagonist

    Modified-release oral theophylline

    Modified-release oral beta$_2$ agonist

### Step 4: high-dose inhaled corticosteroid + regular bronchodilators
Inhaled short-acting beta$_2$ agonist as required
*with*
Regular high-dose[3] inhaled corticosteroid
*plus*
Inhaled long-acting beta$_2$ agonist
*plus*
In adults 6-week sequential therapeutic trial of one or more of

    Leukotriene receptor antagonist

    Modified-release oral theophylline

    Modified-release oral beta$_2$ agonist

### Step 5: regular corticosteroid tablets
Refer to a respiratory specialist
Inhaled short-acting beta$_2$ agonist as required
*with*
Regular high-dose[3] inhaled corticosteroid
*and*
One or more long-acting bronchodilators (see step 4)
*plus*
Regular prednisolone tablets (as single daily dose)
**Note** In addition to regular prednisolone, continue high-dose inhaled corticosteroid (in exceptional cases may exceed licensed doses); these patients should normally be referred to an asthma clinic

### Stepping down
Review treatment every 3 months; if control achieved stepwise reduction may be possible; reduce dose of *inhaled* corticosteroid slowly (consider reduction every 3 months, decreasing dose by up to 50% each time)

## Child under 5 years[4]

### Step 1: occasional relief bronchodilator
Short-acting beta$_2$ agonist as required (not more than once daily)
**Note** Preferably by inhalation (less effective and more side-effects when given by mouth)
Move to step 2 if needed more than twice a week, or if night-time symptoms more than once a week, or if exacerbation in the last 2 years

### Step 2: regular preventer therapy
Inhaled short-acting beta$_2$ agonist as required
*plus*
*Either* regular standard-dose[1] inhaled corticosteroid
*Or* (if inhaled corticosteroid cannot be used) leukotriene receptor antagonist

### Step 3: add-on therapy
**Child under 2 years:**
Refer to respiratory paediatrician
**Child 2–5 years:**
Inhaled short-acting beta$_2$ agonist as required
*plus*
Regular inhaled corticosteroid in standard dose[1]
*plus*
Leukotriene receptor antagonist

### Step 4: persistent poor control
Refer to respiratory paediatrician

### Stepping down
Regularly review need for treatment

---

1. Standard-dose inhaled corticosteroids (given through a metered-dose inhaler and in children a large-volume spacer):

    **Beclometasone dipropionate** or **budesonide** 100–400 micrograms twice daily; CHILD under 12 years 100–200 micrograms twice daily

    **Fluticasone propionate** 50–200 micrograms twice daily; CHILD 4–12 years 50–100 micrograms twice daily

    **Mometasone furoate** (given through a dry-powder inhaler) 200 micrograms twice daily

2. Alternatives to inhaled corticosteroid are leukotriene receptor antagonists, theophylline, inhaled cromoglicate, or inhaled nedocromil

3. High-dose inhaled corticosteroids (given through a metered-dose inhaler and a large-volume spacer):

    **Beclometasone dipropionate** or **budesonide** 0.4–1 mg twice daily; CHILD 5–12 years 200–400 micrograms twice daily

    **Fluticasone propionate** 200–500 micrograms twice daily; CHILD 5–12 years 100–200 micrograms twice daily

    **Mometasone furoate** (given through a dry powder inhaler) 200–400 micrograms twice daily

    **Note.** Doses of inhaled corticosteroids here are for CFC-free metered-dose inhalers; dose adjustments may be required for other inhaler devices, see under individual preparations, section 3.2.
    Failure to achieve control with these doses is unusual, see also Side-effects of Inhaled Corticosteroids, section 3.2

4. Lung-function measurements cannot be used to guide management in those under 5 years

Advice on the management of chronic asthma is based on the recommendations of the British Thoracic Society and Scottish Intercollegiate Guidelines Network (updated June 2009); updates available at www.brit-thoracic.org.uk

**3**

**Respiratory system**

## Management of acute asthma

**Important** Patients with severe or life-threatening acute asthma may not be distressed and may not have all of these abnormalities; the presence of any should alert the doctor. Regard each emergency consultation as being for **severe acute asthma** until shown otherwise

| Moderate acute asthma | Severe acute asthma | Life-threatening acute asthma |
|---|---|---|
| • Able to talk<br>• Respiration (breaths/minute) < 25; CHILD 2–5 years ≤ 40, 5–12 years ≤ 30<br>• Pulse (beats/minute) < 110; CHILD 2–5 years ≤ 140, 5–12 years ≤ 125<br>• Arterial oxygen saturation ≥ 92%<br>• Peak flow > 50% of predicted or best; CHILD 5–12 years ≥ 50%<br><br>*Treat at home or in surgery and assess response to treatment* | • Cannot complete sentences in one breath; CHILD too breathless to talk or feed<br>• Respiration (breaths/minute) ≥ 25; CHILD 2–5 years > 40; 5–12 years > 30<br>• Pulse (beats/minute) ≥ 110; CHILD 2–5 years > 140; 5–12 years > 125<br>• Arterial oxygen saturation < 92%<br>• Peak flow 33–50% of predicted or best; CHILD 5–12 years 33–50%<br><br>*Send immediately to hospital* | • Silent chest, feeble respiratory effort, cyanosis<br>• Hypotension, bradycardia, arrhythmia, exhaustion, agitation (in children), or reduced level of consciousness<br>• Arterial oxygen saturation < 92%<br>• Peak flow < 33% of predicted or best; CHILD 5–12 years < 33%<br><br>*Send immediately to hospital; consult with senior medical staff and refer to intensive care* |
| **Treatment**<br>• Inhaled **short-acting beta₂ agonist** via a large-volume spacer or oxygen-driven nebuliser (if available); give 4–10 puffs of **salbutamol** 100 micrograms/metered inhalation each inhaled separately, and repeat at 10–20 minute intervals if necessary *or give nebulised **salbutamol** 5 mg (CHILD under 5 years 2.5 mg, 5–12 years 2.5–5 mg) or **terbutaline** 10 mg (CHILD under 5 years 5 mg, 5–12 years 5–10 mg), and repeat at 10–20 minute intervals if necessary<br>• **Prednisolone** 40–50 mg by mouth for at least 5 days; CHILD 1–2 mg/kg by mouth for 3–5 days, if the child has been taking an oral corticosteroid for more than a few days, give prednisolone 2 mg/kg (CHILD under 2 years max. 40 mg, over 2 years max. 50 mg)<br><br>*Monitor response for 15–30 minutes*<br><br>*If response is poor or a relapse occurs in 3–4 hours, send immediately to hospital for assessment and further treatment* | **Treatment**<br>• High-flow **oxygen** (if available)<br>• Inhaled **short-acting beta₂ agonist** via a large-volume spacer or oxygen-driven nebuliser (if available); give 4–10 puffs of **salbutamol** 100 micrograms/metered inhalation each inhaled separately, and repeat at 10–20 minute intervals or as necessary *or give nebulised **salbutamol** 5 mg (CHILD under 5 years 2.5 mg, 5–12 years 2.5–5 mg) or **terbutaline** 10 mg (CHILD under 5 years 5 mg, 5–12 years 5–10 mg), and repeat at 10–20 minute intervals or as necessary<br>• **Prednisolone** by mouth as for moderate acute asthma *or* intravenous **hydrocortisone** (preferably as sodium succinate) 100 mg every 6 hours until conversion to oral prednisolone is possible; CHILD 4 mg/kg (under 2 years max. 25 mg, 2–5 years 50 mg, 6–12 years 100 mg)<br><br>*Monitor response for 15–30 minutes*<br><br>*If response is poor:*<br>• Inhaled **ipratropium bromide** via oxygen-driven nebuliser (if available) 500 micrograms (CHILD under 12 years 250 micrograms)<br><br>*Refer those who fail to respond and require ventilatory support to an intensive care or high-dependency unit*<br><br>• Consider intravenous **beta₂ agonists**, **aminophylline** (p. 161) or **magnesium sulphate** [unlicensed indication] (p. 153) only after consultation with senior medical staff | **Treatment**<br>• High-flow **oxygen** (if available)<br>• **Short-acting beta₂ agonist** via oxygen-driven nebuliser (if available); give **salbutamol** 5 mg (CHILD under 5 years 2.5 mg, 5–12 years 2.5–5 mg) or **terbutaline** 10 mg (CHILD under 5 years 5 mg, 5–12 years 5–10 mg), and repeat at 10–20 minute intervals or as necessary; reserve intravenous beta₂ agonists for those in whom inhaled therapy cannot be used reliably<br>• **Prednisolone** by mouth as for moderate acute asthma *or* intravenous **hydrocortisone** (preferably as sodium succinate) 100 mg every 6 hours until conversion to oral prednisolone is possible; CHILD 4 mg/kg (under 2 years max. 25 mg, 2–5 years 50 mg, 6–12 years 100 mg)<br>• Inhaled **ipratropium bromide** via oxygen-driven nebuliser (if available) 500 micrograms (CHILD under 12 years 250 micrograms)<br><br>*Monitor response for 15–30 minutes*<br>• Consider **aminophylline** (p. 161) or **magnesium sulphate** [unlicensed indication] (p. 153) only after consultation with senior medical staff |

**Follow up in all cases**
Monitor symptoms and peak flow. Set up asthma action plan and check inhaler technique
Review by general practitioner or asthma nurse within 48 hours; modify treatment according to the Management of Chronic Asthma table, p. 151

Advice on the management of acute asthma is based on the recommendations of the British Thoracic Society and Scottish Intercollegiate Guidelines Network (updated June 2009); updates available at www.brit-thoracic.org.uk

fetus. Inhaled drugs, theophylline, and prednisolone can be taken as normal during pregnancy and breast-feeding. Women planning to become pregnant should be counselled about the importance of taking their asthma medication regularly to maintain good control.

Severe acute exacerbations of asthma can have an adverse effect on pregnancy and should be treated promptly in hospital with conventional therapy, including oral or parenteral administration of a corticosteroid and nebulisation of a beta$_2$ agonist; prednisolone is the preferred corticosteroid for oral administration since very little of the drug reaches the fetus. Oxygen should be given immediately to maintain arterial oxygen saturation of 94–98% and prevent maternal and fetal hypoxia.

## Management of severe acute asthma

> **Important**
> Regard each emergency consultation as being for severe acute asthma until shown otherwise.
> Failure to respond adequately at any time requires immediate transfer to hospital.

Severe acute asthma can be fatal and **must** be treated promptly and energetically. All patients with severe acute asthma should be given high-flow **oxygen** (if available) and an inhaled **short-acting beta$_2$ agonist** via a large-volume spacer or nebuliser; give 4–10 puffs of **salbutamol** 100 micrograms/metered inhalation, each puff inhaled separately via a large-volume spacer, and repeat at 10–20 minute intervals or as necessary. If there are life-threatening features, give salbutamol or **terbutaline** via an oxygen-driven nebuliser every 10–20 minutes or as necessary, see p. 156 and p. 158. In all cases, a systemic **corticosteroid** (section 6.3.2) should be given. For adults, give prednisolone 40–50 mg by mouth for at least 5 days, or intravenous hydrocortisone 100 mg (preferably as sodium succinate) every 6 hours until conversion to oral prednisolone is possible. For children, give prednisolone 1–2 mg/kg by mouth (max. 40 mg) for 3–5 days or intravenous hydrocortisone 4 mg/kg (under 2 years max. 25 mg, 2–5 years 50 mg, 6–12 years 100 mg) (preferably as sodium succinate) every 6 hours until conversion to oral prednisolone is possible. If the child has been taking an oral corticosteroid for more than a few days, then give prednisolone 2 mg/kg (CHILD under 2 years max. 40 mg, over 2 years max. 50 mg). In life-threatening asthma, also consider initial treatment with **ipratropium** by nebuliser (section 3.1.2).

Most patients do not require and do not benefit from the addition of **intravenous aminophylline** or of **intravenous beta$_2$ agonist**; both cause more adverse effects than nebulised beta$_2$ agonists. Nevertheless, an occasional patient who has not been taking theophylline may benefit from aminophylline infusion (see p. 161). Patients with severe acute asthma may be helped by **magnesium sulphate** [unlicensed indication] 1.2–2 g given by intravenous infusion over 20 minutes, but evidence of benefit is limited.

Treatment of severe acute asthma is safer in hospital where resuscitation facilities are immediately available. Treatment should **never** be delayed for investigations, patients should **never** be sedated, and the possibility of a pneumothorax should be considered.

If the patient's condition deteriorates despite pharmacological treatment, intermittent positive pressure ventilation may be needed.

For a table outlining the management of acute asthma, see p. 152.

## Chronic obstructive pulmonary disease

Smoking cessation (section 4.10) reduces the progressive decline in lung function in chronic obstructive pulmonary disease (COPD, chronic bronchitis, or emphysema). Infection can complicate chronic obstructive pulmonary disease and may be prevented by vaccination (pneumococcal vaccine and influenza vaccine, section 14.4).

A trial of a high-dose inhaled corticosteroid *or* an oral corticosteroid is recommended for patients with moderate airflow obstruction to ensure that asthma has not been overlooked.

Symptoms of chronic obstructive pulmonary disease may be alleviated by an inhaled **short-acting beta$_2$ agonist** (section 3.1.1.1) or a **short-acting antimuscarinic bronchodilator** (section 3.1.2) used as required.

When the airways obstruction is more severe, an inhaled **short-acting antimuscarinic bronchodilator** (section 3.1.2) given regularly should be added. In those who remain symptomatic or have two or more exacerbations in a year, a **long-acting beta$_2$ agonist** or a **long-acting antimuscarinic bronchodilator** given regularly should be added; a short-acting antimuscarinic bronchodilator should be discontinued when a long-acting antimuscarinic bronchodilator is started. If symptoms persist or if the patient is unable to use an inhaler, oral modified-release **aminophylline** or **theophylline** (section 3.1.3) can be used.

In moderate or severe chronic obstructive pulmonary disease, either a combination of a long-acting beta$_2$ agonist with an **inhaled corticosteroid** (section 3.2) or a long-acting antimuscarinic bronchodilator should be tried.

A **mucolytic** drug (section 3.7) may be considered for a patient with a chronic productive cough.

Long-term **oxygen** therapy (section 3.6) prolongs survival in patients with severe chronic obstructive pulmonary disease and hypoxaemia.

During an exacerbation of chronic obstructive pulmonary disease, bronchodilator therapy can be administered through a nebuliser if necessary and oxygen given if appropriate. **Aminophylline** can be given intravenously if response to nebulised bronchodilators is poor. A short course of **oral corticosteroid** (section 6.3.2), such as prednisolone 30 mg daily for 7–14 days, should be given if increased breathlessness interferes with daily activities. **Antibacterial** treatment (Table 1, section 5.1) is required when sputum becomes purulent or if there are other signs of infection.

Patients who have had an episode of hypercapnic respiratory failure should be given a 24% or 28% Venturi mask and an *oxygen alert card* (see p. 154) endorsed with the oxygen saturations required during previous exacerbations. Patients and their carers should be instructed to show the card to emergency healthcare providers in the event of an exacerbation, see also section 3.6.

**3**

**Respiratory system**

---

### Oxygen alert card

Name: _____

I am at risk of type II respiratory failure with a raised $CO_2$ level.

Please use my ____% Venturi mask to achieve an oxygen saturation of ____% to ____% during exacerbations.

Use compressed air to drive nebulisers (with nasal oxygen at 2 litres/minute). If compressed air not available, limit oxygen-driven nebulisers to 6 minutes.

Oxygen alert card based on British Thoracic Society guideline for emergency oxygen use in adult patients (October 2008); available at www.brit-thoracic.org.uk

---

## Croup

Mild croup is largely self-limiting, but treatment with a single dose of a corticosteroid (e.g. dexamethasone 150 micrograms/kg) by mouth may be of benefit.

More severe croup (or mild croup that might cause complications) calls for hospital admission; a single dose of a corticosteroid (e.g. dexamethasone 150 micrograms/kg or prednisolone 1–2 mg/kg by mouth, section 6.3.2) should be administered before transfer to hospital. In hospital, dexamethasone 150 micrograms/kg (by mouth or by injection) or budesonide 2 mg (by nebulisation, section 3.2) will often reduce symptoms; the dose may need to be repeated after 12 hours if necessary.

For severe croup not effectively controlled with corticosteroid treatment, nebulised adrenaline solution 1 in 1000 (1 mg/mL) should be given with close clinical monitoring in a dose of 400 micrograms/kg (max. 5 mg) repeated after 30 minutes if necessary; the effects of nebulised adrenaline last 2–3 hours and the child needs to be monitored carefully for recurrence of the obstruction

## 3.1.1 Adrenoceptor agonists (Sympathomimetics)

**3.1.1.1 Selective beta₂ agonists**

**3.1.1.2 Other adrenoceptor agonists**

The selective beta₂ agonists (selective beta₂-adrenoceptor agonists, selective beta₂ stimulants) (section 3.1.1.1) such as salbutamol or terbutaline are the safest and most effective short-acting beta₂ agonists for asthma. Less selective beta₂ agonists such as orciprenaline (section 3.1.1.2) should be avoided whenever possible.

Adrenaline (epinephrine) (which has both alpha- and beta-adrenoceptor agonist properties) is used in the emergency management of allergic and anaphylactic reactions (section 3.4.3) and in the management of croup (see above).

## 3.1.1.1 Selective beta₂ agonists

Selective beta₂ agonists produce bronchodilation. A short-acting beta₂ agonist is used for immediate relief of asthma symptoms while a long-acting beta₂ agonist is

added to an inhaled corticosteroid in patients requiring prophylactic treatment.

Chronic Asthma table, see p. 151
Acute Asthma table, see p. 152.

**Short-acting beta₂ agonists** Mild to moderate symptoms of asthma respond rapidly to the inhalation of a selective short-acting beta₂ agonist such as **salbutamol** or **terbutaline**. If beta₂ agonist inhalation is needed more often than once daily, prophylactic treatment should be considered, using a stepped approach as outlined in the Management of Chronic Asthma table, p. 151. Regular treatment with an inhaled short-acting beta₂ agonist is less effective than 'as required' inhalation and is not appropriate prophylactic treatment.

A short-acting beta₂ agonist inhaled immediately before exertion reduces *exercise-induced asthma*; however, frequent exercise-induced asthma probably reflects poor overall control and calls for reassessment of asthma treatment.

**Long-acting beta₂ agonists** Formoterol (eformoterol) and **salmeterol** are longer-acting beta₂ agonists which are administered by inhalation. Added to regular inhaled corticosteroid treatment, they have a role in the long-term control of chronic asthma (see Chronic Asthma table, p. 151) and they can be useful in nocturnal asthma. Salmeterol should not be used for the relief of an asthma attack; it has a slower onset of action than salbutamol or terbutaline. Formoterol is licensed for short-term symptom relief and for the prevention of exercise-induced bronchospasm; its speed of onset of action is similar to that of salbutamol.

### CHM advice

To ensure safe use, the CHM has advised that for the management of chronic asthma, long-acting beta₂ agonists (formoterol and salmeterol) should:
- be added only if regular use of standard-dose inhaled corticosteroids has failed to control asthma adequately;
- not be initiated in patients with rapidly deteriorating asthma;
- be introduced at a low dose and the effect properly monitored before considering dose increase;
- be discontinued in the absence of benefit;
- be reviewed as clinically appropriate: stepping down therapy should be considered when good long-term asthma control has been achieved.

Patients should be advised to report any deterioration in symptoms following initiation of treatment with a long-acting beta₂ agonist, see Management of Chronic Asthma table, p. 151.

**Inhalation** *Pressurised-metered dose inhalers* are an effective and convenient method of drug administration in mild to moderate asthma. A spacer device (section 3.1.5) may improve drug delivery. At recommended inhaled doses the duration of action of salbutamol, terbutaline and fenoterol is about 3 to 5 hours and for salmeterol and formoterol 12 hours. The **dose**, the frequency, and the maximum number of inhalations in 24 hours of the beta₂ agonist should be **stated explicitly** to the patient. The patient should be advised to seek medical advice when the prescribed dose of beta₂ agonist fails to provide the usual degree of symptomatic relief because this usually indicates a worsening of the asthma and the patient may require a prophylactic drug such as an inhaled corticosteroid (see Chronic Asthma table, p. 151).

*Nebuliser (or respirator) solutions* of salbutamol and terbutaline are used for the treatment of severe acute asthma in hospital or in general practice. Patients with a severe attack of asthma should preferably have oxygen during nebulisation since beta$_2$ agonists can increase arterial hypoxaemia. For the use of nebulisers in chronic obstructive pulmonary disease, see section 3.1.5. The dose given by nebuliser is substantially higher than that given by inhaler. Patients should therefore be warned that it is dangerous to exceed the prescribed dose and they should seek medical advice if they fail to respond to the usual dose of the respirator solution, see also section 3.1.5.

**CFC-free inhalers** Chlorofluorocarbon (CFC) propellants in pressurised metered-dose inhalers are being replaced by hydrofluoroalkane (HFA) propellants. Patients receiving CFC-free inhalers should be reassured about the efficacy of the new inhalers and counselled that the aerosol may feel and taste different; any difficulty with the new inhaler should be discussed with the doctor or pharmacist.

**Oral** Oral preparations of beta$_2$ agonists may be used by patients who cannot manage the inhaled route. They are sometimes used for children and the elderly, but inhaled beta$_2$ agonists are more effective and have fewer side-effects. The longer-acting oral preparations, including bambuterol, may be of value in nocturnal asthma but they have a limited role and inhaled long-acting beta$_2$ agonists are usually preferred.

**Parenteral** Salbutamol or terbutaline are given by slow intravenous injection or intravenous infusion for severe acute asthma; patients should be carefully monitored and the dose adjusted according to response and heart rate. The regular use of beta$_2$ agonists by the subcutaneous route is not recommended since the evidence of benefit is uncertain and it may be difficult to withdraw such treatment once started. Beta$_2$ agonists may also be given by intramuscular injection.

**Children** Selective beta$_2$ agonists are useful even in children under the age of 18 months. They are most effective by the inhaled route; a pressurised metered-dose inhaler should be used with a spacer device in children under 5 years (see NICE guidance, section 3.1.5). A beta$_2$ agonist may also be given by mouth but administration by inhalation is preferred; a long-acting inhaled beta$_2$ agonist may be used where appropriate (see Chronic Asthma table, p. 151). In severe attacks nebulisation using a selective beta$_2$ agonist or ipratropium is advisable (see also Asthma tables, p. 151 and p. 152).

**Cautions** Beta$_2$ agonists should be used with caution in hyperthyroidism, cardiovascular disease, arrhythmias, susceptibility to QT-interval prolongation, and hypertension. If high doses are needed during pregnancy they should be given by inhalation because a parenteral beta$_2$ agonist can affect the myometrium (section 7.1.3) and possibly cause cardiac problems; see also Pregnancy and Breast-feeding, section 3.1. Beta$_2$ agonists should be used with caution in diabetes—monitor blood glucose

(risk of ketoacidosis, especially when beta$_2$ agonist given intravenously). **Interactions:** Appendix 1 (sympathomimetics, beta$_2$).

**Hypokalaemia** The CSM has advised that potentially serious hypokalaemia may result from beta$_2$ agonist therapy. Particular caution is required in severe asthma, because this effect may be potentiated by concomitant treatment with theophylline and its derivatives, corticosteroids, and diuretics, and by hypoxia. Plasma-potassium concentration should therefore be monitored in severe asthma.

**Side-effects** Side-effects of the beta$_2$ agonists include fine tremor (particularly in the hands), nervous tension, headache, muscle cramps, and palpitation. Other side-effects include tachycardia, arrhythmias, peripheral vasodilation, myocardial ischaemia, and disturbances of sleep and behaviour. Paradoxical bronchospasm (occasionally severe), urticaria, angioedema, hypotension, and collapse have also been reported. High doses of beta$_2$ agonists are associated with hypokalaemia (for CSM advice, see Hypokalaemia above).

### ▌ BAMBUTEROL HYDROCHLORIDE

**Note** Bambuterol is a pro-drug of terbutaline

**Indications** asthma and other conditions associated with reversible airways obstruction

**Cautions** see notes above; hepatic impairment (avoid if severe); renal impairment (Appendix 3); pregnancy (Appendix 4 and notes above)

**Side-effects** see notes above

**Dose**

- 20 mg once daily at bedtime if patient has previously tolerated beta$_2$ agonists; other patients, initially 10 mg once daily at bedtime, increased if necessary after 1–2 weeks to 20 mg once daily; CHILD not recommended

**Bambec®** (AstraZeneca) ▨PoM▨
Tablets, both scored, bambuterol hydrochloride 10 mg, net price 28-tab pack = £12.05; 20 mg, 28-tab pack = £13.14

### ▌ FENOTEROL HYDROBROMIDE

**Indications** reversible airways obstruction
**Cautions** see notes above
**Side-effects** see notes above

◢Compound preparations
For **compound preparation** containing fenoterol, see section 3.1.4

### ▌ FORMOTEROL FUMARATE
(Eformoterol fumarate)

**Indications** reversible airways obstruction (including nocturnal asthma and prevention of exercise-induced bronchospasm) in patients requiring long-term regular bronchodilator therapy, see also Chronic Asthma table, p. 151; chronic obstructive pulmonary disease

**Cautions** see notes above; hepatic impairment (Appendix 2); pregnancy (Appendix 4 and notes above); breast-feeding (Appendix 5)

**Side-effects** see notes above; taste disturbances, nausea, dizziness, rash, and pruritus also reported

**Respiratory system** 3

**Dose**

- See under preparations below

  Counselling Advise patients not to exceed prescribed dose, and to follow manufacturer's directions; if a previously effective dose of inhaled formoterol fails to provide adequate relief, a doctor's advice should be obtained as soon as possible

**Formoterol** (Non-proprietary) PoM

Dry powder for inhalation, formoterol fumarate 12 micrograms/metered inhalation, net price 120-dose unit = £24.11. Counselling, dose

Brands include *Easyhaler® Formoterol*

Dose  by inhalation of powder, asthma, ADULT and CHILD over 6 years, 12 micrograms twice daily, increased to 24 micrograms twice daily in more severe airways obstruction

Chronic obstructive pulmonary disease, 12 micrograms twice daily

**Atimos Modulite®** (Chiesi) ▼ PoM

Aerosol inhalation, formoterol fumarate 12 micrograms/metered inhalation, net price 100-dose unit = £30.06. Counselling, dose

Excipients include HFA-134a (a non-CFC propellant)

Dose  by aerosol inhalation, asthma, ADULT and CHILD over 12 years, 12 micrograms twice daily, increased to max. 24 micrograms twice daily in more severe airways obstruction

Chronic obstructive pulmonary disease, ADULT over 18 years, 12 micrograms twice daily; for symptom relief additional doses may be taken to total max. 48 micrograms daily (max. single dose 24 micrograms)

**Foradil®** (Novartis) PoM

Dry powder for inhalation, formoterol fumarate 12 micrograms/capsule, net price 60-cap pack (with inhaler device) = £30.06. Counselling, dose

Dose  by inhalation of powder, asthma, ADULT and CHILD over 5 years, 12 micrograms twice daily, increased to 24 micrograms twice daily in more severe airways obstruction

Chronic obstructive pulmonary disease, 12 micrograms twice daily

**Oxis®** (AstraZeneca) PoM

Turbohaler® (= dry powder inhaler), formoterol fumarate 6 micrograms/metered inhalation, net price 60-dose unit = £24.80; 12 micrograms/metered inhalation, 60-dose unit = £24.80. Counselling, dose

Dose  by inhalation of powder, chronic asthma, 6–12 micrograms 1–2 times daily, increased up to 24 micrograms twice daily if necessary; occasionally up to 72 micrograms daily may be needed (max. single dose 36 micrograms); reassess treatment if additional doses required on more than 2 days a week; CHILD 6–18 years, 6–12 micrograms 1–2 times daily; occasionally up to 48 micrograms daily may be needed (max. single dose 12 micrograms)

Relief of bronchospasm, ADULT and CHILD over 6 years, 6–12 micrograms

Prevention of exercise-induced bronchospasm, 12 micrograms before exercise; CHILD 6–18 years, 6–12 micrograms before exercise

Chronic obstructive pulmonary disease, 12 micrograms 1–2 times daily; for symptom relief additional doses can be taken to total max. 48 micrograms daily (max. single dose 24 micrograms)

◢Compound preparations

For **compound preparations** containing formoterol, see section 3.2

▌ **SALBUTAMOL**
    (Albuterol)

**Indications** asthma and other conditions associated with reversible airways obstruction; premature labour (section 7.1.3)

**Cautions** see notes above

**Side-effects** see notes above

**Dose**

- By mouth (but use by inhalation preferred), 4 mg (elderly and sensitive patients initially 2 mg) 3–4 times daily; max. single dose 8 mg (but unlikely to provide much extra benefit or to be tolerated); CHILD under 2 years 100 micrograms/kg 4 times daily [unlicensed]; 2–6 years 1–2 mg 3–4 times daily, 6–12 years 2 mg 3–4 times daily

- By subcutaneous *or* intramuscular injection, 500 micrograms, repeated every 4 hours if necessary

- By slow intravenous injection (but see also Management of Acute Asthma table, p. 152), (dilute to a concentration of 50 micrograms/mL), 250 micrograms, repeated if necessary; CHILD see *BNF for Children*

- By intravenous infusion (but see also Management of Acute Asthma table, p. 152), initially 5 micrograms/minute, adjusted according to response and heart-rate usually in range 3–20 micrograms/minute, or more if necessary; CHILD see *BNF for Children*

- By aerosol inhalation (but see also Management of Acute Asthma table, p. 152, *or* Management of Chronic Asthma table, p. 151), 100–200 micrograms (1–2 puffs); for persistent symptoms up to 4 times daily; CHILD 100 micrograms (1 puff), increased to 200 micrograms (2 puffs) if necessary; for persistent symptoms up to 4 times daily

  Prophylaxis of allergen- or exercise-induced bronchospasm, 200 micrograms (2 puffs); CHILD 100 micrograms (1 puff), increased to 200 micrograms (2 puffs) if necessary

- By inhalation of powder (but see also Management of Chronic Asthma table, p. 151), 200–400 micrograms; for persistent symptoms up to 4 times daily; CHILD over 5 years 200 micrograms; for persistent symptoms up to 4 times daily (for *Asmasal Clickhaler®*, *Salbulin Novolizer®*, and *Ventolin Accuhaler®* doses, see under preparations)

  Prophylaxis of allergen- or exercise-induced bronchospasm, 400 micrograms; CHILD 200 micrograms

- By inhalation of nebulised solution (but see also Management of Acute Asthma table, p. 152) ADULT and CHILD over 18 months 2.5–5 mg, repeated up to 4 times daily or more frequently in severe cases; max. 40 mg daily; CHILD under 18 months (transient hypoxaemia may occur—consider supplemental oxygen), 2.5 mg up to 4 times daily or more frequently in severe cases

◢Oral

**Salbutamol** (Non-proprietary) PoM

Tablets, salbutamol (as sulphate) 2 mg, net price 28-tab pack = £13.27; 4 mg, 28-tab pack = £12.18

Oral solution, salbutamol (as sulphate) 2 mg/5 mL, net price 150 mL = £1.35

Brands include *Salapin®* (sugar-free)

**Ventmax® SR** (Chiesi) PoM

Capsules, m/r, salbutamol (as sulphate) 4 mg (green/grey), net price 56-cap pack = £8.24; 8 mg (white), 56-cap pack = £9.88. Label: 25

Dose  8 mg twice daily; CHILD 3–12 years 4 mg twice daily

**Ventolin®** (A&H) PoM

Syrup, sugar-free, salbutamol (as sulphate) 2 mg/5 mL, net price 150 mL = 60p

◢**Parenteral**

**Ventolin®** (A&H) [PoM]

Injection, salbutamol (as sulphate) 500 micrograms/ mL, net price 1-mL amp = 38p

Solution for intravenous infusion, salbutamol (as sulphate) 1 mg/mL. Dilute before use. Net price 5-mL amp = £2.48

◢**Inhalation**

Counselling Advise patients not to exceed prescribed dose and to follow manufacturer's directions; if a previously effective dose of inhaled salbutamol fails to provide at least 3 hours relief, a doctor's advice should be obtained as soon as possible.

Patients receiving CFC-free inhalers should be reassured about their efficacy and counselled that aerosol may feel and taste different

**Salbutamol** (Non-proprietary) [PoM]

Aerosol inhalation, salbutamol 100 micrograms/ metered inhalation, net price 200-dose unit = £2.88. Counselling, dose
Excipients include CFC propellants

Aerosol inhalation, salbutamol (as sulphate) 100 micrograms/metered inhalation, net price 200-dose unit = £2.99. Counselling, dose, change to CFC-free inhaler
Excipients include HFA-134a (a non-CFC propellant)
Brands include Salamol®
Note Can be supplied against a generic prescription but if CFC-free not specified will be reimbursed at price for CFC-containing inhaler

Dry powder for inhalation, salbutamol 100 micrograms/metered inhalation, net price 200-dose unit = £3.46; 200 micrograms/metered inhalation, 100-dose unit = £4.85, 200-dose unit = £6.92. Counselling, dose
Brands include Easyhaler® Salbutamol, Pulvinal® Salbutamol

Inhalation powder, hard capsule (for use with Cyclohaler® device), salbutamol 200 micrograms, net price 120-cap pack = £8.99; 400 micrograms, 120-cap pack = £12.99. Counselling, dose
Brands include Salbutamol Cyclocaps®

Nebuliser solution, salbutamol (as sulphate) 1 mg/ mL, net price 20 × 2.5 mL (2.5 mg) = £1.91; 2 mg/mL, 20 × 2.5 mL (5 mg) = £3.82. May be diluted with sterile sodium chloride 0.9%
Brands include Salamol Steri-Neb®

**Airomir®** (IVAX) [PoM]

Aerosol inhalation, salbutamol (as sulphate) 100 micrograms/metered inhalation, net price 200-dose unit = £1.97. Counselling, dose, change to CFC-free inhaler
Excipients include HFA-134a (a non-CFC propellant)
Note Can be supplied against a generic prescription but if 'CFC-free' not specified will be reimbursed at price for CFC-containing inhaler

Autohaler (breath-actuated aerosol inhalation), salbutamol (as sulphate) 100 micrograms/metered inhalation, net price 200-dose unit = £6.02. Counselling, dose, change to CFC-free inhaler
Excipients include HFA-134a (a non-CFC propellant)

**Asmasal Clickhaler®** (UCB Pharma) [PoM]

Dry powder for inhalation, salbutamol (as sulphate) 95 micrograms/metered inhalation, net price 200-dose unit = £5.65. Counselling, dose
Dose acute bronchospasm, by inhalation of powder, ADULT and CHILD over 5 years, 1–2 puffs; for persistent symptoms up to 4 times daily (but see also Management of Chronic Asthma, p. 151)
Prophylaxis of allergen- or exercise-induced bronchospasm, by inhalation of powder, ADULT and CHILD over 5 years, 1–2 puffs

**Salamol Easi-Breathe®** (IVAX) [PoM]

Aerosol inhalation, salbutamol 100 micrograms/ metered inhalation, net price 200-dose breath-actuated unit = £6.30. Counselling, dose
Excipients include HFA-134a (a non-CFC propellant)

**Salbulin Novolizer®** (Meda) [PoM]

Dry powder for inhalation, salbutamol (as sulphate) 100 micrograms/metered inhalation, net price refillable 200-dose unit = £4.95; 200-dose refill = £2.75. Counselling, dose
Dose acute bronchospasm, by inhalation of powder, ADULT 100–200 micrograms; for persistent symptoms up to 800 micrograms daily (but see also Management of Chronic Asthma, p. 151); CHILD 6–12 years 100–200 micrograms; for persistent symptoms up to 400 micrograms daily (but see also Management of Chronic Asthma, p. 151)
Prophylaxis of allergen- or exercise-induced bronchospasm, by inhalation of powder, ADULT 200 micrograms; CHILD 6–12 years 100–200 micrograms

**Ventolin®** (A&H) [PoM]

Accuhaler® (dry powder for inhalation), disk containing 60 blisters of salbutamol (as sulphate) 200 micrograms/blister with Accuhaler® device, net price = £4.92. Counselling, dose
Dose acute bronchospasm, by inhalation of powder, ADULT and CHILD over 5 years, 200 micrograms; for persistent symptoms up to 4 times daily (but see also Management of Chronic Asthma, p. 151)
Prophylaxis of allergen- or exercise-induced bronchospasm, by inhalation of powder, ADULT and CHILD over 5 years, 200 micrograms

Evohaler® (aerosol inhalation), salbutamol (as sulphate) 100 micrograms/metered inhalation, net price 200-dose unit = £1.50. Counselling, dose, change to CFC-free inhaler
Excipients include HFA-134a (a non-CFC propellant)
Note Can be supplied against a generic prescription but if CFC-free not specified will be reimbursed at price for CFC-containing inhaler

Nebules® (for use with nebuliser), salbutamol (as sulphate) 1 mg/mL, net price 20 × 2.5 mL (2.5 mg) = £1.68; 2 mg/mL, 20 × 2.5 mL (5 mg) = £2.83. May be diluted with sterile sodium chloride 0.9% if administration time in excess of 10 minutes is required

Respirator solution (for use with a nebuliser or ventilator), salbutamol (as sulphate) 5 mg/mL. Net price 20 mL = £2.18 (hosp. only). May be diluted with sterile sodium chloride 0.9%

◢**Compound preparations**

For **compound preparations** containing salbutamol, see section 3.1.4

Chronic Asthma table, see p. 151
Acute Severe Asthma table, see p. 152.

## ▌ SALMETEROL

**Indications** reversible airways obstruction (including nocturnal asthma and prevention of exercise-induced bronchospasm) in patients requiring long-term regular bronchodilator therapy, see also Chronic Asthma table, p. 151; chronic obstructive pulmonary disease
Note Not for immediate relief of acute asthma attacks; existing corticosteroid therapy should not be reduced or withdrawn

**Cautions** see notes above

**Side-effects** see notes above; nausea, dizziness, arthralgia, and rash also reported

**3 Respiratory system**

### Dose

- By inhalation, asthma, 50 micrograms (2 puffs or 1 blister) twice daily; up to 100 micrograms (4 puffs or 2 blisters) twice daily in more severe airways obstruction; CHILD 5–12 years, 50 micrograms (2 puffs or 1 blister) twice daily

Chronic obstructive pulmonary disease 50 micrograms (2 puffs or 1 blister) twice daily

**Counselling** Advise patients that salmeterol should **not** be used for relief of acute attacks, not to exceed prescribed dose, and to follow manufacturer's directions; if a previously effective dose of inhaled salmeterol fails to provide adequate relief, a doctor's advice should be obtained as soon as possible

**Serevent®** (A&H) [PoM]

Accuhaler® (dry powder for inhalation), disk containing 60 blisters of salmeterol (as xinafoate) 50 micrograms/blister with *Accuhaler®* device, net price = £29.26. Counselling, dose

Evohaler® aerosol inhalation ▼, salmeterol (as xinafoate) 25 micrograms/metered inhalation, net price 120-dose unit = £29.26. Counselling, dose, change to CFC-free inhaler
Excipients include HFA-134a (a non-CFC propellant)

Diskhaler® (dry powder for inhalation), disks containing 4 blisters of salmeterol (as xinafoate) 50 micrograms/blister, net price 15 disks with *Diskhaler®* device = £35.79, 15-disk refill = £35.15. Counselling, dose

◀ **Compound preparations**

For **compound preparations** containing salmeterol, see section 3.2

---

## TERBUTALINE SULPHATE

**Indications** asthma and other conditions associated with reversible airways obstruction; premature labour (section 7.1.3)

**Cautions** see notes above

**Side-effects** see notes above

### Dose

- By mouth (but use by inhalation preferred), initially 2.5 mg 3 times daily for 1–2 weeks, then up to 5 mg 3 times daily; CHILD 1 month–7 years 75 micrograms/kg 3 times daily; 7–15 years 2.5 mg 2–3 times daily

- By subcutaneous *or* slow intravenous injection, 250–500 micrograms up to 4 times daily; CHILD 2–15 years 10 micrograms/kg to a max. of 300 micrograms

- By continuous intravenous infusion as a solution containing 3–5 micrograms/mL, 90–300 micrograms/hour for 8–10 hours; CHILD 1 month–18 years, initially 2–4 micrograms/kg as a loading dose, then 1–10 micrograms/kg/hour according to response and heart rate (max. 300 micrograms/hour); high doses with close monitoring

- By inhalation of powder (*Turbohaler®*), ADULT and CHILD over 5 years, 500 micrograms (1 inhalation); for persistent symptoms up to 4 times daily (but see Management of Chronic Asthma table, p. 151)

- By inhalation of nebulised solution (but see also Management of Acute Asthma table, p. 152, 5–10 mg 2–4 times daily; additional doses may be necessary in severe acute asthma; CHILD under 5 years 5 mg 2–4 times daily, 5–12 years 5–10 mg 2–4 times daily [unlicensed dose]

◀ **Oral and parenteral**

**Bricanyl®** (AstraZeneca) [PoM]

Tablets, scored, terbutaline sulphate 5 mg, net price 20 = 82p

Syrup, sugar-free, terbutaline sulphate 1.5 mg/5 mL, net price 100 mL = £2.00

Injection, terbutaline sulphate 500 micrograms/mL, net price 1-mL amp = 30p; 5-mL amp = £1.40

◀ **Inhalation**

**Counselling** Advise patients not to exceed prescribed dose and to follow manufacturer's directions; if a previously effective dose of inhaled terbutaline fails to provide at least 3 hours relief, a doctor's advice should be obtained as soon as possible

**Bricanyl®** (AstraZeneca) [PoM]

Turbohaler® (= dry powder inhaler), terbutaline sulphate 500 micrograms/metered inhalation, net price 100-dose unit = £6.92. Counselling, dose

Respules® (= single-dose units for nebulisation), terbutaline sulphate 2.5 mg/mL, net price 20 × 2-mL units (5-mg) = £4.04

---

### 3.1.1.2 Other adrenoceptor agonists

Ephedrine and the partially selective beta agonist, orciprenaline, are less suitable and less safe for use as bronchodilators than the selective beta$_2$ agonists, because they are more likely to cause arrhythmias and other side-effects. They should be avoided whenever possible.

**Adrenaline (epinephrine) injection** (1 in 1000) is used in the emergency treatment of acute allergic and anaphylactic reactions (section 3.4.3), in angioedema (section 3.4.3), and in cardiopulmonary resuscitation (section 2.7.3). Adrenaline solution (1 in 1000) is used by nebulisation in the management of severe croup (section 3.1).

---

## EPHEDRINE HYDROCHLORIDE

**Indications** reversible airways obstruction, but see notes above

**Cautions** hyperthyroidism, diabetes mellitus, ischaemic heart disease, hypertension, renal impairment, elderly; prostatic hypertrophy (risk of acute retention); interaction with MAOIs a disadvantage; **interactions**: Appendix 1 (sympathomimetics)

**Side-effects** tachycardia, anxiety, restlessness, insomnia common; also tremor, arrhythmias, dry mouth, cold extremities

### Dose

- 15–60 mg 3 times daily; CHILD up to 1 year 7.5 mg 3 times daily, 1–5 years 15 mg 3 times daily, 6–12 years 30 mg 3 times daily

[1]**Ephedrine Hydrochloride** (Non-proprietary) [PoM]
Tablets, ephedrine hydrochloride 15 mg, net price 28 = £4.59; 30 mg, 28 = £6.95

1. For exemptions see *Medicines, Ethics and Practice*, No. 33, London, Pharmaceutical Press, 2009 (and subsequent editions as available)

## ■ ORCIPRENALINE SULPHATE ◢

**Indications** reversible airways obstruction, but see notes above

**Cautions** see section 3.1.1.1 and notes above; **interactions:** Appendix 1 (sympathomimetics)

**Side-effects** see section 3.1.1.1 and notes above

**Dose**

- 20 mg 4 times daily; CHILD up to 1 year 5–10 mg 3 times daily, 1–3 years 5–10 mg 4 times daily, 3–12 years 40–60 mg daily in divided doses

**Alupent®** (Boehringer Ingelheim) PoM ◢
Syrup, sugar-free, orciprenaline sulphate 10 mg/5 mL, net price 300 mL = £2.00

---

## 3.1.2 Antimuscarinic bronchodilators

**Ipratropium** can provide short-term relief in chronic asthma, but short-acting beta₂ agonists act more quickly and are preferred. Ipratropium by nebulisation can be added to other standard treatment in life-threatening asthma or if acute asthma fails to improve with standard therapy (see Acute Asthma table, p. 152).

The aerosol inhalation of ipratropium can be used for short-term relief in mild chronic obstructive pulmonary disease in patients who are not using a long-acting antimuscarinic drug. Its maximal effect occurs 30–60 minutes after use; its duration of action is 3 to 6 hours and bronchodilation can usually be maintained with treatment 3 times a day.

**Tiotropium,** a long-acting antimuscarinic bronchodilator, is effective for the management of chronic obstructive pulmonary disease; it is not suitable for the relief of acute bronchospasm.

**Cautions** Antimuscarinic bronchodilators should be used with caution in patients with prostatic hyperplasia, bladder outflow obstruction, and those susceptible to angle-closure glaucoma (see below); **interactions:** Appendix 1 (antimuscarinics)

Glaucoma *Acute angle-closure glaucoma* reported with nebulised ipratropium, particularly when given with nebulised salbutamol (and possibly other beta₂ agonists); care needed to protect patient's eyes from nebulised drug or from drug powder.

**Side-effects** Dry mouth is the most common side-effect of antimuscarinic bronchodilators; less commonly nausea and headache occur. Constipation, tachycardia, palpitation, paradoxical bronchospasm, urinary retention, blurred vision, angle-closure glaucoma, and hypersensitivity reactions including rash, urticaria, pruritus, and angioedema occur rarely.

---

## ■ IPRATROPIUM BROMIDE

**Indications** reversible airways obstruction, particularly in chronic obstructive pulmonary disease; rhinitis (section 12.2.2)

**Cautions** see notes above; pregnancy (see p. 153 and Appendix 4); breast-feeding (see p. 153 and Appendix 5)

**Side-effects** see notes above

**Dose**

- By aerosol inhalation, 20–40 micrograms, 3–4 times daily; CHILD up to 6 years 20 micrograms 3 times daily, 6–12 years 20–40 micrograms 3 times daily
- By inhalation of powder, ADULT and CHILD over 12 years, 40 micrograms 3–4 times daily (may be doubled in less responsive patients)
- By inhalation of nebulised solution, reversible airways obstruction in chronic obstructive pulmonary disease, 250–500 micrograms 3–4 times daily
  Acute bronchospasm (see also Acute Asthma table, p. 152), 500 micrograms repeated as necessary; CHILD under 5 years 125–250 micrograms, max. 1 mg daily; 6–12 years 250 micrograms, max. 1 mg daily
  **Counselling** Advise patient not to exceed prescribed dose and to follow manufacturer's directions

**Ipratropium Bromide** (Non-proprietary) PoM
Nebuliser solution, ipratropium bromide 250 micrograms/mL, net price 20 × 1-mL (250-microgram) unit-dose vials = £6.75, 60 × 1-mL = £21.78; 20 × 2-mL (500-microgram) = £7.43, 60 × 2-mL = £26.97. If dilution is necessary use only sterile sodium chloride 0.9%

**Atrovent®** (Boehringer Ingelheim) PoM
Aerocaps® (dry powder for inhalation; for use with *Atrovent Aerohaler®*), green, ipratropium bromide 40 micrograms, net price pack of 100 caps with *Aerohaler®* = £14.53; 100 caps = £10.53. Counselling, dose
Note One *Atrovent Aerocap®* is equivalent to 2 puffs of *Atrovent®* metered aerosol inhalation

Aerosol inhalation ▼, ipratropium bromide 20 micrograms/metered inhalation, net price 200-dose unit = £5.05. Counselling, dose, change to CFC-free inhaler
Excipients include HFA-134a (a non-CFC propellant)

Nebuliser solution, isotonic, ipratropium bromide 250 micrograms/mL, net price 20 × 1-mL unit-dose vials = £4.14, 60 × 1-mL vials = £12.44; 20 × 2-mL vials = £4.87, 60 × 2-mL vials = £14.59. If dilution is necessary use only sterile sodium chloride 0.9%

**Ipratropium Steri-Neb®** (IVAX) PoM
Nebuliser solution, isotonic, ipratropium bromide 250 micrograms/mL, net price 20 × 1-mL (250-microgram) unit-dose vials = £8.72; 20 × 2-mL (500-microgram) = £9.94. If dilution is necessary use only sterile sodium chloride 0.9%

**Respontin®** (A&H) PoM
Nebuliser solution, isotonic, ipratropium bromide 250 micrograms/mL, net price 20 × 1-mL (250-microgram) unit-dose vials = £4.87; 20 × 2-mL (500-microgram) = £5.72. If dilution is necessary use only sterile sodium chloride 0.9%

◢Compound ipratropium preparations
Section 3.1.4

---

## ■ TIOTROPIUM

**Indications** maintenance treatment of chronic obstructive pulmonary disease

**Cautions** see notes above; renal impairment (Appendix 3); pregnancy (Appendix 4); breast-feeding (Appendix 5)

**Side-effects** see notes above; *less commonly* taste disturbance, dysphonia, and dizziness; *rarely* gastrointestinal reflux, and epistaxis

**3**
**Respiratory system**

**Respiratory system**

**3**

**Dose**
• See under preparations below

**Spiriva®** (Boehringer Ingelheim) PoM
Inhalation powder, hard capsule (for use with *HandiHaler®* device), green, tiotropium (as tiotropium bromide monohydrate) 18 micrograms, net price 30-cap pack with *HandiHaler®* device = £36.27, 30-cap refill = £33.17
Dose by inhalation of powder, ADULT over 18 years, 18 micrograms once daily

Respimat® (solution for inhalation)▼, tiotropium (as tiotropium bromide monohydrate) 2.5 micrograms/metered inhalation, net price 60-dose unit = £36.27
Dose by inhalation, ADULT over 18 years, 5 micrograms (2 puffs) once daily
Note The *Scottish Medicines Consortium* has advised (November 2007) that *Spiriva Respimat®* is restricted for use in chronic obstructive pulmonary disease in patients who have poor manual dexterity and difficulty using the *HandiHaler®* device

## 3.1.3 Theophylline

**Theophylline** is a xanthine used as a bronchodilator in *asthma* and stable *chronic obstructive pulmonary disease*; it is not generally effective in exacerbations of chronic obstructive pulmonary disease. It may have an additive effect when used in conjunction with small doses of beta₂ agonists; the combination may increase the risk of side-effects, including hypokalaemia (for CSM advice see p. 155).

Theophylline is metabolised in the liver; there is considerable variation in plasma-theophylline concentration particularly in smokers, in patients with hepatic impairment or heart failure, or if certain drugs are taken concurrently. The plasma-theophylline concentration is *increased* in heart failure, cirrhosis, viral infections, in the elderly, and by drugs that inhibit its metabolism. The plasma-theophylline concentration is *decreased* in smokers and in chronic alcoholism and by drugs that induce liver metabolism. For other interactions of theophylline see Appendix 1.

Differences in the half-life of theophylline are important because its toxic dose is close to the therapeutic dose; particular care is required when introducing or withdrawing drugs that interact with theophylline. In most individuals a plasma-theophylline concentration of between 10–20 mg/litre is required for satisfactory bronchodilation, although a plasma-theophylline concentration of 10 mg/litre (or less) may be effective. Adverse effects can occur within the range 10–20 mg/litre and both the frequency and severity increase at concentrations above 20 mg/litre.

Theophylline is given by injection as **aminophylline**, a mixture of theophylline with ethylenediamine, which is 20 times more soluble than theophylline alone. Aminophylline injection is needed rarely for severe attacks of asthma. It must be given by **very slow** intravenous injection (over at least 20 minutes); it is too irritant for intramuscular use. Measurement of plasma theophylline concentration may be helpful, and is **essential** if aminophylline is to be given to patients who have been taking theophylline, because serious side-effects such as convulsions and arrhythmias can occasionally precede other symptoms of toxicity.

**Caffeine** is a xanthine derivative used as a respiratory stimulant in neonatal apnoea, see section 3.5.1.

## THEOPHYLLINE

**Indications** reversible airways obstruction, acute severe asthma; see also Management of Chronic and Acute Asthma (p. 151 and p. 152)

**Cautions** cardiac disease, hypertension, hyperthyroidism; peptic ulcer; epilepsy; elderly; fever; **CSM** advice on hypokalaemia risk, p. 155; avoid in acute porphyria (section 9.8.2); monitor plasma-theophylline concentration (see notes above); hepatic impairment (Appendix 2); pregnancy (see p. 153 and Appendix 4); breast-feeding (see p. 153 and Appendix 5); **interactions:** Appendix 1 (theophylline) and notes above

**Side-effects** tachycardia, palpitation, nausea and other gastro-intestinal disturbances, headache, CNS stimulation, insomnia, arrhythmias, and convulsions especially if given rapidly by intravenous injection; **overdosage:** see Emergency Treatment of Poisoning, p. 33

**Dose**
• See below
Note Plasma-theophylline concentration for optimum response 10–20 mg/litre (55–110 micromol/litre); 4–6 hours after a dose and at least 5 days after starting treatment; narrow margin between therapeutic and toxic dose, see also notes above

**◢Modified release**
Note The rate of absorption from modified-release preparations can vary between brands. The Council of the Royal Pharmaceutical Society of Great Britain advises pharmacists that if a general practitioner prescribes a modified-release oral theophylline preparation without specifying a brand name, the pharmacist should contact the prescriber and agree the brand to be dispensed. Additionally, it is essential that a patient discharged from hospital should be maintained on the brand on which that patient was stabilised as an in-patient.

**Nuelin SA®** (3M)
SA tablets, m/r, theophylline 175 mg, net price 60-tab pack = £3.19. Label: 21, 25
Dose 175–350 mg every 12 hours; CHILD 6–12 years 175 mg every 12 hours

SA 250 tablets, m/r, scored, theophylline 250 mg, net price 60-tab pack = £4.46. Label: 21, 25
Dose 250–500 mg every 12 hours; CHILD 6–12 years 125–250 mg every 12 hours

**Slo-Phyllin®** (Merck)
Capsules, m/r, theophylline 60 mg (white/clear, enclosing white pellets), net price 56-cap pack = £2.76; 125 mg (brown/clear, enclosing white pellets), 56-cap pack = £3.48; 250 mg (blue/clear, enclosing white pellets), 56-cap pack = £4.34. Label: 25, or counselling, see below
Dose 250–500 mg every 12 hours; CHILD 2–6 years 60–120 mg every 12 hours, 6–12 years 125–250 mg every 12 hours
Counselling Swallow whole with fluid or swallow enclosed granules with soft food (e.g. yoghurt)

**Uniphyllin Continus®** (Napp)
Tablets, m/r, scored, theophylline 200 mg, net price 56-tab pack = £3.00; 300 mg, 56-tab pack = £4.77; 400 mg, 56-tab pack = £5.42. Label: 25
Dose 200 mg every 12 hours, increased according to response to 400 mg every 12 hours; CHILD 2–12 years, 9 mg/kg (up to 200 mg) every 12 hours; some children with chronic asthma may require 10–16 mg/kg (max. 400 mg) every 12 hours
Note May be appropriate to give larger evening or morning dose to achieve optimum therapeutic effect when symptoms most severe; in patients whose night or daytime symptoms persist despite other therapy, who are not currently receiving theophylline, total daily requirement may be added as single evening or morning dose

## ■ AMINOPHYLLINE

**Note** Aminophylline is a stable mixture or combination of theophylline and ethylenediamine; the ethylenediamine confers greater solubility in water

**Indications** reversible airways obstruction, acute severe asthma

**Cautions** see under Theophylline

**Side-effects** see under Theophylline; also allergy to ethylenediamine can cause urticaria, erythema, and exfoliative dermatitis

**Dose**

- See under preparations, below

  **Note** Plasma-theophylline concentration for optimum response 10–20 mg/litre (55–110 micromol/litre); measure plasma-theophylline concentration 4–6 hours after dose by mouth and at least 5 days after starting oral treatment; measure plasma-theophylline concentration 4–6 hours after the start of intravenous infusion; narrow margin between therapeutic and toxic dose, see also notes above

> To avoid excessive dosage in obese patients, dose should be calculated on the basis of ideal weight for height

**Aminophylline** (Non-proprietary) [PoM]

Injection, aminophylline 25 mg/mL, net price 10-mL amp = 90p

Brands include *Minijet® Aminophylline*

**Dose** acute severe asthma or acute exacerbation of chronic obstructive pulmonary disease **not** previously treated with theophylline, by slow intravenous injection over at least 20 minutes (with close monitoring), 250–500 mg (5 mg/kg), then see below; CHILD 5 mg/kg, then see below

Acute severe asthma or acute exacerbation of chronic obstructive pulmonary disease, by intravenous infusion (with close monitoring), 500 micrograms/kg/hour, adjusted according to plasma-theophylline concentration; CHILD 6 months–9 years 1 mg/kg/hour, 10–16 years 800 micrograms/kg/hour, adjusted according to plasma-theophylline concentration

**Note** Patients taking oral theophylline or aminophylline should not normally receive intravenous aminophylline unless plasma-theophylline concentration is available to guide dosage

### ◢ Modified release

**Note** Advice about modified-release theophylline preparations on p. 160 also applies to modified-release aminophylline preparations

**Phyllocontin Continus®** (Napp)

Tablets, m/r, yellow, f/c, aminophylline hydrate 225 mg, net price 56-tab pack = £2.44. Label: 25

**Dose** ADULT and CHILD body-weight over 40 kg initially 1 tablet twice daily, increased after 1 week to 2 tablets twice daily according to plasma-theophylline concentration

**Note** Brands of modified-release tablets containing aminophylline 225 mg include *Norphyllin® SR*

Forte tablets, m/r, yellow, f/c, aminophylline hydrate 350 mg, net price 56-tab pack = £4.22. Label: 25

**Dose** initially 1 tablet twice daily, increased after 1 week to 2 tablets twice daily if necessary

**Note** *Phyllocontin Continus® Forte* tablets are for smokers and other patients with shorter theophylline half-life (see notes above)

<br>

## 3.1.4 Compound bronchodilator preparations

In general, patients are best treated with single-ingredient preparations, such as a selective beta$_2$ agonist (section 3.1.1.1) or ipratropium bromide (section 3.1.2), so that the dose of each drug can be adjusted.

This flexibility is lost with compound bronchodilator preparations. However, a combination product may be appropriate for patients stabilised on individual components in the same proportion.

For **cautions, contra-indications** and **side-effects** see under individual drugs.

**Combivent®** (Boehringer Ingelheim) [PoM] ◢

Nebuliser solution, isotonic, ipratropium bromide 500 micrograms, salbutamol (as sulphate) 2.5 mg/2.5-mL vial, net price 60 unit-dose vials = £24.10

**Dose** bronchospasm in chronic obstructive pulmonary disease, by inhalation of nebulised solution, ADULT and CHILD over 12 years, 1 vial (2.5 mL) 3–4 times daily

**Glaucoma** In addition to other potential side-effects acute angle-closure glaucoma has been reported with nebulised ipratropium—for details, see p. 159

**Duovent®** (Boehringer Ingelheim) [PoM] ◢

Nebuliser solution, isotonic, fenoterol hydrobromide 1.25 mg, ipratropium bromide 500 micrograms/4-mL vial, net price 20 unit-dose vials = £8.00

**Dose** acute severe asthma or acute exacerbation of chronic asthma, by inhalation of nebulised solution, ADULT and CHILD over 14 years, 1 vial (4 mL); may be repeated up to max. 4 vials in 24 hours

**Glaucoma** In addition to other potential side-effects acute angle-closure glaucoma has been reported with nebulised ipratropium—for details, see p. 159

<br>

## 3.1.5 Peak flow meters, inhaler devices and nebulisers

### Peak flow meters

Measurement of peak flow is particularly helpful for patients who are 'poor perceivers' and hence slow to detect deterioration in their asthma, and for those with moderate or severe asthma.

Standard-range peak flow meters are suitable for both adults and children; low-range peak flow meters are appropriate for severely restricted airflow in adults and children. Patients must be given clear guidelines as to the action they should take if their peak flow falls below a certain level. Patients can be encouraged to adjust some of their own treatment (within specified limits) according to changes in peak flow rate.

### Standard Range Peak Flow Meter

Conforms to standard EN 13826

MicroPeak®, range 60–800 litres/minute, net price = £6.50, replacement mouthpiece = 38p (Micro Medical)

Mini-Wright®, range 60–800 litres/minute, net price = £6.86, replacement mouthpiece = 38p (Clement Clarke)

Personal Best®, range 60–800 litres/minute, net price = £6.48, replacement mouthpiece = 25p (Respironics)

Piko-1®, range 15–999 litres/minute, net price = £9.50, replacement mouthpiece = 38p (nSPIRE Health)

Pocketpeak®, range 60–800 litres/minute, net price = £6.53, replacement mouthpiece = 38p (nSPIRE Health)

Vitalograph®, range 50–800 litres/minute, net price = £4.50 (children's coloured version also available), replacement mouthpiece = 40p (Vitalograph)

**Note** Readings from new peak flow meters are often lower than those obtained from old Wright-scale peak flow meters and the correct recording chart should be used

**Low Range Peak Flow Meter**

Compliant to standard EN 13826 except for scale range
Mini-Wright®, range 30–400 litres/minute, net price = £6.90,
replacement mouthpiece = 38p (Clement Clarke)

Pocketpeak®, range 50–400 litres/minute, net price = £6.53,
replacement mouthpiece = 38p (nSPIRE Health)

**Note** Readings from new peak flow meters are often lower than
those obtained from old Wright-scale peak flow meters and the
correct recording chart should be used

# Drug delivery devices

**Inhaler devices** These include *pressurised metered-dose inhalers*, *breath-actuated inhalers*, and *dry powder inhalers*. Many patients can be taught to use a pressurised metered-dose inhaler effectively but some patients, particularly the elderly and children, find them difficult to use. *Spacer devices* (see below) can help such patients because they remove the need to coordinate actuation with inhalation. Dry powder inhalers may be useful in adults and children over 5 years who are unwilling or unable to use a pressurised metered-dose inhaler. Alternatively, breath-actuated inhalers are suitable for adults and older children provided they can use the device effectively.

On changing from a pressurised metered-dose inhaler to a dry powder inhaler, patients may notice a lack of sensation in the mouth and throat previously associated with each actuation. Coughing may also occur.

The patient should be instructed carefully on the use of the inhaler and it is important to check that the inhaler continues to be used correctly because inadequate inhalation technique may be mistaken for a lack of response to the drug.

| **NICE guidance** |
| --- |
| **Inhaler devices for children with chronic asthma (children under 5 years, August 2000; children 5–15 years, March 2002)** |
| A child's needs, ability to develop and maintain effective technique, and likelihood of good compliance should govern the choice of inhaler and spacer device; only then should cost be considered. |
| For children aged under 5 years: |
| • corticosteroid and bronchodilator therapy should be delivered by pressurised metered-dose inhaler and spacer device, with a facemask if necessary; |
| • if this is not effective, and depending on the child's condition, nebulised therapy may be considered and, in children over 3 years, a dry powder inhaler may also be considered [but see notes above]. |
| For children aged 5–15 years: |
| • corticosteroid therapy should be routinely delivered by a pressurised metered-dose inhaler and spacer device; |
| • children and their carers should be trained in the use of the chosen device; suitability of the device should be reviewed at least annually. Inhaler technique and compliance should be monitored. |

**Spacer devices** Spacer devices remove the need for co-ordination between actuation of a pressurised metered-dose inhaler and inhalation. The spacer device reduces the velocity of the aerosol and subsequent impaction on the oropharynx and allows more time

for evaporation of the propellant so that a larger proportion of the particles can be inhaled and deposited in the lungs. Spacer devices are particularly useful for patients with poor inhalation technique, for children, for patients requiring high doses of inhaled corticosteroids (see Management of Chronic Asthma table, p. 151), for nocturnal asthma, and for patients prone to candidiasis with inhaled corticosteroids. The size of the spacer is important, the larger spacers with a one-way valve (*Volumatic®*) being most effective. It is important to prescribe a spacer device that is compatible with the metered-dose inhaler, see devices below. Spacer devices should not be regarded as interchangeable; patients should be advised not to switch between spacer devices.

**Use and care of spacer devices** Patients should inhale from the spacer device as soon as possible after actuation because the drug aerosol is very short-lived; single-dose actuation is recommended. Tidal breathing is as effective as single breaths. The device should be cleansed once a month by washing in mild detergent and then allowed to dry in air; the mouthpiece should be wiped clean of detergent before use. More frequent cleaning should be avoided since any electrostatic charge may affect drug delivery. Spacer devices should be replaced every 6–12 months.

**Able Spacer®** (Clement Clarke)

Spacer device, small-volume device. For use with all pressurised (aerosol) inhalers, net price standard device = £4.20; with infant, child or adult mask = £6.86

**AeroChamber® Plus** (GSK)

Spacer device, medium-volume device. For use with all pressurised (aerosol) inhalers, net price standard device (blue) = £4.43, with mask (blue) = £7.40; infant device (orange) with mask = £7.40; child device (yellow) with mask = £7.40

**Babyhaler®** (A&H) (NHS)

Spacer device, for paediatric use with *Flixotide®*, *Seretide®*, *Serevent®*, and *Ventolin®* inhalers, net price = £11.34

**Haleraid®** (A&H) (NHS)

Inhalation aid, device to place over pressurised (aerosol) inhalers to aid when strength in hands is impaired (e.g. in arthritis). For use with *Flixotide®*, *Seretide®*, *Serevent®*, and *Ventolin®* inhalers. Available as *Haleraid®-120* for 120-dose inhalers and *Haleraid®-200* for 200-dose inhalers, net price = 80p

**Nebuchamber®** (AstraZeneca)

Spacer device, for use with *Pulmicort®* aerosol inhalers, net price = £8.56

**Optichamber®** (Respironics)

Spacer device, for use with all pressurised (aerosol) inhalers, net price = £4.28; with small or medium mask = £7.40 (NHS)

**PARI Vortex Spacer®** (Pari)

Spacer device, medium-volume device. For use with all pressurised (aerosol) inhalers, net price with mouthpiece = £6.07 (NHS); with mask for infant or child = £7.91; with adult mask = £9.97 (NHS)

**Pocket Chamber®** (nSPIRE Health)

Spacer device, small-volume device. For use with all pressurised (aerosol) inhalers, net price = £4.18; with infant, small, medium, or large mask = £9.75

**Volumatic®** (A&H)

Spacer inhaler, large-volume device. For use with *Clenil Modulite®*, *Flixotide®*, *Seretide®*, *Serevent®*, and *Ventolin®* inhalers, net price = £2.75; with paediatric mask = £2.75

**3 Respiratory system**

# Nebulisers

> In England and Wales nebulisers and compressors are not available on the NHS (but they are free of VAT); some nebulisers (but not compressors) are available on form GP10A in Scotland (for details consult Scottish Drug Tariff).

A nebuliser converts a solution of a drug into an aerosol for inhalation. It is used to deliver higher doses of drug to the airways than is usual with standard inhalers. The main indications for use of a nebuliser are:

- to deliver a beta$_2$ agonist or ipratropium to a patient with an *acute exacerbation* of asthma or of chronic obstructive pulmonary disease;
- to deliver a beta$_2$ agonist or ipratropium on a *regular basis* to a patient with severe asthma or reversible airways obstruction who has been shown to benefit from regular treatment with higher doses;
- to deliver *prophylactic medication* such as a corticosteroid to a patient unable to use other inhalational devices (particularly to a young child);
- to deliver an antibiotic (such as colistin) to a patient with chronic purulent infection (as in cystic fibrosis or bronchiectasis);
- to deliver budesonide to a child with severe croup;
- to deliver pentamidine for the prophylaxis and treatment of pneumocystis pneumonia.

The proportion of a nebuliser solution that reaches the lungs depends on the type of nebuliser and although it can be as high as 30%, it is more frequently close to 10% and sometimes below 10%. The remaining solution is left in the nebuliser as residual volume or it is deposited in the mouthpiece and tubing. The extent to which the nebulised solution is deposited in the airways or alveoli depends on particle size. Particles with a mass median diameter of 1–5 microns are deposited in the airways and are therefore appropriate for asthma whereas a particle size of 1–2 microns is needed for alveolar deposition of pentamidine to combat pneumocystis infection. The type of nebuliser is therefore chosen according to the deposition required and according to the viscosity of the solution (antibiotic solutions usually being more viscous).

Some jet nebulisers are able to increase drug output during inspiration and hence increase efficiency.

The patient should be aware that the dose of a bronchodilator given by nebulisation is usually **much higher** than that from an aerosol inhaler.

The British Thoracic Society has advised that nebulised bronchodilators are appropriate for patients with chronic persistent asthma or those with severe acute asthma. In chronic persistent asthma, nebulised bronchodilators should only be used to relieve persistent daily wheeze (see Chronic Asthma table p. 151). The British Thoracic Society has recommended that the use of nebulisers in chronic persistent asthma should be considered only:

- after a review of the diagnosis;
- if the airflow obstruction is significantly reversible by bronchodilators without unacceptable side-effects;
- after the patient has been using the usual hand-held inhaler correctly;

- after a larger dose of bronchodilator from a hand-held inhaler (with a spacer if necessary) has been tried for at least 2 weeks;
- if the patient is complying with the prescribed dose and frequency of anti-inflammatory treatment including regular use of high-dose inhaled corticosteroid.

Before prescribing a nebuliser, a home trial should preferably be undertaken to monitor peak flow for up to 2 weeks on standard treatment and up to 2 weeks on nebulised treatment. If prescribed, patients must:

- have clear instructions from doctor, specialist nurse or pharmacist on the use of the nebuliser and on peak-flow monitoring;
- be instructed not to treat acute attacks at home without also seeking help;
- receive an education program;
- have regular follow up including peak-flow monitoring and be seen by doctor, specialist nurse or physiotherapist.

## ◢ Jet nebulisers

Jet nebulisers are more widely used than ultrasonic nebulisers. Most jet nebulisers require an optimum gas flow rate of 6–8 litres/minute and in hospital can be driven by piped air or oxygen; in acute asthma the nebuliser should be driven by oxygen. Domiciliary oxygen cylinders do not provide an adequate flow rate therefore an electrical compressor is required for domiciliary use.

For patients with *chronic obstructive pulmonary disease and hypercapnia*, oxygen can be dangerous and the nebuliser should be driven by air (see also p. 155). In exacerbations of chronic obstructive pulmonary disease, the nebuliser should be driven by compressed air in hypercapnia or acidosis. If oxygen is required, it should be given simultaneously by nasal cannula.

> **Important:** the Department of Health has reminded users of the need to use the correct grade of tubing when connecting a nebuliser to a medical gas supply or compressor.

**Medix Lifecare Nebuliser Chamber®** (Medix) ⟨NHS⟩
Jet nebuliser, disposable; for use with bronchodilators, antimuscarinics, corticosteroids, and antibacterials, replacement recommended every 2–3 months if used 4 times a day. Compatible with *AC 2000 Hi Flo®* ⟨NHS⟩, *World Traveller Hi Flo®* ⟨NHS⟩ and *Econoneb®* ⟨NHS⟩, net price = £1.00

**Medix Lifecare Nebuliser System®** (Medix) ⟨NHS⟩
Jet nebuliser, consisting of mouthpiece, tubing, and nebuliser chamber, net price = £2.00; mask kits with tubing and nebuliser chamber also available, net price (adult) = £2.00; (child) = £2.10

**PARI LC® SPRINT** (Pari) ⟨NHS⟩
Jet nebuliser, non-disposable, for hospital or home use; for use with bronchodilators, antibacterials, and corticosteroids, replacement recommended yearly if used 4 times a day. Compatible with *PARI TurboBOY® S* ⟨NHS⟩, *PARI JuniorBOY® S* ⟨NHS⟩, *PARI BOY® Mobile S* ⟨NHS⟩, and *PARI WALK BOY®* ⟨NHS⟩ compressors, net price = £16.05

**PARI LC® SPRINT BABY** (Pari) ⟨NHS⟩
Jet nebuliser, non-disposable, for hospital or home use; for use with bronchodilators, antibacterials and corticosteroids; replacement recommended yearly if used 4 times a day. Compatible with *PARI TurboBOY® S* ⟨NHS⟩, *PARI JuniorBOY® S* ⟨NHS⟩, *PARI BOY® Mobile S* ⟨NHS⟩, *PARI WALK BOY®* ⟨NHS⟩ compressors. Available separately for children aged less than 1 year, 1–4 years or 4–7 years, net price (with mask and connection tube) = £32.15

**3**

**Respiratory system**

**Sidestream Durable®** (Profile Respiratory) ⓝⒽⓈ
Jet nebuliser, non-disposable, for home use; for use with bronchodilators; yearly replacement recommended if 4 six-minute treatments used per day. Compatible with *Freeway Freedom®* ⓝⒽⓈ and *Porta-Neb®* ⓝⒽⓈ, net price year pack = £20.40 (*Porta-Neb®*), £29.00 (*Freeway Freedom®*). Disposable *Sidestream®* ⓝⒽⓈ nebuliser also available

**Ventstream®** (Profile Respiratory) ⓝⒽⓈ
Jet nebuliser, closed-system, for use with low flow compressors, compatible with *Porta-Neb®* ⓝⒽⓈ and *Freeway Freedom®* ⓝⒽⓈ compressors; for use with antibacterials, bronchodilators, and corticosteroids, replacement recommended yearly if used 3 times a day, net price year pack with filter = £39.00 (*Porta-Neb®*), £41.00 (*Freeway Freedom®*)

◢ **Home compressors with nebulisers**

**AC 2000 HI FLO®** (Medix) ⓝⒽⓈ
Home and hospital use, containing 1 *Jet Nebuliser®* ⓝⒽⓈ set with mouthpiece, 1 adult and 1 child mask, 1 spare inlet filter, filter spanner. Mains operated. Nebulises bronchodilators, corticosteroids, and antibacterials, net price = £117.00; carrying case available

**AC 4000®** (Medix) ⓝⒽⓈ
Home and hospital use, containing 1 *Jet Nebuliser®* ⓝⒽⓈ set with mouthpiece, 1 adult and 1 child face mask, 1 spare inlet filter, filter spanner. Mains operated. Nebulises bronchodilators, corticosteroids, and antibacterials, net price = £80.10

**Aquilon®** (Henleys) ⓝⒽⓈ
Portable, home use, with 1 adult or 1 child mask and tubing. Mains operated; for use with bronchodilators, corticosteroids and antibacterials, net price = £82.50

**Econoneb®** (Medix) ⓝⒽⓈ
Home, clinic and hospital use, used with 1 *Jet Nebuliser®* ⓝⒽⓈ set with mouthpiece, 1 adult and 1 child mask, 1 spare inlet filter, filter spanner. Nebulises bronchodilators, corticosteroids, and antibacterials. Mains operated, net price = £99.00

**Freeway Freedom®** (Profile Respiratory) ⓝⒽⓈ
Portable, containing *Sidestream Durable®* ⓝⒽⓈ nebuliser, 1 adult mask, 1 child mask, 1 angled mouthpiece, 1 coiled *Duratube®*, 4 inlet filters, charger and power lead, net price = £203.20; with *Ventstream®* ⓝⒽⓈ nebuliser, 1 straight mouthpiece, 1 coiled *Duratube®*, 4 inlet filters, 1 aerosol hose, charger and power lead, net price = £203.20

**PARI JuniorBOY® S** (Pari) ⓝⒽⓈ
Portable, for hospital or home use, containing *PARI LC® SPRINT Junior* ⓝⒽⓈ nebuliser with child mouthpiece, mask, connection tube, and mains cable. Filter replacement recommended every 12 months. Compatible with *PARI LC® SPRINT* ⓝⒽⓈ, and *PARI LC® SPRINT BABY* ⓝⒽⓈ nebulisers, net price = £70.00

**PARI TurboBOY® S** (Pari) ⓝⒽⓈ
Portable, for hospital or home use, containing *PARI SPRINT* ⓝⒽⓈ nebuliser with adult mouthpiece, mask, connection tube and mains cable. Filter replacement recommended every 12 months. Compatible with *PARI LC® SPRINT* ⓝⒽⓈ, and *PARI LC® SPRINT BABY* ⓝⒽⓈ nebulisers, net price = £65.00

**PARI BOY® Mobile S** (Pari) ⓝⒽⓈ
Portable, containing *PARI LC® SPRINT* ⓝⒽⓈ nebuliser with connection tube, mains cable, rechargeable battery, car battery adaptor, and carrying case. Compatible with *PARI LC® SPRINT BABY* ⓝⒽⓈ nebuliser. Nebulises bronchodilators, corticosteroids, and antibacterials, net price = £180.00

**Porta-Neb®** (Profile Respiratory) ⓝⒽⓈ
Portable, containing *Sidestream Durable®* ⓝⒽⓈ nebuliser, 1 adult mask, 1 child mask, 1 angled mouthpiece, 1 coiled *Duratube®*, 4 inlet filters. Mains operated, net price = £94.00; with *Ventstream®* ⓝⒽⓈ nebuliser, 1 straight mouthpiece, 1 coiled *Duratube®*, 4 inlet filters, aerosol hose. Mains operated, net price = £104.80

**De Vilbiss 5650®** (De Vilbiss) ⓝⒽⓈ
Home, clinic use, containing disposable nebuliser set, mouthpiece, mask, mains lead, tubing, thumb-valve. For use with bronchodilators, net price = £142.14

**De Vilbiss 4650®** (De Vilbiss) ⓝⒽⓈ
Home, clinic and hospital use, with mouthpiece. Mains operated, net price = £93.95

**Tourer®** (Henleys) ⓝⒽⓈ
Portable, home use, mains/car battery operated; for use with bronchodilators, corticosteroids and antibacterials, net price = £101.25

**Ultima®** (Henleys) ⓝⒽⓈ
Portable, home use, rechargable or mains/car battery operated. Nebulises bronchodilators and corticosteroids, net price = £156.00 (includes case)

**World Traveller HI FLO®** (Medix) ⓝⒽⓈ
Portable, containing 1 *Jet Nebuliser®* ⓝⒽⓈ set with mouthpiece, 1 adult and 1 child mask, 1 spare inlet filter, filter spanner. Battery, car, and mains operated; rechargeable battery pack available. Nebulises bronchodilators, corticosteroids, and antibacterials, net price excluding battery = £166.00; with battery = £216.00; carrying case available

◢ **Compressors**

**Omron CX3®** (Omron) ⓝⒽⓈ
Home and hospital use, mains operated, net price = £48.75

**Omron compAIR CX**ᴾʳᵒ® (Omron) ⓝⒽⓈ
Home and hospital use, mains operated, net price = £56.78 (includes 1 adult mask, child mask, 5 spare filters, and carrying case)

**System 22 CR60®** (Profile Respiratory) ⓝⒽⓈ
Hospital use, high flow compressor. Mains operated, net price = £199.90. Also compatible with *System 22 Antibiotic Tee®* ⓝⒽⓈ for nebulisation of high viscosity drugs such as antibacterials

**Turboneb®** (Medix) ⓝⒽⓈ
Hospital use, high flow compressor. Nebulises bronchodilators, corticosteroids, antibacterials, and pentamidine. Mains operated, net price = £125.00

◢ **Ultrasonic nebulisers**

Ultrasonic nebulisers produce an aerosol by ultrasonic vibration of the drug solution and therefore do not require a gas flow

**F16 Wave®** (Parkside) ⓝⒽⓈ
Portable, adjustable delivery rate. Mains/car battery operated or rechargeable battery pack (supplied), net price = £130.00

**Liberty®** (Medix) ⓝⒽⓈ
Portable, home and clinic use, containing disposable mouthpiece and chamber cover. Mains and car battery operated. Nebulises bronchodilators and antibacterials, net price £112.49

**Omron MicroAIR®** (Omron) ⓝⒽⓈ
Portable, battery operated, net price = £149.96 (includes 1 adult mask, 1 child mask, and carrying case; mains adaptor also available)

**Omron NE-U17®** (Omron) ⓝⒽⓈ
Clinic and hospital use, mains operated, net price = £650.17

**Ultra Neb 2000®** (De Vilbiss) ⓝⒽⓈ
Hospital, clinic, and home use, delivery rate adjustable. Supplied with stand, net price = £1205.00

---

## Nebuliser diluent

Nebulisation may be carried out using an undiluted nebuliser solution or it may require dilution beforehand. The usual diluent is sterile sodium chloride 0.9% (physiological saline).

**Sodium Chloride** (Non-proprietary) ⓅⓄⓂ
Nebuliser solution, sodium chloride 0.9%, net price 20 × 2.5 mL = £8.95
Brands include *Saline Steripoule®*, *Saline Steri-Neb®*

# 3.2 Corticosteroids

Corticosteroids are used for the management of reversible and irreversible airways disease. An inhaled corticosteroid used for 3–4 weeks may help to distinguish asthma from chronic obstructive pulmonary disease; clear improvement over 3–4 weeks suggests asthma.

**Asthma** Corticosteroids are effective in *asthma*; they reduce airway inflammation (and hence reduce oedema and secretion of mucus into the airway).

An inhaled corticosteroid is used regularly for prophylaxis of asthma when patients require a beta₂ agonist more than twice a week, or if symptoms disturb sleep more than once a week, or if the patient has suffered exacerbations in the last 2 years requiring a systemic corticosteroid or a nebulised bronchodilator (see Management of Chronic Asthma table, p. 151). *Regular use* of inhaled corticosteroids reduces the risk of exacerbation of asthma.

Current and previous smoking reduces the effectiveness of inhaled corticosteroids and higher doses may be necessary.

Corticosteroid inhalers must be used regularly for maximum benefit; alleviation of symptoms usually occurs 3 to 7 days after initiation. **Beclometasone dipropionate** (beclomethasone dipropionate), **budesonide**, **fluticasone propionate**, and **mometasone furoate** appear to be equally effective. Preparations that combine a corticosteroid with a long-acting beta₂ agonist may be helpful for patients stabilised on the individual components in the same proportion.

In adults using an inhaled corticosteroid and a long-acting beta₂ agonist for the prophylaxis of asthma, but who are poorly controlled, (see step 3 of the table on p. 151) *Symbicort*® (budesonide with formoterol) can be used as a reliever (instead of a short-acting beta₂ agonist), in addition to its regular use for the prophylaxis of asthma. *Symbicort*® can also be used in this way in adults using an inhaled corticosteroid with a dose greater than beclometasone dipropionate 400 micrograms daily[1], but who are poorly controlled (see step 2 of the table on p. 151). When starting this treatment, the total regular daily dose of inhaled corticosteroid should not be reduced. Patients must be carefully instructed on the appropriate dose and management of exacerbations before initiating this therapy, see *Symbicort*® p. 168. Patients using budesonide with formoterol as a reliever once a day or more should have their treatment reviewed regularly. This management approach has not been investigated with combination inhalers containing other corticosteroids and long-acting beta₂ agonists.

Patients taking long-term oral corticosteroids for asthma can often be transferred to an inhaled corticosteroid but the transfer must be slow, with gradual reduction in the dose of the oral corticosteroid, and at a time when the asthma is well controlled.

High doses of inhaled corticosteroid can be prescribed for patients who respond only partially to standard doses with a long-acting beta₂ agonist or another

---

1. For standard doses of other inhaled corticosteroids, see Management of Chronic Asthma table, p. 151.

long-acting bronchodilator (see Management of Chronic Asthma table, p. 151). High doses should be continued only if there is clear benefit over the lower dose. The recommended maximum dose of an inhaled corticosteroid should not generally be exceeded. However, if a higher dose is required, then it should be initiated and supervised by a specialist. The use of high doses of inhaled corticosteroid can minimise the requirement for an oral corticosteroid.

Systemic corticosteroid therapy may be necessary during episodes of infection or if the asthma is worsening, when higher doses are needed and access of inhaled drug to small airways may be reduced; patients may need a reserve supply of tablets.

**Chronic obstructive pulmonary disease** In *chronic obstructive pulmonary disease* inhaled corticosteroid treatment may reduce exacerbations. An inhaled corticosteroid [unlicensed indication] should be considered (in addition to bronchodilator treatment) if the forced expiratory volume in 1 second ($FEV_1$) is less than 50% of the predicted value and if the patient has had 2 or more exacerbations in a year which require antibacterial treatment or an oral corticosteroid.

**Cautions of inhaled corticosteroids** Systemic therapy may be required during periods of stress or when either airways obstruction or mucus prevent drug access to smaller airways. For advice on the use of corticosteroids in women with asthma who are pregnant or breast-feeding, see p. 153, and Appendix 4 and Appendix 5; **interactions:** Appendix 1 (corticosteroids)

**Paradoxical bronchospasm** The potential for paradoxical bronchospasm (calling for discontinuation and alternative therapy) should be borne in mind—mild bronchospasm may be prevented by inhalation of a short-acting beta₂ agonist beforehand (or by transfer from an aerosol inhalation to a dry powder inhalation).

**CFC-free inhalers** Chlorofluorocarbon (CFC) propellants in pressurised aerosol inhalers are being replaced by hydrofluoroalkane (HFA) propellants. Patients receiving CFC-free inhalers should be reassured about the efficacy of the new inhalers and counselled that the aerosol may feel and taste different; any difficulty with the new inhaler should be discussed with the doctor or pharmacist.

Doses for CFC-free corticosteroid inhalers may be different from those that contain CFCs, see also MHRA/CHM advice below.

> **MHRA/CHM advice (July 2008)**
> - Beclometasone dipropionate CFC-free pressurised metered-dose inhalers (*Qvar*® and *Clenil Modulite*®) are **not** interchangeable and should be prescribed by brand name; *Qvar*® has extra-fine particles, is more potent than traditional CFC-containing inhalers, and is approximately twice as potent as *Clenil Modulite*®;
> - *Fostair*® is a combination beclometasone dipropionate and formoterol fumarate CFC-free pressurised metered-dose inhaler; *Fostair*® has extra-fine particles and is more potent than traditional beclometasone dipropionate CFC-free inhalers.

**Side-effects of inhaled corticosteroids** Inhaled corticosteroids have considerably fewer systemic effects than oral corticosteroids (section 6.3.2), but adverse effects have been reported.

High doses of inhaled corticosteroids (see Management of Chronic Asthma table, p. 151) used for prolonged periods can induce adrenal suppression. Inhaled corticosteroids have been associated with adrenal crisis and coma in children; excessive doses should be avoided. Patients using high doses of inhaled corticosteroids should be given a 'steroid card' (section 6.3.2) and specific written advice to consider corticosteroid replacement during an episode of stress, such as severe intercurrent illness or an operation.

High doses of inhaled corticosteroid have been associated with lower respiratory tract infections, including pneumonia, in older patients with chronic obstructive pulmonary disease.

Bone mineral density may be reduced following long-term inhalation of higher doses of corticosteroids, predisposing patients to osteoporosis (section 6.6). It is therefore sensible to ensure that the dose of an inhaled corticosteroid is no higher than necessary to keep a patient's asthma under good control. Treatment with an inhaled corticosteroid can usually be stopped after a mild exacerbation as long as the patient knows that it is necessary to reinstate it should the asthma deteriorate or the peak flow rate fall.

In children, growth restriction associated with systemic corticosteroid therapy does not seem to occur with recommended doses of inhaled therapy; although initial growth velocity may be reduced, there appears to be no effect on achieving normal adult height. However, the CSM has recommended that the height of children receiving prolonged treatment of inhaled corticosteroid is monitored; if growth is slowed, referral to a paediatrician should be considered. Large-volume spacer devices should be used for administering inhaled corticosteroids in children under 5 years (see NICE guidance, section 3.1.5); they are also useful in older children and adults, particularly if high doses are required. Spacer devices increase airway deposition and reduce oropharyngeal deposition.

A small risk of glaucoma with prolonged high doses of inhaled corticosteroids has been reported; cataracts have also been reported with inhaled corticosteroids. Hoarseness and candidiasis of the mouth or throat have been reported, usually only with large doses (see also below). Hypersensitivity reactions (including rash and angioedema) have been reported rarely. Other side-effects that have been reported very rarely include paradoxical bronchospasm, anxiety, depression, sleep disturbances, and behavioural changes including hyperactivity and irritability.

Candidiasis The risk of oral candidiasis can be reduced by using a spacer device with the corticosteroid inhaler; rinsing the mouth with water (or cleaning a child's teeth) after inhalation of a dose may also be helpful. Antifungal oral suspension or lozenges (section 12.3.2) can be used to treat oral candidiasis without discontinuing therapy.

Oral An acute attack of asthma should be treated with a short course of an oral corticosteroid starting with a high dose, e.g. prednisolone 40–50 mg daily for a few days. Patients whose asthma has deteriorated rapidly usually respond quickly to corticosteroids. The dose can usually be stopped abruptly in a mild exacerbation of

asthma (see also Withdrawal of Corticosteroids, section 6.3.2) but it should be reduced gradually in those with poorer asthma control, to reduce the possibility of serious relapse. For the use of corticosteroids in the emergency treatment of acute severe asthma, see Management of Acute Asthma table, p. 152.

In chronic continuing asthma, when the response to other drugs has been inadequate, longer term administration of an oral corticosteroid may be necessary; in such cases high doses of an inhaled corticosteroid should be continued to minimise oral corticosteroid requirements. In chronic obstructive pulmonary disease prednisolone 30 mg daily should be given for 7–14 days; treatment can be stopped abruptly. Prolonged treatment with oral prednisolone is of no benefit and maintenance treatment is not normally recommended.

An oral corticosteroid should normally be taken as a single dose in the morning to reduce the disturbance to circadian cortisol secretion. Dosage should always be titrated to the lowest dose that controls symptoms. Regular peak-flow measurements help to optimise the dose.

Parenteral For the use of hydrocortisone injection in the emergency treatment of acute severe asthma, see Management of Acute Asthma table, p. 152.

## BECLOMETASONE DIPROPIONATE
### (Beclomethasone Dipropionate)

**Indications** prophylaxis of asthma (see also Management of Chronic Asthma table, p. 151)

**Cautions** see notes above

**Side-effects** see notes above

**Dose**

- By aerosol inhalation, see Management of Chronic Asthma table, p. 151 (important: for *Clenil Modulite*® and *Qvar*®, see under preparations)

- By inhalation of dry powder (important: for *Asmabec*® and *Becodisks*®, see under preparations), 200–400 micrograms twice daily; adjusted as necessary up to 800 micrograms twice daily; CHILD over 5 years 100–200 micrograms twice daily, adjusted as necessary

**Beclometasone** (Non-proprietary) [PoM]
Aerosol inhalation, beclometasone dipropionate 50 micrograms/metered inhalation, net price 200-dose unit = £4.57; 100 micrograms/metered inhalation, 200-dose unit = £5.95; 200 micrograms/metered inhalation, 200-dose unit = £16.58; 250 micrograms/metered inhalation, 200-dose unit = £12.58. Label: 8, counselling, dose; also 10 and steroid card with high doses
Excipients include CFC propellants
Brands include *Beclazone*®

Dry powder for inhalation, beclometasone dipropionate 100 micrograms/metered inhalation, net price 100-dose unit = £5.36; 200 micrograms/metered inhalation, 100-dose unit = £9.89, 200-dose unit = £15.60; 400 micrograms/metered inhalation, 100-dose unit = £19.61. Label: 8, counselling, dose; also 10 and steroid card with high doses
Brands include *Pulvinal*® *Beclometasone Dipropionate*, *Easyhaler*® *Beclometasone Dipropionate*

Inhalation powder, hard capsule (for use with *Cyclohaler®* device), beclometasone dipropionate 100 micrograms, net price 120-cap pack = £15.99; 200 micrograms, 120-cap pack = £25.00; 400 micrograms, 120-cap pack = £32.25. Label: 8, counselling, dose; also 10 and steroid card with high doses
Brands include *Beclometasone Cyclocaps®*

**Asmabec Clickhaler®** (UCB Pharma) (PoM)
Dry powder for inhalation, beclometasone dipropionate 50 micrograms/metered inhalation, net price 200-dose unit = £6.42; 100 micrograms/metered inhalation, 200-dose unit = £9.43; 250 micrograms/metered inhalation, 100-dose unit = £11.83. Label: 8, counselling, dose; also 10 and steroid card with high doses
Dose by inhalation of powder, prophylaxis of asthma, 100–400 micrograms twice daily, adjusted as necessary; max. 1 mg twice daily; CHILD 6–12 years 50–200 micrograms twice daily, adjusted as necessary

**Becodisks®** (A&H) (PoM)
Dry powder for inhalation, disks containing 8 blisters of beclometasone dipropionate 100 micrograms/blister, net price 15 disks with *Diskhaler®* device = £11.53, 15-disk refill = £10.97; 200 micrograms/blister, 15 disks with *Diskhaler®* device = £21.98, 15-disk refill = £21.41; 400 micrograms/blister, 15 disks with *Diskhaler®* device = £43.38, 15-disk refill = £42.83. Label: 8, counselling, dose; also 10 and steroid card with high doses
Dose by inhalation of powder, prophylaxis of asthma, 400 micrograms twice daily, adjusted as necessary to 800 micrograms twice daily; CHILD 5–12 years 100–200 micrograms twice daily, adjusted as necessary

**Clenil Modulite®** (Chiesi) ▼ (PoM)
Aerosol inhalation, beclometasone dipropionate 50 micrograms/metered inhalation, net price 200-dose unit = £3.70; 100 micrograms/metered inhalation = £7.42; 200 micrograms/metered inhalation = £16.17; 250 micrograms/metered inhalation = £16.29. Label: 8, counselling, dose; also 10 and steroid card with high doses
Excipients include HFA-134a (a non-CFC propellant)
Dose by aerosol inhalation, 200–400 micrograms twice daily, adjusted as necessary up to 1 mg twice daily; CHILD under 12 years 100–200 micrograms twice daily
Note *Clenil Modulite®* is not interchangeable with other CFC-free beclometasone dipropionate inhalers; the MHRA has advised (August 2006 and July 2008) that CFC-free beclometasone dipropionate inhalers should be prescribed by brand name
Dental prescribing on NHS *Clenil Modulite®* 50 micrograms/metered inhalation may be prescribed

**Qvar®** (IVAX) (PoM)
Aerosol inhalation, beclometasone dipropionate 50 micrograms/metered inhalation, net price 200-dose unit = £7.87; 100 micrograms/metered inhalation, 200-dose unit = £17.21. Label: 8, counselling, dose; also 10 and steroid card with high doses
Excipients include HFA-134a (a non-CFC propellant)
Autohaler® (breath-actuated aerosol inhalation), beclometasone dipropionate 50 micrograms/metered inhalation, net price 200-dose unit = £7.87; 100 micrograms/metered inhalation, 200-dose unit = £17.21. Label: 8, counselling, dose; also 10 and steroid card with high doses
Excipients include HFA-134a (a non-CFC propellant)
Easi-Breathe® (breath-actuated aerosol inhalation), beclometasone dipropionate 50 micrograms/metered inhalation, net price 200-dose = £7.74; 100 micrograms/metered inhalation, 200-dose = £16.95.

Label: 8, counselling, dose; also 10 and steroid card with high doses
Excipients include HFA-134a (a non-CFC propellant)
Dose by aerosol inhalation, prophylaxis of asthma, ADULT and CHILD over 12 years, 50–200 micrograms twice daily, increased if necessary to max. 400 micrograms twice daily
Important When switching a patient with well-controlled asthma from another corticosteroid inhaler, initially a 100-microgram metered dose of *Qvar®* should be prescribed for:

- 200–250 micrograms of beclometasone dipropionate or budesonide

- 100 micrograms of fluticasone propionate

When switching a patient with poorly controlled asthma from another corticosteroid inhaler, initially a 200-microgram metered dose of *Qvar®* should be prescribed for 100 micrograms of beclometasone dipropionate, budesonide, or fluticasone propionate; the dose of *Qvar®* should be adjusted according to response
Note The MHRA has advised (August 2006 and July 2008) that beclometasone dipropionate CFC-free inhalers should be prescribed by brand name

◢**Compound preparations**
**Fostair®** (Chiesi) ▼ (PoM)
Aerosol inhalation, beclometasone dipropionate 100 micrograms, formoterol fumarate 6 micrograms/metered inhalation, net price 120-dose unit = £29.32. Label: 8, counselling, dose, 10, steroid card
Excipients include HFA-134a (a non-CFC propellant)
Dose by aerosol inhalation, asthma, ADULT over 18 years, 1–2 puffs twice daily; max. 4 puffs daily
When switching patients from other beclometasone dipropionate and formoterol fumarate inhalers, *Fostair®* 100/6 can be prescribed for patients already using beclometasone dipropionate 250 micrograms in a CFC-containing inhaler; the dose of *Fostair®* should be adjusted according to response
Note The MHRA has advised (August 2006 and July 2008) that beclometasone dipropionate CFC-free inhalers should be prescribed by brand name

## BUDESONIDE

**Indications** prophylaxis of asthma (see also Management of Chronic Asthma table, p. 151); croup

**Cautions** see notes above

**Side-effects** see notes above

**Dose**
- See preparations below

**Budesonide** (Non-proprietary) (PoM)
Dry powder for inhalation, budesonide 100 micrograms/metered inhalation, net price 200-dose unit = £9.25; 200 micrograms/metered inhalation, 200-dose unit = £18.50; 400 micrograms/metered inhalation, 100-dose unit = £18.50. Label: 8, counselling, dose; also 10 and steroid card with high doses
Brands include *Easyhaler® Budesonide*

Inhalation powder, hard capsule (for use with *Cyclohaler®* device), budesonide 200 micrograms, net price 100-cap pack = £15.48; 400 micrograms, 50-cap pack = £15.48. Label: 8, counselling, dose; also 10 and steroid card with high doses
Brands include *Budesonide Cyclocaps®*
Dose by inhalation of powder, ADULT and CHILD over 12 years, 100–800 micrograms twice daily, adjusted as necessary; alternatively, in mild to moderate asthma, for patients previously stabilised on a twice daily dose, 200–400 micrograms (max. 800 micrograms) as a single dose in the evening; CHILD 6–12 years 100–400 micrograms twice daily, adjusted as necessary; alternatively, in mild to moderate asthma, for patients previously stabilised on a twice daily dose, 200–400 micrograms as a single dose in the evening

**3**

**Respiratory system**

**Novolizer®** (Viatris) ▼ PoM

Dry powder for inhalation, budesonide 200 micrograms, net price refillable inhaler device and 100-dose cartridge = £14.86; 100-dose refill cartridge = £9.59. Label: 8, counselling, dose; also 10 and steroid card with high doses

Dose by inhalation of powder, ADULT and CHILD over 12 years, 200–800 micrograms twice daily, adjusted as necessary; alternatively, in mild to moderate asthma, for patients previously stabilised on a twice daily dose, 200–400 micrograms (max. 800 micrograms) as a single dose in the evening; CHILD 6–12 years 200–400 micrograms twice daily, adjusted as necessary; alternatively, in mild to moderate asthma, for patients previously stabilised on a twice daily dose, 200–400 micrograms as a single dose in the evening

**Pulmicort®** (AstraZeneca) PoM

Aerosol inhalation ▼, budesonide 100 micrograms/metered inhalation, net price 120-dose unit = £9.60; 200 micrograms/metered inhalation, 120-dose unit = £13.20. Label: 8, counselling, dose, change to CFC-free inhaler; also 10 and steroid card with high doses
Excipients include HFA–134a (a non-CFC propellant)

Dose by aerosol inhalation, ADULT and CHILD over 12 years, 100–400 micrograms twice daily, adjusted as necessary; max. 800 micrograms daily; CHILD 2–12 years, 100–400 micrograms twice daily adjusted as necessary

Turbohaler® (= dry powder inhaler), budesonide 100 micrograms/metered inhalation, net price 200-dose unit = £18.50; 200 micrograms/metered inhalation, 100-dose unit = £18.50; 400 micrograms/metered inhalation, 50-dose unit = £18.50. Label: 8, counselling, dose; also 10 and steroid card with high doses

Dose by inhalation of powder, ADULT and CHILD over 12 years, 100–800 micrograms twice daily, adjusted as necessary; alternatively, in mild to moderate asthma, for patients previously stabilised on a twice daily dose, 200–400 micrograms (max. 800 micrograms) as a single dose in the evening; CHILD 5–12 years 100–400 micrograms twice daily, adjusted as necessary; alternatively, in mild to moderate asthma, for patients previously stabilised on a twice daily dose, 200–400 micrograms as a single dose in the evening

Respules® (= single-dose units for nebulisation), budesonide 250 micrograms/mL, net price 20 × 2-mL (500-microgram) unit = £32.00; 500 micrograms/mL, 20 × 2-mL (1-mg) unit = £44.64. May be diluted with sterile sodium chloride 0.9%. Label: 8, counselling, dose, 10, steroid card

Dose prophylaxis of asthma, by inhalation of nebulised suspension, ADULT and CHILD over 12 years, 1–2 mg twice daily, reduced to 0.5–1 mg twice daily; CHILD 3 months–12 years, 0.5–1 mg twice daily, reduced to 250–500 micrograms twice daily
Croup, by inhalation of nebulised solution, 2 mg as a single dose (or as two 1-mg doses separated by 30 minutes)

◀**Compound preparations**

**Symbicort®** (AstraZeneca) PoM

Symbicort 100/6 Turbohaler® (= dry powder inhaler), budesonide 100 micrograms, formoterol fumarate 6 micrograms/metered inhalation, net price 120-dose unit = £33.00. Label: 8, counselling, dose

Dose by inhalation of powder, asthma maintenance therapy, 1–2 puffs twice daily increased if necessary to max. 4 puffs twice daily, reduced to 1 puff once daily if control maintained; CHILD 6–12 years, 2 puffs twice daily reduced to 1 puff once daily if control maintained; 12–17 years, 1–2 puffs twice daily reduced to 1 puff once daily if control maintained

Asthma, maintenance and reliever therapy, (but see notes above, p. 165) ADULT over 18 years, 2 puffs daily in 1–2 divided doses; for relief of symptoms, 1 puff as needed up to max. 6 puffs at a time; max. 8 puffs daily; up to 12 puffs can be used for a limited time but medical assessment should be considered

Symbicort 200/6 Turbohaler® (= dry powder inhaler), budesonide 200 micrograms, formoterol fumarate 6 micrograms/metered inhalation, net price 120-dose unit = £38.00. Label: 8, counselling, dose; also 10 and steroid card with high doses

Dose by inhalation of powder, asthma maintenance therapy, 1–2 puffs twice daily increased if necessary to max. 4 puffs twice daily, reduced to 1 puff once daily if control maintained; CHILD 12–17 years 1–2 puffs twice daily reduced to 1 puff once daily if control maintained

Asthma, maintenance and reliever therapy, (but see notes above, p. 165) ADULT over 18 years, 2 puffs daily in 1–2 divided doses, increased if necessary to 2 puffs twice daily; for relief of symptoms, 1 puff as needed up to max. 6 puffs at a time; max. 8 puffs daily; up to 12 puffs can be used for a limited time but medical assessment should be considered

Chronic obstructive pulmonary disease, 2 puffs twice daily

Symbicort 400/12 Turbohaler® (= dry powder inhaler), budesonide 400 micrograms, formoterol fumarate 12 micrograms/metered inhalation, net price 60-dose unit = £38.00. Label: 8, counselling, dose; also 10 and steroid card with high doses

Dose by inhalation of powder, asthma maintenance therapy, 1 puff twice daily increased if necessary to max. 2 puffs twice daily, reduced to 1 puff once daily if control maintained; CHILD 12–17 years 1 puff twice daily reduced to 1 puff once daily if control maintained

Chronic obstructive pulmonary disease, 1 puff twice daily

## CICLESONIDE

**Indications** prophylaxis of asthma

**Cautions** see notes above

**Side-effects** see notes above

**Dose**

● By aerosol inhalation, ADULT and CHILD over 12 years, 160 micrograms daily as a single dose reduced to 80 micrograms daily if control maintained

**Alvesco®** (Nycomed) ▼ PoM

Aerosol inhalation, ciclesonide 80 micrograms/metered inhalation, net price 120-dose unit = £28.56; 160 micrograms/metered inhalation, 60-dose unit = £16.80, 120-dose unit = £33.60. Label: 8, counselling, dose
Excipients include HFA-134a (a non-CFC propellant)

## FLUTICASONE PROPIONATE

**Indications** prophylaxis of asthma (see also Management of Chronic Asthma table, p. 151)

**Cautions** see notes above

**Side-effects** see notes above; also *very rarely* dyspepsia, hyperglycaemia, and arthralgia

**Dose**

● See preparations below

**Flixotide®** (A&H) PoM

Accuhaler® (dry powder for inhalation), disk containing 60 blisters of fluticasone propionate 50 micrograms/blister with *Accuhaler®* device, net price = £6.38; 100 micrograms/blister with *Accuhaler®* device = £8.93; 250 micrograms/blister with *Accuhaler®* device = £21.26; 500 micrograms/blister with *Accuhaler®* device = £36.14. Label: 8, counselling, dose; also label 10 and steroid card with high doses
Note *Flixotide Accuhaler®* 250 micrograms and 500 micrograms are not indicated for children

Dose by inhalation of powder, prophylaxis of asthma, ADULT and CHILD over 16 years, 100–500 micrograms twice daily, increased according to severity of asthma (max. 1 mg twice daily); CHILD 5–16 years, 50–100 micrograms twice daily adjusted as necessary; max. 200 micrograms twice daily

Diskhaler® (dry powder for inhalation), fluticasone propionate 100 micrograms/blister, net price 15 disks of 4 blisters with Diskhaler® device = £12.71, 15-disk refill = £12.18; 250 micrograms/blister, 15 disks of 4 blisters with Diskhaler® device = £24.11, 15-disk refill = £23.58; 500 micrograms/blister, 15 disks of 4 blisters with Diskhaler® device = £40.05, 15-disk refill = £39.52. Label: 8, counselling, dose; also label 10 and steroid card with high doses

Note Flixotide Diskhaler® 250 micrograms and 500 micrograms are not indicated for children

Dose by inhalation of powder, prophylaxis of asthma, ADULT and CHILD over 16 years, 100–500 micrograms twice daily, increased according to severity of asthma (max. 1 mg twice daily); CHILD 5–16 years, 100–200 micrograms twice daily

Evohaler® aerosol inhalation, fluticasone propionate 50 micrograms/metered inhalation, net price 120-dose unit = £5.44; 125 micrograms/metered inhalation, 120-dose unit = £21.26; 250 micrograms/metered inhalation, 120-dose unit = £36.14. Label: 8, counselling, dose, change to CFC-free inhaler; also label 10 and steroid card with high doses

Excipients include HFA-134a (a non-CFC propellant)

Note Flixotide Evohaler® 125 micrograms and 250 micrograms not indicated for children

Dose by aerosol inhalation, prophylaxis of asthma, ADULT and CHILD over 16 years, 100–500 micrograms twice daily, increased according to severity of asthma (max. 1 mg twice daily); CHILD 4–16 years, 50–100 micrograms twice daily adjusted as necessary; max. 200 micrograms twice daily

Nebules® (= single-dose units for nebulisation), fluticasone propionate 250 micrograms/mL, net price 10 × 2-mL (500-microgram) unit = £9.34; 1 mg/mL, 10 × 2-mL (2-mg) unit = £37.35. May be diluted with sterile sodium chloride 0.9%. Label: 8, counselling, dose, 10, steroid card

Dose by inhalation of nebulised suspension, prophylaxis of asthma, ADULT and CHILD over 16 years, 0.5–2 mg twice daily; CHILD 4–16 years, 1 mg twice daily

◢Compound preparations
**Seretide®** (A&H) [PoM]

Seretide 100 Accuhaler® (dry powder for inhalation), disk containing 60 blisters of fluticasone propionate 100 micrograms, salmeterol (as xinafoate) 50 micrograms/blister with Accuhaler® device, net price = £31.19. Label: 8, counselling, dose

Dose by inhalation of powder, prophylaxis of asthma, ADULT and CHILD over 5 years, 1 blister twice daily, reduced to 1 blister once daily if control maintained

Seretide 250 Accuhaler® (dry powder for inhalation), disk containing 60 blisters of fluticasone propionate 250 micrograms, salmeterol (as xinafoate) 50 micrograms/blister with Accuhaler® device, net price = £35.00. Label: 8, counselling, dose, 10, steroid card

Dose by inhalation of powder, prophylaxis of asthma, ADULT and CHILD over 12 years, 1 blister twice daily

Seretide 500 Accuhaler® (dry powder for inhalation), disk containing 60 blisters of fluticasone propionate 500 micrograms, salmeterol (as xinafoate) 50 micrograms/blister with Accuhaler® device, net price = £40.92. Label: 8, counselling, dose, 10, steroid card

Dose by inhalation of powder, prophylaxis of asthma, ADULT and CHILD over 12 years, 1 blister twice daily
Chronic obstructive pulmonary disease, ADULT 1 blister twice daily

Note The Scottish Medicines Consortium has advised (February 2008) that Seretide 500 Accuhaler® is not recommended for use within NHS Scotland for chronic obstructive pulmonary disease in patients with a forced expiratory volume in 1 second (FEV₁) less

than 60% and greater than 50% of the predicted normal value, with significant symptoms despite regular bronchodilator therapy, and a history of repeated exacerbations

Seretide 50 Evohaler® (aerosol inhalation), fluticasone propionate 50 micrograms, salmeterol (as xinafoate) 25 micrograms/metered inhalation, net price 120-dose unit = £18.00. Label: 8, counselling, dose, change to CFC-free inhaler

Excipients include HFA-134a (a non-CFC propellant)

Dose by aerosol inhalation, prophylaxis of asthma, ADULT and CHILD over 5 years, 2 puffs twice daily, reduced to 2 puffs once daily if control maintained

Seretide 125 Evohaler® (aerosol inhalation), fluticasone propionate 125 micrograms, salmeterol (as xinafoate) 25 micrograms/metered inhalation, net price 120-dose unit = £35.00. Label: 8, counselling, dose, change to CFC-free inhaler, 10, steroid card

Excipients include HFA-134a (a non-CFC propellant)

Dose by aerosol inhalation, prophylaxis of asthma, ADULT and CHILD over 12 years, 2 puffs twice daily

Seretide 250 Evohaler® (aerosol inhalation), fluticasone propionate 250 micrograms, salmeterol (as xinafoate) 25 micrograms/metered inhalation, net price 120-dose unit = £59.48. Label: 8, counselling, dose, change to CFC-free inhaler, 10, steroid card

Excipients include HFA-134a (a non-CFC propellant)

Dose by aerosol inhalation, prophylaxis of asthma, ADULT and CHILD over 12 years, 2 puffs twice daily

## ▌ MOMETASONE FUROATE

**Indications** prophylaxis of asthma (see also Management of Chronic Asthma table, p. 151)

**Cautions** see notes above

**Side-effects** see notes above; also pharyngitis, headache; less commonly palpitation

**Dose**

• By inhalation of powder, 200–400 micrograms as a single dose in the evening or in 2 divided doses; dose increased to 400 micrograms twice daily if necessary; CHILD not recommended

**Asmanex®** (Schering-Plough) ▼ [PoM]
Twisthaler (= dry powder inhaler), mometasone furoate 200 micrograms/metered inhalation, net price 30-dose unit = £15.70, 60-dose unit = £23.54; 400 micrograms/metered inhalation, 30-dose unit = £21.78, 60-dose unit = £36.05. Label: 8, counselling, dose, 10, steroid card

Note The Scottish Medicines Consortium has advised (November 2003) that Asmanex® is restricted for use following failure of first-line inhaled corticosteroids

## 3.3 Cromoglicate and related therapy and leukotriene receptor antagonists

3.3.1 Cromoglicate and related therapy
3.3.2 Leukotriene receptor antagonists

## 3.3.1 Cromoglicate and related therapy

The mode of action of **sodium cromoglicate** and **nedocromil** is not completely understood. They may be of value in asthma with an allergic basis, but, in practice, it is difficult to predict who will benefit; they could probably be given for 4 to 6 weeks to assess response. Dose frequency is adjusted according to response but is usually 3 to 4 times a day initially; this may subsequently be reduced.

In general, *prophylaxis* with sodium cromoglicate is less effective than prophylaxis with corticosteroid inhalations (see Chronic Asthma table, p. 151). There is evidence of efficacy of nedocromil in children aged 5–12 years. Sodium cromoglicate is of no value in the treatment of acute attacks of asthma.

Sodium cromoglicate can prevent exercise-induced asthma. However, exercise-induced asthma may reflect poor overall control and the patient should be assessed.

If inhalation of sodium cromoglicate causes bronchospasm, a selective beta₂ agonist such as salbutamol or terbutaline should be inhaled a few minutes beforehand.

## SODIUM CROMOGLICATE
### (Sodium Cromoglycate)

**Indications** prophylaxis of asthma (see also Management of Chronic Asthma table, p. 151); food allergy (section 1.5.4); allergic conjunctivitis (section 11.4.2); allergic rhinitis (section 12.2.1)

**Cautions** discontinue if eosinophilic pneumonia occurs

**Side-effects** coughing, transient bronchospasm, and throat irritation; *very rarely* hypersensitivity reactions (including angioedema); rhinitis and headache also reported

**Dose**

- By aerosol inhalation, ADULT and CHILD over 5 years, 10 mg (2 puffs) 4 times daily, increased if necessary to 6–8 times daily; or additional dose may also be taken before exercise; maintenance, 5 mg (1 puff) 4 times daily

**Intal®** (Sanofi-Aventis) PoM
Aerosol inhalation, sodium cromoglicate 5 mg/metered inhalation, net price 112-dose unit = £14.84. Label: 8, counselling, change to CFC-free inhaler
Excipients include HFA-227 (a non-CFC propellant)

## NEDOCROMIL SODIUM

**Indications** prophylaxis of asthma (see also Management of Chronic Asthma table, p. 151)

**Side-effects** see under Sodium Cromoglicate; also headache, nausea, vomiting, dyspepsia and abdominal pain; bitter taste (masked by mint flavour)

**Dose**

- By aerosol inhalation, ADULT and CHILD over 6 years 4 mg (2 puffs) 4 times daily, when control achieved may be possible to reduce to twice daily
Counselling Regular use is necessary

**Tilade CFC-free Inhaler®** (Sanofi-Aventis) ▼ PoM
Aerosol inhalation, mint-flavoured, nedocromil sodium 2 mg/metered inhalation. Net price 112-dose unit = £39.94. Label: 8, counselling, change to CFC-free inhaler
Excipients include HFA-227 (a non-CFC propellant)

## 3.3.2 Leukotriene receptor antagonists

The leukotriene receptor antagonists, **montelukast** and **zafirlukast**, block the effects of cysteinyl leukotrienes in the airways. They are effective in asthma when used alone or with an inhaled corticosteroid (see Chronic Asthma table, p. 151). Montelukast has not been shown to be more effective than a standard dose of inhaled corticosteroid but the two drugs appear to have an additive effect. The leukotriene receptor antagonists may be of benefit in exercise-induced asthma and in those with concomitant rhinitis but they are less effective in those with severe asthma who are also receiving high doses of other drugs.

Churg-Strauss syndrome has occurred very rarely in association with the use of leukotriene receptor antagonists; in many of the reported cases the reaction followed the reduction or withdrawal of oral corticosteroid therapy. The CSM has advised that prescribers should be alert to the development of eosinophilia, vasculitic rash, worsening pulmonary symptoms, cardiac complications, or peripheral neuropathy.

## MONTELUKAST

**Indications** prophylaxis of asthma, see notes above and Chronic Asthma table, p. 151; symptomatic relief of seasonal allergic rhinitis in patients with asthma

**Cautions** pregnancy (see p. 150 and Appendix 4); breast-feeding (see p. 150 and Appendix 5); **interactions**: Appendix 1 (leukotriene receptor antagonists)

**Side-effects** abdominal pain, thirst; hyperkinesia (in young children); headache; *very rarely* Churg-Strauss syndrome (see notes above); dry mouth, diarrhoea, dyspepsia, nausea, vomiting, hepatic disorders, palpitation, oedema, increased bleeding, hypersensitivity reactions (including anaphylaxis and skin reactions), depression, suicidal thoughts and behaviour, tremor, asthenia, dizziness, hallucinations, paraesthesia, hypoaesthesia, sleep disturbances, abnormal dreams, agitation, aggression, seizures, arthralgia, and myalgia, also reported

**Dose**

- Prophylaxis of asthma, ADULT and CHILD over 15 years, 10 mg once daily in the evening; CHILD 6 months–6 years 4 mg once daily in the evening, 6–15 years 5 mg once daily in the evening

- Seasonal allergic rhinitis, ADULT and CHILD over 15 years, 10 mg once daily in the evening

**Singulair®** (MSD) PoM
Chewable tablets, pink, cherry-flavoured, montelukast (as sodium salt) 4 mg, net price 28-tab pack = £25.69; 5 mg, 28-tab pack = £25.69. Label: 23, 24
Excipients include aspartame equivalent to phenylalanine 674 micrograms/4-mg tablet and 842 micrograms/5-mg tablet (section 9.4.1)

Granules, montelukast (as sodium salt) 4 mg, net price 28-sachet pack = £25.69. Counselling, administration
Counselling Granules may be swallowed or mixed with cold food (but not fluid) and taken immediately

Tablets, beige, f/c, montelukast (as sodium salt) 10 mg, net price 28-tab pack = £26.97
**Note** The *Scottish Medicines Consortium* has advised (June 2007) that *Singulair®* chewable tablets and granules are restricted for use as an alternative to low-dose inhaled corticosteroids for children 2–14 years with mild persistent

asthma who have not recently had serious asthma attacks that required oral corticosteroid use and who are not capable of using inhaled corticosteroids; *Singulair*® chewable tablets and granules should be initiated by a specialist in paediatric asthma

### ZAFIRLUKAST

**Indications** prophylaxis of asthma, see notes above and Chronic Asthma table, p. 151

**Cautions** elderly, renal impairment (Appendix 3); pregnancy (see p. 153 and Appendix 4); **interactions:** Appendix 1 (leukotriene receptor antagonists)

*Hepatic disorders* Patients or their carers should be told how to recognise development of liver disorder and advised to seek medical attention if symptoms or signs such as persistent nausea, vomiting, malaise, or jaundice develop

**Contra-indications** hepatic impairment; breast-feeding (see p. 153 and Appendix 5)

**Side-effects** gastro-intestinal disturbances, headache, insomnia, malaise; *rarely* bleeding disorders, hypersensitivity reactions including angioedema and skin reactions, arthralgia, myalgia, hepatitis, hyperbilirubinaemia, thrombocytopenia; *very rarely* Churg-Strauss syndrome (see notes above), agranulocytosis

**Dose**

• ADULT and CHILD over 12 years, 20 mg twice daily

**Accolate**® (AstraZeneca) [PoM]
Tablets, f/c, zafirlukast 20 mg, net price 56-tab pack = £17.75. Label: 23

## 3.4 Antihistamines, hyposensitisation, and allergic emergencies

3.4.1 Antihistamines
3.4.2 Allergen Immunotherapy
3.4.3 Allergic emergencies

## 3.4.1 Antihistamines

All antihistamines are of potential value in the treatment of nasal allergies, particularly seasonal allergic rhinitis (hay fever), and they may be of some value in vasomotor rhinitis. They reduce rhinorrhoea and sneezing but are usually less effective for nasal congestion. Antihistamines are used topically in the eye (section 11.4.2), in the nose (section 12.2.1), and on the skin (section 13.3).

Oral antihistamines are also of some value in preventing urticaria and are used to treat urticarial rashes, pruritus, and insect bites and stings; they are also used in drug allergies. Injections of chlorphenamine (chlorpheniramine) or promethazine are used as an adjunct to adrenaline (epinephrine) in the emergency treatment of anaphylaxis and angioedema (section 3.4.3). For the use of antihistamines (including cinnarizine, cyclizine, and promethazine teoclate) in nausea and vomiting, see section 4.6. Buclizine is included as an anti-emetic in a preparation for migraine (section 4.7.4.1). For reference to the use of antihistamines for occasional insomnia, see section 4.1.1.

All older antihistamines cause sedation but **alimemazine** (trimeprazine) and **promethazine** may be more sedating whereas **chlorphenamine** and **cyclizine** (section 4.6) may be less so. This sedating activity is sometimes used to manage the pruritus associated with some allergies. There is little evidence that any one of the older, 'sedating' antihistamines is superior to another and patients vary widely in their response.

Non-sedating antihistamines such as **cetirizine**, **desloratadine** (an active metabolite of loratadine), **fexofenadine** (an active metabolite of terfenadine), **levocetirizine** (an isomer of cetirizine), **loratadine**, and **mizolastine** cause less sedation and psychomotor impairment than the older antihistamines because they penetrate the blood brain barrier only to a slight extent.

**Cautions and contra-indications** Sedating antihistamines have significant antimuscarinic activity and they should therefore be used with caution in prostatic hypertrophy, urinary retention, susceptibility to angle-closure glaucoma, and pyloroduodenal obstruction. Antihistamines should be used with caution in hepatic disease (Appendix 2). Caution may be required in epilepsy. Children and the elderly are more susceptible to side-effects. Many antihistamines should be avoided in acute porphyria but some are thought to be safe, see section 9.8.2. **Interactions:** Appendix 1 (antihistamines).

**Side-effects** Drowsiness is a significant side-effect with most of the older antihistamines although paradoxical stimulation may occur rarely, especially with high doses or in children and the elderly. Drowsiness may diminish after a few days of treatment and is considerably less of a problem with the newer antihistamines (see also notes above). Side-effects that are more common with the older antihistamines include headache, psychomotor impairment, and antimuscarinic effects such as urinary retention, dry mouth, blurred vision, and gastro-intestinal disturbances.

Other rare side-effects of antihistamines include hypotension, palpitation, arrhythmias, extrapyramidal effects, dizziness, confusion, depression, sleep disturbances, tremor, convulsions, hypersensitivity reactions (including bronchospasm, angioedema, and anaphylaxis, rashes, and photosensitivity reactions), blood disorders, liver dysfunction, and angle-closure glaucoma.

## Non-sedating antihistamines

**Driving** Although drowsiness is rare, nevertheless patients should be advised that it can occur and may affect performance of skilled tasks (e.g. driving); excess alcohol should be avoided.

### CETIRIZINE HYDROCHLORIDE

**Indications** symptomatic relief of allergy such as hay fever, chronic idiopahtic urticaria

**Cautions** see notes above; also renal impairment (Appendix 3)

**Contra-indications** see notes above; also pregnancy (Appendix 4); breast-feeding (Appendix 5)

**Side-effects** see notes above

**3 Respiratory system**

**Dose**

- ADULT and CHILD over 6 years, 10 mg once daily *or* 5 mg twice daily; CHILD 1–2 years see *BNF for Children*, 2–6 years, hay fever, 5 mg once daily *or* 2.5 mg twice daily

**Cetirizine** (Non-proprietary)

Tablets, cetirizine hydrochloride 10 mg, net price 30-tab pack = 97p. Counselling, driving

Dental prescribing on NHS Cetirizine 10 mg tablets may be prescribed

Oral solution, cetirizine hydrochloride 5 mg/5 mL, net price 200 mL = £2.20. Counselling, driving

## DESLORATADINE

Note Desloratadine is a metabolite of loratadine

**Indications** symptomatic relief of allergic rhinitis and urticaria

**Cautions** see notes above; also renal impairment (Appendix 3)

**Contra-indications** see notes above; also hypersensitivity to loratadine; pregnancy (Appendix 4); breast-feeding (Appendix 5)

**Side-effects** see notes above; *rarely* myalgia; *very rarely* hallucinations

**Dose**

- 5 mg once daily; CHILD 1–6 years 1.25 mg once daily, 6–12 years 2.5 mg once daily

**Neoclarityn®** (Schering-Plough) ℞

Tablets, blue, f/c, desloratadine 5 mg, net price 30-tab pack = £6.90. Counselling, driving

Oral solution, desloratadine 2.5 mg/5 mL, net price 100 mL (bubblegum-flavour) = £6.90, 150 mL = £10.35. Counselling, driving

## FEXOFENADINE HYDROCHLORIDE

Note Fexofenadine is a metabolite of terfenadine

**Indications** see under Dose

**Cautions** see notes above; also pregnancy (Appendix 4)

**Contra-indications** see notes above; also breast-feeding (Appendix 5)

**Side-effects** see notes above

**Dose**

- Seasonal allergic rhinitis, 120 mg once daily; CHILD 6–12 years, 30 mg twice daily

- Chronic idiopathic urticaria, ADULT and CHILD over 12 years, 180 mg once daily

**Fexofenadine** (Non-proprietary) ℞

Tablets, f/c, fexofenadine hydrochloride 120 mg, net price 30-tab pack = £6.00; 180 mg, 30-tab pack = £7.60. Label: 5, counselling, driving

**Telfast®** (Aventis Pharma) ℞

Tablets, f/c, peach, fexofenadine hydrochloride 30 mg, net price 60-tab pack = £5.46; 120 mg, 30-tab pack = £5.99; 180 mg, 30-tab pack = £7.58. Label: 5, counselling, driving

## LEVOCETIRIZINE HYDROCHLORIDE

Note Levocetirizine is an isomer of cetirizine

**Indications** symptomatic relief of allergy such as hay fever, urticaria

**Cautions** see notes above; also renal impairment (avoid if eGFR less than 10 mL/minute/1.73 m²; Appendix 3); pregnancy (Appendix 4) and breast-feeding (Appendix 5)

**Contra-indications** see notes above

**Side-effects** see notes above; *very rarely* weight gain

**Dose**

- ADULT and CHILD over 6 years, 5 mg once daily; CHILD 2–6 years 1.25 mg twice daily

**Xyzal®** (UCB Pharma) ℞

Tablets, f/c, levocetirizine hydrochloride 5 mg, net price 30-tab pack = £4.39. Counselling, driving

Oral solution, levocetirizine hydrochloride 2.5 mg/5 mL, net price 200 mL = £6.00. Counselling, driving

## LORATADINE

**Indications** symptomatic relief of allergy such as hay fever, chronic idiopathic urticaria

**Cautions** see notes above

**Contra-indications** see notes above; also pregnancy (Appendix 4) and breast-feeding (Appendix 5)

**Side-effects** see notes above

**Dose**

- ADULT and CHILD over 6 years 10 mg once daily; CHILD 2–6 years 5 mg once daily

**Loratadine** (Non-proprietary)

Tablets, loratadine 10 mg, net price 30-tab pack = £1.28. Counselling, driving

Dental prescribing on NHS Loratadine 10 mg may be prescribed

Syrup, loratadine 5 mg/5 mL, net price 100 mL = £5.16. Counselling, driving

## MIZOLASTINE

**Indications** symptomatic relief of allergy such as hay fever, urticaria

**Cautions** see notes above

**Contra-indications** see notes above; also susceptibility to QT-interval prolongation (including cardiac disease and hypokalaemia); significant hepatic impairment; pregnancy (Appendix 4) and breast-feeding (Appendix 5)

**Side-effects** see notes above; weight gain; anxiety, asthenia; *less commonly* arthralgia and myalgia

**Dose**

- ADULT and CHILD over 12 years, 10 mg once daily

**Mizollen®** (Sanofi-Aventis) ℞

Tablets, m/r, f/c, scored, mizolastine 10 mg, net price 30-tab pack = £5.77. Label: 25, counselling, driving

## Sedating antihistamines

**Driving** Drowsiness may affect performance of skilled tasks (e.g. driving); sedating effects enhanced by alcohol.

### ▌ ALIMEMAZINE TARTRATE
(Trimeprazine tartrate)

**Indications** urticaria and pruritus, premedication

**Cautions** see notes above; pregnancy (Appendix 4); see also section 4.2.1

**Contra-indications** see notes above; also renal impairment; breast-feeding (Appendix 5); see also section 4.2.1

**Side-effects** see notes above; see also section 4.2.1

**Dose**

- Urticaria and pruritus, 10 mg 2–3 times daily, in severe cases up to max. 100 mg daily has been used; ELDERLY 10 mg 1–2 times daily; CHILD under 2 years, see *BNF for Children*, 2–5 years 2.5 mg 3–4 times daily, 5–12 years 5 mg 3–4 times daily
- Premedication, CHILD 2–7 years up to 2 mg/kg 1–2 hours before operation

**Vallergan®** (Sanofi-Aventis) [PoM]

Tablets, blue, f/c, alimemazine tartrate 10 mg, net price 28-tab pack = £4.28. Label: 2

Syrup, straw-coloured, alimemazine tartrate 7.5 mg / 5 mL, net price 100 mL = £4.88. Label: 2

Syrup forte, alimemazine tartrate 30 mg/5 mL, net price 100 mL = £7.55. Label: 2

### ▌ CHLORPHENAMINE MALEATE
(Chlorpheniramine maleate)

**Indications** symptomatic relief of allergy such as hay fever, urticaria; emergency treatment of anaphylactic reactions (section 3.4.3)

**Cautions** see notes above; also pregnancy (Appendix 4) and breast-feeding (Appendix 5)

**Contra-indications** see notes above

**Side-effects** see notes above; also exfoliative dermatitis and tinnitus reported; injections may cause transient hypotension or CNS stimulation and may be irritant

**Dose**

- By mouth, 4 mg every 4–6 hours, max. 24 mg daily; CHILD under 1 year see *BNF for Children*, 1–2 years 1 mg twice daily; 2–6 years 1 mg every 4–6 hours, max. 6 mg daily; 6–12 years 2 mg every 4–6 hours, max. 12 mg daily
- By intramuscular injection *or* by intravenous injection over 1 minute, 10 mg, repeated if required up to 4 times in 24 hours; CHILD under 6 months 250 micrograms/kg (max. 2.5 mg), repeated if required up to 4 times in 24 hours; 6 months–6 years 2.5 mg, repeated if required up to 4 times in 24 hours; 6–12 years 5 mg, repeated if required up to 4 times in 24 hours

**Chlorphenamine** (Non-proprietary)

Tablets, chlorphenamine maleate 4 mg, net price 28 = £1.09. Label: 2

*Dental prescribing on NHS* Chlorphenamine tablets may be prescribed

Oral solution, chlorphenamine maleate 2 mg/5 mL, net price 150 mL = £2.39. Label: 2

*Dental prescribing on NHS* Chlorphenamine oral solution may be prescribed

Injection [PoM][1], chlorphenamine maleate 10 mg/mL, net price 1-mL amp = £1.62

1. [PoM] restriction does not apply where administration is for saving life in emergency

**Piriton®** (GSK Consumer Healthcare)

Tablets, yellow, scored, chlorphenamine maleate 4 mg, net price 28 = £1.62. Label: 2

Syrup, chlorphenamine maleate 2 mg/5 mL, net price 150 mL = £2.39. Label: 2

### ▌ CLEMASTINE

**Indications** symptomatic relief of allergy such as hay fever, urticaria

**Cautions** see notes above; also pregnancy (Appendix 4) and breast-feeding (Appendix 5)

**Contra-indications** see notes above

**Side-effects** see notes above

**Dose**

- 1 mg twice daily, increased up to 6 mg daily if required; INFANT under 1 year not recommended, CHILD 1–3 years 250–500 micrograms twice daily; 3–6 years 500 micrograms twice daily; 6–12 years 0.5– 1 mg twice daily

**Tavegil®** (Novartis Consumer Health)

Tablets, scored, clemastine (as hydrogen fumarate) 1 mg. Net price 60-tab pack = £2.35. Label: 2

### ▌ CYPROHEPTADINE HYDROCHLORIDE

**Indications** symptomatic relief of allergy such as hay fever, urticaria; migraine (section 4.7.4.2)

**Cautions** see notes above; also pregnancy (Appendix 4)

**Contra-indications** see notes above; also breast-feeding (Appendix 5)

**Side-effects** see notes above

**Dose**

- Allergy, usual dose 4 mg 3–4 times daily; usual range 4–20 mg daily, max. 32 mg daily; INFANT under 2 years not recommended, CHILD 2–6 years 2 mg 2–3 times daily, max. 12 mg daily; 7–14 years 4 mg 2–3 times daily, max. 16 mg daily
- Migraine, 4 mg with a further 4 mg after 30 minutes if necessary; maintenance, 4 mg every 4–6 hours

**Periactin®** (MSD)

Tablets, scored, cyproheptadine hydrochloride 4 mg, net price 30-tab pack = 86p. Label: 2

### ▌ HYDROXYZINE HYDROCHLORIDE

**Indications** pruritus; anxiety (short-term)

**Cautions** see notes above

**Contra-indications** see notes above; also pregnancy (Appendix 4) and breast-feeding (Appendix 5)

**Side-effects** see notes above

**Dose**

- Pruritus, initially 25 mg at night increased if necessary to 25 mg 3–4 times daily; CHILD 1–6 years initially 5– 15 mg at night increased if necessary to 50 mg daily in 3–4 divided doses; 6–12 years initially 15–25 mg at night increased if necessary to 50–100 mg daily in 3–4 divided doses; CHILD under 1 year see *BNF for Children*
- Anxiety (but not recommended), 50–100 mg 4 times daily; CHILD not recommended

**3** Respiratory system

**Atarax®** (Alliance) (PoM)
Tablets, both s/c, hydroxyzine hydrochloride 10 mg (orange), net price 84-tab pack = £2.18; 25 mg (green), 28-tab pack = £1.17. Label: 2

**Ucerax®** (UCB Pharma) (PoM)
Tablets(JHS), f/c, scored, hydroxyzine hydrochloride 25 mg, net price 25-tab pack = £1.22. Label: 2
Syrup, hydroxyzine hydrochloride 10 mg/5 mL, net price 200-mL pack = £1.78. Label: 2

### ◼ KETOTIFEN

**Indications** allergic rhinitis
**Cautions** see notes above
**Contra-indications** pregnancy (Appendix 4); breast-feeding (Appendix 5)
**Side-effects** see notes above; also excitation, irritability, nervousness; *less commonly* cystitis; *rarely* weight gain; *very rarely* Stevens-Johnson syndrome
**Dose**
* 1 mg twice daily with food increased if necessary to 2 mg twice daily; initial treatment in readily sedated patients 0.5–1 mg at night; CHILD 3 years and over, 1 mg twice daily

**Zaditen®** (Novartis) (PoM)
Tablets, scored, ketotifen (as hydrogen fumarate) 1 mg, net price 60-tab pack = £10.75. Label: 2, 21
Elixir, ketotifen (as hydrogen fumarate), 1 mg/5 mL, net price 300 mL (strawberry-flavoured) = £12.73. Label: 2, 21

### ◼ PROMETHAZINE HYDROCHLORIDE

**Indications** symptomatic relief of allergy such as hay fever and urticaria; emergency treatment of anaphylactic reactions; sedation (section 4.1.1); nausea and vomiting (section 4.6)
**Cautions** see notes above; severe coronary artery disease; pregnancy (Appendix 4); breast-feeding (Appendix 5)
**Contra-indications** see notes above
**Side-effects** see notes above; also restlessness; intramuscular injection may be painful
**Dose**
* By mouth, 10–20 mg 2–3 times daily; CHILD under 2 years not recommended, 2–5 years 5–15 mg daily in 1–2 divided doses, 5–10 years 10–25 mg daily in 1–2 divided doses
* By deep intramuscular injection, 25–50 mg; max. 100 mg; CHILD 5–10 years 6.25–12.5 mg
* By slow intravenous injection in emergencies, 25–50 mg as a solution containing 2.5 mg/mL in water for injections; max. 100 mg

**Phenergan®** (Sanofi-Aventis)
Tablets, both blue, f/c, promethazine hydrochloride 10 mg, net price 56-tab pack = £2.85; 25 mg, 56-tab pack = £4.34. Label: 2
Dental prescribing on NHS May be prescribed as Promethazine Hydrochloride Tablets 10 mg or 25 mg
Elixir, golden, promethazine hydrochloride 5 mg/ 5 mL, net price 100 mL = £2.67. Label: 2
Dental prescribing on NHS May be prescribed as Promethazine Hydrochloride Oral Solution 5 mg/5 mL

Injection (PoM)[1], promethazine hydrochloride 25 mg/ mL, net price 1-mL amp = 67p
Promethazine hydrochloride injection 25 mg/mL (1-mL and 2-mL ampoules) also available from Antigen
1. (PoM) restriction does not apply where administration is for saving life in emergency

## 3.4.2 Allergen Immunotherapy

Immunotherapy using allergen vaccines containing house dust mite, animal dander (cat or dog), or extracts of grass and tree pollen can reduce symptoms of asthma and allergic rhinoconjunctivitis. A vaccine containing extracts of wasp and bee venom is used to reduce the risk of severe anaphylaxis and systemic reactions in individuals with hypersensitivity to wasp and bee stings. Those requiring immunotherapy must be referred to a hospital specialist for accurate diagnosis, assessment, and treatment.

> In view of concerns about the safety of desensitising vaccines, it is recommended that they are used by specialists and only for the following indications:
> * seasonal allergic hay fever (caused by pollen) that has not responded to anti-allergic drugs;
> * hypersensitivity to wasp and bee venoms.
> Desensitising vaccines should generally be avoided or used with particular care in patients with asthma.

Desensitising vaccines should be avoided in pregnant women, in children under five years old, and in those taking beta-blockers (adrenaline may be ineffective in case of a hypersensitivity reaction), or ACE inhibitors (risk of severe anaphylactoid reactions).

Hypersensitivity reactions to immunotherapy (especially to wasp and bee venom extracts) can be life-threatening; bronchospasm usually develops within 1 hour and anaphylaxis within 30 minutes of injection. Therefore patients need to be monitored for 1 hour after injection. If symptoms or signs of hypersensitivity develop (e.g. rash, urticaria, bronchospasm, faintness), **even when mild**, the patient should be observed until these have **resolved completely**.

For details of the management of anaphylactic shock, see section 3.4.3.

Each set of allergen extracts usually contains vials for the administration of graded amounts of allergen to patients undergoing hyposensitisation. Maintenance sets containing vials at the highest strength are also available. Product literature must be consulted for details of allergens, vial strengths, and administration.

### ◼ BEE AND WASP ALLERGEN EXTRACTS

**Indications** hypersensitivity to wasp or bee venom (see notes above)
**Cautions** see notes above and consult product literature
CSM advice The CSM has advised that facilities for cardiopulmonary resuscitation must be immediately available and patients monitored closely for one hour after each injection
**Contra-indications** see notes above and consult product literature
**Side-effects** consult product literature

**Dose**

- By subcutaneous injection, consult product literature

**Pharmalgen®** (ALK-Abelló) [PoM]

Bee venom extract (*Apis mellifera*) or wasp venom extract (*Vespula* spp.), net price initial treatment set = £59.77 (bee), £73.28 (wasp); maintenance treatment set = £69.54 (bee), £89.45 (wasp)

---

## ▌ GRASS AND TREE POLLEN EXTRACTS

**Indications** treatment of seasonal allergic hay fever due to grass or tree pollen in patients who have failed to respond to anti-allergy drugs (see notes above)

**Cautions** see notes above and consult product literature

CSM advice The CSM has advised that facilities for cardiopulmonary resuscitation must be immediately available and patients monitored closely for one hour after each injection

**Contra-indications** see notes above and consult product literature

**Side-effects** see notes above and consult product literature

**Dose**

- See under preparations, below

**Pollinex®** (Allergy) [PoM]

Grasses and rye or tree pollen extract, net price initial treatment set (3 vials) and extension course treatment (1 vial) = £320.00

Dose By subcutaneous injection, consult product literature

◀Grass pollen extract

**Grazax®** (ALK-Abelló) ▼ [PoM]

Oral lyophilisates (= freeze-dried tablets), grass pollen extract 75 000 units, net price 30-tab pack = £67.50. Counselling, administration

Dose ADULT and CHILD over 5 years, 1 tablet daily; start treatment at least 4 months before start of pollen season and continue for up to 3 years

Counselling Tablets should be placed under the tongue and allowed to disperse

---

## Omalizumab

Omalizumab is a monoclonal antibody that binds to immunoglobulin E (IgE). It is used as additional therapy in individuals with proven IgE-mediated sensitivity to inhaled allergens, whose severe persistent allergic asthma cannot be controlled adequately with high-dose inhaled corticosteroid together with a long-acting beta$_2$ agonist. Omalizumab should be initiated by physicians in specialist centres experienced in the treatment of severe persistent asthma.

Churg-Strauss syndrome has occurred rarely in patients given omalizumab; the reaction is usually associated with the reduction of oral corticosteroid therapy. Churg-Strauss syndrome can present as eosinophilia, vasculitic rash, cardiac complications, worsening pulmonary symptoms, or peripheral neuropathy. Hypersensitivity reactions can also occur immediately following treatment with omalizumab or sometimes more than 24 hours after the first injection.

For details on the management of anaphylactic shock, see section 3.4.3.

---

**NICE guidance**

**Omalizumab for severe persistent allergic asthma (November 2007)**

Omalizumab is recommended as additional therapy for the prophylaxis of severe persistent allergic asthma in adults and children over 12 years, who cannot be controlled adequately with high-dose inhaled corticosteroids and long-acting beta$_2$ agonists in addition to leukotriene receptor antagonists, theophylline, oral corticosteroids, oral beta$_2$ agonists, and smoking cessation where clinically appropriate. The following conditions apply:

- confirmation of IgE-mediated allergy to a perennial allergen by clinical history and allergy skin testing;
- either 2 or more severe exacerbations of asthma requiring hospital admission within the previous year, or 3 or more severe exacerbations of asthma within the previous year, at least one of which required hospital admission, and a further 2 which required treatment or monitoring in excess of the patient's usual regimen, in an accident and emergency unit.

Omalizumab should be initiated and monitored by a physician experienced in both allergy and respiratory medicine in a specialist centre, and discontinued at 16 weeks in patients who have not shown an adequate response to therapy.

---

## ▌ OMALIZUMAB

**Indications** prophylaxis of allergic asthma (see notes above)

**Cautions** autoimmune disease; susceptibility to helminth infection—discontinue if infection does not respond to anthelmintic; hepatic impairment; renal impairment; pregnancy (Appendix 4)

**Contra-indications** breast-feeding (Appendix 5)

**Side-effects** headache; injection-site reactions; *less commonly* nausea, diarrhoea, dyspepsia, flushing, fatigue, dizziness, drowsiness, paraesthesia, weight gain, influenza-like symptoms, photosensitivity, hypersensitivity reactions (including hypotension, bronchospasm, laryngoedema, rash, pruritus, serum sickness, and anaphylaxis); Churg-Strauss syndrome (see notes above), thrombocytopenia, arthralgia, myalgia, and alopecia also reported

**Dose**

- By subcutaneous injection, ADULT and CHILD over 12 years, according to immunoglobulin E concentration and body-weight, consult product literature

**Xolair®** (Novartis) ▼ [PoM]

Injection, powder for reconstitution, omalizumab, net price 150-mg vial = £256.15 (with solvent)

Excipients include sucrose 108 mg/vial

---

## 3.4.3 Allergic emergencies

Adrenaline (epinephrine) provides physiological reversal of the immediate symptoms (such as laryngeal oedema, bronchospasm, and hypotension) associated with hypersensitivity reactions such as *anaphylaxis* and *angioedema*.

# Anaphylaxis

*Anaphylactic shock* requires prompt treatment of *laryngeal oedema, bronchospasm,* and *hypotension.* Atopic individuals are particularly susceptible. Insect stings are a recognised risk (in particular wasp and bee stings). Latex and certain foods, including eggs, fish, cow's milk protein, peanuts, and tree nuts may also precipitate anaphylaxis. Medicinal products particularly associated with anaphylaxis include blood products, vaccines, hyposensitising (allergen) preparations, antibacterials, aspirin and other NSAIDs, heparin, and neuromuscular blocking drugs. In the case of drugs, anaphylaxis is more likely after parenteral administration; resuscitation facilities must always be available for injections associated with special risk. Anaphylactic reactions may also be associated with *additives and excipients* in foods and medicines. Refined arachis (peanut) oil, which may be present in some medicinal products, is unlikely to cause an allergic reaction—nevertheless it is wise to check the full formula of preparations which may contain allergenic fats or oils.

*First-line treatment of anaphylaxis* includes securing the airway, restoration of blood pressure (laying the patient flat and raising the legs, or in the recovery position if unconscious or nauseated and at risk of vomiting) and administration of **adrenaline** (epinephrine) injection. Adrenaline is given **intramuscularly** in a dose of 500 micrograms (0.5 mL adrenaline injection 1 in 1000); a dose of 300 micrograms (0.3 mL adrenaline injection 1 in 1000) may be appropriate for *immediate self-administration.* The dose is repeated if necessary at 5-minute intervals according to blood pressure, pulse, and respiratory function (**important:** possible need for *intravenous route* using *dilute solution,* see below). High-flow **oxygen** administration (section 3.6) and intravenous fluids (section 9.2.2) are also of primary importance. An antihistamine (e.g. **chlorphenamine,** given by slow intravenous injection or intramuscular injection in a dose of 10 mg, see p. 173) is a useful adjunctive treatment, given after adrenaline injection and continued for 24 to 48 hours according to clinical response to prevent relapse. Patients receiving beta-blockers require special consideration (see under Adrenaline, p. 177).

*Continuing respiratory deterioration* requires further treatment with **bronchodilators** including inhaled or intravenous salbutamol (see p. 156), inhaled ipratropium (see p. 159), intravenous aminophylline (see p. 161), or intravenous magnesium sulphate [unlicensed indication] (see under Acute Severe Asthma, p. 153); in addition to oxygen, assisted respiration and possibly emergency tracheotomy may be necessary.

An intravenous corticosteroid e.g. **hydrocortisone** (as sodium succinate) in a dose of 200 mg (section 6.3.2) is of secondary value in the initial management of anaphylactic shock because the onset of action is delayed for several hours, but should be given to prevent further deterioration in severely affected patients and continued for 24 to 48 hours according to clinical response.

When a patient is so ill that there is doubt about the adequacy of the circulation, the initial injection of adrenaline may need to be given as a *dilute solution by the intravenous route*; for details of cautions, dose, and strength, see under Intravenous Adrenaline (Epinephrine), below.

Cardiopulmonary arrest may follow an anaphylactic reaction; resuscitation should be started immediately (see p. 125).

For advice on the management of medical emergencies in dental practice, see p. 21.

Patients who are suspected of having had an anaphylactic reaction should be referred to a specialist for specific allergy diagnosis; avoidance of the allergen is the principal treatment.

## Intramuscular adrenaline (epinephrine)

The *intramuscular route* is the *first choice route* for the administration of adrenaline (epinephrine) in the management of anaphylactic shock. Adrenaline has a rapid onset of action after intramuscular administration and in the shocked patient its absorption from the intramuscular site is faster and more reliable than from the subcutaneous site (the intravenous route should be reserved for extreme emergency when there is doubt about the adequacy of the circulation; for details of cautions, dose and strength see under Intravenous Adrenaline (Epinephrine), below).

Patients with severe allergy should ideally be instructed in the self-administration of adrenaline by intramuscular injection (for details see under Self-administration of Adrenaline (Epinephrine), below).

*Prompt injection* of adrenaline is of paramount importance. The following adrenaline doses are based on the revised recommendations of the Working Group of the Resuscitation Council (UK).

| Dose of intramuscular injection of adrenaline (epinephrine) for anaphylactic shock | | |
|---|---|---|
| Age | Dose | Volume of adrenaline **1 in 1000** (1 mg/mL) |
| Child under 6 years | 150 micrograms | 0.15 mL[1] |
| Child 6–12 years | 300 micrograms | 0.3 mL |
| Adult and child 12–18 years | 500 micrograms | 0.5 mL[2] |
| These doses may be repeated several times if necessary at 5-minute intervals according to blood pressure, pulse, and respiratory function. | | |

1. Use suitable syringe for measuring small volume
2. 300 micrograms (0.3 mL) if child is small or prepubertal

## Intravenous adrenaline (epinephrine)

When the patient is severely ill and there is real doubt about the adequacy of the circulation and absorption after intramuscular injection, adrenaline (epinephrine) can be given by *slow intravenous injection* in a dose of 50 micrograms (0.5 mL of the dilute 1 in 10 000 adrenaline injection) repeated according to response; if multiple doses are required, adrenaline should be given as a **slow** intravenous infusion *stopping when a response has been obtained;* children may respond to as little as 1 microgram/kg (0.01 mL/kg of the dilute 1 in 10 000 adrenaline injection) by **slow** *intravenous injection* over several minutes.

Intravenous adrenaline should be given only by those experienced in its use, in a setting where patients can be carefully monitored; it should only be given to children when intravenous access is already available.

Great vigilance is needed to ensure that the *correct strength* of adrenaline injection is used; anaphylactic shock kits need to make a *very clear distinction* between the 1 in 10 000 strength and the 1 in 1000 strength. It is also important that, where intramuscular injection might still succeed, time should not be wasted seeking intravenous access.

For reference to the use of the intravenous route for *cardiac resuscitation*, see section 2.7.3.

## Self-administration of adrenaline (epinephrine)

Individuals at considerable risk of anaphylaxis need to carry adrenaline (epinephrine) at all times and need to be *instructed in advance* how to inject it. In addition, the packs need to be labelled so that in the case of rapid collapse someone else is able to administer the adrenaline. It is important to ensure that an adequate supply is provided to treat symptoms until medical assistance is available.

Adrenaline for administration by intramuscular injection is available in 'auto-injectors', pre-assembled syringes fitted with a needle suitable to administer for very rapid administration (if necessary by a bystander or a healthcare provider if it is the only preparation available). *Anapen®* and *EpiPen®* consist of a fully assembled syringe and needle delivering a dose of 300 micrograms of adrenaline by *intramuscular injection*; 150 microgram versions (*Anapen® Junior, EpiPen® Jr*) are also available for use in children.

## ADRENALINE/EPINEPHRINE

**Indications** emergency treatment of acute anaphylaxis; angioedema; cardiopulmonary resuscitation (section 2.7.3); priapism [unlicensed indication] (section 7.4.5)

**Cautions** heart disease, hypertension, arrhythmias, cerebrovascular disease, phaeochromocytoma; diabetes mellitus, hyperthyroidism; susceptibility to angle-closure glaucoma; elderly

Interactions Severe anaphylaxis in patients taking non-cardioselective beta-blockers may not respond to adrenaline, calling for intravenous salbutamol (see p. 156); adrenaline can cause severe hypertension and bradycardia in those taking non-cardioselective beta-blockers. Other **interactions**, see Appendix 1 (sympathomimetics).

**Side-effects** nausea, vomiting; tachycardia, arrhythmias, palpitation, cold extremities, hypertension (risk of cerebral haemorrhage); dyspnoea, pulmonary oedema (on excessive dosage or extreme sensitivity); anxiety, tremor, restlessness, headache, weakness, dizziness; hyperglycaemia; urinary retention; sweating; tissue necrosis at injection site and angle-closure glaucoma also reported

### Dose

- Acute anaphylaxis, by intramuscular injection (preferably midpoint in anterolateral thigh) of 1 in 1000 (1 mg/mL) solution, see notes and table above
- Acute anaphylaxis when there is doubt as to the adequacy of the circulation, by slow intravenous injection of 1 in 10 000 (100 micrograms/mL) solution (extreme caution—specialist use only), see notes above

Important Intravenous route should be used with **extreme care** by specialists only, see p. 176

◢**Intramuscular or subcutaneous**

[1]**Adrenaline/Epinephrine 1 in 1000** (Non-proprietary) [PoM]

Injection, adrenaline (as acid tartrate) 1 mg/mL, net price 0.5-mL amp = 49p; 1-mL amp = 52p

[1]**Minijet® Adrenaline 1 in 1000** (UCB Pharma) [PoM]

Injection, adrenaline (as hydrochloride) 1 in 1000 (1 mg/mL), net price 1 mL (with 25 gauge × 0.25 inch needle for subcutaneous injection) = £10.79, 1 mL (with 21 gauge × 1.5 inch needle for intramuscular injection) = £6.36 (both disposable syringes)
Excipients include sulphites

◢**Intravenous**

**Extreme caution**, see notes above

**Adrenaline/Epinephrine 1 in 10 000, Dilute** (Non-proprietary) [PoM]

Injection, adrenaline (as acid tartrate) 100 micrograms/mL, 10-mL amp, 1-mL and 10-mL prefilled syringe

**Minijet® Adrenaline 1 in 10 000** (UCB Pharma) [PoM]

Injection, adrenaline (as hydrochloride) 1 in 10 000 (100 micrograms/mL), net price 3-mL prefilled syringe = £6.27; 10-mL prefilled syringe = £6.15
Excipients include sulphites

◢**Intramuscular injection for self-administration**

**Anapen®** (Lincoln Medical) [PoM]

[1]Anapen® 0.3 mg solution for injection (delivering a single dose of adrenaline 300 micrograms), adrenaline 1 mg/mL (1 in 1000), net price 1.05-mL auto-injector device = £30.67
Excipients include sulphites
Note 0.75 mL of the solution remains in the auto-injector device after use
Dose by intramuscular injection, ADULT and CHILD over 30 kg, 300 micrograms repeated after 10–15 minutes as necessary

Anapen® Junior 0.15 mg solution for injection (delivering a single dose of adrenaline 150 micrograms), adrenaline 500 micrograms/mL (1 in 2000), net price 1.05-mL auto-injector device = £30.67
Excipients include sulphites
Note 0.75 mL of the solution remains in the auto-injector device after use
Dose by intramuscular injection, CHILD 15–30 kg, 150 micrograms repeated after 10–15 minutes as necessary

**EpiPen®** (ALK-Abelló) [PoM]

[1]EpiPen® Auto-injector 0.3 mg (delivering a single dose of adrenaline 300 micrograms), adrenaline 1 mg/mL (1 in 1000), net price 2-mL auto-injector = £29.15
Excipients include sulphites
Note 1.7 mL of the solution remains in the *Auto-injector* after use
Dose by intramuscular injection, ADULT and CHILD over 30 kg, 300 micrograms repeated after 5–15 minutes as necessary

Epipen® Jr Auto-injector 0.15 mg (delivering a single dose of adrenaline 150 micrograms), adrenaline 500 micrograms/mL (1 in 2000), net price 2-mL auto-injector = £29.18
Excipients include sulphites
Note 1.7 mL of the solution remains in the *Auto-injector* after use
Dose by intramuscular injection, CHILD 15–30 kg, 150 micrograms (but on the basis of a dose of 10 micrograms/kg, 300 micrograms may be more appropriate for some children) repeated after 5–15 minutes as necessary

---

1. [PoM] restriction does not apply to adrenaline injection 1 mg/mL where administration is for saving life in emergency

**3**

**Respiratory system**

## Angioedema

*Angioedema* is dangerous if *laryngeal oedema* is present. In this circumstance **adrenaline (epinephrine)** injection and **oxygen** should be given as described under Anaphylaxis (see p. 176 ); antihistamines and corticosteroids should also be given. Tracheal intubation may be necessary.

**Hereditary angioedema** The administration of **C1-esterase inhibitor**, an endogenous complement blocker derived from human plasma, (in fresh frozen plasma or in partially purified form) can terminate acute attacks of *hereditary angioedema*, but is not practical for long-term prophylaxis. **Icatibant** is licensed for the treatment of acute attacks of hereditary angioedema in adults with C1-esterase inhibitor deficiency.

**Tranexamic acid** (section 2.11) and **danazol** (section 6.7.2) [unlicensed indication] are used for short-term and long-term prophylaxis of hereditary angioedema. Short-term prophylaxis is started several days before planned procedures (e.g. dental work) and continued for 2–5 days afterwards. Danazol should be avoided in children because of its androgenic effects.

### C1-ESTERASE INHIBITOR

**Indications** acute attacks of hereditary angioedema

**Cautions** pregnancy (Appendix 4); breast-feeding (Appendix 5)

**Side-effects** *rarely* injection-site reactions, hypersensitivity reactions (including anaphylaxis)

**Dose**

- By slow intravenous injection or intravenous infusion, ADULT and CHILD 20 units/kg

**Berinert®** (CSL Behring) ▼ PoM
Injection, powder for reconstitution C1-esterase inhibitor, net price 500-unit vial = £550.00
Electrolytes Na⁺ 2.1 mmol/10 mL vial

### ICATIBANT

**Indications** acute attacks of hereditary angioedema in patients with C1-esterase inhibitor deficiency

**Cautions** ischaemic heart disease, stroke; pregnancy (Appendix 4); breast-feeding (Appendix 5)

**Side-effects** nausea, abdominal pain; nasal congestion; headache, dizziness; asthenia; rash, injection-site reactions; *less commonly* vomiting, weight gain, cough, asthma, fatigue, pyrexia, pharyngitis, flushing, and pruritus

**Dose**

- By subcutaneous injection, ADULT over 18 years, 30 mg as a single dose, repeated after 6 hours if necessary; a third dose may be given after a further 6 hours (max. 3 doses in 24 hours)

**Firazyr®** (Jerini) ▼ PoM
Injection, icatibant (as acetate) 10 mg/mL, net price 3-mL prefilled syringe = £1395.00

## 3.5 Respiratory stimulants and pulmonary surfactants

### 3.5.1 Respiratory stimulants
### 3.5.2 Pulmonary surfactants

## 3.5.1 Respiratory stimulants

Respiratory stimulants (analeptic drugs) have a limited place in the treatment of ventilatory failure in patients with chronic obstructive pulmonary disease. They are effective only when given by intravenous injection or infusion and have a short duration of action. Their use has largely been replaced by ventilatory support including nasal intermittent positive pressure ventilation. However, occasionally when ventilatory support is contra-indicated and in patients with hypercapnic respiratory failure who are becoming drowsy or comatose, respiratory stimulants in the short term may arouse patients sufficiently to co-operate and clear their secretions.

Respiratory stimulants can also be harmful in respiratory failure since they stimulate non-respiratory as well as respiratory muscles. They should only be given under **expert supervision** in hospital and must be combined with active physiotherapy. There is at present no oral respiratory stimulant available for long-term use in chronic respiratory failure.

**Doxapram** is given by continuous intravenous infusion. Frequent arterial blood gas and pH measurements are necessary during treatment to ensure correct dosage.

For the use of **caffeine** in the management of neonatal apnoea, see *BNF for Children*.

### DOXAPRAM HYDROCHLORIDE

**Indications** see under Dose

**Cautions** give with oxygen in severe irreversible airways obstruction or severely decreased lung compliance (because of increased work load of breathing); give with beta₂ agonist in bronchoconstriction; hypertension (avoid if severe), impaired cardiac reserve; hepatic impairment, pregnancy (compelling reasons only); **interactions:** Appendix 1 (doxapram)

**Contra-indications** severe hypertension, status asthmaticus, coronary artery disease, thyrotoxicosis, epilepsy, physical obstruction of respiratory tract

**Side-effects** perineal warmth, dizziness, sweating, moderate increase in blood pressure and heart rate; side-effects reported in postoperative period (causal effect not established) include muscle fasciculation, hyperactivity, confusion, hallucinations, cough, dyspnoea, laryngospasm, bronchospasm, sinus tachycardia, bradycardia, extrasystoles, nausea, vomiting and salivation

**Respiratory system**

**3**

**Dose**

- Postoperative respiratory depression, by intravenous injection over at least 30 seconds, 1–1.5 mg/kg repeated if necessary after intervals of 1 hour *or* alternatively by intravenous infusion, 2–3 mg/minute adjusted according to response; CHILD not recommended
- Acute respiratory failure, by intravenous infusion, 1.5–4 mg/minute adjusted according to response (given concurrently with oxygen and whenever possible monitor with frequent measurement of blood gas tensions); CHILD not recommended
- Neonatal apnoea, see *BNF for Children*

**Dopram®** (Anpharm) PoM
Injection, doxapram hydrochloride 20 mg/mL. Net price 5-mL amp = £3.00

Intravenous infusion, doxapram hydrochloride 2 mg/mL in glucose 5%. Net price 500-mL bottle = £21.33

## 3.5.2 Pulmonary surfactants

Pulmonary surfactants are used in the management of respiratory distress syndrome (hyaline membrane disease) in neonates and preterm neonates. They may also be given prophylactically to those considered at risk of developing the syndrome.

**Cautions** Continuous monitoring is required to avoid hyperoxaemia caused by rapid improvement in arterial oxygen concentration.

**Side-effects** Pulmonary haemorrhage has been rarely associated with pulmonary surfactants, especially in more preterm neonates; obstruction of the endotracheal tube by mucous secretions has also been reported.

### BERACTANT

**Indications** treatment of respiratory distress syndrome in preterm neonates over 700 g; prophylaxis of respiratory distress syndrome in preterm neonates less than 32 weeks post-menstrual age

**Cautions** see notes above

**Side-effects** see notes above

**Dose**

- By endotracheal tube, phospholipid 100 mg/kg equivalent to a volume of 4 mL/kg, preferably within 8 hours of birth; may be repeated within 48 hours at intervals of at least 6 hours for up to 4 doses

**Survanta®** (Abbott) PoM
Suspension, beractant (bovine lung extract) providing phospholipid 25 mg/mL, with lipids and proteins, net price 8-mL vial = £306.43

### PORACTANT ALFA

**Indications** treatment of respiratory distress syndrome or hyaline membrane disease in neonates over 700 g; prophylaxis of respiratory distress syndrome in preterm neonates

**Cautions** see notes above

**Side-effects** see notes above

**Dose**

- By endotracheal tube, treatment, 100–200 mg/kg; further doses of 100 mg/kg may be repeated 12 hours later and after further 12 hours if still intubated; max. total dose 300–400 mg/kg; prophylaxis, 100–200 mg/kg soon after birth (preferably within 15 minutes); further doses of 100 mg/kg may be repeated 6–12 hours later and after further 12 hours if still intubated; max. total dose 300–400 mg/kg

**Curosurf®** (Chiesi) PoM
Suspension, poractant alfa (porcine lung phospholipid fraction) 80 mg/mL, net price 1.5-mL vial = £298.74; 3-mL vial = £580.64

## 3.6 Oxygen

Oxygen should be regarded as a drug. It is prescribed for hypoxaemic patients to increase alveolar oxygen tension and decrease the work of breathing. The concentration of oxygen required depends on the condition being treated; the administration of an inappropriate concentration of oxygen can have serious or even fatal consequences.

Oxygen is probably the most common drug used in medical emergencies. It should be prescribed initially to achieve a normal or near–normal oxygen saturation; in most acutely ill patients with a normal or low arterial carbon dioxide ($P_a CO_2$), oxygen saturation should be 94–98% oxygen saturation. However, in some clinical situations such as cardiac arrest and carbon monoxide poisoning (see also Emergency Treatment of Poisoning, p. 35) it is more appropriate to aim for the highest possible oxygen saturation until the patient is stable. A lower target of 88–92% oxygen saturation is indicated for patients at risk of hypercapnic respiratory failure, see below.

*High concentration oxygen therapy*, with concentrations of up to 60%, is safe in uncomplicated cases of conditions such as pneumonia, pulmonary thromboembolism, pulmonary fibrosis, shock, severe trauma, sepsis, or anaphylaxis. In such conditions low arterial oxygen ($P_a O_2$) is usually associated with low or normal arterial carbon dioxide ($P_a CO_2$), and therefore there is little risk of hypoventilation and carbon dioxide retention.

In acute severe asthma, the arterial carbon dioxide ($P_a CO_2$) is usually subnormal but as asthma deteriorates it may rise steeply (particularly in children). These patients usually require high concentrations of oxygen and if the arterial carbon dioxide ($P_a CO_2$) remains high despite other treatment, intermittent positive-pressure ventilation needs to be considered urgently. Where facilities for blood gas measurement are not immediately available, for example while transferring the patient to hospital, 40–60% oxygen delivered through a high-flow mask is recommended.

*Low concentration oxygen therapy* (controlled oxygen therapy) is reserved for patients at risk of hypercapnic respiratory failure, which is more likely in those with:

- chronic obstructive pulmonary disease;
- cystic fibrosis;
- non-cystic fibrosis bronchiectasis;

**3**

**Respiratory system**

- severe kyphoscoliosis or severe ankylosing spondylitis;
- severe lung scarring caused by tuberculsosis;
- musculoskeletal disorders with respiratory weakness, especially if on home ventilation;
- an overdose of opioids, benzodiazepines, or other drugs causing respiratory depression.

Treatment should be initiated in hospital because repeated blood gas measurements are required to determine the correct concentration. Until blood gases can be measured, initial oxygen should be given using a controlled concentration of 28% or less, titrated towards a target oxygen saturation of 88–92%. The aim is to provide the patient with enough oxygen to achieve an acceptable arterial oxygen tension without worsening carbon dioxide retention and respiratory acidosis. Patients may carry an *oxygen alert card*, see section 3.1.

**Domiciliary oxygen**   Oxygen should only be prescribed for use in the home after careful evaluation in hospital by respiratory experts.

Patients should be advised of the risks of continuing to smoke when receiving oxygen therapy, including the risk of fire. Smoking cessation therapy (section 4.10) should be tried before home oxygen prescription.

**Air travel**   Some patients with arterial hypoxaemia require supplementary oxygen for air travel. The patient's requirement should be discussed with the airline before travel.

## Long-term oxygen therapy

*Long-term* administration of oxygen (usually at least 15 hours daily) prolongs survival in some patients with chronic obstructive pulmonary disease.

Assessment for long-term oxygen therapy requires measurement of arterial blood gas tensions. Measurements should be taken on 2 occasions at least 3 weeks apart to demonstrate clinical stability, and not sooner than 4 weeks after an acute exacerbation of the disease. Long-term oxygen therapy should be considered for patients with:

- chronic obstructive pulmonary disease with $P_aO_2 < 7.3$ kPa when breathing air during a period of clinical stability;
- chronic obstructive pulmonary disease with $P_aO_2$ 7.3–8 kPa in the presence of secondary polycythaemia, nocturnal hypoxaemia, peripheral oedema, or evidence of pulmonary hypertension;
- severe chronic asthma with $P_aO_2 < 7.3$ kPa or persistent disabling breathlessness;
- interstitial lung disease with $P_aO_2 < 8$ kPa and in patients with $P_aO_2 > 8$ kPa with disabling dyspnoea;
- cystic fibrosis when $P_aO_2 < 7.3$ kPa *or* if $P_aO_2$ 7.3–8 kPa in the presence of secondary polycythaemia, nocturnal hypoxaemia, pulmonary hypertension, or peripheral oedema;
- pulmonary hypertension, without parenchymal lung involvement when $P_aO_2 < 8$ kPa;
- neuromuscular or skeletal disorders, after specialist assessment;

- obstructive sleep apnoea despite continuous positive airways pressure therapy, after specialist assessment;
- pulmonary malignancy or other terminal disease with disabling dyspnoea;
- heart failure with daytime $P_aO_2 < 7.3$ kPa when breathing air or with nocturnal hypoxaemia;
- paediatric respiratory disease, after specialist assessment.

Increased respiratory depression is seldom a problem in patients with stable respiratory failure treated with low concentrations of oxygen although it may occur during exacerbations; patients and relatives should be warned to call for medical help if drowsiness or confusion occur.

## Short-burst oxygen therapy

Oxygen is occasionally prescribed for short-burst (intermittent) use for episodes of breathlessness not relieved by other treatment in patients with severe chronic obstructive pulmonary disease, interstitial lung disease, heart failure, and in palliative care. It is important, however, that the patient does not rely on oxygen instead of obtaining medical help or taking more specific treatment. Short-burst oxygen therapy can be used to improve exercise capacity and recovery; it should only be continued if there is proven improvement in breathlessness or exercise tolerance.

## Ambulatory oxygen therapy

Ambulatory oxygen is prescribed for patients on long-term oxygen therapy who need to be away from home on a regular basis. Patients who are not on long-term oxygen therapy can be considered for ambulatory oxygen therapy if there is evidence of exercise-induced oxygen desaturation and of improvement in blood oxygen saturation and exercise capacity with oxygen. Ambulatory oxygen therapy is not recommended for patients with heart failure or those who smoke.

## Oxygen therapy equipment

Under the NHS oxygen may be supplied as **oxygen cylinders**. Oxygen flow can be adjusted as the cylinders are equipped with an oxygen flow meter with 'medium' (2 litres/minute) and 'high' (4 litres/minute) settings.

**Oxygen concentrators** are more economical for patients who require oxygen for long periods, and in England and Wales can be ordered on the NHS on a regional tendering basis (see p. 181). A concentrator is recommended for a patient who requires oxygen for more than 8 hours a day (or 21 cylinders per month). Exceptionally, if a higher concentration of oxygen is required the output of 2 oxygen concentrators can be combined using a 'Y' connection.

A nasal cannula is usually preferred for long-term oxygen therapy from an oxygen concentrator. It can, however, produce dermatitis and mucosal drying in sensitive individuals.

Giving oxygen by nasal cannula allows the patient to talk, eat, and drink, but the concentration of oxygen is not controlled; this may not be appropriate for acute respiratory failure. When oxygen is given through a nasal cannula at a rate of 1–2 litres/minute the inspiratory oxygen concentration is usually low, but it varies with ventilation and can be high if the patient is underventilating.

## Arrangements for supplying oxygen

The following oxygen services may be ordered in England and Wales:

- emergency oxygen;
- short-burst (intermittent) oxygen therapy;
- long-term oxygen therapy;
- ambulatory oxygen.

The type of oxygen service (or combination of services) should be ordered on a Home Oxygen Order Form (HOOF); the amount of oxygen required (hours per day) and flow rate should be specified. The supplier will determine the appropriate equipment to be provided. Special needs or preferences should be specified on the HOOF.

The clinician should obtain the patient's consent to pass on the patient's details to the supplier and the fire brigade. The supplier will contact the patient to make arrangements for delivery, installation, and maintenance of the equipment. The supplier will also train the patient to use the equipment.

The clinician should send order forms to the supplier by facsimile (see below); a copy of the HOOF should be sent to the Primary Care Trust or Local Health Board. The supplier will continue to provide the service until a revised order is received, or until notified that the patient no longer requires the home oxygen service.

| | |
|---|---|
| England | BOC Medical |
| Eastern | *to order*: |
| South West | Tel: 0800 136 603 |
| | Fax: 0800 169 9989 |
| | |
| North East | Air Liquide |
| South East London | *to order*: |
| Kent, Surrey and Sussex | Tel: 0500 823 773 |
| South West London | Fax: 0800 781 4610 |
| Thames Valley, Hampshire | |
| and Isle of Wight | |
| | |
| North West | Air Products |
| Yorkshire and Humberside | *to order*: |
| East Midlands | Tel: 0800 373 580 |
| West Midlands | Fax: 0800 214 709 |
| North London | |
| Wales | |

In **Scotland** refer the patient for assessment by a respiratory consultant. If the need for a concentrator is confirmed the consultant will arrange for the provision of a concentrator through the Common Services Agency. In **Northern Ireland** oxygen concentrators and cylinders should be prescribed on form HS21; oxygen concentrators are supplied by a local contractor. In **Scotland** and **Northern Ireland** prescriptions for oxygen cylinders and accessories can be dispensed by pharmacists contracted to provide domiciliary oxygen services.

## 3.7 Mucolytics

Mucolytics are prescribed to facilitate expectoration by reducing sputum viscosity. In some patients with chronic obstructive pulmonary disease and a chronic productive cough, mucolytics can reduce exacerbations; mucolytic therapy should be stopped if there is no benefit after a 4-week trial. Steam inhalation with postural drainage is effective in bronchiectasis and in some cases of chronic bronchitis.

Mucolytics should be used with caution in those with a history of peptic ulceration because they may disrupt the gastric mucosal barrier.

For reference to dornase alfa and hypertonic saline, see below.

### ■ CARBOCISTEINE

**Indications** reduction of sputum viscosity, see notes above

**Cautions** see notes above; pregnancy (Appendix 4)

**Contra-indications** active peptic ulceration

**Side-effects** *rarely* gastro-intestinal bleeding; hypersensitivity reactions (including rash and anaphylaxis) also reported

**Dose**

- Initially 2.25 g daily in divided doses, then 1.5 g daily in divided doses as condition improves; CHILD 2–5 years 62.5–125 mg 4 times daily, 5–12 years 250 mg 3 times daily

**Carbocisteine** (Sanofi-Aventis) ⓅⓄⓂ
Capsules, carbocisteine 375 mg, net price 120-cap pack = £16.03
Brands include *Mucodyne®*

Oral liquid, carbocisteine 125 mg/5 mL, net price 300 mL = £4.39; 250 mg/5 mL, 300 mL = £5.61
Brands include *Mucodyne® Paediatric* 125 mg/5 mL (cherry- and raspberry-flavoured) and *Mucodyne®* 250 mg/5 mL (cinnamon-and rum-flavoured)

### ■ ERDOSTEINE

**Indications** symptomatic treatment of acute exacerbations of chronic bronchitis

**Cautions** see notes above; hepatic impairment (avoid if severe—Appendix 2); renal impairment (Appendix 3); pregnancy (Appendix 4)

**Contra-indications** breast-feeding (Appendix 5)

**Side-effects** *very rarely* nausea, vomiting, diarrhoea, abdominal pain, taste disturbance, headache, rash, and urticaria

**Dose**

- ADULT over 18 years, 300 mg twice daily for up to 10 days

**Erdotin®** (KoGEN) ▼ ⓅⓄⓂ
Capsules, yellow/green, erdosteine 300 mg, net price 20-cap pack = £5.75
Note The *Scottish Medicines Consortium* (October 2007) has advised that erdosteine (*Erdotin®*) is not recommended for the symptomatic treatment of acute exacerbations of chronic bronchitis

**3**

**Respiratory system**

**Respiratory system**

**3**

## MECYSTEINE HYDROCHLORIDE
(Methyl Cysteine Hydrochloride)

**Indications** reduction of sputum viscosity

**Cautions** see notes above

**Contra-indications** pregnancy; breast-feeding

**Dose**

- 200 mg 4 times daily for 2 days, then 200 mg 3 times daily for 6 weeks, then 200 mg twice daily; CHILD 5–12 years 100 mg 3 times daily

**Visclair®** (Ranbaxy)
Tablets, yellow, s/c, e/c, mecysteine hydrochloride 100 mg, net price 100 = £17.65. Label: 5, 22, 25

## Dornase alfa

Dornase alfa is a genetically engineered version of a naturally occurring human enzyme which cleaves extra-cellular deoxyribonucleic acid (DNA). It is used in cystic fibrosis and is administered by inhalation using a jet nebuliser (section 3.1.5).

## DORNASE ALFA
Phosphorylated glycosylated recombinant human deoxyribonuclease 1 (rhDNase)

**Indications** management of cystic fibrosis patients with a forced vital capacity (FVC) of greater than 40% of predicted to improve pulmonary function

**Cautions** pregnancy (Appendix 4); breast-feeding (Appendix 5)

**Side-effects** pharyngitis, voice changes, chest pain; occasionally laryngitis, rashes, urticaria, conjunctivitis

**Dose**

- ADULT and CHILD over 5 years, by inhalation of neb-ulised solution (by jet nebuliser), 2500 units (2.5 mg) once daily (patients over 21 years may benefit from twice daily dosage)

**Pulmozyme®** (Roche) [PoM]
Nebuliser solution, dornase alfa 1000 units (1 mg)/mL. Net price 2.5-mL (2500 units) vial = £16.88
Note For use undiluted with jet nebulisers only; ultrasonic nebu-lisers are unsuitable

## Hypertonic sodium chloride

Nebulised hypertonic sodium chloride solution is used to mobilise lower respiratory tract secretions in mucous consolidation (e.g. cystic fibrosis).

**MucoClear 6%®** (Pari)
Nebuliser solution, sodium chloride 6%, net price 20 × 4 mL = £12.98; 60 × 4 mL = £29.98
Dose by inhalation of nebulised solution, 4 mL twice daily

## 3.8 Aromatic inhalations

Inhalations containing volatile substances such as eucalyptus oil are traditionally used and although the vapour may contain little of the additive it encourages deliberate inspiration of warm moist air which is often comforting in bronchitis; boiling water should not be used owing to the risk of scalding. Inhalations are also used for the relief of nasal obstruction in acute rhinitis or sinusitis. Menthol and eucalyptus inhalation is used to relieve sinusitis affecting the maxillary antrum (section 12.2.2)

**Children** The use of strong aromatic decongestants (applied as rubs or to pillows) is not advised for infants under the age of 3 months. Carers of young infants in whom nasal obstruction with mucus is a problem can readily be taught appropriate techniques of suction aspiration but sodium chloride 0.9% given as nasal drops is preferred.

**Benzoin Tincture, Compound, BP**
(Friars' Balsam)
Tincture, balsamic acids approx. 4.5%. Label: 15
Dose add one teaspoonful to a pint of hot, not boiling, water and inhale the vapour

**Menthol and Eucalyptus Inhalation, BP 1980**
Inhalation, racementhol or levomenthol 2 g, eucalyptus oil 10 mL, light magnesium carbonate 7 g, water to 100 mL
Dose add one teaspoonful to a pint of hot, not boiling, water and inhale the vapour
Dental prescribing on the NHS Menthol and Eucalyptus Inhala-tion BP, 1980 may be prescribed

**Karvol®** (Crookes) [JHS]
Inhalation capsules, levomenthol 35.55 mg, with chlorobutanol, pine oils, terpineol, and thymol, net price 10-cap pack = £2.25; 20-cap pack = £4.06
Inhalation solution, levomenthol 7.9%, with chloro-butanol, pine oils, terpineol, and thymol, net price 12-mL dropper bottle = £1.90
Dose express into handkerchief or add to a pint of hot, not boiling, water the contents of 1 capsule or 6 drops of solution; avoid in infants under 3 months

## 3.9 Cough preparations

**3.9.1** Cough suppressants

**3.9.2** Expectorant and demulcent cough preparations

## 3.9.1 Cough suppressants

Cough may be a symptom of an underlying disorder, such as asthma (section 3.1.1), gastro-oesophageal reflux disease (section 1.1), or rhinitis (section 12.2.1), which should be addressed before prescribing cough suppressants. Cough may be a side-effect of another drug, such as an ACE inhibitor (section 2.5.5.1), or it can be associated with smoking or environmental pollutants. Cough can also have a significant habit component. When there is no identifiable cause, cough suppressants may be useful, for example if sleep is disturbed. They may cause sputum retention and this may be harmful in patients with chronic bronchitis and bronchiectasis.

**Codeine** may be effective but it is constipating and can cause dependence; **dextromethorphan** and **phol-codine** have fewer side-effects.

**Sedating antihistamines** are used as the cough sup-pressant component of many compound cough prepara-tions on sale to the public; all tend to cause drowsiness which may reflect their main mode of action.

**Children** The use of cough suppressants containing codeine or similar opioid analgesics is not generally recommended in children and should be avoided altogether in children under 6 years.

> **MHRA/CHM advice (March 2008 and February 2009) Over-the-counter cough and cold medicines for children**
>
> Children under 6 years should not be given over-the-counter cough and cold medicines containing the following ingredients:
> - brompheniramine, chlorphenamine, diphenhydramine, doxylamine, promethazine, or triprolidine (antihistamines);
> - dextromethorphan or pholcodine (cough suppressants);
> - guaifenesin or ipecacuanha (expectorants);
> - phenylephrine, pseudoephedrine, ephedrine, oxymetazoline, or xylometazoline (decongestants).
>
> Over-the-counter cough and cold medicines can be considered for children aged 6–12 years after basic principles of best care have been tried. Children should not be given more than 1 cough or cold preparation at a time because different brands may contain the same active ingredient; care should be taken to give the correct dose.

### ■ CODEINE PHOSPHATE

**Indications** dry or painful cough; diarrhoea (section 1.4.2); pain (section 4.7.2)

**Cautions** see notes above and section 4.7.2

**Contra-indications** see section 4.7.2

**Side-effects** see section 4.7.2

#### ¹Codeine Linctus, BP [PoM]

Linctus (= oral solution), codeine phosphate 15 mg/ 5 mL. Net price 100 mL = 62p (diabetic, 33p)
Brands include *Galcodine®*

Dose 5–10 mL 3–4 times daily; CHILD (but not generally recommended) 5–12 years, 2.5–5 mL

Note BP directs that when Diabetic Codeine Linctus is prescribed, Codeine Linctus formulated with a vehicle appropriate for administration to diabetics, whether or not labelled 'Diabetic Codeine Linctus', shall be dispensed or supplied

1. Can be sold to the public provided the maximum single dose does not exceed 5 mL

#### Codeine Linctus, Paediatric, BP

Linctus (= oral solution), codeine phosphate 3 mg/ 5 mL. Net price 100 mL = 18p
Brands include *Galcodine® Paediatric* (sugar-free)

Dose CHILD (but not generally recommended) 2–5 years 5 mL 3– 4 times daily

Note BP directs that Paediatric Codeine Linctus may be prepared extemporaneously by diluting Codeine Linctus with a suitable vehicle in accordance with the manufacturer's instructions

◢Other preparations
Tablets, syrup, and injection section 4.7.2

### ■ PHOLCODINE

**Indications** dry or painful cough

**Cautions** see under Codeine Phosphate

**Contra-indications** see under Codeine Phosphate

**Side-effects** see under Codeine Phosphate

#### Pholcodine Linctus, BP

Linctus (= oral solution), pholcodine 5 mg/5 mL in a suitable flavoured vehicle, containing citric acid monohydrate 1%. Net price 100 mL = 43p
Brands include *Pavacol-D®* (sugar-free), *Galenphol®* (sugar-free)

Dose 5–10 mL 3–4 times daily; CHILD (but not generally recommended, see notes above) 6–12 years 2.5–5 mL

#### Pholcodine Linctus, Strong, BP

Linctus (= oral solution), pholcodine 10 mg/5 mL in a suitable flavoured vehicle, containing citric acid monohydrate 2%. Net price 100 mL = 38p

Dose 5 mL 3–4 times daily
Brands include *Galenphol®*

#### Galenphol® (Thornton & Ross)

Paediatric linctus (= oral solution), orange, sugar-free, pholcodine 2 mg/5 mL. Net price 90-mL pack = £1.11

Dose CHILD (but not generally recommended, see notes above) 6–12 years 10 mL 3 times daily

## Palliative care

Diamorphine and methadone have been used to control distressing cough in terminal lung cancer although morphine is now preferred (see p. 17). In other circumstances they are contra-indicated because they induce sputum retention and ventilatory failure as well as causing opioid dependence. Methadone linctus should be avoided because it has a long duration of action and tends to accumulate.

### ■ METHADONE HYDROCHLORIDE

**Indications** cough in terminal disease

**Cautions** see notes in section 4.7.2

**Contra-indications** see notes in section 4.7.2

**Side-effects** see notes in section 4.7.2; longer-acting than morphine therefore effects may be cumulative

**Dose**
- See below

#### Methadone Linctus [CD] ◢

Linctus (= oral solution), methadone hydrochloride 2 mg/5 mL in a suitable vehicle with a tolu flavour. Label: 2

Dose 2.5–5 mL every 4–6 hours, reduced to twice daily on prolonged use

### ■ MORPHINE HYDROCHLORIDE

**Indications** cough in terminal disease (see also Prescribing in Palliative Care p. 17)

**Cautions** see notes in section 4.7.2

**Contra-indications** see notes in section 4.7.2

**Side-effects** see notes in section 4.7.2

**Dose**
- Initially 5 mg every 4 hours

◢Preparation
Section 4.7.2

**3**

**Respiratory system**

## 3.9.2 Expectorant and demulcent cough preparations

**Expectorants** are claimed to promote expulsion of bronchial secretions but there is no evidence that any drug can specifically facilitate expectoration. The assumption that sub-emetic doses of expectorants, such as ammonium chloride, ipecacuanha, and squill promote expectoration is a myth. However, a simple expectorant mixture may serve a useful placebo function and has the advantage of being inexpensive.

**Demulcent cough preparations** contain soothing substances such as syrup or glycerol and some patients believe that such preparations relieve a dry irritating cough. Preparations such as **simple linctus** have the advantage of being harmless and inexpensive; **paediatric simple linctus** is particularly useful in children.

**Compound preparations** are on sale to the public for the treatment of cough and colds but should not be used in children under 6 years; the rationale for some is dubious. Care should be taken to give the correct dose and to not use more than one preparation at a time, see MHRA/CHM advice, p. 183.

**Ammonia and Ipecacuanha Mixture, BP**

Mixture, ammonium bicarbonate 200 mg, liquorice liquid extract 0.5 mL, ipecacuanha tincture 0.3 mL, concentrated camphor water 0.1 mL, concentrated anise water 0.05 mL, double-strength chloroform water 5 mL, water to 10 mL. It should be recently prepared
Dose ADULT and CHILD over 12 years, 10–20 mL up to 4 times daily

**Simple Linctus, BP**

Linctus (= oral solution), citric acid monohydrate 2.5% in a suitable vehicle with an anise flavour. Net price 200 mL = 42p
Dose ADULT and CHILD over 12 years 5 mL 3–4 times daily
A sugar-free version is also available

**Simple Linctus, Paediatric, BP**

Linctus (= oral solution), citric acid monohydrate 0.625% in a suitable vehicle with an anise flavour. Net price 200 mL = 72p
Dose CHILD 1 month–12 years 5–10 mL 3–4 times daily
A sugar-free version is also available

## 3.10 Systemic nasal decongestants

Nasal decongestants for administration by mouth may not be as effective as preparations for local application (section 12.2.2) but they do not give rise to rebound nasal congestion on withdrawal. **Pseudoephedrine** is available over the counter; it has few sympathomimetic effects.

Systemic decongestants should be used with **caution** in diabetes, hypertension, hyperthyroidism, susceptibility to angle-closure glaucoma, prostatic hypertrophy, renal impairment (Appendix 3), pregnancy (Appendix 4), and ischaemic heart disease, and should be **avoided** in patients taking monoamine oxidase inhibitors; **interactions:** Appendix 1 (sympathomimetics).

## PSEUDOEPHEDRINE HYDROCHLORIDE

**Indications** see notes above
**Cautions** see notes above

**Side-effects** tachycardia, anxiety, restlessness, insomnia; *rarely* hallucinations, rash; *very rarely* angle-closure glaucoma; urinary retention also reported

**Dose**

- 60 mg 3–4 times daily; CHILD 6–12 years 30 mg 3–4 times daily

¹**Galpseud®** (Thornton & Ross)
Tablets, pseudoephedrine hydrochloride 60 mg, net price 20 = £1.06

Linctus, orange, sugar-free, pseudoephedrine hydrochloride 30 mg/5 mL, net price 100 mL = 69p

¹**Sudafed®** (Pfizer Consumer)
Tablets, red, f/c, pseudoephedrine hydrochloride 60 mg, net price 24 = £2.12

Elixir, red, pseudoephedrine hydrochloride 30 mg/5 mL, net price 100 mL = £1.55

---

1. Can be sold to the public provided no more than 720 mg of pseudoephedrine salts are supplied, and ephedrine base (or salts) are not supplied at the same time; for details see *Medicines, Ethics and Practice*, No. 33, London, Pharmaceutical Press, 2009 (and subsequent editions as available)

**Respiratory system**

**3**

# 4 Central nervous system

**4.1 Hypnotics and anxiolytics** 185

4.1.1 Hypnotics 186

4.1.2 Anxiolytics 190

4.1.3 Barbiturates 193

**4.2 Drugs used in psychoses and related disorders** 193

4.2.1 Antipsychotic drugs 194

4.2.2 Antipsychotic depot injections 204

4.2.3 Antimanic drugs 206

**4.3 Antidepressant drugs** 208

4.3.1 Tricyclic and related antidepressant drugs 209

4.3.2 Monoamine-oxidase inhibitors 213

4.3.3 Selective serotonin re-uptake inhibitors 215

4.3.4 Other antidepressant drugs 218

**4.4 CNS stimulants and drugs used for attention deficit hyperactivity disorder** 220

**4.5 Drugs used in the treatment of obesity** 223

4.5.1 Anti-obesity drugs acting on the gastro-intestinal tract 223

4.5.2 Centrally acting appetite suppressants 224

**4.6 Drugs used in nausea and vertigo** 225

**4.7 Analgesics** 232

4.7.1 Non-opioid analgesics 233

4.7.2 Opioid analgesics 237

4.7.3 Neuropathic pain 246

4.7.4 Antimigraine drugs 247

4.7.4.1 Treatment of acute migraine 247

4.7.4.2 Prophylaxis of migraine 251

4.7.4.3 Cluster headache 252

**4.8 Antiepileptic drugs** 252

4.8.1 Control of epilepsy 252

4.8.2 Drugs used in status epilepticus 265

4.8.3 Febrile convulsions 268

**4.9 Drugs used in parkinsonism and related disorders** 268

4.9.1 Dopaminergic drugs used in parkinsonism 268

4.9.2 Antimuscarinic drugs used in parkinsonism 276

4.9.3 Drugs used in essential tremor, chorea, tics, and related disorders 277

**4.10 Drugs used in substance dependence** 279

**4.11 Drugs for dementia** 285

## 4.1 Hypnotics and anxiolytics

**4.1.1 Hypnotics**

**4.1.2 Anxiolytics**

**4.1.3 Barbiturates**

Most anxiolytics ('sedatives') will induce sleep when given at night and most hypnotics will sedate when given during the day. Prescribing of these drugs is widespread but dependence (both physical and psychological) and tolerance occurs. This may lead to difficulty in withdrawing the drug after the patient has been taking it regularly for more than a few weeks (see Dependence and Withdrawal, below). Hypnotics and anxiolytics should therefore be reserved for short courses to alleviate acute conditions after causal factors have been established.

Benzodiazepines are the most commonly used anxiolytics and hypnotics; they act at benzodiazepine receptors which are associated with gamma-aminobutyric acid (GABA) receptors. Older drugs such as meprobamate and barbiturates (section 4.1.3) are **not** recommended—they have more side-effects and interactions than benzodiazepines and are much more dangerous in overdosage.

**Paradoxical effects** A paradoxical increase in hostility and aggression may be reported by patients taking benzodiazepines. The effects range from talkativeness and excitement to aggressive and antisocial acts. Adjustment of the dose (up or down) sometimes attenuates the impulses. Increased anxiety and perceptual disorders are other paradoxical effects. Increased hostility and aggression after barbiturates and alcohol usually indicates intoxication.

**Driving** Hypnotics and anxiolytics may impair judgement and increase reaction time, and so affect ability to drive or operate machinery; they increase the effects of alcohol. Moreover the hangover effects of a night dose may impair driving on the following day. See also Drugs and Driving under General Guidance, p. 3.

**Dependence and withdrawal** Withdrawal of a benzodiazepine should be gradual because abrupt withdrawal may produce confusion, toxic psychosis, convulsions, or a condition resembling delirium tremens. Abrupt withdrawal of a barbiturate (section 4.1.3) is even more likely to have serious effects.

4 Central nervous system

The benzodiazepine withdrawal syndrome may develop at any time up to 3 weeks after stopping a long-acting benzodiazepine, but may occur within a day in the case of a short-acting one. It is characterised by insomnia, anxiety, loss of appetite and of body-weight, tremor, perspiration, tinnitus, and perceptual disturbances. Some symptoms may be similar to the original complaint and encourage further prescribing; some symptoms may continue for weeks or months after stopping benzodiazepines.

A benzodiazepine can be withdrawn in steps of about one-eighth (range one-tenth to one-quarter) of the daily dose every fortnight. A suggested withdrawal protocol for patients who have difficulty is as follows:

1. Transfer patient to equivalent daily dose of diazepam[1] preferably taken at night

2. Reduce diazepam dose every 2–3 weeks in steps of 2 or 2.5 mg; if withdrawal symptoms occur, maintain this dose until symptoms improve

3. Reduce dose further, if necessary in smaller steps;[2] it is better to reduce too slowly rather than too quickly

4. Stop completely; time needed for withdrawal can vary from about 4 weeks to a year or more

Counselling may help; beta-blockers should **only** be tried if other measures fail; antidepressants should be used **only** where depression or panic disorder co-exist or emerge; **avoid** antipsychotics (which may aggravate withdrawal symptoms).

> **CSM advice**
> 1. Benzodiazepines are indicated for the short-term relief (two to four weeks only) of anxiety that is severe, disabling, or subjecting the individual to unacceptable distress, occurring alone or in association with insomnia or short-term psychosomatic, organic, or psychotic illness.
> 2. The use of benzodiazepines to treat short-term 'mild' anxiety is inappropriate and unsuitable.
> 3. Benzodiazepines should be used to treat insomnia only when it is severe, disabling, or subjecting the individual to extreme distress.

## 4.1.1 Hypnotics

Before a hypnotic is prescribed the cause of the insomnia should be established and where, possible, underlying factors should be treated. However, it should be noted that some patients have unrealistic sleep expectations, and others understate their alcohol consumption which is often the cause of the insomnia.

1. Approximate equivalent doses, diazepam 5 mg
≡ chlordiazepoxide 15 mg
≡ loprazolam 0.5–1 mg
≡ lorazepam 500 micrograms
≡ lormetazepam 0.5–1 mg
≡ nitrazepam 5 mg
≡ oxazepam 15 mg
≡ temazepam 10 mg
2. Steps may be adjusted according to initial dose and duration of treatment and can range from diazepam 500 micrograms (one-quarter of a 2-mg tablet) to 2.5 mg

*Transient insomnia* may occur in those who normally sleep well and may be due to extraneous factors such as noise, shift work, and jet lag. If a hypnotic is indicated one that is rapidly eliminated should be chosen, and only one or two doses should be given.

*Short-term insomnia* is usually related to an emotional problem or serious medical illness. It may last for a few weeks and may recur; a hypnotic can be useful but should not be given for more than three weeks (preferably only one week). Intermittent use is desirable with omission of some doses. A rapidly eliminated drug is generally appropriate.

*Chronic insomnia* is rarely benefited by hypnotics and is sometimes due to mild dependence caused by injudicious prescribing of hypnotics. Psychiatric disorders such as anxiety, depression, and abuse of drugs and alcohol are common causes. Sleep disturbance is very common in depressive illness and early wakening is often a useful pointer. The underlying psychiatric complaint should be treated, adapting the drug regimen to alleviate insomnia. For example, clomipramine or mirtazapine prescribed for depression will also help to promote sleep if taken at night. Other causes of insomnia include daytime cat-napping and physical causes such as pain, pruritus, and dyspnoea.

Hypnotics should **not** be prescribed indiscriminately and routine prescribing is undesirable. They should be reserved for short courses in the acutely distressed. Tolerance to their effects develops within 3 to 14 days of continuous use and long-term efficacy cannot be assured. A major drawback of long-term use is that withdrawal can cause rebound insomnia and a withdrawal syndrome (section 4.1).

Where prolonged administration is unavoidable hypnotics should be discontinued as soon as feasible and the patient warned that sleep may be disturbed for a few days before normal rhythm is re-established; broken sleep with vivid dreams may persist for several weeks.

**Children** The prescribing of hypnotics to children, except for occasional use such as for night terrors and somnambulism (sleep-walking), is not justified.

**Elderly** Hypnotics should be avoided in the elderly, because the elderly are at greater risk of becoming ataxic and confused and so liable to fall and injure themselves.

**Dental procedures** Some anxious patients may benefit from the use of a hypnotic for 1 to 3 nights before the dental appointment. Hypnotics do not relieve pain, and if pain interferes with sleep an appropriate analgesic should be given. **Diazepam** (section 4.1.2), **nitrazepam** or **temazepam** are used at night for dental patients. Temazepam is preferred when it is important to minimise any residual effect the following day. For information on anxiolytics for dental procedures, see section 15.1.4.1.

## Benzodiazepines

Benzodiazepines used as hypnotics include **nitrazepam** and **flurazepam** which have a prolonged action and may give rise to residual effects on the following day; repeated doses tend to be cumulative.

Loprazolam, lormetazepam, and temazepam act for a shorter time and they have little or no hangover effect. Withdrawal phenomena are more common with the short-acting benzodiazepines.

If insomnia is associated with daytime anxiety then the use of a long-acting benzodiazepine anxiolytic such as diazepam given as a single dose at night may effectively treat both symptoms.

For general guidelines on benzodiazepine prescribing see section 4.1.2 and for benzodiazepine withdrawal see section 4.1.

## NITRAZEPAM

**Indications** insomnia (short-term use; see CSM advice, p. 186)

**Cautions** respiratory disease, muscle weakness and myasthenia gravis, history of drug or alcohol abuse, marked personality disorder, pregnancy (Appendix 4), breast-feeding (Appendix 5); reduce dose in elderly and debilitated, and in hepatic impairment (avoid if severe; Appendix 2) and renal impairment (Appendix 3); avoid prolonged use (and abrupt withdrawal thereafter); acute porphyria (section 9.8.2); **interactions:** Appendix 1 (anxiolytics and hypnotics)
Driving Drowsiness may persist the next day and affect performance of skilled tasks (e.g. driving); effects of alcohol enhanced

**Contra-indications** respiratory depression; marked neuromuscular respiratory weakness including unstable myasthenia gravis; acute pulmonary insufficiency; severe hepatic impairment; sleep apnoea syndrome; not for use alone to treat depression (or anxiety associated with depression) or chronic psychosis

**Side-effects** drowsiness and lightheadedness the next day; confusion and ataxia (especially in the elderly); amnesia may occur; dependence; see also under Diazepam (section 4.1.2); **overdosage:** see Emergency Treatment of Poisoning, p. 32

**Dose**
- 5–10 mg at bedtime; ELDERLY (or debilitated) 2.5–5 mg; CHILD 1 month–2 years (infantile spasms) see *BNF for Children*

**Nitrazepam** (Non-proprietary) PoM
Tablets, nitrazepam 5 mg, net price 28 = 96p. Label: 19
Brands include *Mogadon®* JHS, *Remnos®* JHS
Dental prescribing on NHS Nitrazepam Tablets may be prescribed

Oral suspension, nitrazepam 2.5 mg/5 mL. Net price 150 mL = £5.09. Label: 19
Brands include *Somnite®* JHS

## FLURAZEPAM

**Indications** insomnia (short-term use; see CSM advice, p. 186)

**Cautions** see under Nitrazepam

**Contra-indications** see under Nitrazepam

**Side-effects** see under Nitrazepam

**Dose**
- 15–30 mg at bedtime; ELDERLY (or debilitated) 15 mg; CHILD not recommended

**Dalmane®** (Valeant) PoM JHS
Capsules, flurazepam (as hydrochloride), 15 mg (grey/yellow), net price 30-cap pack = £5.44; 30 mg (black/grey), 30-cap pack = £6.98. Label: 19

## LOPRAZOLAM

**Indications** insomnia (short-term use; see CSM advice, p. 186)

**Cautions** see under Nitrazepam

**Contra-indications** see under Nitrazepam

**Side-effects** see under Nitrazepam; shorter acting

**Dose**
- 1 mg at bedtime, increased to 1.5 or 2 mg if required; ELDERLY (or debilitated) 0.5 or 1 mg; CHILD not recommended

**Loprazolam** (Non-proprietary) PoM
Tablets, loprazolam 1 mg (as mesilate). Net price 28-tab pack = £18.00. Label: 19

## LORMETAZEPAM

**Indications** insomnia (short-term use; see CSM advice, p. 186)

**Cautions** see under Nitrazepam

**Contra-indications** see under Nitrazepam

**Side-effects** see under Nitrazepam; shorter acting

**Dose**
- 0.5–1.5 mg at bedtime; ELDERLY (or debilitated) 500 micrograms; CHILD not recommended

**Lormetazepam** (Non-proprietary) PoM
Tablets, lormetazepam 500 micrograms, net price 30-tab pack = £61.76; 1 mg, 30-tab pack = £68.23. Label: 19

## TEMAZEPAM

**Indications** insomnia (short-term use; see CSM advice, p. 186); see also section 15.1.4.1 for perioperative use

**Cautions** see under Nitrazepam

**Contra-indications** see under Nitrazepam

**Side-effects** see under Nitrazepam; shorter acting

**Dose**
- 10–20 mg at bedtime, exceptional circumstances 30–40 mg; ELDERLY (or debilitated) 10 mg at bedtime, exceptional circumstances 20 mg; CHILD not recommended

**Temazepam** (Non-proprietary) CD
Tablets, temazepam 10 mg, net price 28-tab pack = £4.62; 20 mg, 28-tab pack = £1.60. Label: 19

Oral solution, sugar-free, temazepam 10 mg/5 mL, net price 300 mL = £24.02. Label: 19
Dental prescribing on NHS Temazepam Tablets or Oral Solution may be prescribed

## Zaleplon, zolpidem, and zopiclone

Zaleplon, zolpidem and zopiclone are non-benzodiazepine hypnotics, but they act at the benzodiazepine receptor. Zolpidem and zopiclone have a short duration of action; zaleplon is very short acting. All three drugs are not licensed for long-term use; dependence has been reported in a small number of patients.

**4**

**Central nervous system**

**4 Central nervous system**

## ZALEPLON

**Indications** insomnia (short-term use—up to 2 weeks)

**Cautions** respiratory insufficiency (avoid if severe); muscle weakness and myasthenia gravis, history of drug or alcohol abuse; depression (risk of suicidal ideation); avoid prolonged use (risk of tolerance and withdrawal symptoms); hepatic impairment (avoid if severe; Appendix 2); pregnancy (Appendix 4); breast-feeding (Appendix 5); **interactions:** Appendix 1 (anxiolytics and hypnotics)

**Contra-indications** sleep apnoea syndrome, marked neuromuscular respiratory weakness including unstable myasthenia gravis

**Side-effects** amnesia, paraesthesia, drowsiness; dysmenorrhea; *less commonly* nausea, anorexia, asthenia, incoordination, confusion, impaired concentration, depression, depersonalisation, dizziness, hallucinations, disturbances of smell, hearing, speech, and vision; photosensitivity; paradoxical effects (see p. 185) and sleep-walking also reported

**Dose**

- ADULT over 18 years, 10 mg at bedtime or after going to bed if difficulty falling asleep; ELDERLY 5 mg
  
  Note Patients should be advised not to take a second dose during a single night

**Sonata®** (Meda) PoM

Capsules, zaleplon 5 mg (white/light brown), net price 14-cap pack = £2.46; 10 mg (white), 14-cap pack = £2.86. Label: 2

## ZOLPIDEM TARTRATE

**Indications** insomnia (short-term use—up to 4 weeks)

**Cautions** depression, muscle weakness and myasthenia gravis, history of drug or alcohol abuse, hepatic impairment (avoid if severe; Appendix 2); renal impairment; elderly; avoid prolonged use (and abrupt withdrawal thereafter); **interactions:** Appendix 1 (anxiolytics and hypnotics)

Driving Drowsiness may persist the next day and affect performance of skilled tasks (e.g. driving); effects of alcohol enhanced

**Contra-indications** obstructive sleep apnoea, acute or severe respiratory depression, marked neuromuscular respiratory weakness including unstable myasthenia gravis, severe hepatic impairment, psychotic illness, pregnancy (Appendix 4); breast-feeding (Appendix 5)

**Side-effects** diarrhoea, nausea, vomiting, vertigo, dizziness, headache, drowsiness, asthenia, amnesia; dependence, memory disturbances, nightmares, nocturnal restlessness, depression, confusion, perceptual disturbances or diplopia, tremor, ataxia, falls, skin reactions, changes in libido; paradoxical effects (see p. 185) and sleep-walking also reported

**Dose**

- ADULT over 18 years, 10 mg at bedtime; ELDERLY (or debilitated) 5 mg

**Zolpidem** (Non-proprietary) PoM

Tablets, zolpidem tartrate 5 mg, net price 28-tab pack = £1.63; 10 mg, 28-tab pack = £1.65. Label: 19

**Stilnoct®** (Sanofi-Synthelabo) PoM

Tablets, both f/c, zolpidem tartrate 5 mg, net price 28-tab pack = £2.96; 10 mg, 28-tab pack = £4.31. Label: 19

## ZOPICLONE

**Indications** insomnia (short-term use—up to 4 weeks)

**Cautions** elderly; muscle weakness and myasthenia gravis, history of drug abuse, psychiatric illness; avoid prolonged use (risk of tolerance and withdrawal symptoms); hepatic impairment (avoid if severe; Appendix 2); renal impairment (Appendix 3); pregnancy (Appendix 4); **interactions:** Appendix 1 (anxiolytics and hypnotics)

Driving Drowsiness may persist the next day and affect performance of skilled tasks (e.g. driving); effects of alcohol enhanced

**Contra-indications** marked neuromuscular respiratory weakness including unstable myasthenia gravis, respiratory failure, severe sleep apnoea syndrome; breast-feeding (Appendix 5)

**Side-effects** taste disturbance; *less commonly* nausea, vomiting; dizziness, drowsiness, dry mouth, headache; *rarely* amnesia, confusion, depression, hallucinations, nightmares; *very rarely* light headedness, incoordination; paradoxical effects (see p. 185) and sleep-walking also reported

**Dose**

- ADULT over 18 years, 7.5 mg at bedtime; ELDERLY initially 3.75 mg at bedtime increased if necessary

**Zopiclone** (Non-proprietary) PoM

Tablets, zopiclone 3.75 mg, net price 28-tab pack = £1.56; 7.5 mg, 28-tab pack = £1.54. Label: 19

**Zimovane®** (Rhône-Poulenc Rorer) PoM

Tablets, f/c, zopiclone 3.75 mg (*Zimovane® LS*), net price 28-tab pack = £2.24; 7.5 mg (scored), 28-tab pack = £3.26. Label: 19

## Chloral and derivatives

Chloral hydrate and derivatives were formerly popular hypnotics for children (but the use of hypnotics in children is not usually justified). There is no convincing evidence that they are particularly useful in the elderly and their role as hypnotics is now very limited. Triclofos causes fewer gastro-intestinal disturbances than chloral hydrate.

## CHLORAL HYDRATE

**Indications** insomnia (short-term use)

**Cautions** reduce dose in elderly and debilitated; avoid prolonged use (and abrupt withdrawal thereafter); avoid contact with skin and mucous membranes; hepatic impairment (avoid if severe—Appendix 2); **interactions:** Appendix 1 (anxiolytics and hypnotics)

Driving Drowsiness may persist the next day and affect performance of skilled tasks (e.g. driving); effects of alcohol enhanced

**Contra-indications** severe cardiac disease, gastritis, severe renal impairment; pregnancy; breast-feeding (Appendix 5); acute porphyria (section 9.8.2)

**Side-effects** gastric irritation (nausea and vomiting reported), abdominal distention, flatulence, headache, tolerance, dependence, excitement, delirium (especially on abrupt withdrawal), ketonuria, and rash

**Dose**

- See under preparations below

### Chloral Mixture, BP 2000 (PoM)
(Chloral Oral Solution)

Mixture, chloral hydrate 500 mg/5 mL in a suitable vehicle. Label: 19, 27

Dose 5–20 mL; CHILD 1–12 years 30–50 mg/kg (max. 1 g), taken well diluted with water at bedtime

Available from 'special-order' manufacturers or specialist importing companies, see p. 969

### Chloral Elixir, Paediatric, BP 2000 (PoM)
(Chloral Oral Solution, Paediatric)

Elixir, chloral hydrate 200 mg/5 mL (4%) in a suitable vehicle with a black currant flavour. Label: 1, 27

Dose CHILD 1 month–1 year 30–50 mg/kg, taken well diluted with water at bedtime

Available from 'special-order' manufacturers or specialist importing companies, see p. 969

◄Cloral betaine

**Welldorm®** (Alphashow) (PoM)

Tablets, blue-purple, f/c, cloral betaine 707 mg (≡ chloral hydrate 414 mg). Net price 30-tab pack = £12.10. Label: 19, 27

Dose ADULT and CHILD over 12 years, 1–2 tablets with water or milk at bedtime, max. 5 tablets (chloral hydrate 2 g) daily

Elixir, red, chloral hydrate 143.3 mg/5 mL. Net price 150-mL pack = £8.70. Label: 19, 27

Dose 15–45 mL (chloral hydrate 0.4–1.3 g) with water or milk, at bedtime, max. 70 mL (chloral hydrate 2 g) daily; CHILD 2–12 years, 1–1.75 mL/kg (chloral hydrate 30–50 mg/kg), max. 35 mL (chloral hydrate 1 g) daily

## ■ TRICLOFOS SODIUM

**Indications** insomnia (short-term use)

**Cautions** avoid prolonged use (and abrupt withdrawal thereafter); elderly; hepatic impairment (Appendix 2); renal impairment (Appendix 3); **interactions**: Appendix 1 (anxiolytics and hypnotics)
Driving Drowsiness may persist the next day and affect performance of skilled tasks (e.g. driving); effects of alcohol enhanced

**Contra-indications** cardiac disease; gastritis; acute porphyria (section 9.8.2); pregnancy; breast-feeding (Appendix 5)

**Side-effects** abdominal distension, flatulence, gastric irritation including nausea and vomiting, dependence, malaise, ataxia, drowsiness, headache, lightheadedness, vertigo, confusion, paranoia, excitement, nightmares, delirium (especially on abrupt withdrawal), ketonuria, blood disorders, skin reactions, and urticaria

**Dose**
● See under preparation below

### Triclofos Oral Solution, BP (PoM)
(Triclofos Elixir)

Oral solution, triclofos sodium 500 mg/5 mL. Net price 300 mL = £28.23. Label: 19

Dose 10–20 mL (1–2 g triclofos sodium) at bedtime; CHILD up to 1 year 25–30 mg/kg, 1–5 years 2.5–5 mL (250–500 mg triclofos sodium), 6–12 years 5–10 mL (0.5–1 g triclofos sodium)

## Clomethiazole

**Clomethiazole** (chlormethiazole) may be a useful hypnotic for elderly patients because of its freedom from hangover but, as with all hypnotics, routine administration is undesirable and dependence occurs. It is licensed

for use as a hypnotic only in the elderly (and for *very short-term use* in younger adults to attenuate alcohol withdrawal symptoms, section 4.10).

## ■ CLOMETHIAZOLE
(Chlormethiazole)

**Indications** see under Dose; alcohol withdrawal (section 4.10)

**Cautions** cardiac and respiratory disease (confusional state may indicate hypoxia), chronic pulmonary insufficiency, sleep apnoea syndrome; history of drug abuse; avoid prolonged use (and abrupt withdrawal thereafter); marked personality disorder; elderly; excessive sedation may occur (particularly with higher doses); hepatic impairment (especially if severe because sedation can mask hepatic coma; Appendix 2); renal impairment (Appendix 3); pregnancy (Appendix 4); breast-feeding (Appendix 5); **interactions**: Appendix 1 (anxiolytics and hypnotics)
Driving Drowsiness may persist the next day and affect performance of skilled tasks (e.g. driving); effects of alcohol enhanced

**Contra-indications** acute pulmonary insufficiency; alcohol-dependent patients who continue to drink

**Side-effects** nasal congestion and irritation (increased nasopharyngeal and bronchial secretions), conjunctival irritation, headache; *rarely* gastro-intestinal disturbances, paradoxical excitement, confusion, dependence, rash, urticaria, bullous eruption, anaphylaxis, alterations in liver enzymes

**Dose**
● Severe insomnia in the elderly (short-term use), 1–2 capsules (*or* 5–10 mL syrup) at bedtime; CHILD not recommended
● Restlessness and agitation in the elderly, 1 capsule (*or* 5 mL syrup) 3 times daily
● Alcohol withdrawal, initially 2–4 capsules, if necessary repeated after some hours; day 1 (first 24 hours), 9–12 capsules in 3–4 divided doses; day 2, 6–8 capsules in 3–4 divided doses; day 3, 4–6 capsules in 3–4 divided doses; then gradually reduced over days 4–6; total treatment for not more than 9 days

**Heminevrin®** (AstraZeneca) (PoM)

Capsules, grey-brown, clomethiazole base 192 mg in an oily basis. Net price 60-cap pack = £4.78. Label: 19

Syrup, sugar-free, clomethiazole edisilate 250 mg/5 mL. Net price 300-mL pack = £4.00. Label: 19

Note For an equivalent therapeutic effect 1 capsule ≡ 5 mL syrup

## Antihistamines

Some **antihistamines** (section 3.4.1) such as promethazine are on sale to the public for occasional insomnia; their prolonged duration of action can often cause drowsiness the following day. The sedative effect of antihistamines may diminish after a few days of continued treatment; antihistamines are associated with headache, psychomotor impairment and antimuscarinic effects.

Promethazine is also popular for use in children, but the use of hypnotics in children is not usually justified.

## PROMETHAZINE HYDROCHLORIDE

**Indications** sedation (short-term use); allergy and urticaria (section 3.4.1); nausea and vomiting (section 4.6)
**Cautions** section 3.4.1
**Contra-indications** section 3.4.1
**Side-effects** section 3.4.1
**Dose**
- By mouth, 25–50 mg; CHILD 2–5 years 15–20 mg, 5–10 years 20–25 mg
- By deep intramuscular injection, 25–50 mg; CHILD 5–10 years 6.25–12.5 mg

◢Preparations
Section 3.4.1

## Alcohol

**Alcohol** is a poor hypnotic because the diuretic action interferes with sleep during the latter part of the night. Alcohol also disturbs sleep patterns, and so can worsen sleep disorders; **interactions:** Appendix 1 (alcohol).

## Sodium oxybate

**Sodium oxybate** is a central nervous system depressant that is licensed for the treatment of narcolepsy with cataplexy.

## SODIUM OXYBATE

**Indications** narcolepsy with cataplexy (under specialist supervision)
**Cautions** history of drug abuse or depression; epilepsy; elderly; respiratory disorders; heart failure and hypertension (high sodium content); risk of discontinuation effects including rebound cataplexy and withdrawal symptoms; acute porphyria (section 9.8.2); hepatic impairment (Appendix 2); renal impairment (Appendix 3); breast-feeding (Appendix 5); **interactions:** Appendix 1 (sodium oxybate)
**Contra-indications** pregnancy (Appendix 4)
**Side-effects** nausea, vomiting, diarrhoea, abdominal pain, anorexia; hypertension, peripheral oedema; dyspnoea; sleep disorders, confusion, disorientation, paraesthesia, hypoesthesia, impaired attention, depression, drowsiness, anxiety, dizziness, headache, tremor, asthenia, fatigue; urinary incontinence; nocturnal enuresis; arthralgia, muscle cramps; blurred vision; sweating; *less commonly* faecal incontinence, myoclonus, psychosis, paranoia, hallucination, agitation, amnesia, and rash; respiratory depression, dependence, seizures, suicidal ideation, and urticaria also reported
**Dose**
- ADULT over 18 years, initially 2.25 g on retiring and repeated 2.5–4 hours later, increased according to response in steps of 1.5 g daily in 2 divided doses at intervals of 1–2 weeks; max. 9 g daily in two divided doses
  Note Dose titration should be repeated if restarting after interval of more than 14 days
  Counselling Dilute each dose with 60 mL water; prepare both doses before retiring. Observe the same time interval

(2–3 hours) each night between the last meal and the first dose

**Xyrem®** (UCB Pharma) ▼ PoM
Oral solution, sugar-free, sodium oxybate 500 mg/mL, net price 180 mL = £360.00. Label: 13, 19, counselling, administration
Electrolytes Na⁺ 3.96 mmol/mL

## Melatonin

Melatonin is a pineal hormone; it is licensed for the short-term treatment of insomnia in adults over 55 years.

## MELATONIN

**Indications** insomnia (short-term use)
**Cautions** renal impairment (Appendix 3); **interactions:** Appendix 1 (melatonin)
**Contra-indications** autoimmune disease; hepatic impairment (Appendix 2); pregnancy (Appendix 4); breast-feeding (Appendix 5)
**Side-effects** pharyngitis; back pain, headache, asthenia; *less commonly* abdominal pain, constipation, dry mouth, weight gain, drowsiness, dizziness, sleep disorders, restlessness, nervousness, irritability, and sweating; *rarely* flatulence, halitosis, hypersalivation, vomiting, hypertriglyceridaemia, aggression, agitation, fatigue, impaired memory, mood changes, hot flushes, priapism, increased libido, leucopenia, thrombocytopenia, muscle cramp, skin reaction, lacrimation, and visual disturbances
**Dose**
- ADULT over 55 years, 2 mg once daily 1–2 hours before bedtime for 3 weeks; CHILD 1 month–18 years see *BNF for Children*

**Circadin®** (Lundbeck) ▼ PoM
Tablets, m/r, melatonin 2 mg, net price 21-tab pack = £10.77. Label: 2, 21, 25

## 4.1.2 Anxiolytics

Benzodiazepine anxiolytics can be effective in alleviating anxiety states. Although these drugs are sometimes prescribed for stress-related symptoms, unhappiness, or minor physical disease, their use in such conditions is inappropriate. Benzodiazepine anxiolytics should not be used as sole treatment for chronic anxiety, and they are not appropriate for treating depression or chronic psychosis. In bereavement, psychological adjustment may be inhibited by benzodiazepines. In children, anxiolytic treatment should be used only to relieve acute anxiety (and related insomnia) caused by fear (e.g. before surgery).

Anxiolytic benzodiazepine treatment should be limited to the lowest possible dose for the shortest possible time (see CSM advice, section 4.1). Dependence is particularly likely in patients with a history of alcohol or drug abuse and in patients with marked personality disorders.

Some antidepressants (section 4.3) are licensed for use in anxiety and related disorders; see section 4.3 for a comment on their role in chronic anxiety. Some anti-

*4 Central nervous system*

psychotics, in low doses, are also sometimes used in severe anxiety for their sedative action, but long-term use should be avoided because of the risk of adverse effects (section 4.2.1). The use of antihistamines (e.g. hydroxyzine, section 3.4.1) for their sedative effect in anxiety is not appropriate.

**Beta-blockers** (section 2.4) do not affect psychological symptoms of anxiety, such as worry, tension, and fear, but they do reduce autonomic symptoms, such as palpitation and tremor; they do not reduce non-autonomic symptoms, such as muscle tension. Beta-blockers are therefore indicated for patients with predominantly somatic symptoms; this, in turn, may prevent the onset of worry and fear.

# Benzodiazepines

**Benzodiazepines** are indicated for the *short-term relief of severe anxiety*; long-term use should be avoided (see CSM advice, p. 186). Diazepam, alprazolam, chlordiazepoxide, and clobazam have a sustained action. Shorter-acting compounds such as **lorazepam** and **oxazepam** may be preferred in patients with hepatic impairment but they carry a greater risk of withdrawal symptoms.

In *panic disorders* (with or without agoraphobia) resistant to antidepressant therapy (section 4.3), a benzodiazepine (lorazepam 3–5 mg daily or clonazepam 1–2 mg daily (section 4.8.1) [both unlicensed]) may be used; alternatively, a benzodiazepine may be used as short-term adjunctive therapy at the start of antidepressant treatment to prevent the initial worsening of symptoms.

Diazepam or lorazepam are very occasionally administered intravenously for the *control of panic attacks*. This route is the most rapid but the procedure is not without risk (section 4.8.2) but should be used only when alternative measures have failed. The intramuscular route has no advantage over the oral route.

For guidelines on benzodiazepine withdrawal, see p. 185.

## DIAZEPAM

**Indications** short-term use in anxiety or insomnia (see CSM advice, p. 186); adjunct in acute alcohol withdrawal; status epilepticus (section 4.8.2); febrile convulsions (section 4.8.3); muscle spasm (section 10.2.2); peri-operative use (section 15.1.4.1)

**Cautions** respiratory disease, muscle weakness and myasthenia gravis, history of drug or alcohol abuse, marked personality disorder, pregnancy (Appendix 4), breast-feeding (Appendix 5); reduce dose in elderly and debilitated, and in hepatic impairment (avoid if severe; Appendix 2), renal impairment (Appendix 3); avoid prolonged use (and abrupt withdrawal thereafter); special precautions for intravenous injection (section 4.8.2); acute porphyria (section 9.8.2); when given parenterally, close observation required until full recovery from sedation; **interactions:** Appendix 1 (anxiolytics and hypnotics)

*Driving* Drowsiness may affect performance of skilled tasks (e.g. driving); effects of alcohol enhanced

**Contra-indications** respiratory depression; marked neuromuscular respiratory weakness including unstable myasthenia gravis; acute pulmonary insufficiency; sleep apnoea syndrome; severe hepatic

impairment; not for chronic psychosis; should not be used alone in depression or in anxiety with depression; avoid injections containing benzyl alcohol in neonates (see under preparations below)

**Side-effects** drowsiness and lightheadedness the next day; confusion and ataxia (especially in the elderly); amnesia; dependence; paradoxical increase in aggression (see also section 4.1); muscle weakness; *occasionally:* headache, vertigo, hypotension, salivation changes, gastro-intestinal disturbances, visual disturbances, dysarthria, tremor, changes in libido, incontinence, urinary retention; blood disorders and jaundice reported; skin reactions; on intravenous injection, pain, thrombophlebitis, and rarely apnoea; **overdosage:** see Emergency Treatment of Poisoning, p. 32

**Dose**

- By mouth, anxiety, 2 mg 3 times daily increased if necessary to 15–30 mg daily in divided doses; ELDERLY (or debilitated) half adult dose
  Insomnia associated with anxiety, 5–15 mg at bedtime

- By intramuscular injection *or* slow intravenous injection (into a large vein, at a rate of not more than 5 mg/minute), for severe acute anxiety, control of acute panic attacks, and acute alcohol withdrawal, 10 mg, repeated if necessary after not less than 4 hours
  **Note** Only use intramuscular route when oral and intravenous routes not possible; special precautions for intravenous injection section 4.8.2

- By rectum as rectal solution, acute anxiety and agitation, 500 micrograms/kg repeated after 12 hours as required; ELDERLY 250 micrograms/kg; CHILD not recommended
  As suppositories, anxiety when oral route not appropriate, 10–30 mg (higher dose divided); dose form not appropriate for less than 10 mg

**Diazepam** (Non-proprietary) ▱PoM

Tablets, diazepam 2 mg, net price 28 = 96p; 5 mg, 28 = 99p; 10 mg, 28 = £1.03. Label: 2 or 19
Brands include *Rimapam*® ▱JHS▱ *Tensium*® ▱JHS▱

Oral solution, diazepam 2 mg/5 mL, net price 100 mL = £6.75. Label: 2 or 19
Brands include *Dialar*® ▱JHS▱

Strong oral solution, diazepam 5 mg/5 mL, net price 100-mL pack = £6.38. Label: 2 or 19▱JHS▱
Brands include *Dialar*® ▱JHS▱

Injection (solution), diazepam 5 mg/mL. Do not dilute (except for intravenous infusion, see Appendix 6). Net price 2-mL amp = 45p
Excipients may include benzyl alcohol (avoid in neonates, see Excipients, p. 2), ethanol, propylene glycol

Injection (emulsion), diazepam 5 mg/mL. For intravenous injection or infusion, see Appendix 6. Net price 2-mL amp = 92p
Brands include *Diazemuls*®

Rectal tubes (= rectal solution), diazepam 2 mg/mL, net price 1.25-mL (2.5-mg) tube = 90p, 2.5-mL (5-mg) tube = £1.27; 4 mg/mL, 2.5-mL (10-mg) tube = £1.65. Label: 2 or 19
Brands include *Diazepam Rectubes*®, *Stesolid*®

Suppositories, diazepam 10 mg, net price 6 = £10.20. Label: 2 or 19
Brands include *Valclair*®
**Dental prescribing on NHS** Diazepam Tablets or Diazepam Oral Solution 2 mg/5 mL may be prescribed

## ALPRAZOLAM

**Indications** anxiety (short-term use; see CSM advice, p. 186)

**Cautions** see under Diazepam

**Contra-indications** see under Diazepam

**Side-effects** see under Diazepam

**Dose**

- 250–500 micrograms 3 times daily (ELDERLY or debilitated 250 micrograms 2–3 times daily), increased if necessary to a total of 3 mg daily; CHILD not recommended

**Alprazolam** (Non-proprietary) PoM JHS
Tablets, alprazolam 250 micrograms, net price 60-tab pack = £2.97; 500 micrograms, 60-tab pack = £5.69. Label: 2
Brands include *Xanax®* JHS

## CHLORDIAZEPOXIDE HYDROCHLORIDE

**Indications** anxiety (short-term use; see CSM advice, p. 186); adjunct in acute alcohol withdrawal (section 4.10)

**Cautions** see under Diazepam

**Contra-indications** see under Diazepam

**Side-effects** see under Diazepam

**Dose**

- Anxiety, 10 mg 3 times daily increased if necessary to 60–100 mg daily in divided doses; ELDERLY (or debilitated) half adult dose; CHILD not recommended

**Chlordiazepoxide** (Non-proprietary) PoM
Capsules, chlordiazepoxide hydrochloride 5 mg, net price 100-cap pack = £3.60; 10 mg, 100-cap pack = £10.39. Label: 2
Brands include *Librium®* JHS, *Tropium®* JHS

**Chlordiazepoxide Hydrochloride** (Non-proprietary) PoM
Tablets, chlordiazepoxide hydrochloride 5 mg, net price 100 = £4.24; 10 mg, 100 = £11.34. Label: 2

## LORAZEPAM

**Indications** short-term use in anxiety or insomnia (see CSM advice, p. 186); status epilepticus (section 4.8.2); peri-operative (section 15.1.4.1)

**Cautions** see under Diazepam; short acting; when given parenterally, facilities for managing respiratory depression with mechanical ventilation must be at hand

**Contra-indications** see under Diazepam

**Side-effects** see under Diazepam

**Dose**

- By mouth, anxiety, 1–4 mg daily in divided doses; ELDERLY (or debilitated) half adult dose
  Insomnia associated with anxiety, 1–2 mg at bedtime; CHILD not recommended
- By intramuscular *or* slow intravenous injection (into a large vein), acute panic attacks, 25–30 micrograms/kg (usual range 1.5–2.5 mg), repeated every 6 hours if necessary; CHILD not recommended
  Note Only use intramuscular route when oral and intravenous routes not possible

**Lorazepam** (Non-proprietary) PoM
Tablets, lorazepam 1 mg, net price 28-tab pack = £8.14; 2.5 mg, 28-tab pack = £13.72. Label: 2 or 19
Injection, lorazepam 4 mg/mL. Net price 1-mL amp = 35p
Excipients include benzyl alcohol, propylene glycol (see Excipients, p. 2)
Brands include *Ativan®* JHS
Note For intramuscular injection it should be diluted with an equal volume of water for injections or physiological saline (but only use when oral and intravenous routes not possible)

## OXAZEPAM

**Indications** anxiety (short-term use; see CSM advice, p. 186)

**Cautions** see under Diazepam; short acting

**Contra-indications** see under Diazepam

**Side-effects** see under Diazepam

**Dose**

- Anxiety, 15–30 mg (elderly or debilitated 10–20 mg) 3–4 times daily; CHILD not recommended
- Insomnia associated with anxiety, 15–25 mg (max. 50 mg) at bedtime; CHILD not recommended

**Oxazepam** (Non-proprietary) PoM
Tablets, oxazepam 10 mg, net price 28-tab pack = £6.01; 15 mg, 28-tab pack = £6.29. Label: 2

## Buspirone

**Buspirone** is thought to act at specific serotonin ($5HT_{1A}$) receptors. Response to treatment may take up to 2 weeks. It does not alleviate the symptoms of benzodiazepine withdrawal. Therefore a patient taking a benzodiazepine still needs to have the benzodiazepine withdrawn gradually; it is advisable to do this before starting buspirone. The dependence and abuse potential of buspirone is low; it is, however, licensed for short-term use only (but specialists occasionally use it for several months).

## BUSPIRONE HYDROCHLORIDE

**Indications** anxiety (short-term use)

**Cautions** does not alleviate benzodiazepine withdrawal (see notes above); hepatic impairment (Appendix 2); renal impairment (avoid if eGFR less than 20 mL/minute/1.73 m²; Appendix 3); **interactions**: Appendix 1 (anxiolytics and hypnotics)
Driving May affect performance of skilled tasks (e.g. driving); effects of alcohol may be enhanced

**Contra-indications** epilepsy; acute porphyria (section 9.8.2); pregnancy (Appendix 4); breast-feeding (Appendix 5)

**Side-effects** nausea; dizziness, headache, nervousness, excitement; *rarely* dry mouth, tachycardia, palpitation, chest pain, drowsiness, confusion, seizures, fatigue, and sweating

**Dose**

- ADULT over 18 years, 5 mg 2–3 times daily, increased as necessary every 2–3 days; usual range 15–30 mg daily in divided doses; max. 45 mg daily

**Buspirone Hydrochloride** (Non-proprietary) PoM
Tablets, buspirone hydrochloride 5 mg, net price 30-tab pack = £14.81; 10 mg, 30-tab pack = £16.59.
Counselling, driving

**Buspar®** (Bristol-Myers Squibb) PoM
Tablets, buspirone hydrochloride 5 mg, net price 90-tab pack = £25.09; 10 mg, 90-tab pack = £37.64.
Counselling, driving

## Meprobamate

Meprobamate is **less effective** than the benzodiazepines, more hazardous in overdosage, and can also induce dependence. It is **not** recommended.

**Important:** meprobamate is to be withdrawn from the UK market; MHRA/CHM have advised that treatment with meprobamate should **no longer** be initiated.

### ■ MEPROBAMATE ◿

**Indications**  short-term use in anxiety, but see notes above
**Cautions**  respiratory disease, muscle weakness, epilepsy (may induce seizures), history of drug or alcohol abuse, marked personality disorder, pregnancy (Appendix 4); elderly and debilitated; hepatic impairment (Appendix 2), renal impairment (Appendix 3); avoid prolonged use, abrupt withdrawal may precipitate convulsions; **interactions:** Appendix 1 (anxiolytics and hypnotics)
Driving Drowsiness may affect performance of skilled tasks (e.g. driving); effects of alcohol enhanced
**Contra-indications**  acute pulmonary insufficiency; respiratory depression; acute porphyria (section 9.8.2); breast-feeding (Appendix 5)
**Side-effects**  see under Diazepam, but incidence greater and drowsiness most common side-effect; also gastro-intestinal disturbances, hypotension, paraesthesia, weakness, CNS effects including headache, paradoxical excitement, disturbances of vision; rarely agranulocytosis and rashes
**Dose**
• 400 mg 3–4 times daily; elderly patients half adult dose or less; CHILD not recommended
Note Meprobamate treatment should not be initiated in new patients, see notes above

**Meprobamate** (Non-proprietary) CD ◿
Tablets, scored, meprobamate 400 mg. Net price 84-tab pack = £19.95. Label: 2

### 4.1.3 Barbiturates

The intermediate-acting **barbiturates** have a place only in the treatment of severe intractable insomnia in patients **already taking** barbiturates; they should be **avoided** in the elderly. The long-acting barbiturate phenobarbital is still sometimes of value in epilepsy (section 4.8.1) but its use as a sedative is unjustified. The very short-acting barbiturate thiopental is used in anaesthesia (section 15.1.1).

### ■ BARBITURATES

**Indications**  severe intractable insomnia **only** in patients already taking barbiturates; see also notes above
**Cautions**  avoid use where possible; dependence and tolerance readily occur; abrupt withdrawal may precipitate serious withdrawal syndrome (rebound insomnia, anxiety, tremor, dizziness, nausea, convulsions, delirium, and death); repeated doses are cumulative and can cause excessive sedation; depression and suicidal ideation; shock; respiratory disease (avoid if dyspnoea or obstruction present); hepatic impairment (avoid if severe; Appendix 2); renal impairment (Appendix 3); **interactions:** Appendix 1 (barbiturates)
Driving Drowsiness may persist the next day and affect performance of skilled tasks (e.g. driving); effects of alcohol enhanced
**Contra-indications**  insomnia caused by pain; acute porphyria (section 9.8.2); children, young adults, elderly and debilitated patients, also patients with history of drug or alcohol abuse; pregnancy (Appendix 4); breast-feeding (Appendix 5)
**Side-effects**  drowsiness, incoordination; less commonly nausea, vomiting, constipation, liver damage, bradycardia, hypotension, syncope, hypoventilation, apnoea, respiratory depression, agitation, confusion, hyperkinesia, ataxia, CNS depression, sleep disorders, hallucinations, anxiety, dizziness, headache, paradoxical excitement, impaired memory, fever, and megaloblastic anaemia
**Dose**
• See under preparations below

**Sodium Amytal®** (Flynn) CD ◿
Capsules, amobarbital (amylobarbitone) sodium 60 mg, 200 mg. Label: 19
Available from 'special-order' manufacturers or specialist importing companies, see p. 969

**Soneryl®** (Flynn) CD ◿
Tablets, pink, scored, butobarbital (butobarbitone) 100 mg. Net price 56-tab pack = £10.65. Label: 19
Dose 100–200 mg at bedtime (**important:** but see also contra-indications)

**Tuinal®** (Flynn) CD ◿
Capsules, orange/blue, amobarbital (amylobarbitone) sodium 50 mg, secobarbital (quinalbarbitone) sodium 50 mg, net price 100 = £19.40. Label: 19
Dose 1–2 capsules at bedtime (**important:** but see also contra-indications)
Note Prescriptions need only specify 'Tuinal capsules'

## 4.2 Drugs used in psychoses and related disorders

4.2.1 Antipsychotic drugs
4.2.2 Antipsychotic depot injections
4.2.3 Antimanic drugs

**Advice of Royal College of Psychiatrists on doses above BNF upper limit.** Unless otherwise stated, doses in the BNF are licensed doses—any higher dose is therefore **unlicensed** (for an explanation of the significance of this, see p. 1).

1.  Consider alternative approaches including adjuvant therapy and newer or atypical neuroleptics such as clozapine.

2.  Bear in mind risk factors, including obesity—particular caution is indicated in older patients especially those over 70.

3.  Consider potential for drug interactions—see **interactions**: Appendix 1 (antipsychotics).

4.  Carry out ECG to exclude untoward abnormalities such as prolonged QT interval; repeat ECG periodically and reduce dose if prolonged QT interval or other adverse abnormality develops.

5.  Increase dose slowly and not more often than once weekly.

6.  Carry out regular pulse, blood pressure, and temperature checks; ensure that patient maintains adequate fluid intake.

7.  Consider high-dose therapy to be for limited period and review regularly; abandon if no improvement after 3 months (return to standard dosage).

**Important** When prescribing an antipsychotic for administration on an emergency basis, the intramuscular dose should be **lower** than the corresponding oral dose (owing to absence of first-pass effect), particularly if the patient is very active (increased blood flow to muscle considerably increases the rate of absorption). The prescription should specify the dose for **each route** and should **not** imply that the same dose can be given by mouth or by intramuscular injection. The dose of antipsychotic for emergency use should be reviewed at least **daily**.

## 4.2.1 Antipsychotic drugs

Antipsychotic drugs are also known as 'neuroleptics' and (misleadingly) as 'major tranquillisers'. Antipsychotic drugs generally tranquillise without impairing consciousness and without causing paradoxical excitement but they should not be regarded merely as tranquillisers. For conditions such as schizophrenia the tranquillising effect is of secondary importance.

In the short term they are used to calm disturbed patients whatever the underlying psychopathology, which may be schizophrenia, brain damage, mania, toxic delirium, or agitated depression. Antipsychotic drugs are used to alleviate severe anxiety but this too should be a short-term measure.

**Schizophrenia** Antipsychotic drugs relieve florid psychotic symptoms such as thought disorder, hallucinations, and delusions, and prevent relapse. Although they are usually less effective in apathetic withdrawn patients, they sometimes appear to have an activating influence. Patients with acute schizophrenia generally respond better than those with chronic symptoms.

Long-term treatment of a patient with a definite diagnosis of schizophrenia may be necessary even after the first episode of illness in order to prevent the illness from becoming chronic. Withdrawal of drug treatment requires careful surveillance because the patient who appears well on medication may suffer a disastrous relapse if treatment is withdrawn inappropriately. In addition the need for continuation of treatment may not become immediately evident because relapse is often delayed for several weeks after cessation of treatment.

Antipsychotic drugs are considered to act by interfering with dopaminergic transmission in the brain by blocking dopamine $D_2$ receptors, which may give rise to the extrapyramidal effects described below, and also to hyperprolactinaemia. Antipsychotic drugs may also affect cholinergic, alpha-adrenergic, histaminergic, and serotonergic receptors.

**Cautions and contra-indications** Antipsychotic drugs should be used with **caution** in patients with hepatic impairment (Appendix 2), renal impairment (Appendix 3), cardiovascular disease, Parkinson's disease (may be exacerbated by antipsychotics), epilepsy (and conditions predisposing to epilepsy), depression, myasthenia gravis, prostatic hypertrophy, or a susceptibility to angle-closure glaucoma. Caution is also required in severe respiratory disease and in patients with a history of jaundice or who have blood dyscrasias (perform blood counts if unexplained infection or fever develops). As photosensitisation may occur with higher dosages, patients should avoid direct sunlight.

Antipsychotic drugs may be **contra-indicated** in comatose states, CNS depression, and phaeochromocytoma. Most antipsychotic drugs are best avoided during pregnancy, unless essential (Appendix 4) and it is advisable to discontinue breast-feeding during treatment (Appendix 5); **interactions**: Appendix 1 (antipsychotics).

> **Prescribing for the elderly**
> The balance of risks and benefit should be considered before prescribing antipsychotic drugs for elderly patients. In elderly patients with dementia, antipsychotic drugs are associated with a small increased risk of mortality and an increased risk of stroke or transient ischaemic attack. Furthermore, elderly patients are particularly susceptible to postural hypotension and to hyper- and hypothermia in hot or cold weather.
> It is recommended that:
> *   Antipsychotic drugs should not be used in elderly patients to treat mild to moderate psychotic symptoms.
> *   Treatment should be reviewed regularly.

**Driving** Drowsiness may affect performance of skilled tasks (e.g. driving or operating machinery), especially at start of treatment; effects of alcohol are enhanced.

**Withdrawal** Withdrawal of antipsychotic drugs after long-term therapy should always be gradual and closely monitored to avoid the risk of acute withdrawal syndromes or rapid relapse.

**Side-effects** Extrapyramidal symptoms are the most troublesome. They occur most frequently with the piperazine phenothiazines (fluphenazine, perphenazine, prochlorperazine, and trifluoperazine), the butyrophenones (benperidol and haloperidol), and the depot preparations. They are easy to recognise but cannot be predicted accurately because they depend on the dose, the type of drug, and on individual susceptibility.

Extrapyramidal symptoms consist of:

- *parkinsonian symptoms* (including tremor), which may occur more commonly in adults or the elderly and may appear gradually;

- *dystonia* (abnormal face and body movements) and *dyskinesia*, which occur more commonly in children or young adults and appear after only a few doses;

- *akathisia* (restlessness), which characteristically occurs after large initial doses and may resemble an exacerbation of the condition being treated; and

- *tardive dyskinesia* (rhythmic, involuntary movements of tongue, face, and jaw), which usually develops on long-term therapy or with high dosage, but it may develop on short-term treatment with low doses—short-lived tardive dyskinesia may occur after withdrawal of the drug.

*Parkinsonian symptoms* remit if the drug is withdrawn and may be suppressed by the administration of **antimuscarinic** drugs (section 4.9.2). However, routine administration of such drugs is not justified because not all patients are affected and because they may unmask or worsen tardive dyskinesia.

*Tardive dyskinesia* is of particular concern because it may be irreversible on withdrawing therapy and treatment is usually ineffective. However, some manufacturers suggest that drug withdrawal at the earliest signs of tardive dyskinesia (fine vermicular movements of the tongue) may halt its full development. Tardive dyskinesia occurs fairly frequently, especially in the elderly, and treatment must be carefully and regularly reviewed.

*Hypotension and interference with temperature regulation* are dose-related side-effects and are liable to cause dangerous falls and hypothermia or hyperthermia in the elderly.

*Neuroleptic malignant syndrome* (hyperthermia, fluctuating level of consciousness, muscle rigidity, and autonomic dysfunction with pallor, tachycardia, labile blood pressure, sweating, and urinary incontinence) is a rare but potentially fatal side-effect of some drugs. Discontinuation of the antipsychotic is essential because there is no proven effective treatment, but cooling, bromocriptine, and dantrolene have been used. The syndrome, which usually lasts for 5–7 days after drug discontinuation, may be unduly prolonged if depot preparations have been used.

*Other side-effects include:* drowsiness; apathy; agitation, excitement and insomnia; convulsions; dizziness; headache; confusion; gastro-intestinal disturbances; nasal congestion; antimuscarinic symptoms (such as dry mouth, constipation, difficulty with micturition, and blurred vision; *very rarely*, precipitation of angle-closure glaucoma); cardiovascular symptoms (such as hypotension, tachycardia, and arrhythmias); ECG changes (cases of sudden death have occurred); endocrine effects such as menstrual disturbances, galactorrhoea, gynaecomastia, impotence, and weight gain; blood dyscrasias (such as agranulocytosis and leucopenia), photosensitisation, contact sensitisation and rashes, and jaundice (including cholestatic); corneal and lens opacities, and purplish pigmentation of the skin, cornea, conjunctiva, and retina.

**Overdosage:** for poisoning with phenothiazines and related compounds, see Emergency Treatment of Poisoning, p. 33.

**Classification of antipsychotics**   The **phenothiazine** derivatives can be divided into 3 main groups.

*Group 1*: chlorpromazine, levomepromazine (methotrimeprazine), and promazine, generally characterised by pronounced sedative effects and moderate antimuscarinic and extrapyramidal side-effects.

*Group 2*: pericyazine and pipotiazine, generally characterised by moderate sedative effects, marked antimuscarinic effects, but fewer extrapyramidal side-effects than groups 1 or 3.

*Group 3*: fluphenazine, perphenazine, prochlorperazine, and trifluoperazine, generally characterised by fewer sedative effects, fewer antimuscarinic effects, but more pronounced extrapyramidal side-effects than groups 1 and 2.

Drugs of other chemical groups resemble the phenothiazines of *group 3* in their clinical properties. They include the **butyrophenones** (benperidol and haloperidol); **diphenylbutylpiperidines** (pimozide); **thioxanthenes** (flupentixol and zuclopenthixol); and the **substituted benzamides** (sulpiride).

For details of the newer antipsychotic drugs amisulpride, clozapine, olanzapine, quetiapine, risperidone, sertindole, and zotepine, see under Atypical Antipsychotic Drugs, p. 199.

**Choice**   As indicated above, the various drugs differ somewhat in predominant actions and side-effects. Selection is influenced by the degree of sedation required and the patient's susceptibility to extrapyramidal side-effects. However, the differences between antipsychotic drugs are less important than the great variability in patient response; moreover, tolerance to secondary effects such as sedation usually develops. The atypical antipsychotics may be appropriate if extrapyramidal side-effects are a particular concern (see under Atypical Antipsychotics, below). Clozapine is used for schizophrenia when other antipsychotics are ineffective or not tolerated.

Prescribing of more than one antipsychotic drug at the same time is **not** recommended; it may constitute a hazard and there is no significant evidence that side-effects are minimised.

**Chlorpromazine** is still widely used despite the wide range of adverse effects associated with it. It has a marked sedating effect and is useful for treating violent patients without causing stupor. Agitated states in the elderly can be controlled without confusion, a dose of 10 to 25 mg once or twice daily usually being adequate.

**Flupentixol** (flupenthixol) and **pimozide** (see CSM warning, p. 198) are less sedating than chlorpromazine.

**Sulpiride** in high doses controls florid positive symptoms, but in lower doses it can have an alerting effect on apathetic withdrawn schizophrenics.

**Fluphenazine, haloperidol,** and **trifluoperazine** are also of value but their use is limited by the high incidence of extrapyramidal symptoms. Haloperidol may be preferred for the rapid control of hyperactive psychotic states; it causes less hypotension than chlorpromazine and is therefore also popular for agitation and restlessness in the elderly, despite the high incidence of extrapyramidal side-effects.

**4**

**Central nervous system**

Central nervous system

4

**Promazine** is not sufficiently active by mouth to be used as an antipsychotic drug; it has been used to treat agitation and restlessness in the elderly (see Other uses, below).

**Other uses** Nausea and vomiting (section 4.6), choreas, motor tics (section 4.9.3), and intractable hiccup (see under Chlorpromazine Hydrochloride and under Haloperidol). **Benperidol** is used in deviant antisocial sexual behaviour but its value is not established; see also section 6.4.2 for the role of cyproterone acetate.

Psychomotor agitation should be investigated for an underlying cause; it can be managed with low doses of chlorpromazine or haloperidol used for short periods. Antipsychotic drugs can be used with caution for the short-term treatment of severe agitation and restlessness in the elderly (but see p. 194).

### Equivalent doses of oral antipsychotics

These equivalences are intended **only** as an approximate guide; individual dosage instructions should **also** be checked; patients should be carefully monitored after **any** change in medication

| Antipsychotic drug | Daily dose |
|---|---|
| Chlorpromazine | 100 mg |
| Clozapine | 50 mg |
| Haloperidol | 2–3 mg |
| Pimozide | 2 mg |
| Risperidone | 0.5–1 mg |
| Sulpiride | 200 mg |
| Trifluoperazine | 5 mg |

**Important** These equivalences must **not** be extrapolated beyond the maximum dose for the drug. Higher doses require careful titration in specialist units and the equivalences shown here may not be appropriate

#### Dosage
After an initial period of stabilisation, in most patients, the total daily oral dose can be given as a single dose. For the advice of The Royal College of Psychiatrists on doses above the BNF upper limit, see p. 193.

### ▌ BENPERIDOL

**Indications** control of deviant antisocial sexual behaviour (but see notes above)

**Cautions** see notes above; also manufacturer advises regular blood counts and liver function tests during long-term treatment

**Contra-indications** see notes above

**Side-effects** see notes above

**Dose**
- 0.25–1.5 mg daily in divided doses, adjusted according to response; ELDERLY (or debilitated) initially half adult dose; CHILD not recommended

**Anquil®** (Concord) ℞
Tablets, scored, benperidol 250 micrograms, net price 112-tab pack = £124.80. Label: 2
**Note** The proprietary name *Benquil*® has been used for benperidol tablets

### ▌ CHLORPROMAZINE HYDROCHLORIDE

**Warning** Owing to the risk of contact sensitisation, pharmacists, nurses, and other health workers should avoid direct contact with chlorpromazine; tablets should not be crushed and solutions should be handled with care

**Indications** see under Dose; antiemetic in palliative care (section 4.6)

**Cautions** see notes above; also patients should remain supine and the blood pressure monitored for 30 minutes after intramuscular injection

**Contra-indications** see notes above

**Side-effects** see notes above; also intramuscular injection may be painful, cause hypotension and tachycardia, and give rise to nodule formation

**Dose**
- By mouth, schizophrenia and other psychoses, mania, short-term adjunctive management of severe anxiety, psychomotor agitation, excitement, and violent or dangerously impulsive behaviour initially 25 mg 3 times daily (*or* 75 mg at night), adjusted according to response, to usual maintenance dose of 75–300 mg daily (but up to 1 g daily may be required in psychoses); ELDERLY (or debilitated) third to half adult dose; CHILD (childhood schizophrenia and autism) 1–6 years 500 micrograms/kg every 4–6 hours (max. 40 mg daily); 6–12 years 10 mg 3 times daily (max. 75 mg daily)
 Intractable hiccup, 25–50 mg 3–4 times daily
- By deep intramuscular injection, (for relief of acute symptoms but see also Cautions and Side-effects), 25–50 mg every 6–8 hours; CHILD, 1–6 years 500 micrograms/kg every 6–8 hours (max. 40 mg daily); 6–12 years 500 micrograms/kg every 6–8 hours (max. 75 mg daily)
 Induction of hypothermia (to prevent shivering), 25–50 mg every 6–8 hours; CHILD 1–12 years, initially 0.5–1 mg/kg, followed by maintenance 500 micrograms/kg every 4–6 hours
- By rectum in suppositories as chlorpromazine base 100 mg every 6–8 hours [unlicensed]
 **Note** For equivalent therapeutic effect 100 mg chlorpromazine base given *rectally* as a suppository ≡ 20–25 mg chlorpromazine hydrochloride *by intramuscular injection* ≡ 40–50 mg of chlorpromazine base or hydrochloride *by mouth*

**Chlorpromazine** (Non-proprietary) ℞
Tablets, coated, chlorpromazine hydrochloride 25 mg, 28-tab pack = £3.09; 50 mg, 28-tab pack = £3.32; 100 mg, 28-tab pack = £3.43. Label: 2, 11
Brands include *Chloractil*®

Oral solution, chlorpromazine hydrochloride 25 mg/ 5 mL, net price 150 mL = £1.50, 100 mg/5 mL, 150 mL = £3.75. Label: 2, 11

Injection, chlorpromazine hydrochloride 25 mg/mL, net price 1-mL amp = 60p; 2-mL amp = 63p

Suppositories, chlorpromazine 25 mg and 100 mg. Label: 2, 11
Available from 'special-order' manufacturers or specialist importing companies, see p. 969

**Largactil®** (Sanofi-Aventis) ℞
Injection, chlorpromazine hydrochloride 25 mg/mL. Net price 2-mL amp = 60p

## FLUPENTIXOL
(Flupenthixol)

**Indications** schizophrenia and other psychoses, particularly with apathy and withdrawal but not mania or psychomotor hyperactivity; depression (section 4.3.4)

**Cautions** see notes above; avoid in acute porphyria (section 9.8.2)

**Contra-indications** see notes above; also excitable and overactive patients

**Side-effects** see notes above; less sedating but extrapyramidal symptoms frequent

**Dose**
- Psychosis, initially 3–9 mg twice daily adjusted according to the response; max. 18 mg daily; ELDERLY (or debilitated) initially quarter to half adult dose; CHILD not recommended

**Depixol®** (Lundbeck) [PoM]
Tablets, yellow, s/c, flupentixol 3 mg (as dihydrochloride), net price 100 = £9.74. Label: 2

◢Depot preparation
Section 4.2.2

## HALOPERIDOL

**Indications** see under Dose; motor tics (section 4.9.3)

**Cautions** see notes above; also subarachnoid haemorrhage and metabolic disturbances such as hypokalaemia, hypocalcaemia, or hypomagnesaemia

**Contra-indications** see notes above

**Side-effects** see notes above, but less sedating and fewer antimuscarinic or hypotensive symptoms; pigmentation and photosensitivity reactions rare; extrapyramidal symptoms, particularly dystonic reactions and akathisia especially in thyrotoxic patients; rarely weight loss; hypoglycaemia; inappropriate antidiuretic hormone secretion

**Dose**
- Schizophrenia and other psychoses, mania, short-term adjunctive management of psychomotor agitation, excitement, and violent or dangerously impulsive behaviour, ADULT and CHILD over 12 years, by mouth, initially 0.5–3 mg 2–3 times daily *or* 3–5 mg 2–3 times daily in severely affected or resistant patients; in resistant schizophrenia up to 30 mg daily may be needed; adjusted according to response to lowest effective maintenance dose (as low as 5–10 mg daily); ELDERLY (or debilitated) initially half adult dose

  By intramuscular *or* by intravenous injection, ADULT over 18 years, initially 2–10 mg, then every 4–8 hours according to response to total max. 18 mg daily; severely disturbed patients may require initial dose of up to 18 mg; ELDERLY (or debilitated) initially half adult dose
- Agitation and restlessness in the elderly, by mouth, initially 0.5–1.5 mg once or twice daily
- Short-term adjunctive management of severe anxiety, by mouth, ADULT over 18 years, 500 micrograms twice daily
- Intractable hiccup, by mouth, ADULT over 18 years, 1.5 mg 3 times daily adjusted according to response
- Nausea and vomiting, see Prescribing in Palliative Care, p. 17

  By intramuscular *or* intravenous injection, 1–2 mg

**Haloperidol** (Non-proprietary) [PoM]
Tablets, haloperidol 500 micrograms, net price 28-tab pack = 91p; 1.5 mg, 28-tab pack = £1.62; 5 mg, 28-tab pack = £3.93; 10 mg, 28-tab pack = £4.27; 20 mg, 28-tab pack = £11.17. Label: 2

**Dozic®** (Rosemont) [PoM]
Oral liquid, sugar-free, haloperidol 1 mg/mL, net price 100-mL pack = £6.86. Label: 2

**Haldol®** (Janssen-Cilag) [PoM]
Tablets, both scored, haloperidol 5 mg (blue), net price 100 = £7.35; 10 mg (yellow), 100 = £14.37. Label: 2

Oral liquid, sugar-free, haloperidol 2 mg/mL, net price 100-mL pack (with pipette) = £4.54. Label: 2

Injection, haloperidol 5 mg/mL, net price 1-mL amp = 29p

**Serenace®** (IVAX) [PoM]
Capsules, green, haloperidol 500 micrograms, net price 30-cap pack = 98p. Label: 2

Tablets, haloperidol 1.5 mg, net price 30-tab pack = £1.37; 5 mg (pink), 30-tab pack = £3.95; 10 mg (pale pink), 30-tab pack = £6.76. Label: 2

Oral liquid, sugar-free, haloperidol 2 mg/mL, net price 500-mL pack = £34.48. Label: 2

◢Depot preparation
Section 4.2.2

## LEVOMEPROMAZINE
(Methotrimeprazine)

**Indications** see under Dose

**Cautions** see notes above; patients receiving large initial doses should remain supine
Elderly Risk of postural hypotension; not recommended for ambulant patients over 50 years unless risk of hypotensive reaction assessed

**Contra-indications** see notes above

**Side-effects** see notes above; occasionally raised erythrocyte sedimentation rate occurs

**Dose**
- Schizophrenia, by mouth initially 25–50 mg daily in divided doses increased as necessary; bedpatients initially 100–200 mg daily usually in 3 divided doses, increased if necessary to 1 g daily; ELDERLY, see Cautions
- Pain in palliative care, see p. 16
- Restlessness and confusion in palliative care, see p. 18; CHILD 1–18 years, see *BNF for Children*
- Nausea and vomiting in palliative care, by mouth, see p. 17, or by subcutaneous infusion, see p. 18; CHILD 1 month–18 years, see *BNF for Children*

**Nozinan®** (Link) [PoM]
Tablets, scored, levomepromazine maleate 25 mg, net price 84-tab pack = £20.26. Label: 2

Injection, levomepromazine hydrochloride 25 mg/mL, net price 1-mL amp = £2.01

## PERICYAZINE
(Periciazine)

**Indications** see under Dose

**Cautions** see notes above

**Contra-indications** see notes above; renal impairment

**4**

Central nervous system

**Central nervous system**

**4**

**Side-effects** see notes above; more sedating; hypotension common when treatment initiated; respiratory depression

**Dose**

- Schizophrenia and other psychoses, initially 75 mg daily in divided doses increased at weekly intervals by steps of 25 mg according to response; usual max. 300 mg daily (elderly initially 15–30 mg daily); CHILD and INFANT over 1 year (schizophrenia or behavioural disorders only), initially, 500 micrograms daily for 10-kg child, increased by 1 mg for each additional 5 kg body-weight to max. total daily dose of 10 mg; dose may be gradually increased according to response but maintenance should not exceed twice initial dose

- Short-term adjunctive management of severe anxiety, psychomotor agitation, and violent or dangerously impulsive behaviour, initially 15–30 mg (elderly 5–10 mg) daily divided into 2 doses, taking the larger dose at bedtime, adjusted according to response; CHILD not recommended

**Neulactil®** (Winthrop) ℗ℴℳ
Tablets, yellow, scored, pericyazine 2.5 mg, net price 84-tab pack = £9.23; 10 mg, 84-tab pack = £24.95. Label: 2

Syrup forte, brown, pericyazine 10 mg/5 mL. Net price 100-mL pack = £12.08. Label: 2

## ▌ PERPHENAZINE

**Indications** see under Dose; antiemetic (section 4.6)

**Cautions** see notes above

**Contra-indications** see notes above; also agitation and restlessness in the elderly

**Side-effects** see notes above; less sedating; extrapyramidal symptoms, especially dystonia, more frequent, particularly at high dosage; rarely systemic lupus erythematosus

**Dose**

- Schizophrenia and other psychoses, mania, short-term adjunctive management of anxiety, severe psychomotor agitation, excitement, and violent or dangerously impulsive behaviour, initially 4 mg 3 times daily adjusted according to the response; max. 24 mg daily; ELDERLY quarter to half adult dose (but see Cautions); CHILD under 14 years not recommended

**Fentazin®** (Goldshield) ℗ℴℳ
Tablets, s/c, perphenazine 2 mg, net price 100 = £22.38; 4 mg, 100 = £26.34. Label: 2

## ▌ PIMOZIDE

**Indications** see under Dose

**Cautions** see notes above

CSM warning Following reports of sudden unexplained death, the CSM recommends ECG before treatment. The CSM also recommends that patients on pimozide should have an annual ECG (if the QT interval is prolonged, treatment should be reviewed and either withdrawn or dose reduced under close supervision) and that pimozide should **not** be given with other antipsychotic drugs (including depot preparations), tricyclic antidepressants or other drugs which prolong the QT interval, such as certain antimalarials, antiarrhythmic drugs and certain antihistamines and should **not** be given with drugs which cause electrolyte disturbances (especially diuretics)

**Contra-indications** see notes above; history of arrhythmias or congenital QT prolongation

**Side-effects** see notes above; less sedating; serious arrhythmias reported; glycosuria and, rarely, hyponatraemia reported

**Dose**

- Schizophrenia, ADULT and CHILD over 12 years, initially 2 mg daily, increased according to response in steps of 2–4 mg at intervals of not less than 1 week; usual dose range 2–20 mg daily; ELDERLY half usual starting dose

- Monosymptomatic hypochondriacal psychosis, paranoid psychosis, ADULT and CHILD over 12 years, initially 4 mg daily, increased according to response in steps of 2–4 mg at intervals of not less than 1 week; max. 16 mg daily; ELDERLY half usual starting dose

**Orap®** (Janssen-Cilag) ℗ℴℳ
Tablets, scored, green, pimozide 4 mg, net price 100 = £27.41. Label: 2

## ▌ PROCHLORPERAZINE

**Indications** see under Dose; antiemetic (section 4.6)

**Cautions** see notes above; also hypotension more likely after intramuscular injection

**Contra-indications** see notes above; children, but see section 4.6 for use as antiemetic

**Side-effects** see notes above; less sedating; extrapyramidal symptoms, particularly dystonias, more frequent; respiratory depression may occur in susceptible patients

**Dose**

- By mouth, schizophrenia and other psychoses, mania, prochlorperazine maleate or mesilate, 12.5 mg twice daily for 7 days adjusted at intervals of 4–7 days to usual dose of 75–100 mg daily according to response; CHILD not recommended
Short-term adjunctive management of severe anxiety, 15–20 mg daily in divided doses; max. 40 mg daily; CHILD not recommended

- By deep intramuscular injection, psychoses, mania, prochlorperazine mesilate 12.5–25 mg 2–3 times daily; CHILD not recommended

◀Preparations
Section 4.6

## ▌ PROMAZINE HYDROCHLORIDE

**Indications** see under Dose

**Cautions** see notes above; also cerebral arteriosclerosis

**Contra-indications** see notes above

**Side-effects** see notes above; also haemolytic anaemia

**Dose**

- Short-term adjunctive management of psychomotor agitation, 100–200 mg 4 times daily; CHILD not recommended

- Agitation and restlessness in elderly, 25–50 mg 4 times daily

**Promazine** (Non-proprietary) ℗ℴℳ
Tablets, coated, promazine hydrochloride 25 mg, net price 100 = £6.58; 50 mg, 100 = £16.27. Label: 2

Oral solution, promazine hydrochloride 25 mg/5 mL, net price 150 mL = £4.08; 50 mg/5 mL, 150 mL = £4.18. Label: 2

## SULPIRIDE

**Indications** schizophrenia

**Cautions** see notes above; also excited, agitated, or aggressive patients (even low doses may aggravate symptoms); renal impairment (avoid if severe)

**Contra-indications** see notes above; also acute porphyria (section 9.8.2)

**Side-effects** see notes above; also hepatitis

**Dose**

- ADULT and CHILD over 14 years, 200–400 mg twice daily; max. 800 mg daily in predominantly negative symptoms, and 2.4 g daily in mainly positive symptoms; ELDERLY, lower initial dose, increased gradually according to response

**Sulpiride** (Non-proprietary) ᴘᴏᴹ

Tablets, sulpiride 200 mg, net price 30-tab pack = £7.32, 56-tab pack = £6.46; 400 mg, 30-tab pack = £12.55. Label: 2

**Dolmatil®** (Sanofi-Synthelabo) ᴘᴏᴹ

Tablets, both scored, sulpiride 200 mg, net price 100-tab pack = £13.31; 400 mg (f/c), 100-tab pack = £34.87. Label: 2

**Sulpor®** (Rosemont) ᴘᴏᴹ

Oral solution, sugar-free, lemon- and aniseed-flavoured, sulpiride 200 mg/5 mL, net price 150 mL = £25.38. Label: 2

## TRIFLUOPERAZINE

**Indications** see under Dose; antiemetic (section 4.6)

**Cautions** see notes above

**Contra-indications** see notes above

**Side-effects** see notes above; extrapyramidal symptoms more frequent, especially at doses exceeding 6 mg daily; pancytopenia; thrombocytopenia; hyperthermia; anorexia

**Dose**

- Schizophrenia and other psychoses, short-term adjunctive management of psychomotor agitation, excitement, and violent or dangerously impulsive behaviour, ADULT and CHILD over 12 years, initially 5 mg twice daily, increased by 5 mg daily after 1 week, then at intervals of 3 days, according to the response; ELDERLY reduce initial dose by at least half

- Short-term adjunctive management of severe anxiety, ADULT and CHILD over 12 years, 2–4 mg daily in divided doses, increased if necessary to 6 mg daily; CHILD 3–5 years up to 1 mg daily, 6–12 years up to 4 mg daily; ELDERLY reduce initial dose by at least half

**Trifluoperazine** (Non-proprietary) ᴘᴏᴹ

Tablets, coated, trifluoperazine (as hydrochloride) 1 mg, net price 100 = £6.10; 5 mg, 100 = £5.32. Label: 2

Oral solution, trifluoperazine (as hydrochloride) 5 mg/5 mL, net price 150-mL = £9.46. Label: 2

**Stelazine®** (Goldshield) ᴘᴏᴹ

Tablets, both blue, f/c, trifluoperazine (as hydrochloride) 1 mg, net price 112 = £3.43; 5 mg, 112 = £4.89. Label: 2

Syrup, sugar-free, yellow, trifluoperazine (as hydrochloride) 1 mg/5 mL, net price 200-mL pack = £2.95. Label: 2

## ZUCLOPENTHIXOL ACETATE

**Indications** short-term management of acute psychosis, mania, or exacerbations of chronic psychosis

**Cautions** see notes above; avoid in acute porphyria (section 9.8.2)

**Contra-indications** see notes above

**Side-effects** see notes above

**Dose**

- By deep intramuscular injection into the gluteal muscle or lateral thigh, 50–150 mg (ELDERLY 50–100 mg), if necessary repeated after 2–3 days (1 additional dose may be needed 1–2 days after the first injection); max. cumulative dose 400 mg per course and max. 4 injections; max. duration of treatment 2 weeks—if maintenance treatment necessary change to an oral antipsychotic 2–3 days after last injection, or to a longer acting antipsychotic depot injection given concomitantly with last injection of zuclopenthixol acetate; CHILD not recommended

**Clopixol Acuphase®** (Lundbeck) ᴘᴏᴹ

Injection (oily), zuclopenthixol acetate 50 mg/mL, net price 1-mL amp = £3.39; 2-mL amp = £6.53

◀ Depot preparation

Section 4.2.2

## ZUCLOPENTHIXOL

**Indications** schizophrenia and other psychoses

**Cautions** see notes above; avoid in acute porphyria (section 9.8.2)

**Contra-indications** see notes above; apathetic or withdrawn states

**Side-effects** see notes above; urinary frequency or incontinence; weight loss (less common than weight gain)

**Dose**

- By mouth, initially 20–30 mg daily in divided doses, increasing to a max. of 150 mg daily if necessary; usual maintenance dose 20–50 mg daily; ELDERLY (or debilitated) initially quarter to half adult dose; CHILD not recommended

**Clopixol®** (Lundbeck) ᴘᴏᴹ

Tablets, f/c, zuclopenthixol (as dihydrochloride) 2 mg (red), net price 100 = £2.09; 10 mg (light red-brown), 100 = £5.64; 25 mg (red-brown), 100 = £11.28. Label: 2

◀ Depot preparation

Section 4.2.2

## Atypical antipsychotic drugs

The 'atypical' antipsychotic drugs **amisulpride**, **aripiprazole**, **clozapine**, **olanzapine**, **paliperidone**, **quetiapine**, **risperidone**, and **zotepine** may be better tolerated than other antipsychotic drugs; extrapyramidal symptoms may be less frequent than with older antipsychotic drugs.

Aripiprazole, clozapine, olanzapine, quetiapine, and sertindole cause little or no elevation of prolactin concentration; when changing from other antipsychotic drugs, a reduction in prolactin may increase fertility.

**4**

**Central nervous system**

Clozapine is licensed for the treatment of schizophrenia only in patients unresponsive to, or intolerant of, conventional antipsychotic drugs. It can cause agranulocytosis and its use is restricted to patients registered with a clozapine patient monitoring service (see under Clozapine).

**Sertindole** has been reintroduced following an earlier suspension of the drug because of concerns about arrhythmias; its use is restricted to patients who are enrolled in clinical studies and who are intolerant of at least one other antipsychotic.

The *Scottish Medicines Consortium* (p. 3) has advised (March 2008) that paliperidone (*Invega®*) is **not** recommended for use within NHS Scotland.

---

**NICE guidance**

**Atypical antipsychotics for schizophrenia (June 2002)**

NICE has recommended that:

- the atypical antipsychotics (amisulpride, olanzapine, quetiapine, risperidone, and zotepine) should be considered when choosing first-line treatment of *newly diagnosed schizophrenia*;
- an atypical antipsychotic is considered the treatment option of choice for managing an *acute schizophrenic episode* when discussion with the individual is not possible;
- an atypical antipsychotic should be considered for an individual who is suffering unacceptable side-effects from a conventional antipsychotic;
- an atypical antipsychotic should be considered for an individual in relapse whose symptoms were previously inadequately controlled;
- changing to an atypical antipsychotic is not necessary if a conventional antipsychotic controls symptoms adequately and the individual does not suffer unacceptable side-effects;
- clozapine should be introduced if schizophrenia is inadequately controlled despite the sequential use of two or more antipsychotics (one of which should be an atypical antipsychotic) each for at least 6–8 weeks.

---

**Cautions and contra-indications** While atypical antipsychotic drugs have not generally been associated with clinically significant prolongation of the QT interval, they should be used with care if prescribed with other drugs that increase the QT interval. Atypical antipsychotic drugs should be used with caution in patients with cardiovascular disease, or a history of epilepsy; they should be used with great caution in the elderly (see p. 194); **interactions:** Appendix 1 (antipsychotics).

**Driving** Atypical antipsychotic drugs may affect performance of skilled tasks (e.g. driving); effects of alcohol are enhanced.

**Withdrawal** Withdrawal of antipsychotic drugs after long-term therapy should always be gradual and closely monitored to avoid the risk of acute withdrawal syndromes or rapid relapse.

**Side-effects** Side-effects of the atypical antipsychotic drugs include weight gain, dizziness, postural hypotension (especially during initial dose titration) which may be associated with syncope or reflex tachycardia in some patients, extrapyramidal symptoms (usually mild

and transient and which respond to dose reduction or to an antimuscarinic drug), and occasionally tardive dyskinesia on long-term administration (discontinue drug on appearance of early signs). Hyperglycaemia and sometimes diabetes can occur, particularly with clozapine, olanzapine, and risperidone; monitoring weight and plasma-glucose concentration may identify the development of hyperglycaemia. Neuroleptic malignant syndrome has been reported rarely. Hypersalivation associated with clozapine therapy can be treated with hyoscine hydrobromide [unlicensed indication] (p. 231), provided that patients are not at particular risk from the additive antimuscarinic side-effects of hyoscine and clozapine.

---

## ■ AMISULPRIDE

**Indications** schizophrenia

**Cautions** see notes above; also Parkinson's disease; renal impairment (Appendix 3)

**Contra-indications** see notes above; also phaeochromocytoma, prolactin-dependent tumours; pregnancy (Appendix 4); breast-feeding (Appendix 5)

**Side-effects** see notes above; also insomnia, anxiety, agitation, drowsiness, gastro-intestinal disorders such as constipation, nausea, vomiting, and dry mouth; hyperprolactinaemia; *occasionally* bradycardia; *rarely* seizures

**Dose**

- Acute psychotic episode, 400–800 mg daily in 2 divided doses, adjusted according to response; max. 1.2 g daily; CHILD under 15 years not recommended
- Predominantly negative symptoms, 50–300 mg daily; CHILD under 15 years not recommended

**Amisulpride** (Non-proprietary) ▣ﾖﾙ
Tablets, amisulpride 50 mg, net price 60-tab pack = £16.52; 100 mg, 60-tab pack = £33.42; 200 mg, 60-tab pack = £55.87; 400 mg, 60-tab pack = £111.36. Label: 2

**Solian®** (Sanofi-Synthelabo) ▣ﾖﾙ
Tablets, scored, amisulpride 50 mg, net price 60-tab pack = £22.76; 100 mg, 60-tab pack = £35.29; 200 mg, 60-tab pack = £58.99; 400 mg, 60-tab pack = £117.97. Label: 2

Solution, 100 mg/mL, net price 60 mL (caramel flavour) = £33.76. Label: 2

---

## ■ ARIPIPRAZOLE

**Indications** see under Dose

**Cautions** see notes above; cerebrovascular disease; elderly (reduce initial dose); hepatic impairment (Appendix 2); pregnancy (Appendix 4)

**Contra-indications** see notes above; breast-feeding (Appendix 5)

**Side-effects** see notes above; gastro-intestinal disturbances; tachycardia; fatigue, insomnia, akathisia, drowsiness, restlessness, tremor, headache, asthenia; blurred vision; *less commonly* depression; *very rarely* anorexia, dysphagia, oropharyngeal spasm, laryngospasm, hepatitis, jaundice, hypersalivation, pancreatitis, oedema, thromboembolism, arrhythmias, bradycardia, hypertension, chest pain, agitation, anxiety, speech disorder, suicidal ideation, seizures, hyponatraemia, stiffness, myalgia, rhabdomyolysis, priapism, urinary retention and incontinence, blood disorders, sweating, alopecia, photosensitivity reactions, rash, weight loss, and impaired temperature regulation; *with injection*, dry mouth

**Dose**

- Schizophrenia, by mouth, ADULT over 18 years 10–15 mg once daily, usual maintenance 15 mg once daily; max. 30 mg once daily

- Mania, by mouth, ADULT over 18 years, 15 mg once daily, increased if necessary; max. 30 mg once daily

- Control of agitation and disturbed behaviour in schizophrenia, by intramuscular injection, ADULT over 18 years, initially 5.25–15 mg (usual dose 9.75 mg) as a single dose followed by 5.25–15 mg after 2 hours if necessary; max. 3 injections daily; max. daily combined oral and parenteral dose 30 mg

**Abilify®** (Bristol-Myers Squibb) ▸PoM
Tablets, aripiprazole 5 mg (blue), net price 28-tab pack = £97.67; 10 mg (pink), 28-tab pack = £97.67; 15 mg (yellow), 28-tab pack = £97.67; 30 mg (pink), 28-tab pack = £195.33. Label: 2

Orodispersible tablets, aripiprazole 10 mg (pink), net price 28-tab pack = £97.67; 15 mg (yellow), 28-tab pack = £97.67. Label: 2, counselling, administration
Excipients include aspartame (section 9.4.1)
Counselling Tablets should be placed on the tongue and allowed to dissolve, or be dispersed in water and swallowed

Oral solution, aripiprazole 1 mg/mL, net price 150 mL with measuring cup = £104.64. Label: 2

Injection ▾, aripiprazole 7.5 mg/mL, net price 1.3-mL (9.75-mg) vial = £3.49

---

## CLOZAPINE

**Indications** schizophrenia (including psychosis in Parkinson's disease) in patients unresponsive to, or intolerant of, conventional antipsychotic drugs

**Cautions** see notes above; elderly; monitor leucocyte and differential blood counts (see Agranulocytosis, below); prostatic hypertrophy, susceptibility to angle-closure glaucoma; taper off other antipsychotics before starting; close medical supervision during initiation (risk of collapse because of hypotension); hepatic impairment (Appendix 2); pregnancy (Appendix 4)
Withdrawal On planned withdrawal reduce dose over 1–2 weeks to avoid risk of rebound psychosis. If abrupt withdrawal necessary observe patient carefully
Agranulocytosis Neutropenia and potentially fatal agranulocytosis reported. Leucocyte and differential blood counts must be normal before starting; monitor counts every week for 18 weeks then at least every 2 weeks and if clozapine continued and blood count stable after 1 year at least every 4 weeks (and 4 weeks after discontinuation); if leucocyte count below 3000/mm³ or if absolute neutrophil count below 1500/mm³ discontinue permanently and refer to haematologist. Patients who have low white blood cell counts because of benign ethnic neutropenia may be started on clozapine with the agreement of a haematologist. Avoid drugs which depress leucopoiesis; patients should report immediately symptoms of infection, especially influenza-like illness
Myocarditis and cardiomyopathy Fatal myocarditis (most commonly in first 2 months) and cardiomyopathy reported.
- Perform physical examination and take full medical history before starting

- Specialist examination required if cardiac abnormalities or history of heart disease found—clozapine initiated only in absence of severe heart disease and if benefit outweighs risk

- Persistent tachycardia especially in first 2 months should prompt observation for other indicators for myocarditis or cardiomyopathy

- If myocarditis or cardiomyopathy suspected clozapine should be stopped and patient evaluated urgently by cardiologist

- Discontinue permanently in clozapine-induced myocarditis or cardiomyopathy

Gastro-intestinal obstruction Reactions resembling gastro-intestinal obstruction reported. Clozapine should be used cautiously with drugs which cause constipation (e.g. antimuscarinic drugs) or in history of colonic disease or bowel surgery. Monitor for constipation and prescribe laxative if required

**Contra-indications** severe cardiac disorders (e.g. myocarditis; see Cautions); severe renal impairment; history of neutropenia or agranulocytosis (see Cautions); bone-marrow disorders; paralytic ileus (see Cautions); alcoholic and toxic psychoses; history of circulatory collapse; drug intoxication; coma or severe CNS depression; uncontrolled epilepsy; breast-feeding (Appendix 5)

**Side-effects** see notes above; also constipation (see Cautions), hypersalivation, dry mouth, nausea, vomiting, anorexia; tachycardia, ECG changes, hypertension; drowsiness, dizziness, headache, tremor, seizures, fatigue, impaired temperature regulation; urinary incontinence and retention; leucopenia, eosinophilia, leucocytosis; blurred vision; sweating; *less commonly* agranulocytosis (**important:** see Cautions); *rarely* dysphagia, hepatitis, cholestatic jaundice, pancreatitis, circulatory collapse, arrhythmia, myocarditis (**important:** see Cautions), pericarditis, thromboembolism, agitation, confusion, delirium, anaemia; *very rarely* parotid gland enlargement, intestinal obstruction (see Cautions), cardiomyopathy, myocardial infarction, respiratory depression, priapism, interstitial nephritis, thrombocytopenia, thrombocythaemia, hypertriglyceridaemia, hypercholesterolaemia, hyperlipidaemia, angle-closure glaucoma, fulminant hepatic necrosis, and skin reactions

**Dose**

- Schizophrenia, ADULT over 16 years, 12.5 mg once or twice (ELDERLY 12.5 mg once) on first day then 25–50 mg (ELDERLY 25–37.5 mg) on second day then increased gradually (if well tolerated) in steps of 25–50 mg daily (ELDERLY max. increment 25 mg daily) over 14–21 days up to 300 mg daily in divided doses (larger dose at night, up to 200 mg daily may be taken as a single dose at bedtime); if necessary may be further increased in steps of 50–100 mg once (preferably) or twice weekly; usual dose 200–450 mg daily (max. 900 mg daily)
Note *Restarting* after *interval of more than 2 days*, 12.5 mg once or twice on first day (but may be feasible to increase more quickly than on initiation)—extreme caution if previous respiratory or cardiac arrest with initial dosing

- Psychosis in Parkinson's disease, ADULT over 16 years, 12.5 mg at bedtime then increased according to response in steps of 12.5 mg up to twice weekly; usual dose range 25–37.5 mg at bedtime, usual max. 50 mg daily; exceptionally, dose may be increased further in steps of 12.5 mg weekly to max. 100 mg daily in 1–2 divided doses

**Clozaril®** (Novartis) ▸PoM
Tablets, yellow, clozapine 25 mg (scored), net price 28-tab pack = £6.17, 84-tab pack (hosp. only) = £18.49; 100 mg, 28-tab pack = £24.64, 84-tab pack

**4**

**Central nervous system**

Central nervous system

(hosp. only) = £73.92. Label: 2, 10, patient information leaflet

Note Patient, prescriber, and supplying pharmacist must be registered with the Clozaril Patient Monitoring Service—takes several days to do this

### Denzapine® (Merz) PoM

Tablets, yellow, scored, clozapine 25 mg, net price 28-tab pack = £6.17, 84-tab pack = £18.49; 50 mg, 50-tab pack = £22.00; 100 mg, 28-tab pack = £24.64, 84-tab pack = £73.92; 200 mg, 50-tab pack = £88.00. Label: 2, 10, patient information leaflet

Suspension, clozapine 50 mg/mL, net price 100 mL = £44.00. Label: 2, 10, patient information leaflet, counselling, administration

Counselling Shake well for 90 seconds when dispensing or if visibly settled; otherwise shake well for 10 seconds before use

Note May be diluted with water

Note Patient, prescriber, and supplying pharmacist must be registered with the Denzapine Patient Monitoring Service—takes several days to do this

### Zaponex® (IVAX) PoM

Tablets, yellow, scored, clozapine 25 mg, net price 84-tab pack = £8.28; 100 mg, 84-tab pack = £33.88. Label: 2, 10, patient information leaflet

Note Patient, prescriber, and supplying pharmacist must be registered with the Zaponex Treatment Access System—takes several days to do this

## ▌ OLANZAPINE

**Indications** see under Dose

**Cautions** see notes above; also prostatic hypertrophy, susceptibility to angle-closure glaucoma, paralytic ileus, diabetes mellitus (risk of exacerbation or keto-acidosis), low leucocyte or neutrophil count, bone-marrow depression, hypereosinophilic disorders, myeloproliferative disease, Parkinson's disease; hepatic impairment (Appendix 2); renal impairment (Appendix 3); pregnancy (Appendix 4)

CNS and respiratory depression Blood pressure, pulse and respiratory rate should be monitored for at least 4 hours after intramuscular injection, particularly in those also receiving another antipsychotic or benzodiazepine

**Contra-indications** breast-feeding (Appendix 5); *for injection*, acute myocardial infarction, unstable angina, severe hypotension or bradycardia, sick sinus syndrome, recent heart surgery

**Side-effects** see notes above; also mild, transient antimuscarinic effects (*very rarely* precipitation of angle-closure glaucoma); drowsiness, speech difficulty, exacerbation of Parkinson's disease, abnormal gait, hallucinations, akathisia, asthenia, fatigue, increased appetite, increased body temperature, raised triglyceride concentration, oedema, hyperprolactinaemia (but clinical manifestations rare); urinary incontinence; eosinophilia; *less commonly* hypotension, bradycardia, QT interval prolongation, photosensitivity; *rarely* seizures, leucopenia, rash; *very rarely* thromboembolism, hypercholesterolaemia, hypothermia, urinary retention, priapism, thrombocytopenia, neutropenia, rhabdomyolysis, hepatitis, pancreatitis and alopecia; *with injection*, injection-site reactions, sinus pause, hypoventilation

**Dose**

● Schizophrenia, combination therapy for mania, preventing recurrence in bipolar disorder, by mouth, ADULT over 18 years, 10 mg daily adjusted to usual range of 5–20 mg daily; doses greater than 10 mg

daily only after reassessment; max. 20 mg daily; CHILD 12–18 years, see *BNF for Children*

● Monotherapy for mania, by mouth, ADULT over 18 years, 15 mg daily adjusted to usual range of 5–20 mg daily; doses greater than 15 mg only after reassessment; max. 20 mg daily; CHILD 12–18 years, see *BNF for Children*

● Control of agitation and disturbed behaviour in schizophrenia or mania, by intramuscular injection, ADULT over 18 years, initially 5–10 mg (usual dose 10 mg) as a single dose followed by 5–10 mg after 2 hours if necessary; ELDERLY initially 2.5–5 mg as a single dose followed by 2.5–5 mg after 2 hours if necessary; max. 3 injections daily for 3 days; max. daily combined oral and parenteral dose 20 mg

Note When one or more factors present that might result in slower metabolism (e.g. female gender, elderly, non-smoker) consider lower initial dose and more gradual dose increase

### Zyprexa® (Lilly) PoM

Tablets, f/c, olanzapine 2.5 mg, net price 28-tab pack = £21.85; 5 mg, 28-tab pack = £43.70; 7.5 mg, 56-tab pack = £131.10; 10 mg, 28-tab pack = £79.45, 15 mg (blue), 28-tab pack = £119.18; 20 mg (pink), 28-tab pack = £158.90. Label: 2

Orodispersible tablet (*Velotab®*), yellow, olanzapine 5 mg, net price 28-tab pack = £43.70; 10 mg, 28-tab pack = £79.45; 15 mg, 28-tab pack = £119.18; 20 mg, 28-tab pack = £158.90. Label: 2, counselling, administration

Excipients include aspartame (section 9.4.1)

Counselling *Velotab®* may be placed on the tongue and allowed to dissolve or dispersed in water, orange juice, apple juice, milk, or coffee

Injection▼, powder for reconstitution, olanzapine 5 mg/mL, net price 10-mg vial = £3.48

## ▌ PALIPERIDONE

Note Paliperidone is a metabolite of risperidone

**Indications** schizophrenia

**Cautions** see notes above; predisposition to gastro-intestinal obstruction; elderly patients with dementia and risk factors for stroke; Parkinson's disease; severe hepatic impairment; renal impairment (avoid if eGFR less than 10 mL/minute/1.73 m²; Appendix 3); pregnancy (Appendix 4)

**Contra-indications** breast-feeding (Appendix 5)

**Side-effects** see notes above; also abdominal pain, dry mouth, hypersalivation, vomiting; tachycardia, bradycardia, first-degree AV block, bundle branch block; drowsiness, headache, asthenia; *less commonly* palpitation, arrhythmias, ischaemia, oedema, seizures, nightmare, syncope, menstrual disturbances, erectile dysfunction, galactorrhoea, and gynaecomastia

**Dose**

● ADULT over 18 years, 6 mg once daily in the morning, adjusted if necessary in increments of 3 mg over at least 5 days; usual range 3–12 mg daily

Counselling Always take with breakfast or always take on an empty stomach

### Invega® (Janssen-Cilag) ▼ PoM

Tablets, m/r, paliperidone 3 mg (white), net price 28-tab pack = £97.28; 6 mg (beige), 28-tab pack = £97.28; 9 mg (pink), 28-tab pack = £145.92. Label: 2, 25, counselling, administration

## ▲ QUETIAPINE

**Indications** schizophrenia; treatment of episodes of mania either alone or with mood stabilisers

**Cautions** see notes above; also hepatic impairment (Appendix 2); renal impairment (Appendix 3); pregnancy (Appendix 4); cerebrovascular disease

**Contra-indications** breast-feeding (Appendix 5)

**Side-effects** see notes above; also dry mouth, constipation, dyspepsia; tachycardia, elevated plasma-triglyceride and cholesterol concentrations, peripheral oedema; drowsiness, headache, asthenia; leucopenia, neutropenia; rhinitis; *less commonly* seizures, restless legs syndrome, and eosinophilia; *rarely* jaundice and priapism; *very rarely* hepatitis, angioedema, and Stevens-Johnson syndrome

**Dose**

- Schizophrenia, ADULT over 18 years, 25 mg twice daily on day 1, 50 mg twice daily on day 2, 100 mg twice daily on day 3, 150 mg twice daily on day 4, then adjusted according to response, usual range 300–450 mg daily in 2 divided doses; max. 750 mg daily; ELDERLY initially 25 mg daily as a single dose, increased in steps of 25–50 mg daily in 2 divided doses; CHILD 12–18 years, see *BNF for Children*

- Mania, ADULT over 18 years, 50 mg twice daily on day 1, 100 mg twice daily on day 2, 150 mg twice daily on day 3, 200 mg twice daily on day 4, then adjusted according to response in steps of up to 200 mg daily to max. 800 mg daily; usual range 400–800 mg daily in 2 divided doses; ELDERLY initially 25 mg daily as a single dose, increased in steps of 25–50 mg daily in 2 divided doses

**Seroquel®** (AstraZeneca) ⟨PoM⟩
Tablets, f/c, quetiapine (as fumarate) 25 mg (peach), net price 60-tab pack = £33.83; 100 mg (yellow), 60-tab pack = £113.10; 150 mg (pale yellow), 60-tab pack = £113.10; 200 mg (white), 60-tab pack = £113.10; 300 mg (white), 60-tab pack = £170.00. Label: 2

◢Modified release

**Seroquel® XL** (AstraZeneca) ▼ ⟨PoM⟩
Tablets, m/r, quetiapine (as fumarate) 50 mg (peach), net price 60-tab pack = £67.66; 200 mg (yellow), 60-tab pack = £113.10; 300 mg (pale yellow), 60-tab pack = £170.00; 400 mg (white), 60-tab pack = £226.20. Label: 2, 23, 25

Dose schizophrenia, mania, ADULT over 18 years, 300 mg once daily on day 1, then 600 mg once daily on day 2, then adjusted according to response; dose range 400–800 mg once daily; ELDERLY initially 50 mg once daily adjusted according to response in steps of 50 mg daily

## ▲ RISPERIDONE

**Indications** acute and chronic psychoses, mania; short-term treatment (up to 6 weeks) of persistent aggression in patients with moderate to severe Alzheimer's dementia unresponsive to non-pharmacological interventions and when there is a risk of harm to self or others; short-term treatment (up to 6 weeks) of persistent aggression in conduct disorder (under specialist supervision)

**Cautions** see notes above; Parkinson's disease; dementia with Lewy bodies; dehydration; avoid in acute porphyria (section 9.8.2); hepatic impairment (Appendix 2); renal impairment (Appendix 3); pregnancy (Appendix 4); breast-feeding (Appendix 5)

**Side-effects** see notes above; also gastro-intestinal disturbances (including diarrhoea, constipation, nausea and vomiting, dyspepsia, abdominal pain), dry mouth; dyspnoea; drowsiness, asthenia, tremor, sleep disturbances, agitation, anxiety, headache; urinary incontinence; arthralgia, myalgia; abnormal vision; epistaxis; rash; *less commonly* anorexia, ECG changes, hypoaesthesia, impaired concentration, hyperprolactinaemia (with galactorrhoea, menstrual disturbances, gynaecomastia), sexual dysfunction, blood disorders, tinnitus, angioedema; *rarely* intestinal obstruction, pancreatitis, jaundice, seizures, hyponatraemia, abnormal temperature regulation; oedema and priapism also reported

**Dose**

- Psychoses, 2 mg in 1–2 divided doses on first day *then* 4 mg in 1–2 divided doses on second day (slower titration appropriate in some patients); usual dose range 4–6 mg daily; doses above 10 mg daily only if benefit considered to outweigh risk (max. 16 mg daily); ELDERLY initially 500 micrograms twice daily increased in steps of 500 micrograms twice daily to 1–2 mg twice daily; CHILD 12–18 years see *BNF for Children*

- Mania, initially 2 mg once daily, increased if necessary in steps of 1 mg daily; usual dose range 1–6 mg daily; ELDERLY initially 500 micrograms twice daily increased in steps of 500 micrograms twice daily to 1–2 mg twice daily

- Persistent aggression in Alzheimer's dementia, initially 250 micrograms twice daily, increased according to response in steps of 250 micrograms twice daily on alternate days; usual dose 500 micrograms twice daily (up to 1 mg twice daily has been required)

- Persistent aggression in conduct disorder, CHILD over 5 years, body-weight under 50 kg, initially 250 micrograms once daily, increased according to response in steps of 250 micrograms on alternate days; usual dose 500 micrograms daily (up to 750 micrograms once daily has been required); CHILD over 5 years, body-weight over 50 kg, initially 500 micrograms once daily, increased according to response in steps of 500 micrograms on alternate days; usual dose 1 mg daily (up to 1.5 mg once daily has been required)

**Risperidone** (Non-proprietary) ▼ ⟨PoM⟩
Tablets, risperidone 500 micrograms, net price 20-tab pack = £3.08; 1 mg, 20-tab pack = £4.96, 60-tab pack = £14.44; 2 mg, 60-tab pack = £27.84; 3 mg, 60-tab pack = £39.90; 4 mg, 60-tab pack = £54.31; 6 mg, 28-tab pack = £39.55. Label: 2

Orodispersible tablets, risperidone 0.5 mg, net price 28-tab pack = £8.69; 1 mg, 28-tab pack = £18.39; 2 mg, 28-tab pack = £33.30. Label: 2, counselling, administration
**Counselling** Tablets should be placed on the tongue, allowed to dissolve and swallowed

Liquid, risperidone 1 mg/mL, net price 100-mL pack = £55.23. Label: 2, counselling, use of dose syringe
**Note** Liquid may be diluted with mineral water, orange juice or black coffee (should be taken immediately)

**Risperdal®** (Janssen-Cilag) ▼ ⟨PoM⟩
Tablets, f/c, scored, risperidone 500 micrograms (brown-red), net price 20-tab pack = £6.78; 1 mg (white), 20-tab pack = £11.16, 60-tab pack = £33.48; 2 mg (orange), 60-tab pack = £66.01; 3 mg (yellow), 60-tab pack = £97.07; 4 mg (green), 60-tab pack = £128.14; 6 mg (yellow), 28-tab pack = £90.60. Label: 2

Orodispersible tablets (*Quicklet®*), pink, risperidone 500 micrograms, net price 28-tab pack = £10.98; 1 mg, 28-tab pack = £17.67; 2 mg, 28-tab pack = £33.31; 3 mg, 28-tab pack = £48.38; 4 mg, 28-tab pack = £62.31. Label: 2, counselling, administration
Excipients include aspartame (section 9.4.1)
**Counselling** Tablets should be placed on the tongue, allowed to dissolve and swallowed

Liquid, risperidone 1 mg/mL, net price 100 mL = £53.93. Label: 2, counselling, use of dose syringe
**Note** Liquid may be diluted with mineral water, orange juice or black coffee (should be taken immediately)

◀**Depot preparation**
Section 4.2.2

## SERTINDOLE

**Indications** schizophrenia, see also notes above
**Cautions** see notes above; hepatic impairment (Appendix 2); correct hypokalaemia or hypomagnesaemia before treatment; monitor ECG during treatment; monitor blood pressure during dose titration and early maintenance therapy (risk of postural hypotension)
**Contra-indications** see notes above; pregnancy (Appendix 4), breast-feeding (Appendix 5), severe hepatic impairment, QT interval prolongation (ECG required before and during treatment—consult product literature); concomitant administration of drugs which prolong QT interval (see interactions); uncorrected hypokalaemia or hypomagnesaemia
**Side-effects** see notes above; prolonged QT interval, peripheral oedema, dry mouth, rhinitis, nasal congestion, dyspnoea, paraesthesia, abnormal ejaculation (decreased volume); *rarely* seizures, hyperglycaemia
**Dose**
- Initially 4 mg daily increased in steps of 4 mg at intervals of 4–5 days to usual maintenance of 12–20 mg as a single daily dose; max. 24 mg daily; ELDERLY consider slower dose titration and lower maintenance dose; CHILD and ADOLESCENT not recommended

**Serdolect®** (Lundbeck) ▼ PoM
Tablets, f/c, sertindole 4 mg, 30-tab pack; 12 mg 28-tab pack; 16 mg, 28-tab pack; 20 mg 28-tab pack
Available only on named-patient basis (see notes above)

## ZOTEPINE

**Indications** schizophrenia
**Cautions** see notes above; personal or close family history of epilepsy; withdrawal of concomitantly prescribed CNS depressants; QT interval prolongation—ECG required (before treatment and at each dose increase) in patients at risk of arrhythmias; monitor plasma electrolytes particularly before treatment and at each dose increase; hepatic impairment (Appendix 2); renal impairment (Appendix 3); prostatic hypertrophy, urinary retention, susceptibility to angle-closure glaucoma, paralytic ileus, pregnancy (Appendix 4)
**Contra-indications** acute intoxication with CNS depressants; high doses of concomitantly prescribed antipsychotics; acute gout (avoid for 3 weeks after episode resolves), history of nephrolithiasis; breast-feeding (Appendix 5)
**Side-effects** see notes above; constipation, dyspepsia, dry mouth, tachycardia, QT interval prolongation,

rhinitis, agitation, anxiety, depression, asthenia, headache, EEG abnormalities, insomnia, drowsiness, hyperthermia or hypothermia, increased salivation, blood dyscrasias (including leucocytosis, leucopenia), raised erythrocyte sedimentation rate, blurred vision, sweating; *less frequently* anorexia, diarrhoea, nausea and vomiting, abdominal pain, hypertension, influenza-like syndrome, cough, dyspnoea, confusion, convulsions, decreased libido, speech disorder, vertigo, hyperprolactinaemia, anaemia, thrombocythaemia, increased serum creatinine, hypoglycaemia and hyperglycaemia, hyperlipidaemia, hypouricaemia, oedema, thirst, impotence, urinary incontinence, arthralgia, myalgia, conjunctivitis, acne, dry skin, rash; *rarely* bradycardia, epistaxis, abdominal enlargement, amnesia, ataxia, coma, delirium, hypaesthesia, myoclonus, thrombocytopenia, abnormal ejaculation, urinary retention, menstrual irregularities, myasthenia, alopecia, photosensitivity; *very rarely* angle-closure glaucoma
**Dose**
- Initially 25 mg 3 times daily increased according to response at intervals of 4 days to max. 100 mg 3 times daily; ELDERLY initially 25 mg twice daily increased according to response to max. 75 mg twice daily; CHILD and ADOLESCENT under 18 years not recommended

**Zoleptil®** (Healthcare Logistics) PoM
Tablets, s/c, zotepine 25 mg (white), net price 30-tab pack = £21.50, 90-tab pack = £42.98; 50 mg (yellow), 30-tab pack = £28.65, 90-tab pack = £57.30; 100 mg (pink), 30-tab pack = £47.28, 90-tab pack = £94.55. Label: 2

## 4.2.2 Antipsychotic depot injections

Long-acting depot injections are used for maintenance therapy especially when compliance with oral treatment is unreliable. However, depot injections of conventional antipsychotics may give rise to a higher incidence of extrapyramidal reactions than oral preparations; extrapyramidal reactions occur less frequently with atypical antipsychotics such as risperidone.

**Administration** Depot antipsychotics are administered by deep intramuscular injection at intervals of 1 to 4 weeks. When initiating therapy with sustained-release preparations of conventional antipsychotics, patients should first be given a small test-dose as undesirable side-effects are prolonged. In general not more than 2–3 mL of oily injection should be administered at any one site; correct injection technique (including the use of z-track technique) and rotation of injection sites are essential. If the dose needs to be reduced to alleviate side-effects, it is important to recognise that the plasma-drug concentration may not fall for some time after reducing the dose, therefore it may be a month or longer before side-effects subside.

> **Dosage** Individual responses to neuroleptic drugs are very variable and to achieve optimum effect, dosage and dosage interval must be titrated according to the patient's response. For the advice of The Royal College of Psychiatrists on doses above the BNF upper limit, see p. 193.

| **Equivalent doses of depot antipsychotics** | | |
| :--- | :--- | :--- |

These equivalences are intended **only** as an approximate guide; individual dosage instructions should **also** be checked; patients should be carefully monitored after **any** change in medication

| Antipsychotic drug | Dose (mg) | Interval |
| :--- | :--- | :--- |
| Flupentixol decanoate | 40 | 2 weeks |
| Fluphenazine decanoate | 25 | 2 weeks |
| Haloperidol (as decanoate) | 100 | 4 weeks |
| Pipotiazine palmitate | 50 | 4 weeks |
| Zuclopenthixol decanoate | 200 | 2 weeks |

**Important** These equivalences must **not** be extrapolated beyond the maximum dose for the drug

**Choice** There is no clear-cut division in the use of the conventional antipsychotics, but **zuclopenthixol** may be suitable for the treatment of agitated or aggressive patients whereas **flupentixol** can cause over-excitement in such patients. The incidence of extrapyramidal reactions is similar for the conventional antipsychotics.

**Cautions** See section 4.2.1. Treatment requires careful monitoring for optimum effect. When transferring from oral to depot therapy, dosage by mouth should be reduced gradually.

**Contra-indications** See section 4.2.1. Do not use in children.

**Side-effects** See section 4.2.1. Pain may occur at injection site and occasionally erythema, swelling, and nodules. For side-effects of specific antipsychotics see under the relevant drug.

### ▮ FLUPENTIXOL DECANOATE
(Flupenthixol Decanoate)

**Indications** maintenance in schizophrenia and other psychoses

**Cautions** see notes on p. 194 and also under Flupentixol (section 4.2.1) and notes above; an alternative antipsychotic may be necessary if symptoms such as aggression or agitation appear

**Contra-indications** see notes on p. 194 and also under Flupentixol (section 4.2.1) and notes above

**Side-effects** see notes on p. 194 and also under Flupentixol (section 4.2.1) and notes above, but may have a mood elevating effect

**Dose**
- By deep intramuscular injection into the upper outer buttock or lateral thigh, test dose 20 mg, then after at least 7 days 20–40 mg repeated at intervals of 2–4 weeks, adjusted according to response; max. 400 mg weekly; usual maintenance dose 50 mg every 4 weeks to 300 mg every 2 weeks; ELDERLY initially quarter to half adult dose; CHILD not recommended

**Depixol®** (Lundbeck) [PoM]
Injection (oily), flupentixol decanoate 20 mg/mL. Net price 1-mL amp = £1.06; 2-mL amp = £1.78

**Depixol Conc.®** (Lundbeck) [PoM]
Injection (oily), flupentixol decanoate 100 mg/mL. Net price 0.5-mL amp = £2.39; 1-mL amp = £4.38

**Depixol Low Volume®** (Lundbeck) [PoM]
Injection (oily), flupentixol decanoate 200 mg/mL. Net price 1-mL amp = £13.66

### ▮ FLUPHENAZINE DECANOATE

**Indications** maintenance in schizophrenia and other psychoses

**Cautions** see notes on p. 194 and also notes above

**Contra-indications** see notes on p. 194 and also notes above; also marked cerebral atherosclerosis

**Side-effects** see notes on p. 194 and notes above; less sedating and fewer antimuscarinic or hypotensive symptoms, but extrapyramidal symptoms, particularly dystonic reactions and akathisia, more frequent; systemic lupus erythematosus, inappropriate anti-diuretic hormone secretion, oedema, also reported; extrapyramidal symptoms usually appear a few hours after injection and continue for about 2 days but may be delayed

**Dose**
- By deep intramuscular injection into the gluteal muscle, test dose 12.5 mg (6.25 mg in elderly), then after 4–7 days 12.5–100 mg repeated at intervals of 14–35 days, adjusted according to response; CHILD not recommended

**Fluphenazine decanoate** (Non-proprietary) [PoM]
Injection (oily), fluphenazine decanoate 25 mg/mL, net price 1-mL amp = £2.35; 100 mg/mL, 0.5-mL amp = £4.50, 1-mL amp = £8.79
Excipients include sesame oil

**Modecate®** (Sanofi-Synthelabo) [PoM]
Injection (oily), fluphenazine decanoate 25 mg/mL. Net price 0.5-mL amp = £1.30, 1-mL amp = £2.26, 2-mL amp = £4.44
Excipients include sesame oil

**Modecate Concentrate®** (Sanofi-Synthelabo) [PoM]
Injection (oily), fluphenazine decanoate 100 mg/mL. Net price 0.5-mL amp = £4.47, 1-mL amp = £8.75
Excipients include sesame oil

### ▮ HALOPERIDOL

**Indications** maintenance in schizophrenia and other psychoses

**Cautions** see notes on p. 194 and also under Haloperidol (section 4.2.1) and notes above

**Contra-indications** see notes on p. 194 and also under Haloperidol (section 4.2.1) and notes above

**Side-effects** see notes on p. 194 and also under Haloperidol (section 4.2.1) and notes above

**Dose**
- By deep intramuscular injection into the gluteal muscle, initially 50 mg every 4 weeks, if necessary increasing by 50-mg increments to 300 mg every 4 weeks; higher doses may be needed in some patients; ELDERLY, initially 12.5–25 mg every 4 weeks; CHILD not recommended
**Note** If 2-weekly administration preferred, doses should be halved

**Haldol Decanoate®** (Janssen-Cilag) [PoM]
Injection (oily), haloperidol (as decanoate) 50 mg/mL, net price 1-mL amp = £3.89; 100 mg/mL, 1-mL amp = £5.15
Excipients include sesame oil

**4**

**Central nervous system**

4 Central nervous system

## ■ PIPOTIAZINE PALMITATE
### (Pipothiazine Palmitate)

**Indications** maintenance in schizophrenia and other psychoses

**Cautions** see notes on p. 194 and notes above

**Contra-indications** see notes on p. 194 and notes above

**Side-effects** see notes on p. 194 and notes above

**Dose**
- By deep intramuscular injection into the gluteal muscle, test dose 25 mg, then a further 25–50 mg after 4–7 days, then adjusted according to response at intervals of 4 weeks; usual maintenance range 50–100 mg (max. 200 mg) every 4 weeks; ELDERLY initially 5–10 mg; CHILD not recommended

**Piportil Depot®** (Sanofi-Aventis) [PoM]
Injection (oily), pipotiazine palmitate 50 mg/mL. Net price 1-mL amp = £16.29; 2-mL amp = £26.65
Excipients include sesame oil

## ■ RISPERIDONE

**Indications** schizophrenia and other psychoses in patients tolerant to risperidone by mouth

**Cautions** see under Risperidone (section 4.2.1) and notes above

**Side-effects** see under Risperidone (section 4.2.1); also hypertension; depression, paraesthesia; *less commonly* apathy, weight loss, injection-site reactions, and pruritus

**Dose**
- By deep intramuscular injection into the gluteal muscle, patients taking oral risperidone up to 4 mg daily, initially 25 mg every 2 weeks; patients taking oral risperidone over 4 mg daily, initially 37.5 mg every 2 weeks; dose adjusted at intervals of at least 4 weeks in steps of 12.5 mg to max. 50 mg (ELDERLY 25 mg) every 2 weeks; CHILD and ADOLESCENT under 18 years not recommended
**Note** During initiation risperidone by mouth may need to be continued for 4–6 weeks; risperidone by mouth may also be used during dose adjustment of depot injection

**Risperdal Consta®** (Janssen-Cilag) ▼ [PoM]
Injection, powder for reconstitution, risperidone 25-mg vial, net price = £79.69; 37.5-mg vial = £111.32; 50-mg vial = £142.76 (all with diluent)

## ■ ZUCLOPENTHIXOL DECANOATE

**Indications** maintenance in schizophrenia and paranoid psychoses

**Cautions** see notes on p. 194 and notes above; avoid in acute porphyria (section 9.8.2)

**Contra-indications** see notes on p. 194 and notes above

**Side-effects** see notes on p. 194 and notes above

**Dose**
- By deep intramuscular injection into the upper outer buttock or lateral thigh, test dose 100 mg, followed after at least 7 days by 200–500 mg or more, repeated at intervals of 1–4 weeks, adjusted according to response; max. 600 mg weekly; ELDERLY quarter to half usual starting dose; CHILD not recommended

**Clopixol®** (Lundbeck) [PoM]
Injection (oily), zuclopenthixol decanoate 200 mg/mL, net price 1-mL amp = £2.21

**Clopixol Conc.®** (Lundbeck) [PoM]
Injection (oily), zuclopenthixol decanoate 500 mg/mL, net price 1-mL amp = £5.21

## 4.2.3 Antimanic drugs

Drugs are used in mania to control acute attacks and to prevent their recurrence.

### Benzodiazepines

Use of benzodiazepines (section 4.1) may be helpful in the initial stages of treatment until lithium achieves its full effect; they should not be used for long periods because of the risk of dependence.

### Antipsychotic drugs

In an acute attack of mania, treatment with an antipsychotic drug (section 4.2.1) is usually required because it may take a few days for lithium to exert its antimanic effect. Lithium may be given concurrently with the antipsychotic drug, and treatment with the antipsychotic gradually tailed off as lithium becomes effective. Alternatively, lithium therapy may be commenced once the patient's mood has been stabilised with the antipsychotic. The adjunctive use of atypical antipsychotics such as olanzapine (section 4.2.1) and risperidone with either lithium or valproic acid may also be of benefit.

High doses of haloperidol or flupentixol may be hazardous when used with lithium; irreversible toxic encephalopathy has been reported.

### Carbamazepine

Carbamazepine (section 4.8.1) may be used for the prophylaxis of bipolar disorder (manic-depressive disorder) in patients unresponsive to lithium; it seems to be particularly effective in patients with rapid-cycling manic-depressive illness (4 or more affective episodes per year).

### Valproic acid

Valproic acid (as the semisodium salt) is licensed for the treatment of manic episodes associated with bipolar disorder. It may be useful in patients unresponsive to lithium.

Sodium valproate (section 4.8.1) has also been used, but it is unlicensed for this indication.

## ■ VALPROIC ACID

**Indications** treatment of manic episodes associated with bipolar disorder

**Cautions** see Sodium Valproate (section 4.8.1); monitor closely if dose greater than 45 mg/kg daily

**Contra-indications** see Sodium Valproate (section 4.8.1)

**Side-effects** see Sodium Valproate (section 4.8.1)

**Dose**

- Initially 750 mg daily in 2–3 divided doses, increased according to response, usual dose 1–2 g daily; CHILD and ADOLESCENT under 18 years not recommended

**Depakote®** (Sanofi-Aventis) PoM

Tablets, e/c, valproic acid (as semisodium valproate) 250 mg, net price 90-tab pack = £12.17; 500 mg, 90-tab pack = £24.29. Label: 25

Note Semisodium valproate comprises equimolar amounts of sodium valproate and valproic acid

**Convulex®** (Pharmacia) PoM

Section 4.8.1 (epilepsy)

## Lithium

Lithium salts are used in the prophylaxis and treatment of mania, in the prophylaxis of bipolar disorder (manic-depressive disorder) and in the prophylaxis of recurrent depression (unipolar illness or unipolar depression). Lithium is unsuitable for children.

The decision to give prophylactic lithium usually requires *specialist advice*, and must be based on careful consideration of the likelihood of recurrence in the individual patient, and the benefit weighed against the risks. In long-term use lithium has been associated with thyroid disorders and mild cognitive and memory impairment. Long-term treatment should therefore be undertaken only with careful assessment of risk and benefit, and with regular monitoring of thyroid function. The need for continued therapy should be assessed regularly and patients should be maintained on lithium after 3–5 years only if benefit persists.

**Serum concentrations** Lithium salts have a narrow therapeutic/toxic ratio and should therefore not be prescribed unless facilities for monitoring serum-lithium concentrations are available. There seem few if any reasons for preferring one or other of the salts of lithium available. Doses are adjusted to achieve serum-lithium concentration of 0.4–1 mmol/litre (lower end of the range for maintenance therapy and elderly patients) on samples taken 12 hours after the preceding dose. It is important to determine the optimum range for each individual patient.

Overdosage, usually with serum-lithium concentration of over 1.5 mmol/litre, may be fatal and toxic effects include tremor, ataxia, dysarthria, nystagmus, renal impairment, and convulsions. If these potentially hazardous signs occur, treatment should be stopped, serum-lithium concentrations redetermined, and steps taken to reverse lithium toxicity. In mild cases withdrawal of lithium and administration of generous amounts of sodium salts and fluid will reverse the toxicity. Serum-lithium concentration in excess of 2 mmol/litre require urgent treatment as indicated under Emergency Treatment of Poisoning, p. 33.

**Interactions** Lithium toxicity is made worse by sodium depletion, therefore concurrent use of diuretics (particularly thiazides) is hazardous and should be avoided. For other **interactions** with lithium, see Appendix 1 (lithium).

**Withdrawal** While there is no clear evidence of withdrawal or rebound psychosis, abrupt discontinuation of lithium increases the risk of relapse. If lithium is to be discontinued, the dose should be reduced gradually over a period of a few weeks and patients should be warned of possible relapse if it is discontinued abruptly.

> **Lithium cards**
>
> A lithium treatment card available from pharmacies tells patients how to take lithium preparations, what to do if a dose is missed, and what side-effects to expect. It also explains why regular blood tests are important and warns that some medicines and illnesses can change serum-lithium concentration. Cards may be purchased from the National Pharmacy Association.
> Tel: (01727) 858 687
> sales@npa.co.uk

### ■ LITHIUM CARBONATE

**Indications** treatment and prophylaxis of mania, bipolar disorder, and recurrent depression (see also notes above); aggressive or self-mutilating behaviour

**Cautions** measure serum-lithium concentration regularly (every 3 months on stabilised regimens), measure renal function and thyroid function every 6–12 months on stabilised regimens and advise patient to seek attention if symptoms of hypothyroidism develop (women at greater risk) e.g. lethargy, feeling cold; maintain adequate sodium and fluid intake; test renal function before initiating and if evidence of toxicity, avoid in renal impairment (Appendix 3), cardiac disease, and conditions with sodium imbalance such as Addison's disease; reduce dose or discontinue in diarrhoea, vomiting and intercurrent infection (especially if sweating profusely); psoriasis (risk of exacerbation); pregnancy (Appendix 4), breast-feeding (Appendix 5), elderly (reduce dose), diuretic treatment, myasthenia gravis; surgery (section 15.1); avoid abrupt withdrawal (see notes above); **interactions:** Appendix 1 (lithium)

Counselling Patients should maintain adequate fluid intake and avoid dietary changes which reduce or increase sodium intake; lithium treatment cards are available from pharmacies (see above)

**Side-effects** gastro-intestinal disturbances, fine tremor, renal impairment (particularly impaired urinary concentration and polyuria), polydipsia, leucocytosis; also weight gain and oedema (may respond to dose reduction); hyperparathyroidism and hypercalcaemia reported; signs of intoxication are blurred vision, increasing gastro-intestinal disturbances (anorexia, vomiting, diarrhoea), muscle weakness, increased CNS disturbances (mild drowsiness and sluggishness increasing to giddiness with ataxia, coarse tremor, lack of co-ordination, dysarthria), and require withdrawal of treatment; with severe **overdosage** (serum-lithium concentration above 2 mmol/litre) hyperreflexia and hyperextension of limbs, convulsions, toxic psychoses, syncope, renal failure, circulatory failure, coma, and occasionally, death; goitre, raised antidiuretic hormone concentration, hypothyroidism, hypokalaemia, ECG changes, and kidney changes may also occur; see also Emergency Treatment of Poisoning, p. 33

**Dose**

- See under preparations below, adjusted to achieve a serum-lithium concentration of 0.4–1 mmol/litre 12 hours after a dose on days 4–7 of treatment, then

4    Central nervous system

**Central nervous system** 4

every week until dosage has remained constant for 4 weeks and every 3 months thereafter; doses are initially divided throughout the day, but once daily administration is preferred when serum-lithium concentration stabilised

**Note Preparations vary widely in bioavailability**; changing the preparation requires the same precautions as initiation of treatment

Note Lithium carbonate 200 mg ≡ lithium citrate 509 mg

**Camcolit®** (Norgine) [PoM]

Camcolit 250® tablets, f/c, scored, lithium carbonate 250 mg (Li⁺ 6.8 mmol), net price 100-tab pack = £3.09. Label: 10, lithium card, counselling, see above

Camcolit 400® tablets, m/r, f/c, scored, lithium carbonate 400 mg (Li⁺ 10.8 mmol), net price 100-tab pack = £4.13. Label: 10, lithium card, 25, counselling, see above

**Dose** (see Dose above for advice on bioavailability and serum monitoring):
ADULT and CHILD over 12 years, treatment, initially 1–1.5 g daily; prophylaxis, initially 300–400 mg daily
Note Camcolit 400® also available as Lithonate® (TEVA UK)

**Liskonum®** (GSK) [PoM]

Tablets, m/r, f/c, scored, lithium carbonate 450 mg (Li⁺ 12.2 mmol), net price 60-tab pack = £2.88. Label: 10, lithium card, 25, counselling, see above
**Dose** (see Dose above for advice on bioavailability and serum monitoring):
ADULT and CHILD over 12 years, treatment, initially 450–675 mg twice daily (elderly initially 225 mg twice daily); prophylaxis, initially 450 mg twice daily (elderly 225 mg twice daily)

**Priadel®** (Sanofi-Aventis) [PoM]

Tablets, m/r, both scored, lithium carbonate 200 mg (Li⁺ 5.4 mmol), net price 100-tab pack= £2.30; 400 mg (Li⁺ 10.8 mmol), 100-tab pack = £3.35. Label: 10, lithium card, 25, counselling, see above
**Dose** (see Dose above for advice on bioavailability and serum monitoring):
Treatment and prophylaxis, initially 0.4–1.2 g daily as a single dose or in 2 divided doses (elderly or patients less than 50 kg, 400 mg daily); CHILD not recommended

Liquid, see under Lithium Citrate below

---

### ■ LITHIUM CITRATE

**Indications** see under Lithium Carbonate and notes above

**Cautions** see under Lithium Carbonate and notes above
Counselling Patients should maintain an adequate fluid intake and should avoid dietary changes which might reduce or increase sodium intake; lithium treatment cards are available from pharmacies (see above)

**Side-effects** see under Lithium Carbonate and notes above

**Dose**
● See under preparations below, adjusted to achieve serum-lithium concentration of 0.4–1 mmol/litre as described under Lithium Carbonate
Note Preparations vary widely in bioavailability; changing the preparation requires the same precautions as initiation of treatment
Note Lithium carbonate 200 mg ≡ lithium citrate 509 mg

**Li-Liquid®** (Rosemont) [PoM]

Oral solution, lithium citrate 509 mg/5 mL (Li⁺ 5.4 mmol/5 mL), yellow, net price 150-mL pack = £5.79; 1.018 g/5 mL (Li⁺ 10.8 mmol/5 mL), orange,

150-mL pack = £11.58. Label: 10, lithium card, counselling, see above
**Dose** (see Dose above for advice on bioavailability and serum monitoring):
Treatment and prophylaxis, initially 1.018–3.054 g daily in 2 divided doses (elderly or patients less than 50 kg, initially 509 mg twice daily); CHILD not recommended

**Priadel®** (Sanofi-Aventis) [PoM]

Tablets, see under Lithium Carbonate

Liquid, sugar-free, lithium citrate 520 mg/5 mL (approx. Li⁺ 5.4 mmol/5 mL), net price 150-mL pack = £5.61. Label: 10, lithium card, counselling, see above
**Dose** (see Dose above for advice on bioavailability and serum monitoring, see above):
Treatment and prophylaxis, initially 1.04–3.12 g daily in 2 divided doses (elderly or patients less than 50 kg, 520 mg twice daily); CHILD not recommended

## 4.3 Antidepressant drugs

**4.3.1 Tricyclic and related antidepressant drugs**

**4.3.2 Monoamine-oxidase inhibitors**

**4.3.3 Selective serotonin re-uptake inhibitors**

**4.3.4 Other antidepressant drugs**

Antidepressant drugs are effective for treating moderate to severe depression associated with psychomotor and physiological changes such as loss of appetite and sleep disturbance; improvement in sleep is usually the first benefit of therapy. They are also effective for dysthymia (lower grade chronic depression). Antidepressant drugs are not generally effective in mild depression, and cognitive behavioural therapy should be considered initially; however, a trial of antidepressant therapy may be considered in cases refractory to psychological treatments or those associated with psychosocial or medical problems. Drug treatment of mild depression may also be considered in patients with a history of moderate or severe depression.

**Choice** The major classes of antidepressant drugs include the tricyclics and related antidepressants, the selective serotonin re-uptake inhibitors (SSRIs), and the monoamine oxidase inhibitors (MAOIs). A number of antidepressant drugs cannot be accommodated easily into this classification; these are included in section 4.3.4.

There is little to choose between the different classes of antidepressant drugs in terms of efficacy, so choice should be based on the individual patient's requirements, including the presence of concomitant disease, existing therapy, suicide risk, and previous response to antidepressant therapy. Since there may be an interval of 2 weeks before the antidepressant action takes place, electroconvulsive treatment may be required in severe depression when delay is hazardous or intolerable.

SSRIs are better tolerated and are safer in overdose than other classes of antidepressants and should be considered first-line for treating depression. In patients with unstable angina or who have had a recent myocardial infarction, sertraline has been shown to be safe.

Tricyclic antidepressants have similar efficacy to SSRIs but are more likely to be discontinued because of side-effects; toxicity in overdosage is also a problem. See section 4.3.1 for more details.

MAOIs have dangerous interactions with some foods and drugs, and should be reserved for use by specialists.

Although anxiety is often present in depressive illness (and may be the presenting symptom), the use of an antipsychotic or an anxiolytic may mask the true diagnosis. Anxiolytics (section 4.1.2) or antipsychotic drugs (section 4.2.1) should therefore be used with caution in depression but they are useful adjuncts in agitated patients.

See also section 4.2.3 for references to the management of bipolar disorders.

**St John's wort** (*Hypericum perforatum*) is a popular herbal remedy on sale to the public for treating mild depression. However, preparations of St John's wort can induce drug metabolising enzymes and a number of important interactions with conventional drugs have been identified, see Appendix 1 (St John's wort). The amount of active ingredient can vary between different preparations of St John's wort and switching from one to another can change the degree of enzyme induction. Furthermore, when a patient stops taking St John's wort, concentrations of interacting drugs may increase, leading to toxicity. Antidepressant drugs should **not** be used with St John's wort because of the potential for interaction.

---

**Hyponatraemia and antidepressant therapy**
Hyponatraemia (usually in the elderly and possibly due to inappropriate secretion of antidiuretic hormone) has been associated with all types of antidepressants; however, it has been reported more frequently with SSRIs than with other antidepressants. The CSM has advised that hyponatraemia should be considered in all patients who develop drowsiness, confusion, or convulsions while taking an antidepressant.

---

**Suicidal behaviour and antidepressant therapy**
The use of antidepressants has been linked with suicidal thoughts and behaviour; children, young adults, and patients with a history of suicidal behaviour are particularly at risk. Where necessary patients should be monitored for suicidal behaviour, self-harm, or hostility, particularly at the beginning of treatment or if the dose is changed.

---

**Management** Patients should be reviewed every 1–2 weeks at the start of antidepressant treatment. Treatment should be continued for at least 4 weeks (6 weeks in the elderly) before considering whether to switch antidepressant due to lack of efficacy. In cases of partial response, continue for a further 2 weeks (elderly patients may take longer to respond).

Following remission, antidepressant treatment should be continued at the same dose for at least 6 months (about 12 months in the elderly). Patients with a history of recurrent depression should continue to receive maintenance treatment for at least 2 years.

**Failure to respond** Failure to respond to initial treatment with an SSRI may require an increase in the dose, or switching to a different SSRI or mirtazapine; in

patients with atypical depression, an MAOI such as phenelzine may be effective. Other second-line choices include lofepramine, moclobemide, and reboxetine. Other tricyclic antidepressants and venlafaxine should be considered for more severe forms of depression; dosulepin (dothiepin) and irreversible MAOIs should only be prescribed by specialists. Failure to respond to a second antidepressant may require the addition of another antidepressant of a different class, or an augmenting agent such as lithium, but such adjunctive treatment should be initiated only by doctors with special experience of these combinations. Electroconvulsive therapy may be initiated in severe refractory depression.

**Withdrawal** Gastro-intestinal symptoms of nausea, vomiting, and anorexia, accompanied by headache, giddiness, 'chills', and insomnia, and sometimes by hypomania, panic-anxiety, and extreme motor restlessness may occur if an antidepressant (particularly an MAOI) is stopped suddenly after regular administration for 8 weeks or more. The dose should preferably be reduced gradually over about 4 weeks, or longer if withdrawal symptoms emerge (6 months in patients who have been on long-term maintenance treatment). SSRIs have been associated with a specific withdrawal syndrome (section 4.3.3).

**Anxiety disorders and obsessive-compulsive disorder** Management of acute anxiety generally involves the use of a benzodiazepine or buspirone (section 4.1.2). For chronic anxiety (of longer than 4 weeks' duration) it may be appropriate to use an antidepressant. Combined therapy with a benzodiazepine may be required until the antidepressant takes effect. *Generalised anxiety disorder*, a form of chronic anxiety, is treated with an SSRI such as escitalopram or paroxetine; pregabalin and venlafaxine are also licensed for the treatment of generalised anxiety disorder.

*Panic disorder, obsessive-compulsive disorder, post-traumatic stress disorder*, and phobic states such as *social anxiety disorder* are treated with SSRIs. Clomipramine or imipramine can be used second-line in panic disorder [unlicensed]; clomipramine can also be used second-line for obsessive-compulsive disorder. Moclobemide is licensed for the treatment of social anxiety disorder.

---

## 4.3.1 Tricyclic and related antidepressant drugs

This section covers tricyclic antidepressants and also 1-, 2-, and 4-ring structured drugs with broadly similar properties.

Some tricyclic antidepressants are used in the management of *panic disorder* (section 4.3). For reference to the role of some tricyclic antidepressants in some forms of *neuralgia*, see section 4.7.3, and in *nocturnal enuresis* in children, see section 7.4.2.

**Cautions** Tricyclic and related antidepressant drugs should be used with caution in patients with cardiovascular disease (see also Contra-indications, below); because of the risk of arrhythmias, patients with concomitant conditions such as hyperthyroidism and phaeochromocytoma should be treated with care.

**4**

**Central nervous system**

Care is also needed in patients with epilepsy and hepatic impairment (avoid if severe; Appendix 2).

Tricyclic antidepressant drugs have antimuscarinic activity, and therefore caution is needed in patients with prostatic hypertrophy, chronic constipation, increased intra-ocular pressure, urinary retention, or those with a susceptibility to angle-closure glaucoma. Tricyclic and related antidepressant drugs should be used with caution in patients with a history of psychosis or bipolar disorder, because antidepressant therapy may aggravate these conditions; treatment should be stopped if the patient enters a manic phase.

Elderly patients are particularly susceptible to many of the side-effects of tricyclic antidepressants; low initial doses should be used, with close monitoring, particularly for psychiatric and cardiac side-effects.

For use in pregnancy or breast-feeding, see Appendix 4 and Appendix 5.

**Overdosage** Limited quantities of tricyclic antidepressants should be prescribed at any one time because their cardiovascular effects are dangerous in overdosage. In particular, overdosage with dosulepin (dothiepin) and amitriptyline is associated with a relatively high rate of fatality. For advice on **overdosage** see Emergency Treatment of Poisoning, p. 31.

**Withdrawal** If possible tricyclic and related antidepressants should be withdrawn slowly (see also section 4.3).

**Interactions** A tricyclic or related antidepressant (or an SSRI or related antidepressant) should not be started until 2 weeks after stopping an MAOI (3 weeks if starting clomipramine or imipramine). Conversely, an MAOI should not be started until at least 7–14 days after a tricyclic or related antidepressant (3 weeks in the case of clomipramine or imipramine) has been stopped. For guidance relating to the reversible monoamine oxidase inhibitor, moclobemide, see p. 214. For other tricyclic antidepressant **interactions**, see Appendix 1 (antidepressants, tricyclic and antidepressants, tricyclic (related)).

**Driving** Drowsiness may affect the performance of skilled tasks (e.g. driving); effects of alcohol enhanced.

**Contra-indications** Tricyclic and related antidepressants are contra-indicated in the immediate recovery period after myocardial infarction, in arrhythmias (particularly heart block), in the manic phase of bipolar disorder, and in severe liver disease. Avoid treatment with tricyclic antidepressant drugs in acute porphyria (section 9.8.2).

**Side-effects** Arrhythmias and heart block occasionally follow the use of tricyclic antidepressants, particularly amitriptyline, and may be a factor in the sudden death of patients with cardiac disease; other cardiovascular side-effects include postural hypotension, tachycardia, and ECG changes. The tricyclic-related antidepressant drugs may be associated with a lower risk of cardiotoxicity in overdosage.

Central nervous system side-effects are common, particularly in the elderly, and include anxiety, dizziness, agitation, confusion, sleep disturbances, irritability, and paraesthesia; drowsiness is associated with some of the tricyclic antidepressants (see under Choice, below). Convulsions, hallucinations, delusions, mania, and hypomania may occur (see also under Cautions), and, rarely, extrapyramidal symptoms including tremor and dysarthria.

Antimuscarinic side-effects include dry mouth, blurred vision (very rarely precipitation of angle-closure glaucoma), constipation (rarely leading to paralytic ileus, particularly in the elderly), and urinary retention. Tricyclic-related antidepressant drugs have a lower incidence of antimuscarinic side-effects than older tricyclics.

Endocrine effects include breast enlargement, galactorrhoea, and gynaecomastia. Sexual dysfunction may occur. Changes in blood sugar, increased appetite, and weight gain can accompany treatment with tricyclic antidepressant drugs, but anorexia and weight loss are also seen. Hepatic and haematological reactions may occur and have been particularly associated with mianserin. Another side-effect to which the elderly are particularly susceptible is hyponatraemia (see Hyponatraemia and Antidepressant Therapy, p. 209). Other class side-effects include nausea, vomiting, taste disturbance, tinnitus, rash, urticaria, pruritus, photosensitivity, alopecia, and sweating.

The patient should be encouraged to persist with treatment as some tolerance to these side-effects seems to develop. They are reduced if low doses are given initially and then gradually increased, but this must be balanced against the need to obtain a full therapeutic effect as soon as possible.

Neuroleptic malignant syndrome (section 4.2.1) may, very rarely, occur in the course of antidepressant drug treatment.

Suicidal behaviour has been linked with antidepressants (see p. 209).

**Dosage** About 10 to 20% of patients fail to respond to tricyclic and related antidepressant drugs and inadequate dosage may account for some of these failures. It is important to use doses that are sufficiently high for effective treatment but not so high as to cause toxic effects. Low doses should be used for initial treatment in the **elderly** (see under Side-effects, below).

In most patients the long half-life of tricyclic antidepressant drugs allows **once-daily** administration, usually at night; the use of modified-release preparations is therefore unnecessary.

**Choice** Tricyclic and related antidepressants block the re-uptake of both serotonin and noradrenaline, although to different extents. For example, clomipramine is more selective for serotonergic transmission, and imipramine is more selective for noradrenergic transmission. Tricyclic and related antidepressant drugs can be roughly divided into those with additional sedative properties and those that are less sedating. Agitated and anxious patients tend to respond best to the sedative compounds, whereas withdrawn and apathetic patients will often obtain most benefit from the less sedating ones. Those with **sedative** properties include amitriptyline, clomipramine, dosulepin (dothiepin), doxepin, mianserin, trazodone, and trimipramine. Those with **less sedative** properties include imipramine, lofepramine, and nortriptyline.

Tricyclic and related antidepressants also have varying degrees of antimuscarinic side-effects and cardiotoxicity in overdosage, which may be important in individual patients. **Lofepramine** has a lower incidence of side-effects and is less dangerous in overdosage but is infrequently associated with hepatic toxicity. **Imipramine** is also well established, but has more marked antimuscarinic side-effects than other tricyclic and related antidepressants. **Amitriptyline** and **dosulepin** (dothiepin) are effective but they are particularly dangerous in overdosage (see Overdosage, below) and are not recommended for the treatment of depression; dosulepin (dothiepin) should only be prescribed by specialists.

**Children and adolescents** Evidence of the efficacy of tricyclic antidepressants for depression in children has not been established; see also CSM advice, p. 215.

## Tricyclic antidepressants

### ◼ AMITRIPTYLINE HYDROCHLORIDE

**Indications** depressive illness (but not recommended, see notes above); nocturnal enuresis in children (section 7.4.2); neuropathic pain [unlicensed] (section 4.7.3); migraine prophylaxis [unlicensed] (section 4.7.4.2)

**Cautions** see notes above

**Contra-indications** see notes above

**Side-effects** see notes above; also abdominal pain, stomatitis, palpitation, oedema, hypertension, restlessness, fatigue, mydriasis, and increased intra-ocular pressure; high rate of fatality in overdose—see notes above

**Dose**
- Depression (but not recommended, see notes above), ADULT and CHILD over 16 years, initially 75 mg (elderly and adolescents 30–75 mg) daily in divided doses or as a single dose at bedtime increased gradually as necessary to 150–200 mg
- Nocturnal enuresis, CHILD 7–10 years 10–20 mg, 11–16 years 25–50 mg at night; max. period of treatment (including gradual withdrawal) 3 months—full physical examination before further course
- Neuropathic pain [unlicensed indication], initially 10–25 mg daily at night, increased if necessary to 75 mg daily; higher doses under specialist supervision
- Migraine prophylaxis [unlicensed indication], initially 10 mg at night, increased if necessary to maintenance of 50–75 mg at night

**Amitriptyline** (Non-proprietary) [PoM]
Tablets, coated, amitriptyline hydrochloride 10 mg, net price 28-tab pack = 94p; 25 mg, 28-tab pack = 94p; 50 mg, 28-tab pack = £1.13. Label: 2
Oral solution, amitriptyline hydrochloride 25 mg/ 5 mL, net price 150 mL = £13.53; 50 mg/5 mL, 150 mL = £14.72. Label: 2

◀**Compound preparations**
**Triptafen®** (Goldshield) [PoM] ◢
Tablets, pink, s/c, amitriptyline hydrochloride 25 mg, perphenazine 2 mg, net price 100-tab pack = £25.49. Label: 2
Dose depression with anxiety, ADULT and CHILD over 14 years, 1 tablet 3 times daily, increased if necessary to 4 tablets daily (with last dose at bedtime); review treatment if no response within 4 weeks; discontinue after 3 months

**Triptafen-M®** (Goldshield) [PoM] ◢
Tablets, pink, s/c, amitriptyline hydrochloride 10 mg, perphenazine 2 mg, net price 100-tab pack = £22.80. Label: 2
Dose mild to moderate depression with anxiety, ADULT and CHILD over 14 years, 1 tablet 3 times daily, increased if necessary to 4 tablets daily (with last dose at bedtime); review treatment if no response within 4 weeks; discontinue after 3 months

### ◼ CLOMIPRAMINE HYDROCHLORIDE

**Indications** depressive illness, phobic and obsessional states; adjunctive treatment of cataplexy associated with narcolepsy

**Cautions** see notes above

**Contra-indications** see notes above

**Side-effects** see notes above; also abdominal pain, diarrhoea, hypertension, flushing, restlessness, fatigue, aggression, impaired memory, muscle weakness, muscle hypertonia, myoclonus, mydriasis, and yawning; *very rarely* allergic alveolitis

**Dose**
- Depressive illness, ADULT over 18 years, initially 10 mg daily, increased gradually as necessary to 30–150 mg daily in divided doses or as a single dose at bedtime; max. 250 mg daily; ELDERLY initially 10 mg daily increased carefully over approx. 10 days to 30–75 mg daily
- Phobic and obsessional states, ADULT over 18 years, initially 25 mg daily (ELDERLY 10 mg daily) increased over 2 weeks to 100–150 mg daily; max. 250 mg daily
- Adjunctive treatment of cataplexy associated with narcolepsy, ADULT over 18 years, initially 10 mg daily, gradually increased until satisfactory response (range 10–75 mg daily)

**Clomipramine** (Non-proprietary) [PoM]
Capsules, clomipramine hydrochloride 10 mg, net price 28-cap pack = £2.49; 25 mg, 28-cap pack = £2.93; 50 mg, 28-cap pack = £3.75. Label: 2

**Anafranil®** (Novartis) [PoM]
Capsules, clomipramine hydrochloride 10 mg (yellow/caramel), net price 84-cap pack = £3.23; 25 mg (orange/caramel), 84-cap pack = £6.35; 50 mg (grey/caramel), 56-cap pack = £8.06. Label: 2

◀**Modified release**
**Anafranil SR®** (Novartis) [PoM] ◢
Tablets, m/r, grey-red, f/c, clomipramine hydrochloride 75 mg, net price 28-tab pack = £8.83. Label: 2, 25
Dose see above; to be taken once daily

### ◼ DOSULEPIN HYDROCHLORIDE ◢
(Dothiepin hydrochloride)

**Indications** depressive illness, particularly where sedation is required

**Cautions** see notes above

**Contra-indications** see notes above

**Side-effects** see notes above; also increased intra-ocular pressure; high rate of fatality in overdose—see notes above

**Dose**
- Initially 75 mg (ELDERLY 50–75 mg) daily in divided doses or as a single dose at bedtime, increased gradually as necessary to 150 mg daily (ELDERLY 75 mg may be sufficient); up to 225 mg daily in some circumstances (e.g. hospital use); CHILD not recommended

**4　Central nervous system**

**Dosulepin** (Non-proprietary) [PoM] ◿

Capsules, dosulepin hydrochloride 25 mg, net price 28-cap pack = £1.16. Label: 2

Tablets, dosulepin hydrochloride 75 mg, net price 28-tab pack = £1.60. Label: 2

**Prothiaden®** (Teofarma) [PoM] ◿

Capsules, red/red-brown, dosulepin hydrochloride 25 mg, net price 28-cap pack = £1.70. Label: 2

Tablets, red, s/c, dosulepin hydrochloride 75 mg, net price 28-tab pack = £2.97. Label: 2

## DOXEPIN

**Indications** depressive illness, particularly where sedation is required; pruritus in eczema (section 13.3)

**Cautions** see notes above

**Contra-indications** see notes above

**Side-effects** see notes above; also abdominal pain, stomatitis, diarrhoea, flushing, and oedema

**Dose**

- ADULT and CHILD over 12 years, initially 75 mg daily in divided doses or as a single dose at bedtime, adjusted according to response; usual maintenance 30–300 mg daily (doses above 100 mg given in 3 divided doses); ELDERLY initially 10–50 mg daily adjusted according to response (usual maintenance 30–50 mg daily)

**Sinepin®** (Marlborough) [PoM]

Capsules, doxepin (as hydrochloride) 25 mg, net price 28-cap pack = £3.77; 50 mg, 28-cap pack = £5.71. Label: 2

## IMIPRAMINE HYDROCHLORIDE

**Indications** depressive illness; nocturnal enuresis in children (section 7.4.2)

**Cautions** see notes above

**Contra-indications** see notes above

**Side-effects** see notes above; also palpitation, flushing, restlessness, fatigue; very rarely abdominal pain, stomatitis, hypertension, oedema, cardiac decompensation, allergic alveolitis, aggression, myoclonus, peripheral vasospasm, and mydriasis

**Dose**

- Depression, initially up to 75 mg daily in divided doses increased gradually to 150–200 mg (up to 300 mg in hospital patients); up to 150 mg may be given as a single dose at bedtime; ELDERLY initially 10 mg daily, increased gradually to 30–50 mg daily; CHILD not recommended for depression

- Nocturnal enuresis, CHILD 7–8 years 25 mg, 8–11 years 25–50 mg, over 11 years 50–75 mg at bedtime; max. period of treatment (including gradual withdrawal) 3 months—full physical examination before further course

**Imipramine** (Non-proprietary) [PoM]

Tablets, coated, imipramine hydrochloride 10 mg, net price 28-tab pack = £1.15; 25 mg, 28-tab pack = £1.17. Label: 2

## LOFEPRAMINE

**Indications** depressive illness

**Cautions** see notes above

**Contra-indications** see notes above; also severe renal impairment

**Side-effects** see notes above; also oedema and hepatic disorders reported

**Dose**

- 140–210 mg daily in divided doses; ELDERLY may respond to lower doses; CHILD not recommended

**Lofepramine** (Non-proprietary) [PoM]

Tablets, lofepramine 70 mg (as hydrochloride), net price 56-tab pack = £16.28. Label: 2
Brands include *Feprapax®*

Oral suspension, lofepramine 70 mg/5 mL (as hydrochloride), net price 150 mL = £22.22. Label: 2
Brands include *Lomont®* (sugar-free)

## NORTRIPTYLINE

**Indications** depressive illness; nocturnal enuresis in children (section 7.4.2); neuropathic pain [unlicensed] (section 4.7.3)

**Cautions** see notes above; manufacturer advises plasma-nortriptyline concentration monitoring if dose above 100 mg daily, but evidence of practical value uncertain

**Contra-indications** see notes above

**Side-effects** see notes above; also abdominal pain, stomatitis, diarrhoea, hypertension, oedema, flushing, restlessness, fatigue, and mydriasis

**Dose**

- Depression, low dose initially increased as necessary to 75–100 mg daily in divided doses or as a single dose (max. 150 mg daily); ADOLESCENT and ELDERLY 30–50 mg daily in divided doses; CHILD not recommended for depression

- Nocturnal enuresis, CHILD 7 years 10 mg, 8–11 years 10–20 mg, over 11 years 25–35 mg, 30 minutes before bedtime; max period of treatment (including gradual withdrawal) 3 months—full physical examination and ECG before further course

- Neuropathic pain [unlicensed], initially 10–25 mg daily at night, increased if necessary to 75 mg daily; higher doses under specialist supervision

**Allegron®** (King) [PoM]

Tablets, nortriptyline (as hydrochloride) 10 mg, net price 100-tab pack = £12.06; 25 mg (orange, scored), 100-tab pack = £24.02. Label: 2

## TRIMIPRAMINE

**Indications** depressive illness, particularly where sedation required

**Cautions** see notes above

**Contra-indications** see notes above

**Side-effects** see notes above

**Dose**

- Initially 50–75 mg daily in divided doses or as a single dose at bedtime, increased as necessary to 150–300 mg daily; ELDERLY initially 10–25 mg 3 times daily, maintenance half adult dose may be sufficient; CHILD not recommended

**Surmontil®** (Aventis Pharma) [PoM]

Capsules, green/white, trimipramine 50 mg (as maleate), net price 28-cap pack = £7.60. Label: 2

Tablets, trimipramine (as maleate) 10 mg, net price 28-tab pack = £3.43, 84-tab pack = £10.27; 25 mg, 28-tab pack = £4.53, 84-tab pack = £13.55. Label: 2

## Related antidepressants

### ▊ MIANSERIN HYDROCHLORIDE

**Indications** depressive illness, particularly where sedation is required

**Cautions** see notes above

Blood counts A full **blood count** is recommended every 4 weeks during the first 3 months of treatment; clinical monitoring should continue subsequently and treatment should be stopped and a full blood count obtained if *fever, sore throat, stomatitis,* or other signs of infection develop

**Contra-indications** see notes above

**Side-effects** see notes above; also arthritis and arthralgia

**Dose**

- ADULT over 18 years, initially 30–40 mg (elderly 30 mg) daily in divided doses *or* as a single dose at bedtime, increased gradually as necessary; usual dose range 30–90 mg

**Mianserin** (Non-proprietary) ꝖoM

Tablets, mianserin hydrochloride 10 mg, net price 28-tab pack = £7.36; 30 mg, 28-tab pack = £11.58. Label: 2, 25

### ▊ TRAZODONE HYDROCHLORIDE

**Indications** depressive illness, particularly where sedation is required; anxiety

**Cautions** see notes above

**Contra-indications** see notes above

**Side-effects** see notes above; *rarely* priapism (discontinue immediately)

**Dose**

- Depression, initially 150 mg (elderly 100 mg) daily in divided doses after food *or* as a single dose at bedtime; may be increased to 300 mg daily; hospital patients up to max. 600 mg daily in divided doses; CHILD not recommended

- Anxiety, 75 mg daily, increasing if necessary to 300 mg daily; CHILD not recommended

**Trazodone** (Non-proprietary) ꝖoM

Capsules, trazodone hydrochloride 50 mg, net price 84-cap pack = £7.17; 100 mg, 56-cap pack = £7.06. Label: 2, 21

Tablets, trazodone hydrochloride 150 mg, net price 28-tab pack = £6.61. Label: 2, 21

**Molipaxin®** (Sanofi-Aventis) ꝖoM

Capsules, trazodone hydrochloride 50 mg (violet/green), net price 84-cap pack = £23.92; 100 mg (violet/fawn), 56-cap pack = £28.14. Label: 2, 21

Tablets, pink, f/c, trazodone hydrochloride 150 mg, net price 28-tab pack = £16.08. Label: 2, 21

Liquid, sugar-free, trazodone hydrochloride 50 mg/5 mL, net price 120 mL = £13.37. Label: 2, 21

## 4.3.2 Monoamine-oxidase inhibitors
### (MAOIs)

Monoamine-oxidase inhibitors are used much less frequently than tricyclic and related antidepressants, or SSRIs and related antidepressants because of the dangers of dietary and drug interactions and the fact that it is easier to prescribe MAOIs when tricyclic antidepressants have been unsuccessful than vice versa. **Tranylcypromine** is the most **hazardous** of the MAOIs because of its stimulant action. The drugs of choice are **phenelzine** or **isocarboxazid** which are less stimulant and therefore safer.

Phobic patients and depressed patients with atypical, hypochondriacal, or hysterical features are said to respond best to MAOIs. However, MAOIs should be tried in any patients who are refractory to treatment with other antidepressants as there is occasionally a dramatic response. Response to treatment may be delayed for 3 weeks or more and may take an additional 1 or 2 weeks to become maximal.

**Withdrawal** If possible MAOIs should be withdrawn slowly (see also section 4.3).

**Interactions** MAOIs inhibit monoamine oxidase, thereby causing an accumulation of amine neurotransmitters. The metabolism of some amine drugs such as *indirect-acting sympathomimetics* (present in many cough and decongestant preparations, section 3.10) is also inhibited and their pressor action may be potentiated; the pressor effect of tyramine (in some foods, such as mature cheese, pickled herring, broad bean pods, and *Bovril®, Oxo®, Marmite®* or any similar meat or yeast extract or fermented soya bean extract) may also be dangerously potentiated. These interactions may cause a dangerous rise in blood pressure. An early warning symptom may be a throbbing headache. Patients should be advised to eat only fresh foods and avoid food that is suspected of being stale or 'going off'. This is especially important with meat, fish, poultry or offal; game should be avoided. The danger of interaction persists for up to 2 weeks after treatment with MAOIs is discontinued. Patients should also avoid alcoholic drinks or dealcoholised (low alcohol) drinks.

*Other antidepressants* should **not** be started for 2 weeks after treatment with MAOIs has been stopped (3 weeks if starting clomipramine or imipramine). Some psychiatrists use selected tricyclics in conjunction with MAOIs but this is hazardous, indeed potentially lethal, except in experienced hands and there is no evidence that the combination is more effective than when either constituent is used alone. The combination of tranylcypromine with clomipramine is particularly **dangerous**.

Conversely, an MAOI should not be started until at least 7–14 days after a tricyclic or related antidepressant (3 weeks in the case of clomipramine or imipramine) has been stopped.

In addition, an MAOI should not be started for at least 2 weeks after a previous MAOI has been stopped (then started at a reduced dose).

For other interactions with MAOIs including those with opioid analgesics (notably pethidine), see Appendix 1

**4**

**Central nervous system**

(MAOIs). For guidance on interactions relating to the reversible monoamine oxidase inhibitor, moclobemide, see below; for guidance on interactions relating to SSRIs, see p. 215.

## PHENELZINE

**Indications** depressive illness

**Cautions** diabetes mellitus, cardiovascular disease, epilepsy, blood disorders, concurrent electroconvulsive therapy; elderly (great caution); monitor blood pressure (risk of postural hypotension and hypertensive responses—discontinue if palpitations or frequent headaches); if possible avoid abrupt withdrawal; severe hypertensive reactions to certain drugs and foods; avoid in agitated patients; acute porphyria (section 9.8.2); pregnancy (Appendix 4) and breast-feeding; surgery (section 15.1); **interactions:** Appendix 1 (MAOIs)

Driving Drowsiness may affect performance of skilled tasks (e.g. driving)

**Contra-indications** hepatic impairment or abnormal liver function tests (Appendix 2), cerebrovascular disease, phaeochromocytoma; not indicated in manic phase

**Side-effects** commonly postural hypotension (especially in elderly) and dizziness; less common side-effects include drowsiness, insomnia, headache, weakness and fatigue, dry mouth, constipation and other gastro-intestinal disturbances, oedema, myoclonic movement, hyperreflexia, elevated liver enzymes; agitation and tremors, nervousness, euphoria, arrhythmias, blurred vision, nystagmus, difficulty in micturition, sweating, convulsions, rashes, purpura, leucopenia, sexual disturbances, and weight gain with inappropriate appetite may also occur; psychotic episodes with hypomanic behaviour, confusion, and hallucinations may be induced in susceptible persons; suicidal behaviour (see p. 209); jaundice has been reported and, on rare occasions, fatal progressive hepatocellular necrosis; paraesthesia, peripheral neuritis, peripheral neuropathy may be due to pyridoxine deficiency; hyponatraemia (see Hyponatraemia and Antidepressant Therapy, p. 209)

**Dose**
- 15 mg 3 times daily, increased if necessary to 4 times daily after 2 weeks (hospital patients, max. 30 mg 3 times daily), then reduced gradually to lowest possible maintenance dose (15 mg on alternate days may be adequate); CHILD not recommended

**Nardil®** (Concord) ℗oM 📄
Tablets, orange, f/c, phenelzine (as sulphate) 15 mg, net price 100 = £23.94. Label: 3, 10, patient information leaflet

## ISOCARBOXAZID

**Indications** depressive illness
**Cautions** see under Phenelzine
**Contra-indications** see under Phenelzine
**Side-effects** see under Phenelzine
**Dose**
- Initially 30 mg daily in single or divided doses until improvement occurs (increased after 4 weeks if necessary to max. 60 mg daily for 4–6 weeks under close supervision), then reduced to usual maintenance dose 10–20 mg daily (but up to 40 mg daily may

be required); ELDERLY 5–10 mg daily; CHILD not recommended

**Isocarboxazid** (Non-proprietary) ℗oM 📄
Tablets, pink, scored, isocarboxazid 10 mg. Net price 56-tab pack = £50.05. Label: 3, 10, patient information leaflet

## TRANYLCYPROMINE

**Indications** depressive illness
**Cautions** see under Phenelzine
**Contra-indications** see under Phenelzine; hyperthyroidism
**Side-effects** see under Phenelzine; insomnia if given in evening; hypertensive crises with throbbing headache requiring discontinuation of treatment more frequent than with other MAOIs; liver damage less frequent than with phenelzine

**Dose**
- Initially 10 mg twice daily not later than 3 p.m., increasing the second daily dose to 20 mg after 1 week if necessary; doses above 30 mg daily under close supervision only; usual maintenance dose 10 mg daily; CHILD not recommended

**Tranylcypromine** (Non-proprietary) ℗oM 📄
Tablets, tranylcypromine (as sulphate) 10 mg. Net price 28-tab pack = £32.62. Label: 3, 10, patient information leaflet

## Reversible MAOIs

**Moclobemide** is indicated for major depression and social anxiety disorder; it is reported to act by reversible inhibition of monoamine oxidase type A (it is therefore termed a RIMA). It should be reserved as a second-line treatment.

**Interactions** Moclobemide is claimed to cause less potentiation of the pressor effect of tyramine than the traditional (irreversible) MAOIs, but patients should avoid consuming large amounts of tyramine-rich food (such as mature cheese, yeast extracts and fermented soya bean products).

The risk of drug interactions is also claimed to be less but patients still need to avoid sympathomimetics such as ephedrine and pseudoephedrine. In addition, moclobemide should not be given with another antidepressant. Owing to its short duration of action no treatment-free period is required after it has been stopped but it should not be started until at least a week after a tricyclic or related antidepressant or an SSRI or related antidepressant has been stopped (2 weeks in the case of sertraline, and at least 5 weeks in the case of fluoxetine), or for at least a week after an MAOI has been stopped. For other interactions, see Appendix 1 (moclobemide).

## MOCLOBEMIDE

**Indications** depressive illness; social anxiety disorder
**Cautions** avoid in agitated or excited patients (or give with sedative for up to 2–3 weeks), thyrotoxicosis, hepatic impairment (Appendix 2), may provoke manic episodes in bipolar disorders, pregnancy (Appendix 4) and breast-feeding (Appendix 5—patient information leaflet advises avoid); **interactions:** see notes above and Appendix 1 (moclobemide)

**4** Central nervous system

**Contra-indications** acute confusional states, phaeochromocytoma

**Side-effects** sleep disturbances, dizziness, gastrointestinal disorders, headache, restlessness, agitation; paraesthesia, dry mouth, visual disturbances, oedema, skin reactions, confusional states reported; *rarely* raised liver enzymes, galactorrhoea; hyponatraemia (see Hyponatraemia and Antidepressant Therapy, p. 209)

**Dose**

- Depression, initially 300 mg daily usually in divided doses after food, adjusted according to response; usual range 150–600 mg daily; CHILD not recommended

- Social anxiety disorder, initially 300 mg daily increased on fourth day to 600 mg daily in 2 divided doses, continued for 8–12 weeks to assess efficacy; CHILD not recommended

**Moclobemide** (Non-proprietary) PoM

Tablets, moclobemide 150 mg, net price 30-tab pack = £2.52; 300 mg, 30-tab pack = £3.60. Label: 10, patient information leaflet, 21

**Manerix®** (Roche) PoM

Tablets, yellow, f/c, scored, moclobemide 150 mg, net price 30-tab pack = £7.43; 300 mg, 30-tab pack = £13.14. Label: 10, patient information leaflet, 21

## 4.3.3 Selective serotonin re-uptake inhibitors

**Citalopram, escitalopram, fluoxetine, fluvoxamine, paroxetine,** and **sertraline** selectively inhibit the re-uptake of serotonin (5-hydroxytryptamine, 5-HT); they are termed selective serotonin re-uptake inhibitors (SSRIs). For a general comment on the management of depression and on the comparison between *tricyclic and related antidepressants* and the *SSRIs and related antidepressants*, see section 4.3.

> **CSM advice (depressive illness in children and adolescents)**
> The CSM has advised that the balance of risks and benefits for the treatment of depressive illness in individuals under 18 years is considered unfavourable for the SSRIs citalopram, escitalopram, paroxetine, and sertraline, and for mirtazapine and venlafaxine. Clinical trials have failed to show efficacy and have shown an increase in harmful outcomes. However, it is recognised that specialists may sometimes decide to use these drugs in response to individual clinical need; children and adolescents should be monitored carefully for suicidal behaviour, self-harm or hostility, particularly at the beginning of treatment.
> Only fluoxetine has been shown in clinical trials to be effective for treating depressive illness in children and adolescents. However, it is possible that, in common with the other SSRIs, it is associated with a small risk of self-harm and suicidal thoughts. Overall, the balance of risks and benefits for fluoxetine in the treatment of depressive illness in individuals under 18 years is considered favourable, but children and adolescents must be carefully monitored as above.

**Cautions** SSRIs should be used with caution in patients with epilepsy (avoid if poorly controlled, discontinue if convulsions develop), cardiac disease, diabetes mellitus, susceptibility to angle-closure glaucoma, a history of mania or bleeding disorders (especially gastro-intestinal bleeding), and if used with other drugs that increase the risk of bleeding, hepatic impairment (Appendix 2), renal impairment (Appendix 3), pregnancy (Appendix 4), and breast-feeding (Appendix 5). They should also be used with caution in those receiving concurrent electroconvulsive therapy (prolonged seizures reported with fluoxetine). SSRIs may also impair performance of skilled tasks (e.g. driving). **Interactions:** see below and Appendix 1 (antidepressants, SSRI).

**Withdrawal** Gastro-intestinal disturbances, headache, anxiety, dizziness, paraesthesia, sleep disturbances, fatigue, influenza-like symptoms, and sweating are the most common features of abrupt withdrawal of an SSRI or marked reduction of the dose; the dose should be tapered over a few weeks to avoid these effects.

**Interactions** An SSRI or related antidepressant should not be started until 2 weeks after stopping an MAOI. Conversely, an MAOI should not be started until at least a week after an SSRI or related antidepressant has been stopped (2 weeks in the case of sertraline, at least 5 weeks in the case of fluoxetine). For guidance relating to the reversible monoamine oxidase inhibitor, moclobemide, see above. For other SSRI antidepressant interactions, see Appendix 1 (antidepressants, SSRI).

**Contra-indications** SSRIs should not be used if the patient enters a manic phase.

**Side-effects** SSRIs are less sedating and have fewer antimuscarinic and cardiotoxic effects than tricyclic antidepressants (section 4.3). Side-effects of the SSRIs include gastro-intestinal effects (dose-related and fairly common—include nausea, vomiting, dyspepsia, abdominal pain, diarrhoea, constipation), anorexia with weight loss (increased appetite and weight gain also reported) and hypersensitivity reactions including rash (consider discontinuation—may be sign of impending serious systemic reaction, possibly associated with vasculitis); urticaria, angioedema, anaphylaxis, arthralgia, myalgia and photosensitivity; other side-effects include dry mouth, nervousness, anxiety, headache, insomnia, tremor, dizziness, asthenia, hallucinations, drowsiness, convulsions (see Cautions above), galactorrhoea, sexual dysfunction, urinary retention, sweating, hypomania or mania (see Cautions above), movement disorders and dyskinesias, visual disturbances, hyponatraemia (see Hyponatraemia and Antidepressant Therapy, p. 209), and bleeding disorders including ecchymoses and purpura. Suicidal behaviour has been linked with antidepressants (see p. 209). Angle-closure glaucoma may very rarely be precipitated by treatment with SSRIs.

### ▮ CITALOPRAM

**Indications** depressive illness, panic disorder

**Cautions** see notes above

**Contra-indications** see notes above

**Side-effects** see notes above; also palpitation, tachycardia, postural hypotension, coughing, yawning, confusion, impaired concentration, malaise, amnesia, migraine, paraesthesia, abnormal dreams, taste dis-

**4** Central nervous system

turbance, increased salivation, rhinitis, tinnitus, polyuria, micturition disorders, euphoria; paradoxical increased anxiety during initial treatment of panic disorder (reduce dose)

**Dose**

- By mouth as tablets, depressive illness, 20 mg once daily increased if necessary in steps of 20 mg daily at intervals of 3–4 weeks; max. 60 mg daily (ELDERLY over 65 years, max. 40 mg daily); CHILD under 18 years see *BNF for Children* and CSM advice, p. 215

  Panic disorder, ADULT over 18 years, initially 10 mg daily increased gradually if necessary in steps of 10 mg daily, usual dose 20–30 mg daily; max. 60 mg daily (ELDERLY over 65 years, max. 40 mg daily)

- By mouth as oral drops, depressive illness, 16 mg daily as a single dose increased if necessary in steps of 16 mg daily at intervals of 3–4 weeks; max. 48 mg daily (ELDERLY over 65 years, max. 32 mg daily); CHILD under 18 years see *BNF for Children* and CSM advice, p. 215

  Panic disorder, ADULT over 18 years, initially 8 mg daily as a single dose increased gradually if necessary in steps of 8 mg daily, usual dose 16–24 mg daily; max. 48 mg daily (ELDERLY over 65 years, max. 32 mg daily)

**Citalopram** (Non-proprietary) [PoM]

Tablets, citalopram (as hydrobromide) 10 mg, net price 28-tab pack = £1.08; 20 mg, 28-tab pack = £1.26; 40 mg, 28-tab pack = £1.44. Counselling, driving

Oral drops, citalopram (as hydrochloride) 40 mg/mL, net price 15 mL = £19.66. Counselling, driving, administration

Note 4 drops (8 mg) is equivalent in therapeutic effect to 10-mg tablet

Mix with water, orange juice or apple juice before taking

**Cipramil®** (Lundbeck) [PoM]

Tablets, f/c, citalopram (as hydrobromide) 10 mg, net price 28-tab pack = £8.97; 20 mg (scored), 28-tab pack = £14.91; 40 mg, 28-tab pack = £25.20. Counselling, driving

Oral drops, sugar-free, citalopram (as hydrochloride) 40 mg/mL, net price 15 mL = £20.16. Counselling, driving, administration

Excipients include alcohol

Note 4 drops (8 mg ) is equivalent in therapeutic effect to 10-mg tablet

Mix with water, orange juice, or apple juice before taking

## ESCITALOPRAM

Note Escitalopram is the active enantiomer of citalopram

**Indications** see under Dose

**Cautions** see notes above

**Contra-indications** see notes above

**Side-effects** see notes above; also sinusitis, yawning; fatigue, restlessness, abnormal dreams, paraesthesia; pyrexia; *less commonly* taste disturbance, bruxism, syncope, tachycardia, oedema, confusion, menstrual disturbances, epistaxis, mydriasis, tinnitus, pruritus, and alopecia; *rarely* bradycardia, aggression, and depersonalisation; hepatitis, postural hypotension, QT interval prolongation, and thrombocytopenia also reported; paradoxical increased anxiety during initial treatment of panic disorder (reduce dose)

**Dose**

- ADULT over 18 years, depressive illness, generalised anxiety disorder, and obsessive-compulsive disorder, 10 mg once daily increased if necessary to max. 20 mg

daily; ELDERLY initially half adult dose, lower maintenance dose may be sufficient; CHILD not recommended (see CSM advice, p. 215)

- ADULT over 18 years, panic disorder, initially 5 mg once daily increased to 10 mg daily after 7 days; max. 20 mg daily; ELDERLY initially half adult dose, lower maintenance dose may be sufficient

- ADULT over 18 years, social anxiety disorder, initially 10 mg once daily adjusted after 2–4 weeks; usual dose 5–20 mg daily

**Cipralex®** (Lundbeck) [PoM]

Tablets, f/c, escitalopram (as oxalate) 5 mg, net price 28-tab pack = £8.97; 10 mg (scored), 28-tab pack = £14.91; 20 mg (scored), 28-tab pack = £25.20. Counselling, driving

Oral drops, sugar-free, escitalopram (as oxalate) 10 mg/mL, net price 28 mL = £18.82. Counselling, driving, administration

Note Can be mixed with water, orange juice, or apple juice before taking

The *Scottish Medicines Consortium* (p. 3) has advised that escitalopram (*Cipralex®*) is **not** recommended within NHS Scotland for the treatment of social anxiety disorder (April 2008)

## FLUOXETINE

**Indications** see under Dose

**Cautions** see notes above

**Contra-indications** see notes above

**Side-effects** see notes above; also vasodilatation, postural hypotension, pharyngitis, dyspnoea, chills, taste disturbances, sleep disturbances, euphoria, confusion, yawning, impaired concentration, changes in blood sugar, alopecia, urinary frequency; *rarely* pulmonary inflammation and fibrosis; *very rarely* hepatitis, toxic epidermal necrolysis, and neuroleptic malignant syndrome-like event

**Dose**

- Major depression, 20 mg once daily increased after 3–4 weeks if necessary, and at appropriate intervals thereafter; max. 60 mg once daily (ELDERLY usual max. 40 mg once daily but 60 mg can be used); CHILD 8–18 years, 10 mg once daily increased after 1–2 weeks if necessary, max. 20 mg once daily (but see also CSM advice, p. 215)

- Bulimia nervosa, ADULT over 18 years, 60 mg once daily

- Obsessive-compulsive disorder, ADULT over 18 years, 20 mg once daily; if inadequate response after 2 weeks increase gradually to max. 60 mg once daily (ELDERLY usual max. 40 mg once daily but 60 mg can be used)

Long duration of action Consider the long half-life of fluoxetine when adjusting dosage (or in overdosage)

**Fluoxetine** (Non-proprietary) [PoM]

Capsules, fluoxetine (as hydrochloride) 20 mg, net price 30-cap pack = £1.02; 60 mg, 30-cap pack = £55.73. Counselling, driving

Brands include *Oxactin®*

Liquid, fluoxetine (as hydrochloride) 20 mg/5 mL, net price 70 mL = £7.27. Counselling, driving

Brands include *Prozep®*

**Prozac®** (Lilly) [PoM]

Capsules, fluoxetine (as hydrochloride) 20 mg (green/yellow), net price 30-cap pack = £1.53. Counselling, driving

Liquid, fluoxetine (as hydrochloride) 20 mg/5 mL, net price 70 mL = £11.12. Counselling, driving

## FLUVOXAMINE MALEATE

**Indications** depressive illness, obsessive-compulsive disorder

**Cautions** see notes above

**CSM advice** The CSM has advised that concomitant use of fluvoxamine and theophylline or aminophylline should usually be avoided; see also **interactions:** Appendix 1 (antidepressants, SSRIs)

**Contra-indications** see notes above

**Side-effects** see notes above; palpitation, tachycardia (may also cause bradycardia); *rarely* postural hypotension, confusion, ataxia, paraesthesia, malaise, taste disturbance, neuroleptic malignant syndrome-like event, abnormal liver function tests, usually symptomatic (discontinue treatment)

**Dose**

- Depression, ADULT over 18 years, initially 50–100 mg daily in the evening, increased gradually if necessary to max. 300 mg daily (over 150 mg in divided doses); usual maintenance dose 100 mg daily

- Obsessive-compulsive disorder, initially 50 mg in the evening increased gradually if necessary after some weeks to max. 300 mg daily (over 150 mg in divided doses); usual maintenance dose 100–300 mg daily; CHILD over 8 years initially 25 mg daily increased if necessary in steps of 25 mg every 4–7 days to max. 200 mg daily (over 50 mg in 2 divided doses)
  **Note** If no improvement in obsessive-compulsive disorder within 10 weeks, treatment should be reconsidered

**Fluvoxamine** (Non-proprietary) PoM
Tablets, fluvoxamine maleate 50 mg, net price 60-tab pack = £6.17; 100 mg, 30-tab pack = £8.22. Counselling, driving

**Faverin®** (Solvay) PoM
Tablets, f/c, scored, fluvoxamine maleate 50 mg, net price 60-tab pack = £17.10; 100 mg, 30-tab pack = £17.10. Counselling, driving

## PAROXETINE

**Indications** major depression, obsessive-compulsive disorder, panic disorder; social anxiety disorder; post-traumatic stress disorder; generalised anxiety disorder

**Cautions** see notes above; also achlorhydria or high gastric pH (reduced absorption of oral suspension)
**CSM advice** Extrapyramidal reactions (including orofacial dystonias) and withdrawal syndrome are reported to the CSM more commonly with paroxetine than with other SSRIs

**Contra-indications** see notes above

**Side-effects** see notes above; also yawning; raised cholesterol; *less commonly* arrhythmias, transient changes in blood pressure, confusion, urinary incontinence; *rarely* panic attacks and paradoxical increased anxiety during initial treatment of panic disorder (reduce dose), depersonalisation, and neuroleptic malignant syndrome-like event; *very rarely* peripheral oedema, acute glaucoma, hepatic disorders (e.g. hepatitis), and priapism

**Dose**

- Major depression, social anxiety disorder, post-traumatic stress disorder, generalised anxiety disorder, ADULT over 18 years, usually 20 mg each morning, higher doses on specialist advice only (see also CSM advice, below); max. 50 mg daily (ELDERLY 40 mg

daily); CHILD not recommended (see CSM advice, p. 215)

- Obsessive-compulsive disorder, ADULT over 18 years, initially 20 mg each morning, increased gradually in steps of 10 mg to usual dose of 40 mg daily, higher doses on specialist advice only (see also CSM advice, below); max. 60 mg daily (ELDERLY 40 mg daily)

- Panic disorder, ADULT over 18 years, initially 10 mg each morning, increased gradually in steps of 10 mg to usual dose of 40 mg daily, higher doses on specialist advice only (see also CSM advice, below); max. 60 mg daily (ELDERLY 40 mg daily)
  **CSM advice** The recommended dose for the treatment of depression, social anxiety disorder, generalised anxiety disorder, and post-traumatic stress disorder is 20 mg daily and for obsessive-compulsive disorder and panic disorder it is 40 mg daily. There is no evidence that higher doses are more effective

**Paroxetine** (Non-proprietary) PoM
Tablets, paroxetine (as hydrochloride) 20 mg, net price 30-tab pack = £2.84; 30 mg, 30-tab pack = £6.21. Label: 21, counselling, driving

**Seroxat®** (GSK) PoM
Tablets, f/c, scored, paroxetine (as hydrochloride) 10 mg, net price 28-tab pack = £11.84; 20 mg, 30-tab pack = £12.69; 30 mg (blue), 30-tab pack = £22.28. Label: 21, counselling, driving

Oral suspension, orange, sugar-free, paroxetine (as hydrochloride) 10 mg/5 mL. Net price 150-mL pack = £9.12. Label: 5, 21, counselling, driving

## SERTRALINE

**Indications** depressive illness, obsessive-compulsive disorder (under specialist supervision in children), post-traumatic stress disorder in women

**Cautions** see notes above

**Contra-indications** see notes above

**Side-effects** see notes above; pancreatitis, hepatitis, jaundice, liver failure, tachycardia, postural hypotension, amnesia, paraesthesia, aggression, urinary incontinence, and menstrual irregularities also reported

**Dose**

- Depressive illness, initially 50 mg daily, increased if necessary by increments of 50 mg over several weeks to max. 200 mg daily; usual maintenance dose 50 mg daily; CHILD under 18 years, see *BNF for Children* and CSM advice, p. 215

- Obsessive-compulsive disorder, ADULT and CHILD over 12 years initially 50 mg daily, increased if necessary in steps of 50 mg over several weeks; usual dose range 50–200 mg daily; CHILD 6–12 years initially 25 mg daily, increased to 50 mg daily after 1 week, further increased if necessary in steps of 50 mg at intervals of at least 1 week (max. 200 mg daily)

- Post-traumatic stress disorder, ADULT over 18 years, initially 25 mg daily, increased after 1 week to 50 mg daily; if response is partial and if drug tolerated, dose increased in steps of 50 mg over several weeks to max. 200 mg daily

**Sertraline** (Non-proprietary) PoM
Tablets, sertraline (as hydrochloride) 50 mg, net price 28-tab pack = £1.36; 100 mg, 28-tab pack = £1.67. Counselling, driving

**Lustral®** (Pfizer) [PoM]

Tablets, f/c, sertraline (as hydrochloride) 50 mg (scored), net price 28-tab pack = £17.82; 100 mg, 28-tab pack = £29.16. Counselling, driving

## 4.3.4 Other antidepressant drugs

**Agomelatine** is a melatonin receptor agonist and a selective serotonin-receptor antagonist; it does not affect the uptake of serotonin, noradrenaline, or dopamine.

**Duloxetine** inhibits the re-uptake of both serotonin and noradrenaline and is licensed to treat major depressive disorder.

The thioxanthene **flupentixol** (*Fluanxol®*) has antidepressant properties, and low doses (1 to 3 mg daily) are given by mouth for this purpose. Flupentixol is also used for the treatment of psychoses (section 4.2.1 and section 4.2.2)

**Mirtazapine**, a presynaptic alpha₂-adrenoreceptor antagonist, increases central noradrenergic and serotonergic neurotransmission. It has few antimuscarinic effects, but causes sedation during initial treatment.

**Reboxetine**, a selective inhibitor of noradrenaline re-uptake, has been introduced for the treatment of depressive illness.

**Tryptophan** is licensed as adjunctive therapy for depression resistant to standard antidepressants; it has been associated with eosinophilia-myalgia syndrome. Tryptophan should be initiated under specialist supervision.

**Venlafaxine** is a serotonin and noradrenaline re-uptake inhibitor (SNRI); it lacks the sedative and antimuscarinic effects of the tricyclic antidepressants.

### ■ AGOMELATINE

**Indications** major depression

**Cautions** elderly; mania or hypomania; concomitant use of drugs associated with hepatic injury; excessive alcohol consumption; monitor liver function before treatment and after 6, 12 and 24 weeks of treatment, then as appropriate (discontinue if serum transaminases exceed 3 times the upper limit of reference range); pregnancy (Appendix 4); **interactions**: Appendix 1 (agomelatine)

**Contra-indications** dementia; hepatic impairment; breast feeding (Appendix 5)

**Side-effects** nausea, diarrhoea, constipation, abdominal pain, increased serum transaminases (see Cautions); headache, dizziness, drowsiness, insomnia, fatigue, anxiety; back pain; sweating; *less commonly* paraesthesia, blurred vision, and eczema; *rarely* hepatitis and rash; suicidal behaviour (see Suicidal Behaviour and Antidepressant Therapy, p. 209) also reported

**Dose**

● ADULT over 18 years, 25 mg at bedtime, increased if necessary after 2 weeks to 50 mg at bedtime

**Valdoxan®** (Servier) ▼ [PoM]

Tablets, orange-yellow, f/c, agomelatine 25 mg, net price 28-tab pack = £38.53

### ■ DULOXETINE

**Indications** major depressive disorder; generalised anxiety disorder; diabetic neuropathy (section 6.1.5); stress urinary incontinence (section 7.4.2)

**Cautions** section 7.4.2; pregnancy (Appendix 4)

**Contra-indications** section 7.4.2

**Side-effects** section 7.4.2

**Dose**

● Major depression, ADULT over 18 years, 60 mg once daily

● Generalised anxiety disorder, ADULT over 18 years, initially 30 mg daily, increased if necessary to 60 mg once daily; max. 120 mg daily

● Diabetic neuropathy, ADULT over 18 years, 60 mg once daily; max. 120 mg daily in divided doses

Note In diabetic neuropathy, discontinue if inadequate response after 2 months; review treatment at least every 3 months

**Cymbalta®** (Lilly) ▼ [PoM]

Capsules, duloxetine (as hydrochloride) 30 mg (white/blue), net price 28-cap pack = £22.40; 60 mg (green/blue), 28-cap pack = £27.72. Label: 2

Note The *Scottish Medicines Consortium* has advised (September 2006) that duloxetine (*Cymbalta®*) should be restricted for use by specialists when other treatments for diabetic peripheral neuropathic pain are unsuitable or inadequate

**Yentreve®** (Lilly) ▼ [PoM]

Section 7.4.2 (stress urinary incontinence)

### ■ FLUPENTIXOL
(Flupenthixol)

**Indications** depressive illness; psychoses (section 4.2.1)

**Cautions** cardiovascular disease (including cardiac disorders and cerebral arteriosclerosis), QT-interval prolongation (avoid concomitant administration of drugs that prolong QT interval); diabetes; senile confusional states, parkinsonism; elderly; hepatic impairment (Appendix 2); renal impairment (Appendix 3); acute porphyria (section 9.8.2); see also section 4.2.1; **interactions**: Appendix 1 (antipsychotics)

**Contra-indications** excitable and overactive patients; impaired consciousness; circulatory collapse; coma

**Side-effects** section 4.2.1; also hypersalivation, dyspnoea, asthenia, hyperglycaemia, myalgia; torsade de pointes and sudden death also reported

**Dose**

● ADULT over 18 years, initially 1 mg (elderly 500 micrograms) in the morning, increased after 1 week to 2 mg (elderly 1 mg) if necessary; max. 3 mg (elderly 2 mg) daily, doses above 2 mg (elderly 1 mg) being divided in 2 portions, second dose not after 4 p.m. Discontinue if no response after 1 week at max. dosage

Counselling Although drowsiness may occur, can also have an alerting effect so should not be taken in the evening

**Fluanxol®** (Lundbeck) [PoM]

Tablets, yellow, s/c, flupentixol (as dihydrochloride) 500 micrograms, net price 60-tab pack = £2.02; 1 mg, 60-tab pack = £3.40. Label: 2, counselling, administration

## MIRTAZAPINE

**Indications** major depression

**Cautions** elderly, cardiac disorders, hypotension, history of urinary retention, susceptibility to angle-closure glaucoma, diabetes mellitus, psychoses (may aggravate psychotic symptoms), history of seizures or bipolar depression; hepatic impairment; renal impairment (Appendix 3); pregnancy (Appendix 4); breast-feeding (Appendix 5); **interactions:** Appendix 1 (mirtazapine)

**Blood disorders** Patients should be advised to report any fever, sore throat, stomatitis or other signs of infection during treatment. Blood count should be performed and the drug stopped immediately if blood dyscrasia suspected

**Withdrawal** Nausea, vomiting, dizziness, agitation, anxiety, and headache are most common features of withdrawal if treatment stopped abruptly or if dose reduced markedly; dose should be reduced over several weeks

**Side-effects** increased appetite, weight gain, dry mouth; postural hypotension, peripheral oedema; drowsiness, fatigue, tremor, dizziness, abnormal dreams, confusion, anxiety, insomnia; arthralgia, myalgia; *less commonly* syncope, hypotension, mania, hallucinations, movement disorders; *rarely* myoclonus; *very rarely* blood disorders (see Cautions), convulsions, hyponatraemia (see Hyponatraemia and Antidepressant Therapy, p. 209), suicidal behaviour (see p. 209), and angle-closure glaucoma

**Dose**

• Initially 15–30 mg daily at bedtime increased within 2–4 weeks according to response; max. 45 mg daily as a single dose at bedtime or in 2 divided doses; CHILD under 18 years not recommended (see CSM advice, p. 215)

**Mirtazapine** (Non-proprietary) PoM
Tablets, mirtazapine 15 mg, net price 28-tab pack = £17.47; 30 mg, 28-tab pack = £2.69; 45 mg, 28-tab pack = £15.03. Label: 2, 25

Orodispersible tablets, mirtazapine 15 mg, net price 30-tab pack = £11.94; 30 mg, 30-tab pack = £11.94; 45 mg, 30-tab pack = £11.96. Label: 2, counselling, administration

Oral solution, mirtazapine 15 mg/mL, net price 66 mL = £47.00. Label: 2

**Zispin SolTab®** (Organon) PoM
Orodispersible tablets, mirtazapine 15 mg, net price 6-tab pack = £3.84, 30-tab pack = £18.83; 30 mg, 30-tab pack = £18.83; 45 mg, 30-tab pack = £18.83. Label: 2, counselling, administration
Excipients include aspartame (section 9.4.1)
Counselling *Zispin SolTab®* should be placed on the tongue, allowed to disperse and swallowed

## REBOXETINE

**Indications** major depression

**Cautions** history of cardiovascular disease and epilepsy; bipolar disorder; urinary retention; prostatic hypertrophy; susceptibility to angle-closure glaucoma; avoid abrupt withdrawal; hepatic impairment (Appendix 2); renal impairment (Appendix 3); **interactions:** Appendix 1 (reboxetine)

**Contra-indications** pregnancy (Appendix 4); breast-feeding (Appendix 5)

**Side-effects** nausea, dry mouth, constipation, anorexia; tachycardia, palpitation, vasodilation, postural hypotension; headache, insomnia, dizziness; chills;

impotence; urinary retention; impaired visual accommodation; sweating; lowering of plasma-potassium concentration on prolonged administration in the elderly; *very rarely* angle-closure glaucoma; *also reported* vomiting, hypertension, paraesthesia, agitation, anxiety, irritability, hallucinations, aggression, cold extremities, and rash; suicidal behaviour (see p. 209)

**Dose**

• 4 mg twice daily increased if necessary after 3–4 weeks to 10 mg daily in divided doses, max. 12 mg daily; CHILD under 18 years and ELDERLY not recommended

**Edronax®** (Pharmacia) PoM
Tablets, scored, reboxetine (as mesilate) 4 mg, net price 60-tab pack = £18.91. Counselling, driving

## TRYPTOPHAN
(L-Tryptophan)

**Indications** see notes above

**Cautions** eosinophilia-myalgia syndrome has been reported (withhold treatment if increased eosinophil count, myalgia, arthralgia, fever, dyspnoea, neuropathy, oedema or skin lesions develop until possibility of eosinophilia-myalgia syndrome excluded); pregnancy (Appendix 4); breast-feeding (Appendix 5); **interactions:** Appendix 1 (tryptophan)

**Contra-indications** history of eosinophilia-myalgia syndrome following use of tryptophan

**Side-effects** drowsiness, nausea, headache, light-headedness, suicidal behaviour (see p. 209); eosinophilia-myalgia syndrome, see Cautions

**Dose**

• 1 g 3 times daily; max. 6 g daily; ELDERLY lower dose may be appropriate especially in renal or hepatic impairment; CHILD not recommended

**Optimax®** (Merck) PoM
Tablets, scored, tryptophan 500 mg. Net price 84-tab pack = £23.47. Label: 3

## VENLAFAXINE

**Indications** major depression, generalised anxiety disorder

**Cautions** heart disease (monitor blood pressure); history of epilepsy; susceptibility to angle-closure glaucoma; concomitant use of drugs that increase risk of bleeding, history of bleeding disorders; hepatic impairment (avoid if severe—Appendix 2); renal impairment (avoid if eGFR less than 10 mL/minute/ 1.73 m² —Appendix 3); breast-feeding (Appendix 5); **interactions:** Appendix 1 (venlafaxine)

**Driving** May affect performance of skilled tasks (e.g. driving)

**Withdrawal** Gastro-intestinal disturbances, headache, anxiety, dizziness, paraesthesia, tremor, sleep disturbances, and sweating are most common features of withdrawal if treatment stopped abruptly or if dose reduced markedly; dose should be reduced over several weeks

**Contra-indications** conditions associated with high risk of cardiac arrhythmia, uncontrolled hypertension; pregnancy (Appendix 4)

**Side-effects** constipation, nausea, anorexia, weight changes, diarrhoea, dyspepsia, vomiting, abdominal pain; hypertension, palpitation, vasodilatation, changes in serum cholesterol; chills, pyrexia, dyspnoea, yawning; dizziness, dry mouth, insomnia, nervousness, drowsiness, asthenia, headache, abnormal dreams, agitation, anxiety, confusion, hypertonia, paraesthesia, tremor; urinary frequency, sexual dysfunction, menstrual disturbances; arthralgia, myalgia; visual disturbances, mydriasis (very rarely angle-closure glaucoma); tinnitus; sweating, pruritus, rash; *less commonly* bruxism, taste disturbance, hypotension and postural hypotension, arrhythmias, syndrome of inappropriate anti-diuretic hormone secretion (see Hyponatraemia and Antidepressant Therapy, p. 209), apathy, hallucinations, myoclonus, urinary retention, bleeding disorders (including ecchymosis and rarely haemorrhage), alopecia, hypersensitivity reactions including angioedema, urticaria, photosensitivity; *rarely* hepatitis, ataxia, incoordination, speech disorder, mania and hypomania, seizures, and neuroleptic malignant syndrome, Stevens-Johnson syndrome; *very rarely* pancreatitis, QT interval prolongation, aggression, delirium, extrapyramidal symptoms including akathisia, hyperprolactinaemia, blood dyscrasias, rhabdomyolysis; suicidal behaviour (doses over 300 mg under specialist supervision; see also p. 209)

**Dose**

- Depression, ADULT over 18 years, initially 75 mg daily in 2 divided doses increased if necessary after at least 3–4 weeks to 150 mg daily in 2 divided doses; severely depressed or hospitalised patients, increased further if necessary in steps of up to 75 mg every 2–3 days; max. 375 mg daily; CHILD under 18 years not recommended (see CSM advice, p. 215)
- Generalised anxiety disorder and social anxiety disorder, see under preparations below

**Venlafaxine** (Non-proprietary) [PoM]

Tablets, venlafaxine (as hydrochloride) 37.5 mg, net price 56-tab pack = £18.95; 75 mg, 56-tab pack = £30.04. Label: 3, counselling, driving

**Efexor®** (Wyeth) [PoM]

Tablets, peach, venlafaxine (as hydrochloride) 37.5 mg, net price 56-tab pack = £22.50; 75 mg, 56-tab pack = £37.51. Label: 3, counselling, driving

◢**Modified release**

**Efexor® XL** (Wyeth) [PoM]

Capsules, m/r, venlafaxine (as hydrochloride) 75 mg (peach), net price 28-cap pack = £22.50; 150 mg (orange), 28-cap pack = £37.51. Label: 3, 25, counselling, driving

Dose  depression, ADULT over 18 years, 75 mg once daily, increased if necessary after at least 3 weeks to 150 mg once daily; max. 225 mg once daily; CHILD under 18 years not recommended (see CSM advice, p. 215)

Generalised anxiety disorder, ADULT over 18 years, 75 mg once daily; discontinue if no response after 8 weeks

Social anxiety disorder, ADULT over 18 years, 75 mg once daily; discontinue if no response after 12 weeks

**Foraven XL®** (Forum) [PoM]

Capsules, m/r, venlafaxine (as hydrochloride) 75 mg (peach), net price 28-cap pack = £23.41; 150 mg (orange), 28-cap pack = £39.03. Label: 3, 25, counselling, driving

Dose  depression, ADULT over 18 years, 75 mg once daily, increased if necessary after at least 3 weeks to 150 mg once daily; max. 375 mg once daily (doses over 300 mg under specialist supervision); CHILD under 18 years not recommended (see CSM advice, p. 215)

**Tifaxin XL®** (Genus) [PoM]

Capsules, m/r, venlafaxine (as hydrochloride) 75 mg (yellow/transparent), net price 28-cap pack = £16.39; 150 mg (buff/transparent), 28-cap pack = £27.32. Label: 3, 25, counselling, driving

Dose  depression, ADULT over 18 years, 75 mg once daily, increased if necessary after at least 2 weeks to 150 mg once daily; increased according to response, max. 375 mg once daily (doses over 225 mg under specialist supervision); CHILD under 18 years not recommended (see CSM advice, p. 215)

Social anxiety disorder, ADULT over 18 years, 75 mg once daily; increased if necessary in steps of 75 mg after intervals of at least 4 days; max. 225 mg once daily; discontinue if no response after 12 weeks

**Venaxx XL®** (Goldshield) [PoM]

Capsules, m/r, venlafaxine (as hydrochloride) 75 mg (beige), net price 28-cap pack = £10.40; 150 mg (red), 28-cap pack = £17.40. Label: 3, 25, counselling, driving

Dose  depression, ADULT over 18 years, 75 mg once daily, increased if necessary after at least 2 weeks to 150 mg once daily; increased according to response, max. 375 mg once daily (doses over 225 mg under specialist supervision); CHILD under 18 years not recommended (see CSM advice, p. 215)

**Venlalic® XL** (Dallas Burston Ashbourne) [PoM]

Tablets, m/r, venlafaxine (as hydrochloride) 75 mg, net price 30-tab pack = £12.27; 150 mg, 30-tab pack = £19.85; 225 mg 30-tab pack = £36.16. Label: 3, 25, counselling, driving

Dose  depression, ADULT over 18 years, 75 mg once daily, increased if necessary after at least 2 weeks to 150 mg once daily; increased according to response, max. 375 mg once daily (doses over 225 mg under specialist supervision); CHILD under 18 years not recommended (see CSM advice, p. 215)

## 4.4 CNS stimulants and drugs used for attention deficit hyperactivity disorder

Central nervous system stimulants include the **amphetamines** (notably dexamfetamine) **and related drugs** (e.g. methylphenidate). They have very few indications and in particular, should **not** be used to treat depression, obesity, senility, debility, or for relief of fatigue.

CNS stimulants should only be prescribed to children with severe and persistent symptoms of *attention deficit hyperactivity disorder* (ADHD), when the diagnosis has been confirmed by a specialist; treatment may be continued by general practitioners, under a shared-care arrangement. Treatment often needs to be continued into adolescence, and may need to be continued into adulthood.

Drug treatment of ADHD should be part of a comprehensive treatment programme. The choice of medication should take into consideration co-morbid conditions (such as tic disorders, Tourette syndrome and epilepsy), the adverse effect profile, potential for drug misuse, and preferences of the patient and carers. **Methylphenidate** and **atomoxetine** are used for the management of ADHD; **dexamfetamine** (dexamphetamine) is an alternative in children who do not respond to these drugs. Growth is not generally affected by treatment with CNS stimulants but it is advisable to monitor growth during treatment.

**Modafinil** is used for the treatment of daytime sleepiness associated with narcolepsy or obstructive sleep apnoea syndrome; dependence with long-term use cannot be excluded and it should therefore be used with caution.

Dexamfetamine and methylphenidate [unlicensed indication] are also used to treat narcolepsy.

## ATOMOXETINE

**Indications** attention deficit hyperactivity disorder (initiated by a specialist physician experienced in managing the condition)

**Cautions** cardiovascular disease including hypertension and tachycardia; structural cardiac abnormalities; monitor growth in children; QT interval prolongation (avoid concomitant administration of drugs that prolong QT interval); psychosis or mania; history of seizures; aggressive behaviour, hostility, or emotional lability; susceptibility to angle-closure glaucoma; hepatic impairment (see Hepatic Disorders below; Appendix 2); pregnancy (Appendix 4); breast-feeding (Appendix 5); **interactions:** Appendix 1 (atomoxetine)

**Hepatic disorders** Following rare reports of hepatic disorders, the CSM has advised that patients and carers should be advised of the risk and be told how to recognise symptoms; prompt medical attention should be sought in case of abdominal pain, unexplained nausea, malaise, darkening of the urine or jaundice

**Suicidal ideation** Following reports of suicidal thoughts and behaviour, the CSM has advised that patients and their carers should be informed about the risk and told to report clinical worsening, suicidal thoughts or behaviour, irritability, agitation, or depression

**Side-effects** anorexia, dry mouth, nausea, vomiting, abdominal pain, constipation, dyspepsia, flatulence; palpitation, tachycardia, increased blood pressure, postural hypotension, hot flushes; sleep disturbance, dizziness, headache, fatigue, lethargy, depression, psychotic or manic symptoms, aggression, hostility, emotional lability, drowsiness, anxiety, irritability, tremor, rigors; urinary retention, enuresis, prostatitis, sexual dysfunction, menstrual disturbances; mydriasis, conjunctivitis; dermatitis, pruritus, rash, sweating, weight changes; *less commonly* suicidal ideation (see Suicidal Ideation, above), cold extremities; *very rarely* hepatic disorders (see Hepatic Disorders, above), seizures, angle-closure glaucoma, and Raynaud's phenomenon

**Dose**
- ADULT over 18 years, body-weight over 70 kg, initially 40 mg daily for 7 days, increased according to response; usual maintenance 80–100 mg daily, but may be increased to max. 120 mg daily [unlicensed] under the direction of a specialist; CHILD 6–18 years, body-weight over 70 kg, initially 40 mg daily for 7 days, increased according to response; usual maintenance 80 mg daily, but may be increased to max. 120 mg daily [unlicensed] under the direction of a specialist; ADULT and CHILD over 6 years, body-weight under 70 kg, initially 500 micrograms/kg daily for 7 days, increased according to response; usual maintenance 1.2 mg/kg daily, but may be increased to 1.8 mg/kg daily (max. 120 mg daily) [unlicensed] under the direction of a specialist

**Note** Total daily dose may be given *either* as a single dose in the morning *or* in 2 divided doses with last dose no later than early evening

**Strattera®** (Lilly) ▼ PoM
Capsules, atomoxetine (as hydrochloride) 10 mg (white), net price 7-cap pack = £15.02, 28-cap pack = £60.06; 18 mg (gold/white), 7-cap pack = £15.02, 28-cap pack = £60.06; 25 mg (blue/white), 7-cap pack = £15.02, 28-cap pack = £60.06; 40 mg (blue), 7-cap pack = £15.02, 28-cap pack = £60.06; 60 mg (blue/gold), 28-cap pack = £60.06; 80 mg (brown/white), 28-cap pack = £80.08. Label: 3

## DEXAMFETAMINE SULPHATE
(Dexamphetamine sulphate)

**Indications** narcolepsy; refractory attention deficit hyperactivity disorder (under specialist supervision)

**Cautions** anorexia; mild hypertension (contra-indicated if moderate or severe)—monitor blood pressure; psychosis or bipolar disorder; monitor for aggressive behaviour or hostility during initial treatment; renal impairment; history of epilepsy (discontinue if convulsions occur); tics and Tourette syndrome (use with caution)—discontinue if tics occur; monitor growth in children (see also below); susceptibility to angle-closure glaucoma; avoid abrupt withdrawal; data on safety and efficacy of long-term use not complete; acute porphyria (section 9.8.2); **interactions:** Appendix 1 (sympathomimetics)

**Special cautions in children** Monitor height and weight as growth restriction may occur during prolonged therapy (drug-free periods may allow catch-up in growth but withdraw slowly to avoid inducing depression or renewed hyperactivity)

**Driving** May affect performance of skilled tasks (e.g. driving); effects of alcohol unpredictable

**Contra-indications** cardiovascular disease including moderate to severe hypertension, structural cardiac abnormalities, advanced arteriosclerosis, hyperexcitability or agitated states, hyperthyroidism, history of drug or alcohol abuse; pregnancy (Appendix 4); breast-feeding (Appendix 5)

**Side-effects** insomnia, restlessness, irritability and excitability, night terrors, euphoria, tremor, dizziness, aggression, paranoia, anxiety, confusion, depression, fatigue, headache; convulsions (see also Cautions); dependence and tolerance, psychosis; anorexia, gastro-intestinal symptoms, growth restriction in children (see also under Cautions); dry mouth, sweating, tachycardia (and anginal pain), palpitation, myocardial infarction, hypertension, hypotension; impotence; visual disturbances; alopecia, rash; cardiomyopathy reported with chronic use; cardiovascular collapse; cerebral vasculitis; central stimulants have provoked choreoathetoid movements and dyskinesia, tics and Tourette syndrome in predisposed individuals (see also Cautions above); *very rarely* angle-closure glaucoma; **overdosage:** see Emergency Treatment of Poisoning, p. 33

**Dose**
- Narcolepsy, 10 mg (ELDERLY, 5 mg) daily in divided doses increased by 10 mg (ELDERLY, 5 mg) daily at intervals of 1 week to a max. of 60 mg daily
- Refractory attention deficit hyperactivity disorder, ADULT over 18 years [unlicensed use], 5 mg twice daily, increased according to response; max. 60 mg daily; maintenance dose given in 2–4 divided doses; CHILD 4–6 years, 2.5 mg daily, increased if necessary by 2.5 mg daily at intervals of 1 week, usual max. 20 mg daily; CHILD 6–18 years 5–10 mg daily, increased if necessary by 5 mg daily at intervals of 1 week, usual max. 20 mg daily, but up to 40 mg daily occasionally required

4 **Central nervous system**

**Dexedrine®** (UCB Pharma) CD
Tablets, scored, dexamfetamine sulphate 5 mg. Net
price 28-tab pack = £3.00. Counselling, driving

# METHYLPHENIDATE HYDROCHLORIDE

**Indications** attention deficit hyperactivity disorder
(under specialist supervision); narcolepsy [unlicensed
indication]

**Cautions** monitor growth (if prolonged treatment);
blood pressure and full blood count; anxiety or agitation; tics or a family history of Tourette syndrome;
epilepsy (discontinue if increased seizure frequency);
susceptibility to angle-closure glaucoma; avoid abrupt
withdrawal; pregnancy (Appendix 4); **interactions:**
Appendix 1 (sympathomimetics)

**Contra-indications** anxiety or agitation; severe
depression; suicidal ideation; drug or alcohol dependence; psychosis; hyperthyroidism; cardiovascular
disease (including severe hypertension and arrhythmias), structural cardiac abnormalities; breast-feeding
(Appendix 5)

**Side-effects** abdominal pain, nausea, vomiting, dyspepsia, dry mouth, anorexia, reduced weight gain;
tachycardia, palpitation, arrhythmias, changes in
blood pressure; cough, nasopharyngitis; tics (*very
rarely* Tourette syndrome), insomnia, nervousness,
asthenia, depression, irritability, aggression, headache, drowsiness, dizziness, movement disorders;
fever; arthralgia; rash, pruritus, alopecia; *less commonly* diarrhoea, dyspnoea, abnormal dreams, confusion, suicidal ideation, urinary frequency, haematuria, muscle cramps, epistaxis; *rarely* angina, growth
restriction, visual disturbances; *very rarely* hepatic
dysfunction, myocardial infarction, cerebral arteritis,
psychosis, neuroleptic malignant syndrome, tolerance
and dependence, blood disorders including leucopenia and thrombocytopenia, angle-closure glaucoma, exfoliative dermatitis, erythema multiforme

**Dose**

● Attention deficit hyperactivity disorder, ADULT over 18
years [unlicensed use], 5 mg 3 times daily increased if
necessary according to response, max. 100 mg daily;
CHILD 6–18 years, initially 5 mg 1–2 times daily,
increased if necessary at weekly intervals by 5–10 mg
daily; usual max. 60 mg daily in divided doses but may
be increased to 2.1 mg/kg daily (max. 90 mg daily)
under the direction of a specialist; discontinue if no
response after 1 month, also suspend treatment every
1–2 years to assess condition; CHILD 4–6 years see
*BNF for Children*
 **Evening dose** If effect wears off in evening (with rebound
 hyperactivity) a dose at bedtime may be appropriate
 (establish need with trial bedtime dose)
 **Note** Treatment may be started using a modified-release
 preparation

● Narcolepsy [unlicensed indication], 10–60 mg (usually
20–30 mg) daily in divided doses before meals

**Methylphenidate Hydrochloride** (Non-proprietary)
CD
Tablets, methylphenidate hydrochloride 5 mg, net
price 30-tab pack = £2.67; 10 mg, 30-tab pack = £5.80;
20 mg, 30-tab pack = £9.59
Brands include *Equasym®*, *Medikinet®*

**Ritalin®** (Novartis) CD
Tablets, scored, methylphenidate hydrochloride
10 mg, net price 30-tab pack = £5.57

◢**Modified release**

**Concerta® XL** (Janssen-Cilag) CD
Tablets, m/r, methylphenidate hydrochloride 18 mg
(yellow), net price 30-tab pack = £31.19; 27 mg (grey),
30-tab pack = £36.81; 36 mg (white), 30-tab pack =
£42.45. Label: 25
 **Counselling** Tablet membrane may pass through gastro-intestinal
 tract unchanged
 **Cautions** dose form not appropriate for use in dysphagia or if
 gastro-intestinal lumen restricted
 **Dose** CHILD 6–18 years, initially 18 mg once daily (in the morning), increased if necessary in weekly steps of 18 mg according to
 response, usual max. 54 mg once daily, but may be increased to
 2.1 mg/kg daily (max. 108 mg daily) [unlicensed] under the
 direction of a specialist; discontinue if no response after 1 month;
 suspend treatment every 1–2 years to assess condition
 **Note** Total daily dose of 15 mg of standard-release formulation is
 equivalent to *Concerta® XL* 18 mg once daily

**Equasym XL®** (Shire) CD
Capsules, m/r, methylphenidate hydrochloride 10 mg
(white/green), net price 30-cap pack = £25.00; 20 mg
(white/blue), 30-cap pack = £30.00; 30 mg (white/
brown), 30-cap pack = £35.00. Label: 25
 **Dose** ADULT over 18 years [unlicensed use], initially 10 mg once
 daily in the morning before breakfast, increased gradually if
 necessary, max.100 mg daily; CHILD 6–18 years, initially 10 mg
 once daily in the morning before breakfast, increased gradually if
 necessary, usual max. 60 mg daily but may be increased to
 2.1 mg/kg daily (max. 90 mg daily) [unlicensed] under the direction of a specialist; discontinue if no response after 1 month;
 suspend treatment every 1–2 years to assess condition
 **Note** Contents of capsule can be sprinkled on a tablespoon of
 apple sauce (then swallowed immediately without chewing)

**Medikinet XL®** (Flynn) CD
Capsules, m/r, methylphenidate hydrochloride 10 mg
(lilac/white), net price 28-cap pack = £20.18; 20 mg
(lilac), 28-cap pack = £26.91; 30 mg (purple/light
grey), 28-cap pack = £31.39; 40 mg (purple/grey), 28-
cap pack = £43.20. Label: 25
 **Dose** ADULT over 18 years [unlicensed use], initially 10 mg once
 daily in the morning with breakfast, adjusted according to
 response, max. 100 mg daily; CHILD 6–18 years, initially 10 mg
 once daily in the morning with breakfast, adjusted according to
 response, usual max. 60 mg daily but may be increased to 2.1 mg/
 kg daily (max. 90 mg daily) [unlicensed] under the direction of a
 specialist; discontinue if no response after 1 month; suspend
 treatment every 1–2 years to assess condition
 **Note** Contents of capsule can be sprinkled on a tablespoon of
 apple sauce (then swallowed immediately without chewing)

# MODAFINIL

**Indications** daytime sleepiness associated with
narcolepsy, obstructive sleep apnoea syndrome, and
chronic shift work

**Cautions** monitor blood pressure and heart rate in
hypertensive patients (but see Contra-indications);
history of psychosis, depression, mania, alcohol or
drug abuse; discontinue treatment if psychiatric
symptoms develop; possibility of dependence; discontinue treatment if rash develops; hepatic impairment (Appendix 2); renal impairment (Appendix 3);
**interactions:** Appendix 1 (modafinil)

**Contra-indications** moderate to severe uncontrolled
hypertension, arrhythmia; history of left ventricular
hypertrophy, cor pulmonale, or of clinically significant
signs of CNS stimulant-induced mitral valve prolapse
(including ischaemic ECG changes, chest pain and
arrhythmias); pregnancy (Appendix 4); breast-feeding
(Appendix 5)

**Side-effects** dry mouth, appetite changes, gastro-
intestinal disturbances (including nausea, diarrhoea,

constipation, and dyspepsia), abdominal pain; tachycardia, vasodilatation, chest pain, palpitation; headache (uncommonly migraine), anxiety, sleep disturbances, dizziness, drowsiness, depression, confusion, paraesthesia, asthenia; *less commonly* flatulence, reflux, vomiting, mouth ulcers, glossitis, dysphagia, taste disturbance, weight changes, hypertension, hypotension, bradycardia, arrhythmia, peripheral oedema, hypercholesterolaemia, rhinitis, dyspnoea, epistaxis, dyskinesia, amnesia, emotional lability, tremor, decreased libido, agitation, aggression, hyperglycaemia, thirst, urinary frequency, menstrual disturbances, eosinophilia, leucopenia, myasthenia, muscle cramps, hypertonia, myalgia, arthralgia, dry eye, sinusitis, acne, sweating, rash, and pruritus; *also reported* psychosis, mania, delusions, hallucinations, suicidal ideation, Stevens-Johnson syndrome, and toxic epidermal necrolysis

**Dose**

- Narcolepsy and obstructive sleep apnoea syndrome, ADULT over 12 years, initially 200 mg daily, *either* in 2 divided doses morning and at noon *or* as a single dose in the morning, dose adjusted according to response to 200–400 mg daily in 2 divided doses or as a single dose; ELDERLY initiate at 100 mg daily; CHILD 5–12 years, see *BNF for Children*
- Chronic shift work sleep disorder, 200 mg taken 1 hour before the start of the work shift

**Provigil®** (Cephalon) ▼ PoM
Tablets, modafinil 100 mg, net price 30-tab pack = £53.62; 200 mg (scored), 30 tab-pack = £107.25

---

## Cocaine

**Cocaine** is a drug of addiction which causes central nervous stimulation. Its clinical use is mainly as a topical local anaesthetic (section 15.2). It has been included in analgesic elixirs for the relief of pain in palliative care but this use is obsolete. For management of cocaine poisoning, see p. 33.

## 4.5 Drugs used in the treatment of obesity

4.5.1 Anti-obesity drugs acting on the gastro-intestinal tract
4.5.2 Centrally acting appetite suppressants

Obesity is associated with many health problems including cardiovascular disease, diabetes mellitus, gallstones and osteoarthritis. Factors that aggravate obesity may include depression, other psychosocial problems, and some drugs.

The main treatment of the obese individual is a suitable diet, carefully explained to the individual, with appropriate support and encouragement; the individual should also be advised to increase physical activity. Smoking cessation (while maintaining body weight) may be worthwhile before attempting supervised weight loss since cigarette smoking may be more harmful than obesity. Attendance at groups (e.g. 'weight-watchers') helps some individuals.

Obesity should be managed in an appropriate setting by staff who have been trained in the management of obesity; the individual should receive advice on diet and lifestyle modification and be monitored for changes in weight as well as in blood pressure, blood lipids and other associated conditions.

An anti-obesity drug should be considered only for those with a body mass index (BMI, individual's bodyweight divided by the square of the individual's height) of 30 kg/$m^2$ or greater in whom at least 3 months of managed care involving supervised diet, exercise and behaviour modification fails to achieve a realistic reduction in weight. In the presence of risk factors (such as diabetes, coronary heart disease, hypertension, and obstructive sleep apnoea), it may be appropriate to prescribe a drug to individuals with a BMI of 27 kg/$m^2$ or greater, provided that such use is permitted by the drug's marketing authorisation. Drugs should **never** be used as the sole element of treatment. The individual should be monitored on a regular basis; drug treatment should be discontinued if the individual regains weight at any time whilst receiving drug treatment.

Drugs specifically licensed for the management of obesity are **orlistat** (section 4.5.1), **sibutramine** and **rimonabant** (both section 4.5.2). There is little evidence to guide selection between these drugs, but it may be appropriate to choose orlistat for those who have a high intake of fats whereas sibutramine or rimonabant may be chosen for those who cannot control their eating.

Combination therapy involving more than one anti-obesity drug is **contra-indicated** until further information about efficacy and long-term safety is available.

Thyroid hormones have **no** place in the treatment of obesity except in biochemically proven hypothyroid patients. The use of diuretics, chorionic gonadotrophin, or amphetamines is **not** appropriate for weight reduction.

## 4.5.1 Anti-obesity drugs acting on the gastro-intestinal tract

**Orlistat**, a lipase inhibitor, reduces the absorption of dietary fat. It is used in conjunction with a mildly hypocaloric diet in individuals with a body mass index (BMI) of 30 kg/$m^2$ or more *or* in individuals with a BMI of 28 kg/$m^2$ in the presence of other risk factors such as type 2 diabetes, hypertension, or hypercholesterolaemia.

Orlistat should be used in conjunction with other lifestyle measures to manage obesity (section 4.5); treatment should only be continued beyond 12 months after discussing potential benefits and risks with the patient. On stopping orlistat, there may be a gradual reversal of weight loss.

Some of the weight loss in those taking orlistat probably results from individuals reducing their fat intake to avoid severe gastro-intestinal effects including steatorrhoea. Vitamin supplementation (especially of vitamin D) may be considered if there is concern about deficiency of fat-soluble vitamins.

The most commonly used bulk-forming drug is **methylcellulose** (section 1.6.1). It is claimed to reduce intake by producing a feeling of satiety but there is little evidence to support its use in the management of obesity.

**Central nervous system** 4

### ORLISTAT

**Indications** adjunct in obesity (see notes above)

**Cautions** may impair absorption of fat-soluble vitamins; epilepsy; pregnancy (Appendix 4); **interactions:** Appendix 1 (orlistat)

**Multivitamins** If a multivitamin supplement is required, it should be taken at least 2 hours after orlistat dose or at bedtime

**Contra-indications** chronic malabsorption syndrome; cholestasis; breast-feeding (Appendix 5)

**Side-effects** oily leakage from rectum, flatulence, faecal urgency, liquid or oily stools, faecal incontinence, abdominal distension and pain (gastro-intestinal effects minimised by reduced fat intake), tooth and gingival disorders; respiratory infections; fatigue, anxiety, headache; menstrual disturbances, urinary-tract infection; hypoglycaemia; *rarely* rectal bleeding, hypothyroidism; *very rarely* diverticulitis, cholelithiasis, hepatitis, and bullous eruptions; oxalate nephropathy also reported

**Dose**

- ADULT over 18 years, 120 mg taken immediately before, during, or up to 1 hour after each main meal (up to max. 360 mg daily); continue treatment beyond 12 weeks only if weight loss since start of treatment exceeds 5% (target for initial weight loss may be lower in patients with type 2 diabetes); CHILD over 12 years, initiated by specialist only [unlicensed use]

**Note** If a meal is missed or contains no fat, the dose of orlistat should be omitted

**Xenical®** (Roche) ▼ [PoM]

Capsules, turquoise, orlistat 120 mg, net price 84-cap pack = £32.27

---

### 4.5.2 Centrally acting appetite suppressants

**Sibutramine** inhibits the re-uptake of noradrenaline and serotonin. It is used in the adjunctive management of obesity in individuals with a body mass index (BMI) of 30 kg/m$^2$ or more (and no associated co-morbidity) or in individuals with a BMI of 27 kg/m$^2$ or more in the presence of other risk factors such as type 2 diabetes or dyslipidaemia. Sibutramine is not licensed for use for longer than 1 year; on stopping sibutramine, there may be a gradual reversal of weight loss.

**Rimonabant** is a cannabinoid receptor antagonist for the adjunctive management of obesity in individuals with a BMI of 30 kg/m$^2$ or more, or in individuals with a BMI above 27 kg/m$^2$ in the presence of other risk factors such as type 2 diabetes or dyslipidaemia. On stopping rimonabant, there may be a gradual reversal of weight loss.

> **Rimonabant**
> The marketing authorisation for rimonabant has been suspended following a review by the CHMP. The CHMP concluded that the benefits of rimonabant treatment do not outweigh the risks of psychiatric adverse reactions. Prescribers should not issue prescriptions for rimonabant; treatment of patients who are taking rimonabant should be reviewed.

Dexfenfluramine, diethylpropion, fenfluramine, and phentermine have been associated with valvular heart disease and the rare but serious risk of pulmonary hypertension.

### RIMONABANT

**Indications** adjunct in obesity (see notes above)

**Cautions** epilepsy; history of suicidal ideation or of depressive disorder (avoid unless no alternative); elderly—over 75 years; hepatic impairment (avoid if severe—Appendix 2); **interactions:** Appendix 1 (rimonabant)

**Contra-indications** major depressive illness, concomitant treatment with antidepressant; uncontrolled psychiatric illness; severe renal impairment; pregnancy (Appendix 4); breast-feeding (Appendix 5)

**Depression** Patients and carers should be informed of the risk of depression and advised to stop treatment and seek medical attention if symptoms occur

**Side-effects** nausea, vomiting, diarrhoea, dry mouth, anorexia; depression (see above), anxiety, irritability, nervousness, sleep disorders, impaired memory, dizziness, paraesthesia, hypoaesthesia, sciatica, hot flush, asthenia, impaired attention; tendonitis, muscle cramp; pruritus, hyperhidrosis; *less commonly* hiccups, anger, aggression, suicidal ideation; *rarely* hallucinations

**Dose**

- See Rimonabant, above; ADULT over 18 years 20 mg daily before breakfast

**Acomplia®** (Sanofi-Aventis) ▼ [PoM]

Tablets, f/c, rimonabant 20 mg, net price 28-tab pack = £44.00. Counselling, depression (see above)

---

### SIBUTRAMINE HYDROCHLORIDE

**Indications** adjunct in obesity (see notes above)

**Cautions** monitor blood pressure and pulse rate (every 2 weeks for first 3 months *then* monthly for 3 months *then* at least every 3 months)—discontinue if blood pressure exceeds 145/90 mmHg or if systolic or diastolic pressure raised by more than 10 mmHg or if pulse rate raised by 10 beats per minute at 2 consecutive visits; sleep apnoea syndrome (increased risk of hypertension); epilepsy; open-angle glaucoma, susceptibility to angle-closure glaucoma, history of ocular hypertension; monitor for pulmonary hypertension; family history of motor or vocal tics, history of depression; predisposition to bleeding, concomitant use of drugs that increase risk of bleeding; hepatic impairment (avoid if severe; Appendix 2); renal impairment (avoid if eGFR less than 30 mL/minute/1.73 m$^2$; Appendix 3); **interactions:** Appendix 1 (sibutramine)

**Contra-indications** history of major eating disorders; psychiatric illness; Tourette syndrome; history of coronary artery disease, congestive heart failure, tachycardia, peripheral arterial occlusive disease, arrhythmias, and of cerebrovascular disease; uncontrolled hypertension; hyperthyroidism; prostatic hypertrophy; phaeochromocytoma; history of drug or alcohol abuse; pregnancy (Appendix 4); breast-feeding (Appendix 5)

**Side-effects** constipation, dry mouth, nausea, taste disturbances, diarrhoea, vomiting, gastro-intestinal haemorrhage, haemorrhoid aggravation; tachycardia, palpitation, arrhythmias, hypertension, flushing; insomnia, lightheadedness, paraesthesia, headache, anxiety, depression, seizures, transient memory disturbance; sexual dysfunction, menstrual disturbances, urinary retention; thrombocytopenia; blurred vision; sweating, alopecia, cutaneous bleeding disorders, hypersensitivity reactions including Henoch-Schön-lein purpura, rash, urticaria, angioedema and anaphylaxis; interstitial nephritis, glomerulonephritis; *rarely* headache and increased appetite on withdrawal; *very rarely* angle-closure glaucoma

**Dose**

- Initially 10 mg daily in the morning, increased if weight loss less than 2 kg after 4 weeks to 15 mg daily; discontinue if weight loss less than 2 kg after 4 weeks at higher dose (see also Discontinuation of Treatment below); max. period of treatment 1 year; CHILD over 12 years, initiated by specialist only [unlicensed use]; ELDERLY over 65 years not recommended

**Discontinuation of treatment** Discontinue treatment if:

- weight loss after 3 months less than 5% of initial body-weight;
- weight loss stabilises at less than 5% of initial body-weight;
- individuals regain 3 kg or more after previous weight loss

In individuals with co-morbid conditions, treatment should be continued only if weight loss is associated with other clinical benefits

**Reductil®** (Abbott) PoM

Capsules, sibutramine hydrochloride 10 mg (blue/yellow), net price 28-cap pack = £25.00; 15 mg (blue/white), 28-cap pack = £25.00

## 4.6 Drugs used in nausea and vertigo

Antiemetics should be prescribed only when the cause of vomiting is known because otherwise they may delay diagnosis, particularly in children. Antiemetics are unnecessary and sometimes harmful when the cause can be treated, such as in diabetic ketoacidosis, or in digoxin or antiepileptic overdose.

If antiemetic drug treatment is indicated, the drug is chosen according to the aetiology of vomiting.

**Antihistamines** are effective against nausea and vomiting resulting from many underlying conditions. There is no evidence that any one antihistamine is superior to another but their duration of action and incidence of adverse effects (drowsiness and antimuscarinic effects) differ.

The **phenothiazines** are dopamine antagonists and act centrally by blocking the chemoreceptor trigger zone. They are of considerable value for the prophylaxis and treatment of nausea and vomiting associated with diffuse neoplastic disease, radiation sickness, and the emesis caused by drugs such as opioids, general anaesthetics, and cytotoxics. **Prochlorperazine**, **perphenazine**, and **trifluoperazine** are less sedating than **chlorpromazine**; severe dystonic reactions sometimes occur with phenothiazines, especially in children. Some phenothiazines are available as rectal suppositories, which can be useful in patients with persistent vomiting or with severe nausea; prochlorperazine can also be administered as a buccal tablet which is placed between the upper lip and the gum.

**Droperidol** is a butyrophenone, structurally related to haloperidol, which blocks dopamine receptors in the chemoreceptor trigger zone.

Other antipsychotic drugs including **haloperidol** and **levomepromazine** (methotrimeprazine) are used for the relief of nausea and vomiting in terminal illness (see Palliative Care, p. 17).

**Metoclopramide** is an effective antiemetic and its activity closely resembles that of the phenothiazines. Metoclopramide also acts directly on the gastro-intestinal tract and it may be superior to the phenothiazines for emesis associated with gastroduodenal, hepatic, and biliary disease. In postoperative nausea and vomiting, metoclopramide in a dose of 10 mg has limited efficacy. High-dose metoclopramide injection is now less commonly used for cytotoxic-induced nausea and vomiting. As with the phenothiazines, metoclopramide can induce acute dystonic reactions involving facial and skeletal muscle spasms and oculogyric crises. These dystonic effects are more common in the young (especially girls and young women) and the very old; they usually occur shortly after starting treatment with metoclopramide and subside within 24 hours of stopping it. Injection of an antiparkinsonian drug such as procyclidine (section 4.9.2) will abort dystonic attacks.

**Domperidone** acts at the chemoreceptor trigger zone; it is used for the relief of nausea and vomiting, especially when associated with cytotoxic therapy. It has the advantage over metoclopramide and the phenothiazines of being less likely to cause central effects such as sedation and dystonic reactions because it does not readily cross the blood-brain barrier. In Parkinson's disease, it is used to prevent nausea and vomiting during treatment with apomorphine and also to treat nausea caused by other dopaminergic drugs (section 4.9.1). Domperidone is also used to treat vomiting due to emergency hormonal contraception (section 7.3.5).

**Dolasetron, granisetron,** and **ondansetron** are specific $5HT_3$ antagonists which block $5HT_3$ receptors in the gastro-intestinal tract and in the CNS. They are of value in the management of nausea and vomiting in patients receiving cytotoxics and in postoperative nausea and vomiting. **Palonosetron** is licensed for prevention of nausea and vomiting associated with moderately or highly emetogenic cytotoxic chemotherapy.

**Dexamethasone** (section 6.3.2) has antiemetic effects and it is used in vomiting associated with cancer chemotherapy. It can be used alone or with metoclopramide, prochlorperazine, lorazepam, or a $5HT_3$ antagonist (section 8.1).

**Aprepitant** and **fosaprepitant** are neurokinin 1 receptor antagonists licensed for the prevention of acute and delayed nausea and vomiting associated with cisplatin-based cytotoxic chemotherapy; they are given with dexamethasone and a $5HT_3$ antagonist.

**Nabilone** is a synthetic cannabinoid with antiemetic properties. It may be used for nausea and vomiting caused by cytotoxic chemotherapy that is unresponsive to conventional antiemetics. Side-effects such as drowsiness and dizziness occur frequently with standard doses.

## Vomiting during pregnancy

Nausea in the first trimester of pregnancy is generally mild and does not require drug therapy. On rare occasions if vomiting is severe, short-term treatment with an antihistamine, such as **promethazine**, may be required. **Prochlorperazine** or **metoclopramide** may be considered as second-line treatments. If symptoms do not settle in 24 to 48 hours then specialist opinion should be sought. Hyperemesis gravidarum is a more serious condition, which requires intravenous fluid and electrolyte replacement and sometimes nutritional support. Supplementation with thiamine must be considered in order to reduce the risk of Wernicke's encephalopathy.

## Postoperative nausea and vomiting

The incidence of postoperative nausea and vomiting depends on many factors including the anaesthetic used, the type and duration of surgery, and the patient's sex. The aim is to prevent postoperative nausea and vomiting from occurring. Drugs used include some **phenothiazines** (e.g. prochlorperazine), **droperidol**, **metoclopramide** (but 10-mg dose has limited efficacy and higher parenteral doses associated with greater side-effects), **5HT₃ antagonists**, **antihistamines** (such as cyclizine), and **dexamethasone**. A combination of two antiemetic drugs acting at different sites may be needed in resistant postoperative nausea and vomiting.

## Motion sickness

Antiemetics should be given to prevent motion sickness rather than after nausea or vomiting develop. The most effective drug for the prevention of motion sickness is **hyoscine**. A transdermal hyoscine patch provides prolonged activity but it needs to be applied several hours before travelling. The sedating antihistamines are slightly less effective against motion sickness, but are generally better tolerated than hyoscine. If a sedative effect is desired **promethazine** is useful, but generally a slightly less sedating antihistamine such as **cyclizine** or **cinnarizine** is preferred. The 5HT₃ antagonists, domperidone, metoclopramide, and the phenothiazines (except the antihistamine phenothiazine promethazine) are **ineffective** in motion sickness.

## Other vestibular disorders

Management of vestibular diseases is aimed at treating the underlying cause as well as treating symptoms of the balance disturbance and associated nausea and vomiting. Vertigo and nausea associated with Ménière's disease and middle-ear surgery can be difficult to treat.

**Betahistine** is an analogue of histamine and is claimed to reduce endolymphatic pressure by improving the microcirculation. Betahistine is licensed for vertigo, tinnitus, and hearing loss associated with Ménière's disease.

A **diuretic** alone or combined with salt restriction may provide some benefit in vertigo associated with Ménière's disease; **antihistamines** (such as cinnarizine), and **phenothiazines** (such as prochlorperazine) are also used. Where possible, prochlorperazine should be reserved for the treatment of acute symptoms.

For advice to avoid the inappropriate prescribing of drugs (notably phenothiazines) for dizziness in the elderly, see Prescribing for the Elderly, p. 19.

## Cytotoxic chemotherapy

For the management of nausea and vomiting induced by cytotoxic chemotherapy, see section 8.1.

## Palliative care

For the management of nausea and vomiting in palliative care, see p. 17 and p. 18.

## Migraine

For the management of nausea and vomiting associated with migraine, see p. 251.

## Antihistamines

### ▮ CINNARIZINE

**Indications** vestibular disorders, such as vertigo, tinnitus, nausea, and vomiting in Ménière's disease; motion sickness

**Cautions** section 3.4.1; pregnancy (Appendix 4); breast-feeding (Appendix 5)

**Contra-indications** section 3.4.1

**Side-effects** section 3.4.1; also *rarely* weight gain, sweating, lichen planus, and lupus-like skin reactions

**Dose**

- Vestibular disorders, 30 mg 3 times daily; CHILD 5–12 years 15 mg 3 times daily
- Motion sickness, 30 mg 2 hours before travel then 15 mg every 8 hours during journey if necessary; CHILD 5–12 years, 15 mg 2 hours before travel then 7.5 mg every 8 hours during journey if necessary

**Cinnarizine** (Non-proprietary)
Tablets, cinnarizine 15 mg, net price 84-tab pack = £17.35. Label: 2

**Stugeron®** (Janssen-Cilag)
Tablets, scored, cinnarizine 15 mg, net price 15-tab pack = £1.55, 100-tab pack = £3.35. Label: 2

#### ▰With dimenhydrinate
**Arlevert®** (Hampton) [PoM]
Tablets, cinnarizine 20 mg, dimenhydrinate 40 mg, net price 100-tab pack = £24.00. Label: 2
Dose ADULT over 18 years, 1 tablet 3 times daily

### ▮ CYCLIZINE

**Indications** nausea, vomiting, vertigo, motion sickness, labyrinthine disorders

**Cautions** section 3.4.1; severe heart failure; may counteract haemodynamic benefits of opioids; **interactions**: Appendix 1 (antihistamines)

**Contra-indications** section 3.4.1

**Side-effects** section 3.4.1

**Dose**

- By mouth, cyclizine hydrochloride 50 mg up to 3 times daily; CHILD 6–12 years 25 mg up to 3 times daily
- By intramuscular *or* intravenous injection, cyclizine lactate 50 mg 3 times daily

**Valoid®** (Amdipharm)
Tablets, scored, cyclizine hydrochloride 50 mg. Net price 100 = £7.41. Label: 2
Injection [PoM], cyclizine lactate 50 mg/mL. Net price 1-mL amp = 52p

## PROMETHAZINE HYDROCHLORIDE

**Indications** nausea, vomiting, vertigo, labyrinthine disorders, motion sickness; allergy and urticaria (section 3.4.1); sedation (section 4.1.1)

**Cautions** section 3.4.1

**Contra-indications** section 3.4.1

**Side-effects** section 3.4.1 but more sedating

**Dose**

- By mouth, 20–25 mg at bedtime on night before travel, repeat following morning if necessary; CHILD 2–5 years 5 mg at night, and following morning if necessary, 5–10 years 10 mg at night, and following morning if necessary

◢**Preparations**
Section 3.4.1

## PROMETHAZINE TEOCLATE

**Indications** nausea, vertigo, labyrinthine disorders, motion sickness (acts longer than the hydrochloride)

**Cautions** section 3.4.1; also pregnancy (Appendix 4) and breast-feeding (Appendix 5)

**Contra-indications** section 3.4.1

**Side-effects** section 3.4.1

**Dose**

- 25–75 mg, max. 100 mg, daily; CHILD 5–10 years, 12.5–37.5 mg daily
- Motion sickness prevention, ADULT and CHILD over 10 years, 25 mg at bedtime on night before travel *or* 25 mg 1–2 hours before travel; CHILD 5–10 years, 12.5 mg at bedtime on night before travel *or* 12.5 mg 1–2 hours before travel
- Severe vomiting during pregnancy [unlicensed], 25 mg at bedtime, increased if necessary to max. 100 mg daily (but see also Vomiting During Pregnancy, p. 225)

**Avomine®** (Manx)
Tablets, scored, promethazine teoclate 25 mg. Net price 10-tab pack = £1.13; 28-tab pack = £3.13. Label: 2

## Phenothiazines and related drugs

## CHLORPROMAZINE HYDROCHLORIDE

**Indications** nausea and vomiting of terminal illness (where other drugs have failed or are not available); other indications (section 4.2.1 and section 15.1.4.1)

**Cautions** see Chlorpromazine Hydrochloride, section 4.2.1

**Contra-indications** see Chlorpromazine Hydrochloride, section 4.2.1

**Side-effects** see Chlorpromazine Hydrochloride, section 4.2.1

**Dose**

- By mouth, 10–25 mg every 4–6 hours; CHILD 500 micrograms/kg every 4–6 hours (1–5 years max. 40 mg daily, 6–12 years max. 75 mg daily)
- By deep intramuscular injection initially 25 mg then 25–50 mg every 3–4 hours until vomiting stops; CHILD 500 micrograms/kg every 6–8 hours (1–5

years max. 40 mg daily, 6–12 years max. 75 mg daily)

- By rectum in suppositories, chlorpromazine 100 mg every 6–8 hours [unlicensed]

◢**Preparations**
Section 4.2.1

## DROPERIDOL

**Indications** prevention and treatment of postoperative nausea and vomiting

**Cautions** see section 4.2.1 also chronic obstructive pulmonary disease or respiratory failure; electrolyte disturbances; history of alcohol abuse; continuous pulse oximetry required if risk of ventricular arrhythmia—continue for 30 minutes following administration; hepatic impairment (Appendix 2); renal impairment (Appendix 3); pregnancy (Appendix 4); breast-feeding (Appendix 5); **interactions**: Appendix 1 (droperidol)

**Contra-indications** see section 4.2.1; QT-interval prolongation (avoid concomitant administration of drugs that prolong QT-interval); hypokalaemia; hypomagnesaemia; bradycardia

**Side-effects** see section 4.2.1; also anxiety, cardiac arrest, hallucinations, and inappropriate antidiuretic hormone secretion

**Dose**

- Prevention and treatment of postoperative nausea and vomiting, by intravenous injection, 0.625–1.25 mg (ELDERLY 625 micrograms) 30 minutes before end of surgery, repeated every 6 hours as required; CHILD over 2 years (second-line use only) 20–50 micrograms/kg (max. 1.25 mg)
- Prevention of nausea and vomiting caused by opioid analgesics in postoperative patient-controlled analgesia (PCA), by intravenous injection, 15–50 micrograms of droperidol for every 1 mg of morphine in PCA (max. 5 mg droperidol daily); ELDERLY reduce dose

**Xomolix®** (ProStrakan) ▼ [PoM]
Injection, droperidol 2.5 mg/mL, net price 1–mL amp = £3.94

## PERPHENAZINE

**Indications** severe nausea, vomiting (see notes above); other indications (section 4.2.1)

**Cautions** see Perphenazine (section 4.2.1)

**Contra-indications** see Perphenazine (section 4.2.1)

**Side-effects** see Perphenazine (section 4.2.1); extra-pyramidal symptoms particularly in young adults, elderly, and debilitated

**Dose**

- 4 mg 3 times daily, adjusted according to response; max. 24 mg daily (chemotherapy-induced); ELDERLY quarter to half adult dose; CHILD under 14 years not recommended

◢**Preparations**
Section 4.2.1

**4**

**Central nervous system**

Central nervous system

4

## PROCHLORPERAZINE

**Indications** severe nausea, vomiting, vertigo, labyrinthine disorders (see notes above); other indications section 4.2.1

**Cautions** see under Prochlorperazine (section 4.2.1); oral route only for children (avoid if under 10 kg); elderly (see notes above)

**Contra-indications** see under Prochlorperazine (section 4.2.1)

**Side-effects** see under Prochlorperazine (section 4.2.1); extrapyramidal symptoms, particularly in children, elderly, and debilitated

**Dose**

Note Doses are expressed as prochlorperazine maleate or mesilate; 1 mg prochlorperazine maleate ≡ 1 mg prochlorperazine mesilate

- By mouth, nausea and vomiting, acute attack, 20 mg initially then 10 mg after 2 hours; prevention 5–10 mg 2–3 times daily; CHILD (over 10 kg only) 250 micrograms/kg 2–3 times daily

  Labyrinthine disorders, 5 mg 3 times daily, gradually increased if necessary to 30 mg daily in divided doses, then reduced after several weeks to 5–10 mg daily; CHILD not recommended

- By deep intramuscular injection, nausea and vomiting, 12.5 mg when required followed if necessary after 6 hours by an oral dose, as above; CHILD and ADOLESCENT under 18 years, see *BNF for Children*

**Prochlorperazine** (Non-proprietary) PoM

Tablets, prochlorperazine maleate 5 mg, net price 28 = £1.83, 84 = £4.15. Label: 2

**Stemetil®** (Castlemead) PoM

Tablets, prochlorperazine maleate 5 mg (off-white), net price 84-tab pack = £5.94. Label: 2

Syrup, straw-coloured, prochlorperazine mesilate 5 mg/5 mL. Net price 100-mL pack = £3.34. Label: 2

Injection, prochlorperazine mesilate 12.5 mg/mL, net price 1-mL amp = 52p

◢Buccal preparation

¹**Buccastem®** (R&C) PoM

Tablets (buccal), pale yellow, prochlorperazine maleate 3 mg, net price 5 × 10-tab pack = £4.91. Label: 2, counselling, administration, see under Dose below

Dose ADULT and CHILD over 12 years, 1–2 tablets twice daily; tablets are placed high between upper lip and gum and left to dissolve

1. Prochlorperazine maleate can be sold to the public for adults over 18 years (provided packs do not contain more than 24 mg) for the treatment of nausea and vomiting in previously diagnosed migraine only (max. daily dose 12 mg)

## TRIFLUOPERAZINE

**Indications** severe nausea and vomiting (see notes above); other indications (section 4.2.1)

**Cautions** section 4.2.1

**Contra-indications** section 4.2.1

**Side-effects** section 4.2.1; extrapyramidal symptoms, particularly in children, elderly, and debilitated

**Dose**

- 2–4 mg daily in divided doses *or* as a single dose of a modified-release preparation; max. 6 mg daily; CHILD 3–5 years up to 1 mg daily, 6–12 years up to 4 mg daily

◢Preparations

Section 4.2.1

## Domperidone and metoclopramide

## DOMPERIDONE

**Indications** nausea and vomiting, dyspepsia, gastro-oesophageal reflux

**Cautions** children; renal impairment (Appendix 3); breast-feeding (Appendix 5); **interactions**: Appendix 1 (domperidone)

**Contra-indications** prolactinoma, hepatic impairment; where increased gastro-intestinal motility harmful; pregnancy (Appendix 4)

**Side-effects** *rarely* gastro-intestinal disturbances (including cramps) and hyperprolactinaemia; *very rarely* extrapyramidal effects and rashes

**Dose**

- By mouth, ADULT and CHILD body-weight over 35 kg, 10–20 mg 3–4 times daily; max. 80 mg daily; CHILD body-weight up to 35 kg (nausea and vomiting only), 250–500 micrograms/kg 3–4 times daily; max. 2.4 mg/kg daily

- By rectum, ADULT and CHILD body-weight over 35 kg, 60 mg twice daily; CHILD 15–35 kg (nausea and vomiting only), 30 mg twice daily; CHILD body-weight under 15 kg, not recommended

¹**Domperidone** (Non-proprietary) PoM

Tablets, 10 mg (as maleate), net price 30-tab pack = £1.35; 100-tab pack = £2.50

Suspension, domperidone 5 mg/5 mL, net price 200-mL pack = £7.00

1. Domperidone can be sold to the public (provided packs do not contain more than 200 mg) for the relief of postprandial symptoms of excessive fullness, nausea, epigastric bloating and belching occasionally accompanied by epigastric discomfort and heartburn (max. single dose 10 mg, max. daily dose 40 mg)

**Motilium®** (Sanofi-Synthelabo) PoM

Tablets, f/c, domperidone 10 mg (as maleate), net price 30-tab pack = £2.71; 100-tab pack = £9.04

Suppositories domperidone 30 mg, net price 10 = £3.06

## METOCLOPRAMIDE HYDROCHLORIDE

**Indications** adults, nausea and vomiting, particularly in gastro-intestinal disorders (section 1.2) and treatment with cytotoxics or radiotherapy; migraine (section 4.7.4.1)

Patients under 20 years Use restricted to severe intractable vomiting of known cause, vomiting of radiotherapy and cytotoxics, aid to gastro-intestinal intubation, premedication; dose should be determined on the basis of body-weight

**Cautions** elderly, young adults, and children; atopic allergy (including asthma); may mask underlying disorders such as cerebral irritation; acute porphyria (section 9.8.2); epilepsy; hepatic impairment (Appendix 2), renal impairment (Appendix 3); pregnancy (Appendix 4); **interactions**: Appendix 1 (metoclopramide)

**Contra-indications** gastro-intestinal obstruction, perforation or haemorrhage; 3–4 days after gastro-intestinal surgery; phaeochromocytoma; breast-feeding (Appendix 5)

**Side-effects** extrapyramidal effects (especially in children and young adults—see p. 225), hyperprolac-

tinaemia, occasionally tardive dyskinesia on prolonged administration; also reported, anxiety, confusion, drowsiness, restlessness, diarrhoea, depression,
neuroleptic malignant syndrome, rashes, pruritus,
oedema; cardiac conduction abnormalities reported
following intravenous administration; *rarely*
methaemoglobinaemia (more severe in G6PD deficiency)

**Dose**

- By mouth *or* by intramuscular injection *or* by intravenous injection over 1–2 minutes, nausea and
vomiting, 10 mg (5 mg in young adults 15–19 years
under 60 kg) 3 times daily; CHILD up to 1 year (up to
10 kg) 100 micrograms/kg (max. 1 mg) twice daily,
1–3 years (10–14 kg) 1 mg 2–3 times daily, 3–5 years
(15–19 kg) 2 mg 2–3 times daily, 5–9 years (20–
29 kg) 2.5 mg 3 times daily, 9–15 years (30 kg and
over) 5 mg 3 times daily
**Note** Daily dose of metoclopramide should not normally
exceed 500 micrograms/kg, particularly for children and
young adults (restricted use, see above)

For diagnostic procedures, as a single dose 5–10
minutes before examination, 10–20 mg (10 mg in
young adults 15–19 years); CHILD under 3 years 1 mg,
3–5 years 2 mg, 5–9 years 2.5 mg, 9–14 years 5 mg

**Metoclopramide** (Non-proprietary) PoM
Tablets, metoclopramide hydrochloride 10 mg, net
price 28-tab pack = 93p

Oral solution, metoclopramide hydrochloride 5 mg/
5 mL, net price 200-mL pack = £3.83. Counselling, use
of pipette
**Note** Sugar-free versions are available and can be ordered by
specifying 'sugar-free' on the prescription

Injection, metoclopramide hydrochloride 5 mg/mL,
net price 2-mL amp = 26p

**Maxolon®** (Shire) PoM
Tablets, scored, metoclopramide hydrochloride
10 mg, net price 84-tab pack = £5.24

Injection, metoclopramide hydrochloride 5 mg/mL.
Net price 2-mL amp = 27p

◢High-dose (with cytotoxic chemotherapy only)
**Maxolon High Dose®** (Shire) PoM
Injection, metoclopramide hydrochloride 5 mg/mL,
net price 20-mL amp = £2.67.
For dilution and use as an intravenous infusion in nausea and
vomiting associated with cytotoxic chemotherapy only
**Dose** by continuous intravenous infusion (preferred method),
initially (before starting chemotherapy), 2–4 mg/kg over 15–20
minutes, then 3–5 mg/kg over 8–12 hours; max. in 24 hours,
10 mg/kg
By intermittent intravenous infusion, initially (before starting
chemotherapy), up to 2 mg/kg over at least 15 minutes then up to
2 mg/kg over at least 15 minutes every 2 hours; max. in 24 hours,
10 mg/kg

◢Modified release
**Maxolon SR®** (Shire) PoM ◢
Capsules, m/r, clear, enclosing white granules,
metoclopramide hydrochloride 15 mg, net price 56-
cap pack = £7.01. Label: 25
**Dose** patients over 20 years, 1 capsule twice daily

◢Compound preparations (for migraine)
Section 4.7.4.1

# 5HT₃ antagonists

## ■ DOLASETRON MESILATE

**Indications** see under Dose

**Cautions** concomitant administration of drugs that
prolong QT interval, congestive heart failure;
pregnancy (Appendix 4); breast-feeding (Appendix 5);
**interactions**: Appendix 1 (dolasetron)

**Contra-indications** prolonged QT interval, cardiac
conduction disorders

**Side-effects** diarrhoea, constipation, dyspepsia,
abdominal pain, flatulence, anorexia, taste disturbance; tachycardia, bradycardia, ECG changes,
flushing; fever, shivering; headache, sleep disorder,
fatigue, dizziness, drowsiness, hypersensitivity reactions including rash, *rarely* intestinal obstruction,
pancreatitis, jaundice, oedema, cardiac arrhythmia,
bronchospasm, seizures, *very rarely* severe hypotension following intravenous injection

**Dose**

- Prevention of nausea and vomiting induced by cytotoxic chemotherapy, by intravenous injection (over
30 seconds) *or* by intravenous infusion, ADULT over
18 years, 100 mg 30 minutes before treatment

- Prevention of postoperative nausea and vomiting by
intravenous injection (over 30 seconds) *or* by
intravenous infusion, ADULT over 18 years, 12.5 mg
at cessation of anaesthesia,

- Treatment of postoperative nausea and vomiting, by
intravenous injection (over 30 seconds) *or* by
intravenous infusion, ADULT over 18 years, 12.5 mg

**Anzemet®** (Amdipharm) ▼ PoM
Injection, dolasetron mesilate 20 mg/mL, net price
0.625-mL (12.5-mg) amp = £4.00, 5-mL (100-mg) amp
= £13.00

## ■ GRANISETRON

**Indications** see under Dose

**Cautions** pregnancy (Appendix 4); breast-feeding
(Appendix 5)

**Side-effects** constipation, nausea, diarrhoea, vomiting, abdominal pain; headache, drowsiness, asthenia;
fever; *rarely* hepatic dysfunction, chest pain, arrhythmia; *very rarely* anorexia, dizziness, insomnia, agitation, movement disorders, rash

**Dose**

- Nausea and vomiting induced by cytotoxic chemotherapy or radiotherapy, by mouth, 1–2 mg within 1
hour before start of treatment, then 2 mg daily in 1–
2 divided doses during treatment; when intravenous
infusion also used, max. combined total 9 mg in 24
hours; CHILD 20 micrograms/kg (max. 1 mg) within 1
hour before start of treatment, then 20 micrograms/
kg (max. 1 mg) twice daily for up to 5 days during
treatment

By intravenous injection (diluted in 15 mL sodium
chloride 0.9% and given over not less than 30
seconds) *or* by intravenous infusion (over 5 minutes), prevention, 3 mg before start of cytotoxic
therapy (up to 2 additional 3-mg doses may be given
within 24 hours); treatment, as for prevention (the
two additional doses must not be given less than 10
minutes apart); max. 9 mg in 24 hours; CHILD, by
intravenous infusion, (over 5 minutes), prevention,

40 micrograms/kg (max. 3 mg) before start of cytotoxic therapy; treatment, as for prevention—one additional dose of 40 micrograms/kg (max. 3 mg) may be given within 24 hours (not less than 10 minutes after initial dose)

- Postoperative nausea and vomiting, by intravenous injection (diluted to 5 mL and given over 30 seconds), prevention, 1 mg before induction of anaesthesia; treatment, 1 mg, given as for prevention; max. 2 mg in one day; CHILD not recommended

**Granisetron** (Non-proprietary) PoM

Tablets, granisetron (as hydrochloride) 1 mg, net price 10-tab pack = £65.49

Injection, granisetron (as hydrochloride) 1 mg/mL, for dilution before use, net price 1-mL amp = £1.60, 3-mL amp = £4.80

**Kytril®** (Roche) PoM

Tablets, f/c, granisetron (as hydrochloride) 1 mg, net price 10-tab pack = £62.94; 2 mg, 5-tab pack = £62.94

Injection, granisetron (as hydrochloride) 1 mg/mL, for dilution before use, net price 1-mL amp = £8.26, 3-mL amp = £24.78

---

### ■ ONDANSETRON

**Indications** see under Dose

**Cautions** QT interval prolongation (avoid concomitant administration of drugs that prolong QT interval); hepatic impairment (Appendix 2); pregnancy (Appendix 4); breast-feeding (Appendix 5); **interactions:** Appendix 1 (ondansetron)

**Side-effects** constipation; headache; flushing; injection site-reactions; *less commonly* hiccups, hypotension, bradycardia, chest pain, arrhythmias, movement disorders, seizures; *on intravenous administration, rarely* dizziness, transient visual disturbances (*very rarely* transient blindness); suppositories may cause rectal irritation

**Dose**

- Moderately emetogenic chemotherapy or radiotherapy, by mouth, 8 mg 1–2 hours before treatment *or* by rectum, 16 mg 1–2 hours before treatment *or* by intramuscular injection *or* slow intravenous injection, 8 mg immediately before treatment
  *then* by mouth, 8 mg every 12 hours for up to 5 days *or* by rectum, 16 mg daily for up to 5 days; CHILD, by slow intravenous injection *or* by intravenous infusion over 15 minutes, 5 mg/m² immediately before chemotherapy then 4 mg by mouth every 12 hours for up to 5 days
- Severely emetogenic chemotherapy, by intramuscular injection *or* slow intravenous injection, 8 mg immediately before treatment, where necessary followed by 2 further doses of 8 mg at intervals of 2–4 hours (*or* followed by 1 mg/hour by continuous intravenous infusion for up to 24 hours)
  *then* by mouth, 8 mg every 12 hours for up to 5 days *or* by rectum, 16 mg daily for up to 5 days;
  *alternatively,* by intravenous infusion over at least 15 minutes, 32 mg immediately before treatment *or* by rectum, 16 mg 1–2 hours before treatment
  *then* by mouth, 8 mg every 12 hours for up to 5 days *or* by rectum, 16 mg daily for up to 5 days; CHILD, by slow intravenous injection, 5 mg/m² immediately before chemotherapy then 4 mg by mouth every 12 hours for up to 5 days

- Prevention of postoperative nausea and vomiting, by mouth, 16 mg 1 hour before anaesthesia *or* 8 mg 1 hour before anaesthesia followed by 8 mg at intervals of 8 hours for 2 further doses
  *alternatively,* by intramuscular *or* slow intravenous injection, 4 mg at induction of anaesthesia; CHILD over 2 years, by slow intravenous injection, 100 micrograms/kg (max. 4 mg) before, during, or after induction of anaesthesia
- Treatment of postoperative nausea and vomiting, by intramuscular *or* slow intravenous injection, 4 mg; CHILD over 2 years, by slow intravenous injection, 100 micrograms/kg (max. 4 mg)

**Ondansetron** (Non-proprietary) PoM

Tablets, ondansetron (as hydrochloride) 4 mg, net price 30-tab pack = £88.71; 8 mg, 10-tab pack = £59.08
Brands include Ondemet®

Injection, ondansetron (as hydrochloride) 2 mg/mL, net price 2-mL amp = £5.39, 4-mL amp = £10.79
Brands include Ondemet®

**Zofran®** (GSK) PoM

Tablets, yellow, f/c, ondansetron (as hydrochloride) 4 mg, net price 30-tab pack = £107.91; 8 mg, 10-tab pack = £71.94

Oral lyophilisates (Zofran Melt®), ondansetron 4 mg, net price 10-tab pack = £35.97; 8 mg, 10-tab pack = £71.94. Counselling, administration
Excipients include aspartame (section 9.4.1)
Counselling Tablets should be placed on the tongue, allowed to disperse and swallowed

Syrup, sugar-free, strawberry-flavoured, ondansetron (as hydrochloride) 4 mg/5 mL, net price 50-mL pack = £35.97

Injection, ondansetron (as hydrochloride) 2 mg/mL, net price 2-mL amp = £5.99; 4-mL amp = £11.99

Suppositories, ondansetron 16 mg, net price 1 = £14.39

---

### ■ PALONOSETRON

**Indications** prevention of nausea and vomiting induced by moderately and severely emetogenic chemotherapy

**Cautions** history of constipation; intestinal obstruction; concomitant administration of drugs that prolong QT interval; pregnancy (Appendix 4); breast-feeding (Appendix 5)
**Driving** Dizziness or drowsiness may affect performance of skilled tasks (e.g. driving)

**Side-effects** diarrhoea, constipation; headache, dizziness; *less commonly* dyspepsia, abdominal pain, dry mouth, flatulence, changes in blood pressure, tachycardia, bradycardia, arrhythmia, myocardial ischaemia, hiccups, drowsiness, asthenia, insomnia, anxiety, euphoria, paraesthesia, peripheral neuropathy, anorexia, motion sickness, influenza-like symptoms, urinary retention, glycosuria, hyperglycaemia, electrolyte disturbance, arthralgia, eye irritation, amblyopia, tinnitus, rash, pruritus

**Dose**

- By intravenous injection (over 30 seconds), 250 micrograms as a single dose 30 minutes before treatment; do not repeat dose within 7 days; CHILD and ADOLESCENT under 18 years not recommended

**Aloxi®** (IS Pharmaceuticals) ▼ PoM

Injection, palonosetron (as hydrochloride) 50 micrograms/mL, net price 5-mL amp = £55.89

## Neurokinin receptor antagonist

### ▮ APREPITANT

**Indications** adjunct to dexamethasone and a 5HT$_3$ antagonist in preventing nausea and vomiting associated with moderately and highly emetogenic chemotherapy

**Cautions** hepatic impairment (Appendix 2); pregnancy (Appendix 4); **interactions:** Appendix 1 (aprepitant)

**Contra-indications** breast-feeding (Appendix 5)

**Side-effects** hiccups, dyspepsia, diarrhoea, constipation, anorexia; asthenia, headache, dizziness; *less commonly* weight changes, dry mouth, colitis, flatulence, stomatitis, abdominal pain, gastro-oesophageal reflux, duodenal ulcer, oedema, bradycardia, cough, disorientation, euphoria, anxiety, confusion, thirst, abnormal dreams, hyperglycaemia, polyuria, anaemia, dysuria, haematuria, myalgia, conjunctivitis, pharyngitis, sneezing, tinnitus, sweating, oily skin, pruritus, rash, acne, photosensitivity, flushing, hyponatraemia

**Dose**

- ADULT over 18 years 125 mg 1 hour before chemotherapy, then 80 mg daily as a single dose for the next 2 days; consult product literature for dose of concomitant corticosteroid and 5HT$_3$ antagonist

**Emend®** (MSD) (PoM)
Capsules, aprepitant 80 mg (white), net price 2-cap pack = £31.61; 125 mg (white/pink), 5-cap pack = £79.03; 3-day pack of one 125-mg capsule and two 80-mg capsules = £47.42

### ▮ FOSAPREPITANT

Note Fosaprepitant is a prodrug of aprepitant

**Indications** adjunct to dexamethasone and a 5HT$_3$ antagonist in preventing nausea and vomiting associated with moderately and highly emetogenic chemotherapy

**Cautions** hepatic impairment (Appendix 2); pregnancy (Appendix 4); **interactions:** Appendix 1 (aprepitant)

**Contra-indications** breast-feeding (Appendix 5)

**Side-effects** anorexia, constipation, diarrhoea, dyspepsia, hiccups; asthenia, dizziness, headache; *less commonly* weight changes, abdominal pain, colitis, dry mouth, duodenal ulcer, flatulence, gastro-oesophageal reflux, stomatitis, taste disturbances, bradycardia, oedema, cough, abnormal dreams, anxiety, disorientation, confusion, euphoria, thirst, hyperglycaemia, dysuria, polyuria, flushing, neutropenia, anaemia, haematuria, hyponatraemia, myalgia, conjunctivitis, pharyngitis, sneezing, tinnitus, acne, photosensitivity, flushing, pruritus, oily skin, rash, sweating

**Dose**

- By intravenous infusion, over 15 minutes, ADULT over 18 years, 115 mg 30 minutes before chemotherapy on day 1 of cycle (followed by aprepitant on days 2 and 3 of cycle); consult product literature for dose of concomitant corticosteroid and 5HT$_3$ antagonist

**Ivemend®** (MSD) ▼ (PoM)
Injection, powder for reconstitution, fosaprepitant (as dimeglumine), net price 115-mg vial = £20.55
The *Scottish Medicines Consortium* (p. 3) has advised (September 2008) that fosaprepitant (*Ivemend*®) is accepted for restricted use for the prevention of acute and delayed nausea and vomiting associated with highly emetogenic cisplatin-based chemotherapy

## Cannabinoid

### ▮ NABILONE

**Indications** nausea and vomiting caused by cytotoxic chemotherapy, unresponsive to conventional anti-emetics (under close observation, preferably in hospital setting)

**Cautions** history of psychiatric disorder; elderly; hypertension; heart disease; adverse effects on mental state can persist for 48–72 hours after stopping; pregnancy (Appendix 4); **interactions:** Appendix 1 (nabilone)
Driving Drowsiness may affect performance of skilled tasks (e.g. driving); effects of alcohol enhanced

**Contra-indications** severe hepatic impairment; breast-feeding (Appendix 5)

**Side-effects** drowsiness, vertigo, euphoria, dry mouth, ataxia, visual disturbance, concentration difficulties, sleep disturbance, dysphoria, hypotension, headache and nausea; also confusion, disorientation, hallucinations, psychosis, depression, decreased coordination, tremors, tachycardia, decreased appetite, and abdominal pain
Behavioural effects Patients should be made aware of possible changes of mood and other adverse behavioural effects

**Dose**

- Initially 1 mg twice daily, increased if necessary to 2 mg twice daily, throughout each cycle of cytotoxic therapy and, if necessary, for 48 hours after the last dose of each cycle; max. 6 mg daily given in 3 divided doses. The first dose should be taken the night before initiation of cytotoxic treatment and the second dose 1–3 hours before the first dose of cytotoxic drug; ADOLESCENT and CHILD under 18 years consult local treatment protocol [unlicensed use]

**Nabilone** (Valeant) (PoM)
Capsules, blue/white, nabilone 1 mg. Net price 20-cap pack = £125.84. Label: 2, counselling, behavioural effects

## Hyoscine

### ▮ HYOSCINE HYDROBROMIDE
(Scopolamine Hydrobromide)

**Indications** motion sickness; hypersalivation associated with clozapine therapy; premedication (section 15.1.3); excessive respiratory secretions (see Prescribing in Palliative Care, p. 17)

**Cautions** section 1.2

**Contra-indications** section 1.2

**Side-effects** section 1.2

**Dose**

- Motion sickness, by mouth, ADULT and CHILD over 10 years, 150–300 micrograms up to 30 minutes before start of journey repeated every 6 hours if required; max. 900 micrograms daily; CHILD 3–4 years 75 micrograms up to 30 minutes before start of journey repeated after 6 hours if required, max. 150 micrograms daily; 4–10 years 75–150 micrograms up to 30 minutes before start of journey repeated every 6 hours if required; max. 450 micrograms daily

- Hypersalivation associated with clozapine therapy [unlicensed indication], by mouth, 300 micrograms up to 3 times daily; max. 900 micrograms daily; CHILD under 18 years, see *BNF for Children*

**Joy Rides®** (GSK Consumer Healthcare)
Tablets, chewable, raspberry-flavoured, hyoscine hydrobromide 150 micrograms, net price 12-tab pack = £1.49. Label: 2, 24

**Kwells®** (Bayer Consumer Care)
Tablets, chewable, scored, hyoscine hydrobromide 150 micrograms (*Kwells® Kids*) (white), net price 12-tab pack = £1.67; 300 micrograms (pink), 12-tab pack = £1.67. Label: 2

◢Patches
**Scopoderm TTS®** (Novartis Consumer Health) [PoM]
Patch, self-adhesive, pink, releasing hyoscine approx. 1 mg/72 hours when in contact with skin. Net price 2 = £4.30. Label: 19, counselling, see below

**Dose** motion sickness prevention, apply 1 patch to hairless area of skin behind ear 5–6 hours before journey; replace if necessary after 72 hours, siting replacement patch behind other ear; CHILD under 10 years not recommended

**Counselling** Explain accompanying instructions to patient and in particular emphasise advice to wash hands after handling and to wash application site after removing, and to use one patch at a time

◢Parenteral preparations
Section 15.1.3

## Other drugs for Ménière's disease

Betahistine has been promoted as a specific treatment for Ménière's disease.

### ▮ BETAHISTINE DIHYDROCHLORIDE

**Indications** vertigo, tinnitus and hearing loss associated with Ménière's disease
**Cautions** asthma, history of peptic ulcer; pregnancy and breast-feeding; **interactions:** Appendix 1 (betahistine)
**Contra-indications** phaeochromocytoma
**Side-effects** gastro-intestinal disturbances; headache, rashes and pruritus reported
**Dose**
- Initially 16 mg 3 times daily, preferably with food; maintenance 24–48 mg daily; CHILD not recommended

**Betahistine Dihydrochloride** (Non-proprietary) [PoM]
Tablets, betahistine dihydrochloride 8 mg, net price 84-tab pack = £2.58 120-tab pack = £1.47; 16 mg, 84-tab pack = £2.06. Label: 21

**Serc®** (Solvay) [PoM]
Tablets, betahistine dihydrochloride 8 mg (*Serc®-8*), net price 120-tab pack = £9.04; 16 mg (*Serc®-16*) (scored), 84-tab pack = £12.65. Label: 21

## 4.7 Analgesics

> 4.7.1 Non-opioid analgesics
> 4.7.2 Opioid analgesics
> 4.7.3 Neuropathic pain
> 4.7.4 Antimigraine drugs

The non-opioid drugs (section 4.7.1), paracetamol and aspirin (and other NSAIDs), are particularly suitable for pain in musculoskeletal conditions, whereas the opioid analgesics (section 4.7.2) are more suitable for moderate to severe pain, particularly of visceral origin.

**Pain in palliative care** For advice on pain relief in palliative care, see p. 15.

**Pain in sickle-cell disease** The pain of mild sickle-cell crises is managed with paracetamol, a NSAID (section 10.1.1), codeine, or dihydrocodeine. Severe crises may require the use of morphine or diamorphine; concomitant use of a NSAID may potentiate analgesia and allow lower doses of the opioid to be used. Pethidine should be avoided if possible because accumulation of a neurotoxic metabolite can precipitate seizures; the relatively short half-life of pethidine necessitates frequent injections.

**Dental and orofacial pain** Analgesics should be used judiciously in dental care as a **temporary** measure until the cause of the pain has been dealt with.

Dental pain of inflammatory origin, such as that associated with pulpitis, apical infection, localised osteitis (dry socket) or pericoronitis is usually best managed by treating the infection, providing drainage, restorative procedures, and other local measures. Analgesics provide temporary relief of pain (usually for about 1 to 7 days) until the causative factors have been brought under control. In the case of pulpitis, intra-osseous infection or abscess, reliance on analgesics alone is usually inappropriate.

Similarly the pain and discomfort associated with acute problems of the oral mucosa (e.g. acute herpetic gingivostomatitis, erythema multiforme) may be relieved by **benzydamine** mouthwash or spray (p. 617) until the cause of the mucosal disorder has been dealt with. However, where a patient is febrile, the antipyretic action of **paracetamol** (p. 234) or **ibuprofen** (p. 565) is often helpful.

The *choice* of an analgesic for dental purposes should be based on its suitability for the patient. Most dental pain is relieved effectively by non-steroidal anti-inflammatory drugs (NSAIDs). NSAIDs that are used for dental pain include **ibuprofen**, **diclofenac**, and **aspirin**; for further details see section 4.7.1 and section 10.1.1. **Paracetamol** has analgesic and antipyretic effects but no anti-inflammatory effect.

Opioid analgesics (section 4.7.2) such as **dihydrocodeine** and **pethidine** act on the central nervous system and are traditionally used for *moderate to severe pain*. However, opioid analgesics are relatively ineffective in dental pain and their side-effects can be unpleasant. Paracetamol, ibuprofen, or aspirin are adequate for most cases of dental pain and an opioid is rarely required.

Combining a non-opioid with an opioid analgesic can provide greater relief of pain than either analgesic given alone. However, this applies only when an adequate dose of each analgesic is used. Most combination analgesic preparations have not been shown to provide greater relief of pain than an adequate dose of the non-opioid component given alone. Moreover, combination preparations have the disadvantage of an increased number of side-effects.

Any analgesic given before a dental procedure should have a low risk of increasing postoperative bleeding. In the case of pain after the dental procedure, taking an analgesic before the effect of the local anaesthetic has worn off can improve control. Postoperative analgesia with ibuprofen or aspirin is usually continued for about 24 to 72 hours.

*Temporomandibular dysfunction* can be related to anxiety in some patients who may clench or grind their teeth (bruxism) during the day or night. The muscle spasm (which appears to be the main source of pain) may be treated empirically with an overlay appliance which provides a free sliding occlusion and may also interfere with grinding. In addition, **diazepam** (section 4.1.2), which has muscle relaxant as well as anxiolytic properties, may be helpful but it should only be prescribed on a short-term basis during the acute phase. Analgesics such as aspirin (section 4.7.1) or ibuprofen (section 10.1.1) may also be required.

For the management of neuropathic pain, persistent idiopathic facial pain, and trigeminal neuralgia, see section 4.7.3.

**Dysmenorrhoea** Use of an oral contraceptive prevents the pain of dysmenorrhoea which is generally associated with ovulatory cycles. If treatment is necessary paracetamol or a NSAID (section 10.1.1) will generally provide adequate relief of pain. The vomiting and severe pain associated with dysmenorrhoea in women with endometriosis may call for an antiemetic (in addition to an analgesic). Antispasmodics (such as alverine citrate, section 1.2) have been advocated for dysmenorrhoea but the antispasmodic action does not generally provide significant relief.

## 4.7.1 Non-opioid analgesics

**Aspirin** is indicated for headache, transient musculo-skeletal pain, dysmenorrhoea and pyrexia. In inflammatory conditions, most physicians prefer anti-inflammatory treatment with another NSAID which may be better tolerated and more convenient for the patient. Aspirin is used increasingly for its antiplatelet properties (section 2.9). Aspirin tablets or dispersible aspirin tablets are adequate for most purposes as they act rapidly.

Gastric irritation may be a problem; it is minimised by taking the dose after food. Enteric-coated preparations are available, but have a slow onset of action and are therefore unsuitable for single-dose analgesic use (though their prolonged action may be useful for night pain).

Aspirin interacts significantly with a number of other drugs and its interaction with warfarin is a **special hazard**, see **interactions**: Appendix 1 (aspirin).

**Paracetamol** is similar in efficacy to aspirin, but has no demonstrable anti-inflammatory activity; it is less irritant to the stomach and for that reason is now generally preferred to aspirin, particularly in the elderly. **Over-**

**dosage** with paracetamol is particularly dangerous as it may cause hepatic damage which is sometimes not apparent for 4 to 6 days (see Emergency Treatment of Poisoning, p. 29).

**Nefopam** may have a place in the relief of persistent pain unresponsive to other non-opioid analgesics. It causes little or no respiratory depression, but sympathomimetic and antimuscarinic side-effects may be troublesome.

**Non-steroidal anti-inflammatory analgesics** (NSAIDs, section 10.1.1) are particularly useful for the treatment of patients with chronic disease accompanied by pain and inflammation. Some of them are also used in the short-term treatment of mild to moderate pain including transient musculoskeletal pain but paracetamol is now often preferred, particularly in the elderly (see also p. 20). They are also suitable for the relief of pain in *dysmenorrhoea* and to treat pain caused by *secondary bone tumours*, many of which produce lysis of bone and release prostaglandins (see Prescribing in Palliative Care, p. 15). Selective inhibitors of cyclo-oxygenase-2 may be used in preference to non-selective NSAIDs for patients at high risk of developing serious gastro-intestinal side-effects. NSAIDs including ketorolac are also used for peri-operative analgesia (section 15.1.4.2).

A non-opioid analgesic administered by intrathecal infusion (**ziconotide** (*Prialt®* ▼), available from Eisai) is licensed for the treatment of chronic severe pain; ziconotide can be used by a hospital specialist as an adjunct to opioid analgesics.

**Dental and orofacial pain** Most dental pain is relieved effectively by NSAIDs (section 10.1.1). **Aspirin** (p. 234) is effective against mild to moderate dental pain; dispersible tablets provide a rapidly absorbed form of aspirin suitable for most purposes.

The analgesic effect of **paracetamol** in mild to moderate dental pain is probably less than that of aspirin, but it does not affect bleeding time or interact significantly with warfarin. Moreover, it is less irritant to the stomach. Paracetamol is a suitable analgesic for children; sugar-free versions can be requested by specifying 'sugar-free' on the prescription.

For further information on the management of dental and orofacial pain, see p. 232.

## Compound analgesic preparations

Compound analgesic preparations that contain a simple analgesic (such as aspirin or paracetamol) with an opioid component reduce the scope for effective titration of the individual components in the management of pain of varying intensity.

Compound analgesic preparations containing paracetamol or aspirin with a *low dose* of an opioid analgesic (e.g. 8 mg of codeine phosphate per compound tablet) are commonly used, but the advantages have not been substantiated. The low dose of the opioid may be enough to cause opioid side-effects (in particular, constipation) and can complicate the treatment of **overdosage** (see p. 31) yet may not provide significant additional relief of pain.

A *full dose* of the opioid component (e.g. 60 mg codeine phosphate) in compound analgesic preparations effectively augments the analgesic activity but is associated

**4**

**Central nervous system**

with the full range of opioid side-effects (including nausea, vomiting, severe constipation, drowsiness, respiratory depression, and risk of dependence on long-term administration). For details of the **side-effects** of opioid analgesics, see p. 237 (**important**: the elderly are particularly susceptible to opioid side-effects and should receive lower doses).

In general, when assessing pain, it is necessary to weigh up carefully whether there is a need for a non-opioid and an opioid analgesic to be taken simultaneously.

For information on the use of combination analgesic preparations in dental and orofacial pain, see p. 233.

**Caffeine** is a weak stimulant that is often included, in small doses, in analgesic preparations. It is claimed that the addition of caffeine may enhance the analgesic effect, but the added effect, mild habit-forming effect and possible provocation of headache may not always be desirable. Moreover, in excessive dosage or on withdrawal caffeine may itself induce headache.

**Co-proxamol** tablets (dextropropoxyphene in combination with paracetamol) are no longer licensed because of safety concerns, particularly toxicity in overdose. Co-proxamol tablets [unlicensed] may still be prescribed for patients who find it difficult to change, because, for example, alternatives are not effective or suitable.

## ASPIRIN
### (Acetylsalicylic Acid)

**Indications** mild to moderate pain, pyrexia; antiplatelet (section 2.9)

**Cautions** asthma, allergic disease, hepatic impairment (Appendix 2), renal impairment (Appendix 3), dehydration; preferably avoid during fever or viral infection in children (risk of Reye's syndrome, see below); pregnancy (Appendix 4); elderly; G6PD-deficiency (section 9.1.5); concomitant use of drugs that increase risk of bleeding; **interactions:** Appendix 1 (aspirin)

**Contra-indications** children under 16 years and in breast-feeding (Reye's syndrome, see below; Appendix 5); previous or active peptic ulceration, haemophilia; not for treatment of gout
Hypersensitivity Aspirin and other NSAIDs are **contraindicated** in patients with a history of hypersensitivity to aspirin or any other NSAID—*which includes those* in whom attacks of *asthma, angioedema, urticaria or rhinitis* have been precipitated by aspirin or any other NSAID
Reye's syndrome Owing to an association with Reye's syndrome, the CSM has advised that aspirin-containing preparations should not be given to children under 16 years, unless specifically indicated, e.g. for Kawasaki syndrome

**Side-effects** generally mild and infrequent but high incidence of gastro-intestinal irritation with slight asymptomatic blood loss, increased bleeding time, bronchospasm and skin reactions in hypersensitive patients. Prolonged administration, see section 10.1.1. **Overdosage:** see Emergency Treatment of Poisoning, p. 29

**Dose**
• By mouth, 300–900 mg every 4–6 hours when necessary; max. 4 g daily; CHILD under 16 years not recommended (see Reye's Syndrome, above)
• By rectum, 450–900 mg every 4 hours (max. 3.6 g daily); CHILD under 16 years not recommended (see Reye's Syndrome, above)

**Aspirin** (Non-proprietary)
Tablets [PoM][1], aspirin 300 mg. Net price 32-tab pack = 31p. Label: 21, 32
Tablets [PoM][1], e/c, aspirin 300 mg, net price 100-tab pack = £4.72; 75 mg, see section 2.9. Label: 5, 25, 32
Dispersible tablets [PoM][1], aspirin 300 mg, net price 100-tab pack = £5.68; 75 mg, see section 2.9. Label: 13, 21, 32
Note BP directs that when no strength is stated the 300-mg strength should be dispensed, and that when soluble aspirin tablets are prescribed, dispersible aspirin tablets shall be dispensed.
Dental prescribing on NHS Aspirin Dispersible Tablets 300 mg may be prescribed
Suppositories [PoM], aspirin 150 mg, net price 10 = £9.52; 300 mg, 12 = £59.28. Label: 32
Brands include *Resprin*®

**Caprin**® (Pinewood)
Tablets [PoM][1], e/c, f/c, pink, aspirin 300 mg, net price 100-tab pack = £4.89; 75 mg, see section 2.9. Label: 5, 25, 32

**Nu-Seals**® Aspirin (Alliance)
Tablets [PoM][1], e/c, aspirin 300 mg, net price 100-tab pack = £4.15; 75 mg, see section 2.9. Label: 5, 25, 32

◢**With codeine phosphate 8 mg**
[1]**Co-codaprin** (Non-proprietary) [PoM] ◢
Dispersible tablets, co-codaprin 8/400 (codeine phosphate 8 mg, aspirin 400 mg). Net price 100-tab pack = £26.20. Label: 13, 21, 32
Dose 1–2 tablets in water every 4–6 hours; max. 8 tablets daily
When co-codaprin tablets or dispersible tablets are prescribed and no strength is stated, tablets or dispersible tablets, respectively, containing codeine phosphate 8 mg and aspirin 400 mg should be dispensed

◢**Other compound preparations**
**Aspav**® (Alpharma) [PoM]
Dispersible tablets, aspirin 500 mg, papaveretum 7.71 mg (providing the equivalent of 5 mg of anhydrous morphine). Net price 30-tab pack = £5.98. Label: 2, 13, 21, 32
Dose 1–2 tablets in water every 4–6 hours if necessary; max. 8 tablets daily

## PARACETAMOL
### (Acetaminophen)

**Indications** mild to moderate pain, pyrexia

**Cautions** hepatic impairment (Appendix 2); renal impairment (Appendix 3), alcohol dependence; **interactions:** Appendix 1 (paracetamol)

**Side-effects** side-effects rare, but rashes, blood disorders (including thrombocytopenia, leucopenia, neutropenia) reported; hypotension also reported on infusion; **important:** liver damage (and less frequently renal damage) following **overdosage**, see Emergency Treatment of Poisoning, p. 29

**Dose**
• By mouth, 0.5–1 g every 4–6 hours to a max. of 4 g daily; CHILD 2 months 60 mg for post-immunisation pyrexia, repeated once after 6 hours if necessary; otherwise under 3 months, see *BNF for Children*;

1. Can be sold to the public provided packs contain no more than 32 capsules or tablets; pharmacists can sell multiple packs up to a total quantity of 100 capsules or tablets in justifiable circumstances; for details see *Medicines, Ethics and Practice*, No. 33, London, Pharmaceutical Press, 2009 (and subsequent editions as available)

3 months–1 year 60–120 mg, 1–5 years 120–250 mg, 6–12 years 250–500 mg; these doses may be repeated every 4–6 hours when necessary (max. of 4 doses in 24 hours)

- By intravenous infusion over 15 minutes, ADULT and CHILD over 50 kg, 1 g every 4–6 hours, max. 4 g daily; ADULT and CHILD 10–50 kg, 15 mg/kg every 4–6 hours, max. 60 mg/kg daily; NEONATE and CHILD less than 10 kg, 7.5 mg/kg every 4–6 hours, max. 30 mg/kg daily

- By rectum, ADULT and CHILD over 12 years 0.5–1 g every 4–6 hours to a max. of 4 g daily; CHILD under 3 months, see *BNF for Children*, 3 months–1 year 60–125 mg, 1–5 years 125–250 mg, 5–12 years 250–500 mg; these doses may be repeated every 4–6 hours as necessary (max. 4 doses in 24 hours)

**Note** For full Joint Committee on Vaccination and Immunisation recommendation on post-immunisation pyrexia, see section 14.1

**Paracetamol** (Non-proprietary)

Tablets (and caplets) PoM [1], paracetamol 500 mg. Net price 16 = 17p, 32 = £1.18, 100 = £1.65. Label: 29, 30
Brands include *Panadol* JHS

Capsules PoM [1], paracetamol 500 mg, net price 32-cap pack = £1.03. Label: 29, 30
Brands include *Panadol Capsules* JHS

Soluble tablets (= Dispersible tablets) PoM [2], paracetamol 500 mg. Net price 60-tab pack = £3.96. Label: 13, 29, 30
Brands include *Panadol Soluble* JHS (contains Na+ 18.6 mmol/tablet)

Paediatric soluble tablets (= Paediatric dispersible tablets), paracetamol 120 mg. Net price 16-tab pack = 89p. Label: 13, 30
Brands include *Disprol* Soluble *Paracetamol* JHS

Oral suspension 120 mg/5 mL (= Paediatric Mixture), paracetamol 120 mg/5 mL. Net price 100 mL = 42p. Label: 30
**Note** BP directs that when Paediatric Paracetamol Oral Suspension or Paediatric Paracetamol Mixture is prescribed Paracetamol Oral Suspension 120 mg/5 mL should be dispensed; sugar-free versions can be ordered by specifying 'sugar-free' on the prescription
Brands include *Calpol* Paediatric, *Calpol* Paediatric sugar-free, *Disprol* Paediatric, *Medinol* Paediatric sugar-free, *Paldesic*, *Panadol* sugar-free

Oral suspension 250 mg/5 mL (= Mixture), paracetamol 250 mg/5 mL. Net price 100 mL = 66p. Label: 30
Brands include *Calpol* 6 Plus JHS, *Medinol* Over 6 JHS, *Paldesic*

Suppositories, paracetamol 60 mg, net price 10 = £9.96; 125 mg, 10 = £11.50; 250 mg, 10 = £23.00; 500 mg, 10 = £11.17. Label: 30
Brands include *Alvedon*
**Note** Other strengths available from 'special-order' manufacturers or specialist importing companies, see p. 969

**Dental prescribing on NHS** Paracetamol Tablets, Paracetamol Soluble Tablets 500 mg, and Paracetamol Oral Suspension may be prescribed

---

1. Can be sold to the public provided packs contain no more than 32 capsules or tablets; pharmacists can sell multiple packs up to a total quantity of 100 capsules or tablets in justifiable circumstances; for details see *Medicines, Ethics and Practice*, No. 33, London, Pharmaceutical Press, 2009 (and subsequent editions as available)
2. Can be sold to the public in certain circumstances; for exemptions see *Medicines, Ethics and Practice*, No. 33, London, Pharmaceutical Press, 2009 (and subsequent editions as available)

**Perfalgan®** (Bristol-Myers Squibb) ▼ PoM

Intravenous infusion, paracetamol 10 mg/mL, net price 50-mL vial = £1.44, 100-mL vial = £1.59

**◢Co-codamol 8/500**

When co-codamol tablets, dispersible (or effervescent) tablets, or capsules are prescribed and **no strength is stated**, tablets, dispersible (or effervescent) tablets, or capsules, respectively, containing codeine phosphate **8 mg** and paracetamol **500 mg** should be dispensed.

[2]**Co-codamol 8/500** (Non-proprietary) PoM ◢

Tablets, co-codamol 8/500 (codeine phosphate 8 mg, paracetamol 500 mg), net price 30-tab pack = £1.05. Label: 29, 30
Brands include *Panadeine* JHS
**Dose** 1–2 tablets every 4–6 hours; max. 8 tablets daily; CHILD 6–12 years ½–1 tablet, max. 4 tablets daily

Effervescent *or* dispersible tablets, co-codamol 8/500 (codeine phosphate 8 mg, paracetamol 500 mg). Net price 100-tab pack = £4.62. Label: 13, 29, 30
Brands include *Paracodol* JHS
**Note** The Drug Tariff allows tablets of co-codamol labelled 'dispersible' to be dispensed against an order for 'effervescent' and *vice versa*
**Dose** 1–2 tablets in water every 4–6 hours, max. 8 tablets daily; CHILD 6–12 years ½–1 tablet, max. 4 tablets daily

Capsules, co-codamol 8/500 (codeine phosphate 8 mg, paracetamol 500 mg). Net price 10-cap pack = £1.10, 20-cap pack = £1.66. Label: 29, 30
Brands include *Paracodol* JHS
**Dose** 1–2 capsules every 4 hours; max. 8 capsules daily

**◢Co-codamol 15/500**

When co-codamol tablets, dispersible (or effervescent) tablets, or capsules are prescribed and **no strength is stated**, tablets, dispersible (or effervescent) tablets, or capsules, respectively, containing codeine phosphate **8 mg** and paracetamol **500 mg** should be dispensed (see preparations above).

See warnings and notes on p. 233 (**important:** special care in elderly—reduce dose)

**Codipar®** (Goldshield) PoM ◢

Caplets (= tablets), co-codamol 15/500 (codeine phosphate 15 mg, paracetamol 500 mg). Net price 100-tab pack = £8.25. Label: 2, 29, 30
**Dose** 1–2 tablets every 4 hours; max. 8 tablets daily; CHILD not recommended

**◢Co-codamol 30/500**

When co-codamol tablets, dispersible (or effervescent) tablets, or capsules are prescribed and **no strength is stated**, tablets, dispersible (or effervescent) tablets, or capsules, respectively, containing codeine phosphate **8 mg** and on paracetamol **500 mg** should be dispensed (see preparations above).

See warnings and notes on p. 233 (**important:** special care in elderly—reduce dose)

**Co-codamol 30/500** (Non-proprietary) PoM ◢

Tablets (and caplets), co-codamol 30/500 (codeine phosphate 30 mg, paracetamol 500 mg), net price 100-tab pack = £3.97. Label: 2, 29, 30
**Dose** 1–2 tablets every 4 hours; max. 8 tablets daily; CHILD not recommended

**4 Central nervous system**

Capsules, co-codamol 30/500 (codeine phosphate 30 mg, paracetamol 500 mg), net price 100-cap pack = £5.32. Label: 2, 29, 30
Brands include *Medocodene®*, *Zapain®*
Dose 1–2 capsules every 4 hours; max. 8 capsules daily; CHILD not recommended

Effervescent tablets, co-codamol 30/500 (codeine phosphate 30 mg, paracetamol 500 mg), net price 100-tab pack = £9.89. Label: 2, 13, 29, 30
Brands include *Medocodene® Effervescent* (contains Na⁺ 13.6 mmol/tablet)
Dose 1–2 tablets in water every 4 hours; max. 8 tablets daily; CHILD not recommended

**Kapake®** (Galen) PoM ◢
Tablets, scored, co-codamol 30/500 (codeine phosphate 30 mg, paracetamol 500 mg), net price 30-tab pack = £2.26 (hosp. only), 100-tab pack = £7.10. Label: 2, 29, 30
Dose 1–2 tablets every 4 hours; max. 8 tablets daily; CHILD not recommended

Capsules, co-codamol 30/500 (codeine phosphate 30 mg, paracetamol 500 mg), net price 100-cap pack = £7.10. Label: 2, 29, 30
Dose 1–2 capsules every 4 hours; max. 8 capsules daily; CHILD not recommended

**Solpadol®** (Sanofi-Synthelabo) PoM ◢
Caplets (= tablets), co-codamol 30/500 (codeine phosphate 30 mg, paracetamol 500 mg). Net price 100-tab pack = £6.74. Label: 2, 29, 30
Dose 2 tablets every 4 hours; max. 8 tablets daily; CHILD not recommended

Capsules, grey/purple, co-codamol 30/500 (codeine phosphate 30 mg, paracetamol 500 mg). Net price 100-cap pack = £6.74. Label: 2, 29, 30
Dose 1–2 capsules every 4 hours; max. 8 capsules daily; CHILD not recommended

Effervescent tablets, co-codamol 30/500 (codeine phosphate 30 mg, paracetamol 500 mg). Contains Na⁺ 16.9 mmol/tablet; avoid in *renal impairment*. Net price 32-tab pack = £2.59, 100-tab pack = £8.09. Label: 2, 13, 29, 30
Dose 2 tablets in water every 4 hours; max. 8 tablets daily; CHILD not recommended

**Tylex®** (UCB Pharma) PoM ◢
Capsules, co-codamol 30/500 (codeine phosphate 30 mg, paracetamol 500 mg). Net price 100-cap pack = £8.01. Label: 2, 29, 30
Dose 1–2 capsules every 4 hours; max. 8 capsules daily; CHILD not recommended

Effervescent tablets, co-codamol 30/500 (codeine phosphate 30 mg, paracetamol 500 mg). Contains Na⁺ 13.6 mmol/tablet; avoid in *renal impairment*. Net price 100-tab pack = £8.80. Label: 2, 13, 29, 30
Excipients include aspartame 25 mg/tablet (section 9.4.1)
Dose 1–2 tablets in water every 4 hours; max. 8 tablets daily; CHILD not recommended

◢**With methionine (co-methiamol)**

A mixture of methionine and paracetamol; methionine has no analgesic activity but may prevent paracetamol-induced liver toxicity if overdose taken

**Paradote®** (Penn)
Tablets, f/c, co-methiamol 100/500 (DL-methionine 100 mg, paracetamol 500 mg). Net price 24-tab pack = £1.05, 96-tab pack = £2.77. Label: 29, 30
Dose 2 tablets every 4 hours; max. 8 tablets daily; CHILD 12 years and under, not recommended

◢**With dihydrocodeine tartrate 10 mg**
See notes on p. 233

**Co-dydramol** (Non-proprietary) PoM ◢
Tablets, scored, co-dydramol 10/500 (dihydrocodeine tartrate 10 mg, paracetamol 500 mg). Net price 30-tab pack = £1.14. Label: 21, 29, 30
Dose 1–2 tablets every 4–6 hours; max. 8 tablets daily; CHILD not recommended
When co-dydramol tablets are prescribed and no strength is stated tablets containing dihydrocodeine tartrate 10 mg and paracetamol 500 mg should be dispensed.
Note Tablets containing paracetamol 500 mg and dihydrocodeine 7.46 mg (*Paramol®* JHS) are on sale to the public. The name *Paramol®* was formerly applied to a brand of co-dydramol tablets

◢**With dihydrocodeine tartrate 20 or 30 mg**
See warnings and notes on p. 233 (**important: special care in elderly—reduce dose**)

**Remedeine®** (Napp) PoM ◢
Tablets, paracetamol 500 mg, dihydrocodeine tartrate 20 mg. Net price 112-tab pack = £10.79. Label: 2, 21, 29, 30
Dose 1–2 tablets every 4–6 hours; max. 8 tablets daily; CHILD not recommended

Forte tablets, paracetamol 500 mg, dihydrocodeine tartrate 30 mg. Net price 56-tab pack = £6.66. Label: 2, 21, 29, 30
Dose 1–2 tablets every 4–6 hours; max. 8 tablets daily; CHILD not recommended

◢**With isometheptene mucate**
**Isometheptene mucate** (in combination with paracetamol) is licensed for the treatment of acute attacks of migraine; other more effective treatments are available.

¹**Midrid®** (Manx) PoM ◢
Capsules, red, isometheptene mucate 65 mg, paracetamol 325 mg. Net price 30-cap pack = £5.50. Label: 30, counselling, dosage
Dose migraine, 2 capsules at onset of attack, followed by 1 capsule every hour if necessary; max. 5 capsules in 12 hours; CHILD not recommended

1. A pack containing 15 capsules may be sold to the public

---

## NEFOPAM HYDROCHLORIDE

**Indications** moderate pain
**Cautions** hepatic or renal disease, elderly, urinary retention; pregnancy (Appendix 4) and breast-feeding; **interactions:** Appendix 1 (nefopam)
**Contra-indications** convulsive disorders; not indicated for myocardial infarction
**Side-effects** nausea, nervousness, urinary retention, dry mouth, lightheadedness; less frequently vomiting, blurred vision, drowsiness, sweating, insomnia, tachycardia, headache; confusion and hallucinations also reported; may colour urine (pink)
**Dose**
- By mouth, initially 60 mg (elderly, 30 mg) 3 times daily, adjusted according to response; usual range 30–90 mg 3 times daily; CHILD not recommended

**Acupan®** (3M) PoM
Tablets, f/c, nefopam hydrochloride 30 mg. Net price 90-tab pack = £9.58. Label: 2, 14

## 4.7.2 Opioid analgesics

Opioid analgesics are usually used to relieve moderate to severe pain particularly of visceral origin. Repeated administration may cause dependence and tolerance, but this is no deterrent in the control of pain in terminal illness, for guidelines see Prescribing in Palliative Care, p. 15. Regular use of a potent opioid may be appropriate for certain cases of chronic non-malignant pain; treatment should be supervised by a specialist and the patient should be assessed at regular intervals.

**Cautions** Opioids should be used with caution in patients with impaired respiratory function (avoid in chronic obstructive pulmonary disease) and asthma (avoid during an acute attack), hypotension, shock, myasthenia gravis, prostatic hypertrophy, obstructive or inflammatory bowel disorders, diseases of the biliary tract, and convulsive disorders. A reduced dose is recommended in elderly or debilitated patients, in hepatic impairment (avoid if severe; Appendix 2) and renal impairment (avoid if severe; Appendix 3), in hypothyroidism, and in adrenocortical insufficiency. Repeated use of opioid analgesics is associated with the development of psychological and physical dependence; although this is rarely a problem with therapeutic use, caution is advised if prescribing for patients with a history of drug dependence. Avoid abrupt withdrawal after long-term treatment. Transdermal preparations (fentanyl or buprenorphine patches) are not suitable for acute pain or in those patients whose analgesic requirements are changing rapidly because the long time to steady state prevents rapid titration of the dose. For prescribing in pregnancy and breast-feeding, see Appendix 4 and Appendix 5, respectively. Interactions: Appendix 1 (opioid analgesics; **important**: special hazard with *pethidine and possibly other opioids* and MAOIs).

Palliative care In the control of pain in terminal illness, the cautions listed above should not necessarily be a deterrent to the use of opioid analgesics.

**Contra-indications** Opioid analgesics should be avoided in patients with acute respiratory depression and when there is a risk of paralytic ileus. They are also contra-indicated in conditions associated with raised intracranial pressure and in head injury (opioid analgesics interfere with pupillary responses vital for neurological assessment). Comatose patients should not be treated with opioid analgesics.

**Side-effects** Opioid analgesics share many side-effects, although qualitative and quantitative differences exist. The most common side-effects include nausea and vomiting (particularly in initial stages), constipation, dry mouth, and biliary spasm; larger doses produce muscle rigidity, hypotension, and respiratory depression (for reversal of opioid-induced respiratory depression, see section 15.1.7). Other common side-effects of opioid analgesics include bradycardia, tachycardia, palpitation, oedema, postural hypotension, hallucinations, vertigo, euphoria, dysphoria, mood changes, dependence, dizziness, confusion, drowsiness, sleep disturbances, headache, sexual dysfunction, difficulty with micturition, urinary retention, ureteric spasm, miosis, visual disturbances, sweating, flushing, rash, urticaria, and pruritus. **Overdosage**: see Emergency Treatment of Poisoning, p. 31.

**Driving** Drowsiness may affect performance of skilled tasks (e.g. driving); effects of alcohol enhanced.

**Choice** Morphine remains the most valuable opioid analgesic for severe pain although it frequently causes nausea and vomiting. It is the standard against which other opioid analgesics are compared. In addition to relief of pain, morphine also confers a state of euphoria and mental detachment.

Morphine is the opioid of choice for the oral treatment of *severe pain in palliative care*. It is given regularly every 4 hours (or every 12 or 24 hours as modified-release preparations). For guidelines on dosage adjustment in palliative care, see p. 15 .

A modified-release epidural preparation of morphine is available from Flynn Pharma Ltd (*Depodur®* ).

**Buprenorphine** has both opioid agonist and antagonist properties and may precipitate withdrawal symptoms, including pain, in patients dependent on other opioids. It has abuse potential and may itself cause dependence. It has a much longer duration of action than morphine and sublingually is an effective analgesic for 6 to 8 hours. Unlike most opioid analgesics, the effects of buprenorphine are only partially reversed by naloxone.

**Codeine** is used for the relief of mild to moderate pain but is too constipating for long-term use.

**Diphenoxylate** (in combination with atropine, as cophenotrope) is used in acute diarrhoea (section 1.4.2).

**Dipipanone** used alone is less sedating than morphine but the only preparation available contains an antiemetic and is therefore not suitable for regular regimens in palliative care.

**Diamorphine** (heroin) is a powerful opioid analgesic. It may cause less nausea and hypotension than morphine. In *palliative care* the greater solubility of diamorphine allows effective doses to be injected in smaller volumes and this is important in the emaciated patient.

**Dihydrocodeine** has an analgesic efficacy similar to that of codeine. The dose of dihydrocodeine by mouth is usually 30 mg every 4 hours; doubling the dose to 60 mg may provide some additional pain relief but this may be at the cost of more nausea and vomiting. A 40-mg tablet is now also available.

**Alfentanil**, **fentanyl** and **remifentanil** are used by injection for intra-operative analgesia (section 15.1.4.3); fentanyl is available in a transdermal drug delivery system as a self-adhesive patch which is changed every 72 hours.

**Meptazinol** is claimed to have a low incidence of respiratory depression. It has a reported length of action of 2 to 7 hours with onset within 15 minutes.

**Methadone** is less sedating than morphine and acts for longer periods. In prolonged use, methadone should not be administered more often than twice daily to avoid the risk of accumulation and opioid overdosage. Methadone may be used instead of morphine in the occasional patient who experiences excitation (or exacerbation of pain) with morphine.

**Oxycodone** has an efficacy and side-effect profile similar to that of morphine. It is used primarily for control of *pain in palliative care*.

**Papaveretum** is rarely used; morphine is easier to prescribe and less prone to error with regard to the strength and dose.

4

Central nervous system

Pentazocine has both agonist and antagonist properties and precipitates withdrawal symptoms, including pain in patients dependent on other opioids. By injection it is more potent than dihydrocodeine or codeine, but hallucinations and thought disturbances may occur. It is not recommended and, in particular, should be avoided after myocardial infarction as it may increase pulmonary and aortic blood pressure as well as cardiac work.

Pethidine produces prompt but short-lasting analgesia; it is less constipating than morphine, but even in high doses is a less potent analgesic. It is not suitable for severe continuing pain. It is used for analgesia in labour; however, other opioids, such as morphine or diamorphine, are often preferred for obstetric pain.

Tramadol produces analgesia by two mechanisms: an opioid effect and an enhancement of serotonergic and adrenergic pathways. It has fewer of the typical opioid side-effects (notably, less respiratory depression, less constipation and less addiction potential); psychiatric reactions have been reported.

Dose The dose of opioids in the BNF may need to be adjusted individually according to the degree of analgesia and side-effects; patients' response to opioids varies widely.

Postoperative analgesia The use of intra-operative opioids affects the prescribing of postoperative analgesics and in many cases delays the need for a postoperative analgesic. A postoperative opioid analgesic should be given with care since it may potentiate any residual respiratory depression (for the treatment of opioid-induced respiratory depression, see section 15.1.7). Non-opioid analgesics are also used for postoperative pain (section 15.1.4.2).

Morphine is used most widely. Tramadol is not as effective in severe pain as other opioid analgesics. Buprenorphine may antagonise the analgesic effect of previously administered opioids and is generally not recommended. Pethidine is metabolised to norpethidine which may accumulate, particularly in renal impairment; norpethidine stimulates the central nervous system and may cause convulsions.

Opioids are also given epidurally [unlicensed route] in the postoperative period but are associated with side-effects such as pruritus, urinary retention, nausea and vomiting; respiratory depression can be delayed, particularly with morphine.

For details of patient-controlled analgesia (PCA) to relieve postoperative pain, consult hospital protocols. Formulations specifically designed for PCA are available (*Pharma-Ject® Morphine Sulphate*).

Dental and orofacial pain Opioid analgesics are relatively ineffective in dental pain. Like other opioids, dihydrocodeine often causes nausea and vomiting which limits its value in dental pain; if taken for more than a few doses it is also liable to cause constipation. Dihydrocodeine is not very effective in postoperative dental pain.

Pethidine can be taken by mouth, but for optimal effect, it needs to be given by injection. Its efficacy in postoperative dental pain is not proven and its use in dentistry is likely to be minimal. The side-effects of pethidine are similar to those of dihydrocodeine and, apart from constipation, pethidine is also more likely to cause them. Dependence is unlikely if very few tablets

are prescribed on very few occasions; nevertheless, dental surgeons need to be aware of the possibility that addicts may seek to acquire supplies.

For the management of dental and orofacial pain, see p. 232.

Addicts Although caution is necessary, addicts (and ex-addicts) may be treated with analgesics in the same way as other people when there is a real clinical need. Doctors do not require a special licence to prescribe opioid analgesics for addicts for relief of pain due to organic disease or injury.

## BUPRENORPHINE

Indications see under Dose and under Patches; opioid dependence (section 4.10)

Cautions see notes above; also impaired consciousness; effects only partially reversed by naloxone
Fever or external heat Monitor patients using patches for increased side-effects if fever present (increased absorption possible); avoid exposing application site to external heat (may also increase absorption)

Contra-indications see notes above

Side-effects see notes above; can induce mild withdrawal symptoms in patients dependent on opioids; also diarrhoea, abdominal pain, anorexia, dyspepsia; vasodilatation; dyspnoea; paraesthesia, asthenia, fatigue, agitation, anxiety; *less commonly* flatulence, taste disturbance, angina, hypertension, syncope, hypoxia, wheezing, cough, restlessness, depersonalisation; dysarthria, impaired memory, hypoaesthesia, tremor, influenza-like symptoms, pyrexia, rhinitis, rigors, muscle cramp, myalgia, tinnitus, dry eye, and dry skin; *rarely* paralytic ileus, dysphagia, impaired concentration, and psychosis; *very rarely* retching, hyperventilation, hiccups, and muscle fasciculation

Dose
- Moderate to severe pain, by sublingual administration, 200–400 micrograms every 6–8 hours; CHILD over 6 years, 16–25 kg, 100 micrograms every 6–8 hours; 25–37.5 kg, 100–200 micrograms every 6–8 hours; 37.5–50 kg, 200–300 micrograms every 6–8 hours

  By intramuscular *or* slow intravenous injection, 300–600 micrograms every 6–8 hours; CHILD over 6 months 3–6 micrograms/kg every 6–8 hours (max. 9 micrograms/kg)
- Premedication, by sublingual administration, 400 micrograms

  By intramuscular injection, 300 micrograms
- Intra-operative analgesia, by slow intravenous injection, 300–450 micrograms

Temgesic® (Schering-Plough) ▣
Tablets (sublingual), buprenorphine (as hydrochloride), 200 micrograms, net price 50-tab pack = £5.23; 400 micrograms, 50-tab pack = £10.46. Label: 2, 26

Injection, buprenorphine (as hydrochloride) 300 micrograms/mL, net price 1-mL amp = 48p

◢Patches
BuTrans® (Napp) ▣
Patches, self-adhesive, beige, buprenorphine, '5' patch (releasing 5 micrograms/hour for 7 days), net price 2 = £8.80; '10' patch (releasing 10 micrograms/

hour for 7 days), 4 = £32.02; '20' patch (releasing 20 micrograms/hour for 7 days), 4 = £58.31. Label: 2

**Dose** moderate, non-malignant pain unresponsive to non-opioid analgesics, ADULT over 18 years, initially one '5 micrograms/hour' patch; apply to dry, non-irritated, non-hairy skin on upper torso, removing after 7 days and siting replacement patch on a different area (avoid same area for at least 3 weeks)

**Dose adjustment** When starting, analgesic effect should **not** be evaluated until the system has been worn for **72 hours** (to allow for gradual increase in plasma-buprenorphine concentration)—if necessary, dose should be adjusted at 3-day intervals using a patch of the next strength or 2 patches of the same strength (applied at *same time* to avoid confusion). Max. 2 patches can be used at any one time

**Long duration of action** In view of the long duration of action, other opioids should not be administered within 24 hours of patch removal

**Transtec®** (Napp) [CD]

Patches, self-adhesive, skin-coloured, buprenorphine, '35' patch (releasing 35 micrograms/hour for 96 hours), net price 4 = £16.03; '52.5' patch (releasing 52.5 micrograms/hour for 96 hours), 4 = £24.06; '70' patch (releasing 70 micrograms/hour for 96 hours), 4 = £32.06. Label: 2

**Dose** moderate to severe chronic cancer pain and severe pain unresponsive to non-opioid analgesics, ADULT over 18 years, apply to dry, non-irritated, non-hairy skin on upper torso, removing after no longer than 96 hours and siting replacement patch on a different area (avoid same area for at least 6 days). Patients who have not previously received strong opioid analgesic, initially, one '35 micrograms/hour' patch replaced after no longer than 96 hours; patients who have received strong opioid analgesic, initial dose based on previous 24-hour opioid requirement, consult product literature

**Dose adjustment** When starting, analgesic effect should **not** be evaluated until the system has been worn for **24 hours** (to allow for gradual increase in plasma-buprenorphine concentration)—if necessary, dose should be adjusted at intervals of no longer than 96 hours using a patch of the next strength *or* using 2 patches of the same strength (applied at *same time* to avoid confusion). Max. 2 patches can be used at any one time. For breakthrough pain, consider 200–400 micrograms buprenorphine sublingually.

**Important:** it may take approx. 30 hours for the plasma-buprenorphine concentration to decrease by 50% after patch is removed

**Long duration of action** In view of the long duration of action, patients who have severe side-effects should be monitored for up to 30 hours after removing patch

## CODEINE PHOSPHATE

**Indications** mild to moderate pain; diarrhoea (section 1.4.2); cough suppression (section 3.9.1)

**Cautions** see notes above; also cardiac arrhythmias; acute abdomen; gallstones

**Variation in metabolism** The capacity to metabolise codeine can vary considerably and lead to either reduced therapeutic effect or marked increase in side-effects

**Contra-indications** see notes above

**Side-effects** see notes above; also abdominal pain, anorexia, seizures, malaise, hypothermia, and muscle fasciculation; pancreatitis also reported

**Dose**

- By mouth, 30–60 mg every 4 hours when necessary, to a max. of 240 mg daily; CHILD 1–12 years, 3 mg/kg daily in divided doses
- By intramuscular injection, 30–60 mg every 4 hours when necessary

**Codeine Phosphate** (Non-proprietary)

Tablets [PoM], codeine phosphate 15 mg, net price 28 = £1.08; 30 mg, 28 = £1.19; 60 mg, 28 = £1.73. Label: 2

Syrup [PoM], codeine phosphate 25 mg/5 mL. Net price 100 mL = 90p. Label: 2

Injection [CD], codeine phosphate 60 mg/mL. Net price 1-mL amp = £2.44

◢ **Linctus**

Section 3.9.1

## DIAMORPHINE HYDROCHLORIDE
### (Heroin Hydrochloride)

**Indications** see under Dose

**Cautions** see notes above; also severe diarrhoea; toxic psychosis, CNS depression; severe cor pulmonale

**Contra-indications** see notes above; also delayed gastric emptying; phaeochromocytoma

**Side-effects** see notes above; also anorexia, taste disturbance; syncope; asthenia; raised intracranial pressure; myocardial infarction also reported

**Dose**

- Acute pain, by subcutaneous *or* intramuscular injection, 5 mg repeated every 4 hours if necessary (up to 10 mg for heavier well-muscled patients); by slow intravenous injection, quarter to half corresponding intramuscular dose

- Myocardial infarction, by slow intravenous injection (1–2 mg/minute), 5 mg followed by a further 2.5–5 mg if necessary; elderly or frail patients, reduce dose by half

- Acute pulmonary oedema, by slow intravenous injection (1 mg/minute) 2.5–5 mg

- Chronic pain, by mouth *or* by subcutaneous *or* intramuscular injection, 5–10 mg regularly every 4 hours; dose may be increased according to needs; intramuscular dose should be approx. half corresponding oral dose, and approx. one third corresponding oral *morphine* dose—see also Prescribing in Palliative Care, p. 15; by subcutaneous infusion (using syringe driver), see Prescribing in Palliative Care, p. 18

**Diamorphine** (Non-proprietary) [CD]

Tablets, diamorphine hydrochloride 10 mg. Net price 100-tab pack = £14.65. Label: 2

Injection, powder for reconstitution, diamorphine hydrochloride. Net price 5-mg amp = £2.69, 10-mg amp = £3.37, 30-mg amp = £3.60, 100-mg amp = £9.80, 500-mg amp = £42.91

## DIHYDROCODEINE TARTRATE

**Indications** moderate to severe pain

**Cautions** see notes above; also pancreatitis; severe cor pulmonale

**Contra-indications** see notes above

**Side-effects** see notes above; also paralytic ileus, abdominal pain, and paraesthesia

**Dose**

- By mouth, 30 mg every 4–6 hours when necessary (see also notes above); CHILD over 4 years 0.5–1 mg/kg every 4–6 hours

- By deep subcutaneous *or* intramuscular injection, up to 50 mg repeated every 4–6 hours if necessary; CHILD over 4 years 0.5–1 mg/kg every 4–6 hours

**Dihydrocodeine** (Non-proprietary)

Tablets [PoM], dihydrocodeine tartrate 30 mg. Net price 28 = £1.49. Label: 2, 21

**Dental prescribing on NHS** Dihydrocodeine Tablets 30 mg may be prescribed

Oral solution [PoM], dihydrocodeine tartrate 10 mg/ 5 mL. Net price 150 mL = £3.08. Label: 2, 21

Injection [CD], dihydrocodeine tartrate 50 mg/mL. Net price 1-mL amp = £2.58

**DF118 Forte®** (Martindale) [PoM]

Tablets, dihydrocodeine tartrate 40 mg. Net price 100-tab pack = £11.51. Label: 2, 21

**Dose** ADULT and CHILD over 12 years, severe pain, 40–80 mg 3 times daily; max. 240 mg daily

◢**Modified release**

**DHC Continus®** (Napp) [PoM]

Tablets, m/r, dihydrocodeine tartrate 60 mg, net price 56-tab pack = £5.28; 90 mg, 56-tab pack = £8.66; 120 mg, 56-tab pack = £11.11. Label: 2, 25

**Dose** ADULT and CHILD over 12 years, chronic severe pain, 60–120 mg every 12 hours

**Note** Dihydrocodeine is an ingredient of some compound analgesic preparations, section 4.7.1

---

## DIPIPANONE HYDROCHLORIDE

**Indications** moderate to severe pain

**Cautions** see notes above; also diabetes mellitus; phaeochromocytoma

**Contra-indications** see notes above

**Side-effects** see notes above; also psychosis, restlessness, raised intracranial pressure

**Dose**

● See preparation below

**Diconal®** (Amdipharm) [CD]

Tablets, pink, scored, dipipanone hydrochloride 10 mg, cyclizine hydrochloride 30 mg. Net price 50-tab pack = £9.57. Label: 2

**Dose** *acute pain*, 1 tablet gradually increased to 3 tablets every 6 hours; CHILD not recommended

**Caution Not recommended** in palliative care, see Nausea and Vomiting, p. 18

---

## FENTANYL

**Indications** severe chronic pain, breakthrough pain; parenteral indications (section 15.1.4.3)

**Cautions** see notes above; also diabetes mellitus, impaired consciousness, cerebral tumour

> **Transdermal fentanyl**
> **Fever or external heat** Monitor patients using patches for increased side-effects if fever present (increased absorption possible); avoid exposing application site to external heat (may also increase absorption)
> **Respiratory depression** Risk of fatal respiratory depression, particularly in patients not previously treated with a strong opioid analgesic; manufacturer recommends use only in opioid tolerant patients

**Contra-indications** see notes above

**Side-effects** see notes above; also abdominal pain, anorexia, dyspepsia, dysphagia, mouth ulceration, taste disturbance, dry mouth; vasodilatation; apnoea; anxiety; myoclonus; *less commonly* flatulence, diarrhoea, laryngospasm, dyspnoea, hypoventilation, depersonalisation, dysarthria, amnesia, incoordination, paraesthesia, malaise, agitation, tremor, thirst and muscle weakness; *rarely* hiccups and arrhythmia;

*very rarely* paralytic ileus, haemoptysis, psychosis, and seizures; shock, asystole, pyrexia, ataxia, and muscle fasciculation also reported

**Dose**

● Chronic intractable pain, by transdermal route, apply to dry, non-irritated, non-irradiated, non-hairy skin on torso or upper arm, removing after 72 hours and siting replacement patch on a different area (avoid using the same area for several days). ADULT over 16 years **not currently treated** with a strong opioid analgesic (but see Cautions), initial dose, one '12' or '25 micrograms/hour' patch replaced after 72 hours; ADULT and CHILD over 2 years **currently treated** with a strong opioid analgesic, initial dose based on previous 24-hour opioid requirement (consult product literature)

**Dose adjustment** When starting, evaluation of the analgesic effect should **not** be made before the system has been worn for **24 hours** (to allow for the gradual increase in plasma-fentanyl concentration)—previous analgesic therapy should be phased out gradually from time of first patch application; if necessary dose should be adjusted at 72-hour intervals in steps of 12–25 micrograms/hour. More than one patch may be used at a time for doses greater than 100 micrograms/hour (but applied at the *same time* to avoid confusion)—consider additional or alternative analgesic therapy if dose required exceeds 300 micrograms/hour (**important:** it may take up to 25 hours for the plasma-fentanyl concentration to decrease by 50%—replacement opioid therapy should be initiated at a low dose and increased gradually).

**Long duration of action** In view of the long duration of action, patients who have had severe side-effects should be monitored for up to 24 hours after patch removal

● Breakthrough pain, see under oral preparations

**Conversion** (from oral morphine to transdermal fentanyl) see Prescribing in Palliative Care, p. 16

◢**Tablets**

**Abstral®** (ProStrakan) ▼ [CD]

Tablets (sublingual), fentanyl (as citrate) 100 micrograms, net price 10-tab pack = £49.99, 30-tab pack = £149.70; 200 micrograms, 10-tab pack = £49.99, 30-tab pack = £149.70; 300 micrograms, 10-tab pack = £49.99, 30-tab pack = £149.70; 400 micrograms, 10-tab pack = £49.99, 30-tab pack = £149.70; 600 micrograms, 30-tab pack = £149.70. Label: 2, 26

**Dose** breakthrough pain in patients receiving opioid therapy for chronic cancer pain, ADULT over 18 years, initially 100 micrograms repeated if necessary after 15–30 minutes; adjust dose according to response; no more than 2 dose units, 15–30 minutes apart, for each pain episode; max. 800 micrograms per episode of breakthrough pain

**Note** If more than 4 episodes of breakthrough pain each day, adjust background analgesia

The *Scottish Medicines Consortium* (p. 3) has advised (January 2009) that *Abstral®* sublingual tablets should be restricted for the management of breakthrough pain in adult patients using opioid therapy for chronic cancer pain, when other short-acting opioids are unsuitable

**Effentora®** (Cephalon) ▼ [CD]

Tablets (buccal), fentanyl (as citrate) 100 micrograms, net price 4-tab pack = £20.56; 200 micrograms, 4-tab pack = £20.56; 400 micrograms, 4-tab pack = £20.56; 600 micrograms, 4-tab pack = £20.56; 800 micrograms, 4-tab pack = £20.56. Label: 2, counselling, administration

**Electrolytes** Na$^+$ 0.35 mmol/100 microgram tablet, Na$^+$ 0.70 mmol/ tablet (all other strengths)

**Dose** breakthrough pain in patients receiving opioid therapy for chronic cancer pain, ADULT over 18 years, initially 100 micrograms repeated if necessary 30 minutes after first dose (no more than 2 dose units for each pain episode); adjust dose according to response; max. 800 micrograms per episode of breakthrough pain;

leave at least 4 hours between treatment of episodes of break-through pain during titration

**Counselling** Place tablet between cheek and gum above upper molar and leave to dissolve; if more than 1 tablet required, place second tablet on the other side of the mouth

The *Scottish Medicines Consortium* (p. 3) has advised that *Effentora®* buccal tablets should be restricted for the management of breakthrough pain in adult patients using opioid therapy for chronic cancer pain, when other short-acting opioids are unsuitable

◢**Lozenges**

**Actiq®** (Cephalon) ☐CD☐

Lozenge (buccal), with oromucosal applicator, fentanyl (as citrate) 200 micrograms, net price 3 = £17.86, 30 = £178.55; 400 micrograms, 3 = £17.86, 30 = £178.55; 600 micrograms, 3 = £17.86, 30 = £178.55; 800 micrograms, 3 = £17.86, 30 = £178.55; 1.2 mg, 3 = £17.86, 30 = £178.55; 1.6 mg, 3 = £17.86, 30 = £178.55. Label: 2

**Dose** breakthrough pain in patients receiving opioid therapy for chronic cancer pain, initially 200 micrograms (over 15 minutes) repeated if necessary 15 minutes after first dose (no more than 2 dose units for each pain episode); adjust dose according to response; max. 4 dose units daily

**Note** If more than 4 episodes of breakthrough pain each day, adjust background analgesia

◢**Patches**

**Prescriptions** Prescriptions for fentanyl patches can be written to show the strength in terms of the release rate and it is acceptable to write '*Fentanyl 25 patches*' to prescribe patches that release fentanyl 25 micrograms per hour. The dosage should be expressed in terms of the interval between applying a patch and replacing it with a new one, e.g. '*one patch to be applied every 72 hours*'. The total quantity of patches to be supplied should be written in words and figures.

**Fentanyl** (Non-proprietary) ☐CD☐

Patches, self-adhesive, fentanyl, '12' patch (releasing approx. 12 micrograms/hour for 72 hours), net price 5 = £18.11; '25' patch (releasing approx. 25 micrograms/hour for 72 hours), 5 = £25.89; '50' patch (releasing approx. 50 micrograms/hour for 72 hours), 5 = £48.36; '75' patch (releasing approx. 75 micrograms/hour for 72 hours), 5 = £67.41; '100' patch (releasing approx. 100 micrograms/hour for 72 hours), 5 = £83.09. Label: 2, counselling, administration

Brands include *Fentalis®*, *Matrifen®*, *Mezolar®*, *Osmanil®*, *Tilofyl®*, *Victanyl®*

**Durogesic DTrans®** (Janssen-Cilag) ☐CD☐

Patches, self-adhesive, transparent, fentanyl, '12' patch (releasing approx. 12 micrograms/hour for 72 hours), net price 5 = £18.11; '25' patch (releasing approx. 25 micrograms/hour for 72 hours), 5 = £25.89; '50' patch (releasing approx. 50 micrograms/hour for 72 hours), 5 = £48.36; '75' patch (releasing approx. 75 micrograms/hour for 72 hours), 5 = £67.41; '100' patch (releasing approx. 100 micrograms/hour for 72 hours), 5 = £83.09. Label: 2, counselling, administration

## ■ HYDROMORPHONE HYDROCHLORIDE

**Indications** severe pain in cancer

**Cautions** see notes above; also pancreatitis; toxic psychosis

**Contra-indications** see notes above; also acute abdomen

**Side-effects** see notes above; also paralytic ileus, peripheral oedema, seizures, asthenia, dyskinesia, agitation, and tremor

**Dose**

● See under preparations below

**Palladone®** (Napp) ☐CD☐

Capsules, hydromorphone hydrochloride 1.3 mg (orange/clear), net price 56-cap pack = £8.82; 2.6 mg (red/clear), 56-cap pack = £17.64. Label: 2, counselling, see below

**Dose** 1.3 mg every 4 hours, increased if necessary according to severity of pain; CHILD under 12 years not recommended

**Counselling** Swallow whole or open capsule and sprinkle contents on soft food

◢**Modified release**

**Palladone® SR** (Napp) ☐CD☐

Capsules, m/r, hydromorphone hydrochloride 2 mg (yellow/clear), net price 56-cap pack = £20.98; 4 mg (pale blue/clear), 56-cap pack = £28.75; 8 mg (pink/clear), 56-cap pack = £56.08; 16 mg (brown/clear), 56-cap pack = £106.53; 24 mg (dark blue/clear), 56-cap pack = £159.82. Label: 2, counselling, see below

**Dose** 4 mg every 12 hours, increased if necessary according to severity of pain; CHILD under 12 years not recommended

**Counselling** Swallow whole or open capsule and sprinkle contents on soft food

## ■ MEPTAZINOL

**Indications** moderate to severe pain, including post-operative and obstetric pain and renal colic; peri-operative analgesia, section 15.1.4.3

**Cautions** see notes above; effects only partially reversed by naloxone

**Contra-indications** see notes above; also myocardial infarction; phaeochromocytoma

**Side-effects** see notes above; can induce withdrawal symptoms in patients dependent on opioids; also diarrhoea, abdominal pain, dyspepsia, and hypothermia

**Dose**

● By mouth, 200 mg every 3–6 hours as required; CHILD not recommended

● By intramuscular injection, 75–100 mg every 2–4 hours if necessary; obstetric analgesia, 100–150 mg according to patient's weight (2 mg/kg); CHILD not recommended

● By slow intravenous injection, 50–100 mg every 2–4 hours if necessary; CHILD not recommended

**Meptid®** (Almirall) ☐PoM☐

Tablets, orange, f/c, meptazinol 200 mg, net price 112-tab pack = £22.11. Label: 2

Injection, meptazinol 100 mg (as hydrochloride)/mL, net price 1-mL amp = £1.92

## ■ METHADONE HYDROCHLORIDE

**Indications** severe pain, see notes above; cough in terminal disease (section 3.9.1); adjunct in treatment of opioid dependence (section 4.10)

**Cautions** see notes above; also history of cardiac conduction abnormalities, family history of sudden

**4 Central nervous system**

death (ECG monitoring recommended; see also QT Interval Prolongation, below)

**QT interval prolongation** The CHM has recommended that patients with the following risk factors for QT interval prolongation are carefully monitored while taking methadone: heart or liver disease, electrolyte abnormalities, or concomitant treatment with drugs that can prolong QT interval; patients requiring more than 100 mg daily should also be monitored

**Contra-indications** see notes above; also phaeochromocytoma

**Side-effects** see notes above; also QT interval prolongation, torsade de pointes, hypothermia, restlessness, raised intracranial pressure, dysmenorrhoea, dry eyes, and hyperprolactinaemia

**Dose**

- By mouth *or* by subcutaneous *or* intramuscular injection, 5–10 mg every 6–8 hours, adjusted according to response; on prolonged use not to be given more frequently than every 12 hours; CHILD not recommended

**Methadone** (Non-proprietary) ⃝CD
Tablets, methadone hydrochloride 5 mg. Net price 50 = £2.88. Label: 2
Brands include *Physeptone*®

Injection ▼, methadone hydrochloride, 10 mg/mL, net price 1-mL amp = 90p, 2-mL amp = £1.51, 3.5-mL amp = £1.90, 5-mL amp = £2.05
Brands include *Physeptone*®, *Synastone*®

◀Linctus
Section 3.9.1

◀Oral solution and oral concentrate
Section 4.10

## ▮ MORPHINE SALTS

**Indications** see notes above and under Dose; acute diarrhoea (section 1.4.2); cough in terminal care (section 3.9.1)

**Cautions** see notes above; also pancreatitis, cardiac arrhythmias, severe cor pulmonale

**Contra-indications** see notes above; also delayed gastric emptying, acute abdomen; heart failure secondary to chronic lung disease; phaeochromocytoma

**Side-effects** see notes above; also paralytic ileus, abdominal pain, anorexia, dyspepsia, exacerbation of pancreatitis, taste disturbance; hypertension, hypothermia, syncope, bronchospasm, inhibition of cough reflex; restlessness, seizures, paraesthesia, asthenia, malaise, disorientation, excitation, agitation, delirium, raised intracranial pressure; amenorrhoea, myoclonus, muscle fasciculation, and rhabdomyolysis

**Dose**

The patient should be closely monitored for pain relief as well as for side-effects especially respiratory depression. See also notes above.

- Acute pain, by subcutaneous injection (not suitable for oedematous patients) *or* by intramuscular injection, initially 10 mg (ELDERLY or frail 5 mg) every 4 hours (or more frequently during titration), adjusted according to response; NEONATE initially 100 micrograms/kg every 6 hours, adjusted according to response; CHILD 1–6 months initially 100–200 micrograms/kg every 6 hours, adjusted according to response; CHILD 6 months–2 years initially 100–200 micrograms/kg every 4 hours,

adjusted according to response; CHILD 2–12 years initially 200 micrograms/kg every 4 hours, adjusted according to response; CHILD 12–18 years initially 2.5–10 mg every 4 hours, adjusted according to response

By slow intravenous injection, initially 2.5 mg (reduce dose in ELDERLY or frail) every 4 hours (or more frequently during titration), adjusted according to response; NEONATE initially 40–100 micrograms/kg every 6 hours, adjusted according to response; CHILD 1–6 months initially 100–200 micrograms/kg every 6 hours, adjusted according to response; CHILD 6 months–12 years initially 100–200 micrograms/kg every 4 hours, adjusted according to response

- Premedication, by subcutaneous *or* intramuscular injection, up to 10 mg 60–90 minutes before operation; CHILD, by intramuscular injection, 150 micrograms/kg

- Patient controlled analgesia (PCA), consult hospital protocols

- Myocardial infarction, by slow intravenous injection (2 mg/minute), 10 mg followed by a further 5–10 mg if necessary; ELDERLY or frail patients, reduce dose by half

- Acute pulmonary oedema, by slow intravenous injection (2 mg/minute) 5–10 mg; ELDERLY or frail patients, reduce dose by half

- Chronic pain, by mouth *or* by subcutaneous injection (not suitable for oedematous patients) *or* by intramuscular injection, initially 5–20 mg every 4 hours, adjusted according to response; see also Prescribing in Palliative Care, p. 15

By rectum, initially 15–30 mg every 4 hours, adjusted according to response

**Note** The doses stated above refer equally to morphine hydrochloride and sulphate

◀Oral solutions
**Note** For advice on transfer from oral solutions of morphine to modified-release preparations of morphine, see Prescribing in Palliative Care, p. 15

### Morphine Oral Solutions
⃝PoM or ⃝CD

Oral solutions of morphine can be prescribed by writing the formula:
Morphine hydrochloride 5 mg
Chloroform water to 5 mL
**Note** The proportion of morphine hydrochloride may be altered when specified by the prescriber; if above 13 mg per 5 mL the solution becomes ⃝CD. For sample prescription see Controlled Drugs and Drug Dependence, p. 7. It is usual to adjust the strength so that the dose volume is 5 or 10 mL.

### Oramorph® (Boehringer Ingelheim)
Oramorph® oral solution ⃝PoM, morphine sulphate 10 mg/5 mL. Net price 100-mL pack = £1.78; 300-mL pack = £4.95; 500-mL pack = £7.47. Label: 2
Oramorph® concentrated oral solution ⃝CD, sugar-free, morphine sulphate 100 mg/5 mL. Net price 30-mL pack = £4.98; 120-mL pack = £18.59 (both with calibrated dropper). Label: 2

◀Tablets
**Sevredol**® (Napp) ⃝CD
Tablets, f/c, scored, morphine sulphate 10 mg (blue), net price 56-tab pack = £5.61; 20 mg (pink), 56-tab pack = £11.21; 50 mg (pale green), 56-tab pack = £28.02. Label: 2

◢ **Modified-release 12-hourly oral preparations**

**Morphgesic® SR** (Amdipharm) ⒸⒹ

Tablets, m/r, f/c, morphine sulphate 10 mg (buff), net price 60-tab pack = £3.91; 30 mg (violet), 60-tab pack = £9.37; 60 mg (orange), 60-tab pack = £18.30; 100 mg (grey), 60-tab pack = £28.98. Label: 2, 25

**Dose** every 12 hours, dose adjusted according to daily morphine requirements; for further advice on determining dose, see Prescribing in Palliative Care, p. 15; dosage requirements should be reviewed if the brand is altered

**Note** Prescriptions must also specify 'tablets' (i.e. Morphgesic SR tablets)

**MST Continus®** (Napp) ⒸⒹ

Tablets, m/r, f/c, morphine sulphate 5 mg (white), net price 60-tab pack = £3.29; 10 mg (brown), 60-tab pack = £5.26; 15 mg (green), 60-tab pack = £9.61; 30 mg (purple), 60-tab pack = £12.65; 60 mg (orange), 60-tab pack = £24.68; 100 mg (grey), 60-tab pack = £39.07; 200 mg (green), 60-tab pack = £78.16. Label: 2, 25

Suspension (= sachet of granules to mix with water), m/r, pink, morphine sulphate 20 mg/sachet, net price 30-sachet pack = £24.58; 30 mg/sachet, 30-sachet pack = £25.54; 60 mg/sachet, 30-sachet pack = £51.09; 100 mg/sachet, 30-sachet pack = £85.15; 200 mg/sachet pack, 30-sachet pack = £170.30. Label: 2, 13

**Dose** every 12 hours, dose adjusted according to daily morphine requirements; for further advice on determining dose, see Prescribing in Palliative Care, p. 15; dosage requirements should be reviewed if the brand is altered

**Note** Prescriptions must also specify 'tablets' or 'suspension' (i.e. 'MST Continus tablets' or 'MST Continus suspension')

**Zomorph®** (Link) ⒸⒹ

Capsules, m/r, morphine sulphate 10 mg (yellow/clear enclosing pale yellow pellets), net price 60-cap pack = £4.08; 30 mg (pink/clear enclosing pale yellow pellets), 60-cap pack = £9.77; 60 mg (orange/clear enclosing pale yellow pellets), 60-cap pack = £19.06; 100 mg (white/clear enclosing pale yellow pellets), 60-cap pack = £30.18; 200 mg (clear enclosing pale yellow pellets), 60-cap pack = £60.35. Label: 2, counselling, see below

**Dose** every 12 hours, dose adjusted according to daily morphine requirements; for further advice on determining doses, see Prescribing in Palliative Care, p. 15; dosage requirements should be reviewed if the brand is altered

**Counselling** Swallow whole or open capsule and sprinkle contents on soft food

**Note** Prescriptions must also specify 'capsules' (i.e. 'Zomorph capsules')

◢ **Modified-release 24-hourly oral preparations**

**MXL®** (Napp) ⒸⒹ

Capsules, m/r, morphine sulphate 30 mg (light blue), net price 28-cap pack = £10.91; 60 mg (brown), 28-cap pack = £14.95; 90 mg (pink), 28-cap pack = £22.04; 120 mg (green), 28-cap pack = £29.15; 150 mg (blue), 28-cap pack = £36.43; 200 mg (red-brown), 28-cap pack = £46.15. Label: 2, counselling, see below

**Dose** every 24 hours, dose adjusted according to daily morphine requirements; for further advice on determining dose, see Prescribing in Palliative Care, p. 15; dosage requirements should be reviewed if the brand is altered

**Counselling** Swallow whole or open capsule and sprinkle contents on soft food

**Note** Prescriptions must also specify 'capsules' (i.e. 'MXL capsules')

◢ **Suppositories**

**Morphine** (Non-proprietary) ⒸⒹ

Suppositories, morphine hydrochloride or sulphate 10 mg, net price 12 = £8.69; 15 mg, 12 = £8.50; 20 mg, 12 = £33.22; 30 mg, 12 = £12.36. Label: 2

Available from Aurum, Martindale

**Note** Both the strength of the suppositories and the morphine salt contained in them must be specified by the prescriber

◢ **Injections**

**Morphine Sulphate** (Non-proprietary) ⒸⒹ

Injection, morphine sulphate 10, 15, 20, and 30 mg/mL, net price 1- and 2-mL amp (all) = 72p–£1.40

Intravenous infusion, morphine sulphate 1 mg/mL, net price 50-mL vial = £5.00; 2 mg/mL, 50-mL vial = £5.89

**Minijet® Morphine Sulphate** (UCB Pharma) ⒸⒹ

Injection, morphine sulphate 1 mg/mL, net price 10-mL disposable syringe = £8.34

◢ **Injection with antiemetic**

**Caution** In myocardial infarction cyclizine may aggravate severe heart failure and counteract the haemodynamic benefits of opioids, section 4.6. **Not recommended** in palliative care, see Nausea and Vomiting, p. 17

**Cyclimorph®** (Amdipharm) ⒸⒹ

Cyclimorph-10® Injection, morphine tartrate 10 mg, cyclizine tartrate 50 mg/mL. Net price 1-mL amp = £1.75

**Dose** ADULT and CHILD over 12 years, moderate to severe pain (short-term use only) by subcutaneous, intramuscular, or intravenous injection, 1 mL, repeated not more often than every 4 hours; max. 3 doses in any 24-hour period

Cyclimorph-15® Injection, morphine tartrate 15 mg, cyclizine tartrate 50 mg/mL. Net price 1-mL amp = £1.82

**Dose** ADULT and CHILD over 12 years, moderate to severe pain (short-term use only) by subcutaneous, intramuscular, or intravenous injection, 1 mL, repeated not more often than every 4 hours; max. 3 doses in any 24-hour period

## OXYCODONE HYDROCHLORIDE

**Indications** moderate to severe pain in patients with cancer; postoperative pain; severe pain

**Cautions** see notes above; also toxic psychosis; pancreatitis

**Contra-indications** see notes above; also acute abdomen; delayed gastric emptying; chronic constipation; cor pulmonale; acute porphyria (section 9.8.2)

**Side-effects** see notes above; also diarrhoea, abdominal pain, anorexia, dyspepsia; bronchospasm, dyspnoea, impaired cough reflex; asthenia, anxiety; chills; muscle fasciculation; *less commonly* paralytic ileus, gastritis, flatulence, dysphagia, taste disturbance, belching, hiccups, vasodilatation, supraventricular tachycardia, syncope, amnesia, hypoaesthesia, restlessness, seizures, pyrexia, amenorrhoea, hypotonia, paraesthesia, disorientation, malaise, agitation, speech disorder, tremor, and dry skin

**Dose**

- By mouth, initially 5 mg every 4–6 hours, increased if necessary according to severity of pain, usual max. 400 mg daily, but some patients may require

**4**

**Central nervous system**

higher doses; CHILD under 18 years, see *BNF for Children*

- By slow intravenous injection, 1–10 mg every 4 hours when necessary; CHILD under 18 years, not recommended
- By intravenous infusion, initially 2 mg/hour, adjusted according to response; CHILD under 18 years not recommended
- By subcutaneous injection, initially 5 mg every 4 hours when necessary; CHILD under 18 years, not recommended
- By subcutaneous infusion, initially 7.5 mg/24 hours adjusted according to response; CHILD under 18 years, not recommended
- Patient controlled analgesia (PCA), consult hospital protocols

Note 2 mg oral oxycodone is approximately equivalent to 1 mg parenteral oxycodone

**OxyNorm®** (Napp) CD

Capsules, oxycodone hydrochloride 5 mg (orange/beige), net price 56-cap pack = £11.59; 10 mg (white/beige), 56-cap pack = £23.19; 20 mg (pink/beige), 56-cap pack = £46.38. Label: 2

Liquid (= oral solution), sugar-free, oxycodone hydrochloride 5 mg/5 mL, net price 250 mL = £9.85. Label: 2

Concentrate (= concentrated oral solution), sugar-free, oxycodone hydrochloride 10 mg/mL, net price 120 mL = £47.32. Label: 2

Injection, oxycodone hydrochloride 10 mg/mL, net price 1-mL amp = £1.60, 2-mL amp = £3.20

Note The *Scottish Medicines Consortium* has advised (October 2004) that *OxyNorm®* injection is used only in patients with cancer who have difficulty in tolerating morphine or diamorphine

◢Modified release
**OxyContin®** (Napp) CD

Tablets, f/c, m/r, oxycodone hydrochloride 5 mg (blue), net price 28-tab pack = £12.71; 10 mg (white), 56-tab pack = £25.41; 20 mg (pink), 56-tab pack = £50.82; 40 mg (yellow), 56-tab pack = £101.67; 80 mg (green), 56-tab pack = £203.35. Label: 2, 25

Dose initially, 10 mg every 12 hours, increased if necessary according to severity of pain, usual max. 200 mg every 12 hours, but some patients may require higher doses; CHILD under 18 years, see *BNF for Children*

◢With naloxone
**Targinact®** (Napp) ▼ CD

Tablets 10 mg/5 mg, f/c, m/r, oxycodone hydrochloride 10 mg, naloxone hydrochloride 5 mg (white), net price 56-tab pack = £35.11. Label: 2, 25

Tablets 20 mg/10 mg, f/c, m/r, oxycodone hydrochloride 20 mg, naloxone hydrochloride 10 mg (pink), net price 56-tab pack = £70.22. Label: 2, 25

Dose severe pain responsive only to opioid analgesics, ADULT over 18 years not currently treated with opioid analgesics, initially 10 mg/5 mg every 12 hours, increased according to response; patients already receiving opioid analgesics may start with 20 mg/10 mg every 12 hours; max. *Targinact®* 20 mg/10 mg every 12 hours

Note Supplemental modified-release oxycodone (without naloxone) can be prescribed for patients that need higher doses—consult product literature

The *Scottish Medicines Consortium* (p. 3) has advised (February 2009) that *Targinact®* is not recommended for use within NHS Scotland

---

## PAPAVERETUM

**Important** Do **not** confuse with papaverine (section 7.4.5)
A mixture of 253 parts of morphine hydrochloride, 23 parts of papaverine hydrochloride and 20 parts of codeine hydrochloride

The CSM has advised that to avoid confusion the figures of 7.7 mg/ml or 15.4 mg/ml should be used for prescribing purposes

**Indications** premedication; enhancement of anaesthesia (but see section 15.1.4.3); postoperative analgesia; severe chronic pain

**Cautions** see notes above; supraventricular tachycardia

**Contra-indications** see notes above; heart failure secondary to chronic lung disease; phaeochromocytoma

**Side-effects** see notes above; also hypothermia

**Dose**

- By subcutaneous, intramuscular, *or* intravenous injection, 7.7–15.4 mg repeated every 4 hours if necessary (ELDERLY initially 7.7 mg); CHILD up to 1 month 115 micrograms/kg, 1–12 months 154 micrograms/kg, 1–5 years 1.93–3.85 mg, 6–12 years, 3.85–7.7 mg

Intravenous dose In general the intravenous dose should be 25–50% of the corresponding subcutaneous or intramuscular dose

**Papaveretum** (Non-proprietary) CD

Injection, papaveretum 15.4 mg/mL (providing the equivalent of 10 mg of anhydrous morphine/mL), net price 1-mL amp = £1.64

Note The name *Omnopon®* was formerly used for papaveretum preparations

◢With hyoscine
**Papaveretum and Hyoscine Injection** (Non-proprietary) CD

Injection, papaveretum 15.4 mg (providing the equivalent of 10 mg of anhydrous morphine), hyoscine hydrobromide 400 micrograms/mL. Net price 1-mL amp = £3.57

Dose premedication, by subcutaneous or intramuscular injection, 0.5–1 mL

◢With aspirin
Section 4.7.1

---

## PENTAZOCINE

**Indications** moderate to severe pain, but see notes above

**Cautions** see notes above; also pancreatitis, arterial or pulmonary hypertension, cardiac arrhythmias, myocardial infarction, phaeochromocytoma; effects only partially reversed by naloxone

**Contra-indications** see notes above; patients dependent on opioids (can precipitate withdrawal); heart failure secondary to chronic lung disease; acute porphyria (section 9.8.2)

**Side-effects** see notes above; also abdominal pain, hypertension, syncope, seizures, paraesthesia, tremor, raised intracranial pressure, disorientation, hypothermia, chills, blood disorders, myalgia, and toxic epidermal necrolysis

**Dose**

- By mouth, pentazocine hydrochloride 50 mg every 3–4 hours preferably after food (range 25–100 mg); max. 600 mg daily; CHILD 6–12 years 25 mg

- By subcutaneous, intramuscular, or intravenous injection, moderate pain, pentazocine 30 mg, severe pain 45–60 mg every 3–4 hours when necessary; CHILD over 1 year, by subcutaneous *or* intramuscular injection, up to 1 mg/kg, by intravenous injection up to 500 micrograms/kg

**Pentazocine** (Non-proprietary) ⒸⒹ ◢▰

Capsules, pentazocine hydrochloride 50 mg. Net price 28-cap pack = £13.84. Label: 2, 21
Brands include *Fortral®* ⒩ⒽⓈ

Tablets, pentazocine hydrochloride 25 mg. Net price 28-tab pack = £11.99. Label: 2, 21
Brands include *Fortral®* ⒩ⒽⓈ

Injection, pentazocine 30 mg (as lactate)/mL. Net price 1-mL amp = £1.67; 2-mL amp = £3.21
Brands include *Fortral®* ⒩ⒽⓈ

---

## PETHIDINE HYDROCHLORIDE

**Indications** moderate to severe pain, obstetric analgesia; peri-operative analgesia

**Cautions** see notes above; not suitable for severe continuing pain; accumulation of metabolites may result in neurotoxicity; cardiac arrhythmias, severe cor pulmonale

**Contra-indications** see notes above; phaeochromocytoma

**Side-effects** see notes above; also restlessness and hypothermia; convulsions reported in **overdosage**

**Dose**

- Acute pain, by mouth, 50–150 mg every 4 hours; CHILD 0.5–2 mg/kg

  By subcutaneous *or* intramuscular injection, 25–100 mg, repeated after 4 hours; CHILD, by intramuscular injection, 0.5–2 mg/kg

  By slow intravenous injection, 25–50 mg, repeated after 4 hours

- Obstetric analgesia, by subcutaneous *or* intramuscular injection, 50–100 mg, repeated 1–3 hours later if necessary; max. 400 mg in 24 hours

- Premedication, by intramuscular injection, 25–100 mg 1 hour before operation; CHILD 0.5–2 mg/kg

- Postoperative pain, by subcutaneous *or* intramuscular injection, 25–100 mg, every 2–3 hours if necessary; CHILD, by intramuscular injection, 0.5–2 mg/kg

**Note** In the postoperative period, the patient should be closely monitored for pain relief as well as for side-effects especially respiratory depression

**Pethidine** (Non-proprietary) ⒸⒹ

Tablets, pethidine hydrochloride 50 mg, net price 50 = £5.86. Label: 2

Injection, pethidine hydrochloride 50 mg/mL, net price 1-mL amp = 53p, 2-mL amp = 56p; 10 mg/mL, 5-mL amp = £3.17, 10-mL amp = £2.18

◢**With promethazine**
**Pamergan P100®** (Martindale) ⒸⒹ ◢▰

Injection, pethidine hydrochloride 50 mg, promethazine hydrochloride 25 mg/mL. Net price 2-mL amp = £1.44

**Dose** by intramuscular injection, premedication, 2 mL 60–90 minutes before operation; CHILD 8–12 years 0.75 mL, 13–16 years 1 mL

Obstetric analgesia, 1–2 mL every 4 hours if necessary
Severe pain, 1–2 mL every 4–6 hours if necessary

**Note** Although usually given intramuscularly, may be given intravenously after dilution to at least 10 mL with water for injections

---

## TRAMADOL HYDROCHLORIDE

**Indications** moderate to severe pain

**Cautions** see notes above; impaired consciousness; excessive bronchial secretions; not suitable as a substitute in opioid-dependent patients
**General anaesthesia** Not recommended for analgesia during potentially light planes of general anaesthesia (possibly increased intra-operative recall reported)

**Contra-indications** see notes above; uncontrolled epilepsy; acute porphyria (section 9.8.2)

**Side-effects** see notes above; also diarrhoea; fatigue; *less commonly* retching, gastritis, and flatulence; *rarely* anorexia, syncope, hypertension, bronchospasm, dyspnoea, wheezing, seizures, paraesthesia, and muscle weakness; blood disorders also reported

**Dose**

- ADULT and CHILD over 12 years, by mouth, 50–100 mg not more often than every 4 hours; total of more than 400 mg daily not usually required

- ADULT and CHILD over 12 years, by intramuscular injection *or* by intravenous injection (over 2–3 minutes) *or* by intravenous infusion, 50–100 mg every 4–6 hours

  Postoperative pain, 100 mg initially then 50 mg every 10–20 minutes if necessary during first hour to total max. 250 mg (including initial dose) in first hour, *then* 50–100 mg every 4–6 hours; max. 600 mg daily

**Tramadol Hydrochloride** (Non-proprietary) ⓅⓄⓂ

Capsules, tramadol hydrochloride 50 mg. Net price 30-cap pack = £1.39, 100-cap pack = £2.41. Label: 2
Brands include *Tramake®*

Injection, tramadol hydrochloride 50 mg/mL. Net price 2-mL amp = 98p

**Zamadol®** (Meda) ⓅⓄⓂ

Capsules, tramadol hydrochloride 50 mg, net price 100-cap pack = £8.00. Label: 2

Orodispersible tablets (*Zamadol Melt®*), tramadol hydrochloride 50 mg, net price 60-tab pack = £7.12. Label: 2, counselling, administration
**Excipients** include aspartame (section 9.4.1)
**Counselling** *Zamadol Melt®* should be sucked and then swallowed. May also be dispersed in water

Injection, tramadol hydrochloride 50 mg/mL, net price 2-mL amp = £1.10

**Zydol®** (Grünenthal) ⓅⓄⓂ

Capsules, green/yellow, tramadol hydrochloride 50 mg, net price 30-cap pack = £3.22, 100-cap pack = £10.71. Label: 2

Soluble tablets, tramadol hydrochloride 50 mg, net price 20-tab pack = £2.95, 100-tab pack = £13.95. Label: 2, 13

Injection, tramadol hydrochloride 50 mg/mL. Net price 2-mL amp = 90p

◢**Modified-release 12-hourly preparations**
**Dromadol® SR** (IVAX) ⓅⓄⓂ

Tablets, m/r, tramadol hydrochloride 100 mg (white), net price 60-tab pack = £12.78; 150 mg (beige), 60-tab pack = £19.17; 200 mg (orange), 60-tab pack = £25.56. Label: 2, 25

**Dose** ADULT and CHILD over 12 years, initially 100 mg twice daily increased if necessary; usual max. 200 mg twice daily

**Larapam® SR** (Sandoz) (PoM)

Tablets, m/r, tramadol hydrochloride 100 mg, net price 60-tab pack = £17.55; 150 mg, 60-tab pack = £27.35; 200 mg, 60-tab pack = £36.50. Label: 2, 25

Dose ADULT and CHILD over 12 years, initially 100 mg twice daily increased if necessary; usual max. 200 mg twice daily

**Mabron®** (Morningside) (PoM)

Tablets, m/r, tramadol hydrochloride 100 mg, net price 60-tab pack = £18.26; 150 mg, 60-tab pack = £27.39; 200 mg, 60-tab pack = £36.52. Label: 2, 25

Dose ADULT and CHILD over 12 years, 100 mg twice daily increased if necessary; usual max. 200 mg twice daily

**Maxitram SR®** (Chiesi) (PoM)

Capsules, m/r, tramadol hydrochloride 50 mg (white), net price 60-cap pack = £4.55; 100 mg (yellow), 60-cap pack = £12.14; 150 mg (yellow), 60-cap pack = £18.21; 200 mg (yellow), 60-cap pack = £24.28. Label: 2, 25

Dose ADULT and CHILD over 12 years, 100–200 mg twice daily; total of more than 400 mg daily not usually required

**Tramquel® SR** (Meda) (PoM)

Capsules, m/r, tramadol hydrochloride 50 mg (dark green), net price 60-cap pack = £7.64; 100 mg (white), 60-cap pack = £15.28; 150 mg (dark green), 60-cap pack = £22.92; 200 mg (yellow), 60-cap pack = £30.55. Label: 2, counselling, administration

Dose ADULT and CHILD over 12 years, 50–100 mg twice daily increased if necessary to 150–200 mg twice daily; total of more than 400 mg daily not usually required

Counselling Swallow whole or open capsule and swallow contents immediately without chewing

**Zamadol® SR** (Meda) (PoM)

Capsules, m/r, tramadol hydrochloride 50 mg (green), net price 60-cap pack = £7.64; 100 mg, 60-cap pack = £15.28; 150 mg (dark green), 60-cap pack = £22.92; 200 mg (yellow), 60-cap pack = £30.55. Label: 2, counselling, administration

Dose ADULT and CHILD over 12 years, 50–100 mg twice daily increased if necessary to 150–200 mg twice daily; total of more than 400 mg daily not usually required

Counselling Swallow whole or open capsule and swallow contents without chewing

**Zeridame® SR** (Actavis) (PoM)

Tablets, m/r, tramadol hydrochloride 100 mg, net price 60-tab pack = £18.26; 150 mg, 60-tab pack = £27.39; 200 mg, 60-tab pack = £36.52. Label: 2, 25

Dose ADULT and CHILD over 12 years, 100 mg twice daily increased if necessary to 150–200 mg twice daily; usual max. 400 mg daily

**Zydol SR®** (Grünenthal) (PoM)

Tablets, m/r, f/c, tramadol hydrochloride 100 mg, net price 60-tab pack = £18.26; 150 mg (beige), 60-tab pack = £27.39; 200 mg (orange), 60-tab pack = £36.52. Label: 2, 25

Dose ADULT and CHILD over 12 years, 100 mg twice daily increased if necessary to 150–200 mg twice daily; total of more than 400 mg daily not usually required

◢Modified-release 24-hourly preparations

**Tradorec XL®** (Labopharm) (PoM)

Tablets, m/r, tramadol hydrochloride 100 mg, net price 30-tab pack = £14.10; 200 mg, 30-tab pack = £14.98; 300 mg, 30-tab pack = £22.47. Label: 2, 25

Dose ADULT and CHILD over 12 years, initially 100 mg once daily, increased if necessary; usual max. 400 mg once daily

**Zamadol® 24hr** (Meda) (PoM)

Tablets, all f/c, all m/r, tramadol hydrochloride 150 mg, net price 28-tab pack = £10.70; 200 mg, 28-

tab pack = £14.26; 300 mg, 28-tab pack = £21.39; 400 mg, 28-tab pack = £28.51. Label: 2, 25

Dose ADULT and CHILD over 12 years, 150 mg once daily increased if necessary; max. 400 mg once daily

**Zydol XL®** (Grünenthal) (PoM)

Tablets, m/r, f/c, tramadol hydrochloride 150 mg, net price 30-tab pack = £12.18; 200 mg, 30-tab pack = £17.98; 300 mg, 30-tab pack = £24.94; 400 mg, 30-tab pack = £32.47. Label: 2, 25

Dose ADULT and CHILD over 12 years, 150 mg once daily increased if necessary; usual max. 400 mg once daily

◢With paracetamol

**Tramacet®** (Janssen-Cilag) (PoM)

Tablets, f/c, yellow, tramadol hydrochloride 37.5 mg, paracetamol 325 mg, net price 60-tab pack = £9.68. Label: 2, 25, 29, 30

Dose 2 tablets not more than every 6 hours; max. 8 tablets daily; CHILD under 12 years not recommended

## 4.7.3 Neuropathic pain

Neuropathic pain, which occurs as a result of damage to neural tissue, includes *postherpetic neuralgia* (see below), *phantom limb pain, complex regional pain syndrome* (reflex sympathetic dystrophy, causalgia) *compression neuropathies, peripheral neuropathies* (e.g. due to diabetes, haematological malignancies, rheumatoid arthritis, alcoholism, drug misuse), *trauma, central pain* (e.g. pain following stroke, spinal cord injury and syringomyelia) and *idiopathic neuropathy*. The pain occurs in an area of sensory deficit and may be described as burning, shooting or scalding and is often accompanied by pain that is evoked by a non-noxious stimulus (allodynia).

*Trigeminal neuralgia* is also caused by dysfunction of neural tissue, but its management (see below) is distinct from other forms of neuropathic pain.

Neuropathic pain is generally managed with a tricyclic antidepressant and certain antiepileptic drugs. Neuropathic pain may respond only partially to opioid analgesics. Of the opioids, methadone, tramadol, and oxycodone are probably the most effective for neuropathic pain and they may be considered when other measures fail. Nerve blocks, transcutaneous electrical nerve stimulation (TENS) and, in selected cases, central electrical stimulation may help. Many patients with chronic neuropathic pain require multidisciplinary management, including physiotherapy and psychological support.

**Gabapentin** (p. 256) and **pregabalin** (p. 257) are effective for the treatment of neuropathic pain. **Amitriptyline** (p. 211) is also prescribed frequently [unlicensed indication]; **nortriptyline** [unlicensed indication] (p. 212) may be better tolerated than amitriptyline.

**Capsaicin** (section 10.3.2) is licensed for neuropathic pain (but the intense burning sensation during initial treatment may limit use). **Ketamine** (section 15.1.1), an NMDA antagonist, or **lidocaine (lignocaine)** by intravenous infusion may also be useful in some forms of neuropathic pain [both unlicensed indication; specialist use only].

A **corticosteroid** may help to relieve pressure in compression neuropathy and thereby reduce pain. The management of trigeminal neuralgia and postherpetic neuralgia are outlined below; for the management of neuropathic pain in *palliative care* see p. 16; for the management of diabetic neuropathy, see section 6.1.5.

## Trigeminal neuralgia

Surgery may be the treatment of choice in many patients; a neurological assessment will identify those who stand to benefit. **Carbamazepine** (section 4.8.1) taken during the acute stages of trigeminal neuralgia, reduces the frequency and severity of attacks. It is very effective for the severe pain associated with trigeminal neuralgia and (less commonly) glossopharyngeal neuralgia. Blood counts and electrolytes should be monitored when high doses are given. Small doses should be used initially to reduce the incidence of side-effects e.g. dizziness. **Oxcarbazepine** [unlicensed indication] is an alternative to carbamazepine. **Lamotrigine** [unlicensed indication] and **gabapentin** are also used in trigeminal neuralgia. Some cases respond to **phenytoin** (section 4.8.1); the drug may be given by intravenous infusion (possibly as fosphenytoin) in a crisis (specialist use only).

## Postherpetic neuralgia

Postherpetic neuralgia can follow acute herpes zoster infection (shingles), particularly in the elderly. If **amitriptyline** [unlicensed indication] fails to manage the pain adequately, **gabapentin** may improve control. A topical analgesic preparation containing **capsaicin** 0.075% (section 10.3.2) is licensed for use in postherpetic neuralgia. Application of topical local anaesthetic preparations such as lidocaine medicated plasters (section 15.2) may be helpful in some patients.

## Chronic facial pain

Chronic oral and facial pain including persistent idiopathic facial pain (also termed 'atypical facial pain') and temporomandibular dysfunction (previously termed temporomandibular joint pain dysfunction syndrome) may call for prolonged use of analgesics or for other drugs. Tricyclic antidepressants (section 4.3.1) may be useful for facial pain [unlicensed indication], but are not on the Dental Practitioners' List. Disorders of this type require specialist referral and psychological support to accompany drug treatment. Patients on long-term therapy need to be monitored both for progress and for side-effects.

## 4.7.4 Antimigraine drugs

**4.7.4.1** Treatment of acute migraine
**4.7.4.2** Prophylaxis of migraine
**4.7.4.3** Cluster headache

### 4.7.4.1 Treatment of acute migraine

Treatment of a migraine attack should be guided by response to previous treatment and the severity of the attacks. A **simple analgesic** such as aspirin, paracetamol (preferably in a soluble or dispersible form) or a

NSAID is often effective; concomitant **antiemetic** treatment may be required. If treatment with an analgesic is inadequate, an attack may be treated with a specific antimigraine compound such as a **5HT₁ agonist** ('triptan'). **Ergot alkaloids** are rarely required now; oral and rectal preparations are associated with many side-effects and they should be avoided in cerebrovascular or cardiovascular disease.

Excessive use of acute treatments for migraine (opioid and non-opioid analgesics, 5HT₁ agonists, and ergotamine) is associated with medication-overuse headache (analgesic-induced headache); therefore, increasing consumption of these medicines needs careful management.

## Analgesics

Most migraine headaches respond to analgesics such as **aspirin** or **paracetamol** (section 4.7.1) but because peristalsis is often reduced during migraine attacks the medication may not be sufficiently well absorbed to be effective; dispersible or effervescent preparations are therefore preferred.

The NSAID **tolfenamic acid** is licensed specifically for the treatment of an acute attack of migraine; **diclofenac potassium**, **flurbiprofen**, **ibuprofen**, and **naproxen sodium** (section 10.1.1) are also licensed for use in migraine.

### ▌ ANALGESICS

◢**Aspirin**
Section 4.7.1

◢**Paracetamol**
Section 4.7.1

◢**Non-steroidal anti-inflammatory drugs (NSAIDs)**
Section 10.1.1

◢**With antiemetics**
**Migraleve®** (McNeil) ◢
  Tablets, all f/c, *pink tablets*, buclizine hydrochloride 6.25 mg, paracetamol 500 mg, codeine phosphate 8 mg; *yellow tablets*, paracetamol 500 mg, codeine phosphate 8 mg. Net price 48-tab *Migraleve* [PoM] (32 pink + 16 yellow) = £5.10; 48 pink (*Migraleve Pink*) = £5.56; 48 yellow (*Migraleve Yellow*) = £4.70. Label: 2, (*Migraleve Pink*), 17, 30
  Dose 2 pink tablets at onset of attack, or if it is imminent, then 2 yellow tablets every 4 hours if necessary; max. in 24 hours 2 pink and 6 yellow; CHILD under 10 years, only under close medical supervision; 10–14 years, half adult dose

**MigraMax®** (Zeneus) [PoM]
  Oral powder, aspirin (as lysine acetylsalicylate) 900 mg, metoclopramide hydrochloride 10 mg/ sachet, net price 6-sachet pack = £6.73, 20-sachet pack = £22.42. Label: 13, 21, 32
  Dose ADULT over 20 years 1 sachet in water at onset of attack, repeated after 2 hours if necessary (max. 3 sachets in 24 hours); YOUNG ADULT (under 20 years) and CHILD not recommended
  Important Metoclopramide can cause **severe extrapyramidal effects**, particularly in children and young adults (for further details, see p. 225)
  Excipients include aspartame (section 9.4.1)

**4** **Central nervous system**

**Paramax®** (Sanofi-Synthelabo) ▣PoM▣

Tablets, scored, paracetamol 500 mg, metoclopramide hydrochloride 5 mg. Net price 42-tab pack = £9.64. Label: 17, 30

Sachets, effervescent powder, sugar-free, the contents of 1 sachet = 1 tablet; to be dissolved in ¼ tumblerful of liquid before administration. Net price 42-sachet pack = £12.52. Label: 13, 17, 30

Dose (tablets or sachets): 2 at onset of attack then every 4 hours when necessary to max. of 6 in 24 hours; YOUNG ADULT 12–19 years, 1 at onset of attack then 1 every 4 hours when necessary to max. of 3 in 24 hours (max. dose of metoclopramide 500 micrograms/kg daily)

Important Metoclopramide can cause severe extrapyramidal effects, particularly in children and young adults (for further details, see p. 225)

## ■ TOLFENAMIC ACID

**Indications** treatment of acute migraine

**Cautions** see NSAIDs, section 10.1.1

**Contra-indications** see NSAIDs, section 10.1.1

**Side-effects** see NSAIDs, section 10.1.1; also dysuria (most commonly in men), confusion, malaise, hallucination, paraesthesia, tremor, euphoria, fatigue, and visual disturbances reported

**Dose**

- ADULT over 18 years, 200 mg at onset repeated once after 1–2 hours if necessary

**Clotam Rapid®** (Galen) ▣PoM▣

Tablets, tolfenamic acid 200 mg. Net price 10-tab pack = £15.00. Label: 21

## 5HT₁ agonists

A 5HT₁ agonist is of considerable value in the treatment of an acute migraine attack. The 5HT₁ agonists ('triptans') act on the 5HT (serotonin) 1B/1D receptors and they are therefore sometimes referred to as $5HT_{1B/1D}$-receptor agonists. A 5HT₁ agonist may be used during the established headache phase of an attack and is the preferred treatment in those who fail to respond to conventional analgesics.

The 5HT₁ agonists available for treating migraine are **almotriptan**, **eletriptan**, **frovatriptan**, **naratriptan**, **rizatriptan**, **sumatriptan**, and **zolmitriptan**. Sumatriptan is also of value in cluster headache (section 4.7.4.3).

**Cautions** 5HT₁ agonists should be used with caution in conditions which predispose to coronary artery disease (pre-existing cardiac disease, see Contra-indications below); hepatic impairment (see Appendix 2); pregnancy (see Appendix 4) and breast-feeding (see Appendix 5). 5HT₁ agonists are recommended as monotherapy and should not be taken concurrently with other therapies for acute migraine; see also **interactions**: Appendix 1 (5HT₁ agonists). Little information is available on the use of these drugs in the elderly (over 65 years).

**Contra-indications** 5HT₁ agonists are contra-indicated in ischaemic heart disease, previous myocardial infarction, coronary vasospasm (including Prinzmetal's angina), and uncontrolled or severe hypertension.

**Side-effects** Side-effects of the 5HT₁ agonists include sensations of tingling, heat, heaviness, pressure, or tightness of any part of the body (including throat and chest—discontinue if intense, may be due to coronary vasoconstriction or to anaphylaxis; see also CSM advice under Sumatriptan); flushing, dizziness, feeling of weakness; fatigue; nausea and vomiting also reported.

## ■ ALMOTRIPTAN

**Indications** treatment of acute migraine

**Cautions** see under 5HT₁ agonists above; sensitivity to sulphonamides; hepatic impairment (avoid if severe—Appendix 2); renal impairment (Appendix 3); **inter-actions**: Appendix 1 (5HT₁ agonists)

**Contra-indications** see under 5HT₁ agonists above; previous cerebrovascular accident or transient ischaemic attack; peripheral vascular disease

**Side-effects** see under 5HT₁ agonists above; also transient increase in blood pressure, drowsiness; *less commonly* diarrhoea, dyspepsia, dry mouth, chest pain, palpitation, paraesthesia, headache, myalgia, bone pain, tinnitus; *very rarely* myocardial infarction, and tachycardia

**Dose**

- 12.5 mg as soon as possible after onset repeated after 2 hours if migraine recurs (patient not responding should not take second dose for same attack); max. 25 mg in 24 hours; CHILD and ADOLESCENT under 18 years not recommended

**Almogran®** (Organon) ▣PoM▣

Tablets, f/c, almotriptan (as hydrogen malate) 12.5 mg, net price 3-tab pack = £9.07; 6-tab pack = £18.14; 9-tab pack = £27.20. Label: 3

## ■ ELETRIPTAN

**Indications** treatment of acute migraine

**Cautions** see under 5HT₁ agonists above; renal impairment (avoid if severe—Appendix 3); **interactions**: Appendix 1 (5HT₁ agonists)

**Contra-indications** see under 5HT₁ agonists above; previous cerebrovascular accident or transient ischaemic attack; arrhythmias; heart failure; peripheral vascular disease; severe hepatic impairment

**Side-effects** see under 5HT₁ agonists above; also abdominal pain, dry mouth, dyspepsia; tachycardia, palpitation; drowsiness, headache; pharyngitis, rhinitis, chills; myasthenia, myalgia; sweating; *less commonly* diarrhoea, glossitis, thirst, anorexia, taste disturbance; dyspnoea, yawning, oedema, agitation, confusion, euphoria, depression, insomnia, depersonalisation, tremor, dysarthria, stupor, movement disorders, hypertonia, urinary frequency, arthralgia, photophobia, visual disturbances, tinnitus, rash, and pruritus; *rarely* constipation, oesophagitis, bradycardia, asthma, syncope, lymphadenopathy, and menorrhagia; ischaemic colitis and hypertension also reported

**Dose**

- ADULT over 18 years, 40 mg repeated after 2 hours if migraine recurs (patient not responding to initial dose should not take second dose for same attack); increase to 80 mg for subsequent attacks if 40-mg dose inadequate; max. 80 mg in 24 hours

**Relpax®** (Pfizer) ▼ ▣PoM▣

Tablets, f/c, orange, eletriptan (as hydrobromide) 20 mg, net price 6-tab pack = £22.50; 40 mg, 6-tab pack = £22.50. Label: 3

## FROVATRIPTAN

**Indications**  treatment of acute migraine

**Cautions**  see under 5HT$_1$ agonists above; **interactions**: Appendix 1 (5HT$_1$ agonists)

**Contra-indications**  see under 5HT$_1$ agonists above; severe hepatic impairment; previous cerebrovascular attack or transient ischaemic attack; peripheral vascular disease

**Side-effects**  see under 5HT$_1$ agonists above; also dry mouth, dyspepsia, abdominal pain, paraesthesia, drowsiness, headache, visual disturbances, sweating; *less commonly* diarrhoea, dysphagia, flatulence, tachycardia, palpitation, hypertension, rhinitis, pharyngitis, sinusitis, laryngitis, tremor, anxiety, asthenia, insomnia, confusion, nervousness, impaired concentration, agitation, depression, depersonalisation, taste disturbances, micturition disorders, thirst, dehydration, arthralgia, muscle stiffness, tinnitus, vertigo, pruritus; *rarely* constipation, gastro-oesophageal reflux, irritable bowel syndrome, hiccup, peptic ulcer, stomatitis, bradycardia, hyperventilation, amnesia, abnormal dreams, hypertonia, hypotonia, breast tenderness, hypocalcaemia, hypoglycaemia, bilirubinaemia, epistaxis, urticaria, pyrexia, and purpura

**Dose**

● 2.5 mg as soon as possible after onset repeated after 2 hours if migraine recurs (patient not responding should not take second dose for same attack); max. 5 mg in 24 hours; CHILD and ADOLESCENT under 18 years not recommended

**Migard®** (Menarini) PoM

Tablets, f/c, frovatriptan (as succinate) 2.5 mg, net price 6-tab pack = £16.67. Label: 3

## NARATRIPTAN

**Indications**  treatment of acute migraine

**Cautions**  see under 5HT$_1$ agonists above; sensitivity to sulphonamides; renal impairment (avoid if eGFR less than 15 mL/minute/1.73 m²; Appendix 3); **interactions**: Appendix 1 (5HT$_1$ agonists)

Driving Drowsiness may affect performance of skilled tasks (e.g. driving)

**Contra-indications**  see under 5HT$_1$ agonists above; previous cerebrovascular accident or transient ischaemic attack; peripheral vascular disease

**Side-effects**  see under 5HT$_1$ agonists above; also *less commonly* bradycardia, tachycardia, palpitation, and visual disturbance; *rarely* ischaemic colitis

**Dose**

● 2.5 mg, repeated after at least 4 hours if migraine recurs (patient not responding should not take second dose for same attack); max. 5 mg in 24 hours; CHILD and ADOLESCENT under 18 years not recommended

**Naramig®** (GSK) PoM

Tablets, f/c, green, naratriptan (as hydrochloride) 2.5 mg, net price 6-tab pack = £24.55, 12-tab pack = £49.10. Label: 3

## RIZATRIPTAN

**Indications**  treatment of acute migraine

**Cautions**  see under 5HT$_1$ agonists above; renal impairment (avoid in severe impairment; Appendix 3); **interactions**: Appendix 1 (5HT$_1$ agonists)

Driving Drowsiness may affect performance of skilled tasks (e.g. driving)

**Contra-indications**  see under 5HT$_1$ agonists above; previous cerebrovascular accident or transient ischaemic attack; peripheral vascular disease

**Side-effects**  see under 5HT$_1$ agonists above; drowsiness, palpitation, tachycardia, dry mouth, diarrhoea, dyspepsia, thirst, pharyngeal discomfort, dyspnoea, headache, paraesthesia, decreased alertness, insomnia, tremor, ataxia, nervousness, vertigo, confusion, myalgia and muscle weakness, sweating, urticaria, pruritus, blurred vision; *rarely* syncope, hypertension; hypersensitivity reactions (including rash, angioedema, and toxic epidermal necrolysis) and taste disturbance reported

**Dose**

● 10 mg as soon as possible after onset repeated after 2 hours if migraine recurs (patient not responding should not take second dose for same attack); max. 20 mg in 24 hours; CHILD and ADOLESCENT under 18 years not recommended

**Maxalt®** (MSD) PoM

Tablets, pink, rizatriptan (as benzoate) 5 mg, net price 6-tab pack = £26.74; 10 mg, 3-tab pack = £13.37, 6-tab pack = £26.74. Label: 3

Oral lyophilisate (*Maxalt® Melt Wafers*), rizatriptan (as benzoate) 10 mg, net price 3-wafer pack = £13.37, 6-wafer pack = £26.74. Label: 3, counselling, administration

Counselling *Maxalt® Melt* wafers should be placed on the tongue and allowed to dissolve

Excipients include aspartame equivalent to phenylalanine 2.1 mg (section 9.4.1)

## SUMATRIPTAN

**Indications**  treatment of acute migraine; cluster headache (subcutaneous injection only)

**Cautions**  see under 5HT$_1$ agonists above; history of seizures; renal impairment; sensitivity to sulphonamides; **interactions**: Appendix 1 (5HT$_1$ agonists)

Driving Drowsiness may affect performance of skilled tasks (e.g. driving)

**Contra-indications**  see under 5HT$_1$ agonists above; previous cerebrovascular accident or transient ischaemic attack; peripheral vascular disease; moderate and severe hypertension

**Side-effects**  see under 5HT$_1$ agonists above; also drowsiness, transient increase in blood pressure; *very rarely* ischaemic colitis, hypotension, bradycardia or tachycardia, palpitation, arrhythmias, myocardial infarction, Raynaud's syndrome, seizures, tremor, dystonia, nystagmus, and visual disturbances; erythema at injection site; nasal irritation and epistaxis with nasal spray

CSM advice Following reports of chest pain and tightness (coronary vasoconstriction) CSM has emphasised that sumatriptan should **not** be used in ischaemic heart disease or Prinzmetal's angina, and that use with ergotamine should be **avoided** (see also Cautions).

4

Central nervous system

### Dose

- By mouth, 50 mg (some patients may require 100 mg); dose may be repeated after at least 2 hours if migraine recurs; max. 300 mg in 24 hours; CHILD and ADOLESCENT under 18 years, see *BNF for Children*
- By subcutaneous injection using auto-injector, 6 mg; dose may be repeated once after at least 1 hour if migraine recurs; max. 12 mg in 24 hours; CHILD and ADOLESCENT under 18 years not recommended

  **Important** Not for intravenous injection which may cause coronary vasospasm and angina

- Intranasally, 10–20 mg (ADOLESCENT 12–17 years 10 mg) into one nostril; dose may be repeated once after at least 2 hours if migraine recurs; max. 40 mg (ADOLESCENT 12–17 years 20 mg) in 24 hours

**Note** Patient not responding to initial dose should not take second dose for same attack

### ¹Sumatriptan (Non-proprietary) PoM

Tablets, sumatriptan (as succinate) 50 mg, net price 6-tab pack = £8.99; 100 mg, 6-tab pack = £13.60. Label: 3, 10, patient information leaflet

1. Sumatriptan 50 mg tablets can be sold to the public to treat previously diagnosed migraine; max. daily dose 100 mg

### Imigran® (GSK) PoM

Tablets, sumatriptan (as succinate) 50 mg, net price 6-tab pack = £26.54, 12-tab pack = £50.43; 100 mg, 6-tab pack = £42.90, 12-tab pack = £85.80. Label: 3, 10, patient information leaflet

Injection, sumatriptan (as succinate) 12 mg/mL (= 6 mg/0.5-mL syringe), net price, treatment pack (2 × 0.5-mL prefilled syringes and auto-injector) = £42.47; refill pack 2 × 0.5-mL prefilled cartridges = £40.41. Label: 3, 10, patient information leaflet

Nasal spray, sumatriptan 10 mg/0.1-mL actuation, net price 2 unit-dose spray device = £11.80; 20 mg/0.1-mL actuation, 2 unit-dose spray device = £11.80, 6 unit-dose spray device = £35.39. Label: 3, 10, patient information leaflet

### Imigran® Radis (GSK) PoM

Tablets, f/c, sumatriptan (as succinate) 50 mg (pink), net price 6-tab pack = £23.90, 12-tab pack = £47.83; 100 mg (white), 6-tab pack = £42.90, 12-tab pack = £85.80. Label: 3, 10, patient information leaflet

## ▌ ZOLMITRIPTAN

**Indications** treatment of acute migraine

**Cautions** see under $5HT_1$ agonists above; should not be taken within 12 hours of any other $5HT_1$ agonist; **interactions:** Appendix 1 ($5HT_1$ agonists)

**Contra-indications** see under $5HT_1$ agonists above; Wolff-Parkinson-White syndrome or arrhythmias associated with accessory cardiac conduction pathways; previous cerebrovascular accident or transient ischaemic attack

**Side-effects** see under $5HT_1$ agonists above; also dry mouth, drowsiness, paraesthesia, myalgia, muscle weakness; *rarely* palpitation, tachycardia, angio-edema, headache, urticaria; *very rarely* abdominal pain, gastro-intestinal and splenic infarction, ischaemic colitis, angina, myocardial infarction, polyuria, transient increase in blood pressure; *with nasal spray*, taste disturbance and nasal discomfort

### Dose

- By mouth, ADULT over 18 years, 2.5 mg repeated after not less than 2 hours if migraine persists or recurs

(increase to 5 mg for subsequent attacks in patients not achieving satisfactory relief with 2.5-mg dose); max. 10 mg in 24 hours

- Intranasally, ADULT over 18 years, 5 mg (1 spray) into one nostril as soon as possible after onset repeated after not less than 2 hours if migraine persists or recurs; max. 10 mg in 24 hours

### Zomig® (AstraZeneca) PoM

Tablets, f/c, yellow, zolmitriptan 2.5 mg, net price 6-tab pack = £18.00, 12-tab pack = £36.00

Orodispersible tablets (*Zomig Rapimelt®*), zolmitriptan 2.5 mg, net price 6-tab pack = £17.90; 5 mg, 6-tab pack = £22.80 Counselling, administration

Counselling *Zomig Rapimelt®* should be placed on the tongue, allowed to disperse and swallowed

Excipients include aspartame equivalent to phenylalanine 2.81 mg/tablet (section 9.4.1)

Nasal spray, zolmitriptan 5 mg/0.1-mL unit-dose spray device, net price 6 unit-dose sprays = £36.50

## Ergot alkaloids

The value of **ergotamine** for migraine is limited by difficulties in absorption and by its side-effects, particularly nausea, vomiting, abdominal pain, and *muscular cramps*; it is best avoided. The recommended doses of ergotamine preparations should **not** be exceeded and treatment should **not** be repeated at intervals of less than 4 days.

To avoid habituation the frequency of administration of ergotamine should be limited to **no more than** twice a month. It should **never** be prescribed prophylactically but in the management of cluster headache a low dose (e.g. ergotamine 1 mg at night for 6 nights in 7) is occasionally given for 1 to 2 weeks [unlicensed indication].

## ▌ ERGOTAMINE TARTRATE

**Indications** treatment of acute migraine and migraine variants unresponsive to analgesics

**Cautions** risk of peripheral vasospasm (see below); elderly; dependence (see Ergot Alkaloids above); cardiac disease; anaemia; **interactions:** Appendix 1 (ergot alkaloids)

Peripheral vasospasm Warn patient to stop treatment immediately if numbness or tingling of extremities develops and to contact doctor.

**Contra-indications** peripheral vascular disease, coronary heart disease, obliterative vascular disease and Raynaud's syndrome, temporal arteritis, hepatic impairment (Appendix 2), renal impairment (Appendix 3), sepsis, severe or inadequately controlled hypertension, hyperthyroidism, pregnancy (Appendix 4), breast-feeding (Appendix 5), acute porphyria (section 9.8.2)

**Side-effects** abdominal pain, nausea, vomiting; dizziness; *less commonly* diarrhoea, pain and weakness in extremities, cyanosis, peripheral vasoconstriction, paraesthesia, and hypoesthesia; *rarely* intestinal ischaemia, arrhythmias, increased blood pressure, bradycardia, tachycardia, dyspnoea, ergotism (including absence of pulse and numbness in extremities), myalgia, rash, and urticaria; *very rarely* myocardial ischaemia, myocardial infarction, heart-valve fibrosis, and gangrene; constipation, dry mouth, cerebral ischaemia, thrombosis, drowsiness, sleep disturbances, tremor, seizures, extrapyramidal effects, anxiety, depression, confusion, hallucinations, renal artery spasm, urinary retention, blood disorders, blurred vision, and arthralgia also reported; *with suppositories* rectal and anal ulcers on prolonged use

**Dose**

● See under preparations below

**Cafergot®** (Alliance) [PoM] ▱◩

Tablets, s/c, ergotamine tartrate 1 mg, caffeine 100 mg, net price 30-tab pack = £4.02. Label: 18, counselling, dosage

**Dose** ADULT and CHILD over 12 years, 1–2 tablets at onset; max. 4 tablets in 24 hours; not to be repeated at intervals of less than 4 days; max. 8 tablets in one week (but see also notes above)

Suppositories, ergotamine tartrate 2 mg, caffeine 100 mg, net price 30 = £8.10. Label: 18, counselling, dosage

**Dose** ADULT and CHILD over 12 years, 1 suppository at onset; max. 2 in 24 hours; max. 4 suppositories in one week (but see also notes above)

**Migril®** (CP) [PoM] ▱◩

Tablets, scored, ergotamine tartrate 2 mg, cyclizine hydrochloride 50 mg, caffeine hydrate 100 mg, net price 100 = £51.00. Label: 2, 18, counselling, dosage

**Dose** 1 tablet at onset, followed after 30 minutes by ½–1 tablet, repeated every 30 minutes if necessary; max. 3 tablets in 24 hours, 4 tablets per attack, 6 tablets in one week (but see also notes above); CHILD not recommended

---

## Antiemetics

Antiemetics (section 4.6), such as **metoclopramide** or **domperidone**, or phenothiazine and antihistamine antiemetics, relieve the nausea associated with migraine attacks. Antiemetics may be given by intramuscular injection or rectally if vomiting is a problem. Metoclopramide and domperidone have the added advantage of promoting gastric emptying and normal peristalsis; a single dose should be given at the onset of symptoms. Oral analgesic preparations containing metoclopramide are a convenient alternative (**important**: for warnings relating to extrapyramidal effects of metoclopramide particularly in children and young adults, see p. 225).

### 4.7.4.2 Prophylaxis of migraine

Where migraine attacks are frequent, possible provoking factors such as stress, irregular life-style (e.g. lack of sleep), or chemical triggers (e.g. alcohol and nitrates) should be sought; combined oral contraceptives may also provoke migraine, see section 7.3.1 for advice.

Preventive treatment for migraine should be considered for patients who:

● suffer at least two attacks a month;

● suffer an increasing frequency of headaches;

● suffer significant disability despite suitable treatment for migraine attacks;

● cannot take suitable treatment for migraine attacks.

Prophylaxis is also necessary in some rare migraine subtypes and those at risk of migrainous infarction.

The **beta-blockers** propranolol, metoprolol, nadolol, and timolol (section 2.4) are all effective. Propranolol is the most commonly used.

**Pizotifen** is an antihistamine and serotonin antagonist structurally related to the tricyclic antidepressants. It affords good prophylaxis but may cause weight gain. To avoid undue drowsiness treatment may be started at a low dose and gradually increased.

**Sodium valproate** (section 4.8.1) may be effective for migraine prophylaxis [unlicensed indication] in a starting dose of 300 mg twice daily, increased if necessary to 1.2 g daily in divided doses. **Valproic acid** (as semisodium valproate) (section 4.2.3) is similarly effective [unlicensed indication] in a starting dose of 250 mg twice daily, increased if necessary to 1 g daily in divided doses.

**Topiramate** (section 4.8.1) is effective for migraine prophylaxis. Treatment should be supervised by a specialist.

Tricyclic antidepressants (section 4.3.1) (e.g. **amitriptyline**) are also used for preventing migraine [unlicensed indication].

**Cyproheptadine** (section 3.4.1), an antihistamine with serotonin-antagonist and calcium channel-blocking properties, may also be tried in refractory cases.

**Clonidine** (*Dixarit®*) is **not** recommended and may aggravate depression or produce insomnia. **Methysergide**, a semi-synthetic ergot alkaloid, has dangerous side-effects (retroperitoneal fibrosis and fibrosis of the heart valves and pleura); **important**: it should only be administered under hospital supervision.

### ▮ PIZOTIFEN

**Indications** prevention of vascular headache including classical migraine, common migraine, and cluster headache

**Cautions** urinary retention; susceptibility to angle-closure glaucoma; renal impairment; pregnancy; breast-feeding (Appendix 5); **interactions**: Appendix 1 (pizotifen)

**Driving** Drowsiness may affect performance of skilled tasks (e.g. driving); effects of alcohol enhanced

**Side-effects** antimuscarinic effects (*very rarely* angle-closure glaucoma), drowsiness, increased appetite and weight gain; occasionally nausea, dizziness; *rarely* anxiety, aggression, and depression; CNS stimulation may occur in children

**Dose**

● Initially 500 micrograms at night increased gradually to usual dose of 1.5 mg at night *or* in 3 divided doses; may be further increased up to max. daily dose 4.5 mg (but rarely necessary), max. single dose 3 mg; CHILD over 5 years, up to 1.5 mg daily in divided doses; max. single dose at night 1 mg

**Pizotifen** (Non-proprietary) [PoM]

Tablets, pizotifen (as hydrogen malate), 500 micrograms, net price 28-tab pack = £1.34; 1.5 mg, 28-tab pack = £2.47. Label: 2

**Sanomigran®** (Novartis) [PoM]

Tablets, both ivory-yellow, s/c, pizotifen (as hydrogen malate), 500 micrograms, net price 60-tab pack = £2.57; 1.5 mg, 28-tab pack = £4.28. Label: 2

Elixir, pizotifen (as hydrogen malate) 250 micrograms/5 mL, net price 300 mL = £4.51. Label: 2

**Central nervous system** 4

## CLONIDINE HYDROCHLORIDE

**Indications** prevention of recurrent migraine (but see notes above), vascular headache, menopausal flushing; hypertension (section 2.5.2)

**Cautions** depressive illness, concurrent antihypertensive therapy; acute porphyria (section 9.8.2); **interactions**: Appendix 1 (clonidine)

**Side-effects** dry mouth, sedation, dizziness, nausea, nocturnal restlessness; occasionally rashes

**Dose**

- 50 micrograms twice daily, increased after 2 weeks to 75 micrograms twice daily if necessary; CHILD not recommended

**Clonidine** (Non-proprietary) PoM
Tablets, clonidine hydrochloride 25 micrograms. Net price 112-tab pack = £10.29

**Dixarit®** (Boehringer Ingelheim) PoM
Tablets, blue, s/c, clonidine hydrochloride 25 micrograms. Net price 112-tab pack = £6.75

**Catapres®** PoM
Section 2.5.2 (hypertension)

## METHYSERGIDE

**Indications** prevention of severe recurrent migraine, cluster headache and other vascular headaches in patients who are refractory to other treatment and whose lives are seriously disrupted (**important:** hospital supervision only, see notes above); diarrhoea associated with carcinoid syndrome

**Cautions** history of peptic ulceration; avoid abrupt withdrawal of treatment; after 6 months withdraw (gradually over 2 to 3 weeks) for reassessment for at least 1 month (see also notes above); **interactions**: Appendix 1 (ergot alkaloids)

**Contra-indications** renal, hepatic, pulmonary, and cardiovascular disease, severe hypertension, collagen disease, cellulitis, urinary-tract disorders, cachectic or septic conditions, pregnancy, breast-feeding

**Side-effects** nausea, vomiting, heartburn, abdominal discomfort, drowsiness, and dizziness occur frequently in initial treatment; mental and behavioural disturbances, insomnia, oedema, weight gain, rashes, loss of scalp hair, cramps, arterial spasm (including coronary artery spasm with angina and possible myocardial infarction), paraesthesias of extremities, postural hypotension, and tachycardia also occur; retroperitoneal and other abnormal fibrotic reactions may occur on prolonged administration, requiring immediate withdrawal of treatment

**Dose**

- Initially 1 mg at bedtime, increased gradually over about 2 weeks to 1–2 mg 3 times daily with food (see notes above); CHILD not recommended
- Diarrhoea associated with carcinoid syndrome, usual range, 12–20 mg daily (hospital supervision); CHILD not recommended

**Deseril®** (Alliance) PoM
Tablets, s/c, methysergide (as maleate) 1 mg, net price 60-tab pack = £12.45. Label: 2, 21

### 4.7.4.3 Cluster headache

Cluster headache rarely responds to standard analgesics. **Sumatriptan** given by subcutaneous injection is the drug of choice for the *treatment* of cluster headache. Alternatively, 100% **oxygen** at a rate of 7–12 litres/minute is useful in aborting an attack.

*Prophylaxis* of cluster headache is considered if the attacks are frequent, or last over 3 weeks, or if the attacks cannot be treated effectively. **Verapamil** or **lithium** [both unlicensed use] are used for prophylaxis. **Ergotamine**, used on an intermittent basis is an alternative for patients with short bouts, but it should **not** be used for prolonged periods. **Methysergide** is effective but must be used with extreme caution (section 4.7.4.2) and only if other drugs cannot be used or if they are not effective.

## 4.8 Antiepileptic drugs

**4.8.1** Control of epilepsy
**4.8.2** Drugs used in status epilepticus
**4.8.3** Febrile convulsions

## 4.8.1 Control of epilepsy

The object of treatment is to prevent the occurrence of seizures by maintaining an effective dose of one or more antiepileptic drugs. Careful adjustment of doses is necessary, starting with low doses and increasing gradually until seizures are controlled or there are significant adverse effects.

When choosing an antiepileptic drug, the seizure type, concomitant medication, co-morbidity, age, and sex should be taken into account. For women of childbearing age, see Pregnancy and Breast-feeding, p. 253.

The dose frequency is often determined by the plasma-drug half-life, and should be kept as low as possible to encourage adherence with the prescribed regimen. Most antiepileptics, when used in the usual dosage, may be given twice daily. Lamotrigine, phenobarbital, and phenytoin, which have long half-lives, can be given once daily at bedtime. However, with large doses, some antiepileptics may need to be given more frequently to avoid adverse effects associated with high peak plasma-drug concentration. Young children metabolise antiepileptics more rapidly than adults and therefore require more frequent doses and a higher dose in proportion to their body-weight.

**Management** When monotherapy with a first-line antiepileptic drug has failed, monotherapy with a second drug should be tried; the diagnosis should be checked before starting an alternative drug if the first drug showed lack of efficacy. The changeover from one antiepileptic drug to another should be cautious, slowly withdrawing the first drug only when the new regimen has been established. Combination therapy with 2 or more antiepileptic drugs may be necessary, but the concurrent use of antiepileptic drugs increases the risk of adverse effects and drug interactions (see below). If combination therapy does not bring about worthwhile benefits, revert to the regimen (monotherapy or combination therapy) that provided the best balance between tolerability and efficacy.

**Interactions** Interactions between antiepileptic drugs are complex and may enhance toxicity without a corresponding increase in antiepileptic effect. Interactions are usually caused by *hepatic enzyme induction* or *hepatic enzyme inhibition*; *displacement from protein binding sites* is not usually a problem. These interactions are highly variable and unpredictable.

Significant interactions that occur **between antiepileptics** themselves are as follows:

> Note Check under each drug for possible interactions when two or more antiepileptic drugs are used

**Carbamazepine**
*often lowers* plasma concentration of clobazam, clonazepam, lamotrigine, an active metabolite of oxcarbazepine, and of phenytoin (but may also raise phenytoin concentration), tiagabine, topiramate, valproate, and zonisamide

*sometimes lowers* plasma concentration of ethosuximide, and primidone (but tendency for corresponding increase in phenobarbital level)

**Ethosuximide**
*sometimes raises* plasma concentration of phenytoin

**Gabapentin**
no interactions with gabapentin reported

**Lamotrigine**
*sometimes raises* plasma concentration of an active metabolite of carbamazepine (but evidence is conflicting)

**Levetiracetam**
no interactions with levetiracetam reported

**Oxcarbazepine**
*sometimes lowers* plasma concentration of carbamazepine (but may raise concentration of an active metabolite of carbamazepine)

*sometimes raises* plasma concentration of phenytoin

*often raises* plasma concentration of phenobarbital

**Phenobarbital** *or* **Primidone**
*often lowers* plasma concentration of carbamazepine, clonazepam, lamotrigine, and of phenytoin (but may also raise phenytoin concentration), tiagabine, valproate, and zonisamide

*sometimes lowers* plasma concentration of ethosuximide

**Phenytoin**
*often lowers* plasma concentration of clonazepam, carbamazepine, lamotrigine, an active metabolite of oxcarbazepine, and of tiagabine, topiramate, valproate, and zonisamide

*often raises* plasma concentration of phenobarbital

*sometimes lowers* plasma concentration of ethosuximide, and primidone (by increasing conversion to phenobarbital)

**Pregabalin**
no interactions with pregabalin reported

**Rufinamide**
*sometimes raises* plasma concentration of phenytoin

**Topiramate**
*sometimes raises* plasma concentration of phenytoin

**Valproate**
*sometimes lowers* plasma concentration of an active metabolite of oxcarbazepine

*often raises* plasma concentration of an active metabolite of carbamazepine, and of lamotrigine, primidone, phenobarbital, and phenytoin (but may also lower)

*sometimes raises* plasma concentration of ethosuximide, primidone, (and tendency for significant increase in phenobarbital level), and rufinamide

**Vigabatrin**
*often lowers* plasma concentration of phenytoin

*sometimes lowers* plasma concentration of phenobarbital, and primidone

For other important interactions see **Appendix 1**; for advice on hormonal contraception and enzyme-inducing drugs (including antiepileptics), see section 7.3.1 and section 7.3.2.

**Withdrawal** Antiepileptic drugs should be withdrawn under specialist supervision. Abrupt withdrawal, particularly of the barbiturates and benzodiazepines, should be avoided because this may precipitate severe rebound seizures. Reduction in dosage should be gradual and, in the case of barbiturates, withdrawal of the drug may take months.

The decision to withdraw antiepileptic drugs from a seizure-free patient, and its timing, is often difficult and depends on individual circumstances. Even in patients who have been seizure-free for several years, there is a significant risk of seizure recurrence on drug withdrawal.

In patients receiving several antiepileptic drugs, only one drug should be withdrawn at a time.

**Driving** Patients suffering from epilepsy may drive a motor vehicle (but not a heavy goods or public service vehicle) provided that they have had a seizure-free period of one year or, if subject to attacks only while asleep, have established a 3-year period of asleep attacks without awake attacks. Patients affected by drowsiness should not drive or operate machinery.

Guidance issued by the Drivers Medical Unit of the Driver and Vehicle Licensing Agency (DVLA) recommends that patients should be advised not to drive during withdrawal of antiepileptic drugs, or for 6 months afterwards (see also Drugs and Driving under General Guidance, p. 3).

**Pregnancy and breast-feeding** There is an increased risk of teratogenicity associated with the use of antiepileptic drugs (reduced if treatment is limited to a single drug). In view of the increased risk of neural tube and other defects associated, in particular, with **carbamazepine**, **lamotrigine**, **oxcarbazepine**, **phenytoin**, and **valproate**, women taking antiepileptic drugs who *may become pregnant* should be **informed of the possible consequences**. Those who *wish to become pregnant* should be referred to an appropriate specialist for advice. Women who become pregnant should be **counselled** and offered **antenatal screening** (alpha-fetoprotein measurement and a second trimester ultrasound scan).

To counteract the risk of neural tube defects, adequate folate supplements are advised for women before and during pregnancy (section 9.1.2).

The concentration of antiepileptic drugs in the blood can change during pregnancy, particularly in the later stages. The dose of antiepileptic drugs should be monitored carefully during pregnancy and after birth, and adjustments made on a clinical basis.

**4**

**Central nervous system**

Routine injection of vitamin K (section 9.6.6) at birth effectively counteracts any antiepileptic-associated risk of neonatal haemorrhage.

Breast-feeding is acceptable with all antiepileptic drugs, taken in normal doses, with the possible exception of the barbiturates, and also some of the more recently introduced ones, see Appendix 5.

## Partial seizures with or without secondary generalisation

Carbamazepine, lamotrigine, oxcarbazepine, and sodium valproate are the drugs of choice for partial (focal) seizures; second-line drugs include clobazam, gabapentin, levetiracetam, pregabalin, tiagabine, topiramate, and zonisamide.

## Generalised seizures

Tonic-clonic seizures  The drugs of choice for tonic-clonic seizures are carbamazepine, lamotrigine, and sodium valproate. Clobazam, levetiracetam, oxcarbazepine, and topiramate are second-line drugs.

Absence seizures  Ethosuximide and sodium valproate are the drugs of choice in typical absence seizures; alternatives include clonazepam and lamotrigine. Sodium valproate is also highly effective in treating the generalised tonic-clonic seizures which can co-exist with absence seizures in idiopathic primary generalised epilepsy.

Myoclonic seizures  Myoclonic seizures (myoclonic jerks) occur in a variety of syndromes, and response to treatment varies considerably. Sodium valproate is the drug of choice; clonazepam and levetiracetam can also be used. Alternatives include lamotrigine and topiramate, but lamotrigine may occasionally exacerbate myoclonic seizures. For reference to the adjunctive use of piracetam, see section 4.9.3.

Sodium valproate and levetiracetam are effective in treating the generalised tonic-clonic seizures that co-exist with myoclonic seizures in idiopathic generalised epilepsy.

Atypical absence, atonic, and tonic seizures  Atypical absence, atonic, and tonic seizures are usually seen in childhood, in specific epilepsy syndromes, or associated with cerebral damage or mental retardation. They may respond poorly to the traditional drugs. Sodium valproate, lamotrigine, and clonazepam can be tried. Second-line drugs that are occasionally helpful include clobazam, ethosuximide, levetiracetam, and topiramate.

## Epilepsy syndromes

Some drugs are licensed for use in particular epilepsy syndromes, such as lamotrigine and rufinamide in Lennox-Gastaut syndrome. The epilepsy syndromes are specific types of epilepsy that are characterised according to a number of features including seizure type, age of onset, and EEG characteristics.

For more information on epilepsy syndromes in children, see *BNF for Children*, section 4.8.1. Prescribing

information for stiripentol (*Diacomit®*) in severe myoclonic epilepsy of infancy (Dravet syndrome) can also be found in *BNF for Children*.

## Carbamazepine and oxcarbazepine

Carbamazepine is a drug of choice for simple and complex partial seizures and for tonic-clonic seizures secondary to a focal discharge. It is essential to initiate carbamazepine therapy at a low dose and build this up slowly with increments of 100–200 mg every two weeks. Reversible blurring of vision, dizziness, and unsteadiness are dose-related, and may be dose-limiting. These side-effects may be reduced by altering the timing of medication; use of modified-release tablets also significantly lessens the incidence of dose-related side-effects.

Oxcarbazepine is licensed for the treatment of partial seizures with or without secondarily generalised tonic-clonic seizures. Oxcarbazepine induces hepatic enzymes to a lesser extent than carbamazepine.

### ▌ CARBAMAZEPINE

Indications  partial and secondary generalised tonic-clonic seizures, primary generalised tonic-clonic seizures; trigeminal neuralgia; prophylaxis of bipolar disorder unresponsive to lithium

Cautions  hepatic impairment (Appendix 2) or renal impairment; cardiac disease (see also Contra-indications); skin reactions (see also Blood, Hepatic or Skin disorders, below and under Side-effects); test for HLA-B*1502 allele in individuals of Han Chinese or Thai origin—risk of Stevens-Johnson syndrome in presence of HLA-B*1502 allele; history of haematological reactions to other drugs; manufacturer recommends blood counts and hepatic and renal function tests (but evidence of practical value unsatisfactory); may exacerbate absence and myoclonic seizures; consider vitamin D supplementation in patients that are immobilized for long periods or who have inadequate sun exposure or dietary intake of calcium; susceptibility to angle-closure glaucoma; pregnancy (important: see p. 253 and Appendix 4 (neural tube screening)), breast-feeding (see p. 253 and Appendix 5); avoid abrupt withdrawal; interactions: see p. 253 and Appendix 1 (carbamazepine)

Blood, hepatic or skin disorders  Patients or their carers should be told how to recognise signs of blood, liver, or skin disorders, and advised to seek immediate medical attention if symptoms such as fever, sore throat, rash, mouth ulcers, bruising, or bleeding develop. Leucopenia which is severe, progressive or associated with clinical symptoms requires withdrawal (if necessary under cover of suitable alternative).

Contra-indications  AV conduction abnormalities (unless paced); history of bone marrow depression; acute porphyria (section 9.8.2)

Side-effects  nausea and vomiting, dizziness, drowsiness, headache, ataxia, confusion and agitation (elderly), visual disturbances (especially diplopia and often associated with peak plasma concentrations); constipation or diarrhoea, anorexia; mild transient generalised erythematous rash may occur in a large number of patients (withdraw if worsens or is accompanied by other symptoms); leucopenia and other blood disorders (including thrombocytopenia, agranulocytosis and aplastic anaemia); other side-effects include cholestatic jaundice, hepatitis and acute renal failure, Stevens-Johnson syndrome, toxic epidermal necrolysis, alopecia, thromboembolism, arthralgia, fever, proteinuria, lymph node enlargement, cardiac conduction disturbances (sometimes arrhythmias), dyskinesias, paraesthesia, depression, impotence (and impaired fertility), gynaecomastia, galactorrhoea, aggression, activation of psychosis; *very rarely* angle-closure glaucoma; photosensitivity, pulmonary hypersensitivity (with dyspnoea and pneumonitis), hyponatraemia, oedema, and disturbances of bone metabolism (with osteomalacia) also reported (see Cautions); suicidal ideation

### Dose

Note Different preparations may vary in bioavailability; to avoid reduced effect or excessive side-effects, it may be prudent to avoid changing the formulation (see also notes above on how side-effects may be reduced)

- By mouth, epilepsy, initially, 100–200 mg 1–2 times daily, increased slowly (see notes above) to usual dose of 0.4–1.2 g daily in divided doses; in some cases 1.6–2 g daily in divided doses, may be needed; ELDERLY reduce initial dose; CHILD daily in divided doses, up to 1 year 100–200 mg, 1–5 years 200–400 mg, 5–10 years 400–600 mg, 10–15 years 0.4–1 g

 Trigeminal neuralgia, initially 100 mg 1–2 times daily (but some patients may require higher initial dose), increased gradually according to response; usual dose 200 mg 3–4 times daily, up to 1.6 g daily in some patients

 Prophylaxis of bipolar disorder unresponsive to lithium (see also section 4.2.3), initially 400 mg daily in divided doses increased until symptoms controlled; usual range 400–600 mg daily; max. 1.6 g daily

- By rectum, epilepsy, for short-term use (max. 7 days) when oral therapy temporarily not possible; 125-mg suppository approx. equivalent to 100-mg tablet, but final adjustment should always depend on clinical response (plasma concentration monitoring recommended); max. 1 g daily in 4 divided doses

 Note Plasma concentration for optimum response 4–12 mg/litre (20–50 micromol/litre)

### Carbamazepine (Non-proprietary) PoM

Tablets, carbamazepine 100 mg, net price 28 = £5.64; 200 mg, 28 = £4.90; 400 mg, 28 = £6.59. Label: 3, 8, counselling, blood, hepatic or skin disorder symptoms (see above), driving (see above)

Brands include *Epimaz*®

Dental prescribing on NHS Carbamazepine Tablets may be prescribed

### Tegretol® (Novartis) PoM

Tablets, all scored, carbamazepine 100 mg, net price 84-tab pack = £2.43; 200 mg, 84-tab pack = £4.50; 400 mg, 56-tab pack = £5.90. Label: 3, 8, counselling, blood, hepatic or skin disorder symptoms (see above), driving (see notes above)

Chewtabs, orange, carbamazepine 100 mg, net price 56-tab pack = £3.72; 200 mg, 56-tab pack = £6.92. Label: 3, 8, 21, 24, counselling, blood, hepatic or skin disorder symptoms (see above), driving (see notes above)

Liquid, sugar-free, carbamazepine 100 mg/5 mL. Net price 300-mL pack = £7.20. Label: 3, 8, counselling, blood, hepatic or skin disorder symptoms (see above), driving (see notes above)

Suppositories, carbamazepine 125 mg, net price 5 = £9.45; 250 mg, 5 = £12.60. Label: 3, 8, counselling,

blood, hepatic or skin disorder symptoms (see above), driving (see notes above)

### ◀ Modified release

### Carbagen® SR (Generics) PoM

Tablets, m/r, f/c, both scored, carbamazepine 200 mg, net price 56-tab pack = £4.88; 400 mg, 56-tab pack = £9.63. Label: 3, 8, 25, counselling, blood, hepatic or skin disorder symptoms (see above), driving (see notes above)

Dose epilepsy (ADULT and CHILD over 5 years), as above; trigeminal neuralgia, as above; total daily dose given in 1–2 divided doses; bipolar disorder, as above

### Tegretol® Retard (Novartis) PoM

Tablets, m/r, both scored, carbamazepine 200 mg (beige-orange), net price 56-tab pack = £5.30; 400 mg (brown-orange), 56-tab pack = £10.44. Label: 3, 8, 25, counselling, blood, hepatic or skin disorder symptoms (see above), driving (see notes above)

Dose epilepsy (ADULT and CHILD over 5 years), as above; trigeminal neuralgia, as above; total daily dose given in 2 divided doses

## OXCARBAZEPINE

**Indications** monotherapy and adjunctive treatment of partial seizures with or without secondarily generalised tonic-clonic seizures; trigeminal neuralgia [unlicensed indication] (section 4.7.3)

**Cautions** hypersensitivity to carbamazepine; avoid abrupt withdrawal; hyponatraemia (monitor plasma-sodium concentration in patients at risk), heart failure (monitor body-weight), cardiac conduction disorders; avoid in acute porphyria (section 9.8.2); hepatic impairment (Appendix 2); renal impairment (Appendix 3); pregnancy (see p. 253 and Appendix 4); breast-feeding (Appendix 5); **interactions:** Appendix 1 (oxcarbazepine)

Blood, hepatic or skin disorders Patients or their carers should be told how to recognise signs of blood, liver, or skin disorders, and advised to seek immediate medical attention if symptoms such as lethargy, confusion, muscular twitching, fever, sore throat, rash, blistering, mouth ulcers, bruising, or bleeding develop

**Side-effects** nausea, vomiting, constipation, diarrhoea, abdominal pain; dizziness, headache, drowsiness, agitation, amnesia, asthenia, ataxia, confusion, impaired concentration, depression, tremor; hyponatraemia; acne, alopecia, rash, nystagmus, visual disorders including diplopia; *less commonly* urticaria, leucopenia; *very rarely* hepatitis, pancreatitis, arrhythmias, hypersensitivity reactions, blood disorders, systemic lupus erythematosus, Stevens-Johnson syndrome, and toxic epidermal necrolysis; suicidal ideation

### Dose

- Initially 300 mg twice daily increased according to response in steps of up to 600 mg daily at weekly intervals; usual dose range 0.6–2.4 g daily in divided doses; CHILD 6–18 years, 8–10 mg/kg daily in 2 divided doses increased according to response in steps of up to 10 mg/kg daily at weekly intervals (in adjunctive therapy, maintenance dose approx. 30 mg/kg daily); max. 46 mg/kg daily in divided doses

 Note In adjunctive therapy, the dose of concomitant antiepileptics may need to be reduced when using high doses of oxcarbazepine

### Oxcarbazepine (Non-proprietary) PoM

Tablets, oxcarbazepine 150 mg, net price 50-tab pack = £10.00; 300 mg, 50-tab pack = £19.96; 600 mg, 50-

4

Central nervous system

tab pack = £39.81. Label: 3, 8, counselling, blood, hepatic, or skin disorders (see above), driving (see notes above)

**Trileptal®** (Novartis) [PoM]

Tablets, f/c, scored, oxcarbazepine 150 mg (green), net price 50-tab pack = £10.00; 300 mg (yellow), 50-tab pack = £20.00; 600 mg (pink), 50-tab pack = £40.00. Label: 3, 8, counselling, blood, hepatic or skin disorders (see above), driving (see notes above)

Oral suspension, sugar-free, oxcarbazepine 300 mg/5 mL, net price 250 mL (with oral syringe) = £40.00. Label: 3, 8, counselling, blood, hepatic or skin disorders (see above), driving (see notes above)

Excipients include propylene glycol (see Excipients, p. 2)

## Ethosuximide

**Ethosuximide** is used in typical absence seizures; it may also be used in atypical absence seizures. Ethosuximide is rarely used for myoclonic or tonic seizures.

### ■ ETHOSUXIMIDE

**Indications** see notes above

**Cautions** avoid abrupt withdrawal; hepatic impairment; renal impairment; pregnancy (see p. 253 and Appendix 4); breast-feeding (Appendix 5); avoid in acute porphyria (section 9.8.2); **interactions:** Appendix 1 (ethosuximide)

Blood disorders Patients or their carers should be told how to recognise signs of blood disorders, and advised to seek immediate medical attention if symptoms such as fever, sore throat, mouth ulcers, bruising, or bleeding develop

**Side-effects** gastro-intestinal disturbances (including nausea, vomiting, diarrhoea, abdominal pain, anorexia, weight loss); *less frequently* headache, fatigue, drowsiness, dizziness, hiccup, ataxia, mild euphoria, irritability, aggression, impaired concentration; *rarely* tongue swelling, sleep disturbances, night terrors, depression, psychosis, photophobia, dyskinesia, increased libido, vaginal bleeding, myopia, gingival hypertrophy, and rash; also reported, hyperactivity, increase in seizure frequency, blood disorders such as leucopenia, agranulocytosis, pancytopenia, and aplastic anaemia (blood counts required if features of infection), systemic lupus erythematosus, and Stevens-Johnson syndrome; suicidal ideation

**Dose**

• ADULT and CHILD over 6 years, initially 500 mg daily, increased by 250 mg at intervals of 4–7 days to usual dose of 1–1.5 g daily; occasionally up to 2 g daily may be needed; CHILD up to 6 years initially 250 mg daily, increased gradually to usual dose of 20 mg/kg daily; max. 1 g daily

**Ethosuximide** (Non-proprietary) [PoM]

Capsules, ethosuximide 250 mg, net price 56-cap pack = £38.23. Label: 8, counselling, blood disorders (see above), driving (see notes above)

**Emeside®** (Chemidex) [PoM]

Syrup, black currant, ethosuximide 250 mg/5 mL, net price 200-mL pack = £6.60. Label: 8, counselling, blood disorders (see above), driving (see notes above)

**Zarontin®** (Pfizer) [PoM]

Syrup, yellow, ethosuximide 250 mg/5 mL, net price 200-mL pack = £4.31. Label: 8, counselling, blood disorders (see above), driving (see notes above)

## Gabapentin and pregabalin

**Gabapentin** and **pregabalin** are used for the treatment of partial seizures with or without secondary generalisation. They are also licensed for the treatment of neuropathic pain (p. 246). Pregabalin is licensed for the treatment of generalised anxiety disorder (p. 209).

The *Scottish Medicines Consortium* (p. 3) has advised (July 2007) that pregabalin (*Lyrica®*) is not recommended for the treatment of central neuropathic pain.

The *Scottish Medicines Consortium* (p. 3) has advised (April 2009) that pregabalin (*Lyrica®*) is accepted for restricted use within NHS Scotland for the treatment of peripheral neuropathic pain in adults who have not achieved adequate pain relief with, or have not tolerated, first- or second-line treatments; discontinue treatment if sufficient benefit is not achieved within 8 weeks of reaching the maximum tolerated dose.

### ■ GABAPENTIN

**Indications** monotherapy and adjunctive treatment of partial seizures with or without secondary generalisation; peripheral neuropathic pain (section 4.7.3)

**Cautions** avoid abrupt withdrawal (may cause anxiety, insomnia, nausea, pain, and sweating—taper off over at least 1 week); elderly; renal impairment (Appendix 3); diabetes mellitus; false positive readings with some urinary protein tests; pregnancy (see p. 253 and Appendix 4); breast-feeding (see p. 253 and Appendix 5); **interactions:** Appendix 1 (gabapentin)

**Side-effects** diarrhoea, dry mouth, dyspepsia, nausea, vomiting, constipation, abdominal pain, flatulence, appetite changes, gingivitis, weight gain; hypertension, vasodilation, oedema; dyspnoea, cough, rhinitis; confusion, depression, hostility, sleep disturbances, headache, dizziness, anxiety, amnesia, ataxia, dysarthria, nystagmus, tremor, asthenia, paraesthesia, hyperkinesia; influenza-like symptoms; impotence, urinary incontinence; leucopenia; myalgia, arthralgia; diplopia, amblyopia; rash, purpura, pruritus, acne; *rarely* pancreatitis, hepatitis, jaundice, palpitation, hallucinations, movement disorders, thrombocytopenia, blood-glucose fluctuations in patients with diabetes, tinnitus, acute renal failure, Stevens-Johnson syndrome, and alopecia; suicidal ideation

**Dose**

• Epilepsy, 300 mg once daily on day 1, then 300 mg twice daily on day 2, then 300 mg 3 times daily on day 3 *or* initially 300 mg 3 times daily on day 1; then increased according to response in steps of 300 mg daily (in 3 divided doses) every 2–3 days; usual dose 0.9–3.6 g daily in 3 divided doses; CHILD 6–12 years (adjunctive therapy only) 10–15 mg/kg once daily initially, then increased according to response over 3 days to usual maintenance dose 25–35 mg/kg daily in 3 divided doses; max. 50 mg/kg daily in 3 divided doses; CHILD 2–6 years see BNF for Children

• Neuropathic pain, ADULT over 18 years, 300 mg once daily on day 1, then 300 mg twice daily on day 2, then 300 mg 3 times daily (approx. every 8 hours) on day 3 *or* initially 300 mg 3 times daily on day 1, then increased according to response in steps of 300 mg daily (in 3 divided doses) every 2–3 days to max. 3.6 g daily

4 Central nervous system

**Gabapentin** (Non-proprietary) [PoM]

Capsules, gabapentin 100 mg, net price 100-cap pack = £5.35; 300 mg, 100-cap pack = £7.39; 400 mg, 100-cap pack = £7.74. Label: 3, 5, 8, counselling, driving (see notes above)

Tablets, gabapentin 600 mg, net price 100-tab pack = £99.26; 800 mg, 100-tab pack = £65.05. Label: 3, 5, 8, counselling, driving (see notes above)

**Neurontin®** (Pfizer) [PoM]

Capsules, gabapentin 100 mg (white), net price 100-cap pack = £18.29; 300 mg (yellow), 100-cap pack = £42.40; 400 mg (orange), 100-cap pack = £49.06. Label: 3, 5, 8, counselling, driving (see notes above)

Tablets, f/c, gabapentin 600 mg, net price 100-tab pack = £84.80; 800 mg, 100-tab pack = £98.13. Label: 3, 5, 8, counselling, driving (see notes above)

---

### ■ PREGABALIN

**Indications** peripheral and central neuropathic pain; adjunctive therapy for partial seizures with or without secondary generalisation; generalised anxiety disorder

**Cautions** avoid abrupt withdrawal (taper over at least 1 week); severe congestive heart failure; renal impairment (Appendix 3); pregnancy (Appendix 4)

**Contra-indications** breast-feeding (Appendix 5)

**Side-effects** dry mouth, constipation, nausea, vomiting, flatulence; oedema; dizziness, drowsiness, irritability, attention disturbance, disturbances in muscle control and movement, memory impairment, paraesthesia, euphoria, confusion, fatigue, appetite changes, weight gain; changes in sexual function; visual disturbances and ocular disorders (including blurred vision, diplopia, eye strain and eye irritation); *less commonly* abdominal distension, increased salivation, gastro-oesophageal reflux disease, taste disturbance, thirst, hot flushes, tachycardia, syncope, dyspnoea, chest tightness, nasal dryness, stupor, depersonalisation, depression, insomnia, abnormal dreams, hallucinations, agitation, mood swings, panic attacks, asthenia, speech disorder, dysuria, urinary incontinence, thrombocytopenia, joint swelling, muscle cramp, myalgia, arthralgia, sweating, and rash; *rarely* ascites, dysphagia, pancreatitis, hypotension, hypertension, cold extremities, first-degree AV block, arrhythmia, bradycardia, nasopharyngitis, cough, epistaxis, rhinitis, parosmia, pyrexia, rigors, disinhibition, weight loss, hypoglycaemia or hyperglycaemia, renal failure, menstrual disturbances, breast pain, breast discharge, breast hypertrophy, neutropenia, rhabdomyolysis, hyperacusis, hypokalaemia, and leucocytosis; diarrhoea, congestive heart failure, angioedema, loss of consciousness, headache, Stevens-Johnson syndrome, and pruritus also reported; suicidal ideation

**Dose**

- Neuropathic pain, ADULT over 18 years, initially 150 mg daily in 2–3 divided doses, increased if necessary after 3–7 days to 300 mg daily in 2–3 divided doses, increased further if necessary after 7 days to max. 600 mg daily in 2–3 divided doses

- Epilepsy, ADULT over 18 years, initially 25 mg twice daily, increased at 7-day intervals in steps of 50 mg daily to 300 mg daily in 2–3 divided doses, increased further if necessary after 7 days to max. 600 mg daily in 2–3 divided doses

- Generalised anxiety disorder, ADULT over 18 years, initially 150 mg daily in 2–3 divided doses, increased if necessary at 7-day intervals in steps of 150 mg daily; max. 600 mg daily in 2–3 divided doses

**Note** Pregabalin doses in BNF may differ from those in product literature

**Lyrica®** (Pfizer) ▼ [PoM]

Capsules, pregabalin 25 mg (white), net price 56-cap pack = £64.40, 84-cap pack = £96.60; 50 mg (white), 84-cap pack = £96.60; 75 mg (white/orange), 56-cap pack = £64.40; 100 mg (orange), 84-cap pack = £96.60; 150 mg (white), 56-cap pack = £64.40; 200 mg (orange), 84-cap pack = £96.60; 225 mg (white/orange), 56-cap pack = £64.40; 300 mg (white/orange), 56-cap pack = £64.40. Label: 3, 8, counselling, driving (see notes above)

---

## Lacosamide

**Lacosamide** is licensed for adjunctive treatment of partial seizures with or without secondary generalisation.

The *Scottish Medicines Consortium* (p. 3) has advised (January 2009) that lacosamide (*Vimpat®*) is accepted for restricted use within NHS Scotland as adjunctive treatment for partial seizures with or without secondary generalisation in patients from 16 years. It is restricted for specialist use in refractory epilepsy.

### ■ LACOSAMIDE

**Indications** see notes above

**Cautions** conduction problems or severe cardiac disease (increased risk of PR-interval prolongation), elderly; hepatic impairment (Appendix 2); renal impairment (Appendix 3); pregnancy (see p. 253 and Appendix 4); breast-feeding (see p. 253 and Appendix 5); **interactions:** Appendix 1 (lacosamide)

**Contra-indications** second- or third-degree AV block

**Side-effects** nausea, vomiting, flatulence, constipation; dizziness, headache, depression, diplopia, nystagmus, impaired coordination, impaired memory, cognitive disorder, drowsiness, tremor, asthenia, fatigue; pruritus; *less commonly* PR-interval prolongation; suicidal ideation

**Dose**

- By intravenous infusion over 15–60 minutes (for up to 5 days) or by mouth, ADULT and CHILD over 16 years, initially 50 mg twice daily, increased weekly by 50 mg twice daily to max. 200 mg twice daily

**Vimpat®** (UCB Pharma) ▼ [PoM]

Tablets, f/c, lacosamide 50 mg (pink), net price 14-tab pack = £9.01; 100 mg (yellow), 14-tab pack = £18.02, 56-tab pack = £72.08; 150 mg (pink), 14-tab pack = £27.03, 56-tab pack £108.12; 200 mg (blue), 56-tab pack = £144.16. Label: 8, counselling, driving (see notes above)

Syrup, lacosamide 15 mg/mL, net price 200 mL = £38.61. Label: 8, counselling, driving (see notes above)
Electrolytes Na⁺ 0.4 mmol/5 mL
Excipients include aspartame (section 9.4.1)

Intravenous infusion, lacosamide 10 mg/mL, net price 200-mg vial = £29.70
Electrolytes Na⁺ 2.6 mmol/vial

## Lamotrigine

**Lamotrigine** is an antiepileptic for partial seizures and primary and secondarily generalised tonic-clonic seizures. Lamotrigine may cause serious skin rash especially in children; dose recommendations should be adhered to closely.

Lamotrigine is used either as sole treatment or as an adjunct to treatment with other antiepileptic drugs. Valproate increases plasma-lamotrigine concentration whereas the enzyme inducing antiepileptics reduce it; care is therefore required in choosing the appropriate initial dose and subsequent titration. Where the potential for interaction is not known, treatment should be initiated with lower doses such as those used with valproate.

### ▌ LAMOTRIGINE

**Indications** monotherapy and adjunctive treatment of partial seizures and primary and secondarily generalised tonic-clonic seizures; seizures associated with Lennox-Gastaut syndrome; trigeminal neuralgia [unlicensed indication] (section 4.7.3)

**Cautions** closely monitor and consider withdrawal if rash, fever, or other signs of hypersensitivity syndrome develop; avoid abrupt withdrawal (taper off over 2 weeks or longer) unless serious skin reaction occurs; hepatic impairment (Appendix 2); renal impairment (Appendix 3 and Appendix 4); breast-feeding (Appendix 5); **interactions:** see p. 253 and Appendix 1 (lamotrigine)
**Blood disorders** The CSM has advised prescribers to be alert for symptoms and signs suggestive of bone-marrow failure such as anaemia, bruising, or infection. Aplastic anaemia, bone-marrow depression and pancytopenia have been associated rarely with lamotrigine.

**Side-effects** rash (see Skin Reactions, below); hypersensitivity syndrome (possibly including rash, fever, lymphadenopathy, hepatic dysfunction, blood disorders, disseminated intravascular coagulation and multi-organ dysfunction); nausea, vomiting, diarrhoea, hepatic dysfunction; headache, fatigue, dizziness, sleep disturbances, tremor, movement disorders, agitation, confusion, hallucinations, occasional increase in seizure frequency; blood disorders (including leucopenia, thrombocytopenia, pancytopenia—see Blood Disorders, above); arthralgia; lupus erythematosus-like effect; photosensitivity; nystagmus, diplopia, blurred vision, conjunctivitis; suicidal ideation
**Skin reactions** Serious skin reactions including Stevens-Johnson syndrome and toxic epidermal necrolysis (rarely with fatalities) have developed especially in children; most rashes occur in the first 8 weeks. Rash is sometimes associated with hypersensitivity syndrome (see Side-effects, above) and is more common in patients with history of allergy or rash from other antiepileptic drugs. Consider withdrawal if rash or signs of hypersensitivity syndrome develop. The CSM has advised that factors associated with increased risk of serious skin reactions include concomitant use of valproate, initial lamotrigine dosing higher than recommended, and more rapid dose escalation than recommended.
**Counselling** Warn patients to see their doctor immediately if rash or signs or symptoms of hypersensitivity syndrome develop

### Dose

**Important** Do not confuse the different combinations; see also notes above
**Note** Dose titration should be repeated if restarting after an interval of more than 5 days

- Monotherapy, ADULT and CHILD over 12 years, initially 25 mg once daily for 14 days, increased to 50 mg once daily for further 14 days, then increased by max. 50–100 mg daily every 7–14 days; usual maintenance 100–200 mg daily in 1–2 divided doses (up to 500 mg daily has been required)
- Adjunctive therapy *with valproate*, initially 25 mg on alternate days for 14 days then 25 mg once daily for further 14 days, thereafter increased by max. 25–50 mg daily every 7–14 days; usual maintenance, 100–200 mg daily in 1–2 divided doses; CHILD 2–12 years initially 150 micrograms/kg once daily for 14 days (those weighing under 13 kg may receive 2 mg on alternate days for first 14 days) then 300 micrograms/kg once daily for further 14 days, thereafter increased by max. 300 micrograms/kg daily every 7–14 days; usual maintenance 1–5 mg/kg daily in 1–2 divided doses (max. single dose 100 mg)
- Adjunctive therapy (with enzyme inducing drugs) *without valproate*, initially 50 mg once daily for 14 days then 50 mg twice daily for further 14 days, thereafter increased by max. 100 mg daily every 7–14 days; usual maintenance 200–400 mg daily in 1–2 divided doses (up to 700 mg daily has been required); CHILD 2–12 years initially 600 micrograms/kg daily in 2 divided doses for 14 days then 1.2 mg/kg daily in 2 divided doses for further 14 days, thereafter increased by max. 1.2 mg/kg daily every 7–14 days; usual maintenance 5–15 mg/kg daily in 2 divided doses (max. single dose 200 mg)
- Adjunctive therapy *with oxcarbazepine*, initially 25 mg once daily for 14 days, increased to 50 mg once daily for further 14 days, then increased by max. 50–100 mg daily every 7–14 days; usual maintenance 100–200 mg daily in 1–2 divided doses; CHILD 2–12 years initially 300 micrograms/kg daily in 2 divided doses for 14 days then 600 micrograms/kg daily in 1–2 divided doses for further 14 days, thereafter increased by max. 600 micrograms/kg daily every 7–14 days; usual maintenance 1–10 mg/kg daily in 1–2 divided doses; max. 200 mg daily

**Lamotrigine** (Non-proprietary) ⓟⓞⓜ
Tablets, lamotrigine 25 mg, net price 56-tab pack = £3.06; 50 mg, 56-tab pack = £3.82; 100 mg, 56-tab pack = £5.26; 200 mg, 30-tab pack = £27.53, 56-tab pack = £9.43. Label: 8, counselling, driving (see notes above), skin reactions (see above)

Dispersible tablets, lamotrigine 5 mg, net price 28-tab pack = £2.83; 25 mg, 56-tab pack = £3.80; 100 mg, 56-tab pack = £6.96. Label: 8, 13, counselling, driving (see notes above), skin reactions (see above)

**Lamictal®** (GSK) ⓟⓞⓜ
Tablets, yellow, lamotrigine 25 mg, net price 21-tab pack ('*Valproate Add-on therapy' Starter Pack*) = £7.35, 42-tab pack ('*Monotherapy' Starter Pack*) = £14.70, 56-tab pack = £19.61; 50 mg, 42-tab pack ('*Non-valproate Add-on therapy' Starter Pack*) = £25.01, 56-tab pack = £33.35; 100 mg, 56-tab pack = £57.53; 200 mg, 56-tab pack = £97.79. Label: 8, counselling, driving (see notes above), skin reactions (above)

Dispersible tablets, chewable, lamotrigine 2 mg, net price 30-tab pack = £10.45; 5 mg, 28-tab pack = £7.82; 25 mg, 56-tab pack = £19.61; 100 mg, 56-tab pack = £57.53. Label: 8, 13, counselling, , driving (see notes above), skin reactions (above)

## Levetiracetam

**Levetiracetam** is licensed for monotherapy and adjunctive treatment of partial seizures with or without secondary generalisation, and for adjunctive therapy of myoclonic seizures and primarily generalised tonic-clonic seizures.

### ■ LEVETIRACETAM

**Indications** see notes above

**Cautions** avoid abrupt withdrawal; hepatic impairment (Appendix 2); renal impairment (Appendix 3); pregnancy (see p. 253 and Appendix 4); breast-feeding (Appendix 5); **interactions:** Appendix 1 (levetiracetam)

**Side-effects** nausea, vomiting, dyspepsia, diarrhoea, abdominal pain, anorexia, weight changes; cough; drowsiness, asthenia, amnesia, ataxia, seizures, dizziness, headache, tremor, hyperkinesia, depression, emotional lability, insomnia, anxiety, impaired attention, aggression, irritability; thrombocytopenia; myalgia; visual disturbances; pruritus, rash; *also reported* pancreatitis, hepatic dysfunction, confusion, psychosis, hallucinations, suicidal ideation, paraesthesia, leucopenia, pancytopenia, and alopecia

**Dose**

- Monotherapy of partial seizures with or without secondary generalisation, by mouth *or* by intravenous infusion, ADULT and CHILD over 16 years, initially 250 mg once daily increased according to response in steps of 250 mg twice daily every 2 weeks; max. 1.5 g twice daily

- Adjunctive therapy of partial seizures with or without secondary generalisation, by mouth *or* by intravenous infusion, ADULT and CHILD over 12 years, body-weight over 50 kg, initially 250 mg twice daily, adjusted in steps of 500 mg twice daily every 2–4 weeks; max. 1.5 g twice daily; CHILD 4–18 years body-weight under 50 kg, initially 10 mg/kg once daily, adjusted in steps not exceeding 10 mg/kg twice daily every 2 weeks; max. 30 mg/kg twice daily

- Adjunctive therapy of myoclonic seizures and tonic-clonic seizures, by mouth *or* by intravenous infusion, ADULT and CHILD over 12 years, body-weight over 50 kg, initially 250 mg twice daily, adjusted in steps of 500 mg twice daily every 2–4 weeks; max. 1.5 g twice daily; CHILD 12–18 years, body-weight under 50 kg, initially 10 mg/kg once daily, adjusted in steps not exceeding 10 mg/kg twice daily every 2 weeks; max. 30 mg/kg twice daily

**Keppra®** (UCB Pharma) PoM

Tablets, f/c, levetiracetam 250 mg (blue), net price 60-tab pack = £29.70; 500 mg (yellow), 60-tab pack = £52.30; 750 mg (orange) 60-tab pack = £89.10; 1 g (white), 60-tab pack = £101.10. Label: 8

Oral solution, sugar-free, levetiracetam 100 mg/mL, net price 300 mL = £71.00. Label: 8

Concentrate for intravenous infusion, levetiracetam 100 mg/mL. For dilution before use. Net price 5-mL vial = £13.50
Electrolytes Na⁺<0.5 mmol/vial

## Phenobarbital and other barbiturates

**Phenobarbital** (phenobarbitone) is effective for tonic-clonic and partial seizures but may be sedative in adults and cause behavioural disturbances and hyperkinesia in children. It may be tried for atypical absence, atonic, and tonic seizures. Rebound seizures may be a problem on withdrawal. Monitoring plasma concentrations is less useful than with other drugs because tolerance occurs.

**Primidone** is largely converted to phenobarbital and this is probably responsible for its antiepileptic action. A small starting dose of primidone (125 mg) is essential, and the drug should be introduced over several weeks.

### ■ PHENOBARBITAL
(Phenobarbitone)

**Indications** all forms of epilepsy except absence seizures; status epilepticus (section 4.8.2)

**Cautions** see notes above; elderly; debilitated; children; respiratory depression (avoid if severe); avoid abrupt withdrawal (dependence with prolonged use); history of drug or alcohol abuse; consider vitamin D supplementation in patients that are immobilized for long periods or who have inadequate sun exposure or dietary intake of calcium; avoid in acute porphyria (section 9.8.2); hepatic impairment (avoid if severe—Appendix 2); renal impairment; pregnancy (see p. 253 and Appendix 4); breast-feeding (see p. 253 and Appendix 5); **interactions:** see p. 253 and Appendix 1 (barbiturates)

**Side-effects** hepatitis, cholestasis; hypotension; respiratory depression; behavioural disturbances, nystagmus, irritability, drowsiness, lethargy, depression, ataxia, paradoxical excitement, hallucinations, impaired memory and cognition, hyperactivity particularly in the elderly and in children; osteomalacia (see Cautions); megaloblastic anaemia (may be treated with folic acid), agranulocytosis, thrombocytopenia; allergic skin reactions; *very rarely* Stevens-Johnson syndrome and toxic epidermal necrolysis; suicidal ideation; **overdosage:** see Emergency Treatment of Poisoning, p. 28

**Dose**

- By mouth, 60–180 mg at night; CHILD 5–8 mg/kg daily
  Note For therapeutic purposes phenobarbital and phenobarbital sodium may be considered equivalent in effect. Plasma-phenobarbital concentration for optimum response 15–40 mg/litre (60–180 micromol/litre)

**Phenobarbital** (Non-proprietary) CD

Tablets, phenobarbital 15 mg, net price 28-tab pack = 86p; 30 mg, 28-tab pack = 59p; 60 mg, 28-tab pack = 69p. Label: 2, 8, counselling, driving (see notes above)

Elixir, phenobarbital 15 mg/5 mL in a suitable flavoured vehicle, containing alcohol 38%, net price 100 mL = 77p. Label: 2, 8, counselling, driving (see notes above)
Note Some hospitals supply **alcohol-free** formulations of varying phenobarbital strengths

**◢Injection**
Section 4.8.2

**Central nervous system**

## ■ PRIMIDONE

**Indications** all forms of epilepsy except absence seizures; essential tremor (also section 4.9.3)

**Cautions** see under Phenobarbital; **interactions:** see p. 253 and Appendix 1 (primidone)

**Side-effects** see under Phenobarbital; also nausea and visual disturbances; *less commonly* vomiting, headache, and dizziness; *rarely* arthralgia

**Dose**

- Epilepsy, ADULT and CHILD over 9 years, initially 125 mg daily at bedtime, increased by 125 mg every 3 days to 500 mg daily in 2 divided doses, then increased according to response by 250 mg every 3 days to usual maintenance 0.75–1.5 g daily in 2 divided doses; CHILD under 9 years, initially 125 mg daily at bedtime, increased by 125 mg every 3 days according to response; usual maintenance, CHILD under 2 years, 250–500 mg daily in 2 divided doses; 2–5 years, 500–750 mg daily in 2 divided doses; 5–9 years 0.75–1 g daily in 2 divided doses

- Essential tremor, initially 62.5 mg daily increased gradually over 2–3 weeks according to response; max. 750 mg daily

**Note** Monitor plasma concentrations of derived phenobarbital; optimum range as for phenobarbital. Primidone doses in BNF may differ from those in product literature

**Mysoline®** (Acorus) ℗ₒ𝕄
Tablets, scored, primidone 250 mg, net price 100-tab pack = £12.60. Label: 2, 8, counselling, driving (see notes above)

## Phenytoin

Phenytoin is effective for tonic-clonic and partial seizures. It has a narrow therapeutic index and the relationship between dose and plasma concentration is non-linear; small dosage increases in some patients may produce large rises in plasma concentrations with acute toxic side-effects. Monitoring of plasma concentration greatly assists dosage adjustment. A few missed doses or a small change in drug absorption may result in a marked change in plasma concentration.

Phenytoin may cause coarse facies, acne, hirsutism, and gingival hyperplasia and so may be particularly undesirable in adolescent patients.

When only parenteral administration is possible, **fosphenytoin** (section 4.8.2), a pro-drug of phenytoin, may be convenient to give. Whereas phenytoin can be given intravenously only, fosphenytoin may also be given by intramuscular injection.

## ■ PHENYTOIN

**Indications** all forms of epilepsy except absence seizures; status epilepticus (section 4.8.2); trigeminal neuralgia if carbamazepine inappropriate (see also section 4.7.3)

**Cautions** avoid abrupt withdrawal; manufacturer recommends blood counts (but evidence of practical value unsatisfactory); consider vitamin D supplementation in patients that are immobilized for long periods or who have inadequate sun exposure or dietary intake of calcium; avoid in acute porphyria (section 9.8.2); hepatic impairment (Appendix 2); pregnancy (**important:** see notes above and Appendix 4); breast-feeding (see notes above and Appendix 5); **interactions:** see p. 253 and Appendix 1 (phenytoin)

**Blood or skin disorders** Patients or their carers should be told how to recognise signs of blood or skin disorders, and advised to seek immediate medical attention if symptoms such as fever, sore throat, rash, mouth ulcers, bruising, or bleeding develop. Leucopenia which is severe, progressive, or associated with clinical symptoms requires withdrawal (if necessary under cover of suitable alternative)

**Side-effects** nausea, vomiting, constipation, insomnia, transient nervousness, tremor, paraesthesia, dizziness, headache, anorexia; gingival hypertrophy and tenderness (maintain good oral hygiene); rash (discontinue; if mild re-introduce cautiously but discontinue immediately if recurrence); acne, hirsutism, coarse facies; *rarely* hepatotoxicity, peripheral neuropathy, dyskinesia, lymphadenopathy, osteomalacia (see Cautions); blood disorders (including megaloblastic anaemia (may be treated with folic acid), leucopenia, thrombocytopenia, and aplastic anaemia), polyarteritis nodosa, lupus erythematosus, Stevens-Johnson syndrome, and toxic epidermal necrolysis; also reported pneumonitis and interstitial nephritis; suicidal ideation; *with excessive dosage* nystagmus, diplopia, slurred speech, ataxia, confusion, and hyperglycaemia

**Dose**

- By mouth, initially 3–4 mg/kg daily *or* 150–300 mg daily (as a single dose *or* in 2 divided doses) increased gradually as necessary (with plasma-phenytoin concentration monitoring); usual dose 200–500 mg daily (exceptionally, higher doses may be used); CHILD initially 5 mg/kg daily in 2 divided doses, usual dose range 4–8 mg/kg daily (max. 300 mg daily)

**Note** Plasma concentration for optimum response 10–20 mg/litre (40–80 micromol/litre)

**Counselling** Take preferably with or after food

**Phenytoin** (Non-proprietary) ℗ₒ𝕄
Tablets, coated, phenytoin sodium 100 mg, net price 28-tab pack = £30.00. Label: 8, counselling, administration, blood or skin disorder symptoms (see above), driving (see notes above)

**Note** On the basis of single dose tests there are no clinically relevant differences in bioavailability between available phenytoin sodium tablets and capsules but there may be a pharmacokinetic basis for maintaining the same brand of phenytoin in some patients

**Epanutin®** (Pfizer) ℗ₒ𝕄
Capsules, phenytoin sodium 25 mg (white/purple), net price 28-cap pack = 66p; 50 mg (white/pink), 28-cap pack = 67p; 100 mg (white/orange), 84-cap pack = £2.83; 300 mg (white/green), 28-cap pack = £2.83. Label: 8, counselling, administration, blood or skin disorder symptoms (see above), driving (see notes above)

Infatabs® (= chewable tablets), yellow, scored, phenytoin 50 mg, net price 112 = £7.38. Label: 8, 24, counselling, blood or skin disorder symptoms (see above), driving (see notes above)

**Note** Contain phenytoin 50 mg (as against phenytoin sodium) therefore care is needed on changing to capsules or tablets containing phenytoin sodium

Suspension, red, phenytoin 30 mg/5 mL, net price 500 mL = £4.27. Label: 8, counselling, administration, blood or skin disorder symptoms (see above), driving (see notes above)

Note Suspension of phenytoin 90 mg in 15 mL may be considered to be approximately equivalent in therapeutic effect to capsules or tablets containing phenytoin sodium 100 mg, but nevertheless care is needed in making changes

## Rufinamide

**Rufinamide** is licensed for the adjunctive treatment of seizures in Lennox-Gastaut syndrome.

The *Scottish Medicines Consortium* (p. 3) has advised (October 2008) that rufinamide (*Inovelon*®) is accepted for restricted use within NHS Scotland as adjunctive therapy in the treatment of seizures associated with Lennox-Gastaut syndrome in patients 4 years and above. It is restricted for use when alternative traditional antiepileptic drugs are unsatisfactory.

### ▌ RUFINAMIDE

**Indications** adjunctive treatment of seizures in Lennox-Gastaut syndrome

**Cautions** closely monitor and consider withdrawal if rash, fever, or other signs of hypersensitivity syndrome develop; avoid abrupt withdrawal; hepatic impairment (avoid if severe; Appendix 2); pregnancy (see p. 253 and Appendix 4); **interactions**: see p. 253 and Appendix 1 (rufinamide)

**Contra-indications** breast-feeding (Appendix 5)

**Side-effects** nausea, vomiting, constipation, diarrhoea, dyspepsia, abdominal pain, weight loss, anorexia; rhinitis, epistaxis; dizziness, headache, drowsiness, insomnia, anxiety, fatigue, increase in seizure frequency, impaired coordination, hyperactivity, tremor, gait disturbances; influenza-like symptoms; oligomenorrhoea; back pain; nystagmus, diplopia, blurred vision; rash and acne; hypersensitivity syndrome (possibly including rash, fever, lymphadenopathy, hepatic dysfunction, haematuria, and multiorgan dysfunction) also reported

**Hypersensitivity syndrome** Serious hypersensitivity syndrome (see Side-effects) has developed, especially in children and upon initiation of therapy; consider withdrawal if rash or signs or symptoms of hypersensitivity syndrome develop

**Counselling** Warn patients to seek immediate medical attention if signs or symptoms of hypersensitivity develop

**Dose**

● ADULT and CHILD over 4 years body-weight over 30 kg, initially 200 mg twice daily increased according to response in steps of 200 mg twice daily at intervals of not less than 2 days; body-weight 30–50 kg max. 900 mg twice daily; body-weight 50–70 kg max. 1.2 g twice daily; body-weight over 70 kg max. 1.6 g twice daily; CHILD over 4 years body-weight less than 30 kg, initially 100 mg twice daily increased according to response in steps of 100 mg twice daily at intervals of not less than 2 days; max. 500 mg twice daily (max. 300 mg twice daily if adjunctive therapy *with valproate*)

**Inovelon**® (Eisai) ▼ [PoM]
Tablets, pink, f/c, scored, rufinamide 100 mg, net price 10-tab pack = £8.58; 200 mg, 60-tab pack =

£51.48; 400 mg, 60-tab pack = £85.80. Label: 21, counselling, driving (see notes above), hypersensitivity syndrome (see above)

## Tiagabine

**Tiagabine** is used as adjunctive treatment for partial seizures, with or without secondary generalisation.

### ▌ TIAGABINE

**Indications** adjunctive treatment for partial seizures with or without secondary generalisation not satisfactorily controlled with other antiepileptics

**Cautions** avoid in acute porphyria (section 9.8.2); hepatic impairment (Appendix 2); avoid abrupt withdrawal; **interactions**: Appendix 1 (tiagabine)

**Driving** May impair performance of skilled tasks (e.g. driving)

**Side-effects** diarrhoea; dizziness, tiredness, nervousness, tremor, impaired concentration, emotional lability, speech impairment; *rarely* confusion, depression, drowsiness, psychosis, non-convulsive status epilepticus, bruising, and visual disturbances; suicidal ideation; leucopenia also reported

**Dose**

● Adjunctive therapy, ADULT and CHILD over 12 years, with *enzyme-inducing* drugs, 5 mg twice daily for 1 week, then increased at weekly intervals in steps of 5–10 mg daily; usual maintenance dose 30–45 mg daily (doses above 30 mg given in 3 divided doses); in patients receiving *non-enzyme-inducing* drugs, initial maintenance dose 15–30 mg daily

**Gabitril**® (Cephalon) [PoM]
Tablets, f/c, tiagabine (as hydrochloride) 5 mg, net price 100-tab pack = £41.68; 10 mg, 100-tab pack = £83.36; 15 mg, 100-tab pack = £125.04. Label: 21

## Topiramate

**Topiramate** can be given alone or as adjunctive treatment in generalised tonic-clonic seizures or partial seizures with or without secondary generalisation. It can be used as adjunctive treatment for seizures associated with Lennox-Gastaut syndrome. Topiramate is also licensed for prophylaxis of migraine (section 4.7.4.2).

### ▌ TOPIRAMATE

**Indications** monotherapy and adjunctive treatment of generalised tonic-clonic seizures or partial seizures with or without secondary generalisation; adjunctive treatment of seizures in Lennox-Gastaut syndrome; migraine prophylaxis (under specialist supervision)

**Cautions** avoid abrupt withdrawal; ensure adequate hydration (especially if predisposition to nephrolithiasis or in strenuous activity or warm environment); avoid in acute porphyria (section 9.8.2); hepatic impairment (Appendix 2); renal impairment (Appendix 3); pregnancy (see notes above and

**4**

**Central nervous system**

Appendix 4); **interactions:** see p. 253 and Appendix 1 (topiramate)

**CSM advice** Topiramate has been associated with acute myopia with secondary angle-closure glaucoma, typically occurring within 1 month of starting treatment. Choroidal effusions resulting in anterior displacement of the lens and iris have also been reported. The CSM advises that if raised intra-ocular pressure occurs:

- seek specialist ophthalmological advice;
- use appropriate measures to reduce intra-ocular pressure;
- stop topiramate as rapidly as feasible

**Contra-indications** breast-feeding (Appendix 5)

**Side-effects** nausea, abdominal pain, dyspepsia, diarrhoea, dry mouth, taste disturbance, weight loss, anorexia; paraesthesia, hypoaesthesia, headache, fatigue, dizziness, speech disorder, drowsiness, insomnia, impaired memory and concentration, anxiety, depression; visual disturbances; *less commonly* suicidal ideation; *rarely* reduced sweating mainly in children, metabolic acidosis, and alopecia; *very rarely* leucopenia, thrombocytopenia, and serious skin reactions

**Dose**

- Monotherapy, initially 25 mg at night for 1 week *then* increased in steps of 25–50 mg daily at intervals of 1–2 weeks taken in 2 divided doses; usual dose 100 mg daily in 2 divided doses; max. 400 mg daily; CHILD 6–16 years, initially 0.5–1 mg/kg at night for 1 week *then* increased in steps of 0.5–1 mg/kg daily at intervals of 1–2 weeks taken in 2 divided doses; usual dose 3–6 mg/kg daily in 2 divided doses; max. 15 mg/kg daily

- Adjunctive therapy, initially 25 mg at night for 1 week *then* increased in steps of 25–50 mg daily at intervals of 1–2 weeks taken in 2 divided doses; usual dose 200–400 mg daily in 2 divided doses; max. 800 mg daily; CHILD 2–16 years, initially 25 mg at night for 1 week *then* increased in steps of 1–3 mg/kg daily at intervals of 1–2 weeks taken in 2 divided doses; recommended dose range 5–9 mg/kg daily in 2 divided doses; max. 15 mg/kg daily

- Migraine prophylaxis ADULT and CHILD over 16 years, initially 25 mg at night for 1 week *then* increased in steps of 25 mg daily at intervals of 1 week; usual dose 50–100 mg daily in 2 divided doses

**Note** If patient cannot tolerate titration regimens recommended above then smaller steps or longer interval between steps may be used

**Topamax®** (Janssen-Cilag) ▼ PoM

Tablets, f/c, topiramate 25 mg, net price 60-tab pack = £19.68; 50 mg (light yellow), 60-tab pack = £32.33; 100 mg (yellow), 60-tab pack = £57.91; 200 mg (salmon), 60-tab pack = £112.46. Label: 3, 8, counselling, driving (see notes above)

Sprinkle capsules, topiramate 15 mg, net price 60-cap pack = £15.09; 25 mg, 60-cap pack = £22.63; 50 mg, 60-cap pack = £37.18. Label: 3, 8, counselling, administration, driving (see notes above)

**Counselling** Swallow whole or open capsule and sprinkle contents on soft food

## Valproate

**Sodium valproate** is effective in controlling tonic-clonic seizures, particularly in primary generalised epilepsy. It is a drug of choice in primary generalised epilepsy, generalised absences and myoclonic seizures, and can be tried in atypical absence, atonic, and tonic seizures.

Plasma-valproate concentrations are not a useful index of efficacy, therefore routine monitoring is unhelpful. The drug has widespread metabolic effects, and may have dose-related side-effects.

**Valproic acid** (as semisodium valproate) (section 4.2.3) is licensed for acute mania associated with bipolar disorder.

## ■ SODIUM VALPROATE

**Indications** all forms of epilepsy

**Cautions** monitor liver function before therapy and during first 6 months especially in patients most at risk (see also below); measure full blood count and ensure no undue potential for bleeding before starting and before surgery; systemic lupus erythematosus; false-positive urine tests for ketones; avoid abrupt withdrawal; consider vitamin D supplementation in patients that are immobilized for long periods or who have inadequate sun exposure or dietary intake of calcium; renal impairment (Appendix 3); pregnancy (**important** see notes above and Appendix 4); breast-feeding (Appendix 5); **interactions:** see p. 253 and Appendix 1 (valproate)

**Liver toxicity** Liver dysfunction (including fatal hepatic failure) has occurred in association with valproate (especially in children under 3 years and in those with metabolic or degenerative disorders, organic brain disease or severe seizure disorders associated with mental retardation) usually in first 6 months and usually involving multiple antiepileptic therapy. Raised liver enzymes during valproate treatment are usually transient but patients should be reassessed clinically and liver function (including prothrombin time) monitored until return to normal—discontinue if abnormally prolonged prothrombin time (particularly in association with other relevant abnormalities).

**Blood or hepatic disorders** Patients or their carers should be told how to recognise signs and symptoms of blood or liver disorders and advised to seek immediate medical attention if symptoms develop

**Pancreatitis** Patients or their carers should be told how to recognise signs and symptoms of pancreatitis and advised to seek immediate medical attention if symptoms such as abdominal pain, nausea and vomiting develop; discontinue if pancreatitis is diagnosed

**Contra-indications** active liver disease, family history of severe hepatic dysfunction; acute porphyria (section 9.8.2)

**Side-effects** nausea, gastric irritation, diarrhoea; weight gain; hyperammonaemia, thrombocytopenia; transient hair loss (regrowth may be curly); *less frequently* increased alertness, aggression, hyperactivity, behavioural disturbances, ataxia, tremor, and vasculitis; *rarely* hepatic dysfunction (see under Cautions; withdraw treatment immediately if persistent vomiting and abdominal pain, anorexia, jaundice, oedema, malaise, drowsiness, or loss of seizure control), lethargy, drowsiness, confusion, stupor, hallucinations, menstrual disturbances, anaemia, leucopenia, pancytopenia, hearing loss, and rash; *very rarely* pancreatitis (see under Cautions), peripheral oedema, increase in bleeding time, extrapyramidal symptoms, dementia, encephalopathy, coma, gynaecomastia, Fanconi's syndrome, hirsutism, acne, enuresis, hyponatraemia, toxic epidermal necrolysis, and Stevens-Johnson syndrome; suicidal ideation; reduced bone mineral density (see Cautions)

**Dose**

- By mouth, initially 600 mg daily in 2 divided doses, preferably after food, increased by 200 mg daily every 3 days to max. 2.5 g daily, usual maintenance dose 1–2 g daily (20–30 mg/kg daily); CHILD body-weight up to 20 kg, initially 20 mg/kg daily in divided doses, may be increased provided plasma concentration monitored (dose above 40 mg/kg daily also monitor clinical chemistry and haematological parameters); CHILD under 12 years body-weight over 20 kg, initially 400 mg daily in divided doses increased according to response (usual range 20–30 mg/kg daily); max. 35 mg/kg daily

- By intravenous injection (over 3–5 minutes) *or* by intravenous infusion, continuation of valproate treatment, same as current dose by oral route

Initiation of valproate therapy, by intravenous injection (over 3–5 minutes), 400–800 mg (up to 10 mg/kg) followed by intravenous infusion up to max. 2.5 g daily; CHILD under 12 years, usually 20–30 mg/kg daily, may be increased provided plasma concentration monitored (dose above 40 mg/kg daily also monitor clinical chemistry and haematological parameters)

◢**Oral**

**Sodium Valproate** (Non-proprietary) [PoM]
Tablets (crushable), scored, sodium valproate 100 mg, net price 100-tab pack = £5.60. Label: 8, counselling, pancreatitis, blood or hepatic disorder symptoms (see above), driving (see notes above)

Tablets, e/c, sodium valproate 200 mg, net price 100-tab pack = £5.78; 500 mg, 100-tab pack = £11.56. Label: 5, 8, 25, counselling, pancreatitis, blood or hepatic disorder symptoms (see above), driving (see notes above)
Brands include *Orlept*®

Oral solution, sodium valproate 200 mg/5 mL, net price 300-mL pack = £6.57. Label: 8, counselling, pancreatitis, blood or hepatic disorder symptoms (see above), driving (see notes above)
Brands include *Orlept*® sugar-free

**Epilim**® (Sanofi-Synthelabo) [PoM]
Tablets (crushable), scored, sodium valproate 100 mg, net price 100 = £5.60. Label: 8, counselling, pancreatitis, blood or hepatic disorder symptoms (see above), driving (see notes above)

Tablets, both e/c, lilac, sodium valproate 200 mg, net price 100 = £7.70; 500 mg, 100 = £19.25. Label: 5, 8, 25, counselling, pancreatitis, blood or hepatic disorder symptoms (see above), driving (see notes above)

Liquid, red, sugar-free, sodium valproate 200 mg/5 mL, net price 300-mL pack = £9.33. Label: 8, counselling, pancreatitis, blood or hepatic disorder symptoms (see above), driving (see notes above)

Syrup, red, sodium valproate 200 mg/5 mL, net price 300-mL pack = £7.78. Label: 8, counselling, pancreatitis, blood or hepatic disorder symptoms (see above), driving (see notes above)

◢**Modified release**

**Epilim Chrono**® (Sanofi-Synthelabo) [PoM]
Tablets, m/r, lilac, sodium valproate 200 mg (as sodium valproate and valproic acid), net price 100-tab pack = £11.65; 300 mg, 100-tab pack = £17.47; 500 mg, 100-tab pack = £29.10. Label: 8, 25, counselling, pancreatitis, blood or hepatic disorder symptoms (see above), driving (see notes above)
Dose ADULT and CHILD over 20 kg, as above, total daily dose given in 1–2 divided doses

**Epilim Chronosphere**® (Sanofi-Aventis) [PoM]
Granules, m/r, sodium valproate 50 mg (as sodium valproate and valproic acid), net price 30-sachet pack = £30.00; 100 mg, 30-sachet pack = £30.00; 250 mg, 30-sachet pack = £30.00; 500 mg, 30-sachet pack = £30.00; 750 mg, 30-sachet pack = £30.00; 1000 mg, 30-sachet pack = £30.00. Label: 8, 25, counselling, administration, pancreatitis, blood or hepatic disorder symptoms (see above), driving (see notes above)
Dose ADULT and CHILD, as above, total daily dose given in 1–2 divided doses
Counselling Granules may be mixed with cold food or drink and swallowed immediately without chewing

**Episenta**® (Beacon) [PoM]
Capsules, enclosing m/r granules, sodium valproate 150 mg, net price 100-cap pack = £5.70; 300 mg, 100-cap pack = £10.90. Label: 8, 25, counselling, administration, pancreatitis, blood or hepatic disorder symptoms (see above), driving (see notes above)
Dose ADULT and CHILD, as above, total daily dose given in 1–2 divided doses
Counselling Contents of capsule may be mixed with cold food or drink and swallowed immediately without chewing

Granules, m/r, sodium valproate 500 mg, net price 100-sachet pack = £18.00; 1 g, 100-sachet pack = £35.50. Label: 8, 25, counselling, administration, pancreatitis, blood or hepatic disorder symptoms (see above), driving (see notes above)
Dose ADULT and CHILD, as above, total daily dose given in 1–2 divided doses
Counselling Granules may be mixed with cold food or drink and swallowed immediately without chewing

◢**Parenteral**

**Epilim**® **Intravenous** (Sanofi-Synthelabo) [PoM]
Injection, powder for reconstitution, sodium valproate, net price 400-mg vial (with 4-mL amp water for injections) = £11.58

**Episenta**® (Beacon) [PoM]
Injection, sodium valproate 100 mg/mL, net price 3-mL amp = £7.00, 10-mL amp = £23.33

◢**Valproic acid**

**Convulex**® (Pharmacia) [PoM]
Capsules, e/c, valproic acid 150 mg, net price 100-cap pack = £3.68; 300 mg, 100-cap pack = £7.35; 500 mg, 100-cap pack = £12.25. Label: 8, 25, counselling, pancreatitis, blood or hepatic disorder symptoms (see above), driving (see notes above)
Dose epilepsy, ADULT and CHILD as for sodium valproate, total daily dose given in 2–4 divided doses
Equivalence to sodium valproate Manufacturer advises that *Convulex*® has a 1:1 dose relationship with products containing sodium valproate, but nevertheless care is needed in making changes

**Depakote**® (Sanofi-Synthelabo) [PoM]
Section 4.2.3 (bipolar disorder)

# Vigabatrin

For partial epilepsy with or without secondary generalisation, **vigabatrin** is given in combination with other antiepileptic treatment; its use is restricted to patients in whom all other combinations are inadequate or are not tolerated. It can be used as sole therapy in the management of infantile spasms in West's syndrome.

**4**

**Central nervous system**

About one-third of patients treated with vigabatrin have suffered visual field defects; counselling and **careful monitoring** for this side-effect are required (see also Visual Field Defects under Cautions below). Vigabatrin has prominent behavioural side-effects in some patients.

### ▌ VIGABATRIN

**Indications** initiated and supervised by appropriate specialist, adjunctive treatment of partial seizures with or without secondary generalisation not satisfactorily controlled with other antiepileptics; monotherapy for management of infantile spasms (West's syndrome)

**Cautions** renal impairment (Appendix 3); elderly; closely monitor neurological function; avoid sudden withdrawal (taper off over 2–4 weeks); history of psychosis, depression or behavioural problems; pregnancy (see p. 253 and Appendix 4) and breast-feeding (Appendix 5); absence seizures (may be exacerbated); **interactions**: see p. 253 and Appendix 1 (vigabatrin)

Visual field defects Vigabatrin is associated with visual field defects. The CSM has advised that onset of symptoms varies from 1 month to several years after starting. In most cases, visual field defects have persisted despite discontinuation. Product literature advises visual field testing before treatment and at 6-month intervals; a procedure for testing visual fields in those with a developmental age of less than 9 years is available from the manufacturers. Patients should be warned to report any new visual symptoms that develop and those with symptoms should be referred for an urgent ophthalmological opinion. Gradual withdrawal of vigabatrin should be considered.

**Contra-indications** visual field defects

**Side-effects** nausea, abdominal pain; oedema; drowsiness (rarely encephalopathic symptoms including marked sedation, stupor, and confusion with non-specific slow wave EEG—reduce dose or withdraw), fatigue, excitation, and agitation (especially in children), dizziness, headache, nervousness, depression, aggression, paranoia, impaired concentration, memory disturbances, tremor, paraesthesia, weight gain; visual field defects (see also under Cautions), blurred vision, nystagmus, diplopia; *less commonly* ataxia, psychosis, mania, and rash; occasional increase in seizure frequency (especially if myoclonic); *rarely* suicidal ideation and retinal disorders (including peripheral retinal neuropathy); *very rarely* hepatitis, optic neuritis and optic atrophy; also reported, decrease in liver enzymes and speech disorder

**Dose**
- With current antiepileptic therapy, initially 1 g daily in single or 2 divided doses then increased according to response in steps of 500 mg at weekly intervals; usual range 2–3 g daily (max. 3 g daily); CHILD initially 40 mg/kg daily in single or 2 divided doses then adjusted according to body-weight 10–15 kg, 0.5–1 g daily; body-weight 15–30 kg, 1–1.5 g daily; body-weight 30–50 kg, 1.5–3 g daily; body-weight over 50 kg, 2–3 g daily
- Infantile spasms (West's syndrome), *monotherapy*, 50 mg/kg daily, adjusted according to response over 7 days; up to 150 mg/kg daily used with good tolerability

**Sabril®** (Aventis Pharma) (PoM)
Tablets, f/c, scored, vigabatrin 500 mg, net price 100-tab pack = £30.84. Label: 3, 8, counselling, driving (see notes above)

Powder, sugar-free, vigabatrin 500 mg/sachet. Net price 50-sachet pack = £17.08. Label: 3, 8, 13, counselling, driving (see notes above)

Note The contents of a sachet should be dissolved in water or a soft drink immediately before taking

## Zonisamide

**Zonisamide** can be used as adjunctive treatment for refractory partial seizures with or without secondary generalisation.

### ▌ ZONISAMIDE

**Indications** adjunctive therapy for refractory partial seizures with or without secondary generalisation

**Cautions** elderly; ensure adequate hydration (especially if predisposition to nephrolithiasis or in strenuous activity or warm environment); concomitant use of drugs that increase risk of hyperthermia or nephrolithiasis; avoid abrupt withdrawal; hepatic impairment (avoid if severe—Appendix 2); renal impairment (Appendix 3); pregnancy (Appendix 4); **interactions**: see p. 253 and Appendix 1 (zonisamide)

**Contra-indications** hypersensitivity to sulphonamides; breast-feeding (Appendix 5)

**Side-effects** nausea, diarrhoea, abdominal pain, anorexia, weight loss; drowsiness, dizziness, confusion, agitation, irritability, depression, ataxia, speech disorder, impaired memory and attention, pyrexia; diplopia; rash (consider withdrawal); *less commonly* vomiting, cholelithiasis, cholecystitis, aggression, suicidal ideation, convulsions, psychosis, urinary calculus, hypokalaemia; *very rarely* hepatitis, pancreatitis, dyspnoea, hallucinations, insomnia, amnesia, coma, myasthenic syndrome, neuroleptic malignant syndrome, heat stroke, hydronephrosis, renal impairment, metabolic acidosis, blood disorders, rhabdomyolysis, impaired sweating, pruritus, and Stevens-Johnson syndrome; suicidal ideation

**Dose**
- ADULT over 18 years, initially 50 mg daily in 2 divided doses, increased after 7 days to 100 mg daily in 2 divided doses; then increase if necessary by 100 mg every 7 days; usual maintenance 300–500 mg daily in 1–2 divided doses

**Zonegran®** (Eisai) ▼ (PoM)
Capsules, zonisamide 25 mg (white), net price 14-cap pack = £8.82; 50 mg (white/grey), 56-cap pack = £47.04; 100 mg (white/red), 56-cap pack = £62.72. Label: 3

## Benzodiazepines

**Clonazepam** is occasionally used in tonic-clonic or partial seizures, but its sedative side-effects may be prominent. **Clobazam** may be used as adjunctive therapy in the treatment of epilepsy (section 4.1.2), but the effectiveness of these and other **benzodiazepines** may wane considerably after weeks or months of continuous therapy.

**4 Central nervous system**

## CLOBAZAM

**Indications** adjunct in epilepsy; anxiety (short-term use)

**Cautions** see under Diazepam (section 4.1.2)

**Contra-indications** see under Diazepam (section 4.1.2)

**Side-effects** see under Diazepam (section 4.1.2)

**Dose**

- Epilepsy, 20–30 mg daily; max. 60 mg daily; CHILD over 3 years, not more than half adult dose
- Anxiety, 20–30 mg daily in divided doses or as a single dose at bedtime, increased in severe anxiety (in hospital patients) to a max. of 60 mg daily in divided doses; ELDERLY (or debilitated) 10–20 mg daily

¹**Clobazam** (Non-proprietary) ℙ𝕠𝕄 𝕁𝕙𝕊
Tablets, clobazam 10 mg. Net price 30-tab pack = £4.68. Label: 2 or 19, 8, counselling, driving (see notes above)
Brands include *Frisium®* 𝕁𝕙𝕊

1. 𝕁𝕙𝕊 except for epilepsy and endorsed 'SLS'

## CLONAZEPAM

**Indications** all forms of epilepsy; myoclonus; status epilepticus (section 4.8.2)

**Cautions** see notes above; elderly and debilitated, respiratory disease, spinal or cerebellar ataxia, history of alcohol or drug abuse, depression or suicidal ideation; avoid sudden withdrawal; myasthenia gravis (avoid if unstable); acute porphyria (section 9.8.2); hepatic impairment (avoid if severe; Appendix 2); renal impairment (see notes above and Appendix 4); breast-feeding (see notes above and Appendix 5); **interactions:** Appendix 1 (anxiolytics and hypnotics)

Driving Drowsiness may affect performance of skilled tasks (e.g. driving); effects of alcohol enhanced

**Contra-indications** respiratory depression; acute pulmonary insufficiency; sleep apnoea syndrome; marked neuromuscular respiratory weakness including unstable myasthenia gravis

**Side-effects** drowsiness, fatigue, dizziness, muscle hypotonia, co-ordination disturbances; also poor concentration, restlessness, confusion, amnesia, dependence, and withdrawal; salivary or bronchial hypersecretion in infants and small children; *rarely* gastro-intestinal symptoms, respiratory depression, headache, paradoxical effects including aggression and anxiety, sexual dysfunction, urinary incontinence, urticaria, pruritus, reversible hair loss, skin pigmentation changes; dysarthria, and visual disturbances on long-term treatment; blood disorders reported; **overdosage:** see Emergency Treatment of Poisoning, p. 32

**Dose**

- 1 mg (ELDERLY 500 micrograms) initially at night for 4 nights, increased according to response over 2–4 weeks to usual maintenance dose of 4–8 mg usually at night (may be given in 3–4 divided doses if necessary); CHILD up to 1 year, initially 250 micrograms increased as above to usual maintenance dose of 0.5–1 mg, 1–5 years, initially 250 micrograms increased as above to 1–3 mg, 5–12 years, initially 500 micrograms increased as above to 3–6 mg

Note Clonazepam doses in BNF may differ from those in product literature

**Rivotril®** (Roche) ℙ𝕠𝕄
Tablets, both scored, clonazepam 500 micrograms (beige), net price 100 = £3.77; 2 mg (white), 100 = £5.03. Label: 2, 8, counselling, driving (see notes above)

Injection, section 4.8.2

## Other drugs

**Acetazolamide** (section 11.6), a carbonic anhydrase inhibitor, has a specific role in treating epilepsy associated with menstruation. It can also be used with other antiepileptics for tonic-clonic and partial seizures. It is occasionally helpful in atypical absence, atonic, and tonic seizures.

**Piracetam** (section 4.9.3) is used as adjunctive treatment for cortical myoclonus.

## 4.8.2 Drugs used in status epilepticus

Immediate measures to manage status epilepticus include positioning the patient to avoid injury, supporting respiration including the provision of oxygen, maintaining blood pressure, and the correction of any hypoglycaemia. Parenteral **thiamine** should be considered if alcohol abuse is suspected; **pyridoxine** (section 9.6.2) should be given if the status epilepticus is caused by pyridoxine deficiency.

Convulsive status epilepticus should be treated urgently with intravenous **lorazepam**, repeated once after 10 minutes if seizures recur. Intravenous diazepam is effective but it is associated with a high risk of thrombophlebitis (reduced by using an emulsion formulation). Absorption of diazepam from intramuscular injection or from suppositories is too slow for treatment of status epilepticus. **Clonazepam** can also be used as an alternative.

Where facilities for resuscitation are not immediately available, **diazepam** can be administered as a rectal solution or **midazolam** [unlicensed use] can be given into the buccal cavity.

> **Important**
> If seizures recur or fail to respond within 30 minutes, phenytoin sodium, fosphenytoin, or phenobarbital sodium should be used.
> If these measures fail to control seizure within 60 minutes, anaesthesia with thiopental (section 15.1.1), midazolam (section 15.1.4), or in adults, a non-barbiturate anaesthetic such as propofol [unlicensed indication] (section 15.1.1), should be instituted with full intensive care support.

**Phenytoin sodium** may be given by slow intravenous injection, with ECG monitoring, followed by the maintenance dosage. Intramuscular use of phenytoin is not recommended (absorption is slow and erratic).

Alternatively, **fosphenytoin**, a pro-drug of phenytoin, can be given more rapidly and when given intravenously causes fewer injection-site reactions than phenytoin. Intravenous administration requires ECG monitoring. Although it can also be given intramuscularly, absorp-

**4**

**Central nervous system**

tion is too slow by this route for treatment of status epilepticus. Doses of fosphenytoin should be expressed in terms of phenytoin sodium.

**Paraldehyde** also remains a valuable drug. Given rectally it causes little respiratory depression and is therefore useful where facilities for resuscitation are poor.

For advice on the management of epileptic seizures in dental practice, see p. 22.

**Non-convulsive status epilepticus** The urgency to treat non-convulsive status epilepticus depends upon the severity of the patient's condition. If there is incomplete loss of awareness, usual oral antiepileptic therapy should be continued or restarted. Patients who fail to respond to oral antiepileptic therapy or have complete lack of awareness can be treated in the same way as for convulsive status epilepticus, although anaesthesia is rarely needed.

## CLONAZEPAM

**Indications** status epilepticus; other forms of epilepsy, and myoclonus (section 4.8.1)

**Cautions** see section 4.8.1; facilities for reversing respiratory depression with mechanical ventilation must be at hand (but see also notes above)
**Intravenous infusion** Intravenous infusion of clonazepam is potentially hazardous (especially if prolonged), calling for close and constant observation and best carried out in specialist centres with intensive care facilities. Prolonged infusion may lead to accumulation and delay recovery

**Contra-indications** see section 4.8.1; avoid injections containing benzyl alcohol in neonates (see under preparations below)

**Side-effects** see section 4.8.1; hypotension and apnoea

**Dose**
- By intravenous injection into a large vein (over at least 2 minutes) *or* by intravenous infusion, 1 mg, repeated if necessary; CHILD all ages, 500 micrograms

**Rivotril®** (Roche) PoM
Injection, clonazepam 1 mg/mL in solvent, for dilution with 1 mL water for injections immediately before injection or as described in Appendix 6. Net price 1-mL amp (with 1 mL water for injections) = 61p
Excipients include benzyl alcohol (avoid in neonates unless there is no safer alternative available, see Excipients, p. 2), ethanol, propylene glycol

◢Oral preparations
Section 4.8.1

## DIAZEPAM

**Indications** status epilepticus; febrile convulsions; convulsions due to poisoning (see p. 28); other indications (section 4.1.2, section 10.2.2, and section 15.1.4.1)

**Cautions** see section 4.1.2; when given intravenously facilities for reversing respiratory depression with mechanical ventilation must be at hand (but see also notes above)

**Contra-indications** see section 4.1.2

**Side-effects** see section 4.1.2; hypotension and apnoea

**Dose**
- Status epilepticus (but see notes above), febrile convulsions, and convulsions due to poisoning, by intravenous injection, 10 mg at a rate of 1 mL (5 mg) per minute, repeated once after 10 minutes if necessary; CHILD under 12 years, 300–400 micrograms/kg [unlicensed dose], repeated once after 10 minutes if necessary

  By rectum as rectal solution, ADULT over 18 years, 10–20 mg (max. 30 mg), repeated once after 10–15 minutes if necessary; ELDERLY 10 mg (max. 15 mg); NEONATE 1.25–2.5 mg; CHILD 1 month–2 years, 5 mg; 2–12 years, 5–10 mg; 12–18 years, 10 mg

**Diazepam** (Non-proprietary) PoM
Injection (solution), diazepam 5 mg/mL. See Appendix 6. Net price 2-mL amp = 45p
Excipients may include benzyl alcohol (avoid in neonates, see Excipients, p. 2), ethanol, propylene glycol

Injection (emulsion), diazepam 5 mg/mL (0.5%). See Appendix 6. Net price 2-mL amp = 92p
Brands include *Diazemuls®*

Rectal tubes (= rectal solution), diazepam 2 mg/mL, net price 1.25-mL (2.5-mg) tube = 90p, 2.5-mL (5-mg) tube = £1.27; 4 mg/mL, 2.5-mL (10-mg) tube = £1.65
Brands include *Diazepam Rectubes®*, *Stesolid®*

◢Oral preparations
Section 4.1.2

## FOSPHENYTOIN SODIUM

Note Fosphenytoin is a pro-drug of phenytoin

**Indications** status epilepticus; seizures associated with neurosurgery or head injury; when phenytoin by mouth not possible

**Cautions** see Phenytoin Sodium; liver impairment (Appendix 2); renal impairment (Appendix 3); resuscitation facilities must be available; **interactions**: see p. 253 and Appendix 1 (phenytoin)

**Contra-indications** see Phenytoin Sodium

**Side-effects** see Phenytoin Sodium
CSM advice Intravenous infusion of fosphenytoin has been associated with severe cardiovascular reactions including asystole, ventricular fibrillation, and cardiac arrest. Hypotension, bradycardia, and heart block have also been reported. The CSM advises:

- monitor heart rate, blood pressure, and respiratory function for duration of infusion

- observe patient for at least 30 minutes after infusion

- if hypotension occurs, reduce infusion rate or discontinue

- reduce dose or infusion rate in elderly, and in renal or hepatic impairment.

**Dose**

> Note Prescriptions for fosphenytoin sodium should state the dose in terms of phenytoin sodium equivalent (PE); fosphenytoin sodium 1.5 mg ≡ phenytoin sodium 1 mg

- Status epilepticus, by intravenous infusion (at a rate of 100–150 mg(PE)/minute), initially 20 mg(PE)/kg then by intravenous infusion (at a rate of 50–100 mg(PE)/minute), 4–5 mg(PE)/kg daily in 1–2 divided doses, dose adjusted according to response and trough plasma-phenytoin concentration

  CHILD 5 years and over, by intravenous infusion (at a rate of 2–3 mg(PE)/kg/minute), initially 20 mg(PE)/kg then by intravenous infusion (at a rate of 1–2 mg(PE)/kg/minute), 4–5 mg(PE)/kg daily in 1–4 divided doses, dose adjusted according to response and trough plasma-phenytoin concentration

- Prophylaxis or treatment of seizures associated with neurosurgery or head injury, by intramuscular injection *or* by intravenous infusion (at a rate of 50–100 mg(PE)/minute), initially 10–15 mg(PE)/kg then by intramuscular injection *or* by intravenous infusion (at a rate of 50–100 mg(PE)/minute), 4–5 mg(PE)/kg daily (in 1–2 divided doses), dose adjusted according to response and trough plasma-phenytoin concentration

  CHILD 5 years and over, by intravenous infusion (at a rate of 1–2 mg(PE)/kg/minute), initially 10–15 mg(PE)/kg then 4–5 mg(PE)/kg daily in 1–4 divided doses, dose adjusted according to response and trough plasma-phenytoin concentration

- Temporary substitution for oral phenytoin, by intramuscular injection *or* by intravenous infusion (at a rate of 50–100 mg(PE)/minute), same dose and dosing frequency as oral phenytoin therapy; CHILD 5 years and over, by intravenous infusion (at a rate of 1–2 mg(PE)/kg/minute), same dose and dosing frequency as oral phenytoin therapy

**Note** ELDERLY consider 10–25% reduction in dose or infusion rate

**Note** Fosphenytoin sodium doses in BNF may differ from those in product literature

**Pro-Epanutin®** (Pfizer) PoM
Injection, fosphenytoin sodium 75 mg/mL (equivalent to phenytoin sodium 50 mg/mL), net price 10-mL vial = £40.00
Electrolytes phosphate 3.7 micromol/mg fosphenytoin sodium (phosphate 5.6 micromol/mg phenytoin sodium)

## LORAZEPAM

**Indications** status epilepticus; other indications (section 4.1.2)

**Cautions** see section 4.1.2

**Contra-indications** see under Diazepam (section 4.1.2)

**Side-effects** see under Diazepam (section 4.1.2)

**Dose**

- By slow intravenous injection (into large vein), 4 mg repeated once after 10 minutes if necessary; CHILD under 12 years 100 micrograms/kg (max. 4 mg) repeated once after 10 minutes if necessary

◢Preparations
Section 4.1.2

## MIDAZOLAM

**Indications** status epilepticus [unlicensed indication]; other indications (section 15.1.4)

**Cautions** section 15.1.4

**Contra-indications** section 15.1.4

**Side-effects** section 15.1.4

**Dose**

- By buccal administration [unlicensed], ADULT and CHILD over 10 years, 10 mg repeated once after 10 minutes if necessary; CHILD up to 6 months, 300 micrograms/kg (max. 2.5 mg); 6 months–1 year, 2.5 mg; 1–5 years, 5 mg; 5–10 years, 7.5 mg
**Note** Midazolam injection solution may be given by buccal administration

**Midazolam** (Non-proprietary) CD
Buccal liquid, midazolam 10 mg/mL
Available from 'special-order' manufacturers or specialist importing companies, see p. 969

◢Injection
Section 15.1.4

## PARALDEHYDE

**Indications** status epilepticus

**Cautions** bronchopulmonary disease, hepatic impairment; pregnancy (Appendix 4) and breast-feeding (Appendix 5); **interactions:** Appendix 1 (paraldehyde)

**Contra-indications** gastric disorders; rectal administration in colitis

**Side-effects** rashes; rectal irritation after enema

**Dose**

- By rectum (doses expressed as undiluted paraldehyde), ADULT and CHILD over 12 years, 20 mL; CHILD up to 3 months 0.5 mL, 3–6 months 1 mL, 6–12 months 1.5 mL, 1–2 years 2 mL, 2–5 years 3–4 mL, 5–12 years 5–10 mL
**Administration** for *rectal administration*, do not administer paraldehyde undiluted

**Paraldehyde** (Non-proprietary) PoM
Enema, 8–50%, available from 'special-order' manufacturers or specialist importing companies, see p. 969

## PHENOBARBITAL SODIUM
### (Phenobarbitone sodium)

**Indications** status epilepticus; other forms of epilepsy except absence seizures (section 4.8.1)

**Cautions** see under Phenobarbital (section 4.8.1)

**Side-effects** see under Phenobarbital (section 4.8.1)

**Dose**

- Status epilepticus, by intravenous injection (dilute injection 1 in 10 with water for injections), 10 mg/kg at a rate of not more than 100 mg/minute; max. 1 g
**Note** For therapeutic purposes phenobarbital and phenobarbital sodium may be considered equivalent in effect

**Phenobarbital** (Non-proprietary) CD
Injection, phenobarbital sodium 200 mg/mL, net price 1-mL amp = £2.00
Excipients include propylene glycol 90% (see Excipients, p. 2)
**Note** Must be diluted before intravenous administration (see under Dose)

◢Oral preparations
Section 4.8.1

## PHENYTOIN SODIUM

**Indications** status epilepticus; seizures in neurosurgery; arrhythmias, but now obsolete (section 2.3.2)

**Cautions** hypotension and heart failure; resuscitation facilities must be available; injection solutions alkaline (irritant to tissues); see also p. 260; **interactions:** see p. 253 and Appendix 1 (phenytoin)

**Contra-indications** sinus bradycardia, sino-atrial block, and second- and third-degree heart block; Stokes-Adams syndrome; acute porphyria (section 9.8.2)

**Side-effects** intravenous injection may cause cardio-vascular and CNS depression (particularly if injection too rapid) with arrhythmias, hypotension, and cardiovascular collapse; alterations in respiratory function (including respiratory arrest); injection site reactions; see also p. 260

**Dose**

● By slow intravenous injection *or* infusion (with blood pressure and ECG monitoring), status epilepticus, 18 mg/kg at a rate not exceeding 50 mg per minute, as a loading dose (see also notes above); maintenance doses of about 100 mg should be given thereafter at intervals of every 6–8 hours, monitored by measurement of plasma concentrations; rate and dose reduced according to weight; CHILD 18 mg/kg as a loading dose (NEONATE 15–20 mg/kg at rate of 1–3 mg/kg/minute)

Ventricular arrhythmias (but use now obsolete), by intravenous injection via caval catheter, 3.5–5 mg/kg at a rate not exceeding 50 mg/minute, with blood pressure and ECG monitoring; repeated once if necessary

Note To avoid local venous irritation each injection or infusion should be preceded and followed by an injection of sterile physiological saline through the same needle or catheter

● By intramuscular injection, not recommended (see notes above)

Note Phenytoin sodium doses in BNF may differ from those in product literature

**Phenytoin** (Non-proprietary) ℗oM

Injection, phenytoin sodium 50 mg/mL with propylene glycol 40% and alcohol 10% in water for injections, net price 5-mL amp = £3.40

**Epanutin® Ready-Mixed Parenteral** (Pfizer) ℗oM

Injection, phenytoin sodium 50 mg/mL with propylene glycol 40% and alcohol 10% in water for injections, net price 5-mL amp = £4.88

Electrolytes 1.1 mmol Na⁺ per 5 mL ampoule

◢Oral preparations

Section 4.8.1

## 4.8.3 Febrile convulsions

*Brief febrile convulsions* need no specific treatment; antipyretic medication, e.g. **paracetamol** (section 4.7.1) is commonly used to reduce fever and prevent further convulsions but evidence to support this practice is lacking. *Prolonged febrile convulsions* (those lasting 15 minutes or longer), *recurrent convulsions*, or those occurring in a child at known risk must be treated more actively, as there is the possibility of resulting brain damage. **Diazepam** is the drug of choice given either by slow intravenous injection or preferably rectally in solution (section 4.8.2). The rectal route is preferred as satisfactory absorption is achieved within minutes and administration is much easier. Suppositories are not suitable because absorption is too slow.

Intermittent prophylaxis (i.e. the anticonvulsant administered at the onset of fever) is possible in only a small proportion of children. Again **diazepam** is the treatment of choice, orally or rectally.

Long-term anticonvulsant prophylaxis for febrile convulsions is rarely indicated. Anticonvulsant treatment needs to be considered only for children at risk from prolonged or complex febrile convulsions, including those whose first seizure occurred at under 14 months or who have neurological abnormalities or who have had previous prolonged or focal convulsions.

## 4.9 Drugs used in parkinsonism and related disorders

4.9.1 Dopaminergic drugs used in parkinsonism

4.9.2 Antimuscarinic drugs used in parkinsonism

4.9.3 Drugs used in essential tremor, chorea, tics, and related disorders

In idiopathic Parkinson's disease, the progressive degeneration of pigmented neurones in the substantia nigra leads to a deficiency of the neurotransmitter dopamine. The resulting neurochemical imbalance in the basal ganglia causes the characteristic signs and symptoms of the illness. Drug therapy does not prevent disease progression, but it improves most patients' quality of life.

Patients with suspected Parkinson's disease should be referred to a specialist to confirm the diagnosis; the diagnosis should be reviewed every 6–12 months.

Features resembling those of Parkinson's disease can occur in diseases such as progressive supranuclear palsy and multiple system atrophy, but they do not normally show a sustained response to the drugs used in the treatment of idiopathic Parkinson's disease.

When initiating treatment, patients should be advised about its limitations and possible side-effects. About 5–10% of patients with Parkinson's disease respond poorly to treatment.

Treatment is usually not started until symptoms cause significant disruption of daily activities. Therapy with two or more antiparkinsonian drugs may be necessary as the disease progresses. Most patients eventually require **levodopa** and subsequently develop motor complications.

Antiparkinsonian drug therapy should never be stopped abruptly as this carries a small risk of neuroleptic malignant syndrome.

**Elderly** Antiparkinsonian drugs can cause confusion in the elderly. It is particularly important to initiate treatment with low doses and to increase the dose gradually.

## 4.9.1 Dopaminergic drugs used in parkinsonism

### Dopamine receptor agonists

The dopamine receptor agonists, **bromocriptine**, **cabergoline**, **pergolide**, **pramipexole**, **ropinirole**, and **rotigotine** have a direct action on dopamine receptors. The treatment of new patients is often started with dopamine receptor agonists. They are also used with levodopa in more advanced disease. Rotigotine is licensed for use as monotherapy in early-stage Parkinson's disease.

When used alone, dopamine receptor agonists cause fewer motor complications in long-term treatment compared with levodopa treatment but the overall motor performance improves slightly less. The dopamine receptor agonists are associated with more neuropsychiatric side-effects than levodopa. The ergot-derived dopamine receptor agonists, bromocriptine, cabergoline, and pergolide, have been associated with fibrotic reactions (see notes below). Patients should be monitored for signs of cardiac fibrosis, before and at regular intervals during treatment with cabergoline or pergolide. In most cases, non-ergot-derived dopamine agonists are preferred over ergot-derived dopamine agonists.

Dopamine receptor agonists can cause excessive daytime sleepiness and sudden onset of sleep, see Sudden Onset of Sleep, p. 272.

**Hypotensive reactions** Hypotensive reactions can occur in some patients taking dopamine agonists; these can be particularly problematic during the first few days of treatment and care should be exercised when driving or operating machinery.

Doses of dopamine receptor agonists should be increased slowly according to response and tolerability. Treatment with dopamine receptor agonists should not be withdrawn abruptly.

> ### Fibrotic reactions
> Ergot-derived dopamine receptor agonists, bromocriptine, cabergoline, and pergolide, have been associated with pulmonary, retroperitoneal, and pericardial fibrotic reactions.
> Exclude cardiac valvulopathy with echocardiography before starting treatment with these ergot derivatives for Parkinson's disease or chronic endocrine disorders (excludes suppression of lactation); it may also be appropriate to measure the erythrocyte sedimentation rate and serum creatinine and to obtain a chest X-ray. Patients should be monitored for dyspnoea, persistent cough, chest pain, cardiac failure, and abdominal pain or tenderness. If long-term treatment is expected, then lung-function tests may also be helpful. Patients taking cabergoline or pergolide should be regularly monitored for cardiac fibrosis by echocardiography (within 3–6 months of initiating treatment and subsequently at 6–12 month intervals).

**Apomorphine** is a potent dopamine agonist that is sometimes helpful in advanced disease for patients experiencing unpredictable 'off' periods with levodopa treatment. Apomorphine is highly emetogenic; patients must receive domperidone for at least 2 days before starting treatment. Specialist supervision is advisable throughout apomorphine treatment.

## ■ APOMORPHINE HYDROCHLORIDE

**Indications** refractory motor fluctuations in Parkinson's disease ('off' episodes) inadequately controlled by levodopa with dopa-decarboxylase inhibitor or other dopaminergics (for capable and motivated patients under specialist supervision)

**Cautions** see notes above; pulmonary or cardiovascular disease, history of postural hypotension (special care on initiation); neuropsychiatric problems or dementia; hepatic, haemopoietic, renal, and cardiovascular monitoring; *on administration with levodopa* test initially and every 6 months for haemolytic anaemia (development calls for specialist haematological care with dose reduction and possible discontinuation); renal impairment; pregnancy; **interactions:** Appendix 1 (apomorphine)

**Contra-indications** respiratory depression, hypersensitivity to opioids; not suitable if 'on' response to levodopa marred by severe dyskinesia, hypotonia or psychiatric effects; hepatic impairment; breast-feeding; not for intravenous administration

**Side-effects** nausea, vomiting (see below under Dose); drowsiness (including sudden onset of sleep), confusion, hallucinations, injection-site reactions (including nodule formation and ulceration)—change injection sites in rotation; *less commonly* postural hypotension, breathing difficulties, dykinesias during 'on' periods (may require discontinuation), haemolytic anaemia with levodopa (see Cautions), and rash; *rarely* eosinophilia; pathological gambling, increased libido, and hypersexuality also reported

**Dose**

- By subcutaneous injection, usual range (after initiation as below) 3–30 mg daily in divided doses; subcutaneous infusion may be preferable in those requiring division of injections into more than 10 doses daily; max. single dose 10 mg; CHILD and ADOLESCENT under 18 years not recommended

- By continuous subcutaneous infusion (those requiring division into more than 10 injections daily) initially 1 mg/hour daily increased according to response (not more often than every 4 hours) in max. steps of 500 micrograms/hour, to usual rate of 1–4 mg/hour (14–60 micrograms/kg/hour); change infusion site every 12 hours and give during waking hours only (24-hour infusions not advised unless severe night-time symptoms)—intermittent bolus boosts also usually needed; CHILD and ADOLESCENT under 18 years not recommended

**Note** Total daily dose by either route (or combined routes) max. 100 mg

**Requirements for initiation** *Hospital admission* and at least 2 days of pretreatment with domperidone for nausea and vomiting, *after at least 3 days* withhold existing antiparkinsonian medication overnight to provoke 'off' episode, *determine* threshold dose, *re-establish* other antiparkinsonian drugs, *determine* effective apomorphine regimen, *teach* to administer by subcutaneous injection into lower abdomen or outer thigh at first sign of 'off' episode, *discharge* from hospital, *monitor* frequently and *adjust* dosage regimen as appropriate (domperidone may normally be withdrawn over several weeks or longer)—for full details of initiation requirements, consult product literature

**APO-go®** (Forum) (PoM)
Injection, apomorphine hydrochloride 10 mg/mL, net price 2-mL amp = £7.59, 5-mL amp = £14.62
Excipients include sulphites

Injection (APO-go® Pen), apomorphine hydrochloride 10 mg/mL, net price 3-mL pen injector = £24.78
Excipients include sulphites

Injection (APO-go® PFS), apomorphine hydrochloride 5 mg/mL, net price 10-mL prefilled syringe = £14.62
Excipients include sulphites

**4**

**Central nervous system**

## ▋ BROMOCRIPTINE

**Indications** parkinsonism (but not drug-induced extrapyramidal symptoms); endocrine disorders (section 6.7.1)

**Cautions** see section 6.7.1 and notes above

**Contra-indications** section 6.7.1

**Side-effects** section 6.7.1

**Dose**

- First week 1–1.25 mg at night, second week 2–2.5 mg at night, third week 2.5 mg twice daily, fourth week 2.5 mg 3 times daily then increasing by 2.5 mg every 3–14 days according to response to a usual range of 10–30 mg daily; taken with food

◢**Preparations**
Section 6.7.1

## ▋ CABERGOLINE

**Indications** alone or as adjunct to levodopa with dopa-decarboxylase inhibitor in Parkinson's disease where dopamine receptor agonists other than ergot derivative not appropriate; endocrine disorders (section 6.7.1)

**Cautions** see section 6.7.1 and notes above

**Contra-indications** section 6.7.1

**Side-effects** section 6.7.1

**Dose**

- Initially 1 mg daily, increased by increments of 0.5–1 mg at 7 or 14 day intervals; usual range 2–3 mg daily
  **Note** Concurrent dose of levodopa may be decreased gradually while dose of cabergoline is increased

**Cabergoline** (Non-proprietary) [PoM]
Tablets, scored, cabergoline 1 mg, net price 20-tab pack = £52.97; 2 mg, 20-tab pack = £63.79. Label: 21, counselling, hypotensive reactions, driving, see notes above
**Note** Dispense in original container (contains desiccant)

## ▋ PERGOLIDE

**Indications** alone or as adjunct to levodopa with dopa-decarboxylase inhibitor in Parkinson's disease where dopamine receptor agonists other than ergot derivative not appropriate

**Cautions** see notes above; arrhythmias or underlying cardiac disease; history of confusion, psychosis, or hallucinations, dyskinesia (may exacerbate); acute porphyria (section 9.8.2); pregnancy (Appendix 4); breast-feeding (Appendix 5); **interactions:** Appendix 1 (pergolide)

**Contra-indications** history of fibrotic disorders; cardiac valvulopathy (exclude before treatment, see Fibrotic Reactions, p. 269)

**Side-effects** see notes above; also nausea, vomiting, dyspepsia, abdominal pain; dyspnoea, rhinitis; hallucinations, dyskinesia, drowsiness (including sudden onset of sleep); diplopia; also reported constipation, diarrhoea, tachycardia, atrial premature contractions, palpitation, hypotension, syncope, Raynaud's phenomenon, cardiac valvulopathy, pericarditis, pericardial effusion, pleuritis, pleural effusion, pleural fibrosis, insomnia, confusion, dizziness, pathological gambling, neuroleptic malignant syndrome, fever, increased libido, hypersexuality, and rash

**Dose**

- Monotherapy, 50 micrograms at night on day 1, then 50 micrograms twice daily on days 2–4, then increased by 100–250 micrograms daily every 3–4 days to 1.5 mg daily in 3 divided doses at day 28; after day 30, further increases every 3–4 days of up to 250 micrograms daily; usual maintenance dose 2.1–2.5 mg daily; max. 3 mg daily
- Adjunctive therapy with levodopa, 50 micrograms daily for 2 days, increased gradually by 100–150 micrograms every 3 days over next 12 days, usually given in 3 divided doses; further increases of 250 micrograms every 3 days; max. 3 mg daily; during pergolide titration levodopa dose may be reduced cautiously

**Pergolide** (Non-proprietary) [PoM]
Tablets, pergolide (as mesilate) 50 micrograms, net price 100-tab pack = £14.41; 250 micrograms, 100-tab pack = £10.52; 1 mg, 100-tab pack = £21.58. Counselling, hypotensive reactions, driving, see notes above

**Celance®** (Lilly) [PoM]
Tablets, all scored, pergolide (as mesilate) 50 micrograms (ivory), net price 100-tab pack = £20.70; 250 micrograms (green), 100-tab pack = £16.91; 1 mg (pink), 100-tab pack = £43.44. Counselling, hypotensive reactions, driving, see notes above

## ▋ PRAMIPEXOLE

**Indications** Parkinson's disease, used alone or as an adjunct to levodopa with dopa-decarboxylase inhibitor; moderate to severe restless legs syndrome

**Cautions** see notes above; psychotic disorders; ophthalmological testing recommended (risk of visual disorders); severe cardiovascular disease; renal impairment (Appendix 3); pregnancy (Appendix 4); **interactions:** Appendix 1 (pramipexole)

**Contra-indications** breast-feeding (Appendix 5)

**Side-effects** see notes above; also nausea, constipation; postural hypotension, hypotension, headache, confusion, drowsiness (including sudden onset of sleep), fatigue, insomnia, dizziness, hallucinations (mostly visual), dyskinesia, peripheral oedema; hyperkinesia, delusions, abnormal dreams, paradoxical worsening of restless legs syndrome, and behavioural changes including pathological gambling, binge eating, hypersexuality, and changes in libido also reported

**Dose**
**Important** Doses and strengths are stated in terms of pramipexole (base); equivalent strengths in terms of pramipexole dihydrochloride monohydrate (salt) are as follows:
88 micrograms base ≡ 125 micrograms salt;
180 micrograms base ≡ 250 micrograms salt;
350 micrograms base ≡ 500 micrograms salt;
700 micrograms base ≡ 1 mg salt

- Parkinson's disease, initially 88 micrograms 3 times daily, dose doubled every 5–7 days if tolerated to 350 micrograms 3 times daily; further increased if necessary by 180 micrograms 3 times daily at weekly intervals; max. 3.3 mg daily in 3 divided doses
  **Note** During pramipexole dose titration and maintenance, levodopa dose may be reduced
- Restless legs syndrome, initially 88 micrograms once daily 2–3 hours before bedtime, dose doubled every 4–7 days if necessary to 350 micrograms daily; max. 540 micrograms daily; CHILD under 18 years not recommended

**Mirapexin®** (Boehringer Ingelheim) ▼ [PoM]
Tablets, pramipexole 88 micrograms, net price 30-tab pack = £9.55; 180 micrograms (scored), 30-tab pack = £19.10, 100-tab pack = £63.67; 350 micrograms (scored), 30-tab pack = £38.20, 100-tab pack = £127.34; 700 micrograms (scored), 30-tab pack = £76.40, 100-tab pack = £254.69. Counselling, hypotensive reactions, driving, see notes above

## ROPINIROLE

**Indications** Parkinson's disease, either used alone or as an adjunct to levodopa with a dopa-decarboxylase inhibitor; moderate to severe restless legs syndrome

**Cautions** see notes above; severe cardiovascular disease, major psychotic disorders; hepatic impairment (Appendix 2); renal impairment (Appendix 3); **interactions:** Appendix 1 (ropinirole)

**Contra-indications** pregnancy (Appendix 4); breast-feeding (Appendix 5)

**Side-effects** see notes above; also nausea, vomiting, abdominal pain, dyspepsia, constipation; hypotension; syncope, peripheral oedema; drowsiness (including sudden onset of sleep, see p. 272), dizziness, nervousness, fatigue, dyskinesia, hallucinations, confusion; *less commonly* psychosis, pathological gambling, hypersexuality, and increased libido; *very rarely* hepatic disorders; *also reported* paradoxical worsening of restless legs syndrome

**Dose**
● Parkinson's disease, initially 750 micrograms daily in 3 divided doses, increased by increments of 750 micrograms at weekly intervals to 3 mg daily; further increased by increments of up to 3 mg at weekly intervals according to response; usual range 9–16 mg daily (but higher doses may be required if used with levodopa); max. 24 mg daily
Note When administered as adjunct to levodopa, concurrent dose of levodopa may be reduced by approx. 20%; ropinirole doses in the BNF may differ from those in product literature

● Restless legs syndrome, ADULT over 18 years initially 250 micrograms at night for 2 days, increased if tolerated to 500 micrograms at night for 5 days and then to 1 mg at night for 7 days; further increased at weekly intervals in steps of 500 micrograms daily according to response; usual dose 2 mg at night; max. 4 mg daily
Note Repeat dose titration if restarting after interval of more than a few days

**Ropinirole** (Non-proprietary) [PoM]
Tablets, ropinirole (as hydrochloride) 250 microgram, net price 12-tab pack = £3.94; 500 microgram, 28-tab pack = £15.75; 1 mg, 84-tab pack = £47.26; 2 mg, 84-tab pack = £94.53; 5 mg, 84-tab pack = £163.27. Label: 21, counselling, driving, see notes above

**Adartrel®** (GSK) [PoM]
Tablets, f/c, ropinirole (as hydrochloride) 250 micrograms (white), net price 12-tab pack = £3.94; 500 micrograms (yellow), 28-tab pack = £15.75, 84-tab pack = £47.26; 2 mg (pink), 28-tab pack = £31.51, 84-tab pack = £94.53. Label: 21, counselling, driving, see notes above
Note Licensed for use in restless legs syndrome only
The *Scottish Medicines Consortium* has advised (June 2006) that *Adartrel®* should be restricted for use in patients with a baseline score of 24 points or more on the International Restless Legs Scale

**Requip®** (GSK) [PoM]
Tablets, f/c, ropinirole (as hydrochloride) 1 mg (green), net price 84-tab pack = £47.26; 2 mg (pink),

84-tab pack = £94.53; 5 mg (blue), 84-tab pack = £163.27; 28-day starter pack of 42 × 250-microgram (white) tablets, 42 × 500-microgram (yellow) tablets, and 21 × 1-mg (green) tablets = £40.10; 28-day follow-on pack of 42 × 500-microgram (yellow) tablets, 42 × 1-mg (green) tablets, and 63 × 2-mg (pink) tablets = £74.40. Label: 21, counselling, driving, see notes above
Note Licensed for use in Parkinson's disease only

◢**Modified release**
**Requip® XL** (GSK) ▼ [PoM]
Tablets, m/r, ropinirole (as hydrochloride) 2 mg (pink), net price 28-tab pack = £31.36; 4 mg (brown), 28-tab pack = £62.72; 8 mg (red), 28-tab pack = £105.28. Label: 25, counselling, driving, see notes above
Dose stable Parkinson's disease in patients transferring from ropinirole immediate-release tablets, initially *Requip® XL* once daily substituted for total daily dose equivalent of ropinirole immediate-release tablets; if control not maintained after switching, *in patients receiving less than 8 mg once daily*, increase in steps of 2 mg at intervals of at least 1 week to 8 mg once daily according to response; *in patients receiving 8 mg once daily or more*, increase in steps of 2 mg at intervals of at least 2 weeks according to response; max. 24 mg once daily
Note When administered as adjunct to levodopa, concurrent dose of levodopa may be reduced

## ROTIGOTINE

**Indications** Parkinson's disease, either used alone or as an adjunct to levodopa with dopa-decarboxylase inhibitor

**Cautions** see notes above; ophthalmic testing recommended; avoid exposure of patch to heat; hepatic impairment (Appendix 2); **interactions:** Appendix 1 (rotigotine)

**Contra-indications** pregnancy (Appendix 4); breast-feeding (Appendix 5); remove patch (aluminium-containing) before magnetic resonance imaging or cardioversion

**Side-effects** nausea, vomiting, constipation, dry mouth, diarrhoea, dyspepsia, weight changes; postural hypotension, peripheral oedema; confusion, drowsiness (including sudden onset of sleep), sleep disorders, dizziness, headache, dyskinesia, asthenia, hallucinations; hyperhidrosis, rash (including local reactions to patch), and pruritus; *less commonly* abdominal pain, anorexia, taste disturbance, palpitation, tachycardia, hypotension, hypertension, atrial fibrillation, syncope, dyspnoea, cough, hiccup, tremor, psychosis, pathological gambling, anxiety, impaired attention, dystonia, paraesthesia, impaired memory, erectile dysfunction, increased libido, arthralgia, and visual disturbances; *rarely* convulsions and loss of consciousness

**Dose**
● Monotherapy, apply '2 mg/24 hours' patch to dry, non-irritated skin on torso, thigh, or upper arm, removing after 24 hours and siting replacement patch on a different area (avoid using the same area for 14 days); increased in steps of 2 mg/24 hours at weekly intervals if required; max. 8 mg/24 hours

● Adjunctive therapy with levodopa, apply '4 mg/24 hours' patch to dry, non-irritated skin on torso, thigh, or upper arm, removing after 24 hours and siting replacement patch on a different area (avoid using the same site for 14 days); increased in steps of 2 mg/24 hours at weekly intervals if required; max. 16 mg/24 hours

4

Central nervous system

**Neupro®** (UCB Pharma) ▼ PoM

Patches, self-adhesive, beige, rotigotine 2 mg/24 hours, net price 28 = £77.24; 4 mg/24 hours, 28 = £117.71; 6 mg/24 hours, 28 = £142.79; 8 mg/24 hours, 28 = £142.79; 28-day starter pack of 7 × 2 mg/24 hours, 7 × 4 mg/24 hours, 7 × 6 mg/24 hours, and 7 × 8 mg/24 hours patches = £142.79. Counselling, hypotensive reactions, driving, see notes above

Note The *Scottish Medicines Consortium* has advised that *Neupro®* is accepted as monotherapy for the treatment of early-stage idiopathic Parkinson's disease (June 2007) and for restricted use for the treatment of advanced Parkinson's disease in combination with levodopa where the transdermal route would facilitate treatment (July 2007)

## Levodopa

**Levodopa**, the amino-acid precursor of dopamine, acts by replenishing depleted striatal dopamine; it is given with an extracerebral **dopa-decarboxylase inhibitor** that reduces the peripheral conversion of levodopa to dopamine, thereby limiting side-effects such as nausea, vomiting and cardiovascular effects. Additionally, effective brain-dopamine concentrations can be achieved with lower doses of levodopa. The extracerebral dopa-decarboxylase inhibitors used with levodopa are benserazide (in **co-beneldopa**) and carbidopa (in **co-careldopa**).

Levodopa, in combination with a dopa-decarboxylase inhibitor, is useful in the elderly or frail, in patients with other significant illnesses, and in those with more severe symptoms. It is effective and well tolerated in the majority of patients.

Levodopa therapy should be initiated at a low dose and increased in small steps; the final dose should be as low as possible. Intervals between doses should be chosen to suit the needs of the individual patient.

Note When co-careldopa is used, the total daily dose of carbidopa should be at least 70 mg. A lower dose may not achieve full inhibition of extracerebral dopa-decarboxylase, with a resultant increase in side-effects.

Nausea and vomiting with co-beneldopa or co-careldopa are rarely dose-limiting but domperidone (section 4.6) may be useful in controlling these effects.

Levodopa treatment is associated with the development of potentially troublesome motor complications including response fluctuations and dyskinesias. Response fluctuations are characterised by large variations in motor performance, with normal function during the 'on' period, and weakness and restricted mobility during the 'off' period. 'End-of-dose' deterioration also occurs, where the duration of benefit after each dose becomes progressively shorter. Modified-release preparations may help with 'end-of-dose' deterioration or nocturnal immobility and rigidity. Motor complications are particularly problematic in young patients treated with levodopa.

**Cautions** Levodopa should be used with caution in severe cardiovascular or pulmonary disease, psychiatric illness (avoid if severe), endocrine disorders (including hyperthyroidism, Cushing's syndrome, diabetes mellitus, osteomalacia, and phaeochromocytoma), and in those with a history of convulsions, malignant melanoma, or peptic ulcer. Levodopa should be used with caution in open-angle glaucoma and patients susceptible to angle-closure glaucoma, and in hepatic or renal impairment. Patients should be advised to avoid abrupt withdrawal (risk of neuroleptic malignant

syndrome and rhabdomyolysis), and to be aware of the potential for excessive drowsiness and sudden onset of sleep (see Sudden Onset of Sleep, below). Levodopa should be used with caution in pregnancy (Appendix 4); **interactions:** Appendix 1 (levodopa).

**Contra-indications** Levodopa should be avoided in breast-feeding (Appendix 5).

**Side-effects** Side-effects of levodopa include nausea, vomiting, taste disturbances, dry mouth, anorexia, arrhythmias, postural hypotension, syncope, drowsiness (including sudden onset of sleep), fatigue, dementia, psychoses, hallucinations, confusion, euphoria, abnormal dreams, insomnia, depression (*very rarely* with suicidal ideation), anxiety, dizziness, dystonia, dyskinesia, and chorea.

*Less commonly* weight loss or gain, constipation, diarrhoea, hypersalivation, dysphagia, flatulence, hypertension, chest pain, oedema, hoarseness, ataxia, increased hand tremor, malaise, muscle cramps, and reddish discoloration of the urine and other body fluids may occur. *Rare* side-effects include abdominal pain, gastro-intestinal bleeding, dyspepsia, phlebitis, dyspnoea, agitation, paraesthesia, bruxism, trismus, hiccups, neuroleptic malignant syndrome (associated with abrupt withdrawal), convulsions, reduced mental acuity, disorientation, headache, urinary retention, urinary incontinence, priapism, activation of malignant melanoma, leucopenia, haemolytic and non-haemolytic anaemia, thrombocytopenia, agranulocytosis, blurred vision, blepharospasm, diplopia, activation of Horner's syndrome, pupil dilatation, oculogyric crisis, angio-edema, rash, urticaria, pruritus, flushing, alopecia, exanthema, Henoch-Schönlein purpura, and increased sweating. *Very rarely* angle-closure glaucoma may occur; pathological gambling, increased libido, hypersexuality, and false positive tests for urinary ketones have also been reported.

> ### Sudden onset of sleep
>
> Excessive daytime sleepiness and sudden onset of sleep can occur with co-careldopa, co-beneldopa, and dopamine receptor agonists.
>
> Patients starting treatment with these drugs should be warned of the possibility of these effects and of the need to exercise caution when driving or operating machinery.
>
> Patients who have suffered excessive sedation or sudden onset of sleep, should refrain from driving or operating machines until those effects have stopped recurring.

## ■ CO-BENELDOPA

A mixture of benserazide hydrochloride and levodopa in mass proportions corresponding to 1 part of benserazide and 4 parts of levodopa

**Indications** parkinsonism (but not drug-induced extrapyramidal symptoms), see notes above

**Cautions** see notes above

**Contra-indications** see notes above

**Side-effects** see notes above

**Dose**

● See preparations

**Madopar®** (Roche) PoM

Capsules 62.5, blue/grey, co-beneldopa 12.5/50 (benserazide 12.5 mg (as hydrochloride), levodopa

50 mg). Net price 100-cap pack = £5.96. Label: 14, counselling, driving, see notes above

Capsules 125, blue/pink, co-beneldopa 25/100 (benserazide 25 mg (as hydrochloride), levodopa 100 mg). Net price 100-cap pack = £8.30. Label: 14, counselling, driving, see notes above

Capsules 250, blue/caramel, co-beneldopa 50/200 (benserazide 50 mg (as hydrochloride), levodopa 200 mg). Net price 100-cap pack = £14.16. Label: 14, counselling, driving, see notes above

Dispersible tablets 62.5, scored, co-beneldopa 12.5/50 (benserazide 12.5 mg (as hydrochloride), levodopa 50 mg). Net price 100-tab pack = £7.08. Label: 14, counselling, administration, see below, driving, see notes above

Dispersible tablets 125, scored, co-beneldopa 25/100 (benserazide 25 mg (as hydrochloride) levodopa 100 mg). Net price 100-tab pack = £12.55. Label: 14, counselling, administration, see below, driving, see notes above

Note The tablets can be dispersed in water or orange squash (not orange juice) or swallowed whole

Dose expressed as levodopa, initially 50 mg 3–4 times daily (100 mg 3 times daily in advanced disease), increased by 100 mg daily once or twice weekly according to response; usual maintenance dose 400–800 mg daily in divided doses; ELDERLY initially 50 mg once or twice daily, increased by 50 mg daily every 3–4 days according to response

Note When transferring patients from another levodopa/dopa-decarboxylase inhibitor preparation, the previous preparation should be discontinued 12 hours before (although interval can be shorter)

◢Modified release
**Madopar®** CR (Roche) PoM
Capsules 125, m/r, dark green/light blue, co-beneldopa 25/100 (benserazide 25 mg (as hydrochloride), levodopa 100 mg). Net price 100-cap pack = £15.34. Label: 5, 14, 25, counselling, driving, see notes above

Dose Patients not taking levodopa/dopa-decarboxylase inhibitor therapy, initially 1 capsule 3 times daily (max. initial dose 6 capsules daily)

Patients transferring from immediate-release levodopa/dopa-decarboxylase inhibitor preparations, initially 1 capsule substituted for every 100 mg of levodopa and given at same dosage frequency, increased every 2–3 days according to response; average increase of 50% needed over previous levodopa dose and titration may take up to 4 weeks

Supplementary dose of immediate-release *Madopar®* may be needed with first morning dose; if response still poor to total daily dose of *Madopar®* CR plus *Madopar®* corresponding to 1.2 g levodopa, consider alternative therapy

## CO-CARELDOPA

A mixture of carbidopa and levodopa; the proportions are expressed in the form $x/y$ where $x$ and $y$ are the strengths in milligrams of carbidopa and levodopa respectively

**Indications** parkinsonism (but not drug-induced extrapyramidal symptoms), see notes above

**Cautions** see notes above

**Contra-indications** see notes above

**Side-effects** see notes above

**Dose**
- Expressed as levodopa, initially 100 mg (with carbidopa 25 mg) 3 times daily, increased by 50–100 mg (with carbidopa 12.5–25 mg) daily or on alternate days according to response, up to 800 mg (with carbidopa 200 mg) daily in divided doses

- Alternatively, initially 50–100 mg (with carbidopa 10–12.5 mg) 3–4 times daily, increased by 50–100 mg daily or on alternate days according to response, up to 800 mg (with carbidopa 80–100 mg) daily in divided doses

- Alternatively, initially 125 mg (with carbidopa 12.5 mg, as ½ tablet of co-careldopa 25/250) 1–2 times daily, increased by 125 mg (with carbidopa 12.5 mg) daily or on alternate days according to response

Note At least 70 mg carbidopa daily is necessary to achieve full inhibition of peripheral dopa-decarboxylase. When transferring patients from another levodopa/dopa-decarboxylase inhibitor preparation, the previous preparation should be discontinued at least 12 hours before

**Co-careldopa** (Non-proprietary) PoM
Tablets, co-careldopa 10/100 (carbidopa 10 mg (anhydrous), levodopa 100 mg), net price 100-tab pack = £17.38. Label: 14, counselling, driving, see notes above

Tablets, co-careldopa 25/100 (carbidopa 25 mg (anhydrous), levodopa 100 mg), net price 100-tab pack = £21.86. Label: 14, counselling, driving, see notes above

Tablets, co-careldopa 25/250 (carbidopa 25 mg (anhydrous), levodopa 250 mg), net price 100-tab pack = £29.27. Label: 14, counselling, driving, see notes above

**Sinemet®** (Bristol-Myers Squibb) PoM
Sinemet-62.5 tablets, yellow, scored, co-careldopa 12.5/50 (carbidopa 12.5 mg (anhydrous), levodopa 50 mg), net price 90-tab pack = £6.28. Label: 14, counselling, driving, see notes above

Note 2 tablets *Sinemet-62.5®* = 1 tablet *Sinemet Plus®*

Sinemet-110 tablets, blue, scored, co-careldopa 10/100 (carbidopa 10 mg (anhydrous), levodopa 100 mg), net price 90-tab pack = £6.57. Label: 14, counselling, driving, see notes above

Sinemet-Plus tablets, yellow, scored, co-careldopa 25/100 (carbidopa 25 mg (anhydrous), levodopa 100 mg), net price 90-tab pack = £9.66. Label: 14, counselling, driving, see notes above

Note Co-careldopa 25/100 provides an adequate dose of carbidopa when low doses of levodopa are needed

Sinemet-275 tablets, blue, scored, co-careldopa 25/250 (carbidopa 25 mg (anhydrous), levodopa 250 mg), net price 90-tab pack = £13.72. Label: 14, counselling, driving, see notes above

◢For use with enteral tube
**Duodopa®** (Solvay) ▼ PoM
Intestinal gel, co-careldopa 5/20 (carbidopa 5 mg as monohydrate, levodopa 20 mg)/mL, net price 100 mL cassette (for use with *Duodopa®* portable pump) = £77.00. Label: 14, counselling, driving, see notes above

Dose Severe Parkinson's disease inadequately controlled by other preparations, consult product literature

◢Modified release
**Caramet®** CR (TEVA UK) PoM
Tablets, m/r, orange-brown, co-careldopa 25/100 (carbidopa 25 mg (as monohydrate), levodopa 100 mg), net price 60-tab pack = £11.47; co-careldopa 50/200 (carbidopa 50 mg (as monohydrate), levodopa

**Central nervous system** (4)

200 mg), 60-tab pack = £11.47. Label: 14, 25, counselling, driving, see notes above

**Dose** patients not receiving levodopa/dopa-decarboxylase inhibitor preparations, expressed as levodopa, initially 100–200 mg twice daily (at least 6 hours between doses); dose adjusted according to response at intervals of at least 2 days

Patients transferring from immediate-release levodopa/dopa-decarboxylase inhibitor preparations, discontinue previous preparation at least 12 hours before first dose of *Caramet® CR*; substitute *Caramet® CR* to provide a similar amount of levodopa daily and extend dosing interval by 30–50%; dose then adjusted according to response at intervals of at least 2 days

### Half Sinemet® CR (Bristol-Myers Squibb) [PoM]

Tablets, m/r, pink, co-careldopa 25/100 (carbidopa 25 mg (anhydrous), levodopa 100 mg), net price 60-tab pack = £11.60. Label: 14, 25, counselling, driving, see notes above

**Dose** For fine adjustment of *Sinemet® CR* dose (see below)

### Sinemet® CR (Bristol-Myers Squibb) [PoM]

Tablets, m/r, peach, scored, co-careldopa 50/200 (carbidopa 50 mg (anhydrous), levodopa 200 mg), net price 60-tab pack = £11.60. Label: 14, 25, counselling, driving, see notes above

**Dose** Patients not receiving levodopa/dopa-decarboxylase inhibitor therapy, initially, 1 *Sinemet® CR* tablet twice daily; both dose and interval then adjusted according to response at intervals of not less than 3 days

Patients transferring from immediate-release levodopa/dopa-decarboxylase inhibitor preparations, 1 *Sinemet® CR* tablet twice daily can be substituted for a daily dose of levodopa 300–400 mg in immediate-release *Sinemet®* tablets (substitute *Sinemet® CR* to provide approx. 10% more levodopa per day and extend dosing interval by 30–50%); dose and interval then adjusted according to response at intervals of not less than 3 days

### ◢With entacapone

**Note** For Parkinson's disease and end-of-dose motor fluctuations not adequately controlled with levodopa and dopa-decarboxylase inhibitor treatment

### Stalevo® (Orion) [PoM]

Stalevo 50 mg/12.5 mg/200 mg tablets, f/c, brown, levodopa 50 mg, carbidopa 12.5 mg, entacapone 200 mg, net price 30-tab pack = £21.11, 100-tab pack = £70.37. Label: 14 (urine reddish-brown), 25, counselling, driving, see notes above, avoid iron-containing preparations at the same time of day

**Dose** only 1 tablet to be taken for each dose; max. 10 tablets daily

Stalevo 75 mg/18.75 mg/200 mg tablets, f/c, brown, levodopa 75 mg, carbidopa 18.75 mg, entacapone 200 mg, net price 30-tab pack = £21.11, 100-tab pack = £70.37. Label: 14 (urine reddish-brown), 25, counselling, driving, see notes above, avoid iron containing preparations at the same time of day

**Dose** only 1 tablet to be taken for each dose; max. 10 tablets daily

Stalevo 100 mg/25 mg/200 mg tablets, f/c, brown, levodopa 100 mg, carbidopa 25 mg, entacapone 200 mg, net price 30-tab pack = £21.11, 100-tab pack = £70.37. Label: 14 (urine reddish-brown), 25, counselling, driving, see notes above, avoid iron-containing preparations at the same time of day

**Dose** only 1 tablet to be taken for each dose; max. 10 tablets daily

Stalevo 125 mg/31.25 mg/200 mg tablets, f/c, brown, levodopa 125 mg, carbidopa 31.25 mg, entacapone 200 mg, net price 30-tab pack = £21.11, 100-tab pack = £70.37. Label: 14 (urine reddish-brown), 25, counselling, driving, see notes above, avoid iron-containing preparations at the same time of day

**Dose** only 1 tablet to be taken for each dose; max. 10 tablets daily

Stalevo 150 mg/37.5 mg/200 mg tablets, f/c, brown, levodopa 150 mg, carbidopa 37.5 mg, entacapone 200 mg, net price 30-tab pack = £21.11, 100-tab pack = £70.37. Label: 14 (urine reddish-brown), 25, counselling, driving, see notes above, avoid iron-containing preparations at the same time of day

**Dose** only 1 tablet to be taken for each dose; max. 10 tablets daily

Stalevo 200 mg/50 mg/200 mg tablets, f/c, brown, levodopa 200 mg, carbidopa 50 mg, entacapone 200 mg, net price 30-tab pack = £21.11, 100-tab pack = £70.37. Label: 14 (urine reddish-brown), 25, counselling, driving, see notes above, avoid iron containing preparations at the same time of day

**Dose** only 1 tablet to be taken for each dose; max. 7 tablets daily

**Note** Patients receiving standard-release co-careldopa or co-beneldopa alone, initiate *Stalevo®* at a dose that provides similar (or slightly lower) amount of levodopa

Patients with dyskinesia or receiving more than 800 mg levodopa daily, introduce entacapone before transferring to *Stalevo®* (levodopa dose may need to be reduced by 10–30% initially)

Patients receiving entacapone and standard-release co-careldopa or co-beneldopa, initiate *Stalevo®* at a dose that provides similar (or slightly higher) amount of levodopa

## Monoamine-oxidase-B inhibitors

**Rasagiline**, a monoamine-oxidase-B inhibitor, is licensed for the management of Parkinson's disease used alone or as an adjunct to levodopa for 'end-of-dose' fluctuations.

**Selegiline** is a monoamine-oxidase-B inhibitor used in conjunction with levodopa to reduce 'end-of-dose' deterioration in advanced Parkinson's disease. Early treatment with selegiline alone can delay the need for levodopa therapy. When combined with levodopa, selegiline should be avoided or used with great caution in postural hypotension.

### RASAGILINE

**Indications** Parkinson's disease, used alone or as adjunct to levodopa with dopa-decarboxylase inhibitor

**Cautions** avoid abrupt withdrawal; hepatic impairment (Appendix 2); pregnancy (Appendix 4); breast-feeding (Appendix 5); **interactions:** Appendix 1 (rasagiline)

**Side-effects** dry mouth, dyspepsia, constipation; angina; headache, depression, anorexia, weight loss, abnormal dreams, vertigo, hallucinations; influenza-like symptoms; urinary urgency; leucopenia; arthralgia; conjunctivitis; rash; *less commonly* myocardial infarction, and cerebrovascular accident

**Dose**
● 1 mg daily

**Azilect®** (Teva) [PoM]
Tablets, rasagiline (as mesilate) 1 mg, net price 28-tab pack = £70.72

### SELEGILINE HYDROCHLORIDE

**Indications** Parkinson's disease, used alone or as adjunct to levodopa with dopa-decarboxylase inhibitor

**Cautions** avoid abrupt withdrawal; gastric and duodenal ulceration (avoid in active ulceration), uncontrolled hypertension, arrhythmias, angina, psychosis, side-effects of levodopa may be increased, concurrent levodopa dosage can be reduced by 10–20%; **interactions**: Appendix 1 (selegiline)

**Contra-indications** pregnancy (Appendix 4); breast-feeding (Appendix 5)

**Side-effects** nausea, constipation, diarrhoea, dry mouth; postural hypotension; dyskinesia, vertigo, sleeping disorders, confusion, hallucinations; arthralgia, myalgia; mouth ulcers with oral lyophilisate; *rarely* arrhythmias, agitation, headache, micturition difficulties, skin reactions; also reported chest pain

**Dose**

- 10 mg in the morning, or 5 mg at breakfast and midday; ELDERLY see below

    **Elderly** To avoid initial confusion and agitation, it may be appropriate to start treatment with a dose of 2.5 mg daily, particularly in the elderly

**Selegiline Hydrochloride** (Non-proprietary) [PoM]

Tablets, selegiline hydrochloride 5 mg, net price 56-tab pack = £4.99; 10 mg, 30-tab pack = £7.91

**Eldepryl®** (Orion) [PoM]

Tablets, both scored, selegiline hydrochloride 5 mg, net price 60-tab pack = £10.06; 10 mg, 30-tab pack = £9.82

Oral liquid, selegiline hydrochloride 10 mg/5 mL, net price 200 mL = £18.20

◢**Oral lyophilisate**

**Zelapar®** (Cephalon) [PoM]

Oral lyophilisates (= freeze-dried tablets), yellow, selegiline hydrochloride 1.25 mg, net price 30-tab pack = £47.96. Counselling, administration

Excipients include aspartame (section 9.4.1)

**Dose** 1.25 mg daily before breakfast

**Counselling** Tablets should be placed on the tongue and allowed to dissolve. Advise patient not to drink, rinse, or wash mouth out for 5 minutes after taking the tablet

**Note** Patients receiving 10 mg conventional selegiline hydrochloride tablets can be switched to *Zelapar®* 1.25 mg

## Catechol-*O*-methyltransferase inhibitors

**Entacapone** and **tolcapone** prevent the peripheral breakdown of levodopa, by inhibiting catechol-*O*-methyltransferase, allowing more levodopa to reach the brain. They are licensed for use as an adjunct to co-beneldopa or co-careldopa for patients with Parkinson's disease who experience 'end-of-dose' deterioration and cannot be stabilised on these combinations. Due to the risk of hepatotoxicity, tolcapone should be prescribed under specialist supervision only, when other catechol-*O*-methyltransferase inhibitors combined with co-beneldopa or co-careldopa are ineffective.

### ENTACAPONE

**Indications** adjunct to levodopa with dopa-decarboxylase inhibitor in Parkinson's disease and 'end-of-dose' motor fluctuations

**Cautions** avoid abrupt withdrawal; concurrent levodopa dose may need to be reduced by about 10–30%; **interactions**: Appendix 1 (entacapone)

**Contra-indications** pregnancy (Appendix 4); breast-feeding (Appendix 5); hepatic impairment; phaeochromocytoma; history of neuroleptic malignant syndrome or non-traumatic rhabdomyolysis

**Side-effects** nausea, vomiting, abdominal pain, constipation, diarrhoea, urine may be coloured reddish-brown, dry mouth; confusion, dizziness, abnormal dreams, fatigue, insomnia, dystonia, dyskinesia, hallucinations; increased sweating; *very rarely* hepatic dysfunction and rash; *very rarely* anorexia, weight loss, agitation, and urticaria; also reported colitis, neuroleptic malignant syndrome, rhabdomyolysis, and skin, hair, and nail discoloration

**Dose**

- 200 mg with each dose of levodopa with dopa-decarboxylase inhibitor; max. 2 g daily

**Comtess®** (Orion) [PoM]

Tablets, f/c, brown/orange, entacapone 200 mg, net price 30-tab pack = £17.50, 100-tab pack = £58.32. Label: 14, (urine reddish-brown), counselling, driving, see notes above, avoid iron-containing products at the same time of day

### TOLCAPONE

**Indications** adjunct to levodopa with dopa-decarboxylase inhibitor in Parkinson's disease and 'end-of-dose' motor fluctuations if another inhibitor of peripheral catechol-*O*-methyltransferase inappropriate (under specialist supervision)

**Cautions** avoid abrupt withdrawal; most patients receiving more than 600 mg levodopa daily require reduction of levodopa dose by about 30%; renal impairment (Appendix 3); pregnancy (Appendix 4); **interactions**: Appendix 1 (tolcapone)

**Hepatotoxicity** Potentially life-threatening hepatotoxicity including fulminant hepatitis reported rarely, usually in females and during the first 6 months, but late-onset liver injury has also been reported; test liver function before treatment, and monitor every 2 weeks for first year, every 4 weeks for next 6 months and every 8 weeks thereafter (restart monitoring schedule if dose increased); discontinue if abnormal liver function tests or symptoms of liver disorder (counselling, see below); do not re-introduce tolcapone once discontinued

**Counselling** Patients should be told how to recognise signs of liver disorder and advised to seek immediate medical attention if symptoms such as anorexia, nausea, vomiting, fatigue, abdominal pain, dark urine, or pruritus develop

**Contra-indications** hepatic impairment or raised liver enzymes (see Hepatotoxicity above); severe dyskinesia, phaeochromocytoma, previous history of neuroleptic malignant syndrome, rhabdomyolysis, or hyperthermia; breast-feeding (Appendix 5)

**Side-effects** diarrhoea, constipation, dyspepsia, abdominal pain, nausea, anorexia, xerostomia, hepatotoxicity (see above); chest pain; confusion, dystonia, dyskinesia, drowsiness, headache, dizziness, sleep disturbances, excessive dreaming, hallucinations; syncope; urine discoloration; sweating; neuroleptic malignant syndrome and rhabdomyolysis reported on dose reduction or withdrawal

**Dose**

- 100 mg 3 times daily, leave 6 hours between each dose; max. 200 mg 3 times daily in exceptional circumstances; first daily dose should be taken at the same time as levodopa with dopa-decarboxylase inhibitor

    **Note** Continue beyond 3 weeks **only** if substantial improvement

**Tasmar®** (Meda) ▼ [PoM]

Tablets, f/c, yellow, tolcapone 100 mg, net price 100-tab pack = £95.20. Label: 14, 25

**4**

**Central nervous system**

**4 Central nervous system**

## Amantadine

**Amantadine** is a weak dopamine agonist with modest antiparkinsonian effects. It improves mild bradykinetic disabilities as well as tremor and rigidity. It may also be useful for dyskinesias in more advanced disease. Tolerance to its effects may develop and confusion and hallucinations may occasionally occur. Withdrawal of amantadine should be gradual irrespective of the patient's response to treatment.

### ◼ AMANTADINE HYDROCHLORIDE

**Indications** Parkinson's disease (but not drug-induced extrapyramidal symptoms); antiviral (section 5.3.4)

**Cautions** hepatic impairment; renal impairment (avoid if eGFR less than 15 mL/minute/1.73 m²; Appendix 3), congestive heart disease (may exacerbate oedema), confused or hallucinatory states, elderly; avoid abrupt withdrawal in Parkinson's disease; **interactions:** Appendix 1 (amantadine)

Driving May affect performance of skilled tasks (e.g. driving)

**Contra-indications** epilepsy; history of gastric ulceration; pregnancy (Appendix 4), breast-feeding (Appendix 5)

**Side-effects** anorexia, nausea, nervousness, inability to concentrate, insomnia, dizziness, convulsions, hallucinations or feelings of detachment, blurred vision, gastro-intestinal disturbances, livedo reticularis and peripheral oedema; rarely leucopenia, rashes

**Dose**
- Parkinson's disease, 100 mg daily increased after one week to 100 mg twice daily, usually in conjunction with other treatment; some patients may require higher doses, max. 400 mg daily; ELDERLY 65 years and over, 100 mg daily adjusted according to response
- Post-herpetic neuralgia, 100 mg twice daily for 14 days, continued for a further 14 days if necessary

**Symmetrel®** (Alliance) PoM
Capsules, red-brown, amantadine hydrochloride 100 mg. Net price 56-cap pack = £16.22. Counselling, driving, see Cautions

Syrup, amantadine hydrochloride 50 mg/5 mL. Net price 150-mL pack = £5.33. Counselling, driving, see Cautions

**Lysovir®** (Alliance) PoM
See p. 355

### 4.9.2 Antimuscarinic drugs used in parkinsonism

Antimuscarinic drugs exert their antiparkinsonian action by reducing the effects of the relative central cholinergic excess that occurs as a result of dopamine deficiency. Antimuscarinic drugs can be useful in drug-induced parkinsonism, but they are generally not used in idiopathic Parkinson's disease because they are less effective than dopaminergic drugs and they are associated with cognitive impairment.

The antimuscarinic drugs **orphenadrine**, **procyclidine**, and **trihexyphenidyl** (benzhexol), reduce the symptoms of parkinsonism induced by antipsychotic drugs, but there is no justification for giving them routinely in the absence of parkinsonian side-effects. Tardive dyskinesia is not improved by antimuscarinic drugs and may be made worse.

In idiopathic Parkinson's disease, antimuscarinic drugs reduce tremor and rigidity but they have little effect on bradykinesia. They may be useful in reducing sialorrhoea.

No important differences exist between the antimuscarinic drugs, but some patients tolerate one better than another.

Procyclidine may be given parenterally and it is effective emergency treatment for acute drug-induced dystonic reactions.

**Cautions** Antimuscarinics should be used with caution in cardiovascular disease, hypertension, psychotic disorders, prostatic hypertrophy, pyrexia, in those susceptible to angle-closure glaucoma, and in the elderly. Antimuscarinics should not be withdrawn abruptly in patients receiving long-term treatment. Antimuscarinics are liable to abuse. They should also be used with caution in hepatic impairment, renal impairment, pregnancy (Appendix 4), and breast-feeding (Appendix 5). **Interactions:** Appendix 1 (Antimuscarinics)

**Driving** May affect performance of skilled tasks (e.g. driving)

**Contra-indications** Antimuscarinics should be avoided in gastro-intestinal obstruction and myasthenia gravis.

**Side-effects** Side-effects of antimuscarinics include constipation, dry mouth, nausea, vomiting, tachycardia, dizziness, confusion, euphoria, hallucinations, impaired memory, anxiety, restlessness, urinary retention, blurred vision, and rash. Angle-closure glaucoma may occur very rarely

### ◼ ORPHENADRINE HYDROCHLORIDE

**Indications** parkinsonism; drug-induced extrapyramidal symptoms (but not tardive dyskinesia, see notes above)

**Cautions** see notes above

**Contra-indications** see notes above; also acute porphyria (section 9.8.2)

**Side-effects** see notes above; *less commonly* insomnia and impaired coordination

**Dose**
- Initially 150 mg daily in divided doses, increased gradually in steps of 50 mg every 2–3 days according to response; usual dose range 150–300 mg daily in divided doses; max. 400 mg daily; ELDERLY preferably lower end of range

**Orphenadrine Hydrochloride** (Non-proprietary) PoM
Tablets, orphenadrine hydrochloride 50 mg, net price 20 = £11.13. Counselling, driving, see notes above

Oral solution, orphenadrine hydrochloride 50 mg/5 mL, net price 200 mL = £9.47. Counselling, driving, see notes above

**Biorphen®** (Alliance) PoM
Liquid, sugar-free, orphenadrine hydrochloride 25 mg/5 mL, net price 200 mL = £8.48. Counselling, driving, see notes above

**Disipal®** (Astellas) PoM
Tablets, yellow, s/c, orphenadrine hydrochloride 50 mg, net price 20 = 69p. Counselling, driving, see notes above
Excipients include tartrazine

## PROCYCLIDINE HYDROCHLORIDE

**Indications**   parkinsonism; drug-induced extrapyramidal symptoms (but not tardive dyskinesia, see notes above)

**Cautions**   see notes above

**Contra-indications**   see notes above

**Side-effects**   see notes above, but causes sedation rather than stimulation; also gingivitis

**Dose**

- By mouth, 2.5 mg 3 times daily, increased gradually in steps of 2.5–5 mg daily every 2–3 days if necessary; usual max. 30 mg daily in 2–4 divided doses (60 mg daily in exceptional circumstances); ELDERLY preferably lower end of range

- By intramuscular *or* intravenous injection, acute dystonia, 5–10 mg (occasionally more than 10 mg), usually effective in 5–10 minutes but may need 30 minutes for relief; ELDERLY preferably lower end of range

**Procyclidine** (Non-proprietary) ⓅⓄⓂ
Tablets, procyclidine hydrochloride 5 mg, net price 28-tab pack = £6.10. Counselling, driving, see notes above

**Arpicolin®** (Rosemont) ⓅⓄⓂ
Syrup, sugar-free, procyclidine hydrochloride 2.5 mg/ 5 mL, net price 150 mL = £4.22; 5 mg/5 mL, 150 mL pack = £7.54. Counselling, driving, see notes above

**Kemadrin®** (GSK) ⓅⓄⓂ
Tablets, scored, procyclidine hydrochloride 5 mg, net price 20 = 94p. Counselling, driving, see notes above

**Kemadrin®** (Auden Mckenzie) ⓅⓄⓂ
Injection, procyclidine hydrochloride 5 mg/mL, net price 2-mL amp = £1.49

## TRIHEXYPHENIDYL HYDROCHLORIDE
(Benzhexol hydrochloride)

**Indications**   parkinsonism; drug-induced extrapyramidal symptoms (but not tardive dyskinesia, see notes above)

**Cautions**   see notes above

**Contra-indications**   see notes above

**Side-effects**   see notes above

**Dose**

- 1 mg daily, increased gradually; usual maintenance dose 5–15 mg daily in 3–4 divided doses (max. 20 mg daily); ELDERLY preferably lower end of range

**Trihexyphenidyl** (Non-proprietary) ⓅⓄⓂ
Tablets, trihexyphenidyl hydrochloride 2 mg, net price 84-tab pack = £25.53; 5 mg, 100-tab pack = £15.60. Counselling, with or after food, driving, see notes above

**Broflex®** (Alliance) ⓅⓄⓂ
Syrup, pink, black currant, trihexyphenidyl hydrochloride 5 mg/5 mL, net price 200 mL = £7.44. Counselling, driving, see notes above

## 4.9.3 Drugs used in essential tremor, chorea, tics, and related disorders

**Tetrabenazine** is mainly used to control movement disorders in Huntington's chorea and related disorders. It may act by depleting nerve endings of dopamine. It has useful action in only a proportion of patients and its use may be limited by the development of depression.

**Haloperidol** may be useful in improving motor tics and symptoms of Tourette syndrome and related choreas. **Pimozide** [unlicensed indication] (see section 4.2.1 for CSM warning), **clonidine** [unlicensed indication] (section 4.7.4.2), and **sulpiride** [unlicensed indication] (section 4.2.1) are also used in Tourette syndrome. **Trihexyphenidyl (benzhexol)** (section 4.9.2) in high dosage can also improve some movement disorders; it is sometimes necessary to build the dose up over many weeks, to 20 to 30 mg daily or higher. **Chlorpromazine** and **haloperidol** are used to relieve intractable hiccup (section 4.2.1).

**Propranolol** or another beta-adrenoceptor blocking drug (section 2.4) may be useful in treating essential tremor or tremors associated with anxiety or thyrotoxicosis. Propranolol is given in a dosage of 40 mg 2 or 3 times daily, increased if necessary; 80 to 160 mg daily is usually required for maintenance.

**Primidone** (section 4.8.1) in some cases provides relief from benign essential tremor; the dose is increased slowly to reduce side-effects.

**Piracetam** is used as an adjunctive treatment for myoclonus of cortical origin.

**Riluzole** is used to extend life in patients with motor neurone disease who have amyotrophic lateral sclerosis.

> **NICE guidance**
> **Riluzole for motor neurone disease (January 2001)**
> Riluzole is recommended for treating the amyotrophic lateral sclerosis (ALS) form of motor neurone disease (MND). Treatment should be initiated by a specialist in MND but it can then be supervised under a shared-care arrangement involving the general practitioner.

## HALOPERIDOL

**Indications**   motor tics, adjunctive treatment in choreas and Tourette syndrome; other indications, section 4.2.1

**Cautions**   section 4.2.1

**Contra-indications**   section 4.2.1

**Side-effects**   section 4.2.1

**Dose**

- By mouth, 0.5–1.5 mg 3 times daily adjusted according to the response; 10 mg daily or more may occasionally be necessary in Tourette syndrome; CHILD 5–12 years, Tourette syndrome, 12.5–

**4**

**Central nervous system**

25 microgram/kg twice daily, adjusted according to response up to max. 10 mg daily

◄**Preparations**
Section 4.2.1

## PIRACETAM

**Indications** adjunctive treatment of cortical myoclonus

**Cautions** avoid abrupt withdrawal; elderly; haemostasis, major surgery, or severe haemorrhage; renal impairment (avoid if eGFR less than 20 mL/minute; Appendix 3)

**Contra-indications** cerebral haemorrhage; hepatic impairment; pregnancy; breast-feeding

**Side-effects** weight gain, nervousness, hyperkinesia; *less commonly* drowsiness, depression, asthenia,; *also reported* abdominal pain, nausea, vomiting, diarrhoea, headache, anxiety, confusion, hallucination, vertigo, ataxia, insomnia, and rash

**Dose**

* Initially 7.2 g daily in 2–3 divided doses, increased according to response by 4.8 g daily every 3–4 days to max. 20 g daily (subsequently, attempts should be made to reduce dose of concurrent therapy); CHILD under 16 years not recommended
  **Oral solution** Follow the oral solution with a glass of water (or soft drink) to reduce bitter taste.

**Nootropil®** (UCB Pharma) [PoM]
Tablets, f/c, scored, piracetam 800 mg, net price 90-tab pack = £11.75; 1.2 g, 60-tab pack = £10.97. Label: 3

Oral solution, piracetam, 333.3 mg/mL, net price 300-mL pack = £16.31. Label: 3

## RILUZOLE

**Indications** to extend life in patients with amyotrophic lateral sclerosis, initiated by specialists experienced in the management of motor neurone disease

**Cautions** history of abnormal hepatic function (consult product literature for details)
**Blood disorders** Patients or their carers should be told how to recognise signs of neutropenia and advised to seek immediate medical attention if symptoms such as fever occur; white blood cell counts should be determined in febrile illness; neutropenia requires discontinuation of riluzole
**Driving** Dizziness or vertigo may affect performance of skilled tasks (e.g. driving)

**Contra-indications** hepatic impairment; renal impairment (Appendix 3); pregnancy (Appendix 4); breast-feeding (Appendix 5)

**Side-effects** nausea, vomiting, diarrhoea, abdominal pain; tachycardia; asthenia, headache, dizziness, drowsiness, oral paraesthesia; *less commonly* pancreatitis and anaemia; *rarely* neutropenia; *very rarely* hepatitis

**Dose**

* 50 mg twice daily; CHILD not recommended

**Rilutek®** (Aventis Pharma) [PoM]
Tablets, f/c, riluzole 50 mg. Net price 56-tab pack = £242.39. Counselling, blood disorders, driving, see Cautions

## TETRABENAZINE

**Indications** see under Dose

**Cautions** pregnancy (Appendix 4); avoid in breast-feeding; **interactions:** Appendix 1 (tetrabenazine)
Driving May affect performance of skilled tasks (e.g. driving)

**Side-effects** drowsiness, gastro-intestinal disturbances, depression, extrapyramidal dysfunction, hypotension; *rarely* parkinsonism; neuroleptic malignant syndrome reported

**Dose**

* Movement disorders due to Huntington's chorea, hemiballismus, senile chorea, and related neurological conditions, initially 12.5 mg twice daily (elderly 12.5 mg daily) gradually increased to 12.5–25 mg 3 times daily; max. 200 mg daily

* Moderate to severe tardive dyskinesia, initially 12.5 mg daily, gradually increased according to response

**Xenazine® 25** (Cambridge) [PoM]
Tablets, yellow, scored, tetrabenazine 25 mg. Net price 112-tab pack = £100.00. Label: 2

# Torsion dystonias and other involuntary movements

Botulinum toxin type A should be used under specialist supervision. *Botox®* and *Dysport®* are licensed for the treatment of focal spasticity (including arm symptoms in conjunction with physiotherapy, dynamic equinus foot deformity caused by spasticity in ambulant paediatric cerebral palsy patients over 2 years of age, hand and wrist disability associated with stroke), blepharospasm, hemifacial spasm, and spasmodic torticollis. *Botox®* is also licensed for severe hyperhidrosis of the axillae.

*Vistabel®* is licensed for the temporary improvement of moderate to severe wrinkles between the eyebrows.

*Xeomin®* is licensed for the treatment of blepharospasm and spasmodic torticollis.

## BOTULINUM TOXIN TYPE A

**Indications** see notes above; preparations are **not** interchangeable and should be used under specialist supervision

**Cautions** history of dysphagia or aspiration; neurological disorders (can lead to increased sensitivity and exaggerated muscle weakness); pregnancy (Appendix 4); breast-feeding (Appendix 5)
**Specific cautions for blepharospasm or hemifacial spasm** Caution if risk of angle-closure glaucoma; reduced blinking can lead to corneal exposure, persistent epithelial defect and corneal ulceration (especially in those with VIIth nerve disorders)—careful testing of corneal sensation in previously operated eyes, avoidance of injection in lower lid area to avoid ectropion, and vigorous treatment of epithelial defect needed

**Contra-indications** generalised disorders of muscle activity (e.g. myasthenia gravis)

**Side-effects** increased electrophysiologic jitter in some distant muscles; misplaced injections may paralyse nearby muscle groups and excessive doses may paralyse distant muscles; influenza-like symptoms; *rarely* arrhythmias, myocardial infarction, seizures, hypersensitivity reactions including rash, pruritus and anaphylaxis, antibody formation (substantial deterioration in response), and injection-site reactions; *very rarely* exaggerated muscle weakness, dysphagia, and aspiration (seek medical attention if swallowing, speech, or respiratory disorders)

**Specific side-effects for blepharospasm or hemifacial spasm** Ptosis; keratitis, lagophthalmos, dry eye, irritation, photophobia, lacrimation; facial oedema; *less commonly* dry mouth, facial weakness (including drooping), dizziness, tiredness, ectropion, entropion, diplopia, visual disturbances, conjunctivitis; *rarely* eyelid bruising and swelling (minimised by applying gentle pressure at injection site immediately after injection); *very rarely* angle-closure glaucoma, corneal ulceration

**Specific side-effects in paediatric cerebral palsy** Drowsiness, paraesthesia, urinary incontinence, myalgia

**Specific side-effects for temporary improvement of moderate to severe wrinkles between the eyebrows** Headache; ptosis; *less commonly* nausea, dry mouth, facial oedema, dizziness, asthenia, anxiety, paraesthesia, visual disturbances, blepharitis, photosensitivity reactions, and dry skin

**Specific side-effects in spasmodic torticollis** Dysphagia and pooling of saliva (occurs most frequently after injection into sternomastoid muscle), nausea, dry mouth, rhinitis, drowsiness, headache, dizziness, hypertonia, stiffness; *less commonly* dyspnoea, voice alteration, diplopia, and ptosis

**Specific side-effects in axillary hyperhidrosis** Non-axillary sweating, hot flushes; *less commonly* myalgia and joint pain

**Specific side-effects in focal upper-limb spasticity associated with stroke** Dysphagia; hypertonia; *less commonly* arthralgia and bursitis

**Dose**

* Consult product literature (**important:** specific to **each individual preparation** and **not interchangeable**)

**Botox®** (Allergan) (PoM)
Injection, powder for reconstitution, botulinum toxin type A complex, net price 50-unit vial = £77.50, 100-unit vial = £138.20

**Dysport®** (Ipsen) (PoM)
Injection, powder for reconstitution, botulinum toxin-haemagglutinin complex type A , net price 500-unit vial = £157.00

**Vistabel®** (Allergan) (PoM)
Injection, powder for reconstitution, botulinum toxin type A, net price 50-unit vial = £85.00

**Xeomin®** (Merz) ▼ (PoM)
Injection, powder for reconstitution, botulinum toxin type A, net price 100-unit vial = £119.90

---

## ▌ BOTULINUM TOXIN TYPE B

**Indications** spasmodic torticollis (cervical dystonia)—specialist use only

**Cautions** history of dysphagia or aspiration; inadvertent injection into a blood vessel; tolerance may occur

**Contra-indications** neuromuscular or neuromuscular junctional disorders; pregnancy (Appendix 4) and breast-feeding (Appendix 5)

**Side-effects** increased electrophysiologic jitter in some distant muscles; dry mouth, dyspepsia, worsening torticollis, neck pain, myasthenia, voice changes, taste disturbances; *very rarely* exaggerated muscle weakness, dysphagia, and aspiration (seek medical attention if swallowing, speech, or respiratory disorders)

**Dose**

* By intramuscular injection, initially 5000–10 000 units divided between 2–4 most affected muscles; adjust dose and frequency according to response; **important: not** interchangeable with other botulinum toxin preparations

**NeuroBloc®** (Eisai) (PoM)
Injection, botulinum toxin type B 5000 units/mL, net price 0.5-mL vial = £111.20; 1-mL vial = £148.27; 2-mL vial = £197.69
Note May be diluted with sodium chloride 0.9%

---

## ▌4.10 Drugs used in substance dependence

This section includes drugs used in alcohol dependence, cigarette smoking, and opioid dependence.

The health departments of the UK have produced a report, *Drug Misuse and Dependence* which contains guidelines on clinical management.

*Drug Misuse and Dependence*, London, The Stationery Office, 1999 can be obtained from:

The Publications Centre
PO Box 276
London, SW8 5DT
Tel: (087) 0600 5522
Fax: (087) 0600 5533

*or* from The Stationery Office bookshops and through all good booksellers.

It is **important** to be aware that *people who misuse drugs* may be at risk not only from the intrinsic toxicity of the drug itself but also from the practice of injecting preparations intended for administration by mouth. Excipients used in the production of oral dose forms are usually insoluble and may lead to *abscess formation at the site of injection*, or even to *necrosis and gangrene*; moreover, deposits in the heart or lungs may lead to *severe cardiac or pulmonary toxicity*. Additional hazards include *infection* following the use of a dirty needle or an unsterilised diluent.

---

### Alcohol dependence

**Disulfiram** is used as an adjunct to the treatment of alcohol dependence. It gives rise to extremely unpleasant systemic reactions after the ingestion of even a small amount of alcohol because it leads to accumulation of acetaldehyde in the body. Reactions include flushing of the face, throbbing headache, palpitation, tachycardia, nausea, vomiting, and, with large doses of alcohol, arrhythmias, hypotension, and collapse. Small amounts of alcohol included in many oral medicines may be sufficient to precipitate a reaction (even toiletries and mouthwashes that contain alcohol should be avoided). It may be advisable for patients to carry a card warning of the danger of administration of alcohol.

Long-acting **benzodiazepines** (section 4.1) are used to attenuate withdrawal symptoms but they also have a dependence potential. To minimise the risk of dependence, administration should be for a limited period only (e.g. **chlordiazepoxide** 10–50 mg 4 times daily, gradually reducing over 7–14 days). Benzodiazepines should not be prescribed if the patient is likely to continue drinking alcohol.

**Clomethiazole** (chlormethiazole) (section 4.1.1) should be used for the management of withdrawal in an **inpatient setting only**. It is associated with a risk of dependence and should not be prescribed if the patient is likely to continue drinking alcohol.

**Acamprosate**, in combination with counselling, may be helpful in maintaining abstinence in alcohol-dependent patients. It should be initiated as soon as possible *after* abstinence has been achieved and should be maintained if the patient relapses. Continued alcohol abuse, however, negates the therapeutic benefit of acamprosate.

### ACAMPROSATE CALCIUM

**Indications** maintenance of abstinence in alcohol dependence

**Cautions** continued alcohol abuse (risk of treatment failure)

**Contra-indications** severe hepatic impairment; renal impairment (avoid if serum creatinine over 120 micromol/litre; Appendix 3); pregnancy; breast-feeding

**Side-effects** diarrhoea, nausea, vomiting, abdominal pain; fluctuation in libido; pruritus, maculopapular rash; *rarely* bullous skin reactions

**Dose**

● ADULT 18–65 years, body-weight 60 kg and over, 666 mg 3 times daily; body-weight less than 60 kg, 666 mg at breakfast, 333 mg at midday and 333 mg at night

**Treatment course** Treatment should be initiated as soon as possible after alcohol withdrawal period and maintained if patient relapses; recommended treatment period 1 year

**Campral EC®** (Merck) (PoM)
Tablet, e/c, acamprosate calcium 333 mg, net price 168-tab pack = £24.00. Label: 21, 25
Electrolytes Ca²⁺ 0.8 mmol/tablet

### DISULFIRAM

**Indications** adjunct in the treatment of chronic alcohol dependence (under specialist supervision)

**Cautions** ensure that alcohol not consumed for at least 24 hours before initiating treatment; see also notes above; alcohol challenge **not** recommended on routine basis (if considered essential—specialist units only with resuscitation facilities); hepatic or renal impairment, respiratory disease, diabetes mellitus, epilepsy; **interactions**: Appendix 1 (disulfiram)
**Alcohol reaction** Patients should be warned of unpredictable and occasionally severe nature of disulfiram-alcohol interactions. Reactions can occur within 10 minutes and last several hours (may require intensive supportive therapy—oxygen should be available). Patients should not ingest alcohol at all and should be warned of possible presence of alcohol in liquid medicines, remedies, tonics, foods and even in toiletries (alcohol should also be avoided for at least 1 week after stopping)

**Contra-indications** cardiac failure, coronary artery disease, history of cerebrovascular accident, hypertension, psychosis, severe personality disorder, suicide risk, pregnancy (Appendix 4), breast-feeding (Appendix 5)

**Side-effects** initially drowsiness and fatigue; nausea, vomiting, halitosis, reduced libido; rarely psychotic reactions (depression, paranoia, schizophrenia,

mania), allergic dermatitis, peripheral neuritis, hepatic cell damage

**Dose**

● 800 mg as a single dose on first day, reducing over 5 days to 100–200 mg daily; should not be continued for longer than 6 months without review; CHILD not recommended

**Antabuse®** (Actavis) (PoM)
Tablets, scored, disulfiram 200 mg. Net price 50-tab pack = £25.26. Label: 2, counselling, alcohol reaction

---

## Cigarette smoking

Smoking cessation interventions are a cost-effective way of reducing ill health and prolonging life. Smokers should be advised to stop and offered help if interested in doing so, with follow-up when appropriate.

When possible, smokers should have access to a smoking cessation clinic for behavioural support. **Nicotine replacement therapy** and **bupropion** are effective aids to smoking cessation for those smoking more than 10 cigarettes a day. **Bupropion** has been used as an antidepressant but its mode of action in smoking cessation is not clear and may involve an effect on noradrenaline and dopamine neurotransmission. **Varenicline** is a selective nicotine receptor partial agonist used as an aid for smoking cessation. Nicotine replacement therapy is regarded as the pharmacological treatment of choice in the management of smoking cessation.

Cigarette smoking should stop completely before starting nicotine replacement therapy. If complete smoking cessation is not possible some nicotine preparations are licensed for use as part of a programme to reduce smoking before stopping completely; the smoking cessation regimen can be followed during a quit attempt.

**NICE guidance**
**Nicotine replacement therapy and bupropion for smoking cessation (March 2002)**
Nicotine replacement therapy or bupropion should be prescribed only for a smoker who commits to a target stop date. The smoker should be offered advice and encouragement to aid smoking cessation.
Therapy to aid smoking cessation is chosen according to the smoker's likely compliance, availability of counselling and support, previous experience of smoking-cessation aids, contra-indications and adverse effects of the products, and the smoker's preferences.
Initial supply of the prescribed smoking-cessation therapy should be sufficient to last only 2 weeks after the target stop date; normally this will be 2 weeks of nicotine replacement therapy or 3–4 weeks of bupropion. A second prescription should be issued only if the smoker demonstrates a continuing attempt to stop smoking.
If an attempt to stop smoking is unsuccessful, the NHS should not normally fund a further attempt within 6 months.
There is currently insufficient evidence to recommend the combined use of nicotine replacement therapy and bupropion.

NICE guidance
Varenicline for smoking cessation (July 2007)
Varenicline is recommended as an adjunct to smoking cessation for smokers who have expressed a desire to quit smoking; it should normally be prescribed only as a part of a programme of behavioural support.

### CSM advice (bupropion)
The CSM has issued a reminder that bupropion is contra-indicated in patients with a history of seizures or of eating disorders, a CNS tumour, or who are experiencing acute symptoms of alcohol or benzodiazepine withdrawal. Bupropion should not be prescribed to patients with other risk factors for seizures unless the potential benefit of smoking cessation clearly outweighs the risk. Factors that increase the risk of seizures include concomitant administration of drugs that can lower the seizure threshold (e.g. antidepressants, antimalarials [such as mefloquine and chloroquine], antipsychotics, quinolones, sedating antihistamines, systemic corticosteroids, theophylline, tramadol), alcohol abuse, history of head trauma, diabetes, and use of stimulants and anorectics.

## BUPROPION HYDROCHLORIDE
(Amfebutamone hydrochloride)

**Indications** see notes above

**Cautions** elderly; predisposition to seizures (see CSM advice above); measure blood pressure before and during treatment (monitor weekly if used with nicotine products); hepatic impairment (Appendix 2), renal impairment (Appendix 3); **interactions**: Appendix 1 (bupropion)
Driving May impair performance of skilled tasks (e.g. driving)

**Contra-indications** see CSM advice above; history of bipolar disorder; pregnancy (Appendix 4); breast-feeding (Appendix 5)

**Side-effects** dry mouth, gastro-intestinal disturbances, taste disturbance; insomnia (reduced by avoiding dose at bedtime), tremor, impaired concentration, headache, dizziness, depression, agitation, anxiety; fever; rash; pruritus; sweating; *less commonly* chest pain, tachycardia, hypertension, flushing, confusion, tinnitus, asthenia, and visual disturbances; *rarely* jaundice, hepatitis, palpitation, postural hypotension, hallucinations, depersonalisation, seizures, dystonia, ataxia, abnormal dreams, memory impairment, paraesthesia, blood-glucose disturbances, urinary retention, urinary frequency, Stevens-Johnson syndrome, and exacerbation of psoriasis; *very rarely* delusions, and aggression

**Dose**
• ADULT over 18 years, start 1–2 weeks before target stop date, initially 150 mg daily for 6 days then 150 mg twice daily (max. single dose 150 mg, max. daily dose 300 mg; minimum 8 hours between doses); period of treatment 7–9 weeks; discontinue if abstinence not achieved at 7 weeks; consider max. 150 mg daily in patients with risk factors for seizures (see CSM advice above); ELDERLY max. 150 mg daily

**Zyban®** (GSK) PoM
Tablets, m/r, f/c, bupropion hydrochloride 150 mg, net price 60-tab pack = £47.82. Label: 25, counselling, driving, see Cautions

## NICOTINE

**Indications** see notes above

**Cautions** severe or unstable cardiovascular disease (including hospitalisation for severe arrhythmias, recent myocardial infarction, or recent cerebrovascular accident)—initiate under medical supervision; uncontrolled hyperthyroidism; diabetes mellitus (monitor blood-glucose concentration closely when initiating treatment); phaeochromocytoma; *oral preparations*, oesophagitis, gastritis, peptic ulcers; *patches*, skin disorders (patches should not be placed on broken skin); hepatic impairment (Appendix 2); renal impairment (Appendix 3); pregnancy (Appendix 4); breast-feeding (Appendix 5)
Note Most warnings under Cautions also apply to continuation of cigarette smoking

**Side-effects** gastro-intestinal disturbances (including nausea, vomiting, dyspepsia); headache, dizziness; influenza-like symptoms; dry mouth; rash; *less frequently* palpitation; *rarely* atrial fibrillation; *with nasal spray*, sneezing, epistaxis, watering eyes, ear sensations; *with lozenges*, thirst, paraesthesia of mouth, taste disturbances; *with patches*, skin reactions (discontinue if severe)—vasculitis also reported, blood pressure changes; *with patches or lozenges*, sleep disturbances, nightmares, chest pain; *with gum or lozenges*, mouth ulceration, increased salivation; *with gum, lozenge, sublingual tablets*, or *inhalator*, hiccups, throat irritation

**Dose**
• See under preparations, below

**Nicopass®** (Fabre)
Lozenges, sugar-free, fresh mint- or liquorice mint-flavoured, nicotine (as resinate complex) 1.5 mg, net price pack of 12 = £1.68, pack of 36 = £4.18, pack of 96 = £8.94. Label: 24
Excipients include aspartame (section 9.4.1)
Dose smoking cessation, ADULT over 18 years (not heavily dependent on nicotine), initially suck 1 lozenge when urge to smoke occurs (max. 20 lozenges daily); withdraw gradually after 3 months; max. period of treatment 6 months

**Nicopatch®** (Fabre)
Patches, self-adhesive, nicotine '*7 mg*' *patch* (releasing approx. 7 mg/24 hours), net price 7 = £8.95; '*14 mg*' *patch* (releasing approx. 14 mg/24 hours), 7 = £8.95; '*21 mg*' *patch* (releasing approx. 21 mg/24 hours), 7 = £8.95
Dose smoking cessation, ADULT over 18 years, apply to dry, non-hairy skin site, removing after 24 hours and siting replacement patch on a different area (avoid using same area for 24 hours); individuals smoking *less than 20 cigarettes daily*, initially '14-mg' or '21-mg' patch daily (depending on severity of withdrawal symptoms); individuals smoking *20 or more cigarettes daily*, initially '21-mg' patch daily; withdraw gradually, reducing dose every 3–4 weeks; review treatment if abstinence not achieved within 3 months; max. period of treatment should not exceed 6 months

**Nicorette®** (McNeil)
Microtab (sublingual), nicotine (as a cyclodextrin complex) 2 mg, net price starter pack of 2 × 15-tablet discs with dispenser = £4.46; refill pack of 7 × 15-tablet discs = £12.04. Label: 26
Dose smoking cessation, individuals smoking *20 cigarettes or less daily*, sublingually, 2 mg each hour; for patients who fail to stop smoking or have significant withdrawal symptoms, consider

*4 Central nervous system*

Central nervous system

**4**

increasing to 4 mg each hour; individuals smoking *more than 20 cigarettes daily*, sublingually, 4 mg each hour; max. 80 mg daily; treatment continued for at least 3 months followed by a gradual reduction in dose; review treatment if abstinence not achieved within 9 months; CHILD 12–18 years, treatment continued for up to 8 weeks followed by gradual reduction over 4 weeks; review treatment if abstinence not achieved within 3 months

**Chewing gum**, sugar-free, nicotine (as resin) 2 mg, net price pack of 15 = £1.71, pack of 30 = £3.25, pack of 105 = £8.89; 4 mg, net price pack of 15 = £2.11, pack of 30 = £3.99, pack of 105 = £10.83
Note Also available in mint, freshfruit, freshmint, and icy white flavours

**Dose** smoking cessation, individuals smoking *20 cigarettes or less daily*, initially chew one 2-mg piece slowly (chew gum until taste becomes strong, then rest gum between cheek and gum, when taste fades start chewing again) for approx. 30 minutes when urge to smoke occurs; individuals smoking *more than 20 cigarettes daily* or needing more than 15 pieces of 2-mg gum daily should use the 4-mg strength; max. 15 pieces of 4-mg strength daily; withdraw gradually after 3 months; review treatment if abstinence not achieved within 9 months; CHILD 12–18 years, treatment continued for up to 8 weeks followed by gradual reduction over 4 weeks; review treatment if abstinence not achieved within 3 months

Smoking reduction, chew 1 piece when urge to smoke occurs between smoking episodes; reduce smoking within 6 weeks and attempt smoking cessation within 6 months; review treatment if abstinence not achieved within 9 months
Note Children under 18 years should consult a healthcare professional before starting smoking-reduction regimen

**Patches**, self-adhesive, beige, nicotine, *'5 mg' patch* (releasing approx. 5 mg/16 hours), net price 7 = £9.07; *'10 mg' patch* (releasing approx. 10 mg/16 hours), 7 = £9.07; *'15 mg' patch* (releasing approx. 15 mg/16 hours), 2 = £2.85, 7 = £9.07

**Dose** smoking cessation, ADULT and CHILD over 12 years, apply on waking to dry, non-hairy skin on hip, chest or upper arm, removing after approx. 16 hours, usually when retiring to bed; site next patch on different area (avoid using same area on consecutive days); initially '15-mg' patch for 16 hours daily for 8 weeks then if abstinence achieved '10-mg' patch for 16 hours daily for 2 weeks then '5-mg' patch for 16 hours daily for 2 weeks; review treatment if abstinence not achieved within 3 months—further courses may be given if considered beneficial

**Nicorette Invisi patches**, self-adhesive, beige, nicotine, *'10 mg' patch* (releasing approx. 10 mg/16 hours), net price 7 = £14.83; *'15 mg' patch* (releasing approx. 15 mg/16 hours), 7 = £14.83; *'25 mg' patch* (releasing approx. 25 mg/16 hours), 7 = £14.83

**Dose** smoking cessation, ADULT and CHILD over 12 years, apply on waking to dry, non-hairy skin on hip, chest or upper arm, removing after approx. 16 hours, usually when retiring to bed; site next patch on different area (avoid using same area on consecutive days); individuals smoking 10 or more cigarettes daily, initially '25-mg' patch for 16 hours daily for 8 weeks then if abstinence achieved '15-mg' patch for 16 hours daily for 2 weeks then '10-mg' patch for 16 hours daily for 2 weeks; individuals smoking less than 10 cigarettes daily, initially '15-mg' patch for 16 hours daily for 8 weeks then '10-mg' patch for 16 hours daily for 4 weeks; review treatment if abstinence not achieved within 3 months—further courses may be given if considered beneficial

Note Patients using the '25-mg' patch who experience excessive side-effects that do not resolve within a few days should change to '15-mg' patch for the remainder of the initial 8-week course before switching to the '10-mg' patch for the final 4 weeks

**Nasal spray**, nicotine 500 micrograms/metered spray, net price 200-spray unit = £13.30

**Dose** smoking cessation, ADULT and CHILD over 12 years, apply 1 spray into each nostril as required to max. twice an hour for 16 hours daily (max. 64 sprays daily) for 8 weeks, then reduce gradually over next 4 weeks (reduce by half at end of first 2 weeks, stop altogether at end of next 2 weeks); review treatment if abstinence not achieved within 3 months

**Inhalator** (nicotine-impregnated plug for use in inhalator mouthpiece), nicotine 10 mg/cartridge, net price

6-cartridge (starter) pack = £4.46, 42-cartridge (refill) pack = £14.02

**Dose** smoking cessation, ADULT and CHILD over 12 years, inhale when urge to smoke occurs; initially use between 6 and 12 cartridges daily for up to 8 weeks, then reduce number of cartridges used by half over next 2 weeks and then stop altogether at end of further 2 weeks; review treatment if abstinence not achieved within 3 months

Smoking reduction, ADULT and CHILD over 12 years, inhale when urge to smoke occurs between smoking episodes; reduce smoking within 6 weeks and attempt smoking cessation within 6 months; review treatment if abstinence not achieved within 9 months
Note Children under 18 years should consult a healthcare professional before starting a smoking-reduction regimen

**Nicotinell®** (Novartis Consumer Health)
**Chewing gum**, sugar-free, nicotine (as polacrilin complex) 2 mg, net price pack of 12 = £1.71, pack of 24 = £3.01, pack of 96 = £8.26, pack of 204 = £14.23; 4 mg, pack of 12 = £1.70, pack of 24 = £3.30, pack of 96 = £10.26
Note Also available in fruit, liquorice and mint flavours

**Dose** smoking cessation, individuals smoking *20 cigarettes or less daily*, initially chew one 2-mg piece slowly (chew gum until taste becomes strong, then rest gum between cheek and gum, when taste fades start chewing again) for approx. 30 minutes, when urge to smoke occurs; individuals smoking *more than 20 cigarettes daily* should use the 4-mg strength; max. 60 mg daily; withdraw gradually after 3 months; max. period of treatment should not usually exceed 6 months; CHILD 12–18 years, withdraw gradually and review treatment if abstinence not achieved within 3 months

**Mint lozenge**, sugar-free, nicotine (as bitartrate) 1 mg, net price pack of 12 = £1.71, pack of 36 = £4.27, pack of 96 = £9.12; 2 mg, net price pack of 12 = £1.99, pack of 36 = £4.95, pack of 96 = £10.60. Label: 24
Excipients include aspartame (section 9.4.1)

**Dose** smoking cessation, individuals smoking *30 cigarettes or less daily*, initially suck one 1-mg lozenge every 1–2 hours, when urge to smoke occurs; individuals smoking *more than 30 cigarettes daily* should use the 2-mg strength; max. 30 mg daily; withdraw gradually after 3 months; max. period of treatment should not usually exceed 6 months; CHILD 12–18 years, withdraw gradually and review treatment if abstinence not achieved within 3 months

**TTS Patches**, self-adhesive, all yellowish-ochre, nicotine, *'10' patch* (releasing approx. 7 mg/24 hours), net price 7 = £9.12; *'20' patch* (releasing approx. 14 mg/24 hours), net price 2 = £2.57, 7 = £9.40; *'30' patch* (releasing approx. 21 mg/24 hours), net price 2 = £2.85, 7 = £9.97, 21 = £24.51

**Dose** smoking cessation, ADULT and CHILD over 12 years, apply to dry, non-hairy skin on trunk or upper arm, removing after 24 hours and siting replacement patch on a different area (avoid using the same area for several days); individuals smoking *less than 20 cigarettes daily*, initially '20' patch daily; individuals smoking *20 or more cigarettes daily*, initially '30' patch daily; withdraw gradually, reducing dose every 3–4 weeks; review treatment if abstinence not achieved within 3 months

**NiQuitin®** (GSK Consumer Healthcare)
**Chewing gum**, sugar-free, mint-flavour, nicotine 2 mg (white), net price pack of 12 = £1.71, pack of 24 = £2.85, pack of 96 = £8.55; 4 mg (yellow), net price pack of 12 = £1.71, pack of 24 = £2.85, pack of 96 = £8.55

**Dose** smoking cessation, initially chew 1 piece slowly (chew gum until taste becomes strong, then rest gum between cheek and gum, when taste fades start chewing again) for approx. 30 minutes, when urge to smoke occurs; max. 15 pieces daily; withdraw gradually after 3 months; review treatment if abstinence not achieved within 9 months; CHILD 12–18 years, withdraw gradually and review treatment if abstinence not achieved within 3 months

Smoking reduction, chew 1 piece when urge to smoke occurs between smoking episodes (max. 15 pieces daily); reduce smoking within 6 weeks and attempt cessation within 6 months; review treatment if abstinence not achieved within 9 months
Note Children under 18 years should consult a healthcare professional before starting smoking-reduction regimen

Temporary abstinence, chew 1 piece when urge to smoke occurs between smoking episodes (max. 15 pieces daily); review treatment if unable to undertake permanent quit attempt within 6 months

Lozenges, sugar-free, nicotine (as polacrilex) 2 mg, net price pack of 36 = £5.12, pack of 72 = £9.97; 4 mg, pack of 36 = £5.12, pack of 72 = £9.97. Contains 0.65 mmol Na$^+$/lozenge. Label: 24

Excipients include aspartame (section 9.4.1)

Note Also available as *Pre-Quit 4 mg Lozenges*

Dose smoking cessation, initially suck 1 lozenge every 1–2 hours when urge to smoke occurs (max. 15 lozenges daily) for 6 weeks, then 1 lozenge every 2–4 hours for 3 weeks, then 1 lozenge every 4–8 hours for 3 weeks; withdraw gradually after 3 months; review treatment if abstinence not achieved within 9 months; CHILD 12–18 years, withdraw gradually and review treatment if abstinence not achieved within 3 months

Smoking reduction, suck 1 lozenge when urge to smoke occurs between smoking episodes (max. 15 lozenges daily); reduce smoking within 6 weeks and attempt cessation within 6 months; review treatment if abstinence not achieved within 9 months

Note Children under 18 years should consult a healthcare professional before starting smoking-reduction regimen

Temporary abstinence, suck 1 lozenge every 1–2 hours when urge to smoke occurs between smoking episodes (max. 15 lozenges daily); review treatment if unable to undertake permanent quit attempt within 6 months

Patches, self-adhesive, pink/beige, nicotine *'7 mg' patch* (releasing approx. 7 mg/24 hours), net price 7 = £9.97; *'14 mg' patch* (releasing approx. 14 mg/24 hours), 7 = £9.97; *'21 mg' patch* (releasing approx. 21 mg/24 hours), 7 = £9.97, 14 = £18.79

Note Also available as a clear patch

Dose smoking cessation, apply on waking to dry, non-hairy skin site, removing after 24 hours and siting replacement patch on different area (avoid using same area for 7 days); individuals smoking *10 or more cigarettes daily*, initially '21-mg' patch daily for 6 weeks then '14-mg' patch daily for 2 weeks then '7-mg' patch daily for 2 weeks; individuals smoking *less than 10 cigarettes daily*, initially '14-mg' patch daily for 6 weeks then '7-mg' patch daily for 2 weeks; review treatment if abstinence not achieved within 9 months; CHILD 12–18 years, withdraw gradually and review if abstinence not achieved within 3 months

Note Patients using the '21-mg' patch who experience excessive side-effects, which do not resolve within a few days, should change to '14-mg' patch for the remainder of the initial 6 weeks before switching to the '7-mg' patch for the final 2 weeks

## VARENICLINE

Indications see notes above

Cautions risk of relapse, irritability, depression, and insomnia on discontinuation (consider dose tapering on completion of 12-week course); history of psychiatric illness (may exacerbate underlying illness including depression); renal impairment (Appendix 3); breast-feeding (Appendix 5)

### MHRA/CHM advice
Suicidal behaviour and varenicline
Patients should be advised to discontinue treatment and seek prompt medical advice if they develop agitation, depressed mood, or suicidal thoughts. Patients with a history of psychiatric illness should be monitored closely while taking varenicline

Contra-indications pregnancy (Appendix 4)

Side-effects gastro-intestinal disturbances, appetite changes, dry mouth, taste disturbance; headache, drowsiness, dizziness, sleep disorders, abnormal dreams; *less commonly* thirst, weight gain, aphthous stomatitis, gingival pain, chest pain, hypertension,

tachycardia, atrial fibrillation, palpitation, panic attack, abnormal thinking, mood swings, dysarthria, asthenia, tremor, incoordination, hypertonia, restlessness, hypoaesthesia, impaired temperature regulation, menorrhagia, vaginal discharge, sexual dysfunction, dysuria, arthralgia, muscle spasm, visual disturbances, eye pain, lacrimation, tinnitus, acne, sweating, rash, and pruritus; myocardial infarction, depression, suicidal ideation (see MHRA/CHM advice above), and hypersensitivity reactions (angio-edema and facial swelling) also reported

Dose
- ADULT over 18 years, start 1–2 weeks before target stop date, initially 500 micrograms once daily for 3 days, increased to 500 micrograms twice daily for 4 days, then 1 mg twice daily for 11 weeks (reduce to 500 micrograms twice daily if not tolerated); 12-week course can be repeated in abstinent individuals to reduce risk of relapse

Champix® (Pfizer) ▼ PoM
Tablets, f/c, varenicline (as tartrate) 500 micrograms (white), net price 56-tab pack = £54.60; 1 mg (blue) 28-tab pack = £27.30, 56-tab pack = £54.60; starter pack of 11 × 500-microgram tabs with 14 × 1-mg tabs = £27.30. Label: 3

# Opioid dependence

The management of opioid dependence requires medical, social, and psychological treatment; access to a multidisciplinary team is valuable. Treatment with opioid substitutes or with naltrexone is best initiated under the supervision of an appropriately qualified physician.

Methadone, an opioid *agonist*, can be substituted for opioids such as diamorphine, preventing the onset of withdrawal symptoms; it is itself addictive and should only be prescribed for those who are physically dependent on opioids. It is administered in a single daily dose usually as methadone oral solution 1 mg/mL. The dose is adjusted according to the degree of dependence.

Buprenorphine is an opioid partial agonist. Because of its abuse and dependence potential it should be prescribed only for those who are already physically dependent on opioids. It can be used as substitution therapy for patients with moderate opioid dependence. In patients dependent on high doses of opioids, buprenorphine may precipitate withdrawal due to its partial antagonist properties; in these patients, the daily opioid dose should be reduced gradually before initiating therapy with buprenorphine.

Naltrexone, an opioid *antagonist*, blocks the action of opioids and precipitates withdrawal symptoms in opioid-dependent subjects. Because the euphoric action of opioid agonists is blocked by naltrexone it is given to former addicts as an aid to prevent relapse.

Lofexidine is used for the alleviation of symptoms in individuals whose opioid use is well controlled and are undergoing opioid withdrawal. Like clonidine it is an alpha-adrenergic agonist and appears to act centrally to produce a reduction in sympathetic tone, but reduction in blood pressure is less marked.

4

Central nervous system

## NICE guidance
### Methadone and buprenorphine for the management of opioid dependence (January 2007)

Oral methadone and buprenorphine are recommended for maintenance therapy in the management of opioid dependence. Patients should be committed to a supportive care programme including a flexible dosing regimen administered under supervision for at least 3 months, until compliance is assured. Selection of methadone or buprenorphine should be made on a case-by-case basis, but methadone should be prescribed if both drugs are equally suitable.

## NICE guidance
### Naltrexone for the management of opioid dependence (January 2007)

Naltrexone is recommended for the prevention of relapse in detoxified formerly opioid-dependent patients who are motivated to remain in a supportive care abstinence programme. Naltrexone should be administered under supervision and its effectiveness in preventing opioid misuse reviewed regularly.

## BUPRENORPHINE

**Indications** adjunct in the treatment of opioid dependence; premedication, peri-operative analgesia, analgesia in other situations (section 4.7.2)

**Cautions** see section 4.7.2 and notes above; effects only partially reversed by naloxone

**Contra-indications** see section 4.7.2; breast-feeding (Appendix 5)

**Side-effects** see section 4.7.2

**Dose**

- By sublingual administration, initially, 0.8–4 mg as a single daily dose, adjusted according to response; max. 32 mg daily; withdraw gradually; CHILD under 16 years not recommended

Note In patients who have not undergone opioid withdrawal, buprenorphine should be given at least 6 hours after last use of opioid or when signs of withdrawal appear
In patients receiving methadone, dose of methadone should be reduced to max. 30 mg daily before starting buprenorphine

**Buprenorphine** (Non-proprietary) ⒸⒹ

Tablets (sublingual), buprenorphine (as hydrochloride) 400 micrograms, net price 7-tab pack = £1.57; 2 mg, 7-tab pack = £6.71; 8 mg, 7-tab pack = £19.76. Label: 2, 26

**Subutex®** (Schering-Plough) ⒸⒹ

Tablets (sublingual), buprenorphine (as hydrochloride) 400 micrograms, net price 7-tab pack = £1.57; 2 mg, 7-tab pack = £6.59; 8 mg, 7-tab pack = £19.78. Label: 2, 26

◀With naloxone

**Suboxone®** (Schering-Plough) ▼ ⒸⒹ

Suboxone 2 mg/500 micrograms tablets (sublingual), buprenorphine (as hydrochloride) 2 mg, naloxone (as hydrochloride) 500 micrograms, net price 28-tab pack = £26.37. Label: 2, 26

Suboxone 8 mg/2 mg tablets (sublingual), buprenorphine (as hydrochloride) 8 mg, naloxone (as hydrochloride) 2 mg, net price 28-tab pack = £79.11. Label: 2, 26

Dose expressed as buprenorphine, ADULT and CHILD over 15 years, initially 2-8 mg once daily, increased in steps of 2–8 mg according to response; max. 24 mg daily; total weekly dose may be divided and given on alternate days or 3 times weekly (but max. daily dose 24 mg)

Note In patients who have not undergone opioid withdrawal, Suboxone® should be given when signs of withdrawal appear, at least 6 hours after last use of opioid

In patients receiving methadone, dose of methadone should be reduced to max. 30 mg daily before starting Suboxone®; first dose of Suboxone® should be given when signs of withdrawal appear, at least 24 hours after last dose of methadone

Note The Scottish Medicines Consortium has advised (February 2007) that Suboxone® should be restricted for use in patients in whom methadone is not suitable

## LOFEXIDINE HYDROCHLORIDE

**Indications** management of symptoms of opioid withdrawal

**Cautions** severe coronary insufficiency, recent myocardial infarction, cerebrovascular disease, marked bradycardia (monitor pulse rate); history of QT prolongation, concomitant administration of drugs that prolong QT interval; withdraw gradually over 2–4 days (or longer) to minimise risk of rebound hypertension and associated symptoms; renal impairment (Appendix 3); pregnancy (Appendix 4); breast-feeding (Appendix 5); interactions: Appendix 1 (lofexidine)

**Side-effects** dry mucous membranes, hypotension, bradycardia, rebound hypertension on withdrawal, drowsiness

**Dose**

- Initially, 800 micrograms daily in divided doses, increased as necessary in steps of 400–800 micrograms daily to max. 2.4 mg daily in divided doses; max. single dose 800 micrograms; recommended duration of treatment 7–10 days if no opioid use (but longer may be required); CHILD under 18 years not recommended

**BritLofex®** (Forum) ⒫ⓄⓂ

Tablets, peach, f/c, lofexidine hydrochloride 200 micrograms, net price 60-tab pack = £61.79. Label: 2

## METHADONE HYDROCHLORIDE

**Indications** adjunct in treatment of opioid dependence, see notes above; analgesia (section 4.7.2); cough in terminal disease (section 3.9.1)

**Cautions** section 4.7.2

**Contra-indications** section 4.7.2

**Side-effects** section 4.7.2; **overdosage:** see Emergency Treatment of Poisoning, p. 31

Important Methadone, even in low doses is a **special hazard** for children; non-dependent adults are also at risk of toxicity; dependent adults are at risk if tolerance is incorrectly assessed during induction

Incompatibility Syrup preserved with hydroxybenzoate (parabens) esters may be incompatible with methadone hydrochloride.

**Dose**

- Initially 10–40 mg daily, increased by up to 10 mg daily (max. weekly increase 30 mg) until no signs of withdrawal or intoxication; usual dose range 60–120 mg daily; CHILD not recommended (see also important note above)

Note Methadone hydrochloride doses in the BNF may differ from those in the product literature

**Methadone** (Non-proprietary) [CD]

Oral solution 1 mg/mL, methadone hydrochloride 1 mg/mL, net price 20 mL = 29p, 30 mL = 62p, 40 mL = 58p, 50 mL = £1.04, 60 mL = 87p, 100 mL = £1.31, 500 mL = £9.18. Label: 2

Brands include *Eptadone®*, *Metharose®* (sugar-free), *Physeptone®* (sugar-free)

Important Methadone oral solution 1 mg/mL is 2½ times the strength of Methadone Linctus (section 3.9.1). Many preparations of Methadone oral solution are licensed for opioid drug addiction only but some are also licensed for analgesia in severe pain

Oral solution 5 mg/mL, methadone hydrochloride 5 mg/mL, net price 20 mL = £1.47, 1 litre = £73.33. Label: 2

Brands include *Eptadone®*

Note Care is required in prescribing and dispensing the *correct strength* since any confusion could lead to an overdose

Injection, methadone hydrochloride 25 mg/mL, net price 2-mL amp = £2.05; 50 mg/mL, 1-mL amp = £2.05

Brands include *Synastone®*

**Methadose®** (Rosemont) [CD]

Oral concentrate, methadone hydrochloride 10 mg/mL (blue), net price 150 mL = £12.01; 20 mg/mL (brown), 150 mL = £24.02. Label: 2

Note The final strength of the methadone mixture to be dispensed to the patient must be specified on the prescription

Important Care is required in prescribing and dispensing the **correct strength** since any confusion could lead to an overdose; this preparation should be dispensed only **after dilution** as appropriate with *Methadose®* Diluent (life of diluted solution 3 months) and is for drug dependent persons (see also p. 7)

---

### ■ NALTREXONE HYDROCHLORIDE

**Indications** adjunct to prevent relapse in detoxified formerly opioid-dependent patients (who have remained opioid-free for at least 7–10 days)

**Cautions** liver function tests needed before and during treatment; test for opioid dependence with naloxone before treatment; avoid concomitant use of opioids but increased dose of opioid analgesic may be required for pain (monitor for opioid intoxication); hepatic impairment (Appendix 2); renal impairment (Appendix 3); pregnancy (Appendix 4); breast-feeding (Appendix 5)

Note Patients should be warned that an attempt to overcome the blockade of opioid receptors by overdosing could result in acute opioid intoxication

**Contra-indications** patients currently dependent on opioids

**Side-effects** nausea, vomiting, abdominal pain, diarrhoea, constipation, reduced appetite, increased thirst; chest pain; anxiety, sleep disorders, headache, reduced energy, increased energy, irritability, emotional lability, dizziness; chills; urinary retention; delayed ejaculation, decreased potency; arthralgia, myalgia; increased lacrimation; rash, and increased sweating; *rarely* hepatic dysfunction, suicidal ideation,

and speech disorders; *very rarely* hallucinations, tremor, and idiopathic thrombocytopenia

**Dose**

- ADULT over 18 years (initiate in specialist clinics only), 25 mg initially then 50 mg daily; total weekly dose (350 mg) may be divided and given on 3 days of the week for improved compliance (e.g. 100 mg on Monday and Wednesday, and 150 mg on Friday)

**Nalorex®** (Bristol-Myers Squibb) [PoM]

Tablets, yellow, f/c, scored, naltrexone hydrochloride 50 mg, net price 28-tab pack = £22.79

**Opizone®** (Genus) [PoM]

Tablets, beige, f/c, scored, naltrexone hydrochloride 50 mg, net price 28-tab pack = £23.00

---

## 4.11 Drugs for dementia

Acetylcholinesterase inhibiting drugs are used in the treatment of Alzheimer's disease, specifically for mild to moderate disease. Rivastigmine is also licensed for mild to moderate dementia associated with Parkinson's disease. The evidence to support the use of these drugs relates to their cognitive enhancement.

Treatment with drugs for dementia should be initiated and supervised only by a specialist experienced in the management of dementia.

Benefit is assessed by repeating the cognitive assessment at around 3 months. Such assessment cannot demonstrate how the disease may have progressed in the absence of treatment but it can give a good guide to response. Up to half the patients given these drugs will show a slower rate of cognitive decline. Drugs for dementia should be discontinued in those thought not to be responding. Many specialists repeat the cognitive assessment 4 to 6 weeks after discontinuation to assess deterioration; if significant deterioration occurs during this short period, consideration should be given to restarting therapy.

**Donepezil** is a reversible inhibitor of acetylcholinesterase. **Galantamine** is a reversible inhibitor of acetylcholinesterase and it also has nicotinic receptor agonist properties. **Rivastigmine** is a reversible non-competitive inhibitor of acetylcholinesterases; it is also licensed for treating mild to moderate dementia in Parkinson's disease.

Acetylcholinesterase inhibitors can cause unwanted dose-related cholinergic effects and should be started at a low dose and the dose increased according to response and tolerability.

**Memantine** is a NMDA-receptor antagonist that affects glutamate transmission; it is licensed for treating moderate to severe Alzheimer's disease.

**4**

**Central nervous system**

## NICE guidance

Donepezil, galantamine, rivastigmine, and memantine for Alzheimer's disease (September 2007)

Donepezil, galantamine, and rivastigmine are recommended for the adjunctive treatment of moderate Alzheimer's disease in those whose mini mental-state examination (MMSE) score is 10–20 points under the following conditions:

- Alzheimer's disease must be diagnosed in a specialist clinic; the clinic should also assess cognitive, global, and behavioural functioning, activities of daily living, and the likelihood of compliance with treatment;
- treatment should be initiated by specialists but can be continued by general practitioners under a shared-care protocol;
- the carers' views of the condition should be sought before and during drug treatment;
- the patient should be assessed every 6 months and drug treatment should normally continue only if the MMSE score remains at or above 10 points and if treatment is considered to have a worthwhile effect on the global, functional, and behavioural condition.
- Patients receiving acetylcholinesterase inhibitors for mild Alzheimer's disease can continue treatment until they, their carers, or their specialist consider it appropriate to stop.

Healthcare professionals should not rely solely on the MMSE score to assess the severity of Alzheimer's disease when the patient has learning or other disabilities, or other communication difficulties.

NICE does not recommend memantine for moderately severe to severe Alzheimer's disease except as part of well designed clinical studies; patients already receiving memantine can continue treatment until they, their carers, or their specialist consider it appropriate to stop.

## ■ DONEPEZIL HYDROCHLORIDE

**Indications** mild to moderate dementia in Alzheimer's disease

**Cautions** sick sinus syndrome or other supraventricular conduction abnormalities; susceptibility to peptic ulcers; asthma, chronic obstructive pulmonary disease; hepatic impairment (Appendix 2); pregnancy (Appendix 4); **interactions:** Appendix 1 (parasympathomimetics)

**Contra-indications** breast-feeding

**Side-effects** nausea, vomiting, anorexia, diarrhoea; fatigue, insomnia, headache, dizziness, syncope, hallucinations, agitation, aggression; muscle cramps; urinary incontinence; rash, pruritus; *less commonly* gastric and duodenal ulcers, gastro-intestinal haemorrhage, bradycardia, seizures; *rarely* sino-atrial block, AV block, hepatitis, extrapyramidal symptoms; potential for bladder outflow obstruction

**Dose**

- Initially 5 mg once daily at bedtime, increased if necessary after one month to max. 10 mg daily

**Aricept®** (Pfizer, Eisai) PoM

Tablets, f/c, donepezil hydrochloride 5 mg (white), net price 28-tab pack = £63.54; 10 mg (yellow), 28-tab pack = £89.06.

**Aricept Evess®** (Pfizer, Eisai) PoM

Orodispersible tablets, donepezil hydrochloride 5 mg (white), net price 28-tab pack = £63.54; 10 mg (yellow), 28-tab pack = £89.06. Counselling, administration

Counselling *Aricept Evess®* should be placed on the tongue, allowed to disperse, and swallowed

## ■ GALANTAMINE

**Indications** mild to moderate dementia in Alzheimer's disease

**Cautions** cardiac disease (including sick sinus syndrome or other supraventricular conduction abnormalities, unstable angina, congestive heart failure); electrolyte disturbances; susceptibility to peptic ulcers; asthma, chronic obstructive pulmonary disease, pulmonary infection; avoid in urinary retention and gastro-intestinal obstruction; hepatic impairment (Appendix 2—avoid if severe); pregnancy (Appendix 4); **interactions:** Appendix 1 (parasympathomimetics)

**Contra-indications** renal impairment (Appendix 3); breast-feeding (Appendix 5)

**Side-effects** nausea, vomiting, diarrhoea, abdominal pain, dyspepsia; syncope; rhinitis; sleep disturbances, dizziness, confusion, depression, headache, fatigue, anorexia, tremor; fever; weight loss; *less commonly* arrythmias, palpitation, myocardial infarction, cerebrovascular disease, paraesthesia, tinnitus, and leg cramps; *rarely* bradycardia, seizures, hallucinations, agitation, aggression, dehydration, hypokalaemia, and rash; *very rarely* gastrointestinal bleeding, dysphagia, hypotension, exacerbation of Parkinson's disease, and sweating

**Dose**

- Initially 4 mg twice daily for 4 weeks increased to 8 mg twice daily for 4 weeks; maintenance 8–12 mg twice daily

**Reminyl®** (Shire) PoM

Tablets, all f/c, galantamine (as hydrobromide) 8 mg (pink), net price 56-tab pack = £68.32; 12 mg (orange-brown), 56-tab pack = £84.00 Label: 3, 21

Oral solution, galantamine (as hydrobromide) 4 mg/mL, net price 100 mL with pipette = £120.00. Label: 3, 21

◢ **Modified release**

**Reminyl® XL** (Shire) PoM

Capsules, m/r, galantamine (as hydrobromide) 8 mg (white), net price 28-cap pack = £51.88; 16 mg (pink), 28-cap pack = £64.90; 24 mg (beige), 28-cap pack = £79.80. Label: 3, 21, 25

Dose initially 8 mg once daily for 4 weeks increased to 16 mg once daily for 4 weeks; maintenance 16–24 mg daily

## ■ MEMANTINE HYDROCHLORIDE

**Indications** moderate to severe dementia in Alzheimer's disease

**Cautions** history of convulsions; renal impairment (avoid if eGFR less than 5 mL/minute; Appendix 3); pregnancy (Appendix 4); **interactions:** Appendix 1 (memantine)

**Contra-indications** breast-feeding

**Side-effects** constipation; hypertension; headache, dizziness, drowsiness; *less commonly* vomiting, thrombosis, heart failure, confusion, fatigue, hallucinations, and abnormal gait; *very rarely* seizures; pancreatitis, psychosis, depression, and suicidal ideation also reported

**Dose**

- Initially 5 mg once daily, increased in steps of 5 mg at weekly intervals; max. 20 mg daily

**Ebixa®** (Lundbeck) PoM

Tablets, f/c, scored, memantine hydrochloride 10 mg, net price 28-tab pack = £34.50, 56-tab pack = £69.01, 112-tab pack = £138.01; 20 mg, 28-tab pack = £69.01; treatment initiation pack, 7 × 5 mg, 7 × 10 mg, 7 × 15 mg, and 7 × 20 mg = £43.13

Oral drops, memantine hydrochloride 10 mg/g, net price 50 g = £61.61, 100 g = £123.23

Note 5 mg ≡ 10 drops of memantine hydrochloride oral drops

---

## ■ RIVASTIGMINE

**Indications** mild to moderate dementia in Alzheimer's disease or in Parkinson's disease

**Cautions** gastric or duodenal ulcers (or susceptibility to ulcers); monitor body-weight; sick sinus syndrome, conduction abnormalities; history of asthma or chronic obstructive pulmonary disease; history of seizures; bladder outflow obstruction; hepatic impairment (avoid if severe—Appendix 2); renal impairment (Appendix 3); pregnancy (Appendix 4); interactions: Appendix 1 (parasympathomimetics)

Note If treatment interrupted for more than several days, re-introduce with initial dose and increase gradually (see Dose)

**Contra-indications** breast-feeding (Appendix 5)

**Side-effects** nausea, vomiting, diarrhoea, dyspepsia, anorexia, abdominal pain; dizziness, headache, drowsiness, tremor, asthenia, malaise, agitation, confusion; sweating; weight loss; *less commonly* gastric or duodenal ulceration, bradycardia, syncope, depression, insomnia; *rarely* angina pectoris, seizures; *very rarely* gastro-intestinal haemorrhage, pancreatitis, cardiac arrhythmias, hypertension, hallucinations, extrapyramidal symptoms (including worsening of Parkinson's disease), and rash; *with patches* application-site reactions

Note Gastro-intestinal side-effects more common in women

**Dose**

- See under preparations below

**Exelon®** (Novartis) ▼ PoM

Capsules, rivastigmine (as hydrogen tartrate) 1.5 mg (yellow), net price 28-cap pack = £33.25, 56-cap pack = £66.51; 3 mg (orange), 28-cap pack = £33.25, 56-cap pack = £66.51; 4.5 mg (red), 28-cap pack = £33.25, 56-cap pack = £66.51; 6 mg (red/orange), 28-cap pack = £33.25, 56-cap pack = £66.51. Label: 21, 25

Oral solution, rivastigmine (as hydrogen tartrate) 2 mg/mL, net price 120 mL (with oral syringe) = £99.14. Label: 21

Dose initially 1.5 mg twice daily, increased in steps of 1.5 mg twice daily at intervals of at least 2 weeks according to response and tolerance; usual range 3–6 mg twice daily; max. 6 mg twice daily

Patches, self-adhesive, beige, rivastigmine 4.6 mg/24 hours, net price 30 = £77.97; 9.5 mg/24 hours, 30 = £77.97

Dose initially apply 4.6 mg/24 hours patch to clean, dry, non-hairy, non-irritated skin on back, upper arm, or chest, removing after 24 hours and siting a replacement patch on a different area (avoid using the same area for 14 days); if well tolerated increase to 9.5 mg/24 hours patch daily after no less than 4 weeks; if patch

not applied for more than several days, treatment should be restarted with 4.6 mg/24 hours patch

Note When switching a patient from oral to transdermal therapy, patients taking 3–6 mg daily should be prescribed the 4.6 mg/24 hours patch; patients taking 9 mg daily who do not tolerate the dose well should be prescribed the 4.6 mg/24 hours patch, while those taking 9 mg daily who tolerate the dose well should be prescribed the 9.5 mg/24 hours patch; patients taking 12 mg daily should be prescribed the 9.5 mg/24 hours patch. The first patch should be applied on the day following the last oral dose

Note The *Scottish Medicines Consortium* has advised (October 2007) that *Exelon®* patches should be restricted for use in patients with moderately severe Alzheimer's disease under the conditions of the NICE guidance (September 2007) and when a transdermal patch is an appropriate choice of formulation

# 5 Infections

**5.1 Antibacterial drugs** **289**

**5.1.1** Penicillins  295

**5.1.1.1** Benzylpenicillin and phenoxy-methylpenicillin  295

**5.1.1.2** Penicillinase-resistant penicillins  296

**5.1.1.3** Broad-spectrum penicillins  298

**5.1.1.4** Antipseudomonal penicillins  301

**5.1.1.5** Mecillinams  302

**5.1.2** Cephalosporins, carbapenems, and other beta-lactams  302

**5.1.2.1** Cephalosporins  302

**5.1.2.2** Carbapenems  306

**5.1.2.3** Other beta-lactam antibiotics  307

**5.1.3** Tetracyclines  308

**5.1.4** Aminoglycosides  310

**5.1.5** Macrolides  312

**5.1.6** Clindamycin  315

**5.1.7** Some other antibacterials  315

**5.1.8** Sulphonamides and trimethoprim  320

**5.1.9** Antituberculosis drugs  321

**5.1.10** Antileprotic drugs  326

**5.1.11** Metronidazole and tinidazole  327

**5.1.12** Quinolones  328

**5.1.13** Urinary-tract infections  331

**5.2 Antifungal drugs** **332**

**5.3 Antiviral drugs** **339**

**5.3.1** HIV infection  339

**5.3.2** Herpesvirus infections  348

**5.3.2.1** Herpes simplex and varicella–zoster infection  348

**5.3.2.2** Cytomegalovirus infection  351

**5.3.3** Viral hepatitis  352

**5.3.4** Influenza  354

**5.3.5** Respiratory syncytial virus  356

**5.4 Antiprotozoal drugs** **357**

**5.4.1** Antimalarials  357

**5.4.2** Amoebicides  366

**5.4.3** Trichomonacides  367

**5.4.4** Antigiardial drugs  367

**5.4.5** Leishmaniacides  367

**5.4.6** Trypanocides  367

**5.4.7** Drugs for toxoplasmosis  368

**5.4.8** Drugs for pneumocystis pneumonia  368

**5.5 Anthelmintics** **369**

**5.5.1** Drugs for threadworms  369

**5.5.2** Ascaricides  370

**5.5.3** Drugs for tapeworm infections  370

**5.5.4** Drugs for hookworms  371

**5.5.5** Schistosomicides  371

**5.5.6** Filaricides  371

**5.5.7** Drugs for cutaneous larva migrans  371

**5.5.8** Drugs for strongyloidiasis  371

This chapter also includes advice on the drug management of the following:
anthrax, p. 328
*Clostridium difficile* infection, p. 290
bacterial infections: table 1, summary of antibacterial treatment, p. 290–293
bacterial infections: table 2, summary of antibacterial prophylaxis, p. 293–295
Lyme disease, p. 298
MRSA infections, p. 297
oral infections, p. 289, p. 292, p. 332

## Notifiable diseases

Doctors must notify the Proper Officer of the local authority (usually the consultant in communicable disease control) when attending a patient suspected of suffering from any of the diseases listed below; a form is available from the Proper Officer.

| | |
|---|---|
| Anthrax | Ophthalmia neonatorum |
| Cholera | Paratyphoid fever |
| Diphtheria | Plague |
| Dysentery (amoebic or bacillary) | Poliomyelitis, acute |
| | Rabies |
| Encephalitis, acute | Relapsing fever |
| Food poisoning | Rubella |
| Haemorrhagic fever (viral) | Scarlet fever |
| Hepatitis, viral | Smallpox |
| Leprosy | Tetanus |
| Leptospirosis | Tuberculosis |
| Malaria | Typhoid fever |
| Measles | Typhus |
| Meningitis | Whooping cough |
| Meningococcal septicaemia (without meningitis) | Yellow fever |
| Mumps | |

**Note** It is good practice for doctors to also inform the consultant in communicable disease control of instances of other infections (e.g. psittacosis) where there could be a public health risk.

# 5.1 Antibacterial drugs

**Choice of a suitable drug** Before selecting an antibacterial the clinician must first consider two factors—the patient and the known or likely causative organism. Factors related to the patient which must be considered include history of allergy, renal and hepatic function, susceptibility to infection (i.e. whether immunocompromised), ability to tolerate drugs by mouth, severity of illness, ethnic origin, age, whether taking other medication and, if female, whether pregnant, breast-feeding or taking an oral contraceptive.

The known or likely organism and its antibacterial sensitivity, in association with the above factors, will suggest one or more antibacterials, the final choice depending on the microbiological, pharmacological, and toxicological properties.

An example of a rational approach to the selection of an antibacterial is treatment of a urinary-tract infection in a patient complaining of nausea and symptoms of a urinary-tract infection in early pregnancy. The organism is reported as being resistant to ampicillin but sensitive to nitrofurantoin (can cause nausea), gentamicin (can be given only by injection and best avoided in pregnancy), tetracycline (causes dental discoloration) and trimethoprim (folate antagonist therefore theoretical teratogenic risk), and cefalexin. The safest antibiotics in pregnancy are the penicillins and cephalosporins; therefore, cefalexin would be indicated for this patient.

The principles involved in selection of an antibacterial must allow for a number of variables including changing renal and hepatic function, increasing bacterial resistance, and new information on side-effects. Duration of therapy, dosage, and route of administration depend on site, type and severity of infection and response.

**Antibacterial policies** Local policies often limit the antibacterials that may be used to achieve reasonable economy consistent with adequate cover, and to reduce the development of resistant organisms. A policy may indicate a range of drugs for general use, and permit other drugs only on the advice of the microbiologist or physician responsible for the control of infectious diseases.

**Before starting therapy** The following precepts should be considered before starting:

- Viral infections should not be treated with antibacterials. However, antibacterials are occasionally helpful in controlling secondary bacterial infection (e.g. acute necrotising ulcerative gingivitis secondary to herpes simplex infection);

- Samples should be taken for culture and sensitivity testing; **'blind'** antibacterial prescribing for unexplained pyrexia usually leads to further difficulty in establishing the diagnosis;

- Knowledge of **prevalent organisms** and their current sensitivity is of great help in choosing an antibacterial before bacteriological confirmation is available. Generally, narrow-spectrum antibacterials are preferred to broad-spectrum antibacterials unless there is a clear clinical indication (e.g. life-threatening sepsis);

- The **dose** of an antibacterial varies according to a number of factors including age, weight, hepatic function, renal function, and severity of infection. The prescribing of the so-called 'standard' dose in serious infections may result in failure of treatment or even death of the patient; therefore it is important to prescribe a dose appropriate to the condition. An inadequate dose may also increase the likelihood of antibacterial resistance. On the other hand, for an antibacterial with a narrow margin between the toxic and therapeutic dose (e.g. an aminoglycoside) it is also important to avoid an excessive dose and the concentration of the drug in the plasma may need to be monitored;

- The **route** of administration of an antibacterial often depends on the severity of the infection. Life-threatening infections require intravenous therapy. Antibacterials that are well absorbed may be given by mouth even for some serious infections. Parenteral administration is also appropriate when the oral route cannot be used (e.g. because of vomiting) or if absorption is inadequate. Whenever possible, painful intramuscular injections should be avoided in children;

- **Duration** of therapy depends on the nature of the infection and the response to treatment. Courses should not be unduly prolonged because they encourage resistance, they may lead to side-effects and they are costly. However, in certain infections such as tuberculosis or osteomyelitis it may be necessary to treat for prolonged periods. Conversely a single dose of an antibacterial may cure uncomplicated urinary-tract infections.

**Oral bacterial infections** Antibacterial drugs should only be prescribed for the *treatment* of oral infections on the basis of defined need. They may be used in conjunction with (but not as an alternative to) other appropriate measures, such as providing drainage or extracting a tooth.

The 'blind' prescribing of an antibacterial for unexplained pyrexia, cervical lymphadenopathy, or facial swelling can lead to difficulty in establishing the diagnosis. In severe oral infections, a sample should always be taken for bacteriology.

Oral infections which may require antibacterial treatment include acute periapical or periodontal abscess, cellulitis, acutely created oral-antral communication (and acute sinusitis), severe pericoronitis, localised osteitis, acute necrotising ulcerative gingivitis, and destructive forms of chronic periodontal disease. Most of these infections are readily resolved by the early establishment of drainage and removal of the cause (typically an infected necrotic pulp). Antibacterials may be indicated if treatment has to be delayed and they are essential in immunocompromised patients or in those with conditions such as diabetes or Paget's disease. Certain rarer infections including bacterial sialadenitis, osteomyelitis, actinomycosis, and infections involving fascial spaces such as Ludwig's angina, require antibiotics and specialist hospital care.

Antibacterial drugs may also be useful after dental surgery in some cases of spreading infection. Infection may spread to involve local lymph nodes, to fascial spaces (where it can cause airway obstruction), or into the bloodstream (where it can lead to cavernous sinus thrombosis and other serious complications). Extension of an infection can also lead to maxillary sinusitis; osteomyelitis is a complication, which usually arises when host resistance is reduced.

If the oral infection fails to respond to antibacterial treatment within 48 hours the antibacterial should be

**5**

**Infections**

changed, preferably on the basis of bacteriological investigation. Failure to respond may also suggest an incorrect diagnosis, lack of essential additional measures (such as drainage), poor host resistance, or poor patient compliance.

Combination of a penicillin (or erythromycin) with metronidazole may sometimes be helpful for the treatment of severe oral infections or oral infections that have not responded to initial antibacterial treatment.

See also **Penicillins** (section 5.1.1), **Cephalosporins** (section 5.1.2), **Tetracyclines** (section 5.1.3), **Macrolides** (section 5.1.5), **Clindamycin** (section 5.1.6), **Metronidazole** (section 5.1.11), **Fusidic acid** (section 13.10.1.2) .

**Superinfection** In general, broad-spectrum antibacterial drugs such as the cephalosporins are more likely to be associated with adverse reactions related to the selection of resistant organisms e.g. *fungal infections* or *antibiotic-associated colitis* (pseudomembranous colitis); other problems associated with superinfection include vaginitis and pruritus ani.

**Therapy** Suggested treatment is shown in table 1. When the pathogen has been isolated treatment may be changed to a more appropriate antibacterial if necessary. If no bacterium is cultured the antibacterial can be continued or stopped on clinical grounds. Infections for which prophylaxis is useful are listed in table 2.

## Table 1. Summary of antibacterial therapy

> If treating a patient suspected of suffering from a notifiable disease, the consultant in communicable disease control should be informed (see p. 288)

### Gastro-intestinal system

**Gastro-enteritis**
Antibacterial not usually indicated
Frequently self-limiting and may not be bacterial

**Campylobacter enteritis**
Ciprofloxacin *or* erythromycin
Frequently self-limiting; treat severe infection

**Invasive salmonellosis**
Ciprofloxacin *or* cefotaxime
Includes severe infections which may be invasive

**Shigellosis**
Ciprofloxacin *or* azithromycin [unlicensed indication]
Amoxicillin or trimethoprim can be used if organism sensitive. Antibacterial not indicated for mild cases

**Typhoid fever**
Ciprofloxacin *or* cefotaxime
Infections from Indian subcontinent, Middle-East, and South-East Asia may be multiple-antibacterial-resistant and sensitivity should be tested; azithromycin [unlicensed indication] may be an option in mild or moderate disease caused by multiple antibacterial-resistant organisms

*Clostridium difficile* infection
Oral metronidazole *or* oral vancomycin
Treat for 10–14 days. Use vancomycin for third or subsequent episode of infection, for severe infection, for infection not responding to metronidazole, or in patients intolerant of metronidazole. For infection not responding to vancomycin or for life-threatening infection, use oral vancomycin + intravenous metronidazole

**Biliary-tract infection**
Ciprofloxacin *or* gentamicin *or* a cephalosporin

**Peritonitis**
A cephalosporin + metronidazole *or* gentamicin + metronidazole *or* gentamicin + clindamycin *or* piperacillin with tazobactam

**Peritoneal dialysis-associated peritonitis**
*Either* vancomycin[1] + ceftazidime added to dialysis fluid *or* vancomycin added to dialysis fluid + ciprofloxacin by mouth
Treat for 14 days or longer

### Cardiovascular system

**Endocarditis: initial 'blind' therapy**
Flucloxacillin (*or* benzylpenicillin if symptoms less severe) + gentamicin
Substitute flucloxacillin (or benzylpenicillin) with vancomycin + rifampicin if cardiac prostheses present, or if penicillin-allergic, or if meticillin-resistant *Staphylococcus aureus* suspected

**Endocarditis caused by staphylococci**
Flucloxacillin (*or* vancomycin + rifampicin if penicillin-allergic or if meticillin-resistant *Staphylococcus aureus*)
Treat for at least 4 weeks; treat prosthetic valve endocarditis for at least 6 weeks and if using flucloxacillin add rifampicin for at least 2 weeks

**Endocarditis caused by streptococci** (e.g. viridans streptococci)
Benzylpenicillin (*or* vancomycin[1] if penicillin- allergic or highly penicillin-resistant) + gentamicin
Treat endocarditis caused by fully sensitive streptococci with benzylpenicillin or vancomycin alone for 4 weeks *or* (if no intracardiac abscess or infected emboli) with benzylpenicillin + gentamicin for 2 weeks. Treat more resistant organisms for 4–6 weeks (stopping gentamicin after 2 weeks for organisms moderately sensitive to penicillin); if aminoglycoside cannot be used and if streptococci moderately sensitive to penicillin, treat with benzylpenicillin alone for 4 weeks. Treat prosthetic valve endocarditis for at least 6 weeks (stopping gentamicin after 2 weeks if organisms fully sensitive to penicillin)

**Endocarditis caused by enterococci** (e.g. *Enterococcus faecalis*)
Amoxicillin[2] (*or* vancomycin[1] if penicillin-allergic or penicillin-resistant) + gentamicin
Treat for at least 4 weeks (at least 6 weeks for prosthetic valve endocarditis); if gentamicin-resistant, substitute gentamicin with streptomycin

**Endocarditis caused by haemophilus, actinobacillus, cardiobacterium, eikenella, and kingella species** ('HACEK' organisms)
Amoxicillin[2] (*or* ceftriaxone if amoxicillin-resistant) + low-dose gentamicin
Treat for 4 weeks (6 weeks for prosthetic valve endocarditis); stop gentamicin after 2 weeks

### Respiratory system

***Haemophilus influenzae* epiglottitis**
Cefotaxime *or* chloramphenicol
Give intravenously

**Exacerbations of chronic bronchitis**
Amoxicillin[2] *or* tetracycline (*or* erythromycin[3])
Some pneumococci and *Haemophilus influenzae* strains tetracycline-resistant; approx. 20% *H. influenzae* strains amoxicillin-resistant

**Uncomplicated community-acquired pneumonia**
Amoxicillin[2] (*or* benzylpenicillin if previously healthy chest *or* erythromycin[3] if penicillin-allergic)
Add flucloxacillin if staphylococci suspected, e.g. in influenza or measles (or vancomycin[1] if meticillin-resistant *Staphylococcus aureus* suspected); treat for 7 days (14–21 days

---

1. Where vancomycin is suggested teicoplanin may be used.
2. Where amoxicillin is suggested ampicillin may be used.
3. Where erythromycin is suggested another macrolide (e.g. azithromycin or clarithromycin) may be used.

for infections caused by staphylococci); pneumococci with decreased penicillin sensitivity being isolated but not yet common in UK; add erythromycin[1] if hospitalised for clinical reasons or if atypical pathogens suspected

### Severe community-acquired pneumonia of unknown aetiology
Cefuroxime + erythromycin[1] or cefotaxime + erythromycin[1] or co-amoxiclav + erythromycin[1]

Add vancomycin[2] if meticillin-resistant *Staphylococcus aureus* suspected; treat for 10 days (14–21 days if staphylococci, legionella, or Gram-negative enteric bacilli suspected)

### Pneumonia possibly caused by atypical pathogens
Erythromycin[1]

Severe Legionella infections may require addition of rifampicin; tetracycline is an alternative for chlamydial and mycoplasma infections; treat for at least 14 days (14–21 days for legionella)

### Hospital-acquired pneumonia
*Early-onset infection* (less than 5 days after admission to hospital), co-amoxiclav or cefuroxime

Treat for 7 days. If life threatening infection, or if recent history of antibacterial treatment, or if resistant organisms suspected, treat as for late-onset hospital-acquired pneumonia

*Late-onset infection* (more than 5 days after admission to hospital), an antipseudomonal penicillin (e.g. piperacillin with tazobactam) or a broad-spectrum cephalosporin (e.g. ceftazidime) or another antipseudomonal beta-lactam or a quinolone (e.g. ciprofloxacin)

Treat for 7 days (longer if *Pseudomonas aeruginosa* confirmed). Add vancomycin if MRSA suspected. Consider adding an aminoglycoside for severe illness caused by *Pseudomonas aeruginosa*

## Central nervous system

### Meningitis: initial empirical therapy
- Transfer patient urgently to hospital

- If bacterial meningitis and especially if *meningococcal disease* suspected, general practitioners should give benzylpenicillin (see p. 296 for dose) before urgent transfer to hospital; cefotaxime (section 5.1.2) may be an alternative in penicillin allergy; chloramphenicol (section 5.1.7) may be used if history of immediate hypersensitivity reaction to penicillin or to cephalosporins

- Consider adjunctive treatment with dexamethasone (particularly if pneumococcal meningitis suspected in adults; section 6.3.2) starting before or with first dose of antibacterial; avoid dexamethasone in septic shock, meningococcal septicaemia, or if immunocompromised, or in meningitis following surgery

### Meningitis caused by meningococci
Benzylpenicillin or cefotaxime

Treat for at least 5 days; substitute chloramphenicol if history of immediate hypersensitivity reaction to penicillin or to cephalosporins. To eliminate nasopharyngeal carriage give rifampicin for 2 days (see Table 2, section 5.1)

### Meningitis caused by pneumococci
Cefotaxime

Treat for 10–14 days; substitute benzylpenicillin if organism penicillin-sensitive; if organism highly penicillin- and cephalosporin-resistant, add vancomycin and if necessary rifampicin. Consider adjunctive treatment with dexamethasone (section 6.3.2) starting before or with first dose of antibacterial (but may reduce penetration of vancomycin into cerebrospinal fluid)

### Meningitis caused by *Haemophilus influenzae*
Cefotaxime

Treat for at least 10 days; substitute chloramphenicol if history of immediate hypersensitivity reaction to penicillin or to cephalosporins, or if organism resistant to cefotaxime. Consider adjunctive treatment with dexamethasone (section 6.3.2) starting before or with first dose of antibacterial. For *H. influenzae* type b give rifampicin for 4 days before hospital discharge (see Table 2, section 5.1)

### Meningitis caused by Listeria
Amoxicillin[3] + gentamicin

Treat for 10–14 days

## Urinary tract

### Acute pyelonephritis
A broad-spectrum cephalosporin or a quinolone

Treat for 10–14 days; longer treatment may be necessary in complicated pyelonephritis

### Acute prostatitis
A quinolone or trimethoprim

Treat for 28 days

### 'Lower' urinary-tract infection
Trimethoprim or nitrofurantoin or amoxicillin[3] or oral cephalosporin

Treat for 7 days but a short course (e.g. 3 days) is usually adequate for uncomplicated urinary-tract infections in women. See also section 5.1.13

## Genital system

### Syphilis
Benzathine benzylpenicillin [unlicensed] or doxycycline or erythromycin

Treat early syphilis (infection of less than 2 years) with benzathine benzylpenicillin as a single dose (repeat dose after 7 days for women in the third trimester of pregnancy) or with doxycycline or erythromycin for 14 days. Treat late latent syphilis (asymptomatic infection of more than 2 years) with doxycycline for 28 days or with benzathine benzylpenicillin once weekly for 2 weeks. Treat asymptomatic contacts of patients with infectious syphilis with doxycycline for 14 days. Contact tracing recommended.

### Uncomplicated gonorrhoea
Cefixime [unlicensed indication] or ciprofloxacin

Single-dose treatment in uncomplicated infection. Choice depends on locality where infection acquired. Pharyngeal infection requires treatment with ceftriaxone. Use ciprofloxacin only if organism sensitive. Contact tracing recommended; remember chlamydia

### Uncomplicated genital chlamydial infection, non-gonococcal urethritis and non-specific genital infection
Doxycycline or azithromycin

Treat with doxycycline for 7 days or with azithromycin as a single dose; alternatively, treat with erythromycin for 14 days. Contact tracing recommended

### Pelvic inflammatory disease
Doxycycline + metronidazole + i/m ceftriaxone or ofloxacin + metronidazole

Treat for at least 14 days (use i/m ceftriaxone as a single dose). In severely ill patients initial treatment with doxycycline + i/v ceftriaxone (as a single dose) + i/v metronidazole, then switch to oral treatment with doxycycline + metronidazole to complete 14 days' treatment. Contact tracing recommended

### Bacterial vaginosis
Oral or topical metronidazole or topical clindamycin

Oral treatment for 5–7 days (or with high-dose metronidazole as a single dose); topical treatment for 5 days (7 days with clindamycin)

---

1. Where erythromycin is suggested another macrolide (e.g. azithromycin or clarithromycin) may be used.
2. Where vancomycin is suggested teicoplanin may be used.

3. Where amoxicillin is suggested ampicillin may be used.

5 Infections

## Blood

### Community-acquired septicaemia

A broad-spectrum antipseudomonal penicillin (e.g. *Tazocin®*, *Timentin®*) *or* a broad-spectrum cephalosporin (e.g. cefuroxime)

Add aminoglycoside if pseudomonas suspected, or if severe sepsis, or if patient recently discharged from hospital. Add vancomycin[1] if meticillin-resistant *Staphylococcus aureus* suspected. Add metronidazole to broad-spectrum cephalosporin if anaerobic infection suspected

### Hospital-acquired septicaemia

A broad-spectrum antipseudomonal beta-lactam antibacterial (e.g. *Tazocin®*, *Timentin®*, ceftazidime, imipenem (with cilastatin as *Primaxin®*) *or* meropenem)

Add aminoglycoside if pseudomonas suspected, or if multiple-resistant organisms suspected, or if severe sepsis. Add vancomycin[1] if meticillin-resistant *Staphylococcus aureus* suspected. Add metronidazole to broad-spectrum cephalosporin if anaerobic infection suspected

### Septicaemia related to vascular catheter

Vancomycin[1]

Add a broad-spectrum antipseudomonal beta-lactam if Gram-negative sepsis suspected, especially in the immunocompromised. Consider removing vascular catheter, particularly if infection caused by *Staphylococcus aureus*, pseudomonas, or candida

### Meningococcal septicaemia

Benzylpenicillin *or* cefotaxime

If meningococcal disease suspected, general practitioners advised to give a single dose of benzylpenicillin (see p. 296 for dose) before urgent transfer to hospital; cefotaxime (section 5.1.2) may be an alternative in penicillin allergy; chloramphenicol may be used if history of immediate hypersensitivity reaction to penicillin or to cephalosporins. To eliminate nasopharyngeal carriage give rifampicin for 2 days (see Table 2, section 5.1)

## Musculoskeletal system

### Osteomyelitis

Flucloxacillin *or* clindamycin if penicillin-allergic (*or* vancomycin[1] if resistant *Staphylococcus epidermidis* or meticillin-resistant *Staph. aureus*)

Treat acute infection for 4–6 weeks and chronic infection for at least 12 weeks. Combine vancomycin[1] with either fusidic acid or rifampicin if prostheses present or if life-threatening condition

### Septic arthritis

Flucloxacillin *or* clindamycin if penicillin-allergic (*or* vancomycin[1] if resistant *Staphylococcus epidermidis* or meticillin-resistant *Staph. aureus*) (*or* cefotaxime if gonococcal arthritis or Gram-negative infection)

Treat usually for 6 weeks (longer if infection complicated or if prosthesis present; treat for 2 weeks if gonococcal infection). Combine vancomycin[1] with either fusidic acid or rifampicin if prostheses present or if life-threatening condition

## Eye

### Purulent conjunctivitis

Chloramphenicol *or* gentamicin eye-drops

## Ear, nose, and oropharynx

### Pericoronitis

Metronidazole *or* amoxicillin

Antibacterial required only in presence of systemic features of infection or of trismus or persistent swelling despite local treatment; treat for 3 days or until symptoms resolve

### Acute necrotising ulcerative gingivitis

Metronidazole *or* amoxicillin

Antibacterial required only if systemic features of infection; treat for 3 days or until symptoms resolve

### Periapical or periodontal abscess

Amoxicillin *or* metronidazole

Antibacterial required only in severe disease with cellulitis or if systemic features of infection; treat for 5 days

### Periodontitis

Metronidazole *or* doxycycline

Antibacterial required for severe disease or disease unresponsive to local treatment

### Throat infections

Phenoxymethylpenicillin (*or* erythromycin[2] if penicillin-allergic)

Most throat infections are caused by viruses and many do not require antibacterial treatment. Consider antibacterial, if history of valvular heart disease, if marked systemic upset, if peritonsillar cellulitis or abscess, or if at increased risk from acute infection (e.g. in immunosuppression, cystic fibrosis); prescribe antibacterial for beta-haemolytic streptococcal pharyngitis; treat for 10 days. **Avoid** amoxicillin if possibility of glandular fever, see section 5.1.1.3. Initial parenteral therapy (in severe infection) with benzylpenicillin, then oral therapy with phenoxymethylpenicillin or amoxicillin[3]

### Sinusitis

Amoxicillin[3] *or* doxycycline *or* erythromycin[2]

Antibacterial should usually be used only for persistent symptoms and purulent discharge lasting at least 7 days or if severe symptoms. Also, consider antibacterial for those at high risk of serious complications (e.g. in immunosuppression, cystic fibrosis). Treat for 7 days

### Otitis externa

Flucloxacillin (*or* erythromycin[2] if penicillin-allergic)

Consider systemic antibacterial if spreading cellulitis or patient systemically unwell. Use ciprofloxacin (or an aminoglycoside) if pseudomonas suspected. For topical preparations see section 12.1.1

### Otitis media

Amoxicillin[3] (*or* erythromycin[2] if penicillin-allergic)

Many infections caused by viruses. Most uncomplicated cases resolve without antibacterial treatment. In children without systemic features, antibacterial treatment may be started after 72 hours if no improvement. Consider earlier treatment if deterioration, if systemically unwell, if at high risk of serious complications (e.g. in immunosuppression, cystic fibrosis), if mastoiditis present, or in children under 2 years of age with bilateral otitis media. Treat for 5 days (longer if severely ill); initial parenteral therapy in severe infections; consider co-amoxiclav or ceftriaxone if no improvement after 24–48 hours

## Skin

### Impetigo

Topical fusidic acid (*or* mupirocin if meticillin-resistant *Staphylococcus aureus*); oral flucloxacillin *or* erythromycin[2] if widespread

Topical treatment for 7 days usually adequate; max. duration of topical treatment 10 days; seek local microbiology advice before using topical treatment in hospital; oral treatment for 7 days; add phenoxymethylpenicillin to flucloxacillin if streptococcal infection suspected

### Erysipelas

Phenoxymethylpenicillin (*or* erythromycin[2] if penicillin-allergic)

Treat for at least 7 days; add flucloxacillin to phenoxymethylpenicillin if staphylococcus suspected; substitute benzylpenicillin for phenoxymethylpenicillin if parenteral treatment required

### Cellulitis

Benzylpenicillin + flucloxacillin (*or* erythromycin[2] alone if penicillin-allergic)

Substitute phenoxymethylpenicillin for benzylpenicillin if oral treatment appropriate. Discontinue flucloxacillin if streptococcal infection confirmed. Substitute treatment with

---

1. Where vancomycin is suggested teicoplanin may be used.

2. Where erythromycin is suggested another macrolide (e.g. azithromycin or clarithromycin) may be used.

3. Where amoxicillin is suggested ampicillin may be used.

broad-spectrum antibacterials if Gram-negative bacteria or anaerobes suspected

**Animal and human bites**

Co-amoxiclav alone (or doxycycline + metronidazole if penicillin-allergic)

Cleanse wound thoroughly. For tetanus-prone wound, give human tetanus immunoglobulin (with a tetanus-containing vaccine if necessary, according to immunisation history and risk of infection), see under Tetanus Vaccines, section 14.4. Consider rabies prophylaxis (section 14.4) for bites from animals in endemic countries; assess risk of blood-borne viruses

**Acne**

See section 13.6

## Table 2. Summary of antibacterial prophylaxis

### Prevention of recurrence of rheumatic fever

Phenoxymethylpenicillin 250 mg twice daily or sulfadiazine 1 g daily (500 mg daily for patients under 30 kg)

### Prevention of secondary case of invasive group A *streptococcal infection*[1]

Phenoxymethylpenicillin 250–500 mg every 6 hours for 10 days; CHILD under 1 year 62.5 mg every 6 hours, 1–5 years 125 mg every 6 hours, 6–12 years 250 mg every 6 hours

Patients who are penicillin allergic,

*either* erythromycin ADULT and CHILD over 8 years, 250–500 mg every 6 hours for 10 days; CHILD under 2 years 125 mg every 6 hours, 2–8 years 250 mg every 6 hours

*or* azithromycin [unlicensed indication] 500 mg once daily for 5 days; CHILD over 6 months, 12 mg/kg (max. 500 mg) once daily

### Prevention of secondary case of meningococcal meningitis[2]

Rifampicin 600 mg every 12 hours for 2 days; CHILD 10 mg/kg (under 1 year, 5 mg/kg) every 12 hours for 2 days

*or* ciprofloxacin 500 mg as a single dose; CHILD [unlicensed] 2–5 years 125 mg; 5–12 years 250 mg

*or* i/m ceftriaxone [unlicensed indication] 250 mg as a single dose; CHILD under 12 years 125 mg

### Prevention of secondary case of Haemophilus influenzae type b disease[2]

Rifampicin 600 mg once daily for 4 days (regimen of choice for adults); CHILD 1–3 months 10 mg/kg once daily for 4 days, over 3 months 20 mg/kg once daily for 4 days (max. 600 mg daily)

### Prevention of secondary case of diphtheria in non-immune patient

Erythromycin 500 mg every 6 hours for 7 days; CHILD up to 2 years 125 mg every 6 hours, 2–8 years 250 mg every 6 hours

Treat for further 10 days if nasopharyngeal swabs positive after first 7 days' treatment

### Prevention of secondary case of pertussis in non-immune patient or partially immune patient

Erythromycin[3] ADULT and CHILD over 8 years, 250–500 mg every 6 hours for 7 days; CHILD under 2 years 125 mg every 6 hours, 2–8 years 250 mg every 6 hours

### Prevention of pneumococcal infection in asplenia or in patients with sickle-cell disease

Phenoxymethylpenicillin 500 mg every 12 hours; CHILD under 5 years 125 mg every 12 hours, 6–12 years 250 mg every 12 hours—if cover also needed for *H. influenzae* in CHILD give amoxicillin instead (under 5 years 125 mg every 12 hours, over 5 years 250 mg every 12 hours)

Note Antibiotic prophylaxis is not fully reliable; for vaccines in asplenia see p. 670

### Prevention of gas-gangrene in high lower-limb amputations or following major trauma

Benzylpenicillin 300–600 mg every 6 hours for 5 days or if penicillin-allergic metronidazole 400–500 mg every 8 hours

### Prevention of tuberculosis in susceptible close contacts or those who have become tuberculin positive[4]

Isoniazid 300 mg daily for 6 months; CHILD 5 mg/kg daily (max. 300 mg daily)

*or* isoniazid 300 mg daily + rifampicin 600 mg daily (450 mg if less than 50 kg) for 3 months; CHILD isoniazid 5 mg/kg daily (max. 300 mg daily) + rifampicin 10 mg/kg daily (max. 450 mg daily if body-weight less than 50 kg; max. 600 mg daily if body-weight over 50 kg)

*or* (if isoniazid-resistant tuberculosis in patients under 35 years) rifampicin 600 mg daily (450 mg if less than 50 kg) for 6 months; CHILD 10 mg/kg daily (max. 450 mg daily if body-weight less than 50 kg; max. 600 mg daily if body-weight over 50 kg)

### Prevention of infection in gastro-intestinal procedures

**Operations on stomach or oesophagus**

Single dose[5] of i/v gentamicin *or* i/v cefuroxime

Add teicoplanin[6] if high risk of meticillin-resistant *Staphylococcus aureus*

---

1. For details of those who should receive chemoprophylaxis contact a consultant in communicable disease control (or a consultant in infectious diseases or the local Health Protection Agency Laboratory).
2. For details of those who should receive chemoprophylaxis contact a consultant in communicable disease control (or a consultant in infectious diseases or the local Health Protection Agency laboratory). Unless there has been direct exposure of the mouth or nose to infectious droplets from a patient with meningococcal disease who has received less than 24 hours of antibacterial treatment, healthcare workers do not generally require chemoprophylaxis.

3. Where erythromycin is suggested another macrolide (e.g. azithromycin or clarithromycin) may be used.
4. For details of those who should receive chemoprophylaxis contact the lead clinician for local tuberculosis services (or a consultant in communicable disease control). See also section 5.1.9, for advice on immunocompromised patients and on prevention of tuberculosis.
5. Additional intra-operative or postoperative doses of antibacterial may be given for prolonged procedures or if there is major blood loss.
6. Where teicoplanin is suggested vancomycin may be used

**5**

**Infections**

**Open biliary surgery**

Single dose[1] of i/v cefuroxime + i/v metronidazole[2] *or* i/v gentamicin + i/v metronidazole[2]

> Add teicoplanin[3] if high risk of meticillin-resistant *Staphylococcus aureus*

**Resections of colon and rectum for carcinoma, and resections in inflammatory bowel disease, and appendicectomy**

Single dose[1] of i/v gentamicin + i/v metronidazole[2] *or* i/v cefuroxime + i/v metronidazole[2] *or* i/v co-amoxiclav alone

> Add teicoplanin[3] if high risk of meticillin-resistant *Staphylococcus aureus*

**Endoscopic retrograde cholangiopancreatography**

Single dose of i/v gentamicin *or* oral *or* i/v ciprofloxacin

> Prophylaxis recommended if pancreatic pseudocyst, immunocompromised, history of liver transplantation, or risk of incomplete biliary drainage

**Percutaneous endoscopic gastrostomy or jejunostomy**

Single dose of i/v co-amoxiclav *or* i/v cefuroxime

> Use i/v teicoplanin[3] if history of allergy to penicillins or cephalosporins, or if high risk of meticillin-resistant *Staphylococcus aureus*

## Prevention of infection in orthopaedic surgery

**Joint replacement including hip and knee and management of fractures**

Single dose[1] of i/v cefuroxime *or* i/v flucloxacillin

> Substitute i/v teicoplanin[3] if history of allergy to penicillins or to cephalosporins or if high risk of meticillin-resistant *Staphylococcus aureus*; use cefuroxime + metronidazole for complex open fractures with extensive soft-tissue damage; prophylaxis continued for 24 hours in open fractures (longer if complex open fractures)

## Prevention of infection in urological procedures

**Transrectal prostate biopsy**

Single dose[1] of oral ciprofloxacin + oral metronidazole *or* i/v gentamicin + i/v metronidazole[2]

**Transurethral resection of prostate**

Single dose[1] of oral ciprofloxacin *or* i/v gentamicin *or* i/v cefuroxime

## Prevention of infection in obstetric and gynaecological surgery

**Caesarean section**

Single dose[1] of i/v cefuroxime

> Administer immediately after umbilical cord is clamped; substitute i/v clindamycin if history of allergy to penicillins or cephalosporins

**Hysterectomy**

Single dose[1] of i/v cefuroxime + i/v metronidazole[2] *or* i/v gentamicin + i/v metronidazole[2] *or* i/v co-amoxiclav alone

**Termination of pregnancy**

Single dose[1] of oral metronidazole

> If genital chlamydial infection cannot be ruled out, give doxycycline (section 5.1.3) postoperatively

---

1. Additional intra-operative or postoperative doses of antibacterial may be given for prolonged procedures or if there is major blood loss.
2. Metronidazole may alternatively be given by suppository but to allow adequate absorption, it should be given 2 hours before surgery.
3. Where teicoplanin is suggested vancomycin may be used

## Prevention of infection in vascular surgery

**Reconstructive arterial surgery of abdomen, pelvis or legs**

Single dose[1] of i/v cefuroxime *or* i/v ciprofloxacin

> Add i/v metronidazole for patients at risk from anaerobic infections including those with diabetes, gangrene, or undergoing amputation; add i/v teicoplanin[3] if high risk of meticillin-resistant *Staphylococcus aureus*

## Prevention of endocarditis

> ### NICE guidance
> ### Antimicrobial prophylaxis against infective endocarditis in adults and children undergoing interventional procedures (March 2008)
>
> Antibacterial prophylaxis and chlorhexidine mouthwash are **not** recommended for the prevention of endocarditis in patients undergoing dental procedures.
>
> Antibacterial prophylaxis is **not** recommended for the prevention of endocarditis in patients undergoing procedures of the:
> - upper and lower respiratory tract (including ear, nose, and throat procedures and bronchoscopy);
> - genito-urinary tract (including urological, gynaecological, and obstetric procedures);
> - upper and lower gastro-intestinal tract.
>
> Whilst these procedures can cause bacteraemia, there is no clear association with the development of infective endocarditis. Prophylaxis may expose patients to the adverse effects of antimicrobials when the evidence of benefit has not been proven.
>
> Any infection in patients at risk of endocarditis[4] should be investigated promptly and treated appropriately to reduce the risk of endocarditis.
>
> If patients at risk of endocarditis[4] are undergoing a gastro-intestinal or genito-urinary tract procedure at a site where infection is suspected, they should receive appropriate antibacterial therapy that includes cover against organisms that cause endocarditis.
>
> Patients at risk of endocarditis[4] should be:
> - advised to maintain good oral hygiene;
> - told how to recognise signs of infective endocarditis, and advised when to seek expert advice.

> ### Dermatological procedures
> Advice of a Working Party of the British Society for Antimicrobial Chemotherapy is that patients who undergo dermatological procedures[5] do not require antibacterial prophylaxis against endocarditis.

---

4. Patients at risk of endocarditis include those with valve replacement, acquired valvular heart disease with stenosis or regurgitation, structural congenital heart disease (including surgically corrected or palliated structural conditions, but excluding isolated atrial septal defect, fully repaired ventricular septal defect, fully repaired patent ductus arteriosus, and closure devices considered to be endothelialised), hypertrophic cardiomyopathy, or a previous episode of infective endocarditis.
5. The British Association of Dermatologists Therapy Guidelines and Audit Subcommittee advise that such dermatological procedures include skin biopsies and excision of moles or of malignant lesions.

## Joint prostheses and dental treatment

**Joint prostheses and dental treatment**
Advice of a Working Party of the British Society for Antimicrobial Chemotherapy is that patients with prosthetic joint implants (including total hip replacements) do not require antibiotic prophylaxis for dental treatment. The Working Party considers that it is unacceptable to expose patients to the adverse effects of antibiotics when there is no evidence that such prophylaxis is of any benefit, but that those who develop any intercurrent infection require prompt treatment with antibiotics to which the infecting organisms are sensitive.
The Working Party has commented that joint infections have rarely been shown to follow dental procedures and are even more rarely caused by oral streptococci.

## Immunosuppression and indwelling intraperitoneal catheters

**Immunosuppression and indwelling intraperitoneal catheters**
Advice of a Working Party of the British Society for Antimicrobial Chemotherapy is that patients who are immunosuppressed (including transplant patients) and patients with indwelling intraperitoneal catheters do not require antibiotic prophylaxis for dental treatment provided there is no other indication for prophylaxis.
The Working Party has commented that there is little evidence that dental treatment is followed by infection in immunosuppressed and immunodeficient patients nor is there evidence that dental treatment is followed by infection in patients with indwelling intraperitoneal catheters.

## 5.1.1 Penicillins

| 5.1.1.1 | Benzylpenicillin and phenoxymethylpenicillin |
| 5.1.1.2 | Penicillinase-resistant penicillins |
| 5.1.1.3 | Broad-spectrum penicillins |
| 5.1.1.4 | Antipseudomonal penicillins |
| 5.1.1.5 | Mecillinams |

The penicillins are bactericidal and act by interfering with bacterial cell wall synthesis. They diffuse well into body tissues and fluids, but penetration into the cerebrospinal fluid is poor except when the meninges are inflamed. They are excreted in the urine in therapeutic concentrations.

**Hypersensitivity reactions** The most important side-effect of the penicillins is hypersensitivity which causes rashes and anaphylaxis and can be fatal. Allergic reactions to penicillins occur in 1–10% of exposed individuals; anaphylactic reactions occur in fewer than 0.05% of treated patients. Patients with a history of atopic allergy (e.g. asthma, eczema, hay fever) are at a higher risk of anaphylactic reactions to penicillins. Individuals with a history of anaphylaxis, urticaria, or rash immediately after penicillin administration are at risk of immediate hypersensitivity to a penicillin; these indivi-

duals should not receive a penicillin. Patients who are allergic to one penicillin will be allergic to all because the hypersensitivity is related to the basic penicillin structure. As patients with a history of immediate hypersensitivity to penicillins may also react to the cephalosporins and other beta-lactam antibiotics, they should not receive these antibiotics; aztreonam may be less likely to cause hypersensitivity in penicillin-sensitive patients and can be used with caution. If a penicillin (or another beta-lactam antibiotic) is essential in an individual with immediate hypersensitivity to penicillin then specialist advice should be sought on hypersensitivity testing or using a beta-lactam antibiotic with a different structure to the penicillin that caused the hypersensitivity (see also p. 302).

Individuals with a history of a minor rash (i.e. non-confluent, non-pruritic rash restricted to a small area of the body) or a rash that occurs more than 72 hours after penicillin administration are probably not allergic to penicillin and in these individuals a penicillin should not be withheld unnecessarily for serious infections; the possibility of an allergic reaction should, however, be borne in mind. Other beta-lactam antibiotics (including cephalosporins) can be used in these patients.

A rare but serious toxic effect of the penicillins is encephalopathy due to cerebral irritation. This may result from excessively high doses or in patients with severe renal failure. The penicillins should **not** be given by intrathecal injection because they can cause encephalopathy which may be fatal.

Another problem relating to high doses of penicillin, or normal doses given to patients with renal failure, is the accumulation of electrolyte since most injectable penicillins contain either sodium or potassium.

Diarrhoea frequently occurs during oral penicillin therapy. It is most common with broad-spectrum penicillins, which can also cause antibiotic-associated colitis.

### 5.1.1.1 Benzylpenicillin and phenoxymethylpenicillin

**Benzylpenicillin sodium** (Penicillin G) remains an important and useful antibiotic but is inactivated by bacterial beta-lactamases. It is effective for many streptococcal (including pneumococcal), gonococcal, and meningococcal infections and also for anthrax (section 5.1.12), diphtheria, gas-gangrene, leptospirosis, and treatment of Lyme disease (section 5.1.3). Pneumococci, meningococci, and gonococci which have decreased sensitivity to penicillin have been isolated; benzylpenicillin is no longer the drug of first choice for pneumococcal meningitis. Although benzylpenicillin is effective in the treatment of tetanus, metronidazole (section 5.1.11) is preferred. Benzylpenicillin is inactivated by gastric acid and absorption from the gut is low; therefore it is best given by injection.

**Benzathine benzylpenicillin** (available from 'special-order' manufacturers or specialist importing companies, see p. 969) is used for the treatment of early syphilis and late latent syphilis; it is given by intramuscular injection.

**Phenoxymethylpenicillin** (Penicillin V) has a similar antibacterial spectrum to benzylpenicillin, but is less active. It is gastric acid-stable, so is suitable for oral administration. It should not be used for serious infections because absorption can be unpredictable and plasma concentrations variable. It is indicated principally for respiratory-tract infections in children, for streptococcal tonsillitis, and for continuing treatment after one or more injections of benzylpenicillin when clinical response has begun. It should not be used for meningococcal or gonococcal infections. Phenoxymethylpenicillin is used for prophylaxis against streptococcal infections following rheumatic fever and against pneumococcal infections following splenectomy or in sickle-cell disease.

**Oral infections** Phenoxymethylpenicillin is effective for dentoalveolar abscess.

### ◾ BENZYLPENICILLIN SODIUM
(Penicillin G)

**Indications** throat infections, otitis media, endocarditis, meningococcal disease, pneumonia, cellulitis (Table 1, section 5.1); anthrax; prophylaxis in limb amputation (Table 2, section 5.1); see also notes above

**Cautions** history of allergy; false-positive urinary glucose (if tested for reducing substances); renal impairment (Appendix 3); **interactions:** Appendix 1 (penicillins)

**Contra-indications** penicillin hypersensitivity

**Side-effects** hypersensitivity reactions including urticaria, fever, joint pains, rashes, angioedema, anaphylaxis, serum sickness-like reaction; *rarely* CNS toxicity including convulsions (especially with high doses or in severe renal impairment), interstitial nephritis, haemolytic anaemia, leucopenia, thrombocytopenia, and coagulation disorders; also reported diarrhoea (including antibiotic-associated colitis)

**Dose**

- By intramuscular *or* by slow intravenous injection *or* by infusion, 2.4–4.8 g daily in 4 divided doses, increased if necessary in more serious infections (single doses over 1.2 g intravenous route only; see also below); PRETERM NEONATE and NEONATE under 1 week, 50 mg/kg daily in 2 divided doses; NEONATE 1–4 weeks, 75 mg/kg daily in 3 divided doses; CHILD 1 month–12 years, 100 mg/kg daily in 4 divided doses (higher doses may be required, see also below); intravenous route recommended in neonates and infants
- Endocarditis (in combination with another antibacterial if necessary, see Table 1, section 5.1), by slow intravenous injection *or* by infusion, 7.2 g daily in 6 divided doses, increased if necessary (e.g. in enterococcal endocarditis or if benzylpenicillin used alone) to 14.4 g daily in 6 divided doses
- Anthrax (in combination with other antibacterials, see also section 5.1.12), by slow intravenous injection *or* by infusion, 2.4 g every 4 hours; CHILD 150 mg/kg daily in 4 divided doses
- Intrapartum prophylaxis against group B streptococcal infection, by slow intravenous injection *or* by infusion, initially 3 g then 1.5 g every 4 hours until delivery
- Meningitis, meningococcal disease, by slow intravenous injection *or* by infusion, 2.4 g every 4 hours; PRETERM NEONATE and NEONATE, 225 mg/kg daily in 3 divided doses; CHILD 1 month–12 years, 180–300 mg/kg daily in 4–6 divided doses

**Important.** If bacterial meningitis and especially if meningococcal disease is suspected general practitioners are advised to give a single injection of benzylpenicillin by

intravenous injection (or by intramuscular injection) before transferring the patient urgently to hospital. Suitable doses are: ADULT 1.2 g; INFANT under 1 year 300 mg; CHILD 1–9 years 600 mg, 10 years and over as for adult. In **penicillin allergy**, cefotaxime (section 5.1.2) may be an alternative; chloramphenicol may be used if there is a history of anaphylaxis to penicillins

- By intrathecal injection, **not** recommended
Note Benzylpenicillin doses in BNF may differ from those in product literature

**Crystapen®** (Genus) ᴾᵒᴹ
Injection, powder for reconstitution, benzylpenicillin sodium (unbuffered), net price 600-mg vial = 95p, 2-vial 'GP pack' = £2.64; 1.2-g vial = £1.89
Electrolytes Na⁺ 1.68 mmol/600-mg vial; 3.36 mmol/1.2-g vial

### ◾ PHENOXYMETHYLPENICILLIN
(Penicillin V)

**Indications** oral infections (see notes above); tonsillitis, otitis media, erysipelas, cellulitis; group A streptococcal infection, rheumatic fever and pneumococcal infection prophylaxis (Table 2, section 5.1)

**Cautions** see under Benzylpenicillin; **interactions:** Appendix 1 (penicillins)

**Contra-indications** see under Benzylpenicillin

**Side-effects** see under Benzylpenicillin

**Dose**

- 500 mg every 6 hours increased up to 1 g every 6 hours in severe infections; CHILD up to 1 year 62.5 mg every 6 hours, increased up to 12.5 mg/kg every 6 hours in severe infections; 1–6 years, 125 mg every 6 hours, increased up to 12.5 mg/kg every 6 hours in severe infections; 6–12 years, 250 mg every 6 hours, increased up to 12.5 mg/kg every 6 hours in severe infections
Note Phenoxymethylpenicillin doses in the BNF may differ from those in product literature

**Phenoxymethylpenicillin** (Non-proprietary) ᴾᵒᴹ
Tablets, phenoxymethylpenicillin (as potassium salt) 250 mg, net price 28-tab pack = £1.25. Label: 9, 23

Oral solution, phenoxymethylpenicillin (as potassium salt) for reconstitution with water, net price 125 mg/5 mL, 100 mL = £1.90; 250 mg/5 mL, 100 mL = £2.59. Label: 9, 23
Dental prescribing on NHS Phenoxymethylpenicillin Tablets and Oral Solution may be prescribed

### 5.1.1.2 Penicillinase-resistant penicillins

Most staphylococci are now resistant to benzylpenicillin because they produce penicillinases. **Flucloxacillin**, however, is not inactivated by these enzymes and is thus effective in infections caused by penicillin-resistant staphylococci, which is the sole indication for its use. Flucloxacillin is acid-stable and can, therefore, be given by mouth as well as by injection.

Flucloxacillin is well absorbed from the gut. For CSM warning on hepatic disorders see under Flucloxacillin.

**Temocillin** is active against Gram-negative bacteria and is stable against a wide range of beta-lactamases. It should be reserved for the treatment of infections caused by beta-lactamase-producing strains of Gram-negative bacteria, including those resistant to third-generation cephalosporins. Temocillin is not active against *Pseudomonas aeruginosa* or *Acinetobacter* spp.

**MRSA** Infection from *Staphylococcus aureus* strains resistant to meticillin [now discontinued] (meticillin-resistant *Staph. aureus*, MRSA) and to flucloxacillin can be difficult to manage. Treatment is guided by the sensitivity of the infecting strain.

**Rifampicin** (section 5.1.9) or **sodium fusidate** (section 5.1.7) should **not** be used alone because resistance may develop rapidly. A **tetracycline** alone or a combination of rifampicin and sodium fusidate can be used for *skin* and *soft-tissue infections* caused by MRSA; **clindamycin** alone is an alternative. A **glycopeptide** (e.g. vancomycin, section 5.1.7) can be used for severe skin and soft-tissue infections associated with MRSA; if a glycopeptide is unsuitable, **linezolid** (section 5.1.7) can be used on expert advice. As linezolid is **not** active against Gram-negative organisms, it can be used for mixed skin and soft-tissue infections only when other treatments are not available; linezolid must be given with other antibacterials if the infection also involves Gram-negative organisms. A combination of a glycopeptide and sodium fusidate *or* a glycopeptide and rifampicin can be considered for skin and soft-tissue infections that have failed to respond to a single antibacterial.

The combination of the streptogramin antibiotics **quinupristin** and **dalfopristin** (section 5.1.7) should be reserved for skin and soft-tissue infections that have not responded to other antibacterials or for patients who cannot tolerate other antibacterials. **Tigecycline** (section 5.1.3) and **daptomycin** (section 5.1.7) are licensed for the treatment of complicated skin and soft-tissue infections involving MRSA.

A **tetracycline** or **clindamycin** can be used for *bronchiectasis* caused by MRSA. A **glycopeptide** can be used for *pneumonia* associated with MRSA; if a glycopeptide is unsuitable, **linezolid** can be used on expert advice. Linezolid must be given with other antibacterials if the infection also involves Gram-negative organisms. **Quinupristin** and **dalfopristin** should be reserved for hospital acquired pneumonia that has not responded to other antibacterials or for patients who cannot tolerate other antibacterials.

A **tetracycline** can be used for *urinary-tract infections* caused by MRSA; **trimethoprim** or **nitrofurantoin** are alternatives. A **glycopeptide** can be used for urinary-tract infections that are severe or resistant to other antibacterials.

A **glycopeptide** can be used for *septicaemia* associated with MRSA.

For the management of *endocarditis*, *osteomyelitis*, or *septic arthritis* associated with MRSA, see Table 1, section 5.1.

Prophylaxis with vancomycin or teicoplanin (alone or in combination with another antibacterial active against other pathogens) is appropriate for patients undergoing surgery if:

- there is a history of MRSA colonisation or infection without documented eradication;

- there is a risk that the patient's MRSA carriage has recurred;

- the patient comes from an area with a high prevalence of MRSA.

For eradication of nasal carriage of MRSA, see section 12.2.3.

## FLUCLOXACILLIN

**Indications** infections due to beta-lactamase-producing staphylococci including otitis externa; adjunct in pneumonia, impetigo, cellulitis, osteomyelitis and in staphylococcal endocarditis (Table 1, section 5.1)

**Cautions** see under Benzylpenicillin (section 5.1.1.1); also hepatic impairment (see CSM advice below); risk of kernicterus in jaundiced neonates when high doses given parenterally

> **CSM advice (hepatic disorders)**
> CSM has advised that very rarely cholestatic jaundice and hepatitis may occur up to several weeks after treatment with flucloxacillin has been stopped. Administration for more than 2 weeks and increasing age are risk factors. CSM has reminded that:
> - flucloxacillin should not be used in patients with a history of hepatic dysfunction associated with flucloxacillin;
> - flucloxacillin should be used with caution in patients with hepatic impairment;
> - careful enquiry should be made about hypersensitivity reactions to beta-lactam antibacterials.

**Contra-indications** see under Benzylpenicillin (section 5.1.1.1)

**Side-effects** see under Benzylpenicillin (section 5.1.1.1); also gastro-intestinal disturbances; *very rarely* hepatitis and cholestatic jaundice (see also CSM advice above)

**Dose**

- By mouth, 250–500 mg every 6 hours, at least 30 minutes before food; CHILD under 2 years quarter adult dose; 2–10 years half adult dose

- By intramuscular injection, 250–500 mg every 6 hours; CHILD under 2 years quarter adult dose; 2–10 years half adult dose

- By slow intravenous injection *or* by intravenous infusion, 0.25–2 g every 6 hours; CHILD under 2 years quarter adult dose; 2–10 years half adult dose
  Endocarditis (in combination with another antibacterial, see Table 1, section 5.1), body-weight under 85 kg, 8 g daily in 4 divided doses; body-weight over 85 kg, 12 g daily in 6 divided doses
  Osteomyelitis (see Table 1, section 5.1), up to 8 g daily in 3–4 divided doses

- Surgical prophylaxis, by slow intravenous injection *or* by intravenous infusion, 1–2 g at induction; up to 4 further doses of 500 mg may be given every 6 hours by mouth, *or* by intramuscular injection, *or* by slow intravenous injection *or* by intravenous infusion for high risk procedures

Note Flucloxacillin doses in BNF may differ from those in product literature

**Flucloxacillin** (Non-proprietary) PoM
Capsules, flucloxacillin (as sodium salt) 250 mg, net price 28 = £1.93; 500 mg, 28 = £3.90. Label: 9, 23
Brands include *Floxapen®*, *Fluclomix®*, *Ladropen®*

Oral solution (= elixir or syrup), flucloxacillin (as sodium salt) for reconstitution with water, 125 mg/5 mL, net price 100 mL = £3.07; 250 mg/5 mL, 100 mL = £8.51. Label: 9, 23
Brands include *Ladropen®*

Injection, powder for reconstitution, flucloxacillin (as sodium salt). Net price 250-mg vial = £1.23; 500-mg vial = £2.45; 1-g vial = £4.90

**5**

**Infections**

**Floxapen®** (GSK) PoM

Suspension (= syrup), flucloxacillin (as magnesium salt) for reconstitution with water, 125 mg/5 mL, net price 100 mL = £4.03; 250 mg/5 mL, 100 mL = £8.02. Label: 9, 23

### TEMOCILLIN

**Indications** septicaemia, urinary-tract infections, lower respiratory-tract infections caused by susceptible Gram-negative bacteria

**Cautions** see under Benzylpenicillin (section 5.1.1.1); renal impairment (Appendix 3); pregnancy (Appendix 4); breast-feeding (Appendix 5)

**Contra-indications** see under Benzylpenicillin (section 5.1.1.1)

**Side-effects** see under Benzylpenicillin (section 5.1.1.1)

**Dose**

• By intramuscular injection *or* by intravenous injection over 3–4 minutes, *or* by intravenous infusion, ADULT and CHILD over 12 years (body-weight over 45 kg), 1–2 g every 12 hours

Uncomplicated urinary-tract infections, ADULT and CHILD over 12 years (body-weight over 45 kg), 1 g daily as a single daily dose or in divided doses

**Negaban®** (Eumedica) PoM

Injection, powder for reconstitution, temocillin (as sodium salt), net price 1-g vial = £25.45
Electrolytes Na+ 4.35 mmol/g

### 5.1.1.3 Broad-spectrum penicillins

**Ampicillin** is active against certain Gram-positive and Gram-negative organisms but is inactivated by penicillinases including those produced by *Staphylococcus aureus* and by common Gram-negative bacilli such as *Escherichia coli*. Almost all staphylococci, approx. 60% of *E. coli* strains and approx. 20% of *Haemophilus influenzae* strains are now resistant. The likelihood of resistance should therefore be considered before using ampicillin for the 'blind' treatment of infections; in particular, it should not be used for hospital patients without checking sensitivity.

Ampicillin is well excreted in the bile and urine. It is principally indicated for the treatment of exacerbations of chronic bronchitis and middle ear infections, both of which may be due to *Streptococcus pneumoniae* and *H. influenzae*, and for urinary-tract infections (section 5.1.13).

Ampicillin can be given by mouth but less than half the dose is absorbed, and absorption is further decreased by the presence of food in the gut.

Maculopapular rashes commonly occur with ampicillin (and amoxicillin) but are not usually related to true penicillin allergy. They almost always occur in patients with glandular fever; broad-spectrum penicillins should not therefore be used for 'blind' treatment of a sore throat. Rashes are also common in patients with acute or chronic lymphocytic leukaemia or in cytomegalovirus infection.

**Amoxicillin** (amoxycillin) is a derivative of ampicillin and has a similar antibacterial spectrum. It is better absorbed than ampicillin when given by mouth, producing higher plasma and tissue concentrations; unlike ampicillin, absorption is not affected by the presence of food in the stomach. Amoxicillin may also be used for the treatment of Lyme disease [not licensed], see below.

**Co-amoxiclav** consists of amoxicillin with the beta-lactamase inhibitor clavulanic acid. Clavulanic acid itself has no significant antibacterial activity but, by inactivating beta-lactamases, it makes the combination active against beta-lactamase-producing bacteria that are resistant to amoxicillin. These include resistant strains of *Staph. aureus*, *E. coli*, and *H. influenzae*, as well as many *Bacteroides* and *Klebsiella* spp. Co-amoxiclav should be reserved for infections likely, or known, to be caused by amoxicillin-resistant beta-lactamase-producing strains; for CSM warning on cholestatic jaundice see under Co-amoxiclav.

A combination of ampicillin with flucloxacillin (as co-fluampicil) is available to treat infections involving either streptococci or staphylococci (e.g. cellulitis).

**Lyme disease**  Lyme disease should generally be treated by those experienced in its management. **Doxycycline** (p. 309), **amoxicillin** [unlicensed indication] or **cefuroxime axetil** are the antibacterials of choice for *early Lyme disease* or *Lyme arthritis*. If these antibacterials are contra-indicated, a **macrolide** (e.g. erythromycin) can be used for early Lyme disease. Intravenous administration of **ceftriaxone, cefotaxime** (p. 302), or **benzylpenicillin** (p. 296) is recommended for Lyme disease associated with cardiac or neurological complications. The duration of treatment is usually 2–4 weeks; Lyme arthritis may require further treatment.

**Oral infections**  Amoxicillin or ampicillin are as effective as phenoxymethylpenicillin (section 5.1.1.1) but they are better absorbed; however, they may encourage emergence of resistant organisms. Like phenoxymethylpenicillin, amoxicillin and ampicillin are ineffective against bacteria that produce beta-lactamases. Amoxicillin may be useful for short-course oral regimens. Co-amoxiclav is active against beta-lactamase-producing bacteria that are resistant to amoxicillin. Co-amoxiclav may be used for severe dental infection with spreading cellulitis or dental infection not responding to first-line antibacterial treatment.

### AMOXICILLIN
(Amoxycillin)

**Indications** see under Ampicillin; oral infections (see notes above); also endocarditis treatment (Table 1, section 5.1); anthrax (section 5.1.12); adjunct in listerial meningitis (Table 1, section 5.1); *Helicobacter pylori* eradication (section 1.3)

**Cautions** see under Ampicillin; maintain adequate hydration with high doses (particularly during parenteral therapy)

**Contra-indications** see under Ampicillin

**Side-effects** see under Ampicillin

**Dose**

• By mouth, 250 mg every 8 hours, doubled in severe infections; CHILD up to 10 years, 125 mg every 8 hours, doubled in severe infections

Otitis media, 1 g every 8 hours; CHILD 40 mg/kg daily in 3 divided doses (max. 3 g daily)

Pneumonia, 0.5–1 g every 8 hours

Anthrax (treatment and post-exposure prophylaxis—see also section 5.1.12), 500 mg every

8 hours; CHILD body-weight under 20 kg, 80 mg/kg daily in 3 divided doses, body-weight over 20 kg, adult dose

- *Short-course oral therapy*

Dental abscess, 3 g repeated after 8 hours

Urinary-tract infections, 3 g repeated after 10–12 hours

- By intramuscular injection, 500 mg every 8 hours; CHILD, 50–100 mg/kg daily in divided doses
- By intravenous injection or infusion, 500 mg every 8 hours increased to 1 g every 6 hours in severe infections; CHILD 50–100 mg/kg daily in divided doses
- Listerial meningitis (in combination with another antibiotic, see Table 1, section 5.1), by intravenous infusion, 2 g every 4 hours for 10–14 days
- Endocarditis (in combination with another antibiotic if necessary, see Table 1, section 5.1), by intravenous infusion, 2 g every 6 hours, increased to 2 g every 4 hours e.g. in enterococcal endocarditis or if amoxicillin used alone

**Note** Amoxicillin doses in BNF may differ from those in product literature

**Amoxicillin** (Non-proprietary) [PoM]

Capsules, amoxicillin (as trihydrate) 250 mg, net price 21 = £1.16; 500 mg, 21 = £1.53. Label: 9
Brands include *Amix®*, *Amoram®*, *Amoxident®*, *Galenamox®*, *Rimoxallin®*

Oral suspension, amoxicillin (as trihydrate) for reconstitution with water, 125 mg/5 mL, net price 100 mL = £1.34; 250 mg/5 mL, 100 mL = £1.48. Label: 9
**Note** Sugar-free versions are available and can be ordered by specifying 'sugar-free' on the prescription
Brands include *Amoram®*, *Galenamox®*, *Rimoxallin®*

Sachets, sugar-free, amoxicillin (as trihydrate) 3 g/sachet, net price 2-sachet pack = £5.43, 14-sachet pack = £31.94. Label: 9, 13

Injection, powder for reconstitution, amoxicillin (as sodium salt), net price 250-mg vial = 32p; 500-mg vial = 66p; 1-g vial = £1.16
**Dental prescribing on NHS** Amoxicillin Capsules and Oral Suspension may be prescribed. Amoxicillin Sachets may be prescribed as Amoxicillin Oral Powder

**Amoxil®** (GSK) [PoM]

Capsules, both maroon/gold, amoxicillin (as trihydrate), 250 mg, net price 21-cap pack = £3.45; 500 mg, 21-cap pack = £6.91. Label: 9

Paediatric suspension, amoxicillin 125 mg (as trihydrate)/1.25 mL when reconstituted with water, net price 20 mL (peach- strawberry- and lemon-flavoured) = £3.25. Label: 9, counselling , use of pipette
Excipients include sucrose 600 mg/1.25 mL

Sachets SF, powder, sugar-free, amoxicillin (as trihydrate) 3 g/sachet, 2-sachet pack (peach- strawberry- and lemon-flavoured) = £2.99. Label: 9, 13

Injection, powder for reconstitution, amoxicillin (as sodium salt), net price 500-mg vial = 56p; 1-g vial = £1.12
Electrolytes Na⁺ 3.3 mmol/g

## AMPICILLIN

**Indications** urinary-tract infections, otitis media, sinusitis, oral infections (see notes above), bronchitis, uncomplicated community-acquired pneumonia (Table 1, section 5.1), *Haemophilus influenzae* infec-

tions, invasive salmonellosis; listerial meningitis (Table 1, section 5.1)

**Cautions** history of allergy; renal impairment (Appendix 3); erythematous rashes common in glandular fever, cytomegalovirus infection, and acute or chronic lymphocytic leukaemia (see notes above); **interactions**: Appendix 1 (penicillins)

**Contra-indications** penicillin hypersensitivity

**Side-effects** nausea, vomiting, diarrhoea; rashes (discontinue treatment); rarely, antibiotic-associated colitis; see also under Benzylpenicillin (section 5.1.1.1)

**Dose**

- By mouth, 0.25–1 g every 6 hours, at least 30 minutes before food; CHILD under 10 years, half adult dose

Urinary-tract infections, 500 mg every 8 hours; CHILD under 10 years, half adult dose

- By intramuscular injection or intravenous injection or infusion, 500 mg every 4–6 hours; CHILD under 10 years, half adult dose
- Endocarditis (in combination with another antibiotic if necessary), by intravenous infusion, 2 g every 6 hours, increased to 2 g every 4 hours e.g. in enterococcal endocarditis or if ampicillin used alone
- Listerial meningitis (in combination with another antibiotic), by intravenous infusion, 2 g every 4 hours for 10–14 days; NEONATE 50 mg/kg every 6 hours; INFANT 1–3 months, 50–100 mg/kg every 6 hours; CHILD 3 months–12 years, 100 mg/kg every 6 hours (max. 12 g daily)

**Note** Ampicillin doses in BNF may differ from those in product literature

**Ampicillin** (Non-proprietary) [PoM]

Capsules, ampicillin 250 mg, net price 28 = £3.88; 500 mg, 28 = £19.68. Label: 9, 23
Brands include *Rimacillin®*

Oral suspension, ampicillin 125 mg/5 mL when reconstituted with water, net price 100 mL = £3.38; 250 mg/5 mL, 100 mL = £6.61. Label: 9, 23
Brands include *Rimacillin®*

Injection, powder for reconstitution, ampicillin (as sodium salt), net price 500-mg vial = £7.83
**Dental prescribing on NHS** Ampicillin Capsules and Oral Suspension may be prescribed

**Penbritin®** (Chemidex) [PoM]

Capsules, grey/red, ampicillin (as trihydrate) 250 mg, net price 28-cap pack = £2.10; 500 mg, 28-cap pack = £5.28. Label: 9, 23

Syrup, apricot- caramel- and peppermint-flavoured, ampicillin (as trihydrate) for reconstitution with water, 125 mg/5 mL, net price 100 mL = £3.78; 250 mg/5 mL, 100 mL = £7.39. Label: 9, 23
Excipients include sucrose 3.6 g/5 mL

◢**With flucloxacillin**
See Co-fluampicil

## CO-AMOXICLAV

A mixture of amoxicillin (as the trihydrate or as the sodium salt) and clavulanic acid (as potassium clavulanate); the proportions are expressed in the form $x/y$ where $x$ and $y$ are the strengths in milligrams of amoxicillin and clavulanic acid respectively

**Indications** infections due to beta-lactamase-producing strains (where amoxicillin alone not appropriate) including respiratory-tract infections, genito-urinary

**5**
**Infections**

and abdominal infections, cellulitis, animal bites, severe dental infection with spreading cellulitis or dental infection not responding to first-line anti-bacterial

**Cautions** see under Ampicillin and notes above; also caution in hepatic impairment (monitor hepatic function), pregnancy; maintain adequate hydration with high doses (particularly during parenteral therapy)

Cholestatic jaundice CSM has advised that cholestatic jaundice can occur either during or shortly after the use of co-amoxiclav. An epidemiological study has shown that the risk of acute liver toxicity was about 6 times greater with co-amoxiclav than with amoxicillin. Cholestatic jaundice is more common in patients above the age of 65 years and in men; these reactions have only rarely been reported in children. Jaundice is usually self-limiting and very rarely fatal. The duration of treatment should be appropriate to the indication and should not usually exceed 14 days

**Contra-indications** penicillin hypersensitivity, history of co-amoxiclav-associated or penicillin-associated jaundice or hepatic dysfunction

**Side-effects** see under Ampicillin; hepatitis, cholestatic jaundice (see above); Stevens-Johnson syndrome, toxic epidermal necrolysis, exfoliative dermatitis, vasculitis reported; rarely prolongation of bleeding time, dizziness, headache, convulsions (particularly with high doses or in renal impairment); superficial staining of teeth with suspension; phlebitis at injection site

**Dose**

- By mouth, expressed as co-amoxiclav, one *250/125* strength tablet every 8 hours, increased in severe infections to one *500/125* strength tablet every 8 hours; CHILD see under preparations below (under 6 years *Augmentin® '125/31 SF'* suspension; 6–12 years *Augmentin® '250/62 SF'* suspension *or* for short-term treatment with twice daily dosage in CHILD 2 months–12 years *Augmentin-Duo® 400/57* suspension)

  Severe dental infections (but not generally first-line, see notes above), expressed as co-amoxiclav, one *250/125* strength tablet every 8 hours for 5 days

- By intravenous injection over 3–4 minutes or by intravenous infusion, expressed as co-amoxiclav, 1.2 g every 8 hours increased in more serious infections to 1.2 g every 6 hours; INFANTS up to 3 months 30 mg/kg every 8 hours (every 12 hours in the perinatal period and in premature infants); CHILD 3 months–12 years, 30 mg/kg every 8 hours increased in more serious infections to 30 mg/kg every 6 hours

  Surgical prophylaxis, expressed as co-amoxiclav, 1.2 g at induction; for high risk procedures (e.g. colorectal surgery) up to 2–3 further doses of 1.2 g may be given every 8 hours

**Co-amoxiclav** (Non-proprietary) PoM

Tablets, co-amoxiclav 250/125 (amoxicillin 250 mg as trihydrate, clavulanic acid 125 mg as potassium salt), net price 21-tab pack = £2.59. Label: 9
Dental prescribing on NHS Co-amoxiclav 250/125 Tablets may be prescribed

Tablets, co-amoxiclav 500/125 (amoxicillin 500 mg as trihydrate, clavulanic acid 125 mg as potassium salt), net price 21-tab pack = £6.17. Label: 9

Oral suspension, co-amoxiclav 125/31 (amoxicillin 125 mg as trihydrate, clavulanic acid 31.25 mg as

potassium salt)/5 mL when reconstituted with water, net price 100 mL = £3.26. Label: 9
Dental prescribing on NHS Co-amoxiclav 125/31 Suspension may be prescribed

Oral suspension, co-amoxiclav 250/62 (amoxicillin 250 mg as trihydrate, clavulanic acid 62.5 mg as potassium salt)/5 mL when reconstituted with water, net price 100 mL = £4.04. Label: 9
Dental prescribing on NHS Co-amoxiclav 250/62 Suspension may be prescribed

Injection 500/100, powder for reconstitution, co-amoxiclav 500/100 (amoxicillin 500 mg as sodium salt, clavulanic acid 100 mg as potassium salt), net price per vial = £1.21

Injection 1000/200, powder for reconstitution, co-amoxiclav 1000/200 (amoxicillin 1 g as sodium salt, clavulanic acid 200 mg as potassium salt), net price per vial = £2.42

**Augmentin®** (GSK) PoM

Tablets 375 mg, f/c, co-amoxiclav 250/125 (amoxicillin 250 mg as trihydrate, clavulanic acid 125 mg as potassium salt), net price 21-tab pack = £4.28. Label: 9

Tablets 625 mg, f/c, co-amoxiclav 500/125 (amoxicillin 500 mg as trihydrate, clavulanic acid 125 mg as potassium salt). Net price 21-tab pack = £8.16. Label: 9

Dispersible tablets, sugar-free, co-amoxiclav 250/125 (amoxicillin 250 mg as trihydrate, clavulanic acid 125 mg as potassium salt). Net price 21-tab pack = £9.82. Label: 9, 13

Suspension '125/31 SF', sugar-free, co-amoxiclav 125/31 (amoxicillin 125 mg as trihydrate, clavulanic acid 31.25 mg as potassium salt)/5 mL when reconstituted with water. Net price 100 mL (raspberry-and orange-flavoured) = £4.08. Label: 9
Excipients include aspartame 12.5 mg/5 mL (section 9.4.1)
Dose CHILD 1–6 years (10–18 kg) 5 mL every 8 hours or INFANT and CHILD up to 6 years 0.8 mL/kg daily in 3 divided doses; in severe infections dose increased to 1.6 mL/kg daily in 3 divided doses

Suspension '250/62 SF', sugar-free, co-amoxiclav 250/62 (amoxicillin 250 mg as trihydrate, clavulanic acid 62.5 mg as potassium salt)/5 mL when reconstituted with water. Net price 100 mL (raspberry-and orange-flavoured) = £5.74. Label: 9
Excipients include aspartame 12.5 mg/5 mL (section 9.4.1)
Dose CHILD 6–12 years (18–40 kg) 5 mL every 8 hours or 0.4 mL/kg daily in 3 divided doses; in severe infections dose increased to 0.8 mL/kg daily in 3 divided doses

Injection 600 mg, powder for reconstitution, co-amoxiclav 500/100 (amoxicillin 500 mg as sodium salt, clavulanic acid 100 mg as potassium salt). Net price per vial = £1.33
Electrolytes Na⁺ 1.35 mmol, K⁺ 0.5 mmol/600-mg vial

Injection 1.2 g, powder for reconstitution, co-amoxiclav 1000/200 (amoxicillin 1 g as sodium salt, clavulanic acid 200 mg as potassium salt). Net price per vial = £2.65
Electrolytes Na⁺ 2.7 mmol, K⁺ 1 mmol/1.2-g vial

**Augmentin-Duo®** (GSK) PoM

Suspension '400/57', sugar-free, strawberry-flavoured, co-amoxiclav 400/57 (amoxicillin 400 mg as trihydrate, clavulanic acid 57 mg as potassium salt)/5 mL when reconstituted with water. Net price 35 mL = £4.21, 70 mL = £5.91. Label: 9
Excipients include aspartame 12.5 mg/5 mL (section 9.4.1)
Dose CHILD 2 months–2 years 0.15 mL/kg twice daily, 2–6 years (13–21 kg) 2.5 mL twice daily, 7–12 years (22–40 kg) 5 mL twice daily, doubled in severe infections

# CO-FLUAMPICIL

A mixture of equal parts by mass of flucloxacillin and ampicillin

**Indications** mixed infections involving beta-lactamase-producing staphylococci

**Cautions** see under Ampicillin and Flucloxacillin

**Contra-indications** see under Ampicillin and Flucloxacillin

**Side-effects** see under Ampicillin and Flucloxacillin

**Dose**

- By mouth, co-fluampicil, 250/250 every 6 hours, dose doubled in severe infections; CHILD under 10 years half adult dose, dose doubled in severe infections

- By intramuscular or slow intravenous injection or by intravenous infusion, co-fluampicil 250/250 every 6 hours, dose doubled in severe infections; CHILD under 2 years quarter adult dose, 2–10 years half adult dose, dose doubled in severe infections

**Co-fluampicil** (Non-proprietary) [PoM]

Capsules, co-fluampicil 250/250 (flucloxacillin 250 mg as sodium salt, ampicillin 250 mg as trihydrate), net price 28-cap pack = £15.85. Label: 9, 22
Brands include *Flu-Amp®*

**Magnapen®** (Wockhardt) [PoM]

Capsules, black/turquoise, co-fluampicil 250/250 (flucloxacillin 250 mg as sodium salt, ampicillin 250 mg as trihydrate), net price 20-cap pack = £4.00. Label: 9, 22

Syrup, co-fluampicil 125/125 (flucloxacillin 125 mg as magnesium salt, ampicillin 125 mg as trihydrate)/ 5 mL when reconstituted with water, net price 100 mL = £4.99. Label: 9, 22
Excipients include sucrose 3.14 g/5 mL

Injection 500 mg, powder for reconstitution, co-fluampicil 250/250 (flucloxacillin 250 mg as sodium salt, ampicillin 250 mg as sodium salt), net price per vial = £1.33
Electrolytes Na+ 1.3 mmol/vial

## 5.1.1.4 Antipseudomonal penicillins

The carboxypenicillin, **ticarcillin**, is principally indicated for serious infections caused by *Pseudomonas aeruginosa* although it also has activity against certain other Gram-negative bacilli including *Proteus* spp. and *Bacteroides fragilis*.

Ticarcillin is now available only in combination with clavulanic acid (section 5.1.1.3); the combination (*Timentin®*) is active against beta-lactamase-producing bacteria resistant to ticarcillin.

The ureidopenicillin, **piperacillin**, is more active than ticarcillin against *Ps. aeruginosa*. Piperacillin is now available only in combination with the beta-lactamase inhibitor tazobactam. The spectrum of activity of piperacillin with tazobactam is comparable to that of the carbapenems, imipenem and meropenem (section 5.1.2).

For pseudomonas septicaemias (especially in neutropenia or endocarditis) these antipseudomonal penicillins should be given with an aminoglycoside (e.g. gentamicin section 5.1.4) since they have a synergistic effect.

Owing to the sodium content of many of these antibiotics, high doses may lead to hypernatraemia.

# PIPERACILLIN WITH TAZOBACTAM

**Indications** see under Dose

**Cautions** see under Benzylpenicillin (section 5.1.1.1); renal impairment (Appendix 3); pregnancy (Appendix 4); breast-feeding (Appendix 5)

**Contra-indications** see under Benzylpenicillin (section 5.1.1.1)

**Side-effects** see under Benzylpenicillin (section 5.1.1.1); also nausea, vomiting, diarrhoea; *less commonly* stomatitis, dyspepsia, constipation, jaundice, hypotension, headache, insomnia, and injection-site reactions; *rarely* abdominal pain, hepatitis, oedema, fatigue, and eosinophilia; *very rarely* hypoglycaemia, hypokalaemia, pancytopenia, Stevens-Johnson syndrome, and toxic epidermal necrolysis

**Dose**

**Note** Expressed as a combination of piperacillin and tazobactam (both as sodium salts) in a ratio of 8:1

- Lower respiratory-tract, urinary-tract, intra-abdominal and skin infections, and septicaemia, ADULT and CHILD over 12 years, by intravenous injection over 3–5 minutes or by intravenous infusion, 2.25–4.5 g every 6–8 hours, usually 4.5 g every 8 hours

- Complicated appendicitis, by intravenous injection over 3–5 minutes or by intravenous infusion, CHILD 2–12 years, 112.5 mg/kg (max. 4.5 g) every 8 hours for 5–14 days; CHILD under 2 years, not recommended

- Infections in neutropenic patients (in combination with an aminoglycoside), by intravenous injection over 3–5 minutes or by intravenous infusion, ADULT and CHILD over 50 kg, 4.5 g every 6 hours; CHILD less than 50 kg, 90 mg/kg every 6 hours

**Piperacillin with tazobactam** (Non-proprietary) [PoM]

Injection 2.25 g, powder for reconstitution, piperacillin 2 g (as sodium salt), tazobactam 250 mg (as sodium salt), net price 2.25-g vial = £7.16

Injection 4.5 g, powder for reconstitution, piperacillin 4 g (as sodium salt), tazobactam 500 mg (as sodium salt), net price 4.5-g vial = £14.21

**Tazocin®** (Wyeth) [PoM]

Injection 2.25 g, powder for reconstitution, piperacillin 2 g (as sodium salt), tazobactam 250 mg (as sodium salt), net price 2.25-g vial = £7.65
Electrolytes Na+ 5.58 mmol/2.25-g vial

Injection 4.5 g, powder for reconstitution, piperacillin 4 g (as sodium salt), tazobactam 500 mg (as sodium salt), net price 4.5-g vial = £15.17
Electrolytes Na+ 11.16 mmol/4.5-g vial

# TICARCILLIN

**Indications** infections due to *Pseudomonas* and *Proteus* spp, see notes above

**Cautions** see under Benzylpenicillin (section 5.1.1.1)

**Contra-indications** see under Benzylpenicillin (section 5.1.1.1)

**Side-effects** see under Benzylpenicillin (section 5.1.1.1); also nausea, vomiting, coagulation disorders, haemorrhagic cystitis (more frequent in children), injection-site reactions, Stevens-Johnson syndrome, toxic epidermal necrolysis, hypokalaemia, eosinophilia

**Dose**

- See under preparation

5

Infections

◀With clavulanic acid

**Note** For a CSM warning on cholestatic jaundice possibly associated with clavulanic acid, see under Co-amoxiclav p. 300.

**Timentin** (GSK) PoM

Injection 3.2 g, powder for reconstitution, ticarcillin 3 g (as sodium salt), clavulanic acid 200 mg (as potassium salt). Net price per vial = £5.44
Electrolytes Na⁺ 16 mmol, K⁺ 1 mmol /3.2-g vial

**Dose** by intravenous infusion, 3.2 g every 6–8 hours increased to every 4 hours in more severe infections; CHILD 1 month–18 years, body-weight under 40 kg, 80 mg/kg every 8 hours, increased to every 6 hours in more severe infections; body weight over 40 kg, adult dose

### 5.1.1.5 Mecillinams

**Pivmecillinam** has significant activity against many Gram-negative bacteria including *Escherichia coli*, klebsiella, enterobacter, and salmonellae. It is not active against *Pseudomonas aeruginosa* or enterococci. Pivmecillinam is hydrolysed to mecillinam, which is the active drug.

### PIVMECILLINAM HYDROCHLORIDE

**Indications** see under Dose below

**Cautions** see under Benzylpenicillin (section 5.1.1.1); also liver and renal function tests required in long-term use; avoid in acute porphyria (section 9.8.2); pregnancy; **interactions**: Appendix 1 (penicillins)

**Contra-indications** see under Benzylpenicillin (section 5.1.1.1); also carnitine deficiency, oesophageal strictures, gastro-intestinal obstruction, infants under 3 months

**Side-effects** see under Benzylpenicillin (section 5.1.1.1); nausea, vomiting, dyspepsia; also reduced serum and total body carnitine (especially with long-term or repeated use)

**Dose**

• Acute uncomplicated cystitis, ADULT and CHILD over 40 kg, initially 400 mg then 200 mg every 8 hours for 3 days

• Chronic or recurrent bacteriuria, ADULT and CHILD over 40 kg, 400 mg every 6–8 hours

• Urinary-tract infections, CHILD under 40 kg, 20–40 mg/kg daily in 3–4 divided doses

• Salmonellosis, not recommended therefore no dose stated

**Counselling** Tablets should be swallowed whole with plenty of fluid during meals while sitting or standing

**Selexid®** (LEO) PoM

Tablets, f/c, pivmecillinam hydrochloride 200 mg, net price 10-tab pack = £4.50. Label 9, 21, 27, counselling, posture (see Dose above)

### 5.1.2 Cephalosporins, carbapenems, and other beta-lactams

Antibiotics in this section include the **cephalosporins**, such as cefotaxime, ceftazidime, cefuroxime, cefalexin and cefradine, the **monobactam**, aztreonam, and the **carbapenems**, imipenem (a thienamycin derivative), meropenem, doripenem, and ertapenem.

### 5.1.2.1 Cephalosporins

The cephalosporins are broad-spectrum antibiotics which are used for the treatment of septicaemia, pneumonia, meningitis, biliary-tract infections, peritonitis, and urinary-tract infections. The pharmacology of the cephalosporins is similar to that of the penicillins, excretion being principally renal. Cephalosporins penetrate the cerebrospinal fluid poorly unless the meninges are inflamed; cefotaxime is a suitable cephalosporin for infections of the CNS (e.g meningitis).

The principal side-effect of the cephalosporins is hypersensitivity and about 0.5–6.5% of penicillin-sensitive patients will also be allergic to the cephalosporins. Patients with a history of immediate hypersensitivity to penicillin should not receive a cephalosporin. If a cephalosporin is essential in these patients because a suitable alternative antibacterial is not available, then cefixime, cefotaxime, ceftazidime, ceftriaxone, or cefuroxime can be used with caution; cefaclor, cefadroxil, cefalexin, and cefradine should be avoided.

Antibiotic-associated colitis may occur with the use of broad-spectrum cephalosporins.

**Cefradine** (cephradine) has generally been replaced by the newer cephalosporins.

**Cefuroxime** is a 'second generation' cephalosporin that is less susceptible than the earlier cephalosporins to inactivation by beta-lactamases. It is, therefore, active against certain bacteria which are resistant to the other drugs and has greater activity against *Haemophilus influenzae* and *Neisseria gonorrhoeae*.

**Cefotaxime**, **ceftazidime** and **ceftriaxone** are 'third generation' cephalosporins with greater activity than the 'second generation' cephalosporins against certain Gram-negative bacteria. However, they are less active than cefuroxime against Gram-positive bacteria, most notably *Staphylococcus aureus*. Their broad antibacterial spectrum may encourage superinfection with resistant bacteria or fungi.

**Ceftazidime** has good activity against pseudomonas. It is also active against other Gram-negative bacteria.

**Ceftriaxone** has a longer half-life and therefore needs to be given only once daily. Indications include serious infections such as septicaemia, pneumonia, and meningitis. The calcium salt of ceftriaxone forms a precipitate in the gall bladder which may rarely cause symptoms but these usually resolve when the antibiotic is stopped.

**Orally active cephalosporins** The orally active 'first generation' cephalosporins, **cefalexin** (cephalexin), **cefradine**, and **cefadroxil** and the 'second generation' cephalosporin, **cefaclor**, have a similar antimicrobial spectrum. They are useful for urinary-tract infections which do not respond to other drugs or which occur in pregnancy, respiratory-tract infections, otitis media, sinusitis, and skin and soft-tissue infections. Cefaclor has good activity against *H. influenzae*, but it is associated with protracted skin reactions especially in children. Cefadroxil has a long duration of action and can be given twice daily; it has poor activity against *H. influenzae*. **Cefuroxime axetil**, an ester of the 'second generation' cephalosporin cefuroxime, has the same antibacterial spectrum as the parent compound; it is poorly absorbed.

**Cefixime** has a longer duration of action than the other cephalosporins that are active by mouth. It is only licensed for acute infections.

**Cefpodoxime proxetil** is more active than the other oral cephalosporins against respiratory bacterial pathogens and it is licensed for upper and lower respiratory-tract infections.

For treatment of Lyme disease, see section 5.1.1.3.

**Oral infections**  The cephalosporins offer little advantage over the penicillins in dental infections, often being less active against anaerobes. Infections due to oral streptococci (often termed viridans streptococci) which become resistant to penicillin are usually also resistant to cephalosporins. This is of importance in the case of patients who have had rheumatic fever and are on long-term penicillin therapy. Cefalexin and cefradine have been used in the treatment of oral infections.

## ▌ CEFACLOR

**Indications** infections due to sensitive Gram-positive and Gram-negative bacteria, but see notes above
**Cautions** sensitivity to beta-lactam antibacterials (avoid if history of immediate hypersensitivity reaction, see also notes above and p. 295); renal impairment (Appendix 3); pregnancy and breast-feeding (but appropriate to use); false positive urinary glucose (if tested for reducing substances) and false positive Coombs' test; **interactions**: Appendix 1 (cephalosporins)
**Contra-indications** cephalosporin hypersensitivity
**Side-effects** diarrhoea and rarely antibiotic-associated colitis (CSM has warned both more likely with higher doses), nausea and vomiting, abdominal discomfort, headache; allergic reactions including rashes, pruritus, urticaria, serum sickness-like reactions with rashes, fever and arthralgia, and anaphylaxis; Stevens-Johnson syndrome, toxic epidermal necrolysis reported; disturbances in liver enzymes, transient hepatitis and cholestatic jaundice; other side-effects reported include eosinophilia and blood disorders (including thrombocytopenia, leucopenia, agranulocytosis, aplastic anaemia and haemolytic anaemia); reversible interstitial nephritis, hyperactivity, nervousness, sleep disturbances, hallucinations, confusion, hypertonia, and dizziness
**Dose**

* 250 mg every 8 hours, doubled for severe infections; max. 4 g daily; CHILD over 1 month, 20 mg/kg daily in 3 divided doses, doubled for severe infections, max. 1 g daily; or 1 month–1 year, 62.5 mg every 8 hours; 1–5 years, 125 mg; over 5 years, 250 mg; doses doubled for severe infections

**Cefaclor** (Non-proprietary) ℗ℴℳ
Capsules, cefaclor (as monohydrate) 250 mg, net price 21-cap pack = £4.52; 500 mg, 50-cap pack = £22.76. Label: 9
Brands include *Keftid®*

Suspension, cefaclor (as monohydrate) for reconstitution with water, 125 mg/5 mL, net price 100 mL = £5.45; 250 mg/5 mL, 100 mL = £6.58. Label: 9
Note Sugar-free versions are available and can be ordered by specifying 'sugar-free' on the prescription
Brands include *Keftid®*

**Distaclor®** (Flynn) ℗ℴℳ
Capsules, cefaclor (as monohydrate) 500 mg (violet/grey), net price 20 = £17.33. Label: 9

Suspension, both pink, cefaclor (as monohydrate) for reconstitution with water, 125 mg/5 mL, net price 100 mL = £4.13; 250 mg/5 mL, 100 mL = £8.26. Label: 9

**Distaclor MR®** (Flynn) ℗ℴℳ
Tablets, m/r, both blue, cefaclor (as monohydrate) 375 mg. Net price 14-tab pack = £8.31. Label: 9, 21, 25
Dose 375 mg every 12 hours with food, dose doubled for pneumonia
Lower urinary-tract infections, 375 mg every 12 hours with food

## ▌ CEFADROXIL

**Indications** see under Cefaclor; see also notes above
**Cautions** see under Cefaclor
**Contra-indications** see under Cefaclor
**Side-effects** see under Cefaclor
**Dose**

* Patients over 40 kg, 0.5–1 g twice daily; skin, soft tissue, and simple urinary-tract infections, 1 g daily; CHILD under 1 year, 25 mg/kg daily in divided doses; 1–6 years, 250 mg twice daily; over 6 years, 500 mg twice daily

**Cefadroxil** (Non-proprietary) ℗ℴℳ
Capsules, cefadroxil (as monohydrate) 500 mg, net price 20-cap pack = £5.25. Label: 9

**Baxan®** (Bristol-Myers Squibb) ℗ℴℳ
Capsules, cefadroxil (as monohydrate) 500 mg, net price 20-cap pack = £5.05. Label: 9

Suspension, cefadroxil (as monohydrate) for reconstitution with water, 125 mg/5 mL, net price 60 mL = £1.57; 250 mg/5 mL, 60 mL = £3.11; 500 mg/5 mL, 60 mL = £4.66. Label: 9

## ▌ CEFALEXIN
(Cephalexin)

**Indications** see under Cefaclor
**Cautions** see under Cefaclor
**Contra-indications** see under Cefaclor
**Side-effects** see under Cefaclor
**Dose**

* 250 mg every 6 hours or 500 mg every 8–12 hours increased to 1–1.5 g every 6–8 hours for severe infections; CHILD 25 mg/kg daily in divided doses, doubled for severe infections, max. 100 mg/kg daily; or under 1 year 125 mg every 12 hours, 1–5 years 125 mg every 8 hours, 5–12 years 250 mg every 8 hours
* Prophylaxis of recurrent urinary-tract infection, ADULT 125 mg at night

**Cefalexin** (Non-proprietary) ℗ℴℳ
Capsules, cefalexin 250 mg, net price 28-cap pack = £1.86; 500 mg, 21-cap pack = £2.49. Label: 9

Tablets, cefalexin 250 mg, net price 28-tab pack = £2.17; 500 mg, 21-tab pack = £2.70. Label: 9

Oral suspension, cefalexin for reconstitution with water, 125 mg/5 mL, net price 100 mL = £1.76; 250 mg/5 mL, 100 mL = £2.08. Label: 9
Dental prescribing on NHS Cefalexin Capsules, Tablets, and Oral Suspension may be prescribed

**5**
**Infections**

**Ceporex®** (Galen) [PoM]

Capsules, both caramel/grey, cefalexin 250 mg, net price 28-cap pack = £4.02; 500 mg, 28-cap pack = £7.85. Label: 9

Tablets, all pink, f/c, cefalexin 250 mg, net price 28-tab pack = £4.02; 500 mg, 28-tab pack = £7.85. Label: 9

Syrup, all orange, cefalexin for reconstitution with water, 125 mg/5 mL, net price 100 mL = £1.43; 250 mg/5 mL, 100 mL = £2.87; 500 mg/5 mL, 100 mL = £5.57. Label: 9

**Keflex®** (Flynn) [PoM]

Capsules, cefalexin 250 mg (green/white), net price 28-cap pack = £1.46; 500 mg (pale green/dark green), 21-cap pack = £1.98. Label: 9

Tablets, both peach, cefalexin 250 mg, net price 28-tab pack = £1.60; 500 mg (scored), 21-tab pack = £2.08. Label: 9

Suspension, cefalexin for reconstitution with water, 125 mg/5 mL, net price 100 mL = 84p; 250 mg/5 mL, 100 mL = £1.40. Label: 9

### ▌ CEFIXIME

**Indications** see under Cefaclor (acute infections only); gonorrhoea [unlicensed indication] (Table 1, section 5.1)

**Cautions** see under Cefaclor

**Contra-indications** see under Cefaclor

**Side-effects** see under Cefaclor

**Dose**

- ADULT and CHILD over 10 years, 200–400 mg daily in 1–2 divided doses; CHILD over 6 months 8 mg/kg daily in 1–2 divided doses *or* 6 months–1 year 75 mg daily; 1–4 years 100 mg daily; 5–10 years 200 mg daily
- Gonorrhoea [unlicensed indication], 400 mg as a single dose

**Suprax®** (Rhône-Poulenc Rorer) [PoM]

Tablets, f/c, scored, cefixime 200 mg. Net price 7-tab pack = £13.23. Label: 9

Paediatric oral suspension, cefixime 100 mg/5 mL when reconstituted with water, net price 50 mL (with double-ended spoon for measuring 3.75 mL or 5 mL since dilution not recommended) = £10.53, 100 mL = £18.91. Label: 9

### ▌ CEFOTAXIME

**Indications** see under Cefaclor; gonorrhoea; surgical prophylaxis; Haemophilus epiglottitis and meningitis (Table 1, section 5.1); see also notes above

**Cautions** see under Cefaclor

**Contra-indications** see under Cefaclor

**Side-effects** see under Cefaclor; rarely arrhythmias following rapid injection reported

**Dose**

- By intramuscular *or* intravenous injection *or* by intravenous infusion, 1 g every 12 hours increased in severe infections (e.g. meningitis) to 8 g daily in 4 divided doses; higher doses (up to 12 g daily in 3–4 divided doses) may be required; NEONATE 50 mg/kg daily in 2–4 divided doses increased to 150–200 mg/kg daily in severe infections; CHILD 100–150 mg/kg daily in 2–4 divided doses increased up to 200 mg/kg daily in very severe infections Gonorrhoea, 500 mg as a single dose

**Important.** If bacterial meningitis and especially if

meningococcal disease is suspected the patient should be transferred urgently to hospital. If benzylpenicillin cannot be given (e.g. because of an allergy), a single dose of cefotaxime may be given (if available) before urgent transfer to hospital. Suitable doses of cefotaxime by intravenous injection (or by intramuscular injection) are ADULT and CHILD over 12 years 1 g; CHILD under 12 years 50 mg/kg; chloramphenicol (section 5.1.7) may be used if there is a history of anaphylaxis to penicillins or cephalosporins

**Cefotaxime** (Non-proprietary) [PoM]

Injection, powder for reconstitution, cefotaxime (as sodium salt), net price 500-mg vial = £2.14; 1-g vial = £4.31; 2-g vial = £8.57

### ▌ CEFPODOXIME

**Indications** see under Dose

**Cautions** see under Cefaclor

**Contra-indications** see under Cefaclor

**Side-effects** see under Cefaclor

**Dose**

- Upper respiratory-tract infections (but in pharyngitis and tonsillitis reserved for infections which are recurrent, chronic, or resistant to other antibacterials), 100 mg twice daily (200 mg twice daily in sinusitis); CHILD 15 days–6 months 4 mg/kg every 12 hours, 6 months–2 years 40 mg every 12 hours, 3–8 years 80 mg every 12 hours, over 9 years 100 mg every 12 hours
- Lower respiratory-tract infections (including bronchitis and pneumonia), 100–200 mg twice daily; CHILD 15 days–6 months 4 mg/kg every 12 hours, 6 months–2 years 40 mg every 12 hours, 3–8 years 80 mg every 12 hours, over 9 years 100 mg every 12 hours
- Skin and soft-tissue infections, 200 mg twice daily; CHILD 15 days–6 months 4 mg/kg every 12 hours, 6 months–2 years 40 mg every 12 hours, 3–8 years 80 mg every 12 hours, over 9 years 100 mg every 12 hours
- Uncomplicated urinary-tract infections, 100 mg twice daily (200 mg twice daily in uncomplicated upper urinary-tract infections); CHILD 15 days–6 months 4 mg/kg every 12 hours, 6 months–2 years 40 mg every 12 hours, 3–8 years 80 mg every 12 hours, over 9 years 100 mg every 12 hours
- Uncomplicated gonorrhoea, 200 mg as a single dose

**Orelox®** (Hoechst Marion Roussel) [PoM]

Tablets, f/c, cefpodoxime 100 mg (as proxetil), net price 10-tab pack = £9.78. Label: 5, 9, 21

Oral suspension, cefpodoxime (as proxetil) for reconstitution with water, 40 mg/5 mL, net price 100 mL = £11.50. Label: 5, 9, 21

Excipients include aspartame (section 9.4.1)

### ▌ CEFRADINE
(Cephradine)

**Indications** see under Cefaclor; surgical prophylaxis

**Cautions** see under Cefaclor

**Contra-indications** see under Cefaclor

**Side-effects** see under Cefaclor

**Dose**

- By mouth, 250–500 mg every 6 hours *or* 0.5–1 g every 12 hours; up to 1 g every 6 hours in severe infections; CHILD, 25–50 mg/kg daily in 2–4 divided doses

- By deep intramuscular injection *or* by intravenous injection over 3–5 minutes *or* by intravenous infusion, 0.5–1 g every 6 hours, increased to 8 g daily in severe infections; CHILD 50–100 mg/kg daily in 4 divided doses
- Surgical prophylaxis, by deep intramuscular injection *or* by intravenous injection over 3–5 minutes, 1–2 g at induction

**Cefradine** (Non-proprietary) [PoM]
Capsules, cefradine 250 mg, net price 20-cap pack = £3.71; 500 mg, 20-cap pack = £5.78. Label: 9
Brands include *Nicef*®
Dental prescribing on NHS Cefradine Capsules may be prescribed

**Velosef**® (Squibb) [PoM]
Capsules, cefradine 250 mg (orange/blue), net price 20-cap pack = £3.17; 500 mg (blue), 20-cap pack = £6.26. Label: 9
Syrup, cefradine 250 mg/5 mL when reconstituted with water. Net price 100 mL = £3.77. Label: 9
Dental prescribing on NHS *Velosef*® syrup may be prescribed as Cefradine Oral Solution
Injection, powder for reconstitution, cefradine. Net price 500-mg vial = 89p; 1-g vial = £1.74

## ▍CEFTAZIDIME

**Indications** see under Cefaclor; see also notes above
**Cautions** see under Cefaclor
**Contra-indications** see under Cefaclor
**Side-effects** see under Cefaclor
**Dose**

- By deep intramuscular injection *or* intravenous injection *or* infusion, 1 g every 8 hours *or* 2 g every 12 hours; 2 g every 8–12 hours *or* 3 g every 12 hours in severe infections; single doses over 1 g intravenous route only; ELDERLY usual max. 3 g daily; CHILD, up to 2 months 25–60 mg/kg daily in 2 divided doses, over 2 months 30–100 mg/kg daily in 2–3 divided doses; up to 150 mg/kg daily (max. 6 g daily) in 3 divided doses if immunocompromised or meningitis; intravenous route recommended for children

Urinary-tract and less serious infections, 0.5–1 g every 12 hours

Pseudomonal lung infection in cystic fibrosis, ADULT 100–150 mg/kg daily in 3 divided doses; CHILD up to 150 mg/kg daily (max. 6 g daily) in 3 divided doses; intravenous route recommended for children

Surgical prophylaxis, prostatic surgery, 1 g at induction of anaesthesia repeated if necessary when catheter removed

**Ceftazidime** (Non-proprietary) [PoM]
Injection, powder for reconstitution, ceftazidime (as pentahydrate), with sodium carbonate, net price 1-g vial = £8.50; 2-g vial = £17.90

**Fortum**® (GSK) [PoM]
Injection, powder for reconstitution, ceftazidime (as pentahydrate), with sodium carbonate, net price 250-mg vial = £2.20, 500-mg vial = £4.40, 1-g vial = £8.79, 2-g vial = £17.59, 3-g vial = £25.76; *Monovial*, 2 g vial (with transfer needle) = £17.59
Electrolytes Na⁺ 2.3 mmol/g

**Kefadim**® (Flynn) [PoM]
Injection, powder for reconstitution, ceftazidime (as pentahydrate), with sodium carbonate, net price 1-g vial = £7.92; 2-g vial = £15.84
Electrolytes Na⁺ 2.3 mmol/g

## ▍CEFTRIAXONE

**Indications** see under Cefaclor and notes above; surgical prophylaxis; prophylaxis of meningococcal meningitis [unlicensed indication] (Table 2, section 5.1)

**Cautions** see under Cefaclor; severe renal impairment (Appendix 3); hepatic impairment if accompanied by renal impairment (Appendix 2); premature neonates; may displace bilirubin from serum albumin, administer over 60 minutes in neonates (see also Contra-indications); treatment longer than 14 days, renal failure, dehydration—risk of ceftriaxone precipitation in gall bladder

**Contra-indications** see under Cefaclor; neonates with jaundice, hypoalbuminaemia, acidosis or impaired bilirubin binding; concomitant treatment with calcium in children—risk of precipitation in urine and lungs of neonates (and possibly infants and older children)

**Side-effects** see under Cefaclor; calcium ceftriaxone precipitates in urine (particularly in very young, dehydrated or those who are immobilised) or in gall bladder—consider discontinuation if symptomatic; rarely prolongation of prothrombin time, pancreatitis

**Dose**

- By deep intramuscular injection, *or* by intravenous injection over at least 2–4 minutes, *or* by intravenous infusion, 1 g daily; 2–4 g daily in severe infections; intramuscular doses over 1 g divided between more than one site; single intravenous doses above 1 g by intravenous infusion only
NEONATE by intravenous infusion over 60 minutes, 20–50 mg/kg daily (max. 50 mg/kg daily) INFANT and CHILD under 50 kg, by deep intramuscular injection, *or* by intravenous injection over 2–4 minutes, *or* by intravenous infusion, 20–50 mg/kg daily; up to 80 mg/kg daily in severe infections; doses of 50 mg/kg and over by intravenous infusion only; 50 kg and over, adult dose
- Endocarditis caused by haemophilus, actinobacillus, cardiobacterium, eikenella, and kingella species ('HACEK organisms') (in combination with another antibacterial, see Table 1, section 5.1; [unlicensed indication]), by intravenous infusion, 2–4 g daily
- Early syphilis [unlicensed indication], by deep intramuscular injection, 500 mg daily for 10 days
- Uncomplicated gonorrhoea, by deep intramuscular injection, 250 mg as a single dose
- Surgical prophylaxis, by deep intramuscular injection *or* by intravenous injection over at least 2–4 minutes, 1 g at induction; colorectal surgery, by deep intramuscular injection *or* by intravenous infusion, 2 g at induction; intramuscular doses over 1 g divided between more than one site

**Ceftriaxone** (Non-proprietary) [PoM]
Injection, powder for reconstitution, ceftriaxone (as sodium salt), net price 1-g vial = £10.17; 2-g vial = £20.36

**5**

**Infections**

**Rocephin®** (Roche) [PoM]

Injection, powder for reconstitution, ceftriaxone (as sodium salt), net price 250-mg vial = £2.45; 1-g vial = £9.77; 2-g vial = £19.57

Electrolytes Na⁺ 3.6 mmol /g

---

## CEFUROXIME

**Indications** see under Cefaclor; surgical prophylaxis; more active against *Haemophilus influenzae* and *Neisseria gonorrhoeae*; Lyme disease

**Cautions** see under Cefaclor

**Contra-indications** see under Cefaclor

**Side-effects** see under Cefaclor

**Dose**

- By mouth (as cefuroxime axetil), 250 mg twice daily in most infections including mild to moderate lower respiratory-tract infections (e.g. bronchitis); doubled for more severe lower respiratory-tract infections or if pneumonia suspected

  Urinary-tract infection, 125 mg twice daily, doubled in pyelonephritis

  Gonorrhoea, 1 g as a single dose

  CHILD over 3 months, 125 mg twice daily, if necessary doubled in child over 2 years with otitis media

  Lyme disease, ADULT and CHILD over 12 years, 500 mg twice daily for 20 days

- By intramuscular injection *or* intravenous injection *or* infusion, 750 mg every 6–8 hours; 1.5 g every 6–8 hours in severe infections; single doses over 750 mg intravenous route only

  CHILD usual dose 60 mg/kg daily (range 30–100 mg/kg daily) in 3–4 divided doses (2–3 divided doses in neonates)

- Gonorrhoea, 1.5 g as a single dose by intramuscular injection (divided between 2 sites)

- Surgical prophylaxis, 1.5 g by intravenous injection at induction; up to 3 further doses of 750 mg may be given by intramuscular *or* intravenous injection every 8 hours for high-risk procedures

- Meningitis, 3 g intravenously every 8 hours; CHILD, 200–240 mg/kg daily (in 3–4 divided doses) reduced to 100 mg/kg daily after 3 days or on clinical improvement; NEONATE, 100 mg/kg daily reduced to 50 mg/kg daily

**Cefuroxime** (Non-proprietary) [PoM]

Tablets, cefuroxime (as axetil) 250 mg, net price 14-tab pack = £9.01. Label: 9, 21, 25

**Zinacef®** (GSK) [PoM]

Injection, powder for reconstitution, cefuroxime (as sodium salt). Net price 250-mg vial = 94p; 750-mg vial = £2.34; 1.5-g vial = £4.70

Electrolytes Na⁺ 1.8 mmol/750-mg vial

**Zinnat®** (GSK) [PoM]

Tablets, both f/c, cefuroxime (as axetil) 125 mg, net price 14-tab pack = £4.65; 250 mg, 14-tab pack = £9.29. Label: 9, 21, 25

Suspension, cefuroxime (as axetil) 125 mg/5 mL when reconstituted with water, net price 70 mL (tutti-frutti-flavoured) = £5.30. Label: 9, 21

Excipients include aspartame (section 9.4.1), sucrose 3.1 g/5 mL

---

**5.1.2.2 Carbapenems**

The carbapenems are beta-lactam antibacterials with a broad-spectrum of activity which includes many Gram-positive and Gram-negative bacteria, and anaerobes; **imipenem**, **meropenem**, and **doripenem** have good activity against *Pseudomonas aeruginosa*. The carbapenems are not active against meticillin-resistant *Staphylococcus aureus* and *Enterococcus faecium*.

Imipenem and meropenem are used for the treatment of severe hospital-acquired infections and polymicrobial infections including septicaemia, hospital-acquired pneumonia, intra-abdominal infections, skin and soft-tissue infections, and complicated urinary-tract infections. Doripenem is an alternative for hospital-acquired pneumonia, complicated intra-abdominal infections, and complicated urinary-tract infections.

**Ertapenem** is licensed for treating abdominal and gynaecological infections and for community-acquired pneumonia, but it is not active against atypical respiratory pathogens and it has limited activity against penicillin-resistant pneumococci. It is also licensed for treating foot infections of the skin and soft tissue in patients with diabetes. Unlike the other carbapenems, ertapenem is not active against *Pseudomonas* or against *Acinetobacter* spp.

Imipenem is partially inactivated in the kidney by enzymatic activity and is therefore administered in combination with **cilastatin**, a specific enzyme inhibitor, which blocks its renal metabolism. Meropenem, doripenem, and ertapenem are stable to the renal enzyme which inactivates imipenem and therefore can be given without cilastatin.

Side-effects of imipenem with cilastatin are similar to those of other beta-lactam antibiotics; neurotoxicity has been observed at very high dosage, in renal failure, or in patients with CNS disease. Ertapenem has been associated with seizures uncommonly. Meropenem has less seizure-inducing potential and can be used to treat central nervous system infection.

---

## DORIPENEM

**Indications** hospital-acquired pneumonia; complicated intra-abdominal infections; complicated urinary-tract infections

**Cautions** sensitivity to beta-lactam antibacterials (avoid if history of immediate hypersensitivity reaction, see also p. 295); renal impairment (Appendix 3); pregnancy (Appendix 4); breast-feeding (Appendix 5); **interactions:** Appendix 1 (doripenem)

**Side-effects** nausea, diarrhoea; headache; phlebitis, pruritus, rash; *less commonly* antibiotic-associated colitis; also reported, neutropenia

**Dose**

- By intravenous infusion, ADULT over 18 years, 500 mg every 8 hours; max. duration of treatment 14 days

**Doribax®** (Janssen-Cilag) ▼ [PoM]

Intravenous infusion, powder for reconstitution, doripenem (as monohydrate), net price 500-mg vial = £14.52

# ERTAPENEM

**Indications** abdominal infections; acute gynaecological infections; community-acquired pneumonia; diabetic foot infections of the skin and soft-tissue; prophylaxis for colorectal surgery

**Cautions** sensitivity to beta-lactam antibacterials (avoid if history of immediate hypersensitivity reaction, see also p. 295); elderly; renal impairment (Appendix 3), CNS disorders—risk of seizures; pregnancy (Appendix 4); **interactions:** Appendix 1 (ertapenem)

**Contra-indications** breast-feeding (Appendix 5)

**Side-effects** diarrhoea, nausea, vomiting, headache, injection-site reactions, rash, pruritus, raised platelet count; *less commonly* dry mouth, taste disturbances, dyspepsia, abdominal pain, anorexia, constipation, melaena, antibiotic-associated colitis, bradycardia, hypotension, chest pain, oedema, pharyngeal discomfort, dyspnoea, dizziness, sleep disturbances, confusion, asthenia, seizures, vaginitis, raised glucose, petechiae; *rarely* dysphagia, cholecystitis, liver disorder (including jaundice), arrhythmia, increase in blood pressure, syncope, nasal congestion, cough, wheezing, anxiety, depression, agitation, tremor, pelvic peritonitis, renal impairment, muscle cramp, scleral disorder, blood disorders (including neutropenia, thrombocytopenia, haemorrhage), hypoglycaemia, electrolyte disturbances; *very rarely* hallucinations

**Dose**
- By intravenous infusion, ADULT and ADOLESCENT over 13 years, 1 g once daily; CHILD 3 months–13 years, 15 mg/kg every 12 hours (max. 1 g daily)
Surgical prophylaxis, colorectal surgery, ADULT over 18 years, 1 g completed within 1 hour before surgery

**Invanz®** (MSD) ℗oM
Intravenous infusion, powder for reconstitution, ertapenem (as sodium salt), net price 1-g vial = £31.65
Electrolytes Na⁺ 6 mmol/1-g vial

# IMIPENEM WITH CILASTATIN

**Indications** aerobic and anaerobic Gram-positive and Gram-negative infections; surgical prophylaxis; hospital-acquired septicaemia (Table 1, section 5.1); not indicated for CNS infections

**Cautions** sensitivity to beta-lactam antibacterials (avoid if history of immediate hypersensitivity reaction, see also p. 295); renal impairment (Appendix 3); CNS disorders (e.g. epilepsy); pregnancy (Appendix 4); breast-feeding (Appendix 5); **interactions:** Appendix 1 (imipenem with cilastatin)

**Side-effects** nausea, vomiting, diarrhoea (antibiotic-associated colitis reported), taste disturbances, tooth or tongue discoloration, hearing loss; blood disorders, positive Coombs' test; allergic reactions (with rash, pruritus, urticaria, Stevens-Johnson syndrome, fever, anaphylactic reactions, rarely toxic epidermal necrolysis, exfoliative dermatitis); myoclonic activity, convulsions, confusion and mental disturbances reported; slight increases in liver enzymes and bilirubin reported, rarely hepatitis; increases in serum creatinine and blood urea; red coloration of urine in children reported; local reactions: erythema, pain and induration, and thrombophlebitis

**Dose**
- By intravenous infusion, in terms of imipenem, 1–2 g daily (in 3–4 divided doses); less sensitive organisms, up to 50 mg/kg daily (max. 4 g daily) in 3–4 divided doses; CHILD 3 months and older, 60 mg/kg (up to max. of 2 g) daily in 4 divided doses; over 40 kg, adult dose
Surgical prophylaxis, 1 g at induction repeated after 3 hours, supplemented in high risk (e.g. colorectal) surgery by doses of 500 mg 8 and 16 hours after induction

**Primaxin®** (MSD) ℗oM
Intravenous infusion, powder for reconstitution, imipenem (as monohydrate) 500 mg with cilastatin (as sodium salt) 500 mg, net price per vial = £12.00
Electrolytes Na⁺ 1.72 mmol/vial

# MEROPENEM

**Indications** aerobic and anaerobic Gram-positive and Gram-negative infections

**Cautions** sensitivity to beta-lactam antibacterials (avoid if history of immediate hypersensitivity reaction, see also p. 295); hepatic impairment (monitor liver function; Appendix 2); renal impairment (Appendix 3); pregnancy (Appendix 4); breast-feeding (Appendix 5); **interactions:** Appendix 1 (meropenem)

**Side-effects** nausea, vomiting, diarrhoea (antibiotic-associated colitis reported), abdominal pain, disturbances in liver function tests; headache; thrombocythaemia, positive Coombs' test; rash, pruritus, injection-site reactions; *less commonly* eosinophilia, thrombocytopenia; *rarely* convulsions; also reported paraesthesia, leucopenia, haemolytic anaemia, reduction in partial thromboplastin time, Stevens-Johnson syndrome, and toxic epidermal necrolysis

**Dose**
- By intravenous injection over 5 minutes *or* by intravenous infusion, 500 mg every 8 hours, dose doubled in hospital-acquired pneumonia, peritonitis, septicaemia and infections in neutropenic patients; CHILD 3 months–12 years [not licensed for infection in neutropenia] 10–20 mg/kg every 8 hours, over 50 kg body weight adult dose
Meningitis, 2 g every 8 hours; CHILD 3 months–12 years 40 mg/kg every 8 hours, over 50 kg body weight adult dose

Exacerbations of chronic lower respiratory-tract infection in cystic fibrosis, up to 2 g every 8 hours; CHILD 4–18 years 25–40 mg/kg every 8 hours

**Meronem®** (AstraZeneca) ℗oM
Injection, powder for reconstitution, meropenem (as trihydrate), net price 500-mg vial = £8.60; 1-g vial = £17.19
Electrolytes Na⁺ 3.9 mmol/g

## 5.1.2.3 Other beta-lactam antibiotics

**Aztreonam** is a monocyclic beta-lactam ('monobactam') antibiotic with an antibacterial spectrum limited to Gram-negative aerobic bacteria including *Pseudomonas aeruginosa*, *Neisseria meningitidis*, and *Haemophilus influenzae*; it should not be used alone for 'blind' treatment since it is not active against Gram-positive organisms. Aztreonam is also effective against *Neisseria gonorrhoeae* (but not against concurrent chlamydial infection). Side-effects are similar to those of the other beta-lactams although aztreonam may be less likely to cause hypersensitivity in penicillin-sensitive patients.

5

Infections

**5 Infections**

## ▨ AZTREONAM

**Indications** Gram-negative infections including *Pseudomonas aeruginosa*, *Haemophilus influenzae*, and *Neisseria meningitidis*

**Cautions** hypersensitivity to beta-lactam antibiotics; hepatic impairment; renal impairment (Appendix 3); breast-feeding (Appendix 5); **interactions:** Appendix 1 (aztreonam)

**Contra-indications** aztreonam hypersensitivity; pregnancy (Appendix 4)

**Side-effects** nausea, vomiting, diarrhoea, abdominal cramps; mouth ulcers, altered taste; jaundice and hepatitis; flushing; hypersensitivity reactions; blood disorders (including thrombocytopenia and neutropenia); rashes, injection-site reactions; rarely hypotension, seizures, asthenia, confusion, dizziness, headache, halitosis, and breast tenderness; very rarely antibiotic-associated colitis, gastro-intestinal bleeding, and toxic epidermal necrolysis

**Dose**

- By deep intramuscular injection *or* by intravenous injection over 3–5 minutes *or* by intravenous infusion, 1 g every 8 hours *or* 2 g every 12 hours; 2 g every 6–8 hours for severe infections (including systemic *Pseudomonas aeruginosa* and lung infections in cystic fibrosis); single doses over 1 g intravenous route only

 Urinary-tract infections, 0.5–1 g every 8–12 hours

- CHILD over 1 week, by intravenous injection *or* infusion, 30 mg/kg every 6–8 hours increased in severe infections for child of 2 years or older to 50 mg/kg every 6–8 hours; max. 8 g daily

- Gonorrhoea, cystitis, by intramuscular injection, 1 g as a single dose

**Azactam®** (Squibb) ⟨PoM⟩
Injection, powder for reconstitution, aztreonam. Net price 500-mg vial = £4.81; 1-g vial = £9.59; 2-g vial = £19.20

## 5.1.3 Tetracyclines

The tetracyclines are broad-spectrum antibiotics whose value has decreased owing to increasing bacterial resistance. They remain, however, the treatment of choice for infections caused by chlamydia (trachoma, psittacosis, salpingitis, urethritis, and lymphogranuloma venereum), rickettsia (including Q-fever), brucella (doxycycline with either streptomycin or rifampicin), and the spirochaete, *Borrelia burgdorferi* (Lyme disease—see section 5.1.1.3). They are also used in respiratory and genital mycoplasma infections, in acne, in destructive (refractory) periodontal disease, in exacerbations of chronic bronchitis (because of their activity against *Haemophilus influenzae*), and for leptospirosis in penicillin hypersensitivity (as an alternative to erythromycin).

For the role of tetracyclines in the management of meticillin-resistant *Staphylococcus aureus* (MRSA) infection, see p. 297.

Microbiologically, there is little to choose between the various tetracyclines, the only exception being **minocycline** which has a broader spectrum; it is active against *Neisseria meningitidis* and has been used for meningococcal prophylaxis but is no longer recommended because of side-effects including dizziness and vertigo (see section 5.1, table 2 for current recommendations). Compared to other tetracyclines, minocycline is associated with a greater risk of lupus-erythematosus-like syndrome. Minocycline sometimes causes irreversible pigmentation.

**Oral infections** In adults, tetracyclines can be effective against oral anaerobes but the development of resistance (especially by oral streptococci) has reduced their usefulness for the treatment of acute oral infections; they may still have a role in the treatment of destructive (refractory) forms of periodontal disease. Doxycycline has a longer duration of action than tetracycline or oxytetracycline and need only be given once daily; it is reported to be more active against anaerobes than some other tetracyclines.

For the use of doxycycline in the treatment of recurrent aphthous ulceration, oral herpes, or as an adjunct to gingival scaling and root planing for periodontitis, see section 12.3.1 and section 12.3.2.

**Cautions** Tetracyclines should be used with caution in patients with hepatic impairment (Appendix 2) or those receiving potentially hepatotoxic drugs. Tetracyclines may increase muscle weakness in patients with myasthenia gravis, and exacerbate systemic lupus erythematosus. Antacids, and aluminium, calcium, iron, magnesium and zinc salts decrease the absorption of tetracyclines; milk also reduces the absorption of demeclocycline, oxytetracycline, and tetracycline. Other **interactions:** Appendix 1 (tetracyclines).

**Contra-indications** Deposition of tetracyclines in growing bone and teeth (by binding to calcium) causes staining and occasionally dental hypoplasia, and they should **not** be given to children under 12 years, or to pregnant (Appendix 4) or breast-feeding women (Appendix 5). However, doxycycline may be used in children for treatment and post-exposure prophylaxis of anthrax when an alternative antibacterial cannot be given [unlicensed indication]. With the exception of **doxycycline** and **minocycline**, the tetracyclines may exacerbate renal failure and should **not** be given to patients with kidney disease (Appendix 3). Tetracyclines should not be given to patients with acute porphyria (section 9.8.2)

**Side-effects** Side-effects of the tetracyclines include nausea, vomiting, diarrhoea (antibiotic-associated colitis reported occasionally), dysphagia, and oesophageal irritation. Other rare side-effects include hepatotoxicity, pancreatitis, blood disorders, photosensitivity (particularly with demeclocycline), and hypersensitivity reactions (including rash, exfoliative dermatitis, Stevens-Johnson syndrome, urticaria, angioedema, anaphylaxis, pericarditis). Headache and visual disturbances may indicate benign intracranial hypertension (discontinue treatment); bulging fontanelles have been reported in infants.

## ▨ TETRACYCLINE

**Indications** see notes above; acne vulgaris, rosacea (section 13.6)

**Cautions** see notes above

**Contra-indications** see notes above

**Side-effects** see notes above; also acute renal failure, skin discoloration

**Dose**

- 250 mg every 6 hours, increased in severe infections to 500 mg every 6–8 hours
- Acne, see section 13.6.2
- Non-gonococcal urethritis, 500 mg every 6 hours for 7–14 days (21 days if failure or relapse after first course)

  **Counselling** Tablets should be swallowed whole with plenty of fluid while sitting or standing

**Tetracycline** (Non-proprietary) ⒫ᴼᴹ

Tablets, coated, tetracycline hydrochloride 250 mg, net price 28-tab pack = £9.09. Label: 7, 9, 23, counselling, posture

Dental prescribing on NHS Tetracycline Tablets may be prescribed

---

### DEMECLOCYCLINE HYDROCHLORIDE

**Indications** see notes above; also inappropriate secretion of antidiuretic hormone, section 6.5.2

**Cautions** see notes above, but photosensitivity more common (avoid exposure to sunlight or sun lamps)

**Contra-indications** see notes above

**Side-effects** see notes above; also reversible nephrogenic diabetes insipidus, acute renal failure

**Dose**

- 150 mg every 6 hours *or* 300 mg every 12 hours

**Ledermycin®** (Goldshield) ⒫ᴼᴹ

Capsules, red, demeclocycline hydrochloride 150 mg, net price 28-cap pack = £15.10. Label: 7, 9, 11, 23

---

### DOXYCYCLINE

**Indications** see notes above; chronic prostatitis; sinusitis, syphilis, pelvic inflammatory disease (Table 1, section 5.1); treatment and prophylaxis of anthrax [unlicensed indication]; malaria treatment and prophylaxis (section 5.4.1); recurrent aphthous ulceration, adjunct to gingival scaling and root planing for periodontitis (section 12.3.1); oral herpes simplex (section 12.3.2); rosacea [unlicensed indication], acne vulgaris (section 13.6)

**Cautions** see notes above, but may be used in renal impairment; alcohol dependence; photosensitivity reported (avoid exposure to sunlight or sun lamps)

**Contra-indications** see notes above

**Side-effects** see notes above; also anorexia, flushing, and tinnitus

**Dose**

- 200 mg on first day, then 100 mg daily; severe infections (including refractory urinary-tract infections), 200 mg daily
- Early syphilis, 100 mg twice daily for 14 days; late latent syphilis, 100 mg twice daily for 28 days; neurosyphilis, 200 mg twice daily for 28 days
- Uncomplicated genital chlamydia, non-gonococcal urethritis, 100 mg twice daily for 7 days (14 days in pelvic inflammatory disease, see also Table 1, section 5.1)
- Anthrax (treatment or post-exposure prophylaxis; see also section 5.1.12), 100 mg twice daily; CHILD (only if alternative antibacterial cannot be given) [unlicensed dose] 5 mg/kg daily in 2 divided doses (max. 200 mg daily)

  **Counselling** Capsules should be swallowed whole with plenty of fluid during meals while sitting or standing

Note Doxycycline doses in BNF may differ from those in product literature

**Doxycycline** (Non-proprietary) ⒫ᴼᴹ

Capsules, doxycycline (as hyclate) 50 mg, net price 28-cap pack = £1.76; 100 mg, 8-cap pack = £1.14. Label: 6, 9, 11, 27, counselling, posture

Brands include *Doxylar®*

Dental prescribing on NHS Doxycycline Capsules 100 mg may be prescribed

**Vibramycin-D®** (Pfizer) ⒫ᴼᴹ

Dispersible tablets, yellow, scored, doxycycline 100 mg, net price 8-tab pack = £4.91. Label: 6, 9, 11, 13

---

### LYMECYCLINE

**Indications** see notes above

**Cautions** see notes above

**Contra-indications** see notes above

**Side-effects** see notes above

**Dose**

- 408 mg every 12 hours, increased to 1.224–1.632 g daily in severe infections
- Acne, 408 mg daily for at least 8 weeks

**Tetralysal 300®** (Galderma) ⒫ᴼᴹ

Capsules, red/yellow, lymecycline 408 mg (= tetracycline 300 mg), net price 28-cap pack = £7.77, 56-cap pack = £14.97. Label: 6, 9

---

### MINOCYCLINE

**Indications** see notes above; meningococcal carrier state; acne vulgaris (section 13.6.2)

**Cautions** see notes above, but may be used in renal impairment; if treatment continued for longer than 6 months, monitor every 3 months for hepatotoxicity, pigmentation and for systemic lupus erythematosus—discontinue if these develop or if pre-existing systemic lupus erythematosus worsens

**Contra-indications** see notes above

**Side-effects** see notes above; also dizziness and vertigo (more common in women); *rarely* anorexia, tinnitus, impaired hearing, hyperaesthesia, paraesthesia, acute renal failure, pigmentation (sometimes irreversible), and alopecia; *very rarely* systemic lupus erythematosus, discoloration of conjunctiva, tears, and sweat

**Dose**

- 100 mg twice daily
- Acne, see section 13.6.2 and under preparations, below
- Prophylaxis of asymptomatic meningococcal carrier state (but no longer recommended, see notes above), 100 mg twice daily for 5 days usually followed by rifampicin

  **Counselling** Tablets or capsules should be swallowed whole with plenty of fluid while sitting or standing

**Minocycline** (Non-proprietary) ⒫ᴼᴹ

Capsules, minocycline (as hydrochloride) 50 mg, net price 56-cap pack = £15.27; 100 mg, 28-cap pack = £13.09. Label: 6, 9, counselling, posture

Brands include *Aknemin®*

Tablets, minocycline (as hydrochloride) 50 mg, net price 28-tab pack = £3.76, 100 mg, 28-tab pack = £7.27. Label: 6, 9, counselling, posture

◢ Modified release

**Acnamino® MR** (Dexcel) [PoM]
Capsules, m/r, buff/brown (enclosing pink and peach tablets), minocycline (as hydrochloride) 100 mg, net price 56-cap pack = £21.14. Label: 6, 25
Dose acne, 1 capsule daily

**Minocin MR®** (Meda) [PoM]
Capsules, m/r, orange/brown (enclosing yellow and white pellets), minocycline (as hydrochloride) 100 mg. Net price 56-cap pack = £20.08. Label: 6, 25
Dose acne, 1 capsule daily

**Sebomin MR®** (Actavis) [PoM]
Capsules, m/r, orange, minocycline (as hydrochloride) 100 mg, net price 56-cap pack = £20.32. Label: 6, 25
Dose acne, 1 capsule daily

### ▮ OXYTETRACYCLINE

**Indications** see notes above; acne vulgaris, rosacea (section 13.6)
**Cautions** see notes above
**Contra-indications** see notes above
**Side-effects** see notes above
**Dose**
● 250–500 mg every 6 hours
● Acne, see section 13.6.2

**Oxytetracycline** (Non-proprietary) [PoM]
Tablets, coated, oxytetracycline dihydrate 250 mg, net price 28-tab pack = £1.08. Label: 7, 9, 23
Brands include *Oxymycin®*
Dental prescribing on NHS Oxtetracycline Tablets may be prescribed

## Tigecycline

**Tigecycline** is a glycylcycline antibacterial structurally related to the tetracyclines; side-effects similar to those of the tetracyclines can potentially occur. Tigecycline is active against Gram-positive and Gram-negative bacteria, including tetracycline-resistant organisms, and some anaerobes. It is also active against meticillin-resistant *Staphylococcus aureus* and vancomycin-resistant enterococci, but *Pseudomonas aeruginosa* and many strains of *Proteus spp* are resistant to tigecycline. Tigecycline should be reserved for the treatment of complicated skin and soft-tissue infections and complicated abdominal infections caused by multiple-antibacterial resistant organisms.

### ▮ TIGECYCLINE

**Indications** complicated intra-abdominal infections; complicated skin and soft-tissue infections
**Cautions** cholestasis, hepatic impairment (Appendix 2); breast-feeding (Appendix 5); **interactions:** Appendix 1 (tigecycline)
**Contra-indications** hypersensitivity to tetracyclines; pregnancy (Appendix 4)
**Side-effects** see notes above; also nausea, vomiting, abdominal pain, dyspepsia, diarrhoea, anorexia, bilirubinaemia, dizziness, headache, prolonged

prothrombin time, prolonged activated partial thromboplastin time, rash, pruritus, and injection-site reactions; *less commonly* pancreatitis and hypo-proteinaemia; also reported, antibiotic-associated colitis and thrombocytopenia
**Dose**
● By intravenous infusion, ADULT over 18 years, initially 100 mg, then 50 mg every 12 hours for 5–14 days

**Tygacil®** (Wyeth) ▼ [PoM]
Intravenous infusion, powder for reconstitution, tigecycline, net price 50-mg vial = £32.31

## 5.1.4 Aminoglycosides

These include amikacin, gentamicin, neomycin, streptomycin, and tobramycin. All are bactericidal and active against some Gram-positive and many Gram-negative organisms. Amikacin, gentamicin, and tobramycin are also active against *Pseudomonas aeruginosa*; streptomycin is active against *Mycobacterium tuberculosis* and is now almost entirely reserved for tuberculosis (section 5.1.9).

The aminoglycosides are not absorbed from the gut (although there is a risk of absorption in inflammatory bowel disease and liver failure) and must therefore be given by injection for systemic infections.

Excretion is principally via the kidney and accumulation occurs in renal impairment.

Most side-effects of this group of antibiotics are dose-related therefore care must be taken with dosage and whenever possible treatment should not exceed 7 days. The important side-effects are ototoxicity, and nephrotoxicity; they occur most commonly in the elderly and in patients with renal failure.

If there is impairment of renal function (or high pre-dose serum concentrations) the interval between doses must be increased; if the renal impairment is severe the dose itself should be reduced as well.

Aminoglycosides may impair neuromuscular transmission and should not be given to patients with myasthenia gravis; large doses given during surgery have been responsible for a transient myasthenic syndrome in patients with normal neuromuscular function.

Aminoglycosides should preferably not be given with potentially ototoxic diuretics (e.g. furosemide (frusemide)); if concurrent use is unavoidable administration of the aminoglycoside and of the diuretic should be separated by as long a period as practicable.

**Once daily dosage** *Once daily administration* of aminoglycosides is more convenient, provides adequate serum concentrations, and in many cases has largely superseded *multiple daily dose regimens* (given in 2–3 divided doses during the 24 hours). Local guidelines on dosage and serum concentrations should be consulted. A once-daily, high-dose regimen of an aminoglycoside should be avoided in patients with endocarditis, extensive burns of more than 20% of the total body surface area, or creatinine clearance less than 20 mL/minute.

**Serum concentrations** Serum concentration monitoring avoids both excessive and subtherapeutic concentrations thus preventing toxicity and ensuring efficacy. In patients with normal renal function, aminoglycoside concentrations should be measured after 3 or 4 doses of a multiple daily dose regimen; patients with renal impairment may require earlier and more frequent measurement of aminoglycoside concentration.

For multiple daily dose regimens, blood samples should be taken approximately 1 hour after intramuscular or intravenous administration ('peak' concentration) and also just before the next dose ('trough' concentration). For once daily dose regimens, consult local guidelines on serum concentration monitoring.

Serum-aminoglycoside concentrations should be measured in all patients and **must** be determined in infants, in the elderly, in obesity, and in cystic fibrosis, *or* if high doses are being given, *or* if there is renal impairment.

**Endocarditis** Gentamicin is used in combination with other antibiotics for the treatment of bacterial endocarditis (Table 1, section 5.1). Serum-gentamicin concentration should be determined twice each week (more often in renal impairment). **Streptomycin** may be used as an alternative in gentamicin-resistant enterococcal endocarditis.

**Gentamicin** is the aminoglycoside of choice in the UK and is used widely for the treatment of serious infections. It has a broad spectrum but is inactive against anaerobes and has poor activity against haemolytic streptococci and pneumococci. When used for the 'blind' therapy of undiagnosed serious infections it is usually given in conjunction with a penicillin or metronidazole (or both). Gentamicin is used together with another antibiotic for the treatment of endocarditis (see above and Table 1, section 5.1).

Loading and maintenance doses of gentamicin may be calculated on the basis of the patient's weight and renal function (e.g. using a nomogram); adjustments are then made according to serum-gentamicin concentrations. High doses are occasionally indicated for serious infections, especially in the neonate, in the patient with cystic fibrosis, or in the immunocompromised patient. Whenever possible treatment should not exceed 7 days.

**Amikacin** is more stable than gentamicin to enzyme inactivation. Amikacin is used in the treatment of serious infections caused by gentamicin-resistant Gram-negative bacilli.

**Tobramycin** has similar activity to gentamicin. It is slightly more active against *Ps. aeruginosa* but shows less activity against certain other Gram-negative bacteria. Tobramycin may be administered by nebuliser on a cyclical basis (28 days of tobramycin followed by a 28-day tobramycin-free interval) for the treatment of chronic pulmonary *Ps. aeruginosa* infection in cystic fibrosis; however, resistance may develop and some patients do not respond to treatment.

**Neomycin** is too toxic for parenteral administration and can only be used for infections of the skin or mucous membranes or to reduce the bacterial population of the colon prior to bowel surgery or in hepatic failure. Oral administration may lead to malabsorption. Small amounts of neomycin may be absorbed from the gut in patients with hepatic failure and, as these patients

may also be uraemic, cumulation may occur with resultant ototoxicity.

## GENTAMICIN

**Indications** septicaemia and neonatal sepsis; meningitis and other CNS infections; biliary-tract infection, acute pyelonephritis or prostatitis, endocarditis (see notes above); pneumonia in hospital patients, adjunct in listerial meningitis (Table 1, section 5.1); eye (section 11.3.1); ear (section 12.1.1)

**Cautions** pregnancy (Appendix 4), renal impairment, neonates, infants and elderly (adjust dose and monitor renal, auditory and vestibular function together with serum gentamicin concentrations); avoid prolonged use; conditions characterised by muscular weakness; obesity (use ideal weight for height to calculate dose and monitor serum-gentamicin concentration closely); see also notes above; **interactions:** Appendix 1 (aminoglycosides)

**Contra-indications** myasthenia gravis

**Side-effects** vestibular and auditory damage, nephrotoxicity; rarely, hypomagnesaemia on prolonged therapy, antibiotic-associated colitis, stomatitis; also reported, nausea, vomiting, rash, blood disorders; see also notes above

**Dose**

- Multiple daily dose regimen, by intramuscular *or* by slow intravenous injection over at least 3 minutes *or* by intravenous infusion, 3–5 mg/kg daily (in divided doses every 8 hours), see also notes above; CHILD under 18 years see *BNF for Children*

  Endocarditis (in combination with other antibacterials, see Table 1, section 5.1), ADULT 1 mg/kg every 8 hours

- Once daily dose regimen (see notes above and also consult local guidelines), by intravenous infusion, initially 5–7 mg/kg, then adjust according to serum-gentamicin concentration

- By intrathecal injection, seek specialist advice, 1 mg daily (increased if necessary to 5 mg daily)

Note For multiple daily dose regimen, one-hour ('peak') serum concentration should be 5–10 mg/litre (3–5 mg/litre for endocarditis); pre-dose ('trough') concentration should be less than 2 mg/litre (less than 1 mg/litre for endocarditis). For once-daily dose regimen, consult local guidelines on monitoring serum-gentamicin concentration

**Gentamicin** (Non-proprietary) ℗ℴℳ

Injection, gentamicin (as sulphate), net price 40 mg/mL, 1-mL amp = £1.40, 2-mL amp = £1.54, 2-mL vial = £1.48

Paediatric injection, gentamicin (as sulphate) 10 mg/mL, net price 2-mL vial = £1.80

Intrathecal injection, gentamicin (as sulphate) 5 mg/mL, net price 1-mL amp = 74p

**Cidomycin®** (Sanofi-Aventis) ℗ℴℳ

Injection, gentamicin (as sulphate) 40 mg/mL. Net price 2-mL amp or vial = £1.48

**Genticin®** (Amdipharm) ℗ℴℳ

Injection, gentamicin (as sulphate) 40 mg/mL. Net price 2-mL amp = £1.40

**Isotonic Gentamicin Injection** (Baxter) ℗ℴℳ

Intravenous infusion, gentamicin (as sulphate) 800 micrograms/mL in sodium chloride intravenous infusion 0.9%. Net price 100-mL (80-mg) *Viaflex®* bag = £1.61

Electrolytes Na⁺ 15.4 mmol/100-mL bag

**5**

**Infections**

## AMIKACIN

**Indications** serious Gram-negative infections resistant to gentamicin

**Cautions** see under Gentamicin

**Contra-indications** see under Gentamicin

**Side-effects** see under Gentamicin

**Dose**

- By intramuscular *or* by slow intravenous injection *or* by infusion, 15 mg/kg daily in 2 divided doses, increased to 22.5 mg/kg daily in 3 divided doses in severe infections; max. 1.5 g daily for up to 10 days (max. cumulative dose 15 g); CHILD under 18 years see *BNF for Children*

  Note One-hour ('peak') serum concentration should not exceed 30 mg/litre; pre-dose ('trough') concentration should be less than 10 mg/litre

**Amikacin** (Non-proprietary) [PoM]
Injection, amikacin (as sulphate) 250 mg/mL. Net price 2-mL vial = £10.14
Electrolytes Na+ 0.56 mmol/500-mg vial

**Amikin®** (Bristol-Myers Squibb) [PoM]
Paediatric injection, amikacin (as sulphate) 50 mg/mL. Net price 2-mL vial = £2.11
Electrolytes Na+ < 0.5 mmol/vial

## NEOMYCIN SULPHATE

**Indications** bowel sterilisation before surgery, see also notes above

**Cautions** see under Gentamicin but too toxic for systemic use, see notes above

**Contra-indications** see under Gentamicin; intestinal obstruction; renal impairment (Appendix 3)

**Side-effects** see under Gentamicin but poorly absorbed on oral administration; increased salivation, stomatitis, impaired intestinal absorption with steatorrhoea and diarrhoea

**Dose**

- By mouth, pre-operative bowel sterilisation, 1 g every hour for 4 hours, then 1 g every 4 hours for 2–3 days

  Hepatic coma, up to 4 g daily in divided doses usually for 5–7 days

**Neomycin** (Non-proprietary) [PoM]
Tablets, neomycin sulphate 500 mg. Net price 20 = £4.13
Brands include *Nivemycin®*

## TOBRAMYCIN

**Indications** see under Gentamicin and notes above

**Cautions** see under Gentamicin
Specific cautions for inhaled treatment Other inhaled drugs should be administered before tobramycin; monitor for bronchospasm with initial dose, measure peak flow before and after nebulisation—if bronchospasm occurs, repeat test using bronchodilator; monitor renal function before treatment and then annually; severe haemoptysis

**Contra-indications** see under Gentamicin

**Side-effects** see under Gentamicin; *on inhalation,* mouth ulcers, taste disturbances, voice alteration, cough, bronchospasm (see Cautions)

**Dose**

- By intramuscular injection *or* by slow intravenous injection *or* by intravenous infusion, 3 mg/kg daily in divided doses every 8 hours, see also notes above; in severe infections up to 5 mg/kg daily in

divided doses every 6–8 hours (reduced to 3 mg/kg as soon as clinically indicated); CHILD under 18 years see *BNF for Children*

- Urinary-tract infection, by intramuscular injection, 2–3 mg/kg daily as a single dose
  Note One-hour ('peak') serum concentration should not exceed 10 mg/litre; pre-dose ('trough') concentration should be less than 2 mg/litre

- Chronic pulmonary *Pseudomonas aeruginosa* infection in patients with cystic fibrosis, by inhalation of nebulised solution, ADULT and CHILD over 6 years, 300 mg every 12 hours for 28 days, subsequent courses repeated after 28-day interval without tobramycin nebuliser solution

◢**Parenteral**

**Tobramycin** (Non-proprietary) [PoM]
Injection, tobramycin (as sulphate) 40 mg/mL, net price 1-mL (40-mg) vial = £4.00, 2-mL (80-mg) vial = £4.16, 6-mL (240-mg) vial = £19.20

◢**Inhalation**

**Bramitob®** (Chiesi) [PoM]
Nebuliser solution, tobramycin 75 mg/mL, net price 56 × 4-mL (300-mg) unit = £1187.00

**Tobi®** (Chiron) [PoM]
Nebuliser solution, tobramycin 60 mg/mL, net price 56 × 5-mL (300-mg) unit = £1187.20

## 5.1.5 Macrolides

**Erythromycin** has an antibacterial spectrum that is similar but not identical to that of penicillin; it is thus an alternative in penicillin-allergic patients.

Indications for erythromycin include respiratory infections, whooping cough, legionnaires' disease, and campylobacter enteritis. It is active against many penicillin-resistant staphylococci but some are now also resistant to erythromycin; it has poor activity against *Haemophilus influenzae*. Erythromycin is also active against chlamydia and mycoplasmas.

Erythromycin causes nausea, vomiting, and diarrhoea in some patients; in mild to moderate infections this can be avoided by giving a lower dose (250 mg 4 times daily) but if a more serious infection, such as Legionella pneumonia, is suspected higher doses are needed.

**Azithromycin** is a macrolide with slightly less activity than erythromycin against Gram-positive bacteria but enhanced activity against some Gram-negative organisms including *H. influenzae*. Plasma concentrations are very low but tissue concentrations are much higher. It has a long tissue half-life and once daily dosage is recommended. For treatment of Lyme disease, see section 5.1.1.3. Azithromycin is also used in the treatment of trachoma [unlicensed indication] (section 11.3.1).

**Clarithromycin** is an erythromycin derivative with slightly greater activity than the parent compound. Tissue concentrations are higher than with erythromycin. It is given twice daily.

Azithromycin and clarithromycin cause fewer gastro-intestinal side-effects than erythromycin.

**Spiramycin** is also a macrolide (section 5.4.7).

The ketolide **telithromycin** is a derivative of erythromycin. The antibacterial spectrum of telithromycin is similar to that of macrolides and it is also active against penicillin- and erythromycin-resistant *Streptococcus pneumoniae*. Telithromycin should only be used to treat beta-haemolytic streptococcal pharyngitis and tonsillitis, sinusitis, community-acquired pneumonia, and exacerbations of chronic bronchitis if caused by organisms resistant to beta-lactam antibacterials and other macrolides, or if conventional treatment is contra-indicated.

**Oral infections** Erythromycin is an alternative for oral infections in penicillin-allergic patients or where a beta-lactamase producing organism is involved. However, many organisms are now resistant to erythromycin or rapidly develop resistance; its use should therefore be limited to short courses. Metronidazole (section 5.1.11) may be preferred as an alternative to a penicillin.

## ERYTHROMYCIN

**Indications** susceptible infections in patients with penicillin hypersensitivity; oral infections (see notes above); campylobacter enteritis, syphilis, non-gonococcal urethritis, respiratory-tract infections (including Legionnaires' disease), skin infections (Table 1, section 5.1); chronic prostatitis; prophylaxis of diphtheria, group A streptococcal infection, and whooping cough (Table 2, section 5.1); acne vulgaris and rosacea (section 13.6)

**Cautions** neonate under 2 weeks (risk of hypertrophic pyloric stenosis); predisposition to QT interval prolongation (including electrolyte disturbances, concomitant use of drugs that prolong QT interval); avoid in acute porphyria (section 9.8.2); hepatic impairment (Appendix 2); renal impairment (Appendix 3); pregnancy (not known to be harmful) and breast-feeding (only small amounts in milk); **interactions**: Appendix 1 (macrolides)

**Side-effects** nausea, vomiting, abdominal discomfort, diarrhoea (antibiotic-associated colitis reported); less frequently urticaria, rashes and other allergic reactions; reversible hearing loss reported after large doses; cholestatic jaundice, pancreatitis, cardiac effects (including chest pain and arrhythmias), myasthenia-like syndrome, Stevens-Johnson syndrome, and toxic epidermal necrolysis also reported

**Dose**

- By mouth, ADULT and CHILD over 8 years, 250–500 mg every 6 hours *or* 0.5–1 g every 12 hours (see notes above); up to 4 g daily in divided doses in severe infections; NEONATE 12.5 mg/kg every 6 hours; CHILD 1 month–2 years 125 mg every 6 hours, 2–8 years 250 mg every 6 hours, doses doubled for severe infections

Early syphilis, 500 mg 4 times daily for 14 days

Uncomplicated genital chlamydia, non-gonococcal urethritis, 500 mg twice daily for 14 days

- By intravenous infusion, ADULT and CHILD severe infections, 50 mg/kg daily by continuous infusion *or* in divided doses every 6 hours; mild infections (oral treatment not possible), 25 mg/kg daily; NEONATE see *BNF for Children*

**Erythromycin** (Non-proprietary) ℗ℴℳ

Capsules, enclosing e/c microgranules, erythromycin 250 mg, net price 28-cap pack = £5.95. Label: 5, 9, 25
Brands include *Tiloryth®*

Tablets, e/c, erythromycin 250 mg, net price 28 = £1.78. Label: 5, 9, 25
Dental prescribing on NHS Erythromycin Tablets e/c may be prescribed

**Erythromycin Ethyl Succinate** (Non-proprietary) ℗ℴℳ

Oral suspension, erythromycin (as ethyl succinate) for reconstitution with water 125 mg/5 mL, net price 100 mL = £1.83; 250 mg/5 mL, 100 mL = £2.49; 500 mg/5 mL, 100 mL = £3.96. Label: 9
Note Sugar-free versions are available and can be ordered by specifying 'sugar-free' on the prescription
Brands include *Primacine®*
Dental prescribing on NHS Erythromycin Ethyl Succinate Oral Suspension may be prescribed

**Erythromycin Lactobionate** (Non-proprietary) ℗ℴℳ

Intravenous infusion, powder for reconstitution, erythromycin (as lactobionate), net price 1-g vial = £9.98

**Erymax®** (Zeneus) ℗ℴℳ

Capsules, opaque orange/clear orange, enclosing orange and white e/c pellets, erythromycin 250 mg, net price 28-cap pack = £5.72, 112-cap pack = £22.87. Label: 5, 9, 25
Dose 1 capsule every 6 hours *or* 2 capsules every 12 hours; acne, 1 capsule twice daily for 1 month then 1 capsule daily

**Erythrocin®** (Abbott) ℗ℴℳ

Tablets, both f/c, erythromycin (as stearate), 250 mg, net price 20 = £3.64; 500 mg, 20 = £7.28. Label: 9
Dental prescribing on NHS May be prescribed as Erythromycin Stearate Tablets

**Erythroped®** (Abbott) ℗ℴℳ

Suspension SF, sugar-free, banana-flavoured, erythromycin (as ethyl succinate) for reconstitution with water, 125 mg/5 mL (*Suspension PI SF*), net price 140 mL = £3.06; 250 mg/5 mL, 140 mL = £5.95; 500 mg/5 mL (*Suspension SF Forte*), 140 mL = £10.56. Label: 9

**Erythroped A®** (Abbott) ℗ℴℳ

Tablets, yellow, f/c, erythromycin 500 mg (as ethyl succinate). Net price 28-tab pack = £10.78. Label: 9
Dental prescribing on NHS May be prescribed as Erythromycin Ethyl Succinate Tablets

## AZITHROMYCIN

**Indications** respiratory-tract infections; otitis media; skin and soft-tissue infections; uncomplicated genital chlamydial infections and non-gonococcal urethritis (Table 1, section 5.1); mild or moderate typhoid due to multiple-antibacterial-resistant organisms [unlicensed indication]; prophylaxis of group A streptococcal infection (Table 2, section 5.1)

**Cautions** see under Erythromycin; pregnancy (Appendix 4) and breast-feeding (Appendix 5); **interactions**: Appendix 1 (macrolides)

**Contra-indications** severe hepatic impairment (Appendix 2)

**Side-effects** see under Erythromycin; also anorexia, dyspepsia, flatulence, dizziness, headache, drowsiness, convulsions, arthralgia, and disturbances in taste and smell; *rarely* constipation, hepatitis, hepatic failure, syncope, insomnia, agitation, anxiety, asthenia, paraesthesia, hyperactivity, thrombocytopenia, haemolytic anaemia, interstitial nephritis, acute renal failure, photosensitivity, tooth and tongue discoloration

**5**

**Infections**

**Infections 5** (left margin)

**Dose**

- 500 mg once daily for 3 days *or* 500 mg on first day then 250 mg once daily for 4 days; CHILD over 6 months 10 mg/kg once daily for 3 days; *or* body-weight 15–25 kg, 200 mg once daily for 3 days; body-weight 26–35 kg, 300 mg once daily for 3 days; body-weight 36–45 kg, 400 mg once daily for 3 days
- Uncomplicated genital chlamydial infections and non-gonococcal urethritis, 1 g as a single dose
- Typhoid [unlicensed indication], 500 mg once daily for 7 days

**Azithromycin** (Non-proprietary) ℗⊙M

Capsules, azithromycin (as dihydrate) 250 mg, net price 4-cap pack = £8.96, 6-cap pack = £13.45. Label: 5, 9, 23

[1]Tablets, azithromycin (as monohydrate hemi-ethanolate) 250 mg, net price 4-tab pack = £8.82; 500 mg, 3-tab pack = £9.16. Label: 5, 9

1. Azithromycin tablets can be sold to the public for the treatment of confirmed, asymptomatic *Chlamydia trachomatis* genital infection in those over 16 years of age, and for the epidemiological treatment of their sexual partners, subject to max. single dose of 1 g, max. daily dose 1 g, and a pack size of 1 g

**Zithromax®** (Pfizer) ℗⊙M

Capsules, azithromycin (as dihydrate) 250 mg, net price 4-cap pack = £8.95, 6-cap pack = £13.43. Label: 5, 9, 23

Oral suspension, cherry/banana-flavoured, azithromycin (as dihydrate) 200 mg/5 mL when reconstituted with water. Net price 15-mL pack = £5.08, 22.5-mL pack = £7.62, 30-mL pack = £13.80. Label: 5, 9
Dental prescribing on NHS May be prescribed as Azithromycin Oral Suspension 200 mg/5 mL

## ■ CLARITHROMYCIN

**Indications** respiratory-tract infections, mild to moderate skin and soft tissue infections, otitis media; *Helicobacter pylori* eradication (section 1.3)

**Cautions** see under Erythromycin; renal impairment (Appendix 3); pregnancy (Appendix 4); breast-feeding (Appendix 5); **interactions:** Appendix 1 (macrolides)

**Side-effects** see under Erythromycin; also dyspepsia, tooth and tongue discoloration, smell and taste disturbances, stomatitis, glossitis, and headache; *less commonly* hepatitis, arthralgia, and myalgia; *rarely* tinnitus; *very rarely* pancreatitis, dizziness, insomnia, nightmares, anxiety, confusion, psychosis, paraesthesia, convulsions, hypoglycaemia, renal failure, leucopenia, and thrombocytopenia; on intravenous infusion, local tenderness, phlebitis

**Dose**

- By mouth, 250 mg every 12 hours for 7 days, increased in severe infections to 500 mg every 12 hours for up to 14 days; CHILD body-weight under 8 kg, 7.5 mg/kg twice daily; 8–11 kg (1–2 years), 62.5 mg twice daily; 12–19 kg (3–6 years), 125 mg twice daily; 20–29 kg (7–9 years), 187.5 mg twice daily; 30–40 kg (10–12 years), 250 mg twice daily
- By intravenous infusion into larger proximal vein, 500 mg twice daily; CHILD under 12 years see *BNF for Children*

**Clarithromycin** (Non-proprietary) ℗⊙M

Tablets, clarithromycin 250 mg, net price 14-tab pack = £3.28; 500 mg, 14-tab pack = £6.60. Label: 9

**Klaricid®** (Abbott) ℗⊙M

Tablets, both yellow, f/c, clarithromycin 250 mg, net price 14-tab pack = £7.14; 500 mg, 14-tab pack = £11.53, 20-tab pack = £16.47. Label: 9

Paediatric suspension, clarithromycin for reconstitution with water 125 mg/5 mL, net price 70 mL = £5.36, 100 mL = £9.23; 250 mg/5 mL, 70 mL = £10.72. Label: 9

Granules, clarithromycin 250 mg/sachet, net price 14-sachet pack = £11.68. Label: 9, 13

Intravenous infusion, powder for reconstitution, clarithromycin. Net price 500-mg vial = £9.45
Electrolytes Na+< 0.5 mmol/500-mg vial

**Klaricid XL®** (Abbott) ℗⊙M

Tablets, m/r, yellow, clarithromycin 500 mg, net price 7-tab pack = £6.46, 14-tab pack = £12.71. Label: 9, 21, 25
Dose 500 mg once daily (doubled in severe infections) for 7–14 days

## ■ TELITHROMYCIN

**Indications** see notes above

**Cautions** hepatic impairment (Appendix 2; see also Hepatic Disorders below); renal impairment (Appendix 3); pregnancy (Appendix 4); coronary heart disease, ventricular arrhythmias, bradycardia, hypokalaemia, hypomagnesaemia—risk of QT interval prolongation; concomitant administration of drugs that prolong QT-interval; avoid in acute porphyria (section 9.8.2); **interactions:** Appendix 1 (telithromycin)
Hepatic disorders Patients should be told how to recognise signs of liver disorder, and advised to discontinue treatment and seek prompt medical attention if symptoms such as anorexia, nausea, vomiting, abdominal pain, jaundice, or dark urine develop
Driving Visual disturbances or transient loss of consciousness may affect performance of skilled tasks (e.g. driving); effects may occur after the first dose. Administration at bedtime may reduce these side-effects. Patients should be advised not to drive or operate machinery if affected

**Contra-indications** myasthenia gravis; history of telithromycin-associated hepatitis or jaundice; prolongation of QT interval; congenital or family history of QT interval prolongation (if not excluded by ECG); breast-feeding (Appendix 5)

**Side-effects** diarrhoea, nausea, vomiting, flatulence, abdominal pain, taste disturbances; dizziness, headache; *less commonly* constipation, stomatitis, anorexia, hepatitis, flushing, palpitations, drowsiness, insomnia, nervousness, eosinophilia, blurred vision, rash, urticaria, and pruritus; *rarely* cholestatic jaundice, arrhythmias, hypotension, transient loss of consciousness, paraesthesia, and diplopia; *very rarely* antibiotic-associated colitis, altered sense of smell, muscle cramp, erythema multiforme; also reported pancreatitis, confusion, hallucinations and arthralgia

**Dose**

- 800 mg once daily for 5 days for sinusitis or exacerbation of chronic bronchitis *or* for 7–10 days in community-acquired pneumonia; CHILD under 18 years safety and efficacy not established
- Tonsillitis or pharyngitis caused by *Streptococcus pyogenes*, ADULT and CHILD over 12 years, 800 mg once daily for 5 days

**Ketek®** (Sanofi-Aventis) ▼ PoM
Tablets, orange, f/c, telithromycin 400 mg, net price
10-tab pack = £18.56. Label: 9, counselling , driving,
hepatic disorders

## 5.1.6 Clindamycin

Clindamycin is active against Gram-positive cocci,
including streptococci and penicillin-resistant staphylococci, and also against many anaerobes, especially *Bacteroides fragilis*. It is well concentrated in bone and
excreted in bile and urine.

Clindamycin is recommended for staphylococcal joint
and bone infections such as osteomyelitis, and intra-
abdominal sepsis; it is an alternative to macrolides for
erysipelas or cellulitis in penicillin-allergic patients.
Clindamycin can also be used for infections associated
with meticillin-resistant *Staphylococcus aureus* (MRSA) in
bronchiectasis, bone and joint infections, and skin and
soft-tissue infections.

Clindamycin has been associated with antibiotic-associated colitis (section 1.5), which may be fatal; it is most
common in middle-aged and elderly women, especially
following an operation. Although antibiotic-associated
colitis can occur with most antibacterials, it occurs more
frequently with clindamycin. Patients should therefore
discontinue treatment immediately if diarrhoea develops.

**Oral infections** Clindamycin should not be used
routinely for the treatment of oral infections because it
may be no more effective than penicillins against anaerobes and there may be cross-resistance with erythromycin-resistant bacteria. Clindamycin can be used for
the treatment of dentoalveolar abscess that has not
responded to penicillin or to metronidazole.

### CLINDAMYCIN

**Indications** see notes above; staphylococcal bone and
joint infections, peritonitis; falciparum malaria (section 5.4.1)

**Cautions** discontinue immediately if diarrhoea or colitis develops; monitor liver and renal function on
prolonged therapy and in neonates and infants;
pregnancy (Appendix 4); breast-feeding (Appendix 5);
avoid rapid intravenous administration; avoid in acute
porphyria (section 9.8.2); **interactions:** Appendix 1
(clindamycin)

**Contra-indications** diarrhoeal states; avoid injections
containing benzyl alcohol in neonates (see under
preparations below)

**Side-effects** diarrhoea (discontinue treatment),
abdominal discomfort, oesophagitis, oesophageal
ulcers, taste disturbances, nausea, vomiting, antibiotic-associated colitis; jaundice; leucopenia, eosinophilia, and thrombocytopenia reported; polyarthritis
reported; rash, pruritus, urticaria, anaphylactoid
reactions, Stevens-Johnson syndrome, toxic epidermal necrolysis, exfoliative and vesiculobullous
dermatitis reported; pain, induration, and abscess
after intramuscular injection; thrombophlebitis after
intravenous injection

**Dose**
● By mouth, 150–300 mg every 6 hours; up to 450 mg
every 6 hours in severe infections; CHILD, 3–6 mg/kg
every 6 hours
  **Counselling** Patients should discontinue immediately and
  contact doctor if diarrhoea develops; capsules should be
  swallowed with a glass of water.
● By deep intramuscular injection *or* by intravenous
infusion, 0.6–2.7 g daily (in 2–4 divided doses); life-
threatening infection, up to 4.8 g daily; single doses
above 600 mg by intravenous infusion only; single
doses by intravenous infusion not to exceed 1.2 g;
CHILD over 1 month, 15–40 mg/kg daily in 3–4
divided doses; severe infections, at least 300 mg
daily regardless of weight

**Clindamycin** (Non-proprietary) PoM
Capsules, clindamycin (as hydrochloride) 150 mg, net
price 24-cap pack = £21.51. Label: 9, 27, counselling,
see above (diarrhoea)
**Dental prescribing on NHS** Clindamycin Capsules may be
prescribed

**Dalacin C®** (Pharmacia) PoM
Capsules, clindamycin (as hydrochloride) 75 mg
(lavender), net price 24-cap pack = £7.45; 150 mg,
(lavender/maroon), 24-cap pack = £13.72. Label: 9,
27, counselling, see above (diarrhoea)
**Dental prescribing on NHS** May be prescribed as Clindamycin Capsules

Injection, clindamycin (as phosphate) 150 mg/mL,
net price 2-mL amp = £6.20; 4-mL amp = £12.35
Excipients include benzyl alcohol (avoid in neonates, see Excipients,
p. 2)

## 5.1.7 Some other antibacterials

Antibacterials discussed in this section include chloramphenicol, fusidic acid, glycopeptide antibiotics
(vancomycin and teicoplanin), linezolid, the streptogra-
mins (quinupristin and dalfopristin) and the polymyxin,
colistin.

### Chloramphenicol

**Chloramphenicol** is a potent broad-spectrum antibiotic; however, it is associated with serious haematological
side-effects when given systemically and should therefore be reserved for the treatment of life-threatening
infections, particularly those caused by *Haemophilus
influenzae*, and also for typhoid fever.

Chloramphenicol eye drops (section 11.3.1) and chloramphenicol ear drops (section 12.1.1) are also available.

### CHLORAMPHENICOL

**Indications** see notes above

**Cautions** avoid repeated courses and prolonged
treatment; reduce doses in hepatic impairment
(Appendix 2); renal impairment (Appendix 3); blood
counts required before and periodically during treatment; monitor plasma-chloramphenicol concentration in neonates (see below); **interactions:** Appendix
1 (chloramphenicol)

**Contra-indications** pregnancy (Appendix 4), breast-
feeding (Appendix 5), acute porphyria (section 9.8.2)

5

Infections

**Side-effects** blood disorders including reversible and irreversible aplastic anaemia (with reports of resulting leukaemia), peripheral neuritis, optic neuritis, headache, depression, urticaria, erythema multiforme, nausea, vomiting, diarrhoea, stomatitis, glossitis, dry mouth; nocturnal haemoglobinuria reported; grey syndrome (abdominal distension, pallid cyanosis, circulatory collapse) may follow excessive doses in neonates with immature hepatic metabolism

**Dose**

* By mouth *or* by intravenous injection *or* infusion, 50 mg/kg daily in 4 divided doses (exceptionally, can be doubled for severe infections such as septicaemia and meningitis, providing high doses reduced as soon as clinically indicated); CHILD, haemophilus epiglottitis and pyogenic meningitis, 50–100 mg/kg daily in divided doses (high dosages decreased as soon as clinically indicated); NEONATE under 2 weeks 25 mg/kg daily (in 4 divided doses); INFANT 2 weeks–1 year 50 mg/kg daily (in 4 divided doses)

Note Plasma concentration monitoring required in neonates and preferred in those under 4 years of age, in the elderly, and in hepatic impairment; recommended peak plasma concentration (approx. 1 hour after intravenous injection or infusion) 15–25 mg/litre; pre-dose ('trough') concentration should not exceed 15 mg/litre

**Chloramphenicol** (Non-proprietary) PoM
Capsules, chloramphenicol 250 mg. Net price 60 = £377.00

**Kemicetine®** (Pharmacia) PoM
Injection, powder for reconstitution, chloramphenicol (as sodium succinate). Net price 1-g vial = £1.39
Electrolytes Na+ 3.14 mmol/g

---

# Fusidic acid

**Fusidic acid** and its salts are narrow-spectrum antibiotics. The only indication for their use is in infections caused by penicillin-resistant staphylococci, especially osteomyelitis, as they are well concentrated in bone; they are also used for staphylococcal endocarditis. A second antistaphylococcal antibiotic is usually required to prevent emergence of resistance.

## SODIUM FUSIDATE

**Indications** penicillin-resistant staphylococcal infection including osteomyelitis; staphylococcal endocarditis in combination with other antibacterials (Table 1, section 5.1)

**Cautions** monitor liver function with high doses, on prolonged therapy or in hepatic impairment (Appendix 2); elimination may be reduced in hepatic impairment or biliary disease or biliary obstruction; pregnancy (Appendix 4); breast-feeding (Appendix 5); **interactions:** Appendix 1 (fusidic acid)

**Side-effects** nausea, vomiting, reversible jaundice, especially after high dosage or rapid infusion (withdraw therapy if persistent); rarely hypersensitivity reactions, acute renal failure (usually with jaundice), blood disorders

**Dose**

* See under Preparations, below

**Sodium fusidate** (LEO) PoM
Intravenous infusion, powder for reconstitution, sodium fusidate 500 mg (= fusidic acid 480 mg), with buffer, net price per vial (with diluent) = £70.04
Electrolytes Na+ 3.1 mmol/vial when reconstituted with buffer
Dose as sodium fusidate, by intravenous infusion, ADULT over 50 kg, 500 mg 3 times daily; ADULT under 50 kg and CHILD, 6–7 mg/kg 3 times daily

**Fucidin®** (LEO) PoM
Tablets, f/c, sodium fusidate 250 mg, net price 10-tab pack = £6.02. Label: 9
Dose as sodium fusidate, 500 mg every 8 hours, doubled for severe infections
Skin infection, as sodium fusidate, 250 mg every 12 hours for 5–10 days

Suspension, off-white, banana- and orange-flavoured, fusidic acid 250 mg/5 mL, net price 50 mL = £6.73. Label: 9, 21
Dose as fusidic acid, ADULT 750 mg every 8 hours; CHILD up to 1 year 50 mg/kg daily (in 3 divided doses), 1–5 years 250 mg every 8 hours, 5–12 years 500 mg every 8 hours
Note Fusidic acid is incompletely absorbed and doses recommended for suspension are proportionally higher than those for sodium fusidate tablets

---

# Vancomycin and teicoplanin

The glycopeptide antibiotics vancomycin and teicoplanin have bactericidal activity against aerobic and anaerobic Gram-positive bacteria including multi-resistant staphylococci. However, there are reports of *Staphylococcus aureus* with reduced susceptibility to glycopeptides. There are increasing reports of glycopeptide-resistant enterococci.

**Vancomycin** is used *by the intravenous route* in the treatment of endocarditis and other serious infections caused by Gram-positive cocci. It has a long duration of action and can therefore be given every 12 hours. Vancomycin (added to dialysis fluid) is also used in the treatment of peritonitis associated with peritoneal dialysis [unlicensed route] (Table 1 section 5.1).

Vancomycin given *by mouth* is effective in the treatment of *Clostridium difficile* infection (see also section 1.5); a dose of 125 mg every 6 hours for 10 to 14 days is considered adequate (up to 500 mg every 6 hours can be considered if the infection fails to respond or if it is life-threatening). Vancomycin should **not** be given by mouth for systemic infections since it is not significantly absorbed.

**Teicoplanin** is similar to vancomycin but has a significantly longer duration of action allowing once-daily administration. Unlike vancomycin, teicoplanin can be given by intramuscular as well as by intravenous injection; it is not given by mouth.

## VANCOMYCIN

**Indications** see notes above

**Cautions** avoid rapid infusion (risk of anaphylactoid reactions, see Side-effects); rotate infusion sites; renal impairment (Appendix 3); elderly; avoid if history of deafness; all patients require plasma-vancomycin measurement (after 3 or 4 doses if renal function normal, earlier if renal impairment), blood counts, urinalysis, and renal function tests; monitor auditory function in elderly or if renal impairment; pregnancy (Appendix 4) and breast-feeding (Appendix 5); teicoplanin sensitivity; systemic absorption may follow oral administration especially in inflammatory bowel disorders or following multiple doses; **interactions:** Appendix 1 (vancomycin)

**Side-effects** after parenteral administration: nephrotoxicity including renal failure and interstitial nephritis; ototoxicity (discontinue if tinnitus occurs); blood disorders including neutropenia (usually after 1 week or cumulative dose of 25 g), rarely agranulocytosis and thrombocytopenia; nausea; chills, fever; eosinophilia, anaphylaxis, rashes (including exfoliative dermatitis, Stevens-Johnson syndrome, toxic epidermal necrolysis, and vasculitis); phlebitis (irritant to tissue); on rapid infusion, severe hypotension (including shock and cardiac arrest), wheezing, dyspnoea, urticaria, pruritus, flushing of the upper body ('red man' syndrome), pain and muscle spasm of back and chest

**Dose**

- By mouth, *Clostridium difficile* infection, 125 mg every 6 hours for 10–14 days, see notes above; CHILD 5 mg/kg every 6 hours, over 5 years, half adult dose
  Note Oral paediatric dose is lower than that on product literature but is adequate

- By intravenous infusion, 1–1.5 g every 12 hours; ELDERLY over 65 years, 500 mg every 12 hours *or* 1 g once daily; CHILD over 1 month, 15 mg/kg every 8 hours (max. 2 g daily)
  Note Plasma concentration monitoring required (see Cautions above); pre-dose ('trough') concentration should be 10–15 mg/litre (15–20 mg/litre for less sensitive strains of meticillin-resistant *Staphylococcus aureus*); vancomycin doses in BNF may differ from those in product literature

**Vancomycin** (Non-proprietary) PoM

Capsules, vancomycin (as hydrochloride) 125 mg, net price 28-cap pack = £132.47; 250 mg, 28-cap pack = £132.47. Label: 9

Injection, powder for reconstitution, vancomycin (as hydrochloride), for use as an infusion, net price 500-mg vial = £7.25; 1-g vial = £14.50
Note Can be used to prepare solution for oral administration

**Vancocin®** (Flynn) PoM

Matrigel capsules, vancomycin (as hydrochloride) 125 mg, net price 28-cap pack = £88.31. Label: 9

Injection, powder for reconstitution, vancomycin (as hydrochloride), for use as an infusion, net price 500-mg vial = £8.05; 1-g vial = £16.11
Note Can be used to prepare solution for oral administration

## TEICOPLANIN

**Indications** potentially serious Gram-positive infections including endocarditis, dialysis-associated peritonitis, and serious infections due to *Staphylococcus aureus*; prophylaxis in orthopaedic surgery at risk of infection with Gram-positive organisms

**Cautions** vancomycin sensitivity; blood counts and liver and kidney function tests required; monitor plasma-teicoplanin concentration if severe sepsis or burns, deep-seated staphylococcal infection (including bone and joint infection), endocarditis, renal impairment, in elderly, and in intravenous drug abusers; monitor renal and auditory function during prolonged treatment in renal impairment (Appendix 3) or if other nephrotoxic or neurotoxic drugs given; pregnancy (Appendix 4) and breast-feeding; **interactions:** Appendix 1 (teicoplanin)

**Side-effects** nausea, vomiting, diarrhoea; rash, pruritus, fever, bronchospasm, rigors, urticaria, angioedema, anaphylaxis; dizziness, headache; blood disorders including eosinophilia, leucopenia, neutropenia, and thrombocytopenia; disturbances in liver enzymes, transient increase of serum creatinine, renal failure; tinnitus, mild hearing loss, and vestibular disorders also reported; rarely exfoliative dermatitis, Stevens-Johnson syndrome, toxic epidermal necrolysis; local reactions include erythema, pain, thrombophlebitis, injection site abscess and rarely flushing with infusion

**Dose**

- By intramuscular injection *or* by intravenous injection *or* infusion, initially 400 mg (for severe infections, by intravenous injection *or* infusion, initially 400 mg every 12 hours for 3 doses), then 200 mg once daily (400 mg once daily for severe infections); higher doses may be required in patients over 85 kg and in severe burns, or meticillin-resistant *Staphylococcus aureus* infection (consult product literature)

- CHILD over 2 months by intravenous injection *or* infusion, initially 10 mg/kg every 12 hours for 3 doses, subsequently 6 mg/kg once daily (severe infections or in neutropenia, 10 mg/kg once daily); subsequent doses can be given by intramuscular injection (but intravenous administration preferred in children); NEONATE by intravenous infusion, initially a single dose of 16 mg/kg, subsequently 8 mg/kg once daily

- Streptococcal endocarditis (in combination with another antibacterial if necessary, see Table 1, section 5.1), by intravenous injection *or* infusion, ADULT initially 6 mg/kg every 12 hours for 3 doses, then 6 mg/kg once daily

- Enterococcal endocarditis (in combination with another antibacterial, see Table 1, section 5.1), by intravenous injection *or* infusion, ADULT initially 10 mg/kg every 12 hours for 3 doses, then 10 mg/kg once daily

- Orthopaedic surgery prophylaxis, by intravenous injection, 400 mg at induction of anaesthesia
  Note Plasma-teicoplanin concentration is not measured routinely because a relationship between plasma concentration and toxicity has not been established. However, the plasma-teicoplanin concentration can be used to optimise treatment in some patients (see Cautions). Pre-dose ('trough') concentrations should be greater than 10 mg/litre (greater than 15–20 mg/litre in endocarditis) but less than 60 mg/litre

**Targocid®** (Sanofi-Aventis) PoM

Injection, powder for reconstitution, teicoplanin, net price 200-mg vial (with diluent) = £3.57; 400-mg vial (with diluent) = £6.10
Electrolytes Na$^+$< 0.5 mmol/200- and 400-mg vial

## Daptomycin

**Daptomycin** is a lipopeptide antibacterial with a spectrum of activity similar to vancomycin but its efficacy against enterococci has not been established. Daptomycin should be reserved for complicated skin and soft-tissue infections caused by resistant Gram-positive bacteria including meticillin-resistant *Staphylococcus aureus* (MRSA). It needs to be given with other antibacterials for mixed infections involving Gram-negative bacteria and some anaerobes.

The *Scottish Medicines Consortium* (p. 3) has advised (February 2008) that daptomycin (*Cubicin®*) is accepted for restricted use within NHS Scotland for the treatment

5

Infections

of MRSA bacteraemia associated with right-sided endocarditis or with complicated skin and soft-tissue infections.

## DAPTOMYCIN

**Indications** see under Dose

**Cautions** interference with assay for prothrombin time and INR—take blood sample immediately before daptomycin dose; hepatic impairment (Appendix 2); renal impairment (Appendix 3); pregnancy (Appendix 4); **interactions:** Appendix 1 (daptomycin)
**Muscle effects** Myalgia, muscle weakness, and myositis may occur uncommonly; rhabdomyolysis is very rare. Monitor creatine kinase before treatment and then weekly during treatment (more frequently if creatine kinase elevated more than 5 times upper limit of normal before treatment, or if receiving another drug known to cause myopathy (preferably avoid concomitant use), or if eGFR less than 30 mL/minute/1.73 m²). If unexplained muscle pain, tenderness, weakness, or cramps develop during treatment, measure creatine kinase every 2 days; discontinue if unexplained muscular symptoms and creatine kinase elevated markedly

**Contra-indications** breast-feeding (Appendix 5)

**Side-effects** nausea, vomiting, diarrhoea; headache; rash, injection-site reactions; *less commonly* constipation, abdominal pain, dyspepsia, anorexia, taste disturbance, jaundice, hypertension, hypotension, flushing, arrhythmias, anxiety, insomnia, dizziness, fatigue, paraesthesia, hyperglycaemia, vaginitis, renal failure, anaemia, eosinophilia, thrombocythaemia, electrolyte disturbances, muscle effects (see Cautions); arthralgia, glossitis, and pruritus; also reported syncope, wheezing, and peripheral neuropathy

**Dose**
- By intravenous infusion, complicated skin and soft-tissue infections caused by Gram-positive bacteria, ADULT over 18 years, 4 mg/kg once daily; increased to 6 mg/kg once daily if associated with *Staphylococcus aureus* bacteraemia

  Right-sided endocarditis caused by *Staphylococcus aureus*, ADULT over 18 years, 6 mg/kg once daily

**Cubicin®** (Novartis) ▼ PoM
Intravenous infusion, powder for reconstitution, daptomycin, net price 350-mg vial = £62.00; 500-mg vial = £88.57

## Linezolid

**Linezolid**, an oxazolidinone antibacterial, is active against Gram-positive bacteria including meticillin-resistant *Staphylococcus aureus* (MRSA), and vancomycin-resistant enterococci. Resistance to linezolid can develop with prolonged treatment or if the dose is less than that recommended. Linezolid is an option if a glycopeptide, such as vancomycin, cannot be used to treat pneumonia or severe skin and soft-tissue infections caused by MRSA. Linezolid is **not** active against Gram-negative organisms and must be given with other antibacterials if the infection also involves Gram-negative organisms (the combination should be used for mixed skin and soft tissue infections only when other treatments are not available). A higher incidence of blood disorders and optic neuropathy have been reported in patients receiving linezolid for more than the maximum recommended duration of 28 days.

## LINEZOLID

**Indications** pneumonia, complicated skin and soft-tissue infections caused by Gram-positive bacteria (initiated under expert supervision)

**Cautions** monitor full blood count (including platelet count) weekly (see also CSM Advice below); history of seizures; unless close observation and blood-pressure monitoring possible, avoid in uncontrolled hypertension, phaeochromocytoma, carcinoid tumour, thyrotoxicosis, bipolar depression, schizophrenia, or acute confusional states; hepatic impairment (Appendix 2); renal impairment (Appendix 3); pregnancy (Appendix 4); **interactions:** Appendix 1 (MAOIs)

> **CSM advice (blood disorders)**
> Haematopoietic disorders (including thrombocytopenia, anaemia, leucopenia, and pancytopenia) have been reported in patients receiving linezolid. It is recommended that full blood counts are monitored weekly. Close monitoring is recommended in patients who:
> - receive treatment for more than 10–14 days;
> - have pre-existing myelosuppression;
> - are receiving drugs that may have adverse effects on haemoglobin, blood counts, or platelet function;
> - have severe renal impairment.
>
> If significant myelosuppression occurs, treatment should be stopped unless it is considered essential, in which case intensive monitoring of blood counts and appropriate management should be implemented.

> **CHM advice (optic neuropathy)**
> Severe optic neuropathy may occur rarely, particularly if linezolid is used for longer than 28 days. The CHM recommends that:
> - patients should be warned to report symptoms of visual impairment (including blurred vision, visual field defect, changes in visual acuity and colour vision) immediately;
> - patients experiencing new visual symptoms (regardless of treatment duration) should be evaluated promptly, and referred to an ophthalmologist if necessary;
> - visual function should be monitored regularly if treatment is required for longer than 28 days.

**Monoamine oxidase inhibition** Linezolid is a reversible, non-selective monoamine oxidase inhibitor (MAOI). Patients should avoid consuming large amounts of tyramine-rich foods (such as mature cheese, yeast extracts, undistilled alcoholic beverages, and fermented soya bean products). In addition, linezolid should not be given with another MAOI or within 2 weeks of stopping another MAOI. Unless close observation and blood-pressure monitoring is possible, avoid in those receiving SSRIs, 5HT₁ agonists ('triptans'), tricyclic antidepressants, sympathomimetics, dopaminergics, buspirone, pethidine and possibly other opioid analgesics. For other interactions see Appendix 1 (MAOIs)

**Contra-indications** breast-feeding (Appendix 5); see also Monoamine oxidase inhibition above

**Side-effects** diarrhoea (antibiotic-associated colitis reported), nausea, vomiting, taste disturbances; headache; *less commonly* thirst, dry mouth, glossitis, stomatitis, tongue discoloration, abdominal pain, dyspepsia, gastritis, constipation, pancreatitis, hypertension, fever, fatigue, dizziness, insomnia, hypoaesthesia, paraesthesia, tinnitus, polyuria, anaemia, leucopenia, thrombocytopenia, eosinophilia, electrolyte disturbances, blurred vision, rash, pruritus, diaphoresis, and injection-site reactions; *very rarely* transient ischaemic attacks, renal failure, pancytopenia and Stevens-Johnson syndrome; also reported convulsions, lactic acidosis; peripheral and optic neuropathy reported on prolonged therapy (see also CHM advice above)

**Dose**

- By mouth, 600 mg every 12 hours usually for 10–14 days (max. duration of treatment 28 days); CHILD [unlicensed] 1 week–12 years, 10 mg/kg every 8 hours; 12–18 years, adult dose
- By intravenous infusion over 30–120 minutes, 600 mg every 12 hours; CHILD [unlicensed] 1 week–12 years, 10 mg/kg every 8 hours; 12–18 years, adult dose

**Zyvox®** (Pharmacia) ▼ PoM
Tablets, f/c, linezolid 600 mg, net price 10-tab pack = £445.00. Label: 9, 10, patient information leaflet

Suspension, yellow, linezolid 100 mg/5 mL when reconstituted with water, net price 150 mL (orange-flavoured) = £222.50. Label: 9, 10 patient information leaflet
Excipients include aspartame 20 mg/5 mL (section 9.4.1)

Intravenous infusion, linezolid 2 mg/mL, net price 300-mL *Excel®* bag = £44.50
Excipients include Na+ 5 mmol/300-mL bag, glucose 13.71 g/300-mL bag

---

# Quinupristin and dalfopristin

A combination of the streptogramin antibiotics, **quinupristin** and **dalfopristin** (as *Synercid®*) is licensed for infections due to Gram-positive bacteria. The combination should be reserved for treating infections which have failed to respond to other antibacterials (e.g. meticillin-resistant *Staphylococcus aureus*, MRSA) or for patients who cannot be treated with other antibacterials. Quinupristin and dalfopristin are not active against *Enterococcus faecalis* and they need to be given in combination with other antibacterials for mixed infections which also involve Gram-negative organisms.

**QUINUPRISTIN WITH DALFOPRISTIN**
A mixture of quinupristin and dalfopristin (both as mesilate salts) in the proportions 3 parts to 7 parts

**Indications** serious Gram-positive infections where no alternative antibacterial is suitable including hospital-acquired pneumonia, skin and soft-tissue infections, infections due to vancomycin-resistant *Enterococcus faecium*

**Cautions** hepatic impairment (avoid if severe; Appendix 2); pregnancy (Appendix 4); predisposition to cardiac arrhythmias (including congenital QT syndrome, concomitant use of drugs that prolong QT interval, cardiac hypertrophy, dilated cardiomyopathy, hypokalaemia, hypomagnesaemia, bradycardia); **interactions**: Appendix 1 (quinupristin with dalfopristin)

**Contra-indications** plasma-bilirubin concentration greater than 3 times upper limit of reference range; breast-feeding (Appendix 5)

**Side-effects** nausea, vomiting, diarrhoea; headache, asthenia; anaemia, leucopenia, eosinophilia, raised urea and creatinine; arthralgia, myalgia; rash, pruritus; injection-site reactions on peripheral venous administration; *less commonly* stomatitis, constipation, abdominal pain, antibiotic-associated colitis, hepatitis,

jaundice, pancreatitis, anorexia, peripheral oedema, hypotension, chest pain, arrhythmias, dyspnoea, insomnia, anxiety, confusion, dizziness, paraesthesia, hypertonia, myasthenia, and gout; *rarely* electrolyte disturbances; *very rarely* thrombocytopenia and pancytopenia

**Dose**
Note Expressed as a combination of quinupristin and dalfopristin (in a ratio of 3:7)

- ADULT over 18 years, by intravenous infusion into central vein, 7.5 mg/kg every 8 hours for 7 days in skin and soft-tissue infections; for 10 days in hospital-acquired pneumonia; duration of treatment in *E. faecium* infection depends on site of infection
Note In emergency, first dose may be administered *via* peripheral line until central venous catheter in place

**Synercid®** (Nordic) PoM
Intravenous infusion, powder for reconstitution, quinupristin (as mesilate) 150 mg, dalfopristin (as mesilate) 350 mg, net price 500-mg vial = £37.00
Electrolytes Na+ approx. 16 mmol/500-mg vial

---

## Polymyxins

The polymyxin antibiotic, **colistin**, is active against Gram-negative organisms including *Pseudomonas aeruginosa*, *Acinetobacter baumanii*, and *Klebsiella pneumoniae*. It is **not** absorbed by mouth and thus needs to be given by injection for a systemic effect. Intravenous administration of colistin should be reserved for Gram-negative infections resistant to other antibacterials; its major adverse effects are dose-related neurotoxicity and nephrotoxicity.

Colistin is used by mouth in bowel sterilisation regimens in neutropenic patients (usually with nystatin); it is **not** recommended for gastro-intestinal infections. It is also given by inhalation of a nebulised solution as an adjunct to standard antibacterial therapy in patients with cystic fibrosis.

Both colistin and polymyxin B are included in some preparations for topical application.

**COLISTIN**

**Indications** see notes above

**Cautions** renal impairment (Appendix 3); acute porphyria (section 9.8.2); risk of bronchospasm on inhalation—may be prevented or treated with a selective beta₂ agonist; **interactions**: Appendix 1 (polymyxins)

**Contra-indications** myasthenia gravis; pregnancy (Appendix 4); breast-feeding (Appendix 5)

**Side-effects** neurotoxicity reported especially with excessive doses (including apnoea, perioral and peripheral paraesthesia, vertigo; *rarely* vasomotor instability, slurred speech, confusion, psychosis, visual disturbances); nephrotoxicity; hypersensitivity reactions including rash; injection-site reactions; inhalation may cause sore throat, sore mouth, cough, bronchospasm

**Dose**

- By mouth, bowel sterilisation, 1.5–3 million units every 8 hours
- By slow intravenous injection into a totally implantable venous access device, *or* by

intravenous infusion (but see notes above), ADULT and CHILD body-weight under 60 kg, 50 000–75 000 units/kg daily in 3 divided doses; body-weight over 60 kg, 1–2 million units every 8 hours
Note Plasma concentration monitoring required in neonates, renal impairment, and in cystic fibrosis; recommended 'peak' plasma-colistin concentration (approx. 30 minutes after intravenous injection or infusion) 10–15 mg/litre (125–200 units/mL)

- By inhalation of nebulised solution, ADULT and CHILD over 2 years, 1–2 million units every 12 hours; CHILD under 2 years, 0.5–1 million units every 12 hours

**Colomycin®** (Forest) PoM
Tablets, scored, colistin sulphate 1.5 million units. Net price 50 = £58.28

Syrup, colistin sulphate 250 000 units/5 mL when reconstituted with water. Net price 80 mL = £3.48

Injection, powder for reconstitution, colistimethate sodium (colistin sulphomethate sodium). Net price 1 million-unit vial = £1.68; 2 million-unit vial = £3.09
Electrolytes (before reconstitution) Na⁺< 0.5 mmol/500 000-unit, 1 million-unit, and 2 million-unit vial
Note *Colomycin®* Injection (dissolved in physiological saline) may be used for nebulisation

**Promixin®** (Profile) PoM
Powder for nebuliser solution, colistimethate sodium (colistin sulphomethate sodium), net price 1 million-unit vial = £4.60

Injection, powder for reconstitution, colistimethate sodium (colistin sulphomethate sodium), net price 1 million unit-vial = £2.30
Electrolytes (before reconstitution) Na⁺< 0.5 mmol/1 million-unit vial

## 5.1.8 Sulphonamides and trimethoprim

The importance of the sulphonamides has decreased as a result of increasing bacterial resistance and their replacement by antibacterials which are generally more active and less toxic.

Sulfamethoxazole (sulphamethoxazole) and trimethoprim are used in combination (as **co-trimoxazole**) because of their synergistic activity. However, co-trimoxazole is associated with rare but serious side-effects (e.g. Stevens-Johnson syndrome and blood dyscrasias, notably bone marrow depression and agranulocytosis) especially in the elderly (see CSM recommendations below).

> **CSM recommendations.**
> Co-trimoxazole should be limited to the role of drug of choice in *Pneumocystis jirovecii* (*Pneumocystis carinii*) pneumonia; it is also indicated for *toxoplasmosis* and *nocardiasis*. It should now only be considered for use in *acute exacerbations of chronic bronchitis* and *infections of the urinary tract* when there is good bacteriological evidence of sensitivity to co-trimoxazole and good reason to prefer this combination to a single antibacterial; similarly it should only be used in *acute otitis media in children* when there is good reason to prefer it.

**Trimethoprim** can be used alone for urinary- and respiratory-tract infections and for prostatitis, shigellosis, and invasive salmonella infections. Trimethoprim has

side-effects similar to co-trimoxazole but they are less severe and occur less frequently.

For *topical preparations* of sulphonamides used in the treatment of burns see section 13.10.1.1.

## ■ CO-TRIMOXAZOLE

A mixture of trimethoprim and sulfamethoxazole in the proportions of 1 part to 5 parts

**Indications** see CSM recommendations above

**Cautions** maintain adequate fluid intake; avoid in blood disorders (unless under specialist supervision); monitor blood counts on prolonged treatment; discontinue immediately if blood disorders or rash develop; predisposition to folate deficiency or hyperkalaemia; elderly (see CSM recommendations above); asthma; G6PD deficiency (section 9.1.5); avoid in infants under 6 weeks (except for treatment or prophylaxis of pneumocystis pneumonia); hepatic impairment (avoid if severe); renal impairment (avoid if eGFR less than 15 mL/minute/1.73 m²; Appendix 3); pregnancy (Appendix 4); breast-feeding (Appendix 5); **interactions:** Appendix 1 (trimethoprim, sulfamethoxazole)

**Contra-indications** acute porphyria (section 9.8.2)

**Side-effects** nausea, diarrhoea; headache; hyperkalaemia; rash (very rarely including Stevens-Johnson syndrome, toxic epidermal necrolysis, photosensitivity)—discontinue immediately; *less commonly* vomiting; *very rarely* glossitis, stomatitis, anorexia, liver damage (including jaundice and hepatic necrosis), pancreatitis, antibiotic-associated colitis, myocarditis, cough and shortness of breath, pulmonary infiltrates, aseptic meningitis, depression, convulsions, peripheral neuropathy, ataxia, tinnitus, vertigo, hallucinations, hypoglycaemia, blood disorders (including leucopenia, thrombocytopenia, megaloblastic anaemia, eosinophilia), hyponatraemia, renal disorders including interstitial nephritis, arthralgia, myalgia, vasculitis, systemic lupus erythematosus and uveitis; rhabdomyolysis reported in HIV-infected patients

**Dose**

- By mouth, 960 mg every 12 hours; CHILD, every 12 hours, 6 weeks–5 months, 120 mg; 6 months–5 years, 240 mg; 6–12 years, 480 mg
- By intravenous infusion, 960 mg every 12 hours increased to 1.44 g every 12 hours in severe infections; CHILD 36 mg/kg daily in 2 divided doses increased to 54 mg/kg daily in severe infections
- Treatment of *Pneumocystis jirovecii* (*Pneumocystis carinii*) infections (undertaken where facilities for appropriate monitoring available—consult microbiologist and product literature), by mouth *or* by intravenous infusion, ADULT and CHILD over 4 weeks, 120 mg/kg daily in 2–4 divided doses for 14 days
- Prophylaxis of *Pneumocystis jirovecii* (*Pneumocystis carinii*) infections, by mouth, 960 mg once daily (may be reduced to 480 mg once daily to improve tolerance) *or* 960 mg on alternate days (3 times a week) *or* 960 mg twice daily on alternate days (3 times a week); CHILD 6 weeks–5 months, 120 mg twice daily on 3 consecutive or alternate days per week *or* on 7 days per week; 6 months–5 years, 240 mg; 6–12 years, 480 mg
Note 480 mg of co-trimoxazole consists of sulfamethoxazole 400 mg and trimethoprim 80 mg

**Co-trimoxazole** (Non-proprietary) PoM
Tablets, co-trimoxazole 480 mg, net price 28-tab pack
= £12.22, 960 mg, 20 = £4.69. Label: 9
Brands include *Fectrim®*, *Fectrim® Forte*

Paediatric oral suspension, co-trimoxazole 240 mg/
5 mL, net price 100 mL = £1.12. Label: 9

Oral suspension, co-trimoxazole 480 mg/5 mL. Net
price 100 mL = £4.41. Label: 9

**Septrin®** (GSK) PoM
Tablets, co-trimoxazole 480 mg. Net price 20 = £3.10.
Label: 9

Forte tablets, scored, co-trimoxazole 960 mg. Net
price 20 = £4.69. Label: 9

Adult suspension, co-trimoxazole 480 mg/5 mL. Net
price 100 mL (vanilla-flavoured) = £4.41. Label: 9

Paediatric suspension, sugar-free, co-trimoxazole
240 mg/5 mL. Net price 100 mL (banana- and vanilla-
flavoured) = £2.45. Label: 9

Intravenous infusion, co-trimoxazole 96 mg/mL. To
be diluted before use. Net price 5-mL amp = £1.78
Excipients include propylene glycol, sulphites

---

### ■ SULFADIAZINE
(Sulphadiazine)

**Indications**  prevention of rheumatic fever recurrence,
toxoplasmosis [unlicensed]—see section 5.4.7

**Cautions**  see under Co-trimoxazole; renal impairment
(avoid if severe; Appendix 3); pregnancy (Appendix 4);
breast-feeding (Appendix 5); **interactions:** Appendix
1 (sulphonamides)

**Contra-indications**  see under Co-trimoxazole

**Side-effects**  see under Co-trimoxazole

**Dose**
- Prevention of rheumatic fever, *by mouth*, 1 g daily
  (500 mg daily for patients less than 30 kg)

**Sulfadiazine** (Non-proprietary) PoM
Tablets, sulfadiazine 500 mg, net price 56-tab pack =
£37.50. Label: 9, 27

---

### ■ TRIMETHOPRIM

**Indications**  urinary-tract infections, acute and chronic
bronchitis; pneumocystis pneumonia (section 5.4.8)

**Cautions**  renal impairment (Appendix 3); pregnancy
(Appendix 4); breast-feeding (Appendix 5); predisposition to folate deficiency; elderly; manufacturer
recommends blood counts on long-term therapy (but
evidence of practical value unsatisfactory); neonates
(specialist supervision required); acute porphyria
(section 9.8.2); **interactions:** Appendix 1 (trimethoprim)
Blood disorders On long-term treatment, patients and their
carers should be told how to recognise signs of blood
disorders and advised to seek immediate medical attention if
symptoms such as fever, sore throat, rash, mouth ulcers,
purpura, bruising or bleeding develop

**Contra-indications**  blood dyscrasias

**Side-effects**  gastro-intestinal disturbances including
nausea and vomiting, pruritus, rashes, hyperkalaemia,
depression of haematopoiesis; rarely erythema multiforme, toxic epidermal necrolysis, photosensitivity
and other allergic reactions including angioedema
and anaphylaxis; aseptic meningitis and uveitis
reported

**Dose**
- Acute infections, 200 mg every 12 hours; CHILD 1
  month–12 years, 4 mg/kg (max. 200 mg) every 12
  hours; *or* 6 weeks–6 months 25 mg every 12 hours, 6
  months–6 years 50 mg every 12 hours, 6–12 years
  100 mg every 12 hours
- Prophylaxis, 100 mg at night; CHILD under 12 years,
  2 mg/kg (max.100 mg) at night

**Trimethoprim** (Non-proprietary) PoM
Tablets, trimethoprim 100 mg, net price 28 = 95p;
200 mg, 14-tab pack = 88p. Label: 9
Brands include *Trimopan®*

Suspension, trimethoprim 50 mg/5 mL, net price
100 mL = £1.62. Label: 9

---

## 5.1.9 Antituberculosis drugs

Tuberculosis is treated in two phases—an *initial phase*
using 4 drugs and a *continuation phase* using 2 drugs in
fully sensitive cases. Treatment requires specialised
knowledge, particularly where the disease involves
resistant organisms or non-respiratory organs.

The regimens given below are recommended for the
treatment of tuberculosis in the UK; variations occur in
other countries. Either the unsupervised regimen or the
supervised regimen described below should be used; the
two regimens should **not** be used concurrently.

**Initial phase**  The concurrent use of 4 drugs during the
initial phase is designed to reduce the bacterial population as rapidly as possible and to prevent the emergence
of drug-resistant bacteria. The drugs are best given as
combination preparations unless one of the components
cannot be given because of resistance or intolerance.
The treatment of choice for the initial phase is the daily
use of isoniazid, rifampicin, pyrazinamide and ethambutol. Treatment should be started without waiting for
culture results if clinical features or histology results are
consistent with tuberculosis; treatment should be continued even if initial culture results are negative. The
initial phase drugs should be continued for 2 months.
Where a positive culture for *M. tuberculosis* has been
obtained, but susceptibility results are not available after
2 months, treatment with rifampicin, isoniazid, pyrazinamide and ethambutol should be continued until full
susceptibility is confirmed, even if this is for longer than
2 months.

Streptomycin is rarely used in the UK but it may be used
in the initial phase of treatment if resistance to isoniazid
has been established before therapy is commenced.

**Continuation phase**  After the initial phase, treatment
is continued for a further 4 months with isoniazid and
rifampicin (preferably given as a combination preparation). Longer treatment is necessary for meningitis,
direct spinal cord involvement, and for resistant organisms which may also require modification of the regimen.

**Unsupervised treatment**  The following regimen
should be used for patients who are likely to take antituberculous drugs reliably **without supervision.**
Patients who are unlikely to comply with daily administration of antituberculous drugs should be treated with
the regimen described under Supervised Treatment.

**5** **Infections**

*Recommended dosage for standard unsupervised 6-month treatment*

**Rifater®** [rifampicin, isoniazid, and pyrazinamide] (for 2-month initial phase only)
ADULT under 40 kg 3 tablets daily, 40–49 kg 4 tablets daily, 50–64 kg 5 tablets daily, over 65 kg 6 tablets daily

**Ethambutol** (for 2-month initial phase only)
ADULT AND CHILD 15 mg/kg daily

**Rifinah®** [rifampicin and isoniazid] (for 4-month continuation phase following initial treatment with *Rifater®*)
ADULT under 50 kg 3 tablets daily of *Rifinah®-150*, 50 kg and over, 2 tablets daily of *Rifinah®-300*

*or* (if combination preparations not appropriate):

**Isoniazid** (for 2-month initial and 4-month continuation phases)
ADULT 300 mg daily; CHILD 5–10 mg/kg (max. 300 mg) daily

**Rifampicin** (for 2-month initial and 4-month continuation phases)
ADULT under 50 kg 450 mg daily, 50 kg and over 600 mg daily; CHILD 10 mg/kg (max. 600 mg) daily

**Pyrazinamide** (for 2-month initial phase only)
ADULT under 50 kg 1.5 g daily, 50 kg and over 2 g daily; CHILD 35 mg/kg daily

**Ethambutol** (for 2-month initial phase only)
ADULT AND CHILD 15 mg/kg daily

**Pregnancy and breast-feeding** The standard regimen (above) may be used during pregnancy and breast-feeding. Streptomycin should not be given in pregnancy.

**Children** Children are given isoniazid, rifampicin, pyrazinamide, and ethambutol for the first 2 months followed by isoniazid and rifampicin during the next 4 months. However, care is needed in young children receiving ethambutol because of the difficulty in testing eyesight and in obtaining reports of visual symptoms (see below).

**Supervised treatment** Drug administration needs to be **fully supervised** (directly observed therapy, DOT) in patients who cannot comply reliably with the treatment regimen. These patients are given isoniazid, rifampicin, pyrazinamide and ethambutol (or streptomycin) 3 times a week under supervision for the first 2 months followed by isoniazid and rifampicin 3 times a week for a further 4 months.

*Recommended dosage for intermittent supervised 6-month treatment*

**Isoniazid** (for 2-month initial and 4-month continuation phases)
ADULT AND CHILD 15 mg/kg (max. 900 mg) 3 times a week

**Rifampicin** (for 2-month initial and 4-month continuation phases)
ADULT 600–900 mg 3 times a week; CHILD 15 mg/kg (max. 900 mg) 3 times a week

**Pyrazinamide** (for 2-month initial phase only)
ADULT under 50 kg 2 g 3 times a week, 50 kg and over 2.5 g 3 times a week; CHILD 50 mg/kg 3 times a week

**Ethambutol** (for 2-month initial phase only)
ADULT AND CHILD 30 mg/kg 3 times a week

**Immunocompromised patients** Multi-resistant *Mycobacterium tuberculosis* may be present in immunocompromised patients. The organism should always be cultured to confirm its type and drug sensitivity. Confirmed *M. tuberculosis* infection sensitive to first-line drugs should be treated with a standard 6-month regimen; after completing treatment, patients should be closely monitored. The regimen may need to be mod-

ified if infection is caused by resistant organisms, and specialist advice is needed.

Specialist advice should be sought about tuberculosis treatment or chemoprophylaxis in a HIV-positive individual; care is required in choosing the regimen and in avoiding potentially hazardous interactions. Starting antiretroviral treatment in the first 2 months of anti-tuberculosis treatment increases the risk of immune reconstitution syndrome.

Infection may also be caused by other mycobacteria e.g. *M. avium* complex in which case specialist advice on management is needed.

**Corticosteroids** In meningeal or pericardial tuberculosis, a corticosteroid should be started at the same time as antituberculosis therapy.

**Prevention of tuberculosis** Some individuals may develop tuberculosis owing to reactivation of previously latent disease. Chemoprophylaxis may be required in those who have evidence of latent tuberculosis and are receiving treatment with immunosuppressants (including cytotoxics and possibly long-term treatment with systemic corticosteroids). In these cases, chemoprophylaxis involves use of either isoniazid alone for 6 months or of isoniazid and rifampicin for 3 months, see Table 2, section 5.1; longer chemoprophylaxis is not recommended.

For prevention of tuberculosis in susceptible close contacts or those who have become tuberculin-positive, see Table 2, section 5.1. For advice on immunisation against tuberculosis, see section 14.4.

**Monitoring** Since isoniazid, rifampicin and pyrazinamide are associated with liver toxicity (see Appendix 2), *hepatic function* should be checked before treatment with these drugs. Those with pre-existing liver disease or alcohol dependence should have frequent checks particularly in the first 2 months. If there is no evidence of liver disease (and pre-treatment liver function is normal), further checks are only necessary if the patient develops fever, malaise, vomiting, jaundice or unexplained deterioration during treatment. In view of the need to comply fully with antituberculous treatment on the one hand and to guard against serious liver damage on the other, patients and their carers should be informed carefully how to recognise signs of liver disorders and advised to discontinue treatment and seek **immediate** medical attention should symptoms of liver disease occur.

*Renal function* should be checked before treatment with antituberculous drugs and appropriate dosage adjustments made. Streptomycin or ethambutol should preferably be avoided in patients with renal impairment, but if used, the dose should be reduced and the plasma-drug concentration monitored.

*Visual acuity* should be tested before ethambutol is used (see below).

> Major causes of treatment failure are incorrect prescribing by the physician and inadequate compliance by the patient. Monthly tablet counts and urine examination (rifampicin imparts an orange-red coloration) may be useful indicators of compliance with treatment. Avoid both excessive and inadequate dosage. Treatment should be supervised by a specialist physician.

**Infections**

**5**

Isoniazid is cheap and highly effective. Like rifampicin it should always be included in any antituberculous regimen unless there is a specific contra-indication. Its only common side-effect is peripheral neuropathy which is more likely to occur where there are pre-existing risk factors such as diabetes, alcohol dependence, chronic renal failure, malnutrition and HIV infection. In these circumstances pyridoxine 10 mg daily (or 20 mg daily if suitable product not available) (section 9.6.2) should be given prophylactically from the start of treatment. Other side-effects such as hepatitis (important: see Monitoring above) and psychosis are rare.

Rifampicin, a rifamycin, is a key component of any antituberculous regimen. Like isoniazid it should always be included unless there is a specific contra-indication.

During the first two months ('initial phase') of rifampicin administration transient disturbance of liver function with elevated serum transaminases is common but generally does not require interruption of treatment. Occasionally more serious liver toxicity requires a change of treatment particularly in those with pre-existing liver disease (important: see Monitoring above).

On intermittent treatment six toxicity syndromes have been recognised—influenza-like, abdominal, and respiratory symptoms, shock, renal failure, and thrombocytopenic purpura—and can occur in 20 to 30% of patients.

Rifampicin induces hepatic enzymes which accelerate the metabolism of several drugs including oestrogens, corticosteroids, phenytoin, sulphonylureas, and anticoagulants; interactions: Appendix 1 (rifamycins). Important: the effectiveness of hormonal contraceptives is reduced and alternative family planning advice should be offered (section 7.3.1).

Rifabutin, a newly introduced rifamycin, is indicated for prophylaxis against M. avium complex infections in patients with a low CD4 count; it is also licensed for the treatment of non-tuberculous mycobacterial disease and pulmonary tuberculosis. Important: as with rifampicin it induces hepatic enzymes and the effectiveness of hormonal contraceptives is reduced requiring alternative family planning methods.

Pyrazinamide [unlicensed] is a bactericidal drug only active against intracellular dividing forms of Mycobacterium tuberculosis; it exerts its main effect only in the first two or three months. It is particularly useful in tuberculous meningitis because of good meningeal penetration. It is not active against M. bovis. Serious liver toxicity may occasionally occur (important: see Monitoring above).

Ethambutol is included in a treatment regimen if isoniazid resistance is suspected; it can be omitted if the risk of resistance is low.

Side-effects of ethambutol are largely confined to visual disturbances in the form of loss of acuity, colour blindness, and restriction of visual fields. These toxic effects are more common where excessive dosage is used or if the patient's renal function is impaired. The earliest features of ocular toxicity are subjective and patients should be advised to discontinue therapy immediately if they develop deterioration in vision and promptly seek further advice. Early discontinuation of the drug is almost always followed by recovery of eyesight. Patients who cannot understand warnings about visual side-effects should, if possible, be given an alternative drug. In particular, ethambutol should be used with caution in children until they are at least 5 years old and capable of reporting symptomatic visual changes accurately.

Visual acuity should be tested by Snellen chart before treatment with ethambutol.

Streptomycin [unlicensed] is now rarely used in the UK except for resistant organisms. It is given intramuscularly in a dose of 15 mg/kg (max. 1 g) daily; the dose is reduced in those under 50 kg, those over 40 years or those with renal impairment. Plasma-drug concentration should be measured in patients with impaired renal function in whom streptomycin must be used with great care. Side-effects increase after a cumulative dose of 100 g, which should only be exceeded in exceptional circumstances.

Drug-resistant tuberculosis should be treated by a specialist physician with experience in such cases, and where appropriate facilities for infection-control exist. Second-line drugs available for infections caused by resistant organisms, or when first-line drugs cause unacceptable side-effects, include amikacin, capreomycin, cycloserine, newer macrolides (e.g. azithromycin and clarithromycin), moxifloxacin and protionamide (prothionamide; no longer on UK market).

## CAPREOMYCIN

**Indications** in combination with other drugs, tuberculosis resistant to first-line drugs

**Cautions** hepatic impairment; renal impairment (Appendix 3); auditory impairment; monitor renal, hepatic, auditory, and vestibular function and electrolytes; pregnancy (teratogenic in animals; Appendix 4) and breast-feeding (Appendix 5); **interactions:** Appendix 1 (capreomycin)

**Side-effects** hypersensitivity reactions including urticaria and rashes; leucocytosis or leucopenia, rarely thrombocytopenia; changes in liver function tests; nephrotoxicity, electrolyte disturbances; hearing loss with tinnitus and vertigo; neuromuscular block after large doses, pain and induration at injection site

**Dose**

• By deep intramuscular injection, 1 g daily (not more than 20 mg/kg) for 2–4 months, then 1 g 2–3 times each week

**Capastat®** (King) ℗o̱M̱
Injection, powder for reconstitution, capreomycin sulphate 1 million units (= capreomycin approx. 1 g). Net price per vial = £22.89

## CYCLOSERINE

**Indications** in combination with other drugs, tuberculosis resistant to first-line drugs

**Cautions** reduce dose in renal impairment (avoid if severe); monitor haematological, renal, and hepatic function; pregnancy (Appendix 4); breast-feeding (Appendix 5); **interactions:** Appendix 1 (cycloserine)

**Contra-indications** epilepsy, depression, severe anxiety, psychotic states, alcohol dependence, acute porphyria (section 9.8.2)

**Side-effects** mainly neurological, including headache, dizziness, vertigo, drowsiness, tremor, convulsions, confusion, psychosis, depression (discontinue or reduce dose if symptoms of CNS toxicity); rashes, allergic dermatitis (discontinue or reduce dose);

megaloblastic anaemia; changes in liver function tests; heart failure at high doses reported

**Dose**

- Initially 250 mg every 12 hours for 2 weeks increased according to blood concentration and response to max. 500 mg every 12 hours; CHILD initially 10 mg/kg daily adjusted according to blood concentration and response

Note Blood concentration monitoring required especially in renal impairment or if dose exceeds 500 mg daily or if signs of toxicity; blood concentration should not exceed 30 mg/litre

**Cycloserine** (King) ℞

Capsules, red/grey cycloserine 250 mg, net price 100-cap pack = £303.45. Label: 2, 8

## ETHAMBUTOL HYDROCHLORIDE

**Indications** tuberculosis, in combination with other drugs

**Cautions** reduce dose in renal impairment and if creatinine clearance less than 30 mL/minute, also monitor plasma-ethambutol concentration (Appendix 3); elderly; pregnancy; test visual acuity before treatment and warn patients to report visual changes—see notes above; young children (see notes above)—routine ophthalmological monitoring recommended

**Contra-indications** optic neuritis, poor vision

**Side-effects** optic neuritis, red/green colour blindness, peripheral neuritis, rarely rash, pruritus, urticaria, thrombocytopenia

**Dose**

- See notes above

Note 'Peak' concentration (2–2.5 hours after dose) should be 2–6 mg/litre (7–22 micromol/litre); 'trough' (pre-dose) concentration should be less than 1 mg/litre (4 micromol/litre); see Cautions above; for advice on laboratory assay of ethambutol contact the Poisons Unit at New Cross Hospital (Tel (020) 7771 5360)

**Ethambutol** (Non-proprietary) ℞

Tablets, ethambutol hydrochloride 100 mg (yellow), net price 56-tab pack = £11.51; 400 mg (grey), 56-tab pack = £42.74. Label: 8

## ISONIAZID

**Indications** tuberculosis, in combination with other drugs; prophylaxis—Table 2, section 5.1

**Cautions** hepatic impairment (Appendix 2; see also below); renal impairment (Appendix 3); slow acetylator status (increased risk of side-effects); epilepsy; history of psychosis; alcohol dependence, malnutrition, diabetes mellitus, HIV infection (risk of peripheral neuritis); pregnancy (Appendix 4) and breastfeeding (Appendix 5); acute porphyria (section 9.8.2); **interactions:** Appendix 1 (isoniazid)

Hepatic disorders Patients or their carers should be told how to recognise signs of liver disorder, and advised to discontinue treatment and seek immediate medical attention if symptoms such as persistent nausea, vomiting, malaise or jaundice develop

**Contra-indications** drug-induced liver disease

**Side-effects** nausea, vomiting, constipation, dry mouth; peripheral neuritis with high doses (pyridoxine prophylaxis, see notes above), optic neuritis, convulsions, psychotic episodes, vertigo; hypersensitivity reactions including fever, erythema multiforme, purpura; blood disorders including agranulocytosis, haemolytic anaemia, aplastic anaemia; hepatitis

(especially over age of 35 years); systemic lupus erythematosus-like syndrome, pellagra, hyperreflexia, difficulty with micturition, hyperglycaemia, and gynaecomastia reported; hearing loss and tinnitus (in patients with end-stage renal impairment)

**Dose**

- By mouth or by intramuscular or intravenous injection, see notes above

**Isoniazid** (Non-proprietary) ℞

Tablets, isoniazid 50 mg, net price 56-tab pack = £8.34; 100 mg, 28-tab pack = £8.29. Label: 8, 22

Elixir (BPC), isoniazid 50 mg, citric acid monohydrate 12.5 mg, sodium citrate 60 mg, concentrated anise water 0.05 mL, compound tartrazine solution 0.05 mL, glycerol 1 mL, double-strength chloroform water 2 mL, water to 5 mL. Label: 8, 22

'Special order' [unlicensed] product; contact Martindale, Rosemont, or regional hospital manufacturing unit

Injection, isoniazid 25 mg/mL, net price 2-mL amp = £11.04

## PYRAZINAMIDE

**Indications** tuberculosis in combination with other drugs [unlicensed]

**Cautions** pregnancy (Appendix 4); hepatic impairment (monitor hepatic function, see also below and Appendix 2); diabetes; gout (avoid in acute attack); **interactions:** Appendix 1 (pyrazinamide)

Hepatic disorders Patients or their carers should be told how to recognise signs of liver disorder, and advised to discontinue treatment and seek immediate medical attention if symptoms such as persistent nausea, vomiting, malaise or jaundice develop

**Contra-indications** acute porphyria (section 9.8.2)

**Side-effects** hepatotoxicity including fever, anorexia, hepatomegaly, splenomegaly, jaundice, liver failure; nausea, vomiting, flushing, dysuria, arthralgia, sideroblastic anaemia, rash and occasionally photosensitivity

**Dose**

- See notes above

**Pyrazinamide** (Non-proprietary) ℞

Tablets, scored, pyrazinamide 500 mg. Label: 8

Available from 'special order' manufacturers or specialist-importing companies, see p. 969

## RIFABUTIN

**Indications** see under Dose

**Cautions** see under Rifampicin; hepatic impairment (Appendix 2); renal impairment (Appendix 3); pregnancy (Appendix 4); breast-feeding (Appendix 5); acute porphyria (section 9.8.2)

**Side-effects** nausea, vomiting; leucopenia, thrombocytopenia, anaemia, rarely haemolysis; raised liver enzymes, jaundice, rarely hepatitis; uveitis following high doses or administration with drugs which raise plasma concentration—see also **interactions:** Appendix 1 (rifamycins); arthralgia, myalgia, influenza-like syndrome, dyspnoea; also hypersensitivity reactions including fever, rash, eosinophilia, bronchospasm, shock; skin, urine, saliva and other body secretions coloured orange-red; asymptomatic corneal opacities reported with long-term use

## Dose

- Prophylaxis of *Mycobacterium avium* complex infections in immunosuppressed patients with low CD4 count (see product literature), 300 mg daily as a single dose
- Treatment of non-tuberculous mycobacterial disease, in combination with other drugs, 450–600 mg daily as a single dose for up to 6 months after cultures negative
- Treatment of pulmonary tuberculosis, in combination with other drugs, 150–450 mg daily as a single dose for at least 6 months
- CHILD not recommended

**Mycobutin®** (Pharmacia) PoM

Capsules, red-brown, rifabutin 150 mg. Net price 30-cap pack = £90.38. Label: 8, 14, counselling, lenses, see under Rifampicin

---

## ▌ RIFAMPICIN

**Indications** see under Dose

**Cautions** hepatic impairment (Appendix 2; liver function tests and blood counts in hepatic disorders, alcohol dependence, and on prolonged therapy, see also below); renal impairment (if above 600 mg daily); pregnancy and breast-feeding (see notes above and Appendix 4 and Appendix 5); acute porphyria (section 9.8.2); **important**: advise patients on hormonal contraceptives to use additional means (see also section 7.3.1); discolours soft contact lenses; see also notes above; **interactions**: Appendix 1 (rifamycins)

Note If treatment interrupted re-introduce with low dosage and increase gradually; discontinue permanently if serious side-effects develop

**Hepatic disorders** Patients or their carers should be told how to recognise signs of liver disorder, and advised to discontinue treatment and seek immediate medical attention if symptoms such as persistent nausea, vomiting, malaise or jaundice develop

**Contra-indications** jaundice

**Side-effects** gastro-intestinal symptoms including anorexia, nausea, vomiting, diarrhoea (antibiotic-associated colitis reported); headache, drowsiness; those occurring mainly on intermittent therapy include influenza-like symptoms (with chills, fever, dizziness, bone pain), respiratory symptoms (including shortness of breath), collapse and shock, haemolytic anaemia, thrombocytopenic purpura, disseminated intravascular coagulation, and acute renal failure; alterations of liver function, jaundice; flushing, urticaria, and rashes; other side-effects reported include oedema, psychoses, adrenal insufficiency, muscular weakness and myopathy, exfoliative dermatitis, toxic epidermal necrolysis, Stevens-Johnson syndrome, pemphigoid reactions, leucopenia, eosinophilia, menstrual disturbances; urine, saliva, and other body secretions coloured orange-red; thrombophlebitis reported if infusion used for prolonged period

## Dose

- Brucellosis, legionnaires' disease, endocarditis and serious staphylococcal infections, in combination with other drugs, by mouth *or* by intravenous infusion, 0.6–1.2 g daily (in 2–4 divided doses)
- Tuberculosis, in combination with other drugs, see notes above
- Leprosy, section 5.1.10

- Prophylaxis of meningococcal meningitis and *Haemophilus influenzae* (type b) infection, section 5.1, table 2

**Rifampicin** (Non-proprietary) PoM

Capsules, rifampicin 150 mg, net price 20 = £3.85; 300 mg, 20 = £8.38. Label: 8, 14, 22, counselling, see lenses above

**Rifadin®** (Aventis Pharma) PoM

Capsules, rifampicin 150 mg (blue/red), net price 20 = £3.66; 300 mg (red), 20 = £7.33. Label: 8, 14, 22, counselling, see lenses above

Syrup, red, rifampicin 100 mg/5 mL (raspberry-flavoured). Net price 120 mL = £3.56. Label: 8, 14, 22, counselling, see lenses above

Intravenous infusion, powder for reconstitution, rifampicin. Net price 600-mg vial (with solvent) = £7.67
Electrolytes Na⁺< 0.5 mmol/vial

**Rimactane®** (Sandoz) PoM

Capsules, rifampicin 150 mg (red), net price 60-cap pack = £11.35; 300 mg (red/brown), 60-cap pack = £22.69. Label: 8, 14, 22, counselling, see lenses above

## ◢ Combined preparations

**Rifater®** (Aventis Pharma) PoM

Tablets, pink, s/c, rifampicin 120 mg, isoniazid 50 mg, pyrazinamide 300 mg. Net price 20 = £4.39. Label: 8, 14, 22, counselling, see lenses above

Dose initial treatment of pulmonary tuberculosis, patients up to 40 kg 3 tablets daily preferably before breakfast, 40–49 kg 4 tablets daily, 50–64 kg 5 tablets daily, 65 kg or more, 6 tablets daily; not suitable for use in children

**Rifinah 150®** (Aventis Pharma) PoM

Tablets, pink, s/c, rifampicin 150 mg, isoniazid 100 mg, net price 84-tab pack = £15.91. Label: 8, 14, 22, counselling, see lenses above

Dose ADULT under 50 kg, 3 tablets daily, preferably before breakfast

**Rifinah 300®** (Aventis Pharma) PoM

Tablets, orange, s/c, rifampicin 300 mg, isoniazid 150 mg, net price 56-tab pack = £21.02. Label: 8, 14, 22, counselling, see lenses above

Dose ADULT 50 kg and over, 2 tablets daily, preferably before breakfast

---

## ▌ STREPTOMYCIN

**Indications** tuberculosis, in combination with other drugs; adjunct to doxycycline in brucellosis; enterococcal endocarditis (Table 1, section 5.1)

**Cautions** see under Aminoglycosides, section 5.1.4; **interactions**: Appendix 1 (aminoglycosides)

**Contra-indications** see under Aminoglycosides, section 5.1.4

**Side-effects** see under Aminoglycosides, section 5.1.4; also hypersensitivity reactions, paraesthesia of mouth

## Dose

- By deep intramuscular injection, tuberculosis [unlicensed], see notes above; brucellosis, expert advice essential

Note One-hour ('peak') concentration should be 15–40 mg/litre; pre-dose ('trough') concentration should be less than 5 mg/litre (less than 1 mg/litre in renal impairment or in those over 50 years)

**5**

**Infections**

**Streptomycin Sulphate** (Non-proprietary) [PoM]
Injection, powder for reconstitution, streptomycin (as sulphate), net price 1-g vial = £8.25
Available as an unlicensed preparation from UCB Pharma

## 5.1.10 Antileprotic drugs

Advice from a member of the Panel of Leprosy Opinion is essential for the treatment of leprosy (Hansen's disease). Details of the Panel can be obtained from the Department of Health telephone (020) 7972 4480.

The World Health Organization has made recommendations to overcome the problem of dapsone resistance and to prevent the emergence of resistance to other antileprotic drugs. Drugs recommended are **dapsone**, **rifampicin** (section 5.1.9), and **clofazimine**. Other drugs with significant activity against *Mycobacterium leprae* include ofloxacin, minocycline and clarithromycin, but none of these are as active as rifampicin; at present they should be reserved as second-line drugs for leprosy.

A three-drug regimen is recommended for *multibacillary leprosy* (lepromatous, borderline-lepromatous, and borderline leprosy) and a two-drug regimen for *paucibacillary leprosy* (borderline-tuberculoid, tuberculoid, and indeterminate). The following regimens are widely used throughout the world (with minor local variations):

*Multibacillary leprosy (3-drug regimen)*

| | |
|---|---|
| Rifampicin | 600 mg once-monthly, supervised (450 mg for adults weighing less than 35 kg) |
| Dapsone | 100 mg daily, self-administered (50 mg daily or 1–2 mg/kg daily for adults weighing less than 35 kg) |
| Clofazimine | 300 mg once-monthly, supervised, *and* 50 mg daily (or 100 mg on alternate days), self-administered |

Multibacillary leprosy should be treated for at least 2 years. Treatment should be continued unchanged during both type I (reversal) or type II (erythema nodosum leprosum) reactions. During reversal reactions neuritic pain or weakness can herald the rapid onset of permanent nerve damage. Treatment with prednisolone (initially 40–60 mg daily) should be instituted at once. Mild type II reactions may respond to aspirin. Severe type II reactions may require corticosteroids; thalidomide [unlicensed] is also useful in men and post-menopausal women who have become corticosteroid dependent, but it should be used under **specialist supervision** and it should **never** be used in women of child-bearing potential (significant teratogenic risk—for CSM guidance on prescribing, see *Current Problems in Pharmacovigilance* 1994; **20**, 8). Increased doses of clofazimine 100 mg 3 times daily for the first month with subsequent reductions, are also useful but may take 4–6 weeks to attain full effect.

*Paucibacillary leprosy (2-drug regimen)*

| | |
|---|---|
| Rifampicin | 600 mg once-monthly, supervised (450 mg for those weighing less than 35 kg) |
| Dapsone | 100 mg daily, self-administered (50 mg daily or 1–2 mg/kg daily for adults weighing less than 35 kg) |

Paucibacillary leprosy should be treated for 6 months. If treatment is interrupted the regimen should be recommenced where it was left off to complete the full course.

Neither the multibacillary nor the paucibacillary antileprosy regimen is sufficient to treat tuberculosis.

### ▌ DAPSONE

**Indications** leprosy, dermatitis herpetiformis; *Pneumocystis jirovecii* (*Pneumocystis carinii*) pneumonia (section 5.4.8)

**Cautions** cardiac or pulmonary disease; anaemia (treat severe anaemia before starting); susceptibility to haemolysis including G6PD deficiency (section 9.1.5)—susceptible breast-feeding infants also at risk (Appendix 5); pregnancy (Appendix 4); avoid in acute porphyria (section 9.8.2); **interactions:** Appendix 1 (dapsone)

**Blood disorders** On long-term treatment, patients and their carers should be told how to recognise signs of blood disorders and advised to seek immediate medical attention if symptoms such as fever, sore throat, rash, mouth ulcers, purpura, bruising or bleeding develop

**Side-effects** (dose-related and uncommon at doses used for leprosy), haemolysis, methaemoglobinaemia, neuropathy, allergic dermatitis (rarely including toxic epidermal necrolysis and Stevens-Johnson syndrome), anorexia, nausea, vomiting, tachycardia, headache, insomnia, psychosis, hepatitis, agranulocytosis; dapsone syndrome (rash with fever and eosinophilia)—discontinue immediately (may progress to exfoliative dermatitis, hepatitis, hypoalbuminaemia, psychosis and death)

**Dose**
- Leprosy, 1–2 mg/kg daily, see notes above
- Dermatitis herpetiformis, see specialist literature

**Dapsone** (Non-proprietary) [PoM]
Tablets, dapsone 50 mg, net price 28-tab pack = £24.22; 100 mg, 28-tab pack = £35.11. Label: 8

### ▌ CLOFAZIMINE

**Indications** leprosy

**Cautions** hepatic and renal impairment; pregnancy; breast-feeding (Appendix 5); may discolour soft contact lenses; avoid if persistent abdominal pain and diarrhoea

**Side-effects** nausea, vomiting (hospitalise if persistent), abdominal pain; headache, tiredness; brownish-black discoloration of lesions and skin including areas exposed to light; reversible hair discoloration; dry skin; red discoloration of faeces, urine and other body fluids; also rash, pruritus, photosensitivity, acne-like eruptions, anorexia, eosinophilic enteropathy, bowel obstruction, dry eyes, dimmed vision, macular and subepithelial corneal pigmentation; elevation of blood sugar, weight loss, splenic infarction, lymphadenopathy

**Dose**
- Leprosy, see notes above
- Lepromatous lepra reactions, dosage increased to 300 mg daily for max. of 3 months

**Clofazimine** (Non-proprietary) [PoM]
Capsules, clofazimine 100 mg. Label: 8, 14, 21
Available on named-patient basis

## 5.1.11 Metronidazole and tinidazole

**Metronidazole** is an antimicrobial drug with high activity against anaerobic bacteria and protozoa; indications include trichomonal vaginitis (section 5.4.3), bacterial vaginosis (notably *Gardnerella vaginalis* infections), and *Entamoeba histolytica* and *Giardia lamblia* infections (section 5.4.2). It is also used for surgical and gynaecological sepsis in which its activity against colonic anaerobes, especially *Bacteroides fragilis*, is important. Metronidazole by the rectal route is an effective alternative to the intravenous route when oral administration is not possible. Intravenous metronidazole is used for the treatment of established cases of tetanus; diazepam (section 10.2.2) and tetanus immunoglobulin (section 14.5.2) are also used.

Metronidazole by mouth is effective for the treatment of *Clostridium difficile* infection , see also section 1.5; it can be given by intravenous infusion if oral treatment is inappropriate.

Topical metronidazole (section 13.10.1.2) reduces the odour produced by anaerobic bacteria in fungating tumours; it is also used in the management of rosacea (section 13.6).

**Tinidazole** is similar to metronidazole but has a longer duration of action.

**Oral infections** Metronidazole is an alternative to a penicillin for the treatment of many oral infections where the patient is allergic to penicillin or the infection is due to beta-lactamase-producing anaerobes (Table 1, section 5.1). It is the drug of first choice for the treatment of acute necrotising ulcerative gingivitis (Vincent's infection) and pericoronitis; suitable alternatives are amoxicillin (section 5.1.1.3) and erythromycin (section 5.1.5). For these purposes metronidazole in a dose of 200 mg 3 times daily for 3 days is sufficient, but the duration of treatment may need to be longer in pericoronitis. Tinidazole is licensed for the treatment of acute ulcerative gingivitis.

### METRONIDAZOLE

**Indications** anaerobic infections (including dental), see under Dose below; protozoal infections (section 5.4.2); *Helicobacter pylori* eradication (section 1.3); skin (section 13.10.1.2)

**Cautions** disulfiram-like reaction with alcohol, hepatic impairment and hepatic encephalopathy (Appendix 2); pregnancy (Appendix 4) and breast-feeding (Appendix 5); avoid in acute porphyria (section 9.8.2); clinical and laboratory monitoring advised if treatment exceeds 10 days; **interactions**: Appendix 1 (metronidazole)

**Side-effects** gastro-intestinal disturbances (including nausea and vomiting), taste disturbances, furred tongue, oral mucositis, anorexia; *very rarely* hepatitis, jaundice, pancreatitis, drowsiness, dizziness, headache, ataxia, psychotic disorders, darkening of urine, thrombocytopenia, pancytopenia, myalgia, arthralgia, visual disturbances, rash, pruritus, and erythema multiforme; on prolonged or intensive therapy peripheral neuropathy, transient epileptiform seizures, and leucopenia

**Dose**

- Anaerobic infections (usually treated for 7 days and for 10–14 days in *Clostridium difficile* infection), by mouth, *either* 800 mg initially then 400 mg every 8 hours *or* 500 mg every 8 hours, CHILD 7.5 mg/kg every 8 hours; by rectum, 1 g every 8 hours for 3 days, then 1 g every 12 hours, CHILD every 8 hours for 3 days, then every 12 hours, age up to 1 year 125 mg, 1–5 years 250 mg, 5–10 years 500 mg, over 10 years, adult dose; by intravenous infusion over 20 minutes, 500 mg every 8 hours; CHILD 7.5 mg/kg every 8 hours

- Leg ulcers and pressure sores, by mouth, 400 mg every 8 hours for 7 days

- Bacterial vaginosis, by mouth, 400–500 mg twice daily for 5–7 days *or* 2 g as a single dose

- Pelvic inflammatory disease (see also Table 1, section 5.1), by mouth, 400 mg twice daily for 14 days

- Acute ulcerative gingivitis, by mouth, 200–250 mg every 8 hours for 3 days; CHILD 1–3 years 50 mg every 8 hours for 3 days; 3–7 years 100 mg every 12 hours; 7–10 years 100 mg every 8 hours

- Acute oral infections, by mouth, 200 mg every 8 hours for 3–7 days (see also notes above); CHILD 1–3 years 50 mg every 8 hours for 3–7 days; 3–7 years 100 mg every 12 hours; 7–10 years 100 mg every 8 hours

- Surgical prophylaxis, by mouth, 400–500 mg 2 hours before surgery; up to 3 further doses of 400–500 mg may be given every 8 hours for high-risk procedures; CHILD 7.5 mg/kg 2 hours before surgery; up to 3 further doses of 7.5 mg/kg may be given every 8 hours for high-risk procedures

  By rectum, 1 g 2 hours before surgery; up to 3 further doses of 1 g may be given every 8 hours for high-risk procedures; CHILD 5–10 years 500 mg 2 hours before surgery; up to 3 further doses of 500 mg may be given every 8 hours for high-risk procedures

  By intravenous infusion (if rectal administration inappropriate), 500 mg at induction; up to 3 further doses of 500 mg may be given every 8 hours for high-risk procedures; CHILD 7.5 mg/kg at induction; up to 3 further doses of 7.5 mg/kg may be given every 8 hours for high-risk procedures

**Note** Metronidazole doses in BNF may differ from those in product literature

**Metronidazole** (Non-proprietary) ▣PoM▣

Tablets, metronidazole 200 mg, net price 21-tab pack = £1.08; 400 mg, 21-tab pack = £1.22. Label: 4, 9, 21, 25, 27
Brands include *Vaginyl*®

Tablets, metronidazole 500 mg, net price 21-tab pack = £28.03. Label: 4, 9, 21, 25, 27

Suspension, metronidazole (as benzoate) 200 mg/5 mL. Net price 100 mL = £8.15. Label: 4, 9, 23
Brands include *Norzol*®

Intravenous infusion, metronidazole 5 mg/mL. Net price 20-mL amp = £1.56, 100-mL container = £3.41
**Dental prescribing on NHS** Metronidazole Tablets and Oral Suspension may be prescribed

**Flagyl**® (Winthrop) ▣PoM▣

Tablets, both f/c, ivory, metronidazole 200 mg, net price 21-tab pack = £4.49; 400 mg, 14-tab pack = £6.34. Label: 4, 9, 21, 25, 27

**5**

**Infections**

Suppositories, metronidazole 500 mg, net price 10 = £15.18; 1 g, 10 = £23.06. Label: 4, 9

**Flagyl S®** (Winthrop) ℞
Suspension, orange- and lemon-flavoured, metronidazole (as benzoate) 200 mg/5 mL. Net price 100 mL = £11.18. Label: 4, 9, 23

**Metrolyl®** (Sandoz) ℞
Intravenous infusion, metronidazole 5 mg/mL, net price 100-mL Steriflex® bag = £1.22
Electrolytes Na⁺ 14.53 mmol/100-mL bag

Suppositories, metronidazole 500 mg, net price 10 = £12.34; 1 g, 10 = £18.34. Label: 4, 9

## TINIDAZOLE

**Indications** anaerobic infections, see under Dose below; protozoal infections (section 5.4.2); *Helicobacter pylori* eradication (section 1.3)

**Cautions** see under Metronidazole; pregnancy (manufacturer advises avoid in first trimester); avoid in acute porphyria (section 9.8.2); **interactions:** Appendix 1 (tinidazole)

**Side-effects** see under Metronidazole

**Dose**

* Anaerobic infections, 2 g initially, followed by 1 g daily *or* 500 mg twice daily, usually for 5–6 days

* Bacterial vaginosis and acute ulcerative gingivitis, a single 2-g dose

* Abdominal surgery prophylaxis, a single 2-g dose approximately 12 hours before surgery

**Fasigyn®** (Pfizer) ℞
Tablets, f/c, tinidazole 500 mg. Net price 20-tab pack = £13.80. Label: 4, 9, 21, 25

## 5.1.12 Quinolones

**Nalidixic acid** and **norfloxacin** are effective in uncomplicated urinary-tract infections.

**Ciprofloxacin** is active against both Gram-positive and Gram-negative bacteria. It is particularly active against Gram-negative bacteria, including salmonella, shigella, campylobacter, neisseria, and pseudomonas. Ciprofloxacin has only moderate activity against Gram-positive bacteria such as *Streptococcus pneumoniae* and *Enterococcus faecalis*; it should not be used for pneumococcal pneumonia. It is active against chlamydia and some mycobacteria. Most anaerobic organisms are not susceptible. Ciprofloxacin can be used for respiratory tract infections (but not for pneumococcal pneumonia), urinary-tract infections, infections of the gastro-intestinal system (including typhoid fever), bone and joint infections, gonorrhoea and septicaemia caused by sensitive organisms.

**Ofloxacin** is used for urinary-tract infections, lower respiratory-tract infections, gonorrhoea, and non-gonococcal urethritis and cervicitis.

**Levofloxacin** is active against Gram-positive and Gram-negative organisms. It has greater activity against pneumococci than ciprofloxacin. Levofloxacin is licensed for community-acquired pneumonia but it is considered to be **second-line treatment** for this indication.

Although ciprofloxacin, levofloxacin and ofloxacin are licensed for skin and soft-tissue infections, many staphylococci are resistant to the quinolones and their use should be avoided in MRSA infections.

**Moxifloxacin** should be reserved for the treatment of sinusitis, community-acquired pneumonia, or exacerbations of chronic bronchitis which have failed to respond to other antibacterials or for patients who cannot be treated with other antibacterials. It has been associated with life-threatening hepatotoxicity. Moxifloxacin is active against Gram-positive and Gram-negative organisms. It has greater activity against Gram-positive organisms, including pneumococci, than ciprofloxacin. Moxifloxacin is not active against *Pseudomonas aeruginosa* or meticillin-resistant *Staphylococcus aureus* (MRSA).

**Anthrax** *Inhalation* or *gastro-intestinal anthrax* should be treated initially with either **ciprofloxacin** or **doxycycline** [unlicensed indication] (section 5.1.3) combined with one or two other antibacterials (such as amoxicillin, benzylpenicillin, chloramphenicol, clarithromycin, clindamycin, imipenem with cilastatin, rifampicin [unlicensed indication], and vancomycin). When the condition improves and the sensitivity of the *Bacillus anthracis* strain is known, treatment may be switched to a single antibacterial. Treatment should continue for 60 days because germination may be delayed.

*Cutaneous anthrax* should be treated with either ciprofloxacin [unlicensed indication] or doxycycline [unlicensed indication] (section 5.1.3) for 7 days. Treatment may be switched to amoxicillin (section 5.1.1.3) if the infecting strain is susceptible. Treatment may need to be extended to 60 days if exposure is due to aerosol. A combination of antibacterials for 14 days is recommended for cutaneous anthrax with systemic features, extensive oedema, or lesions of the head or neck.

Ciprofloxacin or doxycycline may be given for *post-exposure prophylaxis*. If exposure is confirmed, antibacterial prophylaxis should continue for 60 days. Antibacterial prophylaxis may be switched to amoxicillin after 10–14 days if the strain of *B. anthracis* is susceptible. Vaccination against anthrax (section 14.4) may allow the duration of antibacterial prophylaxis to be shortened.

**Cautions** Quinolones should be used with caution in patients with a history of epilepsy or conditions that predispose to seizures, in G6PD deficiency (section 9.1.5), myasthenia gravis (risk of exacerbation), in renal impairment (Appendix 3); pregnancy (Appendix 4), during breast-feeding (Appendix 5), and in children or adolescents (arthropathy has developed in weight-bearing joints in young *animals*—see below). Exposure to excessive sunlight should be avoided (discontinue if photosensitivity occurs). The CSM has warned that quinolones may induce **convulsions** in patients with or without a history of convulsions; taking NSAIDs at the same time may also induce them. Other **interactions:** Appendix 1 (quinolones).

**Use in children** Quinolones cause arthropathy in the weight-bearing joints of immature *animals* and are therefore generally not recommended in children and growing adolescents. However, the significance of this effect in humans is uncertain and in some specific circumstances short-term use of either ciprofloxacin or nalidixic acid may be justified in children. For further details see *BNF for Children*.

> **Tendon damage**
>
> Tendon damage (including rupture) has been reported rarely in patients receiving quinolones. Tendon rupture may occur within 48 hours of starting treatment; cases have also been reported several months after stopping a quinolone. Healthcare professionals are reminded that:
>
> - quinolones are contra-indicated in patients with a history of tendon disorders related to quinolone use;
> - patients over 60 years of age are more prone to tendon damage;
> - kidney, heart, or lung transplant recipients are more prone to tendon damage;
> - the risk of tendon damage is increased by the concomitant use of corticosteroids;
> - if tendinitis is suspected, the quinolone should be discontinued immediately.

**Side-effects** Side-effects of the quinolones include nausea, vomiting, dyspepsia, abdominal pain, diarrhoea (rarely antibiotic-associated colitis), headache, dizziness, rash (very rarely Stevens-Johnson syndrome and toxic epidermal necrolysis). Less frequent side-effects include anorexia, sleep disturbances, asthenia, confusion, anxiety, depression, hallucinations, tremor, blood disorders (including eosinophilia, leucopenia, thrombocytopenia), arthralgia, myalgia, disturbances in vision and taste. Other side-effects reported rarely or very rarely include hepatic dysfunction (including jaundice and hepatitis), hypotension, vasculitis, dyspnoea (more frequent with moxifloxacin), convulsions, psychoses, paraesthesia, renal failure, interstitial nephritis, tendon inflammation and damage (see also Tendon Damage above), photosensitivity, disturbances in hearing and smell. The drug should be **discontinued** if psychiatric, neurological or hypersensitivity reactions (including severe rash) occur.

## CIPROFLOXACIN

**Indications** see notes above and under Dose; eye infections (section 11.3.1)

**Cautions** see notes above; avoid excessive alkalinity of urine and ensure adequate fluid intake (risk of crystalluria); **interactions:** Appendix 1 (quinolones)

Driving May impair performance of skilled tasks (e.g. driving); effects enhanced by alcohol

**Side-effects** see notes above; also flatulence, pain and phlebitis at injection site; *rarely* dysphagia, pancreatitis, chest pain, tachycardia, syncope, oedema, hot flushes, abnormal dreams, sweating, hyperglycaemia, and erythema nodosum; *very rarely* movement disorders, tinnitus, and tenosynovitis

**Dose**

- By mouth, respiratory-tract infections, 500–750 mg twice daily (750 mg twice daily in pseudomonal lower respiratory-tract infection in cystic fibrosis)

  Urinary-tract infections, 250–750 mg twice daily (250 mg twice daily for 3 days usually adequate for acute uncomplicated cystitis in women)

  Acute or chronic prostatitis, 500 mg twice daily for 28 days

  Gonorrhoea, 500 mg as a single dose

  Most other infections, 500 mg twice daily (increased to 750 mg twice daily in severe or deep-seated infection)

Surgical prophylaxis [unlicensed], 750 mg 60 minutes before procedure

Prophylaxis of meningococcal meningitis, Table 2, section 5.1

- By intravenous infusion over 60 minutes, 400 mg every 8–12 hours

- Anthrax (treatment and post-exposure prophylaxis, see notes above), by mouth, 500 mg twice daily

  By intravenous infusion over 60 minutes, 400 mg every 12 hours

- CHILD under 18 years see *BNF for Children*

**Ciprofloxacin** (Non-proprietary) ▣ⓅⓄⓂ

Tablets, ciprofloxacin (as hydrochloride) 100 mg, net price 6-tab pack = £1.21; 250 mg, 10-tab pack = £1.10, 20-tab pack = £1.18; 500 mg, 10-tab pack = £1.17, 20-tab pack = £1.26; 750 mg, 10-tab pack = £1.90. Label: 7, 9, 25, counselling, driving

Intravenous infusion, ciprofloxacin (as lactate) 2 mg/mL, net price 50-mL bottle = £8.00, 100-mL bottle = £15.00, 200-mL bottle = £22.00

**Ciproxin®** (Bayer) ▣ⓅⓄⓂ

Tablets, all f/c, ciprofloxacin (as hydrochloride) 100 mg, net price 6-tab pack = £2.69; 250 mg (scored), 10-tab pack = £7.21, 20-tab pack = £14.42; 500 mg (scored), 10-tab pack = £13.65, 20-tab pack = £27.29; 750 mg, 10-tab pack = £19.22. Label: 7, 9, 25, counselling, driving

Suspension, strawberry-flavoured, ciprofloxacin for reconstitution with diluent provided, 250 mg/5 mL, net price 100 mL = £16.50. Label: 7, 9, 25, counselling, driving

Intravenous infusion, ciprofloxacin (as lactate) 2 mg/mL, in sodium chloride 0.9%, net price 50-mL bottle = £8.31, 100-mL bottle = £16.23, 200-mL bottle = £24.70

Electrolytes Na$^+$ 15.4 mmol/100-mL bottle

## LEVOFLOXACIN

**Indications** see under Dose

**Cautions** see notes above; predisposition to QT interval prolongation (including cardiac disease, congenital long QT syndrome, electrolyte disturbances, concomitant use with other drugs known to prolong QT interval); **interactions:** Appendix 1 (quinolones)

Driving May impair performance of skilled tasks (e.g. driving)

**Side-effects** see notes above; also flatulence, constipation; *rarely* tachycardia; *very rarely* pneumonitis, peripheral neuropathy, and hypoglycaemia; also reported, rhabdomyolysis and potentially life-threatening hepatic failure; local reactions and transient hypotension reported with infusion

**Dose**

- By mouth, acute sinusitis, 500 mg daily for 10–14 days

  Exacerbation of chronic bronchitis, 250–500 mg daily for 7–10 days

  Community-acquired pneumonia, 500 mg once or twice daily for 7–14 days

  Urinary-tract infections, 250 mg daily for 7–10 days (for 3 days in uncomplicated infection)

  Chronic prostatitis, 500 mg once daily for 28 days

  Skin and soft tissue infections, 250 mg daily *or*

**5**

**Infections**

500 mg once or twice daily for 7–14 days
- By intravenous infusion (over at least 60 minutes for 500 mg), community-acquired pneumonia, 500 mg once or twice daily

Complicated urinary-tract infections, 250 mg daily, increased in severe infections

Skin and soft tissue infections, 500 mg twice daily

**Tavanic®** (Sanofi-Aventis) (PoM)

Tablets, yellow-red, f/c, scored, levofloxacin 250 mg, net price 5-tab pack = £7.23, 10-tab pack = £14.45; 500 mg, 5-tab pack = £12.93, 10-tab pack = £25.85. Label: 6, 9, 25, counselling, driving

Intravenous infusion, levofloxacin 5 mg/mL, net price 100-mL bottle = £26.40
Electrolytes Na⁺ 15.4 mmol/100-mL bottle

## ■ MOXIFLOXACIN

**Indications** sinusitis, community-acquired pneumonia, or exacerbations of chronic bronchitis which have failed to respond to other antibacterials or for patients who cannot be treated with other antibacterials

**Cautions** see notes above; conditions pre-disposing to arrhythmias, including myocardial ischaemia; **interactions**: Appendix 1 (quinolones)
Driving May impair performance of skilled tasks (e.g. driving)

**Contra-indications** see notes above; severe hepatic impairment; history of QT-interval prolongation, bradycardia, history of symptomatic arrhythmias, heart failure with reduced left ventricular ejection fraction, electrolyte disturbances, concomitant use with other drugs known to prolong QT-interval

**Side-effects** see notes above; also gastritis, flatulence, constipation, arrhythmias, palpitation, angina, vasodilatation, hyperlipidaemia, and sweating; *rarely* oedema, hypertension, syncope, dysphagia, abnormal dreams, incoordination, amnesia, hyperglycaemia, hyperuricaemia, and stomatitis; *very rarely* potentially life-threatening hepatic failure

**Dose**
- 400 mg once daily for 10 days in community-acquired pneumonia, for 5–10 days in exacerbation of chronic bronchitis, for 7 days in sinusitis

**Avelox®** (Bayer) ▼ (PoM)

Tablets, red, f/c, moxifloxacin (as hydrochloride) 400 mg, net price 5-tab pack = £11.95. Label: 6, 9, counselling, driving

## ■ NALIDIXIC ACID

**Indications** urinary-tract infections

**Cautions** see notes above; avoid in acute porphyria (section 9.8.2); liver disease; false positive urinary glucose (if tested for reducing substances); monitor blood counts, renal and liver function if treatment exceeds 2 weeks; **interactions**: Appendix 1 (quinolones)

**Side-effects** see notes above; also reported toxic psychosis, increased intracranial pressure, cranial nerve palsy, metabolic acidosis

**Dose**
- 900 mg every 6 hours for 7 days, reduced in chronic infections to 600 mg every 6 hours; CHILD 3 months–18 years see *BNF for Children*

**Uriben®** (Rosemont) (PoM)

Suspension, pink, nalidixic acid 300 mg/5 mL, net price 150 mL (raspberry- and strawberry-flavoured) = £11.42. Label: 9, 11
Excipients include sucrose 450 mg/5 mL

## ■ NORFLOXACIN

**Indications** see under Dose

**Cautions** see notes above; **interactions**: Appendix 1 (quinolones)
Driving May impair performance of skilled tasks (e.g. driving)

**Side-effects** see notes above; also tinnitus, epiphora; *rarely* pancreatitis; *very rarely* arrhythmias; also reported, polyneuropathy and exfoliative dermatitis

**Dose**
- 'Lower' urinary-tract infections, 400 mg twice daily for 7–10 days (for 3 days for uncomplicated infections in women)
- Chronic relapsing 'lower' urinary-tract infections, 400 mg twice daily for up to 12 weeks; may be reduced to 400 mg once daily if adequate suppression within first 4 weeks
- Chronic prostatitis, 400 mg twice daily for 28 days

**Norfloxacin** (Non-proprietary) (PoM)

Tablets, norfloxacin 400 mg, net price 6-tab pack = £2.30, 14-tab pack = £3.17. Label: 7, 9, 23, counselling, driving

**Utinor®** (MSD) (PoM)

Tablets, scored, norfloxacin 400 mg. Net price 7-tab pack = £2.56, 14-tab pack = £5.11. Label: 7, 9, 23, counselling, driving

## ■ OFLOXACIN

**Indications** see under Dose

**Cautions** see notes above; hepatic impairment (Appendix 2); history of psychiatric illness; **interactions**: Appendix 1 (quinolones)
Driving May affect performance of skilled tasks (e.g. driving); effects enhanced by alcohol

**Side-effects** see notes above; also tachycardia; *rarely* abnormal dreams, unsteady gait, neuropathy, and extrapyramidal symptoms; *very rarely* changes in blood sugar; isolated cases of pneumonitis and rhabdomyolysis; on intravenous infusion, hypotension and local reactions (including thrombophlebitis)

**Dose**
- By mouth, urinary-tract infections, 200–400 mg daily preferably in the morning, increased if necessary in upper urinary-tract infections to 400 mg twice daily

Acute or chronic prostatitis, 200 mg twice daily for 28 days

Lower respiratory-tract infections, 400 mg daily preferably in the morning, increased if necessary to 400 mg twice daily

Skin and soft-tissue infections, 400 mg twice daily

Uncomplicated gonorrhoea, 400 mg as a single dose

Uncomplicated genital chlamydial infection, non-gonococcal urethritis, 400 mg daily in single or divided doses for 7 days

Pelvic inflammatory disease (see also section 5.1, table 1), 400 mg twice daily for 14 days

- By intravenous infusion (over at least 30 minutes for each 200 mg), complicated urinary-tract infection, 200 mg daily

  Lower respiratory-tract infection, 200 mg twice daily

  Septicaemia, 200 mg twice daily

  Skin and soft-tissue infections, 400 mg twice daily

  Severe or complicated infections, dose may be increased to 400 mg twice daily

**Ofloxacin** (Non-proprietary) PoM

Tablets, ofloxacin 200 mg, net price 10-tab pack = £4.96; 400 mg, 5-tab pack = £3.24, 10-tab pack = £5.52. Label: 6, 9, 11, counselling, driving

**Tarivid®** (Aventis Pharma) PoM

Tablets, f/c, scored, ofloxacin 200 mg, net price 10-tab pack = £7.53, 20-tab pack = £15.05; 400 mg (yellow), 5-tab pack = £7.52, 10-tab pack = £14.99. Label: 6, 9, 11, counselling, driving

Intravenous infusion, ofloxacin (as hydrochloride) 2 mg/mL, net price 100-mL bottle = £16.16 (hosp. only)

## 5.1.13 Urinary-tract infections

Urinary-tract infection is more common in women than in men; when it occurs in men there is frequently an underlying abnormality of the renal tract. Recurrent episodes of infection are an indication for radiological investigation especially in children in whom untreated pyelonephritis may lead to permanent kidney damage.

*Escherichia coli* is the most common cause of urinary-tract infection; *Staphylococcus saprophyticus* is also common in sexually active young women. Less common causes include Proteus and Klebsiella spp. *Pseudomonas aeruginosa* infections usually occur in the hospital setting and may be associated with functional or anatomical abnormalities of the renal tract. *Staphylococcus epidermidis* and *Enterococcus faecalis* infection may complicate catheterisation or instrumentation.

> Whenever possible a specimen of urine should be collected for culture and sensitivity testing before starting antibacterial therapy. The antibacterial chosen should reflect current local bacterial sensitivity to antibacterials.

*Uncomplicated lower urinary-tract infections* often respond to trimethoprim, nitrofurantoin, amoxicillin, or nalidixic acid given for 7 days (3 days may be adequate for infections in women); those caused by fully sensitive bacteria respond to two 3-g doses of amoxicillin (section 5.1.1.3). Widespread bacterial resistance, especially to ampicillin, amoxicillin, and trimethoprim has increased the importance of urine culture before therapy. Alternatives for resistant organisms include co-amoxiclav (amoxicillin with clavulanic acid), an oral cephalosporin, pivmecillinam, or a quinolone.

Long-term low dose therapy may be required in selected patients to prevent *recurrence of infection*; indications include frequent relapses and significant kidney damage. Trimethoprim, nitrofurantoin and cefalexin have been recommended for long-term therapy.

**Methenamine** (hexamine) should **not** generally be used because it requires an acidic urine for its antimicrobial activity and it is ineffective for upper urinary-tract infec-

tions; it may, however, have a role in the prophylaxis and treatment of chronic or recurrent uncomplicated lower urinary-tract infections.

*Acute pyelonephritis* can lead to septicaemia and is treated initially by injection of a broad-spectrum antibacterial such as cefuroxime or a quinolone if the patient is severely ill; gentamicin can also be used.

*Prostatitis* can be difficult to cure and requires treatment for several weeks with an antibacterial which penetrates prostatic tissue such as trimethoprim, or some quinolones.

Where infection is localised and associated with an indwelling *catheter* a bladder instillation is often effective (section 7.4.4).

Urinary-tract infection in *pregnancy* may be asymptomatic and requires prompt treatment to prevent progression to acute pyelonephritis. Penicillins and cephalosporins are suitable for treating urinary-tract infection during pregnancy. Nitrofurantoin may also be used but it should be avoided at term. Sulphonamides, quinolones, and tetracyclines should be avoided during pregnancy; trimethoprim should also preferably be avoided particularly in the first trimester.

In *renal failure* antibacterials normally excreted by the kidney accumulate with resultant toxicity unless the dose is reduced. This applies especially to the aminoglycosides which should be used with great caution; tetracyclines, methenamine, and nitrofurantoin should be avoided altogether.

**Children**  Urinary-tract infections in children require prompt antibacterial treatment to minimise the risk of renal scarring. Uncomplicated 'lower' urinary-tract infections in *children over 3 months of age* can be treated with trimethoprim, nitrofurantoin, a first generation cephalosporin (e.g. cefalexin), or amoxicillin for 3 days; children should be reassessed if they continue to be unwell 24–48 hours after the initial assessment. Amoxicillin should only be used if the organism causing the infection is sensitive to it.

Acute pyelonephritis in children over 3 months of age can be treated with a first generation cephalosporin or co-amoxiclav for 7–10 days. If the patient is severely ill, then the infection is best treated initially by injection of a broad-spectrum antibacterial such as cefotaxime or co-amoxiclav; gentamicin is an alternative.

*Children under 3 months of age* should be transferred to hospital and treated initially with intravenous antibacterial drugs such as ampicillin with gentamicin, or cefotaxime alone, until the infection responds; full doses of oral antibacterials are then given for a further period.

Recurrent episodes of infection are an indication for imaging tests. *Antibacterial prophylaxis* with low doses of trimethoprim or nitrofurantoin may be considered for children with recurrent infection, significant urinary-tract anomalies, or significant kidney damage.

## ◾ NITROFURANTOIN

**Indications**  urinary-tract infections

**Cautions**  anaemia; diabetes mellitus; electrolyte imbalance; vitamin B and folate deficiency; pulmonary disease; hepatic impairment; monitor lung and liver function on long-term therapy, especially in the elderly (discontinue if deterioration in lung function); susceptibility to peripheral neuropathy; false positive urinary glucose (if tested for reducing substances); urine may be coloured yellow or brown; **interactions:** Appendix 1 (nitrofurantoin)

**Contra-indications** renal impairment (Appendix 3); infants less than 3 months old, G6PD deficiency (including pregnancy at term, and breast-feeding of affected infants, see section 9.1.5 and Appendix 4 and Appendix 5), acute porphyria (section 9.8.2)

**Side-effects** anorexia, nausea, vomiting, and diarrhoea; acute and chronic pulmonary reactions (pulmonary fibrosis reported; possible association with lupus erythematosus-like syndrome); peripheral neuropathy; also reported, hypersensitivity reactions (including angioedema, anaphylaxis, sialadenitis, urticaria, rash and pruritus); rarely, cholestatic jaundice, hepatitis, exfoliative dermatitis, erythema multiforme, pancreatitis, arthralgia, blood disorders (including agranulocytosis, thrombocytopenia, and aplastic anaemia), benign intracranial hypertension, and transient alopecia

**Dose**
- Acute uncomplicated infection, 50 mg every 6 hours with food for 7 days (3 days usually adequate in women); CHILD over 3 months, 3 mg/kg daily in 4 divided doses
- Severe chronic recurrent infection, 100 mg every 6 hours with food for 7 days (dose reduced or discontinued if severe nausea)
- Prophylaxis (but see Cautions), 50–100 mg at night; CHILD over 3 months, 1 mg/kg at night

**Nitrofurantoin** (Non-proprietary) (PoM)
Tablets, nitrofurantoin 50 mg, net price 28-tab pack = £1.84; 100 mg, 28-tab pack = £4.34. Label: 9, 14, 21

Oral suspension, nitrofurantoin 25 mg/5 mL, net price 300 mL = £65.00. Label: 9, 14, 21

**Furadantin®** (Goldshield) (PoM)
Tablets, all yellow, scored, nitrofurantoin 50 mg, net price 20 = £1.96; 100 mg, 20 = £3.62. Label: 9, 14, 21

**Macrobid®** (Goldshield) (PoM)
Capsules, m/r, blue/yellow, nitrofurantoin 100 mg (as nitrofurantoin macrocrystals and nitrofurantoin monohydrate). Net price 14-cap pack = £4.89. Label: 9, 14, 21, 25
Dose uncomplicated urinary-tract infection, 1 capsule twice daily with food
Genito-urinary surgical prophylaxis, 1 capsule twice daily on day of procedure and for 3 days after

**Macrodantin®** (Goldshield) (PoM)
Capsules, nitrofurantoin 50 mg (yellow/white), net price 30-cap pack = £2.49; 100 mg (yellow/white), 20 = £3.21. Label: 9, 14, 21

### ◼ METHENAMINE HIPPURATE ◱
(Hexamine hippurate)

**Indications** prophylaxis and long-term treatment of chronic or recurrent lower urinary-tract infections

**Cautions** pregnancy; avoid concurrent administration with sulphonamides (risk of crystalluria) or urinary alkalinising agents; **interactions:** Appendix 1 (methenamine)

**Contra-indications** hepatic impairment, renal impairment (avoid if eGFR less than 10 mL/minute/1.73 m²; Appendix 3), severe dehydration, gout, metabolic acidosis

**Side-effects** gastro-intestinal disturbances, bladder irritation, rash

**Dose**
- 1 g every 12 hours (may be increased in patients with catheters to 1 g every 8 hours); CHILD 6–12 years 500 mg every 12 hours

**Hiprex®** (3M) ◱
Tablets, scored, methenamine hippurate 1 g. Net price 60-tab pack = £6.58. Label: 9

## 5.2 Antifungal drugs

## Treatment of fungal infections

The systemic treatment of common fungal infections is outlined below; specialist treatment is required in most forms of systemic or disseminated fungal infections. For local treatment of fungal infections, see section 7.2.2 (genital), section 7.4.4 (bladder), section 11.3.2 (eye), section 12.1.1 (ear), section 12.3.2 (oropharynx), and section 13.10.2 (skin).

**Aspergillosis** Aspergillosis most commonly affects the respiratory tract but in severely immunocompromised patients, invasive forms can affect the sinuses, heart, brain, and skin. **Amphotericin** (liposomal formulation preferred if toxicity or renal impairment are concerns) or **voriconazole** can be used for the treatment of aspergillosis. **Caspofungin** or **itraconazole** are alternatives in patients who are refractory to, or intolerant of amphotericin. Itraconazole is also used as an adjunct for the treatment of allergic bronchopulmonary aspergillosis [unlicensed indication]. The *Scottish Medicines Consortium* (March 2003) does not recommend the use of caspofungin because of a lack of robust data on efficacy and safety in the treatment of invasive aspergillosis.

**Candidiasis** Many superficial candidal infections including infections of the skin (section 13.10.2) are treated locally; widespread or intractable infection requires systemic antifungal treatment. Vaginal candidiasis (section 7.2.2) may be treated with locally acting antifungals or with fluconazole given by mouth; for resistant organisms, itraconazole can be given by mouth.

*Oropharyngeal candidiasis* generally responds to topical therapy (section 12.3.2); fluconazole is given by mouth for unresponsive infections; it is effective and is reliably absorbed. Itraconazole may be used for fluconazole-resistant infections. Topical therapy may not be adequate in immunocompromised patients and an oral triazole antifungal is preferred.

For *deep and disseminated candidiasis*, **amphotericin** can be given by intravenous infusion. **Fluconazole** is an alternative for *Candida albicans* infection in clinically stable patients who have not received an azole antifungal recently. **Caspofungin** or **voriconazole** can be used for infections caused by fluconazole-resistant *Candida* spp. that have not responded to amphotericin, or in patients intolerant of amphotericin. In refractory cases, **flucytosine** can be used with intravenous amphotericin.

**Cryptococcosis** Cryptococcosis is uncommon but infection in the immunocompromised, especially in AIDS patients, can be life-threatening; cryptococcal meningitis is the most common form of fungal meningitis. The treatment of choice in cryptococcal meningitis is **amphotericin** by intravenous infusion and **flucytosine** by intravenous infusion for 2 weeks, followed by **fluconazole** by mouth for 8 weeks or until cultures are negative. In cryptococcosis, **fluconazole** is sometimes given alone as an alternative in AIDS patients with mild, localised infections or in those who cannot tolerate amphotericin. Following successful treatment, fluconazole can be used for prophylaxis against relapse until immunity recovers.

**Histoplasmosis** Histoplasmosis is rare in temperate climates; it can be life-threatening, particularly in HIV-infected persons. **Itraconazole** can be used for the treatment of immunocompetent patients with indolent non-meningeal infection, including chronic pulmonary histoplasmosis. **Amphotericin** by intravenous infusion is preferred in patients with fulminant or severe infections. Following successful treatment, itraconazole can be used for prophylaxis against relapse.

**Skin and nail infections** Mild localised fungal infections of the skin (including tinea corporis, tinea cruris, and tinea pedis) respond to topical therapy (section 13.10.2). Systemic therapy is appropriate if topical therapy fails, if many areas are affected, or if the site of infection is difficult to treat such as in infections of the nails (onychomycosis) and of the scalp (tinea capitis). Oral imidazole or triazole antifungals (particularly **itraconazole**) and **terbinafine** are used more frequently than griseofulvin because they have a broader spectrum of activity and require a shorter duration of treatment.

*Tinea capitis* is treated systemically; additional topical application of an antifungal (section 13.10.2) may reduce transmission. **Griseofulvin** is used for tinea capitis in adults and children; it is effective against infections caused by *Trichophyton tonsurans* and *Microsporum* spp. **Terbinafine** is used for tinea capitis caused by *T. tonsurans* [unlicensed indication]. The role of terbinafine in the management of *Microsporum* infections is uncertain.

*Pityriasis versicolor* (section 13.10.2) may be treated with **itraconazole** by mouth if topical therapy is ineffective; **fluconazole** by mouth is an alternative. Oral **terbinafine** is **not** effective for pityriasis versicolor.

Antifungal treatment may not be necessary in asymptomatic patients with tinea infection of the nails. If treatment is necessary, a systemic antifungal is more effective than topical therapy. **Terbinafine** and **itraconazole** have largely replaced griseofulvin for the systemic treatment of *onychomycosis*, particularly of the toenail; terbinafine is considered to be the drug of choice. Itraconazole can be administered as intermittent 'pulse' therapy. For the role of topical antifungals in the treatment of onychomycosis, see section 13.10.2.

**Immunocompromised patients** Immunocompromised patients are at particular risk of fungal infections and may receive antifungal drugs prophylactically; oral imidazole or triazole antifungals are the drugs of choice for prophylaxis. **Fluconazole** is more reliably absorbed than itraconazole and ketoconazole and is considered less toxic than ketoconazole for long-term use.

Amphotericin by intravenous infusion is used for the empirical *treatment* of serious fungal infections. Fluconazole is used for treating *Candida albicans* infection. Caspofungin is licensed for the empirical treatment of systemic fungal infections (such as those involving *Candida* spp. or *Aspergillus* spp.) in patients with neutropenia.

# Drugs used in fungal infections

**Polyene antifungals** The polyene antifungals include amphotericin and nystatin; neither drug is absorbed when given by mouth. They are used for oral, oropharyngeal, and perioral infections by local application in the mouth (section 12.3.2).

**Amphotericin** by intravenous infusion is used for the treatment of systemic fungal infections and is active against most fungi and yeasts. It is highly protein bound and penetrates poorly into body fluids and tissues. When given parenterally amphotericin is toxic and side-effects are common. Lipid formulations of amphotericin (*Abelcet®*, *AmBisome®*, and *Amphocil®*) are significantly less toxic and are recommended when the conventional formulation of amphotericin is contra-indicated because of toxicity, especially nephrotoxicity or when response to conventional amphotericin is inadequate; lipid formulations are more expensive.

**Nystatin** is used principally for *Candida albicans* infections of the skin and mucous membranes, including oesophageal and intestinal candidiasis.

**Imidazole antifungals** The imidazole antifungals include clotrimazole, econazole, ketoconazole, sulconazole, and tioconazole. They are used for the local treatment of vaginal candidiasis (section 7.2.2) and for dermatophyte infection (section 13.10.2).

**Ketoconazole** is better absorbed by mouth than other imidazoles. It has been associated with fatal hepatotoxicity; the CSM has advised that prescribers should weigh the potential benefits of ketoconazole treatment against the risk of liver damage and should carefully monitor patients both clinically and biochemically. It should not be used by mouth for superficial fungal infections.

**Miconazole** (section 12.3.2) can be used locally for oral infections; it is also effective in intestinal infections. Systemic absorption may follow use of miconazole oral gel and may result in significant drug interactions.

**Triazole antifungals** **Fluconazole** is very well absorbed after oral administration. It also achieves good penetration into the cerebrospinal fluid to treat fungal meningitis.

**Itraconazole** is active against a wide range of dermatophytes. Itraconazole capsules require an acid environment in the stomach for optimal absorption.

Itraconazole has been associated with liver damage and should be avoided or used with caution in patients with liver disease; fluconazole is less frequently associated with hepatotoxicity.

**Posaconazole** is licensed for the treatment of invasive fungal infections unresponsive to conventional treatment.

**Voriconazole** is a broad-spectrum antifungal drug which is licensed for use in life-threatening infections.

**Echinocandin antifungals** Caspofungin is active against *Aspergillus* spp. and *Candida* spp. **Anidulafungin** and **micafungin** are licensed for the treatment of invasive candidiasis.

**Other antifungals** Flucytosine is used with amphotericin in a synergistic combination. Bone marrow depression can occur which limits its use, particularly in AIDS patients; weekly blood counts are necessary during prolonged therapy. Resistance to flucytosine can develop during therapy and sensitivity testing is essential before and during treatment.

**Griseofulvin** is effective for widespread or intractable dermatophyte infections but has been superseded by newer antifungals, particularly for nail infections. It is the drug of choice for trichophyton infections in children. Duration of therapy is dependent on the site of the infection and may extend to a number of months.

**Terbinafine** is the drug of choice for fungal nail infections and is also used for ringworm infections where oral treatment is considered appropriate.

## AMPHOTERICIN
(Amphotericin B)

**Indications** See under Dose

**Cautions** when given parenterally, toxicity common (close supervision necessary and test dose required; see Anaphylaxis below); renal impairment (Appendix 3); hepatic and renal function tests, blood counts, and plasma electrolyte (including plasma-potassium and magnesium concentration) monitoring required; corticosteroids (avoid except to control reactions); pregnancy (Appendix 4); breast-feeding (Appendix 5); avoid rapid infusion (risk of arrhythmias); **interactions:** Appendix 1 (amphotericin)

Anaphylaxis The CSM has advised that anaphylaxis occurs rarely with any intravenous amphotericin product and a test dose is advisable before the first infusion; the patient should be carefully observed for at least 30 minutes after the test dose. Prophylactic antipyretics or hydrocortisone should only be used in patients who have previously experienced acute adverse reactions (in whom continued treatment with amphotericin is essential)

**Side-effects** when given parenterally, anorexia, nausea and vomiting, diarrhoea, epigastric pain; febrile reactions, headache, muscle and joint pain; anaemia; disturbances in renal function (including hypokalaemia and hypomagnesaemia) and renal toxicity; also cardiovascular toxicity (including arrhythmias, blood pressure changes), blood disorders, neurological disorders (including hearing loss, diplopia, convulsions, peripheral neuropathy, encephalopathy), abnormal liver function (discontinue treatment), rash, anaphylactoid reactions (see Anaphylaxis, above); pain and thrombophlebitis at injection site

**Dose**
- Oral and perioral infections, see section 12.3.2
- By intravenous infusion, see preparations
  Note Different preparations of intravenous amphotericin vary in their pharmacodynamics, pharmacokinetics, dosage, and administration; these preparations should **not** be considered interchangeable. To avoid confusion, prescribers should specify the brand to be dispensed.

**Fungizone®** (Squibb) [PoM]
Intravenous infusion, powder for reconstitution, amphotericin (as sodium deoxycholate complex), net price 50-mg vial = £3.96
Electrolytes Na⁺ < 0.5 mmol/vial
Dose by intravenous infusion, systemic fungal infections, initial test dose of 1 mg over 20–30 minutes then 250 micrograms/kg daily, gradually increased over 2–4 days, if tolerated, to 1 mg/kg daily; max. (severe infection) 1.5 mg/kg daily or on alternate days; CHILD under 18 years see *BNF for Children*
Note Prolonged treatment usually necessary; if interrupted for longer than 7 days recommence at 250 micrograms/kg daily and increase gradually

### ◢Lipid formulations

**Abelcet®** (Cephalon) [PoM]
Intravenous infusion, amphotericin 5 mg/mL as lipid complex with L-α-dimyristoylphosphatidylcholine and L-α-dimyristoylphosphatidylglycerol, net price 20-mL vial = £82.13 (hosp. only)
Dose by intravenous infusion, severe invasive candidiasis; severe systemic fungal infections in patients not responding to conventional amphotericin or to other antifungal drugs or where toxicity or renal impairment precludes conventional amphotericin, including invasive aspergillosis, cryptococcal meningitis and disseminated cryptococcosis in HIV patients, initial test dose 1 mg over 15 minutes then 5 mg/kg once daily for at least 14 days; CHILD under 18 years see *BNF for Children*

**AmBisome®** (Gilead) [PoM]
Intravenous infusion, powder for reconstitution, amphotericin 50 mg encapsulated in liposomes, net price 50-mg vial = £96.69
Electrolytes Na⁺ < 0.5 mmol/vial
Excipients include sucrose 900 mg/vial
Dose by intravenous infusion, severe systemic or deep mycoses where toxicity (particularly nephrotoxicity) precludes use of conventional amphotericin, initial test dose 1 mg over 10 minutes then 1 mg/kg once daily increased gradually if necessary to 3 mg/kg once daily; max. 5 mg/kg once daily [unlicensed dose]; CHILD under 18 years see *BNF for Children*
Suspected or proven infection in febrile neutropenic patients unresponsive to broad-spectrum antibacterials, initial test dose 1 mg over 10 minutes then 3 mg/kg once daily until afebrile for 3 consecutive days; max. period of treatment 42 days; max. 5 mg/kg once daily [unlicensed dose]; CHILD under 18 years see *BNF for Children*
Visceral leishmaniasis, see section 5.4.5 and product literature

**Amphocil®** (Beacon) [PoM]
Intravenous infusion, powder for reconstitution, amphotericin as a complex with sodium cholesteryl sulphate, net price 50-mg vial = £104.10, 100-mg vial = £190.05
Electrolytes Na⁺ < 0.5 mmol/vial
Dose by intravenous infusion, severe systemic or deep mycoses where toxicity or renal failure preclude use of conventional amphotericin, initial test dose 2 mg over 10 minutes then 1 mg/kg once daily increased gradually if necessary to 3–4 mg/kg once daily; max. 6 mg/kg once daily; CHILD under 18 years see *BNF for Children*

## ANIDULAFUNGIN

**Indications** invasive candidiasis

**Cautions** pregnancy (Appendix 4); breast-feeding (Appendix 5)

**Side-effects** diarrhoea, nausea, vomiting; flushing; convulsion, headache; coagulopathy, hypokalaemia, raised serum creatinine; rash, pruritus; *less commonly* abdominal pain, cholestasis, hypertension, hyperglycaemia, urticaria, and injection-site pain; also reported, hepatitis

**Dose**
- By intravenous infusion, ADULT over 18 years, 200 mg on first day then 100 mg once daily

**Ecalta®** (Pfizer) ▼ PoM

Intravenous infusion, powder for reconstitution, anidulafungin, net-price 100-mg vial = £299.99 (with solvent)

Excipients include alcohol 24%

## █ CASPOFUNGIN

**Indications** invasive aspergillosis either unresponsive to amphotericin or itraconazole or in patients intolerant of amphotericin or itraconazole; invasive candidiasis (see notes above); empirical treatment of systemic fungal infections in patients with neutropenia

**Cautions** hepatic impairment (Appendix 2); pregnancy (Appendix 4); **interactions**: Appendix 1 (caspofungin)

**Contra-indications** breast-feeding (Appendix 5)

**Side-effects** nausea, vomiting, abdominal pain, diarrhoea; tachycardia, flushing; dyspnoea; fever, headache; anaemia, decrease in serum potassium, hypomagnesaemia; rash, pruritus, sweating; injection-site reactions; *less commonly* hypercalcaemia; also reported, hepatic dysfunction, oedema, adult respiratory distress syndrome, hypersensitivity reactions (including anaphylaxis); in children, also hypotension

**Dose**

- By intravenous infusion, 70 mg on first day then 50 mg once daily (70 mg once daily if body-weight over 80 kg); CHILD 1–18 years see *BNF for Children*

**Cancidas®** (MSD) ▼ PoM

Intravenous infusion, powder for reconstitution, caspofungin (as acetate), net price 50-mg vial = £327.67; 70-mg vial = £416.78

## █ FLUCONAZOLE

**Indications** see under Dose

**Cautions** renal impairment (Appendix 3); pregnancy (Appendix 4) and breast-feeding (Appendix 5); concomitant use with hepatotoxic drugs, monitor liver function with high doses or extended courses—discontinue if signs or symptoms of hepatic disease (risk of hepatic necrosis); susceptibility to QT interval prolongation; **interactions**: Appendix 1 (antifungals, triazole)

**Contra-indications** acute porphyria (section 9.8.2)

**Side-effects** nausea, abdominal discomfort, diarrhoea, flatulence, headache, rash (discontinue treatment or monitor closely if infection invasive or systemic); *less frequently* dyspepsia, vomiting, taste disturbance, hepatic disorders, hypersensitivity reactions, anaphylaxis, dizziness, seizures, alopecia, pruritus, toxic epidermal necrolysis, Stevens-Johnson syndrome (severe cutaneous reactions more likely in AIDS patients), hyperlipidaemia, leucopenia, thrombocytopenia, and hypokalaemia reported

**Dose**

- Vaginal candidiasis (see also Recurrent Vulvovaginal Candidiasis, section 7.2.2) and candidal balanitis, ADULT and CHILD over 16 years, by mouth, a single dose of 150 mg
- Mucosal candidiasis (except genital), by mouth, 50 mg daily (100 mg daily in unusually difficult infections) given for 7–14 days in oropharyngeal candidiasis (max. 14 days except in severely immunocompromised patients); for 14 days in atrophic oral candidiasis associated with dentures;

for 14–30 days in other mucosal infections (e.g. oesophagitis, candiduria, non-invasive bronchopulmonary infections); CHILD by mouth *or* by intravenous infusion, 3–6 mg/kg on first day then 3 mg/kg daily (every 72 hours in NEONATE up to 2 weeks old, every 48 hours in neonate 2–4 weeks old)

- Tinea pedis, corporis, cruris, pityriasis versicolor, and dermal candidiasis, by mouth, 50 mg daily for 2–4 weeks (for up to 6 weeks in tinea pedis); max. duration of treatment 6 weeks
- Invasive candidal infections (including candidaemia and disseminated candidiasis) and cryptococcal infections (including meningitis), by mouth *or* intravenous infusion, 400 mg on first day then 200–400 mg daily; max. 800 mg daily in severe infections [unlicensed dose]; treatment continued according to response (at least 8 weeks for cryptococcal meningitis); CHILD 6–12 mg/kg daily (every 72 hours in NEONATE up to 2 weeks old, every 48 hours in NEONATE 2–4 weeks old); max. 800 mg daily [unlicensed dose]
- Prevention of relapse of cryptococcal meningitis in AIDS patients after completion of primary therapy, by mouth *or* by intravenous infusion, 200 mg daily
- Prevention of fungal infections in immunocompromised patients, by mouth *or* by intravenous infusion, 50–400 mg daily adjusted according to risk; 400 mg daily if high risk of systemic infections e.g. following bone-marrow transplantation; commence treatment before anticipated onset of neutropenia and continue for 7 days after neutrophil count in desirable range; CHILD according to extent and duration of neutropenia, 3–12 mg/kg daily (every 72 hours in NEONATE up to 2 weeks old, every 48 hours in NEONATE 2–4 weeks old); max. 400 mg daily

**Fluconazole** (Non-proprietary) PoM
[1] Capsules, fluconazole 50 mg, net price 7-cap pack = £1.00; 150 mg, single-capsule pack = 94p; 200 mg, 7-cap pack = £1.90. Label: 9, (50 and 200 mg)
**Dental prescribing on NHS** Fluconazole Capsules 50 mg may be prescribed

Intravenous infusion, fluconazole 2 mg/mL, net price 25-mL bottle = £7.32; 100-mL bottle = £29.28

**Diflucan®** (Pfizer) PoM
[1] Capsules, fluconazole 50 mg (blue/white), net price 7-cap pack = £16.61; 150 mg (blue), single-capsule pack = £7.12; 200 mg (purple/white), 7-cap pack = £66.42. Label: 9, (50 and 200 mg)

Oral suspension, orange-flavoured, fluconazole for reconstitution with water, 50 mg/5 mL, net price 35 mL = £16.61; 200 mg/5 mL, 35 mL = £66.42. Label: 9
**Dental prescribing on NHS** May be prescribed as Fluconazole Oral Suspension 50 mg/5 mL

Intravenous infusion, fluconazole 2 mg/mL in sodium chloride intravenous infusion 0.9%, net price 25-mL bottle = £7.32; 100-mL bottle = £29.28
Electrolytes Na⁺ 15 mmol/100-mL bottle

## █ FLUCYTOSINE

**Indications** systemic yeast and fungal infections; adjunct to amphotericin in cryptococcal meningitis

---

1. Capsules can be sold to the public for vaginal candidiasis and associated candidal balanitis in those aged 16–60 years, in a container or packaging containing not more than 150 mg and labelled to show a max. dose of 150 mg

*(side tab)* **5** **Infections**

(see Cryptococcosis, p. 333), adjunct to amphotericin in severe systemic candidiasis and in other severe or long-standing infections

**Cautions** renal impairment (Appendix 3); elderly; blood disorders; liver- and kidney-function tests and blood counts required (weekly in renal impairment or blood disorders); pregnancy (Appendix 4), breast-feeding (Appendix 5); **interactions**: Appendix 1 (flucytosine)

**Side-effects** nausea, vomiting, diarrhoea, rashes; less frequently cardiotoxicity, confusion, hallucinations, convulsions, headache, sedation, vertigo, alterations in liver function tests (hepatitis and hepatic necrosis reported), and toxic epidermal necrolysis; blood disorders including thrombocytopenia, leucopenia, and aplastic anaemia reported

**Dose**

• By intravenous infusion over 20–40 minutes, 200 mg/kg daily in 4 divided doses usually for not more than 7 days; extremely sensitive organisms, 100–150 mg/kg daily may be sufficient; CHILD under 18 years see *BNF for Children*

Cryptococcal meningitis (adjunct to amphotericin, see Cryptococcosis, p. 333) 100 mg/kg daily in 4 divided doses for 2 weeks [unlicensed duration]; CHILD under 18 years see *BNF for Children*

Note For plasma concentration monitoring, blood should be taken shortly before starting the next infusion; plasma concentration for optimum response 25–50 mg/litre (200–400 micromol/litre)—should not be allowed to exceed 80 mg/litre (620 micromol/litre)

**Ancotil®** (Valeant) [PoM]
Intravenous infusion, flucytosine 10 mg/mL, net price 250-mL infusion bottle = £30.33 (hosp. only)
Electrolytes Na+ 34.5 mmol/250-mL bottle

Note Flucytosine tablets [unlicensed] may be available from 'special-order' manufacturers or specialist-importing companies, see p. 969

## GRISEOFULVIN

**Indications** dermatophyte infections of the skin, scalp, hair and nails where topical therapy has failed or is inappropriate

**Cautions** **interactions**: Appendix 1 (griseofulvin)
Driving May impair performance of skilled tasks (e.g. driving); effects of alcohol enhanced

**Contra-indications** severe liver disease; systemic lupus erythematosus (risk of exacerbation); acute porphyria (section 9.8.2); pregnancy (**avoid** pregnancy **during** and for **1 month after** treatment (Appendix 4); men should not father children within 6 months of treatment); breast-feeding (Appendix 5)

**Side-effects** nausea, vomiting, diarrhoea; headache; less frequently hepatotoxicity, dizziness, confusion, fatigue, sleep disturbances, impaired co-ordination, peripheral neuropathy, leucopenia, systemic lupus erythematosus, rash (including rarely erythema multiforme, toxic epidermal necrolysis), and photosensitivity

**Dose**

• Dermatophyte infections, 500 mg once daily or in divided doses; in severe infection dose may be doubled, reducing when response occurs; CHILD under 50 kg, 10 mg/kg once daily or in divided doses

• Tinea capitis caused by *Trichophyton tonsurans*, 1 g once daily or in divided doses; CHILD under 50 kg, 15–20 mg/kg once daily or in divided doses

Note Griseofulvin doses in BNF may differ from those in product literature

**Griseofulvin** (Non-proprietary) [PoM]
Tablets, griseofulvin 125 mg, net price 20 = £6.76; 500 mg, 20 = £17.52. Label: 9, 21, counselling, driving

## ITRACONAZOLE

**Indications** see under Dose

**Cautions** absorption reduced in AIDS and neutropenia (monitor plasma-itraconazole concentration and increase dose if necessary); susceptibility to congestive heart failure (see also CSM advice, below); renal impairment (Appendix 3); pregnancy (Appendix 4) and breast-feeding (Appendix 5); **interactions**: Appendix 1 (antifungals, triazole)
**Hepatotoxicity** Potentially life-threatening hepatotoxicity reported very rarely—discontinue if signs of hepatitis develop. Avoid or use with caution if history of hepatotoxicity with other drugs or in active liver disease (Appendix 2). Monitor liver function if treatment continues for longer than one month, if receiving other hepatotoxic drugs, if history of hepatotoxicity with other drugs, or in hepatic impairment
**Counselling** Patients should be told how to recognise signs of liver disorder and advised to seek prompt medical attention if symptoms such as anorexia, nausea, vomiting, fatigue, abdominal pain or dark urine develop

> **CSM advice (heart failure)**
> Following rare reports of heart failure, the CSM has advised caution when prescribing itraconazole to patients at high risk of heart failure. Those at risk include:
> • patients receiving high doses and longer treatment courses;
> • older patients and those with cardiac disease;
> • patients receiving treatment with negative inotropic drugs, e.g. calcium channel blockers.

**Contra-indications** acute porphyria (section 9.8.2)

**Side-effects** *very rarely* nausea, vomiting, dyspepsia, abdominal pain, diarrhoea, constipation, jaundice, hepatitis (see also Hepatotoxicity above), heart failure (see CSM advice above), pulmonary oedema, headache, dizziness, peripheral neuropathy (discontinue treatment), menstrual disorder, hypokalaemia, rash, pruritus, Stevens-Johnson syndrome, and alopecia; *with intravenous injection, very rarely* hypertension and hyperglycaemia

**Dose**

• By mouth, oropharyngeal candidiasis, 100 mg once daily (200 mg once daily in AIDS or neutropenia) for 15 days; see also under *Sporanox®* oral liquid below

Vulvovaginal candidiasis, 200 mg twice daily for 1 day

Pityriasis versicolor, 200 mg once daily for 7 days

Tinea corporis and tinea cruris, *either* 100 mg once daily for 15 days *or* 200 mg once daily for 7 days

Tinea pedis and tinea manuum, *either* 100 mg once daily for 30 days *or* 200 mg twice daily for 7 days

Onychomycosis, *either* 200 mg once daily for 3 months *or* course ('pulse') of 200 mg twice daily for 7 days, subsequent courses repeated after 21-day interval; fingernails 2 courses, toenails 3 courses

Histoplasmosis, 200 mg 1–2 times daily

Systemic aspergillosis, candidiasis and cryptococcosis including cryptococcal meningitis where other antifungal drugs inappropriate or ineffective, 200 mg once daily (candidiasis 100–200 mg once daily) increased in invasive or disseminated disease and in cryptococcal meningitis to 200 mg twice daily

Maintenance in AIDS patients to prevent relapse of underlying fungal infection and prophylaxis in neutropenia when standard therapy inappropriate, 200 mg once daily, increased to 200 mg twice daily if low plasma-itraconazole concentration (see Cautions) Prophylaxis in patients with haematological malignancy or undergoing bone-marrow transplant, see under *Sporanox®* oral liquid below

- By intravenous infusion, systemic aspergillosis, candidiasis and cryptococcosis including cryptococcal meningitis where other antifungal drugs inappropriate or ineffective, histoplasmosis, 200 mg every 12 hours for 2 days, then 200 mg once daily for max. 12 days
- CHILD under 18 years see *BNF for Children*
- ELDERLY safety and efficacy not established

**Itraconazole** (Non-proprietary) ▣PoM

Capsules, enclosing coated beads, itraconazole 100 mg, net price 15-cap pack = £10.78. Label: 5, 9, 21, 25, counselling, hepatotoxicity

**Sporanox®** (Janssen-Cilag) ▣PoM

Capsules, blue/pink, enclosing coated beads, itraconazole 100 mg, net price 4-cap pack = £3.75; 15-cap pack = £14.05; 28-cap pack (*Sporanox®-Pulse*) = £26.24; 60-cap pack = £56.21. Label: 5, 9, 21, 25, counselling, hepatotoxicity

Oral liquid, sugar-free, cherry-flavoured, itraconazole 10 mg/mL, net price 150 mL (with 10-mL measuring cup) = £46.72. Label: 9, 23, counselling, administration, hepatotoxicity

Dose oral or oesophageal candidiasis in HIV-positive or other immunocompromised patients, 20 mL (2 measuring cups) daily in 1–2 divided doses for 1 week (continue for another week if no response)

Fluconazole-resistant oral or oesophageal candidiasis, 10–20 mL (1–2 measuring cups) twice daily for 2 weeks (continue for another 2 weeks if no response; the higher dose should not be used for longer than 2 weeks if no signs of improvement)

Prophylaxis of deep fungal infections (when standard therapy is inappropriate) in patients with haematological malignancy or undergoing bone-marrow transplantation who are expected to become neutropenic, 5 mg/kg daily in 2 divided doses; starting before transplantation or before chemotherapy (taking care to avoid interaction with cytotoxic drugs) and continued until neutrophil count recovers; CHILD and ELDERLY safety and efficacy not established

Counselling Do not take with food; swish around mouth and swallow, do not rinse afterwards

Concentrate for intravenous infusion, itraconazole 10 mg/mL. For dilution before use. Net price 25-mL amp (with infusion bag and filter) = £63.84
Excipients include propylene glycol

### ▮ KETOCONAZOLE

**Indications** see CSM recommendations, p. 333; dermatophytoses and *Malassezia* folliculitis *either* resistant to fluconazole, terbinafine, or itraconazole *or* in patients intolerant of these antifungals; chronic mucocutaneous, cutaneous, and oropharyngeal candidiasis *either* resistant to fluconazole or itraconazole *or* in patients intolerant of these antifungals

**Cautions** predisposition to adrenocortical insufficiency; pregnancy (Appendix 4); **interactions:** Appendix 1 (antifungals, imidazole)
Hepatotoxicity Potentially life-threatening hepatotoxicity reported very rarely; risk of hepatotoxicity greater if given for longer than 10 days. Monitor liver function before treatment, then on weeks 2 and 4 of treatment, then every month. Avoid or use with caution if abnormal liver function tests (avoid in active liver disease) or if history of hepatotoxicity with other drugs. For CSM advice see p. 333
Counselling Patients should be told how to recognise signs of liver disorder and advised to seek prompt medical atten-

tion if symptoms such as anorexia, nausea, vomiting, fatigue, abdominal pain, jaundice, or dark urine develop

**Contra-indications** acute porphyria (section 9.8.2); hepatic impairment; breast-feeding

**Side-effects** nausea, vomiting, abdominal pain; pruritus; *less commonly* diarrhoea, headache, dizziness, drowsiness, and rash; also reported fatal liver damage (see Hepatotoxicity above), dyspepsia, raised intracranial pressure, paraesthesia, adrenocortical insufficiency, erectile dysfunction, menstrual disorders, azoospermia (with high doses), gynaecomastia, thrombocytopenia, photophobia, photosensitivity, and alopecia

**Dose**
- 200 mg once daily, increased if response inadequate to 400 mg once daily; continued until symptoms have cleared and cultures negative, but see Cautions (max. duration of treatment 4 weeks for *Malassezia* infection); CHILD body-weight 15–30 kg, 100 mg once daily; body-weight over 30 kg, adult dose

**Nizoral®** (Janssen-Cilag) ▣PoM

Tablets, scored, ketoconazole 200 mg. Net price 30-tab pack = £14.02. Label: 5, 9, 21, counselling, hepatotoxicity

### ▮ MICAFUNGIN

**Indications** see under Dose

**Cautions** monitor renal function; renal impairment (Appendix 3); pregnancy (Appendix 4); breast-feeding (Appendix 5); **interactions:** Appendix 1 (micafungin)
Hepatotoxicity Potentially life-threatening hepatotoxicity reported. Monitor liver function—discontinue if significant and persistent abnormalities in liver function tests develop. Use with caution in hepatic impairment (avoid if severe; Appendix 2) or if receiving other hepatotoxic drugs. Risk of hepatic side-effects greater in children under 1 year of age

**Side-effects** nausea, vomiting, diarrhoea, abdominal pain; headache, fever; hypokalaemia, hypomagnesaemia, hypocalcaemia, leucopenia, anaemia; rash, phlebitis; *less commonly* dyspepsia, constipation, hepatomegaly, hepatitis and cholestasis (see also Hepatotoxicity above), taste disturbances, anorexia, tachycardia, palpitation, bradycardia, blood pressure changes, flushing, dyspnoea, sleep disturbances, anxiety, confusion, dizziness, tremor, pancytopenia, thrombocytopenia, eosinophilia, hyponatraemia, hypophosphataemia, hyperkalaemia, hyperhidrosis, and pruritus; *rarely* haemolytic anaemia; also reported renal failure (more frequent in children)

**Dose**
- By intravenous infusion, invasive candidiasis, ADULT body-weight over 40 kg, 100 mg once daily (increased to 200 mg daily if inadequate response) for at least 14 days; body-weight under 40 kg, 2 mg/kg once daily (increased to 4 mg/kg daily if inadequate response) for at least 14 days; CHILD under 18 years see *BNF for Children*

Oesophageal candidiasis, ADULT body-weight over 40 kg, 150 mg once daily; body-weight under 40 kg, 3 mg/kg once daily; CHILD 16–18 years see *BNF for Children*

Prophylaxis of candidiasis in patients undergoing bone-marrow transplantation or who are expected to become neutropenic for over 10 days, ADULT body-weight over 40 kg, 50 mg once daily; body-weight under 40 kg, 1 mg/kg once daily; continue for at least 7 days after neutrophil count in desirable range; CHILD under 18 years see *BNF for Children*

5 Infections

**Mycamine®** (Astellas) ▼ PoM
Intravenous infusion, powder for reconstitution, micafungin (as sodium), net price 50-mg vial = £196.08; 100-mg vial = £341.00

## NYSTATIN

**Indications** candidiasis; oral infection (section 12.3.2); skin infection (section 13.10.2)

**Side-effects** nausea, vomiting, diarrhoea at high doses; oral irritation and sensitisation; rash (including urticaria) and rarely Stevens-Johnson syndrome reported

**Dose**
- By mouth, intestinal candidiasis 500 000 units every 6 hours, doubled in severe infection; NEONATE 100 000 units 4 times daily; CHILD 1 month–12 years, 100 000 units 4 times daily; immunocompromised children may require higher doses (e.g. 500 000 units 4 times daily)

Note Unlicensed for treatment of candidiasis in NEONATE. Nystatin doses in BNF may differ from those in product literature

**Nystan®** (Squibb) PoM
Oral suspension, yellow, nystatin 100 000 units/mL, net price 30 mL with pipette = £1.91. Label: 9, counselling, use of pipette

## POSACONAZOLE

**Indications** invasive aspergillosis either unresponsive to, or in patients intolerant of, amphotericin or itraconazole; fusariosis either unresponsive to, or in patients intolerant of, amphotericin; chromoblastomycosis and mycetoma either unresponsive to, or in patients intolerant of, itraconazole; coccidioidomycosis either unresponsive to, or in patients intolerant of, amphotericin, itraconazole, or fluconazole; see also under Dose

**Cautions** cardiomyopathy, bradycardia, symptomatic arrhythmias, history of QT interval prolongation, concomitant use with other drugs known to cause QT-interval prolongation; monitor electrolytes (including potassium, magnesium, and calcium) before and during therapy, monitor liver function—consider discontinuing if impairment suspected (Appendix 2); pregnancy (ensure effective contraception during treatment; Appendix 4); **interactions:** Appendix 1 (antifungals, triazole)

**Contra-indications** acute porphyria (section 9.8.2); breast-feeding (Appendix 5)

**Side-effects** gastro-intestinal disturbances (including nausea, vomiting, abdominal pain, diarrhoea, dyspepsia, and flatulence); dizziness, headache, paraesthesia, drowsiness, fatigue, fever, anorexia; blood disorders (including anaemia, neutropenia, and thrombocytopenia), electrolyte disturbances; dry mouth; rash; *less commonly* pancreatitis, hepatic disorders, arrhythmias, palpitation, changes in blood pressure, oedema, convulsions, neuropathy, tremor, hyperglycaemia, menstrual disorders, renal failure, musculoskeletal pain, visual disturbances, mouth ulcers, and alopecia; *rarely* ileus, cardiac failure, myocardial infarction, stroke, thrombosis, syncope, pneumonitis, psychosis, depression, encephalopathy, adrenal insufficiency, breast pain, hearing impairment, and Stevens-Johnson syndrome

**Dose**
- 400 mg twice daily with food *or* if food not tolerated, 200 mg 4 times daily
- Oropharyngeal candidiasis (severe infection or in immunocompromised patients only), 200 mg with food on first day, then 100 mg once daily with food for 13 days
- Prophylaxis of invasive fungal infections in patients undergoing bone-marrow transplantation or receiving chemotherapy for acute myeloid leukaemia and myelodysplastic syndrome who are expected to become neutropenic, and who are intolerant of fluconazole and itraconazole, 200 mg 3 times daily with food, starting before transplantation or before chemotherapy and continued until neutrophil count recovers
- CHILD under 18 years not recommended

**Noxafil®** (Schering-Plough) ▼ PoM
Suspension, posaconazole 200 mg/5 mL, net price 105 mL (cherry-flavoured) = £491.20. Label: 9, 21

## TERBINAFINE

**Indications** dermatophyte infections of the nails, ringworm infections (including tinea pedis, cruris, and corporis) where oral therapy appropriate (due to site, severity or extent)

**Cautions** psoriasis (risk of exacerbation); autoimmune disease (risk of lupus-erythematosus-like effect); hepatic impairment (Appendix 2); renal impairment (Appendix 3); pregnancy (Appendix 4); breast-feeding (Appendix 5); **interactions:** Appendix 1 (terbinafine)

**Side-effects** abdominal discomfort, anorexia, nausea, diarrhoea; headache; rash and urticaria occasionally with arthralgia or myalgia; *less commonly* taste disturbance; *rarely* liver toxicity (including jaundice, cholestasis and hepatitis)—discontinue treatment; angioedema, dizziness, malaise, paraesthesia, hypoaesthesia, photosensitivity, serious skin reactions (including Stevens-Johnson syndrome and toxic epidermal necrolysis)—discontinue treatment if progressive skin rash; *very rarely* psychiatric disturbances, blood disorders (including leucopenia and thrombocytopenia), lupus erythematosus-like effect, and exacerbation of psoriasis

**Dose**
- By mouth, 250 mg daily usually for 2–6 weeks in tinea pedis, 2–4 weeks in tinea cruris, 4 weeks in tinea corporis, 6 weeks–3 months in nail infections (occasionally longer in toenail infections); CHILD [unlicensed] usually for 4 weeks, tinea capitis, over 1 year, body-weight 10–20 kg, 62.5 mg once daily; body-weight 20–40 kg, 125 mg once daily; body-weight over 40 kg, 250 mg once daily

**Terbinafine** (Non-proprietary) PoM
Tablets, terbinafine (as hydrochloride) 250 mg, net price 14-tab pack = £2.74, 28-tab pack = £3.44. Label: 9

**Lamisil®** (Novartis) PoM
Tablets, off-white, scored, terbinafine (as hydrochloride) 250 mg, net price 14-tab pack = £23.16, 28-tab pack = £44.66. Label: 9

## ▌ VORICONAZOLE

**Indications** invasive aspergillosis; serious infections caused by *Scedosporium* spp., *Fusarium* spp., or invasive fluconazole-resistant *Candida* spp. (including *C. krusei*)

**Cautions** electrolyte disturbances, cardiomyopathy, bradycardia, symptomatic arrhythmias, history of QT interval prolongation, concomitant use with other drugs that prolong QT interval; avoid exposure to sunlight; patients at risk of pancreatitis; monitor liver function before treatment and during treatment; haematological malignancy (increased risk of hepatic reactions); hepatic impairment (Appendix 2); monitor renal function; renal impairment (Appendix 3); pregnancy (ensure effective contraception during treatment—Appendix 4); **interactions**: Appendix 1 (antifungals, triazole)

**Contra-indications** acute porphyria (section 9.8.2); breast-feeding (Appendix 5)

**Side-effects** gastro-intestinal disturbances (including nausea, vomiting, abdominal pain, diarrhoea), jaundice; oedema, hypotension, chest pain; respiratory distress syndrome, sinusitis; headache, dizziness, asthenia, anxiety, depression, confusion, agitation, hallucinations, paraesthesia, tremor; influenza-like symptoms; hypoglycaemia; haematuria; blood disorders (including anaemia, thrombocytopenia, leucopenia, pancytopenia), acute renal failure, hypokalaemia; visual disturbances including altered perception, blurred vision, and photophobia; rash, pruritus, photosensitivity, alopecia, cheilitis; injection-site reactions; *less commonly* cholecystitis, pancreatitis, hepatitis, constipation, arrhythmias (including QT interval prolongation), syncope, raised serum cholesterol, hypersensitivity reactions (including flushing), ataxia, nystagmus, hypoaesthesia, adrenocortical insufficiency, arthritis, blepharitis, optic neuritis, scleritis, glossitis, gingivitis, psoriasis, and Stevens-Johnson syndrome; *rarely* pseudomembranous colitis, convulsions, sleep disturbances, tinnitus, hearing disturbances, extrapyramidal effects, hypertonia, hypothyroidism, hyperthyroidism, discoid lupus erythematosus, toxic epidermal necrolysis, retinal haemorrhage, optic atrophy, and taste disturbances

**Dose**

- By mouth, ADULT and CHILD over 12 years, body-weight over 40 kg, 400 mg every 12 hours for 2 doses then 200 mg every 12 hours, increased if necessary to 300 mg every 12 hours; body-weight under 40 kg, 200 mg every 12 hours for 2 doses then 100 mg every 12 hours, increased if necessary to 150 mg every 12 hours; CHILD 2–12 years, (oral suspension recommended) 200 mg every 12 hours

- By intravenous infusion, 6 mg/kg every 12 hours for 2 doses, then 4 mg/kg every 12 hours (reduced to 3 mg/kg every 12 hours if not tolerated) for max. 6 months; CHILD 2–18 years see *BNF for Children*

**Vfend®** (Pfizer) ⓟⓞⓜ

Tablets, f/c, voriconazole 50 mg, net price 28-tablet pack = £275.68; 200 mg, 28-tab pack = £1102.74. Label: 9, 11, 23

Oral suspension, voriconazole 200 mg/5 mL when reconstituted with water, net price 75 mL (orange-flavoured) = £551.37. Label: 9, 11, 23

Intravenous infusion, powder for reconstitution, voriconazole, net price 200-mg vial = £77.14
Excipients include sulphobutylether beta cyclodextrin sodium (risk of accumulation in renal impairment)
Electrolytes Na⁺ 9.47 mmol/vial

# 5.3 Antiviral drugs

### 5.3.1 HIV infection
### 5.3.2 Herpesvirus infections
### 5.3.3 Viral hepatitis
### 5.3.4 Influenza
### 5.3.5 Respiratory syncytial virus

The majority of virus infections resolve spontaneously in immunocompetent subjects. A number of specific treatments for viral infections are available, particularly for the immunocompromised. This section includes notes on herpes simplex and varicella-zoster, human immunodeficiency virus, cytomegalovirus, respiratory syncytial virus, viral hepatitis and influenza.

# 5.3.1 HIV infection

There is no cure for infection caused by the human immunodeficiency virus (HIV) but a number of drugs slow or halt disease progression. Drugs for HIV infection (antiretrovirals) increase life expectancy considerably but they may be associated with serious side-effects. Treatment should be undertaken only by those experienced in their use.

**Principles of treatment** Treatment is aimed at reducing the plasma viral load as much as possible and for as long as possible; it should be started before the immune system is irreversibly damaged. The need for early drug treatment should, however, be balanced against the risk of toxicity. Commitment to treatment and strict adherence over many years are required; the regimen chosen should take into account convenience and patient tolerance. The development of drug resistance is reduced by using a combination of drugs; such combinations should have synergistic or additive activity while ensuring that their toxicity is not additive. It is recommended that viral sensitivity to antiretroviral drugs is established before starting treatment or before switching drugs if the infection is not responding.

**Initiation of treatment** The optimum time for initiating antiretroviral treatment depends primarily on the CD4 cell count; the plasma viral load and clinical symptoms may also help. The timing and choice of treatment should also take account of the possible effects of antiretroviral drugs on factors such as the risk of cardiovascular events. Treatment includes a combination of drugs known as 'highly active antiretroviral therapy'. Treatment is initiated with 2 nucleoside reverse transcriptase inhibitors and a non-nucleoside reverse transcriptase inhibitor; the regimens of choice contain *either* tenofovir, emtricitabine, and efavirenz *or* abacavir, lamivudine, and efavirenz. Regimens containing 2 nucleoside reverse transcriptase inhibitors and a boosted protease inhibitor are reserved for patients with resistance to first-line regimens, women wishing to become pregnant, or patients with psychiatric illness. Patients who require treatment for both HIV and chronic hepatitis B should be treated with antivirals active against both diseases (section 5.3.3).

**Switching therapy** Deterioration of the condition (including clinical and virological changes) may require a change in therapy. The choice of an alternative regimen depends on factors such as the response to previous treatment, tolerance and the possibility of cross-resistance.

**Pregnancy and breast-feeding** Treatment of HIV infection in pregnancy aims to reduce the risk of toxicity to the fetus (although the teratogenic potential of most antiretroviral drugs is unknown), to minimise the viral load and disease progression in the mother, and to prevent transmission of infection to the neonate. **All treatment options require careful assessment by a specialist.** Zidovudine monotherapy reduces transmission of infection to the neonate. However, combination antiretroviral therapy maximises the chance of preventing transmission and represents optimal therapy for the mother. Combination antiretroviral therapy may be associated with a greater risk of preterm delivery.

Breast-feeding by HIV-positive mothers may cause HIV infection in the infant and should be avoided.

**Children** HIV disease in children has a different natural progression to adults. Children infected with HIV should be managed within a formal paediatric HIV clinical network by specialists with access to guidelines and information on antiretroviral drugs for children.

**Post-exposure prophylaxis** Prophylaxis with antiretroviral drugs [unlicensed indication] may be appropriate following exposure to HIV-contaminated material. Immediate expert advice should be sought in such cases; national guidelines on post-exposure prophylaxis for healthcare workers have been developed (by the Chief Medical Officer's Expert Advisory Group on AIDS, www.dh.gov.uk) and local ones may also be available. Antiretrovirals for prophylaxis are chosen on the basis of efficacy and potential for toxicity. Prompt prophylaxis with antiretroviral drugs [unlicensed indication] is also appropriate following potential sexual exposure to HIV; recommendations have been developed by the British Association for Sexual Health and HIV, www.bashh.org

**Drugs for HIV infection** Zidovudine, a nucleoside reverse transcriptase inhibitor (or 'nucleoside analogue'), was the first anti-HIV drug to be introduced. Other nucleoside reverse transcriptase inhibitors include **abacavir, didanosine, emtricitabine, lamivudine, stavudine,** and **tenofovir**.

The protease inhibitors include **atazanavir, darunavir, fosamprenavir** (a pro-drug of amprenavir), **indinavir, lopinavir, nelfinavir, ritonavir, saquinavir,** and **tipranavir**. Ritonavir in low doses boosts the activity of atazanavir, darunavir, fosamprenavir, indinavir, lopinavir, saquinavir, and tipranavir increasing the persistence of plasma concentrations of these drugs; at such a low dose, ritonavir has no intrinsic antiviral activity. A combination of lopinavir with low-dose ritonavir is available. The protease inhibitors are metabolised by cytochrome P450 enzyme systems and therefore have a significant potential for drug interactions. Protease inhibitors are associated with lipodystrophy and metabolic effects (see below).

The non-nucleoside reverse transcriptase inhibitors **efavirenz, etravirine,** and **nevirapine** are active against the subtype HIV-1 but not HIV-2, a subtype that is rare in the UK. These drugs may interact with a number of drugs metabolised in the liver. Nevirapine is associated with a high incidence of rash (including Stevens-Johnson syndrome) and occasionally fatal hepatitis. Rash is also associated with efavirenz and etravirine but it is usually milder. Psychiatric or CNS disturbances are common with efavirenz. CNS disturbances are often self-limiting and can be reduced by taking the dose at bedtime (especially in the first 2–4 weeks of treatment). Efavirenz has also been associated with an increased plasma cholesterol concentration. Etravirine is used in regimens containing a boosted protease inhibitor for HIV infection resistant to other non-nucleoside reverse transcriptase inhibitors and protease inhibitors.

**Enfuvirtide,** which inhibits the fusion of HIV to the host cell, is licensed for managing infection that has failed to respond to a regimen of other antiretroviral drugs; enfuvirtide should be combined with other potentially active antiretroviral drugs.

**Maraviroc** is an antagonist of the CCR5 chemokine receptor. It is licensed for patients exclusively infected with CCR5-tropic HIV. The *Scottish Medicines Consortium* (p. 3) has advised (March 2008) that maraviroc (*Celsentri*®) is **not** recommended for use within NHS Scotland.

**Raltegravir** is an inhibitor of HIV integrase. It is licensed for the treatment of HIV infection resistant to multiple antiretrovirals. The *Scottish Medicines Consortium* (p. 3) has advised (April 2008) that raltegravir (*Isentress*®) is accepted for restricted use within NHS Scotland for the treatment of patients with HIV infection resistant to 3 classes of antiretrovirals.

**Immune reconstitution syndrome** Improvement in immune function as a result of antiretroviral treatment may provoke a marked inflammatory reaction against residual opportunistic organisms.

**Lipodystrophy syndrome** Metabolic effects associated with antiretroviral treatment include *fat redistribution, insulin resistance,* and *dyslipidaemia*; collectively these have been termed *lipodystrophy syndrome*. The usual risk factors for cardiovascular disease should be taken into account before starting antiretroviral therapy and patients should be advised about lifestyle changes to reduce their cardiovascular risk. Plasma lipids and blood glucose should be measured before starting antiretroviral therapy, after 3–6 months of treatment, and then annually.

Fat redistribution (with loss of subcutaneous fat, increased abdominal fat, 'buffalo hump' and breast enlargement) is associated with regimens containing protease inhibitors and nucleoside reverse transcriptase inhibitors. Stavudine (especially in combination with didanosine), and to a lesser extent zidovudine, are associated with a higher risk of lipoatrophy and should be used only if alternative regimens are not suitable.

Dyslipidaemia is associated with antiretroviral treatment, particularly with protease inhibitors. Protease inhibitors and nucleoside reverse transcriptase inhibitors are associated with insulin resistance and hyperglycaemia. Of the protease inhibitors, atazanavir and darunavir may be less likely to cause dyslipidaemia, while saquinavir and atazanavir may be less likely to impair glucose tolerance.

**Osteonecrosis** Osteonecrosis has been reported in patients with advanced HIV disease or following long-term exposure to combination antiretroviral therapy.

## Nucleoside reverse transcriptase inhibitors

**Cautions** Nucleoside reverse transcriptase inhibitors should be used with caution in patients with chronic hepatitis B or C (greater risk of hepatic side-effects), in hepatic impairment (see also Lactic Acidosis below and Appendix 2), in renal impairment (Appendix 3), and in pregnancy (see also p. 340 and Appendix 4).

**Lactic acidosis** Life-threatening lactic acidosis associated with hepatomegaly and hepatic steatosis has been reported with nucleoside reverse transcriptase inhibitors. They should be used with caution in patients (particularly obese women) with hepatomegaly, hepatitis (especially hepatitis C treated with interferon alfa and ribavirin), liver-enzyme abnormalities and with other risk factors for liver disease and hepatic steatosis (including alcohol abuse). Treatment with the nucleoside reverse transcriptase inhibitor should be **discontinued** in case of symptomatic hyperlactataemia, lactic acidosis, progressive hepatomegaly or rapid deterioration of liver function. Stavudine, especially with didanosine, is associated with a higher risk of lactic acidosis and should be used only if alternative regimens are not suitable.

**Side-effects** Side-effects of the nucleoside reverse transcriptase inhibitors include gastro-intestinal disturbances (such as nausea, vomiting, abdominal pain, flatulence and diarrhoea), anorexia, pancreatitis, liver damage (see also Lactic Acidosis, above), dyspnoea, cough, headache, insomnia, dizziness, fatigue, blood disorders (including anaemia, neutropenia, and thrombocytopenia), myalgia, arthralgia, rash, urticaria, and fever. See notes above for metabolic effects and lipodystrophy (Lipodystrophy Syndrome), and Osteonecrosis.

### ABACAVIR

**Indications** HIV infection in combination with other antiretroviral drugs

**Cautions** see notes above; also test for HLA-B*5701 allele before treatment—risk of hypersensitivity reaction in presence of HLA-B*5701 allele; HIV load greater than 100 000 copies/mL; patients at high risk of cardiovascular disease; **interactions**: Appendix 1 (abacavir)

Hypersensitivity reactions Life-threatening hypersensitivity reactions reported—characterised by fever or rash and possibly nausea, vomiting, diarrhoea, abdominal pain, dyspnoea, cough, lethargy, malaise, headache, and myalgia; less frequently mouth ulceration, oedema, hypotension, sore throat, acute respiratory distress syndrome, anaphylaxis, paraesthesia, arthralgia, conjunctivitis, lymphadenopathy, lymphocytopenia and renal failure (CSM has identified hypersensitivity reactions presenting as sore throat, influenza-like illness, cough, and breathlessness); rarely myolysis; laboratory abnormalities may include raised liver function tests (see Lactic Acidosis above) and creatine kinase; symptoms usually appear in the first 6 weeks, but may occur at any time; monitor for symptoms every 2 weeks for 2 months; discontinue immediately if any symptom of hypersensitivity develops and do not rechallenge (risk of more severe hypersensitivity reaction); discontinue if hypersensitivity cannot be ruled out, even when other diagnoses possible—if rechallenge necessary it must be carried out in hospital setting; if abacavir is stopped for any reason other than hypersensitivity, exclude hypersensitivity reaction as the cause and rechallenge only if medical assistance is readily available; care needed with concomitant use of drugs which cause skin toxicity

Counselling Patients should be told the importance of regular dosing (intermittent therapy may increase the risk of sensitisation), how to recognise signs of hypersensitivity, and advised to seek immediate medical attention if symptoms develop or before re-starting treatment; patients should be advised to keep Alert Card with them at all times

**Contra-indications** breast-feeding (Appendix 5)

**Side-effects** see notes above; also hypersensitivity reactions (see above); *very rarely* Stevens-Johnson syndrome and toxic epidermal necrolysis; rash and gastro-intestinal disturbances more common in children

**Dose**

- 600 mg daily in 1–2 divided doses; CHILD 3 months–12 years, 8 mg/kg every 12 hours (max. 600 mg daily) or body-weight 14–21 kg, 150 mg every 12 hours; body-weight 21–30 kg, 150 mg in the morning and 300 mg in the evening; body-weight over 30 kg, 300 mg every 12 hours

**Ziagen®** (GSK) ▒PoM▒
Tablets, yellow, f/c, scored, abacavir (as sulphate) 300 mg, net price 60-tab pack = £221.81. Counselling, hypersensitivity reactions

Oral solution, sugar-free, banana and strawberry flavoured, abacavir (as sulphate) 20 mg/mL, net price 240-mL = £59.15. Counselling, hypersensitivity reactions

◢**With lamivudine**

For **cautions, contra-indications** and **side-effects** see under individual drugs

**Kivexa®** (GSK) ▒PoM▒
Tablets, orange, f/c, abacavir (as sulphate) 600 mg, lamivudine 300 mg, net price 30-tab pack = £373.94. Counselling, hypersensitivity reactions
Dose ADULT and CHILD over 12 years, body-weight over 40 kg, 1 tablet once daily

◢**With lamivudine and zidovudine**

Note For patients stabilised (for 6–8 weeks) on the individual components in the same proportions. For **cautions, contra-indications** and **side-effects** see under individual drugs

**Trizivir®** (GSK) ▒PoM▒
Tablets, blue-green, f/c, abacavir (as sulphate) 300 mg, lamivudine 150 mg, zidovudine 300 mg, net price 60-tab pack = £540.40. Counselling, hypersensitivity reactions
Dose ADULT over 18 years, 1 tablet twice daily

### DIDANOSINE
(ddI, DDI)

**Indications** HIV infection in combination with other antiretroviral drugs

**Cautions** see notes above; also history of pancreatitis (preferably avoid, otherwise extreme caution, see also below); peripheral neuropathy or hyperuricaemia (see under Side-effects); ophthalmic examination

5

Infections

(including visual acuity, colour vision, and dilated fundus examination) recommended annually or if visual changes occur; **interactions:** Appendix 1 (didanosine)

**Pancreatitis** Suspend treatment if serum lipase raised (even if asymptomatic) or if symptoms of pancreatitis develop; discontinue if pancreatitis confirmed. Whenever possible avoid concomitant treatment with other drugs known to cause pancreatic toxicity (e.g. intravenous pentamidine isetionate); monitor closely if concomitant therapy unavoidable. Since significant elevations of triglycerides cause pancreatitis monitor closely if elevated

**Contra-indications** breast-feeding (Appendix 5)

**Side-effects** see notes above; also pancreatitis (see also under cautions), liver failure, anaphylactic reactions, peripheral neuropathy (switch to another antiretroviral if peripheral neuropathy develops), diabetes mellitus, hypoglycaemia, acute renal failure, rhabdomyolysis, dry eyes, retinal and optic nerve changes, dry mouth, parotid gland enlargement, sialadenitis, alopecia, hyperuricaemia (suspend if raised significantly)

**Dose**

● ADULT under 60 kg 250 mg daily in 1–2 divided doses; 60 kg and over 400 mg daily in 1–2 divided doses; CHILD over 3 months (under 6 years *Videx*® tablets only), 240 mg/m² daily (180 mg/m² daily in combination with zidovudine) in 1–2 divided doses

**Videx®** (Bristol-Myers Squibb) [PoM]

Tablets, with calcium and magnesium antacids, didanosine 25 mg, net price 60-tab pack = £25.56. Label: 23, counselling, administration, see below

Excipients include aspartame equivalent to phenylalanine 36.5 mg per tablet (section 9.4.1)

Note Antacids in formulation may affect absorption of other drugs—see **interactions:** Appendix 1 (antacids)

Counselling To ensure sufficient antacid, each dose to be taken as at least 2 tablets (CHILD under 1 year 1 tablet) chewed thoroughly, crushed or dispersed in water; clear apple juice may be added for flavouring; tablets to be taken 2 hours after lopinavir with ritonavir capsules and oral solution or atazanavir with ritonavir

Videx® EC capsules, enclosing e/c granules, didanosine 125 mg, net price 30-cap pack = £49.16; 200 mg, 30-cap pack = £78.65; 250 mg, 30-cap pack = £98.31; 400 mg, 30-cap pack = £157.30. Label: 25, counselling, administration, see below

Counselling Capsules to be taken at least 2 hours before or 2 hours after food

## EMTRICITABINE

**Indications** HIV infection in combination with other antiretroviral drugs

**Cautions** see notes above; also on discontinuation, monitor patients with hepatitis B (risk of exacerbation of hepatitis); **interactions:** Appendix 1 (emtricitabine)

**Contra-indications** breast-feeding (Appendix 5)

**Side-effects** see notes above; also abnormal dreams, pruritus, and hyperpigmentation

**Dose**

● See preparations

**Emtriva®** (Gilead) [PoM]

Capsules, white/blue, emtricitabine 200 mg, net price 30-cap pack = £163.50

Dose ADULT and CHILD body-weight over 33 kg, 200 mg once daily

Oral solution, orange, emtricitabine 10 mg/mL, net price 170-mL pack (candy-flavoured) = £46.50

Dose ADULT and CHILD body-weight over 33 kg, 240 mg once daily; CHILD 4 months–18 years, body-weight under 33 kg, 6 mg/kg once daily

Electrolytes Na⁺ 460 micromol/mL

Note 240 mg oral solution ≡ 200 mg capsule; where appropriate the capsule may be used instead of the oral solution

◢**With tenofovir**
See under Tenofovir

◢**With efavirenz and tenofovir**
See under Tenofovir

## LAMIVUDINE
### (3TC)

**Indications** see preparations below

**Cautions** see notes above; **interactions:** Appendix 1 (lamivudine)

**Chronic Hepatitis B** Recurrent hepatitis in patients with chronic hepatitis B may occur on discontinuation of lamivudine. When treating chronic hepatitis B with lamivudine, monitor liver function tests every 3 months, and viral and serological markers of hepatitis B every 3–6 months, more frequently in patients with advanced liver disease or following transplantation (monitoring to continue after discontinuation)—consult product literature

**Contra-indications** breast-feeding (Appendix 5)

**Side-effects** see notes above; also peripheral neuropathy, muscle disorders including rhabdomyolysis, nasal symptoms, alopecia

**Dose**

● See preparations below

**Epivir®** (GSK) [PoM]

Tablets, f/c, lamivudine 150 mg (scored, white), net price 60-tab pack = £152.14; 300 mg (grey), 30-tab pack = £167.21

Oral solution, banana- and strawberry-flavoured, lamivudine 50 mg/5 mL, net price 240-mL pack = £41.41

Excipients include sucrose 1 g/5 mL

Dose HIV infection in combination with other antiretroviral drugs, 150 mg every 12 hours or 300 mg once daily; CHILD 3 months–12 years, 4 mg/kg (max. 150 mg) every 12 hours or body-weight 14–21 kg, 75 mg twice daily; body-weight 21–30 kg, 75 mg in the morning and 150 mg in the evening; body-weight over 30 kg, 150 mg twice daily

**Zeffix®** (GSK) [PoM]

Tablets, brown, f/c, lamivudine 100 mg, net price 28-tab pack = £78.09

Oral solution, banana and strawberry flavoured, lamivudine 25 mg/5 mL, net price 240-mL pack = £22.79

Excipients include sucrose 1 g/5 mL

Dose chronic hepatitis B infection with either compensated liver disease (with evidence of viral replication and histology of active liver inflammation or fibrosis), or decompensated liver disease, 100 mg daily; CHILD [unlicensed indication] 2–11 years, 3 mg/kg once daily (max. 100 mg daily); 12–17 years, adult dose

Note Patients receiving lamivudine for concomitant HIV infection should continue to receive lamivudine in a dose appropriate for HIV infection

◢**With abacavir**
See under Abacavir

◢**With zidovudine**
See under Zidovudine

◢**With abacavir and zidovudine**
See under Abacavir

## ■ STAVUDINE
(d4T)

**Indications** HIV infection in combination with other antiretroviral drugs

**Cautions** see notes above; also history of peripheral neuropathy (see under Side-effects); history of pancreatitis or concomitant use with other drugs associated with pancreatitis; **interactions:** Appendix 1 (stavudine)

**Contra-indications** breast-feeding (Appendix 5)

**Side-effects** see notes above; also peripheral neuropathy (switch to another antiretroviral if peripheral neuropathy develops), abnormal dreams, cognitive dysfunction, drowsiness, depression, pruritus; *less commonly* anxiety, gynaecomastia

**Dose**

- ADULT under 60 kg, 30 mg every 12 hours preferably at least 1 hour before food; 60 kg and over, 40 mg every 12 hours; NEONATE under 2 weeks, 500 micrograms/kg every 12 hours; CHILD over 2 weeks, body-weight under 30 kg, 1 mg/kg every 12 hours; body-weight 30 kg and over, adult dose

**Zerit®** (Bristol-Myers Squibb) (PoM)
Capsules, stavudine 20 mg (brown), net price 56-cap pack = £142.28; 30 mg (light orange/dark orange), 56-cap pack = £149.20; 40 mg (dark orange), 56-cap pack = £153.70 (all hosp. only)

Oral solution, cherry-flavoured, stavudine for reconstitution with water, 1 mg/mL, net price 200 mL = £23.40

## ■ TENOFOVIR DISOPROXIL

**Indications** HIV infection in combination with other antiretroviral drugs; chronic hepatitis B infection with compensated liver disease, evidence of viral replication, and histologically documented active liver inflammation or fibrosis

**Cautions** see notes above; also test renal function and serum phosphate before treatment, then every 4 weeks (more frequently if at increased risk of renal impairment) for 1 year and then every 3 months, interrupt treatment if renal function deteriorates or serum phosphate decreases; concomitant or recent use of nephrotoxic drugs; on discontinuation, monitor patients with hepatitis B (risk of exacerbation of hepatitis); **interactions:** Appendix 1 (tenofovir)

**Contra-indications** breast-feeding (Appendix 5)

**Side-effects** see notes above; hypophosphataemia; *rarely* renal failure; also reported nephrogenic diabetes insipidus, reduced bone density, hypokalaemia, myopathy, and rhabdomyolysis

**Dose**

- ADULT over 18 years, 245 mg once daily

**Viread®** (Gilead) ▼ (PoM)
Tablets, f/c, blue, tenofovir disoproxil (as fumarate) 245 mg, net price 30-tab pack = £255.00. Label: 21, counselling, administration
**Counselling** Patients with swallowing difficulties may disperse tablet in half a glass of water, orange juice, or grape juice (but bitter taste)

◢With emtricitabine

For **cautions, contra-indications,** and **side-effects** see under individual drugs

**Truvada®** (Gilead) (PoM)
Tablets, blue, f/c, tenofovir disoproxil (as fumarate) 245 mg, emtricitabine 200 mg, net price 30-tab pack = £418.50. Label: 21, counselling, administration
**Counselling** Patients with swallowing difficulties may disperse tablet in half a glass of water, orange juice, or grape juice (but bitter taste)
**Dose** ADULT over 18 years, 1 tablet once daily

◢With efavirenz and emtricitabine

For **cautions, contra-indications,** and **side-effects** see under individual drugs

**Atripla®** (Gilead) (PoM)
Tablets, pink, f/c, efavirenz 600 mg, emtricitabine 200 mg, tenofovir disoproxil (as fumarate) 245 mg, net price 30-tab pack = £626.90. Label: 23, 25
**Dose** HIV infection stabilised on antiretroviral therapy for more than 3 months, ADULT over 18 years, 1 tablet once daily

## ■ ZIDOVUDINE
(Azidothymidine, AZT)

**Note** The abbreviation AZT which is sometimes used for zidovudine has also been used for another drug

**Indications** HIV infection in combination with other antiretroviral drugs; prevention of maternal-fetal HIV transmission (see notes above under Pregnancy and Breast-feeding)

**Cautions** see notes above; also haematological toxicity particularly with high dose and advanced disease—monitor full blood count after 4 weeks of treatment, then every 3 months; vitamin $B_{12}$ deficiency (increased risk of neutropenia); if anaemia or myelosuppression occur, reduce dose or interrupt treatment according to product literature, or consider other treatment; elderly; **interactions:** Appendix 1 (zidovudine)

**Contra-indications** abnormally low neutrophil counts or haemoglobin concentration (consult product literature); neonates with hyperbilirubinaemia requiring treatment other than phototherapy, or with raised transaminase (consult product literature); acute porphyria (section 9.8.2); breast-feeding (Appendix 5)

**Side-effects** see notes above; also anaemia (may require transfusion), taste disturbance, chest pain, influenza-like symptoms, paraesthesia, neuropathy, convulsions, dizziness, drowsiness, anxiety, depression, loss of mental acuity, myopathy, gynaecomastia, urinary frequency, sweating, pruritus, pigmentation of nails, skin and oral mucosa

**Dose**

- By mouth, ADULT and CHILD body-weight over 30 kg, 250–300 mg twice daily; CHILD body-weight 4–9 kg, 12 mg/kg twice daily; body-weight 9–30 kg, 9 mg/kg twice daily *or* body-weight 8–14 kg, 100 mg twice daily; body-weight 14–21 kg, 100 mg in the morning and 200 mg in the evening; body-weight 21–28 kg, 200 mg twice daily; body-weight 28–30 kg, 200–250 mg twice daily
- Prevention of maternal-fetal HIV transmission, seek specialist advice (combination therapy preferred)
- Patients temporarily unable to take zidovudine by mouth, by intravenous infusion over 1 hour, 1–2 mg/kg every 4 hours (approximating to 1.5–3 mg/kg every 4 hours by mouth) usually for not more than 2 weeks; CHILD 3 months–12 years, 80–160 mg/m² every 6 hours (120 mg/m² every 6

**5**
**Infections**

hours approximates to 180 mg/m$^2$ every 6 hours by mouth)

**Retrovir®** (GSK) [PoM]

Capsules, zidovudine 100 mg (white/blue band), net price 100-cap pack = £110.98; 250 mg (blue/white/dark blue band), 40-cap pack = £110.98

Oral solution, sugar-free, strawberry-flavoured, zidovudine 50 mg/5 mL, net price 200-mL pack with 10-mL oral syringe = £22.20

Injection, zidovudine 10 mg/mL. For dilution and use as an intravenous infusion. Net price 20-mL vial = £11.14

◢**With lamivudine**

For **cautions**, **contra-indications**, and **side-effects** see under individual drugs

**Combivir®** (GSK) [PoM]

Tablets, f/c, scored, zidovudine 300 mg, lamivudine 150 mg, net price 60-tab pack = £318.60

Dose ADULT and CHILD body-weight over 30 kg, 1 tablet twice daily; CHILD body-weight 14–21 kg, half a tablet twice daily; body-weight 21–30 kg, half a tablet in the morning and one tablet in the evening

Note Tablets may be crushed and mixed with semi-solid food or liquid just before administration

◢**With abacavir and lamivudine**

See under Abacavir

---

## Protease inhibitors

**Cautions** Protease inhibitors are associated with hyperglycaemia and should be used with caution in diabetes (see Lipodystrophy Syndrome, p. 340). Caution is also needed in patients with haemophilia who may be at increased risk of bleeding. Protease inhibitors should be used with caution in hepatic impairment (Appendix 2); the risk of hepatic side-effects is increased in patients with chronic hepatitis B or C. Atazanavir, darunavir, fosamprenavir, and tipranavir may be used at usual doses in patients with renal impairment, but other protease inhibitors should be used with caution in renal impairment (Appendix 3). Protease inhibitors should also be used with caution during pregnancy (Appendix 4).

**Contra-indications** Protease inhibitors should not be given to patients with acute porphyria (but see section 9.8.2) or to women who are breast-feeding (Appendix 5).

**Side-effects** Side-effects of the protease inhibitors include gastro-intestinal disturbances (including diarrhoea, nausea, vomiting, abdominal pain, flatulence), anorexia, hepatic dysfunction, pancreatitis; blood disorders including anaemia, neutropenia, and thrombocytopenia; sleep disturbances, fatigue, headache, dizziness, paraesthesia, myalgia, myositis, rhabdomyolysis; taste disturbances; rash, pruritus, Stevens-Johnson syndrome, hypersensitivity reactions including anaphylaxis; see also notes above for lipodystrophy and metabolic effects (Lipodystrophy Syndrome), and Osteonecrosis.

### ▮ ATAZANAVIR

**Indications** HIV infection in combination with other antiretroviral drugs

**Cautions** see notes above; also concomitant use with drugs that prolong PR interval; cardiac conduction disorders; predisposition to QT interval prolongation (including electrolyte disturbances, concomitant use of drugs that prolong QT interval); interactions: Appendix 1 (atazanavir)

**Contra-indications** see notes above

**Side-effects** see notes above; also mouth ulcers, dry mouth, hypertension, syncope, chest pain, dyspnoea, peripheral neuropathy, abnormal dreams, amnesia, disorientation, depression, anxiety, weight changes, increased appetite, gynaecomastia, nephrolithiasis, urinary frequency, haematuria, proteinuria, arthralgia, and alopecia; *rarely* hepatosplenomegaly, oedema, palpitation, and abnormal gait; also reported, cholelithiasis, cholecystitis, and torsade de pointes

**Dose**

● With low-dose ritonavir and food, ADULT over 18 years, 300 mg once daily with ritonavir 100 mg once daily

**Reyataz®** (Bristol-Myers Squibb) [PoM]

Capsules, atazanavir (as sulphate) 150 mg (dark blue/light blue), net price 60-cap pack = £303.38; 200 mg (dark blue), 60-cap pack = £303.38; 300 mg (red/blue), 30-cap pack = £303.38. Label: 5, 21

### ▮ DARUNAVIR

**Indications** HIV infection in combination with other antiretroviral drugs

**Cautions** see notes above; also sulphonamide sensitivity; interactions: Appendix 1 (darunavir)

**Contra-indications** see notes above

**Side-effects** see notes above; also haematemesis, myocardial infarction, angina, QT interval prolongation, syncope, bradycardia, tachycardia, palpitation, hypertension, flushing, peripheral oedema, dyspnoea, cough, peripheral neuropathy, anxiety, confusion, memory impairment, depression, abnormal dreams, convulsions, increased appetite, weight changes, pyrexia, hypothyroidism, osteoporosis, gynaecomastia, erectile dysfunction, reduced libido, dysuria, polyuria, nephrolithiasis, renal failure, arthralgia, visual disturbances, dry eyes, conjunctival hyperaemia, rhinorrhoea, throat irritation, dry mouth, stomatisis, nail discoloration, acne, seborrhoeic dermatitis, eczema, increased sweating, and alopecia

**Dose**

● With low-dose ritonavir, ADULT over 18 years previously treated with antiretroviral therapy, 600 mg twice daily

● With low-dose ritonavir, ADULT over 18 years not previously treated with antiretroviral therapy, 800 mg once daily

Missed dose If a dose is more than 6 hours late on the twice daily regimen (or more than 12 hours late on the once daily regimen), the missed dose should not be taken and the next dose should be taken at the normal time

**Prezista®** (Janssen-Cilag) ▼ [PoM]

Tablets, f/c, darunavir (as ethanolate) 300 mg (orange), net price 120-tab pack = £446.70; 400 mg (light orange), 60-tab pack = £297.80; 600 mg (orange), 60-tab pack = £446.70. Label: 21

## FOSAMPRENAVIR

Note Fosamprenavir is a pro-drug of amprenavir

**Indications** HIV infection in combination with other antiretroviral drugs

**Cautions** see notes above; **interactions:** Appendix 1 (fosamprenavir)

Rash Rash may occur, usually in the second week of therapy; discontinue permanently if severe rash with systemic or allergic symptoms or, mucosal involvement; if rash mild or moderate, may continue without interruption—usually resolves within 2 weeks and may respond to antihistamines

**Contra-indications** see notes above

**Side-effects** see notes above; also reported, rash including rarely Stevens-Johnson syndrome (see also Rash above)

**Dose**

- With low-dose ritonavir, ADULT and CHILD over 6 years, body-weight over 39 kg, 700 mg twice daily; CHILD over 6 years, body-weight 25–39 kg, 18 mg/kg twice daily

  Note 700 mg fosamprenavir is equivalent to approx. 600 mg amprenavir

**Telzir®** (GSK) PoM

Tablets, f/c, pink, fosamprenavir (as calcium) 700 mg, net price 60-tab pack = £274.92

Oral suspension, fosamprenavir (as calcium) 50 mg/mL, net price 225-mL pack (grape-bubblegum-and peppermint-flavoured) (with 10-mL oral syringe) = £73.31. Counselling, administration

Counselling In adults, oral suspension should be taken on an empty stomach; in children under 18 years, oral suspension should be taken with food

## INDINAVIR

**Indications** HIV infection in combination with nucleoside reverse transcriptase inhibitors

**Cautions** see notes above; also ensure adequate hydration (risk of nephrolithiasis especially in children); patients at risk of nephrolithiasis (monitor for nephrolithiasis); **interactions:** Appendix 1 (indinavir)

**Contra-indications** see notes above

**Side-effects** see notes above; also reported, dry mouth, hypoaesthesia, dry skin, hyperpigmentation, alopecia, paronychia, interstitial nephritis (with medullary calcification and cortical atrophy in asymptomatic severe leucocyturia), nephrolithiasis (may require interruption or discontinuation; more frequent in children), dysuria, haematuria, crystalluria, proteinuria, pyuria (in children), pyelonephritis; haemolytic anaemia

**Dose**

- 800 mg every 8 hours; CHILD and ADOLESCENT 4–17 years, 500 mg/m² every 8 hours (max. 800 mg every 8 hours); CHILD under 4 years, safety and efficacy not established

**Crixivan®** (MSD) PoM

Capsules, indinavir (as sulphate), 200 mg, net price 360-cap pack = £226.28; 400 mg, 180-cap pack = £226.28. Label: 27, counselling, administration

Counselling Administer 1 hour before or 2 hours after a meal; may be administered with a low-fat light meal; in combination with didanosine tablets, allow 1 hour between each drug (antacids in didanosine tablets reduce absorption of indinavir); in combination with low-dose ritonavir, give with food

Note Dispense in original container (contains desiccant)

## LOPINAVIR WITH RITONAVIR

**Indications** HIV infection in combination with other antiretroviral drugs

**Cautions** see notes above; concomitant use with drugs that prolong QT or PR interval; cardiac conduction disorders, structural heart disease; pancreatitis (see below); **interactions:** Appendix 1 (lopinavir, ritonavir)

Pancreatitis Signs and symptoms suggestive of pancreatitis (including raised serum lipase) should be evaluated—discontinue if pancreatitis diagnosed

**Contra-indications** see notes above

**Side-effects** see notes and Cautions above; also electrolyte disturbances in children; *less commonly* dysphagia, appetite changes, weight changes, cholecystitis, hypertension, myocardial infarction, palpitation, thrombophlebitis, vasculitis, chest pain, oedema, dyspnoea, cough, agitation, anxiety, amnesia, ataxia, hypertonia, confusion, depression, abnormal dreams, extrapyramidal effects, neuropathy, influenza-like syndrome, Cushing's syndrome, hypothyroidism, menorrhagia, amenorrhoea, sexual dysfunction, breast enlargement, dehydration, nephritis, hypercalciuria, lactic acidosis, arthralgia, hyperuricaemia, abnormal vision, otitis media, tinnitus, dry mouth, sialadenitis, mouth ulceration, periodontitis, acne, alopecia, dry skin, sweating, skin discoloration, nail disorders, *rarely* prolonged PR interval

**Dose**

- See preparations below

**Kaletra®** (Abbott) PoM

Tablets, pale yellow, f/c, lopinavir 100 mg, ritonavir 25 mg, net price 60-tab pack = £76.85. Label: 25

Dose CHILD over 2 years with body-weight under 40 kg and body surface area 0.5–0.9 m², 2 tablets twice daily; body surface area 0.9–1.4 m², 3 tablets twice daily

Tablets, yellow, f/c, lopinavir 200 mg, ritonavir 50 mg, net price 120-tab pack = £307.39. Label: 25

Dose ADULT and CHILD with body surface area greater than 1.4 m² or body-weight 40 kg and over, 2 tablets twice daily

Oral solution, lopinavir 400 mg, ritonavir 100 mg/5 mL, net price 5×60-mL packs = £307.39. Label: 21

Excipients include propylene glycol 153 mg/mL (see Excipients, p. 2), alcohol 42%

Dose 5 mL twice daily with food; CHILD 2–12 years 2.9 mL/m² twice daily with food, max. 5 mL twice daily

## NELFINAVIR

**Indications** HIV infection in combination with other antiretroviral drugs

**Cautions** see notes above; **interactions:** Appendix 1 (nelfinavir)

**Contra-indications** see notes above

**Side-effects** see notes above; also reported, fever

**Dose**

- 1.25 g twice daily *or* 750 mg 3 times daily; CHILD 3–13 years, initially 50–55 mg/kg twice daily (max. 1.25 g twice daily) *or* 25–30 mg/kg 3 times daily (max. 750 mg 3 times daily)

**Viracept®** (Roche) PoM

Tablets, blue, f/c, nelfinavir (as mesilate) 250 mg, net price 300-tab pack = £262.51. Label: 21

## RITONAVIR

**Indications** HIV infection in combination with other antiretroviral drugs; low doses used to increase effect of some protease inhibitors

**Cautions** see notes above; concomitant use with drugs that prolong PR interval; cardiac conduction disorders, structural heart disease; pancreatitis (see below); **interactions:** Appendix 1 (ritonavir)
Pancreatitis Signs and symptoms suggestive of pancreatitis (including raised serum lipase) should be evaluated—discontinue if pancreatitis diagnosed

**Contra-indications** see notes above

**Side-effects** see notes and Cautions above; also diarrhoea (may impair absorption—close monitoring required), vasodilatation, cough, throat irritation, anxiety, perioral and peripheral paraesthesia, hyperaesthesia, fever, decreased blood thyroxine concentration, electrolyte disturbances, raised uric acid, dry mouth, mouth ulcers, and sweating; *less commonly* increased prothrombin time and dehydration; syncope, postural hypotension, seizures, menorrhagia, and renal failure also reported

**Dose**

- Initially 300 mg every 12 hours for 3 days, increased in steps of 100 mg every 12 hours over not longer than 14 days to 600 mg every 12 hours; CHILD over 2 years initially 250 mg/m² every 12 hours, increased by 50 mg/m² at intervals of 2–3 days to 350 mg/m² every 12 hours (max. 600 mg every 12 hours)
- Low-dose booster to increase effect of other protease inhibitors, 100–200 mg once or twice daily

**Norvir®** (Abbott) [PoM]
Capsules, ritonavir 100 mg, net price 84-cap pack = £94.35. Label 21
Excipients include alcohol 12%

Oral solution, sugar-free, ritonavir 400 mg/5 mL, net price 5 × 90-mL packs (with measuring cup) = £403.20. Label: 21, counselling, administration
Counselling Oral solution contains 43% alcohol; bitter taste can be masked by mixing with chocolate milk; do not mix with water, measuring cup must be dry

◄With lopinavir
See under Lopinavir with ritonavir

## SAQUINAVIR

**Indications** HIV infection in combination with other antiretroviral drugs

**Cautions** see notes above; concomitant use of garlic (avoid garlic capsules—reduces plasma-saquinavir concentration); **interactions:** Appendix 1 (saquinavir)

**Contra-indications** see notes above

**Side-effects** see notes above; also dyspnoea, increased appetite, peripheral neuropathy, convulsions, changes in libido, renal impairment, dry mouth, and alopecia

**Dose**

- With low-dose ritonavir, ADULT and ADOLESCENT over 16 years, 1 g every 12 hours

**Invirase®** (Roche) [PoM]
Capsules, brown/green, saquinavir (as mesilate) 200 mg, net price 270-cap pack = £230.70. Label: 21
Tablets, orange, f/c, saquinavir (as mesilate) 500 mg, net price 120-tab pack = £256.33. Label: 21

## TIPRANAVIR

**Indications** HIV infection resistant to other protease inhibitors, in combination with other antiretroviral drugs in patients previously treated with antiretrovirals

**Cautions** see notes above; also patients at risk of increased bleeding from trauma, surgery or other pathological conditions; concomitant use of drugs that increase risk of bleeding; **interactions:** Appendix 1 (tipranavir)
Hepatotoxicity Potentially life-threatening hepatotoxicity reported; monitor liver function before treatment then every 2 weeks for 1 month, then every 3 months. Discontinue if signs or symptoms of hepatitis develop or if liver-function abnormality develops (consult product literature)

**Contra-indications** see notes above

**Side-effects** see notes above; also dyspnoea, anorexia, peripheral neuropathy, influenza-like symptoms, renal impairment and photosensitivity; *rarely* dehydration

**Dose**

- With low-dose ritonavir, ADULT over 18 years, 500 mg twice daily

**Aptivus®** (Boehringer Ingelheim) ▼ [PoM]
Capsules, pink, tipranavir 250 mg, net price 120–cap pack = £441.00. Label: 5, 21
Excipients include ethanol 100 mg per capsule

# Non-nucleoside reverse transcriptase inhibitors

## EFAVIRENZ

**Indications** HIV infection in combination with other antiretroviral drugs

**Cautions** chronic hepatitis B or C (greater risk of hepatic side-effects), hepatic impairment (avoid if severe; Appendix 2); severe renal impairment (Appendix 3); pregnancy (Appendix 4); elderly; history of mental illness or seizures; **interactions:** Appendix 1 (efavirenz)
Rash Rash, usually in the first 2 weeks, is the most common side-effect; discontinue if severe rash with blistering, desquamation, mucosal involvement or fever; if rash mild or moderate, may continue without interruption—usually resolves within 1 month
Psychiatric disorders Patients or their carers should be advised to seek immediate medical attention if symptoms such as severe depression, psychosis or suicidal ideation occur

**Contra-indications** acute porphyria (but see section 9.8.2); breast-feeding (Appendix 5)

**Side-effects** rash including Stevens-Johnson syndrome (see Rash above); abdominal pain, diarrhoea, nausea, vomiting; anxiety, depression, sleep disturbances, abnormal dreams, dizziness, headache, fatigue, impaired concentration (administration at bedtime especially in first 2–4 weeks reduces CNS effects); pruritus; *less commonly* pancreatitis, hepatitis, psychosis, mania, suicidal ideation, amnesia, ataxia, convulsions, and blurred vision; also reported hepatic failure, raised serum cholesterol (see Lipodystrophy Syndrome, p. 340), gynaecomastia, photosensitivity; see also Osteonecrosis, p. 341

**Dose**

- See preparations below

**Sustiva®** (Bristol-Myers Squibb) `PoM`

Capsules, efavirenz 50 mg (yellow/white), net price 30-cap pack = £16.73; 200 mg (yellow), 90-cap pack = £200.27. Label: 23

Dose ADULT and CHILD over 3 years, body-weight 13–15 kg, 200 mg once daily; body-weight 15–20 kg, 250 mg once daily; body-weight 20–25 kg, 300 mg once daily; body-weight 25–32.5 kg, 350 mg once daily; body-weight 32.5–40 kg, 400 mg once daily; body-weight 40 kg and over, 600 mg once daily

Tablets, f/c, yellow, efavirenz 600 mg, net price 30-tab pack = £200.27. Label: 23

Dose ADULT and CHILD, body-weight over 40 kg, 600 mg once daily

Oral solution, sugar-free, strawberry and mint flavour, efavirenz 30 mg/mL, net price 180-mL pack = £53.84

Dose ADULT and CHILD over 5 years, body-weight 13–15 kg, 270 mg once daily; body-weight 15–20 kg, 300 mg once daily; body-weight 20–25 kg, 360 mg once daily; body-weight 25–32.5 kg, 450 mg once daily; body-weight 32.5–40 kg, 510 mg once daily; body-weight 40 kg and over, 720 mg once daily; CHILD 3–5 years, body-weight 13–15 kg, 360 mg once daily; body-weight 15–20 kg, 390 mg once daily; body-weight 20–25 kg, 450 mg once daily; body-weight 25–32.5 kg, 510 mg once daily

Note The bioavailability of *Sustiva®* oral solution is lower than that of the capsules and tablets; the oral solution is **not** interchangeable with either capsules or tablets on a milligram-for-milligram basis

◢**With emtricitabine and tenofovir**

See under Tenofovir

## ETRAVIRINE

**Indications** in combination with other antiretroviral drugs (including a boosted protease inhibitor) for HIV infection resistant to other non-nucleoside reverse transcriptase inhibitors and protease inhibitors

**Cautions** chronic hepatitis B or C (greater risk of hepatic side-effects); hepatic impairment (avoid if severe; Appendix 2); pregnancy (Appendix 4); **interactions**: Appendix 1 (etravirine)
Rash Rash, usually in the second week, is the most common side-effect and appears more frequently in women; discontinue if severe rash; if rash mild or moderate, may continue without interruption—usually resolves within 2 weeks

**Contra-indications** acute porphyria (but see section 9.8.2); breast-feeding (Appendix 5)

**Side-effects** rash (rarely including Stevens-Johnson syndrome; see also Rash above); gastro-oesophageal reflux, nausea, abdominal pain, flatulence, gastritis; myocardial infarction, hypertension; peripheral neuropathy; diabetes, hyperlipidaemia (see also Lipodystrophy Syndrome, p. 340); renal failure; anaemia; *less commonly* pancreatitis, haematemesis, hepatitis, angina, bronchospasm, drowsiness, malaise, gynaecomastia, blurred vision, dry mouth, and sweating; also reported, haemorrhagic stroke; see also Osteonecrosis, p. 341

### Dose

● ADULT over 18 years, 200 mg twice daily after food
Missed dose If a dose is more than 6 hours late, the missed dose should not be taken and the next dose should be taken at the normal time

**Intelence®** (Janssen-Cilag) ▼ `PoM`

Tablets, etravirine 100 mg, net price 120-tab pack = £307.35. Label: 21
Note Dispense in original container (contains desiccant). Patients with swallowing difficulties may disperse tablets in a glass of water just before administration

## ■ NEVIRAPINE

**Indications** HIV infection in combination with other antiretroviral drugs

**Cautions** hepatic impairment (see below and Appendix 2); chronic hepatitis B or C, high CD4 cell count, and women (all at greater risk of hepatic side-effects—manufacturer advises avoid in women with CD4 cell count greater than 250 cells/mm³ or in men with CD4 cell count greater than 400 cells/mm³ unless potential benefit outweighs risk); pregnancy (Appendix 4); **interactions**: Appendix 1 (nevirapine)
Hepatic disease Potentially life-threatening hepatotoxicity including fatal fulminant hepatitis reported usually in first 6 weeks; close monitoring required during first 18 weeks; monitor liver function before treatment then every 2 weeks for 2 months then after 1 month and then regularly; discontinue permanently if abnormalities in liver function tests accompanied by hypersensitivity reaction (rash, fever, arthralgia, myalgia, lymphadenopathy, hepatitis, renal impairment, eosinophilia, granulocytopenia); suspend if severe abnormalities in liver function tests but no hypersensitivity reaction—discontinue permanently if significant liver function abnormalities recur; monitor patient closely if mild to moderate abnormalities in liver function tests with no hypersensitivity reaction
Rash Rash, usually in first 6 weeks, is most common side-effect; incidence reduced if introduced at low dose and dose increased gradually; monitor closely for skin reactions during first 18 weeks; discontinue permanently if severe rash or if rash accompanied by blistering, oral lesions, conjunctivitis, facial oedema, general malaise or hypersensitivity reactions; if rash mild or moderate may continue without interruption but dose should not be increased until rash resolves
Counselling Patients should be told how to recognise hypersensitivity reactions and advised to discontinue treatment and seek immediate medical attention if severe skin reaction, hypersensitivity reactions, or symptoms of hepatitis develop

**Contra-indications** acute porphyria (but see section 9.8.2); breast-feeding (Appendix 5); severe hepatic impairment; post-exposure prophylaxis

**Side-effects** rash including Stevens-Johnson syndrome and rarely, toxic epidermal necrolysis (see also Cautions above); nausea, hepatitis (see also Hepatic Disease above), headache; *less commonly* vomiting, abdominal pain, fatigue, fever, and myalgia; *rarely* diarrhoea, angioedema, anaphylaxis, hypersensitivity reactions (may involve hepatic reactions and rash, see Hepatic Disease above), arthralgia, anaemia, and granulocytopenia (more frequent in children); *very rarely* neuropsychiatric reactions; see also Osteonecrosis, p. 341

### Dose

● ADULT and CHILD over 16 years, 200 mg once daily for first 14 days then (if no rash present) 200 mg twice daily; NEONATE and CHILD under 8 years, 150 mg/m² (max. 200 mg) once daily for first 14 days, then (if no rash present) 150 mg/m² (max. 200 mg) twice daily or 4 mg/kg (max. 200 mg) once daily for first 14 days then (if no rash present) 7 mg/kg (max. 200 mg) twice daily; CHILD 8–16 years, 150 mg/m² (max. 200 mg) once daily for first 14 days then (if no rash present) 150 mg/m² (max. 200 mg) twice daily or 4 mg/kg (max. 200 mg) once daily for first 14 days then (if no rash present) 4 mg/kg (max. 200 mg) twice daily
Note Dose titration should be repeated if treatment interrupted for more than 7 days

**Viramune®** (Boehringer Ingelheim) `PoM`

Tablets, nevirapine 200 mg, net price 60-tab pack = £170.00. Counselling, hypersensitivity reactions

Suspension, nevirapine 50 mg/5 mL, net price 240-mL pack = £50.40. Counselling, hypersensitivity reactions

**Infections**

**5**

## Other antiretrovirals

### ENFUVIRTIDE

**Indications** HIV infection in combination with other antiretroviral drugs for resistant infection or for patients intolerant to other antiretroviral regimens

**Cautions** chronic hepatitis B or C (possibly greater risk of hepatic side-effects); hepatic impairment (Appendix 2); pregnancy (Appendix 4)

Hypersensitivity reactions Hypersensitivity reactions including rash, fever, nausea, vomiting, chills, rigors, low blood pressure, respiratory distress, glomerulonephritis, and raised liver enzymes reported; discontinue immediately if any signs or symptoms of systemic hypersensitivity develop and do not rechallenge

Counselling Patients should be told how to recognise signs of hypersensitivity, and advised to discontinue treatment and seek immediate medical attention if symptoms develop

**Contra-indications** breast-feeding (Appendix 5)

**Side-effects** injection-site reactions; pancreatitis, gastro-oesophageal reflux disease, anorexia, weight loss; hypertriglyceridaemia; peripheral neuropathy, asthenia, tremor, anxiety, nightmares, irritability, impaired concentration, vertigo; pneumonia, sinusitis, influenza-like illness; diabetes mellitus; haematuria; renal calculi, lymphadenopathy; myalgia; conjunctivitis; dry skin, acne, erythema, skin papilloma; *less commonly* hypersensitivity reactions (see Cautions); see also Osteonecrosis, p. 341

**Dose**

- By subcutaneous injection, ADULT and ADOLESCENT over 16 years, 90 mg twice daily; CHILD 6–15 years, 2 mg/kg twice daily (max. 90 mg twice daily)

**Fuzeon®** (Roche) [PoM]
Injection, powder for reconstitution, enfuvirtide 108 mg (= enfuvirtide 90 mg/mL when reconstituted with 1.1 mL Water for Injections), net price 108-mg vial = £18.39 (with solvent, syringe, and alcohol swabs). Counselling, hypersensitivity reactions

### MARAVIROC

**Indications** CCR5-tropic HIV infection in combination with other antiretroviral drugs in patients previously treated with antiretrovirals

**Cautions** cardiovascular disease; chronic hepatitis B or C; hepatic impairment (Appendix 2); renal impairment (Appendix 3); pregnancy (Appendix 4); **interactions**: Appendix 1 (maraviroc)

**Contra-indications** breast-feeding (Appendix 5)

**Side-effects** nausea, vomiting, abdominal pain, dyspepsia, constipation, diarrhoea; cough; dizziness, paraesthesia, asthenia, sleep disturbances, headache, weight loss; muscle spasms, back pain; taste disturbances; rash, pruritus; *less commonly* pancreatitis, hepatic cirrhosis, rectal bleeding, myocardial infarction, myocardial ischaemia, bronchospasm, seizures, hallucinations, loss of consciousness, polyneuropathy, pancytopenia, neutropenia, lymphadenopathy, renal failure, polyuria, and myositis; see also Osteonecrosis, p. 341

**Dose**

- ADULT over 18 years, 300 mg twice daily

**Celsentri®** (Pfizer) ▼ [PoM]
Tablets, blue, f/c, maraviroc, 150 mg, net-price 60-tab pack = £551.10; 300 mg, 60-tab pack = £551.10

### RALTEGRAVIR

**Indications** in combination with other antiretroviral drugs for HIV infection resistant to multiple antiretrovirals

**Cautions** risk factors for myopathy or rhabdomyolysis; chronic hepatitis B or C (greater risk of hepatic side-effects); hepatic impairment (Appendix 2); pregnancy (Appendix 4); **interactions**: Appendix 1 (raltegravir)

**Contra-indications** breast-feeding (Appendix 5)

**Side-effects** diarrhoea, nausea, vomiting, abdominal pain, flatulence, constipation; hypertriglyceridaemia; dizziness, headache, insomnia, asthenia; arthralgia; pruritus, hyperhidrosis, rash (Stevens-Johnson syndrome reported); *less commonly* gastritis, hepatitis, pancreatitis, dry mouth, gastro-oesophageal reflux, glossitis, taste disturbances, pain on swallowing, peptic ulcer, rectal bleeding, lipodystrophy (see Lipodystrophy Syndrome, p. 340), palpitation, ventricular extrasystoles, chest pain, facial oedema, dysphonia, epistaxis, nasal congestion, pharyngeal erythema, drowsiness, abnormal dreams, anxiety, appetite changes, depression, pyrexia, chills, carpal tunnel syndrome, tremor, peripheral neuropathy, erectile dysfunction, gynaecomastia, menopausal symptoms, renal failure, polyuria, anaemia, neutropenia, musculoskeletal pain, visual disturbances, acne, and dry skin; *also reported* suicidal ideation; see also Osteonecrosis, p. 341

**Dose**

- ADULT and CHILD over 16 years, 400 mg twice daily

**Isentress®** (MSD) ▼ [PoM]
Tablets, pink, f/c, raltegravir (as potassium salt) 400 mg, net price 60-tab pack = £647.29. Label: 25

## 5.3.2 Herpesvirus infections

### 5.3.2.1 Herpes simplex and varicella–zoster infection

The two most important herpesvirus pathogens are herpes simplex virus (herpesvirus hominis) and varicella–zoster virus.

**Herpes simplex infections** Herpes infection of the mouth and lips and in the eye is generally associated with herpes simplex virus serotype 1 (HSV-1); other areas of the skin may also be infected, especially in immunodeficiency. Genital infection is most often associated with HSV-2 and also HSV-1. Treatment of herpes simplex infection should start as early as possible and usually within 5 days of the appearance of the infection.

In individuals with good immune function, mild infection of the eye (ocular herpes, section 11.3.3) and of the lips (herpes labialis or cold sores, section 13.10.3) is treated with a topical antiviral drug. Primary herpetic gingivostomatitis is managed by changes to diet and with analgesics (section 12.3.2). Severe infection, neonatal herpes infection or infection in immunocompromised individuals requires treatment with a systemic antiviral drug. Primary or recurrent genital herpes simplex infection is treated with an antiviral drug given by mouth. Persistence of a lesion or recurrence in an immunocompromised patient may signal the development of resistance.

Specialist advice should be sought for systemic treatment of herpes simplex infection in pregnancy.

**Varicella-zoster infections** Regardless of immune function and the use of any immunoglobulins, neonates with *chickenpox* should be treated with a parenteral antiviral to reduce the risk of severe disease. Chickenpox in otherwise healthy children between 1 month and 12 years is usually mild and antiviral treatment is not usually required.

Chickenpox is more severe in adolescents and adults than in children; antiviral treatment started within 24 hours of the onset of rash may reduce the duration and severity of symptoms in otherwise healthy adults and adolescents. Antiviral treatment is generally recommended in immunocompromised patients and those at special risk (e.g. because of severe cardiovascular or respiratory disease or chronic skin disorder); in such cases, an antiviral is given for 10 days with at least 7 days of parenteral treatment.

Pregnant women who develop severe chickenpox may be at risk of complications, especially varicella pneumonia. Specialist advice should be sought for the treatment of chickenpox during pregnancy.

Those who have been exposed to chickenpox and are at special risk of complications may require prophylaxis with varicella-zoster immunoglobulin (see under Disease Specific Immunoglobulins, section 14.5.2).

In *herpes zoster* (shingles) systemic antiviral treatment can reduce the severity and duration of pain, reduce complications, and reduce viral shedding. Treatment with the antiviral should be started within 72 hours of the onset of rash and is usually continued for 7–10 days. Immunocompromised patients at high risk of disseminated or severe infection should be treated with a parenteral antiviral drug.

Chronic pain which persists after the rash has healed (postherpetic neuralgia) requires specific management (section 4.7.3).

**Choice** Aciclovir is active against herpesviruses but does not eradicate them. Uses of aciclovir include systemic treatment of varicella–zoster and the systemic and topical treatment of herpes simplex infections of the skin and mucous membranes (section 13.10.3). It is used by mouth for severe herpetic stomatitis (see also p. 620). Aciclovir eye ointment (section 11.3.3) is used for herpes simplex infections of the eye; it is combined with systemic treatment for ophthalmic zoster.

**Famciclovir**, a prodrug of penciclovir, is similar to aciclovir and is licensed for use in herpes zoster and genital herpes. Penciclovir itself is used as a cream for herpes simplex labialis (section 13.10.3).

**Valaciclovir** is an ester of aciclovir, licensed for herpes zoster and herpes simplex infections of the skin and mucous membranes (including genital herpes); it is also licensed for preventing cytomegalovirus disease following renal transplantation. Famciclovir or valaciclovir are suitable alternatives to aciclovir for oral lesions associated with herpes zoster. Valaciclovir once daily may reduce the risk of transmitting genital herpes to heterosexual partners—specialist advice should be sought.

**Idoxuridine** (section 13.10.3) has been used topically for treating herpes simplex infections of the skin and external genitalia with variable results. Its value in the treatment of shingles is unclear.

**Inosine pranobex** has been used by mouth for herpes simplex infections; its effectiveness remains unproven.

## ACICLOVIR
(Acyclovir)

**Indications** herpes simplex and varicella–zoster (see also under Dose)

**Cautions** maintain adequate hydration (especially with infusion or high doses, or during renal impairment (Appendix 3)); elderly (risk of neurological reactions); pregnancy (Appendix 4); breast-feeding (Appendix 5); **interactions:** Appendix 1 (aciclovir)

**Side-effects** nausea, vomiting, abdominal pain, diarrhoea, headache, fatigue, rash, urticaria, pruritus, photosensitivity; *very rarely* hepatitis, jaundice, dyspnoea, neurological reactions (including dizziness, confusion, hallucinations, convulsions, ataxia, dysarthria, and drowsiness), acute renal failure, anaemia, thrombocytopenia and leucopenia; on *intravenous infusion*, severe local inflammation (sometimes leading to ulceration), and *very rarely* agitation, tremors, psychosis and fever

**Dose**

- By mouth, non-genital herpes simplex, treatment, 200 mg (400 mg in the immunocompromised or if absorption impaired) 5 times daily, usually for 5 days (longer if new lesions appear during treatment or if healing incomplete); CHILD 1 month–2 years, half adult dose, over 2 years, adult dose

  Genital herpes simplex, treatment, 200 mg 5 times daily *or* 400 mg 3 times daily usually for 5 days (longer if new lesions appear during treatment or if healing is incomplete); increased in immunocompromised or HIV-positive patients to 400 mg 5 times daily for 7–10 days during *first episode or* 400 mg 3 times daily for 5–10 days during *recurrent infection*

  Herpes simplex, prevention of recurrence, 200 mg 4 times daily *or* 400 mg twice daily, possibly reduced to 200 mg 2 or 3 times daily; increased to 400 mg 3 times daily if recurrences occur on standard suppressive therapy; therapy interrupted every 6–12 months to reassess recurrence frequency—consider restarting after two or more recurrences

  Herpes simplex, prophylaxis in the immunocompromised, 200–400 mg 4 times daily; CHILD 1 month–2 years, half adult dose, over 2 years, adult dose

  Varicella and herpes zoster, treatment, 800 mg 5 times daily for 7 days; CHILD, varicella, 1 month–2 years 200 mg 4 times daily for 5 days; 2–6 years 400 mg 4 times daily for 5 days; 6–12 years 800 mg 4 times daily for 5 days

  Attenuation of chickenpox (if varicella–zoster immunoglobulin not indicated) [unlicensed use], ADULT and CHILD 40 mg/kg daily in 4 divided doses for 7 days starting 1 week after exposure

- By intravenous infusion, treatment of herpes simplex in the immunocompromised, severe initial genital herpes, and varicella–zoster, 5 mg/kg every 8 hours usually for 5 days, doubled to 10 mg/kg every 8 hours in varicella–zoster in the immunocompromised and in simplex encephalitis (usually given for at least 10 days in encephalitis, possibly for

**5**

**Infections**

14–21 days); prophylaxis of herpes simplex in the immunocompromised, 5 mg/kg every 8 hours
**Note** To avoid excessive dosage in obese patients, parenteral dose should be calculated on the basis of ideal weight for height

NEONATE and INFANT up to 3 months, herpes simplex, 20 mg/kg every 8 hours for 14 days (21 days if CNS involvement); varicella–zoster [unlicensed use] 10–20 mg/kg every 8 hours for at least 7 days; CHILD 3 months–12 years, herpes simplex or varicella–zoster, 250 mg/m² every 8 hours usually for 5 days, doubled to 500 mg/m² every 8 hours for varicella–zoster in the immunocompromised and in simplex encephalitis (usually given for at least 10 days in encephalitis, possibly for 14–21 days)

- By topical application, see section 13.10.3 (skin) and section 11.3.3 (eye)

**Note** Aciclovir doses in BNF may differ from those in product literature

**Aciclovir** (Non-proprietary) (PoM)
Tablets, aciclovir 200 mg, net price 25-tab pack = £4.01; 400 mg, 56-tab pack = £9.28; 800 mg, 35-tab pack = £11.42. Label: 9
Brands include *Virovir®*
**Dental prescribing on NHS** Aciclovir Tablets 200 mg or 800 mg may be prescribed

Dispersible tablets, aciclovir 200 mg, net price 25-tab pack = £2.20; 400 mg, 56-tab pack = £6.80; 800 mg, 35-tab pack = £6.70. Label: 9

Suspension, aciclovir 200 mg/5 mL, net price 125 mL = £31.33; 400 mg/5 mL, 100 mL = £35.25. Label: 9
**Dental prescribing on NHS** Aciclovir Oral Suspension 200 mg/5 mL may be prescribed

Intravenous infusion, powder for reconstitution, aciclovir (as sodium salt), net price 250-mg vial = £9.13; 500-mg vial = £20.22
Electrolytes Na⁺ 1.1 mmol/250-mg vial

Intravenous infusion, aciclovir (as sodium salt), 25 mg/mL, net price 10-mL (250-mg) vial = £10.37; 20-mL (500-mg) vial = £19.21; 40-mL (1-g) vial = £40.44
Electrolytes Na⁺ 1.16 mmol/250-mg vial

**Zovirax®** (GSK) (PoM)
Tablets, all dispersible, f/c, aciclovir 200 mg, net price 25-tab pack = £18.07; 800 mg (scored, *Shingles Treatment Pack*), 35-tab pack = £67.13. Label: 9

Suspension, both off-white, sugar-free, aciclovir 200 mg/5 mL (banana-flavoured), net price 125 mL = £29.53; 400 mg/5 mL (*Double Strength Suspension*, orange-flavoured) 100 mL = £33.01. Label: 9

Intravenous infusion, powder for reconstitution, aciclovir (as sodium salt), net price 250-mg vial = £9.75; 500-mg vial = £18.07
Electrolytes Na⁺ 1.1 mmol/250-mg vial

## FAMCICLOVIR

**Note** Famciclovir is a pro-drug of penciclovir

**Indications** treatment of herpes zoster, acute genital herpes simplex and suppression of recurrent genital herpes

**Cautions** hepatic impairment (Appendix 2); renal impairment (Appendix 3); pregnancy (Appendix 4) and breast-feeding (Appendix 5); **interactions:** Appendix 1 (famciclovir)

**Side-effects** *rarely* nausea, headache, confusion; *very rarely* vomiting, jaundice, dizziness, drowsiness, hal-

lucinations, rash (including Stevens-Johnson syndrome), and pruritus; abdominal pain and fever have been reported in immunocompromised patients

**Dose**

- Herpes zoster, 250 mg 3 times daily for 7 days *or* 750 mg once daily for 7 days (in immunocompromised, 500 mg 3 times daily for 10 days)
- Genital herpes, *first episode*, 250 mg 3 times daily for 5 days (longer if new lesions appear during treatment or if healing incomplete); *recurrent infection*, 125 mg twice daily for 5 days (in immunocompromised or HIV-positive patients, all episodes, 500 mg twice daily for 5–10 days)
- Genital herpes, suppression, 250 mg twice daily (in HIV patients, 500 mg twice daily); therapy interrupted every 6–12 months to reassess recurrence frequency—consider restarting after two or more recurrences
- CHILD not recommended

**Famvir®** (Novartis) (PoM)
Tablets, all f/c, famciclovir 125 mg, net price 10-tab pack = £37.12; 250 mg, 15-tab pack = £111.35, 21-tab pack = £155.87; 56-tab pack = £415.67; 500 mg, 14-tab pack = £207.86, 30-tab pack = £445.28, 56-tab pack = £831.46; 750 mg, 7-tab pack = £148.79. Label: 9

## INOSINE PRANOBEX ◢
(Inosine acedoben dimepranol)

**Indications** see under Dose

**Cautions** renal impairment (Appendix 3); history of gout or hyperuricaemia

**Contra-indications** pregnancy

**Side-effects** reversible increase in serum and urinary uric acid; *less commonly* nausea, vomiting, epigastric discomfort, headache, vertigo, fatigue, arthralgia, rashes and itching; *rarely* diarrhoea, constipation, anxiety, sleep disturbances, and polyuria

**Dose**

- Mucocutaneous herpes simplex, 1 g 4 times daily for 7–14 days
- Adjunctive treatment of genital warts, 1 g 3 times daily for 14–28 days
- Subacute sclerosing panencephalitis, 50–100 mg/kg daily in 6 divided doses

**Imunovir®** (Ardern) (PoM) ◢
Tablets, scored, inosine pranobex 500 mg, net price 100-tab pack = £39.50. Label: 9

## VALACICLOVIR
**Note** Valaciclovir is a pro-drug of aciclovir

**Indications** treatment of herpes zoster; treatment of initial and suppression of recurrent herpes simplex infections of skin and mucous membranes including initial and recurrent genital herpes; reduction of transmission of genital herpes; prevention of cytomegalovirus disease following renal transplantation

**Cautions** see under Aciclovir; hepatic impairment (Appendix 2); renal impairment (Appendix 3)

**Side-effects** see under Aciclovir but neurological reactions more frequent with high doses

**Dose**

- Herpes zoster, 1 g 3 times daily for 7 days; CHILD 12–18 years, see *BNF for Children*

- Herpes simplex, *first episode*, 500 mg twice daily for 5 days, longer if new lesions appear during treatment or if healing incomplete (1 g twice daily for 10 days for genital herpes in immunocompromised or HIV-positive patients); *recurrent infection*, 500 mg twice daily for 5 days (1 g twice daily for 5–10 days for genital herpes in immunocompromised or HIV-positive patients); CHILD 12–18 years, see *BNF for Children*
- Herpes simplex, suppression, 500 mg daily in 1–2 divided doses (in immunocompromised or HIV positive patients, 500 mg twice daily); therapy interrupted every 6–12 months to reassess recurrence frequency—consider restarting after two or more recurrences; CHILD 12–18 years, see *BNF for Children*
- Reduction of transmission of genital herpes, seek specialist advice, 500 mg once daily to be taken by the infected partner
- Prevention of cytomegalovirus disease following renal transplantation (preferably starting within 72 hours of transplantation), ADULT and CHILD over 12 years, 2 g 4 times daily usually for 90 days

**Valtrex® (GSK)** PoM

Tablets, f/c, valaciclovir (as hydrochloride) 250 mg, net price 60-tab pack = £130.87; 500 mg, 10-tab pack = £21.86, 42-tab pack = £91.61. Label: 9

### 5.3.2.2 Cytomegalovirus infection

Recommendations for the optimum maintenance therapy of cytomegalovirus (CMV) infections and the duration of treatment are subject to rapid change.

**Ganciclovir** is related to aciclovir but it is more active against cytomegalovirus; it is also much more toxic than aciclovir and should therefore be prescribed only when the potential benefit outweighs the risks. Ganciclovir is administered by intravenous infusion for the *initial treatment* of CMV infection. Ganciclovir causes profound myelosuppression when given with zidovudine; the two should not normally be given together particularly during initial ganciclovir therapy. The likelihood of ganciclovir resistance increases in patients with a high viral load or in those who receive the drug over a long duration; cross-resistance to cidofovir is common.

**Valaciclovir** (see p. 350) is licensed for prevention of cytomegalovirus disease following renal transplantation.

**Valganciclovir** is an ester of ganciclovir which is licensed for the *initial treatment* and *maintenance treatment* of CMV retinitis in AIDS patients. Valganciclovir is also licensed for preventing CMV disease following solid organ transplantation from a cytomegalovirus-positive donor.

**Foscarnet** is also active against cytomegalovirus; it is toxic and can cause renal impairment.

**Cidofovir** is given in combination with probenecid for CMV retinitis in AIDS patients when ganciclovir and foscarnet are contra-indicated. Cidofovir is nephrotoxic.

For local treatment of CMV retinitis, see section 11.3.3.

### CIDOFOVIR

**Indications** cytomegalovirus retinitis in AIDS patients for whom other drugs are inappropriate

**Cautions** monitor renal function (serum creatinine and urinary protein) and neutrophil count within 24 hours before each dose; co-treatment with probenecid and prior hydration with intravenous fluids necessary to minimise potential nephrotoxicity (see below); diabetes mellitus (increased risk of ocular hypotony); interactions: Appendix 1 (cidofovir)

Nephrotoxicity Do not initiate treatment in renal impairment (assess creatinine clearance and proteinuria—consult product literature); discontinue treatment and give intravenous fluids if renal function deteriorates—consult product literature

Ocular disorders Regular ophthalmological examinations recommended; iritis and uveitis have been reported which may respond to a topical corticosteroid with or without a cycloplegic drug—discontinue cidofovir if no response to topical corticosteroid or if condition worsens, or if iritis or uveitis recurs after successful treatment

**Contra-indications** renal impairment (creatinine clearance 55 mL/minute or less); concomitant administration of potentially nephrotoxic drugs (discontinue potentially nephrotoxic drugs at least 7 days before starting cidofovir); pregnancy (avoid pregnancy during and for 1 month after treatment, men should not father a child during or within 3 months of treatment; Appendix 4), breast-feeding (Appendix 5)

**Side-effects** nephrotoxicity (see Cautions above); nausea, vomiting; dyspnoea; headache, fever, asthenia; neutropenia; decreased intra-ocular pressure, iritis, uveitis (see Cautions above); alopecia, rash; *less commonly* Fanconi syndrome; also reported, hearing impairment and pancreatitis

**Dose**

- Initial (induction) treatment, ADULT over 18 years, by intravenous infusion over 1 hour, 5 mg/kg once weekly for 2 weeks (give probenecid and intravenous fluids with each dose, see below)
- Maintenance treatment, beginning 2 weeks after completion of induction, ADULT over 18 years, by intravenous infusion over 1 hour, 5 mg/kg once every 2 weeks (give probenecid and intravenous fluids with each dose, see below)

Probenecid co-treatment By mouth (preferably after food), probenecid 2 g 3 hours before cidofovir infusion followed by probenecid 1 g at 2 hours and 1 g at 8 hours after the end of cidofovir infusion (total probenecid 4 g); for cautions, contraindications and side-effects of probenecid see section 10.1.4

Prior hydration Sodium chloride 0.9%, by intravenous infusion, 1 litre over 1 hour immediately before cidofovir infusion (if tolerated an additional 1 litre may be given over 1–3 hours, starting at the same time as the cidofovir infusion or immediately afterwards)

**Vistide® (Gilead)** PoM

Intravenous infusion, cidofovir 75 mg/mL, net price 5-mL vial = £653.22

Caution in handling Cidofovir is toxic and personnel should be adequately protected during handling and administration; if solution comes into contact with skin or mucosa, wash off immediately with water

### GANCICLOVIR

**Indications** life-threatening or sight-threatening cytomegalovirus infections in immunocompromised patients only; prevention of cytomegalovirus disease during immunosuppressive therapy following organ transplantation; local treatment of CMV retinitis (section 11.3.3)

**Cautions** close monitoring of full blood count (severe deterioration may require correction and possibly treatment interruption); history of cytopenia; low platelet count; potential carcinogen and teratogen; renal impairment (Appendix 3); radiotherapy; ensure

5

Infections

adequate hydration during intravenous administration; vesicant—infuse into vein with adequate flow preferably using plastic cannula; children (possible risk of long-term carcinogenic or reproductive toxicity—not for neonatal or congenital cytomegalovirus disease); **interactions:** Appendix 1 (ganciclovir)

**Contra-indications** pregnancy (ensure effective contraception during treatment and barrier contraception for men during and for at least 90 days after treatment; Appendix 4); breast-feeding; hypersensitivity to ganciclovir or aciclovir; abnormally low haemoglobin, neutrophil, or platelet counts (consult product literature)

**Side-effects** diarrhoea, nausea, vomiting, dyspepsia, abdominal pain, constipation, flatulence, dysphagia, hepatic dysfunction; dyspnoea, chest pain, cough; headache, insomnia, convulsions, dizziness, neuropathy, depression, anxiety, confusion, abnormal thinking, fatigue, weight loss, anorexia; infection, fever, night sweats; anaemia, leucopenia, thrombocytopenia, pancytopenia, renal impairment; myalgia, arthralgia; macular oedema, retinal detachment, vitreous floaters, eye pain; ear pain, taste disturbance; dermatitis, pruritus; injection-site reactions; *less commonly* mouth ulcers, pancreatitis, arrhythmias, hypotension, anaphylactic reactions, psychosis, tremor, male infertility, haematuria, disturbances in hearing and vision, and alopecia

**Dose**
- By intravenous infusion, initially (induction) 5 mg/kg every 12 hours for 14–21 days for treatment or for 7–14 days for prevention; maintenance (for patients at risk of relapse of retinitis) 6 mg/kg daily on 5 days per week *or* 5 mg/kg daily until adequate recovery of immunity; if retinitis progresses initial induction treatment may be repeated; CHILD under 18 years, see *BNF for Children*

**Cymevene®** (Roche) ▼PoM
Intravenous infusion, powder for reconstitution, ganciclovir (as sodium salt). Net price 500-mg vial = £30.37
Electrolytes Na⁺ 2 mmol/500-mg vial
Caution in handling Ganciclovir is toxic and personnel should be adequately protected during handling and administration; if solution comes into contact with skin or mucosa, wash off immediately with soap and water

## ▌FOSCARNET SODIUM

**Indications** cytomegalovirus retinitis in AIDS patients; mucocutaneous herpes simplex virus infections unresponsive to aciclovir in immunocompromised patients

**Cautions** renal impairment (reduce dose; consult product literature; monitor electrolytes, particularly calcium and magnesium; monitor serum creatinine every second day during induction and every week during maintenance; ensure adequate hydration; avoid rapid infusion; **interactions:** Appendix 1 (foscarnet)

**Contra-indications** pregnancy; breast-feeding (Appendix 5)

**Side-effects** nausea, vomiting, diarrhoea (occasionally constipation and dyspepsia), abdominal pain, anorexia; changes in blood pressure and ECG; headache, fatigue, mood disturbances (including psychosis), asthenia, paraesthesia, convulsions, tremor, dizziness, and other neurological disorders; rash;

impairment of renal function including acute renal failure; hypocalcaemia (sometimes symptomatic) and other electrolyte disturbances; abnormal liver function tests; decreased haemoglobin concentration, leucopenia, granulocytopenia, thrombocytopenia; thrombophlebitis if given undiluted by peripheral vein; genital irritation and ulceration (due to high concentrations excreted in urine); isolated reports of pancreatitis

**Dose**
- CMV retinitis, by intravenous infusion, induction 60 mg/kg every 8 hours for 2–3 weeks then maintenance, 60 mg/kg daily, increased to 90–120 mg/kg if tolerated; if retinitis progresses on maintenance dose, repeat induction regimen
- Mucocutaneous herpes simplex infection, by intravenous infusion, 40 mg/kg every 8 hours for 2–3 weeks or until lesions heal

**Foscavir®** (AstraZeneca) PoM
Intravenous infusion, foscarnet sodium hexahydrate 24 mg/mL, net price 250-mL bottle = £34.49

## ▌VALGANCICLOVIR

Note Valganciclovir is a pro-drug of ganciclovir

**Indications** induction and maintenance treatment of cytomegalovirus retinitis in AIDS patients; prevention of cytomegalovirus disease following solid organ transplantation from a cytomegalovirus-positive donor.

**Cautions** see under Ganciclovir

**Side-effects** see under Ganciclovir

**Dose**
- CMV retinitis, induction, 900 mg twice daily for 21 days then 900 mg once daily; induction regimen may be repeated if retinitis progresses
- Prevention of cytomegalovirus disease following solid organ transplantation (starting within 10 days of transplantation), 900 mg once daily for 100 days
- CHILD under 18 years not recommended
Note Oral valganciclovir 900 mg twice daily is equivalent to intravenous ganciclovir 5 mg/kg twice daily

**Valcyte®** (Roche) PoM
Tablets, pink, f/c, valganciclovir (as hydrochloride) 450 mg, net price 60-tab pack = £1103.28. Label: 21
Caution in handling Valganciclovir is a potential teratogen and carcinogen and caution is advised for handling of broken tablets; if broken tablets come into contact with skin or mucosa, wash off immediately with water

## 5.3.3 Viral hepatitis

Treatment for viral hepatitis should be initiated by a specialist. The management of uncomplicated acute viral hepatitis is largely symptomatic. Early treatment of acute hepatitis C with interferon alfa [unlicensed indication] may reduce the risk of chronic infection. Hepatitis B and hepatitis C viruses are major causes of chronic hepatitis. For details on immunisation against hepatitis A and B infections, see section 14.4 (active immunisation), section 14.5.1 (passive immunisation against hepatitis A), and section 14.5.2 (passive immunisation against hepatitis B).

**Chronic Hepatitis B**   Peginterferon alfa-2a (section 8.2.4) is an option for the initial treatment of chronic hepatitis B (see NICE guidance below) and may be preferable to **interferon alfa**. The use of peginterferon alfa-2a and interferon alfa is limited by a response rate of 30–40% and relapse is frequent. Treatment should be discontinued if no improvement occurs after 4 months. The manufacturers of peginterferon alfa-2a and interferon alfa contraindicate use in decompensated liver disease but low doses can be used with great caution in these patients. Although interferon alfa is contra-indicated in patients receiving immunosuppressant treatment (or who have received it recently), cautious use of peginterferon alfa-2a may be justified in some cases.

**Adefovir dipivoxil, entecavir, lamivudine** (see p. 342), **telbivudine**, or **tenofovir disoproxil** (see p. 343) are licensed for the treatment of chronic hepatitis B. Lamivudine or adefovir can also be used in patients with decompensated liver disease. Hepatitis B viruses with reduced susceptibility to lamivudine have emerged following extended therapy. Adefovir is effective in lamivudine-resistant chronic hepatitis B, but telbivudine should not be used because cross-resistance may occur (see also NICE guidance below). Entecavir is effective in patients not previously treated with nucleoside analogues (see NICE guidance below). Resistance to entecavir can occur in patients who have received lamivudine.

If there is no toxicity or loss in efficacy, treatment with adefovir, entecavir, lamivudine, telbivudine, or tenofovir is usually continued until 6 months after adequate seroconversion has occurred. Treatment with lamivudine or adefovir is continued long-term in patients with decompensated liver disease.

Tenofovir, or a combination of tenofovir with either emtricitabine or lamivudine may be used with other antiretrovirals, as part of 'highly active antiretroviral therapy' (section 5.3.1) in patients who require treatment for both HIV and chronic hepatitis B. If patients infected with both HIV and chronic hepatitis B only require treatment for chronic hepatitis B, they should receive antivirals that are not active against HIV, such as peginterferon alfa-2a. Management of these patients should be co-ordinated between HIV and hepatology specialists.

---

**NICE guidance**
**Adefovir dipivoxil and peginterferon alfa-2a for chronic hepatitis B (February 2006)**
Peginterferon alfa-2a is an option for the initial treatment of chronic hepatitis B.
Adefovir dipivoxil is recommended as an option for the treatment of chronic hepatitis B if:
- treatment with interferon alfa or peginterferon alfa-2a has been unsuccessful, or
- a relapse occurs after successful initial therapy, or
- treatment with interferon alfa or peginterferon alfa-2a is poorly tolerated or contra-indicated.

Adefovir dipivoxil should not be given before treatment with lamivudine. It may be used either alone or in combination with lamivudine when treatment with lamivudine has resulted in viral resistance, or if lamivudine resistance is likely to occur rapidly and adversely affect the outcome.

---

**NICE guidance**
**Entecavir and telbivudine for chronic hepatitis B (August 2008)**
Entecavir is an option for the treatment of chronic hepatitis B.
Telbivudine is not recommended for the treatment of chronic hepatitis B. Patients currently receiving telbivudine can continue treatment until they and their clinician consider it appropriate to stop.

---

**Chronic Hepatitis C**   Before starting treatment, the genotype of the infecting hepatitis C virus should be determined and the viral load measured as this may affect the choice and duration of treatment. A combination of **ribavirin** (see p. 356) and **peginterferon alfa** (section 8.2.4) is used for the treatment of chronic hepatitis C (see NICE guidance, below). The combination of ribavirin and interferon alfa is less effective than the combination of peginterferon alfa and ribavirin. Peginterferon alfa alone should be used if ribavirin is contra-indicated or not tolerated. Ribavirin monotherapy is ineffective.

---

**NICE guidance**
**Peginterferon alfa and ribavirin for mild chronic hepatitis C (August 2006)**
The combination of peginterferon alfa and ribavirin can be used for treating mild chronic hepatitis C in patients over 18 years. Alternatively, treatment can be delayed until the disease has reached a moderate stage ('watchful waiting'). Peginterferon alfa alone can be used if ribavirin is contra-indicated or not tolerated.

---

**NICE guidance**
**Peginterferon alfa, interferon alfa, and ribavirin for moderate to severe chronic hepatitis C (January 2004)**
The combination of peginterferon alfa and ribavirin should be used for treating moderate to severe chronic hepatitis C in patients aged over 18 years:
- not previously treated with interferon alfa or peginterferon alfa;
- treated previously with interferon alfa alone or in combination with ribavirin;
- whose condition did not respond to peginterferon alfa alone or responded but subsequently relapsed.

Peginterferon alfa alone should be used if ribavirin is contra-indicated or not tolerated. Interferon alfa for either monotherapy or combined therapy should be used only if neutropenia and thrombocytopenia are a particular risk. Patients receiving interferon alfa may be switched to peginterferon alfa.
Full guidance available at www.nice.org.uk/TA075.

---

### ADEFOVIR DIPIVOXIL

**Indications**   chronic hepatitis B infection with *either* compensated liver disease with evidence of viral replication, and histologically documented active liver inflammation and fibrosis *or* decompensated liver disease

**Cautions**   monitor liver function tests every 3 months, and viral and serological markers for hepatitis B every

3–6 months; discontinue if deterioration in liver function, hepatic steatosis, progressive hepatomegaly or unexplained lactic acidosis; recurrent hepatitis may occur on discontinuation; monitor renal function before treatment then every 3 months, more frequently in renal impairment (Appendix 3) or in patients receiving nephrotoxic drugs; pregnancy (Appendix 4); elderly; HIV infection (particularly if uncontrolled—theoretical risk of HIV resistance)

**Contra-indications** breast-feeding (Appendix 5)

**Side-effects** nausea, vomiting, dyspepsia, abdominal pain, flatulence, diarrhoea; asthenia, headache; renal failure; hypophosphataemia; rash and pruritus; also reported pancreatitis

**Dose**

- ADULT over 18 years, 10 mg once daily

**Hepsera®** (Gilead) [PoM]
Tablets, adefovir dipivoxil 10 mg, net price 30-tab pack = £302.71

## ENTECAVIR

**Indications** chronic hepatitis B infection with compensated liver disease, evidence of viral replication, and histologically documented active liver inflammation or fibrosis

**Cautions** monitor liver function tests every 3 months, and viral and serological markers for hepatitis B every 3–6 months; discontinue if deterioration in liver function, hepatic steatosis, progressive hepatomegaly or unexplained lactic acidosis; recurrent hepatitis may occur on discontinuation; HIV infection—risk of HIV resistance in patients not receiving 'highly active antiretroviral therapy'; renal impairment (Appendix 3); pregnancy (Appendix 4)

**Contra-indications** breast-feeding (Appendix 5)

**Side-effects** nausea, vomiting, dyspepsia, diarrhoea, raised serum amylase and lipase; headache, fatigue, dizziness, sleep disturbances; less commonly thrombocytopenia; also reported, rash

**Dose**

- ADULT over 18 years, not previously treated with nucleoside analogues, 500 micrograms once daily
- ADULT over 18 years with lamivudine-resistant chronic hepatitis B, 1 mg once daily
Counselling To be taken at least 2 hours before or 2 hours after food

**Baraclude®** (Bristol-Myers Squibb) ▼ [PoM]
Tablets, f/c, entecavir (as monohydrate) 500 micrograms (white), net price 30-tab pack = £363.26; 1 mg (pink), 30-tab pack = £363.26. Counselling, administration

Oral solution, entecavir (as monohydrate) 50 micrograms/mL, net price 210-mL pack (orange-flavoured) = £423.80. Counselling, administration

## TELBIVUDINE

**Indications** chronic hepatitis B infection with compensated liver disease, evidence of viral replication, and histologically documented active liver inflammation or fibrosis

**Cautions** monitor liver function tests every 3 months and viral and serological markers of hepatitis B every 3–6 months; discontinue if deterioration in liver function, hepatic steatosis, progressive hepatomegaly

or unexplained lactic acidosis; hepatitis may recur on discontinuation; renal impairment (Appendix 3); pregnancy (Appendix 4); **interactions:** Appendix 1 (telbivudine)

Counselling Patients should be advised to promptly report unexplained muscle pain, tenderness, or weakness, or numbness, tingling or burning sensations

**Contra-indications** breast-feeding (Appendix 5)

**Side-effects** nausea, diarrhoea, abdominal pain, raised serum amylase and lipase; cough; dizziness, headache, fatigue; rash; less commonly; taste disturbance, arthralgia, myalgia, myopathy (discontinue treatment), and peripheral neuropathy

**Dose**

- ADULT and CHILD over 16 years, 600 mg once daily

**Sebivo®** (Novartis) ▼ [PoM]
Tablets, f/c, telbivudine 600 mg, net price 28-tab pack = £290.33. Counselling, muscle effects, peripheral neuropathy

## 5.3.4 Influenza

For advice on immunisation against influenza, see section 14.4.

**Oseltamivir** and **zanamivir** reduce replication of influenza A and B viruses by inhibiting viral neuraminidase. They are most effective for the treatment of influenza if started within a few hours of the onset of symptoms; they are licensed for use within 48 hours (within 36 hours for zanamivir in children) of the first symptoms. In otherwise healthy individuals they reduce the duration of symptoms by about 1–1.5 days. Oseltamivir or zanamivir can reduce the risk of complications from influenza in the elderly and in patients with chronic disease (see also NICE guidance, p. 355).

Oseltamivir and zanamivir are licensed for post-exposure prophylaxis of influenza when influenza is circulating in the community. Oseltamivir should be given within 48 hours of exposure to influenza while zanamivir should be given within 36 hours of exposure to influenza (see also NICE guidance, p. 355). Oseltamivir and zanamivir are also licensed for use in exceptional circumstances (e.g. when vaccination does not cover the infecting strain) to prevent influenza in an epidemic.

There is evidence that some strains of influenza A virus have reduced susceptibility to oseltamivir.

**Amantadine** is licensed for prophylaxis and treatment of influenza A but it is no longer recommended (see NICE guidance).

Information on pandemic influenza, avian influenza, and swine influenza may be found at www.dh.gov.uk/pandemicflu and at www.hpa.org.uk

**Pregnancy and breast-feeding** Although safety data are limited, either oseltamivir or zanamivir can be used in women who are pregnant or breast-feeding when the potential benefit outweighs the risk (e.g. during a pandemic). Zanamivir is the preferred drug during pregnancy; however, oseltamivir is recommended during severe infection or when zanamivir cannot be used. Oseltamivir is the preferred drug in women who are breast-feeding.

**Oseltamivir, zanamivir, and amantadine for prophylaxis and treatment of influenza (September 2008 and February 2009)**
The drugs described here are not a substitute for vaccination, which remains the most effective way of preventing illness from influenza.
- Amantadine is **not** recommended for prophylaxis or treatment of influenza.
- Oseltamivir *or* zanamivir are **not** recommended for seasonal prophylaxis against influenza.
- When influenza is circulating in the community[1], either oseltamivir or zanamivir is recommended (in accordance with UK licensing) for post-exposure prophylaxis in at-risk patients who are not effectively protected by influenza vaccine, and who have been in close contact with someone suffering from influenza-like illness in the same household or residential setting. Oseltamivir should be given within 48 hours of exposure to influenza while zanamivir should be given within 36 hours of exposure to influenza.
- When influenza is circulating in the community[1], either oseltamivir or zanamivir is recommended (in accordance with UK licensing) for the treatment of influenza in at-risk patients who can start treatment within 48 hours (within 36 hours for zanamivir in children) of the onset of symptoms.
- During local outbreaks of influenza-like illness, when there is a high level of certainty that influenza is present, either oseltamivir or zanamivir may be used for post-exposure prophylaxis or treatment in at-risk patients (regardless of influenza vaccination) living in long-term residential or nursing homes.

At risk patients include those aged over 65 years *or* those who have one or more of the following conditions:
- chronic respiratory disease (including asthma and chronic obstructive pulmonary disease);
- chronic heart disease;
- chronic renal disease;
- chronic liver disease;
- chronic neurological disease;
- immunosuppression;
- diabetes mellitus.

This guidance does not cover the circumstances of a pandemic, an impending pandemic, or a widespread epidemic of a new strain of influenza to which there is little or no immunity in the community.

## AMANTADINE HYDROCHLORIDE

**Indications** see under Dose; parkinsonism (section 4.9.1)

**Cautions** see section 4.9.1

**Contra-indications** see section 4.9.1

**Side-effects** see section 4.9.1

1. National surveillance schemes, including those run by the Health Protection Agency, should be used to indicate when influenza is circulating in the community.

**Dose**
- Influenza A (see also notes above), ADULT and CHILD over 10 years, treatment, 100 mg daily for 4–5 days; prophylaxis, 100 mg daily usually for 6 weeks *or* with influenza vaccination for 2–3 weeks after vaccination

**Lysovir®** (Alliance) (PoM)
Capsules, red-brown, amantadine hydrochloride 100 mg, net price 5-cap pack = £2.40, 14-cap pack = £5.76. Counselling, driving

**Symmetrel®** (Alliance) (PoM)
Section 4.9.1

## OSELTAMIVIR

**Indications** see notes above

**Cautions** renal impairment (Appendix 3); pregnancy (see p. 354 and Appendix 4); breast-feeding (see p. 354 and Appendix 5)

**Side-effects** nausea, vomiting, abdominal pain, diarrhoea; headache; conjunctivitis; *less commonly* eczema; also reported hepatitis, gastro-intestinal bleeding, arrhythmias, neuropsychiatric disorders (more frequent in children and adolescents), visual disturbances, Stevens-Johnson syndrome, and toxic epidermal necrolysis

**Dose**
- Prevention of influenza, ADULT and CHILD over 13 years, 75 mg once daily for 10 days for post-exposure prophylaxis; for up to 6 weeks during an epidemic; CHILD under 1 year see *BNF for Children*; 1–13 years, body-weight under 15 kg, 30 mg once daily, body-weight 15–23 kg, 45 mg once daily, body-weight 23–40 kg, 60 mg once daily, body-weight over 40 kg, adult dose
- Treatment of influenza, ADULT and CHILD over 13 years, 75 mg every 12 hours for 5 days; CHILD under 1 year see *BNF for Children*; 1–13 years, body-weight under 15 kg, 30 mg every 12 hours, body-weight 15–23 kg, 45 mg every 12 hours, body-weight 23–40 kg, 60 mg every 12 hours, body-weight over 40 kg, adult dose

[1]**Tamiflu®** (Roche) ▼ (PoM)
Capsules, oseltamivir (as phosphate) 30 mg (yellow), net price 10-cap pack = £7.86; 45 mg (grey), 10-cap pack = £15.72; 75 mg (grey-yellow), 10-cap pack = £15.72. Label: 9
Note If suspension not available, capsules can be opened and the contents mixed with a small amount of sweetened food, such as yoghurt, just before administration

Suspension, sugar-free, tutti-frutti-flavoured, oseltamivir (as phosphate) for reconstitution with water, 60 mg/5 mL, net price 75 mL = £15.72. Label: 9
Excipients include sorbitol 1.7 g/5 mL
Note Solutions prepared by 'special order' manufacturers may be a different concentration

1. (NHS) except for the treatment and prophylaxis of influenza as indicated in the notes above and NICE guidance; endorse prescription 'SLS'

## ZANAMIVIR

**Indications** see notes above

**Cautions** asthma and chronic pulmonary disease (risk of bronchospasm—short-acting bronchodilator should be available; avoid in severe asthma unless

5

Infections

close monitoring possible and appropriate facilities available to treat bronchospasm); uncontrolled chronic illness; other inhaled drugs should be administered before zanamivir; pregnancy (see p. 354 and Appendix 4); breast-feeding (see p. 354 and Appendix 5)

**Side-effects** *very rarely*, bronchospasm, respiratory impairment, angioedema, urticaria, and rash; also reported, neuropsychiatric disorders (especially in children and adolescents)

**Dose**

- By inhalation of powder, post-exposure prophylaxis of influenza, ADULT and CHILD over 5 years, 10 mg once daily for 10 days

  Prevention of influenza during an epidemic, ADULT and CHILD over 5 years, 10 mg once daily for up to 28 days

  Treatment of influenza, ADULT and CHILD over 5 years, 10 mg twice daily for 5 days

¹**Relenza®** (GSK) [PoM]

Dry powder for inhalation disks containing 4 blisters of zanamivir 5 mg/blister, net price 5 disks with *Diskhaler®* device = £16.36

1. [NHS] except for the treatment and prophylaxis of influenza as indicated in the notes above and NICE guidance; endorse prescription 'SLS'

## 5.3.5 Respiratory syncytial virus

**Ribavirin** (tribavirin) inhibits a wide range of DNA and RNA viruses. It is licensed for administration by inhalation for the treatment of severe bronchiolitis caused by the respiratory syncytial virus (RSV) in infants, especially when they have other serious diseases. However, there is no evidence that ribavirin produces clinically relevant benefit in RSV bronchiolitis. Ribavirin is given by mouth with peginterferon alfa or interferon alfa for the treatment of chronic hepatitis C infection (see Viral Hepatitis, p. 352). Ribavirin is also effective in Lassa fever [unlicensed indication].

**Palivizumab** is a monoclonal antibody licensed for preventing serious lower respiratory-tract disease caused by respiratory syncytial virus in children at high risk of the disease; it should be prescribed under specialist supervision and on the basis of the likelihood of hospitalisation. Palivizumab should be considered for children under 6 months with haemodynamically significant left-to-right shunt congenital heart disease or who have pulmonary hypertension. It should also be considered for children under 2 years *either* with chronic lung disease requiring oxygen at home (or have been on prolonged oxygen treatment) *or* with severe congenital immunodeficiency. Palivizumab can also be used for the first 6–12 months of life in a child born at under 35 weeks gestation who is considered by the specialist to be at special risk of hospitalisation.

## PALIVIZUMAB

**Indications** see notes above

**Cautions** moderate to severe acute infection or febrile illness; thrombocytopenia; serum-palivizumab concentration may be reduced after cardiac surgery

**Contra-indications** hypersensitivity to humanised monoclonal antibodies

**Side-effects** fever, injection-site reactions, nervousness; *less commonly* diarrhoea, vomiting, constipation, haemorrhage, rhinitis, cough, wheeze, pain, drowsiness, asthenia, hyperkinesia, leucopenia, and rash; *rarely* apnoea, hypersensitivity reactions (including anaphylaxis)

**Dose**

- By intramuscular injection (preferably in anterolateral thigh), 15 mg/kg once a month during season of RSV risk (child undergoing cardiac bypass surgery, 15 mg/kg as soon as stable after surgery, then once a month during season of risk); injection volume over 1 mL should be divided between more than one site

**Synagis®** (Abbott) ▼ [PoM]

Injection, powder for reconstitution, palivizumab, net price 50-mg vial = £360.40; 100-mg vial = £663.11

## RIBAVIRIN
(Tribavirin)

**Indications** severe respiratory syncytial virus bronchiolitis in infants and children; in combination with peginterferon alfa or interferon alfa for chronic hepatitis C in patients without liver decompensation (see also section 5.3.3)

**Cautions**

**Specific cautions for inhaled treatment** Maintain standard supportive respiratory and fluid management therapy; monitor electrolytes closely; monitor equipment for precipitation; pregnant women (and those planning pregnancy) should avoid exposure to aerosol

**Specific cautions for oral treatment** Exclude pregnancy before treatment; effective contraception essential during treatment and for 4 months after treatment in women and for 7 months after treatment in men; routine monthly pregnancy tests recommended; condoms must be used if partner of male patient is pregnant (ribavirin excreted in semen); severe hepatic dysfunction or decompensated cirrhosis (Appendix 2); renal impairment (Appendix 3); cardiac disease (assessment including ECG recommended before and during treatment—discontinue if deterioration); gout; determine full blood count, platelets, electrolytes, serum creatinine, liver function tests and uric acid before starting treatment and then on weeks 2 and 4 of treatment, then as indicated clinically—adjust dose if adverse reactions or laboratory abnormalities develop (consult product literature); eye examination recommended before treatment; eye examination also recommended during treatment if pre-existing ophthalmological disorder or if decrease in vision reported—discontinue treatment if ophthalmological disorder deteriorates or if new ophthalmological disorder develops; test thyroid function before treatment and then every 3 months in children

**Interactions**: Appendix 1 (ribavirin)

**Contra-indications** pregnancy (**important teratogenic risk**: see Cautions and Appendix 4); breast-feeding

**Specific contra-indications for oral treatment** Severe cardiac disease, including unstable or uncontrolled cardiac disease in previous 6 months; haemoglobinopathies; severe debilitating medical conditions; autoimmune disease (including autoimmune hepatitis); uncontrolled severe psychiatric condition; history of severe psychiatric condition in children

**Side-effects**

**Specific side-effects for inhaled treatment** Worsening respiration, bacterial pneumonia, and pneumothorax reported; rarely non-specific anaemia and haemolysis
**Specific side-effects for oral treatment** Haemolytic anaemia (anaemia may be improved by epoetin); also (in combination with peginterferon alfa or interferon alfa) nausea, vomiting, dyspepsia, abdominal pain, peptic ulcer, flatulence, diarrhoea, constipation, colitis, pancreatitis, appetite changes, weight loss, pulmonary embolism, chest pain, tachycardia, palpitation, syncope, cerebrovascular disease, peripheral oedema, changes in blood pressure, flushing, dyspnoea, cough, interstitial pneumonitis, sleep disturbances, abnormal dreams, asthenia, impaired concentration and memory, psychoses, anxiety, depression, suicidal ideation (more frequent in children), dizziness, tremor, hypertonia, seizures, ataxia, dysphonia, peripheral neuropathy, influenza-like symptoms, headache, hyperglycaemia, thyroid disorders, menstrual disturbances, reduced libido, impotence, prostatitis, micturition disorders, leucopenia, thrombocytopenia, aplastic anaemia, lymphadenopathy, hypocalcaemia, renal failure, hyperuricaemia, myalgia, arthralgia, systemic lupus erythematosus, vasculitis, sarcoidosis, eye changes (including blurred vision and retinopathy), rhinitis, tinnitus, hearing impairment, dry mouth, stomatitis, glossitis, taste disturbance, pharyngitis, gingivitis, rash (including very rarely Stevens-Johnson syndrome and toxic epidermal necrolysis), pruritus, urticaria, photosensitivity, psoriasis, alopecia, dry skin, increased sweating; in children also growth retardation (including decrease in height and weight), Raynaud's disease, hypertriglyceridaemia, hyperkinesia, testicular pain, virilism, tooth disorders, and skin discoloration

**Dose**

- See preparations below

**Copegus®** (Roche) [PoM]

Tablets, f/c, ribavirin 200 mg (pink), net price 42-tab pack = £111.11, 112-tab pack = £296.29, 168-tab pack – £444.43; 400 mg (red-brown), 56-tab pack = £296.29. Label: 21

**Dose** chronic hepatitis C (in combination with interferon alfa or peginterferon alfa), ADULT over 18 years, body-weight under 75 kg, 400 mg in the morning and 600 mg in the evening; body-weight 75 kg and over, 600 mg twice daily

**Note** Chronic hepatitis C genotype 2 or 3, or patients infected with HIV and hepatitis C require a lower dose of Copegus® (in combination with peginterferon alfa), usual dose 400 mg twice daily

**Rebetol®** (Schering-Plough) [PoM]

Capsules, ribavirin 200 mg, net price 84-cap pack = £163.80, 140-cap pack = £273.00, 168-cap pack = £327.60. Label: 21

Oral solution, ribavirin 200 mg/5 mL, net price 100 mL (bubble-gum-flavoured) = £68.38. Label: 21

**Dose** chronic hepatitis C, ADULT over 18 years (in combination with interferon alfa or peginterferon alfa), body-weight under 65 kg, 400 mg twice daily; body-weight 65–86 kg, 400 mg in the morning and 600 mg in the evening; body-weight 86–105 kg, 600 mg twice daily; body-weight over 105 kg, 600 mg in the morning and 800 mg in the evening; CHILD and ADOLESCENT 3–17 years (in combination with interferon alfa), body-weight under 47 kg, 15 mg/kg daily in 2 divided doses; body-weight 47–50 kg, 200 mg in the morning and 400 mg in the evening; body-weight 50–65 kg, 400 mg twice daily; body-weight over 65 kg, as adult

**Virazole®** (Valeant) [PoM]

Inhalation, ribavirin 6 g for reconstitution with 300 mL water for injections. Net price 3 × 6-g vials = £349.00

**Dose** bronchiolitis, by aerosol inhalation or nebulisation (via small particle aerosol generator) of solution containing 20 mg/mL for 12–18 hours for at least 3 days; max. 7 days

## 5.4 Antiprotozoal drugs

5.4.1 Antimalarials

5.4.2 Amoebicides

5.4.3 Trichomonacides

5.4.4 Antigiardial drugs

5.4.5 Leishmaniacides

5.4.6 Trypanocides

5.4.7 Drugs for toxoplasmosis

5.4.8 Drugs for pneumocystis pneumonia

Advice on specific problems available from:

**Advice for healthcare professionals**

HPA (Health Protection Agency) Malaria Reference Laboratory
www.hpa.org.uk/infections/topics_az/malaria
(020) 7636 3924 (prophylaxis only)

National Travel Health Network and Centre
0845 602 6712

Travel Medicine Team, Health Protection Scotland (registered users of Travax only)
www.travax.nhs.uk
(for registered users of the NHS Travax website only)
(0141) 300 1100 (weekdays 2–4 p.m. only)

Birmingham  (0121) 424 0357

Liverpool  (0151) 705 3100

London  0845 155 5000 (treatment)

Oxford  (01865) 225 430

**Advice for travellers**

Hospital for Tropical Diseases Travel Healthline
www.fitfortravel.nhs.uk
020 7950 7799

WHO advice on international travel and health
www.who.int/ith

National Travel Health Network and Centre (NaTHNaC)
www.nathnac.org/travel/index.htm

## 5.4.1 Antimalarials

Recommendations on the prophylaxis and treatment of malaria reflect guidelines agreed by UK malaria specialists.

The centres listed above should be consulted for advice on special problems.

## Treatment of malaria

If the infective species is **not known**, or if the infection is **mixed**, initial treatment should be as for *falciparum malaria* with quinine, Malarone® (proguanil with atovaquone), or Riamet® (artemether with lumefantrine). Falciparum malaria can progress rapidly in unprotected individuals and antimalarial treatment should be considered in those with features of severe malaria and possible exposure, even if the initial blood tests for the organism are negative.

5

Infections

**5  Infections**

## Falciparum malaria (treatment)

Falciparum malaria (malignant malaria) is caused by *Plasmodium falciparum*. In most parts of the world *P. falciparum* is now resistant to chloroquine which should not therefore be given for treatment.

Quinine, *Malarone®* (proguanil with atovaquone), or *Riamet®* (artemether with lumefantrine) can be given *by mouth* if the patient can swallow and retain tablets and there are no serious manifestations (e.g. impaired consciousness); quinine should be given *by intravenous infusion* (see below) if the patient is seriously ill or unable to take tablets. Mefloquine is now rarely used for treatment because of concerns about resistance.

*Oral.* The adult dosage regimen for **quinine** *by mouth* is:

600 mg (of quinine salt[1]) every 8 hours for 5–7 days *together with or followed by*
either doxycycline 200 mg once daily for 7 days
*or* clindamycin 450 mg every 8 hours for 7 days [unlicensed indication].

If the parasite is likely to be sensitive, **pyrimethamine** 75 mg with **sulfadoxine** 1.5 g may be given as a single dose [unlicensed] together with or after a course of quinine.

Alternatively, *Malarone®* or *Riamet®* may be given instead of quinine. It is not necessary to give doxycycline, clindamycin or pyrimethamine with sulfadoxine after *Malarone®* or *Riamet®* treatment.

The adult dose of *Malarone®* *by mouth* is:
4 ('standard') tablets once daily for 3 days.

The dose of *Riamet®* *by mouth* for adult with body-weight over 35 kg is:
4 tablets initially, followed by 5 further doses of 4 tablets each given at 8, 24, 36, 48, and 60 hours (total 24 tablets over 60 hours).

*Parenteral.* If the patient is seriously ill or unable to take tablets, **quinine** should be given *by intravenous infusion* [unlicensed]. The adult dosage regimen for quinine *by infusion* is:

loading dose[2] of 20 mg/kg[3] (up to maximum 1.4 g) of quinine salt[1] infused over 4 hours *then 8 hours after the start of the loading dose,* maintenance dose of 10 mg/kg[4] (up to maximum 700 mg) of quinine salt[1] infused over 4 hours every 8 hours (until patient can swallow tablets to complete the 7-day course *together with or followed by either* doxycycline or clindamycin as above).

Specialist advice should be sought in difficult cases (e.g. very high parasite count, deterioration on optimal doses of quinine, infection acquired in quinine-resistant areas of south east Asia) because intravenous **artesunate** may be available for 'named-patient' use.

1. Valid for quinine hydrochloride, dihydrochloride, and sulphate; not valid for quinine bisulphate which contains a correspondingly smaller amount of quinine.
2. In intensive care units the loading dose can alternatively be given as quinine salt[1] 7 mg/kg infused over 30 minutes followed immediately by 10 mg/kg infused over 4 hours then (after 8 hours) maintenance dose as described.
3. **Important:** the loading dose of 20 mg/kg should **not** be used if the patient has received quinine or mefloquine during the previous 12 hours.
4. Maintenance dose should be reduced to 5–7 mg/kg of quinine salt[1] in patients with severe renal impairment, severe hepatic impairment, or if parenteral treatment is required for more than 48 hours.

### Children

*Oral.* **Quinine** is well tolerated by children although the salts are bitter. The dosage regimen for quinine *by mouth* for children is:

10 mg/kg (of quinine salt[1]; max. 600 mg) every 8 hours for 7 days *together with or followed by*
**Clindamycin** 7–13 mg/kg (max. 450 mg) every 8 hours for 7 days [unlicensed indication]
*or* in children over 12 years, **doxycycline** 200 mg once daily for 7 days
*or* if the parasite is likely to be sensitive, **pyrimethamine** with **sulfadoxine** as a single dose [unlicensed]: up to 4 years and body-weight over 5 kg, pyrimethamine 12.5 mg with sulfadoxine 250 mg; 5–6 years, pyrimethamine 25 mg with sulfadoxine 500 mg; 7–9 years, pyrimethamine 37.5 mg with sulfadoxine 750 mg; 10–14 years, pyrimethamine 50 mg with sulfadoxine 1 g; 14–18 years, pyrimethamine 75 mg with sulfadoxine 1.5 g

Alternatively, *Malarone®* or *Riamet®* may be given instead of quinine; it is not necessary to give clindamycin, doxycycline, or pyrimethamine with sulfadoxine after *Malarone®* or *Riamet®* treatment. The dose regimen for *Malarone®* *by mouth* for children over 40 kg is the same as for adults (see above); the dose regimen for *Malarone®* for smaller children is reduced as follows:

body-weight 5–8 kg, 2 'paediatric' tablets once daily for 3 days; body-weight 9–10 kg, 3 'paediatric' tablets once daily for 3 days; body-weight 11–20 kg, 1 'standard' tablet once daily for 3 days; body-weight 21–30 kg, 2 'standard' tablets once daily for 3 days; body-weight 31–40 kg, 3 'standard' tablets once daily for 3 days.

The dose regimen of *Riamet®* *by mouth* for children over 12 years and body-weight over 35 kg is the same as for adults (see above). The dose regimen for *Riamet®* for children under 12 years is as follows:

body-weight 5–15 kg 1 tablet initially, followed by 5 further doses of 1 tablet each given at 8, 24, 36, 48, and 60 hours (total 6 tablets over 60 hours); body-weight 15–25 kg 2 tablets initially, followed by 5 further doses of 2 tablets each given at 8, 24, 36, 48, and 60 hours (total 12 tablets over 60 hours); body-weight 25–35 kg 3 tablets initially, followed by 5 further doses of 3 tablets each given at 8, 24, 36, 48, and 60 hours (total 18 tablets over 60 hours)

*Parenteral.* The dose regimen for quinine *by intravenous infusion* for children is calculated on a mg/kg basis as for adults (see above).

**Pregnancy** Falciparum malaria is particularly dangerous in pregnancy, especially in the last trimester. The adult treatment doses of oral and intravenous quinine given above (including the loading dose) can safely be given to pregnant women. Clindamycin 450 mg every 8 hours for 7 days [unlicensed indication] should be given with or after quinine. Doxycycline should be avoided in pregnancy (affects teeth and skeletal development); pyrimethamine with sulfadoxine, *Malarone®*, and *Riamet®* are also best avoided until more information is available.

# Benign malarias (treatment)

Benign malaria is usually caused by *Plasmodium vivax* and less commonly by *P. ovule* and *P. malariae*. **Chloroquine**[1] is the drug of choice for the treatment of benign malarias (but chloroquine-resistant *P. vivax* infection has been reported from Indonesia, New Guinea and some adjacent islands).

The adult dosage regimen for **chloroquine** *by mouth* is:

> initial dose of 620 mg of base *then*

> a single dose of 310 mg of base after 6 to 8 hours *then*

> a single dose of 310 mg of base daily for 2 days

> (approximate total cumulative dose of 25 mg/kg of base)

Chloroquine alone is adequate for *P. malariae* infections but in the case of *P. vivax* and *P. ovale*, a *radical cure* (to destroy parasites in the liver and thus prevent relapses) is required. This is achieved with **primaquine**[2] [unlicensed] given after chloroquine; in *P. vivax* infection primaquine is given in an adult dosage of 30 mg daily for 14 days and for *P. ovale* infection it is given in an adult dosage of 15 mg daily for 14 days.

**Children** The dosage regimen of chloroquine for benign malaria in children is:

> initial dose of 10 mg/kg of base (max. 620 mg) *then*

> a single dose of 5 mg/kg of base (max. 310 mg) after 6–8 hours *then*

> a single dose of 5 mg/kg of base (max. 310 mg) daily for 2 days

For a *radical cure*, primaquine[2] [unlicensed] is then given to children over 6 months of age; specialist advice should be sought for children under 6 months of age. In *P. vivax* infection primaquine is given in a dose of 500 micrograms/kg (max. 30 mg) daily for 14 days, and for *P. ovale* infection it is given in a dose of 250 micrograms/kg (max. 15 mg) daily for 14 days.

**Parenteral** If the patient is unable to take oral therapy, **quinine** can be given by *intravenous infusion* [unlicensed]. The dose (for adults and children) is 10 mg/kg[3] (max. 700 mg) of quinine salt[4] infused over 4 hours every 8 hours, changed to oral chloroquine as soon as the patient's condition permits.

**Pregnancy** The adult treatment doses of chloroquine can be given for benign malaria. In the case of *P. vivax* or *P. ovale*, however, the radical cure with primaquine should be **postponed** until the pregnancy is over; instead chloroquine should be continued at a dose of 310 mg each week during the pregnancy.

---

1. For the treatment of chloroquine-resistant benign malaria, *Malarone*® [unlicensed indication], quinine, or *Riamet*® [unlicensed indication] can be used; as with chloroquine, primaquine should be given for radical cure.
2. Before starting primaquine, blood should be tested for glucose-6-phosphate dehydrogenase (G6PD) activity since the drug can cause haemolysis in G6PD-deficient patients. Specialist advice should be obtained in G6PD deficiency; in mild G6PD deficiency primaquine in a dose for adults of 45 mg once a week (children 750 micrograms/kg once a week; max. 45 mg once a week) for 8 weeks, has been found useful and without undue harmful effects.
3. Maintenance dose should be reduced to 5–7 mg/kg of quinine salt[4] in patients with severe renal impairment, severe hepatic impairment, or if parenteral treatment is required for more than 48 hours.
4. Valid for quinine hydrochloride, dihydrochloride, and sulphate; not valid for quinine bisulphate which contains a correspondingly smaller amount of quinine.

# Prophylaxis against malaria

The recommendations on prophylaxis reflect guidelines agreed by UK malaria specialists; the advice is aimed at residents of the UK who travel to endemic areas. The choice of drug for a particular individual should take into account:

> risk of exposure to malaria;

> extent of drug resistance;

> efficacy of the recommended drugs;

> side-effects of the drugs;

> patient-related factors (e.g. age, pregnancy, renal or hepatic impairment, compliance with prophylactic regimen).

**Protection against bites** Prophylaxis is not absolute, and breakthrough infection can occur with any of the drugs recommended. Personal protection against being bitten is very important. Mosquito nets impregnated with permethrin provide the most effective barrier protection against insects; mats and vaporised insecticides are also useful. Diethyltoluamide (DEET) 20–50% in lotions, sprays, or roll-on formulations is safe and effective when applied to the skin of adults and children over 2 months of age. It can also be used during pregnancy and breast-feeding. The duration of protection varies according to the concentration of DEET and is longest for DEET 50%. Long sleeves and trousers worn after dusk also provide protection.

**Length of prophylaxis** In order to determine tolerance and to establish habit, prophylaxis should generally be started one week (preferably 2–3 weeks in the case of mefloquine) before travel into an endemic area (or if not possible at earliest opportunity up to 1 or 2 days before travel); *Malarone*® or doxycycline prophylaxis should be started 1–2 days before travel. Prophylaxis should be continued for **4 weeks after leaving** (except for *Malarone*® prophylaxis which should be stopped 1 week after leaving).

In those requiring long-term prophylaxis, chloroquine and proguanil may be used for periods of over 5 years. Mefloquine is licensed for up to 1 year (although it has been used for up to 3 years without undue problems). Doxycycline can be used for up to 2 years. *Malarone*® is licensed for use for up to 28 days but can be used for up to 1 year (and possibly longer) with caution. Specialist advice should be sought for long-term prophylaxis.

**Return from malarial region** It is important to be aware that **any illness** that occurs within 1 year and **especially within 3 months of return might be malaria** even if all recommended precautions against malaria were taken. Travellers should be **warned** of this and told that if they develop any illness **particularly within 3 months** of their return they should go **immediately** to a doctor and specifically mention their exposure to malaria.

**Children** Prophylactic doses are based on guidelines agreed by UK malaria experts and may differ from advice in product literature. Weight is a better guide than age. If in doubt telephone centres listed on p. 357.

**Epilepsy** Both chloroquine and mefloquine are unsuitable for malaria prophylaxis in individuals with a history of epilepsy. In areas *without chloroquine resistance* proguanil 200 mg daily alone is recommended; in areas *with chloroquine resistance*, doxycycline or *Malarone*® may be considered; the metabolism of doxycycline may be influenced by antiepileptics (see **interactions:** Appendix 1 (tetracyclines)).

**Asplenia** Asplenic individuals (or those with severe splenic dysfunction) are at particular risk of severe malaria. If travel to malarious areas is unavoidable, rigorous precautions are required against contracting the disease.

**Renal impairment** Avoidance (or dosage reduction) of proguanil is recommended since it is excreted by the kidneys. *Malarone*® should not be used for prophylaxis in patients with estimated glomerular filtration rate less than 30 mL/minute/1.73 m². Chloroquine is only partially excreted by the kidneys and reduction of the dose for prophylaxis is not required except in severe impairment. Mefloquine is considered to be appropriate to use in renal impairment and does not require dosage reduction. Doxycycline is also considered to be appropriate.

**Pregnancy** Travel to malarious areas should be avoided during pregnancy; if travel is unavoidable, effective prophylaxis must be used. Chloroquine and proguanil can be given in the usual doses during pregnancy, but these drugs are not appropriate for most areas because their effectiveness has declined, particularly in Sub-Saharan Africa; in the case of proguanil, folic acid 5 mg daily should be given. The centres listed on p. 357 should be consulted for advice on prophylaxis in chloroquine-resistant areas. The manufacturer advises that prophylaxis with mefloquine should be avoided as a matter of principle but studies of mefloquine in pregnancy (including use in the first trimester) indicate that it can be considered for travel to chloroquine-resistant areas. Doxycycline is contra-indicated during pregnancy. *Malarone*® should be avoided during pregnancy unless there is no suitable alternative.

**Breast-feeding** Prophylaxis is required in **breast-fed infants**; although antimalarials are present in milk, the amounts are too variable to give reliable protection.

**Anticoagulants** Travellers taking warfarin should begin chemoprophylaxis at least 1 week (2–3 weeks for mefloquine) before departure. The INR should be stable before departure. It should be measured before starting chemoprophylaxis, 7 days after starting, and after completing the course. For prolonged stays, the INR should be checked at regular intervals.

## Specific recommendations

Where a journey requires two regimens, the regimen for the higher risk area should be used for the whole journey. Those travelling to remote or little-visited areas may require expert advice.

> Risk may vary in different parts of a country—check under all risk levels

> **Important** Settled immigrants (or long-term visitors) to the UK may be unaware that they will have **lost some of their immunity** and also that the areas where they previously lived **may now be malarious**

## North Africa, the Middle East, and Central Asia

**Very low risk** Risk *very low* in Algeria, Egypt (but *low risk* in El Faiyum, see below), Georgia (south-east, July–October), Kyrgystan (but *low risk* in south-west, see below), Libya, rural Morocco, most tourist areas of Turkey (but *low risk* in Adana and border with Syria, see below), Uzbekistan (extreme south-east only):

> chemoprophylaxis not recommended but avoid mosquito bites and consider malaria if fever presents

**Low risk** Risk *low* in Armenia (June–October), Azerbaijan (southern border areas, June–September), Egypt (El Faiyum only, June–October), Iran (northern border with Azerbaijan, May–October; *variable risk* in rural south-east provinces; see below), rural north Iraq (May–November), Kyrgystan (south-west, May–October), north border of Syria (May–October), Turkey (plain around Adana and east of there, border with Syria, March–November), Turkmenistan (south-east only, June–October):

> preferably

> chloroquine *or* (if chloroquine not appropriate) proguanil hydrochloride

**Variable risk** Risk *variable* and *chloroquine resistance present* in Afghanistan (below 2000 m, May–November), Iran (rural south-east provinces, March–November, see also *Low risk* above), Oman (remote rural areas only), Saudi Arabia (south-west and rural areas of western region; no risk in Mecca, Medina, Jeddah, or high-altitude areas of Asir Province), Tajikistan (June–October), Yemen (no risk in Sana'a):

> chloroquine + proguanil hydrochloride *or* (if chloroquine + proguanil not appropriate) doxycycline

## Sub-Saharan Africa

*No chemoprophylaxis recommended* for Cape Verde (some risk on São Tiago) and Mauritius (but avoid mosquito bites and consider malaria if fever presents)

**Very high risk** Risk *very high* (or *locally very high*) and *chloroquine resistance very widespread* in Angola, Benin, Botswana (northern half, November–June), Burkina Faso, Burundi, Cameroon, Central African Republic, Chad, Comoros, Congo, Democratic Republic of the Congo (formely Zaïre), Djibouti, Equatorial Guinea, Eritrea, Ethiopia (below 2000 m; no risk in Addis Ababa), Gabon, Gambia, Ghana, Guinea, Guinea-Bissau, Ivory Coast, Kenya, Liberia, Madagascar, Malawi, Mali, Mauritania (all year in south; July–October in north), Mozambique, Namibia (all year along Kavango and Kunene rivers; November–June in northern third),

Niger, Nigeria, Principe, Rwanda, São Tomé, Senegal, Sierra Leone, Somalia, South Africa (low-altitude areas of Mpumalanga and Limpopo Provinces, Kruger National Park, and north-east KwaZulu-Natal as far south as Jozini), Sudan, Swaziland, Tanzania, Togo, Uganda, Zambia, Zimbabwe (all year in Zambezi valley; November–June in other areas below 1200 m; risk negligible in Harare and Bulawayo):

> mefloquine *or* doxycycline *or Malarone*®

**Note** In Zimbabwe and neighbouring countries, pyrimethamine with dapsone (also known as *Deltaprim*®) prophylaxis is used by local residents (sometimes with chloroquine)—this regimen is not recommended.

## South Asia

**Low risk** Risk low in Bangladesh (but *high risk* in Chittagong Hill Tracts, see below), India (Kerala [southern states], Tamil Nadu, Karnataka, Southern Andhra Pradesh [including Hyderabad and Mumbai], Rajasthan [including Jaipur], Uttar Pradesh [including Agra], Haryana, Uttaranchal, Himachal Pradesh, Jammu, Kashmir, Punjab, Delhi; *variable risk* in other areas, see below; *high risk* in Assam), Sri Lanka (but *variable risk* north of Vavuniya, see below):

> chemoprophylaxis not recommended but avoid mosquito bites and consider malaria if fever present

**Variable risk** Risk *variable* and *chloroquine resistance usually moderate* in southern districts of Bhutan, India (*low risk* in some areas, see above; *high risk* in Assam, see below), Nepal (below 1500 m, especially Terai districts; no risk in Kathmandu), Pakistan (below 2000 m), Sri Lanka (north of Vavuniya; *low risk* in other areas, see above):

> chloroquine + proguanil hydrochloride *or* (if chloroquine + proguanil not appropriate) mefloquine *or* doxycycline *or Malarone*®

**High risk** Risk *high* and *chloroquine resistance high* in Bangladesh (only in Chittagong Hill Tracts; *low risk* in other areas, see above), India (Assam only; see also *low risk* and *variable risk* above):

> mefloquine *or* doxycycline *or Malarone*® *or* (if mefloquine, doxycycline, or *Malarone*® not appropriate) chloroquine + proguanil hydrochloride

## South-East Asia

**Very low risk** Risk *very low* in Bali, Brunei, main tourist areas of China (but *substantial risk* in Yunnan and Hainan, see below; *chloroquine prophylaxis* appropriate for other remote areas), Hong Kong, Korea (both North and South), Malaysia (both East and West including Cameron Highlands, but *substantial risk* in Sabah [except Kota Kinabalu], and *variable risk* in deep forests, see below), Singapore, Thailand (**important:** regional risk exists, see under *Great risk*, below), Vietnam (cities, coast between

Ho Chi Minh and Hanoi, and Mekong River until close to Cambodian border; *substantial risk* in other areas, see below):

> chemoprophylaxis not recommended but avoid mosquito bites and consider malaria if fever presents

**Variable risk** Risk *variable* and *some chloroquine resistance* in Indonesia (*very low risk* in Bali, and cities but *substantial risk* in Irian Jaya [West Papua] and Lombok, see below), rural Philippines below 600 m (no risk in cities, Cebu, Bohol, and Catanduanes), deep forests of peninsular Malaysia and Sarawak (but *substantial risk* in Sabah, see below):

> chloroquine + proguanil hydrochloride *or* (if chloroquine + proguanil not appropriate) mefloquine *or* doxycycline *or Malarone*®

**Substantial risk** Risk *substantial* and *drug resistance common* in Cambodia (no risk in Phnom Penh; for western provinces, see below), China (Yunnan and Hainan; *chloroquine prophylaxis* appropriate for other remote areas; see also *Very low risk* above), East Timor, Irian Jaya [West Papua], Laos (no risk in Vientiane), Lombok, Malaysia (Sabah; see also *Very low risk* and *Variable risk* above), Myanmar (formerly Burma; see also *Great risk* below), Vietnam (*very low risk* in some areas, see above):

> mefloquine *or* doxycycline *or Malarone*®

**Great risk and drug resistance present** Risk *great and widespread chloroquine and mefloquine resistance present* in western provinces of Cambodia, borders of Thailand with Cambodia, Laos and Myanmar (*very low risk* in Chang Rai and Kwai Bridge, see above), Myanmar (eastern Shan State):

> doxycycline *or Malarone*®

## Oceania

**Risk** Risk *high* and *chloroquine resistance high* in Papua New Guinea (below 1800 m), Solomon Islands, Vanuatu:

> doxycycline *or* mefloquine *or Malarone*®

## Central and South America and the Caribbean

**Variable to low risk** Risk *variable to low* in Argentina (rural areas along northern borders only), rural Belize (except Belize district), Costa Rica (Limon Province except Puerto Limon and northern canton of Pococci), Dominican Republic, El Salvador (Santa Ana province in west), Guatemala (below 1500 m), Haiti, Honduras,

Mexico (states of Oaxaca and Chiapas), Nicaragua, Panama (west of Panama Canal but *variable to high risk* east of Panama Canal, see below), rural Paraguay:

> chloroquine *or* (if chloroquine not appropriate) proguanil hydrochloride

---

**Variable to high risk** Risk *variable to high* and *chloroquine resistance present* in rural areas of Bolivia (below 2500 m), Ecuador (below 1500 m; no malaria in Galapagos Islands and Guayaquil; see below for Esmeraldas Province), Panama (east of Panama Canal), Peru (rural areas east of the Andes and west of the Amazon basin area below 1500 m; see below for Amazon basin area), Venezuela (north of Orinoco river; *high risk* south of and including Orinoco river and Amazon basin area, see below; Caracas free of malaria):

> chloroquine + proguanil hydrochloride *or* (if chloroquine + proguanil not appropriate) mefloquine *or* doxycycline *or* Malarone®

---

**High risk** Risk *high* and *marked chloroquine resistance* in Bolivia (Amazon basin area; see also *variable to high risk* above), Brazil (throughout 'Legal Amazon' area which includes the Amazon basin area, Mato Grosso and Maranhao only; elsewhere *very low risk*—no chemoprophylaxis), Colombia (most areas below 800 m), Ecuador (Esmeraldas Province; *variable to high risk* in other areas, see above), French Guiana, all interior regions of Guyana, Peru (Amazon basin area), Suriname (except Paramaribo and coast), Venezuela (Amazon basin area, areas south of and including Orinoco river):

> mefloquine *or* doxycycline *or* Malarone®

---

### Standby treatment

> Travellers visiting remote, malarious areas for prolonged periods should carry standby treatment if they are likely to be more than 24 hours away from medical care. Self-medication should be **avoided** if medical help is accessible.
>
> In order to avoid excessive self-medication, the traveller should be provided with **written instructions** that urgent medical attention should be sought if fever (38°C or more) develops 7 days (or more) after arriving in a malarious area and that self-treatment is indicated if medical help is not available within 24 hours of fever onset.
>
> In view of the continuing emergence of resistant strains and of the different regimens required for different areas expert advice should be sought on the best treatment course for an individual traveller. A drug used for chemoprophylaxis should not be considered for standby treatment for the same traveller.

## Artemether with lumefantrine

Artemether with lumefantrine is licensed for the *treatment of acute uncomplicated falciparum malaria*.

### ▌ARTEMETHER WITH LUMEFANTRINE

**Indications** treatment of acute uncomplicated falciparum malaria; treatment of benign malaria [unlicensed indication]

**Cautions** electrolyte disturbances, concomitant use with other drugs known to cause QT-interval prolongation; hepatic impairment (Appendix 2); renal impairment (Appendix 3); pregnancy (Appendix 4); monitor patients unable to take food (greater risk of recrudescence); **interactions:** Appendix 1 (artemether with lumefantrine)
*Driving* Dizziness may affect performance of skilled tasks (e.g. driving)

**Contra-indications** history of arrhythmias, of clinically relevant bradycardia, and of congestive heart failure accompanied by reduced left ventricular ejection fraction; family history of sudden death or of congenital QT interval prolongation; breast-feeding (Appendix 5)

**Side-effects** abdominal pain, anorexia, diarrhoea, vomiting, nausea; palpitation, prolonged QT interval; cough; headache, dizziness, sleep disturbances, asthenia, paraesthesia; arthralgia, myalgia; pruritus, rash; *less commonly* ataxia, hypoaesthesia, and clonus

**Dose**
* Treatment of malaria, see p. 358

**Riamet®** (Novartis) ▼ PoM
Tablets, yellow, artemether 20 mg, lumefantrine 120 mg, net price 24-tab pack = £22.50. Label: 21, counselling, driving
Note Tablets may be crushed just before administration

---

## Chloroquine

Chloroquine is used for the *prophylaxis of malaria* in areas of the world where the *risk of chloroquine-resistant falciparum malaria is still low*. It is also used with proguanil when chloroquine-resistant falciparum malaria is present but this regimen may not give optimal protection (see specific recommendations by country, p. 360).

Chloroquine is **no longer recommended** for the *treatment of falciparum malaria* owing to widespread resistance, nor is it recommended if the infective species is *not known* or if the infection is *mixed*; in these cases treatment should be with quinine, *Malarone®*, or *Riamet®* (for details, see p. 357). It is still recommended for the *treatment of benign malarias* (for details, see p. 359).

### ▌CHLOROQUINE

**Indications** chemoprophylaxis and treatment of malaria; rheumatoid arthritis and lupus erythematosus (section 10.1.3)

**Cautions** moderate or severe hepatic impairment; renal impairment (see notes above); pregnancy (but for malaria benefit outweighs risk, see Appendix 4, Antimalarials); may exacerbate psoriasis; neurological disorders (avoid for prophylaxis if history of epilepsy, see notes above); may aggravate myasthenia gravis; severe gastro-intestinal disorders; G6PD deficiency (see section 9.1.5); ophthalmic examination and long-term therapy, see under Chloroquine, section 10.1.3; avoid concurrent therapy with hepatotoxic drugs—other **interactions**: Appendix 1 (chloroquine and hydroxychloroquine)

**Side-effects** gastro-intestinal disturbances, headache, also hypotension, convulsions, visual disturbances, depigmentation or loss of hair, skin reactions (rashes, pruritus); rarely, bone-marrow suppression, hypersensitivity reactions such as urticaria and angioedema; other side-effects (not usually associated with malaria prophylaxis or treatment), see under Chloroquine, section 10.1.3; very toxic in **overdosage**—immediate advice from poisons centres essential (see also p. 32)

**Dose**

Note Doses expressed as chloroquine base

● Prophylaxis of malaria, preferably started 1 week before entering endemic area and continued for 4 weeks after leaving (see notes above), 310 mg once weekly; INFANT up to 12 weeks body-weight under 6 kg, 37.5 mg once weekly; 12 weeks–1 year body-weight 6–10 kg, 75 mg once weekly; CHILD 1–4 years body-weight 10–16 kg, 112.5 mg once weekly; 4–8 years body-weight 16–25 kg, 150 mg once weekly (or 155 mg once weekly if tablets used); 8–13 years body-weight 25–45 kg, 225 mg once weekly (or 232.5 mg once weekly if tablets used); over 13 years body-weight over 45 kg, adult dose

● Treatment of benign malarias, see p. 359

Counselling Warn travellers about **importance** of avoiding mosquito bites, **importance** of taking prophylaxis regularly, and **importance** of immediate visit to doctor if ill within 1 year and **especially** within 3 months of return. For details, see notes above

Note Chloroquine doses in BNF may differ from those in product literature

**¹Avloclor®** (AstraZeneca) (PoM)

Tablets, scored, chloroquine phosphate 250 mg (≡ chloroquine base 155 mg). Net price 20-tab pack = £1.22. Label: 5, counselling, prophylaxis, see above

**¹Malarivon®** (Wallace Mfg) (PoM)

Syrup, chloroquine phosphate 80 mg/5 mL (≡ chloroquine base 50 mg/5 mL), net price 75 mL = £8.75. Label: 5, counselling, prophylaxis, see above

**¹Nivaquine®** (Sanofi-Aventis)

Syrup, golden, chloroquine sulphate 68 mg/5 mL (≡ chloroquine base 50 mg/5 mL), net price 100 mL = £4.60. Label: 5, counselling, prophylaxis, see above

◢**With proguanil**

For cautions and side-effects of proguanil see Proguanil; for dose see Chloroquine and Proguanil

**¹Paludrine/Avloclor®** (AstraZeneca)

Tablets, travel pack of 14 tablets of chloroquine phosphate 250 mg (≡ chloroquine base 155 mg) and 98 tablets of proguanil hydrochloride 100 mg, net price 112-tab pack = £8.79. Label: 5, 21, counselling, prophylaxis, see above

1. Can be sold to the public provided it is licensed and labelled for the prophylaxis of malaria. Drugs for malaria prophylaxis not prescribable on the NHS; health authorities may investigate circumstances under which antimalarials are prescribed

## Mefloquine

Mefloquine is used for the *prophylaxis of malaria* in areas of the world where there is a *high risk of chloroquine-resistant falciparum malaria* (for details, see specific recommendations by country, p. 360).

Mefloquine is now rarely used for the *treatment of falciparum malaria* because of increased resistance. It is rarely used for the treatment of benign malarias because better tolerated alternatives are available. Mefloquine should not be used for treatment if it has been used for prophylaxis.

The CSM has advised that travellers should be informed about adverse reactions of mefloquine and, if they occur, medical advice should be sought on alternative antimalarials before the next dose is due; the patient information leaflet, which describes adverse reactions should always be provided when dispensing mefloquine.

### MEFLOQUINE

**Indications** chemoprophylaxis of malaria, treatment of malaria, see notes above

**Cautions** pregnancy (see notes under Prophylaxis against malaria; Appendix 4)—manufacturer advises **avoid** pregnancy during and for 3 months after; breast-feeding (Appendix 5); avoid for chemoprophylaxis in severe hepatic impairment; cardiac conduction disorders; epilepsy (avoid for prophylaxis); not recommended in infants under 3 months (5 kg); **interactions**: Appendix 1 (mefloquine)

Driving Dizziness or a disturbed sense of balance may affect performance of skilled tasks (e.g. driving); effects may persist for up to 3 weeks

**Contra-indications** hypersensitivity to quinine; avoid for prophylaxis if history of psychiatric disorders (including depression) or convulsions

**Side-effects** nausea, vomiting, diarrhoea, abdominal pain; dizziness, loss of balance, headache, sleep disorders (insomnia, drowsiness, abnormal dreams); *less commonly* circulatory disorders (including hypotension and hypertension), chest pain, tachycardia, palpitation, bradycardia, cardiac conduction disorders, dyspnoea, fatigue, fever, loss of appetite, neuropsychiatric reactions (including sensory and motor neuropathies, tremor, ataxia, anxiety, depression, panic attacks, agitation, hallucinations, psychosis, convulsions), leucopenia, leucocytosis, thrombocytopenia, muscle weakness, myalgia, arthralgia, visual disturbances, tinnitus and vestibular disorders, rash (including Stevens-Johnson syndrome), urticaria, pruritus, alopecia; *rarely* suicidal ideation; *very rarely* AV block, pneumonitis, and encephalopathy

**Dose**

● Prophylaxis of malaria, preferably started 2½ weeks before entering endemic area and continued for 4 weeks after leaving (see notes above), ADULT and CHILD body-weight over 45 kg, 250 mg once weekly; body-weight 6–16 kg, 62.5 mg once weekly; body-weight 16–25 kg, 125 mg once weekly; body-weight 25–45 kg, 187.5 mg once weekly

● Treatment of malaria, see notes above

Counselling See CSM advice in notes above. Also warn travellers about **importance** of avoiding mosquito bites, **importance** of taking prophylaxis regularly, and **importance** of immediate visit to doctor if ill within 1 year and **especially** within 3 months of return. For details, see notes above

Note Mefloquine doses in BNF may differ from those in product literature

**5**

**Infections**

[1]**Lariam**® (Roche) PoM
Tablets, scored, mefloquine (as hydrochloride)
250 mg. Net price 8-tab pack = £14.53. Label: 21, 25,
27, counselling, driving, prophylaxis, see above
**Note** Tablet may be crushed and mixed with food such as
jam or honey just before administration

## Primaquine

Primaquine is used to eliminate the liver stages of *P.
vivax or P. ovale following chloroquine treatment* (for
details, see p. 359).

### ▉ PRIMAQUINE

**Indications** adjunct in the treatment of *Plasmodium
vivax* and *P. ovale* malaria (eradication of liver stages)

**Cautions** G6PD deficiency (test blood, see under
Benign Malarias (treatment), p. 359); systemic dis-
eases associated with granulocytopenia (e.g. rheu-
matoid arthritis, lupus erythematosus); pregnancy
(Appendix 4) and breast-feeding; **interactions:**
Appendix 1 (primaquine)

**Side-effects** nausea, vomiting, anorexia, abdominal
pain; less commonly methaemoglobinaemia, haemolytic anaemia especially in G6PD deficiency, leucopenia

**Dose**
● Treatment of benign malarias, see p. 359

**Primaquine** (Non-proprietary)
Tablets, primaquine (as phosphate) 7.5 mg or 15 mg
Available from 'special-order' manufacturers or specialist-
importing companies, see p. 969

## Proguanil

Proguanil is used (usually *with chloroquine*, but occasionally *alone*) for the *prophylaxis of malaria*, (for details,
see specific recommendations by country, p. 360).

Proguanil used alone is not suitable for the *treatment of
malaria*; however, *Malarone*® (a combination of atovaquone with proguanil) is licensed for the treatment of
acute uncomplicated falciparum malaria. *Malarone*® is
also used for the *prophylaxis of falciparum malaria* in
areas of *widespread mefloquine or chloroquine resistance*.
*Malarone*® is also used as an alternative to mefloquine
or doxycycline. *Malarone*® is particularly suitable for
short trips to highly chloroquine-resistant areas because
it needs to be taken only for 7 days after leaving an
endemic area.

### ▉ PROGUANIL HYDROCHLORIDE

**Indications** chemoprophylaxis of malaria

**Cautions** renal impairment (see notes under Prophylaxis against malaria and Appendix 3); pregnancy
(Appendix 4); **interactions:** Appendix 1 (proguanil)

**Side-effects** mild gastric intolerance, diarrhoea, and
constipation; occasionally mouth ulcers and stomat-

---

1. Drugs for malaria prophylaxis not prescribable on the
NHS; health authorities may investigate circumstances
under which antimalarials prescribed

itis; *very rarely* cholestasis, vasculitis, skin reactions,
and hair loss

**Dose**
● Prophylaxis of malaria, preferably started 1 week
before entering endemic area and continued for 4
weeks after leaving (see notes above), 200 mg once
daily; INFANT up to 12 weeks body-weight under 6 kg,
25 mg once daily; 12 weeks–1 year body-weight 6–
10 kg, 50 mg once daily; CHILD 1–4 years body-weight
10–16 kg, 75 mg once daily; 4–8 years body-weight
16–25 kg, 100 mg once daily; 8–13 years, body-weight
25–45 kg, 150 mg once daily; over 13 years body-
weight over 45 kg, adult dose

Counselling Warn travellers about **importance** of avoiding
mosquito bites, **importance** of taking prophylaxis regularly,
and **importance** of immediate visit to doctor if ill within 1
year and **especially** within 3 months of return. For details,
see notes above
**Note** Proguanil doses in BNF may differ from those in
product literature.

[2]**Paludrine**® (AstraZeneca)
Tablets, scored, proguanil hydrochloride 100 mg. Net
price 98-tab pack = £7.43. Label: 21, counselling,
prophylaxis, see above
**Note** Tablet may be crushed and mixed with food such as
milk, jam, or honey just before administration

◢**With chloroquine**
See under Chloroquine

### ▉ PROGUANIL HYDROCHLORIDE WITH ATOVAQUONE

**Indications** treatment of acute uncomplicated falciparum malaria and prophylaxis of falciparum malaria,
particularly where resistance to other antimalarial
drugs suspected; treatment of benign malaria [unli-
censed indication]

**Cautions** diarrhoea or vomiting (reduced absorption
of atovaquone); efficacy not evaluated in cerebral or
complicated malaria (including hyperparasitaemia,
pulmonary oedema or renal failure); renal impairment
(Appendix 3); pregnancy (Appendix 4); breast-feeding
(Appendix 5); **interactions:** see Appendix 1 (proguanil, atovaquone)

**Side-effects** abdominal pain, nausea, vomiting, diarrhoea; cough; headache, dizziness, insomnia, abnormal
dreams, depression, anorexia, fever; rash, pruritus; *less
frequently* stomatitis, anxiety, blood disorders, hyponatraemia, palpitation, and hair loss; also reported,
hepatitis, cholestasis, tachycardia, hallucinations,
vasculitis, mouth ulcers, and Stevens-Johnson
syndrome

**Dose**
● See preparations
Counselling Warn travellers about **importance** of avoiding
mosquito bites, **importance** of taking prophylaxis regularly,
and **importance** of immediate visit to doctor if ill within 1
year and **especially** within 3 months of return. For details,
see notes above

---

2. Can be sold to the public provided it is licensed and
labelled for the prophylaxis of malaria. Drugs for malaria
prophylaxis not prescribable on the NHS; health authorities
may investigate circumstances under which antimalarials
are prescribed

[1]**Malarone®** (GSK) [PoM]
Tablets ('standard'), pink, f/c, proguanil hydro-chloride 100 mg, atovaquone 250 mg. Net price 12-tab pack = £25.21. Label: 21, counselling, prophylaxis, see above

Dose prophylaxis of malaria, started 1–2 days before entering endemic area and continued for 1 week after leaving, ADULT and CHILD over 40 kg, 1 tablet daily

Treatment of malaria, ADULT and CHILD body-weight over 40 kg, 4 tablets once daily for 3 days; CHILD body-weight 11–21 kg 1 tablet daily for 3 days; body-weight 21–31 kg 2 tablets once daily for 3 days; body-weight 31–40 kg 3 tablets once daily for 3 days

[1]**Malarone® Paediatric** (GSK) [PoM]
Paediatric tablets, pink, f/c proguanil hydrochloride 25 mg, atovaquone 62.5 mg, net price 12-tab pack = £6.26. Label: 21, counselling, prophylaxis, see above

Dose prophylaxis of malaria, started 1–2 days before entering endemic area and continued for 1 week after leaving, CHILD body-weight 11–21 kg, 1 tablet daily; body-weight 21–31 kg, 2 tablets once daily; body-weight 31–40 kg, 3 tablets once daily; body-weight over 40 kg use *Malarone®* ('standard') tablets

Treatment of malaria, CHILD body-weight 5–9 kg, 2 tablets once daily for 3 days; body-weight 9–11 kg, 3 tablets once daily for 3 days; body-weight 11 kg and over use *Malarone®* ('standard') tablets

Note Tablets may be crushed and mixed with food or milky drink just before administration

## Pyrimethamine

Pyrimethamine should not be used alone, but is used with sulfadoxine.

Pyrimethamine with sulfadoxine is not recommended for the *prophylaxis of malaria*, but it can be used in the treatment of *falciparum malaria with (or following) quinine.*

### ▌ PYRIMETHAMINE

**Indications** malaria (but used only in combined pre-parations incorporating sulfadoxine); toxoplasmosis—section 5.4.7

**Cautions** hepatic or renal impairment, pregnancy (Appendix 4); breast-feeding (Appendix 5); blood counts required with prolonged treatment; history of seizures—avoid large loading doses; **interactions:** Appendix 1 (pyrimethamine)

**Side-effects** depression of haematopoiesis with high doses, rashes, insomnia

**Dose**

• Malaria, no dose stated because not recommended alone, see Pyrimethamine with Sulfadoxine below

• Toxoplasmosis, section 5.4.7

**Daraprim®** (GSK) [PoM] ▰
Tablets, scored, pyrimethamine 25 mg. Net price 30-tab pack = £2.60

### ▌ PYRIMETHAMINE WITH SULFADOXINE

**Indications** adjunct to quinine in treatment of *Plasmodium falciparum* malaria; **not** recommended for prophylaxis

**Cautions** see under Pyrimethamine and under Co-trimoxazole (section 5.1.8); pregnancy (Appendix 4);

1. Drugs for malaria prophylaxis not prescribable on the NHS; health authorities may investigate circumstances under which antimalarials prescribed

breast-feeding (Appendix 5); not recommended for prophylaxis (severe side-effects on long-term use); **interactions:** Appendix 1 (pyrimethamine, sulphonamides)

**Contra-indications** see under Pyrimethamine and under Co-trimoxazole (section 5.1.8); sulphonamide allergy

**Side-effects** see under Pyrimethamine and under Co-trimoxazole (section 5.1.8); pulmonary infiltrates (e.g. eosinophilic or allergic alveolitis) reported—discontinue if cough or shortness of breath

**Dose**

• Treatment of falciparum malaria, see p. 358

• Prophylaxis, not recommended by UK malaria experts

**Pyrimethamine with sulfadoxine** (Non-proprietary) [PoM]
Tablets, scored, pyrimethamine 25 mg, sulfadoxine 500 mg, net price 3-tab pack = 74p

Note Also known as *Fansidar®*

Available from 'special-order' manufacturers or specialist importing companies, see p. 969

## Quinine

Quinine is not suitable for the *prophylaxis of malaria.*

Quinine is used for the *treatment of falciparum malaria* or if the infective species is *not known* or if the infection is *mixed* (for details see p. 357).

### ▌ QUININE

**Indications** falciparum malaria; nocturnal leg cramps, see section 10.2.2

**Cautions** cardiac disease (including atrial fibrillation, conduction defects, heart block), elderly—monitor ECG during parenteral treatment; hepatic impairment (Appendix 2); renal impairment (Appendix 3); pregnancy (but appropriate for treatment of malaria; Appendix 4); monitor blood glucose and electrolyte concentration during parenteral treatment; G6PD deficiency (see section 9.1.5); **interactions:** Appendix 1 (quinine)

**Contra-indications** haemoglobinuria, myasthenia gravis, optic neuritis, tinnitus

**Side-effects** cinchonism, including tinnitus, headache, hot and flushed skin, nausea, abdominal pain, rashes, visual disturbances (including temporary blindness), confusion; cardiovascular effects (see Cautions); hypersensitivity reactions including angioedema; hypoglycaemia (especially after parenteral administration); blood disorders (including thrombocytopenia and intravascular coagulation); acute renal failure; photosensitivity; very toxic in **overdosage**—immediate advice from poisons centres essential (see also p. 32)

**Dose**

• Treatment of malaria, see p. 358

Note Quinine (anhydrous base) 100 mg ≡ quinine bisulphate 169 mg ≡ quinine dihydrochloride 122 mg ≡ quinine hydrochloride 122 mg ≡ quinine sulphate 121 mg. Quinine bisulphate 300-mg tablets are available but provide less quinine than 300 mg of the dihydrochloride, hydrochloride, or sulphate

**Quinine Sulphate** (Non-proprietary) [PoM]
Tablets, coated, quinine sulphate 200 mg, net price 28-tab pack = £1.86; 300 mg, 28-tab pack = £1.85

**Quinine Dihydrochloride** (Non-proprietary) PoM
Injection, quinine dihydrochloride 300 mg/mL. For
dilution and use as an infusion. 1- and 2-mL amps
Available from 'special-order' manufacturers or specialist
importing companies, see p. 969
Note Intravenous injection of quinine is so hazardous that it has
been superseded by infusion

## Tetracyclines

**Doxycycline** (section 5.1.3) is used for the *prophylaxis of
malaria* in areas of *widespread mefloquine or chloroquine
resistance*. Doxycycline is also used as an alternative to
mefloquine or *Malarone®* (for details, see specific
recommendations by country, p. 360).

**Doxycycline** is also used as an *adjunct to quinine in the
treatment of falciparum malaria* (for details see p. 358).

### ▋ DOXYCYCLINE

**Indications** prophylaxis of malaria; adjunct to quinine
in treatment of *Plasmodium falciparum* malaria; see
also section 5.1.3
**Cautions** section 5.1.3
**Contra-indications** section 5.1.3
**Side-effects** section 5.1.3
**Dose**
● Prophylaxis of malaria, started 1–2 days before
entering endemic area and continued for 4 weeks after
leaving (see notes above), ADULT and CHILD over 12
years, 100 mg once daily
● Treatment of falciparum malaria, see p. 358

◀Preparations
Section 5.1.3

## 5.4.2 Amoebicides

**Metronidazole** is the drug of choice for *acute invasive
amoebic dysentery* since it is very effective against vege-
tative forms of *Entamoeba histolytica* in ulcers; it is given
in an adult dose of 800 mg three times daily for 5 days.
**Tinidazole** is also effective. Metronidazole and tinidazole are also active against amoebae which may have
migrated to the liver. Treatment with metronidazole (or
tinidazole) is followed by a 10-day course of diloxanide
furoate.

**Diloxanide furoate** is the drug of choice for asymptomatic patients with *E. histolytica* cysts in the faeces;
metronidazole and tinidazole are relatively ineffective.
Diloxanide furoate is relatively free from toxic effects
and the usual course is of 10 days, given alone for
chronic infections or following metronidazole or tinidazole treatment.

For *amoebic abscesses* of the liver **metronidazole** is
effective; tinidazole is an alternative. Aspiration of the
abscess is indicated where it is suspected that it may
rupture or where there is no improvement after 72 hours
of metronidazole; the aspiration may need to be
repeated. Aspiration aids penetration of metronidazole
and, for abscesses with more than 100 mL of pus, if
carried out in conjunction with drug therapy, may
reduce the period of disability.

Diloxanide furoate is not effective against hepatic
amoebiasis, but a 10-day course should be given at
the completion of metronidazole or tinidazole treatment
to destroy any amoebae in the gut.

### ▋ DILOXANIDE FUROATE

**Indications** see notes above; chronic amoebiasis and
as adjunct to metronidazole or tinidazole in acute
amoebiasis
**Contra-indications** pregnancy (Appendix 4), breast-
feeding (Appendix 5)
**Side-effects** flatulence, vomiting, urticaria, pruritus
**Dose**
● 500 mg every 8 hours for 10 days; CHILD body-weight
over 25 kg, 20 mg/kg daily in 3 divided doses for 10
days; body-weight under 25 kg, see *BNF for Children*
See also notes above

**Diloxanide** (Sovereign) PoM
Tablets, diloxanide furoate 500 mg, net price 30-tab
pack = £42.95. Label: 9

### ▋ METRONIDAZOLE

**Indications** see under Dose below; anaerobic infections, section 5.1.11
**Cautions** section 5.1.11
**Side-effects** section 5.1.11
**Dose**
● By mouth, invasive intestinal amoebiasis, extra-
intestinal amoebiasis (including liver abcess),
800 mg every 8 hours for 5 days in intestinal infection (for 5–10 days in extra-intestinal infection);
CHILD 1–3 years 200 mg every 8 hours; 3–7 years
200 mg every 6 hours; 7–10 years 400 mg every 8
hours
Urogenital trichomoniasis, 200 mg every 8 hours for 7
days *or* 400–500 mg every 12 hours for 5–7 days, *or*
2 g as a single dose; CHILD 1–3 years 50 mg every 8
hours for 7 days; 3–7 years 100 mg every 12 hours; 7–
10 years 100 mg every 8 hours
Giardiasis, 2 g daily for 3 days *or* 400 mg 3 times daily
for 5 days *or* 500 mg twice daily for 7–10 days; CHILD
1–3 years 500 mg daily for 3 days; 3–7 years 600–
800 mg daily; 7–10 years 1 g daily

◀Preparations
Section 5.1.11

### ▋ TINIDAZOLE

**Indications** see under Dose below; anaerobic infec-
tions, section 5.1.11
**Cautions** section 5.1.11
**Side-effects** section 5.1.11
**Dose**
● Intestinal amoebiasis, 2 g daily for 2–3 days; CHILD 50–
60 mg/kg daily for 3 days
● Amoebic involvement of liver, 1.5–2 g daily for 3–6
days; CHILD 50–60 mg/kg daily for 5 days
● Urogenital trichomoniasis and giardiasis, single 2 g
dose; CHILD single dose of 50–75 mg/kg (repeated
once if necessary)

◀Preparations
Section 5.1.11

5 Infections

## 5.4.3 Trichomonacides

**Metronidazole** (section 5.4.2) is the treatment of choice for *Trichomonas vaginalis* infection. Contact tracing is recommended and sexual contacts should be treated simultaneously. If metronidazole is ineffective, **tinidazole** (section 5.4.2) may be tried.

## 5.4.4 Antigiardial drugs

**Metronidazole** (section 5.4.2) is the treatment of choice for *Giardia lamblia* infections. Alternative treatments are **tinidazole** (section 5.4.2) or **mepacrine hydrochloride**.

### MEPACRINE HYDROCHLORIDE

**Indications** giardiasis; discoid lupus erythematosus (Antimalarials, section 10.1.3)

**Cautions** hepatic impairment, elderly, history of psychosis; avoid in psoriasis; **interactions:** Appendix 1 (mepacrine)

**Side-effects** gastro-intestinal disturbances; dizziness, headache; with large doses nausea, vomiting and occasionally transient acute toxic psychosis and CNS stimulation; on prolonged treatment yellow discoloration of skin and urine, chronic dermatoses (including severe exfoliative dermatitis), hepatitis, aplastic anaemia; also reported blue/black discoloration of palate and nails and corneal deposits with visual disturbances

**Dose**

- Giardiasis [unlicensed], 100 mg every 8 hours for 5–7 days

**Mepacrine Hydrochloride**
Tablets, mepacrine hydrochloride 100 mg. Label: 4, 9, 14, 21
Available from 'special-order' manufacturers or specialist importing companies, see p. 969

## 5.4.5 Leishmaniacides

Cutaneous leishmaniasis frequently heals spontaneously but if skin lesions are extensive or unsightly, treatment is indicated, as it is in visceral leishmaniasis (kala-azar). Leishmaniasis should be treated under specialist supervision.

**Sodium stibogluconate**, an organic pentavalent antimony compound, is used for visceral leishmaniasis. The dose is 20 mg/kg daily (max. 850 mg) by intramuscular or intravenous injection for 28 days in visceral leishmaniasis and for 20 days in cutaneous infection; the dosage varies with different geographical regions and expert advice should be obtained. Some early non-inflamed lesions of cutaneous leishmaniasis can be treated with intralesional injections of sodium stibogluconate under specialist supervision.

**Amphotericin** is used with or after an antimony compound for visceral leishmaniasis unresponsive to the antimonial alone; side-effects may be reduced by using liposomal amphotericin (*AmBisome®*—section 5.2) at a dose of 1–3 mg/kg daily for 10–21 days to a cumulative dose of 21–30 mg/kg *or* at a dose of 3 mg/kg for 5 consecutive days followed by a single dose of 3 mg/kg 6 days later. Other lipid formulations of amphotericin (*Abelcet®* and *Amphocil®*) are also likely to be effective but less information is available.

**Pentamidine isetionate** (pentamidine isethionate) (section 5.4.8) has been used in antimony-resistant visceral leishmaniasis, but although the initial response is often good, the relapse rate is high; it is associated with serious side-effects. Other treatments include paromomycin [unlicensed] (available from 'special-order' manufacturers or specialist importing companies, see p. 969).

### SODIUM STIBOGLUCONATE

**Indications** leishmaniasis

**Cautions** intravenous injections must be given slowly over 5 minutes (to reduce risk of local thrombosis) and stopped if coughing or substernal pain; mucocutaneous disease (see below); monitor ECG before and during treatment; heart disease (withdraw if conduction disturbances occur); treat intercurrent infection (e.g. pneumonia); hepatic impairment; pregnancy (Appendix 4); breast-feeding (Appendix 5)
**Mucocutaneous disease** Successful treatment of mucocutaneous leishmaniasis may induce severe inflammation around the lesions (may be life-threatening if pharyngeal or tracheal involvement)—may require corticosteroid

**Contra-indications** significant renal impairment

**Side-effects** anorexia, nausea, vomiting, abdominal pain, diarrhoea; ECG changes; coughing (see Cautions); headache, lethargy; arthralgia, myalgia; *rarely* jaundice, flushing, bleeding from nose or gum, substernal pain (see Cautions), vertigo, fever, sweating, and rash; also reported pancreatitis and anaphylaxis; pain and thrombosis on intravenous administration, intramuscular injection also painful

**Dose**

- See notes above

**Pentostam®** (GSK) ▼PoM
Injection, sodium stibogluconate equivalent to pentavalent antimony 100 mg/mL. Net price 100-mL bottle = £66.43
**Note** Injection should be filtered immediately before administration using a filter of 5 microns or less

## 5.4.6 Trypanocides

The prophylaxis and treatment of trypanosomiasis is difficult and differs according to the strain of organism. Expert advice should therefore be obtained.

**5**
**Infections**

## 5.4.7 Drugs for toxoplasmosis

Most infections caused by *Toxoplasma gondii* are self-limiting, and treatment is not necessary. Exceptions are patients with eye involvement (toxoplasma choroido-retinitis), and those who are immunosuppressed. Toxoplasmic encephalitis is a common complication of AIDS. The treatment of choice is a combination of pyrimethamine and sulfadiazine (sulphadiazine), given for several weeks (expert advice **essential**). Pyrimethamine is a folate antagonist, and adverse reactions to this combination are relatively common (folinic acid supplements and weekly blood counts needed). Alternative regimens use combinations of pyrimethamine with clindamycin or clarithromycin or azithromycin. Long-term secondary prophylaxis is required after treatment of toxoplasmosis in immunocompromised patients; prophylaxis should continue until immunity recovers.

If toxoplasmosis is acquired in pregnancy, transplacental infection may lead to severe disease in the fetus. Spiramycin [unlicensed] (available from 'special-order' manufacturers or specialist importing companies, see p. 969) may reduce the risk of transmission of maternal infection to the fetus.

## 5.4.8 Drugs for pneumocystis pneumonia

Pneumonia caused by *Pneumocystis jirovecii (Pneumocystis carinii)* occurs in immunosuppressed patients; it is a common cause of pneumonia in AIDS. Pneumocystis pneumonia should generally be treated by those experienced in its management. Blood gas measurement is used to assess disease severity.

### Treatment

**Mild to moderate disease** Co-trimoxazole (section 5.1.8) in high dosage is the drug of choice for the treatment of mild to moderate pneumocystis pneumonia.

**Atovaquone** is licensed for the treatment of mild to moderate pneumocystis infection in patients who cannot tolerate co-trimoxazole. A combination of **dapsone** 100 mg daily (section 5.1.10) with **trimethoprim** 5 mg/kg every 6–8 hours (section 5.1.8) is given by mouth for the treatment of mild to moderate disease [unlicensed indication].

A combination of **clindamycin** 600 mg by mouth every 8 hours (section 5.1.6) and **primaquine** 30 mg daily by mouth (section 5.4.1) is used in the treatment of mild to moderate disease [unlicensed indication]; this combination is associated with considerable toxicity.

Inhaled **pentamidine isetionate** is sometimes used for mild disease. It is better tolerated than parenteral pentamidine but systemic absorption may still occur.

**Severe disease** Co-trimoxazole (section 5.1.8) in high dosage, given by mouth or by intravenous infusion, is the drug of choice for the treatment of severe pneumocystis pneumonia. **Pentamidine isetionate** given by intravenous infusion is an alternative for patients who cannot tolerate co-trimoxazole, or who have not responded to it. Pentamidine isetionate is a potentially toxic drug that can cause severe hypotension during or immediately after infusion.

Corticosteroid treatment can be lifesaving in those with severe pneumocystis pneumonia (see Adjunctive Therapy below).

**Adjunctive therapy** In moderate to severe infections associated with HIV infection, prednisolone 50–80 mg daily is given by mouth for 5 days (alternatively, hydrocortisone may be given parenterally); the dose is then reduced to complete 21 days of treatment. Corticosteroid treatment should ideally be started at the same time as the anti-pneumocystis therapy and certainly no later than 24–72 hours afterwards. The corticosteroid should be withdrawn before anti-pneumocystis treatment is complete.

### Prophylaxis

Prophylaxis against pneumocystis pneumonia should be given to all patients with a history of the infection. Prophylaxis against pneumocystis pneumonia should also be considered for severely immunocompromised patients. Prophylaxis should continue until immunity recovers sufficiently. It should not be discontinued if the patient has oral candidiasis, continues to lose weight, or is receiving cytotoxic therapy or long-term immunosuppressant therapy.

**Co-trimoxazole** by mouth is the drug of choice for prophylaxis against pneumocystis pneumonia. It is given in a dose of 960 mg daily or 960 mg on alternate days (3 times a week); the dose may be reduced to co-trimoxazole 480 mg daily to improve tolerance.

Intermittent inhalation of **pentamidine isetionate** is used for prophylaxis against pneumocystis pneumonia in patients unable to tolerate co-trimoxazole. It is effective but patients may be prone to extrapulmonary infection. Alternatively, **dapsone** 100 mg daily (section 5.1.10) can be used. **Atovaquone** 750 mg twice daily has also been used for prophylaxis [unlicensed indication].

### ▌ ATOVAQUONE

**Indications** treatment of mild to moderate *Pneumocystis jirovecii (Pneumocystis carinii)* pneumonia in patients intolerant of co-trimoxazole

**Cautions** initial diarrhoea and difficulty in taking with food may reduce absorption (and require alternative therapy); other causes of pulmonary disease should be sought and treated; elderly; hepatic impairment (Appendix 2); renal impairment (Appendix 3); pregnancy (Appendix 4); avoid breast-feeding (Appendix 5); **interactions:** Appendix 1 (atovaquone)

**Side-effects** nausea, diarrhoea, vomiting; headache, insomnia; fever; anaemia, neutropenia, hyponatraemia; rash, pruritus; also reported, Stevens-Johnson syndrome

**Dose**
- 750 mg twice daily with food (particularly high fat) for 21 days; CHILD not recommended

**Wellvone®** (GSK) [PoM]
Suspension, sugar-free, atovaquone 750 mg/5 mL,
net price 210 mL (tutti-frutti-flavoured) = £405.31.
Label: 21

◀ **With proguanil hydrochloride**
See section 5.4.1

## ■ PENTAMIDINE ISETIONATE

**Indications**   see under Dose (should only be given by specialists)

**Cautions**   risk of severe hypotension following administration (establish baseline blood pressure and administer with patient lying down; monitor blood pressure closely during administration, and at regular intervals, until treatment concluded); hypokalaemia, hypomagnesaemia, coronary heart disease, bradycardia, history of ventricular arrhythmias, concomitant use with other drugs which prolong QT-interval; hypertension or hypotension; hyperglycaemia or hypoglycaemia; leucopenia, thrombocytopenia, or anaemia; carry out laboratory monitoring according to product literature; care required to protect personnel during handling and administration; hepatic impairment; renal impairment (Appendix 3); pregnancy (Appendix 4); breast-feeding (Appendix 5); **interactions**: Appendix 1 (pentamidine isetionate)

**Side-effects**   severe reactions, sometimes fatal, due to hypotension, hypoglycaemia, pancreatitis, and arrhythmias; also leucopenia, thrombocytopenia, acute renal failure, hypocalcaemia; also reported: azotaemia, abnormal liver-function tests, anaemia, hyperkalaemia, nausea and vomiting, dizziness, syncope, flushing, hyperglycaemia, rash, and taste disturbances; Stevens-Johnson syndrome reported; on inhalation, bronchoconstriction (may be prevented by prior use of bronchodilators), cough, and shortness of breath; discomfort, pain, induration, abscess formation, and muscle necrosis at injection site

**Dose**
- *Pneumocystis jirovecii (Pneumocystis carinii)* pneumonia, by intravenous infusion, 4 mg/kg once daily for at least 14 days (reduced according to product literature in renal impairment)

  By inhalation of nebulised solution (using suitable equipment—consult product literature) 600 mg pentamidine isetionate once daily for 3 weeks; secondary prevention, 300 mg every 4 weeks *or* 150 mg every 2 weeks

- Visceral leishmaniasis (kala-azar, section 5.4.5), by deep intramuscular injection, 3–4 mg/kg on alternate days to max. total of 10 injections; course may be repeated if necessary

- Cutaneous leishmaniasis, by deep intramuscular injection, 3–4 mg/kg once or twice weekly until condition resolves (but see also section 5.4.5)

- Trypanosomiasis, by deep intramuscular injection *or* intravenous infusion, 4 mg/kg daily or on alternate days to total of 7–10 injections

**Note** Direct intravenous injection should be avoided whenever possible and **never** given rapidly; intramuscular injections should be deep and preferably given into the buttock

**Pentacarinat®** (Sanofi-Aventis) [PoM]
Injection, powder for reconstitution, pentamidine isetionate, net price 300-mg vial = £30.45

Nebuliser solution, pentamidine isetionate, net price 300-mg bottle = £32.15

**Caution in handling** Pentamidine isetionate is toxic and personnel should be adequately protected during handling and administration—consult product literature

## 5.5 Anthelmintics

    **5.5.1 Drugs for threadworms**
    **5.5.2 Ascaricides**
    **5.5.3 Drugs for tapeworm infections**
    **5.5.4 Drugs for hookworms**
    **5.5.5 Schistosomicides**
    **5.5.6 Filaricides**
    **5.5.7 Drugs for cutaneous larva migrans**
    **5.5.8 Drugs for strongyloidiasis**

Advice on prophylaxis and treatment of helminth infections is available from:

| | |
|---|---|
| Birmingham | (0121) 424 0357 |
| Scottish Centre for Infection and Environmental Health (registered users of Travax only) | (0141) 300 1100 (weekdays 2–4 p.m. only) |
| Liverpool | (0151) 708 9393 |
| London | (020) 7387 9300 (treatment) |

## 5.5.1 Drugs for threadworms
**(pinworms, *Enterobius vermicularis*)**

Anthelmintics are effective in threadworm infections, but their use needs to be combined with hygienic measures to break the cycle of auto-infection. All members of the family require treatment.

Adult threadworms do not live for longer than 6 weeks and for development of fresh worms, ova must be swallowed and exposed to the action of digestive juices in the upper intestinal tract. Direct multiplication of worms does not take place in the large bowel. Adult female worms lay ova on the perianal skin which causes pruritus; scratching the area then leads to ova being transmitted on fingers to the mouth, often via food eaten with unwashed hands. Washing hands and scrubbing nails before each meal and after each visit to the toilet is essential. A bath taken immediately after rising will remove ova laid during the night.

**Mebendazole** is the drug of choice for treating threadworm infection in patients of all ages over 2 years. It is given as a single dose; as reinfection is very common, a second dose may be given after 2 weeks.

**Piperazine** is available in combination with sennosides as a single-dose preparation.

**5 Infections**

## MEBENDAZOLE

**Indications** threadworm, roundworm, whipworm, and hookworm infections

**Cautions** pregnancy (toxicity in *rats*); breast-feeding (Appendix 5); **interactions**: Appendix 1 (mebendazole)

Note The package insert in the *Vermox®* pack includes the statement that it is not suitable for women known to be pregnant or children under 2 years

**Side-effects** *very rarely* abdominal pain, diarrhoea, convulsions (in infants) and rash (including Stevens-Johnson syndrome and toxic epidermal necrolysis)

**Dose**

- Threadworms, ADULT and CHILD over 2 years, 100 mg as a single dose; if reinfection occurs second dose may be needed after 2 weeks; CHILD under 2 years, see *BNF for Children*
- Whipworms, ADULT and CHILD over 2 years, 100 mg twice daily for 3 days; CHILD under 2 years, see *BNF for Children*
- Roundworms—section 5.5.2
- Hookworms—section 5.5.4

¹**Mebendazole** (Non-proprietary) (PoM)

Tablets, chewable, mebendazole 100 mg

1. Mebendazole tablets can be sold to the public if supplied for oral use in the treatment of enterobiasis in adults and children over 2 years provided its container or package is labelled to show a max. single dose of 100 mg and it is supplied in a container or package containing not more than 800 mg

**Vermox®** (Janssen-Cilag) (PoM)

Tablets, orange, scored, chewable, mebendazole 100 mg. Net price 6-tab pack = £1.36

Suspension, mebendazole 100 mg/5 mL. Net price 30 mL = £1.59

## PIPERAZINE

**Indications** threadworm and roundworm infections

**Cautions** hepatic impairment (Appendix 2); renal impairment (Appendix 3); epilepsy; pregnancy (Appendix 4); packs on sale to the general public carry a warning to avoid in epilepsy, or in liver or kidney disease, and to seek medical advice in pregnancy; breast-feeding (Appendix 5)

**Side-effects** nausea, vomiting, colic, diarrhoea, allergic reactions including urticaria, bronchospasm, and rare reports of arthralgia, fever, Stevens-Johnson syndrome and angioedema; rarely dizziness, muscular incoordination ('worm wobble'); drowsiness, nystagmus, vertigo, blurred vision, confusion and clonic contractions in patients with neurological or renal abnormalities

**Dose**

- See under Preparation, below

◀**With sennosides**

For cautions, contra-indications, side-effects of senna see section 1.6.2

**Pripsen®** (Thornton & Ross)

Oral powder, piperazine phosphate 4 g, total sennosides (calculated as sennoside B) 15.3 mg/sachet. Net price two-dose sachet pack = £1.73. Label: 13

Dose threadworms, stirred into milk or water, ADULT and CHILD over 6 years, content of 1 sachet as a single dose (bedtime in adults or morning in children), repeated after 14 days; INFANT 3 months–1 year, 1 level 2.5-mL spoonful in the morning, repeated

after 14 days; CHILD 1–6 years, 1 level 5-mL spoonful in the morning, repeated after 14 days

Roundworms, first dose as for threadworms; repeat at monthly intervals for up to 3 months if reinfection risk

## 5.5.2 Ascaricides
### (common roundworm infections)

**Mebendazole** (section 5.5.1) is effective against *Ascaris lumbricoides* and is generally considered to be the drug of choice; the usual dose is 100 mg twice daily for 3 days.

**Levamisole** [unlicensed] (available from 'special-order' manufacturers or specialist importing companies, see p. 969) is an alternative. It is very well tolerated; mild nausea or vomiting has been reported in about 1% of treated patients; it is given as a single dose of 120–150 mg in adults.

**Piperazine** may be given in a single adult dose, see Piperazine, above.

## 5.5.3 Drugs for tapeworm infections

### Taenicides

**Niclosamide** [unlicensed] (available from 'special-order' manufacturers or specialist importing companies, see p. 969) is the most widely used drug for tapeworm infections and side-effects are limited to occasional gastro-intestinal upset, lightheadedness, and pruritus; it is not effective against larval worms. Fears of developing cysticercosis in *Taenia solium* infections have proved unfounded. All the same, an antiemetic can be given before treatment and a laxative can be given 2 hours after niclosamide.

**Praziquantel** [unlicensed] (available from 'special-order' manufacturers or specialist importing companies, see p. 969) is as effective as niclosamide and is given as a single dose of 5–10 mg/kg after a light breakfast (a single dose of 25 mg/kg for *Hymenolepis nana*).

### Hydatid disease

Cysts caused by *Echinococcus granulosus* grow slowly and asymptomatic patients do not always require treatment. Surgical treatment remains the method of choice in many situations. **Albendazole** [unlicensed] (available from 'special-order' manufacturers or specialist importing companies, see p. 969) is used in conjunction with surgery to reduce the risk of recurrence or as primary treatment in inoperable cases. Alveolar echinococcosis due to *E. multilocularis* is usually fatal if untreated. Surgical removal with albendazole cover is the treatment of choice, but where effective surgery is impossible, repeated cycles of albendazole (for a year or more) may help. Careful monitoring of liver function is particularly important during drug treatment.

## 5.5.4 Drugs for hookworms
### (ancylostomiasis, necatoriasis)

Hookworms live in the upper small intestine and draw blood from the point of their attachment to their host. An iron-deficiency anaemia may occur and, if present, effective treatment of the infection requires not only expulsion of the worms but treatment of the anaemia.

**Mebendazole** (section 5.5.1) has a useful broad-spectrum activity, and is effective against hookworms; the usual dose is 100 mg twice daily for 3 days. **Albendazole** [unlicensed] (available from 'special-order' manufacturers or specialist importing companies, see p. 969) given as a single dose of 400 mg, is an alternative.

## 5.5.5 Schistosomicides
### (bilharziasis)

Adult *Schistosoma haematobium* worms live in the genito-urinary veins and adult *S. mansoni* in those of the colon and mesentery. *S. japonicum* is more widely distributed in veins of the alimentary tract and portal system.

**Praziquantel** [unlicensed] is available from Merck (*Cysticide®*) and is effective against all human schistosomes. The dose is 20 mg/kg followed after 4–6 hours by one further dose of 20 mg/kg (60 mg/kg in 3 divided doses on one day for *S. japonicum* infections). No serious adverse effects have been reported. Of all the available schistosomicides, it has the most attractive combination of effectiveness, broad-spectrum activity, and low toxicity.

Hycanthone, lucanthone, niridazole, oxamniquine, and sodium stibocaptate have now been superseded.

## 5.5.6 Filaricides

**Diethylcarbamazine** [unlicensed] (available from 'special-order' manufacturers or specialist importing companies, see p. 969) is effective against microfilariae and adults of *Loa loa*, *Wuchereria bancrofti*, and *Brugia malayi*. To minimise reactions treatment is commenced with a dose of diethylcarbamazine citrate 1 mg/kg on the first day and increased gradually over 3 days to 6 mg/kg daily in divided doses (up to 9 mg/kg daily in divided doses for *Loa loa*); this dosage is maintained for a further period. Close medical supervision is necessary particularly in the early phase of treatment.

In heavy infections there may be a febrile reaction, and in heavy *Loa loa* infection there is a small risk of encephalopathy. In such cases treatment must be given under careful in-patient supervision and stopped at the first sign of cerebral involvement (and specialist advice sought).

**Ivermectin** [unlicensed] (available from 'special-order' manufacturers or specialist importing companies, see p. 969) is very effective in *onchocerciasis* and it is now the drug of choice. A single dose of 150 micrograms/kg by mouth produces a prolonged reduction in microfilarial levels. Retreatment at intervals of 6 to 12 months depending on symptoms must be given until the adult worms die out. Reactions are usually slight and most commonly take the form of temporary aggravation of itching and rash. Diethylcarbamazine or suramin should no longer be used for onchocerciasis because of their toxicity.

## 5.5.7 Drugs for cutaneous larva migrans
### (creeping eruption)

Dog and cat hookworm larvae may enter human skin where they produce slowly extending itching tracks usually on the foot. Single tracks can be treated with topical tiabendazole (no commercial preparation available). Multiple infections respond to **ivermectin**, **albendazole** or **tiabendazole** (thiabendazole) by mouth [all unlicensed] and available from 'special-order' manufacturers or specialist importing companies, see p. 969).

## 5.5.8 Drugs for strongyloidiasis

Adult *Strongyloides stercoralis* live in the gut and produce larvae which penetrate the gut wall and invade the tissues, setting up a cycle of auto-infection. **Ivermectin** [unlicensed] (available from 'special-order' manufacturers or specialist importing companies, see p. 969) in a dose of 200 micrograms/kg daily for 2 days is the treatment of choice for chronic *Strongyloides* infection. **Albendazole** [unlicensed] (available from 'special-order' manufacturers or specialist importing companies, see p. 969) is an alternative given in a dose of 400 mg twice daily for 3 days, repeated after 3 weeks if necessary.

5

Infections

# 6 Endocrine system

| 6.1 | Drugs used in diabetes | 372 |
| 6.1.1 | Insulins | 373 |
| 6.1.1.1 | Short-acting insulins | 376 |
| 6.1.1.2 | Intermediate- and long-acting insulins | 377 |
| 6.1.1.3 | Hypodermic equipment | 379 |
| 6.1.2 | Antidiabetic drugs | 380 |
| 6.1.2.1 | Sulphonylureas | 381 |
| 6.1.2.2 | Biguanides | 382 |
| 6.1.2.3 | Other antidiabetic drugs | 384 |
| 6.1.3 | Diabetic ketoacidosis | 387 |
| 6.1.4 | Treatment of hypoglycaemia | 388 |
| 6.1.5 | Treatment of diabetic nephropathy and neuropathy | 389 |
| 6.1.6 | Diagnostic and monitoring agents for diabetes mellitus | 389 |
| 6.2 | Thyroid and antithyroid drugs | 391 |
| 6.2.1 | Thyroid hormones | 391 |
| 6.2.2 | Antithyroid drugs | 392 |
| 6.3 | Corticosteroids | 394 |
| 6.3.1 | Replacement therapy | 394 |
| 6.3.2 | Glucocorticoid therapy | 394 |
| 6.4 | Sex hormones | 400 |
| 6.4.1 | Female sex hormones | 400 |
| 6.4.1.1 | Oestrogens and HRT | 400 |
| 6.4.1.2 | Progestogens | 407 |
| 6.4.2 | Male sex hormones and antagonists | 409 |
| 6.4.3 | Anabolic steroids | 412 |
| 6.5 | Hypothalamic and pituitary hormones and anti-oestrogens | 412 |
| 6.5.1 | Hypothalamic and anterior pituitary hormones and anti-oestrogens | 412 |
| 6.5.2 | Posterior pituitary hormones and antagonists | 417 |
| 6.6 | Drugs affecting bone metabolism | 419 |
| 6.6.1 | Calcitonin and parathyroid hormone | 421 |
| 6.6.2 | Bisphosphonates and other drugs affecting bone metabolism | 422 |
| 6.7 | Other endocrine drugs | 426 |
| 6.7.1 | Bromocriptine and other dopaminergic drugs | 426 |
| 6.7.2 | Drugs affecting gonadotrophins | 428 |
| 6.7.3 | Metyrapone and trilostane | 432 |
| 6.7.4 | Somatomedins | 432 |

This chapter also includes advice on the drug management of the following:
Adrenal suppression during illness, trauma or surgery, p. 395
Serious infections in patients taking corticosteroids, p. 396
Osteoporosis, p. 419
Breast pain (mastalgia), p. 431

For hormonal contraception, see section 7.3.

## 6.1 Drugs used in diabetes

**6.1.1 Insulins**

**6.1.2 Antidiabetic drugs**

**6.1.3 Diabetic ketoacidosis**

**6.1.4 Treatment of hypoglycaemia**

**6.1.5 Treatment of diabetic nephropathy and neuropathy**

**6.1.6 Diagnostic and monitoring agents for diabetes mellitus**

Diabetes mellitus occurs because of a lack of insulin or resistance to its action. It is diagnosed by measuring fasting or random blood-glucose concentration (and occasionally by oral glucose tolerance test). Although there are many subtypes, the two principal classes of diabetes are type 1 diabetes and type 2 diabetes.

*Type 1 diabetes*, (formerly referred to as insulin-dependent diabetes mellitus (IDDM)), occurs as a result of a deficiency of insulin following autoimmune destruction of pancreatic beta cells. Patients with type 1 diabetes require administration of insulin.

*Type 2 diabetes*, (formerly referred to as non-insulin-dependent diabetes (NIDDM)), is due either to reduced secretion of insulin or to peripheral resistance to the action of insulin. Although patients may be controlled on diet alone, many also require oral antidiabetic drugs or insulin (or both) to maintain satisfactory control. In overweight individuals, type 2 diabetes may be prevented by losing weight and increasing physical activity; use of drugs such as orlistat (section 4.5.1) or sibutramine (section 4.5.2) may be considered in obese patients.

**Treatment of diabetes** Treatment of all forms of diabetes should be aimed at alleviating symptoms and minimising the risk of long-term complications (see below); tight control of diabetes is essential.

Endocrine system

6

Diabetes is a strong risk factor for cardiovascular disease (section 2.12). Other risk factors for cardiovascular disease such as smoking (section 4.10), hypertension (section 2.5), obesity (section 4.5), and hyperlipidaemia (section 2.12) should be addressed. Cardiovascular risk in patients with diabetes can be further reduced by the use of an ACE inhibitor (section 2.5.5.1), low-dose aspirin (section 2.9) and a lipid-regulating drug (section 2.12).

**Prevention of diabetic complications**  Optimal glycaemic control in both type 1 diabetes and type 2 diabetes reduces, in the long term, the risk of microvascular complications including retinopathy, development of proteinuria and to some extent neuropathy. However, a temporary deterioration in established diabetic retinopathy may occur when normalising blood-glucose concentration. For reference to the use of an ACE inhibitor or an angiotensin-II receptor antagonist in the management of diabetic nephropathy, see section 6.1.5.

A measure of the total glycosylated (or glycated) haemoglobin (HbA$_1$) or a specific fraction (HbA$_{1c}$) provides a good indication of glycaemic control over the previous 2–3 months. The ideal HbA$_{1c}$ concentration is between 6.5% and 7.5% (48–59 mmol/mol) but this cannot always be achieved, and those on insulin may have significantly increased risks of severe hypoglycaemia. Tight control of blood pressure in hypertensive patients with type 2 diabetes reduces mortality and protects visual acuity (by reducing considerably the risks of maculopathy and retinal photocoagulation) (see also section 2.5).

**Driving**  Drivers with diabetes are required to notify the Driver and Vehicle Licensing Agency (DVLA) of their condition if they are treated with insulin or if they are treated with oral antidiabetic drugs and also have complications. Detailed guidance on eligibility to drive is available from the DVLA (www.dvla.gov.uk/medical.aspx). Driving is not permitted when hypoglycaemic awareness is impaired or frequent hypoglycaemic episodes occur.

Drivers need to be particularly careful to avoid hypoglycaemia (see also above) and should be warned of the problems. Drivers treated with insulin should normally check their blood-glucose concentration before driving and, on long journeys, at 2-hour intervals; these precautions may also be necessary for drivers taking oral antidiabetic drugs who are at particular risk of hypoglycaemia. Drivers treated with insulin should ensure that a supply of sugar is always available in the vehicle and they should avoid driving if their meal is delayed. If hypoglycaemia occurs, or warning signs develop, the driver should:

- stop the vehicle in a safe place;
- switch off the ignition;
- eat or drink a suitable source of sugar;
- wait until recovery is complete before continuing journey; recovery may take 15 minutes or longer and should preferably be confirmed by checking blood-glucose concentration.

## 6.1.1  Insulins

### 6.1.1.1  Short-acting insulins
### 6.1.1.2  Intermediate- and long-acting insulins
### 6.1.1.3  Hypodermic equipment

Insulin plays a key role in the regulation of carbohydrate, fat, and protein metabolism. It is a polypeptide hormone of complex structure. There are differences in the amino-acid sequence of animal insulins, human insulins and the human insulin analogues. Insulin may be extracted from pork pancreas and purified by crystallisation; it may also be extracted from beef pancreas, but beef insulins are now rarely used. Human sequence insulin may be produced semisynthetically by enzymatic modification of porcine insulin (emp) or biosynthetically by recombinant DNA technology using bacteria (crb, prb) or yeast (pyr).

All insulin preparations are to a greater or lesser extent immunogenic in man but immunological resistance to insulin action is uncommon. Preparations of human sequence insulin should theoretically be less immunogenic, but no real advantage has been shown in trials.

Insulin is inactivated by gastro-intestinal enzymes, and must therefore be given by injection; the subcutaneous route is ideal in most circumstances. Insulin is usually injected into the upper arms, thighs, buttocks, or abdomen; absorption from a limb site may be increased if the limb is used in strenuous exercise after the injection. Generally subcutaneous insulin injections cause few problems; fat hypertrophy does, however, occur but can be minimised by using different injection sites in rotation. Local allergic reactions are rare.

Insulin is needed by all patients with ketoacidosis, and it is likely to be needed by most patients with:

- rapid onset of symptoms;
- substantial loss of weight;
- weakness;
- ketonuria;
- a first-degree relative who has type 1 diabetes.

Insulin is required by almost all children with diabetes. It is also needed for type 2 diabetes when other methods have failed to achieve good control, and temporarily in the presence of intercurrent illness or peri-operatively. Pregnant women with type 2 diabetes may be treated with insulin when diet alone fails. For advice on use of oral antidiabetic drugs in the management of diabetes in pregnancy, see section 6.1.2.

**Management of diabetes with insulin**  The aim of treatment is to achieve the best possible control of blood-glucose concentration without making the patient obsessional and to avoid disabling hypoglycaemia; close co-operation is needed between the patient and the medical team because good control reduces the risk of complications.

Mixtures of insulin preparations may be required and appropriate combinations have to be determined for the individual patient. For patients with acute-onset diabetes, treatment should be started with a short-acting insulin (e.g. soluble insulin, insulin aspart) given 3 times daily with intermediate-acting insulin at bedtime. For those less severely ill, treatment is usually started with a mixture of premixed short- and intermediate-acting insulins (most commonly in a proportion of 30% soluble insulin and 70% isophane insulin) given twice daily; 8 units twice daily is a suitable initial dose for most ambulant patients. The proportion of the short-acting soluble component can be increased in those with excessive postprandial hyperglycaemia.

The dose of insulin is increased gradually, taking care to avoid troublesome hypoglycaemic reactions.

Insulin preparations can be divided into 3 types:

- those of **short** duration which have a relatively rapid onset of action, namely soluble insulin and the rapid-acting insulin analogues, insulin aspart, insulin glulisine, and insulin lispro (section 6.1.1.1);

- those with an **intermediate** action, e.g. isophane insulin (section 6.1.1.2); and

- those whose action is slower in onset and lasts for **long** periods, e.g. protamine zinc insulin, insulin detemir, and insulin glargine (section 6.1.1.2).

The duration of action of a particular type of insulin varies considerably from one patient to another, and needs to be assessed individually.

### Examples of recommended insulin regimens

- Short-acting insulin mixed with intermediate-acting insulin: twice daily (before meals);

- Short-acting insulin mixed with intermediate-acting insulin: before breakfast
  Short-acting insulin: before evening meal
  Intermediate-acting insulin: at bedtime;

- Short-acting insulin: three times daily (before breakfast, midday, and evening meal)
  Intermediate-acting insulin: at bedtime;

- Intermediate-acting insulin with or without short-acting insulin: once daily either before breakfast or at bedtime suffices for some patients with type 2 diabetes who need insulin;

- Continuous subcutaneous insulin infusion (see below).

Insulin requirements may be increased by infection, stress, accidental or surgical trauma, and during puberty. Requirements may be decreased in patients with renal impairment (Appendix 3) or hepatic impairment and in those with some endocrine disorders (e.g. Addison's disease, hypopituitarism) or coeliac disease.

**Pregnancy and breast-feeding** During pregnancy and breast-feeding, insulin requirements may alter and doses should be assessed frequently by an experienced diabetes physician. The dose of insulin generally needs to be increased in the second and third trimesters of pregnancy. The short-acting insulin analogues, insulin aspart and insulin lispro, are not known to be harmful, and may be used during pregnancy and lactation. The safety of long-acting insulin analogues in pregnancy has not been established, therefore isophane insulin is recommended where longer-acting insulins are needed.

**Insulin administration** Insulin is generally given by *subcutaneous injection*. Injection devices ('pens') (section 6.1.1.3), which hold the insulin in a cartridge and meter the required dose, are convenient to use. The conventional syringe and needle is still preferred by many and is also required for insulins not available in cartridge form.

For intensive insulin regimens multiple subcutaneous injections (3 to 4 times daily) are usually recommended.

Short-acting injectable insulins (soluble insulin, insulin aspart, insulin glulisine, and insulin lispro) can also be given by *continuous subcutaneous infusion* using a portable infusion pump. This device delivers a continuous basal insulin infusion and patient-activated bolus doses at meal times. This technique is appropriate only for patients who suffer recurrent hypoglycaemia or marked morning rise in blood-glucose concentration despite optimised multiple-injection regimens. Patients on subcutaneous insulin infusion must be highly motivated, able to monitor their blood-glucose concentration, and have expert training, advice and supervision from an experienced healthcare team.

> **NICE guidance**
>
> **Continuous subcutaneous insulin infusion for the treatment of diabetes mellitus (type 1) (July 2008)**
> Continuous subcutaneous insulin infusion is recommended as an option in adults and children over 12 years with type 1 diabetes:
>
> - who suffer repeated or unpredictable hypoglycaemia, whilst attempting to achieve optimal glycaemic control with multiple-injection regimens, **or**
>
> - whose glycaemic control remains inadequate (HbA$_{1c}$ over 8.5%) despite optimised multiple-injection regimens (including the use of long-acting insulin analogues where appropriate).
>
> Continuous subcutaneous insulin infusion is also recommended as an option for children under 12 years with type 1 diabetes for whom multiple-injection regimens are considered impractical or inappropriate. Children on insulin pumps should undergo a trial of multiple-injection therapy between the ages of 12 and 18 years.

Soluble insulin by the *intravenous route* is reserved for urgent treatment, e.g. in diabetic ketoacidosis, and for fine control in serious illness and in the peri-operative period (see under Diabetes and Surgery, below).

**Units** The word 'unit' should **not** be abbreviated.

**Monitoring** Many patients now monitor their own blood-glucose concentration (section 6.1.6). Since blood-glucose concentrations vary substantially throughout the day, 'normoglycaemia' cannot always be achieved throughout a 24-hour period without causing damaging hypoglycaemia. It is therefore best to recommend that patients should maintain a blood-glucose concentration of between 4 and 9 mmol/litre for most of the time (4–7 mmol/litre before meals and less than 9 mmol/litre after meals), while accepting that on occasions, for brief periods, it will be above these values; strenuous efforts should be made to prevent the blood-glucose concentration from falling below 4 mmol/litre. Patients should be advised to look for 'peaks' and 'troughs' of blood glucose, and to adjust their insulin dosage only once or twice weekly. Overall it is ideal to aim for an HbA$_{1c}$ (glycosylated haemoglobin) concentration of 6.5–7.5% (48–59 mmol/mol) or less (reference range 4–6% or 20–42 mmol/mol) but this is not always possible without causing disabling hypoglycaemia; in those at risk of arterial disease, the aim should be to maintain the HbA$_{1c}$ concentration at 6.5% (48 mmol/

mol) or less. HbA$_{1c}$ should be measured every 3–6 months. Fructosamine can also be used for assessment of control; this is simpler and cheaper but the measurement of HbA$_{1c}$ is generally a more reliable method.

> ### Measurement of HbA$_{1c}$
>
> HbA$_{1c}$ values currently expressed as a percentage, are aligned to the assay used in the Diabetes Control and Complications Trial (DCCT). A new standard, specific for HbA$_{1c}$, has been created by the International Federation of Clinical Chemistry and Laboratory Medicine (IFCC), which expresses HbA$_{1c}$ values in *mmol per mol* of unglycosylated haemoglobin. From 1 June 2009, UK laboratories will express results in both IFCC-standardised units (mmol/mol) and DCCT-aligned units (%). From 1 June 2011, results will only be reported in IFCC-standardised units.
>
> ### Equivalent values
>
> | DCCT-HbA$_{1c}$ (%) | IFCC-HbA$_{1c}$ (mmol/mol) |
> |---|---|
> | 6.0 | 42 |
> | 6.5 | 48 |
> | 7.0 | 53 |
> | 7.5 | 59 |
> | 8.0 | 64 |
> | 9.0 | 75 |

The intake of energy and of simple and complex carbohydrates should be adequate to allow normal growth and development but obesity must be avoided. The carbohydrate intake needs to be regulated and should be distributed throughout the day. Fine control of plasma glucose can be achieved by moving portions of carbohydrate from one meal to another without altering the total intake.

**Hypoglycaemia** Hypoglycaemia is a potential problem with insulin therapy. All patients must be carefully instructed on how to avoid it.

Loss of warning of hypoglycaemia is common among insulin-treated patients and can be a serious hazard, especially for drivers and those in dangerous occupations. Very tight control of diabetes lowers the blood-glucose concentration needed to trigger hypoglycaemic symptoms; increase in the frequency of hypoglycaemic episodes reduces the warning symptoms experienced by the patient. Beta-blockers can also blunt hypoglycaemic awareness (and also delay recovery).

To restore the warning signs, episodes of hypoglycaemia must be minimised; this involves appropriate adjustment of insulin type, dose and frequency together with suitable timing and quantity of meals and snacks.

Some patients have reported loss of hypoglycaemia warning after transfer to human insulin. Clinical studies do not confirm that human insulin decreases hypoglycaemia awareness. If a patient believes that human insulin is responsible for the loss of warning it is reasonable to revert to animal insulin and essential to educate the patient about avoiding hypoglycaemia. Great care should be taken to specify whether a human or an animal preparation is required.

Few patients are now treated with beef insulins; when undertaking conversion from beef to human insulin, the total dose should be reduced by about 10% with careful monitoring for the first few days. When changing between pork and human-sequence insulins, a dose change is not usually needed, but careful monitoring is still advised.

**Diabetes and surgery** Perioperative control of blood-glucose concentrations in patients with type 1 diabetes is achieved via an adjustable, continuous, intravenous infusion of insulin. Detailed local protocols should be available to all healthcare professionals involved in the treatment of these patients; in general, the following steps should be followed:

- Give an injection of the patient's usual insulin on the night before the operation;

- Early on the day of the operation, start an intravenous infusion of glucose containing potassium chloride (provided that the patient is not hyperkalaemic) and infuse at a constant rate appropriate to the patient's fluid requirements (usually 125 mL per hour); make up a solution of soluble insulin in sodium chloride 0.9% and infuse intravenously using a syringe pump piggy-backed to the intravenous infusion. Glucose and potassium infusions, and insulin infusions should be made up according to locally agreed protocols;

- The rate of the insulin infusion should be adjusted according to blood-glucose concentration (frequent monitoring necessary) in line with locally agreed protocols. Other factors affecting the rate of infusion include the patient's volume depletion, cardiac function, and age.

Protocols should include specific instructions on how to manage resistant cases (such as patients who are in shock or severely ill or those receiving corticosteroids or sympathomimetics) and those with hypoglycaemia.

If a syringe pump is not available, soluble insulin should be added to the intravenous infusion of glucose and potassium chloride (provided that the patient is not hyperkalaemic), and the infusion run at the rate appropriate to the patient's fluid requirements (usually 125 mL per hour) with the insulin dose adjusted according to blood-glucose concentration in line with locally agreed protocols.

Once the patient starts to eat and drink, give subcutaneous insulin before breakfast and stop intravenous insulin 30 minutes later; the dose may need to be 10–20% more than usual if the patient is still in bed or unwell. If the patient was not previously receiving insulin, an appropriate initial dose is 30–40 units daily in four divided doses using soluble insulin before meals and intermediate-acting insulin at bedtime and the dose adjusted from day to day. Patients with hyperglycaemia often relapse after conversion back to subcutaneous insulin calling for one of the following approaches:

- additional doses of soluble insulin at any of the four injection times (before meals or bedtime) *or*

- temporary addition of intravenous insulin infusion (while continuing the subcutaneous regimen) until blood-glucose concentration is satisfactory *or*

- complete reversion to the intravenous regimen (especially if the patient is unwell).

**6**

**Endocrine system**

## 6.1.1.1 Short-acting insulins

**Soluble insulin** is a short-acting form of insulin. For maintenance regimens it is usual to inject it 15 to 30 minutes before meals.

Soluble insulin is the most appropriate form of insulin for use in diabetic emergencies e.g. diabetic ketoacidosis (section 6.1.3) and at the time of surgery. It can be given intravenously and intramuscularly, as well as subcutaneously.

When injected subcutaneously, soluble insulin has a rapid onset of action (30 to 60 minutes), a peak action between 2 and 4 hours, and a duration of action of up to 8 hours.

When injected intravenously, soluble insulin has a very short half-life of only about 5 minutes and its effect disappears within 30 minutes.

The human insulin analogues, **insulin aspart**, **insulin glulisine**, and **insulin lispro** have a faster onset and shorter duration of action than soluble insulin; as a result, compared to soluble insulin, fasting and preprandial blood-glucose concentrations are a little higher, postprandial blood-glucose concentration is a little lower, and hypoglycaemia occurs slightly less frequently. Subcutaneous injection of insulin analogues may be convenient for those who wish to inject shortly before or, when necessary, shortly after a meal. They can also help those susceptible to hypoglycaemia before lunch and those who eat late in the evening and are prone to nocturnal hypoglycaemia. They can also be administered by subcutaneous infusion (see Insulin Administration, above). Insulin aspart and insulin lispro can be administered intravenously and can be used as alternatives to soluble insulin for diabetic emergencies and at the time of surgery.

## INSULIN
### (Insulin Injection; Neutral Insulin; Soluble Insulin)

A sterile solution of insulin (i.e. bovine or porcine) or of human insulin; pH 6.6–8.0

**Indications** diabetes mellitus; diabetic ketoacidosis (section 6.1.3)

**Cautions** see notes above; pregnancy (Appendix 4); reduce dose in renal impairment (Appendix 3); **interactions:** Appendix 1 (antidiabetics)

**Side-effects** see notes above; transient oedema; local reactions and fat hypertrophy at injection site; *rarely* hypersensitivity reactions including urticaria, rash; overdose causes hypoglycaemia

**Dose**

- By subcutaneous, intramuscular *or* intravenous injection *or* intravenous infusion, according to requirements

◢Highly purified animal
**Counselling** Show container to patient and confirm that patient is expecting the version dispensed

**Hypurin® Bovine Neutral** (Wockhardt) ᴘᴏᴹ
Injection, soluble insulin (bovine, highly purified) 100 units/mL. Net price 10-mL vial = £18.48; cartridges (for *Autopen® Classic*) 5 × 3 mL = £27.72

**Hypurin® Porcine Neutral** (Wockhardt) ᴘᴏᴹ
Injection, soluble insulin (porcine, highly purified) 100 units/mL. Net price 10-mL vial = £16.80; cartridges (for *Autopen® Classic*) 5 × 3 mL = £25.20

◢Human sequence
**Counselling** Show container to patient and confirm that patient is expecting the version dispensed

**Actrapid®** (Novo Nordisk) ᴘᴏᴹ
Injection, soluble insulin (human, pyr) 100 units/mL. Net price 10-mL vial = £7.48
**Note** Not recommended for use in subcutaneous insulin infusion pumps—may precipitate in catheter or needle

**Humulin S®** (Lilly) ᴘᴏᴹ
Injection, soluble insulin (human, prb) 100 units/mL. Net price 10-mL vial = £15.68; 5 × 3-mL cartridge (for most *Autopen® Classic* or *HumaPen®*) = £26.71

**Insuman® Rapid** (Aventis Pharma) ᴘᴏᴹ
Injection, soluble insulin (human, crb) 100 units/mL, net price 5 × 3-mL cartridge (for *OptiPen® Pro 1*) = £22.52; 5 × 3-mL *Insuman® Rapid OptiSet®* prefilled disposable injection devices (range 2–40 units, allowing 2-unit dosage adjustment) = £26.81
**Note** Not recommended for use in subcutaneous insulin infusion pumps

◢Mixed preparations
See Biphasic Isophane Insulin (section 6.1.1.2)

## INSULIN ASPART
### (Recombinant human insulin analogue)

**Indications** diabetes mellitus

**Cautions** see under Insulin; children (use only if benefit likely compared to soluble insulin)

**Side-effects** see under Insulin

**Dose**

- By subcutaneous injection, immediately before meals or when necessary shortly after meals, according to requirements
- By subcutaneous infusion, intravenous injection *or* intravenous infusion, according to requirements

**NovoRapid®** (Novo Nordisk) ᴘᴏᴹ
Injection, insulin aspart (recombinant human insulin analogue) 100 units/mL, net price 10-mL vial = £16.60; *Penfill®* cartridge (for *NovoPen®* devices) 5 × 3-mL = £29.14; 5 × 3-mL *FlexPen®* prefilled disposable injection devices (range 1–60 units, allowing 1-unit dosage adjustment) = £32.00
**Counselling** Show container to patient and confirm that patient is expecting the version dispensed

## INSULIN GLULISINE
### (Recombinant human insulin analogue)

**Indications** diabetes mellitus

**Cautions** see under Insulin

**Side-effects** see under Insulin

**Dose**

- By subcutaneous injection, ADULT and CHILD over 6 years, immediately before meals or when necessary shortly after meals, according to requirements
- By subcutaneous infusion, ADULT and CHILD over 6 years, according to requirements

6 Endocrine system

**Apidra®** (Sanofi-Aventis) ▼ [PoM]
Injection, insulin glulisine (recombinant human insulin analogue) 100 units/mL, net price 10-mL vial = £16.60; 5× 3-mL cartridge (for *OptiPen® Pro 1* and *Autopen® 24*) = £28.30; 5 × 3-mL *OptiClik®* cartridge (for *OptiClik® Pen* [NHS]) = £30.27; 5 × 3-mL *Apidra® Optiset®* prefilled disposable injection devices (range 2–40 units, allowing 2-unit dosage adjustment) = £28.30; 5 × 3-mL *Apidra® SoloStar®* prefilled disposable injection devices (range 1–80 units, allowing 1-unit dosage adjustment) = £25.00
Counselling Show container to patient and confirm that patient is expecting the version dispensed
Note The *Scottish Medicines Consortium* (p. 3) has advised (October 2008) that *Apidra®* is accepted for restricted use within NHS Scotland for the treatment of adults and children over 6 years with diabetes mellitus in whom the use of a short-acting insulin analogue is appropriate

## ▌ INSULIN LISPRO
(Recombinant human insulin analogue)

**Indications** diabetes mellitus
**Cautions** see under Insulin; children (use only if benefit likely compared to soluble insulin)
**Side-effects** see under Insulin
**Dose**
- By subcutaneous injection shortly before meals or when necessary shortly after meals, according to requirements
- By subcutaneous infusion, *or* intravenous injection, *or* intravenous infusion, according to requirements

**Humalog®** (Lilly) [PoM]
Injection, insulin lispro (recombinant human insulin analogue) 100 units/mL. Net price 10-mL vial = £16.61; 5 × 3-mL cartridge (for *Autopen® Classic* or *HumaPen®*) = £28.31; 5 × 3-mL *Humalog®-Pen* prefilled disposable injection devices (range 1–60 units, allowing 1-unit dosage adjustment) = £29.46; 5 × 3-mL *Humalog® KwikPen* prefilled disposable injection devices (range 1–60 units, allowing 1-unit dosage adjustment) = £29.46
Counselling Show container to patient and confirm that patient is expecting the version dispensed

## 6.1.1.2 Intermediate- and long-acting insulins

When given by subcutaneous injection, intermediate- and long-acting insulins have an onset of action of approximately 1–2 hours, a maximal effect at 4–12 hours, and a duration of 16–35 hours. Some are given twice daily in conjunction with short-acting (soluble) insulin, and others are given once daily, particularly in elderly patients. Soluble insulin can be mixed with intermediate and long-acting insulins (except insulin detemir and insulin glargine) in the syringe, essentially retaining the properties of the two components, although there may be some blunting of the initial effect of the soluble insulin component (especially on mixing with protamine zinc insulin, see below).

**Isophane insulin** is a suspension of insulin with protamine; it is of particular value for initiation of twice-daily insulin regimens. Patients usually mix isophane with soluble insulin but ready-mixed preparations may be appropriate (**biphasic isophane insulin, biphasic insulin aspart,** or **biphasic insulin lispro**).

**Insulin zinc suspension** (30% amorphous, 70% crystalline) has a more prolonged duration of action.

**Protamine zinc insulin** is usually given once daily with short-acting (soluble) insulin. It has the drawback of binding with the soluble insulin when mixed in the same syringe and is now rarely used.

**Insulin glargine** and **insulin detemir** are both human insulin analogues with a prolonged duration of action; insulin glargine is given once daily and insulin detemir is given once or twice daily. NICE (December 2002) has recommended that insulin glargine should be available as an option for patients with type 1 diabetes.

NICE (May 2009) has recommended that, if insulin is required in patients with type 2 diabetes, insulin detemir or insulin glargine may be considered for those:

- who require assistance with injecting insulin *or*
- whose lifestyle is significantly restricted by recurrent symptomatic hypoglycaemia *or*
- who would otherwise need twice-daily basal insulin injections in combination with oral antidiabetic drugs *or*
- who cannot use the device needed to inject isophane insulin.

## ▌ INSULIN DETEMIR
(Recombinant human insulin analogue—long acting)

**Indications** diabetes mellitus
**Cautions** see under Insulin (section 6.1.1.1); pregnancy (Appendix 4)
**Side-effects** see under Insulin (section 6.1.1.1)
**Dose**
- By subcutaneous injection, ADULT and CHILD over 6 years, according to requirements

**Levemir®** (Novo Nordisk) [PoM]
Injection, insulin detemir (recombinant human insulin analogue) 100 units/mL, net price 5 × 3-mL cartridge (for *NovoPen®* devices) = £42.00; 5 × 3-mL *FlexPen®* prefilled disposable injection device (range 1–60 units, allowing 1-unit dosage adjustment) = £42.00; 5 × 3-mL *Levemir InnoLet®* prefilled disposable injection devices (range 1–50 units, allowing 1-unit dosage adjustment) = £44.85
Counselling Show container to patient and confirm that patient is expecting the version dispensed

## ▌ INSULIN GLARGINE
(Recombinant human insulin analogue—long acting)

**Indications** diabetes mellitus
**Cautions** see under Insulin (section 6.1.1.1); pregnancy (Appendix 4)
**Side-effects** see under Insulin (section 6.1.1.1)
**Dose**
- By subcutaneous injection, ADULT and CHILD over 6 years, according to requirements

**Lantus®** (Aventis Pharma) [PoM]
Injection, insulin glargine (recombinant human insulin analogue) 100 units/mL, net price 10-mL vial = £26.00; 5 × 3-mL cartridge (for *OptiPen® Pro 1* and *Autopen® 24*) = £39.00; 5 × 3-mL *OptiClik®* cartridge

(for *OptiClik*® *Pen* (JHS)) = £40.36; 5 × 3-mL *Lantus*®
*OptiSet*® prefilled disposable injection devices (range
2–40 units, allowing 2-unit dosage adjustment) =
£39.00; 5 × 3-mL *Lantus*® *SoloStar*® prefilled
disposable injection devices (range 1–80 units, allowing 1-unit dosage adjustment) = £40.36
Note The *Scottish Medicines Consortium* (p. 3) has advised
(October 2002) that insulin glargine is accepted for restricted
use within NHS Scotland for the treatment of type 1 diabetes:

- in those who are at risk of or experience unacceptable
  frequency or severity of nocturnal hypoglycaemia on
  attempting to achieve better hypoglycaemic control
  during treatment with other insulins

- as a once daily insulin therapy for patients who require a
  carer to administer their insulin.

It is **not** recommended for routine use in patients with type 2
diabetes unless they suffer from recurrent episodes of
hypoglycaemia or require assistance with their insulin
injections.
Counselling Show container to patient and confirm that
patient is expecting the version dispensed

## INSULIN ZINC SUSPENSION
### (Insulin Zinc Suspension (Mixed)—long acting)
A sterile neutral suspension of bovine and/or porcine insulin or
of human insulin in the form of a complex obtained by the
addition of a suitable zinc salt; consists of rhombohedral
crystals (10–40 microns) and of particles of no uniform shape
(not exceeding 2 microns)

**Indications** diabetes mellitus

**Cautions** see under Insulin (section 6.1.1.1)

**Side-effects** see under Insulin (section 6.1.1.1)

**Dose**

- By subcutaneous injection, according to requirements

◢Highly purified animal

**Hypurin**® **Bovine Lente** (Wockhardt) (PoM)
   Injection, insulin zinc suspension (bovine, highly
   purified) 100 units/mL. Net price 10-mL vial = £18.48
   Counselling Show container to patient and confirm that
   patient is expecting the version dispensed

## ISOPHANE INSULIN
### (Isophane Insulin Injection; Isophane Prot-
### amine Insulin Injection; Isophane Insulin
### (NPH)—intermediate acting)
A sterile suspension of bovine or porcine insulin or of human
insulin in the form of a complex obtained by the addition of
protamine sulphate or another suitable protamine

**Indications** diabetes mellitus

**Cautions** see under Insulin (section 6.1.1.1)

**Side-effects** see under Insulin (section 6.1.1.1); protamine may cause allergic reactions

**Dose**

- By subcutaneous injection, according to requirements

◢Highly purified animal
   Counselling Show container to patient and confirm that
   patient is expecting the version dispensed

**Hypurin**® **Bovine Isophane** (Wockhardt) (PoM)
   Injection, isophane insulin (bovine, highly purified)
   100 units/mL. Net price 10-mL vial = £18.48; cartridges (for *Autopen*® *Classic*) 5 × 3 mL = £27.72

**Hypurin**® **Porcine Isophane** (Wockhardt) (PoM)
   Injection, isophane insulin (porcine, highly purified)
   100 units/mL. Net price 10-mL vial = £16.80; cartridges (for *Autopen*® *Classic*) 5 × 3 mL = £25.20

◢Human sequence
   Counselling Show container to patient and confirm that
   patient is expecting the version dispensed

**Insulatard**® (Novo Nordisk) (PoM)
   Injection, isophane insulin (human, pyr) 100 units/
   mL. Net price 10-mL vial = £7.48; *Insulatard Penfill*®
   cartridge (for *Novopen*® devices) 5 × 3 mL = £19.08; 5
   × 3-mL *Insulatard InnoLet*® prefilled disposable
   injection devices (range 1–50 units, allowing 1-unit
   dosage adjustment) = £20.40

**Humulin I**® (Lilly) (PoM)
   Injection, isophane insulin (human, prb) 100 units/
   mL. Net price 10-mL vial = £15.68; 5 × 3-mL cartridge
   (for *Autopen*® *Classic* or *HumaPen*®) = £26.71; 5 × 3-
   mL *Humulin I-Pen*® prefilled disposable injection
   devices (range 1–60 units, allowing 1-unit dosage
   adjustment) = £28.44

**Insuman**® **Basal** (Aventis Pharma) (PoM)
   Injection, isophane insulin (human, crb) 100 units/
   mL, net price 5-mL vial = £5.61; 5 × 3-mL cartridge
   (for *OptiPen*® *Pro 1*) = £22.52; 5 × 3-mL *Insuman*®
   *Basal OptiSet*® prefilled disposable injection devices
   (range 2–40 units, allowing 2-unit dosage adjustment)
   = £26.81

◢Mixed preparations
   See Biphasic Isophane Insulin (p. 379)

## PROTAMINE ZINC INSULIN
### (Protamine Zinc Insulin Injection—long acting)
A sterile suspension of insulin in the form of a complex
obtained by the addition of a suitable protamine and zinc
chloride; this preparation was included in BP 1980 but is not
included in BP 1988

**Indications** diabetes mellitus

**Cautions** see under Insulin (section 6.1.1.1); see also
notes above

**Side-effects** see under Insulin (section 6.1.1.1); protamine may cause allergic reactions

**Dose**

- By subcutaneous injection, according to requirements

**Hypurin**® **Bovine Protamine Zinc** (Wockhardt) (PoM)
   Injection, protamine zinc insulin (bovine, highly purified) 100 units/mL. Net price 10-mL vial = £18.48
   Counselling Show container to patient and confirm that
   patient is expecting the version dispensed

## Biphasic insulins

## BIPHASIC INSULIN ASPART
### (Intermediate-acting insulin)

**Indications** diabetes mellitus

**Cautions** see under Insulin and Insulin Aspart (section
6.1.1.1)

**Side-effects** see under Insulin (section 6.1.1.1); protamine may cause allergic reactions

6 Endocrine system

**Dose**

- By subcutaneous injection, up to 10 minutes before or soon after a meal, according to requirements

**NovoMix® 30** (Novo Nordisk) PoM

Injection, biphasic insulin aspart (recombinant human insulin analogue), 30% insulin aspart, 70% insulin aspart protamine, 100 units/mL, net price 5 × 3-mL *Penfill®* cartridges (for *NovoPen®* devices) = £29.43; 5 × 3-mL *FlexPen®* prefilled disposable injection devices (range 1–60 units, allowing 1-unit dosage adjustment) = £32.00

Counselling Show container to patient and confirm that patient is expecting the version dispensed; the proportions of the two components should be checked **carefully** (the order in which the proportions are stated may not be the same in other countries)

---

■ **BIPHASIC INSULIN LISPRO**
(Intermediate-acting insulin)

**Indications** diabetes mellitus

**Cautions** see under Insulin and Insulin Lispro (section 6.1.1.1)

**Side-effects** see under Insulin (section 6.1.1.1); protamine may cause allergic reactions

**Dose**

- By subcutaneous injection, up to 15 minutes before or soon after a meal, according to requirements

**Humalog® Mix25** (Lilly) PoM

Injection, biphasic insulin lispro (recombinant human insulin analogue), 25% insulin lispro, 75% insulin lispro protamine, 100 units/mL, net price 5 × 3-mL cartridge (for *Autopen® Classic* or *HumaPen®*) = £29.46; 5 × 3-mL prefilled disposable injection devices (range 1–60 units, allowing 1-unit dosage adjustment) = £30.98; 5 × 3-mL *Humalog® Mix25 KwikPen* prefilled disposable injection devices (range 1–60 units, allowing 1-unit dosage adjustment) = £30.98

Counselling Show container to patient and confirm that patient is expecting the version dispensed; the proportions of the two components should be checked **carefully** (the order in which the proportions are stated may not be the same in other countries)

**Humalog® Mix50** (Lilly) PoM

Injection, biphasic insulin lispro (recombinant human insulin analogue), 50% insulin lispro, 50% insulin lispro protamine, 100 units/mL, net price 5 × 3-mL cartridge (for *Autopen® Classic* or *HumaPen®*) = £29.46; 5 × 3-mL prefilled disposable injection devices (range 1–60 units, allowing 1-unit dosage adjustment) = £29.46; 5 × 3-mL *Humalog® Mix50 KwikPen* prefilled disposable injection devices (range 1–60 units, allowing 1-unit dosage adjustment) = £30.98

Counselling Show container to patient and confirm that patient is expecting the version dispensed; the proportions of the two components should be checked **carefully** (the order in which the proportions are stated may not be the same in other countries)

---

■ **BIPHASIC ISOPHANE INSULIN**
(Biphasic Isophane Insulin Injection—intermediate acting)

A sterile buffered suspension of either porcine or human insulin complexed with protamine sulphate (or another suitable protamine) in a solution of insulin of the same species

**Indications** diabetes mellitus

**Cautions** see under Insulin (section 6.1.1.1)

**Side-effects** see under Insulin (section 6.1.1.1); protamine may cause allergic reactions

**Dose**

- By subcutaneous injection, according to requirements

◢**Highly purified animal**

Counselling Show container to patient and confirm that patient is expecting the version dispensed; the proportions of the two components should be checked **carefully** (the order in which the proportions are stated may not be the same in other countries)

**Hypurin® Porcine 30/70 Mix** (Wockhardt) PoM

Injection, biphasic isophane insulin (porcine, highly purified), 30% soluble, 70% isophane, 100 units/mL. Net price 10-mL vial = £16.80; cartridges (for *Autopen® Classic*) 5 × 3 mL = £25.20

◢**Human sequence**

Counselling Show container to patient and confirm that patient is expecting the version dispensed; the proportions of the two components should be checked **carefully** (the order in which the proportions are stated may not be the same in other countries)

**Mixtard® 30** (Novo Nordisk) PoM

Injection, biphasic isophane insulin (human, pyr), 30% soluble, 70% isophane, 100 units/mL. Net price 10-mL vial = £7.48; *Mixtard 30 Penfill®* cartridge (for *Novopen®* devices) 5 × 3 mL = £19.08; 5 × 3-mL *Mixtard 30 InnoLet®* prefilled disposable injection devices (range 1–50 units allowing 1-unit dosage adjustment) = £19.87

**Humulin M3®** (Lilly) PoM

Injection, biphasic isophane insulin (human, prb), 30% soluble, 70% isophane, 100 units/mL. Net price 10-mL vial = £15.68; 5 × 3-mL cartridge (for most *Autopen® Classic* or *HumaPen®*) = £26.71

**Insuman® Comb 15** (Aventis Pharma) PoM

Injection, biphasic isophane insulin (human, crb), 15% soluble, 85% isophane, 100 units/mL, net price 5 × 3-mL *Insuman® Comb 15 OptiSet®* prefilled disposable injection devices (range 2–40 units, allowing 2-unit dosage adjustment) = £26.81

**Insuman® Comb 25** (Aventis Pharma) PoM

Injection, biphasic isophane insulin (human, crb), 25% soluble, 75% isophane, 100 units/mL, net price 5-mL vial = £5.61; 5 × 3-mL cartridge (for *OptiPen® Pro 1*) = £22.52; 5 × 3-mL *Insuman® Comb 25 OptiSet®* prefilled disposable injection devices (range 2–40 units, allowing 2-unit dosage adjustment) = £26.81

**Insuman® Comb 50** (Aventis Pharma) PoM

Injection, biphasic isophane insulin (human, crb), 50% soluble, 50% isophane, 100 units/mL, net price 5 × 3-mL cartridge (for *OptiPen® Pro 1*) = £22.52; 5 × 3-mL *Insuman® Comb 50 OptiSet®* prefilled disposable injection devices (range 2–40 units, allowing 2-unit dosage adjustment) = £26.81

---

**6.1.1.3** Hypodermic equipment

Patients should be advised on the safe disposal of lancets, single-use syringes, and needles. Suitable arrangements for the safe disposal of contaminated waste must be made before these products are prescribed for patients who are carriers of infectious diseases.

**6**

Endocrine system

**Endocrine system** 6

### ◢Injection devices

**Autopen®** (Owen Mumford)

Injection device, *Autopen® 24* (for use with Sanofi-Aventis 3-mL insulin cartridges), allowing 1-unit dosage adjustment, max. 21 units (single-unit version) *or* 2-unit dosage adjustment, max. 42 units (2-unit version), net price (both) = £15.55; *Autopen® Classic* (for use with Lilly and Wockhardt 3-mL insulin cartridges), allowing 1-unit dosage adjustment, max. 21 units (single-unit version) *or* 2-unit dosage adjustment, max. 42 units (2-unit version), net price (all) = £15.79

**HumaPen® Luxura** (Lilly)

Injection device, for use with *Humulin®* and *Humalog®* 3-mL cartridges; allowing 1-unit dosage adjustment, max. 60 units, net price = £26.36

**HumaPen® Luxura HD** (Lilly)

Injection device, for use with *Humulin®* and *Humalog®* 3-mL cartridges; allowing 0.5-unit dosage adjustment, max. 30 units, net price = £26.36

**NovoPen®** (Novo Nordisk)

Injection device; for use with *Penfill®* insulin cartridges; *NovoPen® Junior* (for 3-mL cartridges), allowing 0.5-unit dosage adjustment, max. 35 units, net price = £24.60; *NovoPen® 3 Demi* (for 3-mL cartridges), allowing 0.5-unit dosage adjustment, max. 35 units, net price = £25.03; *NovoPen® 4* (for 3-mL cartridges), allowing 1-unit dosage adjustment, max. 60 units, net price = £26.36

**OptiClik®** (Sanofi-Aventis)

Injection device, for use with *Lantus OptiClik®* or *Apidra OptiClik®* insulin cartridges, allowing 1-unit dosage adjustment, max. 80 units, net price = £20.13

**OptiPen® Pro 1** (Aventis Pharma)

Injection device, for use with *Insuman®* insulin cartridges; allowing 1-unit dosage adjustment, max. 60 units, net price = £22.00

**SQ-PEN®** (Medical House)

Needle-free insulin delivery device for use with any 10-mL vial *or* any 3-mL cartridge of insulin, allowing 1-unit dosage adjustment, max. 50 units, net price *starter pack (SQ-PEN® device, 1 practice nozzle, 1 nozzle, 1 3-mL adaptor, 1 10-mL adaptor)* = £147.83, *3-month consumables pack* for 10-mL adaptor (7 nozzles, 5 × 10-mL insulin vial adaptors) = £18.08, for 3-mL adaptor (7 nozzles, 15 × 3-mL insulin cartridge adaptors) = £30.82; *vial adaptor pack* (6 insulin vial adaptors) = £7.66, *cartridge adaptor pack* (6 insulin cartridge adaptors) = £7.66; *nozzle pack* (6 nozzles) = £10.03

### ◢Lancets

**Lancets—sterile, single use** (Drug Tariff)

[1] *Ascensia Microlet®* 100 = £3.69, 200 = £7.03; *BD Micro-Fine®+* 100 = £3.16, 200 = £6.13; *Cleanlet Fine®* 100 = £3.19, 200 = £6.13; [1] *Finepoint®* 100 = £3.48; [1] *FreeStyle®* 200 = £6.89; [1] *GlucoMen®* Fine 100 = £3.55, 200 = £6.88; *Hypoguard Supreme®* 100 = £2.75; [1] *Milward Steri-Let®*, 23 gauge, 100 = £3.00, 200 = £5.70, 28 gauge, 100 = £3.00, 200 = £5.70; [1] *Monolet®* 100 = £3.28, 200 = £6.24; *Monolet Extra®* 100 = £3.28; *MPD Ultra Thin®* 100 = £3.30, 200 = £6.50; *Multiclix®* 204 = £9.02; [1] *One Touch UltraSoft®* 100 = £3.56; [2] *Softclix®* 200 = £7.20; [2] *Softclix XL®* 50 = £1.80; *Thin Lancets* (formerly *MediSense Thin®*), 200 = £7.02; [1] *Unilet ComforTouch®* 100 = £3.60, 200 = £6.83; [1] *Unilet General Purpose Superlite®* 100 = £3.67, 200 = £6.96; *Unistik 3 Comfort®*, 28-gauge, 100 = £6.24, 200 = £12.20; *Unistik 3 Extra®*, 21-gauge, 100 = £6.24, 200 = £12.20; *Unistik 3 Normal®*, 23-gauge, 100 = £6.24, 200 = £12.20; *Universal®* (formerly *VitalCare®*), 100 = £6.37; *Vitrex Soft®*, 23-gauge, 100 = £3.00, 200 = £5.70; *Vitrex Gentle®* 28-gauge, 100 = £3.19, 200 = £6.13; *WaveSense Ultra-Thin®*, 28-gauge, 200 = £6.90, 33-gauge, 200 = £6.90

Compatible finger-pricking devices (unless indicated otherwise, see footnotes): *B-D Optimus®*, *Glucolet®*, *Monoject®*, *Penlet II®*, *Soft Touch®*

1. [NHS] *Autolet®* and [NHS] *Autolet Impression®* are also compatible finger-pricking devices
2. Use [NHS] *Softclix®* finger-pricking device

### ◢Needles

**Hypodermic Needle, Sterile single use** (Drug Tariff)

For use with reusable glass syringe, sizes 0.5 mm (25G), 0.45 mm (26G), 0.4 mm (27G). Net price 100-needle pack = £2.68

Brands include *Microlance®*, *Monoject®*

**Needles for Prefilled and Reusable Pen Injectors** (Drug Tariff)

Screw on, needle length 6.1 mm or less, net price 100-needle pack = £12.53; 6.2–9.9 mm, 100-needle pack = £8.89; 10 mm or more, 100-needle pack = £8.89

Brands include *BD Micro-Fine®* +, *NovoFine®*, *Unifine® Pentips*

Snap on, needle length 6.1 mm or less, net price 100-needle pack = £12.02; 6.2–9.9 mm, 100-needle pack = £8.52; 10 mm or more, 100-needle pack = £8.52

Brands include *Penfine®*

### ◢Syringes

**Hypodermic Syringe** (Drug Tariff)

Calibrated glass with Luer taper conical fitting, for use with U100 insulin. Net price 0.5 mL and 1 mL = £15.18

Brands include *Abcare®*

**Pre-Set U100 Insulin Syringe** (Drug Tariff)

Calibrated glass with Luer taper conical fitting, supplied with dosage chart and strong box, for blind patients. Net price 1 mL = £21.99

**U100 Insulin Syringe with Needle** (Drug Tariff)

Disposable with fixed or separate needle for single use or single patient-use, colour coded orange. Needle length 8 mm, diameters 0.33 mm (29G), 0.3 mm (30G), net price 10 (with needle), 0.3 mL = £1.35, 0.5 mL = £1.40, 1 mL = £1.41; needle length 12 mm, diameters 0.45 mm (26G), 0.4 mm (27G), 0.36 mm (28G), 0.33 mm (29G), net price 10 (with needle), 0.3 mL = £1.45; 0.5 mL = £1.30; 1 mL = £1.29

Brands include *BD Micro-Fine®+*, *Clinipak®*, *Insupak®*, *Monoject® Ultra*, *Omnikan®*, *Plastipak®*

### ◢Accessories

**Needle Clipping (Chopping) Device** (Drug Tariff)

Consisting of a clipper to remove needle from its hub and container from which cut-off needles cannot be retrieved; designed to hold 1500 needles, not suitable for use with lancets. Net price = £1.32

Brands include *BD Safe-Clip®*

**Sharpsguard** (Drug Tariff)

Net price 1-litre sharpsbin = 85p

## 6.1.2 Antidiabetic drugs

### 6.1.2.1 Sulphonylureas
### 6.1.2.2 Biguanides
### 6.1.2.3 Other antidiabetic drugs

Oral antidiabetic drugs are used for the treatment of type 2 diabetes mellitus. They should be prescribed only if the patient fails to respond adequately to at least 3 months' restriction of energy and carbohydrate intake and an increase in physical activity. They should be used to augment the effect of diet and exercise, and not to replace them.

For patients not adequately controlled by diet and oral hypoglycaemic drugs, insulin may be added to the treatment regimen or substituted for oral therapy. When insulin is added to oral therapy, it is generally given at bedtime as isophane insulin, and when insulin replaces an oral regimen it is generally given as twice-daily injections of a biphasic insulin (or isophane insulin mixed with soluble insulin). Weight gain and hypoglycaemia may be complications of insulin therapy but weight gain may be reduced if the insulin is given in combination with metformin.

Exenatide, an incretin mimetic given by subcutaneous injection, is also available for the treatment of type 2 diabetes, see section 6.1.2.3.

**Pregnancy and breast-feeding** During pregnancy, women with either pre-existing or gestational diabetes may be treated with metformin [unlicensed use], either alone or in combination with insulin (section 6.1.1). Women with gestational diabetes should discontinue hypoglycaemic treatment after giving birth. Metformin can be continued during breast-feeding for those with pre-existing diabetes.

Other oral hypoglycaemic drugs (including sulphonylureas) and exenatide are contra-indicated in pregnancy (see also Appendix 4) and in breast-feeding (Appendix 5).

### 6.1.2.1 Sulphonylureas

The sulphonylureas act mainly by augmenting insulin secretion and consequently are effective only when some residual pancreatic beta-cell activity is present; during long-term administration they also have an extrapancreatic action. All may cause hypoglycaemia but this is uncommon and usually indicates excessive dosage. Sulphonylurea-induced hypoglycaemia may persist for many hours and must always be treated in hospital.

Sulphonylureas are considered for patients who are not overweight, or in whom metformin is contra-indicated or not tolerated. Several sulphonylureas are available and choice is determined by side-effects and the duration of action as well as the patient's age and renal function. The long-acting sulphonylureas **chlorpropamide** and **glibenclamide** are associated with a greater risk of hypoglycaemia; for this reason they should be avoided in the elderly and shorter-acting alternatives, such as **gliclazide** or **tolbutamide**, should be used instead. Chlorpropamide also has more side-effects than the other sulphonylureas (see below) and therefore it is no longer recommended.

When the combination of strict diet and sulphonylurea treatment fails other options include:

- combining with metformin (section 6.1.2.2) (reports of increased hazard with this combination remain unconfirmed);
- combining with pioglitazone or rosiglitazone, but see section 6.1.2.3;
- combining with sitagliptin or vildagliptin (section 6.1.2.3);
- combining with acarbose (section 6.1.2.3), which may have a small beneficial effect, but flatulence can be a problem;
- combining with bedtime isophane insulin (section 6.1.1) but weight gain and hypoglycaemia can occur.

The risk of hypoglycaemia associated with sulphonylureas (see notes above) should be discussed with the patient, especially when concomitant glucose-lowering drugs are prescribed.

Insulin therapy should be instituted temporarily during intercurrent illness (such as myocardial infarction,

coma, infection, and trauma). Sulphonylureas should be omitted on the morning of surgery; insulin is required because of the ensuing hyperglycaemia in these circumstances.

**Cautions** Sulphonylureas can encourage weight gain and should be prescribed only if poor control and symptoms persist despite adequate attempts at dieting; metformin (section 6.1.2.2) is considered the drug of choice in obese patients. Caution is needed in the elderly and in those with mild to moderate hepatic impairment (Appendix 2) because of the hazard of hypoglycaemia.

**Renal impairment** Sulphonylureas should be used with care in those with mild to moderate renal impairment, because of the hazard of hypoglycaemia; they should be avoided where possible in severe renal impairment. If necessary, the short-acting tolbutamide can be used in renal impairment, as can gliclazide which is principally metabolised in the liver, but careful monitoring of blood-glucose concentration is essential; care is required to choose the smallest possible dose that produces adequate control of blood glucose. Chlorpropamide should be avoided altogether in those with renal impairment.

See also Appendix 3.

**Contra-indications** Sulphonylureas should be avoided where possible in severe hepatic impairment (Appendix 2) and in acute porphyria (section 9.8.2). They should not be used during pregnancy (Appendix 4) or breast-feeding (Appendix 5)—see section 6.1.2. Sulphonylureas are contra-indicated in the presence of ketoacidosis.

**Side-effects** Side-effects of sulphonylureas are generally mild and infrequent and include gastro-intestinal disturbances such as nausea, vomiting, diarrhoea and constipation.

Chlorpropamide has appreciably more side-effects, mainly because of its very prolonged duration of action and the consequent hazard of hypoglycaemia and it should no longer be used. It may also cause facial flushing after drinking alcohol; this effect does not normally occur with other sulphonylureas. Chlorpropamide may also enhance antidiuretic hormone secretion and very rarely cause hyponatraemia (hyponatraemia is also reported with glimepiride and glipizide).

Sulphonylureas can occasionally cause a disturbance in liver function, which may rarely lead to cholestatic jaundice, hepatitis, and hepatic failure. Hypersensitivity reactions can occur, usually in the first 6–8 weeks of therapy. They consist mainly of allergic skin reactions which progress rarely to erythema multiforme and exfoliative dermatitis, fever, and jaundice; photosensitivity has rarely been reported with chlorpropamide and glipizide. Blood disorders are also rare but may include leucopenia, thrombocytopenia, agranulocytosis, pancytopenia, haemolytic anaemia, and aplastic anaemia.

### CHLORPROPAMIDE

**Indications** type 2 diabetes mellitus (for use in diabetes insipidus, see section 6.5.2)

**Cautions** see notes above; **interactions**: Appendix 1 (antidiabetics)

**Contra-indications** see notes above

**Side-effects** see notes above

**Dose**

- Initially 250 mg daily with breakfast (ELDERLY 100–125 mg but avoid—see notes above), adjusted according to response; max. 500 mg daily

**Chlorpropamide** (Non-proprietary) PoM ◢
Tablets, chlorpropamide 100 mg, net price 20 = £1.70; 250 mg, 20 = £2.00. Label: 4

## ■ GLIBENCLAMIDE

**Indications** type 2 diabetes mellitus
**Cautions** see notes above; **interactions**: Appendix 1 (antidiabetics)
**Contra-indications** see notes above
**Side-effects** see notes above
**Dose**

- Initially 5 mg daily with or immediately after breakfast, dose adjusted according to response (ELDERLY avoid, see notes above); max. 15 mg daily

**Glibenclamide** (Non-proprietary) PoM
Tablets, glibenclamide 2.5 mg, net price 28-tab pack = 85p; 5 mg, 28-tab pack = 87p

## ■ GLICLAZIDE

**Indications** type 2 diabetes mellitus
**Cautions** see notes above; **interactions**: Appendix 1 (antidiabetics)
**Contra-indications** see notes above
**Side-effects** see notes above
**Dose**

- Initially, 40–80 mg daily, adjusted according to response; up to 160 mg as a single dose, with breakfast; higher doses divided; max. 320 mg daily

**Gliclazide** (Non-proprietary) PoM
Tablets, scored, gliclazide 80 mg, net price 28-tab pack = £1.08, 60-tab pack = £1.62
Brands include *DIAGLYK*®

**Diamicron**® (Servier) PoM
Tablets, scored, gliclazide 80 mg, net price 60-tab pack = £4.38

◢ **Modified release**
**Diamicron**® **MR** (Servier) PoM
Tablets, m/r, gliclazide 30 mg, net price 28-tab pack = £2.96, 56-tab pack = £5.92. Label: 25
Dose initially 30 mg daily with breakfast, adjusted according to response every 4 weeks (after 2 weeks if no decrease in blood glucose); max. 120 mg daily
Note *Diamicron*® *MR* 30 mg may be considered to be approximately equivalent in therapeutic effect to standard formulation *Diamicron*® 80 mg

## ■ GLIMEPIRIDE

**Indications** type 2 diabetes mellitus
**Cautions** see notes above; manufacturer recommends regular hepatic and haematological monitoring but limited evidence of clinical value; **interactions**: Appendix 1 (antidiabetics)
**Contra-indications** see notes above
**Side-effects** see notes above
**Dose**

- Initially 1 mg daily, adjusted according to response in 1-mg steps at 1–2 week intervals; usual max. 4 mg daily (exceptionally, up to 6 mg daily may be used); taken shortly before or with first main meal

**Glimepiride** (Non-proprietary) PoM
Tablets, glimepiride 1 mg, net price 30-tab pack = £2.00; 2 mg, 30-tab pack = £2.75; 3 mg, 30-tab pack = £4.10; 4 mg, 30-tab pack = £5.19

**Amaryl**® (Hoechst Marion Roussel) PoM
Tablets, all scored, glimepiride 1 mg (pink), net price 30-tab pack = £4.33; 2 mg (green), 30-tab pack = £7.13; 3 mg (yellow), 30-tab pack = £10.75; 4 mg (blue), 30-tab pack = £14.24

## ■ GLIPIZIDE

**Indications** type 2 diabetes mellitus
**Cautions** see notes above; **interactions**: Appendix 1 (antidiabetics)
**Contra-indications** see notes above
**Side-effects** see notes above; also dizziness, drowsiness
**Dose**

- Initially 2.5–5 mg daily shortly before breakfast or lunch, adjusted according to response; max. 20 mg daily; up to 15 mg may be given as a single dose; higher doses divided

**Glipizide** (Non-proprietary) PoM
Tablets, glipizide 5 mg, net price 56-tab pack = £4.82

**Glibenese**® (Pfizer) PoM
Tablets, scored, glipizide 5 mg, net price 56-tab pack = £4.36

**Minodiab**® (Pharmacia) PoM
Tablets, scored, glipizide 5 mg, net price 28-tab pack = £1.26

## ■ TOLBUTAMIDE

**Indications** type 2 diabetes mellitus
**Cautions** see notes above; **interactions**: Appendix 1 (antidiabetics)
**Contra-indications** see notes above
**Side-effects** see notes above; also headache, tinnitus
**Dose**

- 0.5–1.5 g (max. 2 g) daily in divided doses with or immediately after meals *or* as a single dose with or immediately after breakfast

**Tolbutamide** (Non-proprietary) PoM
Tablets, tolbutamide 500 mg, net price 28-tab pack = £1.40

### 6.1.2.2 Biguanides

**Metformin**, the only available biguanide, has a different mode of action from the sulphonylureas, and is not interchangeable with them. It exerts its effect mainly by decreasing gluconeogenesis and by increasing peripheral utilisation of glucose; since it acts only in the presence of endogenous insulin it is effective only if there are some residual functioning pancreatic islet cells.

Metformin is the drug of first choice in overweight patients in whom strict dieting has failed to control diabetes, if appropriate it may also be considered as an option in patients who are not overweight. It is also used when diabetes is inadequately controlled with sulphonylurea treatment. When the combination of

*Endocrine system*

**6**

strict diet and metformin treatment fails, other options include:

- combining with a sulphonylurea (section 6.1.2.1) (reports of increased hazard with this combination remain unconfirmed);
- combining with pioglitazone or rosiglitazone (section 6.1.2.3);
- combining with repaglinide or nateglinide (section 6.1.2.3);
- combining with sitagliptin or vildagliptin (section 6.1.2.3);
- combining with acarbose (section 6.1.2.3), which may have a small beneficial effect, but flatulence can be a problem;
- combining with insulin (section 6.1.1) but weight gain and hypoglycaemia can be problems (weight gain minimised if insulin given at night).

Insulin treatment is almost always required in medical and surgical emergencies; insulin should also be substituted before elective surgery (omit metformin on the morning of surgery and give insulin if required).

Hypoglycaemia does not usually occur with metformin; other advantages are the lower incidence of weight gain and lower plasma-insulin concentration. It does not exert a hypoglycaemic action in non-diabetic subjects unless given in overdose.

Gastro-intestinal side-effects are initially common with metformin, and may persist in some patients, particularly when very high doses such as 3 g daily are given.

Very rarely, metformin can provoke lactic acidosis, which is most likely to occur in patients with renal impairment, see Lactic Acidosis below.

Metformin is used for the symptomatic management of polycystic ovary syndrome [unlicensed indication]; it improves insulin sensitivity, may aid weight reduction, helps to normalise menstrual cycle (increasing the rate of spontaneous ovulation), and may improve hirsutism.

---

### ■ METFORMIN HYDROCHLORIDE

**Indications** diabetes mellitus (see notes above); polycystic ovary syndrome [unlicensed indication]

**Cautions** see notes above; determine renal function before treatment and once or twice annually (more frequently in the elderly or if deterioration suspected); **interactions:** Appendix 1 (antidiabetics)
**Lactic acidosis** Metformin should be used cautiously in renal impairment because of the increased risk of lactic acidosis: it is contra-indicated in patients with significant renal impairment. NICE[1] recommends that the dose of metformin should be reviewed if estimated glomerular filtration rate (eGFR) falls below 45 mL/minute/1.73 m$^2$ and to avoid if eGFR less than 30 mL/minute/1.73 m$^2$. To reduce the risk of lactic acidosis, metformin should be stopped or temporarily withdrawn in patients at risk of tissue hypoxia or sudden deterioration in renal function, such as those with dehydration, severe infection, shock, sepsis, acute heart failure, respiratory failure or hepatic impairment (Appendix 2), or those who have recently had a myocardial infarction

**Contra-indications** ketoacidosis, see also Lactic Acidosis above; use of iodine-containing X-ray contrast media (do not restart metformin until renal function returns to normal) and use of general anaesthesia (suspend metformin on the morning of surgery and restart when renal function returns to normal); pregnancy (Appendix 4); breast-feeding (Appendix 5)

---

1. NICE clinical guideline 87 (May 2009): Type 2 diabetes: The management of type 2 diabetes

**Side-effects** anorexia, nausea, vomiting, diarrhoea (usually transient), abdominal pain, taste disturbance, *rarely* lactic acidosis (withdraw treatment), decreased vitamin-B$_{12}$ absorption, erythema, pruritus and urticaria; hepatitis also reported

**Dose**

- Diabetes mellitus, ADULT and CHILD over 10 years initially 500 mg with breakfast for at least 1 week then 500 mg with breakfast and evening meal for at least 1 week then 500 mg with breakfast, lunch and evening meal; usual max. 2 g daily in divided doses
- Polycystic ovary syndrome [unlicensed], initially 500 mg with breakfast for 1 week, then 500 mg with breakfast and evening meal for 1 week, then 1.5–1.7 g daily in 2–3 divided doses

**Note** Metformin doses in the BNF may differ from those in the product literature

**Metformin** (Non-proprietary) ▣
Tablets, coated, metformin hydrochloride 500 mg, net price 28-tab pack = 93p, 84-tab pack = £1.37; 850 mg, 56-tab pack = £1.34. Label: 21

Oral solution, sugar-free, metformin hydrochloride 500 mg/5 mL, net price 100 mL = £62.06. Label: 21
Brands include *Metsol*®

**Glucophage**® (Merck) ▣
Tablets, f/c, metformin hydrochloride 500 mg, net price 84-tab pack = £2.88; 850 mg, 56-tab pack = £3.20. Label: 21

Oral powder, sugar-free, metformin hydrochloride 500 mg/sachet, net price 30-sachet pack = £3.29, 60-sachet pack = £6.50; 1 g/sachet, 30-sachet pack = £6.58, 60-sachet pack = £13.16. Label: 13, 21, counselling, administration
Excipients include aspartame (section 9.4.1)
Counselling The contents of each sachet should be mixed with 150 mL of water and taken immediately

### ◢ Modified release

**Bolamyn**® **SR** (TEVA UK) ▣
Tablets, m/r, metformin hydrochloride 500 mg, net price 28 tab-pack = £3.20, 56 tab-pack = £6.40. Label: 21, 25
**Dose** initially 500 mg once daily, increased every 10–15 days, max. 2 g once daily with evening meal; if control not achieved, use 1 g twice daily with meals, and if control still not achieved change to standard-release tablets
**Note** Patients taking up to 2 g daily of the standard-release metformin may start with the same daily dose of *Bolamyn*® *SR*; not suitable if dose of standard-release tablets more than 2 g daily

**Glucophage**® **SR** (Merck) ▣
Tablets, m/r, metformin hydrochloride 500 mg, net price 28-tab pack = £3.07, 56-tab pack = £6.14; 750 mg, 28-tab pack = £3.20, 56-tab pack = £6.40; 1 g, 28-tab pack = £4.26, 56-tab pack = £8.52. Label: 21, 25
**Dose** initially 500 mg once daily, increased every 10–15 days, max. 2 g once daily with evening meal; if control not achieved, use 1 g twice daily with meals, and if control still not achieved change to standard-release tablets
**Note** Patients taking up to 2 g daily of the standard-release metformin may start with the same daily dose of *Glucophage*® *SR*; not suitable if dose of standard-release tablets more than 2 g daily
The *Scottish Medicines Consortium* (p. 3) has advised (December 2005) that *Glucophage*® *SR* is not recommended for the treatment of type 2 diabetes

### ◢ With pioglitazone
See section 6.1.2.3

### ◢ With rosiglitazone
See section 6.1.2.3

### ◢ With vildagliptin
See section 6.1.2.3

## 6.1.2.3 Other antidiabetic drugs

**Acarbose**, an inhibitor of intestinal alpha glucosidases, delays the digestion and absorption of starch and sucrose; it has a small but significant effect in lowering blood glucose. Use of acarbose is usually reserved for when other oral hypoglycaemics are not tolerated or are contra-indicated. Postprandial hyperglycaemia in type 1 diabetes can be reduced by acarbose, but it has been little used for this purpose. Flatulence deters some from using acarbose although this side-effect tends to decrease with time.

**Nateglinide** and **repaglinide** stimulate insulin release. Both drugs have a rapid onset of action and short duration of activity, and should be administered shortly before each main meal. Repaglinide may be given as monotherapy for patients who are not overweight or for those in whom metformin is contra-indicated or not tolerated, or it may be given in combination with metformin. Nateglinide is licensed only for use with metformin.

The thiazolidinediones, **pioglitazone** and **rosiglitazone**, reduce peripheral insulin resistance, leading to a reduction of blood-glucose concentration. Either drug can be used alone or in combination with metformin or with a sulphonylurea (if metformin inappropriate); the combination of a thiazolidinedione plus metformin is preferred to a thiazolidinedione plus sulphonylurea, particularly for obese patients. Inadequate response to a combination of metformin and sulphonylurea may indicate failing insulin release; the introduction of pioglitazone or rosiglitazone has a limited role in these circumstances and the initiation of insulin is often more appropriate. Blood-glucose control may deteriorate temporarily when a thiazolidinedione is substituted for an oral antidiabetic drug that is being used in combination with another. Long-term benefits of the thiazolidinediones have not yet been demonstrated. NICE (May 2009) has recommended that, when glycaemic control is inadequate with existing treatment, a thiazolidinedione can be added to:

- a sulphonylurea, if metformin is contra-indicated or not tolerated;

- metformin, if risks of hypoglycaemia with sulphonylurea are unacceptable or a sulphonylurea is contra-indicated or not tolerated;

- combination of metformin and a sulphonylurea, if insulin is unacceptable because of lifestyle or other personal issues, or the patient is obese.

NICE has recommended that treatment with a thiazolidinedione is continued only if HbA$_{1c}$ concentration is reduced by at least 0.5% within 6 months of starting treatment.

The *Scottish Medicines Consortium* (p. 3) accepts use of a thiazolidinedione (rosiglitazone (June 2006), pioglitazone (February 2007)) with metformin and a sulphonylurea, for patients (especially if overweight) whose glycaemic control is inadequate despite the use of 2 oral hypoglycaemic drugs and who are unable or unwilling to take insulin; treatment should be initiated and monitored by an experienced diabetes physician.

> **MHRA/CHM advice**
> **Rosiglitazone and pioglitazone cardiovascular safety (December 2007 and February 2008)**
> Rosiglitazone and pioglitazone should not be used in patients with heart failure or history of heart failure; incidence of heart failure is increased when rosiglitazone or pioglitazone is combined with insulin. Rosiglitazone should not be used in patients with acute coronary syndrome. Patients should be closely monitored for signs of heart failure. Rosiglitazone may be associated with a small increased risk of cardiac ischaemia particularly in combination with insulin. Rosiglitazone is not recommended for use in patients with ischaemic heart disease or peripheral arterial disease; in patients with history of ischaemic heart disease rosiglitazone should only be used after careful evaluation of the patient's individual risk. The combination of rosiglitazone and insulin should be used only in exceptional cases, and under close supervision.

**Sitagliptin** and **vildagliptin** inhibit dipeptidylpeptidase-4 to increase insulin secretion and lower glucagon secretion. Both drugs are licensed for use in type 2 diabetes in combination with metformin or a sulphonylurea (if metformin inappropriate) or a thiazolidinedione, when treatment with either metformin or a sulphonylurea or a thiazolidinedione fails to achieve adequate glycaemic control. Sitagliptin is also licensed for use in combination with both metformin and a sulphonylurea when dual therapy with these drugs fails to achieve adequate glycaemic control.

NICE (May 2009) has recommended that, when glycaemic control is inadequate with existing treatment:

- sitagliptin or vildagliptin (instead of a sulphonylurea) can be added to metformin, if there is a significant risk of hypoglycaemia *or* if a sulphonylurea is contra-indicated or not tolerated;

- sitagliptin or vildagliptin can be added to a sulphonylurea, if metformin is contra-indicated or not tolerated;

- sitagliptin can be added to both metformin and a sulphonylurea, if insulin is unacceptable because of lifestyle or other personal issues.

NICE has recommended that treatment with sitagliptin or vildagliptin is continued only if HbA$_{1c}$ concentration is reduced by at least 0.5% within 6 months of starting treatment.

The *Scottish Medicines Consortium* (p. 3) has advised (March 2008) that vildagliptin (*Galvus®*) is accepted for restricted use within NHS Scotland for the treatment of type 2 diabetes mellitus in combination with metformin when addition of a sulphonylurea is inappropriate.

**Exenatide**, a synthetic form of exendin-4, is an incretin mimetic which increases insulin secretion, suppresses glucagon secretion, and slows gastric emptying. It is given by subcutaneous injection for the treatment of type 2 diabetes in combination with metformin or a sulphonylurea, or both, in patients who have not achieved adequate glycaemic control with these drugs alone or in combination. Exenatide use is associated with the prevention of weight gain and possible promotion of weight loss which can be beneficial in overweight patients.

NICE (May 2009) has recommended that, when glycaemic control is inadequate with metformin and sulphonylurea treatment, the addition of exenatide may be considered if the patient has:

- a body mass index of $35 \, \text{kg/m}^2$ or over and is of European descent (with appropriate adjustment for other ethnic groups) and weight-related psychological or medical problems *or*

- a body mass index less than $35 \, \text{kg/m}^2$, and insulin would be unacceptable for occupational reasons *or* weight loss would benefit other significant obesity-related comorbidities.

NICE has recommended that treatment with exenatide is continued only if HbA$_{1c}$ concentration is reduced by at least 1% and a weight loss of at least 3% is achieved within 6 months of starting treatment.

The *Scottish Medicines Consortium* (p. 3) has advised (June 2007) that exenatide (*Byetta®*) is accepted for restricted use within NHS Scotland for the treatment of type 2 diabetes in combination with metformin or sulphonylurea (or both), as an alternative to treatment with insulin in patients where treatment with metformin or sulphonylurea (or both) at maximally tolerated doses has been inadequate, and treatment with insulin would be the next option.

## ACARBOSE

**Indications** diabetes mellitus inadequately controlled by diet or by diet with oral antidiabetic drugs

**Cautions** monitor liver function; may enhance hypoglycaemic effects of insulin and sulphonylureas (hypoglycaemic episodes may be treated with oral glucose but not with sucrose); **interactions:** Appendix 1 (antidiabetics)

**Contra-indications** inflammatory bowel disease, predisposition to partial intestinal obstruction; hernia, previous abdominal surgery; hepatic impairment; renal impairment (avoid if eGFR less than 25 mL/minute/1.73 m$^2$; Appendix 3); pregnancy (Appendix 4); breast-feeding (Appendix 5)

**Side-effects** flatulence, soft stools, diarrhoea (may need to reduce dose or withdraw), abdominal distention and pain; *rarely*, nausea, abnormal liver function tests and skin reactions; *very rarely* ileus, oedema, jaundice, and hepatitis

**Note** Antacids unlikely to be beneficial for treating side-effects

**Dose**
- Initially 50 mg daily increased to 50 mg 3 times daily, then increased if necessary after 6–8 weeks to 100 mg 3 times daily; max. 200 mg 3 times daily; CHILD and ADOLESCENT under 18 years not recommended

**Counselling** Tablets should be chewed with first mouthful of food or swallowed whole with a little liquid immediately before food. To counteract possible hypoglycaemia, patients receiving insulin or a sulphonylurea as well as acarbose need to carry glucose (not sucrose—acarbose interferes with sucrose absorption)

**Glucobay®** (Bayer) [PoM]
Tablets, acarbose 50 mg, net price 90-tab pack = £6.27; 100 mg (scored), 90-tab pack = £11.57. Counselling, administration

## EXENATIDE

**Indications** type 2 diabetes mellitus in combination with metformin or sulphonylurea (or with both) when metformin or a sulphonylurea or both inadequate

**Cautions** elderly; renal impairment (avoid if eGFR less than 30 mL/minute/1.73m$^2$; Appendix 3); pancreatitis (see below); **interactions:** Appendix 1 (antidiabetics)

**Pancreatitis** Severe pancreatitis (sometimes fatal), including haemorrhagic or necrotising pancreatitis, has been reported rarely. Patients or their carers should be told how to recognise signs and symptoms of pancreatitis and advised to seek prompt medical attention if symptoms such as abdominal pain, nausea, and vomiting develop; discontinue permanently if pancreatitis is diagnosed

**Contra-indications** ketoacidosis; severe gastro-intestinal disease; pregnancy (Appendix 4); breast-feeding (Appendix 5)

**Side-effects** gastro-intestinal disturbances including nausea, vomiting, diarrhoea, dyspepsia, abdominal pain and distension, gastro-oesophageal reflux disease, decreased appetite; headache, dizziness, agitation, asthenia; hypoglycaemia; increased sweating, injection-site reactions; antibody formation; *less commonly* pancreatitis (see Cautions above); *very rarely* anaphylactic reactions; also reported constipation, flatulence, eructation, dehydration, taste disturbance, renal impairment, drowsiness, rash, pruritus, urticaria, and angioedema

**Dose**
- By subcutaneous injection, ADULT over 18 years, initially 5 micrograms twice daily within 1 hour before 2 main meals (at least 6 hours apart), increased if necessary after at least 1 month to max. 10 micrograms twice daily

**Counselling** If a dose is missed, continue with the next scheduled dose—do not administer after a meal. Some oral medications should be taken at least 1 hour before or 4 hours after exenatide injection—consult product literature for details

**Byetta®** (Lilly) ▼ [PoM]
Injection, exenatide 250 micrograms/mL, net price 5 microgram/dose prefilled pen (60 doses) = £68.24, 10 microgram/dose prefilled pen (60 doses) = £68.24. Counselling, administration

## NATEGLINIDE

**Indications** type 2 diabetes mellitus in combination with metformin (section 6.1.2.2) when metformin alone inadequate

**Cautions** substitute insulin during intercurrent illness (such as myocardial infarction, coma, infection, and trauma) and during surgery (omit nateglinide on morning of surgery and recommence when eating and drinking normally); elderly, debilitated and malnourished patients; moderate hepatic impairment (avoid if severe—Appendix 2); **interactions:** Appendix 1 (antidiabetics)

**Contra-indications** ketoacidosis; pregnancy (Appendix 4) and breast-feeding (Appendix 5)

**Side-effects** hypoglycaemia; hypersensitivity reactions including pruritus, rashes and urticaria

**Dose**
- Initially 60 mg 3 times daily within 30 minutes before main meals, adjusted according to response up to max. 180 mg 3 times daily; CHILD and ADOLESCENT under 18 years not recommended

6

Endocrine system

**Starlix®** (Novartis) [PoM]
Tablets, f/c, nateglinide 60 mg (pink), net price 84-tab pack = £22.71; 120 mg (yellow), 84-tab pack = £25.88; 180 mg (red), 84-tab pack = £25.88

## PIOGLITAZONE

**Indications** type 2 diabetes mellitus (alone or combined with metformin or a sulphonylurea, or with both, or with insulin—see also notes above)

**Cautions** monitor liver function (see below); cardiovascular disease or in combination with insulin (risk of heart failure—see MHRA/CHM advice p. 384); substitute insulin during peri-operative period (omit pioglitazone on morning of surgery and recommence when eating and drinking normally); increased risk of bone fractures in females in feet, lower leg, hands, and lower arms; avoid in acute porphyria (but see section 9.8.2); **interactions:** Appendix 1 (antidiabetics)
**Liver toxicity** Rare reports of liver dysfunction; monitor liver function before treatment, and periodically thereafter; advise patients to seek immediate medical attention if symptoms such as nausea, vomiting, abdominal pain, fatigue and dark urine develop; discontinue if jaundice occurs

**Contra-indications** hepatic impairment, history of heart failure, pregnancy (Appendix 4), breast-feeding (Appendix 5)

**Side-effects** gastro-intestinal disturbances, weight gain, oedema, anaemia, headache, visual disturbances, dizziness, arthralgia, hypoaesthesia, haematuria, impotence; *less commonly* hypoglycaemia, fatigue, insomnia, vertigo, sweating, altered blood lipids, proteinuria; see also Liver Toxicity above

**Dose**
* Initially 15–30 mg once daily increased to 45 mg once daily according to response

**Actos®** (Takeda) ▼ [PoM]
Tablets, pioglitazone (as hydrochloride) 15 mg, net price 28-tab pack = £14.25; 30 mg, 28-tab pack = £33.25; 45 mg, 28-tab pack = £36.96

◢**With metformin**
For cautions, contra-indications, and side-effects of metformin, see section 6.1.2.2

**Competact®** (Takeda) ▼ [PoM]
Tablets, f/c, pioglitazone (as hydrochloride) 15 mg, metformin hydrochloride 850 mg, net price 56-tab pack = £31.56. Label: 21
**Dose** type 2 diabetes not controlled by metformin alone, 1 tablet twice daily; CHILD and ADOLESCENT under 18 years not recommended
**Note** Titration with the individual components (pioglitazone and metformin) desirable before initiating *Competact®*

## REPAGLINIDE

**Indications** type 2 diabetes mellitus (as monotherapy or in combination with metformin when metformin alone inadequate)

**Cautions** substitute insulin during intercurrent illness (such as myocardial infarction, coma, infection, and trauma) and during surgery (omit repaglinide on morning of surgery and recommence when eating and drinking normally); debilitated and malnourished patients; renal impairment; **interactions:** Appendix 1 (antidiabetics)

**Contra-indications** ketoacidosis; severe hepatic impairment; pregnancy (Appendix 4) and breast-feeding (Appendix 5)

**Side-effects** abdominal pain, diarrhoea, constipation, nausea, vomiting; *rarely* hypoglycaemia, hypersensitivity reactions including pruritus, rashes, vasculitis, urticaria, and visual disturbances

**Dose**
* Initially 500 micrograms within 30 minutes before main meals (1 mg if transferring from another oral hypoglycaemic), adjusted according to response at intervals of 1–2 weeks; up to 4 mg may be given as a single dose, max. 16 mg daily; CHILD and ADOLESCENT under 18 years and ELDERLY over 75 years, not recommended

**Prandin®** (Daiichi Sankyo) [PoM]
Tablets, repaglinide 500 micrograms, net price 30-tab pack = £3.92, 90-tab pack = £11.76; 1 mg (yellow), 30-tab pack = £3.92, 90-tab pack = £11.76; 2 mg (peach), 90-tab pack = £11.76
Formerly marketed as *NovoNorm®*

## ROSIGLITAZONE

**Indications** type 2 diabetes mellitus (alone *or* combined with metformin *or* with a sulphonylurea *or* with both—see also notes above)

**Cautions** monitor liver function (see below); cardiovascular disease or in combination with insulin (risk of heart failure and ischaemic heart disease—see MHRA/CHM advice p. 384); substitute insulin during peri-operative period (omit rosiglitazone on morning of surgery and recommence when eating and drinking normally); increased risk of bone fractures in females in feet, hands, and upper arms; avoid in acute porphyria (but see section 9.8.2); renal impairment (Appendix 3); **interactions:** Appendix 1 (antidiabetics)
**Liver toxicity** Rare reports of liver dysfunction reported; monitor liver function before treatment and periodically thereafter; advise patients to seek immediate medical attention if symptoms such as nausea, vomiting, abdominal pain, fatigue, anorexia and dark urine develop; discontinue if jaundice occurs or liver enzymes significantly raised

**Contra-indications** hepatic impairment, history of heart failure or acute coronary syndrome, pregnancy (Appendix 4), breast-feeding (Appendix 5)

**Side-effects** gastro-intestinal disturbances, cardiac ischaemia, headache, anaemia, altered blood lipids, weight gain, oedema, hypoglycaemia, bone fracture; *less commonly* increased appetite, heart failure, fatigue, paraesthesia, alopecia, dyspnoea; *rarely* pulmonary oedema, onset or worsening of macular oedema; *very rarely* angioedema, urticaria; see also Liver Toxicity above

**Dose**
* Initially 4 mg daily; may be increased after 8 weeks to 8 mg daily (in 1–2 divided doses) according to response; CHILD and ADOLESCENT under 18 years not recommended

**Avandia®** (GSK) [PoM]
Tablets, f/c, rosiglitazone (as maleate) 4 mg (orange), net price 28-tab pack = £20.00, 56-tab pack = £40.00; 8 mg (red/brown), 28-tab pack = £30.00

◢**With metformin**

For cautions, contra-indications, and side-effects of metformin, see section 6.1.2.2

**Avandamet®** (GSK) ▼ PoM

Avandamet® 2 mg/500 mg tablets, f/c, pink, rosiglitazone (as maleate) 2 mg, metformin hydrochloride 500 mg, net price 112-tab pack = £30.00.Label: 21

Avandamet® 2 mg/1 g tablets, f/c, yellow, rosiglitazone (as maleate) 2 mg, metformin hydrochloride 1 g, net price 56-tab pack = £20.00. Label: 21

Avandamet® 4 mg/1 g tablets, f/c, pink, rosiglitazone (as maleate) 4 mg, metformin hydrochloride 1 g, net price 56-tab pack = £30.00. Label: 21

**Dose** type 2 diabetes mellitus not controlled by metformin alone, initially one *Avandamet®* 2 mg/1 g tablet twice daily, increased after 8 weeks according to response up to two *Avandamet®* 2 mg/500 mg tablets twice daily or one *Avandamet®* 4 mg/1 g tablet twice daily; max. 8 mg rosiglitazone and 2 g metformin hydrochloride daily; CHILD and ADOLESCENT under 18 years not recommended

**Note** Titration with the individual components (rosiglitazone and metformin) desirable before initiating *Avandamet®*

## ▌ SITAGLIPTIN

**Indications** type 2 diabetes mellitus (in combination with metformin *or* with a thiazolidinedione *or* with a sulphonylurea *or* with metformin and a sulphonylurea—see notes above)

**Cautions** interactions: Appendix 1 (antidiabetics)

**Contra-indications** ketoacidosis; renal impairment (avoid if eGFR less than 50 mL/minute/1.73 m²; Appendix 3); pregnancy (Appendix 4); breast-feeding (Appendix 5)

**Side-effects** gastro-intestinal disturbances; peripheral oedema; upper respiratory tract infection, nasopharyngitis; pain; osteoarthritis; *less commonly* anorexia, headache, drowsiness, dizziness, hypoglycaemia, osteoarthritis

**Dose**

● ADULT over 18 years, 100 mg once daily

**Note** Dose of concomitant sulphonylurea may need to be reduced

**Januvia®** (MSD) ▼ PoM

Tablets, beige, f/c, sitagliptin (as phosphate) 100 mg, net price 28-tab pack = £33.26

## ▌ VILDAGLIPTIN

**Indications** type 2 diabetes mellitus (in combination with metformin *or* with a sulphonylurea *or* with a thiazolidinedione—see also notes above)

**Cautions** elderly; monitor liver function (see below); heart failure (avoid if moderate or severe); **interactions**: Appendix 1 (antidiabetics)

**Liver toxicity** Rare reports of liver dysfunction; monitor liver function before treatment and every 3 months for first year and periodically thereafter; advise patients to seek prompt medical attention if symptoms such as nausea, vomiting, abdominal pain, fatigue, and dark urine develop; discontinue if jaundice or other signs of liver dysfunction occur

**Contra-indications** ketoacidosis; hepatic impairment (Appendix 2); renal impairment (avoid if eGFR less than 50 mL/minute/1.73 m²; Appendix 3); pregnancy (Appendix 4); breast-feeding (Appendix 5)

**Side-effects** nausea; peripheral oedema; headache, tremor, asthenia, dizziness; *less commonly* constipation; hypoglycaemia; *rarely* hepatic dysfunction (see

also Liver Toxicity above); *very rarely* nasopharyngitis; upper respiratory tract infection and arthralgia also reported

**Dose**

● ADULT over 18 years, in combination with metformin or a thiazolidinedione, 50 mg twice daily; in combination with a sulphonylurea, 50 mg daily in the morning

**Galvus®** (Novartis) ▼ PoM

Tablets, pale yellow, vildagliptin 50 mg, net price 56-tab pack = £31.76

◢**With metformin**

For cautions, contra-indications, and side-effects of metformin, see section 6.1.2.2

**Eucreas®** (Novartis) ▼ PoM

Eucreas® 50 mg/850 mg tablets, f/c, yellow, vildagliptin 50 mg, metformin hydrochloride 850 mg, net price 60-tab pack = £31.76. Label: 21

Eucreas® 50 mg/1 g tablets, f/c, dark yellow, vildagliptin 50 mg, metformin hydrochloride 1 g, net price 60-tab pack = £31.76. Label: 21

**Dose** type 2 diabetes mellitus not controlled by metformin alone, ADULT over 18 years, 1 *Eucreas®* tablet twice daily (based on patient's current metformin dose)

The *Scottish Medicines Consortium* (p. 3) has advised (June 2008) that *Eucreas®* is accepted for restricted use within NHS Scotland for the treatment of type 2 diabetes mellitus in patients unable to achieve adequate glycaemic control with metformin alone or those already treated with vildagliptin and metformin as separate tablets

## ▌6.1.3 **Diabetic ketoacidosis**

The management of diabetic ketoacidosis involves the replacement of fluid and electrolytes and the administration of insulin; local guidelines should be followed. **Soluble insulin**, given intravenously, is the most appropriate form of insulin for the management of diabetic ketoacidosis and hyperosmolar non-ketotic state. It is necessary to achieve and to maintain an adequate plasma-insulin concentration until the metabolic disturbance is brought under control.

Soluble insulin is best given by intravenous infusion, using an infusion pump, and diluted to 1 unit/mL (care in mixing, see Appendix 6). Adequate plasma-insulin concentration can usually be maintained with infusion rates of 6 units/hour for adults and 0.1 units/kg/hour for children. Blood glucose is expected to decrease by about 5 mmol/litre/hour; if the response is inadequate the infusion rate can be doubled or quadrupled. When the blood-glucose concentration has fallen to 10 mmol/litre the infusion rate can be reduced to 3 units/hour for adults (about 0.05 units/kg/hour for children) and continued until the patient is ready to take food by mouth. The insulin infusion should not be stopped before subcutaneous insulin has been started.

No matter how large, a bolus intravenous injection of insulin can provide an adequate plasma concentration for a short time only; therefore if facilities for intravenous infusion are not available the insulin is given by *intramuscular injection*. An initial loading dose of 20 units intramuscularly is followed by 6 units intramuscularly every hour until the blood-glucose concentration falls to 10 mmol/litre; intramuscular injections are then given every 2 hours. Although absorption of insulin is usually rapid after intramuscular injection, it may be

**6**

**Endocrine system**

impaired in the presence of hypotension and poor tissue perfusion; moreover insulin may accumulate during treatment and late hypoglycaemia should be watched for and treated appropriately.

Intravenous replacement of fluid and electrolytes (section 9.2.2) with **sodium chloride** intravenous infusion is an essential part of the management of ketoacidosis; **potassium chloride** is included in the infusion as appropriate to prevent the hypokalaemia induced by the insulin. **Sodium bicarbonate** infusion (1.26% or 2.74%) is used only in cases of extreme acidosis and shock since the acid-base disturbance is normally corrected by the insulin. When the blood glucose has fallen to approximately 10 mmol/litre **glucose** 5% is infused (maximum 2 litres in 24 hours), but insulin infusion must continue.

## 6.1.4 Treatment of hypoglycaemia

Initially glucose 10–20 g is given by mouth either in liquid form or as granulated sugar or sugar lumps. Approximately 10 g of glucose is available from 2 teaspoons of sugar, 3 sugar lumps, *GlucoGel*® (formerly known as *Hypostop Gel*®) glucose 10 g/25 g tube, available from BBI Healthcare), *Dextrogel*® (glucose 10 g/25 g tube, available from M & A Pharmachem), and non-diet versions of *Lucozade*® *Energy Original* 55 mL, *Coca-Cola*® 100 mL, *Ribena*® *Blackcurrant* 18 mL (to be diluted). If necessary this may be repeated in 10–15 minutes. After initial treatment, a snack providing sustained availability of carbohydrate (e.g. a sandwich, fruit, milk, and biscuits) or the next meal, if it is due, can prevent blood-glucose concentration from falling again.

Hypoglycaemia which causes unconsciousness is an emergency. **Glucagon**, a polypeptide hormone produced by the alpha cells of the islets of Langerhans, increases plasma-glucose concentration by mobilising glycogen stored in the liver. In hypoglycaemia, if sugar cannot be given by mouth, glucagon can be given by injection. Carbohydrates should be given as soon as possible to restore liver glycogen; glucagon is not appropriate for chronic hypoglycaemia. It may be issued to close relatives of insulin-treated patients for emergency use in hypoglycaemic attacks. It is often advisable to prescribe on an 'if necessary' basis to hospitalised insulin-treated patients, so that it may be given rapidly by the nurses during an hypoglycaemic emergency. If not effective in 10 minutes intravenous glucose should be given.

Alternatively, 50 mL of **glucose intravenous infusion 20%** (section 9.2.2) may be given intravenously into a large vein through a large-gauge needle; care is required since this concentration is irritant especially if extravasation occurs. Alternatively, 25 mL of glucose intravenous infusion 50% may be given, but this higher concentration is more irritant and viscous making administration difficult. Glucose intravenous infusion 10% may also be used but larger volumes are needed. Close monitoring is necessary in the case of an overdose with a long-acting insulin because further administration of glucose may be required. Patients whose hypoglycaemia is caused by an oral antidiabetic drug should be

transferred to hospital because the hypoglycaemic effects of these drugs may persist for many hours.

For advice on the emergency management of hypoglycaemia in dental practice, see p. 23.

### ■ GLUCAGON

**Indications** see notes above and under Dose

**Cautions** see notes above, insulinoma, glucagonoma; ineffective in chronic hypoglycaemia, starvation, and adrenal insufficiency

**Contra-indications** phaeochromocytoma

**Side-effects** nausea, vomiting, abdominal pain, hypokalaemia, hypotension, rarely hypersensitivity reactions

**Dose**

- Insulin-induced hypoglycaemia, by subcutaneous, intramuscular, *or* intravenous injection, ADULT and CHILD over 8 years (or body-weight over 25 kg), 1 mg; CHILD under 8 years (or body-weight under 25 kg), 500 micrograms; if no response within 10 minutes intravenous glucose must be given
- Diagnostic aid, consult product literature
- Beta-blocker poisoning, see p. 32

Note 1 unit of glucagon = 1 mg of glucagon

¹**GlucaGen® HypoKit** (Novo Nordisk) [PoM]
Injection, powder for reconstitution, glucagon (rys) as hydrochloride with lactose, net price 1-mg vial with prefilled syringe containing water for injection = £11.52

1. [PoM] restriction does not apply where administration is for saving life in emergency

## Chronic hypoglycaemia

**Diazoxide**, administered by mouth, is useful in the management of patients with chronic hypoglycaemia from excess endogenous insulin secretion, either from an islet cell tumour or islet cell hyperplasia. It has no place in the management of acute hypoglycaemia.

### ■ DIAZOXIDE

**Indications** chronic intractable hypoglycaemia (for use in hypertensive crisis see section 2.5.1)

**Cautions** ischaemic heart disease, pregnancy (Appendix 4), labour, impaired renal function (Appendix 3); monitor blood pressure; during prolonged use monitor white cell and platelet count, and in children, regularly assess growth, bone, and psychological development; **interactions:** Appendix 1 (diazoxide)

**Side-effects** anorexia, nausea, vomiting, hyperuricaemia, hypotension, oedema, tachycardia, arrhythmias, extrapyramidal effects; hypertrichosis on prolonged treatment

**Dose**

- By mouth, ADULT and CHILD, initially 5 mg/kg daily in 2–3 divided doses

**Eudemine®** (UCB Pharma) [PoM]
Tablets, diazoxide 50 mg. Net price 20 = £8.93

Injection, see section 2.5.1

## 6.1.5 Treatment of diabetic nephropathy and neuropathy

### Diabetic nephropathy

Regular review of diabetic patients should include an annual test for urinary protein (using *Albustix®*) and serum creatinine measurement. If the urinary protein test is negative, the urine should be tested for microalbuminuria (the earliest sign of nephropathy). If reagent strip tests (*Micral-Test II®* [NHS] or *Microbumintest®* [NHS]) are used and prove positive, the result should be confirmed by laboratory analysis of a urine sample. Provided there are no contra-indications, all diabetic patients with nephropathy causing proteinuria or with established microalbuminuria (at least 3 positive tests) should be treated with an ACE inhibitor (section 2.5.5.1) or an angiotensin-II receptor antagonist (section 2.5.5.2) even if the blood pressure is normal; in any case, to minimise the risk of renal deterioration, blood pressure should be carefully controlled (section 2.5).

ACE inhibitors can potentiate the hypoglycaemic effect of insulin and oral antidiabetic drugs; this effect is more likely during the first weeks of combined treatment and in patients with renal impairment.

For the treatment of hypertension in diabetes, see section 2.5.

### Diabetic neuropathy

Optimal diabetic control is beneficial for the management of *painful neuropathy* in patients with type 1 diabetes (see also section 4.7.3). **Paracetamol** or a **non-steroidal anti-inflammatory drug** such as ibuprofen (section 10.1.1) may relieve *mild to moderate pain*.

The **tricyclic antidepressants** amitriptyline and nortriptyline (section 4.3.1) are the drugs of choice for painful diabetic neuropathy [unlicensed use]; amitriptyline is given in a dose of 25–75 mg daily (higher doses under specialist supervision). **Duloxetine** (section 4.3.4) is licensed for the treatment of diabetic neuropathic pain.

**Gabapentin** (section 4.8.1) is licensed for the treatment of neuropathic pain and is an effective alternative to a tricyclic antidepressant.**Carbamazepine** and **phenytoin** [both unlicensed] (section 4.8.1) may be useful for shooting or stabbing pain, but adverse effects are common; carbamazepine 200–800 mg daily in divided doses has been used.

**Capsaicin** cream 0.075% (section 10.3.2) is licensed for painful diabetic neuropathy and may have some effect, but it produces an intense burning sensation during the initial treatment period.

Neuropathic pain may respond partially to some **opioid analgesics**, such as methadone, oxycodone and tramadol, and they may have a role when other treatments have failed.

In *autonomic neuropathy* diabetic diarrhoea can often be managed by 2 or 3 doses of **tetracycline** 250 mg [unlicensed use] (section 5.1.3). Otherwise **codeine phosphate** (section 1.4.2) is the best drug, but other antidiarrhoeal preparations can be tried. An **antiemetic** which promotes gastric transit, such as metoclopramide or domperidone (section 4.6), is helpful for gastroparesis. In rare cases when an antiemetic does not help, erythromycin (especially when given intravenously) may be beneficial but this needs confirmation.

For the management of erectile dysfunction, see section 7.4.5.

In *neuropathic postural hypotension* increased salt intake and the use of the **mineralocorticoid** fludrocortisone 100–400 micrograms daily [unlicensed use] (section 6.3.1) help by increasing plasma volume, but uncomfortable oedema is a common side-effect. Fludrocortisone can also be combined with **flurbiprofen** (section 10.1.1) and **ephedrine hydrochloride** (section 3.1.1.2) [both unlicensed]. **Midodrine** [unlicensed], an alpha agonist, may also be useful in postural hypotension.

*Gustatory sweating* can be treated with an **antimuscarinic** such as propantheline bromide (section 1.2); side-effects are common. For the management of hyperhidrosis, see section 13.12.

In some patients with *neuropathic oedema*, **ephedrine hydrochloride** [unlicensed use] 30–60 mg 3 times daily offers effective relief.

## 6.1.6 Diagnostic and monitoring agents for diabetes mellitus

### Blood monitoring

Blood **glucose** monitoring using a meter gives a direct measure of the glucose concentration at the time of the test and can detect hypoglycaemia as well as hyperglycaemia. Patients should be properly trained in the use of blood glucose monitoring systems and to take appropriate action on the results obtained. Inadequate understanding of the normal fluctuations in blood glucose can lead to confusion and inappropriate action.

For patients treated with insulin, it is ideal to observe the 'peaks' and 'troughs' of blood glucose over 24 hours and make adjustments to their insulin no more than once or twice weekly. Daily alterations to the insulin dose are highly undesirable (except during illness).

Self-monitoring of blood-glucose concentration is appropriate for patients with type 2 diabetes:

- who are treated with insulin;
- who are treated with oral hypoglycaemic drugs e.g. sulphonylureas, to provide information on hypoglycaemia;
- to monitor changes in blood-glucose concentration resulting from changes in lifestyle or medication, and during intercurrent illness;
- to ensure safe blood-glucose concentration during activities, including driving.

Note In the UK blood-glucose concentration is expressed in mmol/litre and Diabetes UK advises that these units should be used for self-monitoring of blood glucose. In other European countries units of mg/100 mL (or mg/dL) are commonly used. It is advisable to check that the meter is pre-set in the correct units.

6

Endocrine system

If the patient is unwell and diabetic ketoacidosis is suspected, blood **ketones** should be measured according to local guidelines (section 6.1.3). Patients and their carers should be trained in the use of blood ketone monitoring systems and to take appropriate action on the results obtained, including when to seek medical attention.

◀ **Test strips**

**Active®** (Roche Diagnostics)

Reagent strips, for blood glucose monitoring, range 0.6–33.3 mmol/litre, for use with *Glucotrend®* and *Accu-Chek® Active* ᴺᴴˢ meters only. Net price 50-strip pack = £14.76

**Advantage Plus®** (Roche Diagnostics)

Sensor strips, for blood glucose monitoring, range 0.6–33.3 mmol/litre, for use with *Accu-Chek® Advantage* ᴺᴴˢ meter only. Net price 50-strip pack = £14.76

**Ascensia® Autodisc** (Bayer Diabetes Care)

Sensor discs, for blood glucose monitoring, range 0.6–33.3 mmol/litre, for use with *Ascensia Breeze®* ᴺᴴˢ and *Ascensia Esprit® 2* ᴺᴴˢ meters only. Net price 5 × 10-disc pack = £14.62

**Aviva®** (Roche Diagnostics)

Sensor strips, for blood glucose monitoring, range 0.6–33.3 mmol/litre, for use with *Accu-Chek® Aviva* ᴺᴴˢ meter only. Net price 50-strip pack = £14.49

**BM-Accutest®** (Roche Diagnostics)

Reagent strips, for blood glucose monitoring, range 1.1–33.3 mmol/litre, for use with *Accutrend®* ᴺᴴˢ meters only. Net price 50-strip pack = £14.31

**Breeze 2®** (Bayer Diabetes Care)

Sensor discs, for blood glucose monitoring, range 0.6–33.3 mmol/litre, for use with the Breeze 2® ᴺᴴˢ meter only. Net price 5 × 10-disc pack = £14.34

**Compact®** (Roche Diagnostics)

Reagent strips, for blood glucose monitoring, range 0.6–33.3 mmol/litre, for use with *Accu-Chek® Compact* and *Accu-Chek® Compact Plus* ᴺᴴˢ meters only. Net price 3 × 17-strip pack = £14.88

**Contour®** (Bayer Diabetes Care)

Sensor strips, for blood glucose monitoring, range 0.6–33.3 mmol/litre, for use with *Contour®* ᴺᴴˢ meter only. Net price 50-strip pack = £14.74

Note Formerly *Ascensia® Microfill*

**FreeStyle®** (Abbott)

Sensor strips, for blood glucose monitoring, range 1.1–27.8 mmol/litre, for use with *FreeStyle®* ᴺᴴˢ meters only. Net price 50-strip pack = £14.62

**FreeStyle Lite®** (Abbott)

Sensor strips, for blood glucose monitoring, range 1.1–27.8 micromol/litre, for use with *FreeStyle® Lite* ᴺᴴˢ meter only. Net price 50-strip pack = £14.62

**GlucoMen®** (Menarini Diagnostics)

Sensor strips, for blood glucose monitoring, range 1.1–33.3 mmol/litre, for use with *GlucoMen® Glycó* ᴺᴴˢ and *GlucoMen® PC* ᴺᴴˢ meters only. Net price 50-strip pack = £13.67

**GlucoMen® LX** (Menarini Diagnostics)

Sensor strips, for blood glucose monitoring, range 1.1–33.3 mmol/litre, for use with *GlucoMen® LX* ᴺᴴˢ meter only. Net price 50-strip pack = £14.33

**GlucoMen® Visio Sensor** (Menarini Diagnostics)

Sensor strips, for blood glucose monitoring, range 1.1–33.3 mmol/litre, for use with *GlucoMen® Visio* ᴺᴴˢ meter. Net price 50-strip pack = £14.53

**Hypoguard® Supreme** (Hypoguard)

Reagent strips, for blood glucose monitoring, range 2.2–27.7 mmol/litre, for use with *Hypoguard® Supreme* ᴺᴴˢ meters. Net price 50-strip pack = £12.00

**MediSense G2®** (Abbott)

Sensor strips, for blood glucose monitoring, range 1.1–33.3 mmol/litre, for use with *MediSense® Precision QID* ᴺᴴˢ meter only. Net price 50-strip pack = £13.67

**MediSense® Soft-Sense Plus** (Abbott)

Sensor strips, for blood glucose monitoring, range 1.7–25 mmol/litre, for use with *Optium Xceed®* ᴺᴴˢ meter only. Net price 50-strip pack = £14.52

**One Touch®** (LifeScan)

Reagent strips, for blood glucose monitoring, range 1.1–33.3 mmol/litre, for use with *One Touch® II, Profile* and *Basic* ᴺᴴˢ meters only. Net price 50-strip pack = £14.37

**One Touch Ultra®** (LifeScan)

Sensor strips, for blood glucose monitoring, range 1.1–33.3 mmol/litre, for use with *One Touch Ultra®* ᴺᴴˢ, *One Touch Ultra 2®* ᴺᴴˢ, *One Touch UltraSmart®* ᴺᴴˢ, and *One Touch UltraEasy®* ᴺᴴˢ meters only. Net price 50-strip pack = £14.53

**One Touch® Vita** (LifeScan)

Sensor strips, for blood glucose monitoring, range 1.1–33.3 mmol/litre for use with *One Touch® Vita* ᴺᴴˢ meter only. Net price 50-strip pack = £14.53

**Optium® β-ketone test strips** (Abbott)

Reagent Strips, for blood ketone monitoring, range 0–8.0 mmol/litre, for use with *Optium®* ᴺᴴˢ or *Optium Xceed®* ᴺᴴˢ meters only. Net price 10-strip pack = £19.55

**Optium Plus®** (Abbott)

Sensor strips (formerly *Medisense® Optium Plus*), for blood glucose monitoring, range 1.1–33.3 mmol/litre, for use with *Optium Xceed* ᴺᴴˢ meter only. Net price 50-strip pack = £14.53

**PocketScan®** (LifeScan)

Sensor strips, for blood glucose monitoring, range 1.1–33.3 mmol/litre, for use with *PocketScan®* ᴺᴴˢ meter only. Net price 50-strip pack = £14.19

**Prestige®** (Home Diagnostics)

Reagent strips, for blood glucose monitoring, range 1.4–33.3 mmol/litre, for use with *Prestige®* ᴺᴴˢ meter only. Net price 50-strip pack = £14.51

**TRUEone®** (Home Diagnostics)

Sensor strips with meter, for blood glucose monitoring, range 1.1–33.3 mmol/litre. Meter built into top of sensor strip pot. Net price 50-strip and meter pack = £14.25

**TRUETrack®** (Home Diagnostics)

Sensor strips, for blood glucose monitoring, range 1.1–33.3 mmol/litre, for use with *TRUETrack®* ᴺᴴˢ meter only. Net price 50-strip pack = £14.25

**WaveSense Jazz®** (WaveSense)

Reagent strips for blood glucose monitoring, range 1.1–33.3 mmol/litre, for use with *WaveSense Jazz®* ᴺᴴˢ meter only. Net price 50-strip pack = £14.45

◀ **Meters**

**Accu-Chek® Aviva** (Roche Diagnostics) ᴺᴴˢ

Meter, for blood glucose monitoring (for use with *Aviva®* test strips). *Accu-Chek® Aviva* system = £12.99

**Accu-Chek® Compact Plus** (Roche Diagnostics) ᴺᴴˢ

Meter, for blood glucose monitoring (for use with *Compact®* test strips). *Accu-Chek® Compact Plus* system = £12.99

**Breeze 2®** (Bayer Diabetes Care) ᴺᴴˢ

Meter, for blood glucose monitoring (for use with *Breeze* 2® Sensor discs) = £10.29

**Contour®** (Bayer Diabetes Care) ᴺᴴˢ

Meter, for blood glucose monitoring (for use with *Ascensia® Microfill* sensor strips) = £10.29

**FreeStyle®** (Abbott) ᴺᴴˢ

Meters, for blood glucose monitoring (for use with *FreeStyle®* and *FreeStyle Lite®* test strips). *FreeStyle Lite®* meter = £7.79; *FreeStyle Freedom Lite®* meter = £5.99

**Endocrine system**

**6**

**GlucoMen® LX** (Menarini Diagnostics) ⟨NHS⟩

Meter, for blood glucose monitoring (for use with *GlucoMen® LX* sensor strips) = £12.99

**GlucoMen® Visio** (Menarini Diagnostics) ⟨NHS⟩

Meter, for blood glucose monitoring (for use with *GlucoMen® Visio Sensor* strips) = £12.99

**Hypoguard® Supreme** (Hypoguard) ⟨NHS⟩

Meters, for blood glucose monitoring (for use with *Hypoguard® Supreme* test strips). *Hypoguard® Supreme Plus* meter = £35.00; *Hypoguard® Supreme Extra* meter = £45.00

**One Touch Ultra® 2** (LifeScan) ⟨NHS⟩

Meter, for blood glucose monitoring (for use with *One Touch Ultra®* sensor strips) = £12.99

**One Touch UltraEasy®** (LifeScan) ⟨NHS⟩

Meter, for blood glucose monitoring (for use with *One Touch Ultra®* sensor strips) = £12.99

**One Touch UltraSmart®** (LifeScan) ⟨NHS⟩

Meter, for blood glucose monitoring (for use with *One Touch Ultra®* sensor strips) = £19.99

**One Touch® Vita** (LifeScan) ⟨NHS⟩

Meter, for blood glucose monitoring (for use with *One Touch® Vita* sensor strips) = £16.99

**Optium® Xceed** (Abbott) ⟨NHS⟩

Meter, for blood glucose monitoring (for use with *MediSense® Soft-Sense*, and *Optium® Plus* test strips) and for blood ketone monitoring (for use with *Optium®* β-ketone test strips). Net price starter pack = £9.00

**Prestige®** (Home Diagnostics) ⟨NHS⟩

Meter, for blood glucose monitoring (for use with *Prestige®* test strips) = £5.63

**TRUETrack®** (Home Diagnostics) ⟨NHS⟩

Meter, for blood glucose monitoring (for use with *TRUETrack®* test strips) = £5.63

**WaveSense Jazz®** (WaveSense) ⟨NHS⟩

Meter, for blood glucose monitoring (for use with *WaveSense Jazz®* reagent strips) = £24.99

## Urinalysis

Tests for glucose range from reagent strips specific to glucose to reagent tablets which detect all reducing sugars. Few patients still use *Clinitest®*; *Clinistix®* is suitable for screening purposes only. Tests for ketones by patients are rarely required unless they become unwell—see also Blood Monitoring, p. 389.

Microalbuminuria can be detected with *Micral-Test II®* ⟨NHS⟩ or *Microbumintest®* ⟨NHS⟩ but this should be followed by confirmation in the laboratory, since false positive results are common.

◢Glucose

**Clinistix®** (Bayer Diabetes Care)

Reagent strips, for detection of glucose in urine. Net price 50-strip pack = £3.25

**Clinitest®** (Bayer Diabetes Care) ⟨NHS⟩

Reagent tablets, for detection of glucose and other reducing substances in urine. Net price 36-tab pack = £2.00

**Diabur-Test 5000®** (Roche Diagnostics)

Reagent strips, for detection of glucose in urine. Net price 50-strip pack = £2.79

**Diastix®** (Bayer Diabetes Care)

Reagent strips, for detection of glucose in urine. Net price 50-strip pack = £2.76

**Medi-Test® Glucose** (BHR)

Reagent strips, for detection of glucose in urine. Net price 50-strip pack = £2.30

◢Ketones

**Ketostix®** (Bayer Diabetes Care)

Reagent strips, for detection of ketones in urine. Net price 50-strip pack = £2.92

**Ketur Test®** (Roche Diagnostics)

Reagent strips, for detection of ketones in urine. Net price 50-strip pack = £2.68

◢Protein

**Albustix®** (Bayer Diagnostics)

Reagent strips, for detection of protein in urine. Net price 50-strip pack = £4.10

**Medi-Test® Protein 2** (BHR)

Reagent strips, for detection of protein in urine. Net price 50-strip pack = £3.22

◢**Other reagent strips available for urinalysis include:**

*Combur-3 Test®* ⟨NHS⟩ (glucose and protein—Roche Diagnostics), *Clinitek Microalbumin®* ⟨NHS⟩ (albumin and creatinine—Bayer Diagnostics), *Ketodiastix®* ⟨NHS⟩ (glucose and ketones—Bayer Diagnostics), *Medi-Test Combi 2®* ⟨NHS⟩ (glucose and protein—BHR), *Micral-Test II®* ⟨NHS⟩ (albumin—Roche Diagnostics), *Microalbustix®* ⟨NHS⟩ (albumin and creatinine—Bayer Diagnostics), *Microbumintest®* ⟨NHS⟩ (albumin—Bayer Diagnostics), *Uristix®* ⟨NHS⟩ (glucose and protein—Bayer Diagnostics)

## Oral glucose tolerance test

The oral glucose tolerance test is now rarely needed for the diagnosis of diabetes when symptoms of hyperglycaemia are present, though it is still required to establish the presence of gestational diabetes. This generally involves giving anhydrous glucose 75 g (equivalent to Glucose BP 82.5 g) by mouth to the fasting patient, and measuring blood-glucose concentrations at intervals.

The appropriate amount of glucose should be given with 200–300 mL fluid. Anhydrous glucose 75 g may alternatively be given as 113 mL *Polycal®* (Nutricia Clinical) with extra fluid to administer a total volume of 200–300 mL.

## 6.2 Thyroid and antithyroid drugs

6.2.1 Thyroid hormones

6.2.2 Antithyroid drugs

## 6.2.1 Thyroid hormones

Thyroid hormones are used in hypothyroidism (myxoedema), and in diffuse non-toxic goitre, Hashimoto's thyroiditis (lymphadenoid goitre), and thyroid carcinoma. Neonatal hypothyroidism requires prompt treatment for normal development. **Levothyroxine sodium** (thyroxine sodium) is the treatment of choice for *maintenance* therapy.

In infants and children with congenital hypothyroidism and juvenile myxoedema, the dose of levothyroxine should be titrated according to clinical response, growth assessment, and measurements of plasma thyroxine and thyroid-stimulating hormone. See *BNF for Children* (section 6.2.1) for suitable dosage regimens.

**Liothyronine sodium** has a similar action to levothyroxine but is more rapidly metabolised and has a more rapid effect; 20 micrograms is equivalent to 100 micrograms of levothyroxine. Its effects develop after a few hours and disappear within 24 to 48 hours of discontinuing treatment. It may be used in *severe hypothyroid states* when a rapid response is desired.

Liothyronine by intravenous injection is the treatment of choice in *hypothyroid coma*. Adjunctive therapy includes intravenous fluids, hydrocortisone, and treatment of infection; assisted ventilation is often required.

### ■ LEVOTHYROXINE SODIUM
(Thyroxine sodium)

**Indications** hypothyroidism; see also notes above

**Cautions** panhypopituarism or predisposition to adrenal insufficiency (initiate corticosteroid therapy before starting levothyroxine), elderly, cardiovascular disorders (including hypertension, myocardial insufficiency or myocardial infarction, see Initial Dosage below), long-standing hypothyroidism, diabetes insipidus, diabetes mellitus (dose of antidiabetic drugs including insulin may need to be increased); pregnancy (Appendix 4); **interactions:** Appendix 1 (thyroid hormones)

**Initial dosage** Baseline ECG is valuable because changes induced by hypothyroidism can be confused with ischaemia. If metabolism increases too rapidly (causing diarrhoea, nervousness, rapid pulse, insomnia, tremors and sometimes anginal pain where there is latent myocardial ischaemia), reduce dose or withhold for 1–2 days and start again at a lower dose

**Contra-indications** thyrotoxicosis

**Side-effects** usually at excessive dosage (see Initial Dosage above) include diarrhoea, vomiting, anginal pain, arrhythmias, palpitation, tachycardia, tremor, restlessness, excitability, insomnia, headache, flushing, sweating, fever, heat intolerance, weight-loss, muscle cramp, and muscular weakness; transient hair loss in children; hypersensitivity reactions including rash, pruritus and oedema also reported

**Dose**

- ADULT, initially 50–100 micrograms once daily, preferably before breakfast, adjusted in steps of 25–50 micrograms every 3–4 weeks according to response (usual maintenance dose 100–200 micrograms once daily); in cardiac disease, severe hypothyroidism, and patients over 50 years, initially 25 micrograms once daily, adjusted in steps of 25 micrograms every 4 weeks according to response; usual maintenance dose 50–200 micrograms once daily; CHILD under 12 years see *BNF for Children* (section 6.2.1)

- Congenital hypothyroidism and juvenile myxoedema, see *BNF for Children* (section 6.2.1)

**Levothyroxine** (Non-proprietary) [PoM]
Tablets, levothyroxine sodium 25 micrograms, net price 28-tab pack = £2.03; 50 micrograms, 28-tab pack = £1.09; 100 micrograms, 28-tab pack = £1.16
Brands include *Eltroxin*®

Oral solution, levothyroxine sodium 25 micrograms/5 mL, net price 100 mL = £42.75; 50 micrograms/5 mL, 100 mL = £44.90; 100 micrograms/5 mL, 100 mL = £52.75
Brands include *Evotrox*® (sugar-free)

### ■ LIOTHYRONINE SODIUM
(L-Tri-iodothyronine sodium)

**Indications** see notes above

**Cautions** see under Levothyroxine Sodium; pregnancy (Appendix 4); breast-feeding (Appendix 5); **interactions:** Appendix 1 (thyroid hormones)

**Contra-indications** see under Levothyroxine Sodium

**Side-effects** see under Levothyroxine Sodium

**Dose**

- By mouth, initially 10–20 micrograms daily gradually increased to 60 micrograms daily in 2–3 divided doses; ELDERLY smaller initial doses; CHILD, adult dose reduced in proportion to body-weight

- By slow intravenous injection, hypothyroid coma, 5–20 micrograms repeated every 12 hours or as often as every 4 hours if necessary; *alternatively* initially 50 micrograms then 25 micrograms every 8 hours reducing to 25 micrograms twice daily

**Liothyronine sodium** (Goldshield) [PoM]
Tablets, scored, liothyronine sodium 20 micrograms, net price 28-tab pack = £23.77

**Triiodothyronine** (Goldshield) [PoM]
Injection, powder for reconstitution, liothyronine sodium (with dextran). Net price 20-microgram amp = £37.92

## 6.2.2 Antithyroid drugs

Antithyroid drugs are used for hyperthyroidism either to prepare patients for thyroidectomy or for long-term management. In the UK carbimazole is the most commonly used drug. Propylthiouracil may be used in patients who suffer sensitivity reactions to carbimazole as sensitivity is not necessarily displayed to both drugs. Both drugs act primarily by interfering with the synthesis of thyroid hormones.

> **CSM warning (neutropenia and agranulocytosis)**
> Doctors are reminded of the importance of recognising bone marrow suppression induced by carbimazole and the need to stop treatment promptly.
> 1. Patient should be asked to report symptoms and signs suggestive of infection, especially sore throat.
> 2. A white blood cell count should be performed if there is any clinical evidence of infection.
> 3. Carbimazole should be stopped promptly if there is clinical or laboratory evidence of neutropenia.

**Carbimazole** is given in a dose of 15 to 40 mg daily; occasionally a larger dose may be required. This dose is continued until the patient becomes euthyroid, usually after 4 to 8 weeks and the dose is then gradually reduced to a maintenance dose of 5 to 15 mg. Therapy is usually given for 12 to 18 months. Children may be given carbimazole in an initial dose of 250 micrograms/kg three times daily, adjusted according to response; treatment in children should be undertaken by a specialist.

Rashes and pruritus are common but they can be treated with antihistamines without discontinuing therapy; alternatively propylthiouracil can be substituted. All patients should be advised to report any sore throat immediately because of the rare complication of agranulocytosis (see CSM warning, above).

**Propylthiouracil** is given in a dose of 200 to 400 mg daily in adults and this dose is maintained until the patient becomes euthyroid; the dose may then be gradually reduced to a maintenance dose of 50 to 150 mg daily.

Antithyroid drugs only need to be given once daily because of their prolonged effect on the thyroid. Overtreatment can result in the rapid development of hypothyroidism and should be avoided particularly during pregnancy because it can cause fetal goitre.

A combination of carbimazole, 40 to 60 mg daily with levothyroxine, 50 to 150 micrograms daily, may be used in a *blocking-replacement regimen*; therapy is usually given for 18 months. The blocking-replacement regimen is **not** suitable during pregnancy.

**Iodine** has been used as an adjunct to antithyroid drugs for 10 to 14 days before partial thyroidectomy; however, there is little evidence of a beneficial effect. Iodine should not be used for long-term treatment because its antithyroid action tends to diminish.

Radioactive sodium iodide ($^{131}$I) solution is used increasingly for the treatment of thyrotoxicosis at all ages, particularly where medical therapy or compliance is a problem, in patients with cardiac disease, and in patients who relapse after thyroidectomy.

**Propranolol** is useful for rapid relief of thyrotoxic symptoms and may be used in conjunction with antithyroid drugs or as an adjunct to radioactive iodine. Beta-blockers are also useful in neonatal thyrotoxicosis and in supraventricular arrhythmias due to hyperthyroidism. Propranolol has been used in conjunction with iodine to prepare mildly thyrotoxic patients for surgery but it is preferable to make the patient euthyroid with carbimazole. Laboratory tests of thyroid function are not altered by beta-blockers. Most experience in treating thyrotoxicosis has been gained with propranolol but **nadolol** is also used. For doses and preparations of beta-blockers see section 2.4.

*Thyrotoxic crisis* ('thyroid storm') requires emergency treatment with intravenous administration of fluids, propranolol (5 mg) and hydrocortisone (100 mg every 6 hours, as sodium succinate), as well as oral iodine solution and carbimazole or propylthiouracil which may need to be administered by nasogastric tube.

**Pregnancy and breast-feeding** Radioactive iodine therapy is contra-indicated during pregnancy. Propylthiouracil and carbimazole can be given but the blocking-replacement regimen (see above) is **not** suitable. Both propylthiouracil and carbimazole cross the placenta and in high doses may cause fetal goitre and hypothyroidism—the lowest dose that will control the hyperthyroid state should be used (requirements in Graves' disease tend to fall during pregnancy). Rarely, carbimazole has been associated with congenital defects, including aplasia cutis of the neonate.

Carbimazole and propylthiouracil appear in breast milk but this does not preclude breast-feeding as long as neonatal development is closely monitored and the lowest effective dose is used.

## CARBIMAZOLE

**Indications** hyperthyroidism

**Cautions** hepatic impairment (avoid if severe; Appendix 2); pregnancy and breast-feeding (see notes above)

**Contra-indications** severe blood disorders

**Side-effects** nausea, mild gastro-intestinal disturbances, taste disturbance, headache; fever, malaise; rash, pruritus, arthralgia; *rarely* myopathy, alopecia, bone marrow suppression (including pancytopenia and agranulocytosis, see **CSM warning** above), and jaundice
Counselling Warn patient to tell doctor **immediately** if sore throat, mouth ulcers, bruising, fever, malaise, or non-specific illness develops

**Dose**
● See notes above

**Carbimazole** (Non-proprietary) [PoM]
Tablets, carbimazole 5 mg, net price 100-tab pack = £5.51; 20 mg, 100-tab pack = £19.12. Counselling, blood disorder symptoms

**Neo-Mercazole®** (Amdipharm) [PoM]
Tablets, both pink, carbimazole 5 mg, net price 100-tab pack = £4.53; 20 mg, 100-tab pack = £16.83. Counselling, blood disorder symptoms

## IODINE AND IODIDE

**Indications** thyrotoxicosis (pre-operative)

**Cautions** pregnancy (Appendix 4); children; not for long-term treatment

**Contra-indications** breast-feeding (Appendix 5)

**Side-effects** hypersensitivity reactions including coryza-like symptoms, headache, lacrimation, conjunctivitis, pain in salivary glands, laryngitis, bronchitis, rashes; on prolonged treatment depression, insomnia, impotence; goitre in infants of mothers taking iodides

**Dose**
● See under preparation

**Aqueous Iodine Oral Solution**
(Lugol's Solution), iodine 5%, potassium iodide 10% in purified water, freshly boiled and cooled, total iodine 130 mg/mL. Net price 100 mL = £1.19. Label: 27
Dose 0.1–0.3 mL 3 times daily well diluted with milk or water

## PROPYLTHIOURACIL

**Indications** hyperthyroidism

**Cautions** see under Carbimazole; hepatic impairment (Appendix 2); renal impairment (Appendix 3); pregnancy and breast-feeding (see notes above)

**Side-effects** see under Carbimazole; leucopenia; rarely cutaneous vasculitis, thrombocytopenia, aplastic anaemia, hypoprothrombinaemia, hepatitis, encephalopathy, hepatic necrosis, nephritis, lupus erythematous-like syndromes

**Dose**
● See notes above

**Propylthiouracil** (Non-proprietary) [PoM]
Tablets, propylthiouracil 50 mg. Net price 56-tab pack = £36.25

6 Endocrine system

# 6.3 Corticosteroids

### 6.3.1 Replacement therapy
### 6.3.2 Glucocorticoid therapy

## 6.3.1 Replacement therapy

The adrenal cortex normally secretes hydrocortisone (cortisol) which has glucocorticoid activity and weak mineralocorticoid activity. It also secretes the mineralocorticoid aldosterone.

In deficiency states, physiological replacement is best achieved with a combination of **hydrocortisone** (section 6.3.2) and the mineralocorticoid **fludrocortisone**; hydrocortisone alone does not usually provide sufficient mineralocorticoid activity for complete replacement.

In *Addison's disease* or following adrenalectomy, **hydrocortisone** 20 to 30 mg daily by mouth is usually required. This is given in 2 doses, the larger in the morning and the smaller in the evening, mimicking the normal diurnal rhythm of cortisol secretion. The optimum daily dose is determined on the basis of clinical response. Glucocorticoid therapy is supplemented by fludrocortisone 50 to 300 micrograms daily.

In *acute adrenocortical insufficiency*, **hydrocortisone** is given intravenously (preferably as sodium succinate) in doses of 100 mg every 6 to 8 hours in sodium chloride intravenous infusion 0.9%.

In *hypopituitarism* glucocorticoids should be given as in adrenocortical insufficiency, but since production of aldosterone is also regulated by the renin-angiotensin system a mineralocorticoid is not usually required. Additional replacement therapy with levothyroxine (section 6.2.1) and sex hormones (section 6.4) should be given as indicated by the pattern of hormone deficiency.

### ■ FLUDROCORTISONE ACETATE

**Indications** mineralocorticoid replacement in adrenocortical insufficiency

**Cautions** section 6.3.2; **interactions:** Appendix 1 (corticosteroids)

**Contra-indications** section 6.3.2

**Side-effects** section 6.3.2

**Dose**

• 50–300 micrograms daily; CHILD 5 micrograms/kg daily

**Florinef®** (Squibb) (PoM)
Tablets, scored, fludrocortisone acetate 100 micrograms. Net price 100-tab pack = £5.15. Label: 10, steroid card

## 6.3.2 Glucocorticoid therapy

In comparing the relative potencies of corticosteroids in terms of their anti-inflammatory (glucocorticoid) effects it should be borne in mind that high glucocorticoid activity in itself is of no advantage unless it is accompanied by relatively low mineralocorticoid activity (see

Disadvantages of Corticosteroids below). The mineralocorticoid activity of **fludrocortisone** (section 6.3.1) is so high that its anti-inflammatory activity is of no clinical relevance. The table below shows equivalent anti-inflammatory doses.

### Equivalent anti-inflammatory doses of corticosteroids

This table takes no account of mineralocorticoid effects, nor does it take account of variations in duration of action

Prednisolone 5 mg

≡ Betamethasone 750 micrograms
≡ Cortisone acetate 25 mg
≡ Deflazacort 6 mg
≡ Dexamethasone 750 micrograms
≡ Hydrocortisone 20 mg
≡ Methylprednisolone 4 mg
≡ Triamcinolone 4 mg

The relatively high mineralocorticoid activity of **cortisone** and **hydrocortisone**, and the resulting fluid retention, make them unsuitable for disease suppression on a long-term basis. However, they can be used for adrenal replacement therapy (section 6.3.1); hydrocortisone is preferred because cortisone requires conversion in the liver to hydrocortisone. Hydrocortisone is used on a short-term basis by intravenous injection for the emergency management of some conditions. The relatively moderate anti-inflammatory potency of hydrocortisone also makes it a useful topical corticosteroid for the management of inflammatory skin conditions because side-effects (both topical and systemic) are less marked (section 13.4); cortisone is not active topically.

**Prednisolone** has predominantly glucocorticoid activity and is the corticosteroid most commonly used by mouth for long-term disease suppression.

**Betamethasone** and **dexamethasone** have very high glucocorticoid activity in conjunction with insignificant mineralocorticoid activity. This makes them particularly suitable for high-dose therapy in conditions where fluid retention would be a disadvantage.

Betamethasone and dexamethasone also have a long duration of action and this, coupled with their lack of mineralocorticoid action makes them particularly suitable for conditions which require suppression of corticotropin (corticotrophin) secretion (e.g. congenital adrenal hyperplasia). Some esters of betamethasone and of **beclometasone** (beclomethasone) exert a considerably more marked topical effect (e.g. on the skin or the lungs) than when given by mouth; use is made of this to obtain topical effects whilst minimising systemic side-effects (e.g. for skin applications and asthma inhalations).

**Deflazacort** has a high glucocorticoid activity; it is derived from prednisolone.

## Use of corticosteroids

Dosages of corticosteroids vary widely in different diseases and in different patients. If the use of a corticosteroid can save or prolong life, as in exfoliative dermatitis, pemphigus, acute leukaemia or acute transplant rejection, high doses may need to be given, because the complications of therapy are likely to be less serious than the effects of the disease itself.

When long-term corticosteroid therapy is used in some chronic diseases, the adverse effects of treatment may become greater than the disabilities caused by the disease. To minimise side-effects the maintenance dose should be kept as low as possible.

When potentially less harmful measures are ineffective corticosteroids are used topically for the treatment of inflammatory conditions of the skin (section 13.4). Corticosteroids should be avoided or used only under specialist supervision in psoriasis (section 13.5).

Corticosteroids are used both topically (by rectum) and systemically (by mouth or intravenously) in the management of ulcerative colitis and Crohn's disease (section 1.5). They are also included in locally applied creams for haemorrhoids (section 1.7.2).

Use can be made of the mineralocorticoid activity of fludrocortisone to treat postural hypotension in autonomic neuropathy (section 6.1.5).

High-dose corticosteroids should be avoided for the management of septic shock. However, there is evidence that administration of lower doses of hydrocortisone (50 mg intravenously every 6 hours) and fludrocortisone (50 micrograms daily by mouth) is of benefit in adrenocortical insufficiency resulting from septic shock.

Dexamethasone and betamethasone have little if any mineralocorticoid action and their long duration of action makes them particularly suitable for suppressing corticotropin secretion in congenital adrenal hyperplasia where the dose should be tailored to clinical response and by measurement of adrenal androgens and 17-hydroxyprogesterone. In common with all glucocorticoids their suppressive action on the hypothalamic-pituitary-adrenal axis is greatest and most prolonged when they are given at night. In most individuals a single dose of 1 mg of dexamethasone at night, is sufficient to inhibit corticotropin secretion for 24 hours. This is the basis of the 'overnight dexamethasone suppression test' for diagnosing Cushing's syndrome.

Betamethasone and dexamethasone are also appropriate for conditions where water retention would be a disadvantage.

A corticosteroid may be used in the management of raised intracranial pressure or cerebral oedema that occurs as a result of malignancy (see also p. 17); high doses of betamethasone or dexamethasone are generally used. However, a corticosteroid should **not** be used for the management of head injury or stroke because it is unlikely to be of benefit and may even be harmful.

In acute hypersensitivity reactions such as angioedema of the upper respiratory tract and anaphylactic shock, corticosteroids are indicated as an adjunct to emergency treatment with adrenaline (epinephrine) (section 3.4.3). In such cases hydrocortisone (as sodium succinate) by intravenous injection in a dose of 100 to 300 mg may be required.

Corticosteroids are preferably used by inhalation in the management of asthma (section 3.2) but systemic therapy in association with bronchodilators is required for the emergency treatment of severe acute asthma (section 3.1.1).

Corticosteroids may also be useful in conditions such as autoimmune hepatitis, rheumatoid arthritis and sarcoidosis; they may also lead to remissions of acquired

haemolytic anaemia (section 9.1.3), and some cases of the nephrotic syndrome (particularly in children) and thrombocytopenic purpura (section 9.1.4).

Corticosteroids can improve the prognosis of serious conditions such as systemic lupus erythematosus, temporal arteritis, and polyarteritis nodosa; the effects of the disease process may be suppressed and symptoms relieved, but the underlying condition is not cured, although it may ultimately remit. It is usual to begin therapy in these conditions at fairly high dose, such as 40 to 60 mg prednisolone daily, and then to reduce the dose to the lowest commensurate with disease control.

For other references to the use of corticosteroids see Prescribing in Palliative Care, section 8.2.2 (immunosuppression), section 10.1.2 (rheumatic diseases), section 11.4 (eye), section 12.1.1 (otitis externa), section 12.2.1 (allergic rhinitis), and section 12.3.1 (aphthous ulcers).

## Administration

Whenever possible *local treatment* with creams, intra-articular injections, inhalations, eye-drops, or enemas should be used in preference to *systemic treatment*. The suppressive action of a corticosteroid on cortisol secretion is least when it is given as a single dose in the morning. In an attempt to reduce pituitary-adrenal suppression further, the total dose for two days can sometimes be taken as a single dose on alternate days; alternate-day administration has not been very successful in the management of asthma (section 3.2). Pituitary-adrenal suppression can also be reduced by means of intermittent therapy with short courses. In some conditions it may be possible to reduce the dose of corticosteroid by adding a small dose of an immunosuppressive drug (section 8.2.1).

## Cautions and contra-indications of corticosteroids

### Adrenal Suppression

During prolonged therapy with corticosteroids, adrenal atrophy develops and can persist for years after stopping. Abrupt withdrawal after a prolonged period can lead to acute adrenal insufficiency, hypotension or death (see Withdrawal of Corticosteroids, below). Withdrawal can also be associated with fever, myalgia, arthralgia, rhinitis, conjunctivitis, painful itchy skin nodules and weight loss.

To compensate for a diminished adrenocortical response caused by prolonged corticosteroid treatment, any significant intercurrent illness, trauma, or surgical procedure requires a temporary increase in corticosteroid dose, or if already stopped, a temporary reintroduction of corticosteroid treatment. To avoid a precipitous fall in blood pressure during anaesthesia or in the immediate postoperative period, anaesthetists **must** know whether a patient is taking or has been taking a corticosteroid. A suitable regimen for corticosteroid replacement, in patients who have taken more than 10 mg prednisolone daily (or equivalent) within 3 months of surgery, is:

● *Minor surgery under general anaesthesia*—usual oral corticosteroid dose on the morning of surgery or hydrocortisone 25–50 mg (usually the sodium succinate) intravenously at induction; the usual oral corticosteroid dose is recommended after surgery

- *Moderate or major surgery*—usual oral corticosteroid dose on the morning of surgery and hydrocortisone 25–50 mg intravenously at induction, followed by hydrocortisone 25–50 mg 3 times a day by intravenous injection for 24 hours after moderate surgery or for 48–72 hours after major surgery; the usual pre-operative oral corticosteroid dose is recommended on stopping hydrocortisone injections

Patients on long-term corticosteroid treatment should carry a Steroid Treatment Card (see p. 397) which gives guidance on minimising risk and provides details of prescriber, drug, dosage and duration of treatment.

### Infections

Prolonged courses of corticosteroids increase susceptibility to infections and severity of infections; clinical presentation of infections may also be atypical. Serious infections e.g. *septicaemia* and *tuberculosis* may reach an advanced stage before being recognised, and *amoebiasis* or *strongyloidiasis* may be activated or exacerbated (exclude before initiating a corticosteroid in those at risk or with suggestive symptoms). Fungal or viral *ocular infections* may also be exacerbated (see also section 11.4.1).

**Chickenpox** Unless they have had chickenpox, patients receiving oral or parenteral corticosteroids for purposes other than replacement should be regarded as being *at risk of severe chickenpox* (see Steroid Treatment Card). Manifestations of fulminant illness include pneumonia, hepatitis and disseminated intravascular coagulation; rash is not necessarily a prominent feature.

Passive immunisation with varicella–zoster immunoglobulin (section 14.5.2) is needed for exposed non-immune patients receiving systemic corticosteroids or for those who have used them within the previous 3 months. Confirmed chickenpox warrants specialist care and urgent treatment (section 5.3.2.1). Corticosteroids should not be stopped and dosage may need to be increased.

Topical, inhaled or rectal corticosteroids are less likely to be associated with an increased risk of severe chickenpox.

**Measles** Patients taking corticosteroids should be advised to take particular care to avoid exposure to measles and to seek immediate medical advice if exposure occurs. Prophylaxis with intramuscular normal immunoglobulin (section 14.5.1) may be needed.

### Withdrawal of corticosteroids

The CSM has recommended that *gradual* withdrawal of systemic corticosteroids should be considered in those whose disease is unlikely to relapse and have:

- recently received repeated courses (particularly if taken for longer than 3 weeks);
- taken a short course within 1 year of stopping long-term therapy;
- other possible causes of adrenal suppression;
- received more than 40 mg daily prednisolone (or equivalent);
- been given repeat doses in the evening;
- received more than 3 weeks' treatment.

Systemic corticosteroids may be stopped abruptly in those whose disease is unlikely to relapse *and* who have received treatment for 3 weeks or less *and* who are not included in the patient groups described above.

During corticosteroid withdrawal the dose may be reduced rapidly down to physiological doses (equivalent to prednisolone 7.5 mg daily) and then reduced more slowly. Assessment of the disease may be needed during withdrawal to ensure that relapse does not occur.

### Psychiatric reactions

Systemic corticosteroids, particularly in high doses, are linked to psychiatric reactions including euphoria, nightmares, insomnia, irritability, mood lability, suicidal thoughts, psychotic reactions, and behavioural disturbances. A serious paranoid state or depression with risk of suicide can be induced, particularly in patients with a history of mental disorder. These reactions frequently subside on reducing the dose or discontinuing the corticosteroid but they may also require specific management. Patients should be advised to seek medical advice if psychiatric symptoms (especially depression and suicidal thoughts) occur and they should also be alert to the rare possibility of such reactions during withdrawal of corticosteroid treatment.

Systemic corticosteroids should be prescribed with care in those predisposed to psychiatric reactions, including those who have previously suffered corticosteroid-induced psychosis, or who have a personal or family history of psychiatric disorders.

---

**Advice to patients**
A patient information leaflet should be supplied to every patient when a systemic corticosteroid is prescribed. Patients should especially be advised of the following (for details, see Infections, Adrenal Suppression, Psychiatric Reactions, and Withdrawal of Corticosteroids above):

- **Immunosuppression** Prolonged courses of corticosteroids can increase susceptibility to infection and serious infections can go unrecognised. Unless already immune, patients are at risk of severe **chickenpox** and should avoid close contact with people who have chickenpox or shingles. Similarly, precautions should also be taken against contracting **measles**;
- **Adrenal suppression** If the corticosteroid is given for longer than 3 weeks, treatment must not be stopped abruptly. Adrenal suppression can last for a year or more after stopping treatment and the patient must mention the course of corticosteroid when receiving treatment for any illness or injury;
- **Mood and behaviour changes** Corticosteroid treatment, especially with high doses, can alter mood and behaviour early in treatment—the patient can become confused, irritable and suffer from delusion and suicidal thoughts. These effects can also occur when corticosteroid treatment is being withdrawn. Medical advice should be sought if worrying psychological changes occur;
- **Other serious effects** Serious gastro-intestinal, musculoskeletal, and ophthalmic effects which require medical help can also occur; for details see Side-effects of Corticosteroids, p. 397.

Endocrine system 6

Steroid treatment cards (see below) should be issued where appropriate. Doctors and pharmacists can obtain supplies of the card from:
England and Wales
3M Security Printing and Systems Limited
Gorse Street, Chadderton
Oldham, OL9 9QH
Tel: (0161) 683 2189
Fax: (0161) 683 2188
nhsforms@spsl.uk.com
Scotland
Banner Business Supplies
Unit 2, Kingsthorne Park, Nettlehill Road, Houston
Industrial Estate
Livingston, EH54 5DB
Tel: (01506) 448 440
Fax: (01506) 448 400
cust.serv.scotland@bbslimited.co.uk

### Pregnancy and breast-feeding

Following a review of the data on the safety of systemic corticosteroids used in pregnancy and breast-feeding the CSM has concluded:

- corticosteroids vary in their ability to cross the placenta; betamethasone and dexamethasone cross the placenta readily while 88% of prednisolone is inactivated as it crosses the placenta;

- there is no convincing evidence that systemic corticosteroids increase the incidence of congenital abnormalities such as cleft palate or lip;

- when administration is prolonged or repeated during pregnancy, systemic corticosteroids increase the risk of intra-uterine growth restriction; there is no evidence of intra-uterine growth restriction following short-term treatment (e.g. prophylactic treatment for neonatal respiratory distress syndrome);

- any adrenal suppression in the neonate following prenatal exposure usually resolves spontaneously after birth and is rarely clinically important;

- prednisolone appears in small amounts in breast milk but maternal doses of up to 40 mg daily are unlikely to cause systemic effects in the infant; infants should be monitored for adrenal suppression if the mothers are taking a higher dose.

See also Appendix 4 and Appendix 5.

### Other cautions and contra-indications

*Other cautions include:* children and adolescents (growth restriction possibly irreversible), elderly (close supervision required particularly on long-term treatment); frequent monitoring required if history of tuberculosis (or X-ray changes), hypertension, recent myocardial infarction (rupture reported), congestive heart failure, hepatic impairment (Appendix 2), renal impairment, diabetes mellitus including family history, osteoporosis (post-menopausal women at special risk), glaucoma (including family history), ocular herpes simplex—risk of corneal perforation, severe affective disorders (particularly if history of steroid-induced psychosis—see also Psychiatric Reactions, p. 396), epilepsy, peptic ulcer, hypothyroidism, history of steroid myopathy, ulcerative colitis, diverticulitis, recent intestinal anastomoses, thromboembolic disorders; myasthenia gravis; **interactions:** Appendix 1 (corticosteroids)

*Other contra-indications include:* systemic infection (unless specific therapy given); avoid live virus vaccines in those receiving immunosuppressive doses (serum antibody response diminished)

## Side-effects of corticosteroids

Overdosage or prolonged use can exaggerate some of the normal physiological actions of corticosteroids leading to mineralocorticoid and glucocorticoid side-effects.

**Mineralocorticoid** side-effects include hypertension, sodium and water retention, and potassium and calcium loss. They are most marked with fludrocortisone, but are significant with cortisone, hydrocortisone, corticotropin, and tetracosactide (tetracosactrin). Mineralocorticoid actions are negligible with the high potency glucocorticoids, betamethasone and dexamethasone, and occur only slightly with methylprednisolone, prednisolone, and triamcinolone.

**Glucocorticoid** side-effects include diabetes and osteoporosis (section 6.6), which is a danger, particularly in the elderly, as it can result in osteoporotic fractures for example of the hip or vertebrae; in addition high doses

---

# STEROID TREATMENT CARD

I am a patient on STEROID treatment which must not be stopped suddenly

- If you have been taking this medicine for more than three weeks, the dose should be reduced gradually when you stop taking steroids unless your doctor says otherwise.

- Read the patient information leaflet given with the medicine.

- Always carry this card with you and show it to anyone who treats you (for example a doctor, nurse, pharmacist or dentist). For one year after you stop the treatment, you must mention that you have taken steroids.

- If you become ill, or if you come into contact with anyone who has an infectious disease, consult your doctor promptly. If you have never had chickenpox, you should avoid close contact with people who have chickenpox or shingles. If you do come into contact with chickenpox, see your doctor urgently.

- Make sure that the information on the card is kept up to date.

6   Endocrine system

are associated with avascular necrosis of the femoral head. Muscle wasting (proximal myopathy) can also occur. Corticosteroid therapy is also weakly linked with peptic ulceration and perforation (the potential advantage of soluble or enteric-coated preparations to reduce the risk is speculative only). See also Psychiatric Reactions, p. 396.

High doses of corticosteroids can cause Cushing's syndrome, with moon face, striae, and acne; it is usually reversible on withdrawal of treatment, but this must always be gradually tapered to avoid symptoms of acute adrenal insufficiency (**important**: see also Adrenal Suppression, p. 395).

In children, administration of corticosteroids may result in suppression of growth. For the effect of corticosteroids given in pregnancy, see Pregnancy and Breast-feeding, p. 397.

Side-effects can be minimised by using lowest effective dose for minimum period possible.

*Other side-effects include: gastro-intestinal effects*: dyspepsia, abdominal distension, acute pancreatitis, oesophageal ulceration and candidiasis; *musculoskeletal effects*: muscle weakness, vertebral and long bone fractures, tendon rupture; *endocrine effects*: menstrual irregularities and amenorrhoea, hirsutism, weight gain, negative nitrogen and calcium balance, increased appetite; increased susceptibility to and severity of infection, reactivation of dormant tuberculosis; *neuropsychiatric effects*: psychological dependence, insomnia, increased intracranial pressure with papilloedema in children (usually after withdrawal), aggravation of schizophrenia, aggravation of epilepsy; *ophthalmic effects*: glaucoma, papilloedema, posterior subcapsular cataracts, corneal or scleral thinning and exacerbation of ophthalmic viral or fungal disease, increased intra-ocular pressure, exophthalmos; *also* impaired healing, petechiae, ecchymoses, facial erythema, suppression of skin test reactions, urticaria, hyperhidrosis, skin atrophy, bruising, telangiectasia, myocardial rupture following recent myocardial infarction, congestive heart failure, leucocytosis, hyperglycaemia, hypersensitivity reactions (including anaphylaxis), thromboembolism, nausea, malaise, hiccups, headache, vertigo.

For other references to the side-effects of corticosteroids see section 3.2 (asthma), section 11.4 (eye) and section 13.4 (skin).

## BETAMETHASONE

**Indications** suppression of inflammatory and allergic disorders; congenital adrenal hyperplasia; see also notes above; ear (section 12.1.1); eye (section 11.4.1); nose (section 12.2.1); oral ulceration (section 12.3.1)

**Cautions** see notes above; transient effect on fetal movements and heart rate

**Contra-indications** see notes above

**Side-effects** see notes above

**Dose**

* By mouth, usual range 0.5–5 mg daily; see also Administration (above)
* By intramuscular injection *or* slow intravenous injection *or* infusion, 4–20 mg, repeated up to 4 times in 24 hours; CHILD, by slow intravenous injection, up to 1 year 1 mg, 1–5 years 2 mg, 6–12 years 4 mg, repeated up to 4 times in 24 hours according to response

**Betnelan®** (UCB Pharma) (PoM)
Tablets, scored, betamethasone 500 micrograms. Net price 100-tab pack = £4.22. Label: 10, steroid card, 21

**Betnesol®** (UCB Pharma) (PoM)
Soluble tablets, pink, scored, betamethasone 500 micrograms (as sodium phosphate). Net price 100-tab pack = £4.97. Label: 10, steroid card, 13, 21

Injection, betamethasone 4 mg (as sodium phosphate) /mL. Net price 1-mL amp = £1.17. Label: 10, steroid card

## CORTISONE ACETATE

**Indications** see under Dose but now superseded, see also notes above

**Cautions** see notes above

**Contra-indications** see notes above

**Side-effects** see notes above

**Dose**

* For replacement therapy, 25–37.5 mg daily in divided doses

**Cortisone** (Non-proprietary) (PoM)
Tablets, cortisone acetate 25 mg, net price 56-tab pack = £10.92. Label: 10, steroid card, 21

## DEFLAZACORT

**Indications** suppression of inflammatory and allergic disorders

**Cautions** see notes above

**Contra-indications** see notes above

**Side-effects** see notes above

**Dose**

* Usual maintenance 3–18 mg daily (acute disorders, initially up to 120 mg daily); see also Administration (above)

  CHILD 0.25–1.5 mg/kg daily (or on alternate days); see also Administration (above)

**Calcort®** (Sanofi-Aventis) (PoM)
Tablets, deflazacort 6 mg, net price 60-tab pack = £15.82. Label: 5, 10, steroid card

## DEXAMETHASONE

**Indications** suppression of inflammatory and allergic disorders; diagnosis of Cushing's disease, congenital adrenal hyperplasia; cerebral oedema associated with malignancy; croup (section 3.1); nausea and vomiting with chemotherapy (section 8.1); rheumatic disease (section 10.1.2); eye (section 11.4.1); see also notes above

**Cautions** see notes above

**Contra-indications** see notes above

**Side-effects** see notes above; also perineal irritation may follow intravenous administration of the phosphate ester

**Dose**

* By mouth, usual range 0.5–10 mg daily; CHILD 10–100 micrograms/kg daily; see also Administration (above)
* By intramuscular injection *or* slow intravenous injection *or* infusion (as dexamethasone phosphate), initially 0.5–24 mg; CHILD 200–400 micrograms/kg daily

**Endocrine system** **6**

Cerebral oedema associated with malignancy (as dexamethasone phosphate), by intravenous injection, 10 mg initially, then 4 mg by intramuscular injection every 6 hours as required for 2–4 days then gradually reduced and stopped over 5–7 days

Adjunctive treatment of bacterial meningitis, (starting before or with first dose of antibacterial treatment, as dexamethasone phosphate) [unlicensed indication], by intravenous injection, 10 mg every 6 hours for 4 days; CHILD 150 micrograms/kg every 6 hours for 4 days

**Note** Dexamethasone 1 mg ≡ dexamethasone phosphate 1.2 mg ≡ dexamethasone sodium phosphate 1.3 mg

**Dexamethasone** (Non-proprietary) PoM
Tablets, dexamethasone 500 micrograms, net price 28-tab pack = £29.50; 2 mg, 50-tab pack = £7.19, 100-tab pack = £13.92. Label: 10, steroid card, 21
Available from Chemidex and Organon

Oral solution, sugar-free, dexamethasone (as dexamethasone sodium phosphate) 2 mg/5 mL, net price 150-mL = £42.30. Label: 10, steroid card, 21
Brands include *Dexsol®*

Injection, dexamethasone phosphate (as dexamethasone sodium phosphate) 4 mg/mL, net price 1-mL amp = £1.00, 2-mL vial = £1.98; 24 mg/mL, 5-mL vial = £16.66. Label: 10, steroid card
Available from Hospira

Injection, dexamethasone (as dexamethasone sodium phosphate) 4 mg/mL, net price 1-mL amp = 91p, 2-mL vial = £1.27. Label: 10, steroid card
Available from Organon

## HYDROCORTISONE

**Indications** adrenocortical insufficiency (section 6.3.1); shock; see also notes above; hypersensitivity reactions e.g. anaphylactic shock and angioedema (section 3.4.3); asthma (section 3.1); severe inflammatory bowel disease (section 1.5); haemorrhoids (section 1.7.2); rheumatic disease (section 10.1.2); eye (section 11.4.1); skin (section 13.4)

**Cautions** see notes above

**Contra-indications** see notes above

**Side-effects** see notes above; also phosphate ester associated with paraesthesia and pain (particularly in the perineal region)

**Dose**

• By mouth, replacement therapy, 20–30 mg daily in divided doses—see section 6.3.1; CHILD 10–30 mg

• By intramuscular injection *or* slow intravenous injection *or* infusion, 100–500 mg, 3–4 times in 24 hours or as required; CHILD by slow intravenous injection up to 1 year 25 mg, 1–5 years 50 mg, 6–12 years 100 mg

**Hydrocortisone** (Non-proprietary) PoM
Tablets, scored, hydrocortisone 10 mg, net price 30-tab pack = £30.50; 20 mg, 30-tab pack = £32.00. Label: 10, steroid card, 21

[1]**Efcortesol®** (Sovereign) PoM ◢
Injection, hydrocortisone 100 mg (as sodium phosphate)/mL, net price 1-mL amp = £1.08, 5-mL amp = £4.89. Label: 10, steroid card
**Note** Paraesthesia and pain (particularly in the perineal region) may follow intravenous injection of the phosphate ester

1. PoM restriction does not apply where administration is for saving life in emergency

[1]**Solu-Cortef®** (Pharmacia) PoM
Injection, powder for reconstitution, hydrocortisone (as sodium succinate). Net price 100-mg vial = 92p, 100-mg vial with 2-mL amp water for injections = £1.16. Label: 10, steroid card

1. PoM restriction does not apply where administration is for saving life in emergency

## METHYLPREDNISOLONE

**Indications** suppression of inflammatory and allergic disorders; severe inflammatory bowel disease (section 1.5); cerebral oedema associated with malignancy; see also notes above; rheumatic disease (section 10.1.2); skin (section 13.4)

**Cautions** see notes above; also rapid intravenous administration of large doses associated with cardiovascular collapse

**Contra-indications** see notes above

**Side-effects** see notes above

**Dose**

• By mouth, usual range 2–40 mg daily; see also Administration (above)

• By intramuscular injection *or* slow intravenous injection *or* infusion, initially 10–500 mg; graft rejection, up to 1 g daily by intravenous infusion for up to 3 days

**Medrone®** (Pharmacia) PoM
Tablets, scored, methylprednisolone 2 mg (pink), net price 30-tab pack = £3.88; 4 mg, 30-tab pack = £6.19; 16 mg, 30-tab pack = £17.17; 100 mg (blue), 20-tab pack = £48.32. Label: 10, steroid card, 21

**Solu-Medrone®** (Pharmacia) PoM
Injection, powder for reconstitution, methylprednisolone (as sodium succinate) (all with solvent). Net price 40-mg vial = £1.58; 125-mg vial = £4.75; 500-mg vial = £9.60; 1-g vial = £17.30; 2-g vial = £32.86. Label: 10, steroid card

◢**Intramuscular depot**
**Depo-Medrone®** (Pharmacia) PoM
Injection (aqueous suspension), methylprednisolone acetate 40 mg/mL. Net price 1-mL vial = £2.87; 2-mL vial = £5.15; 3-mL vial = £7.47. Label: 10, steroid card
**Dose** by deep intramuscular injection into gluteal muscle, 40–120 mg, a second injection may be given after 2–3 weeks if required

## PREDNISOLONE

**Indications** suppression of inflammatory and allergic disorders; see also notes above; inflammatory bowel disease, section 1.5; asthma, section 3.1 and section 3.2; immunosuppression, section 8.2.2; rheumatic disease, section 10.1.2; eye, section 11.4.1; ear, section 12.1.1

**Cautions** see notes above

**Contra-indications** see notes above

**Side-effects** see notes above

**Dose**

• By mouth, initially, up to 10–20 mg daily (severe disease, up to 60 mg daily), preferably taken in the morning after breakfast; can often be reduced within a few days but may need to be continued for several weeks or months

Maintenance, usual range, 2.5–15 mg daily, but higher doses may be needed; cushingoid side-effects increasingly likely with doses above 7.5 mg daily

6

Endocrine system

- By intramuscular injection, prednisolone acetate (section 10.1.2.2), 25–100 mg once or twice weekly

**Prednisolone** (Non-proprietary) PoM

Tablets, prednisolone 1 mg, net price 28-tab pack = 87p; 5 mg, 28-tab pack = £1.00; 25 mg, 56-tab pack = £20.00. Label: 10, steroid card, 21

Tablets, both e/c, prednisolone 2.5 mg (brown), net price 30-tab pack = £4.67; 5 mg (red), 30-tab pack = £4.73. Label: 5, 10, steroid card, 25
Brands include *Deltacortril Enteric*®

Soluble tablets, prednisolone 5 mg (as sodium phosphate), net price 30-tab pack = £7.45. Label: 10, steroid card, 13, 21

Injection, see section 10.1.2.2

## TRIAMCINOLONE

**Indications** suppression of inflammatory and allergic disorders; see also notes above; rheumatic disease, section 10.1.2; mouth, section 12.3.1; skin, section 13.4

**Cautions** see notes above; also high dosage may cause proximal myopathy, avoid in chronic therapy

**Contra-indications** see notes above

**Side-effects** see notes above

**Dose**

- By deep intramuscular injection, into gluteal muscle, 40 mg of acetonide for depot effect, repeated at intervals according to the patient's response; max. single dose 100 mg

**Kenalog**® **Intra-articular/Intramuscular** (Squibb) PoM

Injection (aqueous suspension), triamcinolone acetonide 40 mg/mL, net price 1-mL vial = £1.52; 1-mL prefilled syringe = £1.88. Label: 10, steroid card
**Note** Intramuscular needle with prefilled syringe should be replaced for intra-articular injection

# 6.4 Sex hormones

**6.4.1 Female sex hormones**
**6.4.2 Male sex hormones and antagonists**
**6.4.3 Anabolic steroids**

# 6.4.1 Female sex hormones

**6.4.1.1 Oestrogens and HRT**
**6.4.1.2 Progestogens**

## 6.4.1.1 Oestrogens and HRT

Oestrogens are necessary for the development of female secondary sexual characteristics; they also stimulate myometrial hypertrophy with endometrial hyperplasia.

In terms of oestrogenic activity *natural oestrogens* (estradiol (oestradiol), estrone (oestrone), and estriol (oestriol)) have a more appropriate profile for hormone replacement therapy (HRT) than *synthetic oestrogens* (ethinylestradiol (ethinyloestradiol) and mestranol). Tibolone has oestrogenic, progestogenic and weak androgenic activity.

Oestrogen therapy is given cyclically or continuously for a number of gynaecological conditions. If long-term therapy is required in women with a uterus, a progestogen should normally be added to reduce the risk of cystic hyperplasia of the endometrium (or of endometriotic foci in women who have had a hysterectomy) and possible transformation to cancer.

Oestrogens are no longer used to suppress lactation because of their association with thromboembolism.

## Hormone replacement therapy

Hormone replacement therapy (HRT) with small doses of an oestrogen (together with a progestogen in women with a uterus) is appropriate for alleviating menopausal symptoms such as vaginal atrophy or vasomotor instability. Oestrogen given systemically in the perimenopausal and postmenopausal period or tibolone given in the postmenopausal period also diminish postmenopausal osteoporosis (section 6.6.1) but other drugs (section 6.6) are preferred. Menopausal atrophic vaginitis may respond to a short course of a topical vaginal oestrogen preparation (section 7.2.1) used for a few weeks and repeated if necessary.

Systemic therapy with an oestrogen or drugs with oestrogenic properties alleviates the symptoms of oestrogen deficiency such as vasomotor symptoms. Tibolone combines oestrogenic and progestogenic activity with weak androgenic activity; it is given continuously, without cyclical progestogen.

HRT may be used in women with early natural or surgical menopause (before age 45 years), since they are at high risk of osteoporosis. For early menopause, HRT can be given until the approximate age of natural menopause (i.e. until age 50 years). Alternatives to HRT should be considered if osteoporosis is the main concern (section 6.6).

Clonidine (section 2.5.2 and section 4.7.4.2) may be used to reduce vasomotor symptoms in women who cannot take an oestrogen, but clonidine may cause unacceptable side-effects.

HRT increases the risk of venous thromboembolism, stroke, endometrial cancer (reduced by a progestogen), breast cancer, and ovarian cancer; there is an increased risk of coronary heart disease in women who start combined HRT more than 10 years after menopause. For details of these risks see HRT Risk table below.

The CSM advises that the minimum effective dose of HRT should be used for the shortest duration. Treatment should be reviewed at least annually and for osteoporosis alternative treatments considered (section 6.6). HRT does not prevent coronary heart disease or protect against a decline in cognitive function and it should **not** be prescribed for these purposes. Experience of treating women over 65 years with HRT is limited.

For the treatment of menopausal symptoms the benefits of short-term HRT outweigh the risks in the majority of women, especially in those aged under 60 years.

**Risk of breast cancer** The CSM has estimated that using *all* types of HRT, including tibolone, increases the risk of breast cancer within 1–2 years of initiating treatment, see HRT Risk table below for details. The increased risk is related to the duration of HRT use (but not to the age at which HRT is started) and this excess risk disappears within 5 years of stopping.

Radiological detection of breast cancer can be made more difficult as mammographic density can increase with HRT use; tibolone has only a limited effect on mammographic density.

**Risk of endometrial cancer** The increased risk of endometrial cancer depends on the dose and duration of oestrogen-only HRT, see HRT Risk table below for details.

In women with a uterus, the addition of a progestogen cyclically (for at least 10 days per 28-day cycle) reduces the additional risk of endometrial cancer; this additional risk is eliminated if a progestogen is given continuously. However, this should be weighed against the increased risk of breast cancer.

**Risk of ovarian cancer** Long-term use of combined HRT or oestrogen-only HRT is associated with a small increased risk of ovarian cancer, see HRT Risk table below for details; this excess risk disappears within a few years of stopping.

**Risk of venous thromboembolism** Women using combined or oestrogen-only HRT are at an increased

risk of deep vein thrombosis and of pulmonary embolism especially in the first year of use, see HRT Risk table below for details.

In *women who have predisposing factors* (such as a personal or family history of deep vein thrombosis or pulmonary embolism, severe varicose veins, obesity, trauma, or prolonged bed-rest) it may be prudent to review the need for HRT as in some cases the risks of HRT may exceed the benefits. See below for advice on surgery.

*Travel* involving prolonged immobility further increases the risk of deep vein thrombosis, see under Travel in section 7.3.1.

**Risk of stroke** Risk of stroke increases with age, therefore older women have a greater absolute risk of stroke. Combined HRT or oestrogen-only HRT slightly increases the risk of *stroke*, see HRT Risk table below for details.

**Risk of coronary heart disease** HRT does not prevent *coronary heart disease* and should not be prescribed for this purpose. There is an increased risk of coronary heart disease in women who start combined

## HRT Risk Table

| Risk | Age range (years) | Background incidence per 1000 women in Europe not using HRT | | **Additional** cases per 1000 women using **oestrogen only HRT** (estimated) | | **Additional** cases per 1000 women using **combined (oestrogen-progestogen) HRT** (estimated) | |
|---|---|---|---|---|---|---|---|
| | | Over 5 years | Over 10 years | For 5 years use | For 10 years use | For 5 years use | For 10 years use |
| Breast cancer[1] | 50–59 | 10 | 20 | 2 | 6 | 6 | 24 |
| | 60–69 | 15 | 30 | 3 | 9 | 9 | 36 |
| Endometrial cancer[2,3] | 50–59 | 2 | 4 | 4 | 32 | NS | NS |
| | 60–69 | 3 | 6 | 6 | 48 | NS | NS |
| Ovarian cancer | 50–59 | 2 | 4 | <1 | 1 | <1 | 1 |
| | 60–69 | 3 | 6 | <1 | 2 | <1 | 2 |
| Venous thromboembolism[4,5] | 50–59 | 5 | | 2 | | 7 | |
| | 60–69 | 8 | | 2 | | 10 | |
| Stroke[6] | 50–59 | 4 | | 1 | | 1 | |
| | 60–69 | 9 | | 3 | | 3 | |
| Coronary heart disease[7,8] | 70–79 | 29–44 | | NS | | 15 | |

**Note** Where background incidence or additional cases have not been included in the table, this indicates a lack of available data. NS indicates a non-significant difference.
Taken from MHRA/CHM (*Drug Safety Update* 2007; **1** (2): 2–6) available at www.mhra.gov.uk/mhra/drugsafetyupdate

1. Tibolone increases the risk of breast cancer but to a lesser extent than with combined HRT.
2. Evidence suggests an increased risk of endometrial cancer with tibolone. After 2.7 years of use (in women of average age 68 years), 1 extra case of endometrial hyperplasia and 4 extra cases of endometrial cancer were diagnosed compared with placebo users.
3. The risk of endometrial cancer cannot be reliably estimated in those using combined HRT because the addition of progestogen for at least 10 days per 28-day cycle greatly reduces the additional risk, and addition of a daily progestogen eliminates the additional risk. The risk of endometrial cancer in women who have not used HRT increases with body mass index (BMI); the increased risk of endometrial cancer in users of oestrogen-only HRT or tibolone is more apparent in women who are not overweight.
4. Limited data does not suggest an increased risk of thromboembolism with tibolone compared to combined HRT or women not taking HRT.
5. Although the level of risk of thromboembolism associated with non-oral routes of administration of HRT has not been established, it may be lower for the transdermal route.
6. Tibolone use increases the risk of stroke about 2.2 times from the first year of treatment; risk of stroke is age-dependent and therefore the absolute risk of stroke with tibolone increases with age.
7. Increased risk of coronary heart disease in women who start combined HRT more than 10 years after menopause.
8. There is insufficient data to draw a conclusion on the risk of coronary heart disease with tibolone.

**6**

**Endocrine system**

HRT more than 10 years after menopause, see HRT Risk table below for details. Although very little information is available on the risk of coronary heart disease in younger women who start HRT close to the menopause, studies suggest a lower relative risk compared with older women.

**Choice** The choice of HRT for an individual depends on an overall balance of indication, risk, and convenience. A woman with a uterus normally requires oestrogen with cyclical progestogen for the last 12 to 14 days of the cycle *or* a preparation which involves continuous administration of an oestrogen and a progestogen (*or* one which provides both oestrogenic and progestogenic activity in a single preparation). Continuous combined preparations or tibolone are **not suitable** for use in the perimenopause or within 12 months of the last menstrual period; women who use such preparations may bleed irregularly in the early stages of treatment—if bleeding continues endometrial abnormality should be ruled out and consideration given to changing to cyclical HRT.

An oestrogen alone is suitable for continuous use in women without a uterus. However, in endometriosis, endometrial foci may remain despite hysterectomy and the addition of a progestogen should be considered in these circumstances.

An oestrogen may be given by mouth or it may be given by subcutaneous or transdermal administration, which avoids first-pass metabolism. In the case of subcutaneous implants, recurrence of vasomotor symptoms at supraphysiological plasma concentrations may occur; moreover, there is evidence of prolonged endometrial stimulation after discontinuation (calling for continued cyclical progestogen). For the use of topical HRT preparations see section 7.2.1.

**Contraception** HRT does **not** provide contraception and a woman is considered potentially fertile for 2 years after her last menstrual period if she is under 50 years, and for 1 year if she is over 50 years. A woman who is under 50 years and free of all risk factors for venous and arterial disease can use a low-oestrogen combined oral contraceptive pill (section 7.3.1) to provide both relief of menopausal symptoms and contraception; it is recommended that the oral contraceptive be stopped at 50 years of age since there are more suitable alternatives. If any potentially fertile woman needs HRT, non-hormonal contraceptive measures (such as condoms) are necessary.

Measurement of follicle-stimulating hormone can help to determine fertility, but high measurements alone (particularly in women aged under 50 years) do not necessarily preclude the possibility of becoming pregnant.

**Surgery** Major surgery under general anaesthesia, including orthopaedic and vascular leg surgery, is a predisposing factor for venous thromboembolism and it may be prudent to stop HRT 4–6 weeks before surgery (see Risk of Venous Thromboembolism, above); it should be restarted only after full mobilisation. If HRT is continued or if discontinuation is not possible (e.g. in non-elective surgery), prophylaxis with heparin and graduated compression hosiery is advised. Oestrogenic activity may persist after removing an estradiol implant (see above).

**Reasons to stop HRT** For circumstances in which HRT should be stopped, see p. 446.

## OESTROGENS FOR HRT

**Note** Relates only to small amounts of oestrogens given for hormone replacement therapy

**Indications** see notes above and under preparations

**Cautions** prolonged exposure to unopposed oestrogens may increase risk of developing endometrial cancer (see notes above); migraine (or migraine-like headaches); diabetes (increased risk of heart disease); history of breast nodules or fibrocystic disease—closely monitor breast status (risk of breast cancer, see notes above); risk factors for oestrogen-dependent tumours (e.g. breast cancer in first-degree relative); uterine fibroids may increase in size, symptoms of endometriosis may be exacerbated; factors predisposing to thromboembolism (see notes above); presence of antiphospholipid antibodies (increased risk of thrombotic events); increased risk of gall-bladder disease reported; hypophyseal tumours; acute porphyria (see section 9.8.2); **interactions:** Appendix 1 (oestrogens)

**Other conditions** The product literature advises caution in other conditions including hypertension, renal disease, asthma, epilepsy, sickle-cell disease, melanoma, otosclerosis, multiple sclerosis, and systemic lupus erythematosus (but care required if antiphospholipid antibodies present, see above). Evidence for caution in these conditions is unsatisfactory and many women with these conditions may stand to benefit from HRT.

**Contra-indications** pregnancy; oestrogen-dependent cancer, history of breast cancer, active thrombophlebitis, active or recent arterial thromboembolic disease (e.g. angina or myocardial infarction), venous thromboembolism, or history of recurrent venous thromboembolism (unless already on anticoagulant treatment), liver disease (where liver function tests have failed to return to normal), Dubin-Johnson and Rotor syndromes (or monitor closely), untreated endometrial hyperplasia, undiagnosed vaginal bleeding, breast-feeding

**Side-effects** see notes above for risks of long-term use; nausea and vomiting, abdominal cramps and bloating, weight changes, breast enlargement and tenderness, premenstrual-like syndrome, sodium and fluid retention, cholestatic jaundice, glucose intolerance, altered blood lipids—may lead to pancreatitis, rashes and chloasma, changes in libido, depression, mood changes, headache, migraine, dizziness, leg cramps (rule out venous thrombosis), vaginal candidiasis, contact lenses may irritate; transdermal delivery systems may cause contact sensitisation (possible severe hypersensitivity reaction on continued exposure), and headache has been reported on vigorous exercise

**Withdrawal bleeding** Cyclical HRT (where a progestogen is taken for 12–14 days of each 28-day oestrogen treatment cycle) usually results in *regular withdrawal bleeding* towards the end of the progestogen. The aim of continuous combined HRT (where a combination of oestrogen and progestogen is taken, usually in a single tablet, throughout each 28-day treatment cycle) is to avoid bleeding, but *irregular bleeding* may occur during the early treatment stages (if it continues endometrial abnormality should be excluded and consideration given to cyclical HRT instead)

**Dose**

* See under preparations

**Counselling on patches** Patch should be removed after 3–4 days (or once a week in case of 7-day patch) and replaced with fresh patch on slightly different site; recommended sites: clean, dry, unbroken areas of skin on trunk below waistline; not to be applied on or near breasts or under waistband. If patch falls off in bath allow skin to cool before applying new patch

◀ **Conjugated oestrogens with progestogen**

**Premique®** (Wyeth) [PoM]

Premique® Low Dose tablets, s/c, ivory, conjugated oestrogen (equine) 300 micrograms and medroxy-progesterone acetate 1.5 mg, net price 3 × 28-tab pack = £6.52

**Dose** menopausal symptoms in women with a uterus, 1 tablet daily continuously

Premique® tablets, s/c, blue, conjugated oestrogen (equine) 625 micrograms and medroxyprogesterone acetate 5 mg. Net price 3 × 28-tab pack = £10.61

**Dose** menopausal symptoms and osteoporosis prophylaxis (see section 6.6), in women with a uterus, 1 tablet daily continuously (starting on day 1 of menstruation if cycles have not ceased)

Premique® Cycle Calendar pack, all s/c, 14 white tablets, conjugated oestrogens (equine) 625 micrograms; 14 green tablets, conjugated oestrogens (equine) 625 micrograms and medroxyprogesterone acetate 10 mg, net price 3 × 28-tab pack = £8.05

**Dose** menopausal symptoms and osteoporosis prophylaxis (see section 6.6), 1 white tablet daily for 14 days, starting on day 1 of menstruation (or at any time if cycles have ceased or are infrequent) then 1 green tablet daily for 14 days; subsequent courses are repeated without interval

**Prempak-C®** (Wyeth) [PoM]

Prempak C® 0.625 Calendar pack, s/c, 28 maroon tablets, conjugated oestrogens (equine) 625 micrograms; 12 light brown tablets, norgestrel 150 micrograms (≡ levonorgestrel 75 micrograms). Net price 3 × 40-tab pack = £6.25

**Dose** menopausal symptoms and osteoporosis prophylaxis (see section 6.6), in women with a uterus, 1 maroon tablet daily continuously, starting on day 1 of menstruation (or at any time if cycles have ceased or are infrequent), and 1 brown tablet daily on days 17–28 of each 28-day treatment cycle; subsequent courses are repeated without interval

Prempak C® 1.25 Calendar pack, s/c, 28 yellow tablets, conjugated oestrogens (equine) 1.25 mg; 12 light brown tablets, norgestrel 150 micrograms (≡ levonorgestrel 75 micrograms). Net price 3 × 40-tab pack = £7.40

**Dose** see under 0.625 Calendar pack, but taking 1 yellow tablet daily continuously (instead of 1 maroon tablet) if symptoms not fully controlled with lower strength

◀ **Estradiol with progestogen**

**Angeliq®** (Schering Health) [PoM]

Tablets, f/c, red, estradiol 1 mg, drospirenone 2 mg. Net price 3 × 28-tab pack = £24.79

**Dose** menopausal symptoms and osteoporosis prophylaxis (see section 6.6), in women with a uterus, 1 tablet daily continuously (if changing from cyclical HRT begin treatment the day after finishing oestrogen plus progestogen phase)

**Cautions** use with care if an increased concentration of potassium might be hazardous; renal impairment (Appendix 3)

**Note** Unsuitable for use in perimenopausal women or within 12 months of last menstrual period—see choice above

**Climagest®** (Novartis) [PoM]

Climagest® 1-mg tablets, 16 grey-blue, estradiol valerate 1 mg; 12 white, estradiol valerate 1 mg and norethisterone 1 mg. Net price 28-tab pack = £5.74; 3 × 28-tab pack = £16.69

**Dose** menopausal symptoms, 1 grey-blue tablet daily for 16 days, starting on day 1 of menstruation (or at any time if cycles have ceased or are infrequent) then 1 white tablet for 12 days; subsequent courses are repeated without interval

Climagest® 2-mg tablets, 16 blue, estradiol valerate 2 mg; 12 yellow, estradiol valerate 2 mg and norethi-

sterone 1 mg. Net price 28-tab pack = £5.74; 3 × 28-tab pack = £16.69

**Dose** see *Climagest® 1-mg*, but starting with 1 blue tablet daily (instead of 1 grey-blue tablet) if symptoms not controlled with lower strength

**Climesse®** (Novartis) [PoM]

Tablets, pink, estradiol valerate 2 mg, norethisterone 700 micrograms. Net price 1 × 28-tab pack = £10.34; 3 × 28-tab pack = £31.03

**Dose** menopausal symptoms and osteoporosis prophylaxis (see section 6.6), in women with a uterus, 1 tablet daily continuously

**Note** Unsuitable for use in perimenopausal women or within 12 months of last menstrual period—see Choice above

**Clinorette®** (ReSource Medical) [PoM]

Tablets, f/c, 16 white, estradiol 2 mg; 12 pink, estradiol 2 mg and norethisterone 1 mg, net price 3 × 28-tab pack = £9.23

**Dose** menopausal symptoms, in women with a uterus, 1 white tablet daily for 16 days starting on day 5 of menstruation (or at any time if cycles have ceased or are infrequent), then 1 pink tablet daily for 12 days; subsequent courses repeated without interval

**Cyclo-Progynova®** (Viatris) [PoM]

Cyclo-Progynova® 2-mg tablets, all s/c, 11 white, estradiol valerate 2 mg; 10 brown, estradiol valerate 2 mg and norgestrel 500 micrograms (≡ levonorgestrel 250 micrograms). Net price per pack = £3.11

**Dose** menopausal symptoms and osteoporosis prophylaxis (see section 6.6), in women with a uterus, 1 white tablet daily for 11 days, starting on day 5 of menstruation (or at any time if cycles have ceased or are infrequent), then 1 brown tablet daily for 10 days, followed by a 7-day tablet-free interval

**Elleste-Duet®** (Meda) [PoM]

Elleste-Duet® 1-mg tablets, 16 white, estradiol 1 mg; 12 green, estradiol 1 mg and norethisterone acetate 1 mg. Net price 3 × 28-tab pack = £9.72

**Dose** menopausal symptoms, 1 white tablet daily for 16 days starting on day 1 of menstruation (or at any time if cycles have ceased or are infrequent), then 1 green tablet daily for 12 days; subsequent courses are repeated without interval

Elleste-Duet® 2-mg tablets, 16 orange, estradiol 2 mg; 12 grey, estradiol 2 mg, norethisterone acetate 1 mg. Net price 3 × 28-tab pack = £9.72

**Dose** menopausal symptoms and osteoporosis prophylaxis (see section 6.6), 1 orange tablet daily for 16 days, starting on day 1 of menstruation (or at any time if cycles have ceased or are infrequent) then 1 grey tablet daily for 12 days; subsequent courses are repeated without interval

Elleste-Duet Conti® tablets, f/c, grey, estradiol 2 mg, norethisterone acetate 1 mg. Net price 3 × 28-tab pack = £16.17

**Dose** menopausal symptoms and osteoporosis prophylaxis (see section 6.6), in women with a uterus, 1 tablet daily on a continuous basis (if changing from cyclical HRT begin treatment at the end of scheduled bleed)

**Note** Unsuitable for use in perimenopausal women or within 12 months of last menstrual period—see Choice above

**Evorel®** (Janssen-Cilag) [PoM]

Evorel® Conti patches, self-adhesive, (releasing estradiol approx. 50 micrograms/24 hours and norethisterone acetate approx. 170 micrograms/ 24 hours), net price 8-patch pack = £11.53, 24-patch pack = £34.59. Counselling, administration

**Dose** menopausal symptoms and osteoporosis prophylaxis (see section 6.6), in women with a uterus, 1 patch to be applied twice weekly continuously

Evorel® Sequi combination pack, 4 self-adhesive patches of *Evorel® 50* (releasing estradiol approx. 50 micrograms/24 hours) and 4 self-adhesive patches of *Evorel® Conti* (releasing estradiol approx. 50 micrograms/24 hours and norethisterone acetate approx.

**6**

**Endocrine system**

170 micrograms/24 hours), net price 8-patch pack = £9.83. Counselling, administration

**Dose** menopausal symptoms and osteoporosis prophylaxis (see section 6.6), in women with a uterus, 1 *Evorel® 50* patch to be applied twice weekly for 2 weeks followed by 1 *Evorel® Conti* patch twice weekly for 2 weeks; subsequent courses are repeated without interval

### Femapak® (Solvay) [PoM]

Femapak® 40 combination pack of 8 self-adhesive patches of *Fematrix® 40* (releasing estradiol approx. 40 micrograms/24 hours) and 14 tablets of dydrogesterone 10 mg. Net price per pack = £7.61. Counselling, administration

**Dose** see under *Femapak® 80*

Femapak® 80 combination pack of 8 self-adhesive patches of *Fematrix® 80* (releasing estradiol approx. 80 micrograms/24 hours) and 14 tablets of dydrogesterone 10 mg. Net price per pack = £8.06. Counselling, administration

**Dose** menopausal symptoms (and osteoporosis prophylaxis (see section 6.6) in case of *Femapak® 80* **only**), in women with a uterus, starting within 5 days of onset of menstruation (or any time if cycles have ceased or are infrequent), apply 1 patch twice weekly continuously and take 1 tablet daily on days 15–28 of each 28-day treatment cycle; therapy should be initiated with *Femapak® 40* in those with menopausal symptoms, prolonged oestrogen deficiency or anticipated intolerance to higher strengths, subsequently adjusted to lowest effective dose

### Femoston® (Solvay) [PoM]

Femoston® 1/10 tablets, both f/c, 14 white, estradiol 1 mg; 14 grey, estradiol 1 mg, dydrogesterone 10 mg. Net price 3 × 28-tab pack = £13.47

**Dose** menopausal symptoms and osteoporosis prophylaxis (see section 6.6), in women with a uterus, 1 white tablet daily for 14 days, starting within 5 days of onset of menstruation (or any time if cycles have ceased or are infrequent) then 1 grey tablet for 14 days; subsequent courses repeated without interval

Femoston® 2/10 tablets, both f/c, 14 red, estradiol 2 mg; 14 yellow, estradiol 2 mg, dydrogesterone 10 mg. Net price 3 × 28-tab pack = £13.47

**Dose** menopausal symptoms and osteoporosis prophylaxis (see section 6.6), in women with a uterus, 1 red tablet daily for 14 days, starting within 5 days of onset of menstruation (or any time if cycles have ceased or are infrequent) then 1 yellow tablet daily for 14 days; subsequent courses repeated without interval; where therapy required for menopausal symptoms alone, *Femoston® 1/10* given initially and *Femoston® 2/10* substituted if symptoms not controlled

Femoston®-conti tablets, f/c, salmon, estradiol 1 mg, dydrogesterone 5 mg, net price 3 × 28-tab pack = £22.44

**Dose** menopausal symptoms and osteoporosis prophylaxis (see section 6.6), in women with a uterus, 1 tablet daily continuously (if changing from cyclical HRT begin treatment the day after finishing oestrogen plus progestogen phase)

**Note** Unsuitable for use in perimenopausal women or within 12 months of last menstrual period—see Choice above

### FemSeven® Conti (Merck) [PoM]

Patches, self-adhesive (releasing estradiol approx. 50 micrograms/24 hours and levonorgestrel approx. 7 micrograms/24 hours); net price 4-patch pack = £15.48, 12-patch pack = £ 44.12. Counselling, administration

**Dose** menopausal symptoms in women with a uterus, 1 patch to be applied once a week continuously

**Note** Unsuitable for use in perimenopausal women or within 12 months of last menstrual period—see Choice above

### FemSeven® Sequi (Merck) [PoM]

Combination pack, self-adhesive patches of *FemSeven® Sequi Phase 1* (releasing estradiol approx. 50 micrograms/24 hours) and of *FemSeven® Sequi Phase 2* (releasing estradiol approx. 50 micrograms/

24 hours and levonorgestrel approx. 10 micrograms/24 hours); net price 1-month pack (2 of each) = £13.18, 3-month pack (6 of each) = £37.54. Counselling, administration

**Dose** menopausal symptoms in women with a uterus, 1 *Phase 1* patch applied once a week for 2 weeks followed by 1 *Phase 2* patch once a week for 2 weeks; subsequent courses are repeated without interval

### Indivina® (Orion) [PoM]

Indivina® 1 mg/2.5 mg tablets, estradiol valerate 1 mg, medroxyprogesterone acetate 2.5 mg, net price 3 × 28-tab pack = £20.89

Indivina® 1 mg/5 mg tablets, estradiol valerate 1 mg, medroxyprogesterone acetate 5 mg, net price 3 × 28-tab pack = £20.89

Indivina® 2 mg/5 mg tablets, estradiol valerate 2 mg, medroxyprogesterone acetate 5 mg, net price 3 × 28-tab pack = £20.89

**Dose** menopausal symptoms and osteoporosis prophylaxis (see section 6.6), in women with a uterus, 1 tablet daily continuously; initiate therapy with *Indivina® 1 mg/2.5 mg* tablets and adjust according to response; start at end of scheduled bleed if changing from cyclical HRT

**Note** Less suitable for use in perimenopausal women or within 3 years of last menstrual period—see Choice above

### Kliofem® (Novo Nordisk) [PoM]

Tablets, f/c yellow, estradiol 2 mg, norethisterone acetate 1 mg. Net price 3 × 28-tab pack = £11.43

**Dose** menopausal symptoms and osteoporosis prophylaxis (see section 6.6), in women with a uterus, 1 tablet daily continuously; start at end of scheduled bleed if changing from cyclical HRT

**Note** Unsuitable for use in perimenopausal women or within 12 months of last menstrual period—see Choice above

### Kliovance® (Novo Nordisk) [PoM]

Tablets, f/c, estradiol 1 mg, norethisterone acetate 500 micrograms, net price 3 × 28-tab pack = £13.20

**Dose** menopausal symptoms and osteoporosis prophylaxis (see section 6.6), in women with a uterus, 1 tablet daily continuously; start at end of scheduled bleed if changing from cyclical HRT

**Note** Unsuitable for use in perimenopausal women or within 12 months of last menstrual period—see Choice above

### Novofem® (Novo Nordisk) [PoM]

Tablets, f/c, 16 red, estradiol 1 mg; 12 white, estradiol 1 mg, norethisterone acetate 1 mg, net price 3 × 28-tab pack = £13.50

**Dose** menopausal symptoms and osteoporosis prophylaxis (see section 6.6), in women with a uterus, 1 red tablet daily for 16 days then 1 white tablet daily for 12 days; subsequent courses are repeated without interval; start treatment with red tablet at any time or if changing from cyclical HRT, start treatment the day after finishing oestrogen plus progestogen phase

### Nuvelle® (Schering Health) [PoM]

Nuvelle® tablets, all s/c, 16 white, estradiol valerate 2 mg; 12 pink, estradiol valerate 2 mg and levonorgestrel 75 micrograms. Net price 3 × 28-tab pack = £12.37

**Dose** menopausal symptoms and osteoporosis prophylaxis (see section 6.6), in women with a uterus, 1 white tablet daily for 16 days, starting on day 1 of menstruation (or any time if cycles have ceased or are infrequent) then 1 pink tablet daily for 12 days; subsequent courses are repeated without interval

Nuvelle® Continuous tablets, f/c, pink, estradiol 2 mg, norethisterone acetate 1 mg, net price 3 × 28-tab pack = £16.19

**Dose** menopausal symptoms and osteoporosis prophylaxis (see section 6.6), in women with a uterus, 1 tablet daily continuously; start at end of scheduled bleed if changing from cyclical HRT

**Note** Unsuitable for use in perimenopausal women or within 12 months of last menstrual period—see Choice above

**Tridestra®** (Orion) [PoM]

Tablets, 70 white, estradiol valerate 2 mg; 14 blue, estradiol valerate 2 mg and medroxyprogesterone acetate 20 mg; 7 yellow, inactive. Net price 91-tab pack = £20.80

Dose menopausal symptoms and osteoporosis prophylaxis (see section 6.6), in women with a uterus, 1 white tablet daily for 70 days, then 1 blue tablet daily for 14 days, then 1 yellow tablet daily for 7 days; subsequent courses are repeated without interval

**Trisequens®** (Novo Nordisk) [PoM]

Tablets, 12 blue, estradiol 2 mg; 10 white, estradiol 2 mg, norethisterone acetate 1 mg; 6 red, estradiol 1 mg, net price 3 × 28-tab pack = £11.10

Dose menopausal symptoms and osteoporosis prophylaxis (see section 6.6), in women with a uterus, 1 blue tablet daily, starting on day 5 of menstruation (or at any time if cycles have ceased or are infrequent), then 1 tablet daily in sequence (without interruption)

◀**Conjugated oestrogens only**

**Premarin®** (Wyeth) [PoM]

Tablets, all s/c, conjugated oestrogens (equine) 300 micrograms (green) net price 3 × 28-tab pack = £6.07; 625 micrograms (maroon), 3 × 28-tab pack = £4.02; 1.25 mg (yellow), 3 × 28-tab pack = £3.58

Dose menopausal symptoms, 0.3–1.25 mg daily continuously; osteoporosis prophylaxis (see section 6.6), 0.625–1.25 mg daily continuously; with cyclical progestogen for 12–14 days of each cycle in women with a uterus

◀**Estradiol only**

**Estradiol Implants** (Organon) [PoM]

Implant, estradiol 25 mg, net price each = £12.95; 50 mg, each = £21.08

Dose by implantation, oestrogen replacement, and osteoporosis prophylaxis (see section 6.6) (with cyclical progestogen for 12–14 days of each cycle in women with a uterus, see notes above), 25–100 mg as required (usually every 4–8 months) according to oestrogen levels—check before each implant

Note On cessation of treatment or if implants are removed from those with a uterus, cyclical progestogen should be continued until withdrawal bleed stops

**Bedol®** (ReSource Medical) [PoM]

Tablets, f/c, estradiol 2 mg, net price 3 × 28-tab pack = £5.07

Dose menopausal symptoms, with cyclical progestogen for 12–14 days of each cycle in women with a uterus, 2 mg daily starting on day 1–5 of menstruation (or at any time if cycles have ceased or are infrequent)

**Climaval®** (Novartis) [PoM]

Tablets, estradiol valerate 1 mg (grey-blue), net price 1 × 28-tab pack = £3.06, 3 × 28-tab pack = £9.19; 2 mg (blue), 1 × 28-tab pack = £3.06, 3 × 28-tab pack = £9.19

Dose menopausal symptoms (if patient has had a hysterectomy), 1–2 mg daily

**Elleste-Solo®** (Meda) [PoM]

Elleste-Solo® 1-mg tablets, estradiol 1 mg. Net price 3 × 28-tab pack = £5.07

Dose menopausal symptoms, with cyclical progestogen for 12–14 days of each cycle in women with a uterus, 1 mg daily starting on day 1 of menstruation (or at any time if cycles have ceased or are infrequent)

Elleste-Solo® 2-mg tablets, orange, estradiol 2 mg. Net price 3 × 28-tab pack = £5.07

Dose menopausal symptoms not controlled with lower strength and osteoporosis prophylaxis (see section 6.6), with cyclical progestogen for 12–14 days of each cycle in women with a uterus, 2 mg daily starting on day 1 of menstruation (or at any time if cycles have ceased or are infrequent)

**Elleste Solo® MX** (Meda) [PoM]

Patches, self-adhesive, estradiol, MX 40 patch (releasing approx. 40 micrograms/24 hours), net price 8-patch pack = £4.93; MX 80 patch (releasing approx.

80 micrograms/24 hours), 8-patch pack = £5.69. Counselling, administration.

Dose menopausal symptoms (and osteoporosis prophylaxis in case of Elleste Solo MX 80® only; see section 6.6), 1 patch to be applied twice weekly continuously starting within 5 days of onset of menstruation (or at any time if cycles have ceased or are infrequent); with cyclical progestogen for 12–14 days of each cycle in women with a uterus; therapy should be initiated with MX 40 in those with menopausal symptoms, prolonged oestrogen deficiency or anticipated intolerance to higher strength, dosage may be increased if required, subsequently adjusted to lowest effective dose

**Estraderm MX®** (Novartis) [PoM]

Patches, self-adhesive, estradiol, MX 25 patch (releasing approx. 25 micrograms/24 hours), net price 8-patch pack = £5.72, 24-patch pack = £17.15; MX 50 patch (releasing approx. 50 micrograms/24 hours), 8-patch pack = £5.74, 24-patch pack = £17.15, 20-patch pack (hosp. only) = £13.04; MX 75 patch (releasing approx. 75 micrograms/24 hours), 8-patch pack = £6.69, 24-patch pack = £20.08; MX 100 patch (releasing approx. 100 micrograms/24 hours), 8-patch pack = £6.94, 24-patch pack = £20.83. Counselling, administration

Dose menopausal symptoms (and osteoporosis prophylaxis in case of Estraderm MX® 50 and 75 only; see section 6.6), 1 patch to be applied twice weekly continuously, with cyclical progestogen for 12 days of each cycle in women with a uterus; therapy should be initiated with MX 50 for first month, subsequently adjusted to lowest effective dose

**Estraderm TTS®** (Novartis) [PoM]

Patches, self-adhesive, estradiol, TTS 25 patch (releasing approx. 25 micrograms/24 hours), net price, 8-patch pack = £7.45, 24-patch pack = £22.36; TTS 100 patch (releasing approx. 100 micrograms/24 hours), 8-patch pack = £9.02, 24-patch pack = £27.16, 20-patch pack (hosp. only) = £16.76. Counselling, administration

Dose menopausal symptoms, 1 patch to be applied twice weekly continuously, with cyclical progestogen for 12 days of each cycle in women with a uterus; therapy should be initiated with TTS 25 for first 3 months, subsequently adjusted to lowest effective dose

**Estradot®** (Novartis) [PoM]

Patches, self-adhesive, estradiol, '25' patch (releasing approx. 25 micrograms/24 hours), net price 8-patch pack = £5.20; '37.5' patch (releasing approx. 37.5 micrograms/24 hours), 8-patch pack = £5.21; '50' patch (releasing approx. 50 micrograms/24 hours), 8-patch pack = £5.22; '75' patch (releasing approx. 75 micrograms/24 hours), 8-patch pack = £6.08; '100' patch (releasing approx. 100 micrograms/24 hours), 8-patch pack = £6.31. Counselling, administration

Dose menopausal symptoms (all strengths) and osteoporosis prophylaxis (Estradot® '50', '75', and '100' only; see section 6.6), 1 patch to be applied twice weekly continuously, with cyclical progestogen for 12 days of each cycle in women with a uterus; for osteoporosis prophylaxis therapy should be initiated with '50' patch

**Evorel®** (Janssen-Cilag) [PoM]

Patches, self-adhesive, estradiol, '25' patch (releasing approx. 25 micrograms/24 hours), net price 8-patch pack = £2.75; '50' patch (releasing approx. 50 micrograms/24 hours), 8-patch pack = £3.11, 24-patch pack = £9.34; '75' patch (releasing approx. 75 micrograms/24 hours), 8-patch pack = £3.31; '100' patch (releasing approx. 100 micrograms/24 hours), 8-patch pack = £3.43. Counselling, administration

Dose menopausal symptoms and osteoporosis prophylaxis (except Evorel® 25; see section 6.6), 1 patch to be applied twice weekly continuously, with cyclical progestogen for at least 12 days of each cycle in women with a uterus; therapy should be initiated with '50' patch for first month, subsequently adjusted to lowest effective dose

6

Endocrine system

**Fematrix®** (Solvay) PoM

Fematrix® 40 patch, self-adhesive, estradiol, *'40' patch* (releasing approx. 40 micrograms/24 hours). Net price 8-patch pack = £4.95. Counselling, administration

Dose menopausal symptoms, 1 patch to be applied twice weekly continuously starting within 5 days of onset of menstruation (or at any time if cycles have ceased or are infrequent), with cyclical progestogen for 12–14 days of each cycle in women with a uterus; *'80' patch* may be used if required (subsequently adjusted to lowest effective dose)

Fematrix® 80 patch, self-adhesive, estradiol (releasing approx. 80 micrograms/24 hours). Net price 8-patch pack = £5.40. Counselling, administration

Dose menopausal symptoms and osteoporosis prophylaxis (see section 6.6), as for *Fematrix® 40*; therapy should be initiated with *Fematrix® 40* in those with menopausal symptoms, prolonged oestrogen deficiency or anticipated intolerance to higher strength

**FemSeven®** (Merck) PoM

Patches, self-adhesive, estradiol, *'50' patch* (releasing approx. 50 micrograms/24 hours), net price 4-patch pack = £6.04, 12-patch pack = £18.02; *'75' patch* (releasing approx. 75 micrograms/24 hours), net price 4-patch pack = £6.98; *'100' patch* (releasing approx. 100 micrograms/24 hours), net price 4-patch pack = £7.28. Counselling, administration

Dose menopausal symptoms and osteoporosis prophylaxis (see section 6.6), 1 patch to be applied once a week continuously, with cyclical progestogen for at least 10 days of each cycle in women with a uterus; therapy should be initiated with *FemSeven® 50* patches for the first few months, subsequently adjusted according to response

**Oestrogel®** (Ferring) PoM

Gel, estradiol 0.06%, net price 64-dose pump pack = £4.80. Counselling, administration

Dose menopausal symptoms and osteoporosis prophylaxis (see section 6.6), 2 measures (estradiol 1.5 mg) to be applied over an area twice that of the template provided once daily continuously, starting within 5 days of menstruation (or anytime if cycles have ceased or are infrequent), with cyclical progestogen for 12 days of each cycle in women with a uterus; for menopausal symptoms may be increased if necessary after 1 month to max. 4 measures daily

Counselling Apply gel to clean, dry, intact skin such as arms, shoulders or inner thighs and allow to dry for 5 minutes before covering with clothing. Not to be applied on or near breasts or on vulval region. Avoid skin contact with another person (particularly male) and avoid other skin products or washing the area for at least 1 hour after application

**Progynova®** (Schering Health) PoM

Tablets, both s/c, estradiol valerate 1 mg (beige), net price 3 × 28-tab pack = £6.30; 2 mg (blue), 3 × 28-tab pack = £6.30

Dose menopausal symptoms, 1–2 mg daily continuously; osteoporosis prophylaxis (see section 6.6), 2 mg daily continuously; with cyclical progestogen for 12 days of each cycle in women with a uterus

**Progynova® TS** (Schering Health) PoM

Patches, self-adhesive, *Progynova® TS 50* (releasing estradiol approx. 50 micrograms/24 hours), net price 12-patch pack = £16.06; *Progynova® TS 100* (releasing estradiol approx. 100 micrograms/24 hours), 12-patch pack = £17.67. Counselling, administration

Dose menopausal symptoms and osteoporosis prophylaxis (*Progynova® TS 50* only; see section 6.6), 1 patch to be applied once a week continuously or 1 patch per week for 3 weeks followed by a 7-day patch-free interval (cyclical); with cyclical progestogen for 12–14 days of each cycle in women with a uterus; in those with menopausal symptoms, therapy should be initiated with *Progynova® TS 50*, dosage may be increased if required, subsequently adjusted to lowest effective dose

Note Women receiving *Progynova® TS 100* patches for menopausal symptoms may continue with this strength for osteoporosis prophylaxis (see section 6.6)

**Sandrena®** (Organon) PoM

Gel, estradiol (0.1%), 500 microgram/500 mg sachet, net price 28-sachet pack = £5.18, 1 mg/1 g sachet, 28-sachet pack = £5.96. Counselling, administration

Excipients include propylene glycol (see section 13.1.3)

Dose menopausal symptoms, estradiol 1 mg (1 g gel) to be applied once daily over area 1–2 times size of hand; with cyclical progestogen for 12–14 days of each cycle in women with a uterus; dose may be adjusted after 2–3 cycles to a usual dose of estradiol 0.5–1.5 mg (0.5–1.5 g gel) daily

Counselling Apply gel to intact areas of skin such as lower trunk or thighs, using right and left sides on alternate days. Wash hands after application. Not to be applied on the breasts or face and avoid contact with eyes. Allow area of application to dry for 5 minutes and do not wash area for at least 1 hour

**Zumenon®** (Solvay) PoM

Tablets, f/c, estradiol 1 mg, net price 84-tab pack = £6.89; 2 mg (red), 84-tab pack = £6.89

Dose menopausal symptoms, initially 1 mg daily starting on day 5 of menstruation (or any time if cycles have ceased or are infrequent) adjusted to 1–4 mg daily according to response; osteoporosis prophylaxis (see section 6.6), 2 mg daily; with cyclical progestogen for 10–14 days of each cycle in women with a uterus

◀**Estradiol, estriol and estrone**

**Hormonin®** (Amdipharm) PoM

Tablets, pink, estradiol 600 micrograms, estriol 270 micrograms, estrone 1.4 mg. Net price 84-tab pack = £6.94

Dose menopausal symptoms and osteoporosis prophylaxis (see section 6.6), 1–2 tablets daily, with cyclical progestogen for 12–14 days of each cycle in women with a uterus

Note *Hormonin®* tablets can be given continuously or cyclically (21 days out of 28)

◀**Estriol only**

**Ovestin®** (Organon) PoM

Tablets, scored, estriol 1 mg. Net price 30-tab pack = £3.91. Label: 25

Dose genito-urinary symptoms associated with oestrogen-deficiency states, 0.5–3 mg daily, as single dose, for up to 1 month, then 0.5–1 mg daily until restoration of epithelial integrity (short-term use); infertility due to poor cervical penetration, 0.25–1 mg daily on days 6–15 of cycle

◀**Estropipate only**

**Harmogen®** (Pharmacia) PoM

Tablets, peach, scored, estropipate 1.5 mg. Net price 28-tab pack = £3.77

Dose menopausal symptoms and osteoporosis prophylaxis (see section 6.6), 1.5 mg daily continuously (with cyclical progestogen for 10–13 days of each cycle in women with a uterus); up to 3 mg daily (in single or divided doses) for vasomotor symptoms and menopausal vaginitis

# ▮ TIBOLONE

**Indications** short-term treatment of symptoms of oestrogen deficiency (including women being treated with gonadotrophin releasing hormone analogues); osteoporosis prophylaxis in women at risk of fractures (second-line)

**Cautions** see notes above and under Oestrogens for HRT; vaginal bleeding (investigate for endometrial cancer if bleeding continues beyond 6 months or after stopping treatment); renal impairment, history of liver disease (Appendix 2), epilepsy, migraine, diabetes mellitus, hypercholesterolaemia; withdraw if signs of thromboembolic disease, abnormal liver function tests or cholestatic jaundice; see also Note below; interactions: Appendix 1 (tibolone)

**Contra-indications** see notes above and under Oestrogens for HRT; hormone-dependent tumours, history of cardiovascular or cerebrovascular disease (e.g. thrombophlebitis, thromboembolism), uninvestigated vaginal bleeding, severe liver disease, pregnancy, breast-feeding

**Side-effects** see notes above; also abdominal pain, weight changes, vaginal bleeding, leucorrhoea, facial hair, and *rarely* amnesia; gastro-intestinal disturbances, oedema, dizziness, headache, migraine, depression, breast cancer (see notes above and section 6.4.1.1), arthralgia, myalgia, visual disturbances, seborrhoeic dermatitis, rash and pruritus also reported

**Dose**

- 2.5 mg daily
  **Note** Unsuitable for use in the premenopause (unless being treated with gonadotrophin-releasing hormone analogue) and as (or with) an oral contraceptive; also unsuitable for use within 12 months of last menstrual period (may cause irregular bleeding); induce withdrawal bleed with progestogen if transferring from another form of HRT

**Livial®** (Organon) [PoM]
Tablets, tibolone 2.5 mg. Net price 28-tab pack = £10.56; 3 × 28-tab pack = £31.68

---

## Ethinylestradiol

Ethinylestradiol (ethinyloestradiol) is licensed for short-term treatment of symptoms of oestrogen deficiency, for osteoporosis prophylaxis if other drugs (section 6.6) cannot be used and for the treatment of female hypogonadism and menstrual disorders.

Ethinylestradiol is occasionally used under **specialist supervision** for the management of *hereditary haemorrhagic telangiectasia* (but evidence of benefit is limited). Side-effects include nausea, fluid retention, and thrombosis. Impotence and gynaecomastia have been reported in men.

For use in prostate cancer, see section 8.3.1.

### ETHINYLESTRADIOL
(Ethinyloestradiol)

**Indications** see notes above

**Cautions** cardiovascular disease (sodium retention with oedema, thromboembolism), hepatic impairment (jaundice), see also under Combined Hormonal Contraceptives (section 7.3.1) and under Oestrogens for HRT (p. 402)

**Contra-indications** see under Combined Hormonal Contraceptives (section 7.3.1) and under Oestrogens for HRT (p. 402)

**Side-effects** feminising effects in men; see also under Combined Hormonal Contraceptives (section 7.3.1) and under Oestrogens for HRT (p. 402)

**Dose**

- Menopausal symptoms and osteoporosis prophylaxis, (with progestogen for 12–14 days per cycle in women with intact uterus), 10–50 micrograms daily for 21 days, repeated after 7-day tablet-free period
- Female hypogonadism, 10–50 micrograms daily, usually on cyclical basis; initial oestrogen therapy should be followed by combined oestrogen and progestogen therapy
- Menstrual disorders, 20–50 micrograms daily from day 5 to 25 of each cycle, with progestogen added either throughout the cycle or from day 15 to 25

**Ethinylestradiol** (Non-proprietary) [PoM]
Tablets, ethinylestradiol 10 micrograms, net price 21-tab pack = £25.01; 50 micrograms, 21-tab pack = £30.00; 1 mg, 28-tab pack = £44.00

---

## Raloxifene

Raloxifene is licensed for the treatment and prevention of *postmenopausal osteoporosis*; unlike hormone replacement therapy, raloxifene does not reduce menopausal vasomotor symptoms.

Raloxifene may reduce the incidence of oestrogen-receptor-positive breast cancer but its role in established breast cancer is not yet clear. The manufacturer advises avoiding its use during treatment for breast cancer.

### RALOXIFENE HYDROCHLORIDE

**Indications** treatment and prevention of postmenopausal osteoporosis

**Cautions** risk factors for venous thromboembolism (discontinue if prolonged immobilisation); risk factors for stroke; breast cancer (see notes above); history of oestrogen-induced hypertriglyceridaemia (monitor serum triglycerides); renal impairment (avoid if severe; Appendix 3); **interactions:** Appendix 1 (raloxifene)

**Contra-indications** history of venous thromboembolism, undiagnosed uterine bleeding, endometrial cancer, hepatic impairment, cholestasis: pregnancy and breast-feeding

**Side-effects** hot flushes, leg cramps, peripheral oedema, influenza-like symptoms; *less commonly* venous thromboembolism, thrombophlebitis; *rarely* rashes, gastro-intestinal disturbances, hypertension, arterial thromboembolism, headache (including migraine), breast discomfort, thrombocytopenia

**Dose**

- 60 mg once daily

**Evista®** (Lilly) [PoM]
Tablets, f/c, raloxifene hydrochloride 60 mg, net price 28-tab pack = £17.06; 84-tab pack = £59.59

### 6.4.1.2 Progestogens

There are two main groups of progestogen, progesterone and its analogues (dydrogesterone and medroxyprogesterone) and testosterone analogues (norethisterone and norgestrel). The newer progestogens (desogestrel, norgestimate, and gestodene) are all derivatives of norgestrel; levonorgestrel is the active isomer of norgestrel and has twice its potency. Progesterone and its analogues are less androgenic than the testosterone derivatives and neither progesterone nor dydrogesterone causes virilisation.

Where endometriosis requires drug treatment, it may respond to a progestogen, e.g. norethisterone, administered on a continuous basis. Danazol, gestrinone, and gonadorelin analogues are also available (section 6.7.2).

**6**

**Endocrine system**

Although oral progestogens have been used widely for menorrhagia they are relatively ineffective compared with tranexamic acid (section 2.11) or, particularly where dysmenorrhoea is also a factor, mefenamic acid (section 10.1.1); the levonorgestrel-releasing intra-uterine system (section 7.3.2.3) may be particularly useful for women also requiring contraception. Oral progestogens have been used for severe dys-menorrhoea, but where contraception is also required in younger women the best choice is a combined oral contraceptive (section 7.3.1).

Progestogens have also been advocated for the allevia-tion of premenstrual symptoms, but no convincing physiological basis for such treatment has been shown.

Progestogens have been used for the prevention of spontaneous abortion in women with a history of recur-rent miscarriage (habitual abortion) but there is no evidence of benefit and they are **not** recommended for this purpose. In pregnant women with anti-phospholipid antibody syndrome who have suffered recurrent miscarriage, administration of low-dose aspirin (section 2.9) and a prophylactic dose of a low molecular weight heparin (section 2.8.1) may decrease the risk of fetal loss (use under specialist supervision only).

**Hormone replacement therapy** In women with a uterus a progestogen needs to be added to long-term oestrogen therapy for hormone replacement, to prevent cystic hyperplasia of the endometrium and possible transformation to cancer; it can be added on a cyclical or a continuous basis (see section 6.4.1.1). Combined packs incorporating suitable progestogen tablets are available, see p. 403.

**Oral contraception** Desogestrel, etynodiol (ethyno-diol), gestodene, levonorgestrel, norethisterone, and norgestimate are used in combined oral contraceptives and in progestogen-only contraceptives (section 7.3.1 and section 7.3.2).

**Cancer** Progestogens also have a role in neoplastic disease (section 8.3.2).

**Cautions** Progestogens should be used with caution in conditions that may worsen with fluid retention e.g. epilepsy, hypertension, migraine, asthma, cardiac or renal dysfunction, and in those susceptible to throm-boembolism (particular caution with high dose). Care is also required in liver impairment (avoid if severe), and in those with a history of depression. Progestogens can decrease glucose tolerance and diabetes should be monitored closely. For **interactions** see Appendix 1 (progestogens).

**Contra-indications** Progestogens should be avoided in patients with a history of liver tumours, and in severe liver impairment. They are also contra-indicated in those with genital or breast cancer (unless progestogens are being used in the management of these conditions), severe arterial disease, undiagnosed vaginal bleeding and acute porphyria (section 9.8.2). Progestogens should not be used if there is a history during pregnancy of idiopathic jaundice, severe pruritus, or pemphigoid gestationis.

**Side-effects** Side-effects of progestogens include menstrual disturbances, premenstrual-like syndrome (including bloating, fluid retention, breast tenderness), weight change, nausea, headache, dizziness, insomnia, drowsiness, depression, change in libido; also skin reac-tions (including urticaria, pruritus, rash, and acne); hirsutism and alopecia. Jaundice and anaphylactoid reactions have also been reported.

## DYDROGESTERONE

**Indications** HRT (section 6.4.1.1)

**Cautions** see notes above; breast-feeding (Appendix 5)

**Contra-indications** see notes above

**Side-effects** see notes above

**Dose**

- See under combined preparations (section 6.4.1.1)

## MEDROXYPROGESTERONE ACETATE

**Indications** see under Dose; contraception (section 7.3.2.2); malignant disease (section 8.3.2)

**Cautions** see notes above; breast-feeding (Appendix 5)

**Contra-indications** see notes above; pregnancy (Appendix 4)

**Side-effects** see notes above; indigestion

**Dose**

- By mouth, 2.5–10 mg daily for 5–10 days beginning on day 16 to 21 of cycle, repeated for 2 cycles in dysfunctional uterine bleeding and 3 cycles in sec-ondary amenorrhoea
- Mild to moderate endometriosis, 10 mg 3 times daily for 90 consecutive days, beginning on day 1 of cycle
- Progestogenic opposition of oestrogen HRT, 10 mg daily for the last 14 days of each 28-day oestrogen HRT cycle

**Provera®** (Pharmacia) PoM

Tablets, all scored, medroxyprogesterone acetate 2.5 mg (orange), net price 30-tab pack = £1.84; 5 mg (blue), 10-tab pack = £1.23; 10 mg (white), 10-tab pack = £2.47, 90-tab pack = £22.16

**Climanor®** (ReSource Medical) PoM

Tablets, f/c, medroxyprogesterone acetate 5 mg, net price 28-tab pack = £3.27

◀**Combined preparations**
Section 6.4.1.1

## NORETHISTERONE

**Indications** see under Dose; HRT (section 6.4.1.1); contraception (section 7.3.1 and section 7.3.2); malignant disease (section 8.3.2)

**Cautions** see notes above; breast-feeding (Appendix 5)

**Contra-indications** see notes above; pregnancy (Appendix 4)

**Side-effects** see notes above

**Dose**

- Endometriosis, by mouth, 10–15 mg daily for 4–6 months or longer, starting on day 5 of cycle (if spotting occurs increase dose to 20–25 mg daily, reduced once bleeding has stopped)
- Dysfunctional uterine bleeding, menorrhagia (but see notes above), by mouth, 5 mg 3 times daily for 10 days to arrest bleeding; to prevent bleeding 5 mg twice daily from day 19 to 26

- Dysmenorrhoea (but see notes above), by mouth, 5 mg 3 times daily from day 5 to 24 for 3–4 cycles
- Premenstrual syndrome (but not recommended, see notes above), by mouth, 5 mg 2–3 times daily from day 19 to 26 for several cycles
- Postponement of menstruation, by mouth, 5 mg 3 times daily starting 3 days before expected onset (menstruation occurs 2–3 days after stopping)

**Norethisterone** (Non-proprietary) [PoM]
Tablets, norethisterone 5 mg, net price 30-tab pack = £2.71

**Primolut N®** (Schering Health) [PoM]
Tablets, norethisterone 5 mg. Net price 30-tab pack = £1.93

**Utovlan®** (Pharmacia) [PoM]
Tablets, norethisterone 5 mg, net price 30-tab pack = £1.40, 90-tab pack = £4.21

◢**Combined preparations**
Section 6.4.1.1

## PROGESTERONE

**Indications** see under preparations
**Cautions** see notes above; breast-feeding (Appendix 5)
**Contra-indications** see notes above; missed or incomplete abortion
**Side-effects** see notes above; injection-site reactions; pain, diarrhoea and flatulence can occur with rectal administration
**Dose**
- See under preparations

**Crinone®** (Serono) [PoM]
Vaginal gel, progesterone 90 mg/application (8%), 15 = £31.45
Dose by vagina, infertility due to inadequate luteal phase, insert 1 applicatorful daily starting either after documented ovulation or on day 18–21 of cycle. *In vitro* fertilisation, daily application continued for 30 days after laboratory evidence of pregnancy

**Cyclogest®** (Actavis) [PoM] ◢
Pessaries, progesterone 200 mg, net price 15 = £7.17; 400 mg, 15 = £10.38
Dose by vagina *or* rectum, premenstrual syndrome and post-natal depression, 200 mg daily to 400 mg twice daily; for premenstrual syndrome start on day 12–14 and continue until onset of menstruation (but not recommended, see notes above); rectally if barrier methods of contraception are used, in patients who have recently given birth or in those who suffer from vaginal infection or recurrent cystitis

**Gestone®** (Nordic) [PoM]
Injection, progesterone 50 mg/mL, 1-mL amp = £4.50, 2-mL amp = £4.50
Dose by deep intramuscular injection into buttock, dysfunctional uterine bleeding, 5–10 mg daily for 5–10 days until 2 days before expected onset of menstruation
Recurrent miscarriage due to inadequate luteal phase (but not recommended, see notes above) or following *in vitro* fertilisation *or* gamete intra-fallopian transfer, 25–100 mg 2–7 times a week from day 15, or day of embryo *or* gamete transfer, until 8–16 weeks of pregnancy; max. 200 mg daily

**Utrogestan®** (Ferring) [PoM]
Capsules, progesterone (micronised) 100 mg, net price 30-cap pack = £5.13; 200 mg 15-cap pack = £5.13. Counselling, administration
Excipients include arachis (peanut) oil
Counselling Capsules should be taken at bedtime on an empty stomach
Dose progestogenic opposition of oestrogen HRT 200 mg once daily on days 15–26, *or* 100 mg once daily on days 1–25, of each 28-day oestrogen HRT cycle

## 6.4.2 Male sex hormones and antagonists

Androgens cause masculinisation; they may be used as replacement therapy in castrated adults and in those who are hypogonadal due to either pituitary or testicular disease. In the normal male they inhibit pituitary gonadotrophin secretion and depress spermatogenesis. Androgens also have an anabolic action which led to the development of anabolic steroids (section 6.4.3).

Androgens are useless as a treatment of impotence and impaired spermatogenesis unless there is associated hypogonadism; they should not be given until the hypogonadism has been properly investigated. Treatment should be under expert supervision.

When given to patients with hypopituitarism they can lead to normal sexual development and potency but not to fertility. If fertility is desired, the usual treatment is with gonadotrophins or pulsatile gonadotrophin-releasing hormone (section 6.5.1) which will stimulate spermatogenesis as well as androgen production.

Caution should be used when androgens or chorionic gonadotrophin are used in treating boys with delayed puberty since the fusion of epiphyses is hastened and may result in short stature; skeletal maturation should be monitored.

Intramuscular depot preparations of **testosterone esters** are preferred for replacement therapy. Testosterone enantate, propionate or undecanoate, or alternatively *Sustanon®*, which consists of a mixture of testosterone esters and has a longer duration of action, may be used. Satisfactory replacement therapy can sometimes be obtained with 1 mL of *Sustanon 250®*, given by intramuscular injection once a month, although more frequent dose intervals are often necessary. Implants of testosterone can be used for hypogonadism; the implants are replaced every 4 to 5 months.

Testosterone implants can be used in postmenopausal women as an adjunct to hormone replacement therapy. A testosterone patch is also licensed to improve libido in *surgically induced* menopausal women (receiving concomitant oestrogen therapy).

## TESTOSTERONE AND ESTERS

**Indications** see under preparations
**Cautions** cardiac, renal, or hepatic impairment (Appendix 2), elderly, ischaemic heart disease, hypertension, epilepsy, migraine, diabetes mellitus, skeletal metastases (risk of hypercalcaemia), undertake regular examination of the prostate and breast during treatment; monitor full blood count, lipid profile and liver function; pre-pubertal boys (see notes above and under Side-effects); **interactions:** Appendix 1 (testosterone)
Women Regularly assess for androgenic side-effects; women should be advised to report any signs of virilisation e.g. deepening of the voice or hirsutism
**Contra-indications** breast cancer in men, prostate cancer, history of primary liver tumours, hypercalcaemia, pregnancy (Appendix 4), breast-feeding (Appendix 5), nephrotic syndrome
**Side-effects** prostate abnormalities and prostate cancer, headache, depression, gastro-intestinal bleeding, nausea, vomiting, cholestatic jaundice, changes in libido, gynaecomastia, polycythaemia,

6 Endocrine system

anxiety, irritability, nervousness, asthenia, paraesthesia, hypertension, electrolyte disturbances including sodium retention with oedema and hypercalcaemia, weight gain; increased bone growth, muscle cramps, arthralgia; androgenic effects such as hirsutism, male-pattern baldness, seborrhoea, acne, pruritus, excessive frequency and duration of penile erection, precocious sexual development and premature closure of epiphyses in pre-pubertal males, suppression of spermatogenesis in men and virilism in women; *rarely* liver tumours; sleep apnoea also reported; *with patches, buccal tablets, and gel*, local irritation and allergic reactions (including burn-like lesions with *patches*), and taste disturbances

**Dose**

• See under preparations

◢**Oral**

**Restandol® Testocaps** (Organon) (PoM)

Capsules, orange, testosterone undecanoate 40 mg in oily solution. Net price 30-cap pack = £8.72; 60-cap pack = £17.44. Label: 21, 25

Dose androgen deficiency, 120–160 mg daily for 2–3 weeks; maintenance 40–120 mg daily

◢**Buccal**

**Striant® SR** (Ardana) (PoM)

Mucoadhesive buccal tablets, m/r, testosterone 30 mg, net price 60-tab pack = £45.84. Counselling, see under Dose below

Dose hypogonadism, 30 mg every 12 hours; CHILD and ADOLESCENT under 18 years not recommended

Counselling Place rounded side of tablet on gum above front teeth and hold lip firmly over the gum for 30 seconds. If tablet detaches within 4 hours of next dose, replace with new tablet which is considered the second dose for the day.

◢**Intramuscular**

**Testosterone Enantate** (Cambridge) (PoM)

Injection (oily), testosterone enantate 250 mg/mL. Net price 1-mL amp = £12.11

Dose by slow intramuscular injection, hypogonadism, initially 250 mg every 2–3 weeks; maintenance 250 mg every 3–6 weeks
Breast cancer, 250 mg every 2–3 weeks

**Nebido®** (Bayer) ▼ (PoM)

Injection (oily), testosterone undecanoate 250 mg/mL. Net price 4-mL amp = £76.70

Dose by deep intramuscular injection, hypogonadism in men over 18 years, 1 g every 10–14 weeks; if necessary, second dose may be given after 6 weeks to achieve rapid steady state plasma testosterone levels and then every 10–14 weeks

**Sustanon 100®** (Organon) (PoM)

Injection (oily), testosterone propionate 20 mg, testosterone phenylpropionate 40 mg, and testosterone isocaproate 40 mg/mL. Net price 1-mL amp = £1.09

Excipients include arachis (peanut) oil, benzyl alcohol (see Excipients p. 2)

Dose by deep intramuscular injection, androgen deficiency, 1 mL every 2 weeks

**Sustanon 250®** (Organon) (PoM)

Injection (oily), testosterone propionate 30 mg, testosterone phenylpropionate 60 mg, testosterone isocaproate 60 mg, and testosterone decanoate 100 mg/mL. Net price 1-mL amp = £2.50

Excipients include arachis (peanut) oil, benzyl alcohol (see Excipients p. 2)

Dose by deep intramuscular injection, androgen deficiency, 1 mL usually every 3 weeks

**Virormone®** (Nordic) (PoM)

Injection, testosterone propionate 50 mg/mL. Net price 2-mL amp = 45p

Dose by intramuscular injection, androgen deficiency, 50 mg 2–3 times weekly
Delayed puberty, 50 mg weekly
Breast cancer in women, 100 mg 2–3 times weekly

◢**Implant**

**Testosterone** (Organon) (PoM)

Implant, testosterone 100 mg, net price = £7.40; 200 mg = £13.79

Dose by implantation, male hypogonadism, 100–600 mg; 600 mg usually maintains plasma-testosterone concentration within the normal range for 4–5 months
Postmenopausal women, 50–100 mg every 4–8 months, as an adjunct to oestrogen replacement therapy

◢**Transdermal preparations**

**Andropatch®** (GSK) (PoM)

Patches, self-adhesive, releasing testosterone approx. 2.5 mg/24 hours, net price 60-patch pack = £47.19; releasing testosterone approx. 5 mg/24 hours, net price 30-patch pack = £47.19. Counselling, administration

Dose androgen deficiency in men (over 15 years) associated with primary or secondary hypogonadism, apply to clean, dry, unbroken skin on back, abdomen, upper arms or thighs, removing after 24 hours and siting replacement patch on a different area (with an interval of 7 days before using the same site); initially apply patches equivalent to testosterone 5 mg/24 hours (2.5 mg/24 hours in non-virilised patients) at night (approx. 10 p.m.), then adjust to 2.5 mg to 7.5 mg every 24 hours according to plasma-testosterone concentration (those with a body-weight over 130 kg may require 7.5 mg every 24 hours)

**Intrinsa®** (Procter & Gamble) ▼ (PoM)

Patches, self-adhesive, releasing testosterone approx. 300 micrograms/24 hours, net price 8-patch pack = £26.91. Counselling, administration

Dose hypoactive sexual desire disorder associated with surgically induced menopause (in women receiving concomitant oestrogen therapy (section 6.4.1.1)), apply 1 patch twice weekly continuously to clean, dry, unbroken skin on lower abdomen below waistline; site replacement patch on a different area (avoid using same area for 7 days); assess treatment after 3–6 months, discontinue if no benefit

Note Not recommended for women naturally menopausal or those taking conjugated oestrogens. Safety and efficacy of use beyond 1 year not established

**Testim®** (Ipsen) (PoM)

Gel, testosterone 50 mg/5 g tube, net price 30-tube pack = £32.00. Counselling, administration

Excipients include propylene glycol (see section 13.1.3)

Dose hypogonadism due to testosterone deficiency in men (over 18 years), 50 mg testosterone (5 g gel) applied once daily; subsequent application adjusted according to response; max. 100 mg (10 g gel) daily

Counselling Squeeze entire content of tube on to one palm and apply as a thin layer on clean, dry, healthy skin of shoulder or upper arm, preferably in the morning after washing or bathing (if 2 tubes required use 1 per shoulder or upper arm); rub in and allow to dry before putting on clothing to cover site; wash hands with soap after application; avoid washing application site for at least 6 hours
Avoid skin contact with application sites to prevent testosterone transfer to other people, especially pregnant women and children—consult product literature

**Testogel®** (Schering Health) (PoM)

Gel, testosterone 50 mg/5 g sachet, net price 30-sachet pack = £31.71. Counselling, administration

Dose hypogonadism due to androgen deficiency in men (over 18 years), 50 mg testosterone (5 g gel) to be applied once daily;

Endocrine system

6

subsequent application adjusted according to response in 25-mg (2.5 g gel) increments to max. 100 mg (10 g gel) daily

**Counselling** Apply thin layer of gel on clean, dry, healthy skin such as shoulders, arms or abdomen, immediately after sachet is opened. Not to be applied on genital area as high alcohol content may cause local irritation. Allow to dry for 3–5 minutes before dressing. Wash hands with soap and water after applying gel, avoid shower or bath for at least 6 hours

Avoid skin contact with gel application sites to prevent testosterone transfer to other people, especially pregnant women and children—consult product literature

**Tostran®** (ProStrakan) PoM

Gel, testosterone 2% (10 mg/metered application), net price 60-g multidose dispenser = £26.67. Counselling, administration

Excipients include butylhydroxytoluene, propylene glycol (see section 13.1.3)

**Dose** hypogonadism due to testosterone deficiency in men (over 18 years), initially 60 mg testosterone (3 g gel) applied once daily; subsequent applications adjusted according to response; max. 80 mg (4 g gel) daily

**Counselling** Apply gel on clean, dry, intact skin of abdomen or both inner thighs, preferably in the morning. Gently rub in with a finger until dry before dressing. Wash hands with soap and water after applying gel; avoid washing application site for at least 2 hours. Not to be applied on genital area.

Avoid skin contact with gel application sites to prevent testosterone transfer to other people, especially pregnant women and children—consult product literature

## ◾ MESTEROLONE

**Indications** see under Dose

**Cautions** see under Testosterone and Esters

**Contra-indications** see under Testosterone and Esters

**Side-effects** see under Testosterone and Esters but spermatogenesis unimpaired

**Dose**

- Androgen deficiency and male infertility associated with hypogonadism, 25 mg 3–4 times daily for several months, reduced to 50–75 mg daily in divided doses for maintenance; CHILD not recommended

**Pro-Viron®** (Schering Health) PoM

Tablets, scored, mesterolone 25 mg. Net price 30-tab pack = £4.27

---

## Anti-androgens

### Cyproterone acetate

**Cyproterone acetate** is an anti-androgen used in the treatment of severe hypersexuality and sexual deviation in the male. It inhibits spermatogenesis and produces reversible infertility (but is not a male contraceptive); abnormal sperm forms are produced. Fully informed consent is recommended and an initial spermatogram. As hepatic tumours have been produced in *animal* studies, careful consideration should be given to the risk/benefit ratio before treatment. Cyproterone acetate is also used as an adjunct in prostatic cancer (section 8.3.4.2) and in the treatment of acne and hirsutism in women (section 13.6.2).

## ◾ CYPROTERONE ACETATE

**Indications** see notes above; prostate cancer (section 8.3.4.2)

**Cautions** ineffective for male hypersexuality in chronic alcoholism (relevance to prostate cancer not known); blood counts initially and throughout treatment; monitor hepatic function regularly (liver function tests should be performed before treatment, see

also under Side-effects below); monitor adrenocortical function regularly; diabetes mellitus (see also Contra-indications)

**Driving** Fatigue and lassitude may impair performance of skilled tasks (e.g. driving)

**Contra-indications** (do not apply in prostate cancer) hepatic disease (Appendix 2), severe diabetes (with vascular changes); sickle-cell anaemia, malignant or wasting disease, severe depression, history of thrombo-embolic disorders; youths under 18 years (may arrest bone maturation and testicular development)

**Side-effects** fatigue and lassitude, breathlessness, weight changes, reduced sebum production (may clear acne), changes in hair pattern, gynaecomastia (rarely leading to galactorrhoea and benign breast nodules); rarely hypersensitivity reactions, rash and osteoporosis; inhibition of spermatogenesis (see notes above); hepatotoxicity reported (including jaundice, hepatitis and hepatic failure usually in men given 200–300 mg daily for prostatic cancer, see section 8.3.4.2 for details and warnings)

**Dose**

- Male hypersexuality, 50 mg twice daily after food

**Cyproterone Acetate** (Non-proprietary) PoM

Tablets, cyproterone acetate 50 mg, net price 56-tab pack = £31.54. Label: 21 counselling, driving

**Androcur®** (Schering Health) PoM

Tablets, scored, cyproterone acetate 50 mg. Net price 56-tab pack = £24.88. Label: 21 counselling, driving

---

## Dutasteride and finasteride

**Dutasteride** and **finasteride** are specific inhibitors of the enzyme 5α-reductase, which metabolises testosterone into the more potent androgen, dihydrotestosterone. This inhibition of testosterone metabolism leads to reduction in prostate size, with improvement in urinary flow rate and in obstructive symptoms. Dutasteride and finasteride are alternatives to alpha-blockers (section 7.4.1) particularly in men with a significantly enlarged prostate. Finasteride is also licensed for use with doxazosin in the management of benign prostatic hyperplasia.

A low strength of finasteride is licensed for treating male-pattern baldness in men (section 13.9).

**Cautions** Dutasteride and finasteride decrease serum concentration of prostate cancer markers such as prostate-specific antigen; reference values may need adjustment. Both dutasteride and finasteride are excreted in semen and use of a condom is recommended if sexual partner is pregnant or likely to become pregnant. Women of childbearing potential should avoid handling crushed or broken tablets of finasteride and leaking capsules of dutasteride.

**Contra-indications** Dutasteride and finasteride are contra-indicated in women, children, and adolescents.

**Side-effects** The side-effects of dutasteride and finasteride include impotence, decreased libido, ejaculation disorders, and breast tenderness and enlargement.

## ◾ DUTASTERIDE

**Indications** benign prostatic hyperplasia

**Cautions** see notes above; **interactions:** Appendix 1 (dutasteride)

**6**

**Endocrine system**

**Contra-indications** see notes above; also severe hepatic impairment

**Side-effects** see notes above

**Dose**

- 500 micrograms daily (may require 6 months' treatment before benefit is obtained)

**Avodart®** (GSK) (PoM)

Capsules, yellow, dutasteride 500 micrograms, net price 30-cap pack = £19.80. Label: 25

### ▌ FINASTERIDE

**Indications** benign prostatic hyperplasia; male-pattern baldness in men (section 13.9)

**Cautions** see notes above; also obstructive uropathy

**Contra-indications** see notes above

**Side-effects** see notes above; also testicular pain, hypersensitivity reactions (including lip and face swelling, pruritus and rash)

**Dose**

- 5 mg daily, review treatment after 6 months (may require several months' treatment before benefit is obtained)

**Proscar®** (MSD) (PoM)

Tablets, blue, f/c, finasteride 5 mg. Net price 28-tab pack = £13.94

## 6.4.3 Anabolic steroids

Anabolic steroids have some androgenic activity but they cause less virilisation than androgens in women. They are used in the treatment of some *aplastic anaemias* (section 9.1.3). Anabolic steroids have been given for osteoporosis in women but they are no longer advocated for this purpose.

The protein-building properties of anabolic steroids have not proved beneficial in the clinical setting. Their use as body builders or tonics is quite unjustified; some athletes abuse them.

### ▌ NANDROLONE

**Indications** osteoporosis in postmenopausal women (but not recommended, see notes above); aplastic anaemia (section 9.1.3)

**Cautions** cardiac and renal impairment, hepatic impairment (Appendix 2), hypertension, diabetes mellitus, epilepsy, migraine; monitor skeletal maturation in young patients; skeletal metastases (risk of hypercalcaemia); **interactions**: Appendix 1 (anabolic steroids)

**Contra-indications** severe hepatic impairment, prostate cancer, male breast cancer, pregnancy (Appendix 4) and breast-feeding, acute porphyria (section 9.8.2)

**Side-effects** acne, sodium retention with oedema, virilisation with high doses including voice changes (sometimes irreversible), amenorrhoea, inhibition of spermatogenesis, premature epiphyseal closure; abnormal liver-function tests reported with high doses; liver tumours reported occasionally on prolonged treatment with anabolic steroids

**Dose**

- See below

**Deca-Durabolin®** (Organon) (PoM) ▨

Injection (oily), nandrolone decanoate 50 mg/mL, net price 1-mL amp = £3.23

Excipients include arachis (peanut) oil, benzyl alcohol (see Excipients, p. 2)

**Dose** by deep intramuscular injection, 50 mg every 3 weeks

## 6.5 Hypothalamic and pituitary hormones and anti-oestrogens

**6.5.1** Hypothalamic and anterior pituitary hormones and anti-oestrogens

**6.5.2** Posterior pituitary hormones and antagonists

> Use of preparations in these sections requires detailed prior investigation of the patient and *should be reserved for specialist centres.*

## 6.5.1 Hypothalamic and anterior pituitary hormones and anti-oestrogens

### Anti-oestrogens

The anti-oestrogens **clomifene** (clomiphene) and **tamoxifen** (section 8.3.4.1) are used in the treatment of female infertility due to oligomenorrhoea or secondary amenorrhoea (e.g. associated with polycystic ovarian disease). They induce gonadotrophin release by occupying oestrogen receptors in the hypothalamus, thereby interfering with feedback mechanisms; chorionic gonadotrophin is sometimes used as an adjunct. Patients should be warned that there is a risk of multiple pregnancy (*rarely* more than twins).

### ▌ CLOMIFENE CITRATE
(Clomiphene Citrate)

**Indications** anovulatory infertility—see notes above

**Cautions** see notes above; polycystic ovary syndrome (cysts may enlarge during treatment), ovarian hyperstimulation syndrome, uterine fibroids, ectopic pregnancy, incidence of multiple births increased (consider ultrasound monitoring), visual symptoms (discontinue and initiate ophthalmological examination); breast-feeding (Appendix 5)

**CSM Advice.** The CSM has recommended that clomifene should not normally be used for longer than 6 cycles (possibly increased risk of ovarian cancer)

**Contra-indications** hepatic disease (Appendix 2), ovarian cysts, hormone-dependent tumours or abnormal uterine bleeding of undetermined cause, pregnancy (exclude before treatment; Appendix 4)

**Side-effects** visual disturbances (withdraw), ovarian hyperstimulation (withdraw), hot flushes, abdominal discomfort, occasionally nausea, vomiting, depression, insomnia, breast tenderness, headache, intermenstrual spotting, menorrhagia, endometriosis, convulsions, weight gain, rashes, dizziness, hair loss

## Dose

- 50 mg daily for 5 days, starting within about 5 days of onset of menstruation (preferably on 2nd day) or at any time (normally preceded by a progestogen-induced withdrawal bleed) if cycles have ceased; second course of 100 mg daily for 5 days may be given in absence of ovulation; most patients who are going to respond will do so to first course; 3 courses should constitute adequate therapeutic trial; long-term cyclical therapy not recommended—see CSM advice, above

**Clomifene** (Non-proprietary) [PoM]
Tablets, clomifene citrate 50 mg, net price 30-tab pack = £11.34

**Clomid®** (Aventis Pharma) [PoM]
Tablets, yellow, scored, clomifene citrate 50 mg. Net price 30-tab pack = £8.46

---

# Anterior pituitary hormones

## Corticotrophins

**Tetracosactide** (tetracosactrin), an analogue of corticotropin (ACTH), is used to test adrenocortical function; failure of the plasma cortisol concentration to rise after administration of tetracosactide indicates adrenocortical insufficiency.

Both corticotropin and tetracosactide were formerly used as alternatives to corticosteroids in conditions such as Crohn's disease or rheumatoid arthritis; their value was limited by the variable and unpredictable therapeutic response and by the waning of their effect with time.

### ▮ TETRACOSACTIDE
(Tetracosactrin)

**Indications** see notes above

**Cautions** as for corticosteroids, section 6.3.2; **important**: risk of anaphylaxis (medical supervision; consult product literature); pregnancy (Appendix 4); breast-feeding (Appendix 5); **interactions**: Appendix 1 (corticosteroids)

**Contra-indications** as for corticosteroids, section 6.3.2; avoid injections containing benzyl alcohol in neonates (see under preparations)

**Side-effects** as for corticosteroids, section 6.3.2

**Dose**

- See under preparations below

**Synacthen®** (Alliance) [PoM]
Injection, tetracosactide 250 micrograms (as acetate)/mL. Net price 1-mL amp = £2.70
Dose diagnostic (30-minute test), by intramuscular or intravenous injection, 250 micrograms as a single dose

**Synacthen Depot®** (Alliance) [PoM]
Injection (aqueous suspension), tetracosactide acetate 1 mg/mL, with zinc phosphate complex. Net price 1-mL amp = £3.87
Excipients include benzyl alcohol (avoid in neonates, see Excipients p. 2)
Dose diagnostic (5-hour test), by intramuscular injection, 1 mg as a single dose
Note Formerly used therapeutically by intramuscular injection, in an initial dose of 1 mg daily (or every 12 hours in acute cases), reduced to 1 mg every 2–3 days, then 1 mg weekly (or 500 micrograms every 2–3 days) but value was limited (see notes above)

# Gonadotrophins

Follicle-stimulating hormone (FSH) and luteinising hormone (LH) together (as in **human menopausal gonadotrophin**), follicle-stimulating hormone alone (as in **follitropin**), or chorionic gonadotrophin, are used in the treatment of infertility in women with proven hypopituitarism or who have not responded to clomifene, or in superovulation treatment for assisted conception (such as *in vitro* fertilisation).

The gonadotrophins are also occasionally used in the treatment of hypogonadotrophic hypogonadism and associated oligospermia. There is no justification for their use in primary gonadal failure.

Chorionic gonadotrophin has also been used in delayed puberty in the male to stimulate endogenous testosterone production, but has little advantage over testosterone (section 6.4.2).

### ▮ CHORIONIC GONADOTROPHIN
(Human Chorionic Gonadotrophin; HCG)

A preparation of a glycoprotein fraction secreted by the placenta and obtained from the urine of pregnant women having the action of the pituitary luteinising hormone

**Indications** see notes above

**Cautions** cardiac or renal impairment, asthma, epilepsy, migraine; prepubertal boys (risk of premature epiphyseal closure or precocious puberty)

**Contra-indications** androgen-dependent tumours

**Side-effects** oedema (particularly in males—reduce dose), headache, tiredness, mood changes, gynaecomastia, local reactions; may aggravate ovarian hyperstimulation, multiple pregnancy

**Dose**

- By subcutaneous *or* intramuscular injection, according to patient's response

**Choragon®** (Ferring) [PoM]
Injection, powder for reconstitution, chorionic gonadotrophin. Net price 5000-unit amp (with solvent) = £3.26. For intramuscular injection

**Pregnyl®** (Organon) [PoM]
Injection, powder for reconstitution, chorionic gonadotrophin. Net price 1500-unit amp = £2.16; 5000-unit amp = £3.21 (both with solvent). For subcutaneous or intramuscular injection

### ▮ CHORIOGONADOTROPIN ALFA
(Human chorionic gonadotropin)

**Indications** see notes above

**Cautions** rule out infertility caused by hypothyroidism, adrenocortical deficiency, hyperprolactinaemia, tumours of the pituitary or hypothalamus

**Contra-indications** ovarian enlargement or cyst (unless caused by polycystic ovarian disease); ectopic pregnancy in previous 3 months; active thromboembolic disorders; hypothalamus, pituitary, ovarian, uterine or mammary malignancy

**Side-effects** nausea, vomiting, abdominal pain; headache, tiredness; injection-site reactions; ovarian hyperstimulation syndrome; rarely diarrhoea, depression, irritability, breast pain; ectopic pregnancy and ovarian torsion reported

**Dose**

- By subcutaneous injection, according to patient's response

6

Endocrine system

Endocrine system

6

**Ovitrelle®** (Serono) `PoM`

Injection, choriogonadotropin alfa, net price 6500-unit/0.5 mL (250-micrograms/0.5 mL) prefilled syringe = £32.01

## ■ FOLLITROPIN ALFA and BETA
(Recombinant human follicle stimulating hormone)

**Indications** see notes above

**Cautions** see under Human Menopausal Gonadotrophins; acute porphyria (section 9.8.2)

**Contra-indications** see under Human Menopausal Gonadotrophins

**Side-effects** see under Human Menopausal Gonadotrophins

**Dose**

- By subcutaneous or intramuscular injection, according to patient's response

### ■ Follitropin alfa
**Gonal-F®** (Serono) `PoM`

Injection, powder for reconstitution, follitropin alfa. Net price 75-unit amp = £21.44; 450 units/0.75 mL, multidose vial = £128.64; 1050 units/1.75 mL, multi-dose vial = £300.16 (all with solvent). For subcutaneous injection

Injection, prefilled pen, follitropin alfa 600 units/mL, net price 0.5 mL (300 units) = £97.08, 0.75 mL (450 units) = £145.62, 1.5 mL (900 units) = £291.24. For subcutaneous injection

### ■ Follitropin alfa with lutropin alfa
**Pergoveris®** (Serono) `PoM`

Injection, powder for reconstitution, follitropin alfa 150 units (11 micrograms), lutropin alfa 75 units (3 micrograms), net price per vial (with solvent) = £60.29. For subcutaneous injection
Electrolytes Na⁺<1 mmol/vial

### ■ Follitropin beta
**Puregon®** (Organon) `PoM`

Injection, follitropin beta 100 units/mL, net price 0.5-mL (50-unit) vial = £18.38; 200 units/mL, 0.5-mL (100-unit) vial = £36.76; 300 units/mL, 0.5-mL (150-unit) vial = £50.62; 400 units/mL, 0.5-mL (200-unit) vial = £67.49; 0.36-mL (300-unit) cartridge = £99.30, 0.72-mL (600-unit) cartridge = £198.60, 1.08-mL (900-unit) cartridge = £297.90, (cartridges for use with *Puregon* pen). For subcutaneous (cartridges and vials) or intramuscular injection (vials)
Excipients may include neomycin and streptomycin

## ■ HUMAN MENOPAUSAL GONADOTROPHINS

**Indications** see notes above

**Cautions** rule out infertility caused by hypothyroidism, adrenocortical deficiency, hyperprolactinaemia, or tumours of the pituitary or hypothalamus

**Contra-indications** ovarian cysts (not caused by polycystic ovarian syndrome); tumours of pituitary, hypothalamus, breast, uterus, ovaries, testes or prostate; vaginal bleeding of unknown cause; pregnancy and breast-feeding

**Side-effects** ovarian hyperstimulation, increased risk of multiple pregnancy and miscarriage, hypersensitivity reactions, gastro-intestinal disturbances, headache, joint pain, fever, injection site reactions, *very rarely* thromboembolism; gynaecomastia, acne, and weight gain reported in men

**Dose**

- By deep intramuscular or subcutaneous injection, according to patient's response

### ■ Menotrophin
Purified extract of human post-menopausal urine containing follicle-stimulating hormone (FSH) and luteinising hormone (LH) in a ratio of 1:1

**Merional®** (Pharmasure) `PoM`

Injection, powder for reconstitution, menotrophin as follicle-stimulating hormone 75 units and luteinising hormone 75 units, net price per vial (with solvent) = £13.95; follicle-stimulating hormone 150 units, luteinising hormone 150 units, net price per vial (with solvent) = £27.90. For intramuscular injection

**Menopur®** (Ferring) `PoM`

Injection, powder for reconstitution, menotrophin as follicle-stimulating hormone 75 units and luteinising hormone 75 units, net price per vial (with solvent) = £13.38. For intramuscular or subcutaneous injection

### ■ Urofollitropin
Purified extract of human post-menopausal urine containing follicle-stimulating hormone (FSH)

**Fostimon®** (Pharmasure) `PoM`

Injection, powder for reconstitution, urofollitropin as follicle-stimulating hormone 75 units, net price per vial (with solvent) = £13.95; follicle-stimulating hormone 150 units, net price per vial (with solvent) = £27.90. For intramuscular or subcutaneous injection

## ■ LUTROPIN ALFA
(Recombinant human luteinising hormone)

**Indications** see notes above

**Cautions** rule out infertility caused by hypothyroidism, adrenocortical deficiency, hyperprolactinaemia, tumours of the pituitary or hypothalamus

**Contra-indications** ovarian enlargement or cyst (unless caused by polycystic ovarian disease); undiagnosed vaginal bleeding; tumours of hypothalamus and pituitary; ovarian, uterine or mammary carcinoma

**Side-effects** nausea, vomiting, abdominal and pelvic pain; headache, somnolence; injection-site reactions; ovarian hyperstimulation syndrome, ovarian cyst, breast pain, ectopic pregnancy; thromboembolism, adnexal torsion, and haemoperitoneum

**Dose**

- By subcutaneous injection, in conjunction with follicle-stimulating hormone, according to response

**Luveris®** (Serono) `PoM`

Injection, powder for reconstitution, lutropin alfa, net price 75-unit vial = £32.01 (with solvent)

## Growth hormone

Growth hormone is used to treat deficiency of the hormone in children and in adults (see NICE guidance below). In children it is used in Prader-Willi syndrome, Turner's syndrome and in chronic renal insufficiency; growth hormone has also recently been licensed for use in short children considered small for gestational age at birth.

Growth hormone of human origin (HGH; somatotrophin) has been replaced by a growth hormone of human sequence, **somatropin**, produced using recombinant DNA technology.

### NICE guidance
### Somatropin in children with growth failure (May 2002)

Treatment with somatropin is recommended for children with:

- proven growth-hormone deficiency;
- Turner's syndrome;
- Prader-Willi syndrome;
- chronic renal insufficiency before puberty.

Treatment should be initiated and monitored by a paediatrician with expertise in managing growth-hormone disorders; treatment can be continued under a shared-care protocol by a general practitioner.

Treatment should be discontinued if the response is poor (i.e. an increase in growth velocity of less than 50% from baseline) in the first year of therapy.

In children with chronic renal insufficiency, treatment should be stopped after renal transplantation and not restarted for at least a year

### NICE guidance
### Somatropin for adults with growth hormone deficiency (August 2003)

Somatropin is recommended in adults **only** if the following 3 criteria are fulfilled:

- Severe growth hormone deficiency, established by an appropriate method,
- Impaired quality of life, measured by means of a specific questionnaire,
- Already receiving treatment for another pituitary hormone deficiency.

Somatropin treatment should be discontinued if the quality of life has not improved sufficiently by 9 months.

Severe growth hormone deficiency developing after linear growth is complete but before the age of 25 years should be treated with growth hormone; treatment should continue until adult peak bone mass has been achieved. Treatment for adult-onset growth hormone deficiency should be stopped only when the patient and the patient's physician consider it appropriate.

Treatment with somatropin should be initiated and managed by a physician with expertise in growth hormone disorders; maintenance treatment can be prescribed in the community under a shared-care protocol.

**Mecasermin**, a human insulin-like growth factor-I (rhIGF-I), is licensed to treat growth failure in children and adolescents with severe primary insulin-like growth factor-I deficiency (section 6.7.4).

## ▌ SOMATROPIN
### (Synthetic Human Growth Hormone)

**Indications** see under Dose

**Cautions** diabetes mellitus (adjustment of antidiabetic therapy may be necessary), papilloedema (see under Side-effects), relative deficiencies of other pituitary hormones (notably hypothyroidism—manufacturers recommend periodic thyroid function tests but limited evidence of clinical value), history of malignant disease, disorders of the epiphysis of the hip (monitor for limping), resolved intracranial hypertension (monitor closely), initiation of treatment close to puberty not recommended in child born small for gestational age; Silver-Russell syndrome; rotate subcutaneous injection sites to prevent lipoatrophy; breast-feeding (Appendix 5); **interactions:** Appendix 1 (somatropin)

**Contra-indications** evidence of tumour activity (complete antitumour therapy and ensure intracranial lesions inactive before starting); not to be used after renal transplantation or for growth promotion in children with closed epiphyses (or near closure in Prader-Willi syndrome); severe obesity or severe respiratory impairment in Prader-Willi syndrome; pregnancy (interrupt treatment if pregnancy occurs, Appendix 4)

**Side-effects** headache, funduscopy for papilloedema recommended if severe or recurrent headache, visual problems, nausea and vomiting occur—if papilloedema confirmed consider benign intracranial hypertension (rare cases reported); fluid retention (peripheral oedema), arthralgia, myalgia, carpal tunnel syndrome, paraesthesia, antibody formation, hypothyroidism, insulin resistance, hyperglycaemia, hypoglycaemia, reactions at injection site; leukaemia in children with growth hormone deficiency also reported

**Dose**

- Gonadal dysgenesis (Turner's syndrome), by subcutaneous injection, 45–50 micrograms/kg daily *or* 1.4 mg/m$^2$ daily
- Deficiency of growth hormone in children, by subcutaneous *or* intramuscular injection, 23–39 micrograms/kg daily *or* 0.7–1 mg/m$^2$ daily
- Growth disturbance in short children born small for gestational age whose growth has not caught up by 4 years or later, by subcutaneous injection, 35 micrograms/kg daily *or* 1 mg/m$^2$ daily
- Prader-Willi syndrome, by subcutaneous injection in children with growth velocity greater than 1 cm/year, in combination with energy-restricted diet, 35 micrograms/kg daily *or* 1 mg/m$^2$ daily; max. 2.7 mg daily
- Chronic renal insufficiency in children (renal function decreased to less than 50%), by subcutaneous injection, 45–50 micrograms/kg daily *or* 1.4 mg/m$^2$ daily (higher doses may be needed) adjusted if necessary after 6 months
- Adult growth hormone deficiency, by subcutaneous injection, initially 150–300 micrograms daily, gradually increased if required to max. 1 mg daily; use minimum effective dose (requirements may decrease with age)

**Note** Dose formerly expressed in units; somatropin 1 mg ≡ 3 units

**Genotropin®** (Pharmacia) PoM

Injection, two-compartment cartridge containing powder for reconstitution, somatropin (rbe) and diluent, net price 5.3-mg (16-unit) cartridge = £122.87, 12-mg (36-unit) cartridge = £278.20. For use with *Gen-otropin® Pen* (JHS) device (available free of charge from clinics). For subcutaneous injection

MiniQuick injection, two-compartment single-dose syringe containing powder for reconstitution, soma-tropin (rbe) and diluent, net price 0.2-mg (0.6-unit) syringe = £4.64; 0.4-mg (1.2-unit) syringe = £9.27; 0.6-mg (1.8-unit) syringe = £13.91; 0.8-mg (2.4-unit) syringe = £18.55; 1-mg (3-unit) syringe = £23.18; 1.2-mg (3.6-unit) syringe = £27.82; 1.4-mg (4.2-unit) syringe = £32.46; 1.6-mg (4.8-unit) syringe = £37.09; 1.8-mg (5.4-unit) syringe = £41.73; 2-mg (6-unit) syringe = £46.37. For subcutaneous injection

**Humatrope®** (Lilly) (PoM)
Injection, powder for reconstitution, somatropin (rbe), net price 6-mg (18-unit) cartridge = £108.00; 12-mg (36-unit) cartridge = £216.00; 24-mg (72-unit) cartridge = £432.00; all supplied with diluent. For subcutaneous or intramuscular injection; cartridges for subcutaneous injection

**Norditropin®** (Novo Nordisk) (PoM)
SimpleXx injection, somatropin (epr) 3.3 mg (10 units)/mL, net price 1.5-mL (5-mg, 15-unit) car-tridge = £106.95; 6.7 mg (20 units)/mL, 1.5-mL (10-mg, 30-unit) cartridge = £213.90; 10 mg (30 units)/mL, 1.5-mL (15-mg, 45-unit) cartridge = £320.85. For use with appropriate *NordiPen®* (JHS) device (available free of charge from clinics). For subcutaneous injection

**NutropinAq®** (Ipsen) (PoM)
Injection, somatropin (rbe), net price 10 mg (30 units) 2-ml cartridge = £207.00. For use with *NutropinAq® Pen* (JHS) device (available free of charge from clinics). For subcutaneous injection

**Omnitrope®** (Sandoz) ▼ (PoM)
Injection, somatropin (rbe) 3.3 mg (10 units)/mL, net price 1.5 mL (5-mg, 15-unit) cartridge = £91.33; 6.7 mg (20 units)/mL, 1.5 mL (10-mg, 30-unit) car-tridge = £182.66. For use with *Omnitrope Pen 5®* (JHS) and *Omnitrope Pen 10®* (JHS) devices respectively (available free of charge from clinics). For subcuta-neous injection
Excipients include benzyl alcohol (in 5-mg cartridge) (avoid in neonates, see Excipients, p. 2)
Note Biosimilar medicine, see p. 1

**Saizen®** (Serono) (PoM)
Injection, powder for reconstitution, somatropin (rmc), net price 1.33-mg (4-unit) vial (with diluent) = £29.28; 3.33-mg (10-unit) vial (with diluent) = £73.20. For subcutaneous or intramuscular injection

Click.easy®, powder for reconstitution, somatropin (rmc), net price 8-mg (24-unit) vial (in *Click.easy®* device with diluent) = £185.44. For use with *One.click®* (JHS) autoinjector device or *Cool.Click®* (JHS) needle-free device (both available free of charge from clinics). For subcutaneous injection

**Zomacton®** (Ferring) (PoM)
Injection, powder for reconstitution, somatropin (rbe), net price 4-mg (12-unit) vial (with diluent) = £79.69, for use with *ZomaJet 2® Vision* (JHS) needle-free device or with *Auto-Jector®* (JHS) (both available free of charge from clinics) or with needles and syringes; 10 mg (30-unit) vial (with diluent) = £199.23, for use with *ZomaJet Vision X®* (JHS) needle-free device

(available free of charge from clinics) or with needles and syringes. For subcutaneous injection
Excipients include benzyl alcohol (in 4-mg vial) (avoid in neonates, see Excipients p. 2)

## Growth hormone receptor antagonists

**Pegvisomant** is a genetically modified analogue of human growth hormone and is a highly selective growth hormone receptor antagonist. Pegvisomant is licensed for the treatment of acromegaly in patients with inade-quate response to surgery, radiation, or both, and to treatment with somatostatin analogues. Pegvisomant should be initiated only by physicians experienced in the treatment of acromegaly.

### ▌ PEGVISOMANT

**Indications** see notes above
**Cautions** liver disease (monitor liver enzymes every 4–6 weeks for 6 months or if symptoms of hepatitis develop); diabetes mellitus (adjustment of antidiabetic therapy may be necessary); possible increase in female fertility
**Contra-indications** pregnancy and breast-feeding
**Side-effects** diarrhoea, constipation, nausea, vomi-ting, abdominal distension, dyspepsia, flatulence, elevated liver enzymes; hypertension; headache, asthenia, dizziness, drowsiness, tremor, sleep distur-bances; influenza-like syndrome, weight gain, hyper-glycaemia, hypoglycaemia; arthralgia, myalgia; injec-tion-site reactions, sweating, pruritus, rash; fatigue; hypercholesterolaemia; less commonly thrombocyto-penia, leucopenia, leucocytosis, bleeding tendency
**Dose**
- By subcutaneous injection, initially 80 mg, then 10 mg daily, increased in steps of 5 mg daily according to response; max. 30 mg daily; CHILD not recommended

**Somavert®** (Pfizer) ▼ (PoM)
Injection, powder for reconstitution, pegvisomant, net price 10-mg vial = £50.00; 15-mg vial = £75.00; 20-mg vial = £100.00 (all with solvent)

## Thyrotrophin

**Thyrotropin alfa** is a recombinant form of thyrotrophin (thyroid stimulating hormone). It is licensed for use with or without radioiodine imaging, together with serum thyroglobulin testing, for the detection of thyroid rem-nants and thyroid cancer in post-thyroidectomy patients. It is also licensed to increase radio-iodine uptake for the ablation of thyroid remnant tissue in suitable post-thyroidectomy patients.

### ▌ THYROTROPIN ALFA
### (Recombinant human thyroid stimulating hormone, rhTSH)

**Indications** see notes above and product literature
**Cautions** presence of thyroglobulin autoantibodies may give false negative results
**Contra-indications** hypersensitivity to bovine or human thyrotropin; pregnancy; breast-feeding
**Side-effects** nausea, vomiting; headache, dizziness, fatigue; *less commonly* asthenia, paraesthesia, back pain, influenza-like symptoms, rash, urticaria; *rarely* diarrhoea; *very rarely* palpitation, flushing, dyspnoea, pain at site of metastases, tremor, arthralgia, myalgia,

hyperhidrosis, and injection-site reactions including pain, pruritus, and rash

**Dose**

- By intramuscular injection into the gluteal muscle, 900 micrograms every 24 hours for 2 doses, consult product literature

**Thyrogen®** (Genzyme) PoM
Injection, powder for reconstitution, thyrotropin alfa 900 micrograms/vial, net price = £297.17

## Hypothalamic hormones

**Gonadorelin** when injected intravenously in normal subjects leads to a rapid rise in plasma concentrations of both luteinising hormone (LH) and follicle-stimulating hormone (FSH). It has not proved to be very helpful, however, in distinguishing hypothalamic from pituitary lesions. **Gonadorelin analogues** are indicated in endometriosis and infertility (section 6.7.2) and in breast and prostate cancer (section 8.3.4).

**Protirelin** is a hypothalamic releasing hormone which stimulates the release of thyrotrophin from the pituitary. It is licensed for the diagnosis of mild hyperthyroidism or hypothyroidism, but its use has been superseded by immunoassays for thyroid-stimulating hormone.

### ▌ GONADORELIN
(Gonadotrophin-releasing hormone; GnRH; LH–RH)

**Indications** see preparations below

**Cautions** pituitary adenoma

**Side-effects** rarely, nausea, headache, abdominal pain, increased menstrual bleeding; rarely, hypersensitivity reaction on repeated administration of large doses; irritation at injection site

**Dose**

- See under preparations

**HRF®** (Intrapharm) PoM
Injection, powder for reconstitution, gonadorelin. Net price 100-microgram vial (with diluent) = £13.72 (hosp. only)
Excipients include benzyl alcohol (avoid in neonates, see Excipients p. 2)
Dose for assessment of pituitary function (adults), by subcutaneous or intravenous injection, 100 micrograms

### ▌ PROTIRELIN
(Thyrotrophin-releasing hormone; TRH)

**Indications** assessment of thyroid function and thyroid stimulating hormone reserve

**Cautions** severe hypopituitarism, myocardial ischaemia, bronchial asthma and obstructive airways disease, pregnancy, breast-feeding (Appendix 5)

**Side-effects** after rapid intravenous administration desire to micturate, flushing, dizziness, nausea, strange taste; transient increase in pulse rate and blood pressure; rarely bronchospasm

**Dose**

- By intravenous injection, 200 micrograms; CHILD under 12 years 1 microgram/kg

**Protirelin** (Cambridge) PoM
Injection, protirelin 100 micrograms/mL. Net price 2-mL amp = £15.15

## 6.5.2 Posterior pituitary hormones and antagonists

## Posterior pituitary hormones

**Diabetes insipidus** Vasopressin (antidiuretic hormone, ADH) is used in the treatment of *pituitary* ('cranial') *diabetes insipidus* as is its analogue **desmopressin**. Dosage is tailored to produce a slight diuresis every 24 hours to avoid water intoxication. Treatment may be required for a limited period only in diabetes insipidus following trauma or pituitary surgery.

Desmopressin is more potent and has a longer duration of action than vasopressin; unlike vasopressin it has no vasoconstrictor effect. It is given by mouth or intranasally for maintenance therapy, and by injection in the postoperative period or in unconscious patients. Desmopressin is also used in the differential diagnosis of diabetes insipidus. Following a dose of 2 micrograms intramuscularly or 20 micrograms intranasally, restoration of the ability to concentrate urine after water deprivation confirms a diagnosis of cranial diabetes insipidus. Failure to respond occurs in nephrogenic diabetes insipidus.

In *nephrogenic* and *partial pituitary diabetes insipidus* benefit may be gained from the paradoxical antidiuretic effect of thiazides (section 2.2.1) e.g. chlortalidone 100 mg twice daily reduced to maintenance dose of 50 mg daily.

Chlorpropamide (section 6.1.2.1) is also useful in partial pituitary diabetes insipidus, and probably acts by sensitising the renal tubules to the action of remaining endogenous vasopressin; it is given in doses of up to 350 mg daily in adults and 200 mg daily in children, care being taken to avoid hypoglycaemia. Carbamazepine (section 4.8.1) is also sometimes useful (in a dose of 200 mg once or twice daily) [unlicensed]; its mode of action may be similar to that of chlorpropamide.

**Other uses** Desmopressin is also used to boost factor VIII concentration in mild to moderate haemophilia and in von Willebrand's disease; it is also used to test fibrinolytic response. For a comment on use of desmopressin in nocturnal enuresis see section 7.4.2.

Vasopressin infusion is used to control variceal bleeding in portal hypertension, prior to more definitive treatment and with variable results. Terlipressin, a derivative of vasopressin, is used similarly.

Oxytocin, another posterior pituitary hormone, is indicated in obstetrics (section 7.1.1).

### ▌ VASOPRESSIN

**Indications** pituitary diabetes insipidus; bleeding from oesophageal varices

**Cautions** heart failure, hypertension, asthma, epilepsy, migraine or other conditions which might be aggravated by water retention; renal impairment (see also Contra-indications); pregnancy (Appendix 4); avoid fluid overload

**Contra-indications** vascular disease (especially disease of coronary arteries) unless extreme caution,

6   Endocrine system

chronic nephritis (until reasonable blood nitrogen concentrations attained)

**Side-effects** fluid retention, pallor, tremor, sweating, vertigo, headache, nausea, vomiting, belching, abdominal cramps, desire to defaecate, hypersensitivity reactions (including anaphylaxis), constriction of coronary arteries (may cause anginal attacks and myocardial ischaemia), peripheral ischaemia and rarely gangrene

**Dose**

- By subcutaneous *or* intramuscular injection, diabetes insipidus, 5–20 units every four hours
- By intravenous infusion, initial control of variceal bleeding, 20 units over 15 minutes

◢ **Synthetic vasopressin**

**Pitressin®** (Goldshield) [PoM]
Injection, argipressin (synthetic vasopressin) 20 units/mL. Net price 1-mL amp = £17.14 (hosp. only)

## DESMOPRESSIN

**Indications** see under Dose

**Cautions** see under Vasopressin; less pressor activity, but still considerable caution in renal impairment (Appendix 3), in cardiovascular disease and in hypertension (not indicated for nocturnal enuresis or nocturia in these circumstances); elderly (avoid for nocturnal enuresis and nocturia in those over 65 years); also considerable caution in cystic fibrosis; in nocturia and nocturnal enuresis limit fluid intake to minimum from 1 hour before to 8 hours afterwards; in nocturia periodic blood pressure and weight checks needed to monitor for fluid overload; pregnancy (Appendix 4) **interactions**: Appendix 1 (desmopressin)

Hyponatraemic convulsions The CSM has advised that patients being treated for primary nocturnal enuresis should be warned to avoid fluid overload (including during swimming) and to stop taking desmopressin during an episode of vomiting or diarrhoea (until fluid balance normal). The risk of hyponatraemic convulsions can also be minimised by keeping to the recommended starting doses and by avoiding concomitant use of drugs which increase secretion of vasopressin (e.g. tricyclic antidepressants)

**Contra-indications** cardiac insufficiency and other conditions treated with diuretics; psychogenic polydipsia and polydipsia in alcohol dependence

**Side-effects** fluid retention, and hyponatraemia (in more serious cases with convulsions) on administration without restricting fluid intake; stomach pain, headache, nausea, vomiting, allergic reactions, and emotional disturbance in children also reported; epistaxis, nasal congestion, rhinitis with nasal spray

**Dose**

- By mouth (as desmopressin acetate)

Diabetes insipidus, treatment, ADULT and CHILD initially 300 micrograms daily (in 3 divided doses); maintenance, 300–600 micrograms daily in 3 divided doses; range 0.2–1.2 mg daily

Primary nocturnal enuresis (if urine concentrating ability normal), ADULT (under 65 years) and CHILD over 5 years (preferably over 7 years) 200 micrograms at bedtime, only increased to 400 micrograms if lower dose not effective (**important:** see also Cautions); withdraw for at least 1 week for reassessment after 3 months

Postoperative polyuria or polydipsia, adjust dose according to urine osmolality

- Sublingually (as desmopressin base)

Diabetes insipidus, treatment, ADULT and CHILD initially 180 micrograms daily in 3 divided doses; range 120–720 micrograms daily

Primary nocturnal enuresis (if urine concentrating ability normal), ADULT (under 65 years) and CHILD over 5 years (preferably over 7 years) 120 micrograms at bedtime, only increased to 240 micrograms if lower dose not effective (**important:** see also Cautions); withdraw for at least 1 week for reassessment after 3 months

Polyuria or polydipsia after hypophysectomy, adjust dose according to urine osmolality

- Intranasally (as desmopressin acetate)

Diabetes insipidus, diagnosis, ADULT and CHILD 20 micrograms (limit fluid intake to 500 mL from 1 hour before to 8 hours after administration)

Diabetes insipidus, treatment, ADULT 10–40 micrograms daily (in 1–2 divided doses); CHILD 5–20 micrograms daily; infants may require lower doses

Nocturia associated with multiple sclerosis (when other treatments have failed), ADULT (under 65 years) 10–20 micrograms at bedtime (**important:** see also Cautions), dose not to be repeated within 24 hours

Renal function testing (empty bladder at time of administration and limit fluid intake to 500 mL from 1 hour before until 8 hours after administration), ADULT 40 micrograms, INFANT under 1 year 10 micrograms (restrict fluid intake to 50% at next 2 feeds to avoid fluid overload), CHILD 1–15 years 20 micrograms

Mild to moderate haemophilia and von Willebrand's disease, ADULT 300 micrograms (one 150-microgram spray into each nostril) 30 minutes before surgery or when bleeding; may be repeated at intervals of 12 hours (or at intervals of at least 3 days if self-administered)

Fibrinolytic response testing, ADULT 300 micrograms (one 150-microgram spray into each nostril); blood sampled after 1 hour for fibrinolytic activity

- By injection (as desmopressin acetate)

Diabetes insipidus, diagnosis (subcutaneous *or* intramuscular), ADULT and CHILD 2 micrograms (limit fluid intake to 500 mL from 1 hour before to 8 hours after administration)

Diabetes insipidus, treatment (subcutaneous, intramuscular *or* intravenous), ADULT 1–4 micrograms daily; INFANT and CHILD 400 nanograms

Renal function testing (empty bladder at time of administration and limit fluid intake to 500 mL from 1 hour before until 8 hours after administration) (subcutaneous *or* intramuscular), ADULT and CHILD 2 micrograms; INFANT 400 nanograms (restrict fluid intake to 50% at next 2 feeds)

Mild to moderate haemophilia and von Willebrand's disease, (subcutaneous *or* intravenous), ADULT and CHILD over 1 month 300 nanograms/kg as a single dose immediately before surgery or after trauma; may be repeated at intervals of 12 hours

Fibrinolytic response testing, (subcutaneous *or* intravenous), ADULT and CHILD 300 nanograms/kg; blood sampled after 20 minutes for fibrinolytic activity

Lumbar-puncture-associated headache, consult product literature

Endocrine system

6

**Desmopressin acetate** (Non-proprietary) PoM
Nasal spray, desmopressin acetate 10 micrograms/ metered spray, net price 6-mL unit (60 metered sprays) = £29.81. Counselling, fluid intake, see above
Brands include Presinex®
Note Children requiring dose of less than 10 micrograms should be given DDAVP® intranasal solution

**DDAVP®** (Ferring) ▼ PoM
Tablets, both scored, desmopressin acetate 100 micrograms, net price 90-tab pack = £44.12; 200 micrograms, 90-tab pack = £88.23. Counselling, fluid intake, see above

Sublingual tablets (DDAVP® Melt), desmopressin (as acetate) 60 micrograms, net price 100-tab pack = £50.53; 120 micrograms, 100-tab pack = £101.07; 240 micrograms, 100-tab pack = £202.14. Label: 26, counselling, fluid intake, see above

Intranasal solution, desmopressin acetate 100 micrograms/mL. Net price 2.5-mL dropper bottle and catheter = £9.72. Counselling, fluid intake, see above

Injection, desmopressin acetate 4 micrograms/mL. Net price 1-mL amp = £1.10

**Desmotabs®** (Ferring) PoM
Tablets, scored, desmopressin acetate 200 micrograms, net price 30-tab pack = £29.43. Counselling, fluid intake, see above

**DesmoMelt®** (Ferring) ▼ PoM
Sublingual tablets, desmopressin (as acetate) 120 micrograms, net price 30-tab pack = £30.34; 240 micrograms, 30-tab pack = £60.68. Label: 26, counselling, fluid intake, see above

**Desmospray®** (Ferring) PoM
Nasal spray, desmopressin acetate 10 micrograms/ metered spray. Net price 6-mL unit (60 metered sprays) = £25.02. Counselling, fluid intake, see above
Note Children requiring dose of less than 10 micrograms should be given DDAVP® intranasal solution

**Octim®** (Ferring) PoM
Nasal spray, desmopressin acetate 150 micrograms/ metered spray, net price 2.5-mL unit (25 metered sprays) = £576.60. Counselling, fluid intake, see above

Injection, desmopressin acetate 15 micrograms/mL, net price 1-mL amp = £19.22

■ **TERLIPRESSIN**

**Indications** bleeding from oesophageal varices
**Cautions** see under Vasopressin
**Contra-indications** see under Vasopressin
**Side-effects** see under Vasopressin, but effects milder
**Dose**
• By intravenous injection, 2 mg followed by 1 or 2 mg every 4 to 6 hours until bleeding is controlled, for up to 72 hours

**Glypressin®** (Ferring) PoM
Injection, terlipressin, powder for reconstitution. Net price 1-mg vial with 5 mL diluent = £18.47 (hosp. only)

## Antidiuretic hormone antagonists

**Demeclocycline** (section 5.1.3) can be used in the treatment of hyponatraemia resulting from inappropriate secretion of antidiuretic hormone, if fluid restriction alone does not restore sodium concentration or is not tolerable. Demeclocycline is thought to act by directly blocking the renal tubular effect of antidiuretic hormone. Initially 0.9–1.2 g is given daily in divided doses, reduced to 600–900 mg daily for maintenance.

## 6.6 Drugs affecting bone metabolism

6.6.1 Calcitonin and parathyroid hormone
6.6.2 Bisphosphonates and other drugs affecting bone metabolism

See also calcium (section 9.5.1.1), phosphorus (section 9.5.2), vitamin D (section 9.6.4), and oestrogens in postmenopausal osteoporosis (section 6.4.1.1).

## Osteoporosis

Osteoporosis occurs most commonly in postmenopausal women and in those taking long-term oral corticosteroids (glucocorticosteroids). Other risk factors for osteoporosis include low body weight, cigarette smoking, excess alcohol intake, lack of physical activity, family history of osteoporosis, and early menopause.

> Those at risk of osteoporosis should maintain an adequate intake of **calcium and vitamin D** and any deficiency should be corrected by increasing dietary intake or taking supplements.

Elderly patients, especially those who are housebound or live in residential or nursing homes, are at increased risk of calcium and vitamin D deficiency and may benefit from supplements (section 9.5.1.1 and section 9.6.4). Reversible secondary causes of osteoporosis such as hyperthyroidism, hyperparathyroidism, osteomalacia or hypogonadism should be excluded, in both men and women, before treatment for osteoporosis is initiated.

**Postmenopausal osteoporosis** The **bisphosphonates** (alendronic acid, disodium etidronate, and risedronate, section 6.6.2) are effective for preventing postmenopausal osteoporosis. **Hormone replacement therapy** (HRT section 6.4.1.1) is an option where other therapies are contra-indicated, cannot be tolerated, or if there is a lack of response. The CSM has advised that HRT should **not** be considered first-line therapy for long-term prevention of osteoporosis in women over 50 years of age. HRT is of most benefit for the prophylaxis of postmenopausal osteoporosis if started early in menopause and continued for up to 5 years, but bone loss resumes (possibly at an accelerated rate) on stopping HRT. **Calcitonin** (section 6.6.1) may be considered for those at high risk of osteoporosis for

6
Endocrine system

whom a bisphosphonate is unsuitable. Women of Afro-Caribbean origin appear to be less susceptible to osteoporosis than those who are white or of Asian origin.

Postmenopausal osteoporosis may be *treated* with a **bisphosphonate** (section 6.6.2). The bisphosphonates (such as alendronate, etidronate, and risedronate) decrease the risk of vertebral fracture; alendronate and risedronate have also been shown to reduce non-vertebral fractures. If bisphosphonates are unsuitable **calcitriol** (section 9.6.4), **calcitonin** or **strontium ranelate** (section 6.6.2) may be considered. Calcitonin [unlicensed indication] may also be useful for pain relief for up to 3 months after a vertebral fracture if other analgesics are ineffective. **Parathyroid hormone**, and **teriparatide** (section 6.6.1) have been introduced for the treatment of postmenopausal osteoporosis.

**Raloxifene** (section 6.4.1.1) is licensed for the *prophylaxis* and *treatment* of vertebral fractures in postmenopausal women.

> **NICE guidance**
> **Alendronate, etidronate, risedronate, raloxifene and strontium ranelate for the primary prevention of osteoporotic fragility fractures in postmenopausal women (October 2008)**
>
> **Alendronate** is recommended as a treatment option for the primary prevention of osteoporotic fractures in the following susceptible postmenopausal women:
> - Women over 70 years who have an independent risk factor for fracture (parental history of hip fracture, alcohol intake of 4 or more units per day, or rheumatoid arthritis) *or* an indicator of low bone mineral density (body mass index under 22 kg/m², ankylosing spondylitis, Crohn's disease, prolonged immobility, untreated premature menopause, or rheumatoid arthritis) **and** confirmed osteoporosis
> - Women aged 65–69 years who have an independent risk factor for fracture **and** confirmed osteoporosis
> - Women under 65 years who have an independent risk factor for fracture **and** at least one additional indicator of low bone mineral density **and** confirmed osteoporosis
>
> **Risedronate** or **etidronate** are recommended as alternatives for women:
> - in whom alendronate is contra-indicated or not tolerated **and**
> - who comply with particular combinations of bone mineral density measurement, age, and independent risk factors for fracture, as indicated in the full NICE guidance[1]
>
> **Strontium ranelate** is recommended as an alternative for women:
> - in whom alendronate and either risedronate or editronate are contra-indicated or not tolerated **and**
> - who comply with particular combinations of bone mineral density measurement, age, and independent risk factors for fracture, as indicated in the full NICE guidance[1]
>
> **Raloxifene** is **not** recommended as a treatment option in postmenopausal women for primary prevention of osteoporotic fractures.

> **NICE guidance**
> **Alendronate, etidronate, risedronate, raloxifene, strontium ranelate, and teriparatide for the secondary prevention of osteoporotic fragility fractures in postmenopausal women (October 2008)**
>
> This guideline recommends treatment options for the secondary prevention of osteoporotic fractures in postmenopausal women with confirmed osteoporosis who have also sustained a clinically apparent osteoporotic fracture.
>
> **Alendronate** is recommended as a treatment option for the secondary prevention of osteoporotic fractures in susceptible postmenopausal women.
>
> **Risedronate** or **etidronate** are recommended as alternatives for women:
> - in whom alendronate is contra-indicated or not tolerated **and**
> - who comply with particular combinations of bone mineral density measurement, age, and independent risk factors for fracture (parental history of hip fracture, alcohol intake of 4 or more units per day, or rheumatoid arthritis, as indicated in the full NICE guidance[2]
>
> **Strontium ranelate** or **raloxifene** are recommended as alternatives for women:
> - in whom alendronate and either risedronate or editronate are contra-indicated or not tolerated **and**
> - who comply with particular combinations of bone mineral density measurement, age, and independent risk factors for fracture, as indicated in the full NICE guidance[2]
>
> **Teriparatide** is recommended as an alternative for women:
> - in whom alendronate and either risedronate or editronate, *or* strontium ranelate are contra-indicated or not tolerated, **or** where treatment with alendronate, risedronate or editronate has been unsatisfactory (indicated by another fragility fracture and a decline in bone mineral density despite treatment for 1 year) **and**
> - who comply with particular combinations of bone mineral density measurement, age, and number of fractures, as indicated in the full NICE guidance[2]

**Corticosteroid-induced osteoporosis** To reduce the risk of osteoporosis doses of oral corticosteroids should be as low as possible and courses of treatment as short as possible. The risk of osteoporosis may be related to cumulative dose of corticosteroids; even intermittent courses can therefore increase the risk. The greatest rate of bone loss occurs during the first 6–12 months of corticosteroid use and so early steps to prevent the development of osteoporosis are important. Long-term use of high-dose inhaled corticosteroids may also contribute to corticosteroid-induced osteoporosis (section 3.2).

Patients taking (or who are likely to take) an oral corticosteroid for 3 months or longer should be assessed and where necessary given prophylactic treatment; those aged over 65 years are at greater risk. Patients taking oral corticosteroids who have sustained a low-trauma fracture should receive treatment for osteoporosis. The therapeutic options for *prophylaxis* and *treatment* of corticosteroid-induced osteoporosis are the same:

- a bisphosphonate (section 6.6.2);
- calcitriol [unlicensed indication] (section 9.6.4);
- hormone replacement (HRT in women (section 6.4.1), testosterone in men [unlicensed indication] (section 6.4.2)).

## 6.6.1 Calcitonin and parathyroid hormone

Calcitonin is involved with parathyroid hormone in the regulation of bone turnover and hence in the maintenance of calcium balance and homoeostasis. **Calcitonin (salmon)** (**salcatonin**, synthetic or recombinant salmon calcitonin) is used to lower the plasma-calcium concentration in some patients with hypercalcaemia (notably when associated with malignant disease). Calcitonin is licensed for treatment of Paget's disease of bone. It can also be used in the prevention and treatment of postmenopausal osteoporosis (see section 6.6).

Recombinant **parathyroid hormone** is used for the treatment of postmenopausal osteoporosis. **Teriparatide** (a recombinant fragment of parathyroid hormone) is used for the treatment of postmenopausal osteoporosis, osteoporosis in men at increased risk of fracture, and corticosteroid-induced osteoporosis. *The Scottish Medicines Consortium*, p. 3 has advised (February 2007) that parathyroid hormone (*Preotact®*) should be initiated by specialists experienced in the treatment of osteoporosis; also that the use of teriparatide (*Forsteo®*) (December 2003) in postmenopausal women should be restricted to the treatment of established (severe) osteoporosis and should be initiated by specialists experienced in the treatment of osteoporosis.

**Cinacalcet** (section 9.5.1.2) is licensed for the treatment of hypercalcaemia in parathyroid carcinoma.

### CALCITONIN (SALMON)/ SALCATONIN

**Indications** see under Dose

**Cautions** history of allergy (skin test advised); renal impairment; heart failure; pregnancy (Appendix 4), breast-feeding (Appendix 5)

**Contra-indications** hypocalcaemia

**Side-effects** nausea, vomiting, diarrhoea, abdominal pain; flushing; dizziness, headache, taste disturbances; musculoskeletal pain; with nasal spray nose and throat irritation, rhinitis, sinusitis and epistaxis; *less commonly* diuresis, oedema, cough, visual disturbances, injection-site reactions, rash, hypersensitivity reactions including pruritus

**Dose**

- Hypercalcaemia of malignancy (see also section 9.5.1.2), ADULT over 18 years, by subcutaneous *or* intramuscular injection, 100 units every 6–8 hours adjusted according to response; max. 400 units every 6–8 hours; in severe or emergency cases, by intravenous infusion, up to 10 units/kg over at least 6 hours
- Paget's disease of bone, ADULT over 18 years, by subcutaneous *or* intramuscular injection, 50 units 3

times weekly to 100 units daily adjusted according to response

- Postmenopausal osteoporosis to reduce risk of vertebral fractures, intranasally, 200 units (1 spray) into one nostril daily, with dietary calcium and vitamin D supplements (section 9.5.1.1 and section 9.6.4)
- Prevention of acute bone loss due to sudden immobility, ADULT over 18 years, by subcutaneous *or* intramuscular injection, 100 units daily in 1–2 divided doses for 2–4 weeks, reduced to 50 units daily at start of mobilisation and continued until fully mobile

**Miacalcic®** (Novartis) [PoM]
Nasal spray ▼, calcitonin (salmon) 200 units/metered spray, net price 2-mL unit (approx. 14 metered sprays) = £20.99

Injection, calcitonin (salmon) 50 units/mL, net price 1-mL amp = £4.27; 100 units/mL, 1-mL amp = £8.55; 200 units/mL, 2-mL vial = £30.75
For subcutaneous or intramuscular injection and for dilution and use as an intravenous infusion

### PARATHYROID HORMONE
(Human recombinant parathyroid hormone)

**Indications** treatment of osteoporosis in postmenopausal women at high risk of fractures (to reduce the risk of vertebral fractures) (see also notes above)

**Cautions** monitor serum or urinary calcium concentration at 1, 3 and 6 months after initiation of treatment (consult product literature for guidance if serum-calcium concentration raised); active or previous urolithiasis; concomitant cardiac glycosides

**Contra-indications** previous radiation therapy to skeleton, pre-existing hypercalcaemia, metabolic bone disease (including hyperparathyroidism and Paget's disease), unexplained raised levels of alkaline phosphatase; avoid in severe hepatic impairment; renal impairment (avoid if eGFR less than 30 mL/minute/1.73 m²; Appendix 3); pregnancy; breast-feeding

**Side-effects** nausea, vomiting, dyspepsia, constipation, diarrhoea; palpitation; headache, dizziness, fatigue, asthenia; transient hypercalcaemia, hypercalciuria; muscle cramp, pain in extremities, back pain; injection-site reactions; *less commonly* abdominal pain, altered sense of smell, taste disturbance, anorexia, influenza, hyperuricaemia

**Dose**

- By subcutaneous injection, 100 micrograms daily, max. duration of treatment 24 months

**Preotact®** (Nycomed) ▼ [PoM]
Injection, dual-chamber cartridge containing powder for reconstitution, parathyroid hormone (rdna) and diluent, net price 1.61-mg (14-dose) cartridge = £130.20. For use with *Preotact®* pen device.

### TERIPARATIDE

**Indications** treatment of osteoporosis in postmenopausal women and in men at increased risk of fractures; treatment of corticosteroid-induced osteoporosis; see also notes above

**Cautions** moderate renal impairment (avoid if severe)

**Contra-indications** pre-existing hypercalcaemia, skeletal malignancies or bone metastases, metabolic bone diseases, including Paget's disease and hyper-

Endocrine system    6

parathyroidism, unexplained raised alkaline phosphatase, previous radiation therapy to the skeleton; pregnancy; breast-feeding

**Side-effects** gastro-intestinal disorders (including nausea, reflux and haemorrhoids); palpitation; dyspnoea; headache, fatigue, asthenia, depression, dizziness, vertigo; anaemia, increased sweating, muscle cramps, sciatica, myalgia, arthralgia; *less commonly* urinary disorders, hypercalcaemia; injection-site reactions; *rarely* hypersensitivity reactions

**Dose**

• By subcutaneous injection, 20 micrograms daily; max. duration of treatment 18 months (course not to be repeated)

**Forsteo®** (Lilly) ▼ PoM

Injection, teriparatide 250 micrograms/mL, net price 3-mL prefilled pen = £271.88

Note 3-ml prefilled pen intended for 28 doses

## 6.6.2 Bisphosphonates and other drugs affecting bone metabolism

**Endocrine system 6**

## Bisphosphonates

Bisphosphonates are adsorbed onto hydroxyapatite crystals in bone, slowing both their rate of growth and dissolution, and therefore reducing the rate of bone turnover. Bisphosphonates have an important role in the prophylaxis and treatment of osteoporosis and corticosteroid-induced osteoporosis; **alendronic acid** or **risedronate sodium** are considered the drugs of choice for these conditions, but **disodium etidronate** may be considered if these drugs are unsuitable or not tolerated (see also section 6.6).

Bisphosphonates are also used in the treatment of *Paget's disease*, hypercalcaemia of malignancy (section 9.5.1.2), and in bone metastases in breast cancer (section 8.3.4.1). Disodium etidronate can impair bone mineralisation when used continuously or in high doses (such as in the treatment of *Paget's disease*).

**Osteonecrosis of the jaw** Osteonecrosis of the jaw has been reported in patients receiving intravenous bisphosphonates and, rarely, in those taking oral bisphosphonates. Adequate oral hygiene should be maintained during and after treatment with bisphosphonates. Ideally in patients with concomitant risk factors (such as cancer, chemotherapy treatment, corticosteroid treatment, or poor oral hygiene), remedial dental work should be carried out before starting bisphosphonate treatment.

### ALENDRONIC ACID

**Indications** see under Dose

**Cautions** upper gastro-intestinal disorders (dysphagia, symptomatic oesophageal disease, gastritis, duodenitis, or ulcers—see also under Contra-indications and Side-effects); history (within 1 year) of ulcers, active gastro-intestinal bleeding, or surgery of the upper gastro-intestinal tract; correct disturbances of calcium and mineral metabolism (e.g. vitamin-D deficiency, hypocalcaemia) before starting and monitor serum-calcium concentration during treatment; consider preventive dental treatment before initiating bisphosphonate (risk of osteonecrosis of the jaw, see notes above); exclude other causes of osteoporosis; atypical stress fractures reported (discontinue unless benefits of continued treatment clearly outweigh risks); **interactions:** Appendix 1 (bisphosphonates)

**Contra-indications** abnormalities of oesophagus and other factors which delay emptying (e.g. stricture or achalasia), hypocalcaemia, renal impairment (avoid if eGFR less than 35 mL/minute/1.73m²; Appendix 3), pregnancy (Appendix 4) and breast-feeding (Appendix 5)

**Side-effects** oesophageal reactions (see below), abdominal pain and distension, dyspepsia, regurgitation, melaena, diarrhoea or constipation, flatulence, musculoskeletal pain, headache; *rarely* rash, pruritus, erythema, photosensitivity, uveitis, scleritis, transient decrease in serum calcium and phosphate; nausea, vomiting, gastritis, peptic ulceration, hypersensitivity reactions (including urticaria and angioedema), and atypical stress fractures with long-term use also reported; myalgia, malaise, and fever at initiation of treatment; *very rarely* severe skin reactions (including Stevens-Johnson syndrome), osteonecrosis (see notes above)

**Oesophageal reactions** Severe oesophageal reactions (oesophagitis, oesophageal ulcers, oesophageal stricture and oesophageal erosions) have been reported; patients should be advised to stop taking the tablets and to seek medical attention if they develop symptoms of oesophageal irritation such as dysphagia, new or worsening heartburn, pain on swallowing or retrosternal pain

**Dose**

• Treatment of postmenopausal osteoporosis and osteoporosis in men, 10 mg daily *or* (in postmenopausal osteoporosis) 70 mg once weekly

• Prevention of postmenopausal osteoporosis, 5 mg daily

• Prevention and treatment of corticosteroid-induced osteoporosis, 5 mg daily (postmenopausal women not receiving hormone replacement therapy, 10 mg daily)

**Counselling** Tablets should be swallowed whole with plenty of water while sitting or standing; to be taken on an empty stomach at least 30 minutes before breakfast (or another oral medicine); patient should stand or sit upright for at least 30 minutes after taking tablet

**Alendronic acid** (Non-proprietary) PoM

Tablets, alendronic acid (as sodium alendronate) 10 mg, net price 28-tab pack = £2.35. Counselling, administration

**Fosamax®** (MSD) PoM

Tablets, alendronic acid (as sodium alendronate) 10 mg, 28-tab pack = £23.12. Counselling, administration

**Alendronic Acid Once-Weekly** (Non-proprietary) PoM

Tablets, alendronic acid (as sodium alendronate) 70 mg, net price 4-tab pack = £3.66. Counselling, administration

**Fosamax® Once Weekly** (MSD) PoM

Tablets, alendronic acid (as sodium alendronate) 70 mg, net price 4-tab pack = £22.80. Counselling, administration

◢**With colecalciferol**

For cautions, contra-indications, and side-effects of colecalciferol, see section 9.6.4

**Fosavance®** (MSD) ▼ PoM

Tablets, alendronic acid (as sodium alendronate) 70 mg, colecalciferol 70 micrograms (2 800 units), net price 4-tab pack = £22.80. Counselling, administration

**Dose** treatment of postmenopausal osteoporosis in women at risk of vitamin D deficiency, 1 tablet once weekly

**Counselling** Tablets should be swallowed whole with plenty of water while sitting or standing; to be taken on an empty stomach at least 30 minutes before breakfast (or another oral medicine); patient should stand or sit upright for at least 30 minutes after taking tablet

## ▮ DISODIUM ETIDRONATE

**Indications** see under Dose

**Cautions** consider preventive dental treatment before initiating bisphosphonate (risk of osteonecrosis of the jaw, see notes above); renal impairment (avoid if moderate to severe; Appendix 3); **interactions:** Appendix 1 (bisphosphonates)

**Contra-indications** pregnancy (Appendix 4) and breast-feeding (Appendix 5); not indicated for osteoporosis in presence of hypercalcaemia or hypercalciuria or for osteomalacia

**Side-effects** nausea, diarrhoea or constipation, abdominal pain; increased bone pain in Paget's disease, also increased risk of fractures with high doses in Paget's disease (discontinue if fractures occur); rarely exacerbation of asthma, skin reactions (including angioedema, rash, urticaria and pruritus), transient hyperphosphataemia, headache, paraesthesia, peripheral neuropathy reported; blood disorders (including leucopenia, agranulocytosis and pancytopenia) also reported; *very rarely* osteonecrosis (see notes above)

**Dose**

- Paget's disease of bone, by mouth, 5 mg/kg as a single daily dose for up to 6 months; doses above 10 mg/kg daily for up to 3 months may be used with caution but doses above 20 mg/kg daily are not recommended; after interval of not less than 3 months may be repeated where evidence of reactivation—including biochemical indices (avoid premature retreatment)

  **Monitoring** Serum phosphate, serum alkaline phosphatase and (if possible) urinary hydroxyproline should be measured before starting and at intervals of 3 months—consult product literature for further details

- Osteoporosis, see under *Didronel PMO®*

  **Counselling** Avoid food for at least 2 hours before and after oral treatment, particularly calcium-containing products e.g. milk; also avoid iron and mineral supplements and antacids

**Didronel®** (Procter & Gamble Pharm.) PoM

Tablets, disodium etidronate 200 mg. Net price 60-tab pack = £19.87. Counselling, food and calcium (see above)

◢**With calcium carbonate**

For cautions and side-effects of calcium carbonate see section 9.5.1.1

**Didronel PMO®** (Procter & Gamble Pharm.) PoM

Tablets, 14 white, disodium etidronate 400 mg; 76 pink, effervescent, calcium carbonate 1.25 g (*Cacit®*). Net price per pack = £20.29. Label: 10, patient

information leaflet, counselling, food and calcium (see above)

**Dose** treatment of osteoporosis, prevention of bone loss in postmenopausal women (particularly if hormone replacement therapy inappropriate), and prevention and treatment of corticosteroid-induced osteoporosis, given in 90-day cycles, 1 *Didronel®* tablet daily for 14 days, then 1 *Cacit®* tablet daily for 76 days

## ▮ DISODIUM PAMIDRONATE

Disodium pamidronate was formerly called aminohydroxypropylidenediphosphonate disodium (APD)

**Indications** see under Dose

**Cautions** renal impairment (Appendix 3); assess renal function before each dose; ensure adequate hydration; hepatic impairment (Appendix 2); cardiac disease (especially in elderly); previous thyroid surgery (risk of hypocalcaemia); monitor serum electrolytes, calcium and phosphate—possibility of convulsions due to electrolyte changes; avoid concurrent use with other bisphosphonates; consider preventive dental treatment before initiating bisphosphonate (risk of osteonecrosis of the jaw, see notes above); **interactions:** Appendix 1 (bisphosphonates)

**Driving** Patients should be warned against driving or operating machinery immediately after treatment (somnolence or dizziness can occur)

**Contra-indications** pregnancy (Appendix 4); breast-feeding (Appendix 5)

**Side-effects** hypophosphataemia, fever and influenza-like symptoms (sometimes accompanied by malaise, rigors, fatigue and flushes); nausea, vomiting, anorexia, abdominal pain, diarrhoea, constipation; symptomatic hypocalcaemia (paraesthesia, tetany), hypomagnesaemia, headache, insomnia, drowsiness; hypertension; anaemia, thrombocytopenia, lymphocytopenia; rash; arthralgia, myalgia, bone pain; *rarely* muscle cramps, dyspepsia, agitation, confusion, dizziness, lethargy; leucopenia, hypotension, pruritus, hyperkalaemia or hypokalaemia, and hypernatraemia; osteonecrosis (see notes above), isolated cases of seizures, hallucinations, haematuria, acute renal failure, deterioration of renal disease, conjunctivitis and other ocular symptoms; atrial fibrillation, and reactivation of herpes simplex and zoster also reported; also injection-site reactions

**Dose**

- By slow intravenous infusion (via cannula in a relatively large vein), see also Appendix 6

  Hypercalcaemia of malignancy, according to serum calcium concentration 15–60 mg in single infusion or in divided doses over 2–4 days; max. 90 mg per treatment course

  Osteolytic lesions and bone pain in bone metastases associated with breast cancer or multiple myeloma, 90 mg every 4 weeks (or every 3 weeks to coincide with chemotherapy in breast cancer)

  Paget's disease of bone, 30 mg once a week for 6 weeks (total dose 180 mg) *or* 30 mg in first week then 60 mg every other week (total dose 210 mg); max. total 360 mg (in divided doses of 60 mg) per treatment course; may be repeated every 6 months

- CHILD not recommended

**Calcium and vitamin D supplements** Oral supplements are advised to minimise potential risk of hypocalcaemia for those with mainly lytic bone metastases or multiple myeloma at risk of calcium or vitamin D deficiency (e.g. through malabsorption or lack of exposure to sunlight) and in those with Paget's disease

6

Endocrine system

**Disodium pamidronate** (Non-proprietary) [PoM]
Concentrate for intravenous infusion, disodium pamidronate 3 mg/mL, net price 5-mL vial = £27.50, 10-mL vial = £55.00; 6 mg/mL, 10-mL vial = £95.00; 9 mg/mL, 10-mL vial = £165.00; 15 mg/mL, 1-mL vial = £29.83, 2-mL vial = £59.66, 4-mL vial = £119.32, 6-mL vial £170.46

**Aredia Dry Powder®** (Novartis) [PoM]
Injection, powder for reconstitution, disodium pamidronate, for use as an infusion. Net price 15-mg vial = £29.83; 30-mg vial = £59.66; 90-mg vial = £170.45 (all with diluent)

## IBANDRONIC ACID

**Indications** see under Dose

**Cautions** consider preventive dental treatment before initiating bisphosphonate (risk of osteonecrosis of the jaw, see notes above); renal impairment (Appendix 3); monitor renal function and serum calcium, phosphate and magnesium; cardiac disease (avoid fluid overload); **interactions:** Appendix 1 (bisphosphonates)

**Contra-indications** pregnancy (Appendix 4); breast-feeding (Appendix 5)

**Side-effects** hypocalcaemia, hypophosphataemia, influenza-like symptoms (including fever, chills, and muscle pain), bone pain; oesophageal reactions (see below), diarrhoea, nausea, vomiting, gastritis, abdominal pain, dyspepsia, pharyngitis; headache, asthenia, rash; *rarely* anaemia, hypersensitivity reactions (pruritus, bronchospasm and angioedema reported); urticaria; injection-site reactions; *very rarely* osteonecrosis (see notes above)

Oesophageal reactions Severe oesophageal reactions reported with all oral bisphosphonates; patients should be advised to stop tablets and seek medical attention for symptoms of oesophageal irritation such as dysphagia, pain on swallowing, retrosternal pain, or heartburn

**Dose**
* Reduction of bone damage in bone metastases in breast cancer, by mouth, 50 mg daily, *or* by intravenous infusion, 6 mg every 3–4 weeks

* Hypercalcaemia of malignancy by intravenous infusion, according to serum calcium concentration, 2–4 mg in single infusion

* Treatment of postmenopausal osteoporosis, by mouth, 150 mg once a month *or* by intravenous injection over 15–30 seconds, 3 mg every 3 months

* CHILD not recommended

Counselling Tablets should be swallowed whole with plenty of water while sitting or standing; to be taken on an empty stomach at least 30 minutes (*Bondronat®* tablets, 50 mg) or 1 hour (*Bonviva®* tablets, 150 mg) before breakfast or another oral medicine; patient should continue to fast, and stand or sit upright for at least 30 minutes (50-mg tablet) or 1 hour (150-mg tablet) after taking tablet

**Bondronat®** (Roche) ▼ [PoM]
Tablets, f/c, ibandronic acid 50 mg, net price 28-tab pack = £187.40. Counselling, administration
Concentrate for intravenous infusion, ibandronic acid 1 mg/mL, net price 2-mL amp = £91.16, 6-mL vial = £187.40

**Bonviva®** (Roche) ▼ [PoM]
Tablets, f/c, ibandronic acid 150 mg, net price 1-tab pack = £18.40, 3-tab pack = £55.21. Counselling, administration
Injection, ibandronic acid 1 mg/mL, net price 3-mL prefilled syringe = £68.64

## RISEDRONATE SODIUM

**Indications** see under Dose

**Cautions** oesophageal abnormalities and other factors which delay transit or emptying (e.g. stricture or achalasia—see also under Side-effects); correct hypocalcaemia before starting, correct other disturbances of bone and mineral metabolism (e.g. vitamin-D deficiency) at onset of treatment; consider preventive dental treatment before initiating bisphosphonate (risk of osteonecrosis of the jaw, see notes above); **interactions:** Appendix 1 (bisphosphonates)

**Contra-indications** hypocalcaemia (see Cautions above); renal impairment (avoid if eGFR less than 30 mL/minute/1.73m²; Appendix 3); pregnancy (Appendix 4); breast-feeding (Appendix 5)

**Side-effects** gastro-intestinal disturbances (including abdominal pain, dyspepsia, nausea, diarrhoea, constipation); dizziness, headache, influenza-like symptoms, musculoskeletal pain; *rarely* oesophageal stricture, oesophagitis, oesophageal ulcer, dysphagia, gastritis, duodenitis, glossitis, peripheral oedema, weight loss, myasthenia, arthralgia, apnoea, bronchitis, sinusitis, rash, nocturia, amblyopia, corneal lesion, dry eye, tinnitus, iritis; *very rarely* hypersensitivity reactions including angioedema, osteonecrosis (see notes above)

**Dose**
* Paget's disease of bone, 30 mg daily for 2 months; may be repeated if necessary after at least 2 months

* Treatment of postmenopausal osteoporosis to reduce risk of vertebral or hip fractures, 5 mg daily *or* 35 mg once weekly

* Prevention of osteoporosis (including corticosteroid-induced osteoporosis) in postmenopausal women, 5 mg daily

* CHILD not recommended

Counselling Swallow tablets whole with full glass of water; on rising, take on an empty stomach at least 30 minutes before first food or drink of the day or, if taking at any other time of the day, avoid food and drink for at least 2 hours before or after risedronate (particularly avoid calcium-containing products e.g. milk; also avoid iron and mineral supplements and antacids); stand or sit upright for at least 30 minutes; do not take tablets at bedtime or before rising

**Actonel®** (Procter & Gamble Pharm.) [PoM]
Tablets, f/c, risedronate sodium 5 mg (yellow), net price 28-tab pack = £18.36; 30 mg (white), 28-tab pack = £146.85. Counselling, administration, food and calcium (see above)

**Actonel Once a Week®** (Procter & Gamble Pharm.) [PoM]
Tablets, f/c, risedronate sodium 35 mg (orange), net price 4-tab pack = £19.51. Counselling, administration, food and calcium (see above)

◢With calcium carbonate and colecalciferol
For cautions, contra-indications, and side-effects of calcium carbonate, see section 9.5.1.1 and of colecalciferol, see section 9.6.4

**Actonel® Combi** (Procter & Gamble Pharm.) [PoM]
Tablets, 4 orange, f/c, risedronate sodium 35 mg (*Actonel Once a Week®*);
Granules, 24 sachets, effervescent, lemon flavour, calcium carbonate 2.5 g (calcium 1 g or Ca²⁺ 25 mmol) and colecalciferol 22 micrograms (880 units), net price

per pack = £19.51. Counselling, administration, food and calcium (see above)

**Dose** treatment of postmenopausal osteoporosis to reduce risk of vertebral or hip fractures, given in weekly cycles, 1 *Actonel Once a Week*® tablet on the first day followed by 1 calcium and colecalciferol sachet daily for 6 days

**Counselling** Tablets should be swallowed whole with plenty of water while sitting or standing; to be taken on an empty stomach at least 30 minutes before breakfast (or another oral medicine); patient should stand or sit upright for at least 30 minutes after taking tablet. Granules should be stirred into a glass of water and after dissolution complete taken immediately

## ▮ SODIUM CLODRONATE

**Indications** see under Dose

**Cautions** monitor renal and hepatic function and white cell count; also monitor serum calcium and phosphate periodically; renal dysfunction reported in patients receiving concomitant NSAIDs; maintain adequate fluid intake during treatment; consider preventive dental treatment before initiating bisphosphonate (risk of osteonecrosis of the jaw, see notes above; renal impairment (avoid if eGFR less than 10 mL/minute/1.73 m²; Appendix 3); **interactions:** Appendix 1 (bisphosphonates)

**Contra-indications** acute gastro-intestinal inflammatory conditions; pregnancy (Appendix 4); breast-feeding (Appendix 5)

**Side-effects** nausea, diarrhoea; skin reactions; bronchospasm; *very rarely* osteonecrosis (see notes above)

**Dose**
- Osteolytic lesions, hypercalcaemia and bone pain associated with skeletal metastases in patients with breast cancer or multiple myeloma, by mouth, 1.6 g daily in single or 2 divided doses increased if necessary to a max. of 3.2 g daily

  **Counselling** Avoid food for 1 hour before and after treatment, particularly calcium-containing products e.g. milk; also avoid iron and mineral supplements and antacids; maintain adequate fluid intake

- Hypercalcaemia of malignancy, by slow intravenous infusion, 300 mg daily for max. 7–10 days *or* by single-dose infusion of 1.5 g

**Bonefos**® (Bayer) [PoM]
Capsules, yellow, sodium clodronate 400 mg, net price 120-cap pack = £142.53. Counselling, food and calcium

Tablets, f/c, scored, sodium clodronate 800 mg, net price 60-tab pack = £149.27. Counselling, food and calcium

**Clasteon**® (Beacon) [PoM]
Capsules, blue/white, sodium clodronate 400 mg, net price 30-cap pack = £40.49, 120-cap pack = £161.97. Counselling, food and calcium

**Loron**® (Roche) [PoM]
Loron 520® tablets, f/c, scored, sodium clodronate 520 mg. Net price 60-tab pack = £155.67. Label: 10, patient information leaflet, counselling, food and calcium

**Dose** 2 tablets daily in single or two divided doses; may be increased to max. 4 tablets daily

## ▮ TILUDRONIC ACID

**Indications** Paget's disease of bone

**Cautions** renal impairment (avoid if eGFR less than 30 mL/minute/1.73 m²; Appendix 3); correct disturbances of calcium metabolism (e.g. vitamin D defi-

ciency, hypocalcaemia) before starting; avoid concomitant use of indometacin; consider preventive dental treatment before initiating bisphosphonate (risk of osteonecrosis of the jaw, see notes above; **interactions:** Appendix 1 (bisphosphonates)

**Contra-indications** juvenile Paget's disease, pregnancy (Appendix 4) and breast-feeding (Appendix 5)

**Side-effects** stomach pain, nausea, diarrhoea; rarely asthenia, dizziness, headache and skin reactions; *very rarely* osteonecrosis (see notes above)

**Dose**
- 400 mg daily as a single dose for 12 weeks; may be repeated if necessary after 6 months

  **Counselling** Avoid food for 2 hours before and after treatment, particularly calcium-containing products e.g. milk; also avoid antacids

**Skelid**® (Sanofi-Synthelabo) [PoM]
Tablets, tiludronic acid (as tiludronate disodium) 200 mg. Net price 28-tab pack = £95.14. Counselling, food and calcium

## ▮ ZOLEDRONIC ACID

**Indications** see under Preparations

**Cautions** correct disturbances of calcium metabolism (e.g. vitamin D deficiency, hypocalcaemia) before starting; monitor serum electrolytes, calcium, phosphate and magnesium; assess renal function before each dose; ensure adequate hydration; renal impairment (Appendix 3); severe hepatic impairment (Appendix 2); cardiac disease (avoid fluid overload); consider preventive dental treatment before initiating bisphosphonate (risk of osteonecrosis of the jaw, see notes above; **interactions:** Appendix 1 (bisphosphonates)

**Contra-indications** pregnancy (Appendix 4), breast-feeding (Appendix 5)

**Side-effects** hypophosphataemia, anaemia, influenza-like symptoms including bone pain, myalgia, arthralgia, fever and rigors; gastro-intestinal disturbances; atrial fibrillation; headache, dizziness, conjunctivitis, renal impairment (rarely acute renal failure); *less commonly* anorexia, taste disturbance, dry mouth, stomatitis, chest pain, hypertension, hypotension, dyspnoea, cough, paraesthesia, tremor, anxiety, lethargy, sleep disturbance, blurred vision, weight gain, pruritus, rash, sweating, muscle cramps, haematuria, proteinuria, urinary frequency, hypersensitivity reactions (including angioedema), asthenia, peripheral oedema, thrombocytopenia, leucopenia, hypomagnesaemia, hypokalaemia, also injection-site reactions; *rarely* bradycardia, confusion, hyperkalaemia, hypernatraemia, pancytopenia, osteonecrosis of the jaw (see also notes above; *very rarely* uveitis and episcleritis

**Dose**
- See under Preparations

**Aclasta**® (Novartis) ▼ [PoM]
Intravenous infusion, zoledronic acid 50 micrograms/mL, net price 100-mL bottle = £283.74

**Dose** Treatment of Paget's disease of bone, by intravenous infusion, 5 mg as a single dose over at least 15 minutes

**Note** At least 500 mg elemental calcium twice daily (with vitamin D, section 9.6.4) for at least 10 days is recommended following infusion

Treatment of postmenopausal osteoporosis and osteoporosis in

6

Endocrine system

men, by intravenous infusion, 5 mg over at least 15 minutes once a year

**Note** In patients with a recent low-trauma hip fracture, the dose should be given 2 or more weeks following hip fracture repair; before first infusion give 50 000–125 000 units of vitamin D (section 9.6.4)

**Note** The *Scottish Medicines Consortium* (p. 3) has advised (February 2008) that in postmenopausal women *Aclasta*® is accepted for restricted use within the NHS Scotland for the treatment of osteoporosis in those for whom oral treatment options for osteoporosis are inappropriate and when initiated by a specialist

### Zometa® (Novartis) ⟨PoM⟩

Concentrate for intravenous infusion, zoledronic acid, 800 micrograms/mL, net price 5-mL (4-mg) vial = £195.00

**Dose** Reduction of bone damage in advanced malignancies involving bone, by intravenous infusion, 4 mg every 3–4 weeks

**Note** Calcium 500 mg daily and vitamin D 400 units daily should also be taken

Hypercalcaemia of malignancy, by intravenous infusion, 4 mg as a single dose

CHILD not recommended

**Note** The *Scottish Medicines Consortium* (p. 3) has advised (May 2003) that for the prevention of skeletal related events *Zometa*® is accepted for restricted use within NHS Scotland for the treatment of patients with breast cancer and multiple myeloma if prescribed by an oncologist

## Strontium ranelate

Strontium ranelate stimulates bone formation and reduces bone resorption. It is licensed for the treatment of postmenopausal osteoporosis. The *Scottish Medicines Consortium* has advised (July 2005) that strontium ranelate should be restricted to use when bisphosphonates are contra-indicated or not tolerated and then only in women aged over 75 years with a previous fracture and low bone mineral density or in other women at equivalent risk.

### ▍ STRONTIUM RANELATE

**Indications** treatment of postmenopausal osteoporosis to reduce risk of vertebral and hip fractures

**Cautions** predisposition to thromboembolism; interferes with colorimetric measurements of calcium in blood and urine; **interactions**: Appendix 1 (strontium ranelate)

**Contra-indications** renal impairment (avoid if eGFR less than 30 mL/minute/1.73 m²; Appendix 3); pregnancy, breast-feeding

**Side-effects** nausea, diarrhoea; venous thromboembolism; headache; dermatitis, eczema; *very rarely* vomiting, abdominal pain, stomatitis, and hypersensitivity reactions, including rash, pruritus, urticaria and angioedema—see Severe Allergic Reactions, below

> **Severe allergic reactions**
> Severe allergic reactions, including drug rash with eosinophilia and systemic symptoms (DRESS), have been reported in patients taking strontium ranelate. DRESS starts with rash, fever, swollen glands, and increased white cell count, and it can affect the liver, kidneys and lungs; DRESS can also be fatal.
> Patients should be advised to stop taking strontium ranelate and consult their doctor immediately if skin rash develops. Treatment with strontium ranelate should not be restarted.

**Dose**

- 2 g once daily in water, preferably at bedtime
  **Counselling** Avoid food for 2 hours before and after taking granules, particularly calcium-containing products e.g. milk; also preferably avoid concomitant antacids containing aluminium and magnesium hydroxides for 2 hours after taking granules

**Protelos®** (Servier) ▼ ⟨PoM⟩

Granules, yellow, strontium ranelate, 2 g/sachet, net price 28-sachets = £25.60. Label: 5, 13, counselling, food and calcium

Excipients include aspartame (section 9.4.1)

## 6.7 Other endocrine drugs

6.7.1 **Bromocriptine and other dopaminergic drugs**
6.7.2 **Drugs affecting gonadotrophins**
6.7.3 **Metyrapone and trilostane**
6.7.4 **Somatomedins**

## 6.7.1 Bromocriptine and other dopaminergic drugs

Bromocriptine is a stimulant of dopamine receptors in the brain; it also inhibits release of prolactin by the pituitary. Bromocriptine is used for the treatment of galactorrhoea, and for the treatment of prolactinomas (when it reduces both plasma prolactin concentration and tumour size). Bromocriptine also inhibits the release of growth hormone and is sometimes used in the treatment of acromegaly, but somatostatin analogues (such as octreotide, section 8.3.4.3) are more effective.

Cabergoline has actions and uses similar to those of bromocriptine, but its duration of action is longer. It has similar side-effects to bromocriptine, however patients intolerant of bromocriptine may be able to tolerate cabergoline (and *vice versa*).

Quinagolide is a non-ergot dopamine $D_2$ agonist; it has actions and uses similar to those of ergot-derived dopamine agonists, but its side-effects differ slightly.

**Cautions** see notes below; also bromocriptine and cabergoline should be used with caution in patients with a history of peptic ulcer, particularly in acromegalic patients. Treatment should be withdrawn if gastro-intestinal bleeding occurs. In hyperprolactinaemic patients, the source of the hyperprolactinaemia should be established (i.e. exclude pituitary tumour before treatment). Gynaecological assessment is recommended annually in premenopausal women (postmenopausal, 6 monthly), preferably including cervical and endometrial cytology. Bromocriptine and cabergoline should be used with caution in patients with Raynaud's syndrome and cardiovascular disease (see also Contra-indications under Bromocriptine, below). Monitor for fibrotic disease (see Fibrotic Reactions, below). Caution is also advised in patients with a history of serious mental disorders (especially psychotic disorders) and in those with acute porphyria (see section 9.8.2). Tolerance may be reduced by alcohol

Endocrine system

6

**Contra-indications** Bromocriptine and cabergoline should not be used in patients with hypersensitivity to ergot alkaloids. They are contra-indicated in those with cardiac valvulopathy (exclude before treatment, see Fibrotic Reactions, below). They should also be avoided in pre-eclampsia (see also Contra-indications under Bromocriptine, below).

**Side-effects** Nausea, constipation, and headache are common side-effects of bromocriptine and cabergoline. Paraesthesia has been reported rarely. Other reported side-effects include hypotension (see also Hypotensive Reactions, below), dyskinesia, pathological gambling, increased libido, hypersexuality, leg cramps, allergic skin reactions, alopecia, and peripheral oedema. Bromocriptine and cabergoline have been associated with pleuritis, pleural effusion, cardiac valvulopathy, pericardial effusion, constrictive pericarditis, and retroperitoneal, pleural, and pulmonary fibrosis (see Fibrotic Reactions).

**Hypotensive reactions** Hypotensive reactions can be disturbing in some patients during the first few days of treatment with bromocriptine, cabergoline, or quinagolide—monitor blood pressure for a few days after starting treatment and following dosage increases; particular care should be exercised when driving or operating machinery.

> **Fibrotic reactions**
>
> Ergot-derived dopamine-receptor agonists, bromocriptine, cabergoline, lisuride [discontinued], and pergolide have been associated with pulmonary, retroperitoneal, and pericardial fibrotic reactions. Exclude cardiac valvulopathy with echocardiography before starting treatment with these ergot derivatives for chronic endocrine disorders (excludes suppression of lactation) or Parkinson's disease; it may also be appropriate to measure the erythrocyte sedimentation rate and serum creatinine and to obtain a chest X-ray. Patients should be monitored for dyspnoea, persistent cough, chest pain, cardiac failure, and abdominal pain or tenderness. If long-term treatment is expected, then lung-function tests may also be helpful. Patients taking cabergoline or pergolide should be regularly monitored for cardiac fibrosis, by echocardiography (within 3–6 months of initiating treatment and subsequently at 6–12 month intervals).

> **Sudden onset of sleep**
>
> Excessive daytime sleepiness and sudden onset of sleep can occur with dopaminergic drugs.
> Patients starting treatment with these drugs should be warned of the possibility of these effects and of the need to exercise caution when driving or operating machinery.
> Patients who have suffered excessive sedation or sudden onset of sleep should refrain from driving or operating machines until those effects have stopped recurring.

**Suppression of lactation** Although bromocriptine and cabergoline are licensed to suppress lactation, they are **not** recommended for routine suppression (or for the relief of symptoms of postpartum pain and engorgement) that can be adequately treated with simple analgesics and breast support. If a dopamine-receptor agonist is required, cabergoline is preferred. Quinagolide is not licensed for the suppression of lactation.

# ■ BROMOCRIPTINE

**Indications** see notes above and under Dose; parkinsonism (section 4.9.1)

**Cautions** see notes above; also specialist evaluation—monitor for pituitary enlargement, particularly during pregnancy; monitor visual field to detect secondary field loss in macroprolactinoma; contraceptive advice if appropriate (oral contraceptives may increase prolactin concentration); avoid breast-feeding for about 5 days if lactation prevention fails; hepatic impairment (Appendix 2); **interactions:** Appendix 1 (bromocriptine)

**Contra-indications** see notes above; also hypertension in postpartum women or in puerperium (see also below)

**Postpartum or puerperium** Should not be used postpartum or in puerperium in women with high blood pressure, coronary artery disease, or symptoms (or history) of serious mental disorder; monitor blood pressure carefully (especially during first few days) in postpartum women. Very rarely hypertension, myocardial infarction, seizures or stroke (both sometimes preceded by severe headache or visual disturbances), and mental disorders have been reported in post-partum women given bromocriptine for lactation suppression—caution with antihypertensive therapy and avoid other ergot alkaloids. Discontinue immediately if hypertension, unremitting headache, or signs of CNS toxicity develop

**Side-effects** see notes above; also drowsiness (see also Sudden Onset of Sleep, above), nasal congestion; *less commonly* vomiting, postural hypotension, fatigue, dizziness, dry mouth; also, particularly with *high doses*, confusion, psychomotor excitation, hallucinations; *rarely* diarrhoea, gastro-intestinal bleeding, gastric ulcer, abdominal pain, tachycardia, bradycardia, arrhythmia, insomnia, psychosis, visual disturbances, tinnitus; *very rarely* vasospasm of fingers and toes particularly in patients with Raynaud's syndrome, and effects like neuroleptic malignant syndrome on withdrawal; urinary incontinence, leucopenia, thrombocytopenia, hyponatraemia, reversible hearing loss, increased libido, and hypersexuality also reported

**Dose**

- Prevention or suppression of lactation (but see notes above and under Cautions), 2.5 mg on day 1 (prevention) or daily for 2–3 days (suppression); then 2.5 mg twice daily for 14 days
- Hypogonadism, galactorrhoea, infertility, initially 1–1.25 mg at bedtime, increased gradually; usual dose 7.5 mg daily in divided doses, increased if necessary to max. 30 mg daily, usual dose in infertility without hyperprolactinaemia, 2.5 mg twice daily
- Acromegaly, initially 1–1.25 mg at bedtime, increase gradually to 5 mg every 6 hours
- Prolactinoma, initially 1–1.25 mg at bedtime; increased gradually to 5 mg every 6 hours (occasional patients may require up to 30 mg daily)
- CHILD under 15 years, not recommended

**Bromocriptine** (Non-proprietary) ▢PoM▢
Tablets, bromocriptine (as mesilate) 2.5 mg, net price 30-tab pack = £18.90. Label: 21, counselling, hypotensive reactions, driving, see notes above

**Parlodel®** (Meda) ▢PoM▢
Tablets, both scored, bromocriptine (as mesilate) 1 mg, net price 100-tab pack = £9.90; 2.5 mg, 30-tab

pack = £4.00. Label: 21, counselling, hypotensive reactions, driving, see notes above

Capsules, bromocriptine (as mesilate) 5 mg (blue/white), net price 100-cap pack = £37.57; 10 mg (white), 100-cap pack = £69.50. Label: 21, counselling, hypotensive reactions, driving, see notes above

## CABERGOLINE

**Indications** see notes above and under Dose

**Cautions** see notes above; also severe hepatic impairment (Appendix 2); monthly pregnancy tests during the amenorrhoeic period; advise non-hormonal contraception if pregnancy not desired (see also Contra-indications, below); **interactions:** Appendix 1 (cabergoline)

**Contra-indications** see notes above; history of puerperal psychosis; exclude pregnancy before starting and discontinue 1 month before intended conception (ovulatory cycles persist for 6 months)—discontinue if pregnancy occurs during treatment (specialist advice needed; Appendix 4); avoid breast-feeding if lactation prevention fails (Appendix 5); history of pulmonary, pericardial, or retroperitoneal fibrotic disorders (see Fibrotic Reactions in notes above); cardiac valvulopathy

**Side-effects** see notes above; also drowsiness (see also Sudden Onset of Sleep, above), dyspepsia, gastritis, epigastric and abdominal pain, angina, syncope, depression, confusion, hallucinations, breast pain; *rarely* vomiting, palpitation, epistaxis, digital vasospasm, hot flushes, transient hemianopia, muscle weakness; *also reported* cardiac valvulopathy, erythromelalgia

**Dose**

- Prevention of lactation (but see notes above and under Contra-indications), during first day postpartum, 1 mg as a single dose; suppression of established lactation (but see notes above) 250 micrograms every 12 hours for 2 days
- Hyperprolactinaemic disorders, 500 micrograms weekly (as a single dose *or* as 2 divided doses on separate days) increased at monthly intervals in steps of 500 micrograms until optimal therapeutic response (usually 1 mg weekly, range 0.25–2 mg weekly) with monthly monitoring of serum prolactin levels; reduce initial dose and increase more gradually if patient intolerant; over 1 mg weekly give as divided doses; up to 4.5 mg weekly has been used in hyperprolactinaemic patients
- Parkinsonism, section 4.9.1
- CHILD under 16 years, not recommended

**Cabergoline** (Non-proprietary) ⒫ⓄⓂ
Tablet, scored, cabergoline 500 micrograms, net price 8-tab pack = £30.51. Label: 21, counselling, hypotensive reactions, driving, see notes above
**Note** Dispense in original container (contains desiccant)

**Dostinex®** (Pharmacia) ⒫ⓄⓂ
Tablets, scored, cabergoline 500 micrograms. Net price 8-tab pack = £30.04. Label: 21, counselling, hypotensive reactions, driving, see notes above
**Note** Dispense in original container (contains desiccant)

## QUINAGOLIDE

**Indications** see notes above and under Dose

**Cautions** see notes above; history of psychotic illness; advise non-hormonal contraception if pregnancy not desired; discontinue if pregnancy occurs during treatment (specialist advice needed; Appendix 4); **interactions:** Appendix 1 (quinagolide)

**Contra-indications** hypersensitivity to quinagolide (but not ergot alkaloids); hepatic impairment (Appendix 2); renal impairment (Appendix 3); breast-feeding (Appendix 5)

**Side-effects** nausea, vomiting, anorexia, abdominal pain, constipation or diarrhoea; syncope, hypotension (see also notes above), oedema, flushing, nasal congestion; headache, dizziness, fatigue, insomnia; *rarely* sudden onset of sleep (see notes above); *very rarely* psychosis

**Dose**

- Hyperprolactinaemia, 25 micrograms at bedtime for 3 days; increased at intervals of 3 days in steps of 25 micrograms to usual maintenance dose of 75–150 micrograms daily; for doses higher than 300 micrograms daily increase in steps of 75–150 micrograms at intervals of not less than 4 weeks; CHILD not recommended

**Norprolac®** (Ferring) ⒫ⓄⓂ
Tablets, quinagolide (as hydrochloride) 75 micrograms (white), net price 30-tab pack = £27.00; starter pack of 3 × 25-microgram tabs (pink) with 3 × 50-microgram tabs (blue) = £4.50. Label: 21, counselling, hypotensive reactions, driving, see notes above

## 6.7.2 Drugs affecting gonadotrophins

**Danazol** inhibits pituitary gonadotrophins; it combines androgenic activity with antioestrogenic and antiprogestogenic activity. It is licensed for the treatment of *endometriosis* and for the relief of severe pain and tenderness in *benign fibrocystic breast disease* where other measures have proved unsatisfactory. It may also be effective in the long-term management of *hereditary angioedema* [unlicensed indication].

**Gestrinone** has general actions similar to those of danazol and is indicated for the treatment of endometriosis.

**Cetrorelix** and **ganirelix** are luteinising hormone releasing hormone antagonists, which inhibit the release of gonadotrophins (luteinising hormone and follicle-stimulating hormone). They are used in the treatment of infertility by assisted reproductive techniques.

## CETRORELIX

**Indications** adjunct in the treatment of female infertility (under specialist supervision)

**Contra-indications** moderate to severe hepatic impairment (Appendix 2); moderate to severe renal impairment (Appendix 3); pregnancy; breast-feeding (Appendix 5)

**Side-effects** nausea, headache, injection site reactions; rarely hypersensitivity reactions

**Dose**

• By subcutaneous injection into the lower abdominal wall,

*either* 250 micrograms in the morning, starting on day 5 or 6 of ovarian stimulation with gonadotrophins (*or* each evening starting on day 5 of ovarian stimulation); continue throughout administration of gonadotrophin including day of ovulation induction (*or* evening before ovulation induction)

*or* 3 mg on day 7 of ovarian stimulation with gonadotrophins; if ovulation induction not possible on day 5 after 3-mg dose, additional 250 micrograms once daily until day of ovulation induction

**Cetrotide®** (Serono) ᴘᴏᴹ
Injection, powder for reconstitution, cetrorelix (as acetate), net price 250-micrograms vial = £23.06; 3-mg vial = £161.42 (both with solvent)

---

### ▌ DANAZOL

**Indications** see notes above and under Dose

**Cautions** cardiac, hepatic, or renal impairment (avoid if severe), elderly, polycythaemia, epilepsy, diabetes mellitus, hypertension, migraine, lipoprotein disorder, history of thrombosis or thromboembolic disease; withdraw if virilisation (may be irreversible on continued use); non-hormonal contraceptive methods should be used, if appropriate; **interactions:** Appendix 1 (danazol)

**Contra-indications** pregnancy (Appendix 4), ensure that patients with amenorrhoea are not pregnant; breast-feeding (Appendix 5); severe hepatic, renal or cardiac impairment; thromboembolic disease; undiagnosed genital bleeding; androgen-dependent tumours; acute porphyria (section 9.8.2)

**Side-effects** nausea, dizziness, skin reactions including rashes, photosensitivity and exfoliative dermatitis, fever, backache, nervousness, mood changes, anxiety, changes in libido, vertigo, fatigue, epigastric and pleuritic pain, headache, weight gain; menstrual disturbances, vaginal dryness and irritation, flushing and reduction in breast size; musculo-skeletal spasm, joint pain and swelling, hair loss; androgenic effects including acne, oily skin, oedema, hirsutism, voice changes and rarely clitoral hypertrophy (see also Cautions); temporary alteration in lipoproteins and other metabolic changes, insulin resistance; thrombotic events; leucopenia, thrombocytopenia, eosinophilia, reversible erythrocytosis or polycythaemia reported; headache and visual disturbances may indicate benign intracranial hypertension; rarely cholestatic jaundice, pancreatitis, peliosis hepatis and benign hepatic adenomata

**Dose**

**Note** In women of child-bearing potential, treatment should start during menstruation, preferably on day 1

• Endometriosis, 200–800 mg daily in up to 4 divided doses, adjusted to achieve amenorrhoea, usually for 3–6 months

• Severe pain and tenderness in benign fibrocystic breast disease not responding to other treatment, 300 mg daily in divided doses usually for 3–6 months

• Hereditary angioedema [unlicensed indication], initially 200 mg 2–3 times daily, then reduced according to response

**Danazol** (Non-proprietary) ᴘᴏᴹ
Capsules, danazol 100 mg, net price 28-cap pack = £18.63, 60-cap pack = £17.04; 200 mg, 56-cap pack = £66.75

**Danol®** (Sanofi-Synthelabo) ᴘᴏᴹ
Capsules, danazol 100 mg (grey/white), net price 60-cap pack = £16.38; 200 mg (pink/white), 60-cap pack = £32.43

---

### ▌ GANIRELIX

**Indications** adjunct in the treatment of female infertility (under specialist supervision)

**Contra-indications** moderate hepatic impairment (Appendix 2); moderate to severe renal impairment (Appendix 3); pregnancy (Appendix 4); breast-feeding (Appendix 5)

**Side-effects** nausea, headache, malaise, injection-site reactions; *very rarely* hypersensitivity reactions including rash, facial oedema, and dyspnoea also reported

**Dose**

• By subcutaneous injection preferably into the upper leg (rotate injection sites to prevent lipoatrophy), 250 micrograms in the morning (or each afternoon) starting on day 6 of ovarian stimulation with gonadotrophins; continue throughout administration of gonadotrophin including day of ovulation induction (if administering in afternoon, give last dose in afternoon *before* ovulation induction)

**Orgalutran®** (Organon) ᴘᴏᴹ
Injection, ganirelix, 500 micrograms/mL, net price 0.5-mL prefilled syringe = £21.90

---

### ▌ GESTRINONE

**Indications** endometriosis

**Cautions** cardiac dysfunction; renal impairment (avoid in severe impairment; Appendix 3); **interactions:** Appendix 1 (gestrinone)

**Contra-indications** pregnancy (use non-hormonal method of contraception); breast-feeding (Appendix 5); severe cardiac or hepatic impairment; metabolic or vascular disorders associated with previous sex hormone treatment

**Side-effects** spotting; acne, oily skin, fluid retention, weight gain, hirsutism, voice change; liver enzyme disturbances; headache; gastro-intestinal disturbances; change in libido, flushing, decrease in breast size; nervousness, depression, change in appetite; muscle cramp

**Dose**

• 2.5 mg twice weekly starting on first day of cycle with second dose 3 days later, repeated on same two days preferably at same time each week; duration of treatment usually 6 months

**Missed doses** One missed dose—2.5 mg as soon as possible and maintain original sequence; two or more missed doses—discontinue, re-start on first day of new cycle (following negative pregnancy test)

**Dimetriose®** (Sanofi-Aventis) ᴘᴏᴹ
Capsules, gestrinone 2.5 mg, net price 8-cap pack = £99.86

---

## Gonadorelin analogues

Administration of **gonadorelin analogues** produces an initial phase of stimulation; continued administration is followed by down-regulation of gonadotrophin-releasing hormone receptors, thereby reducing the release of gonadotrophins (follicle stimulating hormone and luteinising hormone) which in turn leads to inhibition of androgen and oestrogen production.

Gonadorelin analogues are used in the treatment of endometriosis, precocious puberty, infertility, anaemia due to uterine fibroids (together with iron supplementation), breast cancer (section 8.3.4.1), prostate cancer (section 8.3.4.2) and before intra-uterine surgery. Use of leuprorelin and triptorelin for 3 to 4 months before surgery reduces the uterine volume, fibroid size and associated bleeding. For women undergoing hysterectomy or myomectomy, a vaginal procedure is made more feasible following the use of a gonadorelin analogue.

**Cautions** Non-hormonal, barrier methods of contraception should be used during entire treatment period with gonadorelin analogues; also use with caution in patients with metabolic bone disease because decrease in bone mineral density can occur.

**Contra-indications** Gonadorelin analogues are contra-indicated for use longer than 6 months in the treatment of endometriosis (do not repeat), where there is undiagnosed vaginal bleeding, in pregnancy (Appendix 4; exclude pregnancy—also give first injection during menstruation or shortly afterwards or use barrier contraception for 1 month beforehand) and in breast-feeding.

**Side-effects** Side-effects of the gonadorelin analogues related to the inhibition of oestrogen production include menopausal-like symptoms (e.g. hot flushes, increased sweating, vaginal dryness, dyspareunia and loss of libido) and a decrease in trabecular bone density; these effects can be reduced by hormone replacement (e.g. with an oestrogen and a progestogen or with tibolone). Side-effects of gonadorelin analogues also include headache (rarely migraine) and hypersensitivity reactions including urticaria, pruritus, rash, asthma and anaphylaxis; when treating uterine fibroids, bleeding associated with fibroid degeneration can occur; spray formulations can cause irritation of the nasal mucosa including nose bleeds; local reactions at injection site can occur; other side-effects also reported with some gonadorelin analogues include palpitation, hypertension, ovarian cysts (may require withdrawal), changes in breast size, musculoskeletal pain or weakness, visual disturbances, paraesthesia, changes in scalp and body hair, oedema of the face and extremities, weight changes, and mood changes including depression.

## BUSERELIN

**Indications** see under Dose; prostate cancer (section 8.3.4.2)

**Cautions** see notes above; polycystic ovarian disease, depression, hypertension, diabetes

**Contra-indications** see notes above; hormone-dependent tumours

**Side-effects** see notes above; initially withdrawal bleeding and subsequently breakthrough bleeding, leucorrhoea; nausea, vomiting, constipation, diarrhoea; anxiety, memory and concentration disturbances, sleep disturbances, nervousness, dizziness, drowsiness; breast tenderness, lactation; abdominal pain; fatigue; increased thirst, changes in appetite;

acne, dry skin, splitting nails, dry eyes; altered blood lipids, leucopenia, thrombocytopenia; hearing disturbances; reduced glucose tolerance

**Dose**

- Endometriosis, intranasally, 300 micrograms (one 150-microgram spray in each nostril) 3 times daily (starting on days 1 or 2 of menstruation); max. duration of treatment 6 months (do not repeat)
- Pituitary desensitisation before induction of ovulation by gonadotrophins for *in vitro* fertilisation (under specialist supervision), by subcutaneous injection, 200–500 micrograms daily given as a single injection (occasionally up to 500 micrograms twice daily may be needed) starting in early follicular phase (day 1) *or*, after exclusion of pregnancy, in midluteal phase (day 21) and continued until down-regulation achieved (usually about 1–3 weeks) then maintained during gonadotrophin administration (stopping gonadotrophin and buserelin on administration of chorionic gonadotrophin at appropriate stage of follicular development)

  Intranasally, 150 micrograms (one spray in one nostril) 4 times daily during waking hours (occasionally up to 300 micrograms 4 times daily may be needed) starting in early follicular phase (day 1) *or*, after exclusion of pregnancy, in midluteal phase (day 21) and continued until down-regulation achieved (usually about 2–3 weeks) then maintained during gonadotrophin administration (stopping gonadotrophin and buserelin on administration of chorionic gonadotrophin at appropriate stage of follicular development)

  **Counselling** Avoid use of nasal decongestants before and for at least 30 minutes after treatment

**Suprecur®** (Aventis Pharma) ▣PoM▣
Nasal spray, buserelin (as acetate) 150 micrograms/metered spray. Net price 2 × 100-dose pack (with metered dose pumps) = £87.63. Counselling, nasal decongestants

Injection, buserelin (as acetate) 1 mg/mL. Net price 5.5-mL vial = £13.76

## GOSERELIN

**Indications** see under Dose; prostate cancer (section 8.3.4.2); early and advanced breast cancer (section 8.3.4.1)

**Cautions** see notes above; polycystic ovarian disease; diabetes

**Contra-indications** see notes above; breast-feeding (Appendix 5)

**Side-effects** see notes above; withdrawal bleeding

**Dose**

- By subcutaneous injection into anterior abdominal wall (as *Zoladex®*)

  Endometriosis, 3.6 mg every 28 days; max. duration of treatment 6 months (do not repeat)

  Endometrial thinning before intra-uterine surgery, 3.6 mg (may be repeated after 28 days if uterus is large or to allow flexible surgical timing)

  Before surgery in women who have anaemia due to uterine fibroids, 3.6 mg every 28 days (with supplementary iron); max. duration of treatment 3 months

  Pituitary desensitisation before induction of ovulation by gonadotrophins for *in vitro* fertilisation (under specialist supervision), after exclusion of pregnancy, 3.6 mg to achieve pituitary down-regulation (usually

1–3 weeks) then gonadotrophin is administered (stopping gonadotrophin on administration of chorionic gonadotrophin at appropriate stage of follicular development)

◀**Preparation**
Section 8.3.4.2

## ▮ LEUPRORELIN ACETATE

**Indications** see under Dose; prostate cancer (section 8.3.4.2)

**Cautions** see notes above; monitor liver function; family history of osteoporosis; chronic use of other drugs which reduce bone density including alcohol and tobacco; diabetes

**Contra-indications** see notes above; pregnancy(Appendix 4); breast-feeding (Appendix 5)

**Side-effects** see notes above; breast tenderness; nausea, vomiting, diarrhoea, anorexia; fever, chills; sleep disturbances, dizziness, fatigue, leucopenia, thrombocytopenia, altered blood lipids, pulmonary embolism; spinal fracture, paralysis, hypotension and worsening of depression also reported

**Dose**
- By subcutaneous *or* intramuscular injection (as *Prostap® SR*)
Endometriosis, 3.75 mg as a single dose in first 5 days of menstrual cycle then every month for max. 6 months (course not to be repeated)
Endometrial thinning before intra-uterine surgery, 3.75 mg as a single dose (given between days 3 and 5 of menstrual cycle) 5–6 weeks before surgery
Reduction of size of uterine fibroids and of associated bleeding before surgery, 3.75 mg as a single dose every month usually for 3–4 months (max. 6 months)
- By intramuscular injection (as *Prostap® 3*)
Endometriosis, 11.25 mg as a single dose in first 5 days of menstrual cycle then every 3 months for max. 6 months (course not to be repeated)

◀**Preparations**
Section 8.3.4.2

## ▮ NAFARELIN

**Indications** see under Dose
**Cautions** see notes above
**Contra-indications** see notes above
**Side-effects** see notes above; acne
**Dose**
- Endometriosis, women over 18 years, 200 micrograms twice daily as one spray in one nostril in the morning and one spray in the other nostril in the evening (starting on days 2–4 of menstruation), max. duration of treatment 6 months (do not repeat)
- Pituitary desensitisation before induction of ovulation by gonadotrophins for *in vitro* fertilisation (under specialist supervision), 400 micrograms (one spray in each nostril) twice daily starting in early follicular phase (day 2) or, after exclusion of pregnancy, in midluteal phase (day 21) and continued until down-regulation achieved (usually within 4 weeks) then maintained (usually for 8–12 days) during gonadotrophin administration (stopping gonadotrophin and nafarelin on administration of chorionic gonadotro-

phin at follicular maturity); discontinue if down-regulation not achieved within 12 weeks
**Counselling** Avoid use of nasal decongestants before and for at least 30 minutes after treatment; repeat dose if sneezing occurs during or immediately after administration

**Synarel®** (Pharmacia) P̲o̲M̲
Nasal spray, nafarelin (as acetate) 200 micrograms/metered spray. Net price 30-dose unit = £32.28; 60-dose unit = £55.66. Label: 10, patient information leaflet, counselling, see above

## ▮ TRIPTORELIN

**Indications** endometriosis, precocious puberty, reduction in size of uterine fibroids; advanced prostate cancer (section 8.3.4.2)

**Cautions** see notes above
**Contra-indications** see notes above
**Side-effects** see notes above; also gastro-intestinal disturbances; in precocious puberty, withdrawal bleeding may occur in the first month of treatment; asthenia
**Dose**
- See under preparations below

**Decapeptyl® SR** (Ipsen) P̲o̲M̲
Injection, (powder for suspension), m/r, triptorelin (as acetate), net price 3-mg vial (with diluent) = £69.00
Dose by intramuscular injection, endometriosis and reduction in size of uterine fibroids, 3 mg every 4 weeks starting during first 5 days of menstrual cycle; for uterine fibroids continue treatment for at least 3 months; max. duration of treatment 6 months (not to be repeated)
Note Each vial includes an overage to allow accurate administration of 3-mg dose

Injection, (powder for suspension), m/r, triptorelin (as acetate), net price 11.25-mg vial (with diluent) = £207.00
Dose by intramuscular injection, endometriosis, 11.25 mg every 3 months starting during first 5 days of menstrual cycle; max. duration of treatment 6 months (not to be repeated)
Precocious puberty, 11.25 mg every 3 months; discontinue when bone maturation consistent with age of 12 years in girls or 13–14 years in boys
Note Each vial includes an overage to allow accurate administration of 11.25-mg dose

**Gonapeptyl Depot®** (Ferring) P̲o̲M̲
Injection, (powder for suspension), triptorelin (as acetate), net price 3.75-mg prefilled syringe (with prefilled syringe of vehicle) = £81.69
Dose by subcutaneous or deep intramuscular injection, endometriosis and reduction in size of uterine fibroids, 3.75 mg every 4 weeks starting during first 5 days of menstrual cycle; max. duration of treatment 6 months (not to be repeated)
Precocious puberty, body-weight over 30 kg, initially 3.75 mg every 2 weeks for 3 doses, then every 3–4 weeks; body-weight 20–30 kg, initially 2.5 mg every 2 weeks for 3 doses, then every 3–4 weeks; body-weight under 20 kg, initially 1.875 mg every 2 weeks for 3 doses, then every 3–4 weeks; discontinue when bone maturation consistent with age over 12 years in girls or over 13 years in boys

## Breast pain (mastalgia)

Once any serious underlying cause for breast pain has been ruled out, most women will respond to reassurance and reduction in dietary fat; withdrawal of an oral contraceptive or of hormone replacement therapy may help to resolve the pain.

Mild, non-cyclical breast pain is treated with simple analgesics (section 4.7.1); moderate to severe pain,

**6**

**Endocrine system**

cyclical pain or symptoms that persist for longer than 6 months may require specific drug treatment.

**Danazol** (section 6.7.2) is licensed for the relief of severe pain and tenderness in benign fibrocystic breast disease which has not responded to other treatment.

**Tamoxifen** (section 8.3.4.1) may be a useful adjunct in the treatment of mastalgia [unlicensed indication] especially when symptoms can definitely be related to cyclic oestrogen production; it may be given on the days of the cycle when symptoms are predicted.

Treatment for breast pain should be reviewed after 6 months and continued if necessary. Symptoms recur in about 50% of women within 2 years of withdrawal of therapy but may be less severe.

### 6.7.3 Metyrapone and trilostane

**Metyrapone** is a competitive inhibitor of 11β-hydroxylation in the adrenal cortex; the resulting inhibition of cortisol (and to a lesser extent aldosterone) production leads to an increase in ACTH production which, in turn, leads to increased synthesis and release of cortisol precursors. It may be used as a test of anterior pituitary function.

Although most types of *Cushing's syndrome* are treated surgically, that which occasionally accompanies carcinoma of the bronchus is not usually amenable to surgery. Metyrapone has been found helpful in controlling the symptoms of the disease; it is also used in other forms of Cushing's syndrome to prepare the patient for surgery. The dosages used are either low, and tailored to cortisol production, or high, in which case corticosteroid replacement therapy is also needed.

**Trilostane** reversibly inhibits 3β-hydroxysteroid dehydrogenase / delta 5–4 isomerase in the adrenal cortex; the resulting inhibition of the synthesis of mineralocorticoids and glucocorticoids used in *Cushing's syndrome* and *primary hyperaldosteronism*. Trilostane appears to be less effective than metyrapone for Cushing's syndrome (where it is tailored to corticosteroid production). It also has a minor role in postmenopausal breast cancer that has relapsed following initial oestrogen antagonist therapy (corticosteroid replacement therapy is also required). **Ketoconazole** (section 5.2) is also used by specialists for the management of *Cushing's syndrome* [unlicensed indication].

#### ▌ METYRAPONE

**Indications** see notes above and under Dose (specialist supervision in hospital)

**Cautions** gross hypopituitarism (risk of precipitating acute adrenal failure); hypertension on long-term administration; hypothyroidism or hepatic impairment (delayed response); many drugs interfere with diagnostic estimation of steroids; avoid in acute porphyria (section 9.8.2)
   **Driving** Drowsiness may affect the performance of skilled tasks (e.g. driving)

**Contra-indications** adrenocortical insufficiency (see Cautions); pregnancy (Appendix 4), breast-feeding (Appendix 5)

**Side-effects** occasional nausea, vomiting, dizziness, headache, hypotension, sedation; rarely abdominal pain, allergic skin reactions, hypoadrenalism, hirsutism

**Dose**

* Differential diagnosis of ACTH-dependent Cushing's syndrome, 750 mg every 4 hours for 6 doses; CHILD 15 mg/kg (minimum 250 mg) every 4 hours for 6 doses

* Management of Cushing's syndrome, range 0.25–6 g daily, tailored to cortisol production; see notes above

* Resistant oedema due to increased aldosterone secretion in cirrhosis, nephrotic syndrome, and congestive heart failure (with glucocorticoid replacement therapy) 3 g daily in divided doses

**Metopirone®** (Alliance) [PoM]
   Capsules, ivory, metyrapone 250 mg. Net price 100-tab pack = £38.88. Label: 21, counselling, driving

#### ▌ TRILOSTANE

**Indications** see notes above and under Dose (specialist supervision)

**Cautions** breast cancer (concurrent corticosteroid replacement therapy needed, see under Dose), adrenal cortical hyperfunction (tailored to cortisol and electrolytes, concurrent corticosteroid therapy may be needed, see under Dose); hepatic and renal impairment; **interactions**: Appendix 1 (trilostane)

**Contra-indications** pregnancy (use non-hormonal method of contraception; Appendix 4); breast-feeding; children

**Side-effects** flushing, tingling and swelling of mouth, rhinorrhoea, nausea, vomiting, diarrhoea, and rashes reported; rarely granulocytopenia

**Dose**

* Adrenal cortical hyperfunction, 240 mg daily in divided doses for at least 3 days then tailored according to response with regular monitoring of plasma electrolytes and circulating corticosteroids (both mineralocorticoid and glucocorticoid replacement therapy may be needed); usual dose: 120–480 mg daily (may be increased to 960 mg)

* Postmenopausal breast cancer (with glucocorticoid replacement therapy) following relapse to initial oestrogen receptor antagonist therapy, initially 240 mg daily increased every 3 days in steps of 240 mg to a maintenance dose of 960 mg daily (720 mg daily if not tolerated)

**Modrenal®** (Bioenvision) [PoM]
   Capsules, trilostane 60 mg (pink/black), net price 100-cap pack = £49.50; 120 mg (pink/yellow), 100-cap pack = £98.50. Label: 21

### 6.7.4 Somatomedins

Somatomedins are a group of polypeptide hormones structurally related to insulin and commonly known as insulin-like growth factors (IGFs). **Mecasermin**, a human insulin-like growth factor-I (rhIGF-I), is the principal mediator of the somatotropic effects of human growth hormone and is used to treat growth failure in children and adolescents with severe primary insulin-like growth factor-I deficiency.

## MECASERMIN
(Recombinant human insulin-like growth factor-I; rhIGF-I)

**Indications** see notes above

**Cautions** correct hypothyroidism before initiating treatment; diabetes mellitus (adjustment of antidiabetic therapy may be necessary), monitor ECG before and on termination of treatment (and during treatment if ECG abnormal), papilloedema (see under Side-effects), monitor for disorders of the epiphysis of the hip (monitor for limping), monitor for signs of tonsillar hypertrophy (snoring, sleep apnoea, and chronic middle ear effusions); pregnancy (Appendix 4)

**Contra-indications** evidence of tumour activity (discontinue treatment), breast-feeding

**Side-effects** headache, funduscopy for papilloedema recommended if severe or recurrent headache, visual problems, nausea and vomiting occur—if papilloedema confirmed consider benign intracranial hypertension (rare cases reported); cardiomegaly, ventricular hypertrophy, tachycardia; convulsions, sleep apnoea, night terrors, dizziness, nervousness; tonsillar hypertrophy (see Cautions above); hypoglycaemia (especially in first month, and in younger children), hyperglycaemia, gynaecomastia; arthralgia, myalgia; visual disturbance, impaired hearing; antibody formation; injection-site reactions (rotate site)

**Dose**

- By subcutaneous injection, ADOLESCENT and CHILD over 2 years, initially 40 micrograms/kg twice daily for 1 week, if tolerated increase dose in steps of 40 micrograms/kg to max. 120 micrograms/kg twice daily; discontinue if no response within 1 year
**Counselling** Dose should be administered just before or after food; do not increase dose if a dose is missed
**Note** Reduce dose if hypoglycaemia occurs despite adequate food intake; withhold injection if patient unable to eat

**Increlex®** (Ipsen) ▼ PoM
Injection, mecasermin 10 mg/mL, net price 4-mL vial = £605.00. Counselling, administration
Excipients include benzyl alcohol (avoid in neonates, see Excipients, p. 2)

**6**

**Endocrine system**

# 7 Obstetrics, gynaecology, and urinary-tract disorders

**7.1 Drugs used in obstetrics** **434**

7.1.1 Prostaglandins and oxytocics 434

7.1.1.1 Ductus arteriosus 437

7.1.2 Mifepristone 438

7.1.3 Myometrial relaxants 439

**7.2 Treatment of vaginal and vulval conditions** **440**

7.2.1 Preparations for vaginal and vulval changes 440

7.2.2 Vaginal and vulval infections 441

**7.3 Contraceptives** **443**

7.3.1 Combined hormonal contraceptives 443

7.3.2 Progestogen-only contraceptives 449

7.3.2.1 Oral progestogen-only contraceptives 449

7.3.2.2 Parenteral progestogen-only contraceptives 450

7.3.2.3 Intra-uterine progestogen-only device 451

7.3.3 Spermicidal contraceptives 452

7.3.4 Contraceptive devices 452

7.3.5 Emergency contraception 454

**7.4 Drugs for genito-urinary disorders** **455**

7.4.1 Drugs for urinary retention 455

7.4.2 Drugs for urinary frequency, enuresis, and incontinence 457

7.4.3 Drugs used in urological pain 460

7.4.4 Bladder instillations and urological surgery 461

7.4.5 Drugs for erectile dysfunction 462

This chapter also includes advice on the drug management of the following:
emergency contraception, p. 454
induction of abortion, below
induction and augmentation of labour, below
nocturnal enuresis, p. 460
premature labour, p. 439
prevention and treatment of post-partum haemorrhage, p. 435
priapism, p. 462

For hormonal therapy of gynaecological disorders see section 6.4.1 (including HRT), section 6.5.1 and section 6.7.2.

## 7.1 Drugs used in obstetrics

**7.1.1 Prostaglandins and oxytocics**

**7.1.2 Mifepristone**

**7.1.3 Myometrial relaxants**

Because of the complexity of dosage regimens in obstetrics, in all cases **detailed specialist literature** should be consulted.

## 7.1.1 Prostaglandins and oxytocics

Prostaglandins and oxytocics are used to induce abortion or induce or augment labour and to minimise blood loss from the placental site. They include oxytocin, carbetocin, ergometrine, and the prostaglandins. All induce uterine contractions with varying degrees of pain according to the strength of contractions induced.

**Induction of abortion** **Gemeprost**, administered vaginally as pessaries is the preferred prostaglandin for the medical induction of late therapeutic abortion. Gemeprost ripens the cervix before surgical abortion, particularly in primigravidas. The prostaglandin **misoprostol** (section 7.1.2) is given by mouth or by vaginal administration to induce medical abortion [unlicensed indication]; intravaginal use ripens the cervix before surgical abortion [unlicensed indication]. Extra-amniotic **dinoprostone** is rarely used nowadays.

Pre-treatment with **mifepristone** (section 7.1.2) can facilitate the process of medical abortion. It sensitises the uterus to subsequent administration of a prostaglandin and, therefore, abortion occurs in a shorter time and with a lower dose of prostaglandin.

**Induction and augmentation of labour** **Dinoprostone** is available as vaginal tablets, pessaries and vaginal gels for the induction of labour. The intravenous solution is rarely used; it is associated with more side-effects.

**Oxytocin** (*Syntocinon®*) is administered by slow intravenous infusion, using an infusion pump, to induce or augment labour, usually in conjunction with amniotomy. Uterine activity must be monitored carefully and hyperstimulation avoided. Large doses of oxytocin may result in excessive fluid retention.

**Misoprostol** is given orally or vaginally for the induction of labour [unlicensed indication].

> **NICE guidance**
> **Induction of labour** (updated July 2008)
> Available at www.nice.org.uk

**Prevention and treatment of haemorrhage** Bleeding due to incomplete abortion can be controlled with **ergometrine** and **oxytocin** (*Syntometrine®*) given intramuscularly, the dose is adjusted according to the patient's condition and blood loss. This is commonly used before surgical evacuation of the uterus, particularly when surgery is delayed. Oxytocin and ergometrine combined are more effective in early pregnancy than either drug alone.

Active management of the third stage of labour reduces the risk of postpartum haemorrhage; ergometrine 500 micrograms with oxytocin 5 units (*Syntometrine®* 1 mL) is given by intramuscular injection on delivery of the anterior shoulder or, at the latest, immediately after the baby is delivered. Alternatively, oxytocin may be given alone by intramuscular injection [unlicensed], particularly if ergometrine is inappropriate (e.g. in pre-eclampsia); oxytocin alone causes less nausea, vomiting, and hypertension than when given with ergometrine.

In excessive uterine bleeding, any placental products remaining in the uterus should be removed. Oxytocic drugs are used to treat postpartum haemorrhage caused by uterine atony; treatment options are as follows:

- oxytocin 5–10 units by slow intravenous injection, followed in severe cases by intravenous infusion of oxytocin 5–30 units in 500 mL infusion fluid at a rate that controls uterine atony *or*

- ergometrine by intramuscular injection *or*

- ergometrine 250–500 micrograms by intravenous injection (use with caution—risk of hypertension) *or*

- ergometrine 500 micrograms with oxytocin 5 units (*Syntometrine®* 1 mL) by intramuscular injection

**Carboprost** has an important role in severe postpartum haemorrhage unresponsive to ergometrine and oxytocin.

**Misoprostol** [unlicensed] may be an alternative in postpartum haemorrhage unresponsive to ergometrine, oxytocin, and carboprost.

### CARBETOCIN

**Indications** prevention of uterine atony after caesarean section

**Cautions** hyponatraemia; cardiovascular disease (avoid if severe); migraine; asthma

**Contra-indications** pre-eclampsia and eclampsia; epilepsy; hepatic impairment; renal impairment

**Side-effects** nausea, vomiting, abdominal pain, metallic taste; flushing, hypotension, chest pain; dyspnoea; headache, tremor, dizziness; anaemia; back pain; pruritus; feeling of warmth, chills; tachycardia and sweating also reported

**Dose**

- By intravenous injection, a single dose of 100 micrograms, as soon as possible after delivery, preferably before removal of placenta

**Pabal®** (Ferring) ▼ PoM
Injection, carbetocin 100 micrograms/mL, net price 1-mL amp = £17.64

### CARBOPROST

**Indications** postpartum haemorrhage due to uterine atony in patients unresponsive to ergometrine and oxytocin

**Cautions** history of glaucoma or raised intra-ocular pressure; asthma, hypertension, hypotension, anaemia, jaundice, diabetes, epilepsy; uterine scars; excessive dosage may cause uterine rupture; **interactions:** Appendix 1 (prostaglandins)

**Contra-indications** untreated pelvic infection; cardiac, renal, pulmonary, or hepatic disease

**Side-effects** nausea, vomiting and diarrhoea, hyperthermia and flushing, bronchospasm; less frequent effects include raised blood pressure, dyspnoea, and pulmonary oedema; chills, headache, diaphoresis, dizziness; cardiovascular collapse also reported; erythema and pain at injection site reported

**Dose**

- By deep intramuscular injection, 250 micrograms repeated if necessary at intervals of 1½ hours (in severe cases the interval may be reduced but should not be less than 15 minutes); total dose should not exceed 2 mg (8 doses)

**Hemabate®** (Pharmacia) PoM
Injection, carboprost as trometamol salt (tromethamine salt) 250 micrograms/mL, net price 1-mL amp = £18.20 (hosp. only)

### DINOPROSTONE

**Indications** see notes above and under preparations below

**Cautions** history of asthma, glaucoma and raised intra-ocular pressure; hypertension; history of epilepsy; uterine scarring; monitor uterine activity and fetal status (particular care if history of uterine hypertony); uterine rupture; see also notes above; monitor for disseminated intravascular coagulation after parturition; risk factors for disseminated intravascular coagulation; effect of oxytocin enhanced (care needed in monitoring uterine activity when used in sequence); **interactions:** Appendix 1 (prostaglandins)

**Contra-indications** active cardiac, pulmonary, renal or hepatic disease; placenta praevia or unexplained vaginal bleeding during pregnancy, ruptured membranes, major cephalopelvic disproportion or fetal malpresentation, history of caesarean section or major uterine surgery, untreated pelvic infection, fetal distress, grand multiparas and multiple pregnancy, history of difficult or traumatic delivery; avoid extra-amniotic route in cervicitis or vaginitis

**7**

**Obstetrics, gynaecology, and urinary-tract disorders**

**Side-effects** nausea, vomiting, diarrhoea; other side-effects include uterine hypertonus, severe uterine contractions, pulmonary or amniotic fluid embolism, abruptio placenta, fetal distress, maternal hypertension, bronchospasm, rapid cervical dilation, fever, backache; uterine hypercontractility with or without fetal bradycardia, low Apgar scores; cardiac arrest, uterine rupture, stillbirth or neonatal death also reported; vaginal symptoms (warmth, irritation, pain); after intravenous administration—flushing, shivering, headache, dizziness, temporary pyrexia and raised white blood cell count; disseminated intravascular coagulation reported; also local tissue reaction and erythema after intravenous administration and possibility of infection after extra-amniotic administration

**Dose**

- See under preparations, below
  **Important** Do not confuse dose of *Prostin E2*® vaginal **gel** with that of *Prostin E2*® vaginal **tablets**—not bioequivalent.

**Propess**® (Ferring) ℗ℴ𝕄
Pessaries (within retrieval device), releasing dinoprostone approx. 10 mg over 24 hours; net price 1-pessary pack = £30.00
Dose by vagina, cervical ripening and induction of labour at term, 1 pessary (in retrieval device) inserted high into posterior fornix and removed when cervical ripening adequate; if oxytocin necessary, remove 30 minutes before oxytocin infusion; remove if cervical ripening inadequate after 24 hours (dose not to be repeated)

**Prostin E2**® (Pharmacia) ℗ℴ𝕄
Intravenous solution ◢ for dilution and use as an infusion, dinoprostone 1 mg/mL, net price 0.75-mL amp = £8.52; 10 mg/mL, 0.5-mL amp = £18.40 (both hosp. only; rarely used, consult product literature for dose and indications)

Extra-amniotic solution ◢ dinoprostone 10 mg/mL. Net price 0.5-mL amp (with diluent) = £18.40 (hosp. only; less commonly used nowadays, consult product literature for dose and indications)

Vaginal gel, dinoprostone 400 micrograms/mL, net price 2.5 mL (1 mg) = £13.28; 800 micrograms/mL, 2.5 mL (2 mg) = £13.28
Dose by vagina, induction of labour, inserted high into posterior fornix (avoid administration into cervical canal), 1 mg (unfavourable primigravida 2 mg), followed after 6 hours by 1–2 mg if required; max. [gel] 3 mg (unfavourable primigravida 4 mg)

Vaginal tablets, dinoprostone 3 mg. Net price 8-vaginal tab pack = £106.23
Dose by vagina, induction of labour, inserted high into posterior fornix, 3 mg, followed after 6–8 hours by 3 mg if labour is not established; max. 6 mg [vaginal tablets]
Note *Prostin E2 Vaginal Gel* and *Vaginal Tablets* are **not** bioequivalent

---

## ◼ ERGOMETRINE MALEATE

**Indications** see notes above

**Cautions** cardiac disease; hypertension; multiple pregnancy; acute porphyria (section 9.8.2); hepatic impairment (avoid if severe; Appendix 2); renal impairment (avoid if severe; Appendix 3); **interactions**: Appendix 1 (ergot alkaloids)

**Contra-indications** induction of labour, first and second stages of labour, vascular disease, severe cardiac disease, sepsis, severe hypertension, eclampsia

**Side-effects** nausea, vomiting, headache, dizziness, tinnitus, abdominal pain, chest pain, palpitation, dyspnoea, bradycardia, transient hypertension, vasoconstriction; stroke, myocardial infarction and pulmonary oedema also reported

**Dose**

- See notes above

**Ergometrine** (Non-proprietary) ℗ℴ𝕄
Injection, ergometrine maleate 500 micrograms/mL. Net price 1-mL amp = 60p

◢**With oxytocin**

**Syntometrine**® (Alliance) ℗ℴ𝕄
Injection, ergometrine maleate 500 micrograms, oxytocin 5 units/mL. Net price 1-mL amp = £1.35
Dose by intramuscular injection, 1 mL; by intravenous injection, no longer recommended

---

## ◼ GEMEPROST

**Indications** see under Dose

**Cautions** obstructive airways disease, cardiovascular insufficiency, raised intra-ocular pressure, cervicitis or vaginitis; **interactions**: Appendix 1 (prostaglandins)
Important For warnings relating to use of gemeprost in a patient undergoing induction of abortion with mifepristone, see under Mifepristone and Note below

**Contra-indications** unexplained vaginal bleeding, uterine scarring, placenta praevia

**Side-effects** vaginal bleeding and uterine pain; nausea, vomiting, or diarrhoea; headache, muscle weakness, dizziness, flushing, chills, backache, dyspnoea, chest pain, palpitation and mild pyrexia; uterine rupture reported (most commonly in multiparas or if history of uterine surgery or if given with intravenous oxytocics); also reported severe hypotension, coronary artery spasm and myocardial infarction

**Dose**

- By vagina, cervical ripening prior to first trimester surgical abortion, 1 mg inserted into posterior fornix 3 hours before surgery

- Second trimester abortion, 1 mg inserted into posterior fornix every 3 hours for max. of 5 administrations; second course may begin 24 hours after start of treatment (if treatment fails pregnancy should be terminated by another method)

- Second trimester intra-uterine death, 1 mg inserted into posterior fornix every 3 hours for max. of 5 administrations only; monitor for coagulopathy
Note If used in combination with mifepristone, carefully monitor blood pressure and pulse for 3 hours

**Gemeprost** (Sanofi-Aventis) ℗ℴ𝕄
Pessaries, gemeprost 1 mg. Net price 5-pessary pack = £215.00

---

## ◼ OXYTOCIN

**Indications** see under Dose and notes above

**Cautions** induction or enhancement of labour—presence of borderline cephalopelvic disproportion (avoid if significant), secondary uterine inertia, mild or moderate pregnancy-induced hypertension or cardiac disease, women over 35 years or with history of lower-uterine segment caesarean section (see also under Contra-indications below); risk factors for disseminated intravascular coagulation; monitor for disseminated intravascular coagulation after parturition; avoid large infusion volumes and restrict fluid intake by mouth (risk of hyponatraemia and water-intoxication—see also Appendix 6); effects enhanced by concomitant prostaglandins (very careful monitoring of uterine activity); caudal block anaesthesia (may enhance hypertensive effects of sympathomimetic vasopressors); see also **interactions**: Appendix 1 (oxytocin)

**Contra-indications** hypertonic uterine contractions, fetal distress; any condition where spontaneous labour or vaginal delivery inadvisable; avoid prolonged administration in oxytocin-resistant uterine inertia, severe pre-eclamptic toxaemia, or severe cardiovascular disease

**Side-effects** nausea, vomiting; arrhythmia; headache; *rarely* disseminated intravascular coagulation, rash, and anaphylactoid reactions (with dyspnoea, hypotension, or shock); uterine spasm (may occur at low doses), uterine hyperstimulation (usually with excessive doses—may cause fetal distress, asphyxia, and death, or may lead to hypertonicity, tetanic contractions, soft-tissue damage or uterine rupture); water intoxication and hyponatraemia associated with high doses with large infusion volumes of electrolyte-free fluid (see also under Dose below); placental abruption and amniotic fluid embolism also reported on overdose

**Dose**

- Induction of labour for medical reasons or stimulation of labour in hypotonic uterine inertia, by intravenous infusion (not to be started for at least 6 hours after administration of vaginal prostaglandin), initially 0.001–0.004 units/minute, increased at intervals of at least 30 minutes until a maximum of 3–4 contractions occur every 10 minutes (0.01 units/minute is often adequate) up to max. 0.02 units/minute; if regular contractions not established after total of 5 units stop induction attempt (may be repeated next day starting again at 0.001–0.004 units/minute)

  **Important** Careful monitoring of fetal heart rate and uterine motility essential for dose titration (**avoid** intravenous injection during labour); discontinue immediately in uterine hyperactivity or fetal distress

- Caesarean section, by slow intravenous injection immediately after delivery, 5 units

- Prevention of postpartum haemorrhage, by slow intravenous injection, 5 units (if infusion used for induction or enhancement of labour, increase rate during third stage and for next few hours).

  **Important** Avoid rapid intravenous injection (may transiently reduce blood pressure)

  **Note** Can be given in a dose of 10 units by intramuscular injection [unlicensed route] instead of oxytocin with ergometrine (*Syntometrine®*), see notes above

- Treatment of postpartum haemorrhage, by slow intravenous injection, 5–10 units, followed in severe cases by intravenous infusion of 5–30 units in 500 mL infusion fluid at a rate sufficient to control uterine atony

  **Important** Avoid rapid intravenous injection (may transiently reduce blood pressure; prolonged administration, see warning below

- Incomplete, inevitable, or missed abortion, by slow intravenous injection, 5 units followed if necessary by intravenous infusion, 0.02–0.04 units/minute or faster

  **Important** Prolonged intravenous administration at high doses with large volume of fluid (as possible in inevitable or missed abortion or postpartum haemorrhage) may cause water intoxication with hyponatraemia. To avoid: use electrolyte-containing diluent (i.e. not glucose), increase oxytocin concentration to reduce fluid, restrict fluid intake by mouth; monitor fluid and electrolytes.

  **Note** Oxytocin doses in the BNF may differ from those in the product literature

**Syntocinon®** (Alliance) [PoM]
Injection, oxytocin, net price 5 units/mL, 1-mL amp = 76p; 10 units/mL, 1-mL amp = 86p

◢**With ergometrine**
See *Syntometrine®*, p. 436

---

**7.1.1.1  Ductus arteriosus**

## Maintenance of patency

**Alprostadil** (prostaglandin E₁) is used to maintain patency of the ductus arteriosus in neonates with congenital heart defects, prior to corrective surgery in centres where intensive care is immediately available. See *BNF for Children* (section 2.14) for further advice on maintaining the patency of the ductus arteriosus.

### ▐ ALPROSTADIL

**Indications** congenital heart defects in neonates prior to corrective surgery; erectile dysfunction (section 7.4.5)

**Cautions** see notes above; history of haemorrhage, avoid in hyaline membrane disease, monitor arterial pressure; **interactions**: Appendix 1 (prostaglandins)

**Side-effects** apnoea (particularly in neonates under 2 kg), flushing, bradycardia, hypotension, tachycardia, cardiac arrest, oedema, diarrhoea, fever, convulsions, disseminated intravascular coagulation, hypokalaemia; cortical proliferation of long bones and weakening of the wall of the ductus arteriosus and of pulmonary artery may follow prolonged use; gastric-outlet obstruction reported

**Dose**

- By intravenous infusion, initially 5–10 nanograms/kg/minute, adjusted according to response in steps of 5–10 nanograms/kg/minute; max. 100 nanograms/kg/minute (but associated with increased side-effects)

  **Note** Alprostadil doses in BNF may differ from those in product literature

**Prostin VR®** (Pharmacia) [PoM]
Intravenous solution, alprostadil 500 micrograms/mL in alcohol. For dilution and use as an infusion. Net price 1-mL amp = £75.19 (hosp. only)

## Closure of ductus arteriosus

**Indometacin** (indomethacin) is used to close a patent ductus arteriosus in premature babies, probably by inhibiting prostaglandin synthesis. See *BNF for Children* (section 2.14) for further advice on closure of the ductus arteriosus.

### ▐ INDOMETACIN
(Indomethacin)

**Indications** patent ductus arteriosus in premature babies (under specialist supervision in neonatal intensive care unit); uncomplicated premature labour [unlicensed indication] (section 7.1.3); rheumatoid disease (section 10.1.1)

**Cautions** may mask symptoms of infection; may reduce urine output by 50% or more (monitor carefully—see also under Anuria or Oliguria, below) and precipitate renal impairment especially if extracellular volume depleted, heart failure, sepsis, or hepatic impairment, or if receiving nephrotoxic drugs; may induce hyponatraemia; monitor renal function and electrolytes; inhibition of platelet aggregation (monitor for bleeding); **interactions:** Appendix 1 (NSAIDs) **Anuria or oliguria** If anuria or marked oliguria (urinary output less than 0.6 mL/kg/hour) at time of scheduled second or third dose, delay until renal function returns to normal

**Contra-indications** untreated infection, bleeding (especially with active intracranial haemorrhage or gastro-intestinal bleeding); thrombocytopenia, coagulation defects, necrotising enterocolitis, renal impairment

**Side-effects** haemorrhagic, renal, gastro-intestinal (including necrotising enterocolitis), metabolic, and coagulation disorders; pulmonary hypertension, intracranial bleeding, fluid retention, and exacerbation of infection

**Dose**
- By intravenous injection, over 20–30 minutes (using a suitable syringe driver), 3 doses at intervals of 12–24 hours (provided urine output remains adequate), NEONATE under 48 hours, 200 micrograms/kg then 100 micrograms/kg then 100 micrograms/kg; NEONATE 2–7 days, 200 micrograms/kg then 200 micrograms/kg then 200 micrograms/kg; NEONATE over 7 days, 200 micrograms/kg then 250 micrograms/kg then 250 micrograms/kg; solution prepared with 1–2 mL sodium chloride 0.9% or water for injections (not glucose and no preservatives)

If ductus arteriosus reopens a second course of 3 injections may be given 48 hours after first course

**Indocid PDA®** (IDIS) [PoM]
Injection, powder for reconstitution, indometacin (as sodium trihydrate). Net price 3 × 1-mg vials = £43.50 (hosp. only)

## 7.1.2 Mifepristone

**Mifepristone**, an antiprogestogenic steroid, sensitises the myometrium to prostaglandin-induced contractions and ripens the cervix. For termination of pregnancy, a single dose of mifepristone is followed by administration of a prostaglandin (gemeprost or misoprostol [unlicensed]). Guidelines of the Royal College of Obstetricians and Gynaecologists (September 2004) include the following [unlicensed] regimens for inducing medical abortion:

- For gestation up to 9 weeks, mifepristone 200 mg by mouth followed 1–3 days later by misoprostol 800 micrograms vaginally; in women at more than 7 weeks gestation (49–63 days), if the abortion has not occurred 4 hours after misoprostol, a further dose of misoprostol 400 micrograms may be given vaginally or by mouth

- For gestation between 9 and 13 weeks, mifepristone 200 mg by mouth followed 36–48 hours later by misoprostol 800 micrograms vaginally followed if necessary by a maximum of 4 further doses at 3-hourly intervals of misoprostol 400 micrograms vaginally or by mouth

- For gestation between 13 and 24 weeks, mifepristone 200 mg by mouth followed 36–48 hours later by misoprostol 800 micrograms vaginally then a maximum of 4 further doses at 3-hourly intervals of misoprostol 400 micrograms by mouth

## MIFEPRISTONE

**Indications** see under dose

**Cautions** asthma (avoid if severe and uncontrolled); haemorrhagic disorders and anticoagulant therapy; prosthetic heart valve or history of endocarditis (see section 5.1 table 2); risk factors for or existing cardiovascular disease; adrenal suppression (may require corticosteroid); **interactions:** Appendix 1 (mifepristone)

Important For warnings relating to use of gemeprost in a patient undergoing induction of abortion with mifepristone, see under Gemeprost

**Contra-indications** uncontrolled severe asthma; suspected ectopic pregnancy (use other specific means of termination); chronic adrenal failure; acute porphyria (section 9.8.2); hepatic impairment; renal impairment; breast-feeding (Appendix 5)

**Side-effects** gastro-intestinal cramps; uterine contractions, vaginal bleeding (sometimes severe) may occur between administration of mifepristone and surgery (and rarely abortion may occur before surgery); *less commonly* hypersensitivity reactions including rash and urticaria; *rarely* hypotension, malaise, headache, fever, hot flushes, dizziness, and chills; infections (including toxic shock syndrome) also reported

**Dose**
- Medical termination of intra-uterine pregnancy of up to 49 days gestation, by mouth, mifepristone 600 mg as a single dose under medical supervision followed 36–48 hours later (unless abortion already complete) by gemeprost 1 mg by vagina or misoprostol 400 micrograms by mouth [unlicensed]; alternative regimen, mifepristone 200 mg by mouth as a single dose followed 36–48 hours later (unless abortion already complete) by gemeprost 1 mg by vagina; observe for at least 3 hours (or until bleeding or pain at acceptable level); follow-up visit within 2 weeks to verify complete expulsion (if treatment fails essential that pregnancy be terminated by another method) and to assess vaginal bleeding

- Medical termination of intra-uterine pregnancy of 50–63 days gestation, by mouth, mifepristone 600 mg (200 mg also effective) as a single dose under medical supervision, followed 36–48 hours later (unless abortion already complete) by gemeprost 1 mg by vagina; observe for at least 3 hours (or until bleeding or pain at acceptable level); follow-up visit within 2 weeks to verify complete expulsion (if treatment fails essential that pregnancy be terminated by another method) and to assess vaginal bleeding

- Cervical ripening before mechanical cervical dilatation for termination of pregnancy of up to 84 days gestation, by mouth, mifepristone 200 mg as a single dose under medical supervision 36–48 hours before procedure

- Termination of pregnancy of 13–24 weeks gestation (in combination with a prostaglandin), by mouth, mifepristone 600 mg (200 mg may be effective) as a single dose under medical supervision followed 36–48 hours later by gemeprost 1 mg by vagina every 3 hours up to max. 5 mg or misoprostol (see above [unlicensed]); if abortion does not occur, 24 hours after start of treatment repeat course of gemeprost 1 mg by vagina up to max. 5 mg (if treatment fails pregnancy should be terminated by another method); follow-up visit after appropriate interval to assess vaginal bleeding recommended

Note Careful monitoring of blood pressure and pulse essential for 3 hours after administration of gemeprost pessary (risk of profound hypotension)

- Labour induction in fetal death *in utero* where prostaglandin or oxytocin inappropriate, by mouth, mifepristone 600 mg daily as a single dose for 2 days under medical supervision; if labour not started within 72 hours of first dose, another method should be used

**Mifegyne®** (Exelgyn) Ⓡᴏᴹ
Tablets, yellow, mifepristone 200 mg. Net price 3-tab pack = £41.83 (supplied to NHS hospitals and premises approved under Abortion Act 1967). Label: 10, patient information leaflet

## 7.1.3 Myometrial relaxants

Tocolytic drugs postpone *premature labour* and they are used with the aim of reducing harm to the child. However, there is no satisfactory evidence that the use of these drugs reduces mortality. The greatest benefit is gained by using the delay to administer corticosteroid therapy or to implement other measures which improve perinatal health (including transfer to a unit with neonatal intensive care facility).

The oxytocin receptor antagonist, **atosiban**, is licensed for the inhibition of uncomplicated premature labour *between 24 and 33 weeks* of gestation. Atosiban may be preferable to a beta₂ agonist because it has fewer side-effects.

The dihydropyridine calcium-channel blocker **nifedipine** (section 2.6.2) also has fewer side-effects than a beta₂ agonist. Nifedipine [unlicensed indication] can be given initially in a dose of 20 mg followed by 10–20 mg 3–4 times daily adjusted according to uterine activity.

A beta₂ agonist (**ritodrine, salbutamol** or **terbutaline**) is used for inhibiting uncomplicated premature labour between 24 and 33 weeks of gestation and it may permit a delay in delivery of at least 48 hours. Prolonged therapy should be avoided since risk to the mother increases after 48 hours and there is a lack of evidence of benefit from further treatment; maintenance treatment is therefore **not recommended**.

Indometacin (indomethacin) (section 10.1.1), a cyclooxygenase inhibitor, also inhibits labour [unlicensed indication] and it can be useful in situations where a beta₂ agonist is not appropriate; however, there are concerns about neonatal complications such as transient impairment of renal function and premature closure of ductus arteriosus.

## Atosiban

### ▌ ATOSIBAN

**Indications** uncomplicated premature labour (see notes above)

**Cautions** monitor blood loss after delivery; intrauterine growth restriction; abnormal placental site; hepatic impairment (Appendix 2); renal impairment (Appendix 3)

**Contra-indications** eclampsia and severe pre-eclampsia, intra-uterine infection, intra-uterine fetal death, antepartum haemorrhage (requiring immediate delivery), placenta praevia, abruptio placenta, intra-uterine growth restriction with abnormal fetal heart rate, premature rupture of membranes after 30 weeks' gestation

**Side-effects** nausea, vomiting, tachycardia, hypotension, headache, dizziness, hot flushes, hyperglycaemia, injection-site reaction; *less commonly* pruritus, rash, fever, insomnia

**Dose**

- By intravenous injection, initially 6.75 mg over 1 minute, then by intravenous infusion 18 mg/hour for 3 hours, then 6 mg/hour for up to 45 hours; max. duration of treatment 48 hours

**Tractocile®** (Ferring) Ⓡᴏᴹ
Injection, atosiban (as acetate) 7.5 mg/mL, net price 0.9-mL (6.75-mg) vial = £18.41

Concentrate for intravenous infusion, atosiban (as acetate) 7.5 mg/mL, net price 5-mL vial = £52.82

## Beta₂ agonists

**Cautions** Beta₂ agonists should be used with caution in patients with suspected cardiovascular disease (such patients should be assessed by a cardiologist before initiating therapy—see also Contra-indications, below), hypertension, mild to moderate pre-eclampsia, hyperthyroidism, and hypokalaemia (particular risk with potassium-depleting diuretics—see also CSM advice, p. 155). It is important to monitor pulse rate (should not exceed 140 beats per minute), ECG (discontinue treatment if signs of myocardial ischaemia develop), and the patient's fluid and electrolyte status (avoid overhydration—discontinue drug immediately and initiate diuretic therapy if pulmonary oedema occurs). Beta₂ agonists should also be used with caution in diabetes—monitor blood glucose (risk of hyperglycaemia and ketoacidosis, especially with intravenous beta₂ agonists).

**Contra-indications** Beta₂ agonists are contra-indicated in cardiac disease and in patients with significant risk factors for myocardial ischaemia; they should also be avoided in antepartum haemorrhage, intra-uterine infection, intra-uterine fetal death, placenta praevia, abruptio placenta, threatened miscarriage, cord compression, and eclampsia or severe pre-eclampsia.

**Side-effects** Side-effects of the beta₂ agonists include nausea, vomiting, pulmonary oedema (see Cautions above and under Ritodrine dose), palpitation, tachycardia, arrhythmias, myocardial ischaemia, peripheral vasodilation, headache, tremor, hyperglycaemia, hypokalaemia (see Cautions), muscle cramps and tension, and hypersensitivity reactions (including angioedema, urticaria, rash, bronchospasm, hypotension, and collapse).

### ▌ RITODRINE HYDROCHLORIDE

**Indications** uncomplicated premature labour (see notes above)

**Cautions** see notes above; **interactions:** Appendix 1 (sympathomimetics *and* sympathomimetics, beta₂)

7 Obstetrics, gynaecology, and urinary-tract disorders

**Contra-indications** see notes above

**Side-effects** see notes above; also reported flushing, sweating; salivary gland enlargement; leucopenia and agranulocytosis on prolonged administration (several weeks); liver function abnormalities (including increased transaminases and hepatitis)

**Dose**

- By intravenous infusion (**important**: minimum fluid volume, see below), initially 50 micrograms/minute, increased gradually according to response by 50 micrograms/minute every 10 minutes until contractions stop or maternal heart rate reaches 140 beats per minute; continue for 12–48 hours after contractions cease (usual rate 150–350 micrograms/minute); max. rate 350 micrograms/minute; or by intramuscular injection, 10 mg every 3–8 hours continued for 12–48 hours after contractions have ceased; then by mouth (but see notes above), 10 mg 30 minutes before termination of intravenous infusion, repeated every 2 hours for 24 hours, followed by 10–20 mg every 4–6 hours, max. oral dose 120 mg daily

**Important** Manufacturer states that although *fatal pulmonary oedema* associated with ritodrine infusion is almost certainly multifactorial in origin, evidence suggests that **fluid overload** may be the most important single factor. The volume of infusion should therefore be kept to a minimum; for further guidance see Appendix 6. For specific guidance on infusion rates, consult product literature

**Yutopar®** (Durbin) [PoM]

Tablets▲ yellow, scored, ritodrine hydrochloride 10 mg, net price 90-tab pack = £30.40

Injection, ritodrine hydrochloride 10 mg/mL, net price 5-mL amp = £3.55

## ▌ SALBUTAMOL
### (Albuterol)

**Indications** uncomplicated premature labour (see notes above); asthma (section 3.1.1)

**Cautions** see notes above; **interactions:** Appendix 1 (sympathomimetics, beta₂)

**Contra-indications** see notes above

**Side-effects** see notes above

**Dose**

- By intravenous infusion, initially 10 micrograms/minute, rate increased gradually according to response at 10-minute intervals until contractions diminish then increase rate slowly until contractions cease (max. rate 45 micrograms/minute); maintain rate for 1 hour after contractions have stopped, then gradually reduce by 50% every 6 hours; then by mouth (but see notes above), 4 mg every 6–8 hours

◀ **Preparations**

Section 3.1.1.1

## ▌ TERBUTALINE SULPHATE

**Indications** uncomplicated premature labour (see notes above); asthma (section 3.1.1)

**Cautions** see notes above; **interactions:** Appendix 1 (sympathomimetics, beta₂)

**Contra-indications** see notes above

**Side-effects** see notes above; also reported sleep disturbances and behavioural disturbances

**Dose**

- By intravenous infusion, 5 micrograms/minute for 20 minutes, increased every 20 minutes in steps of 2.5 micrograms/minute until contractions have ceased (more than 10 micrograms/minute should **seldom** be given—20 micrograms/minute should **not** be exceeded), continue for 1 hour then decrease every 20 minutes in steps of 2.5 micrograms/minute to lowest dose that maintains suppression, continue at this level for 12 hours then by mouth (but see notes above), 5 mg every 8 hours for as long as is desirable to prolong pregnancy (or alternatively follow the intravenous infusion by subcutaneous injection 250 micrograms every 6 hours for a few days then by mouth as above)

◀ **Preparations**

Section 3.1.1.1

## 7.2 Treatment of vaginal and vulval conditions

**7.2.1 Preparations for vaginal and vulval changes**

**7.2.2 Vaginal and vulval infections**

Symptoms are often restricted to the vulva, but infections almost invariably involve the vagina which should also be treated. Applications to the vulva alone are likely to give only symptomatic relief without cure.

*Aqueous medicated douches* may disturb normal vaginal acidity and bacterial flora.

*Topical anaesthetic agents* give only symptomatic relief and may cause sensitivity reactions. They are indicated only in cases of pruritus where specific local causes have been excluded.

*Systemic drugs* are required in the treatment of infections such as gonorrhoea and syphilis (section 5.1).

## 7.2.1 Preparations for vaginal and vulval changes

### Topical HRT for vaginal atrophy

A cream containing an oestrogen may be applied on a short-term basis to improve the vaginal epithelium in *menopausal atrophic vaginitis*. It is **important** to bear in mind that topical oestrogens should be used in the **smallest effective** amount to minimise systemic effects. Modified-release vaginal tablets and an impregnated vaginal ring are now also available.

The risk of endometrial hyperplasia and carcinoma is increased when *systemic* oestrogens are administered alone for prolonged periods (section 6.4.1.1). The endometrial safety of long-term or repeated use of *topical* vaginal oestrogens is uncertain; treatment should be reviewed at least annually, with special consideration given to any symptoms of endometrial hyperplasia or carcinoma.

Topical oestrogens are also used in postmenopausal women before vaginal surgery for prolapse when there is epithelial atrophy.

For a general comment on hormone replacement therapy, including the role of topical oestrogens, see section 6.4.1.1.

## OESTROGENS, TOPICAL

**Indications** see notes above

**Cautions** see notes above; see also Oestrogens for HRT (section 6.4.1.1); interrupt treatment periodically to assess need for continued treatment

**Contra-indications** see notes above; see also Oestrogens for HRT (section 6.4.1.1); pregnancy and breast-feeding

**Side-effects** see notes above; see also Oestrogens for HRT (section 6.4.1.1); local irritation

**Ortho-Gynest®** (Janssen-Cilag) [PoM]
Intravaginal cream, estriol 0.01%. Net price 80 g with applicator = £2.43
Excipients include arachis (peanut) oil
Condoms damages latex condoms and diaphragms
Dose insert 1 applicatorful daily, preferably in evening; reduced to 1 applicatorful twice a week; attempts to reduce or discontinue should be made at 3–6 month intervals with re-examination

Pessaries, estriol 500 micrograms. Net price 15 pessaries = £4.73
Excipients include butylated hydroxytoluene
Condoms damages latex condoms and diaphragms
Dose insert 1 pessary daily, preferably in the evening, until improvement occurs; maintenance 1 pessary twice a week; attempts to reduce or discontinue should be made at 3–6 month intervals with re-examination

**Ovestin®** (Organon) [PoM]
Intravaginal cream, estriol 0.1%. Net price 15 g with applicator = £4.54
Excipients include cetyl alcohol, polysorbates, stearyl alcohol
Condoms effect on latex condoms and diaphragms not yet known
Dose insert 1 applicator-dose daily for 2–3 weeks, then reduce to twice a week (discontinue every 2–3 months for 4 weeks to assess need for further treatment); vaginal surgery, 1 applicator-dose daily for 2 weeks before surgery, resuming 2 weeks after surgery

**Premarin®** (Wyeth) [PoM]
Vaginal cream, conjugated oestrogens (equine) 625 micrograms/g. Net price 42.5 g with calibrated applicator = £2.19
Excipients include cetyl alcohol, propylene glycol
Condoms effect on latex condoms and diaphragms not yet known
Dose insert 1–2 g daily starting on day 5 of cycle (or at any time if cycles have ceased) for 3 weeks, repeated after a 1-week interval

**Vagifem®** (Novo Nordisk) [PoM]
Vaginal tablets, f /c, m /r, estradiol 25 micrograms in disposable applicators. Net price 15-applicator pack = £7.92
Excipients none as listed in section 13.1.3
Condoms no evidence of damage to latex condoms and diaphragms
Dose insert 1 tablet daily for 2 weeks then reduce to 1 tablet twice weekly; discontinue after 3 months to assess need for further treatment

◢**Vaginal ring**
**Estring®** (Pharmacia) [PoM]
Vaginal ring, releasing estradiol approx. 7.5 micrograms/24 hours. Net price 1-ring pack = £31.42.
Label: 10, patient information leaflet
Dose for postmenopausal urogenital conditions (not suitable for vasomotor symptoms or osteoporosis prophylaxis), to be inserted into upper third of vagina and worn continuously; replace after 3 months; max. duration of continuous treatment 2 years

## Non-hormonal preparations for vaginal atrophy

*Replens MD®* and *Sylk®* are acidic, non-hormonal vaginal moisturisers; *Replens MD®* provides a high moisture content for up to 3 days.

## 7.2.2 Vaginal and vulval infections

Effective specific treatments are available for the common vaginal infections.

## Fungal infections

*Candidal vulvitis* can be treated locally with cream but is almost invariably associated with vaginal infection which should also be treated. *Vaginal candidiasis* is treated primarily with antifungal pessaries or cream inserted high into the vagina (including during menstruation). Single-dose preparations offer an advantage when compliance is a problem. Local irritation may occur on application of vaginal antifungal products.

**Imidazole** drugs (clotrimazole, econazole, and miconazole) are effective against candida in short courses of 1 to 14 days according to the preparation used; treatment can be repeated if initial course fails to control symptoms or if symptoms recur. Vaginal applications may be supplemented with antifungal cream for vulvitis and to treat other superficial sites of infection.

Oral treatment of vaginal infection with **fluconazole** or **itraconazole** (section 5.2) is also effective; oral ketoconazole has been associated with fatal hepatotoxicity (see section 5.2 for CSM warning).

**Vulvovaginal candidiasis in pregnancy** Vulvovaginal candidiasis is common during pregnancy and can be treated with vaginal application of an imidazole (such as clotrimazole), and a topical imidazole cream for vulvitis. Pregnant women need a longer duration of treatment, usually about 7 days, to clear the infection. Oral antifungal treatment should be avoided during pregnancy.

**Recurrent vulvovaginal candidiasis** Recurrence of vulvovaginal candidiasis is particularly likely if there are predisposing factors such as antibacterial therapy, pregnancy, diabetes mellitus and possibly oral contraceptive use. Reservoirs of infection may also lead to recontamination and should be treated; these include other skin sites such as the digits, nail beds, and umbilicus as well as the gastro-intestinal tract and the bladder. The partner may also be the source of re-infection and, if symptomatic, should be treated with cream at the same time.

Treatment against candida may need to be extended for 6 months in recurrent vulvovaginal candidiasis. Some recommended regimens [all unlicensed] include:

- fluconazole (section 5.2) by mouth 100 mg (as a single dose) every week for 6 months
- clotrimazole vaginally 500-mg pessary (as a single dose) every week for 6 months
- itraconazole (section 5.2) by mouth 400 mg (as 2 divided doses on one day) every month for 6 months.

**Obstetrics, gynaecology, and urinary-tract disorders** 7

**7 Obstetrics, gynaecology, and urinary-tract disorders**

## PREPARATIONS FOR VAGINAL AND VULVAL CANDIDIASIS

**Side-effects** occasional local irritation

**Clotrimazole** (Non-proprietary)
Cream (topical), clotrimazole 1%, net price 20 g = £1.84, 50 g = £3.81
Condoms check with manufacturer of cream for effect on latex condoms and diaphragms
Dose apply to anogenital area 2–3 times daily

Pessary, clotrimazole 500 mg, net price 1 pessary with applicator = £3.13
Dose insert 1 pessary at night as a single dose; can be repeated once if necessary

**Canesten®** (Bayer Consumer Care)
Cream (topical), clotrimazole 1%. Net price 20 g = £2.14; 50 g = £3.50
Excipients include benzyl alcohol, cetostearyl alcohol, polysorbates
Condoms damages latex condoms and diaphragms
Dose apply to anogenital area 2–3 times daily

Thrush Cream (topical), clotrimazole 2%, net price 20 g = £3.99
Excipients include benzyl alcohol, cetostearyl alcohol, polysorbates
Condoms damages latex condoms and diaphragms
Dose apply to anogenital area 2–3 times daily

Vaginal cream (*10% VC®*) PoM, clotrimazole 10%. Net price 5-g applicator pack = £4.90
Excipients include benzyl alcohol, cetostearyl alcohol, polysorbates
Condoms damages latex condoms and diaphragms
Dose insert 5 g at night as a single dose; can be repeated once if necessary
Note Brands for sale to the public include *Canesten® Internal Cream*

Cream Combi, clotrimazole 10% vaginal cream and 2% topical cream, net price 5-g vaginal cream (with applicator) and 10-g topical cream = £6.81
Excipients include benzyl alcohol, cetostearyl alcohol, polysorbates
Condoms damages latex condoms and diaphragms
Dose see under individual components

Pessaries, clotrimazole 100 mg, net price 6 pessaries with applicator = £3.63; 200 mg, 3 pessaries with applicator = £3.63
Condoms damages latex condoms and diaphragms
Dose insert 200 mg for 3 nights or 100 mg for 6 nights; course can be repeated once if necessary

Pessary, clotrimazole 500 mg. Net price 1 with applicator = £3.18
Excipients none as listed in section 13.1.3
Condoms damages latex condoms and diaphragms
Dose insert 1 pessary at night as a single dose; can be repeated once if necessary

Combi, clotrimazole 500-mg pessary and cream (topical) 2%. Net price 1 pessary and 10-g cream = £5.51
Condoms damages latex condoms and diaphragms
Dose see under individual components

**Ecostatin®** (Squibb)
Cream (topical), econazole nitrate 1%. Net price 15 g = £1.49; 30 g = £2.75
Excipients include butylated hydroxyanisole, fragrance
Condoms damages latex condoms and diaphragms
Dose apply to anogenital area twice daily

Pessaries PoM, econazole nitrate 150 mg. Net price 3 with applicator = £3.00
Excipients none as listed in section 13.1.3
Condoms damages latex condoms and diaphragms
Dose insert 1 pessary for 3 nights; course can be repeated once if necessary

Pessary (*Ecostatin-1®*) PoM, econazole nitrate 150 mg, formulated for single-dose therapy. Net price 1 pessary with applicator = £3.12
Excipients none as listed in section 13.1.3
Condoms damages latex condoms and diaphragms
Dose insert 1 pessary at night as a single dose; can be repeated once if necessary

Twinpack PoM, econazole nitrate 150-mg pessaries and cream 1%. Net price 3 pessaries and 15-g cream = £4.35
Condoms damages latex condoms and diaphragms
Dose see under individual components

**Gyno-Daktarin®** (Janssen-Cilag) PoM
Intravaginal cream, miconazole nitrate 2%. Net price 78 g with applicators = £4.42
Excipients include butylated hydroxyanisole
Condoms damages latex condoms and diaphragms
Dose insert 5-g applicatorful once daily for 10–14 days or twice daily for 7 days; course can be repeated once if necessary; *topical*, apply to anogenital area twice daily

Ovule (= vaginal capsule) (*Gyno-Daktarin 1®*), miconazole nitrate 1.2 g in a fatty basis. Net price 1 ovule = £3.00
Excipients include hydroxybenzoates (parabens)
Condoms damages latex condoms and diaphragms
Dose insert 1 ovule at night as a single dose; can be repeated once if necessary

**Gyno-Pevaryl®** (Janssen-Cilag) PoM
Cream, econazole nitrate 1%. Net price 15 g = £1.35; 30 g = £3.08
Excipients none as listed in section 13.1.3
Condoms damages latex condoms and diaphragms
Dose insert 5-g applicatorful intravaginally and apply to vulva at night for at least 14 nights; course can be repeated once if necessary

Pessaries, econazole nitrate 150 mg. Net price 3 pessaries = £2.83
Excipients none as listed in section 13.1.3
Condoms damages latex condoms and diaphragms
Dose ADULT and ADOLESCENT over 16 years, insert 1 pessary for 3 nights; course can be repeated once if necessary

Pessary (*Gyno-Pevaryl 1®*), econazole nitrate 150 mg, formulated for single-dose therapy. Net price 1 pessary with applicator = £3.01
Excipients none as listed in section 13.1.3
Condoms damages latex condoms and diaphragms
Dose ADULT and ADOLESCENT over 16 years, insert 1 pessary at night as a single dose; can be repeated once if necessary

**Nizoral®** (Janssen-Cilag) PoM
Cream (topical), ketoconazole 2%. Net price 30 g = £3.40
Excipients include polysorbates, propylene glycol, stearyl alcohol
Condoms effect on latex condoms and diaphragms not yet known
Dose apply to anogenital area once or twice daily

## Other infections

Vaginal preparations intended to restore normal acidity may prevent recurrence of vaginal infections and permit the re-establishment of the normal vaginal flora.

*Trichomonal infections* commonly involve the lower urinary tract as well as the genital system and need systemic treatment with metronidazole or tinidazole (section 5.1.11).

*Bacterial infections* with Gram-negative organisms are particularly common in association with gynaecological operations and trauma. Metronidazole is effective against certain Gram-negative organisms, especially *Bacteroides* spp. and can be used prophylactically in gynaecological surgery.

Clindamycin cream and metronidazole gel are indicated for bacterial vaginosis.

The antiviral drugs aciclovir, famciclovir, and valaciclovir can be used in the treatment of genital infection due to *herpes simplex virus*, the HSV type 2 being a major cause of genital ulceration. They have a beneficial effect on virus shedding and healing, generally giving relief from pain and other symptoms. See section 5.3.2.1 for systemic preparations, and section 13.10.3 for topical preparations.

## ▌ PREPARATIONS FOR OTHER VAGINAL INFECTIONS

**Dalacin®** (Pharmacia) PoM
Cream, clindamycin 2% (as phosphate). Net price 40-g pack with 7 applicators = £10.86
Excipients include benzyl alcohol, cetostearyl alcohol, polysorbates, propylene glycol
Condoms damages latex condoms and diaphragms
Side-effects irritation, cervicitis and vaginitis; poorly absorbed into the blood—very low likelihood of systemic effects (section 5.1.6)
Dose bacterial vaginosis, insert 5-g applicatorful at night for 3–7 nights

**Zidoval®** (3M) PoM
Vaginal gel, metronidazole 0.75%. Net price 40-g pack with 5 applicators = £4.31
Excipients include disodium edetate, hydroxybenzoates (parabens), propylene glycol
Cautions not recommended during menstruation; some absorption may occur, see section 5.1.11 for systemic effects
Side-effects local effects including irritation, candidiasis, abnormal discharge, pelvic discomfort
Dose bacterial vaginosis, insert 5-g applicatorful at night for 5 nights

## 7.3  Contraceptives

**7.3.1  Combined hormonal contraceptives**
**7.3.2  Progestogen-only contraceptives**
**7.3.3  Spermicidal contraceptives**
**7.3.4  Contraceptive devices**
**7.3.5  Emergency contraception**

The Fraser Guidelines[1] should be followed when prescribing contraception for women under 16 years. The UK Medical Eligibility Criteria for Contraceptive Use (available at www.ffprhc.org.uk) is published by The Faculty of Sexual and Reproductive Healthcare; it categorises the risks of using contraceptive methods with pre-existing medical conditions.

**Hormonal contraception** is the most effective method of fertility control, but has major and minor side-effects, especially for certain groups of women.

**Intra-uterine devices** are a highly effective method of contraception but may produce undesirable local side-effects. They may be used in women of all ages irrespective of parity, but are less appropriate for those with an increased risk of pelvic inflammatory disease.

1. See Department of Health Guidance (July 2004): Best practice guidance for doctors and other health professionals on the provision of advice and treatment to young people under 16 on contraception, sexual and reproductive health. Available at www.dh.gov.uk

**Barrier methods** alone (condoms, diaphragms, and caps) are less effective but can be very reliable for well-motivated couples if used in conjunction with a **spermicide**. Occasionally sensitivity reactions occur. A female condom (*Femidom®*) is also available; it is prelubricated but does not contain a spermicide.

## 7.3.1  Combined hormonal contraceptives

Oral contraceptives containing an oestrogen and a progestogen ('combined oral contraceptives') are the most effective preparations for general use. Advantages of combined oral contraceptives include:

- reliable and reversible;
- reduced dysmenorrhoea and menorrhagia;
- reduced incidence of premenstrual tension;
- less symptomatic fibroids and functional ovarian cysts;
- less benign breast disease;
- reduced risk of ovarian and endometrial cancer;
- reduced risk of pelvic inflammatory disease.

Combined oral contraceptives containing a fixed amount of an oestrogen and a progestogen in each active tablet are termed 'monophasic'; those with varying amounts of the two hormones according to the stage of the cycle are termed 'phasic'. A transdermal patch and a vaginal ring, both containing an oestrogen with a progestogen, are also available.

**Choice** The majority of combined oral contraceptives contain ethinylestradiol as the oestrogen component; mestranol and estradiol valerate are also used. The ethinylestradiol content of combined oral contraceptives ranges from 20 to 40 micrograms. Generally a preparation with the lowest oestrogen and progestogen content which gives good cycle control and minimal side-effects in the individual woman is chosen.

- *Low strength preparations* (containing ethinylestradiol 20 micrograms) are particularly appropriate for women with risk factors for circulatory disease, provided a combined oral contraceptive is otherwise suitable. It is recommended that the combined oral contraceptive is not continued beyond 50 years of age since more suitable alternatives exist.

- *Standard strength preparations* (containing ethinylestradiol 30 or 35 micrograms or in 30–40 microgram *phased* preparations) are appropriate for standard use—but see Risk of Venous Thromboembolism below. Phased preparations are generally reserved for women who *either* do not have withdrawal bleeding *or* who have breakthrough bleeding with monophasic products.

The progestogens desogestrel, drospirenone, and gestodene (in combination with ethinylestradiol) may be considered for women who have side-effects (such as acne, headache, depression, weight gain, breast symptoms, and breakthrough bleeding) with other progestogens. However, women should be advised that desogestrel and gestodene have also been associated with an increased risk of *venous thromboembolism*. Drospirenone, a derivative of spironolactone, has anti-androgenic and anti-mineralocorticoid activity; it should be used with care if an increased plasma-potassium concentration might be hazardous.

The progestogen norelgestromin is combined with ethinylestradiol in a transdermal patch (*Evra®*).

The vaginal contraceptive ring contains the progestogen etonogestrel combined with ethinylestradiol (*NuvaRing®*).

**Risk of venous thromboembolism**  There is an increased risk of venous thromboembolic disease (particularly during the first year) in users of oral contraceptives but this risk is considerably smaller than that associated with pregnancy (about 60 cases of venous thromboembolic disease per 100 000 pregnancies). In all cases the risk of venous thromboembolism increases with age and in the presence of other risk factors for venous thromboembolism (e.g. obesity).

The incidence of venous thromboembolism in healthy, non-pregnant women who are not taking an oral contraceptive is about 5–10 cases per 100 000 women per year. For those using combined oral contraceptives containing second-generation progestogens, e.g. levonorgestrel, this incidence is about 15 per 100 000 women per year of use. The risk of venous thromboembolism with transdermal patches may be slightly increased compared with combined oral contraceptives that contain levonorgestrel. Some studies have reported a greater risk of venous thromboembolism in women using combined oral contraceptives containing the third-generation progestogens desogestrel and gestodene; the incidence in these women is about 25 per 100 000 women per year of use. The absolute risk of venous thromboembolism in women using combined oral contraceptives containing these third-generation progestogens is very small and well below the risk associated with pregnancy. The incidence of venous thromboembolism in women using a combined oral contraceptive containing drospirenone is in the same range as that for users of combined oral contraceptives containing other progestogens, including levonorgestrel. The risk of venous thromboembolism with vaginal ring use compared to the risk with other combined hormonal contraceptives is unknown.

Provided that women are informed of the relative risks of venous thromboembolism and accept them, the choice of oral contraceptive is for the woman together with the prescriber jointly to make in light of her individual medical history and any contra-indications.

**Travel**  Women taking oral contraceptives or using the patch or vaginal ring are at an increased risk of deep-vein thrombosis during travel involving long periods of immobility (over 5 hours). The risk may be reduced by appropriate exercise during the journey and possibly by wearing graduated compression hosiery.

**Missed pill**  The critical time for loss of contraceptive protection is when a pill is omitted at the *beginning* or *end* of a cycle (which lengthens the pill-free interval).

If a woman forgets to take a pill, it should be taken as soon as she remembers, and the next one taken at the normal time (even if this means taking 2 pills together). A missed pill is one that is 24 or more hours late. If a woman misses only one pill, she should take an active pill as soon as she remembers and then resume normal pill-taking. No additional precautions are necessary.

If a woman misses 2 or more pills (especially from the first 7 in a packet), she may not be protected. She should take an active pill as soon as she remembers and then resume normal pill-taking. In addition, she must either abstain from sex or use an additional method of contraception such as a condom for the next 7 days. If these 7 days run beyond the end of the packet, the next packet should be started at once, omitting the pill-free interval (or, in the case of *everyday* (ED) pills, omitting the 7 inactive tablets).

For information on how to manage missed pills in women taking *Qlaira®*, refer to product literature.

Emergency contraception (section 7.3.5) is recommended if 2 or more combined oral contraceptive tablets are missed from the first 7 tablets in a packet and unprotected intercourse has occurred since finishing the last packet.

Note The Faculty of Sexual and Reproductive Healthcare offers 2 different types of missed pill advice depending on the ethinylestradiol content of the contraceptive pill. The missed pill information above offers the same advice regardless of the ethinylestradiol content of the contraceptive pill; it is a simplified, more cautious version of advice issued by The Faculty of Sexual and Reproductive Healthcare.

**Delayed application or detached patch**  If a patch is partly detached for less than 24 hours, reapply to the same site or replace with a new patch immediately; no additional contraception is needed and the next patch should be applied on the usual change day. If a patch remains detached for more than 24 hours or if the user is not aware when the patch became detached then stop the current contraceptive cycle and start a new cycle by applying a new patch, giving a new 'Day 1'; an additional non-hormonal contraceptive must be used concurrently for the first 7 days of the new cycle.

If application of a new patch at the start of a new cycle is delayed, contraceptive protection is lost. A new patch should be applied as soon as remembered giving a new 'Day 1'; additional non-hormonal methods of contraception should be used for the first 7 days of the new cycle. If intercourse has occurred during this extended patch-free interval, a possibility of fertilisation should be considered. If application of a patch in the middle of the cycle is delayed (i.e. the patch is not changed on day 8 or day 15):

- for up to 48 hours, apply a new patch immediately; next patch change day remains the same and no additional contraception is required.

- for more than 48 hours, contraceptive protection may have been lost. Stop the current cycle and start a new 4-week cycle immediately by applying a new patch giving a new 'Day 1'; additional non-hormonal contraception should be used for the first 7 days of the new cycle.

If the patch is not removed at the end of the cycle (day 22), remove it as soon as possible and start the next cycle on the usual 'change day', the day after day 28; no additional contraception is required.

**Expulsion, delayed insertion or removal, or broken vaginal ring**  If the vaginal ring is expelled for *less than 3 hours*, rinse the ring with cool water and reinsert immediately; no additional contraception is needed.

If the ring remains outside the vagina for *more than 3 hours* or if the user does not know when the ring was expelled, contraceptive protection may be reduced:

- If ring expelled during week 1 or 2 of cycle, rinse ring with cool water and reinsert; use additional precautions (barrier methods) for next 7 days;

- If ring expelled during week 3 of cycle, either insert a new ring to start a new cycle *or* allow a withdrawal bleed and insert a new ring no later than 7 days after ring was expelled; latter option only available if ring was used continuously for at least 7 days prior to expulsion.

If insertion of a new ring at the start of a new cycle is delayed, contraceptive protection is lost. A new ring should be inserted as soon as possible; additional precautions (barrier methods) should be used for the first 7 days of the new cycle. If intercourse occurred during the extended ring-free interval, pregnancy should be considered.

No additional contraception is required if removal of the ring is delayed by up to 1 week (4 weeks of continuous use). The 7-day ring-free interval should be observed and subsequently a new ring should be inserted. Contraceptive protection may be reduced with continuous use of the ring for more than 4 weeks—pregnancy should be ruled out before inserting a new ring.

If the ring breaks during use, remove it and insert a new ring immediately; additional precautions (barrier methods) should be used for the first 7 days of the new cycle.

**Diarrhoea and vomiting** Vomiting and persistent, severe diarrhoea can interfere with the absorption of combined oral contraceptives. If vomiting occurs within 2 hours of taking a combined oral contraceptive another pill should be taken as soon as possible. In cases of persistent vomiting or severe diarrhoea lasting more than 24 hours, additional precautions should be used during and for 7 days (9 days for *Qlaira*®) after recovery (see also under Missed pill, above). If the vomiting and diarrhoea occurs during the last 7 tablets, the next pill-free interval should be omitted (in the case of ED tablets the inactive ones should be omitted).

**Interactions** The effectiveness of both *combined* and *progestogen-only* oral contraceptives can be considerably reduced by interaction with drugs that induce hepatic enzyme activity (e.g. **carbamazepine**, **griseofulvin**, **modafinil**, **nelfinavir**, **nevirapine**, **oxcarbazepine**, **phenytoin**, **phenobarbital**, **primidone**, **ritonavir**, **St John's Wort**, **topiramate**, and, above all, **rifabutin** and **rifampicin**). A condom together with a long-acting method, such as an injectable contraceptive, may be more suitable for patients with HIV infection or at risk of HIV infection; advice on the possibility of interaction with antiretroviral drugs should be sought from HIV specialists.

For a *short course of an enzyme-inducing drug*, the dose of combined oral contraceptives should be adjusted to provide ethinylestradiol 50 micrograms or more daily [unlicensed use]; furthermore, additional contraceptive precautions should be taken whilst taking the enzyme-inducing drug and for 4 weeks after stopping it.

Women requiring a *long-term course of an enzyme-inducing drug* should be encouraged to consider a contraceptive method that is unaffected by the interacting drug. In women unable to use an alternative method of contraception (for rifampicin and rifabutin see also below), a regimen of combined oral contraceptives should be taken which provides a daily intake of ethinylestradiol 50 micrograms or more [unlicensed use]; 'tricycling' (i.e. taking 3 or 4 packets of monophasic tablets without a break followed by a short tablet-free interval of 4 days) is recommended (but women should be warned of uncertainty about the effectiveness of this regimen). **Rifampicin** and **rifabutin** are such potent

enzyme-inducing drugs that an alternative method of contraception (such as an IUD) is **always** recommended. Since enzyme activity does not return to normal for several weeks after stopping an enzyme-inducing drug, appropriate contraceptive measures are required for 4 to 8 weeks after stopping.

The effectiveness of contraceptive patches and vaginal rings can also be reduced by drugs that induce hepatic enzyme activity. Additional contraceptive precautions are required whilst taking the enzyme-inducing drug and for 4 weeks after stopping. If concomitant administration runs beyond the 3 weeks of patch or vaginal ring use, a new treatment cycle should be started immediately without a patch-free or ring-free break. For women taking enzyme-inducing drugs over a long period, another method of contraception should be considered.

Some antibacterials that do not induce liver enzymes (e.g. ampicillin, doxycycline) may reduce the efficacy of *combined* oral contraceptives by impairing the bacterial flora responsible for recycling ethinylestradiol from the large bowel. Additional contraceptive precautions should be taken whilst taking a short course of an antibacterial drug that is not enzyme-inducing and for 7 days after stopping. If these 7 days run beyond the end of a packet the next packet should be started immediately without a break (in the case of ED tablets the inactive ones should be omitted). If the antibacterial course *exceeds 3 weeks*, the bacterial flora develop antibacterial resistance and additional precautions become unnecessary unless a new antibacterial is prescribed; additional precautions are also unnecessary if a woman starting a *combined* oral contraceptive has been on a course of antibacterial therapy for 3 weeks or more.

It is possible that some antibacterials reduce the efficacy of contraceptive patches and vaginal rings. Additional contraceptive precautions are recommended during concomitant use and for 7 days after discontinuation of an antibacterial that is not enzyme-inducing (except tetracycline with contraceptive patch use, and amoxicillin or doxycycline with vaginal ring use). If concomitant administration runs beyond the 3 weeks of patch or vaginal ring use, a new treatment cycle should be started immediately without a patch-free or ring-free break. If the antibacterial course exceeds 3 weeks, additional precautions become unnecessary unless a new antibacterial is prescribed; additional precautions are also unnecessary if a woman starting a contraceptive patch or vaginal ring has been on a course of antibacterial therapy for 3 weeks or more.

**Surgery** Oestrogen-containing contraceptives should preferably be discontinued (and adequate alternative contraceptive arrangements made) 4 weeks before major elective surgery and all surgery to the legs or surgery which involves prolonged immobilisation of a lower limb; they should normally be recommenced at the first menses occurring at least 2 weeks after full mobilisation. A depot injection of a progestogen-only contraceptive may be offered and the oestrogen-containing contraceptive restarted later—if preferred before the next injection would be due. When discontinuation of an oestrogen-containing contraceptive is not possible, e.g. after trauma or if a patient admitted for an elective procedure is still on an oestrogen-containing contraceptive, thromboprophylaxis (with heparin and graduated compression hosiery) is advised. These recommendations do not apply to minor surgery with short duration of anaesthesia, e.g. laparoscopic sterilisation or tooth extraction, or to women using oestrogen-free hormonal contraceptives (whether by mouth or by injection).

**Reason to stop immediately** Combined hormonal contraceptives or hormone replacement therapy (HRT) should be stopped (pending investigation and treatment), if any of the following occur:

- sudden severe chest pain (even if not radiating to left arm);
- sudden breathlessness (or cough with blood-stained sputum);
- unexplained swelling or severe pain in calf of one leg;
- severe stomach pain;
- serious neurological effects including unusual severe, prolonged headache especially if first time or getting progressively worse *or* sudden partial or complete loss of vision *or* sudden disturbance of hearing or other perceptual disorders *or* dysphasia *or* bad fainting attack or collapse *or* first unexplained epileptic seizure *or* weakness, motor disturbances, very marked numbness suddenly affecting one side or one part of body;
- hepatitis, jaundice, liver enlargement;
- blood pressure above systolic 160 mmHg or diastolic 95 mmHg;
- prolonged immobility after surgery or leg injury;
- detection of a risk factor which contra-indicates treatment (see Cautions and Contra-indications under Combined Hormonal Contraceptives below or under Oestrogens for HRT (section 6.4.1.1)).

## COMBINED HORMONAL CONTRACEPTIVES

**Indications** contraception; menstrual symptoms (section 6.4.1.2)

**Cautions** see notes above; also risk factors for venous thromboembolism (see below and also notes above), arterial disease and migraine, see below; personal or family history of hypertriglyceridaemia (increased risk of pancreatitis); hyperprolactinaemia (seek specialist advice); history of severe depression especially if induced by hormonal contraceptive; undiagnosed breast mass; gene mutations associated with breast cancer (e.g. BRCA 1); sickle-cell disease; inflammatory bowel disease including Crohn's disease; reduced efficacy of contraceptive patch in women with body-weight ≥ 90 kg; **interactions:** see above and Appendix 1 (oestrogens, progestogens)

**Risk factors for venous thromboembolism** See also notes above. Use with **caution** if any of following factors present but **avoid** if two or more factors present:

- *family history of venous thromboembolism* in first-degree relative aged under 45 years (avoid contraceptive containing desogestrel or gestodene, *or* avoid if known prothrombotic coagulation abnormality e.g. factor V Leiden or antiphospholipid antibodies (including lupus anticoagulant));
- *obesity*—body mass index above 30 kg/m² (avoid if body mass index above 39 kg/m²);
- *long-term immobilisation* e.g. in a wheelchair (avoid if confined to bed or leg in plaster cast);
- *history of superficial thrombophlebitis;*
- *age* over 35 years (avoid if over 50 years);
- *smoking.*

**Risk factors for arterial disease** Use with **caution** if any one of following factors present but **avoid** if two or more factors present:

- *family history of arterial disease* in first degree relative aged under 45 years (avoid if atherogenic lipid profile);

- *diabetes mellitus* (avoid if diabetes complications present);
- *hypertension*—blood pressure above *systolic 140 mmHg* or *diastolic 90 mmHg* (avoid if blood pressure above *systolic 160 mmHg* or *diastolic 95 mmHg*);
- *smoking* (avoid if smoking 40 or more cigarettes daily);
- *age* over 35 years (avoid if over 50 years);
- *obesity* (avoid if body mass index above 39 kg/m²);
- *migraine without aura* (avoid if *migraine with aura* (focal symptoms), *or* severe migraine frequently lasting over 72 hours despite treatment, *or* migraine treated with ergot derivatives).

**Migraine** Women should report any increase in headache frequency or onset of focal symptoms (discontinue immediately and refer urgently to neurology expert if focal neurological symptoms not typical of aura persist for more than 1 hour—see also Reason to stop immediately in notes above)

**Contra-indications** see notes above; also pregnancy (Appendix 4); personal history of venous or arterial thrombosis, severe or multiple risk factors for arterial disease or for venous thromboembolism (see above), heart disease associated with pulmonary hypertension or risk of embolus; sclerosing treatment for varicose veins; migraine (but see above); transient cerebral ischaemic attacks without headaches; liver disease including disorders of hepatic excretion (e.g. Dubin-Johnson or Rotor syndromes), infective hepatitis (until liver function returns to normal); systemic lupus erythematosus; acute porphyria (section 9.8.2); liver tumour; gallstones; active trophoblastic disease (until return to normal of urine and plasma gonadotrophin concentration); history of haemolytic uraemic syndrome or history during pregnancy of pruritus, cholestatic jaundice, chorea, pemphigoid gestationis; history of breast cancer but can be used after 5 years if no evidence of disease and non-hormonal methods unacceptable; undiagnosed vaginal bleeding; breast-feeding (until weaning or for 6 months after birth—Appendix 5)

**Side-effects** see notes above; also nausea, vomiting, abdominal cramps, changes in body-weight, liver impairment, hepatic tumours; fluid retention, thrombosis (more common when factor V Leiden present or in blood groups A, B, and AB; see also notes above), hypertension, changes in lipid metabolism; headache, depression, chorea, nervousness, irritability; changes in libido, breast tenderness, enlargement, and secretion; reduced menstrual loss, 'spotting' in early cycles, absence of withdrawal bleeding, amenorrhoea after discontinuation, changes in vaginal discharge, cervical erosion; contact lenses may irritate, visual disturbances; leg cramps; skin reactions, chloasma, photosensitivity; rarely gallstones and systemic lupus erythematosus

**Breast cancer** There is a small increase in the risk of having breast cancer diagnosed in women taking the combined oral contraceptive pill; this relative risk may be due to an earlier diagnosis. In users of combined oral contraceptive pills the cancers are more likely to be localised to the breast. The most important factor for diagnosing breast cancer appears to be the age at which the contraceptive is stopped rather than the duration of use; any increase in the rate of diagnosis diminishes gradually during the 10 years after stopping and disappears by 10 years.

**Cervical cancer** Use of combined oral contraceptives for 5 years or longer is associated with a small increased risk of cervical cancer; the risk diminishes after stopping and disappears by about 10 years. The risk of cervical cancer with transdermal patches and vaginal rings is not yet known.

**Note** The possible small increase in the risk of breast cancer and cervical cancer should be weighed against the protective effect against cancers of the ovary and endometrium

## Dose

- By mouth, each tablet should be taken at approximately same time each day; if delayed by longer than 24 hours contraceptive protection may be lost

  *21-day combined (monophasic) preparations*, 1 tablet daily for 21 days; subsequent courses repeated after a 7-day interval (during which withdrawal bleeding occurs); first course usually started on day 1 of cycle—if starting on day 4 of cycle or later, additional precautions (barrier methods) necessary during first 7 days

  *Every day (ED) combined (monophasic) preparations*, 1 *active* tablet starting on day 1 of cycle (see also under preparations below)—if starting on day 4 of cycle or later, additional precautions (barrier methods) necessary during first 7 days; withdrawal bleeding occurs when *inactive* tablets being taken; subsequent courses repeated without interval

  *Phased preparations*, see under individual preparations below

  **Changing to combined preparation containing different progestogen** *21-day combined preparations*: continue current pack until last tablet and start first tablet of new brand the next day. If a 7-day break is taken before starting new brand, additional precautions (barrier methods) should be used during first 7 days (9 days for *Qlaira®*) of taking the new brand.

  *Every Day (ED) combined preparations*: start the new brand (first tablet of a *21-day preparation* or the first *active* tablet of an *ED preparation*) the day after taking the last *active* tablet of previous brand (omitting the *inactive* tablets).

  **Changing from progestogen-only tablet** Start on day 1 of menstruation or any day if amenorrhoea present and pregnancy has been excluded.

  **Secondary amenorrhoea (exclude pregnancy)** Start any day, additional precautions (barrier methods) necessary during first 7 days (9 days for *Qlaira®*).

  **After childbirth (not breast-feeding)** Start 3 weeks after birth (increased risk of thrombosis if started earlier); later than 3 weeks postpartum additional precautions (barrier methods) necessary for first 7 days (9 days for *Qlaira®*). Not recommended if woman breast-feeding—oral progestogen-only contraceptive preferred.

  **After abortion or miscarriage** Start same day.

- By transdermal application, apply first patch on day 1 of cycle, change patch on days 8 and 15; remove third patch on day 22 and apply new patch after 7-day patch-free interval to start subsequent contraceptive cycle

  **Note** If first patch applied later than day 1, additional precautions (abstinence or barrier methods) should be used for the next 7 days

  **Changing from combined oral contraception** Apply patch on the first day of withdrawal bleeding; if no withdrawal bleeding within 5 days of taking last *active* tablet, rule out pregnancy before applying first patch. Unless patch is applied on first day of withdrawal bleeding, additional precautions (barrier methods) should be used concurrently for first 7 days

  **Changing from progestogen-only method** From an implant, apply first patch on the day implant removed; from an injection, apply first patch when next injection due; from oral progestogen, first patch may be started on any day after stopping pill. For all methods additional precautions (barrier methods) should be used concurrently for first 7 days

  **After childbirth (not breast-feeding)** Start 4 weeks after birth; if started later than 4 weeks after birth additional precautions (barrier methods) should be used for first 7 days

  **After abortion or miscarriage** Before 20 weeks' gestation start immediately; no additional contraception required if started immediately. After 20 weeks' gestation start on day 21 after abortion or on the first day of first spontaneous menstruation; additional precautions (barrier methods) should be used for first 7 days after applying the patch

- By vagina, insert ring into vagina on day 1 of cycle and leave in for 3 weeks; remove ring on day 22; subsequent courses repeated after 7-day ring-free interval (during which withdrawal bleeding occurs)

  **Note** If first ring inserted later than day 1, additional precautions (abstinence or barrier methods) should be used for the next 7 days

  **Changing from combined hormonal contraception** Insert ring at the latest on the day after the usual tablet-free, patch-free, or placebo-tablet interval. If previous contraceptive used correctly and pregnancy unlikely, can switch to ring on any day of cycle

  **Changing from progestogen-only method** From an implant or intra-uterine progestogen-only device, insert ring on the day implant or intra-uterine progestogen-only device removed; from an injection, insert ring when next injection due; from oral preparation, first ring may be inserted on any day after stopping pill. For all methods additional precautions (barrier methods) should be used concurrently for first 7 days

  **After first trimester abortion** Start immediately

  **After childbirth (not breast-feeding) or second trimester abortion** Start 4 weeks after birth or abortion; if started later than 4 weeks after birth or abortion, additional precautions (barrier methods) should be used for first 7 days

## Low strength (oral)

◢**Ethinylestradiol with Norethisterone**

**Loestrin 20®** (Galen) ⟨PoM⟩

Tablets, blue, norethisterone acetate 1 mg, ethinylestradiol 20 micrograms. Net price 3 × 21-tab pack = £2.75

**Dose** 1 tablet daily for 21 days; subsequent courses repeated after 7-day tablet-free interval (during which withdrawal bleeding occurs); for starting routines see under Dose above

◢**Ethinylestradiol with Desogestrel**

See Risk of Venous Thromboembolism in notes above before prescribing

**Mercilon®** (Organon) ⟨PoM⟩

Tablets, desogestrel 150 micrograms, ethinylestradiol 20 micrograms. Net price 3 × 21-tab pack = £7.82

**Dose** 1 tablet daily for 21 days; subsequent courses repeated after 7-day tablet-free interval (during which withdrawal bleeding occurs); for starting routines see under Dose above

◢**Ethinylestradiol with Gestodene**

See Risk of Venous Thromboembolism in notes above before prescribing

**Femodette®** (Schering Health) ⟨PoM⟩

Tablets, s/c, gestodene 75 micrograms, ethinylestradiol 20 micrograms, net price 3 × 21-tab pack = £9.08

**Dose** 1 tablet daily for 21 days; subsequent courses repeated after 7-day tablet-free interval (during which withdrawal bleeding occurs); for starting routines see under Dose above

**Sunya 20/75®** (Stragen) ⟨PoM⟩

Tablets, s/c, gestodene 75 micrograms, ethinylestradiol 20 micrograms, net price 3 × 21-tab pack = £6.62

**Dose** 1 tablet daily for 21 days; subsequent courses repeated after 7-day tablet-free interval (during which withdrawal bleeding occurs); for starting routines see under Dose above

## Low strength (vaginal)

◢**Ethinylestradiol with Etonogestrel**

**NuvaRing®** (Organon) ▼ ⟨PoM⟩

Vaginal ring, releasing ethinylestradiol approx. 15 micrograms/24 hours and etonogestrel approx.

120 micrograms/24 hours, net price 3-ring pack = £27.00. Counselling, administration

**Dose** 1 ring to be inserted into the vagina, removed on day 22; subsequent courses repeated after 7-day ring-free interval (during which withdrawal bleeding occurs); for starting routines see under Dose above

**Counselling** The presence of the ring should be checked regularly. In case of expulsion see Expulsion, Delayed Insertion or Removal, or Broken Vaginal Ring, p. 444

## Standard strength (oral)

◢**Ethinylestradiol with Levonorgestrel**

**Logynon®** (Schering Health) PoM

6 light brown tablets, ethinylestradiol 30 micrograms, levonorgestrel 50 micrograms;

5 white tablets, ethinylestradiol 40 micrograms, levonorgestrel 75 micrograms;

10 ochre tablets, ethinylestradiol 30 micrograms, levonorgestrel 125 micrograms.

Net price 3 × 21-tab pack = £3.96

**Dose** 1 tablet daily for 21 days, starting with light brown tablet marked 1 on day 1 of cycle; repeat after 7-day tablet-free interval

**Logynon ED®** (Schering Health) PoM

6 light brown tablets, ethinylestradiol 30 micrograms, levonorgestrel 50 micrograms;

5 white tablets, ethinylestradiol 40 micrograms, levonorgestrel 75 micrograms;

10 ochre tablets, ethinylestradiol 30 micrograms, levonorgestrel 125 micrograms;

7 white, inactive tablets.

Net price 3 × 28-tab pack = £3.96

**Dose** 1 tablet daily for 28 days, starting on day 1 of cycle with active tablet (withdrawal bleeding occurs when inactive tablets being taken); subsequent courses repeated without interval; for starting routines see under Dose above

**Microgynon 30®** (Schering Health) PoM

Tablets, s/c, levonorgestrel 150 micrograms, ethinylestradiol 30 micrograms. Net price 3 × 21-tab pack = £2.87

**Dose** 1 tablet daily for 21 days; subsequent courses repeated after 7-day tablet-free interval (during which withdrawal bleeding occurs); for starting routines see under Dose above

**Microgynon 30 ED®** (Schering Health) PoM

Tablets, beige, levonorgestrel 150 micrograms, ethinylestradiol 30 micrograms, white inactive tablets. Net price 3 × 28-tab (7 are inactive) pack = £2.59

**Dose** 1 tablet daily for 28 days starting on day 1 of cycle with active tablet (withdrawal bleeding occurs when inactive tablets being taken); subsequent courses repeated without interval; for starting routines see also under Dose above

**Ovranette®** (Wyeth) PoM

Tablets, levonorgestrel 150 micrograms, ethinylestradiol 30 micrograms. Net price 3 × 21-tab pack = £2.20

**Dose** 1 tablet daily for 21 days; subsequent courses repeated after 7-day tablet-free interval (during which withdrawal bleeding occurs); for starting routines see under Dose above

◢**Ethinylestradiol with Norethisterone**

**BiNovum®** (Janssen-Cilag) PoM

7 white tablets, ethinylestradiol 35 micrograms, norethisterone 500 micrograms;

14 peach tablets, ethinylestradiol 35 micrograms, norethisterone 1 mg.

Net price 3 × 21-tab pack = £2.00

**Dose** 1 tablet daily for 21 days, starting with white tablet on day 1 of cycle; repeat after 7-day tablet-free interval

**Brevinor®** (Pharmacia) PoM

Tablets, blue, norethisterone 500 micrograms, ethinylestradiol 35 micrograms. Net price 3 × 21-tab pack = £1.99

**Dose** 1 tablet daily for 21 days; subsequent courses repeated after 7-day tablet-free interval (during which withdrawal bleeding occurs); for starting routines see under Dose above

**Loestrin 30®** (Galen) PoM

Tablets, pale green, norethisterone acetate 1.5 mg, ethinylestradiol 30 micrograms. Net price 3 × 21-tab pack = £3.95

**Dose** 1 tablet daily for 21 days; subsequent courses repeated after 7-day tablet-free interval (during which withdrawal bleeding occurs); for starting routines see under Dose above

**Norimin®** (Pharmacia) PoM

Tablets, norethisterone 1 mg, ethinylestradiol 35 micrograms. Net price 3 × 21-tab pack = £2.28

**Dose** 1 tablet daily for 21 days; subsequent courses repeated after 7-day tablet-free interval (during which withdrawal bleeding occurs); for starting routines see under Dose above

**Ovysmen®** (Janssen-Cilag) PoM

Tablets, norethisterone 500 micrograms, ethinylestradiol 35 micrograms. Net price 3 × 21-tab pack = £1.52

**Dose** 1 tablet daily for 21 days; subsequent courses repeated after 7-day tablet-free interval (during which withdrawal bleeding occurs); for starting routines see under Dose above

**Synphase®** (Pharmacia) PoM

7 blue tablets, ethinylestradiol 35 micrograms, norethisterone 500 micrograms;

9 white tablets, ethinylestradiol 35 micrograms, norethisterone 1 mg;

5 blue tablets, ethinylestradiol 35 micrograms, norethisterone 500 micrograms.

Net price 21-tab pack = £1.20

**Dose** 1 tablet daily for 21 days, starting with blue tablet marked 1 on day 1 of cycle; repeat after 7-day tablet-free interval

**TriNovum®** (Janssen-Cilag) PoM

7 white tablets, ethinylestradiol 35 micrograms, norethisterone 500 micrograms;

7 light peach tablets, ethinylestradiol 35 micrograms, norethisterone 750 micrograms;

7 peach tablets, ethinylestradiol 35 micrograms, norethisterone 1 mg.

Net price 3 × 21-tab pack = £2.78

**Dose** 1 tablet daily for 21 days, starting with white tablet on day 1 of cycle; repeat after 7-day tablet-free interval

◢**Ethinylestradiol with Norgestimate**

**Cilest®** (Janssen-Cilag) PoM

Tablets, blue, norgestimate 250 micrograms, ethinylestradiol 35 micrograms. Net price 3 × 21-tab pack = £2.99, 6 × 21-tab pack = £5.97

**Dose** 1 tablet daily for 21 days; subsequent courses repeated after 7-day tablet-free interval (during which withdrawal bleeding occurs); for starting routines see under Dose above

◢**Ethinylestradiol with Desogestrel**

See Risk of Venous Thromboembolism in notes above before prescribing

**Marvelon®** (Organon) PoM

Tablets, desogestrel 150 micrograms, ethinylestradiol 30 micrograms. Net price 3 × 21-tab pack = £6.57

**Dose** 1 tablet daily for 21 days; subsequent courses repeated after 7-day tablet-free interval (during which withdrawal bleeding occurs); for starting routines see under Dose above

◢**Ethinylestradiol with Drospirenone**

**Yasmin®** (Bayer) [PoM]

> Tablets, f/c, yellow, drospirenone 3 mg, ethinylestradiol 30 micrograms. Net price 3 × 21-tab pack = £14.70
>
> **Cautions** use with care if increased plasma-potassium concentration might be hazardous; renal impairment (Appendix 3)
>
> **Dose** 1 tablet daily for 21 days; subsequent courses repeated after 7-day tablet-free interval (during which withdrawal bleeding occurs); for starting routines see under Dose above

◢**Ethinylestradiol with Gestodene**

See Risk of Venous Thromboembolism in notes above before prescribing

**Femodene®** (Schering Health) [PoM]

> Tablets, s/c, gestodene 75 micrograms, ethinylestradiol 30 micrograms. Net price 3 × 21-tab pack = £6.90
>
> **Dose** 1 tablet daily for 21 days; subsequent courses repeated after 7-day tablet-free interval (during which withdrawal bleeding occurs); for starting routines see under Dose above

**Femodene® ED** (Schering Health) [PoM]

> Tablets, s/c, gestodene 75 micrograms, ethinylestradiol 30 micrograms. Net price 3 × 28-tab (7 are inactive) pack = £6.90
>
> **Dose** 1 tablet daily for 28 days, starting on day 1 of cycle with active tablet (withdrawal bleeding occurs when inactive tablets being taken); subsequent courses repeated without interval; for starting routines see under Dose above

**Katya 30/75®** (Stragen) [PoM]

> Tablets, s/c, gestodene 75 micrograms, ethinylestradiol 30 micrograms. Net price 3 × 21-tab pack = £5.03
>
> **Dose** 1 tablet daily for 21 days; subsequent courses repeated after 7-day tablet-free interval (during which withdrawal bleeding occurs); for starting routines see under Dose above

**Triadene®** (Schering Health) [PoM]

> 6 beige tablets, ethinylestradiol 30 micrograms, gestodene 50 micrograms;
>
> 5 dark brown tablets, ethinylestradiol 40 micrograms, gestodene 70 micrograms;
>
> 10 white tablets, ethinylestradiol 30 micrograms, gestodene 100 micrograms.
>
> Net price 3 × 21-tab pack = £9.17
>
> **Dose** 1 tablet daily for 21 days, starting with beige tablet marked 'start' on day 1 of cycle; repeat after 7-day tablet-free interval

◢**Mestranol with Norethisterone**

**Norinyl-1®** (Pharmacia) [PoM]

> Tablets, norethisterone 1 mg, mestranol 50 micrograms. Net price 3 × 21-tab pack = £2.19
>
> **Dose** 1 tablet daily for 21 days; subsequent courses repeated after 7-day tablet-free interval (during which withdrawal bleeding occurs); for starting routines see under Dose above

◢**Ethinylestradiol with cyproterone acetate**

See Co-cyprindiol (section 13.6.2)

◢**Estradiol with Dienogest**

**Qlaira®** (Bayer) ▼ [PoM]

> 2 dark yellow tablets, estradiol valerate 3 mg;
>
> 5 red tablets, estradiol valerate 2 mg, dienogest 2 mg;
>
> 17 light yellow tablets, estradiol valerate 2 mg, dienogest 3 mg;
>
> 2 dark red tablets, estradiol valerate 1 mg;
>
> 2 white, inactive tablets.
>
> Net price 3 × 28-tab pack = £25.18
>
> **Dose** 1 tablet daily for 28 days starting on day 1 of cycle with active tablet (withdrawal bleeding occurs when inactive tablets being taken); subsequent courses repeated without interval; for starting routines see under Dose above

## Standard strength (transdermal)

◢**Ethinylestradiol with Norelgestromin**

**Evra®** (Janssen-Cilag) [PoM]

> Patches, self-adhesive (releasing ethinylestradiol approx. 33.9 micrograms/24 hours and norelgestromin approx. 203 micrograms/24 hours); net price 9-patch pack = £15.63. Counselling, administration
>
> **Dose** 1 patch to be applied once weekly for three weeks, followed by a 7-day patch-free interval; subsequent courses repeated after 7-day patch-free interval (during which withdrawal bleeding occurs); for starting routines see under Dose above
>
> **Note** Adhesives or bandages should not be used to hold patch in place. If patch no longer sticky do not reapply but use a new patch.

The *Scottish Medicines Consortium* has advised (September 2003) that *Evra®* patches should be restricted for use in women who are likely to comply poorly with combined oral contraceptives

---

## 7.3.2   Progestogen-only contraceptives

**7.3.2.1**   Oral progestogen-only contraceptives

**7.3.2.2**   Parenteral progestogen-only contraceptives

**7.3.2.3**   Intra-uterine progestogen-only device

**7.3.2.1**   **Oral progestogen-only contraceptives**

Oral progestogen-only preparations may offer a suitable alternative when oestrogens are contra-indicated (including those patients with venous thrombosis or a past history or predisposition to venous thrombosis), but have a higher failure rate than combined preparations. They are suitable for older women, for heavy smokers, and for those with hypertension, valvular heart disease, diabetes mellitus, and migraine. Menstrual irregularities (oligomenorrhoea, menorrhagia) are more common but tend to resolve on long-term treatment.

**Interactions** Effectiveness of oral progestogen-only preparations is not affected by antibacterials that do not induce liver enzymes. The efficacy of oral progestogen-only preparations is, however, reduced by enzyme-inducing drugs and an additional or alternative contraceptive method is recommended during treatment with an enzyme-inducing drug and for at least 4 weeks afterwards—see p. 445 and Appendix 1 (progestogens).

**Surgery** All progestogen-only contraceptives (including those given by injection) are suitable for use as an alternative to combined oral contraceptives before major elective surgery, before all surgery to the legs, or before surgery which involves prolonged immobilisation of a lower limb.

**Starting routine** One tablet daily, on a continuous basis, starting on day 1 of cycle and taken at the same time each day (if delayed by longer than 3 hours (12 hours for *Cerazette®*) contraceptive protection may be lost). Additional contraceptive precautions are not necessary when initiating treatment.

**Changing from a combined oral contraceptive** Start on the day following completion of the combined oral

**Obstetrics, gynaecology, and urinary-tract disorders**

**7**

contraceptive course without a break (or in the case of ED tablets omitting the inactive ones).

**After childbirth** Start any time after 3 weeks postpartum (increased risk of breakthrough bleeding if started earlier)—lactation is not affected.

**Missed pill** The following advice is now recommended by family planning organisations:

'If you forget a pill, take it as soon as you remember and carry on with the next pill at the right time. If the pill was more than 3 hours (12 hours for *Cerazette*®) overdue you are not protected. Continue normal pill-taking but you must also use another method, such as the condom, for the next 2 days.'

The Faculty of Sexual and Reproductive Healthcare recommends emergency contraception (see p. 454) if one or more progestogen-only contraceptive tablets are missed or taken more than 3 hours (12 hours for *Cerazette*®) late and unprotected intercourse has occurred before 2 further tablets have been correctly taken.

**Diarrhoea and vomiting** Vomiting and persistent, severe diarrhoea can interfere with the absorption of oral progestogen-only contraceptives. If vomiting occurs within 2 hours of taking an oral progestogen-only contraceptive, another pill should be taken as soon as possible. If a replacement pill is not taken within 3 hours (12 hours for *Cerazette*®) of the normal time for taking the progestogen-only pill, or in cases of persistent vomiting or very severe diarrhoea, additional precautions should be used during illness and for 2 days after recovery (see also under Missed pill above).

## ORAL PROGESTOGEN-ONLY CONTRACEPTIVES
(Progestogen-only pill, 'POP')

**Indications** contraception

**Cautions** arterial disease; sex-steroid dependent cancer; past ectopic pregnancy; malabsorption syndromes; active trophoblastic disease (until return to normal of urine- and plasma-gonadotrophin concentration); functional ovarian cysts; active liver disease; recurrent cholestatic jaundice; history of jaundice in pregnancy; breast-feeding (Appendix 5); **interactions:** see notes above and Appendix 1 (progestogens)
Other conditions The product literature advises caution in patients with history of thromboembolism, hypertension, diabetes mellitus and migraine; evidence for caution in these conditions is unsatisfactory

**Contra-indications** pregnancy (Appendix 4); undiagnosed vaginal bleeding; severe arterial disease; liver tumour; acute porphyria (section 9.8.2); history of breast cancer but can be used after 5 years if no evidence of disease and non-hormonal contraceptive methods unacceptable

**Side-effects** menstrual irregularities (see also notes above); nausea, vomiting, headache, dizziness, breast discomfort, depression, skin disorders, disturbance of appetite, weight changes, changes in libido
Breast cancer There is a small increase in the risk of having breast cancer diagnosed in women using, or who have recently used, a progestogen-only contraceptive pill; this relative risk may be due to an earlier diagnosis. The most important risk factor appears to be the age at which the contraceptive is stopped rather than the duration of use; the risk disappears gradually during the 10 years after stopping and there is no excess risk by 10 years. The CSM has advised that a possible small increase in the risk of breast cancer should be weighed against the benefits

**Dose**

- 1 tablet daily at same time each day, starting on day 1 of cycle then continuously; if administration delayed for 3 hours (12 hours for *Cerazette*®) or more it should be regarded as a 'missed pill', see notes above

**Cerazette®** (Organon) ᴾᵒᴹ
Tablets, f/c, desogestrel 75 micrograms. Net price 3 × 28-tab pack = £8.68
The *Scottish Medicines Consortium* has advised (September 2003) that *Cerazette*® should be restricted for use in women who cannot tolerate oestrogen-containing contraceptives or in whom such preparations are contra-indicated

**Femulen®** (Pharmacia) ᴾᵒᴹ
Tablets, etynodiol diacetate 500 micrograms. Net price 3 × 28-tab pack = £3.31

**Micronor®** (Janssen-Cilag) ᴾᵒᴹ
Tablets, norethisterone 350 micrograms. Net price 3 × 28-tab pack = £1.69

**Norgeston®** (Bayer) ᴾᵒᴹ
Tablets, s/c, levonorgestrel 30 micrograms. Net price 35-tab pack = 94p

**Noriday®** (Pharmacia) ᴾᵒᴹ
Tablets, norethisterone 350 micrograms. Net price 3 × 28-tab pack = £2.10

### 7.3.2.2 Parenteral progestogen-only contraceptives

**Medroxyprogesterone acetate** (*Depo-Provera*®) is a long-acting progestogen given by intramuscular injection; it is as effective as the combined oral preparations but because of its prolonged action it should never be given without *full counselling backed by the patient information leaflet*. It may be used as a short-term or long-term contraceptive for women who have been counselled about the likelihood of menstrual disturbance and the potential for a delay in return to full fertility. Delayed return of fertility and irregular cycles may occur after discontinuation of treatment but there is no evidence of permanent infertility. Heavy bleeding has been reported in patients given medroxyprogesterone acetate in the immediate puerperium; delaying the first injection until 6 weeks after birth may minimise bleeding problems. If the woman is not breast-feeding, the first injection may be given within 5 days postpartum (she should be warned that the risk of heavy or prolonged bleeding may be increased). The manufacturer advises that in women who are breast-feeding, the first dose should be delayed until 6 weeks after birth; however, evidence suggests no harmful effect to infant if given earlier. The benefits of using medroxyprogesterone acetate in breast-feeding women outweigh any risks.

Reduction in bone mineral density and, rarely, osteoporosis and osteoporotic fractures have also been reported with medroxyprogesterone acetate. The reduction in bone mineral density occurs in the first 2–3 years of use and then stabilises. See also CSM advice below.

**Norethisterone enantate** (*Noristerat®*) is a long-acting progestogen given as an oily injection which provides contraception for 8 weeks; it is used as short-term interim contraception e.g. before vasectomy becomes effective.

An **etonogestrel-releasing implant** (*Implanon®*), consisting of a single flexible rod, is also available; the rod is inserted subdermally into the lower surface of the upper arm and it provides effective contraception for up to 3 years. The manufacturer advises that in heavier women, blood etonogestrel concentrations are lower and therefore the implant may not provide effective contraception during the third year; they advise that earlier replacement should be considered in such patients—however evidence to support this recommendation is lacking. Local reactions such as bruising and itching can occur at the insertion site. The contraceptive effect of *Implanon®* is rapidly reversed on removal of the implant. *The doctor or nurse administering (or removing) the system should be fully trained in the technique and should provide full counselling reinforced by the patient information leaflet.*

The cautions, contra-indications, and side-effects of oral progestogen-only contraceptives apply to parenteral progestogen-only contraceptives, except that parenteral preparations reliably inhibit ovulation and therefore protect against ectopic pregnancy and functional ovarian cysts.

**Interactions** Effectiveness of parenteral progestogen-only contraceptives is not affected by antibacterials that do not induce liver enzymes. However, effectiveness of norethisterone and etonogestrel (but not medroxyprogesterone acetate) may be reduced by enzyme-inducing drugs; additional contraceptive precautions should be taken whilst taking the enzyme-inducing drug and for 4 weeks after stopping it *or* an alternative contraceptive method should be considered if *long-term* use of the enzyme-inducing drug is contemplated.

## ▌ PARENTERAL PROGESTOGEN-ONLY CONTRACEPTIVES

**Indications** contraception, see also notes above and under preparations (roles vary according to preparation)

**Cautions** see notes above and under preparations; possible risk of breast cancer (see oral progestogen-only contraceptives (section 7.3.2.1); history during pregnancy of pruritus or of deterioration of otosclerosis, disturbances of lipid metabolism; breast-feeding (see under preparations and Appendix 5);

**interactions:** see notes above and Appendix 1 (progestogens)

**Counselling** Full counselling backed by *patient information leaflet* required before administration

**Contra-indications** see notes above; history of breast cancer but can be used after 5 years if no evidence of disease and non-hormonal contraceptive methods unacceptable; pregnancy (Appendix 4)

**Side-effects** see notes above; injection-site reactions

Cervical cancer Use of injectable progestogen-only contraceptives may be associated with a small increased risk of cervical cancer, similar to that seen with combined oral contraceptives, see p. 446. The risk of cervical cancer with other progestogen-only contraceptives is not yet known.

**Dose**
- See under preparations

### ▲Injectable preparations

**Depo-Provera®** (Pfizer) [PoM]
Injection (aqueous suspension), medroxyprogesterone acetate 150 mg/mL, net price 1-mL prefilled syringe = £6.01, 1-mL vial = £6.01. Counselling, see patient information leaflet

Dose by deep intramuscular injection, 150 mg within first 5 days of cycle or within first 5 days after parturition (delay until 6 weeks after parturition if breast-feeding); for long-term contraception, repeated every 12 weeks (if interval greater than 12 weeks and 5 days, rule out pregnancy before next injection and advise patient to use additional contraceptive measures (e.g. barrier) for 14 days after the injection)

**Noristerat®** (Schering Health) [PoM]
Injection (oily), norethisterone enantate 200 mg/mL, net price 1-mL amp = £3.45. Counselling, see patient information leaflet

Dose by deep intramuscular injection given very slowly *into gluteal muscle*, short-term contraception, 200 mg within first 5 days of cycle or immediately after parturition (duration 8 weeks); may be repeated once after 8 weeks (withhold breast-feeding for neonates with severe or persistent jaundice requiring medical treatment)

### ▲Implants

**Implanon®** (Organon) [PoM]
Implant, containing etonogestrel 68 mg in each flexible rod, net price = £79.46. Counselling, see patient information leaflet

Dose by subdermal implantation, no previous hormonal contraceptive, 1 implant inserted during first 5 days of cycle; parturition or abortion in second trimester, 1 implant inserted between days 21–28 after delivery or abortion (if inserted after 28 days additional precautions necessary for next 7 days); abortion in first trimester, 1 implant inserted immediately; changing from other contraceptive, consult product literature; remove within 3 years of insertion

### ▌ 7.3.2.3 Intra-uterine progestogen-only device

The progestogen-only intra-uterine system, *Mirena®*, releases **levonorgestrel** directly into the uterine cavity. It is licensed for use as a contraceptive, for the treatment of primary menorrhagia and for the prevention of endometrial hyperplasia during oestrogen replacement therapy. This may therefore be a contraceptive method of choice for women who have excessively heavy menses.

The effects of the progestogen-only intra-uterine system are mainly local and hormonal including prevention of endometrial proliferation, thickening of cervical mucus, and suppression of ovulation in some women (in some cycles). In addition to the progestogenic activity, the intra-uterine system itself may contribute slightly to the contraceptive effect. Return of fertility after removal is rapid and appears to be complete.

Advantages of the progestogen-only intra-uterine system over copper intra-uterine devices are that there may be an improvement in any dysmenorrhoea and a reduction in blood loss; there is also evidence that the frequency of pelvic inflammatory disease may be reduced (particularly in the youngest age groups who are most at risk).

In primary menorrhagia, menstrual bleeding is reduced significantly within 3–6 months of inserting the progestogen-only intra-uterine system, probably because it prevents endometrial proliferation. Another treatment should be considered if menorrhagia does not improve within this time (section 6.4.1.2).

**Cautions and contra-indications**   Generally the cautions and contra-indications for the progestogen-only intra-uterine system are as for standard intra-uterine devices (section 7.3.4), but the risk of ectopic pregnancy is considerably smaller. Although the progestogen-only intra-uterine system produces little systemic progestogenic activity, it is usually avoided for 5 years after any evidence of breast cancer. However, the system can be considered for a woman in long-term remission from breast cancer who has menorrhagia and requires effective contraception. Since levonorgestrel is released close to the site of the main contraceptive action (on cervical mucus and endometrium) progestogenic side-effects and interactions are less likely; in particular, enzyme-inducing drugs are unlikely to significantly reduce the contraceptive effect of the progestogen-only intra-uterine system and additional contraceptive precautions are not required.

**Side-effects**   Initially, changes in the pattern and duration of menstrual bleeding (spotting or prolonged bleeding) are common; endometrial disorders should be ruled out before insertion and the patient should be fully counselled (and provided with a patient information leaflet). Improvement in progestogenic side-effects, such as mastalgia and mood changes, and in the bleeding pattern usually occurs a few months after insertion and bleeding may often become very light or absent. Functional ovarian cysts (usually asymptomatic) can occur and usually resolve spontaneously (ultrasound monitoring recommended).

### INTRA-UTERINE PROGESTOGEN-ONLY SYSTEM

**Indications**   see under preparation

**Cautions**   see notes above; active liver disease; liver tumour; in case of pregnancy—remove system (teratogenicity cannot be excluded); advanced uterine atrophy; not suitable for emergency contraception; **interactions:** see notes above and Appendix 1 (progestogens)

**Contra-indications**   see notes above

**Side-effects**   see notes above; also abdominal pain; peripheral oedema; nervousness; salpingitis and pelvic inflammatory disease; pelvic pain, back pain; *rarely* hirsutism, hair loss, pruritus, migraine, rash

**Mirena®** (Bayer) [PoM]
Intra-uterine system, T-shaped plastic frame (impregnated with barium sulphate and with threads

attached to base) with polydimethylsiloxane reservoir releasing levonorgestrel 20 micrograms/24 hours. Net price = £87.32. Counselling, see patient information leaflet

**Dose**   Contraception and menorrhagia, insert into uterine cavity within 7 days of onset of menstruation (anytime if replacement) or immediately after first-trimester termination by curettage; postpartum insertions should be delayed until 6 weeks after delivery; effective for 5 years.

Prevention of endometrial hyperplasia during oestrogen replacement therapy, insert during last days of menstruation or withdrawal bleeding or anytime if amenorrhoeic; effective for 4 years

## 7.3.3 Spermicidal contraceptives

Spermicidal contraceptives are useful additional safeguards but do **not** give adequate protection if used alone unless fertility is already significantly diminished (section 6.4.1.1). They have two components: a spermicide and a vehicle which itself may have some inhibiting effect on sperm activity. They are suitable for use with barrier methods, such as diaphragms or caps; however spermicidal contraceptives are not generally recommended for use with condoms, as there is no evidence of any additional protection compared with non-spermicidal lubricants.

Spermicidal contraceptives are not suitable for use in those with or at high risk of sexually transmitted diseases (including HIV); high frequency use of the spermicide nonoxinol '9' has been associated with genital lesions, which may increase the risk of acquiring these infections.

> Products such as petroleum jelly (*Vaseline®*), baby oil and oil-based vaginal and rectal preparations are likely to damage condoms and contraceptive diaphragms made from latex rubber, and may render them less effective as a barrier method of contraception and as a protection from sexually transmitted diseases (including HIV).

**Gygel®** (Marlborough)
Gel, nonoxinol '9' 2%, net price 30 g = £4.25
**Excipients** include hydroxybenzoates (parabens), propylene glycol, sorbic acid
Condoms no evidence of harm to latex condoms and diaphragms

## 7.3.4 Contraceptive devices

### Intra-uterine devices

The intra-uterine device (IUD) is a suitable contraceptive for women of all ages irrespective of parity; however it is less appropriate for those with an increased risk of pelvic inflammatory disease (see below).

Smaller devices have been introduced to minimise side-effects; these consist of a plastic carrier wound with copper wire or fitted with copper bands; some also have a central core of silver to prevent fragmentation of the copper. Fertility declines with age and therefore a copper intra-uterine device which is fitted in a woman over the age of 40, may remain in the uterus until menopause. The intra-uterine device *Gyne-T 380®* (Janssen-Cilag) is no longer available, but some women may have the device in place until 2009. The intra-uterine devices *Multiload® Cu250* and *Multiload® Cu250 Short* (Organon) have been discontinued, but some women may have the devices in place until 2011.

A frameless, copper-bearing intra-uterine device (*GyneFix®*) is also available. It consists of a knotted, polypropylene thread with 6 copper sleeves; the device is anchored in the uterus by inserting the knot into the uterine fundus. *The healthcare professional inserting (or removing) the device should be fully trained in the technique and should provide full counselling backed by the patient information leaflet.*

The timing and technique of fitting an intra-uterine device are critical for its subsequent performance and call for proper training and experience. Devices should not be fitted during the heavy days of the period; they are best fitted after the end of menstruation and before the calculated time of implantation. The main excess risk of infection occurs in the first 20 days after insertion and is believed to be related to existing carriage of a sexually transmitted disease. Women are considered to be at a higher risk of sexually transmitted diseases if:

- they are under 25 years old *or*
- they are over 25 years old *and*

  - have a new partner *or*
  - have had more than one partner in the past year *or*
  - their regular partner has other partners.

In these women, pre-insertion screening (for chlamydia and, depending on sexual history and local prevalence of disease, *Neisseria gonorrhoeae*) should be performed. If results are unavailable at the time of fitting an intra-uterine device for emergency contraception, appropriate prophylactic antibacterial cover should be given. The woman should be advised to attend *as an emergency* if she experiences sustained pain during the next 20 days.

An intra-uterine device should not be removed in mid-cycle unless an additional contraceptive was used for the previous 7 days. If removal is essential post-coital contraception should be considered.

If an intra-uterine device fails and the woman wishes to continue to full-term the device should be removed in the first trimester if possible.

## ■ INTRA-UTERINE CONTRACEPTIVE DEVICES

**Indications** see notes above

**Cautions** see notes above; also anaemia, menorrhagia (progestogen intra-uterine system might be preferable, section 7.3.2.3), endometriosis, severe primary dysmenorrhoea, history of pelvic inflammatory disease, diabetes, fertility problems, nulliparity and young age, severely scarred uterus (including after endometrial resection) or severe cervical stenosis; valvular heart disease or history of endocarditis (Table 2, section 5.1); drug- or disease-induced immuno-suppression (risk of infection—avoid if marked immunosuppression); epilepsy (risk of seizure at time of insertion); increased risk of expulsion if inserted before uterine involution; gynaecological examination before insertion, 6–8 weeks after then annually but counsel women to see doctor promptly in case of significant symptoms, especially pain; anticoagulant therapy (avoid if possible); remove if pregnancy occurs; if pregnancy occurs, increased likelihood that it may be ectopic

**Contra-indications** pregnancy, severe anaemia, recent sexually transmitted infection (if not fully investigated and treated), unexplained uterine bleeding, distorted or small uterine cavity, genital malignancy, active trophoblastic disease (until return to normal of urine- and plasma-gonadotrophin concentration), pelvic inflammatory disease, established or marked immunosuppression; *copper devices:* copper allergy, Wilson's disease, medical diathermy

**Side-effects** uterine or cervical perforation, displacement, expulsion; pelvic infection may be exacerbated, menorrhagia, dysmenorrhoea, allergy; *on insertion:* pain (alleviated by NSAID such as ibuprofen 30 minutes before insertion) and bleeding, occasionally epileptic seizure and vasovagal attack

**Flexi-T® 300** (FP)
Intra-uterine device, copper wire, surface area approx. 300 mm² wound on vertical stem of T-shaped plastic carrier, impregnated with barium sulphate for radio-opacity, monofilament thread attached to base of vertical stem; preloaded in inserter, net price = £9.47
For uterine length over 5 cm; replacement every 5 years (see also notes above)

**Flexi-T® + 380** (FP)
Intra-uterine device, copper wire, surface area approx. 380 mm² wound on vertical stem of T-shaped plastic carrier with copper sleeve on each arm, impregnated with barium sulphate for radio-opacity, monofilament thread attached to base of vertical stem; preloaded in inserter, net price = £10.06
For uterine length over 6 cm; replacement every 5 years (see also notes above)

**GyneFix®** (FP)
Intra-uterine device, 6 copper sleeves with surface area of 330 mm² on polypropylene thread, net price = £26.64
Suitable for all uterine sizes; replacement every 5 years

**Load® 375** (Durbin)
Intra-uterine device, copper wire, surface area approx. 375 mm², wound on vertical stem of U-shaped plastic carrier, impregnated with barium sulphate for radio-opacity, monofilament thread attached to base of vertical stem; preloaded in inserter, net price = £8.00
For uterine length over 7 cm; replacement every 5 years (see notes above)

**Mini TT 380® Slimline** (Durbin)
Intra-uterine device, copper wire, wound on vertical stem of T-shaped plastic carrier with copper sleeves fitted flush on to distal portion of each horizontal arm, total surface area approx. 380 mm², impregnated with barium sulphate for radio-opacity, thread attached to base of vertical stem; easy-loading system, no capsule, net price = £11.70
For minimum uterine length 5 cm; replacement every 5 years (see also notes above)

**Multiload® Cu375** (Organon)
Intra-uterine device, as *Load® 375*, with copper surface area approx. 375 mm² and vertical stem length 3.5 cm, net price = £9.24
For uterine length 6–9 cm; replacement every 5 years (see notes above)

**Nova-T® 380** (Schering Health)
Intra-uterine device, copper wire with silver core, surface area approx. 380 mm² wound on vertical stem of T-shaped plastic carrier, impregnated with barium sulphate for radio-opacity, threads attached to base of vertical stem, net price = £12.97
For uterine length 6.5–9 cm; replacement every 5 years (see notes above)

**T-Safe® CU 380 A** (FP)
Intra-uterine device, copper wire, wound on vertical stem of T-shaped plastic carrier with copper collar on the distal portion of each arm, total surface area approx. 380 mm², impregnated with barium sulphate for radio-opacity, threads attached to base of vertical stem, net price = £10.29
For uterine length 6.5–9 cm; replacement every 10 years (see notes above)

7

Obstetrics, gynaecology, and urinary-tract disorders

**TT 380® Slimline** (Durbin)

Intra-uterine device, copper wire wound on vertical stem of T-shaped plastic carrier, with copper sleeves fitted flush on to distal portion of each horizontal arm, total surface area approx. 380 mm², impregnated with barium sulphate for radio-opacity, thread attached to base of vertical stem; easy-loading system, no capsule, net price = £11.70

For uterine length 6.5–9 cm; replacement every 10 years (see also notes above)

**UT 380 Short®** (Durbin)

Intra-uterine device, copper wire wound on vertical stem of T-shaped plastic carrier, total surface area approx. 380 mm², impregnated with barium sulphate for radio-opacity, thread attached to base of vertical stem; net price = £10.53

For uterine length 5–7 cm; replacement every 5 years (see also notes above)

**UT 380 Standard®** (Durbin)

Intra-uterine device, copper wire, surface area approx. 380 mm², wound on vertical stem of T-shaped plastic carrier, impregnated with barium sulphate for radio-opacity, thread attached to base of vertical stem; net price = £10.53

For uterine length 6.5–9 cm; replacement every 5 years (see also notes above)

## Other contraceptive devices

◢**Rubber contraceptive caps**
**Type A Contraceptive Pessary**

Opaque rubber, sizes 1 (50 mm), 2 (55 mm), 3 (60 mm), 4 (65 mm), 5 (75 mm), net price = £6.85

**Type B Contraceptive Pessary**

Opaque rubber, sizes 22 to 31 mm (rising in steps of 3 mm), net price = £8.46

**Type C Contraceptive Pessary**

Opaque rubber, sizes 1 to 3 (42, 48, and 54 mm), net price = £7.26

◢**Silicone contraceptive caps**
**Silicone Contraceptive Pessary**

Silicone, sizes 22, 26, and 30 mm, net price = £15.00
Brands include *FemCap*®

◢**Rubber contraceptive diaphragms**
**Type A Diaphragm with Flat Metal Spring**

Transparent rubber with flat metal spring, sizes 55–95 mm (rising in steps of 5 mm), net price = £5.78
Brands include *Reflexions*®

**Type B Diaphragm with Coiled Metal Spring**

Opaque rubber with coiled metal spring, sizes 60–100 mm (rising in steps of 5 mm), net price = £6.59

**Type C Arcing Spring Diaphragm**

Opaque rubber with arcing spring, sizes 60–95 mm (rising in steps of 5 mm), net price = £7.49

◢**Silicone contraceptive diaphragms**
**Type B Diaphragm with Coiled Metal Spring**

Silicone with coiled metal spring, sizes 60–90 mm (rising in steps of 5 mm), net price = £8.35
Brands include *Milex Omniflex*®

**Type C Arcing Spring Diaphragm**

Silicone with arcing spring, sizes 60–90 mm (rising in steps of 5 mm), net price = £8.35
Brands include *Milex Arcing Style*®

## 7.3.5 Emergency contraception

## Hormonal methods

Hormonal emergency contraception involves the use of **levonorgestrel**. It is effective if taken within 72 hours (3 days) of unprotected intercourse; taking the dose as soon as possible increases efficacy. Levonorgestrel may also be used between 72 and 120 hours after unprotected intercourse [unlicensed use] but efficacy decreases with time. Hormonal emergency contraception is less effective than insertion of an intra-uterine device (see below).

If vomiting occurs within 2 hours of taking levonorgestrel, a replacement dose should be given. If an anti-emetic is required domperidone is preferred.

When prescribing hormonal emergency contraception the doctor should explain:

- that the next period may be early or late;
- that a barrier method of contraception needs to be used until the next period;
- the need to return promptly if any lower abdominal pain occurs because this could signify an ectopic pregnancy (and also in 3 to 4 weeks if the subsequent menstrual bleed is abnormally light, heavy or brief, or is absent, or if she is otherwise concerned).

**Intra-uterine pregnancy** despite treatment: see Appendix 4 (levonorgestrel).

**Interactions** The effectiveness of hormonal emergency contraception is reduced by enzyme-inducing drugs; a copper intra-uterine device can be offered instead or the dose of levonorgestrel should be increased to a total of 3 mg taken as a single dose [unlicensed dose—advise women accordingly]. There is no need to increase the dose for emergency contraception if the patient is taking antibacterials that are not enzyme inducers.

## ▌ LEVONORGESTREL

**Indications** emergency contraception

**Cautions** see notes above; past ectopic pregnancy; severe malabsorption syndromes; active trophoblastic disease (until return to normal of urine- and plasma-gonadotrophin concentration); pregnancy (see notes above and Appendix 4); breast-feeding (Appendix 5); **interactions:** see notes above and Appendix 1 (progestogens)

**Contra-indications** acute porphyria (section 9.8.2)

**Side-effects** menstrual irregularities (see also notes above), nausea, low abdominal pain, fatigue, headache, dizziness, breast tenderness, vomiting

**Dose**

- 1.5 mg as a single dose as soon as possible after coitus (preferably within 12 hours but no later than after 72 hours)

[1]**Levonelle® One Step** (Schering Health)

Tablets, levonorgestrel 1.5 mg, net price 1-tab pack = £13.83

1. Can be sold to women over 16 years; when supplying emergency contraception to the public, pharmacists should refer to guidance issued by the Royal Pharmaceutical Society of Great Britain

**Levonelle® 1500** (Schering Health) [PoM]
　Tablets, levonorgestrel 1.5 mg, net price 1-tab pack = £5.37

---

## Intra-uterine device

Insertion of an intra-uterine device is more effective than oral levonorgestrel for emergency contraception. A copper intra-uterine contraceptive device (section 7.3.4) can be inserted up to 120 hours (5 days) after unprotected intercourse; sexually transmitted diseases should be tested for and insertion of the device should usually be covered by antibacterial prophylaxis (e.g. azithromycin 1 g as a single dose). If intercourse has occurred more than 5 days previously, the device can still be inserted up to 5 days after the earliest likely calculated ovulation (i.e. within the minimum period before implantation).

## 7.4 Drugs for genito-urinary disorders

　7.4.1　Drugs for urinary retention
　7.4.2　Drugs for urinary frequency, enuresis, and incontinence
　7.4.3　Drugs used in urological pain
　7.4.4　Bladder instillations and urological surgery
　7.4.5　Drugs for erectile dysfunction

For drugs used in the treatment of urinary-tract infections see section 5.1.13.

## 7.4.1 Drugs for urinary retention

*Acute retention* is painful and is treated by catheterisation.

*Chronic retention* is painless and often long-standing. Catheterisation is unnecessary unless there is deterioration of renal function. After the cause has initially been established and treated, drugs may be required to increase detrusor muscle tone.

*Benign prostatic hyperplasia* is treated either surgically or medically with alpha-blockers (see below). Dutasteride and finasteride (section 6.4.2) are alternatives to alpha-blockers, particularly in men with a significantly enlarged prostate.

---

## Alpha-blockers

The alpha₁-selective alpha blockers, **alfuzosin**, **doxazosin**, **indoramin**, **prazosin**, **tamsulosin** and **terazosin** relax smooth muscle in benign prostatic hyperplasia producing an increase in urinary flow-rate and an improvement in obstructive symptoms.

**Cautions** Since alpha₁-selective alpha blockers reduce blood pressure, patients receiving antihypertensive treatment may require reduced dosage and specialist supervision. Caution may be required in the elderly and in patients with hepatic impairment (Appendix 2) and

renal impairment (Appendix 3). For **interactions** see Appendix 1 (alpha-blockers).

**Contra-indications** Alpha-blockers should be avoided in patients with a history of postural hypotension and micturition syncope.

**Side-effects** Side-effects of alpha₁-selective alpha blockers include drowsiness, hypotension (notably postural hypotension), syncope, asthenia, depression, headache, dry mouth, gastro-intestinal disturbances (including nausea, vomiting, diarrhoea, constipation), oedema, blurred vision, rhinitis, erectile disorders (including priapism), tachycardia, and palpitations. Hypersensitivity reactions including rash, pruritus and angioedema have also been reported.

### ALFUZOSIN HYDROCHLORIDE

**Indications** see notes above
**Cautions** see notes above
**Contra-indications** see notes above; severe hepatic impairment
**Side-effects** see notes above; also flushes and chest pain
**Dose**
- 2.5 mg 3 times daily, max. 10 mg daily; ELDERLY initially 2.5 mg twice daily
　**First dose effect** First dose may cause collapse due to hypotensive effect (therefore should be taken on retiring to bed). Patient should be warned to lie down if symptoms such as dizziness, fatigue or sweating develop, and to remain lying down until they abate completely

**Alfuzosin hydrochloride** (Non-proprietary) [PoM]
　Tablets, f/c, alfuzosin hydrochloride 2.5 mg, net price 60-tab pack = £20.37. Label: 3, counselling, see dose above

**Xatral®** (Sanofi-Synthelabo) [PoM]
　Tablets, f/c, alfuzosin hydrochloride 2.5 mg, net price 60-tab pack = £20.37. Label: 3, counselling, see dose above

◢**Modified release**
**Besavar® XL** (Winthrop) [PoM]
　Tablets, m/r, yellow/white, alfuzosin hydrochloride 10 mg, net price 30-tab pack = £12.76. Label: 3, 21, 25, counselling, see above
　Dose benign prostatic hyperplasia 10 mg once daily
　Acute urinary retention associated with benign prostatic hyperplasia in men over 65 years, 10 mg once daily for 2–3 days during catheterisation and for one day after removal; max. 4 days

**Xatral® XL** (Sanofi-Synthelabo) [PoM]
　Tablets, m/r, yellow/white, alfuzosin hydrochloride 10 mg, net price 10-tab pack = £4.25, 30-tab pack = £12.76. Label: 3, 21, 25, counselling, see above
　Dose benign prostatic hyperplasia 10 mg once daily
　Acute urinary retention associated with benign prostatic hyperplasia in men over 65 years, 10 mg once daily for 2–3 days during catheterisation and for one day after removal; max. 4 days

### DOXAZOSIN

**Indications** see notes above and section 2.5.4
**Cautions** see notes above and section 2.5.4
**Contra-indications** see notes above
**Side-effects** see notes above and section 2.5.4

**Dose**
- Initially 1 mg daily; dose may be doubled at intervals of 1–2 weeks according to response, up to max. 8 mg daily; usual maintenance 2–4 mg daily

◢ **Preparations**
Section 2.5.4

## INDORAMIN

**Indications** see notes above and section 2.5.4
**Cautions** see notes above and section 2.5.4
**Contra-indications** see notes above and section 2.5.4
**Side-effects** see notes above and section 2.5.4
**Dose**
- 20 mg twice daily; increased if necessary by 20 mg every 2 weeks to max. 100 mg daily in divided doses; ELDERLY, 20 mg at night may be adequate

**Doralese®** (Chemidex) PoM
Tablets, yellow, f/c, indoramin 20 mg, net price 60-tab pack = £25.85. Label: 2

## PRAZOSIN

**Indications** see notes above and section 2.5.4
**Cautions** see notes above and section 2.5.4
**Contra-indications** see notes above and section 2.5.4
**Side-effects** see notes above and section 2.5.4; also paraesthesia, arthralgia, epistaxis, nervousness, dyspnoea, hallucinations, and alopecia
**Dose**
- Initially 500 micrograms twice daily for 3–7 days, subsequently adjusted according to response; usual maintenance (and max.) 2 mg twice daily; ELDERLY initiate with lowest possible dose
**First dose effect** First dose may cause collapse due to hypotensive effect (therefore should be taken on retiring to bed). Patient should be warned to lie down if symptoms such as dizziness, fatigue or sweating develop, and to remain lying down until they abate completely

◢ **Preparations**
Section 2.5.4

## TAMSULOSIN HYDROCHLORIDE

**Indications** see notes above
**Cautions** see notes above; also cataract surgery (risk of intra-operative floppy iris syndrome)
**Contra-indications** see notes above; severe hepatic impairment
**Side-effects** see notes above
**Dose**
- 400 micrograms daily as a single dose

**Tamsulosin hydrochloride** (Non-proprietary) PoM
Capsules, m/r, tamsulosin hydrochloride 400 micrograms, net price 30-cap pack = £5.20. Label: 25
Brands include *Bazetham® MR, Contiflo® XL, Diffundox® XL, Omnic® MR, Stronazon® MR, Tabphyn® MR*

**Flomaxtra® XL** (Astellas) PoM
Tablets, m/r, tamsulosin hydrochloride 400 micrograms. Net price 30-tab pack = £11.00. Label: 25

## TERAZOSIN

**Indications** see notes above and section 2.5.4
**Cautions** see notes above and section 2.5.4
**Contra-indications** see notes above
**Side-effects** see notes above and section 2.5.4; also weight gain, paraesthesia, dyspnoea, thrombocytopenia, nervousness, decreased libido, back pain and pain in extremities
**Dose**
- Initially 1 mg at bedtime; if necessary dose may be doubled at intervals of 1–2 weeks according to response, up to max. 10 mg once daily; usual maintenance 5–10 mg daily
**First dose effect** First dose may cause collapse due to hypotensive effect (therefore should be taken on retiring to bed). Patient should be warned to lie down if symptoms such as dizziness, fatigue or sweating develop, and to remain lying down until they abate completely

**Terazosin** (Non-proprietary) PoM
Tablets, terazosin (as hydrochloride) 2 mg, net price 28-tab pack = £2.34; 5 mg, 28-tab pack = £2.78; 10 mg, 28-tab pack = £7.06. Label: 3, counselling, see dose above

**Hytrin®** (Amdipharm) PoM
Tablets, terazosin (as hydrochloride) 2 mg (yellow) net price, 28-tab pack = £2.29; 5 mg (tan), 28-tab pack = £4.29; 10 mg (blue), 28-tab pack = £8.57; starter pack (for benign prostatic hyperplasia) of 7 × 1-mg tab with 14 × 2-mg tab and 7 × 5-mg tab = £10.97. Label: 3, counselling, see dose above

## Parasympathomimetics

The parasympathomimetic **bethanechol** increases detrusor muscle contraction. However, it has only a limited role in the relief of urinary retention; its use has been superseded by catheterisation.

**Distigmine** inhibits the breakdown of acetylcholine. It may help patients with an upper motor neurone neurogenic bladder.

## BETHANECHOL CHLORIDE

**Indications** urinary retention, but see notes above
**Cautions** autonomic neuropathy (use lower initial dose); interactions: Appendix 1 (parasympathomimetics)
**Contra-indications** peptic ulcer; intestinal or urinary obstruction; conditions where increased motility of the urinary or gastro-intestinal tract could be harmful; cardiovascular disorders (including recent myocardial infarction, bradycardia, and heart block); hypotension; obstructive airways disease; epilepsy; parkinsonism; hyperthyroidism; pregnancy (Appendix 4); breastfeeding
**Side-effects** nausea, vomiting, diarrhoea, abdominal pain, increased salivation, eructation; flushing, hypotension, bradycardia; bronchoconstriction, rhinorrhoea; headache; increased lacrimation; increased sweating
**Dose**
- 10–25 mg 3–4 times daily half an hour before food

**Myotonine®** (Glenwood) PoM
Tablets, scored, bethanechol chloride 10 mg, net price 20 = £1.01; 25 mg, 20 = £1.30. Label: 22

## ▌ DISTIGMINE BROMIDE

**Indications** postoperative urinary retention (see notes above), neurogenic bladder; myasthenia gravis (section 10.2.1)

**Cautions** peptic ulcer; conditions where increased motility of the urinary or gastro-intestinal tract could be harmful; oesophagitis; cardiovascular disease; bronchospasm; epilepsy; parkinsonism; pregnancy (Appendix 4); breast-feeding; **interactions:** Appendix 1 (parasympathomimetics)

**Contra-indications** intestinal or urinary obstruction; severe circulatory insufficiency; asthma

**Side-effects** abdominal pain, diarrhoea, increased salivation; bradycardia, AV block, hypotension; dyspnoea; muscle twitching; increased lacrimation, miosis; increased sweating

**Dose**

- Urinary retention, 5 mg daily, half an hour before breakfast
- Neurogenic bladder, 5 mg daily or on alternate days, half an hour before breakfast

**Ubretid®** (Rhône-Poulenc Rorer) (PoM)
Tablets, scored, distigmine bromide 5 mg, net price 30-tab pack = £41.22. Label: 22

## 7.4.2 Drugs for urinary frequency, enuresis, and incontinence

## Urinary incontinence

Incontinence in adults which arises from detrusor instability is managed by combining drug therapy with conservative methods for managing urge incontinence such as pelvic floor exercises and bladder training; stress incontinence is generally managed by non-drug methods. **Duloxetine**, an inhibitor of serotonin and noradrenaline re-uptake can be added and is licensed for the treatment of moderate to severe stress incontinence in women; it may be more effective when used as an adjunct to pelvic floor exercises.

Involuntary detrusor contractions cause urgency and urge incontinence, usually with frequency and nocturia. Antimuscarinic drugs reduce these contractions and increase bladder capacity. **Oxybutynin** also has a direct relaxant effect on urinary smooth muscle. Side-effects limit the use of oxybutynin but they may be reduced by starting at a lower dose. A modified-release preparation of oxybutynin is effective and has fewer side-effects; a transdermal patch is also available. The efficacy and side-effects of **tolterodine** are comparable to those of modified-release oxybutynin. **Flavoxate** has less marked side-effects but it is also less effective. **Darifenacin, fesoterodine, propiverine, solifenacin,** and **trospium** are newer antimuscarinic drugs licensed for urinary frequency, urgency, and incontinence. The need for continuing antimuscarinic drug therapy should be reviewed after 3–6 months.

The *Scottish Medicines Consortium* (p. 3) has advised (June 2008) that fesoterodine (*Toviaz®*) is accepted for restricted use within NHS Scotland as a second-line treatment for overactive bladder syndrome.

Propantheline and tricyclic antidepressants were used for urge incontinence but they are little used now because of their side-effects. The use of imipramine is limited by its potential to cause cardiac side-effects.

Purified bovine collagen implant (*Contigen®*, Bard) is indicated for *urinary incontinence* caused by intrinsic sphincter deficiency (poor or non-functioning bladder outlet mechanism). The implant should be inserted only by surgeons or physicians trained in the technique for injection of the implant.

**Cautions** Antimuscarinic drugs should be used with caution in the elderly (especially if frail), in those with autonomic neuropathy, and in those susceptible to angle-closure glaucoma. They should also be used with caution in hiatus hernia with reflux oesophagitis, hepatic impairment (Appendix 2), and renal impairment (Appendix 3). Antimuscarinics can worsen hyperthyroidism, coronary artery disease, congestive heart failure, hypertension, prostatic hyperplasia, arrhythmias, and tachycardia. For **interactions** see Appendix 1 (antimuscarinics).

**Contra-indications** Antimuscarinic drugs should be avoided in patients with myasthenia gravis, significant bladder outflow obstruction or urinary retention, severe ulcerative colitis, toxic megacolon, and in gastro-intestinal obstruction or intestinal atony.

**Side-effects** Side-effects of antimuscarinic drugs include dry mouth, gastro-intestinal disturbances including constipation, flatulence, taste disturbances, blurred vision, dry eyes, drowsiness, dizziness, fatigue, difficulty in micturition (less commonly urinary retention), palpitation, and skin reactions (including dry skin, rash, and photosensitivity); also headache, diarrhoea, angioedema, arrhythmias, and tachycardia. Central nervous system stimulation, such as restlessness, disorientation, hallucination, and convulsion may occur; children are at higher risk of these effects. Antimuscarinic drugs can reduce sweating, leading to heat sensations and fainting in hot environments or in patients with fever, and *very rarely* may precipitate angle-closure glaucoma.

## ▌ DARIFENACIN

**Indications** urinary frequency, urgency, and incontinence

**Cautions** see notes above; breast-feeding (Appendix 5)

**Contra-indications** see notes above; pregnancy (Appendix 4)

**Side-effects** see notes above; also *less commonly* ulcerative stomatitis, oedema, hypertension, dyspnoea, cough, rhinitis, weakness, insomnia, impotence, and vaginitis

**Dose**

- ADULT over 18 years, 7.5 mg once daily, increased if necessary after 2 weeks to 15 mg once daily

**Emselex®** (Novartis) ▼ (PoM)
Tablets, m/r, darifenacin (as hydrobromide) 7.5 mg (white), net price 28-tab pack = £26.13; 15 mg (peach), 28-tab pack = £26.13. Label: 3, 25

**7 Obstetrics, gynaecology, and urinary-tract disorders**

## DULOXETINE

**Indications** moderate to severe stress urinary incontinence in women; major depressive disorder (section 4.3.4); diabetic neuropathy (section 4.3.4); generalised anxiety disorder (section 4.3.4)

**Cautions** elderly; cardiac disease; hypertension (avoid if uncontrolled); history of mania; history of seizures; raised intra-ocular pressure, susceptibility to angle-closure glaucoma; bleeding disorders or concomitant use of drugs that increase risk of bleeding; **interactions**: Appendix 1 (duloxetine)

Withdrawal Nausea, vomiting, headache, anxiety, dizziness, paraesthesia, sleep disturbances, and tremor are the most common features of abrupt withdrawal or marked reduction of the dose; dose should be reduced over at least 1–2 weeks

**Contra-indications** hepatic impairment; renal impairment (avoid if eGFR less than 30 mL/minute/1.73 m²); pregnancy (Appendix 4); breast-feeding (Appendix 5)

**Side-effects** nausea, vomiting, dyspepsia, constipation, diarrhoea, abdominal pain, weight changes, decreased appetite, flatulence, dry mouth; palpitation, hot flush; insomnia, abnormal dreams, paraesthesia, drowsiness, anxiety, headache, dizziness, fatigue, weakness, tremor, nervousness, anorexia; sexual dysfunction; visual disturbances; sweating, pruritus; *less commonly* gastritis, halitosis, hepatitis, bruxism, tachycardia, hypertension, postural hypotension, syncope, raised cholesterol, vertigo, taste disturbance, cold extremities, impaired temperature regulation, impaired attention, movement disorders, muscle twitching, musculoskeletal pain, thirst, stomatitis, hypothyroidism, urinary disorders, and photosensitivity; *rarely* mania and angle-closure glaucoma; *also reported* supraventricular arrhythmia, chest pain, hallucinations, suicidal behaviour (see Suicidal Behaviour and Antidepressant Therapy, p. 209), seizures, hypersensitivity reactions including urticaria, angioedema, rash (including Stevens-Johnson syndrome) and anaphylaxis, hyponatraemia (see Hyponatraemia and Antidepressant Therapy, p. 209)

**Dose**
• ADULT over 18 years, 40 mg twice daily, assess for benefit and tolerability after 2–4 weeks
Note Initial dose of 20 mg twice daily for 2 weeks can minimise side-effects

**Yentreve®** (Lilly) ▼ PoM
Capsules, duloxetine (as hydrochloride) 20 mg (blue), net price 28-cap pack = £15.40, 56-cap pack = £30.80; 40 mg (orange/blue), 56-cap pack = £30.80. Label: 2

**Cymbalta®** (Lilly) ▼ PoM
Section 4.3.4 (major depressive episode, generalised anxiety disorder, and diabetic neuropathy)

## FESOTERODINE

**Indications** urinary frequency, urgency, and urge incontinence

**Cautions** see notes above; gastro-oesophageal reflux

**Contra-indications** see notes above; pregnancy (Appendix 4); breast-feeding (Appendix 5)

**Side-effects** see notes above; also insomnia; *less commonly* nasal dryness, pharyngolaryngeal pain, cough, and vertigo

**Dose**
• ADULT over 18 years, 4 mg once daily, increased if necessary to max. 8 mg once daily; assess for benefit after 8 weeks
Note Max. 4 mg daily with concomitant atazanavir, clarithromycin, indinavir, itraconazole, ketoconazole, nelfinavir, ritonavir, saquinavir, or telithromycin; in patients with hepatic or renal impairment, consult product literature before concomitant use with amprenavir, aprepitant, atazanavir, clarithromycin, diltiazem, erythromycin, fluconazole, fosamprenavir, indinavir, itraconazole, ketoconazole, nelfinavir, ritonavir, saquinavir, telithromycin, verapamil, or grapefruit juice

**Toviaz®** (Pfizer) ▼ PoM
Tablets, m/r, f/c, fesoterodine fumarate 4 mg (light blue), net price 28-tab pack = £25.78; 8 mg (blue), 28-tab pack = £25.78. Label: 3, 25

## FLAVOXATE HYDROCHLORIDE

**Indications** urinary frequency and incontinence, dysuria, urgency; bladder spasms due to catheterisation, cytoscopy, or surgery

**Cautions** see notes above; pregnancy (Appendix 4), breast-feeding (Appendix 5)

**Contra-indications** see notes above; gastro-intestinal haemorrhage

**Side-effects** see notes above; also vertigo, eosinophilia, leucopenia, urticaria, erythema, and pruritus

**Dose**
• ADULT and ADOLESCENT over 12 years, 200 mg 3 times daily

**Urispas 200®** (Recordati) PoM
Tablets, f/c, flavoxate hydrochloride 200 mg, net price 90-tab pack = £11.67

## OXYBUTYNIN HYDROCHLORIDE

**Indications** urinary frequency, urgency and incontinence, neurogenic bladder instability, and nocturnal enuresis associated with overactive bladder

**Cautions** see notes above; pregnancy (Appendix 4); acute porphyria (section 9.8.2)

**Contra-indications** see notes above; breast-feeding (Appendix 5)

**Side-effects** see notes above; also *less commonly* anorexia, facial flushing; *rarely* night terrors; application site reactions with *patches*

**Dose**
• ADULT and CHILD over 12 years, initially 5 mg 2–3 times daily, increased if necessary to max. 5 mg 4 times daily; ELDERLY initially 2.5–3 mg twice daily, increased to 5 mg twice daily according to response and tolerance; CHILD 5–12 years, neurogenic bladder instability, 2.5–3 mg twice daily, increased to 5 mg 2–3 times daily; CHILD under 5 years, see *BNF for Children*; CHILD 7–18 years, nocturnal enuresis associated with overactive bladder, 2.5–3 mg twice daily increased to 5 mg 2–3 times daily (last dose before bedtime)

**Oxybutynin Hydrochloride** (Non-proprietary) PoM
Tablets, oxybutynin hydrochloride 2.5 mg, net price 56-tab pack = £8.23; 3 mg, 56-tab pack = £9.15; 5 mg, 56-tab pack = £7.70, 84-tab pack = £2.96. Label: 3

**Cystrin®** (Sanofi-Synthelabo) PoM
Tablets, oxybutynin hydrochloride 3 mg, net price 56-tab pack = £9.15; 5 mg (scored), 84-tab pack = £21.99. Label: 3

**Ditropan®** (Sanofi-Synthelabo) [PoM]

Tablets, both blue, scored, oxybutynin hydrochloride 2.5 mg, net price 84-tab pack = £6.59; 5 mg, 84-tab pack = £12.82. Label: 3

Elixir, oxybutynin hydrochloride 2.5 mg/5 mL. Net price 150-mL pack = £6.88. Label: 3

◢Modified release

**Lyrinel® XL** (Janssen-Cilag) [PoM]

Tablets, m/r, oxybutynin hydrochloride 5 mg (yellow), net price 30-tab pack = £11.03; 10 mg (pink), 30-tab pack = £22.05. Label: 3, 25

Dose Initially 5 mg once daily, adjusted according to response in steps of 5 mg at weekly intervals; max. 20 mg once daily; CHILD over 6 years, neurogenic bladder instability, initially 5 mg once daily, adjusted according to response in steps of 5 mg at weekly intervals; max. 15 mg once daily

Note Patients taking immediate-release oxybutynin may be transferred to the nearest equivalent daily dose of *Lyrinel® XL*

◢Transdermal preparations

**Kentera®** (Recordati) [PoM]

Patches, self-adhesive, oxybutynin 36 mg (releasing oxybutynin approx. 3.9 mg/24 hours), net price 8-patch pack = £27.20. Label: 3, counselling, administration

Dose ADULT over 18 years, urinary frequency, urgency and incontinence, apply 1 patch twice weekly to clean, dry, unbroken skin on abdomen, hip or buttock, remove after every 3–4 days and site replacement patch on a different area (avoid using same area for 7 days)

Note The *Scottish Medicines Consortium* has advised (July 2005) that *Kentera®* should be restricted for use in patients who benefit from oral oxybutynin but cannot tolerate its side-effects

## ◼ PROPANTHELINE BROMIDE

**Indications** adult enuresis

**Cautions** see notes above; ulcerative colitis, pregnancy (Appendix 4) and breast-feeding (Appendix 5)

**Contra-indications** see notes above

**Side-effects** see notes above; also facial flushing

**Dose**

- Initially 15 mg 3 times daily at least one hour before food and 30 mg at bedtime, subsequently adjusted according to response (max. 120 mg daily)

◢Preparations

Section 1.2

## ◼ PROPIVERINE HYDROCHLORIDE

**Indications** urinary frequency, urgency and incontinence; neurogenic bladder instability

**Cautions** see notes above

**Contra-indications** see notes above; moderate to severe hepatic impairment; pregnancy (Appendix 4) and breast-feeding (Appendix 5)

**Side-effects** see notes above

**Dose**

- 15 mg 1–3 times daily, increased if necessary to max. 15 mg 4 times daily; CHILD not recommended

**Detrunorm®** (Amdipharm) [PoM]

Tablets, pink, s/c, propiverine hydrochloride 15 mg, net price 56-tab pack = £24.45. Label: 3

◢Modified release

**Detrunorm® XL** (Amdipharm) [PoM]

Capsules, orange/white, m/r, propiverine hydrochloride 30 mg, net price 28-cap pack = £24.45. Label: 3, 25

Dose urinary frequency, urgency, and incontinence, 30 mg once daily; CHILD not recommended

## ◼ SOLIFENACIN SUCCINATE

**Indications** urinary frequency, urgency and urge incontinence

**Cautions** see notes above; neurogenic bladder disorder; pregnancy (Appendix 4)

**Contra-indications** see notes above; severe hepatic impairment (Appendix 2); haemodialysis; breast-feeding (Appendix 5)

**Side-effects** see notes above; also gastro-oesophageal reflux; oedema

**Dose**

- 5 mg daily, increased if necessary to 10 mg once daily; CHILD not recommended

Note Max. 5 mg daily with concomitant itraconazole, ketoconazole, nelfinavir, or ritonavir; in patients with moderate hepatic impairment *or* if eGFR less than 30 mL/minute/1.73m², solifenacin is contra-indicated in those already taking itraconazole, ketoconazole, nelfinavir, or ritonavir

**Vesicare®** (Astellas) [PoM]

Tablets, f/c, solifenacin succinate 5 mg (yellow), net price 30-tab pack = £27.62; 10 mg (pink), 30-tab pack = £35.91. Label: 3

## ◼ TOLTERODINE TARTRATE

**Indications** urinary frequency, urgency and incontinence

**Cautions** see notes above; history of QT-interval prolongation; concomitant use with other drugs known to prolong QT interval

**Contra-indications** see notes above; pregnancy (Appendix 4) and breast-feeding (Appendix 5)

**Side-effects** see notes above; also chest pain, peripheral oedema; sinusitis; bronchitis; paraesthesia, fatigue, vertigo, weight gain; flushing also reported

**Dose**

- ADULT over 18 years, 2 mg twice daily; reduce to 1 mg twice daily if necessary to minimise side-effects

**Detrusitol®** (Pharmacia) [PoM]

Tablets, f/c, tolterodine tartrate 1 mg, net price 56-tab pack = £29.03; 2 mg, 56-tab pack = £30.56. Label: 3

◢Modified release

**Detrusitol® XL** (Pharmacia) [PoM]

Capsules, blue, m/r, tolterodine tartrate 4 mg, net price 28-cap pack = £25.78. Label: 3, 25

Dose ADULT over 18 years, 4 mg once daily (dose form not appropriate for hepatic impairment or if eGFR less than 30 mL/minute/1.73 m²)

## ◼ TROSPIUM CHLORIDE

**Indications** urinary frequency, urgency and incontinence

**Cautions** see notes above; pregnancy (Appendix 4); breast-feeding (Appendix 5)

**Contra-indications** see notes above

**7**

**Obstetrics, gynaecology, and urinary-tract disorders**

**Side-effects** see notes above; also chest pain, dyspnoea, rash and asthenia

**Dose**

- 20 mg twice daily before food; CHILD not recommended

**Regurin®** (Galen) [PoM]

Tablets, brown, f/c, trospium chloride 20 mg, net price 60-tab pack = £26.00. Label: 23

## Nocturnal enuresis

*Nocturnal enuresis* is common in young children but persists in as many as 5% by 10 years of age. Treatment is not appropriate in children under 5 years and it is usually not needed in those aged under 7 years and in cases where the child and parents are not anxious about the bedwetting; however, children over 10 years usually require prompt treatment. An **enuresis alarm** should be first-line treatment for well-motivated, well-supported children aged over 7 years because alarms have a lower relapse rate than drug treatment when discontinued. Use of an alarm can be combined with drug therapy if either method alone is unsuccessful.

Drug therapy is not usually appropriate for children under 7 years of age; it can be used when alternative measures have failed, preferably on a short-term basis, for example to cover periods away from home, or if the child and family are anxious about the condition. The possible side-effects of the various drugs should be borne in mind when they are prescribed.

**Desmopressin** (section 6.5.2), an analogue of vasopressin, is used for nocturnal enuresis; it is given by oral or by sublingual administration. Particular care is needed to avoid fluid overload. Treatment should not be continued for longer than 3 months without interrupting treatment for 1 week for full re-assessment. Desmopressin should not be given intranasally for nocturnal enuresis due to an increased incidence of side-effects.

Tricyclic antidepressants (section 4.3.1) such as **amitriptyline**, **imipramine**, and less often **nortriptyline** can be used, but behavioural disturbances can occur and relapse is common after withdrawal. Treatment should not normally exceed 3 months unless a full physical examination is made and the child is fully re-assessed; toxicity following overdosage with tricyclics is of particular concern.

Nocturnal enuresis associated with daytime symptoms (overactive bladder) can be managed by antimuscarinic drugs (see Urinary incontinence, p. 457), with the addition of desmopressin if necessary.

## 7.4.3 Drugs used in urological pain

The acute pain of *ureteric colic* may be relieved with **pethidine** (section 4.7.2). **Diclofenac** by injection or as suppositories (section 10.1.1) is also effective and compares favourably with pethidine; other non-steroidal anti-inflammatory drugs are occasionally given by injection.

**Lidocaine (lignocaine) gel** is a useful topical application in *urethral pain* or to relieve the discomfort of catheterisation (section 15.2).

## Alkalinisation of urine

*Alkalinisation* of urine can be undertaken with **potassium citrate**. The alkalinising action may relieve the discomfort of *cystitis* caused by lower urinary tract infections. **Sodium bicarbonate** is used as a urinary alkalinising agent in some metabolic and renal disorders (section 9.2.1.3).

### ■ POTASSIUM CITRATE

**Indications** relief of discomfort in mild urinary-tract infections; alkalinisation of urine

**Cautions** renal impairment (avoid if severe; Appendix 3), cardiac disease; elderly; **interactions:** Appendix 1 (potassium salts)

**Side-effects** hyperkalaemia on prolonged high dosage, mild diuresis

**Potassium Citrate Mixture BP (Potassium Citrate Oral Solution)**

Oral solution, potassium citrate 30%, citric acid monohydrate 5% in a suitable vehicle with a lemon flavour. Extemporaneous preparations should be recently prepared according to the following formula: potassium citrate 3 g, citric acid monohydrate 500 mg, syrup 2.5 mL, quillaia tincture 0.1 mL, lemon spirit 0.05 mL, double-strength chloroform water 3 mL, water to 10 mL. Contains about 28 mmol $K^+$/10 mL. Label: 27

**Dose** 10 mL 3 times daily well diluted with water

Proprietary brands of potassium citrate are on sale to the public for the relief of discomfort in mild urinary-tract infections

### ■ SODIUM BICARBONATE

**Indications** relief of discomfort in mild urinary-tract infections; alkalinisation of urine

**Cautions** hepatic impairment (Appendix 2); renal impairment (Appendix 3), cardiac disease, pregnancy; patients on sodium-restricted diet; avoid prolonged use; **interactions:** Appendix 1 (antacids)

**Side-effects** belching, alkalosis on prolonged use

**Dose**

- 3 g in water every 2 hours until urinary pH exceeds 7; maintenance of alkaline urine 5–10 g daily

◢**Preparations**

Section 9.2.1.3

### ■ SODIUM CITRATE

**Indications** relief of discomfort in mild urinary-tract infections

**Cautions** renal impairment; cardiac disease; hypertension; pregnancy; patients on a sodium-restricted diet; elderly

**Side-effects** mild diuresis

**Note** Proprietary brands of sodium citrate are on sale to the public for the relief of discomfort in mild urinary-tract infections

## Other preparations for urinary disorders

A terpene mixture (*Rowatinex®*) is claimed to be of benefit in *urolithiasis* for the expulsion of calculi.

**Rowatinex®** (Rowa) [PoM]
Capsules, yellow, e/c, anethol 4 mg, borneol 10 mg, camphene 15 mg, cineole 3 mg, fenchone 4 mg, pinene 31 mg. Net price 50 = £7.35. Label: 25
Dose 1–2 capsules 3–4 times daily before food; CHILD not recommended

## 7.4.4 Bladder instillations and urological surgery

**Bladder infection**  Various solutions are available as irrigations or washouts.

Aqueous **chlorhexidine** (section 13.11.2) can be used in the management of common infections of the bladder but it is ineffective against most *Pseudomonas* spp. Solutions containing chlorhexidine 1 in 5000 (0.02%) are used but they may irritate the mucosa and cause burning and haematuria (in which case they should be discontinued); sterile **sodium chloride solution 0.9%** (physiological saline) is usually adequate and is preferred as a mechanical irrigant.

Continuous bladder irrigation with **amphotericin** 50 micrograms/mL (section 5.2) may be of value in mycotic infections.

**Dissolution of blood clots**  Clot retention is usually treated by irrigation with sterile **sodium chloride solution 0.9%** but sterile **sodium citrate solution for bladder irrigation 3%** may also be helpful.

**Bladder cancer**  Bladder instillations of **doxorubicin** (section 8.1.2), **mitomycin** (section 8.1.2), and **thiotepa** (section 8.1.1) are used for recurrent superficial bladder tumours. Such instillations reduce systemic side-effects; adverse effects on the bladder (e.g. micturition disorders and reduction in bladder capacity) may occur.

Instillation of **epirubicin** (section 8.1.2) is used for treatment and prophylaxis of certain forms of superficial bladder cancer; instillation of **doxorubicin** (section 8.1.2) is also used for some papillary tumours.

Instillation of **BCG** (Bacillus Calmette-Guérin), a live attenuated strain derived from *Mycobacterium bovis* (section 8.2.4), is licensed for the treatment of primary or recurrent bladder carcinoma *in-situ* and for the prevention of recurrence following transurethral resection.

**Interstitial cystitis**  Dimethyl sulfoxide (dimethyl sulphoxide) may be used for symptomatic relief in patients with interstitial cystitis (Hunner's ulcer). 50 mL of a 50% solution (*Rimso-50®*—available on named-patient basis from Forum) is instilled into the bladder, retained for 15 minutes, and voided by the patient. Treatment is repeated at intervals of 2 weeks. Bladder spasm and hypersensitivity reactions may occur and long-term use requires ophthalmic, renal, and hepatic assessment at intervals of 6 months. **Interactions:** see Appendix 1 (dimethyl sulfoxide).

## ▉ SODIUM CITRATE

**Indications**  bladder washouts, see notes above

**Sterile Sodium Citrate Solution for Bladder Irrigation**
sodium citrate 3%, dilute hydrochloric acid 0.2%, in purified water, freshly boiled and cooled, and sterilised

## Urological surgery

There is a high risk of fluid absorption from the irrigant used in endoscopic surgery within the urinary tract; if this occurs in excess, hypervolaemia, haemolysis, and renal failure may result. **Glycine irrigation solution 1.5%** is the irrigant of choice for transurethral resection of the prostate gland and bladder tumours; **sterile sodium chloride solution 0.9%** (physiological saline) is used for percutaneous renal surgery.

## ▉ GLYCINE

**Indications**  bladder irrigation during urological surgery; see notes above

**Cautions**  see notes above

**Side-effects**  see notes above

**Glycine Irrigation Solution** (Non-proprietary)
Irrigation solution, glycine 1.5% in water for injections

## Maintenance of indwelling urinary catheters

The deposition which occurs in catheterised patients is usually chiefly composed of phosphate and to minimise this the catheter (if latex) should be changed at least as often as every 6 weeks. If the catheter is to be left for longer periods a silicone catheter should be used together with the appropriate use of catheter maintenance solutions. Repeated blockage usually indicates that the catheter needs to be changed.

## ▉ CATHETER PATENCY SOLUTIONS

**Chlorhexidine 0.02%**
Brands include *Uriflex C®*, 100-mL sachet = £2.40; *Uro-Tainer Chlorhexidine®*, 100-mL sachet = £2.60

**Sodium chloride 0.9%**
Brands include *OptiFlo S®*, 50- and 100-mL sachets = £3.20; *Uriflex S®*, 100-mL sachet = £2.40; *Uriflex SP®*, with integral drug additive port, 100-mL sachet = £2.40; *Uro-Tainer Sodium Chloride®*, 50- and 100-mL sachets = £3.23; *Uro-Tainer M®*, with integral drug additive port, 50- and 100-mL sachets = £2.90

**Solution G**
Citric acid 3.23%, magnesium oxide 0.38%, sodium bicarbonate 0.7%, disodium edetate 0.01%. Brands include *OptiFlo G®*, 50- and 100-mL sachets = £3.40; *Uriflex G®*, 100-mL sachet = £2.40; *Uro-Tainer® Twin Suby G*, 2 × 30-mL = £4.42

**Solution R**
Citric acid 6%, gluconolactone 0.6%, magnesium carbonate 2.8%, disodium edetate 0.01%. Brands include *OptiFlo R®*, 50- and 100-mL sachets = £3.40; *Uriflex R®*, 100-mL sachet = £2.40; *Uro-Tainer® Twin Solutio R*, 2 × 30-mL = £4.42

## 7.4.5 Drugs for erectile dysfunction

Reasons for failure to produce a satisfactory erection include *psychogenic*, *vascular*, *neurogenic*, and *endocrine abnormalities*; impotence can also be drug-induced. Intracavernosal injection or urethral application of vasoactive drugs under careful medical supervision is used for both diagnostic and therapeutic purposes.

Erectile disorders may also be treated with drugs given by mouth which increase the blood flow to the penis. Drugs should be used with caution if the penis is deformed (e.g. in angulation, cavernosal fibrosis, and Peyronie's disease).

**Priapism** If priapism occurs with alprostadil, treatment should not be delayed more than 6 hours and is as follows:

Initial therapy by penile aspiration—using aseptic technique a 19–21 gauge butterfly needle inserted into the corpus cavernosum and 20–50 mL of blood aspirated; if necessary the procedure may be repeated on the opposite side.

If initial aspiration is unsuccessful a second 19–21 gauge butterfly needle can be inserted into the opposite corpus cavernosum and sterile physiological saline introduced through the first needle and drained through the second.

If aspiration and lavage of corpora are unsuccessful, *cautious* intracavernosal injection of a sympathomimetic (section 2.7.2) with action on alpha-adrenergic receptors, continuously monitoring blood pressure and pulse (*extreme caution:* coronary heart disease, hypertension, cerebral ischaemia or if taking antidepressant) as follows:

- intracavernosal injections of phenylephrine 100–200 micrograms (0.5–1 mL of a 200 microgram/mL solution) every 5–10 minutes; max. total dose 1 mg [unlicensed indication] [*important:* if suitable strength of phenylephrine injection not available may be specially prepared by diluting 0.1 mL of the phenylephrine 1% (10 mg/mL) injection (section 2.7.2) to 5 mL with sodium chloride 0.9%]; *alternatively*

- intracavernosal injections of adrenaline 10–20 micrograms (0.5–1 mL of a 20 microgram/mL solution) every 5–10 minutes; max. total dose 100 micrograms [unlicensed indication] [*important:* if suitable strength of adrenaline not available may be specially prepared by diluting 0.1 mL of the adrenaline 1 in 1000 (1 mg/mL, section 3.4.3) injection to 5 mL with sodium chloride 0.9%]; *alternatively*

- intracavernosal injection of metaraminol (*caution: has been associated with fatal hypertensive crises*); metaraminol 1 mg (0.1 mL of 10 mg/mL metaraminol injection, section 2.7.2) is diluted to 50 mL with sodium chloride injection 0.9% and given carefully by slow injection into the corpora in 5-mL injections every 15 minutes [unlicensed indication].

If necessary the sympathomimetic injections can be followed by further aspiration of blood through the same butterfly needle.

If sympathomimetics unsuccessful, urgent surgical referral for management (possibly including shunt procedure).

**Prescribing on the NHS** Drug treatments for erectile dysfunction may only be prescribed on the NHS under certain circumstances (see individual preparations). The Department of Health (England) has recommended that treatment should also be available from specialist services (commissioned by Health Authorities and Primary Care Groups, and operating under local agreement) when the condition is causing severe distress; specialist centres should use form FP10(HP) or form HBP in Scotland or form WP10HP in Wales and endorse them 'SLS' if the treatment is to be dispensed in the community. The following criteria should be considered when assessing distress:

- significant disruption to normal social and occupational activities;

- a marked effect on mood, behaviour, social and environmental awareness;

- a marked effect on interpersonal relationships.

## Alprostadil

**Alprostadil** (prostaglandin E$_1$) is given by intracavernosal injection or intraurethral application for the management of erectile dysfunction (after exclusion of treatable medical causes); it is also used as a diagnostic test.

### ▌ALPROSTADIL

**Indications** erectile dysfunction (including aid to diagnosis); neonatal congenital heart defects (section 7.1.1.1)

**Cautions** priapism—patients should be instructed to report any erection lasting 4 hours or longer—for management, see section 7.4.5; anatomical deformations of penis (painful erection more likely)—follow up regularly to detect signs of penile fibrosis (consider discontinuation if angulation, cavernosal fibrosis or Peyronie's disease develop); **interactions:** Appendix 1 (prostaglandins)

**Contra-indications** predisposition to prolonged erection (as in sickle cell anaemia, multiple myeloma or leukaemia); not for use with other agents for erectile dysfunction, in patients with penile implants or when sexual activity medically inadvisable; urethral application also contra-indicated in urethral stricture, severe hypospadia, severe curvature, balanitis, urethritis

**Side-effects** hypotension, hypertension; dizziness, headache; penile pain, other localised pain (buttocks, leg, testicular, abdominal); influenza-like syndrome; urethral burning, urethral bleeding; injection site reactions including penile fibrosis, penile oedema, penile rash, haematoma, haemosiderin deposits; *less commonly* nausea, dry mouth, vasodilatation, syncope, supraventricular extrasystole, rapid pulse, asthenia, leg cramps, pelvic pain, scrotal or testicular oedema, scrotal erythema, testicular thickening, micturation difficulties, haematuria, mydriasis, and sweating; local reactions including penile warmth, pruritus, irritation, penile numbness or sensitivity, balantitis, phimosis, priapism (see section 7.4.5 and under Cautions), abnormal ejaculation; *rarely* vertigo, urinary-tract infection, and hypersensitivity reactions (including rash, erythema, urticaria, and anaphylaxis)

**Dose**

• See under preparations below

◢**Intracavernosal injection**

¹**Caverject®** (Pharmacia) ℗ℴℳ ⒩ℋ⒮

Injection, powder for reconstitution, alprostadil, net price 5-microgram vial = £7.73; 10-microgram vial = £9.24; 20-microgram vial = £11.94; 40-microgram vial = £21.58 (all with diluent-filled syringe, needles and swabs)

Caverject® Dual Chamber, double-chamber cartridges (containing alprostadil and diluent), net price 10-microgram cartridge (for doses 2.5–10 micrograms) = £7.35; 20-microgram cartridge (for doses 5–20 micrograms) = £9.50 (both with needles)

**Dose** by direct intracavernosal injection, ADULT over 18 years, erectile dysfunction, first dose 2.5 micrograms, second dose 5 micrograms (if some response to first dose) or 7.5 micrograms (if no response to first dose), increasing in steps of 5–10 micrograms to obtain dose suitable for producing erection lasting not more than 1 hour (neurological dysfunction, first dose 1.25 micrograms, second dose 2.5 micrograms, third dose 5 micrograms, increasing in steps of 5–10 micrograms to obtain suitable dose); if no response to dose then next higher dose can be given within 1 hour, if there is a response the next dose should not be given for at least 24 hours; usual dose 5–20 micrograms; max. 60 micrograms; max. frequency of injection not more than 3 times per week with at least 24 hour interval between injections

**Note** The first dose must be given by medically trained personnel; self-administration may only be undertaken after proper training

Aid to diagnosis, 10–20 micrograms as a single dose (where evidence of neurological dysfunction, initially 5 micrograms and max. 10 micrograms)—consult product literature for details

¹**Viridal® Duo** (UCB Pharma) ℗ℴℳ ⒩ℋ⒮

Starter Pack (hosp. only), contents as for *Continuation Pack* below plus *Duoject* applicator, 10-microgram starter pack = £20.13, 20-microgram starter pack = £24.54, 40-microgram starter pack = £29.83; *Continuation Pack*, 2 double-chamber cartridges (containing alprostadil and diluent), 2 needles, swabs, 10-microgram continuation pack = £16.55, 20-microgram continuation pack = £21.39, 40-microgram continuation pack = £27.22; replacement *Duoject®* applicators available from UCB Pharma

**Dose** by direct intracavernosal injection, ADULT over 18 years, erectile dysfunction, initially 5 micrograms (2.5 micrograms in neurogenic erectile dysfunction) increasing in steps of 2.5–5 micrograms to obtain dose suitable for producing erection not lasting more than 1 hour; usual range 10–20 micrograms; max. 40 micrograms; max. frequency of injection not more than 2–3 times per week with at least 24 hour interval between injections; reduce dose if erection lasts longer than 2 hours

**Note** The first dose must be given by medically trained personnel; self-administration may only be undertaken after proper training

1. ⒩ℋ⒮ except to treat erectile dysfunction in men who:

• have diabetes, multiple sclerosis, Parkinson's disease, poliomyelitis, prostate cancer, severe pelvic injury, single gene neurological disease, spina bifida, or spinal cord injury;

• are receiving dialysis for renal failure;

• have had radical pelvic surgery, prostatectomy (including transurethral resection of the prostate), or kidney transplant;

• were receiving *Caverject®*, *Erecnos®*, *MUSE®*, *Viagra®*, or *Viridal®* for erectile dysfunction, at the expense of the NHS, on 14 September 1998;

• are suffering severe distress as a result of impotence (prescribed in specialist centres only, see notes above).

The prescription must be endorsed 'SLS'.

◢**Urethral application**

**Counselling** If partner pregnant barrier contraception should be used

¹**MUSE®** (Meda) ℗ℴℳ ⒩ℋ⒮

Urethral application, alprostadil, net price 125-microgram single-use applicator = £9.89, 250-microgram single-use applicator = £10.76, 500-microgram single-use applicator = £10.76, 1-mg single-use applicator = £11.01 (all strengths also available in packs of 6 applicators)

**Condoms** no evidence of harm to latex condoms and diaphragms

**Dose** by direct urethral application, ADULT over 18 years, erectile dysfunction, initially 250 micrograms adjusted according to response (usual range 0.125–1 mg); max. 2 doses in 24 hours and 7 doses in 7 days)

**Note** During initiation of treatment *MUSE®* should be used under medical supervision; self-administration may only be undertaken after proper training

Aid to diagnosis, 500 micrograms as a single dose

## Phosphodiesterase type-5 inhibitors

Sildenafil, tadalafil and **vardenafil** are phosphodiesterase type-5 inhibitors licensed for the treatment of erectile dysfunction; they are not recommended for use with other treatments for erectile dysfunction. The patient should be assessed appropriately before prescribing sildenafil, tadalafil or vardenafil. Since these drugs are given by mouth there is a potential for drug interactions.

**Cautions** Sildenafil, tadalafil, and vardenafil should be used with caution in cardiovascular disease, left ventricular outflow obstruction, anatomical deformation of the penis (e.g. angulation, cavernosal fibrosis, Peyronie's disease), and in those with a predisposition to priapism (e.g. in sickle-cell disease, multiple myeloma, or leukaemia). Concomitant treatment with a phosphodiesterase-5 inhibitor and an alpha-blocker (section 2.5.4 and section 7.4.1) can increase the risk of postural hypotension—initiate treatment with a phosphodiesterase type-5 inhibitor (at a low dose) only once the patient is stable on the alpha-blocker; see also **interactions:** Appendix 1 (sildenafil, tadalafil, vardenafil).

**Contra-indications** Sildenafil, tadalafil, and vardenafil are contra-indicated in patients receiving nitrates, in patients in whom vasodilation or sexual activity are inadvisable, or in patients with a previous history of non-arteritic anterior ischaemic optic neuropathy. In the absence of information, manufacturers contra-indicate these drugs in hypotension (avoid if systolic blood pressure below 90 mmHg), recent stroke, unstable angina, and myocardial infarction.

**Side-effects** The side-effects of sildenafil, tadalafil, and vardenafil include dyspepsia, nausea, vomiting, headache (including migraine), flushing, dizziness, myalgia, back pain, visual disturbances (non-arteritic anterior ischaemic optic neuropathy has been reported—stop drug if sudden visual impairment occurs), and nasal congestion. *Less common* side-effects include painful red eyes, palpitation, tachycardia, hypotension, hypertension, epistaxis. Other side-effects reported rarely include syncope, hypersensitivity reactions (including rash, facial oedema, and Stevens-Johnson syndrome), and priapism. Serious cardiovascular events (including

**7**

**Obstetrics, gynaecology, and urinary-tract disorders**

arrhythmia, unstable angina, and myocardial infarction), seizures, sudden hearing loss (discontinue drug and seek medical advice), and retinal vascular occlusion have also been reported.

## ■ SILDENAFIL

**Indications** erectile dysfunction; pulmonary hypertension (section 2.5.1)

**Cautions** see notes above; also bleeding disorders or active peptic ulceration; hepatic impairment (avoid if severe; Appendix 2); renal impairment (Appendix 3); **interactions:** Appendix 1 (sildenafil)

**Contra-indications** see notes above; also hereditary degenerative retinal disorders

**Side-effects** see notes above; also *less commonly* chest pain, drowsiness, hypoaesthesia, vertigo, tinnitus, dry mouth, fatigue; *rarely* cerebrovascular accident and atrial fibrillation

**Dose**

- ADULT over 18 years initially 50 mg approx. 1 hour before sexual activity, subsequent doses adjusted according to response to 25–100 mg as a single dose as needed; max. 1 dose in 24 hours (max. single dose 100 mg)

  Note Onset of effect may be delayed if taken with food

¹**Viagra®** (Pfizer) [PoM] [NHS]
Tablets, all blue, f/c, sildenafil (as citrate), 25 mg, net price 4-tab pack = £16.59, 8-tab pack = £33.19; 50 mg, 4-tab pack = £19.34, 8-tab pack = £38.67; 100 mg, 4-tab pack = £23.50, 8-tab pack = £46.99

**Revatio®** (Pfizer) ▼ [PoM]
Section 2.5.1 (pulmonary hypertension)

## ■ TADALAFIL

**Indications** erectile dysfunction

**Cautions** see notes above; also hepatic impairment (Appendix 2); renal impairment (Appendix 3); **interactions:** Appendix 1 (tadalafil)

**Contra-indications** see notes above; also moderate heart failure, uncontrolled arrhythmias, uncontrolled hypertension

**Side-effects** see notes above; also increased sweating, abdominal pain, and transient amnesia reported

**Dose**

- ADULT over 18 years, initially 10 mg at least 30 minutes before sexual activity, subsequent doses adjusted

---

1. [NHS] except to treat erectile dysfunction in men who:

- have diabetes, multiple sclerosis, Parkinson's disease, poliomyelitis, prostate cancer, severe pelvic injury, single gene neurological disease, spina bifida, or spinal cord injury;
- are receiving dialysis for renal failure;
- have had radical pelvic surgery, prostatectomy (including transurethral resection of the prostate), or kidney transplant;
- were receiving *Caverject®*, *Erecnos®*, *MUSE®*, *Viagra®*, or *Viridal®* for erectile dysfunction, at the expense of the NHS, on 14 September 1998;
- are suffering severe distress as a result of impotence (prescribed in specialist centres only, see notes above).

The prescription must be endorsed 'SLS'.

---

according to response, up to 20 mg as a single dose; max. 1 dose in 24 hours (but daily dose of 10–20 mg not recommended); for patients who anticipate sexual activity at least twice weekly, 5 mg once daily can be taken, reduced to 2.5 mg once daily according to response

Note Effect of intermittent dosing may persist for longer than 24 hours

¹**Cialis®** (Lilly) [PoM] [NHS]
Tablets, f/c, tadalafil 2.5 mg (orange), net price 28-tab pack = £54.99; 5 mg (light yellow), 28-tab pack = £54.99; 10 mg (light yellow), 4-tab pack = £26.99; 20 mg (yellow), 4-tab pack = £26.99; 8-tab pack = £53.98

## ■ VARDENAFIL

**Indications** erectile dysfunction

**Cautions** see notes above; also elderly; bleeding disorders or active peptic ulceration; susceptibility to prolongation of QT interval (including concomitant use of drugs which prolong QT interval); hepatic impairment (avoid if severe Appendix 2); renal impairment (Appendix 3); **interactions:** Appendix 1 (vardenafil)

**Contra-indications** see notes above; also hereditary degenerative retinal disorders

**Side-effects** see notes above; also *less commonly* drowsiness, dyspnoea, increased lacrimation, photosensitivity; *rarely* anxiety, transient amnesia, hypertonia, and raised intra-ocular pressure

**Dose**

- ADULT over 18 years, initially 10 mg (patients on alpha-blocker therapy 5 mg) approx. 25–60 minutes before sexual activity, subsequent doses adjusted according to response up to max. 20 mg as a single dose; max. 1 dose in 24 hours

  Note Onset of effect may be delayed if taken with high-fat meal

¹**Levitra®** (Bayer) [PoM] [NHS]
Tablets, all orange, f/c, vardenafil (as hydrochloride trihydrate) 5 mg, net price 4-tab pack = £16.58, 8-tab pack = £33.19; 10 mg, 4-tab pack = £22.24, 8-tab pack = £44.47; 20 mg, 4-tab pack = £23.50, 8-tab pack = £46.99

---

# Papaverine and phentolamine

Although not licensed the smooth muscle relaxant **papaverine** has also been given by intracavernosal injection for erectile dysfunction. Patients with neurological or psychogenic impotence are more sensitive to the effect of papaverine than those with vascular abnormalities. **Phentolamine** is added if the response is inadequate [unlicensed indication].

Persistence of the erection for longer than 4 hours is an emergency, see advice in section 7.4.5.

# 8 Malignant disease and immunosuppression

| **8.1** Cytotoxic drugs | **465** |
| **8.1.1** Alkylating drugs | 469 |
| **8.1.2** Anthracyclines and other cytotoxic antibiotics | 472 |
| **8.1.3** Antimetabolites | 474 |
| **8.1.4** Vinca alkaloids and etoposide | 479 |
| **8.1.5** Other antineoplastic drugs | 480 |
| **8.2** Drugs affecting the immune response | **493** |
| **8.2.1** Antiproliferative immunosuppressants | 493 |
| **8.2.2** Corticosteroids and other immunosuppressants | 494 |
| **8.2.3** Rituximab and alemtuzumab | 498 |
| **8.2.4** Other immunomodulating drugs | 499 |
| **8.3** Sex hormones and hormone antagonists in malignant disease | **504** |
| **8.3.1** Oestrogens | 504 |
| **8.3.2** Progestogens | 504 |
| **8.3.3** Androgens | 505 |
| **8.3.4** Hormone antagonists | 505 |
| **8.3.4.1** Breast cancer | 505 |
| **8.3.4.2** Gonadorelin analogues and gonadotrophin-releasing hormone antagonists | 508 |
| **8.3.4.3** Somatostatin analogues | 510 |

## 8.1 Cytotoxic drugs

**8.1.1** Alkylating drugs

**8.1.2** Anthracyclines and other cytotoxic antibiotics

**8.1.3** Antimetabolites

**8.1.4** Vinca alkaloids and etoposide

**8.1.5** Other antineoplastic drugs

The chemotherapy of cancer is complex and should be confined to specialists in oncology. Cytotoxic drugs have both anti-cancer activity and the potential to damage normal tissue; most cytotoxic drugs are teratogenic. Chemotherapy may be given with a curative intent or it may aim to prolong life or to palliate symptoms. In an increasing number of cases chemotherapy may be combined with radiotherapy or surgery or both as either neoadjuvant treatment (initial chemotherapy aimed at shrinking the primary tumour, thereby rendering local therapy less destructive or more effective) or as adjuvant treatment (which follows definitive treatment of the primary disease, when the risk of subclinical metastatic disease is known to be high). All chemotherapy drugs cause side-effects and a balance has to be struck between likely benefit and acceptable toxicity.

Guidelines for handling cytotoxic drugs:
1. Trained personnel should reconstitute cytotoxics;
2. Reconstitution should be carried out in designated areas;
3. Protective clothing (including gloves, gowns, and masks) should be worn;
4. The eyes should be protected and means of first aid should be specified;
5. Pregnant staff should avoid exposure to cytotoxic drugs (all females of child-bearing age should be informed of the reproductive hazard);
6. Use local procedures for dealing with spillages and safe disposal of waste material, including syringes, containers, and absorbent material;
7. Staff exposure to cytotoxic drugs should be monitored.

8

Malignant disease and immunosuppression

**Intrathecal chemotherapy**
A Health Service Circular (HSC 2003/010) provides guidance on the introduction of safe practice in NHS Trusts where intrathecal chemotherapy is administered. Support for training programmes is also available.
Copies, and further information may be obtained from:
Department of Health
PO Box 777
London SE1 6XH
Fax: 01623 724524
It is also available from the Department of Health website (www.dh.gov.uk)

Combinations of cytotoxic drugs are frequently more toxic than single drugs but have the advantage in certain tumours of enhanced response, reduced development of drug resistance and increased survival. However for some tumours, single-agent chemotherapy remains the treatment of choice.

Cytotoxic drugs fall into a number of classes, each with characteristic antitumour activity, sites of action, and toxicity. A knowledge of sites of metabolism and excretion is important because impaired drug handling as a result of disease is not uncommon and may result in enhanced toxicity.

**Doses**
Because of the complexity of dosage regimens in the treatment of malignant disease, dose statements have been omitted from some of the drug entries in this chapter. *In all cases detailed specialist literature should be consulted.*
Prescriptions should **not** be repeated except on the instructions of a specialist.

## Side-effects of cytotoxic drugs

Side-effects common to most cytotoxic drugs are discussed below whilst side-effects characteristic of a particular drug or class of drugs (e.g. neurotoxicity with vinca alkaloids) are mentioned in the appropriate sections. Manufacturers' product literature should be consulted for full details of side-effects associated with individual drugs.

**Extravasation of intravenous drugs** A number of cytotoxic drugs will cause severe local tissue necrosis if leakage into the extravascular compartment occurs. To reduce the risk of extravasation injury it is recommended that cytotoxic drugs are administered by appropriately trained staff. For information on the prevention and management of extravasation injury, see section 10.3.

**Oral mucositis** A sore mouth is a common complication of cancer chemotherapy; it is most often associated with fluorouracil, methotrexate, and the anthracyclines. It is best to prevent the complication. Good oral hygiene (rinsing the mouth frequently and effective brushing of the teeth with a soft brush 2–3 times daily) is probably beneficial. For fluorouracil, sucking ice chips during short infusions of the drug is also helpful.

Once a sore mouth has developed, treatment is much less effective. Saline mouthwashes should be used but there is no good evidence to support the use of antiseptic or anti-inflammatory mouthwashes. In general,

mucositis is self-limiting but with poor oral hygiene it can be a focus for blood-borne infection.

**Tumour lysis syndrome** Tumour lysis syndrome occurs secondary to spontaneous or treatment-related rapid destruction of malignant cells. Features include hyperkalaemia, hyperuricaemia (see below), and hyperphosphataemia with hypocalcaemia; renal damage and arrhythmias can follow. Early identification of patients at risk, and initiation of therapy, is essential. Adequate hydration and urine output are important for preventing tumour lysis syndrome.

**Hyperuricaemia** Hyperuricaemia, which may be present in high-grade lymphoma and leukaemia, can be markedly worsened by chemotherapy and is associated with acute renal failure. Allopurinol (section 10.1.4) should be started 24 hours before treating such tumours and patients should be adequately hydrated. The dose of mercaptopurine or azathioprine should be reduced if allopurinol needs to be given concomitantly (see Appendix 1).

Rasburicase (section 10.1.4), a recombinant urate oxidase, is licensed for hyperuricaemia in patients with haematological malignancy, for details, see p. 582. It rapidly reduces plasma uric acid and may be of particular value in preventing complications following treatment of leukaemias or bulky lymphomas.

**Nausea and vomiting** Nausea and vomiting cause considerable distress to many patients who receive chemotherapy and to a lesser extent abdominal radiotherapy, and may lead to refusal of further treatment; prophylaxis of nausea and vomiting is therefore extremely important. Symptoms may be acute (occurring within 24 hours of treatment), delayed (first occurring more than 24 hours after treatment), or anticipatory (occurring prior to subsequent doses). Delayed and anticipatory symptoms are more difficult to control than acute symptoms and require different management.

Patients vary in their susceptibility to drug-induced nausea and vomiting; those affected more often include women, patients under 50 years of age, anxious patients, and those who experience motion sickness. Susceptibility also increases with repeated exposure to the cytotoxic drug.

Drugs may be divided according to their emetogenic potential and some examples are given below, but the symptoms vary according to the dose, to other drugs administered and to individual susceptibility.

*Mildly emetogenic treatment*—fluorouracil, etoposide, methotrexate (less than 100 mg/m²), the vinca alkaloids, and abdominal radiotherapy.

*Moderately emetogenic treatment*—the taxanes, doxorubicin, intermediate and low doses of cyclophosphamide, mitoxantrone (mitozantrone), and high doses of methotrexate (0.1–1.2 g/m²).

*Highly emetogenic treatment*—cisplatin, dacarbazine, and high doses of cyclophosphamide.

**Prevention of acute symptoms.** For patients at *low risk of emesis*, pretreatment with domperidone or with metoclopramide, continued for up to 24 hours after chemotherapy, is often effective (section 4.6). If metoclopramide or domperidone are not sufficiently effective, additional drugs such as dexamethasone (6–10 mg by mouth) or lorazepam (1–2 mg by mouth) may be used.

For patients at *high risk of emesis* or when other treatment is inadequate, a specific (5HT₃) serotonin antagonist (section 4.6), usually given by mouth, is often highly effective, particularly when used with dexamethasone; adding the neurokinin receptor antagonist, aprepitant (section 4.6) can improve control of cisplatin-related nausea and vomiting.

**Prevention of delayed symptoms**. Dexamethasone, given by mouth, is the drug of choice for preventing delayed symptoms; it is used alone or with metoclopramide or prochlorperazine. The $5HT_3$ antagonists may be less effective for delayed symptoms.

**Prevention of anticipatory symptoms**. Good symptom control is the best way to prevent anticipatory symptoms. Lorazepam can be helpful for its amnesic, sedative, and anxiolytic effects.

**Bone-marrow suppression** All cytotoxic drugs except vincristine and bleomycin cause bone-marrow depression. This commonly occurs 7 to 10 days after administration, but is delayed for certain drugs, such as carmustine, lomustine, and melphalan. Peripheral blood counts must be checked before each treatment, and doses should be reduced or therapy delayed if bone-marrow has not recovered.

Fever in a neutropenic patient (neutrophil count less than $1.0 \times 10^9$/litre) requires immediate broad-spectrum antibacterial therapy. Patients at low risk (those receiving chemotherapy for solid tumours, lymphoma or chronic leukaemia) can be treated with oral ciprofloxacin with or without co-amoxiclav (initially in hospital). All other patients should receive parenteral broad-spectrum antibacterial therapy. Appropriate bacteriological investigations should be conducted as soon as possible.

In selected patients, the duration and the severity of neutropenia can be reduced by the use of recombinant human granulocyte-colony stimulating factors, section 9.1.6.

Symptomatic anaemia is usually treated with red blood cell transfusions. For guidance on the use of erythropoietins in patients with cancer, see MHRA/CHM advice (p. 518) and NICE guidance (p. 518).

**Alopecia** Reversible hair loss is a common complication, although it varies in degree between drugs and individual patients. No pharmacological methods of preventing this are available.

**Reproductive function** Most cytotoxic drugs are teratogenic and should not be administered during pregnancy, especially during the first trimester.

Contraceptive advice should be offered where appropriate before cytotoxic therapy begins (and should cover the duration of contraception required after therapy has ended). Regimens that do not contain an alkylating drug may have less effect on fertility, but those with an alkylating drug carry the risk of causing permanent male sterility (there is no effect on potency). Pre-treatment counselling and consideration of sperm storage may be appropriate. Women are less severely affected, though the span of reproductive life may be shortened by the onset of a premature menopause. No increase in fetal abnormalities or abortion-rate has been recorded in patients who remain fertile after cytotoxic chemotherapy.

**Thromboembolism** Venous thromboembolism can be a complication of cancer itself, but chemotherapy increases the risk.

# Drugs for cytotoxic-induced side-effects

## Anthracycline side-effects

**Anthracycline-induced cardiotoxicity** The anthracycline cytotoxic drugs are associated with dose-related, cumulative, and potentially life-threatening cardiotoxic side-effects.

Dexrazoxane, an iron chelator, is licensed for the prevention of chronic cumulative cardiotoxicity caused by doxorubicin or epirubicin treatment in advanced or metastatic cancer patients who have previously received anthracycline therapy. Patients receiving dexrazoxane should still be monitored for cardiac toxicity. The myelosuppressive effects of dexrazoxane may be additive to those of chemotherapy.

**Anthracycline extravasation** Dexrazoxane is licensed for the treatment of anthracycline extravasation. The first dose should be given as soon as possible and within six hours after the injury. For further information on the prevention and management of extravasation injury, see section 10.3.

Local guidelines for the management of extravasation should be followed or specialist advice sought.

## ▌ DEXRAZOXANE

**Indications** see notes above and under preparations

**Cautions** monitor full blood count; hepatic impairment (Appendix 2); renal impairment (Appendix 3)

**Contra-indications** pregnancy (Appendix 4); breast-feeding

**Side-effects** nausea, vomiting, dyspepsia, abdominal pain, diarrhoea, stomatitis, dry mouth, anorexia; dyspnoea; dizziness, syncope, asthenia, paraesthesia, tremor, fatigue, drowsiness; pyrexia; vaginal haemorrhage; myalgia; bone-marrow suppression; conjunctivitis; alopecia, pruritus; peripheral oedema; injection-site reactions including phlebitis

**Dose**
● See under preparations

**Cardioxane®** (Novartis) ▼ PoM
Intravenous infusion, powder for reconstitution, dexrazoxane (as hydrochloride), net price 500-mg vial = £156.57
Dose prevention of anthracycline-induced cardiotoxicity, ADULT over 18 years, by intravenous infusion (30 minutes prior to anthracycline administration), 20 times the doxorubicin-equivalent dose or 10 times the epirubicin-equivalent dose

**Savene®** (TopoTarget) ▼ PoM
Intravenous infusion, powder for reconstitution, dexrazoxane (as hydrochloride), net price 10 x 500-mg vials (with diluent) = £6750.00
Dose anthracycline extravasation, ADULT over 18 years, by intravenous infusion, 1 g/m² (max. 2 g) daily for 2 days, then 500 mg/m² for 1 day
Note Local coolants such as ice packs should be removed at least 15 minutes before administration

8

Malignant disease and immunosuppression

**Malignant disease and immunosuppression**

**8**

## Chemotherapy-induced mucositis and myelosuppression

**Folinic acid** (given as calcium folinate) is used to counteract the folate-antagonist action of methotrexate and thus speed recovery from methotrexate-induced mucositis or myelosuppression ('folinic acid rescue').

Folinic acid is also used in the management of methotrexate overdose, together with other measures to maintain fluid and electrolyte balance, and to manage possible renal failure.

Folinic acid does not counteract the antibacterial activity of folate antagonists such as trimethoprim.

When folinic acid and fluorouracil are used together in metastatic colorectal cancer the response-rate improves compared to that with fluorouracil alone.

The calcium salt of **levofolinic acid**, a single isomer of folinic acid, is also used for rescue therapy following methotrexate administration, for cases of methotrexate overdose, and for use with fluorouracil for colorectal cancer. The dose of calcium levofolinate is generally half that of calcium folinate.

The disodium salts of folinic acid and levofolinic acid are also used for rescue therapy following methotrexate therapy, and for use with fluorouracil for colorectal cancer.

**Palifermin**, a human keratinocyte growth factor, is licensed for the management of oral mucositis in patients with haematological malignancies receiving myeloablative therapy with autologous haematopoietic stem-cell support.

## CALCIUM FOLINATE
### (Calcium leucovorin)

**Indications** see notes above

**Cautions** avoid simultaneous administration of methotrexate; **not** indicated for pernicious anaemia or other megaloblastic anaemias caused by vitamin B₁₂ deficiency; pregnancy (Appendix 4); breast-feeding (Appendix 5); **interactions**: Appendix 1 (folates)
**Important** Intrathecal injection **contra-indicated**

**Side-effects** hypersensitivity reactions; *rarely* pyrexia after parenteral use; insomnia, agitation, and depression after high doses

**Dose**
Note Doses expressed as folinic acid
- Prevention of methotrexate-induced adverse effects, usually started 24 hours after start of methotrexate infusion, by intramuscular injection, *or* by intravenous injection, *or* by intravenous infusion, 15 mg, repeated every 6 hours for 24 hours (may be continued by mouth); consult local treatment protocol for further information
- Suspected methotrexate overdosage, by intravenous injection *or* by intravenous infusion (at a max. rate of 160 mg/minute), initial dose equal to or exceeding dose of methotrexate; consult poisons information service (p. 27) for advice on continuing management
- Adjunct to fluorouracil in colorectal cancer, consult product literature

**Calcium Folinate** (Non-proprietary) PoM
Tablets, scored, folinic acid (as calcium salt) 15 mg, net price 10-tab pack = £39.20, 30-tab pack = £85.74
Brands include *Refolinon®*
Note Not all strengths and pack sizes are available from all manufacturers

Injection, folinic acid (as calcium salt) 3 mg/mL, net price 1-mL amp = £4.00, 10-mL amp = £4.62; 7.5 mg/mL, net price 2-mL amp = £7.80; 10 mg/mL, net price 5-mL vial = £19.41, 10-mL vial = £35.09, 30-mL vial = £94.69, 35-mL vial = £90.98
Note Not all strengths and pack sizes are available from all manufacturers

Injection, powder for reconstitution, folinic acid (as calcium salt), net price 15-mg vial = £4.46; 30-mg vial = £8.36

## CALCIUM LEVOFOLINATE
### (Calcium levoleucovorin)

**Indications** see notes above

**Cautions** see Calcium Folinate

**Side-effects** see Calcium Folinate; also *rarely* seizures, syncope; Stevens-Johnson syndrome also reported

**Dose**
Note Doses expressed as levofolinic acid
- Prevention of methotrexate-induced adverse effects, (usually started 24 hours after beginning of methotrexate infusion), by intramuscular injection, *or* by intravenous injection *or* by intravenous infusion, usually 7.5 mg every 6 hours for 10 doses
- Suspected methotrexate overdosage, by intravenous injection *or* by intravenous infusion (at a max. rate of 160 mg/minute), initial dose at least 50% of the dose of methotrexate; consult poisons information service (p. 27) for advice on continuing management
- Adjunct to fluorouracil in colorectal cancer, consult product literature

**Calcium Levofolinate** (Non-proprietary) PoM
Injection, levofolinic acid (as calcium salt) 10 mg/mL, net price 17.5-mL vial = £84.63

**Isovorin®** (Wyeth) PoM
Injection, levofolinic acid (as calcium salt) 10 mg/mL, net price 2.5-mL vial = £11.62, 5-mL vial = £26.00, 17.5-mL vial = £81.33

## DISODIUM FOLINATE

**Indications** see notes above

**Cautions** see Calcium Folinate

**Side-effects** see Calcium Folinate

**Dose**
- As an antidote to methotrexate, by intravenous injection or infusion, consult product literature
- Adjunct to fluorouracil in colorectal cancer, consult product literature

**Sodiofolin®** (Medac) PoM
Injection, folinic acid (as disodium salt) 50 mg/mL, net price 2-mL vial = £35.09, 8-mL vial = £126.25, 18-mL vial = £284.07

## DISODIUM LEVOFOLINATE

**Indications** see notes above

**Cautions** see Calcium Folinate

**Side-effects** see Calcium Folinate

**Dose**
- As an antidote to methotrexate, by intravenous injection or infusion, consult product literature
- Adjunct to fluorouracil in colorectal cancer, consult product literature

**Levofolinic Acid** (Non-proprietary) (PoM)

Injection, levofolinic acid (as disodium salt) 50 mg/mL, net price 1-mL vial = £24.70, 4-mL vial = £80.40

## PALIFERMIN

**Indications** see notes above

**Cautions** pregnancy (Appendix 4)

**Contra-indications** breast-feeding

**Side-effects** taste disturbance, thickening and discoloration of tongue; fever; oedema; arthralgia; rash, pruritus, erythema

**Dose**

● By intravenous injection, 60 micrograms/kg once daily for 3 doses (third dose given 24–48 hours before myeloablative therapy) then 3 further doses at least 24 hours after myeloablative therapy, and at least 4 days after most recent palifermin injection, starting on same day as (but after) stem-cell infusion; CHILD not recommended

**Kepivance®** (Amgen) ▼ (PoM)

Injection, powder for reconstitution, palifermin, net price 6.25-mg vial = £544.24

### Urothelial toxicity

Haemorrhagic cystitis is a common manifestation of urothelial toxicity which occurs with the oxazaphosphorines, cyclophosphamide and ifosfamide; it is caused by the metabolite acrolein. **Mesna** reacts specifically with this metabolite in the urinary tract, preventing toxicity. Mesna is used routinely (preferably by mouth) in patients receiving ifosfamide, and in patients receiving cyclophosphamide by the intravenous route at a high dose (e.g. more than 2 g) or in those who experienced urothelial toxicity when given cyclophosphamide previously.

## MESNA

**Indications** see notes above

**Contra-indications** hypersensitivity to thiol-containing compounds

**Side-effects** nausea, vomiting, colic, diarrhoea, fatigue, headache, limb and joint pains, depression, irritability, rash, hypotension and tachycardia; rarely hypersensitivity reactions (more common in patients with auto-immune disorders)

**Dose**

Note Doses calculated according to oxazaphosphorine (cyclophosphamide or ifosfamide) treatment—for details consult product literature

● By mouth, dose is given 2 hours *before* oxazaphosphorine treatment and repeated 2 and 6 hours *after* treatment

● By intravenous injection, dose is given *with* oxazaphosphorine treatment and repeated 4 and 8 hours *after* treatment

**Mesna** (Baxter) (PoM)

Tablets, f/c, mesna 400 mg, net price 10-tab pack = £23.20; 600 mg, 10-tab pack = £30.10

Injection, mesna 100 mg/mL. Net price 4-mL amp = £1.95; 10-mL amp = £4.38

Note For oral administration contents of ampoule are taken in a flavoured drink such as orange juice or cola which may be stored in a refrigerator for up to 24 hours in a sealed container

### 8.1.1 Alkylating drugs

Extensive experience is available with these drugs, which are among the most widely used in cancer chemotherapy. They act by damaging DNA, thus interfering with cell replication. In addition to the side-effects common to many cytotoxic drugs (section 8.1), there are two problems associated with prolonged usage. Firstly, gametogenesis is often severely affected (section 8.1). Secondly, prolonged use of these drugs, particularly when combined with extensive irradiation, is associated with a marked increase in the incidence of acute non-lymphocytic leukaemia.

**Cyclophosphamide** is used for the treatment of chronic lymphocytic leukaemia, the lymphomas, soft-tissue and osteogenic sarcoma, and solid tumours. It is given by mouth or intravenously; it is inactive until metabolised by the liver. A urinary metabolite of cyclophosphamide, acrolein, can cause haemorrhagic cystitis; this is a rare but serious complication; increased fluid intake for 24–48 hours after intravenous injection, can prevent this complication. When high-dose therapy (e.g. more than 2 g intravenously) is used or when the patient is considered to be at high risk of cystitis (e.g. because of pelvic irradiation) mesna (given initially intravenously then by mouth) can also help prevent cystitis—see under Urothelial Toxicity (section 8.1).

**Ifosfamide** is related to cyclophosphamide and is given intravenously; mesna (section 8.1) is routinely given with it to reduce urothelial toxicity.

**Chlorambucil** is used to treat chronic lymphocytic leukaemia, non-Hodgkin's lymphoma, Hodgkin's disease, and Waldenstrom's macroglobulinaemia. It is given by mouth. Side-effects, apart from bone-marrow suppression, are uncommon. However, patients occasionally develop severe widespread rashes which can progress to Stevens-Johnson syndrome or to toxic epidermal necrolysis. If a rash occurs further chlorambucil is contra-indicated and cyclophosphamide is substituted.

**Melphalan** is licensed for the treatment of multiple myeloma, advanced ovarian adenocarcinoma, advanced breast cancer, childhood neuroblastoma, and polycythaemia vera. Melphalan is also licensed for regional arterial perfusion in localised malignant melanoma of the extremities and localised soft-tissue sarcoma of the extremities. Interstitial pneumonitis and life-threatening pulmonary fibrosis are rarely associated with melphalan.

**Busulfan** (busulphan) is given by mouth to treat chronic myeloid leukaemia. Busulfan given by mouth or intravenously, followed by cyclophosphamide, is also licensed as conditioning treatment before haematopoietic stem-cell transplantation in adults and children. Frequent blood tests are necessary because excessive myelosuppression may result in irreversible bone-marrow aplasia. Rarely, progressive pulmonary fibrosis is associated with busulfan. Skin hyperpigmentation is a common side-effect of oral therapy.

**Lomustine** is a lipid-soluble nitrosourea and is given by mouth. It is used mainly to treat Hodgkin's disease resistant to conventional therapy, malignant melanoma and certain solid tumours. Bone-marrow toxicity is delayed, and the drug is therefore given at intervals of 4 to 6 weeks. Permanent bone-marrow damage can

**8**

**Malignant disease and immunosuppression**

occur with prolonged use. Nausea and vomiting are common and moderately severe.

**Carmustine** given intravenously has similar activity to lomustine; it is given to patients with multiple myeloma, non-Hodgkin's lymphomas, and brain tumours. Cumulative renal damage and delayed pulmonary fibrosis may occur with intravenous use. Carmustine implants are licensed for intralesional use in adults for the treatment of recurrent glioblastoma multiforme as an adjunct to surgery. Carmustine implants are also licensed for high-grade malignant glioma as adjunctive treatment to surgery and radiotherapy.

> NICE guidance (carmustine implants and temozolomide for the treatment of newly diagnosed high-grade glioma)
> See p. 483

**Estramustine** is a combination of an oestrogen and chlormethine used predominantly in prostate cancer. It is given by mouth and has both an antimitotic effect and (by reducing testosterone concentration) a hormonal effect.

**Treosulfan** is given by mouth or by intravenous or intraperitoneal administration and is used to treat ovarian cancer. Skin pigmentation is a common side-effect and allergic alveolitis, pulmonary fibrosis and haemorrhagic cystitis occur rarely.

**Thiotepa** is usually used as an intracavitary drug for the treatment of malignant effusions or bladder cancer (section 7.4.4). It is also occasionally used to treat breast cancer, but requires parenteral administration.

**Mitobronitol** is occasionally used to treat chronic myeloid leukaemia; it is available on a named-patient basis from specialist importing companies, see p. 969.

### BUSULFAN
(Busulphan)

**Indications** see notes above

**Cautions** see section 8.1 and notes above; monitor cardiac function; previous radiation therapy; avoid in acute porphyria (but see section 9.8.2); hepatic impairment (Appendix 2) (busulfan)

**Contra-indications** pregnancy (Appendix 4); breast-feeding

**Side-effects** see section 8.1 and notes above; also hepatotoxicity (including hepatic veno-occlusive disease, hyperbilirubinaemia, jaundice and fibrosis); cardiac tamponade in thalassaemia; pneumonia; skin hyperpigmentation

**Dose**
- Chronic myeloid leukaemia, induction of remission, by mouth, 60 micrograms/kg daily (max. 4 mg); maintenance, usually 0.5–2 mg daily
- Conditioning treatment before haematopoietic stem-cell transplantation, by mouth *or* by intravenous infusion, consult product literature

**Busilvex®** (Fabre) ▼ PoM
Concentrate for intravenous infusion, busulfan 6 mg/mL, net price 10-mL vial = £201.25

**Myleran®** (GSK) PoM
Tablets, f/c, busulfan 2 mg, net price 25-tab pack = £5.20

### CARMUSTINE

**Indications** see notes above

**Cautions** see section 8.1 and notes above; avoid in acute porphyria (but see section 9.8.2)

**Contra-indications** pregnancy (Appendix 4), breast-feeding

**Side-effects** see section 8.1 and notes above; irritant to tissues

**Gliadel®** (Link) PoM
Implant, carmustine 7.7 mg, net price = £715.41

### CHLORAMBUCIL

**Indications** see notes above

**Cautions** see section 8.1 and notes above; history of epilepsy and children with nephrotic syndrome (increased risk of seizures); avoid in acute porphyria (but see section 9.8.2); hepatic impairment (Appendix 2)

**Contra-indications** pregnancy (Appendix 4), breast-feeding

**Side-effects** see section 8.1 and notes above

**Dose**
- Hodgkin's disease, used alone, 200 micrograms/kg daily for 4–8 weeks
- Non-Hodgkin's lymphoma, used alone, initially 100–200 micrograms/kg daily for 4–8 weeks then dose reduced or given intermittently
- Chronic lymphocytic leukaemia, initially 150 micrograms/kg daily until leucocyte count sufficiently reduced; maintenance (started 4 weeks after end of first course) 100 micrograms/kg daily
- Waldenstrom's macroglobulinaemia, 6–12 mg daily until leucopenia occurs, then reduce to 2–8 mg daily

**Leukeran®** (GSK) PoM
Tablets, f/c, brown, chlorambucil 2 mg, net price 25-tab pack = £8.36

### CYCLOPHOSPHAMIDE

**Indications** see notes above; rheumatoid arthritis (section 10.1.3)

**Cautions** see section 8.1 and notes above; avoid in acute porphyria (but see section 9.8.2); hepatic impairment (Appendix 2); renal impairment (Appendix 3); **interactions:** Appendix 1 (cyclophosphamide)

**Contra-indications** haemorrhagic cystitis; pregnancy (Appendix 4), breast-feeding (Appendix 5)

**Side-effects** see section 8.1 and notes above; also anorexia; cardiotoxicity at high doses; interstitial pulmonary fibrosis; inappropriate secretion of antidiuretic hormone, disturbances of carbohydrate metabolism; urothelial toxicity; pigmentation of palms, nails, and soles

**Cyclophosphamide** (Non-proprietary) PoM
Tablets, s/c, cyclophosphamide (anhydrous) 50 mg, net price 100 = £12.44. Label: 27

Injection, powder for reconstitution, cyclophosphamide, net price 200-mg vial = £1.86; 500-mg vial = £2.88; 1-g vial = £5.04

# ESTRAMUSTINE PHOSPHATE

**Indications** prostate cancer

**Cautions** see section 8.1; congestive heart failure; diabetes; hypertension; epilepsy; hypercalcaemia; avoid in acute porphyria (but see section 9.8.2); hepatic impairment (avoid if severe; Appendix 2); renal impairment (Appendix 3)

**Contra-indications** peptic ulceration, severe cardiovascular disease

**Side-effects** see section 8.1; also diarrhoea; congestive heart failure, ischaemic heart disease, myocardial infarction; oedema (rarely angioneurotic) impotence, gynaecomastia; altered liver function

**Dose**

- 0.14–1.4 g daily in divided doses (usual initial dose 560–840 mg daily)

  **Counselling** Each dose should be taken not less than 1 hour before or 2 hours after meals and should not be taken with dairy products

**Estracyt®** (Pharmacia) ᴘₒᴹ
Capsules, estramustine phosphate 140 mg (as disodium salt). Net price 100-cap pack = £171.28.
Label: 23, counselling, see above

# IFOSFAMIDE

**Indications** see notes above

**Cautions** see section 8.1 and notes above; ensure satisfactory electrolyte balance and renal function before each course (risk of tubular dysfunction, Fanconi's syndrome or diabetes insipidus if renal toxicity not treated promptly); avoid in acute porphyria (but see section 9.8.2); renal impairment (avoid if serum creatinine concentration greater than 120 micromol/litre; Appendix 3); **interactions:** Appendix 1 (ifosfamide)

**Contra-indications** myelosuppression; urinary-tract obstruction; acute infection (including urinary-tract infection); urothelial damage; hepatic impairment; pregnancy (Appendix 4), breast-feeding

**Side-effects** see section 8.1 and notes above; also drowsiness, confusion, disorientation, restlessness, psychosis; urothelial toxicity, renal toxicity (see Cautions, above)

**Ifosfamide** (Non-proprietary) ᴘₒᴹ
Injection, powder for reconstitution, ifosfamide. Net price 1-g vial = £27.03; 2-g vial = £45.49 (hosp. only)

# LOMUSTINE

**Indications** see notes above

**Cautions** see section 8.1 and notes above; avoid in acute porphyria (but see section 9.8.2)

**Contra-indications** severe renal impairment; coeliac disease; pregnancy (Appendix 4); breast-feeding

**Side-effects** see section 8.1 and notes above

**Dose**

- Used alone, 120–130 mg/m² body-surface every 6–8 weeks

**Lomustine** (Medac) ᴘₒᴹ
Capsules, blue/clear, lomustine 40 mg. Net price 20-cap pack = £455.62

**Note** The brand name *CCNU®* has been used for lomustine capsules

# MELPHALAN

**Indications** see notes above

**Cautions** see section 8.1 and notes above; avoid in acute porphyria (but see section 9.8.2); renal impairment (Appendix 3); **interactions:** Appendix 1 (melphalan)

**Contra-indications** pregnancy (Appendix 4); breast-feeding

**Side-effects** see section 8.1 and notes above

**Dose**

- By mouth, multiple myeloma, dose may vary according to regimen; typical dose 150 micrograms/kg daily for 4 days, repeated every 6 weeks

  Ovarian adenocarcinoma, 200 micrograms/kg daily for 5 days, repeated every 4–8 weeks

  Advanced breast cancer, 150 micrograms/kg daily for 5 days, repeated every 6 weeks

  Polycythaemia vera, initially, 6–10 mg daily reduced after 5–7 days to 2–4 mg daily until satisfactory response then further reduce to 2–6 mg **per week**

- By intravenous injection *or* infusion and regional arterial perfusion, consult product literature

**Alkeran®** (GSK) ᴘₒᴹ
Tablets, melphalan 2 mg, net price 25 = £13.75
Injection, powder for reconstitution, melphalan 50 mg (as hydrochloride). Net price 50-mg vial (with solvent-diluent) = £33.13

# THIOTEPA

**Indications** see notes above and section 7.4.4

**Cautions** see section 8.1; avoid in acute porphyria (but see section 9.8.2); **interactions:** Appendix 1 (thiotepa)

**Contra-indications** pregnancy (Appendix 4); breast-feeding

**Side-effects** see section 8.1

**Thiotepa** (Goldshield) ᴘₒᴹ
Injection, powder for reconstitution, thiotepa, net price 15-mg vial = £5.20

# TREOSULFAN

**Indications** see notes above

**Cautions** see section 8.1; avoid in acute porphyria (but see section 9.8.2)

**Contra-indications** pregnancy; breast-feeding

**Side-effects** see section 8.1 and notes above

**Dose**

- Consult product literature

**Treosulfan** (Medac) ᴘₒᴹ
Capsules, treosulfan 250 mg. Net price 20 = £87.01
Label: 25

Injection, powder for reconstitution, treosulfan. Net price 1 g = £39.44; 5 g = £152.41 (both in infusion bottle with transfer needle)

**8**

**Malignant disease and immunosuppression**

## 8.1.2 Anthracyclines and other cytotoxic antibiotics

Drugs in this group are widely used. Many cytotoxic antibiotics act as radiomimetics and simultaneous use of radiotherapy should be **avoided** as it may result in markedly enhanced toxicity.

**Daunorubicin**, **doxorubicin**, **epirubicin** and **idarubicin** are anthracycline antibiotics. Mitoxantrone (mitozantrone) is an anthracycline derivative.

**Doxorubicin** is used to treat the acute leukaemias, Hodgkin's and non-Hodgkin's lymphomas, paediatric malignancies, and some solid tumours including breast cancer. It is given by injection into a fast-running infusion, commonly at 21-day intervals. Extravasation can cause severe tissue necrosis. Doxorubicin is largely excreted in the bile and an elevated bilirubin concentration is an indication for reducing the dose. Diarrhoea, dehydration, and red coloration of the urine can commonly occur, and renal damage has been reported. Supraventricular tachycardia related to drug administration is an uncommon complication. Higher cumulative doses are associated with cardiomyopathy and it is usual to limit total cumulative doses to 450 mg/m² because symptomatic and potentially fatal heart failure is common above this dose. Patients should be assessed before treatment by echocardiography; the elderly, and those with cardiac disease, hypertension, or who have received myocardial irradiation, should be treated cautiously. Cardiac monitoring may assist in determining safe dosage. Some evidence suggests that weekly low-dose administration may be less cardiotoxic. Doxorubicin is also given by bladder instillation for the treatment of transitional cell carcinoma, papillary bladder tumours and carcinoma *in-situ*.

Liposomal formulations of doxorubicin for intravenous use are also available. They may reduce the incidence of cardiotoxicity and lower the potential for local necrosis, but infusion reactions, sometimes severe, may occur. Hand-foot syndrome (painful, macular reddening skin eruptions) occurs commonly with liposomal doxorubicin and may be dose limiting. It can occur after 2–3 treatment cycles and may be prevented by cooling hands and feet and avoiding socks, gloves, or tight-fitting footwear for 4–7 days after treatment.

> **NICE guidance (paclitaxel, pegylated liposomal doxorubicin and topotecan for second-line or subsequent treatment of advanced ovarian cancer)**
> See p. 485

**Epirubicin** is structurally related to doxorubicin and clinical trials suggest that it is as effective in the treatment of breast cancer. A maximum cumulative dose of 0.9–1 g/m² is recommended to help avoid cardiotoxicity. Like doxorubicin it is given intravenously and by bladder instillation. Hyperpigmentation of skin, nails, and oral mucosa, and red coloration of the urine, may occur.

**Idarubicin** has general properties similar to those of doxorubicin; it is mostly used in the treatment of haematological malignancies. Diarrhoea, abdominal pain, haemorrhage, cardiac disorders, rash, and red pigmentation of the urine are commonly reported. Skin and nail hyperpigmentation have been reported less frequently.

Idarubicin is given intravenously and it may also be given by mouth.

**Daunorubicin** also has general properties similar to those of doxorubicin. It should be given by intravenous infusion and is indicated for acute leukaemias. A liposomal formulation for intravenous use is licensed for AIDS-related Kaposi's sarcoma.

> **Use with trastuzumab**
> Concomitant use of anthracyclines with trastuzumab (section 8.1.5) is associated with cardiotoxicity; for details, see p. 492.

**Mitoxantrone (mitozantrone)** is structurally related to doxorubicin; it is used for metastatic breast cancer. Mitoxantrone is also licensed for use in the treatment of non-Hodgkin's lymphoma and adult non-lymphocytic leukaemia. It is given intravenously and is well tolerated but myelosuppression and dose-related cardiotoxicity occur; cardiac examinations are recommended after a cumulative dose of 160 mg/m².

**Bleomycin** is given intravenously or intramuscularly to treat metastatic germ cell cancer and, in some regimens, non-Hodgkin's lymphoma. It causes little bone-marrow suppression but dermatological toxicity is common and increased pigmentation particularly affecting the flexures and subcutaneous sclerotic plaques may occur. Mucositis is also relatively common and an association with Raynaud's phenomenon is reported. Hypersensitivity reactions manifest by chills and fevers commonly occur a few hours after drug administration and may be prevented by simultaneous administration of a corticosteroid, for example hydrocortisone intravenously. The principal problem associated with the use of bleomycin is progressive pulmonary fibrosis. This is dose-related, occurring more commonly at cumulative doses greater than 300 000 units (see Bleomycin, below) and in the elderly. Basal lung crepitations or suspicious chest X-ray changes are an indication to stop therapy with this drug. Patients who have received extensive treatment with bleomycin (e.g. cumulative dose more than 100 000 units—see Bleomycin below) may be at risk of developing respiratory failure if a general anaesthetic is given with high inspired oxygen concentrations. Anaesthetists should be warned of this.

**Dactinomycin** is principally used to treat paediatric cancers; it is given intravenously. Its side-effects are similar to those of doxorubicin, except that cardiac toxicity is not a problem.

**Mitomycin** is given intravenously to treat upper gastrointestinal and breast cancers and by bladder instillation for superficial bladder tumours. It causes delayed bone-marrow toxicity and therefore it is usually administered at 6-weekly intervals. Prolonged use may result in permanent bone-marrow damage. It may also cause lung fibrosis and renal damage.

## BLEOMYCIN

**Indications** squamous cell carcinoma; see also notes above

**Cautions** see section 8.1 and notes above; renal impairment (Appendix 3); caution in handling—irritant to tissues

**Contra-indications** pregnancy (Appendix 4); breast-feeding

**Side-effects** see section 8.1 and notes above

**Bleomycin** (Non-proprietary) (PoM)

Injection, powder for reconstitution, bleomycin (as sulphate). Net price 15 000-unit vial = £15.56

Note To conform to the European Pharmacopoeia vials previously labelled as containing '15 units' of bleomycin are now labelled as containing 15 000 units. The amount of bleomycin in the vial has not changed.

Brands include *Bleo-Kyowa*®

## DACTINOMYCIN
### (Actinomycin D)

**Indications** see notes above

**Cautions** see section 8.1 and notes above; caution in handling—irritant to tissues

**Contra-indications** pregnancy (Appendix 4); breast-feeding

**Side-effects** see section 8.1 and notes above

**Cosmegen Lyovac**® (Ovation) (PoM)

Injection, powder for reconstitution, dactinomycin, net price 500-microgram vial = £6.75

## DAUNORUBICIN

**Indications** see notes above

**Cautions** see section 8.1 and notes above; hepatic impairment (Appendix 2), renal impairment (Appendix 3); caution in handling—irritant to tissues

**Contra-indications** pregnancy (Appendix 4); breast-feeding

**Side-effects** see section 8.1 and notes above

**Daunorubicin** (Non-proprietary) (PoM)

Injection, powder for reconstitution, daunorubicin (as hydrochloride), net price 20-mg vial = £44.76

Note The brand name *Cerubidin*® was formerly used.

◢ Lipid formulation

**DaunoXome**® (Diatos) (PoM)

Concentrate for intravenous infusion, daunorubicin encapsulated in liposomes. For dilution before use. Net price 50-mg vial = £137.67

For advanced AIDS-related Kaposi's sarcoma

## DOXORUBICIN HYDROCHLORIDE

**Indications** see notes above and section 7.4.4

**Cautions** see section 8.1 and notes above; hepatic impairment (Appendix 2); caution in handling—irritant to tissues; **interactions**: Appendix 1 (doxorubicin)

**Contra-indications** see notes above; severe hepatic impairment; severe myocardial insufficiency, recent myocardial infarction, severe arrhythmias; previous treatment with maximum cumulative doses of doxorubicin or other anthracyclines; intravesical use in urinary infections, bladder inflammation, and in urethral stenosis with catheterisation difficulties; pregnancy (Appendix 4); breast-feeding

**Side-effects** see section 8.1 and notes above

**Doxorubicin** (Non-proprietary) (PoM)

Injection, powder for reconstitution, doxorubicin hydrochloride, net price 10-mg vial = £18.72; 50-mg vial = £96.86

Note The brand name *Adriamycin*® was formerly used

Injection, doxorubicin hydrochloride 2 mg/mL, net price 5-mL vial = £20.60, 25-mL vial = £102.00, 100-mL vial = £275.00

◢ Lipid formulation

**Caelyx**® (Schering-Plough) ▼ (PoM)

Concentrate for intravenous infusion, pegylated doxorubicin hydrochloride 2 mg/mL encapsulated in liposomes. For dilution before use. Net price 10-mL vial = £375.24, 25-mL vial = £742.18

For AIDS-related Kaposi's sarcoma in patients with low CD4 count and extensive mucocutaneous or visceral disease, for advanced ovarian cancer when platinum-based chemotherapy has failed, for progressive multiple myeloma (in combination with bortezomib) in patients who have received at least one prior therapy and who have undergone or are unsuitable for bone-marrow transplantation, and as monotherapy for metastatic breast cancer in patients with increased cardiac risk

**Myocet**® (Zeneus) ▼ (PoM)

Injection, powder for reconstitution, doxorubicin hydrochloride (as doxorubicin–citrate complex) encapsulated in liposomes, net price 50-mg vial (with vials of liposomes and buffer) = £464.50

For use with cyclophosphamide for metastatic breast cancer

## EPIRUBICIN HYDROCHLORIDE

**Indications** see notes above and section 7.4.4

**Cautions** see section 8.1 and notes above; hepatic impairment (Appendix 2); caution in handling—irritant to tissues; **interactions**: Appendix 1 (epirubicin)

**Contra-indications** pregnancy (Appendix 4); breast-feeding

**Side-effects** see section 8.1 and notes above

**Epirubicin** (Non-proprietary) (PoM)

Injection, epirubicin hydrochloride 2 mg/mL, net price 5-mL vial = £16.99, 25-mL vial = £84.95, 50-mL vial = £169.92, 100-mL vial = £308.93

**Pharmorubicin**® **Rapid Dissolution** (Pharmacia) (PoM)

Injection, powder for reconstitution, epirubicin hydrochloride, net price 50-mg vial = £96.54

**Pharmorubicin**® **Solution for Injection** (Pharmacia) (PoM)

Injection, epirubicin hydrochloride 2 mg/mL, net price 5-mL vial = £19.31, 25-mL vial = £96.54, 100-mL vial = £386.16

## IDARUBICIN HYDROCHLORIDE

**Indications** acute leukaemias (see notes above); advanced breast cancer after failure of first-line chemotherapy (not including anthracyclines)

**Cautions** see section 8.1 and notes above; hepatic impairment (Appendix 2); renal impairment (avoid if severe; Appendix 3); caution in handling—irritant to tissues

**Contra-indications** severe myocardial insufficiency; recent myocardial infarction; severe arrhythmias; pregnancy (Appendix 4); breast-feeding

**Side-effects** see section 8.1 and notes above

**Dose**

- By mouth, acute non-lymphocytic leukaemia, monotherapy, 30 mg/m² daily for 3 days *or* in combination therapy, 15–30 mg/m² daily for 3 days

  Advanced breast cancer, monotherapy, 45 mg/m² as a single dose *or* 15 mg/m² daily for 3 consecutive days; repeat every 3–4 weeks

  Note Max. cumulative dose by mouth (for all indications) 400 mg/m²

- By intravenous administration, consult product literature

**Zavedos®** (Pharmacia) (PoM)
Capsules, idarubicin hydrochloride, 5 mg (red), net price 1-cap pack = £41.47; 10 mg (red/white), 1-cap pack = £69.12. Label: 25

Injection, powder for reconstitution, idarubicin hydrochloride, net price 5-mg vial = £87.36; 10-mg vial = £174.72

## ▌ MITOMYCIN

**Indications** see notes above and section 7.4.4
**Cautions** see section 8.1 and notes above; caution in handling—irritant to tissues
**Contra-indications** pregnancy (Appendix 4); breast-feeding
**Side-effects** see section 8.1 and notes above

**Mitomycin C Kyowa®** (Kyowa Hakko) (PoM)
Injection, powder for reconstitution, mitomycin. Net price 2-mg vial = £5.88; 10-mg vial = £19.37; 20-mg vial = £36.94; 40-mg vial = £73.88 (hosp. only)

## ▌ MITOXANTRONE
(Mitozantrone)

**Indications** see notes above
**Cautions** see section 8.1 and notes above; intrathecal administration not recommended
**Contra-indications** pregnancy (Appendix 4); breast-feeding
**Side-effects** see section 8.1 and notes above

**Mitoxantrone** (Non-proprietary) (PoM)
Concentrate for intravenous infusion, mitoxantrone (as hydrochloride) 2 mg/mL, net price 10-mL vial = £100.00

**Onkotrone®** (Baxter) (PoM)
Concentrate for intravenous infusion, mitoxantrone (as hydrochloride) 2 mg/mL, net price 10-mL vial = £121.85, 12.5-mL vial = £152.33, 15-mL vial = £203.04

## ▌ 8.1.3 Antimetabolites

Antimetabolites are incorporated into new nuclear material or combine irreversibly with vital cellular enzymes, preventing normal cellular division.

**Methotrexate** inhibits the enzyme dihydrofolate reductase, essential for the synthesis of purines and pyrimidines. It is given by mouth, intravenously, intramuscularly, or intrathecally.

Methotrexate is used as maintenance therapy for childhood acute lymphoblastic leukaemia. Other uses include choriocarcinoma, non-Hodgkin's lymphoma, and a number of solid tumours. Intrathecal methotrexate is used in the CNS prophylaxis of childhood acute lymphoblastic leukaemia, and as a therapy for established meningeal cancer or lymphoma.

Methotrexate causes myelosuppression, mucositis, and rarely pneumonitis. It is **contra-indicated** in significant renal impairment because it is excreted primarily by the kidney. It is also contra-indicated in patients with severe hepatic impairment. It should also be **avoided** in the presence of significant pleural effusion or ascites because it can accumulate in these fluids, and its subsequent return to the circulation may cause myelosup-

pression. Systemic toxicity may follow intrathecal administration and blood counts should be carefully monitored.

Folinic acid (section 8.1) following methotrexate administration helps to prevent methotrexate-induced mucositis or myelosuppression.

**Capecitabine**, which is metabolised to fluorouracil, is given by mouth. It is licensed for adjuvant treatment of advanced colon cancer following surgery, for monotherapy or combination therapy of metastatic colorectal cancer, and for first-line treatment of advanced gastric cancer in combination with a platinum-based regimen. Capecitabine is also licensed for second-line treatment of locally advanced or metastatic breast cancer either in combination with docetaxel (where previous therapy included an anthracycline) or alone (after failure of a taxane and anthracycline regimen or where further anthracycline treatment is not indicated). For the role of capecitabine in the treatment of breast cancer, see section 8.3.4.1.

> **NICE guidance**
> **Capecitabine and oxaliplatin in the adjuvant treatment of stage III (Dukes' C) colon cancer (April 2006)**
> Capecitabine alone *or* oxaliplatin combined with fluorouracil and folinic acid are options for adjuvant treatment following surgery for stage III (Dukes' C) colon cancer.

> **NICE guidance**
> **Capecitabine and tegafur with uracil for metastatic colorectal cancer (May 2003)**
> Capecitabine or tegafur with uracil (in combination with folinic acid) is an option for the first-line treatment of metastatic colorectal cancer.

**Cytarabine** acts by interfering with pyrimidine synthesis. It is given subcutaneously, intravenously, or intrathecally. Its predominant use is in the induction of remission of acute myeloblastic leukaemia. It is a potent myelosuppressant and requires careful haematological monitoring. A liposomal formulation of cytarabine for intrathecal use is licensed for lymphomatous meningitis.

**Fludarabine** is licensed for the initial treatment of advanced B-cell chronic lymphocytic leukaemia (CLL) or after first-line treatment in patients with sufficient bone-marrow reserves; it is given by mouth, by intravenous injection, or by intravenous infusion. Fludarabine is well tolerated but it does cause myelosuppression, which may be cumulative. Immunosuppression is also common (see panel on cladribine and fludarabine below), and co-trimoxazole is used to prevent pneumocystis infection. Immune-mediated haemolytic anaemia, thrombocytopenia, and neutropenia are less common side-effects.

The *Scottish Medicines Consortium* has advised (October 2006) that fludarabine is accepted for restricted use for the treatment of B-cell chronic lymphocytic leukaemia (CLL) in patients with sufficient bone marrow reserves. First-line treatment should only be initiated in patients with advanced disease, Rai stages III/IV (Binet stage C), or Rai stages I/II (Binet stage A/B) where the patient has disease-related symptoms or evidence of progressive disease.

**8 Malignant disease and immunosuppression**

**Cladribine** is given by intravenous infusion for the treatment of hairy cell leukaemia. It is also given for chronic lymphocytic leukaemia in patients who have failed to respond to standard regimens containing an alkylating agent. Cladribine produces severe myelosuppression, with neutropenia, anaemia, and thrombocytopenia; haemolytic anaemia has also been reported. High doses of cladribine have been associated with acute renal failure and severe neurotoxicity.

**Cladribine** and **fludarabine** have a potent and prolonged immunosuppresive effect. Patients treated with cladribine or fludarabine are more prone to serious bacterial, opportunistic fungal, and viral infections, and prophylactic therapy is recommended in those at risk. To prevent potentially fatal transfusion-related graft-versus-host reaction, only irradiated blood products should be administered. Prescribers should consult specialist literature when using highly immunosuppressive drugs.

**Clofarabine** is licensed for the treatment of acute lymphoblastic leukaemia in patients aged 1 to 21 years who have relapsed or are refractory after receiving at least two previous regimens. It is given by intravenous infusion.

**Nelarabine** is licensed for the treatment of T-cell acute lymphoblastic leukaemia and T-cell lymphoblastic lymphoma in patients who have relapsed or who are refractory after receiving at least two previous regimens. It is given by intravenous infusion. Neurotoxicity is common with nelarabine and close monitoring for neurological adverse events is strongly recommended—discontinue if neurotoxicity occurs.

The *Scottish Medicines Consortium* (p. 3) has advised (March 2008) that the use of nelarabine (*Atriance*®) within NHS Scotland is restricted to bridging treatment before stem cell transplantation.

**Gemcitabine** is used intravenously; it is given alone for elderly patients or for palliative treatment, or with cisplatin as first-line treatment for locally advanced or metastatic non-small cell lung cancer. It is also used in the treatment of locally advanced or metastatic pancreatic cancer (see NICE guidance below). Combined with cisplatin, gemcitabine is also licensed for the treatment of advanced bladder cancer. Combined with carboplatin, gemcitabine is licensed for the treatment of locally advanced or metastatic epithelial ovarian cancer which has relapsed after a recurrence-free interval of at least 6 months following previous platinum-based therapy. Combined with paclitaxel, gemcitabine is also licensed for the treatment of metastatic breast cancer which has relapsed after previous chemotherapy including an anthracycline (see NICE guidance below). Gemcitabine is generally well tolerated but it can cause mild gastro-intestinal side-effects, musculoskeletal pain, influenza-like symptoms and rashes; renal impairment and pulmonary toxicity have also been reported.

Haemolytic uraemic syndrome has been reported rarely and gemcitabine should be discontinued if signs of microangiopathic haemolytic anaemia occur.

The *Scottish Medicines Consortium* has advised (November 2006) that gemcitabine is accepted for restricted use for the treatment of metastatic breast cancer, which has relapsed following previous chemotherapy including an anthracycline (unless contra-indicated).

**Fluorouracil** is usually given intravenously because absorption following oral administration is unpredictable. It is used to treat a number of solid tumours, including gastro-intestinal tract cancers and breast cancer. It is commonly used with folinic acid in advanced colorectal cancer. It may also be used topically for certain malignant and pre-malignant skin lesions. Toxicity is unusual, but may include myelosuppression, mucositis, and rarely a cerebellar syndrome. On prolonged infusion, a desquamative hand–foot syndrome may occur.

**Pemetrexed** inhibits thymidylate transferase and other folate-dependent enzymes. It is licensed for use with cisplatin for the treatment of unresectable malignant pleural mesothelioma which has not previously been treated with chemotherapy (see NICE guidance, below). Pemetrexed is also licensed for use with cisplatin for the first-line treatment of locally advanced or metastatic non-small cell lung cancer other than predominantly squamous cell histology, and as monotherapy for its second-line treatment (but see NICE guidance, below). Pemetrexed is given by intravenous infusion. Common adverse effects include myelosuppression, gastro-intestinal toxicity, and skin disorders.

The *Scottish Medicines Consortium* (p. 3) has advised (July 2005) that pemetrexed (*Alimta*®) in combination with cisplatin is accepted for restricted use within NHS Scotland for previously untreated patients with stage III/IV unresectable malignant pleural mesothelioma.

The *Scottish Medicines Consortium* (p. 3) has advised (August 2008) that pemetrexed (*Alimta*®) is accepted for restricted use within NHS Scotland as monotherapy for the second-line treatment of locally advanced or metastatic non-small cell lung cancer without predominantly squamous cell histology; it is restricted for use in

**8**

**Malignant disease and immunosuppression**

patients with good performance status who would otherwise be eligible for docetaxel treatment.

> **NICE guidance**
> **Pemetrexed for the treatment of malignant pleural mesothelioma (January 2008)**
> Pemetrexed is an option for the treatment of malignant pleural mesothelioma only in patients who have a WHO performance status of 0 or 1 [WHO performance status is a measure of the ability to perform ordinary tasks], who are considered to have advanced disease and for whom surgical resection is considered inappropriate.
> Patients currently receiving pemetrexed who do not fall into the patient population defined above, should have the option to continue therapy until they and their clinicians consider it appropriate to stop.

> **NICE guidance**
> **Pemetrexed for the treatment of non-small cell lung cancer (August 2007)**
> Pemetrexed is **not** recommended for the treatment of locally advanced or metastatic non-small cell lung cancer.
> Patients currently receiving pemetrexed should have the option to continue therapy until they and their clinicians consider it appropriate to stop.

**Raltitrexed**, a thymidylate synthase inhibitor, is given intravenously for palliation of advanced colorectal cancer when fluorouracil and folinic acid cannot be used. It is probably of similar efficacy to fluorouracil. Raltitrexed is generally well tolerated, but can cause marked myelosuppression and gastro-intestinal side-effects.

> **NICE guidance (irinotecan, oxaliplatin and raltitrexed for advanced colorectal cancer)**
> See p. 485

**Mercaptopurine** is used as maintenance therapy for the acute leukaemias and in the management of ulcerative colitis and Crohn's disease (section 1.5.3). Azathioprine, which is metabolised to mercaptopurine, is generally used as an immunosuppressant (section 8.2.1 and section 10.1.3). The dose of both drugs should be reduced if the patient is receiving allopurinol since it interferes with their metabolism.

**Tegafur** (in combination with uracil) is given by mouth, together with calcium folinate, in the management of metastatic colorectal cancer. Tegafur is a prodrug of fluorouracil; uracil inhibits the degradation of fluorouracil. Tegafur (with uracil) has been shown to be of similar efficacy as a combination of fluorouracil and folinic acid for metastatic colorectal cancer. For NICE guidance on capecitabine and tegafur with uracil for metastatic colorectal cancer, see above.

**Tioguanine** (thioguanine) is given by mouth for the treatment of acute leukaemias and chronic myeloid leukaemia. It can be given at various stages of treatment in short-term cycles. Tioguanine has a lower incidence of gastro-intestinal side-effects than mercaptopurine. Long-term therapy is no longer recommended because of the high risk of liver toxicity; treatment with tioguanine should be discontinued if liver toxicity develops.

**Azacitidine** is a pyrimidine analogue that is given by subcutaneous injection. It is licensed for the treatment of intermediate-2 and high-risk myelodysplastic syndromes, chronic myelomonocytic leukaemia with 10–29% marrow blasts without myeloproliferative disorder, and acute myeloid leukaemia with 20–30% blasts and multilineage dysplasia, in adults who are not eligible for haemotopoietic stem cell transplantation.

## AZACITIDINE

**Indications** see notes above

**Cautions** see section 8.1; also severe hepatic impairment; history of severe congestive heart failure, unstable cardiac or pulmonary disease; monitor for bleeding; renal impairment (Appendix 3)

**Contra-indications** advanced malignant hepatic tumour; pregnancy (Appendix 4); breast-feeding

**Side-effects** see section 8.1; also gastro-intestinal disturbances (including diarrhoea, constipation, abdominal pain and dyspepsia), anorexia; hypertension, hypotension; dyspnoea, pneumonia; anxiety, insomnia, dizziness, headache, drowsiness; haematuria; hypokalaemia; arthralgia, myalgia; injection-site reactions, rash, haematoma; haemorrhage (including cerebral haemorrhage); *less commonly* hypersensitivity reactions (including anaphylactic reactions); hepatic coma and renal failure also reported

**Vidaza®** (Celgene) ▼ [PoM]
Injection, powder for reconstitution, azacitidine, net price 100-mg vial = £321.00

## CAPECITABINE

**Indications** see notes above

**Cautions** see section 8.1; history of significant cardiovascular disease, arrhythmias; monitor plasma-calcium concentration; diabetes mellitus; renal impairment (avoid if creatinine clearance less than 30 mL/minute; Appendix 3); **interactions:** Appendix 1 (fluorouracil)

**Contra-indications** hepatic impairment (Appendix 2); pregnancy (Appendix 4); breast-feeding

**Side-effects** see section 8.1; hand–foot (desquamative) syndrome; diarrhoea

**Dose**
- Stage III colon cancer, adjuvant following surgery, ADULT over 18 years 1.25 g/m² twice daily for 14 days, followed by a 7-day interval, given as 3-week cycles for a total of 8 cycles
- Metastatic colorectal cancer, monotherapy, ADULT over 18 years 1.25 g/m² twice daily for 14 days; subsequent courses repeated after a 7-day interval
- Metastatic colorectal cancer, in combination therapy, ADULT over 18 years 0.8–1 g/m² twice daily for 14 days, subsequent courses repeated after a 7-day interval *or* 625 mg/m² twice daily given continuously
- Advanced gastric cancer, in combination with a platinum-based regimen, ADULT over 18 years 0.8–1 g/m² twice daily for 14 days, subsequent courses repeated after a 7-day interval *or* 625 mg/m² twice daily given continuously
- Locally advanced or metastatic breast cancer, monotherapy or in combination with docetaxel, ADULT over 18 years 1.25 g/m² twice daily for 14 days; subsequent courses repeated after a 7-day interval

**Note** Adjust dose according to tolerability—consult product literature

**8 Malignant disease and immunosuppression**

**Xeloda®** (Roche) [PoM]

Tablets, f/c, peach, capecitabine 150 mg, net price 60-tab pack = £44.47; 500 mg, 120-tab pack = £295.06. Label: 21

## CLADRIBINE

**Indications** see notes above and under preparation

**Cautions** see section 8.1 and notes above; use irradiated blood only; hepatic impairment (Appendix 2); renal impairment (Appendix 3)

**Contra-indications** pregnancy (Appendix 4); breast-feeding

**Side-effects** see section 8.1 and notes above; also constipation, diarrhoea, abdominal pain, flatulence; oedema, tachycardia; cough, dyspnoea; dizziness, insomnia, anxiety, headache; chills, asthenia, malaise; myalgia, arthralgia; sweating, rash, pruritus, and purpura

**Leustat®** (Janssen-Cilag) [PoM]

Concentrate for intravenous infusion, cladribine 1 mg/mL. For dilution and use as an infusion, net price 10-mL vial = £162.92

For hairy cell leukaemia and for B-cell chronic lymphocytic leukaemia in patients who have failed to respond to standard regimens containing an alkylating agent

**Litak®** (Lipomed) [PoM]

Injection (for subcutaneous use only—no dilution required), cladribine 2 mg/mL, net price 5-mL vial = £165.00

For hairy cell leukaemia

## CLOFARABINE

**Indications** see notes above

**Cautions** see section 8.1 and notes above; cardiac disease; hepatic impairment (Appendix 2); renal impairment (avoid in severe renal impairment; Appendix 3)

**Contra-indications** pregnancy (Appendix 4); breast-feeding

**Side-effects** see section 8.1; also diarrhoea, abdominal pain, jaundice; tachycardia, flushing, hypotension, pericardial effusion, oedema, haematoma; dyspnoea, cough; anxiety, agitation, dizziness, drowsiness, headache, paraesthesia, peripheral neuropathy, restlessness; haematuria; arthralgia, myalgia; rash, pruritus, hand-foot (desquamative) syndrome, sweating; pancreatitis also reported

**Evoltra®** (Genzyme) ▼ [PoM]

Concentrate for intravenous infusion, clofarabine 1 mg/mL, net price 20-mL vial = £1200.00
Electrolytes Na⁺ 3.08 mmol/vial

## CYTARABINE

**Indications** see notes above

**Cautions** see section 8.1 and notes above; hepatic impairment (Appendix 2); **interactions:** Appendix 1 (cytarabine)

**Contra-indications** pregnancy (Appendix 4); breast-feeding

**Side-effects** see section 8.1 and notes above

**Cytarabine** (Non-proprietary) [PoM]

Injection (for intravenous, subcutaneous, or intrathecal use), cytarabine 20 mg/mL, net price 5-mL vial = £4.00

Injection (for intravenous or subcutaneous use), cytarabine 20 mg/mL, net price 5-mL vial = £3.90, 25-mL vial = £19.50; 100 mg/mL, 1-mL vial = £4.00, 5-mL vial = £20.00, 10-mL vial = £39.00, 20-mL vial = £77.50

◀Lipid formulation for intrathecal use

**DepoCyte®** (Napp) ▼ [PoM]

Intrathecal injection, cytarabine encapsulated in liposomes, net price 50-mg vial = £1223.75
For lymphomatous meningitis

**Note** The *Scottish Medicines Consortium* (p. 3) has advised (July 2007) that liposomal cytarabine suspension (*DepoCyte®*) is not recommended for use within NHS Scotland for the intrathecal treatment of lymphomatous meningitis

## FLUDARABINE PHOSPHATE

**Indications** see notes above

**Cautions** see section 8.1 and notes above; monitor for signs of haemolysis; monitor for neurological toxicity; worsening of existing and increased susceptibility to skin cancer; renal impairment (avoid if creatinine clearance less than 30 mL/minute; Appendix 3); **interactions:** Appendix 1 (fludarabine)

**Contra-indications** haemolytic anaemia; pregnancy (Appendix 4); breast-feeding

**Side-effects** see section 8.1 and notes above; also diarrhoea, anorexia; oedema; pneumonia, cough; peripheral neuropathy, visual disturbances; chills, fever, malaise, weakness; rash

**Dose**

- By mouth, ADULT 40 mg/m² for 5 days every 28 days usually for 6 cycles
- By intravenous injection *or* infusion, consult product literature

**Fludarabine** (Non-proprietary) [PoM]

Injection, powder for reconstitution, fludarabine phosphate, net price 50-mg vial = £140.40

**Fludara®** (Bayer) [PoM]

Tablets, f/c, pink, fludarabine phosphate 10 mg, net price 15-tab pack = £268.12, 20-tab pack = £357.49

Injection, powder for reconstitution, fludarabine phosphate, net price 50-mg vial = £149.92

## FLUOROURACIL

**Indications** see notes above; pre-malignant and malignant skin lesions (section 13.8.1)

**Cautions** see section 8.1 and notes above; caution in handling—irritant to tissues; hepatic impairment (Appendix 2); **interactions:** Appendix 1 (fluorouracil)

**Contra-indications** pregnancy (Appendix 4); breast-feeding

**Side-effects** see section 8.1 and notes above; also local irritation with topical preparation

**Dose**

- By mouth, maintenance 15 mg/kg weekly; max. in one day 1 g
- By intravenous injection *or* infusion *or* by intra-arterial infusion, consult product literature

**8**

**Malignant disease and immunosuppression**

**Fluorouracil** (Non-proprietary) [PoM]
Capsules, fluorouracil 250 mg.
Available from Cambridge on a named-patient basis

Injection, fluorouracil (as sodium salt) 25 mg/mL, net price 10-mL vial = £3.20, 20-mL vial = £6.40, 100-mL vial = £32.00; 50 mg/mL, 10-mL vial = £6.40, 20-mL vial = £12.80, 50-mL vial = £32.00, 100-mL vial = £64.00

## GEMCITABINE

**Indications** see notes above

**Cautions** see section 8.1 and notes above; hepatic impairment (Appendix 2); renal impairment (Appendix 3)

**Contra-indications** pregnancy (Appendix 4); breast-feeding

**Side-effects** see section 8.1 and notes above

**Gemcitabine** (Non-proprietary) [PoM]
Injection, powder for reconstitution, gemcitabine (as hydrochloride), net price 200-mg vial = £32.55, 1-g vial = £162.76

**Gemzar®** (Lilly) [PoM]
Injection, powder for reconstitution, gemcitabine (as hydrochloride), net price 200-mg vial = £32.55; 1-g vial = £162.76 (both hosp. only)

## MERCAPTOPURINE

**Indications** acute leukaemias and chronic myeloid leukaemia; inflammatory bowel disease [unlicensed indication] (section 1.5.3)

**Cautions** see section 8.1 and notes above; monitor liver function—hepatic impairment (Appendix 2); renal impairment (Appendix 3); **interactions:** Appendix 1 (mercaptopurine)

**Contra-indications** pregnancy (Appendix 4); breast-feeding

**Side-effects** see section 8.1 and notes above; also hepatotoxicity; *rarely* intestinal ulceration, pancreatitis

**Dose**
• Initially 2.5 mg/kg daily

**Puri-Nethol®** (GSK) [PoM]
Tablets, yellow, scored, mercaptopurine 50 mg, net price 25-tab pack = £22.54

## METHOTREXATE

**Indications** see notes above and under Dose; Crohn's disease [unlicensed indication] (section 1.5.3); rheumatoid arthritis (section 10.1.3); psoriasis (section 13.5.3)

**Cautions** see section 8.1, notes above and section 10.1.3; hepatic impairment (Appendix 2); renal impairment (avoid if severe; Appendix 3); **interactions:** Appendix 1 (methotrexate)

**Contra-indications** pregnancy (Appendix 4); breast-feeding

**Side-effects** see section 8.1, notes above and section 10.1.3

**Dose**
• By mouth, leukaemia in children (maintenance), 15 mg/m² weekly in combination with other drugs

> **Important**
> Note that the above dose is a **weekly** dose. To avoid error with low-dose methotrexate, it is recommended that:
> • the patient is carefully advised of the **dose** and **frequency** of taking methotrexate and any other prescribed medicine (e.g. folic acid);
> • only one strength of methotrexate tablet (usually 2.5 mg) is prescribed and dispensed;
> • the prescription and the dispensing label clearly show the dose and frequency of methotrexate administration;
> • the patient is warned to report immediately the onset of any feature of blood disorders (e.g. sore throat, bruising, and mouth ulcers), liver toxicity (e.g. nausea, vomiting, abdominal discomfort, and dark urine), and respiratory effects (e.g. shortness of breath).

• By intravenous injection *or* infusion, *or* by intra-arterial infusion, *or* by intramuscular injection, *or* intrathecal administration, consult product literature

**Methotrexate** (Non-proprietary) [PoM]
Injection, methotrexate (as sodium salt) 2.5 mg/mL, net price 2-mL vial = £1.68; 25 mg/mL, 2-mL vial = £3.00, 20-mL vial = £30.00

Injection, methotrexate 100 mg/mL (not for intrathecal use), net price 10-mL vial = £78.33, 50-mL vial = £380.07

◄**Oral preparations**
Section 10.1.3

## NELARABINE

**Indications** see notes above

**Cautions** see section 8.1 and notes above; previous or concurrent intrathecal chemotherapy or craniospinal irradiation (increased risk of neurotoxicity)
Driving May affect performance of skilled tasks (e.g. driving)

**Contra-indications** pregnancy (Appendix 4); breast-feeding

**Side-effects** see section 8.1; also abdominal pain, constipation, taste disturbance, anorexia, diarrhoea; hypotension, oedema; pleural effusion, wheezing, dyspnoea, cough; confusion, seizures, amnesia, drowsiness, peripheral neurological disorders, hypoaesthesia, paraesthesia, ataxia, demyelination, tremor, dizziness, headache, asthenia, fatigue; pyrexia; electrolyte disturbances; blurred vision; muscle weakness, myalgia, arthralgia; benign and malignant tumours also reported

**Atriance®** (GSK) ▼ [PoM]
Intravenous infusion, nelarabine 5 mg/mL, net price 50-mL vial = £222.00
Electrolytes Na⁺ 3.75 mmol/vial

## PEMETREXED

**Indications** see notes above

**Cautions** see section 8.1 and notes above; history of cardiovascular disease; diabetes; prophylactic folic acid and vitamin $B_{12}$ supplementation required (consult product literature); renal impairment (avoid if creatinine clearance less than 45 mL/minute; Appendix 3)

**Contra-indications** pregnancy (Appendix 4); breast-feeding (Appendix 5)

**Side-effects** see section 8.1 and notes above; also dehydration, hepatitis, abdominal pain, colitis, myocardial infarction, transient ischaemic attack, interstitial pneumonitis, and acute renal failure also reported

**Alimta®** (Lilly) [PoM]
Injection, powder for reconstitution, pemetrexed 500 mg (as disodium), net price 500-mg vial = £800.00

## RALTITREXED

**Indications** see notes above

**Cautions** see section 8.1 and notes above; hepatic impairment (Appendix 2); renal impairment (avoid if creatinine clearance less than 25 mL/minute; Appendix 3)

**Contra-indications** pregnancy (Appendix 4); breast-feeding

**Side-effects** see section 8.1 and notes above

**Tomudex®** (Hospira) [PoM]
Injection, powder for reconstitution, raltitrexed. Net price 2-mg vial = £121.86

## TEGAFUR WITH URACIL

**Indications** see notes above

**Cautions** see section 8.1; cardiac disease; renal impairment; hepatic impairment (avoid if severe—Appendix 2); **interactions:** Appendix 1 (fluorouracil)

**Contra-indications** pregnancy (Appendix 4); breast-feeding

**Side-effects** see section 8.1 and notes above

**Dose**

- ADULT, tegafur 300 mg/m$^2$ (with uracil 672 mg/m$^2$) daily in 3 divided doses for 28 days; subsequent courses repeated after 7-day interval; for dose adjustment due to toxicity, consult product literature

**Uftoral®** (Merck Serono) [PoM]
Capsules, tegafur 100 mg, uracil 224 mg, net price 36-cap pack = £96.12, 120-cap pack = £320.40. Label: 23

## TIOGUANINE
(Thioguanine)

**Indications** see notes above

**Cautions** see section 8.1 and notes above; monitor liver function weekly—discontinue if liver toxicity develops; hepatic impairment (Appendix 2); renal impairment (Appendix 3); **interactions:** Appendix 1 (tioguanine)

**Contra-indications** pregnancy (Appendix 4); breast-feeding

**Side-effects** see section 8.1; also stomatitis and hepatotoxicity; *rarely* intestinal necrosis and perforation

**Dose**

- 100–200 mg/m$^2$ daily

**Lanvis®** (GSK) [PoM]
Tablets, yellow, scored, tioguanine 40 mg. Net price 25-tab pack = £54.49

## 8.1.4 Vinca alkaloids and etoposide

The vinca alkaloids, **vinblastine**, **vincristine**, and **vindesine**, are used to treat a variety of cancers including leukaemias, lymphomas, and some solid tumours (e.g. breast and lung cancer). **Vinorelbine** is a semi-synthetic vinca alkaloid, it is given intravenously or orally for the treatment of advanced breast cancer and for advanced non-small cell lung cancer. For the role of vinorelbine in the treatment of breast cancer, see section 8.3.4.1.

Neurotoxicity, usually as peripheral or autonomic neuropathy, occurs with all vinca alkaloids and is a limiting side-effect of vincristine; it occurs less often with vindesine, vinblastine, and vinorelbine. Patients with neurotoxicity commonly have peripheral paraesthesia, loss of deep tendon reflexes, abdominal pain, and constipation; ototoxicity has been reported. If symptoms of neurotoxicity are severe, doses should be reduced. Motor weakness can also occur, and increasing motor weakness calls for discontinuation of these drugs. Recovery from neurotoxic effects is usually slow but complete.

Myelosuppression is the dose-limiting side-effect of vinblastine, vindesine, and vinorelbine; vincristine causes negligible myelosuppression. The vinca alkaloids may cause reversible alopecia. They cause severe local irritation and care must be taken to avoid extravasation. Severe bronchospasm has been reported following administration of the vinca alkaloids (more commonly when used in combination with mitomycin-C).

> Vinblastine, vincristine, vindesine, and vinorelbine injections are for **intravenous administration only**. Inadvertent intrathecal administration can cause severe neurotoxicity, which is usually fatal.
> The National Patient Safety Agency has advised (August 2008) that adult and teenage patients treated in an adult or adolescent unit should receive their vinca alkaloid dose in a 50 mL minibag. Teenagers and children treated in a child unit may receive their vinca alkaloid dose in a syringe.

**Etoposide** may be given orally or by slow intravenous infusion, the oral dose being double the intravenous dose. A preparation containing etoposide phosphate can be given by intravenous injection or infusion. Etoposide is usually given daily for 3–5 days and courses should not be repeated more frequently than at intervals of 21 days. It has particularly useful activity in small cell carcinoma of the bronchus, the lymphomas, and testicular cancer. Toxic effects include alopecia, myelosuppression, nausea, and vomiting.

## ETOPOSIDE

**Indications** see notes above

**Cautions** see section 8.1 and notes above; renal impairment (Appendix 3); **interactions:** Appendix 1 (etoposide)

**Contra-indications** see section 8.1 and notes above; severe hepatic impairment; pregnancy (Appendix 4); breast-feeding

**Side-effects** see section 8.1 and notes above; irritant to tissues

**8**

**Malignant disease and immunosuppression**

**Malignant disease and immunosuppression**

**8**

**Dose**
- By mouth, 120–240 mg/m² daily for 5 days
- By intravenous infusion, consult product literature

**Etoposide** (Non-proprietary) [PoM]
Concentrate for intravenous infusion, etoposide 20 mg/mL, net price 5-mL vial = £12.15, 10-mL vial = £29.00, 25-mL vial = £60.75
Brands include *Eposin*®

**Etopophos**® (Bristol-Myers Squibb) [PoM]
Injection, powder for reconstitution, etoposide (as phosphate), net price 100-mg vial = £26.70 (hosp. only)

**Vepesid**® (Bristol-Myers Squibb) [PoM]
Capsules, both pink, etoposide 50 mg, net price 20 = £101.84; 100 mg, 10-cap pack = £88.99 (hosp. only). Label: 23

## VINBLASTINE SULPHATE

**Indications**   see notes above

**Cautions**   see section 8.1 and notes above; hepatic impairment (Appendix 2); caution in handling; **interactions**: Appendix 1 (vinblastine)

**Contra-indications**   see section 8.1 and notes above; pregnancy (Appendix 4); breast-feeding
Important Intrathecal injection **contra-indicated**

**Side-effects**   see section 8.1 and notes above; irritant to tissues

**Vinblastine** (Non-proprietary) [PoM]
Injection, vinblastine sulphate 1 mg/mL. Net price 10-mL vial = £13.09

**Velbe**® (Genus) [PoM]
Injection, powder for reconstitution, vinblastine sulphate. Net price 10-mg amp = £14.15

## VINCRISTINE SULPHATE

**Indications**   see notes above

**Cautions**   see section 8.1 and notes above; hepatic impairment (Appendix 2); neuromuscular disease; caution in handling; **interactions**: Appendix 1 (vincristine)

**Contra-indications**   see section 8.1 and notes above; pregnancy (Appendix 4); breast-feeding
Important Intrathecal injection **contra-indicated**

**Side-effects**   see section 8.1 and notes above; also *rarely* inappropriate secretion of antidiuretic hormone; diarrhoea, intestinal necrosis, paralytic ileus, seizures, urinary retention, muscle wasting, and eye disorders also reported; irritant to tissues

**Vincristine** (Non-proprietary) [PoM]
Injection, vincristine sulphate 1 mg/mL. Net price 1-mL vial = £13.47; 2-mL vial = £26.66; 5-mL vial = £44.16

**Oncovin**® (Genus) [PoM]
Injection, vincristine sulphate 1 mg/mL, net price 1-mL vial = £14.18; 2-mL vial = £28.05

## VINDESINE SULPHATE

**Indications**   see notes above

**Cautions**   see section 8.1 and notes above; hepatic impairment (Appendix 2); neuromuscular disease; caution in handling

**Contra-indications**   see section 8.1 and notes above; pregnancy (Appendix 4); breast-feeding
Important Intrathecal injection **contra-indicated**

**Side-effects**   see section 8.1 and notes above; irritant to tissues

**Eldisine**® (Genus) [PoM]
Injection, powder for reconstitution, vindesine sulphate, net price 5-mg vial = £78.30 (hosp. only)

## VINORELBINE

**Indications**   see notes above

**Cautions**   see section 8.1 and notes above; ischaemic heart disease; hepatic impairment (avoid capsules if severe; Appendix 2); caution in handling

**Contra-indications**   see section 8.1 and notes above; pregnancy (Appendix 4); breast-feeding; *with capsules* previous significant surgical resection of stomach or small bowel, long-term oxygen therapy, concurrent radiotherapy if treating the liver
Important Intrathecal injection **contra-indicated**

**Side-effects**   see section 8.1 and notes above; also stomatitis; *rarely* pancreatitis; *very rarely* inappropriate secretion of antidiuretic hormone; irritant to tissues

**Dose**
- By mouth, 60 mg/m² once weekly for 3 weeks, increased if tolerated to 80 mg/m² once weekly; max. 160 mg once weekly
- By intravenous injection *or* infusion, consult product literature

**Vinorelbine** (Non-proprietary) [PoM]
Concentrate for intravenous infusion, vinorelbine (as tartrate) 10 mg/mL, net price 1-mL vial = £29.00, 5-mL vial = £139.00

**Navelbine**® (Fabre) [PoM]
Concentrate for intravenous infusion, vinorelbine (as tartrate) 10 mg/mL. Net price 1-mL vial = £29.75; 5-mL vial = £139.98

Capsules, vinorelbine (as tartrate) 20 mg (brown), net price 1-cap pack = £43.98; 30 mg (pink), 1-cap pack = £65.98; 80 mg (yellow), 1-cap pack = £175.92. Label: 21, 25

## 8.1.5 Other antineoplastic drugs

### Amsacrine

**Amsacrine** has an action and toxic effects similar to those of doxorubicin (section 8.1.2) and is given *intravenously*. It is occasionally used in acute myeloid leukaemia. Side-effects include myelosuppression and mucositis; electrolytes should be monitored as fatal arrhythmias have occurred in association with hypokalaemia.

# AMSACRINE

**Indications** see notes above

**Cautions** see section 8.1 and notes above; reduce dose in renal or hepatic impairment; also caution in handling—irritant to skin and tissues

**Contra-indications** pregnancy (Appendix 4); breastfeeding

**Side-effects** see section 8.1 and notes above

**Amsidine®** (Goldshield) PoM
Concentrate for intravenous infusion, amsacrine 5 mg (as lactate)/mL, when reconstituted by mixing two solutions. Net price 1.5-mL (75-mg) amp with 13.5-mL diluent vial = £54.08 (hosp. only)
Note Use glass apparatus for reconstitution

---

## Arsenic trioxide

Arsenic trioxide is licensed for acute promyelocytic leukaemia in patients who have relapsed or failed to respond to previous treatment with a retinoid and chemotherapy.

# ARSENIC TRIOXIDE

**Indications** see notes above

**Cautions** see section 8.1; correct electrolyte abnormalities before treatment; ECG required before and during treatment—consult product literature; avoid concomitant administration with drugs causing QT interval prolongation, hypokalaemia, and hypomagnesaemia; previous treatment with anthracyclines (increased risk of QT interval prolongation); hepatic impairment (Appendix 2); renal impairment (Appendix 3)

**Contra-indications** pregnancy (Appendix 4); breastfeeding

**Side-effects** see section 8.1; diarrhoea, leucocyte activation syndrome (unexplained fever, dyspnoea, weight gain, pulmonary infiltrates, pleural or pericardial effusions, with or without leucocytosis—treat with high dose corticosteroids, consult product literature); hyperglycaemia, hypokalaemia, QT interval prolongation, atrial fibrillation, atrial flutter, haemorrhage, pleuritic pain, musculoskeletal pain, paraesthesia, fatigue; *less commonly* hypotension, oedema, pneumonitis, seizures, renal failure, and rash

**Trisenox®** (Cephalon) PoM
Concentrate for intravenous infusion, arsenic trioxide 1 mg/mL, net price 10-mL amp = £250.90

---

## Bevacizumab

Bevacizumab is a monoclonal antibody that inhibits vascular endothelial growth factor. It is licensed for the treatment of metastatic colorectal cancer in combination with fluoropyrimidine-based chemotherapy (but see NICE guidance below). It is also licensed for first-line treatment of metastatic breast cancer in combination with paclitaxel and for advanced or metastatic renal cell carcinoma in combination with interferon alfa-2a. Bevacizumab, in combination with platinum-based chemotherapy, is licensed for first-line treatment of unresectable advanced, metastatic, or recurrent non-small cell lung cancer other than predominantly squamous cell histology. Bevacizumab is given by intravenous infusion.

**NICE guidance**

**Bevacizumab and cetuximab for the treatment of metastatic colorectal cancer (January 2007)**

- Bevacizumab in combination with fluorouracil plus folinic acid, with or without irinotecan, is **not** recommended for the first-line treatment of metastatic colorectal cancer;
- Cetuximab in combination with irinotecan is **not** recommended for the second-line or subsequent treatment of metastatic colorectal cancer after the failure of an irinotecan-containing chemotherapy regimen;
- Patients currently receiving bevacizumab or cetuximab should have the option to continue therapy until they and their consultants consider it appropriate to stop.

# BEVACIZUMAB

**Indications** see notes above

**Cautions** see section 8.1; intra-abdominal inflammation (risk of gastro-intestinal perforation); increased risk of fistulas (discontinue permanently if tracheo-oesophageal or grade 4 fistula develops); withhold treatment for elective surgery and avoid for at least 28 days after major surgery or until wound fully healed; history of hypertension (increased risk of proteinuria—discontinue if nephrotic syndrome); uncontrolled hypertension; monitor blood pressure; history of arterial thromboembolism; history of cardiovascular disease (increased risk of cardiovascular events especially in the elderly); monitor for congestive heart failure; increased risk of haemorrhage (especially tumour-associated haemorrhage); monitor for reversible posterior leucoencephalopathy syndrome (presenting as seizures, headache, altered mental status, visual disturbance or cortical blindness, with or without hypertension); untreated CNS metastases

**Contra-indications** pregnancy (Appendix 4); breastfeeding (Appendix 5)

**Side-effects** see section 8.1; gastro-intestinal perforation, intestinal obstruction, abdominal pain, diarrhoea, constipation, taste disturbances; mucocutaneous bleeding, haemorrhage, hypoxia, arterial thromboembolism, congestive heart failure, syncope, supraventricular tachycardia, hypertension (see also Cautions); dyspnoea, rhinitis; anorexia, drowsiness, headache, peripheral neuropathy, asthenia, lethargy; pyrexia; proteinuria; dehydration; eye disorders; fistulas, pulmonary hypertension, impaired wound healing, hand-foot syndrome, exfoliative dermatitis, dry skin, and skin discoloration also reported

**Avastin®** (Roche) ▼ PoM
Concentrate for intravenous infusion, bevacizumab 25 mg/mL, net price 4-ml (100-mg) vial = £242.66, 16-ml (400-mg) vial = £924.40

---

## Bexarotene

Bexarotene is an agonist at the retinoid X receptor, which is involved in the regulation of cell differentiation and proliferation. It is associated with little myelosuppression or immunosuppression. Bexarotene can cause regression of cutaneous T-cell lymphoma. The main adverse effects are hyperlipidaemia, hypothyroidism, leucopenia, headache, rash, and pruritus.

**8** Malignant disease and immunosuppression

The *Scottish Medicines Consortium* has advised (November 2002) that bexarotene is recommended for restricted use as a second-line treatment for patients with advanced cutaneous T-cell lymphoma.

### ■ BEXAROTENE

**Indications** skin manifestations of cutaneous T-cell lymphoma refractory to previous systemic treatment

**Cautions** see section 8.1 and notes above; hyperlipidaemia (avoid if uncontrolled), hypothyroidism (avoid if uncontrolled); hypersensitivity to retinoids; **interactions:** Appendix 1 (bexarotene)

**Contra-indications** see section 8.1 and notes above; history of pancreatitis, hypervitaminosis A, hepatic impairment; pregnancy (Appendix 4); breast-feeding

**Side-effects** see section 8.1 and notes above

**Dose**

● Initially 300 mg/m² daily as a single dose with a meal; adjust dose according to response

**Targretin®** (Zeneus) (PoM)

Capsules, bexarotene 75 mg in a liquid suspension, net price 100-cap pack = £937.50

## Bortezomib

**Bortezomib**, a proteasome inhibitor, is licensed as monotherapy for the treatment of multiple myeloma that has progressed despite the use of at least one therapy, and where the patient has already had, or is unable to have, bone-marrow transplantation. It is also licensed for use in combination with melphalan and prednisolone for the treatment of previously untreated multiple myeloma in patients who are not eligible for high-dose chemotherapy with bone marrow transplantation. Bortezomib is given by intravenous injection.

> **NICE guidance**
> **Bortezomib monotherapy for relapsed multiple myeloma (October 2007)**
> Bortezomib monotherapy is an option for the treatment of progressive multiple myeloma in patients who are at first relapse having received one prior therapy and who have undergone, or are unsuitable for, bone-marrow transplantation, under the following circumstances:
>
> ● the response to bortezomib is measured using serum M protein after a maximum of four cycles of treatment, and treatment is continued only in patients who have a reduction in serum M protein of 50% or more (where serum M protein is not measurable, an appropriate alternative biochemical measure of response should be used) **and**
> ● the manufacturer rebates the full cost of bortezomib if there is an inadequate response (as defined above) after four cycles of treatment.
>
> Patients currently receiving bortezomib monotherapy who do not meet the above criteria should have the option to continue therapy until they and their clinicians consider it appropriate to stop.

### ■ BORTEZOMIB

**Indications** see notes above

**Cautions** see section 8.1; cardiovascular disease; pulmonary disease (chest x-ray recommended before treatment—discontinue if interstitial lung disease develops); history of seizures; amyloidosis; risk of neuropathy—consult product literature; monitor blood-glucose concentration in patients on oral antidiabetics; hepatic impairment (avoid if severe; Appendix 2); renal impairment (Appendix 3); **interactions:** Appendix 1 (bortezomib)

**Contra-indications** acute diffuse infiltrative pulmonary disease; pericardial disease; pregnancy (Appendix 4); breast-feeding

**Side-effects** see section 8.1; also gastro-intestinal disturbances including constipation (cases of ileus reported), taste disturbance, dry mouth, decreased appetite; postural hypotension, hypertension, haematoma, phlebitis, chest pain, oedema; dyspnoea, cough; confusion, depression, insomnia, anxiety, peripheral neuropathy, paraesthesia, headache, dizziness, tremor, asthenia, fatigue; influenza-like symptoms; renal impairment, dysuria; dehydration, hypokalaemia, hyperglycaemia; muscle cramps, arthralgia, bone pain; blurred vision, eye pain; epistaxis; urticaria, pruritus, erythema, dry skin, eczema, rash, increased sweating

**Velcade®** (Janssen-Cilag) ▼ (PoM)

Injection, powder for reconstitution, bortezomib (as mannitol boronic ester), net price 3.5-mg vial = £762.38

## Cetuximab

**Cetuximab** is licensed for the treatment of metastatic colorectal cancer in patients with tumours expressing epidermal growth factor receptor, as combination therapy, or as monotherapy if oxaliplatin- and irinotecan-based therapy has failed or if irinotecan is not tolerated (but see NICE guidance under Bevacizumab on p. 481). Cetuximab is also licensed, in combination with radiotherapy, for the treatment of locally advanced squamous cell cancer of the head and neck and in combination with platinum-based chemotherapy for recurrent or metastatic squamous cell cancer of the head and neck (but see NICE guidance below).

Cetuximab is given by intravenous infusion. Patients must receive an antihistamine before the first infusion; an antihistamine is also recommended before subsequent infusions of cetuximab. Resuscitation facilities should be available and treatment should be initiated by a specialist.

> **NICE guidance**
> **Cetuximab for the treatment of locally advanced squamous cell cancer of the head and neck (June 2008)**
> Cetuximab in combination with radiotherapy is an option for the treatment of locally advanced squamous cell cancer of the head and neck in patients who have a Karnofsky performance status of 90% or greater and when all forms of platinum-based chemoradiotherapy treatment are contra-indicated. Patients currently receiving cetuximab who do not fall into the patient population defined above have the option to continue therapy until they and their clinicians consider it appropriate to stop.

### CETUXIMAB

**Indications** see notes above and product literature

**Cautions** cardiopulmonary disease, pulmonary disease—discontinue if interstitial lung disease; pregnancy (Appendix 4)

**Contra-indications** breast-feeding (Appendix 5)

**Side-effects** infusion-related side-effects including dyspnoea, dizziness, chills, fever, and hypersensitivity reactions (possibly delayed onset) such as rash, urticaria, airway obstruction, hypotension, and shock; nausea, vomiting, diarrhoea; headache; skin reactions including acne, pruritus, dry skin, desquamation, hypertrichosis, and nail disorders; conjunctivitis; hypomagnesaemia, hypocalcaemia

**Erbitux®** (Merck) ▼ PoM
Intravenous infusion, cetuximab 5 mg/mL, net price 20-mL vial = £159.02, 100-mL vial = £795.10

## Crisantaspase

**Crisantaspase** is the enzyme asparaginase produced by *Erwinia chrysanthemi*. It is given *intramuscularly*, *intravenously*, or *subcutaneously* almost exclusively in acute lymphoblastic leukaemia. Facilities for the management of anaphylaxis should be available. Side-effects also include nausea, vomiting, fever, pancreatitis, CNS depression, neurotoxicity, liver function changes, coagulation disorders, and blood lipid changes; careful monitoring is therefore necessary and the urine is tested for glucose because of a risk of hyperglycaemia.

### CRISANTASPASE

**Indications** see notes above

**Cautions** see notes above

**Contra-indications** pregnancy (Appendix 4); breast-feeding

**Side-effects** see notes above

**Erwinase®** (EUSA Pharma) PoM
Injection, powder for reconstitution, crisantaspase. Net price 10 000-unit vial = £232.88

## Dacarbazine and temozolomide

**Dacarbazine** is used to treat metastatic melanoma and, in combination therapy, soft tissue sarcomas. It is also a component of a commonly used combination for Hodgkin's disease (ABVD—doxorubicin [previously *Adriamycin®*], bleomycin, vinblastine, and dacarbazine). It is given *intravenously*. The predominant side-effects are myelosuppression and severe nausea and vomiting.

**Temozolomide** is structurally related to dacarbazine. It is given by mouth and is licensed for the initial treatment of glioblastoma multiforme (in combination with radiotherapy) and for second-line treatment of malignant glioma.

### DACARBAZINE

**Indications** see notes above

**Cautions** see section 8.1; hepatic impairment (Appendix 2); renal impairment (avoid if severe; Appendix 3); caution in handling

**Contra-indications** pregnancy (Appendix 4); breast-feeding

**Side-effects** see section 8.1 and notes above; *rarely* liver necrosis due to hepatic vein thrombosis; irritant to skin and tissues

**Dacarbazine** (Non-proprietary) PoM
Injection, powder for reconstitution, dacarbazine (as citrate), net price 100-mg vial = £5.05; 200-mg vial = £7.16; 500-mg vial = £16.50; 600-mg vial = £22.50; 1-g vial = £31.80

### TEMOZOLOMIDE

**Indications** see notes above

**Cautions** see section 8.1; severe hepatic impairment and renal impairment; **interactions:** Appendix 1 (temozolomide)

**Contra-indications** pregnancy (Appendix 4); breast-feeding

**Side-effects** see section 8.1

**Dose**
• Consult product literature; CHILD under 3 years not recommended

**Temodal®** (Schering-Plough) PoM
Capsules, temozolomide 5 mg (green/white), net price 5-cap pack = £16.97; 20 mg (yellow/white), 5-cap pack = £67.88; 100 mg (pink/white), 5-cap pack = £339.40; 140 mg (blue/white), 5-cap pack = £475.16; 180 mg (orange/white), 5-cap pack = £610.92 mg (white), 5-cap pack = £848.50. Label: 23, 25

**8**

**Malignant disease and immunosuppression**

# Hydroxycarbamide

**Hydroxycarbamide** (hydroxyurea) is an orally active drug used mainly in the treatment of chronic myeloid leukaemia. It is also licensed for the treatment of cancer of the cervix in conjunction with radiotherapy. It is occasionally used for polycythaemia (the usual treatment is venesection). Myelosuppression, nausea, and skin reactions are the most common toxic effects.

## ■ HYDROXYCARBAMIDE
(Hydroxyurea)

**Indications** see notes above; sickle-cell disease (section 9.1.3)

**Cautions** see section 8.1 and notes above; renal impairment; **interactions**: Appendix 1 (hydroxycarbamide)

**Contra-indications** pregnancy (Appendix 4); breast-feeding

**Side-effects** see section 8.1 and notes above

**Dose**
- 20–30 mg/kg daily *or* 80 mg/kg every third day

**Hydroxycarbamide** (Non-proprietary) ▨PoM▨
Capsules, hydroxycarbamide 500 mg, net price 20 = £2.22

**Hydrea®** (Squibb) ▨PoM▨
Capsules, pink/green, hydroxycarbamide 500 mg. Net price 20 = £2.14

# Mitotane

**Mitotane** is licensed for the symptomatic treatment of advanced or inoperable adrenocortical carcinoma. It selectively inhibits the activity of the adrenal cortex, necessitating corticosteroid replacement therapy (section 6.3.1); the dose of glucocorticoid should be increased in case of shock, trauma, or infection.

Gastro-intestinal side-effects such as anorexia, nausea, and vomiting, and endocrine side-effects, such as hypogonadism and thyroid disorders, are very common with mitotane; neurotoxicity occurs in many patients.

## ■ MITOTANE

**Indications** see notes above

**Cautions** see section 8.1 and notes above; risk of accumulation in overweight patients; monitor plasma-mitotane concentration—consult product literature; hepatic impairment (Appendix 2); renal impairment (avoid if severe;Appendix 3); **interactions**: Appendix 1 (mitotane)
  **Driving** CNS effects may affect performance of skilled tasks (e.g. driving)
  **Counselling** Warn patient to contact doctor immediately if injury, infection, or illness occurs (because of risk of acute adrenal insufficiency)

**Contra-indications** pregnancy (Appendix 4); breast-feeding

**Side-effects** see section 8.1 and notes above; also gastro-intestinal disturbances (including nausea, vomiting, diarrhoea, epigastric discomfort), anorexia, liver disorders; hypercholesterolaemia, hypertriglyceridaemia; ataxia, confusion, asthenia, myasthenia, paraesthesia, drowsiness, neuropathy, cognitive impairment, movement disorder, dizziness, headache;

gynaecomastia; prolonged bleeding time, leucopenia, thrombocytopenia, anaemia; rash; *rarely* hypersalivation, hypertension, postural hypotension, flushing, pyrexia, haematuria, proteinuria, haemorrhagic cystitis, hypouricaemia, visual disturbances, and ocular disorders

**Dose**
- ADULT over 18 years, initially 2–3 g daily, (up to 6 g daily in severe illness) in 2–3 divided doses, adjusted according to plasma-mitotane concentration; reduce dose or interrupt treatment if signs of toxicity; discontinue if inadequate response after 3 months
  **Note** Plasma-mitotane concentration for optimum response 14–20 mg/litre

**Lysodren®** (HRA Pharma) ▨PoM▨
Tablets, scored, mitotane 500 mg, net price 100-tab pack = £460.40. Label: 2, 10, 21, counselling, driving, adrenal suppression

# Panitumumab

**Panitumumab** is a monoclonal antibody that binds to the epidermal growth factor receptor (EGFR). It is indicated as monotherapy for the treatment of EGFR expressing metastatic colorectal cancer with non-mutated *KRAS* gene after failure of fluoropyrimidine-, oxaliplatin-, and irinotecan-containing chemotherapy regimens. Panitumumab is given by intravenous infusion.

The *Scottish Medicines Consortium* (p. 3) has advised (May 2008) that panitumumab (*Vectibix®*) is **not** recommended for use within NHS Scotland for colorectal cancer.

## ■ PANITUMUMAB

**Indications** see notes above

**Cautions** monitor for dermatological reactions (may require temporary or permanent discontinuation—consult product literature); pulmonary disease—discontinue if pneumonitis or lung infiltrates occur; monitor for hypomagnesaemia and hypocalcaemia

**Contra-indications** interstitial pulmonary disease; pregnancy (Appendix 4); breast-feeding (Appendix 5)

**Side-effects** see section 8.1; also infusion-related reactions; diarrhoea, dry mouth and nose; dyspnoea, cough; fatigue, headache; hypomagnesaemia, hypocalcaemia, hypokalaemia, dehydration; ocular disorders (including conjunctivitis, increased lacrimation, dry eyes, ocular hyperaemia); skin reactions (including rash, erythema, pruritus, dry skin, and exfoliation), mucosal inflammation, hypertrichosis, and nail disorders

**Vectibix®** (Amgen) ▼ ▨PoM▨
Concentrate for intravenous infusion, panitumumab 20 mg/mL, net price 5-mL vial = £287.34, 20-mL vial = £1149.36
**Electrolytes** Na$^+$ 0.75 mmol/vial

# Pentostatin

**Pentostatin** is active in hairy cell leukaemia. It is given *intravenously* on alternate weeks and can induce prolonged complete remission. It can cause myelosuppression, immunosuppression, and a number of other side-effects that may be severe. Treatment should be withheld in patients who develop a severe rash, and withheld or discontinued in patients showing signs of neurotoxicity. Its use should be confined to specialist centres.

## ▌ PENTOSTATIN

**Indications** see notes above

**Cautions** see section 8.1 and notes above; hepatic impairment (Appendix 2); **interactions:** Appendix 1 (pentostatin)

**Contra-indications** renal impairment (Appendix 3); pregnancy (Appendix 4); breast-feeding

**Side-effects** see section 8.1 and notes above

**Nipent®** (Hospira) ▢PoM
Injection, powder for reconstitution, pentostatin. Net price 10-mg vial = £863.78

## Platinum compounds

**Carboplatin** is widely used in the treatment of advanced ovarian cancer and lung cancer (particularly the small cell type). It is given *intravenously*. The dose of carboplatin is determined according to renal function rather than body surface area. Carboplatin can be given on an outpatient basis and is better tolerated than cisplatin; nausea and vomiting are reduced in severity and nephrotoxicity, neurotoxicity, and ototoxicity are much less of a problem than with cisplatin. It is, however, more myelosuppressive than cisplatin.

**Cisplatin** is used alone or in combination for the treatment of testicular, lung, cervical, bladder, head and neck, and ovarian cancer (but carboplatin is preferred for ovarian cancer). It is given *intravenously*. Cisplatin requires intensive intravenous hydration and treatment may be complicated by severe nausea and vomiting. Cisplatin is toxic, causing nephrotoxicity (monitoring of renal function is essential), ototoxicity, peripheral neuropathy, hypomagnesaemia and myelosuppression. It is, however, increasingly given in a day-care setting.

**Oxaliplatin** is licensed in combination with fluorouracil and folinic acid, for the treatment of metastatic colorectal cancer and as adjuvant treatment of colon cancer after resection of the primary tumour; it is given by intravenous infusion. Neurotoxic side-effects (including sensory peripheral neuropathy) are dose limiting. Other side-effects include gastro-intestinal disturbances, ototoxicity, and myelosuppression. If unexplained respiratory symptoms occur, oxaliplatin should be discontinued until investigations exclude interstitial lung disease and pulmonary fibrosis.

**NICE guidance**
**Irinotecan, oxaliplatin, and raltitrexed for advanced colorectal cancer (August 2005)**
A combination of fluorouracil and folinic acid with either irinotecan or oxaliplatin are options for first-line treatment for advanced colorectal cancer.
Irinotecan alone or fluorouracil and folinic acid with oxaliplatin are options for patients who require further treatment subsequently.
Raltitrexed is **not** recommended for the treatment of advanced colorectal cancer. Its use should be confined to clinical studies.

**NICE guidance (capecitabine and oxaliplatin in the adjuvant treatment of stage III (Dukes' C) colon cancer)**
See p. 474

**NICE guidance**
**Paclitaxel for ovarian cancer (January 2003)**
*Either* paclitaxel in combination with a platinum compound (cisplatin or carboplatin) *or* a platinum compound alone are alternatives for the first-line treatment of ovarian cancer (usually following surgery).

**NICE guidance**
**Paclitaxel, pegylated liposomal doxorubicin, and topotecan for second-line or subsequent treatment of advanced ovarian cancer (May 2005)**
Paclitaxel, combined with a platinum compound (carboplatin or cisplatin), is an option for advanced cancer that relapses 6 months or more after completing initial platinum-based chemotherapy. Paclitaxel alone is an option for advanced ovarian cancer that does not respond to, or relapses within 6 months of completing initial platinum-based chemotherapy.
Pegylated liposomal doxorubicin is an option for advanced ovarian cancer that does not respond to, or relapses within 12 months of completing initial platinum-based chemotherapy.
Paclitaxel alone or pegylated liposomal doxorubicin are options for advanced ovarian cancer in patients who are allergic to platinum compounds. Topotecan alone is an option only for advanced ovarian cancer that does not respond to, or relapses within 6 months of completing initial platinum-based chemotherapy or in those allergic to platinum compounds *and* for whom paclitaxel alone or pegylated liposomal doxorubicin are inappropriate.

## ▌ CARBOPLATIN

**Indications** see notes above

**Cautions** see section 8.1 and notes above; renal impairment (avoid if creatinine clearance less than 20 mL/minute; Appendix 3); **interactions:** Appendix 1 (platinum compounds)

**Contra-indications** pregnancy (Appendix 4); breast-feeding

**Side-effects** see section 8.1 and notes above

**Carboplatin** (Non-proprietary) ▢PoM
Injection, carboplatin 10 mg/mL, net price 5-mL vial = £22.04, 15-mL vial = £56.29, 45-mL vial = £168.85, 60-mL vial = £260.00

## ▌ CISPLATIN

**Indications** see notes above

**Cautions** see section 8.1 and notes above; **interactions:** Appendix 1 (platinum compounds)

**Contra-indications** renal impairment (Appendix 3); pregnancy (Appendix 4); breast-feeding

**Side-effects** see section 8.1 and notes above

**Cisplatin** (Non-proprietary) [PoM]

Injection, cisplatin 1 mg/mL, net price 10-mL vial = £5.85, 50-mL vial = £24.50, 100-mL vial = £50.22

Injection, powder for reconstitution, cisplatin, net price 50-mg vial = £17.00

### ▐ OXALIPLATIN

**Indications** metastatic colorectal cancer in combination with fluorouracil and folinic acid; colon cancer—see notes above

**Cautions** see section 8.1 and notes above; **interactions:** Appendix 1 (platinum compounds)

**Contra-indications** see section 8.1; peripheral neuropathy with functional impairment; renal impairment (Appendix 3); pregnancy (Appendix 4); breast-feeding

**Side-effects** see section 8.1 and notes above

**Oxaliplatin** (Non-proprietary) [PoM]

Injection, powder for reconstitution, oxaliplatin, net price 50-mg vial = £150.00, 100-mg vial= £299.50

**Eloxatin®** (Sanofi-Aventis) [PoM]

Concentrate for intravenous infusion, oxaliplatin 5 mg/mL, net price 10-mL vial = £158.57, 20-mL vial = £317.13

## Porfimer sodium and temoporfin

**Porfimer sodium** and **temoporfin** are used in the photodynamic treatment of various tumours. The drugs accumulate in malignant tissue and are activated by laser light to produce a cytotoxic effect.

Porfimer sodium is licensed for photodynamic therapy of non-small cell lung cancer and obstructing oesophageal cancer. Temoporfin is licensed for photodynamic therapy of advanced head and neck cancer.

### ▐ PORFIMER SODIUM

**Indications** non-small cell lung cancer; oesophageal cancer; see notes above

**Cautions** see section 8.1; avoid exposure of skin and eyes to direct sunlight or bright indoor light for at least 30 days

**Contra-indications** see section 8.1; severe hepatic impairment; tracheo-oesophageal or broncho-oesophageal fistula; acute porphyria (section 9.8.2); pregnancy (Appendix 4); breast-feeding (Appendix 5)

**Side-effects** see section 8.1; photosensitivity (see Cautions above—sunscreens offer no protection), constipation

**Photofrin®** (Sinclair) ▼ [PoM]

Injection, powder for reconstitution, porfimer sodium, net price 15-mg vial = £154.00; 75-mg vial = £770.00

### ▐ TEMOPORFIN

**Indications** advanced head and neck squamous cell carcinoma refractory to, or unsuitable for, other treatments

**Cautions** see section 8.1; avoid exposure of skin and eyes to direct sunlight or bright indoor light for at least 15 days after administration; avoid prolonged exposure of injection site arm to direct sunlight for 6 months after administration, if extravasation occurs protect area from light for at least 3 months; **interactions:** Appendix 1 (temoporfin)

**Contra-indications** see section 8.1; acute porphyria (section 9.8.2) or other diseases exacerbated by light; elective surgery or ophthalmic slit-lamp examination for 30 days after administration; concomitant photosensitising treatment; pregnancy (Appendix 4); breast-feeding (Appendix 5)

**Side-effects** see section 8.1; also constipation, dysphagia; haemorrhage, oedema; giddiness, trismus, facial pain; injection site pain, blistering, scarring, erythema, skin necrosis, hyperpigmentation, photosensitivity (see Cautions above; sunscreens ineffective)

**Foscan®** (Biolitec) ▼ [PoM]

Injection, temoporfin 4 mg/mL, net price 5-mL vial = £4400.00

## Procarbazine

**Procarbazine** is most often used in Hodgkin's disease. It is given *by mouth*. Toxic effects include nausea, myelosuppression, and a hypersensitivity rash preventing further use of this drug. It is a mild monoamine-oxidase inhibitor and dietary restriction is rarely considered necessary. Alcohol ingestion may cause a disulfiram-like reaction.

### ▐ PROCARBAZINE

**Indications** see notes above

**Cautions** see section 8.1 and notes above; hepatic impairment—avoid if severe; renal impairment (avoid if severe; Appendix 3); **interactions:** Appendix 1 (procarbazine)

**Contra-indications** pregnancy (Appendix 4); breast-feeding

**Side-effects** see section 8.1 and notes above

**Dose**

- Used alone, initially 50 mg daily, increased by 50 mg daily to 250–300 mg daily in divided doses; maintenance (on remission) 50–150 mg daily to cumulative total of at least 6 g

**Procarbazine** (Cambridge) [PoM]

Capsules, ivory, procarbazine (as hydrochloride) 50 mg, net price 50-cap pack = £190.09. Label: 4

## Protein kinase inhibitors

Dasatinib, erlotinib, imatinib, lapatinib, nilotinib, sorafenib, sunitinib, and temsirolimus are protein kinase inhibitors.

**Dasatinib**, a tyrosine kinase inhibitor, is licensed for the treatment of chronic myeloid leukaemia in those who have resistance to or intolerance of previous therapy, including imatinib. It is also licensed for acute lymphoblastic leukaemia (Philadelphia chromosome positive) in those who have resistance to or intolerance of previous therapy.

The *Scottish Medicines Consortium* (p. 3) has advised (April 2007) that the use of dasatinib (*Sprycel®*) in NHS Scotland is restricted to patients in the chronic phase of chronic myeloid leukaemia.

**Erlotinib**, a tyrosine kinase inhibitor, is licensed in combination with gemcitabine for the treatment of metastatic pancreatic cancer. It is also licensed for the treatment of locally advanced or metastatic non-small cell lung cancer after failure of previous chemotherapy. The development of a rash within the first 4–8 weeks of treatment is indicative of improved survival; treatment should be reviewed if a rash does not develop.

The *Scottish Medicines Consortium* (p. 3) has advised (May 2006) that erlotinib (*Tarceva®*) is accepted for restricted use within NHS Scotland for the treatment of locally advanced or metastatic non-small cell lung cancer, after failure of at least one chemotherapy regimen. Erlotinib is restricted to use in patients who would otherwise be eligible for treatment with docetaxel monotherapy.

> **NICE guidance**
> **Erlotinib for non-small-cell lung cancer (November 2008)**
> Erlotinib is recommended, as an alternative to docetaxel, as second-line treatment for locally advanced or metastatic non-small-cell lung cancer after failure of previous chemotherapy, on the basis that it is provided by the manufacturer at an overall treatment cost equal to that of docetaxel. Erlotinib is **not** recommended in patients for whom docetaxel is unsuitable or as third-line treatment after docetaxel. Patients currently receiving erlotinib who do not fall into the patient population defined above, have the option to continue therapy until they and their clinicians consider it appropriate to stop.

**Imatinib**, a tyrosine kinase inhibitor, is licensed for the treatment of newly diagnosed chronic myeloid leukaemia where bone marrow transplantation is not considered first-line treatment, and for chronic myeloid leukaemia in chronic phase after failure of interferon alfa, or in accelerated phase, or in blast crisis (see NICE guidance below). It is also licensed for c-kit (CD117)-positive unresectable or metastatic malignant gastrointestinal stromal tumours (GIST). Imatinib is licensed for the treatment of newly diagnosed acute lymphoblastic leukaemia in combination with other chemotherapy, and as monotherapy for relapsed or refractory acute lymphoblastic leukaemia. Imatinib is also licensed for the treatment of unresectable dermatofibrosarcoma protuberans and for patients with recurrent or metastatic dermatofibrosarcoma protuberans who cannot have surgery.

Imatinib is also licensed for the treatment of myelodysplastic/myeloproliferative diseases associated with platelet-derived growth factor receptor gene rearrangement and for the treatment of advanced hypereosinophilic syndrome and chronic eosinophilic leukaemia.

The *Scottish Medicines Consortium* (p. 3) has advised (March 2002) that imatinib (*Glivec®*) should be used for chronic myeloid leukaemia only under specialist supervision in accordance with British Society of Haematology guidelines (November 2001).

> **NICE guidance**
> **Imatinib for chronic myeloid leukaemia (October 2003)**
> Imatinib is recommended as first-line treatment for Philadelphia-chromosome-positive chronic myeloid leukaemia in the chronic phase and as an option for patients presenting in the accelerated phase or with blast crisis, provided that imatinib has not been used previously.
> Where imatinib has failed to stop disease progression from chronic phase to accelerated phase or to blast crisis, continued use is recommended only as part of further clinical study.

**Lapatinib**, a tyrosine kinase inhibitor, is licensed in combination with capecitabine for the treatment of advanced or metastatic breast cancer in patients with tumours that overexpress human epidermal growth factor receptor-2 (HER2). It is indicated for patients who have had previous treatment with an anthracycline, a taxane, and trastuzumab.

**Nilotinib**, a tyrosine kinase inhibitor, is licensed for the treatment of chronic myeloid leukaemia in those who have resistance to or intolerance of previous therapy, including imatinib.

The *Scottish Medicines Consortium* (p. 3) has advised (February 2008) that nilotinib (*Tasigna®*) is accepted for restricted use within NHS Scotland for the treatment of chronic-phase chronic myeloid leukaemia in adults resistant to or intolerant of at least one previous therapy, including imatinib.

**Sorafenib**, an inhibitor of multiple kinases, is licensed for the treatment of advanced renal cell carcinoma when treatment with interferon alfa or interleukin-2 has failed or is contra-indicated. It is also licensed for the treatment of hepatocellular carcinoma.

**Sunitinib**, a tyrosine kinase inhibitor, is licensed for the treatment of advanced or metastatic renal cell carcinoma (but see NICE Guidance, below). It is also licensed for the treatment of unresectable or metastatic malignant gastro-intestinal stromal tumours, after failure of imatinib.

> **NICE guidance**
> **Sunitinib for advanced or metastatic renal cell carcinoma (March 2009)**
> Sunitinib is recommended as first-line treatment for advanced or metastatic renal cell carcinoma in patients who are suitable for immunotherapy and have an Eastern Cooperative Oncology Group performance status of 0 or 1.
> Patients currently receiving sunitinib who do not fall into the population defined above have the option to continue therapy until they and their clinicians consider it appropriate to stop.

**Temsirolimus** is a protein kinase inhibitor licensed for the first-line treatment of advanced renal cell carcinoma. Hypersensitivity reactions, including some life-threatening and rare fatal reactions, are associated with temsirolimus therapy, usually during administration of the first dose. Symptoms include flushing, chest pain, dyspnoea, apnoea, hypotension, loss of consciousness, and anaphylaxis. Where possible, patients should receive an intravenous dose of antihistamine 30 minutes before starting the temsirolimus infusion. The infusion may have to be stopped temporarily for the treatment of infusion-related effects—consult product literature for appropriate management. If adverse reactions are not managed with dose delays, a dose reduction should be considered—consult product literature.

## DASATINIB

**Indications** see notes above

**Cautions** see section 8.1; susceptibility to QT-interval prolongation (correct hypokalaemia or hypomagnesaemia before starting treatment); hepatic impairment (Appendix 2); pregnancy (Appendix 4 and section 8.1); **interactions**: Appendix 1 (dasatinib)

**Contra-indications** breast-feeding

**Side-effects** see section 8.1; also diarrhoea, anorexia, weight changes, abdominal pain, taste disturbance, constipation, dyspepsia, colitis, gastritis; arrhythmias, congestive heart failure, hypertension, chest pain, flushing, haemorrhage (including gastro-intestinal and CNS haemorrhage); palpitation; dyspnoea, pulmonary hypertension, cough, oedema (more common in patients over 65 years old), pleural effusion; depression, dizziness, headache, insomnia, neuropathy; influenza-like symptoms; musculoskeletal pain; visual disturbances; tinnitus; acne, dry skin, sweating, pruritus, dermatitis, urticaria; *less commonly* pancreatitis, hepatitis, cholestasis, oesophagitis, hypotension, transient ischaemic attack, thrombophlebitis, syncope, asthma, seizures, amnesia, tremor, drowsiness, gynaecomastia, irregular menstruation, urinary frequency, proteinuria, hypocalcaemia, rhabdomyolysis, hypersensitivity reactions (including erythema nodosum), photosensitivity, and pigmentation and nail disorders; *rarely* cor pulmonale

**Dose**
- Chronic phase chronic myeloid leukaemia, ADULT over 18 years 100 mg once daily, increased if necessary to max. 140 mg once daily
- Accelerated and blast phase chronic myeloid leukaemia, acute lymphoblastic leukaemia, ADULT over 18 years 140 mg once daily, increased if necessary to max. 180 mg once daily

**Sprycel®** (Bristol-Myers Squibb) ▼ PoM
Tablets, f/c, dasatinib (as monohydrate) 20 mg, net price 56-tab pack = £1168.99; 50 mg, 56-tab pack = £2337.97; 70 mg, 56-tab pack = £2337.97; 100 mg, 30-tab pack = £2504.96. Label: 25

## ERLOTINIB

**Indications** see notes above

**Cautions** see section 8.1; pre-existing liver disease or concomitant use with hepatotoxic drugs—monitor liver function; hepatic impairment (Appendix 2); **interactions**: Appendix 1 (erlotinib)

**Contra-indications** severe renal impairment; pregnancy (Appendix 4); breast-feeding (Appendix 5)

**Side-effects** see section 8.1; also diarrhoea, abdominal pain, dyspepsia, flatulence; anorexia, depression, neuropathy, headache; fatigue, rigor; conjunctivitis; rash, pruritus, dry skin; *less commonly* interstitial lung disease—discontinue if unexplained symptoms such as dyspnoea, cough or fever occur; *rarely* hepatic failure; gastro-intestinal perforation, Stevens-Johnson syndrome, and toxic epidermal necrolysis also reported.

**Dose**
- Non-small cell lung cancer, 150 mg once daily
- Pancreatic cancer, 100 mg once daily in combination with gemcitabine

**Tarceva®** (Roche) ▼ PoM
Tablets, f/c, white-yellow, erlotinib (as hydrochloride) 25 mg, net price 30-tab pack = £378.33; 100 mg, 30-tab pack = £1324.14; 150 mg, 30-tab pack = £1631.53. Label: 23

## IMATINIB

**Indications** see notes above

**Cautions** see section 8.1; cardiac disease; monitor for fluid retention; monitor liver function; hepatic impairment (Appendix 2); renal impairment (Appendix 3); **interactions**: Appendix 1 (imatinib)

**Contra-indications** pregnancy (Appendix 4 and section 8.1); breast-feeding

**Side-effects** see section 8.1; also abdominal pain, appetite changes, constipation, diarrhoea, flatulence, gastro-oesophageal reflux, taste disturbance, weight changes, dry mouth; oedema (including pulmonary oedema, pleural effusion, and ascites), flushing, haemorrhage; cough, dyspnoea; dizziness, headache, insomnia, hypoaesthesia, paraesthesia, fatigue; influenza-like symptoms; cramps, arthralgia; visual disturbances, increased lacrimation, conjunctivitis, dry eyes; epistaxis; dry skin, sweating, rash, pruritus, photosensitivity; *less commonly* gastric ulceration, pancreatitis, hepatic dysfunction (rarely hepatic failure, hepatic necrosis), dysphagia, heart failure, tachycardia, palpitation, syncope, hypertension, hypotension, cold extremities, cough, acute respiratory failure, depression, drowsiness, anxiety, peripheral neuropathy, tremor, migraine, impaired memory, vertigo, gynaecomastia, menorrhagia, irregular menstruation, sexual dysfunction, electrolyte disturbances, renal failure, urinary frequency, gout, tinnitus, hearing loss; skin hyperpigmentation; *rarely* intestinal obstruction, gastro-intestinal perforation, inflammatory bowel disease, arrhythmia, atrial fibrillation, myocardial infarction, angina, pulmonary fibrosis, pulmonary hypertension, increased intracranial pressure, convulsions, confusion, haemolytic anaemia, aseptic necrosis of bone, cataract, glaucoma, angioedema, exfoliative dermatitis, and Stevens-Johnson syndrome

**Dose**
- Chronic phase chronic myeloid leukaemia, ADULT 400 mg once daily, increased if necessary to max. 800 mg daily (in 2 divided doses); CHILD (chronic and advanced phase) 2–18 years 340 mg/m$^2$ (max. 800 mg) daily (in 1–2 divided doses), increased to 570 mg/m$^2$ (max. 800 mg) daily if necessary (consult product literature)
- Accelerated phase and blast crisis chronic myeloid leukaemia, ADULT 600 mg once daily, increased if necessary to max. 800 mg daily (in 2 divided doses)
- Acute lymphoblastic leukaemia, ADULT 600 mg once daily
- Gastro-intestinal stromal tumours, ADULT 400 mg once daily
- Dermatofibrosarcoma protuberans, ADULT 800 mg daily in 2 divided doses
- Myelodysplastic/myeloproliferative diseases, ADULT 400 mg once daily

- Advanced hypereosinophilic syndrome and chronic eosinophilic leukaemia, ADULT 100–400 mg once daily

**Glivec®** (Novartis) ▼ PoM

Tablets, f/c, imatinib (as mesilate) 100 mg (yellow-brown, scored), net price 60-tab pack = £802.04; 400 mg (yellow), 30-tab pack = £1604.08. Label: 21, 27
Counselling Tablets may be dispersed in water or apple juice

## ▌ LAPATINIB

**Indications** see notes above

**Cautions** see section 8.1; low gastric pH (reduced absorption); monitor left ventricular function; monitor for pulmonary toxicity; monitor liver function before treatment and at monthly intervals; hepatic impairment (Appendix 2); renal impairment (Appendix 3); pregnancy (Appendix 4 and section 8.1); **interactions**: Appendix 1 (lapatinib)

**Contra-indications** breast-feeding

**Side-effects** see section 8.1; anorexia, diarrhoea (treat promptly); decreased left ventricular ejection fraction; fatigue; rash; hyperbilirubinaemia, hepatotoxicity; *less commonly* interstitial lung disease

**Dose**

- ADULT over 18 years, 1.25 g once daily as a single dose
Counselling Always take at the same time in relation to food: either one hour before or one hour after food

**Tyverb®** (GSK) ▼ PoM

Tablets, yellow, f/c, lapatinib 250 mg, net price 70-tab pack = £804.30. Counselling, administration

## ▌ NILOTINIB

**Indications** see notes above

**Cautions** see section 8.1; history of pancreatitis; susceptibility to QT-interval prolongation (including electrolyte disturbances, concomitant use of drugs that prolong QT interval); hepatic impairment (Appendix 2); pregnancy (Appendix 4 and section 8.1); **interactions**: Appendix 1 (nilotinib)

**Contra-indications** breast-feeding (Appendix 5)

**Side-effects** see section 8.1; also abdominal pain, constipation, diarrhoea, dyspepsia, flatulence, anorexia, weight changes; palpitation, QT-interval prolongation, hypertension, oedema, flushing; dyspnoea, cough, dysphonia; headache, fatigue, asthenia, dizziness, paraesthesia, insomnia, vertigo; hypomagnesaemia, hyperkalaemia, blood glucose changes; bone pain, arthralgia, muscle spasm; urticaria, erythema, hyperhidrosis, dry skin, rash, pruritus; *less commonly* hepatitis, pancreatitis, dry mouth, chest pain, cardiac failure, arrhythmias, pericardial effusion, coronary artery disease, cardiomegaly, cardiac murmur, bradycardia, hypertensive crisis, haemorrhage, melaena, haematoma, pleural effusion, interstitial lung disease, migraine, hypoaesthesia, hyperaesthesia, depression, anxiety, tremor, influenza-like symptoms, hyperthyroidism, breast pain, gynaecomastia, erectile dysfunction, dysuria, urinary frequency, hypokalaemia, hyponatraemia, hypocalcaemia, hypophosphataemia, dehydration, decreased visual acuity, conjunctivitis, dry eyes, epistaxis, and ecchymosis

**Dose**

- ADULT over 18 years, 400 mg twice daily

**Tasigna®** (Novartis) ▼ PoM

Capsules, yellow, nilotinib (as hydrochloride monohydrate) 200 mg, net price 112-cap pack = £2432.85. Label: 23, 25, 27

## ▌ SORAFENIB

**Indications** see notes above

**Cautions** major surgical procedures; cardiac ischaemia; hepatic impairment (Appendix 2); pregnancy (Appendix 4); **interactions**: Appendix 1 (sorafenib)

**Contra-indications** breast-feeding

**Side-effects** see section 8.1; also diarrhoea, constipation, dyspepsia, dysphagia, anorexia, hypertension, haemorrhage, flushing, hoarseness, fatigue, asthenia, depression, peripheral neuropathy, fever, erectile dysfunction, hypophosphataemia, arthralgia, myalgia, tinnitus, rash, pruritus, erythema, dry skin, desquamation, acne, hand-foot skin reaction; *less commonly* reversible posterior leucoencephalopathy, myocardial infarction, congestive heart failure, hypertensive crisis, and gastrointestinal perforations

**Dose**

- ADULT over 18 years, 400 mg twice daily

**Nexavar®** (Bayer) ▼ PoM

Tablets, f/c, red, sorafenib (as tosylate) 200 mg, net price 112-tab pack = £2980.47 Label: 23

## ▌ SUNITINIB

**Indications** see notes above

**Cautions** see section 8.1; cardiovascular disease—discontinue if congestive heart failure develops; susceptibility to QT-interval prolongation; hypertension; increased risk of bleeding; monitor for thyroid dysfunction; pregnancy (Appendix 4 and section 8.1); **interactions**: Appendix 1 (sunitinib)

**Contra-indications** breast-feeding

**Side-effects** see section 8.1; also abdominal pain, diarrhoea, constipation, anorexia, taste disturbance, dehydration; hypertension, oedema; dyspnoea, cough; fatigue, dizziness, headache, insomnia, peripheral neuropathy, paraesthesia; hypothyroidism; arthralgia, myalgia; increased lacrimation; epistaxis; skin, hair, and urine discoloration; hand-foot syndrome, dry skin, and rash; gastro-intestinal perforation, pancreatitis, hepatic failure, proteinuria (*rarely* nephrotic syndrome) and seizures reported

**Dose**

- 50 mg daily for 4 weeks, followed by a 2-week treatment-free period to complete 6-week cycle; adjust dose in steps of 12.5 mg according to tolerability; dose range 25–75 mg daily

**Sutent®** (Pfizer) PoM

Capsules, sunitinib (as malate) 12.5 mg (orange), net price 28-cap pack = £784.70; 25 mg (caramel/orange), 28-cap pack = £1569.40; 50 mg (caramel), 28-cap pack = £3138.80. Label: 14

## ▌ TEMSIROLIMUS

**Indications** see notes above

**Cautions** see notes above; monitor respiratory function; monitor blood lipids; hepatic impairment (avoid if severe; Appendix 2); renal impairment (Appendix 3); **interactions**: Appendix 1 (temsirolimus)

**8**

**Malignant disease and immunosuppression**

**Contra-indications** pregnancy (Appendix 4); breast-feeding

**Side-effects** see section 8.1; also abdominal pain, diarrhoea, anorexia, taste disturbance; hypertension, oedema, thrombophlebitis; cough, dyspnoea, chest pain, interstitial lung disease, hypersensitivity reactions (see notes above); asthenia; increased susceptibility to infection (including urinary-tract infection and pneumonia), pyrexia; hyperglycaemia; renal failure; hypophosphataemia, hypokalaemia, hypercholesterolaemia, hyperlipidaemia; arthralgia; eye disorders; rhinitis, epistaxis; skin disorders (including rash and acne), folliculitis, impaired wound healing; *less commonly* intestinal perforation and intracerebral bleeding

**Dose**

• By intravenous infusion (over 30–60 minutes), ADULT over 18 years, 25 mg once weekly

**Torisel®** (Wyeth) ▼ PoM
Concentrate for intravenous infusion, temsirolimus 25 mg/mL, net price 1.2-mL amp (with diluent) = £620.00
Excipients include propylene glycol and ethanol

## Taxanes

**Paclitaxel** is a member of the taxane group of drugs. It is given by *intravenous infusion*. Paclitaxel given with carboplatin or cisplatin is used for the treatment of ovarian cancer (see NICE guidance p. 485); the combination is also considered appropriate for women whose ovarian cancer is initially considered inoperable. Paclitaxel is also used in the secondary treatment of metastatic breast cancer. There is limited evidence to support its use in non-small cell lung cancer. Routine premedication with a corticosteroid, an antihistamine and a histamine H$_2$-receptor antagonist is recommended to prevent severe hypersensitivity reactions; hypersensitivity reactions may occur rarely despite premedication, although more commonly only bradycardia or asymptomatic hypotension occur.

Other side-effects of paclitaxel include myelosuppression, peripheral neuropathy, and cardiac conduction defects with arrhythmias (which are nearly always asymptomatic). It also causes alopecia and muscle pain; nausea and vomiting is mild to moderate.

**Docetaxel** is licensed for use in locally advanced or metastatic breast cancer and non-small cell lung cancer resistant to other cytotoxic drugs or for initial chemotherapy in combination with other cytotoxic drugs. It is also licensed for hormone-resistant prostate cancer, for use with other cytotoxic drugs for gastric adenocarcinoma and head and neck cancer, and for adjuvant treatment of operable node-positive breast cancer. Its side-effects are similar to those of paclitaxel but persistent fluid retention (commonly as leg oedema that worsens during treatment) can be resistant to treatment; hypersensitivity reactions also occur. Dexamethasone by mouth is recommended for reducing fluid retention and hypersensitivity reactions.

For the role of taxanes in the treatment of breast cancer, see section 8.3.4.1.

The *Scottish Medicines Consortium* (p. 3) has advised that docetaxel (*Taxotere®*) in combination with cisplatin and 5-fluorouracil is accepted for restricted use within NHS Scotland for the induction treatment of patients with unresectable (May 2007) and resectable (June 2008) locally advanced squamous cell carcinoma of the head and neck.

---

NICE guidance (paclitaxel, pegylated liposomal doxorubicin and topotecan for second-line or subsequent treatment of advanced ovarian cancer)
See p. 485

---

NICE guidance
Docetaxel for the treatment of hormone-refractory metastatic prostate cancer (June 2006)
Docetaxel is an option for hormone-refractory metastatic prostate cancer and a Karnofsky score of at least 60% [Karnofsky score is a measure of the ability to perform ordinary tasks].

---

### ■ DOCETAXEL

**Indications** adjuvant treatment of operable node-positive breast cancer, in combination with doxorubicin and cyclophosphamide; with doxorubicin for initial chemotherapy of locally advanced or metastatic breast cancer; monotherapy for locally advanced or metastatic breast cancer where cytotoxic chemotherapy with an anthracycline or an alkylating drug has failed; with capecitabine for locally advanced or metastatic breast cancer where cytotoxic chemotherapy with an anthracycline has failed; with trastuzumab for initial chemotherapy of metastatic breast cancer which overexpresses human epidermal growth factor-2; locally advanced or metastatic non-small cell lung cancer where first-line chemotherapy has failed; with cisplatin for unresectable, locally advanced or metastatic non-small cell lung cancer; with prednisolone for hormone-refractory metastatic prostate cancer; with cisplatin and fluorouracil for initial treatment of metastatic gastric adenocarcinoma, including adenocarcinoma of the gastro-oesophageal junction; with cisplatin and fluorouracil for induction treatment of locally advanced squamous cell carcinoma of the head and neck

**Cautions** see section 8.1 and notes above; hepatic impairment (Appendix 2); avoid in acute porphyria (but see section 9.8.2); **interactions:** Appendix 1 (docetaxel)

**Contra-indications** pregnancy (Appendix 4); breast-feeding

**Side-effects** see section 8.1 and notes above

**Taxotere®** (Sanofi-Aventis) PoM
Concentrate for intravenous infusion, docetaxel 40 mg/mL. Net price 0.5-mL vial = £162.75, 2-mL vial = £534.75 (both with diluent) (hosp. only)

### ■ PACLITAXEL

**Indications** ovarian cancer (advanced or residual disease following laparotomy) in combination with cisplatin; metastatic ovarian cancer where platinum-containing therapy has failed; locally advanced or metastatic breast cancer (in combination with other cytotoxics or alone if other cytotoxics have failed or are inappropriate); adjuvant treatment of node-positive breast cancer following treatment with anthracycline and cyclophosphamide; non-small cell lung cancer (in combination with cisplatin) when surgery or radiotherapy not appropriate; advanced AIDS-related Kaposi's sarcoma where liposomal anthracycline therapy has failed

**Cautions** see section 8.1 and notes above; avoid in acute porphyria (but see section 9.8.2); **interactions:** Appendix 1 (paclitaxel)

**Contra-indications** see section 8.1 and notes above; severe hepatic impairment; pregnancy (Appendix 4); breast-feeding

**Side-effects** see section 8.1 and notes above

**Paclitaxel** (Non-proprietary) [PoM]
Concentrate for intravenous infusion, paclitaxel 6 mg/mL, net price 5-mL vial = £66.85, 16.7-mL vial = £200.35, 25-mL vial = £300.52, 50-mL vial = £601.03
Excipients include polyoxyl castor oil (risk of anaphylaxis, see Excipients, p. 2)

**Abraxane®** (Abraxis) [PoM]
Intravenous infusion, powder for reconstitution, paclitaxel, net price 100-mg vial = £246.00
Electrolytes Contains approx. 18.5 mmol Na⁺/dose

**Taxol®** (Bristol-Myers Squibb) [PoM]
Concentrate for intravenous infusion, paclitaxel 6 mg/mL, net price 5-mL vial = £116.05, 16.7-mL vial = £347.82, 25-mL vial = £521.73, 50-mL vial = £1043.46 (hosp. only)
Excipients include polyoxyl castor oil (risk of anaphylaxis, see Excipients, p. 2)

## Topoisomerase I inhibitors

Irinotecan and topotecan inhibit topoisomerase I, an enzyme involved in DNA replication.

**Irinotecan** is licensed for metastatic colorectal cancer in combination with fluorouracil and folinic acid or as monotherapy when treatment containing fluorouracil has failed. It is also licensed in combination with cetuximab for the treatment of epidermal growth factor receptor-expressing metastatic colorectal cancer after failure of chemotherapy that has included irinotecan. Irinotecan is also licensed in combination with 5-fluorouracil, folinic acid and bevacizumab for the first-line treatment of metastatic carcinoma of the colon or rectum. Irinotecan is also licensed in combination with capecitabine with or without bevacizumab for the first-line treatment of metastatic colorectal carcinoma. Irinotecan is given by intravenous infusion.

> **NICE guidance (irinotecan, oxaliplatin and raltitrexed for advanced colorectal cancer)**
> See p. 485

**Topotecan** is given by intravenous infusion or orally in relapsed small-cell lung cancer when retreatment with the first-line regimen is considered inappropriate. Topotecan injection is also licensed for metastatic ovarian cancer when first-line or subsequent treatment has failed. Topotecan injection is licensed in combination with cisplatin for treatment of recurrent carcinoma of the cervix, after radiotherapy, and for patients with stage IVB disease.

In addition to dose-limiting myelosuppression, side-effects of irinotecan and topotecan include gastro-intestinal effects (delayed diarrhoea requiring prompt treat-ment may follow irinotecan treatment), asthenia, alopecia, and anorexia.

The *Scottish Medicines Consortium* (p. 3) has advised (November 2007) that topotecan (*Hycamtin®*) is accepted for restricted use in combination with cisplatin for treatment of recurrent carcinoma of the cervix after radiotherapy and for stage IVB disease; it is restricted to patients who have not previously received cisplatin treatment.

The *Scottish Medicines Consortium* (p. 3) has advised (March 2009) that use of topotecan capsules within NHS Scotland is restricted to patients in whom standard intravenous chemotherapy is inappropriate and who would otherwise receive best supportive care.

> **NICE guidance (paclitaxel, pegylated liposomal doxorubicin and topotecan for second-line or subsequent treatment of advanced ovarian cancer)**
> See p. 485

## ▊ IRINOTECAN HYDROCHLORIDE

**Indications** see notes above

**Cautions** see section 8.1 and notes above; raised plasma-bilirubin concentration (see under Contra-indications and Appendix 2)

**Contra-indications** see section 8.1 and notes above; also chronic inflammatory bowel disease, bowel obstruction; plasma-bilirubin concentration greater than 3 times the upper limit of reference range; renal impairment (Appendix 3); pregnancy (Appendix 4); breast-feeding

**Side-effects** see section 8.1 and notes above; also acute cholinergic syndrome (with early diarrhoea) and delayed diarrhoea (consult product literature), interstitial pulmonary disease

**Irinotecan** (Non-proprietary) [PoM]
Concentrate for intravenous infusion, irinotecan hydrochloride 20 mg/mL, net price 2-mL vial = £53.00, 5-mL vial = £130.00, 25-mL vial = £650.00

**Campto®** (Pfizer) [PoM]
Concentrate for intravenous infusion, irinotecan hydrochloride 20 mg/mL, net price 2-mL vial = £53.00; 5-mL vial = £130.00; 15-mL vial = £390.00

## ▊ TOPOTECAN

**Indications** see notes above

**Cautions** see section 8.1 and notes above; renal impairment (avoid infusion if creatinine clearance less than 20 mL/minute; avoid oral route if creatinine clearance less than 60 mL/minute; Appendix 3)

**Contra-indications** see section 8.1 and notes above; severe hepatic impairment; pregnancy (Appendix 4); breast-feeding

**Side-effects** see section 8.1 and notes above

**Hycamtin®** (GSK) ▼ [PoM]
Capsules, topotecan (as hydrochloride) 250 micrograms (white), net price 10-cap pack = £75.00; 1 mg (pink), 10-cap pack = £300.00. Label: 25

Intravenous infusion, powder for reconstitution, topotecan (as hydrochloride), net price 1-mg vial = £97.65; 4-mg vial = £290.62

## Trabectedin

**Trabectedin** is licensed for the treatment of advanced soft tissue sarcoma when treatment with anthracyclines and ifosfamide has failed or is contra-indicated.

Trabectedin is given by intravenous infusion. Dexamethasone by intravenous infusion should be given concomitantly for its antiemetic and hepatoprotective effects.

The *Scottish Medicines Consortium* (p. 3) has advised (January 2008) that trabectedin (*Yondelis®*) is **not** recommended for use within NHS Scotland for the treatment of advanced soft tissue sarcoma.

### ▌ TRABECTEDIN

**Indications** see notes above

**Cautions** see section 8.1 and notes above; measure creatine phosphokinase, renal function and hepatic function before starting (consult product literature); monitor haematological and hepatic parameters weekly during first 2 cycles and at least once between treatments in subsequent cycles; concomitant use with hepatotoxic drugs (avoid alcohol); hepatic impairment (Appendix 2)

**Contra-indications** raised bilirubin; renal impairment (avoid if creatinine clearance less than 30 mL/minute; Appendix 3); pregnancy (Appendix 4); breast-feeding (Appendix 5)

**Side-effects** see section 8.1; also abdominal pain, constipation, diarrhoea, dyspepsia, taste disturbance, hepatobiliary disorders; hypotension, oedema, flushing; dyspnoea, cough; headache, insomnia, peripheral neuropathy, paraesthesia, dizziness, anorexia, asthenia, fatigue; pyrexia; hypokalaemia, dehydration, increased blood creatine phosphokinase; myalgia, arthralgia, back pain

**Yondelis®** (Pharma Mar) ▼ PoM
Injection, powder for reconstitution, trabectedin, net price 250-microgram vial = £363.00; 1-mg vial = £1366.00

## Trastuzumab

**Trastuzumab** is licensed for the treatment of early breast cancer which overexpresses human epidermal growth factor receptor-2 (HER2).

Trastuzumab is also licensed, in combination with paclitaxel or docetaxel, for metastatic breast cancer in patients with HER2-positive tumours who have not received chemotherapy for metastatic breast cancer and in whom anthracycline treatment is inappropriate.

Trastuzumab is also licensed, in combination with an aromatase inhibitor, for metastatic breast cancer in postmenopausal patients with hormone-receptor positive HER2-positive tumours not previously treated with trastuzumab.

Trastuzumab is also licensed as monotherapy for metastatic breast cancer in patients with tumours that overexpress HER2 who have received at least 2 chemotherapy regimens including, where appropriate, an anthracycline and a taxane; women with oestrogen-receptor-positive breast cancer should also have received hormonal therapy.

Trastuzumab is given by intravenous infusion. Resuscitation facilities should be available and treatment should be initiated by a specialist. See section 8.3.4.1 for the role of trastuzumab in the treatment of breast cancer.

**Use with anthracyclines** Concomitant use of trastuzumab with anthracyclines (section 8.1.2) is associated with cardiotoxicity. The use of anthracyclines even after stopping trastuzumab can increase the risk of cardiotoxicity and if possible should be avoided for up to 24 weeks. If an anthracycline needs to be used, cardiac function should be monitored closely.

### ▌ TRASTUZUMAB

**Indications** see notes above and product literature

**Cautions** see section 8.1 and notes above; symptomatic heart failure, history of hypertension, coronary artery disease, uncontrolled arrhythmias; pregnancy (Appendix 4)

Cardiotoxicity Monitor cardiac function before and during treatment—for details of monitoring and managing cardiotoxicity, consult product literature

**Contra-indications** see section 8.1 and notes above; severe dyspnoea at rest; breast-feeding (Appendix 5)

**Side-effects** infusion-related side-effects including chills, fever, hypersensitivity reactions such as anaphylaxis, urticaria, and angioedema; gastro-intestinal symptoms; cardiotoxicity (see also above), chest pain, hypotension; pulmonary events (possibly delayed onset); headache, taste disturbance, anxiety, malaise, depression, insomnia, drowsiness, dizziness, paraesthesia, tremor, asthenia, peripheral neuropathy, hypertonia; mastitis, urinary-tract infection; leucopenia, ecchymosis, oedema, weight loss; arthralgia, myalgia, arthritis, bone pain, leg cramps; rash, pruritus, sweating, dry skin, alopecia, acne, nail disorders

**Herceptin®** (Roche) ▼ PoM
Intravenous infusion, powder for reconstitution, trastuzumab, net price 150-mg vial = £407.40

## Tretinoin

**Tretinoin** is licensed for the induction of remission in acute promyelocytic leukaemia. It is used in previously untreated patients as well as in those who have relapsed after standard chemotherapy or who are refractory to it.

### ▌ TRETINOIN

Note Tretinoin is the acid form of vitamin A

**Indications** see notes above; acne (section 13.6.1); photodamage (section 13.8.1)

**Cautions** exclude pregnancy before starting treatment and ensure effective contraception is used during and for at least 1 month after treatment; monitor haematological and coagulation profile, liver function, serum calcium and plasma lipids before and during treatment; increased risk of thromboembolism during first month of treatment; hepatic impairment (Appendix 2); renal impairment (Appendix 3); **interactions:** Appendix 1 (retinoids)

**Contra-indications** pregnancy (**important teratogenic risk:** see Cautions and Appendix 4) and breast-feeding

**Side-effects** retinoic acid syndrome (fever, dyspnoea, acute respiratory distress, pulmonary infiltrates, pleural effusion, hyperleukocytosis, hypotension, oedema, weight gain, hepatic, renal and multi-organ failure) requires immediate treatment—consult product literature; gastro-intestinal disturbances, pancreatitis; arrhythmias, flushing, oedema; headache, benign intracranial hypertension (mainly in children—consider dose reduction if intractable headache in children), shivering, dizziness, confusion, anxiety, depression, insomnia, paraesthesia, visual and hearing disturbances; raised liver enzymes, serum creatinine and lipids; bone and chest pain, alopecia, erythema, rash, pruritus, sweating, dry skin and mucous membranes, cheilitis; thromboembolism, hypercalcaemia, and genital ulceration reported

**Dose**

- ADULT and CHILD 45 mg/m² daily in 2 divided doses, max. duration of treatment 90 days (consult product literature for details of concomitant chemotherapy)

**Vesanoid®** (Roche) PoM

Capsules, yellow/brown, tretinoin 10 mg. Net price 100-cap pack = £163.87. Label: 21, 25

---

## 8.2 Drugs affecting the immune response

| 8.2.1 | Antiproliferative immunosuppressants |
| 8.2.2 | Corticosteroids and other immunosuppressants |
| 8.2.3 | Rituximab and alemtuzumab |
| 8.2.4 | Other immunomodulating drugs |

### Immunosuppressant therapy

Immunosuppressants are used to suppress rejection in organ transplant recipients and to treat a variety of chronic inflammatory and autoimmune diseases. Solid organ transplant patients are usually maintained on a corticosteroid combined with a calcineurin inhibitor (ciclosporin or tacrolimus), or with an antiproliferative drug (azathioprine or mycophenolate mofetil), or with both. Specialist management is required and other immunomodulators may be used to initiate treatment or to treat rejection.

> **Bioavailability**
>
> Different formulations of the same immunosuppressant may vary in bioavailability and to avoid reduced effect or excessive side-effects, it is important not to change formulation except on the advice of a transplant specialist.

**Impaired immune responsiveness** Modification of tissue reactions caused by corticosteroids and other immunosuppressants may result in the rapid *spread of infection*. Corticosteroids may suppress clinical signs of infection and allow diseases such as septicaemia or tuberculosis to reach an advanced stage before being recognised—**important:** for advice on measles exposure, see section 14.5.1, and chickenpox (varicella) exposure, see section 14.5.2. For advice on the use of live vaccines in individuals with impaired immune response, see section 14.1. For general comments and warnings relating to corticosteroids and immunosuppressants, see section 6.3.2 (under Prednisolone).

**Pregnancy** Transplant patients immunosuppressed with azathioprine should not discontinue it on becoming pregnant. However, there have been reports of premature birth and low birth-weight following exposure to azathioprine, particularly in combination with corticosteroids. Spontaneous abortion has been reported following maternal or paternal exposure.

There is less experience of ciclosporin in pregnancy but it does not appear to be any more harmful than azathioprine. The use of these drugs during pregnancy needs to be supervised in specialist units.

Manufacturers advise caution in the use of tacrolimus and contra-indicate mycophenolate during pregnancy (Appendix 4).

## 8.2.1 Antiproliferative immunosuppressants

**Azathioprine** is widely used for transplant recipients and it is also used to treat a number of auto-immune conditions, usually when corticosteroid therapy alone provides inadequate control. It is metabolised to mercaptopurine, and doses should be reduced when allopurinol is given concurrently.

Blood tests and monitoring for signs of myelosuppression are essential in long-term treatment with azathioprine. The enzyme thiopurine methyltransferase (TPMT) metabolises azathioprine; the risk of myelosuppression is increased in those with a low activity of the enzyme, particularly in the very few individuals who are homozygous for low TPMT activity.

**Mycophenolate mofetil** is metabolised to mycophenolic acid which has a more selective mode of action than azathioprine. It is licensed for the prophylaxis of acute rejection in renal, hepatic or cardiac transplantation when used in combination with ciclosporin and corticosteroids. There is evidence that compared with similar regimens incorporating azathioprine, mycophenolate mofetil reduces the risk of acute rejection episodes; the risk of opportunistic infections (particularly due to tissue-invasive cytomegalovirus) and the occurrence of blood disorders such as leucopenia may be higher. Cases of pure red cell aplasia have been reported with mycophenolate mofetil. In some patients, dose reduction or discontinuation of mycophenolate can lead to resolution of the condition, but dose changes should be undertaken under specialist supervision.

**Cyclophosphamide** (section 8.1.1) is less commonly prescribed as an immunosuppressant.

### AZATHIOPRINE

**Indications** see notes above; inflammatory bowel disease [unlicensed indication] (section 1.5.3); rheumatoid arthritis (section 10.1.3)

**Cautions** monitor for toxicity throughout treatment; monitor full blood count weekly (more frequently with higher doses or if hepatic or renal impairment) for first 4 weeks (manufacturer advises weekly monitoring for 8 weeks but evidence of practical value unsatisfactory), thereafter reduce frequency of monitoring to at least every 3 months; hepatic impairment (Appendix 2); renal impairment (Appendix 3); reduce dose in elderly; pregnancy (see section 8.2)—treatment should not generally be initiated during pregnancy;

breast-feeding (Appendix 5); **interactions**: Appendix 1 (azathioprine)

**Bone marrow suppression** Patients should be warned to report immediately any signs or symptoms of bone marrow suppression e.g. inexplicable bruising or bleeding, infection

**Contra-indications** hypersensitivity to azathioprine or mercaptopurine

**Side-effects** hypersensitivity reactions (including malaise, dizziness, vomiting, diarrhoea, fever, rigors, myalgia, arthralgia, rash, hypotension and interstitial nephritis—calling for immediate withdrawal); dose-related bone marrow suppression (see also Cautions); liver impairment, cholestatic jaundice, hair loss and increased susceptibility to infections and colitis in patients also receiving corticosteroids; nausea; rarely pancreatitis, pneumonitis, hepatic veno-occlusive disease

**Dose**
- By mouth, *or* (if oral administration not possible—intravenous solution very irritant, see below) by intravenous injection over at least 1 minute (followed by 50 mL sodium chloride intravenous infusion), *or* by intravenous infusion

Autoimmune conditions, 1–3 mg/kg daily, adjusted according to response (consider withdrawal if no improvement in 3 months)

Suppression of transplant rejection, initially up to 5 mg/kg then 1–4 mg/kg daily according to response

**Note** Intravenous injection is alkaline and very irritant, intravenous route should therefore be used **only** if oral route not feasible, see also Appendix 6

**Azathioprine** (Non-proprietary) ▨
Tablets, azathioprine 25 mg, net price 28-tab pack = £8.15; 50 mg, 56-tab pack = £7.52. Label: 21
Brands include *Azamune®*

**Imuran®** (GSK) ▨
Tablets, both f/c, azathioprine 25 mg (orange), net price 100-tab pack = £10.99; 50 mg (yellow), 100-tab pack = £7.99. Label: 21

Injection, powder for reconstitution, azathioprine (as sodium salt). Net price 50-mg vial = £15.38

---

## ▰ MYCOPHENOLATE MOFETIL

**Indications** prophylaxis of acute renal, cardiac, or hepatic transplant rejection (in combination with ciclosporin and corticosteroids) under specialist supervision

**Cautions** full blood counts every week for 4 weeks then twice a month for 2 months then every month in the first year (consider interrupting treatment if neutropenia develops); elderly (increased risk of infection, gastro-intestinal haemorrhage and pulmonary oedema); children (higher incidence of side-effects may call for temporary reduction of dose or interruption); active serious gastro-intestinal disease (risk of haemorrhage, ulceration and perforation); delayed graft function; increased susceptibility to skin cancer (avoid exposure to strong sunlight); **interactions**: Appendix 1 (mycophenolate)

**Bone marrow suppression** Patients should be warned to report immediately any signs or symptoms of bone marrow suppression e.g. infection or inexplicable bruising or bleeding

**Contra-indications** pregnancy (exclude before starting and avoid for 6 weeks after discontinuation) (Appendix 4); breast-feeding (Appendix 5)

**Side-effects** gastro-intestinal disturbances (including diarrhoea, vomiting, and abdominal pain), gastro-intestinal ulceration and bleeding, abnormal liver function tests, hepatitis, jaundice, pancreatitis; oedema, tachycardia, hypertension, hypotension, vasodilatation; cough, dyspnoea; insomnia, agitation, tremor, dizziness, headache; influenza-like syndrome, infections (viral, bacterial, and fungal); hyperglyc-aemia; renal impairment; increased risk of malignancies, particularly of the skin; blood disorders (including leucopenia, anaemia, thrombocytopenia, pancytopenia, and red cell aplasia—see notes above), disturbances of electrolytes and blood lipids; arthralgia; alopecia, acne, and rash; progressive multifocal leucoencephalopathy reported

**Dose**
- Renal transplantation, by mouth, 1 g twice daily starting within 72 hours of transplantation *or* by intravenous infusion, 1 g twice daily starting within 24 hours of transplantation for max. 14 days (then transfer to oral therapy); CHILD and ADOLESCENT 2–18 years, by mouth 600 mg/m² twice daily (max. 2 g daily)
**Note** Tablets and capsules not appropriate for dose titration in children with body surface area less than 1.25 m²
- Cardiac transplantation, by mouth, 1.5 g twice daily starting within 5 days of transplantation
- Hepatic transplantation, by intravenous infusion, 1 g twice daily starting within 24 hours of transplantation for 4 days (up to max. 14 days), then by mouth, 1.5 g twice daily as soon as is tolerated

**CellCept®** (Roche) ▨
Capsules, blue/brown, mycophenolate mofetil 250 mg, net price 100-cap pack = £83.92

Tablets, lavender, mycophenolate mofetil 500 mg, net price 50-tab pack = £83.92

Oral suspension, mycophenolate mofetil 1 g/5 mL when reconstituted with water, net price 175 mL = £117.48.
Excipients include aspartame (section 9.4.1)

Intravenous infusion, powder for reconstitution, mycophenolate mofetil (as hydrochloride), net price 500-mg vial = £9.31

◣**Mycophenolic acid**
**Myfortic®** (Novartis) ▨
Tablets, e/c, mycophenolic acid (as mycophenolate sodium) 180 mg (green), net price 120-tab pack = £99.71; 360 mg (orange), 120-tab pack = £199.41. Label: 25
**Dose** renal transplantation, 720 mg twice daily starting within 72 hours of transplantation
**Equivalence to mycophenolate mofetil** Mycophenolic acid 720 mg is approximately equivalent to mycophenolate mofetil 1 g but avoid unnecessary switching because of pharmacokinetic differences

---

## 8.2.2 Corticosteroids and other immunosuppressants

**Prednisolone** (section 6.3.2) is widely used in oncology. It has a marked antitumour effect in acute lympho-blastic leukaemia, Hodgkin's disease, and the non-Hodgkin lymphomas. It has a role in the palliation of symptomatic end-stage malignant disease when it may enhance appetite and produce a sense of well-being (see also Prescribing in Palliative Care, p. 16).

**8 Malignant disease and immunosuppression**

The corticosteroids are also powerful immunosuppressants. They are used to prevent organ transplant rejection, and in high dose to treat rejection episodes.

**Ciclosporin** (cyclosporin), a calcineurin inhibitor, is a potent immunosuppressant which is virtually non-myelotoxic but markedly nephrotoxic. It has an important role in organ and tissue transplantation, for prevention of graft rejection following bone marrow, kidney, liver, pancreas, heart, lung, and heart-lung transplantation, and for prophylaxis and treatment of graft-versus-host disease.

**Tacrolimus** is also a calcineurin inhibitor. Although not chemically related to ciclosporin it has a similar mode of action and side-effects, but the incidence of neurotoxicity appears to be greater; cardiomyopathy has also been reported. Disturbance of glucose metabolism also appears to be significant; hypertrichosis appears to be less of a problem than with ciclosporin.

**Sirolimus** is a potent non-calcineurin inhibiting immunosuppressant licensed for renal transplantation. It can cause hyperlipidaemia.

**Basiliximab** is a monoclonal antibody that prevents T-lymphocyte proliferation; it is used for prophylaxis of acute rejection in allogeneic renal transplantation. It is given with ciclosporin and corticosteroid immunosuppression regimens; its use should be confined to specialist centres.

**Antithymocyte immunoglobulin** (rabbit) is licensed for the prophylaxis of organ rejection in renal and heart allograft recipients and for the treatment of corticosteroid-resistant allograft rejection in renal transplantation. Tolerability is increased by pretreatment with an intravenous corticosteroid and antihistamine; an antipyretic drug such as paracetamol may also be beneficial.

---

**NICE guidance**

**Immunosuppressive therapy for renal transplantation in adults (September 2004)**
**Immunosuppressive therapy for renal transplantation in children and adolescents (April 2006)**

For induction therapy in the prophylaxis of organ rejection, either basiliximab or daclizumab [discontinued] are options for combining with a calcineurin inhibitor. For each individual, ciclosporin or tacrolimus is chosen as the calcineurin inhibitor on the basis of side-effects.

Mycophenolate mofetil [mycophenolic acid also available but not licensed for use in children, see p. 494] is recommended as part of an immunosuppressive regimen only if:

- the calcineurin inhibitor is not tolerated, particularly if nephrotoxicity endangers the transplanted kidney; or
- there is very high risk of nephrotoxicity from the calcineurin inhibitor, requiring a reduction in the dose of the calcineurin inhibitor or its avoidance.

Sirolimus is recommended as a component of immunosuppressive regimen **only if** intolerance necessitates the withdrawal of a calcineurin inhibitor.

These recommendations may not be consistent with the marketing authorisation of some of the products.

---

## ANTITHYMOCYTE IMMUNOGLOBULIN (RABBIT)

**Indications** see notes above

**Cautions** see notes above; monitor blood count; pregnancy (Appendix 4)

**Contra-indications** infection; breast-feeding (Appendix 5)

**Side-effects** nausea, vomiting, dysphagia, diarrhoea; hypotension; infusion-related reactions (including cytokine release syndrome and anaphylaxis, see notes above), serum sickness; fever, shivering, increased susceptibility to infection; increased susceptibility to malignancy; lymphopenia, neutropenia, thrombocytopenia; myalgia; pruritus, rash

**Dose**

- Heart transplantation, by intravenous infusion over at least 6 hours, 1–2.5 mg/kg daily for 3–5 days
- Renal transplantation, by intravenous infusion over at least 6 hours, 1–1.5 mg/kg daily for 3–9 days
- Corticosteroid-resistant renal graft rejection, by intravenous infusion over at least 6 hours, 1.5 mg/kg daily for 7–14 days

Note To avoid excessive dosage in obese patients, calculate dose on the basis of ideal body weight

**Thymoglobuline®** (Genzyme) ▼ PoM
Intravenous infusion, powder for reconstitution, rabbit anti-human thymocyte immunoglobulin, net price 25-mg vial = £168.18

---

## BASILIXIMAB

**Indications** see notes above

**Contra-indications** pregnancy (Appendix 4) and breast-feeding

**Side-effects** severe hypersensitivity reactions and cytokine release syndrome have been reported

**Dose**

- By intravenous injection or by intravenous infusion, 20 mg within 2 hours before transplant surgery and 20 mg 4 days after surgery; withhold second dose if severe hypersensitivity or graft loss occurs; CHILD and ADOLESCENT 1–17 years, body-weight under 35 kg, 10 mg within 2 hours before transplant surgery and 10 mg 4 days after surgery; body-weight over 35 kg, adult dose

**Simulect®** (Novartis) PoM
Injection, powder for reconstitution, basiliximab, net price 10-mg vial = £758.69, 20-mg vial = £842.38 (both with water for injections) . For intravenous infusion

---

## CICLOSPORIN
(Cyclosporin)

**Indications** see notes above, and under Dose; severe acute ulcerative colitis [unlicensed indication] (section 1.5.3); rheumatoid arthritis (section 10.1.3); atopic dermatitis and psoriasis (section 13.5.3)

**Cautions** monitor kidney function—dose dependent increase in serum creatinine and urea during first few weeks may necessitate dose reduction in transplant patients (exclude rejection if kidney transplant) or discontinuation in non-transplant patients; monitor liver function (dosage adjustment based on bilirubin and liver enzymes may be needed); monitor blood pressure—discontinue if hypertension develops that cannot be controlled by antihypertensives; hyperuricaemia; monitor serum potassium especially in renal dysfunction (risk of hyperkalaemia); monitor serum magnesium; measure blood lipids before treatment and thereafter as appropriate; pregnancy (see p. 493) and breast-feeding (Appendix 5); acute porphyria (section 9.8.2); use with tacrolimus specifically contra-indicated; for patients other than transplant recipients, preferably avoid other immunosuppressants (increased risk of infection and malignancies, including lymphoma and skin cancer); avoid excessive exposure to UV light, including sunlight; **interactions:** Appendix 1 (ciclosporin)

Additional cautions in nephrotic syndrome *Contra-indicated* in uncontrolled hypertension, uncontrolled infections, and malignancy; reduce dose by 25–50% if serum creatinine more than 30% above baseline on more than one measurement; in renal impairment initially 2.5 mg/kg daily; in long-term management, perform renal biopsies at yearly intervals

**Side-effects** gastro-intestinal disturbances, gingival hyperplasia, hepatic dysfunction, anorexia; hypertension; tremor, headache, paraesthesia, fatigue; renal dysfunction (renal structural changes on long-term administration, see also under Cautions), hyperuricaemia, hyperkalaemia, hypomagnesaemia, hyperlipidaemia, hypercholesterolaemia; muscle cramps, myalgia; hypertrichosis; *less commonly* oedema, weight gain, encephalopathy, anaemia, thrombocytopenia, rash; *rarely* pancreatitis, motor polyneuropathy, menstrual disturbances, gynaecomastia, microangiopathic haemolytic anaemia, haemolytic uraemic syndrome, hyperglycaemia, muscle weakness, myopathy; visual disturbances secondary to benign intracranial hypertension (discontinue), also anaphylaxis reported with infusion

**Dose**

- Organ transplantation, used alone, ADULT and CHILD over 3 months 10–15 mg/kg by mouth 4–12 hours before transplantation followed by 10–15 mg/kg daily for 1–2 weeks postoperatively then reduced gradually to 2–6 mg/kg daily for maintenance (dose should be adjusted according to blood-ciclosporin concentration and renal function); dose lower if given concomitantly with other immunosuppressant therapy (e.g. corticosteroids); if necessary one-third corresponding oral dose can be given by intravenous infusion over 2–6 hours

- Bone-marrow transplantation, prevention and treatment of graft-versus-host disease, ADULT and CHILD over 3 months 3–5 mg/kg daily by intravenous infusion over 2–6 hours from day before transplantation to 2 weeks postoperatively (or 12.5–15 mg/kg daily by mouth) then 12.5 mg/kg daily by mouth for 3–6 months then tailed off (may take up to a year after transplantation)

- Nephrotic syndrome, by mouth, 5 mg/kg daily in 2 divided doses; CHILD 6 mg/kg daily in 2 divided doses; maintenance treatment reduce to lowest effective dose according to proteinuria and serum creatinine measurements; discontinue after 3 months if no improvement in glomerulonephritis or glomerulosclerosis (after 6 months in membranous glomerulonephritis)

**Conversion** Any conversion between brands should be undertaken very carefully and the manufacturer contacted for further information. Currently only *Neoral*® remains available for oral use; *Sandimmun*® capsules and oral solution and *SangCya*®

oral solution are available on named-patient basis only for patients who cannot be transferred to another brand of oral ciclosporin

> Because of differences in bioavailability, the brand of oral ciclosporin to be dispensed should be specified by the prescriber

**Neoral**® (Novartis) [PoM]

Capsules, ciclosporin 10 mg (yellow/white), net price 60-cap pack = £18.98; 25 mg (blue/grey), 30-cap pack = £19.10; 50 mg (yellow/white), 30-cap pack = £37.40; 100 mg (blue/grey), 30-cap pack = £70.99. Counselling, administration

Oral solution, yellow, sugar-free, ciclosporin 100 mg/ mL, net price 50 mL = £106.37. Counselling, administration

**Counselling** Total daily dose should be taken in 2 divided doses. Avoid grapefruit or grapefruit juice for 1 hour before dose

Mix solution with orange juice (or squash) or apple juice (to improve taste) or with water immediately before taking (and rinse with more to ensure total dose). Do not mix with grapefruit juice. Keep medicine measure away from other liquids (including water)

**Sandimmun**® (Novartis) [PoM]

Concentrate for intravenous infusion (oily), ciclosporin 50 mg/mL. To be diluted before use. Net price 1-mL amp = £1.94; 5-mL amp = £9.17

**Excipients** include polyoxyl castor oil (risk of anaphylaxis, see Excipients, p. 2)

**Note** Observe patients for signs of anaphylaxis for at least 30 minutes after starting infusion and at frequent intervals thereafter

## ▌ SIROLIMUS

**Indications** prophylaxis of organ rejection in kidney allograft recipients (initially in combination with ciclosporin and corticosteroid, then with corticosteroid only); see also under Dose

**Cautions** monitor kidney function when given with ciclosporin; Afro-Caribbean patients may require higher doses; hepatic impairment (Appendix 2); **interactions:** Appendix 1 (sirolimus)

**Contra-indications** pregnancy (Appendix 4); breast-feeding (Appendix 5)

**Side-effects** abdominal pain, constipation, nausea, diarrhoea, stomatitis; oedema, tachycardia, hypertension, hypercholesterolaemia, hypertriglyceridaemia, venous thromboembolism; pleural effusion, pneumonitis; headache; pyrexia; increased susceptibility to infection (especially urinary-tract infection); proteinuria, haemolytic uraemic syndrome; anaemia, thrombocytopenia, thrombotic thrombocytopenic purpura, leucopenia, neutropenia, hypokalaemia, hypophosphataemia, hyperglycaemia, lymphocele; arthralgia, osteonecrosis; epistaxis; acne, rash, impaired healing; *less commonly* pancreatitis, pulmonary embolism, pulmonary haemorrhage, pericardial effusion, nephrotic syndrome, increased susceptibility to lymphoma and other malignancies particularly of the skin, and pancytopenia; *rarely* interstitial lung disease, hepatic necrosis, lymphoedema, and hypersensitivity reactions including anaphylactic reactions, angioedema, exfoliative dermatitis, and hypersensitivity vasculitis; reversible impairment of male fertility also reported

**Dose**

- Initially 6 mg, after surgery, then 2 mg once daily (dose adjusted according to blood-sirolimus concentration) in combination with ciclosporin and corticosteroid for 2–3 months (sirolimus given 4 hours after ciclosporin); ciclosporin should then be withdrawn over 4–8 weeks (if not possible, sirolimus should be discontinued and an alternate immunosuppressive regimen used)

**Note** Pre-dose ('trough') blood-sirolimus concentration (using chromatographic assay) when used with ciclosporin should be 4–12 micrograms/litre; after withdrawal of ciclosporin pre-dose blood-sirolimus concentration should be 12–20 micrograms/litre; close monitoring of blood-sirolimus concentration required in hepatic impairment, during treatment with potent inducers or inhibitors of metabolism and after discontinuing them

When changing between oral solution and tablets, measurement of serum 'trough' blood-sirolimus concentration after 1–2 weeks is recommended

**Rapamune®** (Wyeth) ▼ PoM

Tablets, coated, sirolimus 1 mg (white), net price 30-tab pack = £86.49; 2 mg (yellow), 30-tab pack = £172.98. Counselling, administration

Oral solution, sirolimus 1 mg/mL, net price 60 mL = £162.41. Counselling, administration

**Counselling** Food may affect absorption (take at the same time with respect to food). Mix solution with at least 60 mL water or orange juice in a glass or plastic container immediately before taking; refill container with at least 120 mL and drink immediately (to ensure total dose). Do not mix with any other liquids

# ■ TACROLIMUS

**Indications** prophylaxis of organ rejection in liver, kidney, and heart allograft recipients and allograft rejection resistant to conventional immunosuppressive regimens, see also notes above; moderate to severe atopic eczema (section 13.5.3)

**Cautions** see under Ciclosporin; also monitor ECG (**important:** also echocardiography, see CSM warning below); visual status, blood glucose, haematological and neurological parameters and whole-blood 'trough' concentrations (especially during episodes of diarrhoea); prolonged QT interval; hepatic impairment (Appendix 2); pregnancy (exclude before starting—if contraception needed non-hormonal methods should be used; Appendix 4); **interactions:** Appendix 1 (tacrolimus)

**Driving** May affect performance of skilled tasks (e.g. driving)

**Contra-indications** hypersensitivity to macrolides; breast-feeding (Appendix 5); avoid concurrent administration with ciclosporin (care if patient has previously received ciclosporin)

**Side-effects** gastro-intestinal disturbances including dyspepsia, and inflammatory and ulcerative disorders; hepatic dysfunction, jaundice, bile-duct and gall-bladder abnormalities; hypertension (*less frequently* hypotension), tachycardia, angina, arrhythmias, thromboembolic and ischaemic events, *rarely* myocardial hypertrophy, cardiomyopathy (**important:** see CSM warning below); dyspnoea, pleural effusion; tremor, headache, insomnia, paraesthesia, confusion, depression, dizziness, anxiety, convulsions, incoordination, encephalopathy, psychosis; visual and hearing abnormalities; haematological effects including anaemia, leucocytosis, leucopenia, thrombocytopenia, coagulation disorders; altered acid-base balance and glucose metabolism, electrolyte disturbances including hyperkalaemia (*less frequently* hypokalaemia); altered renal function including increased serum creatinine; hypophosphataemia, hypercalcaemia, hyperuricaemia; muscle cramps, arthralgia; pruritus, alopecia, rash, sweating, acne, photosensitivity; susceptibility to lymphoma and other malig-

nancies particularly of the skin; *less commonly* ascites, pancreatitis, atelectasis, kidney damage and renal failure, myasthenia, hirsutism; *rarely* Stevens-Johnson syndrome

**CSM Warning** Cardiomyopathy has been reported in children given tacrolimus after transplantation. Patients should be monitored carefully by echocardiography for hypertrophic changes; dose reduction or discontinuation should be considered if these occur

**Dose**
• See under preparations

---

**MHRA/CHM advice (December 2008)**
*Prograf®* and *Advagraf®* (tacrolimus): serious medication errors
It is important to note the correct use of these medicines:
• *Prograf®* is an immediate-release formulation that is taken twice daily, once in the morning and once in the evening;
• *Advagraf®* is a prolonged-release formulation that is taken once daily in the morning
*Prograf®* and *Advagraf®* are not interchangeable; switching between *Prograf®* and *Advagraf®* requires careful therapeutic monitoring. Substitution should be made only under the close supervision of a transplant specialist.

---

**Prograf®** (Astellas) PoM

Capsules, tacrolimus 500 micrograms (yellow), net price 50-cap pack = £63.13; 1 mg (white), 50-cap pack = £81.90, 100-cap pack = £163.78; 5 mg (greyish-red), 50-cap pack = £302.56. Label: 23, counselling, driving

Concentrate for intravenous infusion, tacrolimus 5 mg/mL. To be diluted before use. Net price 1-mL amp = £59.63

**Excipients** include polyoxyl castor oil (risk of anaphylaxis, see Excipients, p. 2)

**Dose** Liver transplantation, starting 12 hours after transplantation, by mouth, 100–200 micrograms/kg daily in 2 divided doses *or* by intravenous infusion over 24 hours, 10–50 micrograms/kg daily for up to max. 7 days (then transfer to oral therapy); CHILD by mouth, 300 micrograms/kg daily in 2 divided doses *or* by intravenous infusion over 24 hours, 50 micrograms/kg daily for up to max. 7 days (then transfer to oral therapy)

Renal transplantation, starting within 24 hours of transplantation, by mouth, 200–300 micrograms/kg daily in 2 divided doses *or* by intravenous infusion over 24 hours, 50–100 micrograms/kg daily for up to max. 7 days (then transfer to oral therapy); CHILD by mouth, 300 micrograms/kg daily in 2 divided doses *or* by intravenous infusion over 24 hours, 75–100 micrograms/kg daily for up to max. 7 days (then transfer to oral therapy)

Heart transplantation (with or without antibody induction) starting within 5 days of transplantation, by mouth, 75 micrograms/kg daily in 2 divided doses *or* by intravenous infusion over 24 hours, 10–20 micrograms/kg daily for up to max. 7 days (then transfer to oral therapy); CHILD, without antibody induction, initially by intravenous infusion over 24 hours, 30–50 micrograms/kg daily, then by mouth, 300 micrograms/kg daily in 2 divided doses as soon as clinically possible (give 8–12 hours after discontinuing intravenous infusion); following antibody induction, by mouth, 100–300 micrograms/kg daily in 2 divided doses

Maintenance treatment, dose adjusted according to response

Rejection therapy, seek specialist advice

**Important** *Prograf®* and *Advagraf®* are not interchangeable (see MHRA/CHM advice, above); tacrolimus trough levels should be measured before conversion and within 2 weeks of conversion to *Advagraf®*, and if necessary dose adjustment made to maintain similar systemic exposure

▲**Modified release**
**Advagraf®** (Astellas) PoM

Capsules, m/r, tacrolimus 500 micrograms (yellow/orange), net price 50-cap pack = £40.57; 1 mg (white/orange), 50-cap pack = £81.14, 100-cap pack =

**8**

**Malignant disease and immunosuppression**

£162.28; 3 mg (orange), 50-cap pack = £243.42; 5 mg (red/orange), 50-cap pack = £405.71. Label: 23, 25, counselling, driving

**Dose** Liver transplantation, starting 12–18 hours after transplantation, by mouth, 100–200 micrograms/kg once daily in the morning

Renal transplantation, starting within 24 hours of transplantation, by mouth, 200–300 micrograms/kg once daily in the morning

Rejection therapy, seek specialist advice

CHILD not recommended

**Important** *Prograf®* and *Advagraf®* are not interchangeable (see MHRA/CHM advice, p. 497); tacrolimus trough levels should be measured before conversion and within 2 weeks of conversion to *Advagraf®*, and if necessary dose adjustment made to maintain similar systemic exposure

## 8.2.3 Rituximab and alemtuzumab

**Rituximab** is a monoclonal antibody which causes lysis of B lymphocytes. It is licensed for the treatment of chemotherapy-resistant or relapsed stage III–IV follicular non-Hodgkin's lymphoma and, in combination with other chemotherapy, for previously untreated stage III–IV follicular lymphoma (see NICE guidance below), and for first-line treatment of chronic lymphocytic leukaemia. Rituximab is also licensed for maintenance therapy in patients with relapsed or refractory follicular non-Hodgkin's lymphoma that has responded to induction therapy with chemotherapy (with or without rituximab) (see NICE guidance below). It is also licensed for use in combination with other chemotherapy for the treatment of diffuse large B-cell non-Hodgkin's lymphoma (see NICE guidance below). Full resuscitation facilities should be at hand and as with other cytotoxics, treatment should be undertaken under the close supervision of a specialist. See section 10.1.3 for the role of rituximab in rheumatoid arthritis.

Rituximab should be used with caution in patients receiving cardiotoxic chemotherapy or with a history of cardiovascular disease because exacerbation of angina, arrhythmia, and heart failure have been reported. Transient hypotension occurs frequently during infusion and antihypertensives may need to be withheld for 12 hours before infusion. Patients should be monitored for neurological deficits; if progressive multifocal leucoencephalopathy is suspected, suspend treatment until excluded.

Infusion-related side-effects (including cytokine release syndrome) are reported commonly with rituximab and occur predominantly during the first infusion; they include fever and chills, nausea and vomiting, allergic reactions (such as rash, pruritus, angioedema, bronchospasm and dyspnoea), flushing and tumour pain. Patients should be given an analgesic and an antihistamine before each dose of rituximab to reduce these effects. Premedication with a corticosteroid should also be considered. The infusion may have to be stopped temporarily and the infusion-related effects treated—consult product literature for appropriate management. Evidence of pulmonary infiltration and features of tumour lysis syndrome should be sought if infusion-related effects occur.

Fatalities following **severe** cytokine release syndrome (characterised by severe dyspnoea) and associated with features of tumour lysis syndrome have occurred 1–2 hours after infusion of rituximab. Patients with a high

tumour burden as well as those with pulmonary insufficiency or infiltration are at increased risk and should be monitored **very closely** (and a slower rate of infusion considered).

> **NICE guidance**
>
> **Rituximab for the treatment of follicular lymphoma (September 2006)**
>
> Rituximab, in combination with cyclophosphamide, vincristine, and prednisolone is an option for the treatment of symptomatic stage III and IV follicular lymphoma in previously untreated patients.

> **NICE guidance**
>
> **Rituximab for the treatment of relapsed or refractory stage III or IV follicular non-Hodgkin's lymphoma (February 2008)**
>
> Rituximab, in combination with chemotherapy, is an option for the induction of remission in patients with relapsed stage III or IV follicular non-Hodgkin's lymphoma.
>
> Rituximab monotherapy as maintenance therapy is an option for the treatment of patients with relapsed stage III or IV follicular non-Hodgkin's lymphoma in remission induced with chemotherapy (with or without rituximab).
>
> Rituximab monotherapy is an option for the treatment of patients with relapsed or refractory stage III or IV follicular non-Hodgkin's lymphoma, when all alternative treatment options have been exhausted (that is, if there is resistance to or intolerance of chemotherapy).

> **NICE guidance**
>
> **Rituximab for aggressive non-Hodgkin's lymphoma (September 2003)**
>
> Rituximab, in combination with cyclophosphamide, doxorubicin, vincristine, and prednisolone, is recommended for first-line treatment of CD20-positive diffuse large-B-cell lymphoma at clinical stage II, III or IV.
>
> The use of rituximab for localised (stage I) disease should be limited to clinical trials.

**Alemtuzumab**, another monoclonal antibody that causes lysis of B lymphocytes, is licensed for use in patients with chronic lymphocytic leukaemia for whom fludarabine treatment is not appropriate. In common with rituximab, it causes infusion-related side-effects including cytokine release syndrome (see above) and premedication with an analgesic, an antihistamine, and a corticosteroid is recommended.

The *Scottish Medicines Consortium* (p. 3) has advised (August 2008) that alemtuzumab is accepted for restricted use within NHS Scotland for the treatment of B-cell chronic lymphocytic leukaemia (B-CLL) when fludarabine combination chemotherapy is not appropriate. Alemtuzumab is restricted to use in patients with previously untreated B-CLL, with the cytogenetic abnormality 17p-deletion.

### ALEMTUZUMAB

**Indications** see notes above

**Cautions** see notes above—for full details consult product literature

**Contra-indications** pregnancy (Appendix 4); breast-feeding (Appendix 5); for full details consult product literature

**Side-effects** see notes above—for full details (including monitoring and management of side-effects) consult product literature

**Dose**

- Consult product literature

**MabCampath®** (Bayer) ▼ PoM
Concentrate for intravenous infusion, alemtuzumab 30 mg/mL, net price 1-mL vial = £264.11

## RITUXIMAB

**Indications** see notes above; severe active rheumatoid arthritis (section 10.1.3)

**Cautions** see notes above—for full details consult product literature; pregnancy (Appendix 4)

**Contra-indications** breast-feeding (Appendix 5)

**Side-effects** see notes above—but for full details (including monitoring and management of side-effects) consult product literature

**MabThera®** (Roche) PoM
Concentrate for intravenous infusion, rituximab 10 mg/mL, net price 10-mL vial = £174.63, 50-mL vial = £873.15

## 8.2.4 Other immunomodulating drugs

### Interferon alfa

Interferon alfa has shown some antitumour effect in certain lymphomas and solid tumours. Interferon alfa preparations are also used in the treatment of chronic hepatitis B, and chronic hepatitis C ideally in combination with ribavirin (section 5.3.3). Side-effects are dose-related, but commonly include anorexia, nausea, diarrhoea, influenza-like symptoms, and lethargy. Ocular side-effects and depression (including suicidal behaviour) have also been reported. Myelosuppression may occur, particularly affecting granulocyte counts. Cardiovascular problems (hypotension, hypertension, palpitation, and arrhythmias), nephrotoxicity and hepatotoxicity have been reported. Hypertriglyceridaemia, sometimes severe, has been observed; monitoring of lipid concentration is recommended. Other side-effects include hypersensitivity reactions, thyroid abnormalities, hyperglycaemia, alopecia, psoriasiform rash, confusion, coma and seizures (usually with high doses in the elderly).

Polyethylene glycol-conjugated ('pegylated') derivatives of interferon alfa (**peginterferon alfa-2a** and **peginterferon alfa-2b**) are available; pegylation increases the persistence of the interferon in the blood. The peginterferons are licensed for the treatment of chronic hepatitis C, ideally in combination with ribavirin (see section 5.3.3). Peginterferon alfa-2a is also licensed for the treatment of chronic hepatitis B.

NICE guidance (adefovir dipivoxil and peginterferon alfa-2a for chronic hepatitis B)
See p. 353

NICE guidance (peginterferon alfa, interferon alfa, and ribavirin for chronic hepatitis C)
See p. 353

## INTERFERON ALFA

**Indications** see under preparations

**Cautions** consult product literature; hepatic impairment (avoid if severe; Appendix 2); renal impairment (avoid if severe; Appendix 3); pregnancy (Appendix 4); interactions: Appendix 1 (interferons)

**Contra-indications** consult product literature; avoid injections containing benzyl alcohol in neonates (see under preparations below); breast-feeding (Appendix 5)

**Side-effects** see notes above and consult product literature

**Dose**

- Consult product literature

**IntronA®** (Schering-Plough) PoM
Injection, interferon alfa-2b (rbe) 10 million units/mL, net price 1-mL vial = £42.35, 2.5-mL vial = £105.95. For subcutaneous injection or intravenous infusion

Injection pen, interferon alfa-2b (rbe), net price 15 million units/mL, 1.5-mL cartridge = £76.28; 25 million units/mL, 1.5-mL cartridge = £127.14; 50 million units/mL, 1.5-mL cartridge = £254.28. For subcutaneous injection

Note Each 1.5-mL multidose cartridge delivers 12 doses of 0.1 mL i.e. a total of 1.2 mL

For chronic myelogenous leukaemia (as monotherapy or in combination with cytarabine), hairy cell leukaemia, follicular lymphoma, lymph or liver metastases of carcinoid tumour, chronic hepatitis B, chronic hepatitis C, adjunct to surgery in malignant melanoma and maintenance of remission in multiple myeloma

**Roferon-A®** (Roche) PoM
Injection, interferon alfa-2a (rbe). Net price 6 million units/mL, 0.5-mL (3 million-unit) prefilled syringe = £14.48; 9 million units/mL, 0.5-mL (4.5 million-unit) prefilled syringe = £21.72; 12 million units/mL, 0.5-mL (6 million-unit) prefilled syringe = £28.95; 18 million units/mL, 0.5-mL (9 million-unit) prefilled syringe = £43.43; 36 million units/mL, 0.5-mL (18 million-unit) prefilled syringe = £86.86; 30 million units/mL, 0.6-mL (18 million-unit) cartridge = £86.86, for use with *Roferon* pen device. For subcutaneous injection (cartridges, vials, and prefilled syringes) and intramuscular injection (cartridges and vials)
Excipients include benzyl alcohol (avoid in neonates, see Excipients, p. 2)

For AIDS-related Kaposi's sarcoma, hairy cell leukaemia, chronic myelogenous leukaemia, recurrent or metastatic renal cell carcinoma, progressive cutaneous T-cell lymphoma, chronic hepatitis B and chronic hepatitis C, follicular non-Hodgkin's lymphoma, adjunct to surgery in malignant melanoma

## PEGINTERFERON ALFA

**Indications** see under preparations

**Cautions** consult product literature; hepatic impairment (Appendix 2); renal impairment (Appendix 3); pregnancy (Appendix 4); interactions: Appendix 1 (interferons)

**Contra-indications** consult product literature; breast-feeding (Appendix 5)

**Side-effects** see notes above and consult product literature

8

Malignant disease and immunosuppression

**Dose**

● Consult product literature

**Pegasys®** (Roche) ▢ᴾᵒᴹ

Injection, peginterferon alfa-2a, net price 135-microgram prefilled syringe = £109.93, 180-microgram prefilled syringe = £126.91. For subcutaneous injection

Excipients include benzyl alcohol (avoid in neonates, see Excipients, p. 2)

Combined with ribavirin for chronic hepatitis C; as monotherapy for chronic hepatitis C if ribavirin not tolerated or contra-indicated (see section 5.3.3); as monotherapy for chronic hepatitis B

**ViraferonPeg®** (Schering-Plough) ▢ᴾᵒᴹ

Injection, powder for reconstitution, peginterferon alfa-2b (rbe), net price 50-microgram vial = £62.78, 80-microgram vial = £100.44, 100-microgram vial = £125.55, 120-microgram vial = £150.66, 150-microgram vial = £188.33 (all with injection equipment and water for injections). For subcutaneous injection

Injection, prefilled pen, powder for reconstitution, peginterferon alfa-2b (rbe), net price 50-microgram pen = £67.75, 80-microgram pen = £108.40, 100-microgram pen = £135.50, 120-microgram pen = £162.60, 150-microgram pen = £203.25 (all with needles and swabs). For subcutaneous injection

Combined with ribavirin for chronic hepatitis C; as monotherapy for chronic hepatitis C if ribavirin not tolerated or contra-indicated (see section 5.3.3)

## Interferon beta

**Interferon beta** is licensed for use in patients with *relapsing, remitting multiple sclerosis* (characterised by at least two attacks of neurological dysfunction over the previous 2 or 3 years, followed by complete or incomplete recovery) who are able to walk unaided. Not all patients respond and a deterioration in the bouts has been observed in some. It is also licensed for use in patients with a single demyelinating event with an active inflammatory process, if it is severe enough to require treatment with an intravenous corticosteroid, and they are at high risk of developing multiple sclerosis. Interferon beta-1b is also licensed for use in patients with *secondary progressive multiple sclerosis* but its role in this condition has not been confirmed.

Interferon beta should not be used in those with severe depressive illness (or suicidal ideation), or in decompensated liver disease. Caution is advised in those with severe hepatic or renal impairment or a history of cardiac disorders, depressive disorders (avoid in severe depression or in those with suicidal ideation), seizures, or severe myelosupression. Patients should be monitored for signs of hepatic injury. Side-effects reported most frequently include irritation at injection site (including inflammation, hypersensitivity, necrosis) and influenza-like symptoms (fever, chills, myalgia, or malaise) but these decrease over time; nausea and vomiting occur occasionally. Other side-effects include hypersensitivity reactions (including anaphylaxis and urticaria), blood disorders, menstrual disorders, mood and personality changes, suicide attempts, confusion and convulsions; alopecia, hepatitis, and thyroid dysfunction have been reported rarely with interferon beta-1b.

**Provision of disease-modifying therapies for multiple sclerosis**
The Department of Health, the National Assembly for Wales, the Scottish Executive, the Northern Ireland Department of Health, Social Services & Public Safety, and the manufacturers have reached agreement on a risk-sharing scheme for the NHS supply of interferon beta and glatiramer acetate for multiple sclerosis. Health Service Circular (HSC 2002/004) explains how patients can participate in the scheme. It is available on the Department of Health website (www.dh.gov.uk)

## ▮ INTERFERON BETA

**Indications** see notes above and under preparations

**Cautions** see notes above and consult product literature; renal impairment (Appendix 3)

**Contra-indications** see notes above and consult product literature; hepatic impairment (Appendix 2); pregnancy (Appendix 4); breast-feeding (Appendix 5)

**Side-effects** see notes above and consult product literature

**Dose**

● Consult product literature

### ◢Interferon beta-1a

**Avonex®** (Biogen) ▢ᴾᵒᴹ

Injection, interferon beta-1a 60 micrograms (12 million units)/mL, net price 0.5-mL (30-microgram, 6 million-unit) prefilled syringe = £163.50. For intramuscular injection

Injection, powder for reconstitution, interferon beta-1a, net price 30-microgram (6 million-unit) vial with diluent = £163.50. For intramuscular injection

For relapsing, remitting multiple sclerosis or for a single demyelinating event with an active inflammatory process (if it is severe enough to require intravenous corticosteroid and patient at high risk of developing multiple sclerosis)

**Rebif®** (Serono) ▢ᴾᵒᴹ

Injection, interferon beta-1a, net price 22-microgram (6 million-unit) prefilled syringe = £48.16; 44-microgram (12 million-unit) prefilled syringe = £57.32; starter pack of 6 × 8.8–microgram (2.4 million-unit) prefilled syringes with 6 × 22–microgram (6 million-unit) prefilled syringes = £586.19. For subcutaneous injection

For relapsing, remitting multiple sclerosis

◀Interferon beta-1b

**Betaferon®** (Schering Health) [PoM]

Injection, powder for reconstitution, interferon beta-1b. Net price 300-microgram (9.6 million-unit) vial with diluent = £39.78. For subcutaneous injection

Note An autoinjector device (*Betaject® Light*) is available from Schering Health

For relapsing, remitting multiple sclerosis, for secondary progressive multiple sclerosis with active disease, or for a single demyelinating event with an active inflammatory process (if severe enough to require intravenous corticosteroid and patient at high risk of developing multiple sclerosis)

**Extavia®** (Novartis) [PoM]

Injection, powder for reconstitution, interferon beta-1b. Net price 300-microgram (9.6 million-unit) vial with diluent = £39.78. For subcutaneous injection

For relapsing, remitting multiple sclerosis, for secondary progressive multiple sclerosis with active disease, or for a single demyelinating event with an active inflammatory process (if severe enough to require intravenous corticosteroid and patient at high risk of developing multiple sclerosis)

## Interferon gamma

Interferon gamma-1b is licensed to reduce the frequency of serious infection in chronic granulomatous disease and in severe malignant osteopetrosis.

### ■ INTERFERON GAMMA-1b
(Immune interferon)

**Indications** see notes above

**Cautions** severe hepatic impairment (Appendix 2), renal impairment (Appendix 3); seizure disorders (including seizures associated with fever); cardiac disease (including ischaemia, congestive heart failure, and arrhythmias); monitor before and during treatment: haematological tests (including full blood count, differential white cell count, and platelet count), blood chemistry tests (including renal and liver function tests) and urinalysis; avoid simultaneous administration of foreign proteins including immunological products (risk of exaggerated immune response); pregnancy (Appendix 4); breast-feeding (Appendix 5); interactions: Appendix 1 (interferons)

Driving May impair ability to drive or operate machinery; effects may be enhanced by alcohol

**Side-effects** nausea, vomiting; headache, fatigue, fever; myalgia, arthralgia; rash, injection-site reactions; *rarely* confusion and systemic lupus erythematosus; also reported, neutropenia, thrombocytopenia, and raised liver enzymes

**Dose**

• See under preparations

**Immukin®** (Boehringer Ingelheim) [PoM]

Injection, recombinant human interferon gamma-1b 200 micrograms/mL, net price 0.5-mL vial = £66.67

Dose By subcutaneous injection, 50 micrograms/m² 3 times a week; patients with body surface area of 0.5 m² or less, 1.5 micrograms/kg 3 times a week; not yet recommended for children under 6 months with chronic granulomatous disease

## Aldesleukin

Aldesleukin (recombinant interleukin-2) is licensed for metastatic renal cell carcinoma; it is usually given by subcutaneous injection. It is now rarely given by intravenous infusion because of an association with a capil-

lary leak syndrome, which can cause pulmonary oedema and hypotension. Aldesleukin produces tumour shrinkage in a small proportion of patients, but it has not been shown to increase survival. Bone-marrow, hepatic, renal, thyroid, and CNS toxicity is common. It is for use in **specialist units only. Interactions:** Appendix 1 (aldesleukin)

**Proleukin®** (Novartis) [PoM]

Injection, powder for reconstitution, aldesleukin. Net price 18-million unit vial = £112.00. For subcutaneous injection

Injection, powder for reconstitution, aldesleukin. Net price 18-million unit vial = £112.00. For intravenous infusion but see notes above

For metastatic renal cell carcinoma, **excluding** patients in whom all three of the following prognostic factors are present: performance status of Eastern Co-operative Oncology Group of 1 or greater, more than one organ with metastatic disease sites, and a period of less than 24 months between initial diagnosis of primary tumour and date of evaluation of treatment.

## BCG bladder instillation

BCG (Bacillus Calmette-Guérin) is a live attenuated strain derived from *Mycobacterium bovis*. It is licensed as a bladder instillation for the treatment of primary or recurrent bladder carcinoma and for the prevention of recurrence following transurethral resection.

### ■ BACILLUS CALMETTE-GUÉRIN

**Indications** see notes above; BCG immunisation (section 14.4)

**Cautions** screen for active tuberculosis (contra-indicated if tuberculosis confirmed); traumatic catheterisation or urethral or bladder injury (delay administration until mucosal damage healed)

**Contra-indications** impaired immune response, HIV infection, urinary-tract infection, severe haematuria, tuberculosis, fever of unknown origin; pregnancy and breast-feeding

**Side-effects** cystitis, dysuria, urinary frequency, haematuria, malaise, fever, influenza-like syndrome; also systemic BCG infection (with fatalities)—consult product literature; rarely hypersensitivity reactions (such as arthralgia and rash), orchitis, transient urethral obstruction, bladder contracture, renal abscess; ocular symptoms reported

**Dose**

• Consult product literature

**ImmuCyst®** (Cambridge) [PoM]

Bladder instillation, freeze-dried powder containing attenuated *Mycobacterium bovis* prepared from the Connaught strain of bacillus of Calmette and Guérin, net price 81-mg vial = £79.23

**OncoTICE®** (Organon) [PoM]

Bladder instillation, freeze-dried powder containing attenuated *Mycobacterium bovis* prepared from the TICE strain of bacillus of Calmette and Guérin, net price 12.5-mg vial = £73.00

## Glatiramer acetate

Glatiramer is an immunomodulating drug comprising synthetic polypeptides. It is licensed for treating initial symptoms in patients at high risk of developing multiple

8

Malignant disease and immunosuppression

Malignant disease and immunosuppression

8

sclerosis, and also for reducing the frequency of relapses in ambulatory patients with relapsing-remitting multiple sclerosis who have had at least 2 clinical relapses in the past 2 years. Initiation of treatment with glatiramer should be supervised by a specialist.

> NICE guidance (interferon beta and glatiramer for multiple sclerosis)
> See p. 500

> Provision of disease-modifying therapies for multiple sclerosis
> See p. 500

## GLATIRAMER ACETATE

**Indications** see notes above

**Cautions** cardiac disorders; renal impairment (Appendix 3); breast-feeding (Appendix 5)

**Contra-indications** pregnancy (Appendix 4)

**Side-effects** hypersensitivity reactions; flushing, chest pain, palpitation, tachycardia, and dyspnoea may occur within minutes of injection; nausea, constipation, dyspepsia; syncope, anxiety, asthenia, depression, headache, tremor, sweating; oedema, lymphadenopathy; hypertonia, back pain, arthralgia, influenza-like symptoms; injection-site reactions, rash; *rarely* seizures

**Dose**

- By subcutaneous injection, ADULT over 18 years, 20 mg daily

**Copaxone®** (Teva) PoM

Injection, glatiramer acetate 20 mg/mL, net price 1-mL prefilled syringe = £18.73

## Lenalidomide and thalidomide

**Lenalidomide** is an immunomodulating drug with antineoplastic, anti-angiogenic, and pro-erythropoietic properties. It is licensed, in combination with dexamethasone, for the treatment of multiple myeloma in patients who have received at least one previous therapy.

The most serious side-effects of lenalidomide are venous thromboembolism and severe neutropenia. Lenalidomide is structurally related to thalidomide and there is a risk of teratogenesis.

> NICE Guidance
> **Lenalidomide for the treatment of multiple myeloma** (June 2009)
> Lenalidomide in combination with dexamethasone is an option for the treatment of multiple myeloma in patients who have received two or more prior therapies. The drug cost of lenalidomide will be met by the manufacturer for patients who remain on treatment for more than 26 cycles.

**Thalidomide** is used in combination with melphalan and prednisolone as first-line treatment for untreated multiple myeloma, in patients aged 65 years and over, or for those not eligible for high-dose chemotherapy (for example, patients with significant co-morbidity such as cardiac risk factors). It has immunomodulatory and anti-

inflammatory activity. Thalidomide can cause drowsiness, constipation, and on prolonged use peripheral neuropathy.

**Pregnancy** For women of child-bearing potential, pregnancy must be excluded before starting treatment (perform pregnancy test on initiation or within 3 days prior to initiation). Women must practise effective contraception at least 1 month before, during, and for at least 1 month after treatment (oral combined hormonal contraceptives and copper-releasing intrauterine devices not recommended) and men should use condoms during treatment and for at least 1 week after stopping. Women must be registered with a pregnancy prevention programme.

## LENALIDOMIDE

**Indications** see notes above

**Cautions** see notes above; monitor full blood count (including differential white cell count and platelet count) before treatment and every week for the first 8 weeks then every 4 weeks (reduce dose or interrupt treatment if neutropenia or thrombocytopenia develop—consult product literature); concomitant drugs that increase the risk of thromboembolism; high tumour burden—risk of tumour lysis syndrome, see p. 466; monitor thyroid function; renal impairment (Appendix 3); **interactions**: Appendix 1 (lenalidomide)

Thromboembolism Patients and their carers should be made aware of the symptoms of thromboembolism and advised to report sudden breathlessness, chest pain, or swelling of a limb

Neutropenia and thrombocytopenia Patients and their carers should be made aware of the symptoms of neutropenia and advised to seek medical advice if symptoms suggestive of neutropenia (such as fever, sore throat) or of thrombocytopenia (such as bleeding) develop

**Contra-indications** pregnancy (**important teratogenic risk**: see notes above and Appendix 4); breast-feeding (Appendix 5)

**Side-effects** hypotension, deep vein thrombosis; pneumonia, dyspnoea; tremor, hypoaesthesia, fatigue, asthenia; neutropenia, thrombocytopenia, anaemia, lymphopenia, leucopenia; muscle cramp; pruritus, rash; *rarely* Stevens-Johnson syndrome and toxic epidermal necrolysis

**Dose**

- ADULT over 18 years, 25 mg once daily for 21 consecutive days of a 28-day cycle; for doses of dexamethasone, consult product literature

**Revlimid®** (Celgene) ▼ PoM

Capsules, lenalidomide, 5 mg (white), net price 21-cap pack = £3570.00; 10 mg (blue/yellow), 21-cap pack = £3780.00; 15 mg (blue/white), 21-cap pack = £3969.00; 25 mg (white), 21-cap pack = £4368.00. Label: 25, counselling, symptoms of thromboembolism, neutropenia, or thrombocytopenia, patient information leaflet

Note Patient, prescriber, and supplying pharmacy must be registered with Celgene Ltd and comply with a pregnancy prevention programme

## THALIDOMIDE

**Indications** see notes above

**Cautions** see notes above; concomitant drugs which increase risk of peripheral neuropathy or thromboembolism; hepatic impairment (Appendix 2); renal impairment (Appendix 3)

**Thromboembolism** Thromboprophylaxis is recommended for at least the first 5 months of treatment, especially in patients with additional thrombotic risk factors. Patients and their carers should be made aware of the symptoms of thromboembolism and advised to report sudden breathlessness, chest pain, or swelling of a limb

**Peripheral neuropathy** Monitor patients for signs and symptoms of peripheral neuropathy; patients and their carers should be advised to seek medical advice if symptoms such as paraesthesia, abnormal coordination, or weakness develop. Dose reduction, dose interruption, or treatment discontinuation may be necessary—consult product literature. Patients with pre-existing peripheral neuropathy should not be treated with thalidomide unless the potential clinical benefits outweigh the risk

**Contra-indications** pregnancy (**important teratogenic risk**: see notes above and Appendix 4); breast-feeding (Appendix 5)

**Side-effects** vomiting, dry mouth, dyspepsia, constipation; bradycardia, cardiac failure, deep vein thrombosis; dyspnoea, interstitial lung disease, pulmonary embolism, peripheral oedema; asthenia, confusion, depression, dizziness, drowsiness, peripheral neuropathy, dysaesthesia, paraesthesia, syncope, tremor; pyrexia; pneumonia; anaemia, leucopenia, neutropenia, lymphopenia, thrombocytopenia; skin reactions including Stevens-Johnson syndrome; *also reported* toxic epidermal necrolysis, intestinal obstruction, hypothyroidism, and sexual dysfunction

**Dose**
- ADULT over 18 years, 200 mg once daily at bedtime for 6-week cycle; max. 12 cycles

**Thalidomide Pharmion®** (Celgene) ▼ [PoM]
Capsules, thalidomide 50 mg, net price 28-cap pack = £298.48. Label: 2, counselling, symptoms of peripheral neuropathy and thromboembolism (see above)
Note Patient, prescriber, and supplying pharmacy must be registered with Celgene Ltd and comply with a pregnancy prevention programme

# Natalizumab

**Natalizumab** is a monoclonal antibody that inhibits the migration of leucocytes into the central nervous system, hence reducing inflammation and demyelination. It is licensed for use in patients with highly active *relapsing-remitting multiple sclerosis* despite treatment with interferon beta or those with rapidly evolving severe relapsing-remitting multiple sclerosis. Treatment with natalizumab should be initiated and supervised by a specialist.

Natalizumab is associated with an increased risk of opportunistic infection and progressive multifocal leucoencephalopathy (PML). Patients should be monitored for new or worsening neurological symptoms or signs of PML—treatment should be suspended until PML has been excluded. If a patient develops an opportunistic infection or PML, natalizumab should be permanently discontinued.

Infusion-related side-effects include nausea, vomiting, flushing, headache, dizziness, fatigue, rigors, pyrexia, arthralgia, urticaria, and pruritus. Patients should be observed for hypersensitivity reactions, including anaphylaxis, during the infusion and for 1 hour after completion of the infusion. Natalizumab should be dis-

continued permanently if hypersensitivity reaction occurs.

The *Scottish Medicines Consortium* has advised (August 2007) that natalizumab is accepted for restricted use as single disease-modifying therapy in highly active relapsing-remitting multiple sclerosis only in patients with rapidly evolving severe relapsing-remitting multiple sclerosis defined by 2 or more disabling relapses in 1 year and with 1 or more gadolinium-enhancing lesions on brain magnetic resonance imaging (MRI) or a significant increase in T2 lesion load compared with a previous MRI.

> **NICE guidance**
> **Natalizumab for the treatment of adults with highly active relapsing-remitting multiple sclerosis (August 2007)**
> Natalizumab is an option for the treatment only of rapidly evolving severe relapsing-remitting multiple sclerosis (RES). RES is defined by 2 or more disabling relapses in 1 year, and 1 or more gadolinium-enhancing lesions on brain magnetic resonance imaging (MRI) or a significant increase in T2 lesion load compared with a previous MRI. Patients currently receiving natalizumab who do not meet the above criteria, should have the option to continue therapy until they and their consultants consider it appropriate to stop.

## ■ NATALIZUMAB

**Indications** see notes above

**Cautions** see notes above and consult product literature; prior treatment with immunosuppressants; monitor liver function (see below)
**Liver toxicity** Liver dysfunction reported; advise patients to seek immediate medical attention if symptoms such as jaundice or dark urine develop; discontinue treatment if significant liver injury occurs
**Progressive multifocal leucoencephalopathy (PML)** Patients should be given an alert card which includes information about the symptoms of PML; see also notes above
**Hypersensitivity reactions** Patients should be told the importance of uninterrupted dosing, particularly in the early months of treatment (intermittent therapy may increase risk of sensitisation)

**Contra-indications** progressive multifocal leucoencephalopathy; active infection (see notes above); concurrent use of interferon beta or glatiramer acetate; immunosuppression; active malignancies (except cutaneous basal cell carcinoma); pregnancy (Appendix 4); breast-feeding (Appendix 5)

**Side-effects** see notes above; also urinary-tract infection, nasopharyngitis, autoantibodies, and arthralgia; *less commonly* hypersensitivity reactions (see above); liver toxicity also reported

**Dose**
- By intravenous infusion, ADULT over 18 years, 300 mg once every 4 weeks; discontinue if no response after 6 months

**Tysabri®** (Biogen) ▼ [PoM]
Concentrate for intravenous infusion, natalizumab 20 mg/mL, net price 15-mL vial = £1130.00. Counselling, liver toxicity, progressive multifocal leucoencephalopathy, and hypersensitivity, patient alert card

# 8.3 Sex hormones and hormone antagonists in malignant disease

8.3.1 Oestrogens
8.3.2 Progestogens
8.3.3 Androgens
8.3.4 Hormone antagonists

Hormonal manipulation has an important role in the treatment of breast, prostate, and endometrial cancer, and a more marginal role in the treatment of hypernephroma. These treatments are not curative, but may provide excellent palliation of symptoms in selected patients, sometimes for a period of years. Tumour response, and treatment toxicity should be carefully monitored and treatment changed if progression occurs or side-effects exceed benefit.

## 8.3.1 Oestrogens

**Diethylstilbestrol** (stilboestrol) is sometimes used to treat prostate cancer, but it is not usually used first-line because of its side-effects. It is occasionally used in postmenopausal women with breast cancer. Toxicity is common and dose-related side-effects include nausea, fluid retention, and venous and arterial thrombosis. Impotence and gynaecomastia always occur in men, and withdrawal bleeding may be a problem in women. Hypercalcaemia and bone pain may also occur in breast cancer.

**Ethinylestradiol** (ethinyloestradiol) is the most potent oestrogen available; unlike other oestrogens it is only slowly metabolised in the liver. Ethinylestradiol is licensed for the palliative treatment of prostate cancer.

### DIETHYLSTILBESTROL
(Stilbestrol)

**Indications** see notes above

**Cautions** cardiovascular disease

**Contra-indications** hepatic impairment (Appendix 2)

**Side-effects** sodium retention with oedema, thromboembolism, jaundice, feminising effects in men; see also notes above

**Dose**
- Breast cancer, 10–20 mg daily
- Prostate cancer, 1–3 mg daily

**Diethylstilbestrol** (Non-proprietary)
Tablets, diethylstilbestrol 1 mg, net price 28 = £39.05; 5 mg, 28 = £192.73

### ETHINYLESTRADIOL
(Ethinyloestradiol)

**Indications** see notes above; other indications (section 6.4.1.1)

**Cautions** see section 6.4.1.1; **interactions:** Appendix 1 (oestrogens)

**Contra-indications** see section 6.4.1.1

**Side-effects** see section 6.4.1.1

**Dose**
- Prostate cancer (palliative), 0.15–1.5 mg daily

**Preparations**
Section 6.4.1.1

## 8.3.2 Progestogens

Progestogens have a role in the treatment of endometrial cancer; their use in breast cancer and renal cell cancer has declined. Progestogens are now rarely used to treat prostate cancer. **Medroxyprogesterone** or **megestrol** are usually chosen and can be given orally; high-dose or parenteral treatment cannot be recommended. Side-effects are mild but may include nausea, fluid retention, and weight gain.

### MEDROXYPROGESTERONE ACETATE

**Indications** see notes above; contraception (section 7.3.2.2); other indications (section 6.4.1.2)

**Cautions** see section 6.4.1.2 and notes above; **interactions:** Appendix 1 (progestogens)

**Contra-indications** see section 6.4.1.2 and notes above

**Side-effects** see section 6.4.1.2 and notes above; glucocorticoid effects at high dose may lead to a cushingoid syndrome

**Dose**
- See preparations below

**Provera®** (Pharmacia)
Tablets, medroxyprogesterone acetate 100 mg (scored), net price 60-tab pack = £29.98, 100-tab pack = £49.94; 200 mg (scored), 30-tab pack = £29.65, 400 mg, 30-tab pack = £58.67
**Dose** endometrial and renal cell cancer, 200–400 mg daily; breast cancer, 400–800 mg daily

Tablets, medroxyprogesterone acetate 2.5 mg, 5 mg and 10 mg, see section 6.4.1.2

### MEGESTROL ACETATE

**Indications** see notes above

**Cautions** see under Medroxyprogesterone acetate (section 6.4.1.2) and notes above; **interactions:** Appendix 1 (progestogens)

**Contra-indications** see under Medroxyprogesterone acetate (section 6.4.1.2) and notes above

**Side-effects** see under Medroxyprogesterone acetate (section 6.4.1.2) and notes above

**Dose**
- Breast cancer, 160 mg daily in single or divided doses
- Endometrial cancer, 40–320 mg daily in divided doses

**Megace®** (Bristol-Myers Squibb)
Tablets, scored, megestrol acetate 160 mg (off-white), 30-tab pack = £19.91

### NORETHISTERONE

**Indications** see notes above; other indications (section 6.4.1.2)

**Cautions** see section 6.4.1.2 and notes above; **interactions:** Appendix 1 (progestogens)

**Contra-indications** see section 6.4.1.2 and notes above

**Side-effects** see section 6.4.1.2 and notes above

**Dose**

- Breast cancer, 40 mg daily, increased to 60 mg daily if required

◢**Preparations**
Section 6.4.1.2

## 8.3.3 Androgens

Testosterone esters (section 6.4.2) have largely been superseded by other drugs for breast cancer.

## 8.3.4 Hormone antagonists

### 8.3.4.1 Breast cancer

The management of patients with breast cancer involves surgery, radiotherapy, drug therapy, or a combination of these.

For operable breast cancer, treatment before surgery (neoadjuvant therapy) reduces the size of the tumour and facilitates breast-conserving surgery; hormone antagonist therapy (e.g. letrozole) is chosen for steroid hormone-receptor-positive breast cancer and chemotherapy for steroid hormone-receptor-negative tumours or for younger women.

**Early breast cancer** All women should be considered for adjuvant therapy following surgical removal of the tumour. Adjuvant therapy is used to eradicate the micrometastases that cause relapses. Choice of adjuvant treatment is determined by the risk of recurrence, steroid hormone-receptor status of the primary tumour, and menopausal status.

Adjuvant therapy comprises either cytotoxic chemotherapy or hormone-antagonist therapy. Women with steroid hormone-receptor-positive breast cancer are considered for hormone-antagonist therapy (preceded by cytotoxic chemotherapy if necessary) whilst women with steroid hormone-receptor-negative breast cancer should be considered for cytotoxic chemotherapy.

The oestrogen-receptor antagonist **tamoxifen** is effective in premenopausal, perimenopausal, and postmenopausal women. The aromatase inhibitors **anastrozole**, **exemestane**, and **letrozole** are effective in postmenopausal women **only**. Adjuvant hormone antagonist therapy reduces the risk of cancer in the other breast and should generally be continued for 5 years following removal of the tumour. In those considered for extended adjuvant therapy, 5 years of tamoxifen is followed by an aromatase inhibitor such as letrozole for a further 3 years.

Trastuzumab is licensed for use in early breast cancer which overexpresses human epidermal growth factor-2 (HER2) in women who have received surgery, chemotherapy and radiotherapy (as appropriate).

Premenopausal women may also benefit from treatment with a gonadorelin analogue or ovarian ablation.

**Advanced breast cancer** Tamoxifen is used in postmenopausal women with oestrogen-receptor-positive tumours, long disease-free interval following treatment for early breast cancer, and disease limited to bone or soft tissues. However, aromatase inhibitors, such as anastrozole or letrozole, may be more effective and are regarded as preferred treatment in postmenopausal women. Ovarian ablation or the gonadorelin analogue goserelin (*Zoladex*®) (section 8.3.4.2) should be considered in premenopausal women.

Progestogens such as medroxyprogesterone acetate continue to have a role in postmenopausal women with advanced breast cancer. They are as effective as tamoxifen, but they are not as well tolerated; they are less effective than the aromatase inhibitors.

Cytotoxic chemotherapy is preferred for advanced steroid hormone-receptor-negative tumours and for aggressive disease, particularly where metastases involve visceral sites (e.g. the liver) or where the disease-free interval following treatment for early breast cancer is short.

**Chemoprevention** Recent evidence suggests that tamoxifen prophylaxis can reduce breast cancer in women at high risk of the disease. However, the adverse effects of tamoxifen preclude its routine use in most women.

**Cytotoxic drugs used in breast cancer** An anthracycline combined with fluorouracil (section 8.1.3) and cyclophosphamide (section 8.1.1), and sometimes also with methotrexate (section 8.1.3) is effective. Cyclophosphamide, methotrexate, and fluorouracil can be useful if an anthracycline is inappropriate (e.g. in cardiac disease).

**Metastatic disease** The choice of chemotherapy regimen will be influenced by whether the patient has previously received adjuvant treatment and the presence of any co-morbidity.

For women who have not previously received chemotherapy, an anthracycline such as doxorubicin or epirubicin combined with cyclophosphamide is the standard initial therapy for metastatic breast disease.

Patients with anthracycline-refractory or resistant disease should be considered for treatment with a taxane (section 8.1.5) either alone or in combination with trastuzumab if they have tumours that overexpress HER2. Other cytotoxic drugs with activity against breast cancer include capecitabine (section 8.1.3), mitoxantrone, mitomycin (both section 8.1.2), and vinorelbine (section 8.1.4). Trastuzumab alone (section 8.1.5) is an option for chemotherapy-resistant cancers that overexpress HER2.

**Oestrogen-receptor antagonists** Tamoxifen is an oestrogen-receptor antagonist that is licensed for breast cancer and anovulatory infertility (section 6.5.1).

**Fulvestrant** is licensed for the treatment of oestrogen-receptor-positive metastatic or locally advanced breast cancer in postmenopausal women in whom disease progresses or relapses while on, or after, other anti-oestrogen therapy.

**Toremifene** is licensed for steroid hormone-receptor-positive metastatic breast cancer in postmenopausal women, but it is not often used.

**Aromatase inhibitors** Aromatase inhibitors act predominantly by blocking the conversion of androgens to oestrogens in the peripheral tissues. They do not inhibit ovarian oestrogen synthesis and should not be used in premenopausal women.

**Anastrozole** and **letrozole** are non-steroidal aromatase inhibitors; **exemestane** is a steroidal aromatase inhibitor. Anastrozole and letrozole are at least as effective as tamoxifen for first-line treatment of metastatic breast cancer in postmenopausal women. However, it is not yet known whether the benefits of aromatase inhibitors persist over the long term.

The *Scottish Medicines Consortium* (p. 3) has advised (August 2005 and October 2006) that anastrozole (*Arimidex®*) is accepted for restricted use within NHS Scotland, within the licensed indications, for early breast cancer and early invasive breast cancer.

The *Scottish Medicines Consortium* (p. 3) has advised (October 2005) that exemestane (*Aromasin®*) is accepted for restricted use within NHS Scotland as an adjuvant treatment in postmenopausal women with oestrogen-receptor-positive invasive early breast cancer, following 2–3 years of initial adjuvant tamoxifen therapy.

**Gonadorelin analogues** Goserelin (section 8.3.4.2), a gonadorelin analogue is licensed for the management of advanced breast cancer in premenopausal women.

**Other drugs used in breast cancer** Trilostane (section 6.7.3) is licensed for postmenopausal breast cancer. It is quite well tolerated but diarrhoea and abdominal discomfort may be a problem. Trilostane causes adrenal hypofunction and corticosteroid replacement therapy is needed.

The use of **bisphosphonates** (section 6.6.2) in patients with metastatic breast cancer may reduce pain and prevent skeletal complications of bone metastases.

## ANASTROZOLE

**Indications** adjuvant treatment of oestrogen-receptor-positive early invasive breast cancer in postmenopausal women; adjuvant treatment of oestrogen-receptor-positive early breast cancer in postmenopausal women following 2–3 years of tamoxifen therapy; advanced breast cancer in postmenopausal women which is oestrogen-receptor-positive or responsive to tamoxifen

**Cautions** laboratory test for menopause if doubt; susceptibility to osteoporosis (assess bone mineral density before treatment and at regular intervals)

**Contra-indications** pregnancy and breast-feeding; moderate or severe hepatic disease; moderate or severe renal impairment; not for premenopausal women

**Side-effects** hot flushes, vaginal dryness, vaginal bleeding, hair thinning, anorexia, nausea, vomiting, diarrhoea, headache, arthralgia, bone fractures, rash (including Stevens-Johnson syndrome); asthenia and drowsiness—may initially affect ability to drive or operate machinery; slight increases in total cholesterol levels reported; very rarely allergic reactions including angioedema and anaphylaxis

**Dose**

- 1 mg daily

**Arimidex®** (AstraZeneca) ▣PoM

Tablets, f/c, anastrozole 1 mg. Net price 28-tab pack = £68.56

## ▉ EXEMESTANE

**Indications** adjuvant treatment of oestrogen-receptor-positive early breast cancer in postmenopausal women following 2–3 years of tamoxifen therapy; advanced breast cancer in postmenopausal women in whom anti-oestrogen therapy has failed

**Cautions** hepatic impairment (Appendix 2); renal impairment (Appendix 3); **interactions:** Appendix 1 (exemestane)

**Contra-indications** pregnancy and breast-feeding; not indicated for premenopausal women

**Side-effects** nausea, vomiting, abdominal pain, dyspepsia, constipation, anorexia; dizziness, fatigue, headache, depression, insomnia; hot flushes, sweating; alopecia, rash; *less commonly* drowsiness, asthenia, and peripheral oedema; *rarely* thrombocytopenia, leucopenia

**Dose**

- 25 mg daily

**Aromasin®** (Pharmacia) ▣PoM

Tablets, s/c, exemestane 25 mg, net price 30-tab pack = £88.80, 90-tab pack = £266.40. Label: 21

## ▉ FULVESTRANT

**Indications** treatment of oestrogen-receptor-positive metastatic or locally advanced breast cancer in postmenopausal women in whom disease progresses or relapses while on, or after, other anti-oestrogen therapy

**Cautions** hepatic impairment (avoid if severe; Appendix 2)

**Contra-indications** pregnancy (Appendix 4); breast-feeding (Appendix 5)

**Side-effects** hot flushes, nausea, vomiting, diarrhoea, anorexia, headache, back pain, rash, asthenia, venous thromboembolism, injection-site reactions, urinary-tract infections; less commonly vaginal haemorrhage, vaginal candidiasis, leucorrhoea, hypersensitivity reactions including angioedema, urticaria

**Dose**

- By deep intramuscular injection, 250 mg into gluteal muscle every 4 weeks

**Faslodex®** (AstraZeneca) ▣PoM

Injection (oily), fulvestrant 50 mg/mL, net price 5-mL (250-mg) prefilled syringe = £348.27

## ▉ LETROZOLE

**Indications** adjuvant treatment of oestrogen-receptor-positive early breast cancer in postmenopausal women; advanced breast cancer in postmenopausal women (including those in whom other anti-oestrogen therapy has failed); early invasive breast cancer in postmenopausal women after standard adjuvant tamoxifen therapy; pre-operative treatment in postmenopausal women with localised hormone-receptor-positive breast cancer to allow subsequent breast conserving surgery

**Cautions** renal impairment (Appendix 3); susceptibility to osteoporosis (assess bone mineral density before treatment and at regular intervals)

**Contra-indications** severe hepatic impairment; not indicated for premenopausal women; pregnancy (Appendix 4) and breast-feeding

**Side-effects** hot flushes, nausea, vomiting, fatigue, dizziness, headache, dyspepsia, constipation, diarrhoea, depression, anorexia, appetite increase, hypercholesterolaemia, alopecia, increased sweating, rash, peripheral oedema, musculoskeletal pain, osteoporosis, bone fracture; *less commonly* hypertension, palpitation, tachycardia, dyspnoea, cough, drowsiness, insomnia, anxiety, memory impairment, dysaesthesia, taste disturbance, pruritus, dry skin, urticaria, thrombophlebitis, abdominal pain, urinary frequency, urinary-tract infection, vaginal bleeding, vaginal discharge, breast pain, pyrexia, mucosal dryness, stomatitis, cataract, eye irritation, blurred vision, tumour pain, arthritis, leucopenia, general oedema; *rarely* pulmonary embolism, arterial thrombosis, cerebrovascular infarction

**Dose**

● 2.5 mg daily

**Femara®** (Novartis) ℗ℴ𝓜

Tablets, f/c, letrozole 2.5 mg. Net price 14-tab pack = £41.58, 28-tab pack = £66.50

### ▌ TAMOXIFEN

**Indications** see under Dose and notes above; mastalgia [unlicensed indication] (section 6.7.2)

**Cautions** occasional cystic ovarian swellings in premenopausal women; increased risk of thromboembolic events, especially when used with cytotoxics (see also below); breast-feeding (Appendix 5); endometrial changes (**important:** see below); porphyria, **interactions:** Appendix 1 (tamoxifen)

Endometrial changes Increased endometrial changes, including hyperplasia, polyps, cancer, and uterine sarcoma reported; prompt investigation required if abnormal vaginal bleeding including menstrual irregularities, vaginal discharge, and pelvic pain or pressure in those receiving (or who have received) tamoxifen.

**Contra-indications** pregnancy (Appendix 4); treatment of infertility contra-indicated if personal or family history of idiopathic venous thromboembolism or genetic predisposition to thromboembolism

**Side-effects** hot flushes, vaginal bleeding and vaginal discharge (**important:** see also Endometrial Changes under Cautions), suppression of menstruation in some premenopausal women, pruritus vulvae, gastrointestinal disturbances, headache, light-headedness, tumour flare, decreased platelet counts; occasionally oedema, rarely hypercalcaemia if bony metastases, alopecia, rashes, uterine fibroids; also visual disturbances (including corneal changes, cataracts, retinopathy); leucopenia (sometimes with anaemia and thrombocytopenia), rarely neutropenia; hypertriglyceridaemia reported rarely (sometimes with pancreatitis); thromboembolic events reported (see below); liver enzyme changes (rarely fatty liver, cholestasis, hepatitis); rarely interstitial pneumonitis, hypersensitivity reactions including angioedema, Stevens-Johnson syndrome, bullous pemphigoid; see also notes above

Risk of thromboembolism Tamoxifen can increase the risk of thromboembolism particularly during and immediately after major surgery or periods of immobility (consider

interrupting treatment to initiate anticoagulant measures). Patients should be made aware of the symptoms of thromboembolism and advised to report sudden breathlessness and any pain in the calf of one leg

**Dose**

● Breast cancer, 20 mg daily

CSM advice The CSM has advised that tamoxifen in a dose of 20 mg daily substantially increases survival in early breast cancer, and that no further benefit has been demonstrated with higher doses. Patients should be told of the small risk of endometrial cancer (see under Cautions above) and encouraged to report relevant symptoms early. They can, however, be reassured that the benefits of treatment far outweigh the risks

● Anovulatory infertility, 20 mg daily on days 2, 3, 4 and 5 of cycle; if necessary the daily dose may be increased to 40 mg then 80 mg for subsequent courses; if cycles irregular, start initial course on any day, with subsequent course starting 45 days later *or* on day 2 of cycle if menstruation occurs

**Tamoxifen** (Non-proprietary) ℗ℴ𝓜

Tablets, tamoxifen (as citrate) 10 mg, net price 30-tab pack = £1.84; 20 mg, 30-tab pack = £1.95; 40 mg, 30-tab pack = £6.71

Oral solution, tamoxifen (as citrate) 10 mg/5 mL, net price 150 mL = £29.61
Brands include *Soltamox®*

**Nolvadex-D®** (AstraZeneca) ℗ℴ𝓜

Tablets, tamoxifen (as citrate) 20 mg, net-price 30-tab pack = £1.90

### ▌ TOREMIFENE

**Indications** hormone-dependent metastatic breast cancer in postmenopausal women

**Cautions** hypercalcaemia may occur (especially if bone metastases and usually at beginning of treatment); avoid in acute porphyria (but see section 9.8.2); history of severe thromboembolic disease; **interactions:** Appendix 1 (toremifene)

Endometrial changes Increased endometrial changes, including hyperplasia, polyps and cancer reported. Abnormal vaginal bleeding including menstrual irregularities, vaginal discharge and symptoms such as pelvic pain or pressure should be promptly investigated

**Contra-indications** endometrial hyperplasia, severe hepatic impairment (Appendix 2); pregnancy and breast-feeding; QT prolongation (avoid concomitant administration of drugs that prolong QT interval), electrolyte disturbances (particularly uncorrected hypokalaemia), bradycardia, heart failure with reduced left-ventricular ejection fraction, history of arrhythmias

**Side-effects** nausea, vomiting; oedema; depression, dizziness, fatigue; sweating, hot flushes, vaginal bleeding or discharge (**important:** see Cautions); rash; *less commonly* anorexia, constipation, increased weight, thromboembolic events, dyspnoea, insomnia, headache, endometrial hypertrophy; *very rarely* jaundice, transient corneal opacity, and alopecia

**Dose**

● 60 mg daily

**Fareston®** (Orion) ℗ℴ𝓜

Tablets, toremifene (as citrate) 60 mg. Net price 30-tab pack = £29.52

**8.3.4.2  Gonadorelin analogues and gonadotrophin-releasing hormone antagonists**

Metastatic cancer of the prostate usually responds to hormonal treatment aimed at androgen depletion. Standard treatments include bilateral subcapsular orchidectomy or use of a gonadorelin analogue (**buserelin**, **goserelin**, **leuprorelin**, or **triptorelin**). The gonadotrophin-releasing hormone antagonist, **degarelix**, (p. 510) is also available. Response in most patients lasts for 12 to 18 months. No entirely satisfactory therapy exists for disease progression despite this treatment (hormone-refractory prostate cancer), but occasional patients respond to other hormone manipulation e.g. with an anti-androgen. Bone disease can often be palliated with irradiation or, if widespread, with strontium or prednisolone (section 6.3.2).

## Gonadorelin analogues

Gonadorelin analogues are as effective as orchidectomy or **diethylstilbestrol** (section 8.3.1) but are expensive and require parenteral administration, at least initially. They cause initial stimulation then depression of luteinising hormone release by the pituitary. During the initial stage (1–2 weeks) increased production of testosterone may be associated with progression of prostate cancer. In susceptible patients this tumour 'flare' may cause spinal cord compression, ureteric obstruction or increased bone pain. When such problems are anticipated, alternative treatments (e.g. orchidectomy) or concomitant use of an anti-androgen such as cyproterone acetate or flutamide (see below) are recommended; anti-androgen treatment should be started 3 days before the gonadorelin analogue and continued for 3 weeks. Gonadorelin analogues are also used in women for breast cancer (section 8.3.4.1) and other indications (section 6.7.2).

**Cautions** Men at risk of tumour 'flare' (see above) should be monitored closely during the first month of therapy. Caution is required in patients with metabolic bone disease because reduced bone mineral density can occur. The injection site should be rotated.

**Side-effects** The gonadorelin analogues cause side-effects similar to the menopause in women and orchidectomy in men and include hot flushes and sweating, sexual dysfunction, vaginal dryness or bleeding, and gynaecomastia or changes in breast size. Signs and symptoms of prostate or breast cancer may worsen initially (managed in prostate cancer with anti-androgens, see above). Other side-effects include hypersensitivity reactions (rashes, pruritus, asthma, and rarely anaphylaxis), injection site reactions (see Cautions), headache (rarely migraine), visual disturbances, dizziness, arthralgia and possibly myalgia, hair loss, peripheral oedema, gastro-intestinal disturbances, weight changes, sleep disorders, and mood changes.

## Anti-androgens

**Cyproterone acetate**, **flutamide** and **bicalutamide** are anti-androgens that inhibit the tumour 'flare' which may occur after commencing gonadorelin analo-

gue administration. Cyproterone acetate and flutamide are also licensed for use alone in patients with metastatic prostate cancer refractory to gonadorelin analogue therapy. Bicalutamide is used for prostate cancer either alone or as an adjunct to other therapy, according to the clinical circumstances.

## ■ BICALUTAMIDE

**Indications**  locally advanced prostate cancer at high risk of disease progression, either alone or as adjuvant treatment to prostatectomy or radiotherapy; locally advanced, non-metastatic prostate cancer when surgical castration or other medical intervention inappropriate; advanced prostate cancer in combination with gonadorelin analogue or surgical castration

**Cautions**  hepatic impairment (Appendix 2), also consider periodic liver function tests; **interactions**: Appendix 1 (bicalutamide)

**Side-effects**  nausea, diarrhoea, cholestasis, jaundice; asthenia, weight gain; gynaecomastia, breast tenderness, hot flushes, impotence, decreased libido; anaemia; alopecia, dry skin, hirsutism, pruritus; *less commonly* vomiting, abdominal pain, dyspepsia, interstitial lung disease, pulmonary fibrosis, depression, haematuria, thrombocytopenia, hypersensitivity reactions including angioneurotic oedema and urticaria; *rarely* cardiovascular disorders (including angina, heart failure, and arrhythmias), and hepatic failure

**Dose**

- Locally advanced prostate cancer at high risk of disease progression, 150 mg once daily
- Locally advanced, non-metastatic prostate cancer when surgical castration or other medical intervention inappropriate, 150 mg once daily
- Advanced prostate cancer, in combination with gonadorelin analogue or surgical castration, 50 mg once daily (started at the same time as surgical castration or at least 3 days before gonadorelin therapy, see also notes above)

Note  The CSM has advised (October 2003) that bicalutamide should no longer be used for the treatment of localised prostate cancer

**Bicalutamide** (Non-proprietary) ▣PoM

Tablets, bicalutamide 50 mg, net price 28-tab pack = £88.66; 150 mg, 28-tab pack = £168.71

**Casodex®** (AstraZeneca) ▣PoM

Tablets, f/c, bicalutamide 50 mg, net price 28-tab pack = £128.00; 150 mg, 28-tab pack = £240.00

## ■ BUSERELIN

**Indications**  advanced prostate cancer; other indications (section 6.7.2)

**Cautions**  depression, see also notes above

**Side-effects**  see notes above; worsening hypertension, palpitation, glucose intolerance, altered blood lipids, thrombocytopenia, leucopenia, nervousness, fatigue, memory and concentration disturbances, anxiety, increased thirst, hearing disorders, musculoskeletal pain; nasal irritation, nose bleeds and altered sense of taste and smell (spray formulation only)

**Dose**

- By subcutaneous injection, 500 micrograms every 8 hours for 7 days, then intranasally, 1 spray into each nostril 6 times daily (see also notes above)

**Counselling** Avoid use of nasal decongestants before and for at least 30 minutes after treatment.

**Suprefact®** (Aventis Pharma) (PoM)
Injection, buserelin (as acetate) 1 mg/mL. Net price 2 × 5.5-mL vial = £23.69

Nasal spray, buserelin (as acetate) 100 micrograms/ metered spray. Net price treatment pack of 4 × 10-g bottle with spray pump = £101.87. Counselling, see above

## ▮ CYPROTERONE ACETATE

**Indications** prostate cancer, see under Dose and also notes above; other indications, see section 6.4.2

**Cautions** in prostate cancer, blood counts initially and throughout treatment; hepatic impairment (Appendix 2; see also under side-effects below); monitor hepatic function (liver function tests should be performed before treatment, see also under Side-effects below); monitor adrenocortical function regularly; risk of recurrence of thromboembolic disease; diabetes mellitus, sickle-cell anaemia, severe depression (in other indications some of these are contra-indicated, see section 6.4.2)

**Driving** Fatigue and lassitude may impair performance of skilled tasks (e.g. driving)

**Contra-indications** none in prostate cancer; for contra-indications relating to other indications see section 6.4.2

**Side-effects** see section 6.4.2

**Hepatotoxicity** Direct hepatic toxicity including jaundice, hepatitis and hepatic failure have been reported (usually after several months) in patients treated with cyproterone acetate 200–300 mg daily. Liver function tests should be performed before and regularly during treatment and whenever symptoms suggestive of hepatotoxicity occur—if confirmed cyproterone should normally be withdrawn unless the hepatotoxicity can be explained by another cause such as metastatic disease (in which case cyproterone should be continued only if the perceived benefit exceeds the risk)

**Dose**

- Flare with initial gonadorelin therapy, 300 mg daily in 2–3 divided doses, reduced to 200 mg daily in 2–3 divided doses if necessary

- Long-term palliative therapy where gonadorelin analogues or orchidectomy contra-indicated, not tolerated, or where oral therapy preferred, 200–300 mg daily in 2–3 divided doses

- Hot flushes with gonadorelin therapy or after orchidectomy, initially 50 mg daily, adjusted according to response to 50–150 mg daily in 1–3 divided doses

**Cyproterone Acetate** (Non-proprietary) (PoM)
Tablets, cyproterone acetate 50 mg, net price 56-tab pack = £31.54; 100 mg, 84-tab pack = £77.50.
Label: 21, counselling, driving

**Cyprostat®** (Bayer) (PoM)
Tablets, scored, cyproterone acetate 50 mg, net price 168-tab pack = £74.65; 100 mg, 84-tab pack = £74.65.
Label: 21, counselling, driving

## ▮ FLUTAMIDE

**Indications** advanced prostate cancer, see also notes above

**Cautions** cardiac disease (oedema reported); hepatic impairment, also liver function tests, monthly for first 4 months, periodically thereafter and at the first sign or symptom of liver disorder (e.g. pruritus, dark urine, persistent anorexia, jaundice, abdominal pain, unexplained influenza-like symptoms); avoid excessive alcohol consumption; **interactions:** Appendix 1 (flutamide)

**Side-effects** gynaecomastia (sometimes with galactorrhoea); nausea, vomiting, diarrhoea, increased appetite, insomnia, tiredness; other side-effects reported include decreased libido, reduced sperm count, gastric and chest pain, hypertension, headache, dizziness, oedema, blurred vision, thirst, rash, pruritus, haemolytic anaemia, systemic lupus erythematosus-like syndrome, and lymphoedema; hepatic injury (with transaminase abnormalities, cholestatic jaundice, hepatic necrosis, hepatic encephalopathy and occasional fatality) reported

**Dose**

- 250 mg 3 times daily (see also notes above)

**Flutamide** (Non-proprietary) (PoM)
Tablets, flutamide 250 mg. Net price 84-tab pack = £21.66

## ▮ GOSERELIN

**Indications** locally advanced prostate cancer as an alternative to surgical castration; adjuvant treatment to radiotherapy or radical prostatectomy in patients with high-risk localised or locally advanced prostate cancer; neoadjuvant treatment prior to radiotherapy in patients with high-risk localised or locally advanced prostate cancer; metastatic prostate cancer; advanced breast cancer; oestrogen-receptor-positive early breast cancer (section 8.3.4.1); endometriosis, endometrial thinning, uterine fibroids, assisted reproduction (section 6.7.2)

**Cautions** see notes above; diabetes; risk of ureteric obstruction and spinal cord compression in men

**Contra-indications** pregnancy (Appendix 4); breast-feeding (Appendix 5); undiagnosed vaginal bleeding

**Side-effects** see notes above; also transient changes in blood pressure, paraesthesia, rarely hypercalcaemia (in patients with metastatic breast cancer)

**Dose**

- See under preparations below

**Zoladex®** (AstraZeneca) (PoM)
Implant, goserelin 3.6 mg (as acetate) in *SafeSystem®* syringe applicator, net price each = £84.14
**Dose** breast cancer and prostate cancer (see indications above) by subcutaneous injection into anterior abdominal wall, 3.6 mg every 28 days

**Zoladex® LA** (AstraZeneca) (PoM)
Implant, goserelin 10.8 mg (as acetate) in *SafeSystem®* syringe applicator, net price each = £267.48
**Dose** prostate cancer (see indications above), by subcutaneous injection into anterior abdominal wall, 10.8 mg every 12 weeks

## ▮ LEUPRORELIN ACETATE

**Indications** locally advanced prostate cancer as an alternative to surgical castration; adjuvant treatment to radiotherapy or radical prostatectomy in patients with high-risk localised or locally advanced prostate cancer; metastatic prostate cancer; endometriosis, endometrial thinning, uterine fibroids (section 6.7.2)

8   Malignant disease and immunosuppression

**Cautions** see notes above and section 6.7.2; risk of ureteric obstruction and spinal cord compression in men

**Contra-indications** pregnancy (Appendix 4); breast-feeding (Appendix 5)

**Side-effects** see notes above and section 6.7.2; also fatigue, muscle weakness, paraesthesia, hypertension, palpitation, alteration of glucose tolerance and of blood lipids; hypotension, jaundice, thrombocytopenia and leucopenia reported

**Dose**

• See under preparations below

**Prostap® SR** (Takeda) [PoM]
Injection (microsphere powder for reconstitution), leuprorelin acetate, net price 3.75-mg vial with 1-mL vehicle-filled syringe = £75.24
Dose prostate cancer (see indications), by subcutaneous or by intramuscular injection, 3.75 mg every 4 weeks

**Prostap® 3** (Takeda) [PoM]
Injection (microsphere powder for reconstitution), leuprorelin acetate, net price 11.25-mg vial with 2-mL vehicle-filled syringe = £225.72
Dose prostate cancer (see indications), by subcutaneous injection, 11.25 mg every three months

## TRIPTORELIN

**Indications** prostate cancer; endometriosis; precocious puberty, reduction in size of uterine fibroids (section 6.7.2)

**Cautions** see notes above; risk of ureteric obstruction and spinal cord compression in men

**Contra-indications** pregnancy (Appendix 4); breast-feeding (Appendix 5)

**Side-effects** see notes above; also dry mouth, transient hypertension, paraesthesia, and increased dysuria

**Dose**

• See under preparations below

**Decapeptyl® SR** (Ipsen) [PoM]
Injection (powder for suspension), m/r, triptorelin (as acetate), net price 3-mg vial (with diluent) = £69.00
Dose locally advanced non-metastatic prostate cancer as an alternative to surgical castration, metastatic prostate cancer, by intramuscular injection, 3 mg every 4 weeks
Note Each vial includes an overage to allow accurate administration of a 3-mg dose

Injection (powder for suspension), m/r, triptorelin (as acetate), net price 11.25-mg vial (with diluent) = £207.00
Dose locally advanced non-metastatic prostate cancer as an alternative to surgical castration, metastatic prostate cancer, by intramuscular injection, 11.25 mg every 3 months (see also notes above)
Note Each vial includes an overage to allow accurate administration of an 11.25-mg dose

**Gonapeptyl Depot®** (Ferring) [PoM]
Injection (powder for suspension), triptorelin (as acetate), net price 3.75-mg prefilled syringe (with prefilled syringe of vehicle) = £81.69
Dose advanced prostate cancer, by subcutaneous or deep intramuscular injection, 3.75 mg every 4 weeks (see also notes above)

# Gonadotrophin-releasing hormone antagonists

**Degarelix** is a gonadotrophin-releasing hormone antagonist used to treat advanced hormone-dependent prostate cancer. It does not induce a testosterone surge or tumour 'flare', therefore anti-androgen therapy is not required.

## ■ DEGARELIX

**Indications** see notes above

**Cautions** susceptibility to QT-interval prolongation (avoid concomitant use of drugs that prolong QT interval); monitor bone density; diabetes; hepatic impairment (Appendix 2); renal impairment (Appendix 3)

**Side-effects** nausea; dizziness, headache, drowsiness, insomnia, asthenia; influenza-like symptoms; hot flushes, sweating (including night sweats), weight gain; injection-site reactions; *less commonly* diarrhoea, vomiting, abdominal discomfort, dry mouth, constipation, anorexia, atrio-ventricular block, QT-interval prolongation, fainting, hypertension, hypersensitivity reactions, depression, anxiety, oedema, gynaecomastia, micturition urgency, renal impairment, sexual dysfunction, pelvic pain, prostatitis, testicular pain, anaemia, musculoskeletal pain, tinnitus, urticaria, alopecia, and rash

**Dose**

• By subcutaneous injection into the abdominal region, ADULT over 18 years, initially 240 mg (administered as 2 injections of 120 mg), then 80 mg every 28 days

**Firmagon®** (Ferring) ▼ [PoM]
Injection, powder for reconstitution, degarelix (as acetate), net price 80-mg vial (with diluent) = £129.37; 2 × 120-mg vials (with diluent) = £260.00

## 8.3.4.3 Somatostatin analogues

**Lanreotide** and **octreotide** are analogues of the hypothalamic release-inhibiting hormone somatostatin. They are indicated for the relief of symptoms associated with neuroendocrine (particularly carcinoid) tumours and acromegaly. Additionally, lanreotide is licensed for the treatment of thyroid tumours and octreotide is also licensed for the prevention of complications following pancreatic surgery; octreotide may also be valuable in reducing vomiting in palliative care (see p. 18) and in stopping variceal bleeding [unlicensed indication]—see also vasopressin and terlipressin (section 6.5.2).

**Cautions** Growth hormone-secreting pituitary tumours can expand causing serious complications; during treatment with somatostatin analogues patients should be monitored for signs of tumour expansion (e.g. visual field defects). Ultrasound examination of the gallbladder is recommended before treatment and at intervals of 6–12 months during treatment (avoid abrupt withdrawal of short-acting octreotide—see Side-effects below). In insulinoma an increase in the depth and duration of hypoglycaemia may occur (observe patients when initiating treatment and changing doses); in diabetes mellitus, insulin or oral antidiabetic requirements may be reduced.

**Side-effects** Gastro-intestinal disturbances including anorexia, nausea, vomiting, abdominal pain and bloating, flatulence, diarrhoea, and steatorrhoea may occur. Postprandial glucose tolerance may be impaired and rarely persistent hyperglycaemia occurs with chronic administration; hypoglycaemia has also been reported. Gallstones have been reported after long-term treatment (abrupt withdrawal of subcutaneous octreotide is associated with biliary colic and pancreatitis). Pain and irritation may occur at the injection site and sites should be rotated. Rarely, pancreatitis has been reported shortly after administration.

## ■ LANREOTIDE

**Indications** see notes above

**Cautions** see notes above; pregnancy (Appendix 4); breast-feeding (Appendix 5); **interactions:** Appendix 1 (lanreotide)

**Side-effects** see notes above; also reported asthenia, fatigue, raised bilirubin; *less commonly* skin nodule, hot flushes, leg pain, malaise, headache, tenesmus, decreased libido, drowsiness, pruritus, increased sweating; *rarely* hypothyroidism (monitor as necessary)

**Dose**

- See under preparations

**Somatuline® LA** (Ipsen) PoM

Injection (copolymer microparticles for aqueous suspension), lanreotide (as acetate) 30-mg vial (with vehicle) = £329.00

Dose by intramuscular injection, acromegaly and neuroendocrine (particularly carcinoid) tumours, initially 30 mg every 14 days, frequency increased to every 7–10 days according to response

Thyroid tumours, 30 mg every 14 days, frequency increased to every 10 days according to response

**Somatuline Autogel®** (Ipsen)

Injection, prefilled syringe, lanreotide (as acetate) 60 mg = £562.00; 90 mg = £750.00; 120 mg = £955.00

Dose by deep subcutaneous injection into the gluteal region, acromegaly (if somatostatin analogue not given previously), initially 60 mg every 28 days, adjusted according to response; for patients treated previously with somatostatin analogue, consult product literature for initial dose

Neuroendocrine (particularly carcinoid) tumours, initially 60–120 mg every 28 days, adjusted according to response

## ■ OCTREOTIDE

**Indications** see under Dose

**Cautions** see notes above; hepatic impairment; pregnancy (Appendix 4); breast-feeding (Appendix 5); monitor thyroid function on long-term therapy; **interactions:** Appendix 1 (octreotide)

**Side-effects** see notes above; *rarely* altered liver function tests, hepatitis and transient alopecia

**Dose**

- Symptoms associated with carcinoid tumours with features of carcinoid syndrome, VIPomas, glucagonomas, by subcutaneous injection, initially 50 micrograms once or twice daily, gradually increased according to response to 200 micrograms 3 times daily (higher doses required exceptionally); maintenance doses variable; in carcinoid tumours discontinue after 1 week if no effect; if rapid response required, initial dose by intravenous injection (with ECG monitoring and after dilution to

a concentration of 10–50% with sodium chloride 0.9% injection)

- Acromegaly, short-term treatment before pituitary surgery *or* long-term treatment in those inadequately controlled by other treatment *or* until radiotherapy becomes fully effective by subcutaneous injection, 100–200 micrograms 3 times daily; discontinue if no improvement within 3 months

- Prevention of complications following pancreatic surgery, consult product literature

**Octreotide** (Non-proprietary) PoM

Injection, octreotide (as acetate) 50 micrograms/mL, net price 1-mL amp = £3.72; 100 micrograms/mL, 1-mL amp = £6.53; 200 micrograms/mL, 5-mL vial = £69.66; 500 micrograms/mL, 1-mL amp = £33.87

**Sandostatin®** (Novartis) PoM

Injection, octreotide (as acetate) 50 micrograms/mL, net price 1-mL amp = £3.72; 100 micrograms/mL, 1-mL amp = £6.53; 200 micrograms/mL 5-mL vial = £69.66; 500 micrograms/mL, 1-mL amp = £33.87

◢Depot preparation

**Sandostatin Lar®** (Novartis) PoM

Injection (microsphere powder for aqueous suspension), octreotide (as acetate) 10-mg vial = £637.50; 20-mg vial = £850.00; 30-mg vial = £1062.50 (all supplied with 2.5-mL diluent-filled syringe)

Dose acromegaly (test dose by subcutaneous injection 50–100 micrograms if subcutaneous octreotide not previously given), neuroendocrine (particularly carcinoid) tumour adequately controlled by subcutaneous octreotide, by deep intramuscular injection into gluteal muscle, initially 20 mg every 4 weeks for 3 months then adjusted according to response; max. 30 mg every 4 weeks

For acromegaly, start depot octreotide 1 day after the last dose of subcutaneous octreotide (for pituitary surgery give last dose of depot octreotide at least 3 weeks before surgery); for neuroendocrine tumours, continue subcutaneous octreotide for 2 weeks after first dose of depot octreotide

**8**

**Malignant disease and immunosuppression**

# 9 Nutrition and blood

**9.1 Anaemias and some other blood disorders** 512
**9.1.1** Iron-deficiency anaemias 512
**9.1.1.1** Oral iron 512
**9.1.1.2** Parenteral iron 514
**9.1.2** Drugs used in megaloblastic anaemias 515
**9.1.3** Drugs used in hypoplastic, haemolytic, and renal anaemias 517
**9.1.4** Drugs used in platelet disorders 523
**9.1.5** G6PD deficiency 524
**9.1.6** Drugs used in neutropenia 525
**9.2 Fluids and electrolytes** 526
**9.2.1** Oral preparations for fluid and electrolyte imbalance 527
**9.2.1.1** Oral potassium 527
**9.2.1.2** Oral sodium and water 528
**9.2.1.3** Oral bicarbonate 529
**9.2.2** Parenteral preparations for fluid and electrolyte imbalance 530
**9.2.2.1** Electrolytes and water 530
**9.2.2.2** Plasma and plasma substitutes 532
**9.3 Intravenous nutrition** 534
**9.4 Oral nutrition** 540
**9.4.1** Foods for special diets 540
**9.4.2** Enteral nutrition 540
**9.5 Minerals** 541
**9.5.1** Calcium and magnesium 541
**9.5.1.1** Calcium supplements 541
**9.5.1.2** Hypercalcaemia and hypercalciuria 542
**9.5.1.3** Magnesium 543
**9.5.2** Phosphorus 544
**9.5.2.1** Phosphate supplements 544
**9.5.2.2** Phosphate-binding agents 544
**9.5.3** Fluoride 545
**9.5.4** Zinc 546
**9.5.5** Selenium 546
**9.6 Vitamins** 547
**9.6.1** Vitamin A 547
**9.6.2** Vitamin B group 547
**9.6.3** Vitamin C 549
**9.6.4** Vitamin D 549
**9.6.5** Vitamin E 551
**9.6.6** Vitamin K 551

**9.6.7** Multivitamin preparations 552
**9.7 Bitters and tonics** 553
**9.8 Metabolic disorders** 553
**9.8.1** Drugs used in metabolic disorders 553
**9.8.2** Acute porphyrias 557

*(left margin) 9 Nutrition and blood*

## 9.1 Anaemias and some other blood disorders

**9.1.1** Iron-deficiency anaemias
**9.1.2** Drugs used in megaloblastic anaemias
**9.1.3** Drugs used in hypoplastic, haemolytic, and renal anaemias
**9.1.4** Drugs used in platelet disorders
**9.1.5** G6PD deficiency
**9.1.6** Drugs used in neutropenia

Before initiating treatment for anaemia it is essential to determine which type is present. Iron salts may be harmful and result in iron overload if given alone to patients with anaemias other than those due to iron deficiency.

## 9.1.1 Iron-deficiency anaemias

**9.1.1.1** Oral iron
**9.1.1.2** Parenteral iron

*Treatment* with an iron preparation is justified only in the presence of a demonstrable iron-deficiency state. Before starting treatment, it is important to exclude any serious underlying cause of the anaemia (e.g. gastric erosion, gastro-intestinal cancer).

*Prophylaxis* with an iron preparation may be appropriate in malabsorption, menorrhagia, pregnancy, after subtotal or total gastrectomy, in haemodialysis patients, and in the management of low birth-weight infants such as preterm neonates.

### 9.1.1.1 Oral iron

Iron salts should be given by mouth unless there are good reasons for using another route.

Ferrous salts show only marginal differences between one another in efficiency of absorption of iron. Haemoglobin regeneration rate is little affected by the type of salt used provided sufficient iron is given, and in most patients the speed of response is not critical. Choice of preparation is thus usually decided by the incidence of side-effects and cost.

The oral dose of **elemental iron** for iron-deficiency anaemia should be 100 to 200 mg daily. It is customary to give this as **dried ferrous sulphate**, 200 mg ($\equiv$ 65 mg elemental iron) three times daily; for prophylaxis of iron-deficiency anaemia, a dose of ferrous sulphate 200 mg once or twice daily may be effective. For treatment of iron-deficiency anaemia in children and for prophylaxis of iron-deficiency anaemia in babies of low birth weight, see *BNF for Children*.

### Iron content of different iron salts

| Iron salt | Amount | Content of ferrous iron |
| --- | --- | --- |
| Ferrous fumarate | 200 mg | 65 mg |
| Ferrous gluconate | 300 mg | 35 mg |
| Ferrous sulphate | 300 mg | 60 mg |
| Ferrous sulphate, dried | 200 mg | 65 mg |

**Therapeutic response** The haemoglobin concentration should rise by about 100–200 mg/100 mL (1–2 g/litre) per day *or* 2 g/100 mL (20 g/litre) over 3–4 weeks. When the haemoglobin is in the reference range, treatment should be continued for a further 3 months to replenish the iron stores. Epithelial tissue changes such as atrophic glossitis and koilonychia are usually improved, but the response is often slow.

**Side-effects** Gastro-intestinal irritation can occur with iron salts. Nausea and epigastric pain are dose-related, but the relationship between dose and altered bowel habit (constipation or diarrhoea) is less clear. Oral iron, particularly modified-release preparations, can exacerbate diarrhoea in patients with inflammatory bowel disease; care is also needed in patients with intestinal strictures and diverticular disease.

Iron preparations taken orally can be constipating, particularly in older patients and occasionally lead to faecal impaction.

If side-effects occur, the dose may be reduced; alternatively, another iron salt may be used, but an improvement in tolerance may simply be a result of a lower content of elemental iron. The incidence of side-effects due to ferrous sulphate is no greater than with other iron salts when compared on the basis of equivalent amounts of elemental iron.

Iron preparations are a common cause of accidental overdose in children. For the treatment of **iron overdose**, see Emergency Treatment of Poisoning, p. 32.

**Counselling** Although iron preparations are best absorbed on an empty stomach they can be taken after food to reduce gastro-intestinal side-effects; they may discolour stools

**Compound preparations** Preparations containing iron and **folic acid** are used during pregnancy in women who are at high risk of developing iron and folic acid deficiency; they should be distinguished from those used for the prevention of neural tube defects in women planning a pregnancy (see p. 516).

It is important to note that the small doses of folic acid contained in these preparations are inadequate for the treatment of megaloblastic anaemias.

Some oral preparations contain **ascorbic acid** to aid absorption of the iron but the therapeutic advantage of such preparations is minimal and cost may be increased.

There is no justification for the inclusion of other ingredients, such as the **B group of vitamins** (except folic acid for pregnant women, see notes above and on p. 516).

**Modified-release preparations** Modified-release preparations of iron are licensed for once-daily dosage, but have no therapeutic advantage and should not be used. These preparations are formulated to release iron gradually; the low incidence of side-effects may reflect the small amounts of iron available for absorption as the iron is carried past the first part of the duodenum into an area of the gut where absorption may be poor.

### ■ FERROUS SULPHATE

**Indications** iron-deficiency anaemia
**Cautions** interactions: Appendix 1 (iron)
**Side-effects** see notes above
**Dose**
• See under preparations below and notes above

**Ferrous Sulphate** (Non-proprietary)
Tablets, coated, dried ferrous sulphate 200 mg (65 mg iron), net price 28-tab pack = £1.30
Dose prophylactic, 1 tablet daily; therapeutic, 1 tablet 2–3 times daily; CHILD, see *BNF for Children*

**Ironorm® Drops** (Wallace Mfg)
Oral drops, ferrous sulphate 125 mg (25 mg iron)/mL. Net price 15-mL = £4.95
Dose ADULT and CHILD over 6 years, prophylactic, 0.6 mL daily; CHILD under 6 years, see *BNF for Children*

#### ▲ Modified-release preparations
**Feospan®** (Intrapharm) [NHS] [▣]
Spansule® (= capsules m/r), clear/red, enclosing green and brown pellets, dried ferrous sulphate 150 mg (47 mg iron). Net price 30-cap pack = £1.65. Label: 25
Dose 1–2 capsules daily; CHILD over 1 year, 1 capsule daily; can be opened and sprinkled on food

**Ferrograd®** (Teofarma) [▣]
Tablets, f/c, m/r, red, dried ferrous sulphate 325 mg (105 mg iron). Net price 30-tab pack = £1.18. Label: 25
Dose ADULT and CHILD over 12 years, prophylactic and therapeutic, 1 tablet daily before food

#### ▲ With folic acid
**Fefol®** (Intrapharm) [NHS] [▣]
Spansule® (= capsules m/r), clear/green, enclosing brown, yellow, and white pellets, dried ferrous sulphate 150 mg (47 mg iron), folic acid 500 micrograms. Net price 30-cap pack = £1.69. Label: 25
Dose 1 capsule daily

**Ferrograd Folic®** (Teofarma) [▣]
Tablets, f/c, red/yellow, dried ferrous sulphate 325 mg (105 mg iron) for sustained release, folic acid 350 micrograms. Net price 30-tab pack = £1.32. Label: 25
Dose ADULT and CHILD over 12 years, 1 tablet daily before food

#### ▲ With ascorbic acid
**Ferrograd C®** (Teofarma) [NHS] [▣]
Tablets, f/c, red, dried ferrous sulphate 325 mg (105 mg iron) for sustained release, ascorbic acid 500 mg (as sodium salt). Net price 30-tab pack = £1.71. Label: 25
Dose ADULT and CHILD over 12 years, 1 tablet daily before food

**9**

**Nutrition and blood**

## ◾ FERROUS FUMARATE

**Indications** iron-deficiency anaemia
**Cautions** interactions: Appendix 1 (iron)
**Side-effects** see notes above
**Dose**

- See under preparations below and notes above

**Fersaday®** (Goldshield)
Tablets, brown, f/c, ferrous fumarate 322 mg (100 mg iron). Net price 28-tab pack = 79p
Dose prophylactic, 1 tablet daily; therapeutic, 1 tablet twice daily

**Fersamal®** (Goldshield)
Tablets, brown, ferrous fumarate 210 mg (68 mg iron), net price 20 = 29p
Dose prophylactic and therapeutic, 1–2 tablets 3 times daily, but see notes above

Syrup, brown, ferrous fumarate approx. 140 mg (45 mg iron)/5 mL, net price 200 mL = £3.11
Dose prophylactic and therapeutic, 10–20 mL twice daily, but see notes above; CHILD see BNF for Children

**Galfer®** (Thornton & Ross)
Capsules, red/green, ferrous fumarate 305 mg (100 mg iron), net price 20 = 36p
Dose ADULT and CHILD over 12 years, prophylactic, 1 capsule daily; therapeutic, 1 capsule twice daily

Syrup, brown, sugar-free ferrous fumarate 140 mg (45 mg iron)/5 mL, net price 300 mL = £4.86
Dose ADULT and CHILD over 12 years, prophylactic, 10 mL once daily; therapeutic, 10 mL 1–2 times daily; PRETERM NEONATE and NEONATE, see BNF for Children; CHILD 1 month–12 years, prophylactic and therapeutic, 0.5 mL/kg daily in 2–3 divided doses; max. 20 mL daily

◢**With folic acid**
**Galfer FA®** (Thornton & Ross)
Capsules, red/yellow, ferrous fumarate 305 mg (100 mg iron), folic acid 350 micrograms. Net price 30-cap pack = £1.10
Dose 1 capsule daily before food

**Pregaday®** (UCB Pharma)
Tablets, brown, f/c, ferrous fumarate equivalent to 100 mg iron, folic acid 350 micrograms. Net price 28-tab pack =£1.20
Dose 1 tablet daily

◢**With vitamins B and C**
**Givitol®** (Galen) 〔NHS〕 ◪
Capsules, red/maroon, ferrous fumarate 305 mg (100 mg iron) with vitamins B group and C. Net price 20 = 88p
Dose 1 capsule daily before food

## ◾ FERROUS GLUCONATE

**Indications** iron-deficiency anaemia
**Cautions** interactions: Appendix 1 (iron)
**Side-effects** see notes above
**Dose**

- See under preparation below and notes above

**Ferrous Gluconate** (Non-proprietary)
Tablets, red, coated, ferrous gluconate 300 mg (35 mg iron). Net price 20 = 72p
Dose prophylactic, 2 tablets daily before food; therapeutic, 4–6 tablets daily in divided doses before food; CHILD 6–12 years, prophylactic and therapeutic, 1–3 tablets daily

## ◾ POLYSACCHARIDE–IRON COMPLEX

**Indications** iron-deficiency anaemia
**Cautions** interactions: Appendix 1 (iron)
**Side-effects** see notes above
**Dose**

- See under preparation below and notes above

**Niferex®** (Tillomed)
Elixir, brown, sugar-free, polysaccharide–iron complex equivalent to 100 mg of iron/5 mL. Net price 240-mL pack = £6.06; 〔NHS〕[1] 30-mL dropper bottle for paediatric use = £2.16. Counselling, use of dropper
Dose prophylactic, 2.5 mL daily; therapeutic, 5 mL 1–2 times daily (once daily if required during second and third trimester of pregnancy); PRETERM NEONATE, NEONATE, and INFANT (from dropper bottle) 1 drop (approx. 500 micrograms iron) per 450 g body-weight 3 times daily; CHILD 2–6 years 2.5 mL daily, 6–12 years 5 mL daily

1. except 30 mL paediatric dropper bottle for prophylaxis and treatment of iron deficiency in infants born prematurely; endorse prescription 'SLS'

## ◾ SODIUM FEREDETATE
(Sodium ironedetate)

**Indications** iron-deficiency anaemia
**Cautions** interactions: Appendix 1 (iron)
**Side-effects** see notes above
**Dose**

- See under preparation below and notes above

**Sytron®** (Link)
Elixir, sugar-free, sodium feredetate 190 mg equivalent to 27.5 mg of iron/5 mL, net price 100 mL = £1.07
Dose therapeutic, 5 mL increasing gradually to 10 mL 3 times daily; CHILD under 1 year, see BNF for Children; CHILD 1–5 years, therapeutic, 2.5 mL 3 times daily, 6–12 years, therapeutic, 5 mL 3 times daily

### 9.1.1.2 Parenteral iron

Iron can be administered parenterally as iron dextran, iron sucrose, or ferric carboxymaltose. Parenteral iron is generally reserved for use when oral therapy is unsuccessful because the patient cannot tolerate oral iron, or does not take it reliably, or if there is continuing blood loss, or in malabsorption. Parenteral iron may also have a role in the management of chemotherapy-induced anaemia, when given with erythropoietins, in specific patient groups (see NICE guidance, p. 518).

Many patients with chronic renal failure who are receiving haemodialysis (and some who are receiving peritoneal dialysis) also require iron by the intravenous route on a regular basis (see also Erythropoietins, section 9.1.3).

With the exception of patients with severe renal failure receiving haemodialysis, parenteral iron does not produce a faster haemoglobin response than oral iron provided that the oral iron preparation is taken reliably and is absorbed adequately.

Anaphylactoid reactions can occur with parenteral administration of iron complexes. Depending on the preparation, patients may be required to have a small test dose initially, see preparations for details; facilities for cardiopulmonary resuscitation must be available.

## FERRIC CARBOXYMALTOSE

A ferric carboxymaltose complex containing 5% (50 mg/mL) of iron

**Indications** iron-deficiency anaemia, see notes above

**Cautions** hypersensitivity can occur with parenteral iron and facilities for cardiopulmonary resuscitation must be available; oral iron should not be given concomitantly; allergic disorders including asthma and eczema; infection (discontinue if ongoing bacteraemia); hepatic impairment (Appendix 2); pregnancy (Appendix 4)

**Side-effects** gastro-intestinal disturbances; headache, dizziness; rash, injection-site reactions; *less commonly* hypotension, flushing, chest pain, peripheral oedema, fatigue, paraesthesia, malaise, pyrexia, rigors, myalgia, arthralgia, back pain, pruritus, and urticaria

**Dose**

- By slow intravenous injection or by intravenous infusion, ADULT and CHILD over 14 years, calculated according to body-weight and iron deficit, consult product literature

**Ferinject®** (Syner-Med) ▼ PoM
Injection, iron (as ferric carboxymaltose) 50 mg/mL, net price 2-mL vial = £21.75, 10-mL vial = £108.75
Electrolytes Na+ 0.24 mmol/mL

## IRON DEXTRAN

A complex of ferric hydroxide with dextran containing 5% (50 mg/mL) of iron

**Indications** iron-deficiency anaemia, see notes above

**Cautions** oral iron not to be given until 5 days after last injection; pregnancy (Appendix 4)
Anaphylaxis Anaphylactic reactions can occur with parenteral iron and a test dose is recommended before *each* dose; the patient should be carefully observed for 60 minutes after the first test dose and for 15 minutes after subsequent test doses (subsequent test doses not necessary for intramuscular administration). Facilities for cardiopulmonary resuscitation must be available; risk of allergic reactions increased in immune or inflammatory conditions

**Contra-indications** history of allergic disorders including asthma and eczema; infection; active rheumatoid arthritis; severe hepatic impairment; acute renal failure

**Side-effects** *less commonly* nausea, vomiting, abdominal pain, flushing, dyspnoea, anaphylactic reactions (see Anaphylaxis above), numbness, cramps, blurred vision, pruritus, and rash; *rarely* diarrhoea, chest pain, hypotension, angioedema, arrhythmias, tachycardia, dizziness, restlessness, fatigue, seizures, tremor, impaired consciousness, myalgia, arthralgia, sweating, and injection-site reactions; *very rarely* hypertension, palpitation, headache, paraesthesia, haemolysis, and transient deafness

**Dose**

- By deep intramuscular injection into the gluteal muscle or by slow intravenous injection or by intravenous infusion, calculated according to body-weight and iron deficit, consult product literature
CHILD under 14 years, not recommended

**CosmoFer®** (Vitaline) PoM
Injection, iron (as iron dextran) 50 mg/mL, net price 2-mL amp = £7.97, 10-mL amp = £39.85

## IRON SUCROSE

A complex of ferric hydroxide with sucrose containing 2% (20 mg/mL) of iron

**Indications** iron-deficiency anaemia, see notes above

**Cautions** oral iron therapy should not be given until 5 days after last injection; infection (discontinue if ongoing bacteraemia); hepatic impairment (Appendix 2); pregnancy (Appendix 4)
Anaphylaxis Anaphylactic reactions can occur with parenteral iron and a test dose is recommended before the first dose; the patient should be carefully observed for 15 minutes. Facilities for cardiopulmonary resuscitation must be available

**Contra-indications** history of allergic disorders including asthma, eczema and anaphylaxis

**Side-effects** taste disturbances; *less commonly* nausea, vomiting, abdominal pain, diarrhoea, hypotension, tachycardia, flushing, palpitation, chest pain, bronchospasm, dyspnoea, headache, dizziness, fever, myalgia, pruritus, rash, and injection-site reactions; rarely peripheral oedema, anaphylactic reactions (see Anaphylaxis above), fatigue, asthenia, and paraesthesia; confusion, arthralgia, and increased sweating also reported

**Dose**

- By slow intravenous injection *or* by intravenous infusion, calculated according to body-weight and iron deficit, consult product literature; CHILD not recommended

**Venofer®** (Syner-Med) PoM
Injection, iron (as iron sucrose) 20 mg/mL, net price 5-mL amp = £7.08

# 9.1.2 Drugs used in megaloblastic anaemias

Most megaloblastic anaemias result from a lack of either vitamin B$_{12}$ or folate, and it is essential to establish in every case which deficiency is present and the underlying cause. In emergencies, when delay might be dangerous, it is sometimes necessary to administer both substances after the bone marrow test while plasma assay results are awaited. Normally, however, appropriate treatment should not be instituted until the results of tests are available.

One cause of megaloblastic anaemia in the UK is *pernicious anaemia* in which lack of gastric intrinsic factor resulting from an autoimmune gastritis causes malabsorption of vitamin B$_{12}$.

Vitamin B$_{12}$ is also needed in the treatment of megaloblastosis caused by *prolonged nitrous oxide anaesthesia*, which inactivates the vitamin, and in the rare syndrome of *congenital transcobalamin II deficiency*.

Vitamin B$_{12}$ should be given prophylactically after *total gastrectomy* or *total ileal resection* (or after *partial gastrectomy* if a vitamin B$_{12}$ absorption test shows vitamin B$_{12}$ malabsorption).

Apart from dietary deficiency, all other causes of vitamin B$_{12}$ deficiency are attributable to malabsorption. There is little place for the use of low-dose vitamin B$_{12}$ orally and none for vitamin B$_{12}$ intrinsic factor complexes given by mouth. Vitamin B$_{12}$ in larger oral doses of 1–2 mg daily [unlicensed] may be effective.

9

Nutrition and blood

**Hydroxocobalamin** has completely replaced cyanocobalamin as the form of vitamin $B_{12}$ of choice for therapy; it is retained in the body longer than cyanocobalamin and thus for maintenance therapy can be given at intervals of up to 3 months. Treatment is generally initiated with frequent administration of intramuscular injections to replenish the depleted body stores. Thereafter, maintenance treatment, which is usually for life, can be instituted. There is no evidence that doses larger than those recommended provide any additional benefit in vitamin $B_{12}$ neuropathy.

**Folic acid** has few indications for long-term therapy since most causes of folate deficiency are self-limiting or will yield to a short course of treatment. It should not be used in undiagnosed megaloblastic anaemia unless vitamin $B_{12}$ is administered concurrently otherwise neuropathy may be precipitated (see above).

In *folate-deficient megaloblastic anaemia* (e.g. because of poor nutrition, pregnancy, or antiepileptic drugs), daily folic acid supplementation for 4 months brings about haematological remission and replenishes body stores.

For prophylaxis in *chronic haemolytic states, malabsorption*, or *in renal dialysis*, folic acid is given daily or sometimes weekly, depending on the diet and the rate of haemolysis.

For *prophylaxis in pregnancy*, see Prevention of Neural Tube Defects below.

**Folinic acid** is also effective in the treatment of folate-deficient megaloblastic anaemia but it is generally used in association with cytotoxic drugs (see section 8.1); it is given as calcium folinate.

**Prevention of neural tube defects** Folic acid supplements taken before and during pregnancy can reduce the occurrence of neural tube defects. The risk of a neural tube defect occurring in a child should be assessed and folic acid given as follows:

> Women at a low-risk of conceiving a child with a neural tube defect should be advised to take folic acid as a medicinal or food supplement at a dose of 400 micrograms daily before conception and until week 12 of pregnancy. Women who have not been taking folic acid and who suspect they are pregnant should start at once and continue until week 12 of pregnancy.

> Couples are at a high-risk of conceiving a child with a neural tube defect if either partner has a neural tube defect (or either partner has a family history of neural tube defects), if they have had a previous pregnancy affected by a neural tube defect, or if the woman has coeliac disease (or other malabsorption state), diabetes mellitus, sickle-cell anaemia, or is taking antiepileptic medicines (see also section 4.8.1).

> Women in the high-risk group who wish to become pregnant (or who are at risk of becoming pregnant) should be advised to take folic acid 5 mg daily and continue until week 12 of pregnancy (women with sickle-cell disease should continue taking their normal dose of folic acid 5 mg daily throughout pregnancy).

> There is **no** justification for prescribing multiple-ingredient vitamin preparations containing vitamin $B_{12}$ or folic acid.

## HYDROXOCOBALAMIN

**Indications** see under dose below

**Cautions** should not be given before diagnosis fully established but see also notes above; **interactions**: Appendix 1 (hydroxocobalamin)

**Side-effects** nausea, headache, dizziness; fever, hypersensitivity reactions (including rash and pruritus); injection-site reactions; hypokalaemia and thrombocytosis during initial treatment; chromaturia

**Dose**

- By intramuscular injection, pernicious anaemia and other macrocytic anaemias without neurological involvement, initially 1 mg 3 times a week for 2 weeks then 1 mg every 3 months

  Pernicious anaemia and other macrocytic anaemias with neurological involvement, initially 1 mg on alternate days until no further improvement, then 1 mg every 2 months

  Prophylaxis of macrocytic anaemias associated with vitamin $B_{12}$ deficiency, 1 mg every 2–3 months

  Tobacco amblyopia and Leber's optic atrophy, initially 1 mg daily for 2 weeks, then 1 mg twice weekly until no further improvement, thereafter 1 mg every 1–3 months

  CHILD see *BNF for Children*

- Cyanide poisoning [not licensed], see p. 34

**Hydroxocobalamin** (Non-proprietary) (PoM)
Injection, hydroxocobalamin 1 mg/mL. Net price 1-mL amp = £2.46
Note The BP directs that when vitamin $B_{12}$ injection is prescribed or demanded hydroxocobalamin injection shall be dispensed or supplied
Brands include *Cobalin-H®* (JHS), *Neo-Cytamen®* (JHS)

## CYANOCOBALAMIN

**Indications** see notes above

**Dose**

- By mouth, vitamin $B_{12}$ deficiency of dietary origin, 50–150 micrograms daily taken between meals; CHILD 50–105 micrograms daily in 1–3 divided doses

- By intramuscular injection, initially 1 mg repeated 10 times at intervals of 2–3 days, maintenance 1 mg every month, but see notes above

**Cyanocobalamin** (Non-proprietary) 
[1]Tablets (JHS), cyanocobalamin 50 micrograms. Net price 50-tab pack = £6.24
Brands include *Cytacon®* (JHS)

Liquid (JHS), cyanocobalamin 35 micrograms/5 mL. Net price 200 mL = £2.77
Brands include *Cytacon®* (JHS)

Injection (PoM), cyanocobalamin 1 mg/mL. Net price 1-mL amp = £1.67
Brands include *Cytamen®* (JHS)

Note The BP directs that when vitamin $B_{12}$ injection is prescribed or demanded hydroxocobalamin injection shall be dispensed or supplied

1. (JHS) except to treat or prevent vitamin $B_{12}$ deficiency in a patient who is a vegan or who has a proven vitamin $B_{12}$ deficiency of dietary origin; endorse prescription 'SLS'; currently available brands may not be suitable for vegans—cyanocobalamin injection may be a suitable alternative

9 Nutrition and blood

## ▌ FOLIC ACID

**Indications**  see notes above and under dose

**Cautions**  should never be given alone for pernicious anaemia and other vitamin $B_{12}$ deficiency states (may precipitate subacute combined degeneration of the spinal cord); **interactions**: Appendix 1 (folates)

**Side-effects**  *rarely* gastro-intestinal disturbances

**Dose**

* Folate-deficient megaloblastic anaemia, by mouth, ADULT and CHILD over 1 year, 5 mg daily for 4 months (until term in pregnant women); up to 15 mg daily may be required in malabsorption states; CHILD under 1 year, 500 micrograms/kg daily (max. 5 mg) for up to 4 months; up to 10 mg daily may be required in malabsorption states
* Prevention of neural tube defects, by mouth, see notes above
* Prevention of methotrexate-induced side-effects in rheumatic disease [unlicensed], by mouth, ADULT over 18 years 5 mg once weekly; CHILD 2–18 years see *BNF for Children*
* Prevention of methotrexate-induced side-effects in severe psoriasis, by mouth, see section 13.5.3
* Prophylaxis in chronic haemolytic states, by mouth, ADULT 5 mg every 1–7 days depending on underlying disease
* Prophylaxis of folate deficiency in dialysis, by mouth, ADULT 5 mg every 1–7 days; CHILD 1–12 years 250 micrograms/kg (max. 10 mg) once daily, CHILD 12–18 years 5–10 mg once daily

**¹Folic Acid** (Non-proprietary) PoM

Tablets, folic acid 400 micrograms, net price 90-tab pack = £2.32; 5 mg, 28-tab pack = 88p

Syrup, folic acid 2.5 mg/5 mL, net price 150 mL = £9.16; 400 micrograms/5 mL, 150 mL = £1.40
Brands include *Folicare®*, *Lexpec®* (sugar-free)

Injection, folic acid 15 mg, net price 1-mL amp = £1.34
Available from 'special-order' manufacturers or specialist importing companies, see p. 969

1. Can be sold to the public provided daily doses do not exceed 500 micrograms

## 9.1.3 Drugs used in hypoplastic, haemolytic, and renal anaemias

Anabolic steroids (section 6.4.3), pyridoxine, antilymphocyte immunoglobulin, and various corticosteroids are used in hypoplastic and haemolytic anaemias.

**Antilymphocyte immunoglobulin** given intravenously through a central line over 12–18 hours each day for 5 days produces a response in about 50% of cases of acquired *aplastic anaemia*; the response rate may be increased when ciclosporin is given as well. Severe reactions are common in the first 2 days and profound

immunosuppression can occur; antilymphocyte immunoglobulin should be given under specialist supervision with appropriate resuscitation facilities. Alternatively, oxymetholone tablets (available from 'special-order' manufacturers or specialist importing companies, see p. 969) can be used in aplastic anaemia at a dose of 1–5 mg/kg daily for 3 to 6 months.

It is unlikely that dietary deprivation of **pyridoxine** (section 9.6.2) produces clinically relevant haematological effects. However, certain forms of *sideroblastic anaemia* respond to pharmacological doses, possibly reflecting its role as a co-enzyme during haemoglobin synthesis. Pyridoxine is indicated in both *idiopathic acquired* and *hereditary sideroblastic anaemias*. Although complete cures have not been reported, some increase in haemoglobin can occur; the dose required is usually high, up to 400 mg daily. *Reversible sideroblastic anaemias* respond to treatment of the underlying cause but in pregnancy, haemolytic anaemias, and alcohol dependence, or during isoniazid treatment, pyridoxine is also indicated.

**Corticosteroids** (see section 6.3) have an important place in the management of a wide variety of haematological disorders. They include conditions with an immune basis such as *autoimmune haemolytic anaemia*, *immune thrombocytopenias* and *neutropenias*, and *major transfusion reactions*. They are also used in chemotherapy schedules for many types of *lymphoma*, *lymphoid leukaemias*, and *paraproteinaemias*, including *multiple myeloma*.

## Erythropoietins

**Epoetins** (recombinant human erythropoietins) are used to treat symptomatic anaemia associated with erythropoietin deficiency in chronic renal failure, to increase the yield of autologous blood in normal individuals and to shorten the period of symptomatic anaemia in patients receiving cytotoxic chemotherapy. Epoetin beta is also used for the prevention of anaemia in preterm neonates of low birth-weight; only unpreserved formulations should be used in neonates because other preparations may contain benzyl alcohol (see Excipients, p. 2).

**Darbepoetin** is a hyperglycosylated derivative of epoetin; it has a longer half-life and can be administered less frequently than epoetin.

**Methoxy polyethylene glycol-epoetin beta** (pegzerepoetin alfa) is a continuous erythropoietin receptor activator that is licensed for the treatment of symptomatic anaemia associated with chronic kidney disease. It has a longer duration of action than epoetin.

Other factors, such as iron or folate deficiency, that contribute to the anaemia of chronic renal failure should be corrected before treatment and monitored during therapy. Supplemental iron may improve the response in resistant patients. Aluminium toxicity, concurrent infection, or other inflammatory disease can impair the response to erythropoietin.

9 Nutrition and blood

**MHRA/CHM advice (December 2007) Erythropoietins—haemoglobin concentration**

Overcorrection of haemoglobin concentration in patients with chronic kidney disease may increase the risk of death and serious cardiovascular events, and in patients with cancer may increase the risk of thrombosis and related complications:

- patients should not be treated with erythropoietins for the licensed indications in chronic kidney disease or cancer in patients receiving chemotherapy *unless* symptoms of anaemia are present;
- the haemoglobin concentration should be maintained within the range 10–12 g/100 mL;
- haemoglobin concentrations higher than 12 g/100 mL should be avoided;
- the aim of treatment is to relieve symptoms of anaemia, and in patients with chronic kidney disease to avoid the need for blood transfusion; the haemoglobin concentration should not be increased beyond that which provides adequate control of symptoms of anaemia (in some patients, this may be achieved at concentrations lower than the recommended range).

See also MHRA/CHM advice below.

**MHRA/CHM advice (December 2007 and July 2008) Erythropoietins—tumour progression and survival in patients with cancer**

Clinical trial data show an unexplained excess mortality and increased risk of tumour progression in patients with anaemia associated with cancer who have been treated with erythropoietins. Many of these trials used erythropoietins *outside* of the licensed indications (i.e. overcorrected haemoglobin concentration or given to patients who have *not* received chemotherapy):

- erythropoietins licensed for the treatment of *symptomatic* anaemia associated with cancer, are licensed only for patients who are receiving chemotherapy;
- the decision to use erythropoietins should be based on an assessment of the benefits and risks for individual patients; blood transfusion may be the preferred treatment for anaemia associated with cancer chemotherapy, particularly in those with a good cancer prognosis.

See also MHRA/CHM advice above.

**CSM advice (pure red cell aplasia)**

There have been very rare reports of pure red cell aplasia in patients treated with epoetin alfa. The CSM has advised that in patients developing lack of efficacy with epoetin alfa, with a diagnosis of pure red cell aplasia, treatment with epoetin alfa must be discontinued and testing for erythropoietin antibodies considered. Patients who develop pure red cell aplasia should **not** be switched to another form of erythropoietin.

**NICE guidance**

**Epoetin alfa, beta and darbepoetin alfa for cancer treatment-induced anaemia (May 2008)**

Erythropoietin analogues are **not** recommended for routine use in the management of cancer treatment-induced anaemia, but may be considered, in combination with intravenous iron, for:

- women receiving platinum-based chemotherapy for ovarian cancer who have symptomatic anaemia with a haemoglobin concentration of 8 g/100 mL or lower (the use of erythropoietin analogues does not preclude the use of existing approaches to the management of anaemia, including blood transfusion when necessary);
- patients who cannot be given blood transfusions and who have profound cancer treatment-related anaemia that is likely to have an impact on survival.

Patients currently treated with erythropoietin analogues for the management of cancer treatment-related anaemia who do not fulfil the criteria outlined above can continue therapy until they and their specialists consider it appropriate to stop.

## ▌ DARBEPOETIN ALFA

**Indications**   see under Dose below

**Cautions**   see Epoetin; hepatic disease; pregnancy (Appendix 4)

**Contra-indications**   see Epoetin; breast-feeding (Appendix 5)

**Side-effects**   see Epoetin; also, oedema, injection-site pain; isolated reports of pure red cell aplasia, particularly following subcutaneous administration in patients with chronic renal failure (discontinue therapy)—see also CSM advice above

**Dose**

- Symptomatic anaemia associated with chronic renal failure in patients on dialysis (see also MHRA/CHM advice, above), ADULT and CHILD over 11 years, by subcutaneous *or* intravenous injection, initially 450 nanograms/kg once weekly, adjusted according to response by approx. 25% at intervals of at least 4 weeks; maintenance dose, given once weekly *or* once every 2 weeks

- Symptomatic anaemia associated with chronic renal failure in patients not on dialysis (see also MHRA/CHM advice, above), ADULT and CHILD over 11 years, by subcutaneous *or* intravenous injection, initially 450 nanograms/kg once weekly *or* by subcutaneous injection, initially 750 nanograms/kg once every 2 weeks; adjusted according to response by approx. 25% at intervals of at least 4 weeks; maintenance dose, given subcutaneously or intravenously once weekly *or* subcutaneously once every 2 weeks *or* subcutaneously once every month

**Note** Subcutaneous route preferred in patients not on haemodialysis. Reduce dose by approximately 25% if rise in haemoglobin concentration exceeds 2 g/100 mL over 4 weeks or if haemoglobin concentration exceeds 12 g/100 mL; if haemoglobin concentration continues to rise, despite dose reduction, suspend treatment until haemoglobin concentration decreases and then restart at a dose approximately 25% lower than the previous dose. When changing route give same dose then adjust according to weekly or fortnightly haemoglobin measurements. Adjust doses not more frequently than every 2 weeks during maintenance treatment

- Symptomatic anaemia in adults with non-myeloid malignancies receiving chemotherapy (see also MHRA/CHM advice, p. 518), by subcutaneous injection, initially 6.75 micrograms/kg once every 3 weeks *or* 2.25 micrograms/kg once weekly (if response inadequate after 9 weeks further treatment may not be effective); if adequate response obtained, reduce dose by 25–50%

Note Reduce dose by approximately 25–50% if rise in haemoglobin concentration exceeds 2 g/100 mL over 4 weeks or if haemoglobin concentration exceeds 12 g/100 mL; if haemoglobin concentration continues to rise, despite dose reduction, suspend treatment until haemoglobin concentration decreases and restart at a dose approximately 25% lower than the previous dose. Discontinue approximately 4 weeks after ending chemotherapy

### Aranesp® (Amgen) [PoM]

Injection, prefilled syringe, darbepoetin alfa, 25 micrograms/mL, net price 0.4 mL (10 micrograms) = £14.98; 40 micrograms/mL, 0.375 mL (15 micrograms) = £22.47, 0.5 mL (20 micrograms) = £29.96; 100 micrograms/mL, 0.3 mL (30 micrograms) = £44.93, 0.4 mL (40 micrograms) = £59.91, 0.5 mL (50 micrograms) = £74.89; 200 micrograms/mL, 0.3 mL (60 micrograms) = £89.86, 0.4 mL (80 micrograms) = £119.82, 0.5 mL (100 micrograms) = £149.77, 0.65 mL (130 micrograms) = £194.70; 500 micrograms/mL, 0.3 mL (150 micrograms) = £224.66, 0.6 mL (300 micrograms) = £449.32, 1 mL (500 micrograms) = £748.86

Injection (*Aranesp® SureClick*), prefilled disposable injection device, darbepoetin alfa, 40 micrograms/mL, net price 0.5 mL (20 micrograms) = £29.95; 100 micrograms/mL, 0.4 mL (40 micrograms) = £59.91; 200 micrograms/mL, 0.3 mL (60 micrograms) = £89.86, 0.4 mL (80 micrograms) = £119.82, 0.5 mL (100 micrograms) = £149.77; 500 micrograms/mL, 0.3 mL (150 micrograms) = £224.66, 0.6 mL (300 micrograms) = £449.32, 1 mL (500 micrograms) = £748.86

---

### ■ EPOETIN ALFA, BETA, and ZETA
#### (Recombinant human erythropoietins)

Note The prescriber must specify which epoetin is required, see also Biosimilar medicines, p. 1

**Indications** see under preparations, below

**Cautions** see notes above; also inadequately treated or poorly controlled blood pressure (monitor closely blood pressure, reticulocyte counts, haemoglobin, and electrolytes), interrupt treatment if blood pressure uncontrolled; sudden stabbing migraine-like pain is warning of hypertensive crisis; sickle-cell disease (lower target haemoglobin concentration may be appropriate); ischaemic vascular disease; thrombocytosis (monitor platelet count for first 8 weeks); epilepsy; malignant disease; chronic liver failure (Appendix 2); increase in heparin dose may be needed; risk of thrombosis may be increased when used for anaemia in adults receiving cancer chemotherapy; risk of thrombosis may be increased when used for anaemia before orthopaedic surgery—avoid in cardiovascular disease including recent myocardial infarction or cerebrovascular accident; pregnancy (Appendix 4) and breast-feeding (Appendix 5)

**Contra-indications** pure red cell aplasia following erythropoietin therapy (see also CSM advice above); uncontrolled hypertension; patients unable to receive thromboprophylaxis; avoid injections containing

benzyl alcohol in neonates (see under preparations, below)

**Side-effects** diarrhoea, nausea, vomiting; dose-dependent increase in blood pressure or aggravation of hypertension; in isolated patients with normal or low blood pressure, hypertensive crisis with encephalopathy-like symptoms and generalised tonic-clonic seizures requiring immediate medical attention; headache; dose-dependent increase in platelet count (but thrombocytosis rare) regressing during treatment; influenza-like symptoms (may be reduced if intravenous injection given over 5 minutes); cardiovascular events; shunt thrombosis especially if tendency to hypotension or arteriovenous shunt complications; *very rarely* sudden loss of efficacy because of pure red cell aplasia, particularly following subcutaneous administration in patients with chronic renal failure (discontinue erythropoietin therapy)—see also CSM advice above, hyperkalaemia, hypersensitivity reactions (including anaphylaxis and angioedema), skin reactions, and peripheral oedema also reported

**Dose**

- See under preparations, below

#### ■ Epoetin alfa

**Binocrit® (Sandoz)** ▼ [PoM]

Injection, prefilled syringe, epoetin alfa, net price 1000 units = £5.09; 2000 units = £10.18; 3000 units = £15.27; 4000 units = £20.36; 5000 units = £25.46; 6000 units = £30.55; 8000 units = £40.73; 10 000 units = £50.91

Note Biosimilar medicine, p. 1

Dose symptomatic anaemia associated with chronic renal failure in patients on haemodialysis (see also MHRA/CHM advice, p. 518), by intravenous injection over 1–5 minutes, initially 50 units/kg 3 times weekly adjusted according to response in steps of 25 units/kg 3 times weekly at intervals of at least 4 weeks; maintenance dose, usually 25–100 units/kg 3 times weekly; CHILD by intravenous injection initially as for adults; maintenance dose, body-weight under 10 kg usually 75–150 units/kg 3 times weekly, body-weight 10–30 kg usually 60–150 units/kg 3 times weekly, body-weight over 30 kg usually 30–100 units/kg 3 times weekly

Symptomatic anaemia associated with chronic renal failure in adults on peritoneal dialysis (see also MHRA/CHM advice, p. 518), by intravenous injection over 1–5 minutes, initially 50 units/kg twice weekly; maintenance dose 25–50 units/kg twice weekly

Severe symptomatic anaemia of renal origin in adults with renal insufficiency not yet on dialysis (see also MHRA/CHM advice, p. 518), by intravenous injection over 1–5 minutes, initially 50 units/kg 3 times weekly increased according to response in steps of 25 units/kg 3 times weekly at intervals of at least 4 weeks; maintenance dose 17–33 units/kg 3 times weekly; max. 200 units/kg 3 times weekly

Note Reduce dose by approximately 25% if rise in haemoglobin concentration exceeds 2 g/100 mL over 4 weeks or if haemoglobin concentration exceeds 12 g/100 mL; if haemoglobin concentration continues to rise, despite dose reduction, suspend treatment until haemoglobin concentration decreases and then restart at a dose approximately 25% lower than the previous dose.

Symptomatic anaemia in adults receiving cancer chemotherapy (see also MHRA/CHM advice, p. 518), by subcutaneous injection (max. 1 mL per injection site), initially 150 units/kg 3 times weekly (or 450 units/kg once weekly), increased if appropriate rise in haemoglobin (or reticulocyte count) not achieved after 4 weeks to 300 units/kg 3 times weekly; discontinue if inadequate response after 4 weeks at higher dose

Note Reduce dose by approximately 25–50% if rise in haemoglobin concentration exceeds 2 g/100 mL over 4 weeks or if haemoglobin concentration exceeds 12 g/100 mL; if haemoglobin concentration continues to rise, despite dose reduction, suspend treatment until haemoglobin concentration decreases and then restart at a dose approximately 25% lower than the previous dose. Discontinue approximately 4 weeks after ending chemotherapy

To increase yield of autologous blood (to avoid homologous blood) in predonation programme in moderate anaemia *either* when large volume of blood required *or* when sufficient blood

**9**

Nutrition and blood

cannot be saved for elective major surgery, by intravenous injection over 1–5 minutes, 600 units/kg twice weekly for 3 weeks before surgery; consult product literature for details and advice on ensuring high iron stores

Moderate anaemia (haemoglobin concentration 10–13 g/100 mL) before elective orthopaedic surgery in adults with expected moderate blood loss to reduce exposure to allogeneic blood transfusion or if autologous transfusion unavailable, by subcutaneous injection (max. 1 mL per injection site), 600 units/kg every week for 3 weeks before surgery and on day of surgery *or* 300 units/kg daily for 15 days starting 10 days before surgery; consult product literature for details

### Eprex® (Janssen-Cilag) PoM

Injection, prefilled syringe, epoetin alfa, net price 1000 units = £5.72; 2000 units = £11.44; 3000 units = £17.16; 4000 units = £22.88; 5000 units = £28.60; 6000 units = £34.32; 8000 units = £45.76; 10 000 units = £57.19; 20 000 units = £114.39; 30 000 units = £205.90; 40 000 units = £274.53. An auto-injector device is available for use with prefilled syringes

**Dose** symptomatic anaemia associated with chronic renal failure in patients on haemodialysis (see also MHRA/CHM advice, p. 518), by intravenous injection over 1–5 minutes *or* by subcutaneous injection (max. 1 mL per injection site), initially 50 units/kg 3 times weekly adjusted according to response in steps of 25 units/kg 3 times weekly at intervals of at least 4 weeks; maintenance dose, usually a total of 75–300 units/kg weekly (as a single dose or in divided doses); CHILD by intravenous injection initially as for adults; maintenance dose, body-weight under 10 kg usually 75–150 units/kg 3 times weekly, body-weight 10–30 kg usually 60–150 units/kg 3 times weekly, body-weight over 30 kg usually 30–100 units/kg 3 times weekly

Symptomatic anaemia associated with chronic renal failure in adults on peritoneal dialysis (see also MHRA/CHM advice, p. 518), by intravenous injection over 1–5 minutes *or* by subcutaneous injection (max. 1 mL per injection site), initially 50 units/kg twice weekly; maintenance dose 25–50 units/kg twice weekly Severe symptomatic anaemia of renal origin in adults with renal insufficiency not yet on dialysis (see also MHRA/CHM advice, p. 518), by intravenous injection over 1–5 minutes *or* by subcutaneous injection (max. 1 mL per injection site), initially 50 units/kg 3 times weekly increased according to response in steps of 25 units/kg 3 times weekly at intervals of at least 4 weeks; maintenance dose 17–33 units/kg 3 times weekly; max. 200 units/kg 3 times weekly

**Note** Intravenous route preferred; reduce dose by approximately 25% if rise in haemoglobin concentration exceeds 2 g/100 mL over 4 weeks or if haemoglobin concentration exceeds 12 g/100 mL; if haemoglobin concentration continues to rise, despite dose reduction, suspend treatment until haemoglobin concentration decreases and then restart at a dose approximately 25% lower than the previous dose.

Symptomatic anaemia in adults receiving cancer chemotherapy (see also MHRA/CHM advice, p. 518), by subcutaneous injection (max. 1 mL per injection site), initially 150 units/kg 3 times weekly (*or* 450 units/kg once weekly), increased if appropriate rise in haemoglobin (or reticulocyte count) not achieved after 4 weeks to 300 units/kg 3 times weekly; discontinue if inadequate response after 4 weeks at higher dose

**Note** Reduce dose by approximately 25–50% if rise in haemoglobin concentration exceeds 2 g/100 mL over 4 weeks or if haemoglobin concentration exceeds 12 g/100 mL; if haemoglobin concentration continues to rise, despite dose reduction, suspend treatment until haemoglobin concentration decreases and then restart at a dose approximately 25% lower than the previous dose. Discontinue approximately 4 weeks after ending chemotherapy

To increase yield of autologous blood (to avoid homologous blood) in predonation programme in moderate anaemia *either* when large volume of blood required *or* when sufficient blood cannot be saved for elective major surgery, by intravenous injection over 1–5 minutes, 600 units/kg twice weekly for 3 weeks before surgery; consult product literature for details and advice on ensuring high iron stores

Moderate anaemia (haemoglobin concentration 10–13 g/100 mL) before elective orthopaedic surgery in adults with expected moderate blood loss to reduce exposure to allogeneic blood transfusion or if autologous transfusion unavailable, by subcutaneous injection (max. 1 mL per injection site), 600 units/kg every week for 3 weeks before surgery and on day of surgery *or* 300 units/kg daily for 15 days starting 10 days before surgery; consult product literature for details

### ◢Epoetin beta
### NeoRecormon® (Roche) PoM

Injection, prefilled syringe, epoetin beta, net price 500 units = £3.75; 1000 units = £7.49; 2000 units = £14.98; 3000 units = £22.47; 4000 units = £29.96; 5000 units = £37.47; 6000 units = £44.94; 10 000 units = £74.90; 20 000 units = £149.79; 30 000 units = £224.69

**Excipients** include phenylalanine up to 300 micrograms/syringe (section 9.4.1)

Multidose injection, powder for reconstitution, epoetin beta, net price 50 000-unit vial = £374.48; 100 000-unit vial = £748.96 (both with solvent)

**Excipients** include phenylalanine up to 5 mg/vial (section 9.4.1), benzyl alcohol (avoid in neonates, see Excipients p. 2)

**Note** Avoid contact of reconstituted injection with glass; use only plastic materials

Reco-Pen, (for subcutaneous use), double-chamber cartridges (containing epoetin beta and solvent), net price 10 000-unit cartridge = £74.89; 20 000-unit cartridge = £149.79; for use with *Reco-Pen* injection device and needles (both available free from Roche)

**Excipients** include phenylalanine up to 500 micrograms/cartridge (section 9.4.1), benzyl alcohol (avoid in neonates, see Excipients, p. 2)

**Dose** symptomatic anaemia associated with chronic renal failure (see also MHRA/CHM advice, p. 518), by subcutaneous injection, ADULT and CHILD, initially 20 units/kg 3 times weekly for 4 weeks, increased according to response at intervals of 4 weeks in steps of 20 units/kg 3 times weekly; total weekly dose may be divided into daily doses; maintenance dose, initially reduce dose by half then adjust according to response at intervals of 1–2 weeks; weekly maintenance dose may be given as a single dose or in 3 or 7 divided doses; max. 720 units/kg weekly

By intravenous injection over 2 minutes, ADULT and CHILD, initially 40 units/kg 3 times weekly for 4 weeks, increased according to response to 80 units/kg 3 times weekly after 4 weeks, with further increases if needed at intervals of 4 weeks in steps of 20 units/kg 3 times weekly; maintenance dose, initially reduce dose by half then adjust according to response at intervals of 1–2 weeks; max. 720 units/kg weekly

**Note** Subcutaneous route preferred in patients not on haemodialysis. Reduce dose by approximately 25% if rise in haemoglobin concentration exceeds 2 g/100 mL over 4 weeks or if haemoglobin concentration approaches or exceeds 12 g/100 mL; if haemoglobin concentration continues to rise, despite dose reduction, suspend treatment until haemoglobin concentration decreases and then restart at a dose approximately 25% lower than the previous dose

Prevention of anaemia of prematurity in neonates with birth-weight of 0.75–1.5 kg and gestational age of less than 34 weeks, by subcutaneous injection (of single-dose, unpreserved injection), 250 units/kg 3 times weekly preferably starting within 3 days of birth and continued for 6 weeks

Symptomatic anaemia in adults with non-myeloid malignancies receiving chemotherapy (see also MHRA/CHM advice, p. 518), by subcutaneous injection, initially 450 units/kg weekly (as a single dose or in 3–7 divided doses), increased if necessary after 4 weeks (if a rise in haemoglobin of at least 1 g/100 mL not achieved) to 900 units/kg weekly (as a single dose or in 3–7 divided doses); if adequate response obtained reduce dose by 25–50%; max. 60 000 units weekly

**Note** Discontinue treatment if haemoglobin concentration does not increase by at least 1 g/100 mL after 8 weeks of therapy (response unlikely). Reduce dose by approximately 25–50% if rise in haemoglobin concentration exceeds 2 g/100 mL over 4 weeks or if haemoglobin concentration exceeds 12 g/100 mL; if haemoglobin concentration continues to rise, despite dose reduction, suspend treatment until haemoglobin concentration decreases and then restart at a dose approximately 25% lower than the previous dose. Discontinue approximately 4 weeks after ending chemotherapy

To increase yield of autologous blood (to avoid homologous blood) in predonation programme in moderate anaemia when blood-conserving procedures are insufficient or unavailable, consult product literature

### ◢Epoetin zeta
### Retacrit® (Hospira) ▼ PoM

Injection, prefilled syringe, epoetin zeta, net price 1000 units = £5.66; 2000 units = £11.31; 3000 units =

9 Nutrition and blood

£16.97; 4000 units = £22.63; 5000 units = £28.28; 6000 units = £33.94; 8000 units = £45.25; 10 000 units = £56.57; 20 000 units = £113.13; 30 000 units = £169.70; 40 000 units = £226.26

Excipients include phenylalanine up to 500 micrograms/syringe (section 9.4.1)

Note Biosimilar medicine, p. 1

Dose symptomatic anaemia associated with chronic renal failure in patients on haemodialysis (see also MHRA/CHM advice, p. 518), by intravenous injection over 1–5 minutes, initially 50 units/kg 3 times weekly adjusted according to response in steps of 25 units/kg 3 times weekly at intervals of at least 4 weeks; maintenance dose, usually 25–100 units/kg 3 times weekly; CHILD by intravenous injection initially as for adults; maintenance dose, body-weight under 10 kg usually 75–150 units/kg 3 times weekly, body-weight 10–30 kg usually 60–150 units/kg 3 times weekly, body-weight over 30 kg usually 30–100 units/kg 3 times weekly

Symptomatic anaemia associated with chronic renal failure in adults on peritoneal dialysis (see also MHRA/CHM advice, p. 518), by intravenous injection over 1–5 minutes, initially 50 units/kg twice weekly; maintenance dose 25–50 units/kg twice weekly

Severe symptomatic anaemia of renal origin in adults with renal insufficiency not yet on dialysis (see also MHRA/CHM advice, p. 518), by intravenous injection over 1–5 minutes, initially 50 units/kg 3 times weekly increased according to response in steps of 25 units/kg 3 times weekly at intervals of at least 4 weeks; maintenance dose 17–33 units/kg 3 times weekly; max. 200 units/kg 3 times weekly

Note Avoid increasing haemoglobin concentration at a rate exceeding 2 g/100 mL over 4 weeks

Symptomatic anaemia in adults receiving cancer chemotherapy (see also MHRA/CHM advice, p. 518), by subcutaneous injection (max. 1 mL per injection site), initially 150 units/kg 3 times weekly (or 450 units/kg once weekly), increased if appropriate rise in haemoglobin (or reticulocyte count) not achieved after 4 weeks to 300 units/kg 3 times weekly; discontinue if inadequate response after 4 weeks at higher dose

Note Reduce dose by approximately 25–50% if rise in haemoglobin concentration exceeds 2 g/100 mL over 4 weeks or if haemoglobin concentration exceeds 12 g/100 mL; if haemoglobin concentration continues to rise, despite dose reduction, suspend treatment until haemoglobin concentration decreases and then restart at a dose approximately 25% lower than the previous dose. Discontinue approximately 4 weeks after ending chemotherapy

To increase yield of autologous blood (to avoid homologous blood) in predonation programme in moderate anaemia either when large volume of blood required or when sufficient blood cannot be saved for elective major surgery, by intravenous injection over 1–5 minutes, 600 units/kg twice weekly for 3 weeks before surgery; consult product literature for details and advice on ensuring high iron stores

### METHOXY POLYETHYLENE GLYCOL-EPOETIN BETA
(Pegzerepoetin alfa)

Indications  see under Dose below

Cautions  see Epoetin; severe liver disease (Appendix 2); pregnancy (Appendix 4); breast-feeding (Appendix 5)

Contra-indications  see Epoetin

Side-effects  see Epoetin; also hot flushes reported

Dose

• Symptomatic anaemia associated with chronic kidney disease in patients not currently treated with erythropoietin (see also MHRA/CHM advice, p. 518), ADULT over 18 years, by subcutaneous or intravenous injection, initially 600 nanograms/kg once every 2 weeks, adjusted according to response at intervals of at least 4 weeks; maintenance dose of double the previous fortnightly dose may be given every 4 weeks

• Symptomatic anaemia associated with chronic kidney disease in patients currently treated with erythropoietin (see also MHRA/CHM advice, p. 518), ADULT over 18 years, by subcutaneous or intravenous injection, consult product literature

Note Subcutaneous route preferred in patients not on haemodialysis. Reduce dose by approximately 25% if rise in haemoglobin concentration exceeds 2 g/100 mL over 4 weeks, or if haemoglobin concentration approaches or exceeds 12 g/100 mL; if haemoglobin concentration continues to rise, despite dose reduction, suspend treatment until haemoglobin concentration decreases and then restart at a dose approximately 25% lower than the previous dose

Mircera® (Roche) ▼ PoM

Injection, prefilled syringe, methoxy polyethylene glycol-epoetin beta, net price 30 micrograms/0.3 mL = £44.94; 50 micrograms/0.3 mL = £74.89; 75 micrograms/0.3 mL = £112.33; 100 micrograms/0.3 mL = £149.77; 120 micrograms/0.3 mL = £179.74; 150 micrograms/0.3 mL = £224.66; 200 micrograms/0.3 mL = £299.54; 250 micrograms/0.3 mL = £374.43; 360 micrograms/0.6 mL = £539.22

## Sickle-cell disease

Sickle-cell disease is caused by a structural abnormality of haemoglobin resulting in deformed, less flexible red blood cells. Acute complications in the more severe forms include *sickle-cell crisis*, where infarction of the microvasculature and blood supply to organs results in severe pain. Sickle-cell crisis requires hospitalisation, intravenous fluids, analgesia (section 4.7), and treatment of any concurrent infection. Chronic complications include skin ulceration, renal failure, and increased susceptibility to infection. Pneumococcal vaccine (section 14.4), haemophilus influenzae type b vaccine (section 14.4), an annual influenza vaccine (section 14.4) and prophylactic penicillin (Table 2, section 5.1) reduce the risk of infection. Hepatitis B vaccine (section 14.4) should be considered if the patient is not immune.

In most forms of sickle-cell disease, varying degrees of haemolytic anaemia are present accompanied by increased erythropoiesis; this may increase folate requirements and folate supplementation may be necessary (section 9.1.2).

Hydroxycarbamide (hydroxyurea) can reduce the frequency of crises and the need for blood transfusions in sickle-cell disease; it should be considered in consultation with a specialist centre. The beneficial effects of hydroxycarbamide may not become evident for several months. Myelosuppression and skin reactions are the most common side-effects.

### HYDROXYCARBAMIDE
(Hydroxyurea)

Indications  sickle-cell disease (see notes above); chronic myeloid leukaemia, cancer of the cervix (section 8.1.5)

Cautions  see section 8.1 and notes above; also monitor renal and hepatic function before and during treatment; monitor full blood count before treatment, then every 2 weeks for the first 2 months and then every 2 months thereafter (or every 2 weeks if on max. dose); leg ulcers (review treatment if cutaneous vasculitic ulcerations develop); hepatic impairment (avoid if severe; Appendix 2); renal impairment (avoid if eGFR less than 30 mL/minute/1.73 m²; Appendix 3); interactions: Appendix 1 (hydroxycarbamide)

Contra-indications  pregnancy (Appendix 4); breast-feeding

9

Nutrition and blood

**Side-effects** see section 8.1 and notes above; also headache; *less commonly* dizziness and rash; *rarely* reduced sperm count and activity; fever, amenorrhoea, skin cancers (in elderly patients), bleeding and hypomagnesaemia also reported

**Dose**

- By mouth, initially 15 mg/kg daily, increased every 12 weeks in steps of 5 mg/kg daily according to response; usual dose 15–30 mg/kg daily (max. 35 mg/kg daily); CHILD under 18 years, see *BNF for Children*

**Siklos®** (Nordic) ▼ PoM
Tablets, scored, f/c, hydroxycarbamide 1 g, net price 30-tab pack = £500.00

# Iron overload

Severe tissue iron overload can occur in aplastic and other refractory anaemias, mainly as the result of repeated blood transfusions. It is a particular problem in refractory anaemias with hyperplastic bone marrow, especially *thalassaemia major*, where excessive iron absorption from the gut and inappropriate iron therapy can add to the tissue siderosis.

Iron overload associated with haemochromatosis can be treated with repeated venesection. Venesection may also be used for patients who have received multiple transfusions and whose bone marrow has recovered. Where venesection is contra-indicated, the long-term administration of the iron chelating compound **desferrioxamine mesilate** is useful. Subcutaneous infusions of desferrioxamine are given over 8–12 hours, 3–7 times a week. The dose should reflect the degree of iron overload. For children starting therapy (and who have low iron overload) the dose should not exceed 30 mg/kg. For established overload the dose is usually between 20 and 50 mg/kg daily. Desferrioxamine (up to 2 g per unit of blood) may also be given at the time of blood transfusion, provided that the desferrioxamine is **not** added to the blood and is **not** given through the same line as the blood (but the two may be given through the same cannula).

Iron excretion induced by desferrioxamine is enhanced by administration of ascorbic acid (vitamin C, section 9.6.3) 200 mg daily by mouth (100 mg in infants); it should be given separately from food since it also enhances iron absorption. Ascorbic acid should not be given to patients with cardiac dysfunction; in patients with normal cardiac function ascorbic acid should be introduced 1 month after starting desferrioxamine.

Desferrioxamine infusion can be used to treat *aluminium overload* in dialysis patients; theoretically 100 mg of desferrioxamine binds with 4.1 mg of aluminium.

**Deferasirox**, an oral iron chelator, is licensed for the treatment of chronic iron overload in adults and children over 6 years with thalassaemia major who receive frequent blood transfusions (more than 7 mL/kg/month of packed red blood cells). It is also licensed for chronic iron overload when desferrioxamine is contra-indicated or inadequate in patients with thalassaemia major who receive infrequent blood transfusions (less than 7 mL/kg/month of packed red blood cells), in patients with other anaemias, and in children aged 2 to 5 years.

The *Scottish Medicines Consortium* has advised (January 2007) that deferasirox is accepted for restricted use for the treatment of chronic iron overload associated with the treatment of rare acquired or inherited anaemias requiring recurrent blood transfusions. It is not recommended for patients with myelodysplastic syndromes.

**Deferiprone**, an oral iron chelator, is licensed for the treatment of iron overload in patients with thalassaemia major in whom desferrioxamine is contra-indicated or is inadequate. Blood dyscrasias, particularly agranulocytosis, have been reported with deferiprone.

## ◼ DEFERASIROX

**Indications** see notes above

**Cautions** eye and ear examinations required before treatment and annually during treatment; monitor body-weight, height, and sexual development in children annually; monitor serum-ferritin concentration monthly; risk of gastro-intestinal ulceration and haemorrhage; consider treatment interruption if unexplained cytopenia occurs; history of liver cirrhosis; test liver function before treatment, then every 2 weeks during the first month, and then monthly; see also hepatic impairment (Appendix 2); measure baseline serum creatinine and monitor renal function weekly during the first month of treatment and monthly thereafter; test for proteinuria monthly; see also renal impairment (Appendix 3); pregnancy (Appendix 4); breast-feeding (Appendix 5); **interactions:** Appendix 1 (deferasirox)

**Side-effects** gastro-intestinal disturbances (including ulceration and haemorrhage); headache; proteinuria; pruritus, rash; *less commonly* hepatitis, cholelithiasis, oedema, fatigue, anxiety, sleep disorder, dizziness, pyrexia, pharyngitis, glucosuria, renal tubulopathy, disturbances of hearing and vision (including lens opacity and maculopathy), and skin pigmentation; hepatic failure, acute renal failure, blood disorders (including agranulocytosis, neutropenia, pancytopenia, and thrombocytopenia), hypersensitivity reactions (including anaphylaxis and angioedema) also reported

**Dose**

- ADULT and CHILD over 2 years initially 10–30 mg/kg once daily according to serum-ferritin concentration and amount of transfused blood (consult product literature); maintenance, adjust dose every 3–6 months in steps of 5–10 mg/kg according to serum-ferritin concentration; max. 30 mg/kg daily

**Exjade®** (Novartis) ▼ PoM
Dispersible tablets, deferasirox 125 mg, net price 28-tab pack = £117.60; 250 mg, 28-tab pack = £235.20; 500 mg, 28-tab pack = £470.40. Label: 13, 22, counselling, administration
**Counselling** Tablets may be dispersed in water, orange juice, or apple juice; if necessary resuspend residue

## ◼ DEFERIPRONE

**Indications** see notes above

**Cautions** monitor neutrophil count weekly and discontinue treatment if neutropenia develops; monitor plasma-zinc concentration; hepatic impairment (Appendix 2); renal impairment (Appendix 3)
**Blood disorders** Patients or their carers should be told how to recognise signs of neutropenia and advised to seek immediate medical attention if symptoms such as fever or sore throat develop

**Contra-indications** history of agranulocytosis or recurrent neutropenia; pregnancy (contraception advised in women of child-bearing potential; **important teratogenic risk**: see Appendix 4); breast-feeding (Appendix 5)

**Side-effects** gastro-intestinal disturbances (reducing dose and increasing gradually may improve tolerance), increased appetite; headache; red-brown urine discoloration; neutropenia, agranulocytosis; zinc deficiency; arthropathy

**Dose**

• ADULT and CHILD over 6 years 25 mg/kg 3 times daily (max. 100 mg/kg daily)

**Ferriprox®** (Swedish Orphan) ⓅⓄⓂ
Tablets, f/c, scored, deferiprone 500 mg, net price 100-tab pack = £152.39. Label: 14, counselling, blood disorders
Oral solution, red, deferiprone 100 mg/mL, net price 500 mL = £152.39. Label: 14, counselling, blood disorders

### ◼ DESFERRIOXAMINE MESILATE
(Deferoxamine Mesilate)

**Indications** see notes above; iron poisoning, see Emergency Treatment of Poisoning, p. 32

**Cautions** renal impairment; eye and ear examinations before treatment and at 3-month intervals during treatment; monitor body-weight and height in children at 3-month intervals—risk of growth retardation with excessive doses; aluminium-related encephalopathy (may exacerbate neurological dysfunction); pregnancy (Appendix 4); breast-feeding (Appendix 5); **interactions**: Appendix 1 (desferrioxamine)

**Side-effects** hypotension (especially when given too rapidly by intravenous injection), disturbances of hearing and vision (including lens opacity and retinopathy); injection-site reactions, gastro-intestinal disturbances, asthma, fever, headache, arthralgia and myalgia; *very rarely* anaphylaxis, acute respiratory distress syndrome, neurological disturbances (including dizziness, neuropathy and paraesthesia), Yersinia and mucormycosis infections, rash, renal impairment, and blood dyscrasias

**Dose**

• See notes above; iron poisoning, see Emergency Treatment of Poisoning, p. 32
Note For full details and warnings relating to administration, consult product literature

**Desferrioxamine mesilate** (Non-proprietary) ⓅⓄⓂ
Injection, powder for reconstitution, desferrioxamine mesilate, net price 500-mg vial = £4.26; 2-g vial = £17.05

**Desferal®** (Novartis) ⓅⓄⓂ
Injection, powder for reconstitution, desferrioxamine mesilate, net price 500-mg vial = £4.44, 2-g vial = £17.77

## Paroxysmal nocturnal haemoglobinuria

Eculizumab, a recombinant monoclonal antibody, inhibits terminal complement activation at the C5 protein and thereby reduces haemolysis. It is used to reduce haemolysis in paroxysmal nocturnal haemoglobinuria, a severe and disabling form of haemolytic anaemia.

### ◼ ECULIZUMAB

**Indications** paroxysmal nocturnal haemoglobinuria, in those with a history of blood transfusions (specialist use only)

**Cautions** active systemic infection; monitor for intravascular haemolysis (including serum-lactate dehydrogenase concentration) for at least 8 weeks after discontinuation; pregnancy (Appendix 4)
**Meningococcal infection** Vaccinate against *Neisseria meningitidis* at least 2 weeks before treatment (tetravalent vaccine against serotypes A, C, W135 and Y recommended); revaccinate according to current medical guidelines. Advise patient to report promptly any signs of meningococcal infection. Other immunisations should also be up to date (section 14.1)

**Contra-indications** unresolved *Neisseria meningitidis* infection; patients unvaccinated against *Neisseria meningitidis* (see Cautions above); known or suspected hereditary complement deficiencies; breast-feeding (Appendix 5)

**Side-effects** gastro-intestinal disturbances; nasopharyngitis, sinusitis, cough, pharyngolaryngeal pain, epistaxis; headache, fatigue, dizziness, insomnia; infection (including meningococcal infection), pyrexia, influenza-like symptoms; muscle cramp, pain in extremities; rash, pruritus

**Dose**

• By intravenous infusion, ADULT over 18 years, initially 600 mg once a week for 4 weeks, then 900 mg on week 5; maintenance, 900 mg once every 12–16 days

**Soliris®** (Alexion) ▼ ⓅⓄⓂ
Concentrate for intravenous infusion, eculizumab 10 mg/mL, net price 30-mL vial = £3150.00. Counselling, meningococcal infection, patient information card
Electrolytes Na⁺ 5 mmol/vial

### 9.1.4 Drugs used in platelet disorders

Acute idiopathic thrombocytopenic purpura is usually self-limiting in children. In adults, idiopathic thrombocytopenic purpura can be treated with a **corticosteroid**, e.g. prednisolone 1 mg/kg daily, gradually reducing the dose over several weeks. Splenectomy is considered if a satisfactory platelet count is not achieved or if there is a relapse on reducing the dose of corticosteroid or withdrawing it.

**Immunoglobulin** preparations (section 14.5.1), are also used in idiopathic thrombocytopenic purpura or where a temporary rapid rise in platelets is needed, as in pregnancy or pre-operatively; they are also used for children often in preference to a corticosteroid. **Anti-D (Rh₀) immunoglobulin** (section 14.5.3) is effective in raising the platelet count in about 80% of unsplenectomised rhesus-positive individuals; its effects may last longer than normal immunoglobulin for intravenous use, but further doses are usually required.

Other therapy that has been tried in refractory idiopathic thrombocytopenic purpura includes azathioprine (section 8.2.1), cyclophosphamide (section 8.1.1), vincristine (section 8.1.4), ciclosporin (section 8.2.2), and danazol (section 6.7.2). Rituximab (section 8.2.3) may also be effective and in some cases induces prolonged remission. For patients with chronic severe thrombocytopenia refractory to other therapy, tranexamic acid (section 2.11) may be given to reduce the severity of haemorrhage.

**Anagrelide** inhibits platelet formation. It is licensed for essential thrombocythaemia in patients at risk of thrombo-haemorrhagic events who have not responded adequately to other drugs or who cannot tolerate other drugs.

### ■ ANAGRELIDE

**Indications** essential thrombocythaemia in at-risk patients who have not responded adequately to other therapy or who are intolerant of it (initiated under specialist supervision)

**Cautions** cardiovascular disease—assess cardiac function before and during treatment; concomitant aspirin in patients at risk of haemorrhage; monitor full blood count (monitor platelet count every 2 days for 1 week, then weekly until maintenance dose established), liver function, serum creatinine and urea; hepatic impairment (Appendix 2); renal impairment (Appendix 3); **interactions:** Appendix 1 (anagrelide) Driving Dizziness may affect performance of skilled tasks (e.g. driving)

**Contra-indications** pregnancy (Appendix 4); breast-feeding (Appendix 5)

**Side-effects** gastro-intestinal disturbances; palpitation, tachycardia, fluid retention; headache, dizziness, fatigue; anaemia; rash; *less commonly* pancreatitis, gastro-intestinal haemorrhage, congestive heart failure, hypertension, arrhythmias, syncope, chest pain, dyspnoea, sleep disturbances, paraesthesia, hypoaesthesia, depression, nervousness, confusion, amnesia, fever, weight changes, impotence, blood disorders, myalgia, arthralgia, epistaxis, dry mouth, alopecia, skin discoloration, and pruritus; *rarely* gastritis, colitis, postural hypotension, angina, myocardial infarction, vasodilatation, pulmonary hypotension, pulmonary infiltrates, migraine, drowsiness, impaired co-ordination, dysarthria, asthenia, tinnitus, renal failure, nocturia, visual disturbances, and gingival bleeding; allergic alveolitis also reported

**Dose**

* Initially 500 micrograms twice daily adjusted according to response in steps of 500 micrograms daily at weekly intervals to max. 10 mg daily (max. single dose 2.5 mg); usual dose range 1–3 mg daily in divided doses

**Xagrid®** (Shire) ▼ PoM
    Capsules, anagrelide (as hydrochloride), 500 micrograms, net price 100-cap pack = £337.14. Counselling, driving, see above

## 9.1.5 G6PD deficiency

Glucose 6-phosphate dehydrogenase (G6PD) deficiency is highly prevalent in individuals originating from most parts of Africa, from most parts of Asia, from Oceania, and from Southern Europe; it can also occur, rarely, in any other individuals. G6PD deficiency is more common in males than it is in females.

Individuals with G6PD deficiency are susceptible to developing acute haemolytic anaemia when they take

a number of common drugs. They are also susceptible to developing acute haemolytic anaemia when they eat fava beans (broad beans, *Vicia faba*); this is termed *favism* and can be more severe in children or when the fresh fava beans are eaten raw.

When prescribing drugs for patients with G6PD deficiency, the following three points should be kept in mind:

* G6PD deficiency is genetically heterogeneous; susceptibility to the haemolytic risk from drugs varies; thus, a drug found to be safe in some G6PD-deficient individuals may not be equally safe in others;

* manufacturers do not routinely test drugs for their effects in G6PD-deficient individuals;

* the risk and severity of haemolysis is almost always dose-related.

The lists below should be read with these points in mind. Ideally, information about G6PD deficiency should be available before prescribing a drug listed below. However, in the absence of this information, the possibility of haemolysis should be considered, especially if the patient belongs to a group in which G6PD deficiency is common.

A very few G6PD-deficient individuals with chronic non-spherocytic haemolytic anaemia have haemolysis even in the absence of an exogenous trigger. These patients must be regarded as being at high risk of severe exacerbation of haemolysis following administration of any of the drugs listed below.

---

**Drugs with definite risk of haemolysis in most G6PD-deficient individuals**
Dapsone and other sulphones (higher doses for dermatitis herpetiformis more likely to cause problems)
Methylthioninium chloride (methylene blue)
Niridazole [not on UK market]
Nitrofurantoin
Pamaquin [not on UK market]
Primaquine (30 mg weekly for 8 weeks has been found to be without undue harmful effects in African and Asian people, see section 5.4.1)
Quinolones (including ciprofloxacin, moxifloxacin, nalidixic acid, norfloxacin, and ofloxacin)
Sulphonamides (including co-trimoxazole; some sulphonamides, e.g. sulfadiazine, have been tested and found not to be haemolytic in many G6PD-deficient individuals)

---

**Drugs with possible risk of haemolysis in some G6PD-deficient individuals**
Aspirin (acceptable up to a dose of at least 1 g daily in most G6PD-deficient individuals)
Chloroquine (acceptable in acute malaria and malaria chemoprophylaxis)
Menadione, water-soluble derivatives (e.g. menadiol sodium phosphate)
Probenecid [not on UK market]
Quinidine (acceptable in acute malaria) [not on UK market]
Quinine (acceptable in acute malaria)
Rasburicase

**Note** Naphthalene in mothballs also causes haemolysis in individuals with G6PD deficiency

---

## 9.1.6 Drugs used in neutropenia

Recombinant human granulocyte-colony stimulating factor (rhG-CSF) stimulates the production of neutrophils and may reduce the duration of chemotherapy-induced neutropenia and thereby reduce the incidence of associated sepsis; there is as yet no evidence that it improves overall survival. **Filgrastim** (unglycosylated rhG-CSF) and **lenograstim** (glycosylated rhG-CSF) have similar effects; both have been used in a variety of clinical settings, but they do not have any clear-cut routine indications. In congenital neutropenia filgrastim usually increases the neutrophil count with an appropriate clinical response. Prolonged use may be associated with an increased risk of myeloid malignancy. **Pegfilgrastim** is a polyethylene glycol-conjugated ('pegylated') derivative of filgrastim; pegylation increases the duration of filgrastim activity.

Treatment with recombinant human growth factors should only be prescribed by those experienced in their use.

**Cautions** Recombinant human growth factors should be used with caution in patients with pre-malignant or malignant myeloid conditions. Full blood counts including differential white cell and platelet counts should be monitored. Treatment should be withdrawn in patients who develop signs of pulmonary infiltration. There have been reports of pulmonary infiltrates leading to acute respiratory distress syndrome—patients with a history of pulmonary infiltrates or pneumonia may be at higher risk. Recombinant human growth factors should be used with caution in patients with sickle-cell disease. Recombinant human growth factors are not recommended in pregnancy (Appendix 4) or breast-feeding (Appendix 5).

**Side-effects** Side-effects of granulocyte-colony stimulating factors include gastro-intestinal disturbances (including nausea, vomiting, and diarrhoea), anorexia, headache, asthenia, fever, musculoskeletal pain, bone pain, rash, alopecia, injection-site reactions, thrombocytopenia, and leucocytosis. *Less commonly* chest pain, hypersensitivity reactions (including anaphylaxis and bronchospasm) and arthralgia can occur. Pulmonary side-effects, particularly interstitial pneumonia (see Cautions above), cutaneous vasculitis and acute febrile neutrophilic dermatosis have *rarely* been reported.

### FILGRASTIM
(Recombinant human granulocyte-colony stimulating factor, G-CSF)

**Indications** (specialist use only) reduction in duration of neutropenia and incidence of febrile neutropenia in cytotoxic chemotherapy for malignancy (except chronic myeloid leukaemia and myelodysplastic syndromes); reduction in duration of neutropenia (and associated sequelae) in myeloablative therapy followed by bone-marrow transplantation; mobilisation of peripheral blood progenitor cells for harvesting and subsequent autologous or allogeneic infusion; severe congenital neutropenia, cyclic neutropenia, or idiopathic neutropenia and history of severe or recurrent infections (distinguish carefully from other haematological disorders, consult product literature); persistent neutropenia in advanced HIV infection

**Cautions** see notes above; also regular morphological and cytogenetic bone-marrow examinations recommended in severe congenital neutropenia (possible risk of myelodysplastic syndromes or leukaemia); secondary acute myeloid leukaemia, sickle-cell disease; monitor spleen size (risk of rupture); osteoporotic bone disease (monitor bone density if given for more than 6 months); **interactions:** Appendix 1 (filgrastim)

**Contra-indications** severe congenital neutropenia (Kostmann's syndrome) with abnormal cytogenetics

**Side-effects** see notes above; also mucositis, splenic enlargement, hepatomegaly, transient hypotension, epistaxis, urinary abnormalities (including dysuria, proteinuria, and haematuria), osteoporosis, exacerbation of rheumatoid arthritis, anaemia, transient decrease in blood glucose, pseudogout, and raised uric acid

**Dose**

- Cytotoxic-induced neutropenia, preferably by subcutaneous injection *or* by intravenous infusion (over 30 minutes), ADULT and CHILD, 500 000 units/kg daily started at least 24 hours after cytotoxic chemotherapy, continued until neutrophil count in normal range, usually for up to 14 days (up to 38 days in acute myeloid leukaemia)

- Myeloablative therapy followed by bone-marrow transplantation, by intravenous infusion over 30 minutes or over 24 hours *or* by subcutaneous infusion over 24 hours, 1 million units/kg daily, started at least 24 hours following cytotoxic chemotherapy (and within 24 hours of bone-marrow infusion), then adjusted according to neutrophil count (consult product literature)

- Mobilisation of peripheral blood progenitor cells for autologous infusion, used alone, by subcutaneous injection *or* by subcutaneous infusion over 24 hours, 1 million units/kg daily for 5–7 days; used following adjunctive myelosuppressive chemotherapy (to improve yield), by subcutaneous injection, 500 000 units/kg daily, started the day after completing chemotherapy and continued until neutrophil count in normal range; for timing of leucopheresis consult product literature

- Mobilisation of peripheral blood progenitor cells in normal donors for allogeneic infusion, by subcutaneous injection, ADULT under 60 years and CHILD over 16 years, 1 million units/kg daily for 4–5 days; for timing of leucopheresis consult product literature

- Severe chronic neutropenia, by subcutaneous injection, ADULT and CHILD, in severe congenital neutropenia, initially 1.2 million units/kg daily in single or divided doses (initially 500 000 units/kg daily in idiopathic or cyclic neutropenia), adjusted according to response (consult product literature)

- Persistent neutropenia in HIV infection, by subcutaneous injection, initially 100 000 units/kg daily, increased as necessary until neutrophil count in normal range (usual max. 400 000 units/kg daily), then adjusted to maintain neutrophil count in normal range (consult product literature)

**Neupogen®** (Amgen) ⓅⓄⓂ
Injection, filgrastim 30 million-units (300 micrograms)/mL, net price 1-mL vial = £65.74

Injection (Singleject®), filgrastim 60 million-units (600 micrograms)/mL, net price 0.5-mL prefilled syringe = £65.74; 96 million-units (960 micrograms)/mL, 0.5-mL prefilled syringe = £104.85

**Ratiograstim®** (Ratiopharm UK) ▼ PoM
Injection, prefilled syringe, filgrastim, net price 30 million-units (300 micrograms)/0.5 mL = £62.25; 48 million-units (480 micrograms)/0.8 mL = £99.29
Note Biosimilar medicine, p. 1

## LENOGRASTIM

(Recombinant human granulocyte-colony sti-mulating factor, rHuG-CSF)

**Indications** (specialist use only) reduction in the duration of neutropenia and associated complications following peripheral stem cells or bone-marrow transplantation for non-myeloid malignancy, or following treatment with cytotoxic chemotherapy associated with a significant incidence of febrile neutropenia; mobilisation of peripheral blood progenitor cells for harvesting and subsequent infusion

**Cautions** see notes above; also sickle cell disease; monitor spleen size (risk of rupture)

**Side-effects** see notes above; also mucositis, splenic rupture, and toxic epidermal necrolysis

**Dose**

- Following bone-marrow transplantation, by intravenous infusion or subcutaneous injection, ADULT and CHILD over 2 years 19.2 million units/m² daily started the day after transplantation, continued until neutrophil count stable in acceptable range (max. 28 days)

- Following peripheral stem cells transplantation, by intravenous infusion or subcutaneous injection, ADULT 19.2 million units/m² daily started the day after transplantation, continued until neutrophil count stable in acceptable range (max. 28 days); CHILD see *BNF for Children*

- Cytotoxic-induced neutropenia, by subcutaneous injection, ADULT 19.2 million units/m² daily started the day after completion of chemotherapy, continued until neutrophil count stable in acceptable range (max. 28 days); CHILD see *BNF for Children*

- Mobilisation of peripheral blood progenitor cells, used alone, by subcutaneous injection, ADULT 1.28 million units/kg daily for 4–6 days (5–6 days in healthy donors); used following adjunctive myelosuppressive chemotherapy (to improve yield), by subcutaneous injection, 19.2 million units/m² daily, started 1–5 days after completion of chemotherapy and continued until neutrophil count in acceptable range; for timing of leucopheresis consult product literature; CHILD see *BNF for Children*

**Granocyte®** (Chugai) PoM
Injection, powder for reconstitution, lenograstim, net price 13.4 million-unit (105-microgram) vial = £40.11; 33.6 million-unit (263-microgram) vial = £64.47 (both with 1-mL prefilled syringe water for injections)
Excipients include phenylalanine (section 9.4.1)

## PEGFILGRASTIM

(Pegylated recombinant methionyl human granulocyte-colony stimulating factor)

**Indications** (specialist use only) reduction in duration of neutropenia and incidence of febrile neutropenia in cytotoxic chemotherapy for malignancy (except chronic myeloid leukaemia and myelodysplastic syndromes)

**Cautions** see notes above; also acute leukaemia and myelosuppressive chemotherapy; sickle-cell disease; monitor spleen size (risk of rupture); **interactions**: Appendix 1 (filgrastim)

**Side-effects** see notes above; also *very rarely* splenic rupture

**Dose**
Note Dose expressed as filgrastim

- By subcutaneous injection, ADULT over 18 years, 6 mg (0.6 mL) for each chemotherapy cycle, starting 24 hours after chemotherapy

**Neulasta®** (Amgen) PoM
Injection, pegfilgrastim (expressed as filgrastim) 10 mg/mL, net price 0.6-mL (6-mg) prefilled syringe = £686.38; *SureClick®* prefilled disposable injection device 0.6 mL (6 mg) = £714.24

---

## 9.2 Fluids and electrolytes

9.2.1 Oral preparations for fluid and electrolyte imbalance
9.2.2 Parenteral preparations for fluid and electrolyte imbalance

The following tables give a selection of useful electrolyte values:

### Electrolyte concentrations—intravenous fluids

| Intravenous infusion | Millimoles per litre | | | | |
|---|---|---|---|---|---|
| | Na⁺ | K⁺ | HCO₃⁻ | Cl⁻ | Ca²⁺ |
| *Normal plasma values* | 142 | 4.5 | 26 | 103 | 2.5 |
| Sodium Chloride 0.9% | 150 | — | — | 150 | — |
| Compound Sodium Lactate (Hartmann's) | 131 | 5 | 29 | 111 | 2 |
| Sodium Chloride 0.18% and Glucose 4% | 30 | — | — | 30 | — |
| Potassium Chloride 0.3% and Glucose 5% | — | 40 | — | 40 | — |
| Potassium Chloride 0.3% and Sodium Chloride 0.9% | 150 | 40 | — | 190 | — |
| *To correct metabolic acidosis* | | | | | |
| Sodium Bicarbonate 1.26% | 150 | — | 150 | — | — |
| Sodium Bicarbonate 8.4% for cardiac arrest | 1000 | — | 1000 | — | — |
| Sodium Lactate (m/6) | 167 | — | 167 | — | — |

### Electrolyte content—gastro-intestinal secretions

| Type of fluid | Millimoles per litre | | | | |
|---|---|---|---|---|---|
| | H⁺ | Na⁺ | K⁺ | HCO₃⁻ | Cl⁻ |
| Gastric | 40–60 | 20–80 | 5–20 | — | 100–150 |
| Biliary | — | 120–140 | 5–15 | 30–50 | 80–120 |
| Pancreatic | — | 120–140 | 5–15 | 70–110 | 40–80 |
| Small bowel | — | 120–140 | 5–15 | 20–40 | 90–130 |

Faeces, vomit, or aspiration should be saved and analysed where possible if abnormal losses are suspected; where this is impracticable the approximations above may be helpful in planning replacement therapy

## 9.2.1 Oral preparations for fluid and electrolyte imbalance

9.2.1.1 Oral potassium
9.2.1.2 Oral sodium and water
9.2.1.3 Oral bicarbonate

Sodium and potassium salts, which may be given by mouth to prevent deficiencies or to treat established deficiencies of mild or moderate degree, are discussed in this section. Oral preparations for removing excess potassium and preparations for oral rehydration therapy are also included here. Oral bicarbonate, for metabolic acidosis, is also described in this section.

For reference to calcium, magnesium, and phosphate, see section 9.5.

### 9.2.1.1 Oral potassium

Compensation for potassium loss is especially necessary:

- in those taking digoxin or anti-arrhythmic drugs, where potassium depletion may induce arrhythmias;

- in patients in whom secondary hyperaldosteronism occurs, e.g. renal artery stenosis, cirrhosis of the liver, the nephrotic syndrome, and severe heart failure;

- in patients with excessive losses of potassium in the faeces, e.g. chronic diarrhoea associated with intestinal malabsorption or laxative abuse.

Measures to compensate for potassium loss may also be required in the elderly since they frequently take inadequate amounts of potassium in the diet (but see below for **warning** on **renal insufficiency**). Measures may also be required during long-term administration of drugs known to induce potassium loss (e.g. corticosteroids). Potassium supplements are **seldom required** with the small doses of diuretics given to treat hypertension; **potassium-sparing diuretics** (rather than potassium supplements) are recommended for prevention of hypokalaemia due to diuretics such as furosemide (fruse-

mide) or the thiazides when these are given to eliminate oedema.

**Dosage** If potassium salts are used for the *prevention of hypokalaemia*, then doses of potassium chloride 2 to 4 g (approx. 25 to 50 mmol) daily (in divided doses) by mouth are suitable in patients taking a normal diet. *Smaller doses* must be used if there is *renal insufficiency (common in the elderly)* to reduce the **risk** of **hyperkalaemia**. Potassium salts cause nausea and vomiting and poor compliance is a major limitation to their effectiveness; when appropriate, potassium-sparing diuretics are preferable (see also above). Regular monitoring of plasma-potassium concentration is essential in those taking potassium supplements. When there is *established potassium depletion* larger doses may be necessary, the quantity depending on the severity of any continuing potassium loss (monitoring of plasma-potassium concentration and specialist advice would be required). Potassium depletion is frequently associated with chloride depletion and with metabolic alkalosis, and these disorders require correction.

**Administration** Potassium salts are preferably given as a liquid (or effervescent) preparation, rather than modified-release tablets; they should be given as the chloride (the use of effervescent potassium tablets BPC 1968 should be restricted to *hyperchloraemic states*, section 9.2.1.3).

**Salt substitutes** A number of salt substitutes which contain significant amounts of potassium chloride are readily available as health food products (e.g. *LoSalt®* and *Ruthmol®*). These should not be used by patients with renal failure as potassium intoxication may result.

## ▮ POTASSIUM CHLORIDE

**Indications** potassium depletion (see notes above)

**Cautions** elderly, renal impairment (avoid if severe; Appendix 3); intestinal stricture, history of peptic ulcer, hiatus hernia (for modified-release preparations); **important:** special hazard if given with drugs liable to raise plasma-potassium concentration such as potassium-sparing diuretics, ACE inhibitors, or ciclosporin, for other **interactions:** Appendix 1 (potassium salts)

**Contra-indications** plasma-potassium concentration above 5 mmol/litre

**Side-effects** nausea and vomiting (severe symptoms may indicate obstruction), oesophageal or small bowel ulceration

**Dose**
- See notes above
  **Note** Do not confuse Effervescent Potassium Tablets BPC 1968 (section 9.2.1.3) with effervescent potassium chloride tablets. Effervescent Potassium Tablets BPC 1968 do not contain chloride ions and their use should be restricted to hyperchloraemic states (section 9.2.1.3).

**Kay-Cee-L®** (Geistlich)
Syrup, sugar-free, red, potassium chloride 7.5% (1 mmol/mL each of K⁺ and Cl⁻), net price 500 mL = £3.74. Label: 21

**Sando-K®** (HK Pharma)
Tablets, effervescent, potassium bicarbonate and chloride equivalent to potassium 470 mg (12 mmol of K⁺) and chloride 285 mg (8 mmol of Cl⁻). Net price 20 = £1.53. Label: 13, 21

**9**

**Nutrition and blood**

◢Modified-release preparations
Avoid unless effervescent tablets or liquid preparations inappropriate

**Slow-K®** (Alliance) ◢
Tablets, m/r, orange, s/c, potassium chloride 600 mg (8 mmol each of K$^+$ and Cl$^-$). Net price 20 = 43p. Label: 25, 27, counselling, swallow whole with fluid during meals while sitting or standing

## Management of hyperkalaemia

*Acute severe hyperkalaemia* (plasma-potassium concentration above 6.5 mmol/L or in the presence of ECG changes) calls for urgent treatment with 10–20 mL of calcium gluconate 10% by slow intravenous injection, titrated and adjusted to ECG improvement, to temporarily protect against myocardial excitability. An intravenous injection of soluble insulin (5–10 units) with 50 mL glucose 50% given over 5–15 minutes, reduces serum-potassium concentration; this is repeated if necessary or a continuous infusion instituted. Salbutamol [unlicensed indication], by nebulisation or slow intravenous injection may also reduce plasma-potassium concentration; it should be used with caution in patients with cardiovascular disease. The correction of causal or compounding acidosis with sodium bicarbonate infusion (section 9.2.2) should be considered (**important:** preparations of sodium bicarbonate and calcium salts should not be administered in the same line—risk of precipitation). Drugs exacerbating hyperkalaemia should be reviewed and stopped as appropriate; occasionally haemodialysis is needed.

Ion-exchange resins may be used to remove excess potassium in *mild hyperkalaemia* or in *moderate hyperkalaemia* when there are no ECG changes.

## ▮ POLYSTYRENE SULPHONATE RESINS

**Indications** hyperkalaemia associated with anuria or severe oliguria, and in dialysis patients
**Cautions** children (impaction of resin with excessive dosage or inadequate dilution); monitor for electrolyte disturbances (stop if plasma-potassium concentration below 5 mmol/litre); pregnancy and breast-feeding; sodium-containing resin in congestive heart failure, hypertension, renal impairment, and oedema; **interactions:** Appendix 1 (polystyrene sulphonate resins)
**Contra-indications** obstructive bowel disease; oral administration or reduced gut motility in neonates; avoid calcium-containing resin in hyperparathyroidism, multiple myeloma, sarcoidosis, or metastatic carcinoma
**Side-effects** rectal ulceration following rectal administration; colonic necrosis reported following enemas containing sorbitol; sodium retention, hypercalcaemia, gastric irritation, anorexia, nausea and vomiting, constipation (discontinue treatment—avoid magnesium-containing laxatives), diarrhoea; calcium-containing resin can cause hypercalcaemia (in dialysed patients and occasionally in those with renal impairment), hypomagnesaemia
**Dose**
• By mouth, 15 g 3–4 times daily in water (not fruit squash which has a high potassium content) or as a paste; CHILD 0.5–1 g/kg daily in divided doses

• By rectum, as an enema, 30 g in methylcellulose solution, retained for 9 hours followed by irrigation to remove resin from colon; NEONATE and CHILD, 0.5–1 g/kg daily

**Calcium Resonium®** (Sanofi-Synthelabo)
Powder, buff, calcium polystyrene sulphonate. Net price 300 g = £68.47. Label: 13

**Resonium A®** (Sanofi-Synthelabo)
Powder, buff, sodium polystyrene sulphonate. Net price 454 g = £67.50. Label: 13

▮**9.2.1.2** Oral sodium and water

Sodium chloride is indicated in states of sodium depletion and usually needs to be given intravenously (section 9.2.2). In chronic conditions associated with mild or moderate degrees of sodium depletion, e.g. in salt-losing bowel or renal disease, oral supplements of sodium chloride or sodium bicarbonate (section 9.2.1.3), according to the acid-base status of the patient, may be sufficient.

## ▮ SODIUM CHLORIDE

**Indications** sodium depletion—see also 9.2.2.1; nebuliser diluent (section 3.1.5); eye (section 11.8.1); oral hygiene (section 12.3.4); wound irrigation (section 13.11.1)

**Slow Sodium®** (HK Pharma)
Tablets, m/r, sodium chloride 600 mg (approx. 10 mmol each of Na$^+$ and Cl$^-$). Net price 100-tab pack = £6.05. Label: 25
Dose prophylaxis of sodium chloride deficiency 4–8 tablets daily with water (in severe depletion up to max. 20 tablets daily)
Chronic renal salt wasting, up to 20 tablets daily with appropriate fluid intake
CHILD see *BNF for Children*

## Oral rehydration therapy (ORT)

As a worldwide problem *diarrhoea* is by far the most important indication for fluid and electrolyte replacement. Intestinal absorption of sodium and water is enhanced by glucose (and other carbohydrates). Replacement of fluid and electrolytes lost through diarrhoea can therefore be achieved by giving solutions containing sodium, potassium, and glucose or another carbohydrate such as rice starch.

Oral rehydration solutions should:

• enhance the absorption of water and electrolytes;

• replace the electrolyte deficit adequately and safely;

• contain an alkalinising agent to counter acidosis;

• be slightly hypo-osmolar (about 250 mmol/litre) to prevent the possible induction of osmotic diarrhoea;

• be simple to use in hospital and at home;

• be palatable and acceptable, especially to children;

• be readily available.

It is the policy of the World Health Organization (WHO) to promote a single oral rehydration solution but to use it flexibly (e.g. by giving extra water between drinks of oral rehydration solution to moderately dehydrated infants).

*9 Nutrition and blood*

Oral rehydration solutions used in the UK are lower in sodium (50–60 mmol/litre) than the WHO formulation since, in general, patients suffer less severe sodium loss.

Rehydration should be rapid over 3 to 4 hours (except in hypernatraemic dehydration in which case rehydration should occur more slowly over 12 hours). The patient should be reassessed after initial rehydration and if still dehydrated rapid fluid replacement should continue.

Once rehydration is complete further dehydration is prevented by encouraging the patient to drink normal volumes of an appropriate fluid and by replacing continuing losses with an oral rehydration solution; in infants, breast-feeding or formula feeds should be offered between oral rehydration drinks.

For intravenous rehydration see section 9.2.2.

## ORAL REHYDRATION SALTS (ORS)

**Indications**   fluid and electrolyte loss in diarrhoea, see notes above

**Dose**

- According to fluid loss, usually 200–400 mL solution after every loose motion; INFANT 1–1½ times usual feed volume; CHILD 200 mL after every loose motion

### ◢UK formulations

Note After reconstitution any unused solution should be discarded no later than 1 hour after preparation unless stored in a refrigerator when it may be kept for up to 24 hours

**Dioralyte®** (Sanofi-Aventis)

Oral powder, sodium chloride 470 mg, potassium chloride 300 mg, disodium hydrogen citrate 530 mg, glucose 3.56 g/sachet, net price 6-sachet pack = £2.11, 20-sachet pack (black currant- or citrus-flavoured or natural) = £6.72

Note Reconstitute 1 sachet with 200 mL of water (freshly boiled and cooled for infants); 5 sachets reconstituted with 1 litre of water provide Na$^+$ 60 mmol, K$^+$ 20 mmol, Cl$^-$ 60 mmol, citrate 10 mmol, and glucose 90 mmol

**Dioralyte® Relief** (Sanofi-Aventis)

Oral powder, sodium chloride 350 mg, potassium chloride 300 mg, sodium citrate 580 mg, cooked rice powder 6 g/sachet, net price 6-sachet pack (apricot-, black currant- or raspberry-flavoured) = £2.35, 20-sachet pack (apricot-flavoured) = £7.13

Note Reconstitute 1 sachet with 200 mL of water (freshly boiled and cooled for infants); 5 sachets when reconstituted with 1 litre of water provide Na$^+$ 60 mmol, K$^+$ 20 mmol, Cl$^-$ 50 mmol and citrate 10 mmol; contains aspartame (section 9.4.1)

**Electrolade®** (Actavis)

Oral powder, sodium chloride 236 mg, potassium chloride 300 mg, sodium bicarbonate 500 mg, anhydrous glucose 4 g/sachet (banana-, black currant-, lemon and lime-, or orange-flavoured). Net price 6-sachet (plain or multiflavoured) pack = £1.33, 20-sachet (single- or multiflavoured) pack = £4.99

Note Reconstitute 1 sachet with 200 mL of water (freshly boiled and cooled for infants); 5 sachets when reconstituted with 1 litre of water provide Na$^+$ 50 mmol, K$^+$ 20 mmol, Cl$^-$ 40 mmol, HCO$_3$$^-$ 30 mmol, and glucose 111 mmol

### ◢WHO formulation

**Oral Rehydration Salts** (Non-proprietary)

Oral powder, sodium chloride 2.6 g, potassium chloride 1.5 g, sodium citrate 2.9 g, anhydrous glucose 13.5 g. To be dissolved in sufficient water to produce

1 litre (providing Na$^+$ 75 mmol, K$^+$ 20 mmol, Cl$^-$ 65 mmol, citrate 10 mmol, glucose 75 mmol/litre)

Note Recommended by the WHO and the United Nations Children's Fund but not commonly used in the UK.

### 9.2.1.3   Oral bicarbonate

**Sodium bicarbonate** is given by mouth for *chronic acidotic states* such as uraemic acidosis or renal tubular acidosis. The dose for correction of metabolic acidosis is not predictable and the response must be assessed; sodium bicarbonate 4.8 g daily (57 mmol each of Na$^+$ and HCO$_3$$^-$) or more may be required. For severe *metabolic acidosis*, sodium bicarbonate can be given intravenously (section 9.2.2).

Sodium bicarbonate may also be used to increase the pH of the urine (see section 7.4.3); for use in dyspepsia see section 1.1.1.

Sodium supplements may increase blood pressure or cause fluid retention and pulmonary oedema in those at risk; hypokalaemia may be exacerbated.

Where *hyperchloraemic acidosis* is associated with potassium deficiency, as in some renal tubular and gastrointestinal disorders it may be appropriate to give oral **potassium bicarbonate**, although acute or severe deficiency should be managed by intravenous therapy.

## SODIUM BICARBONATE

**Indications**   see notes above

**Cautions**   see notes above; avoid in respiratory acidosis; **interactions:** Appendix 1 (antacids)

**Dose**

- See notes above

**Sodium Bicarbonate** (Non-proprietary)

Capsules, sodium bicarbonate 500 mg (approx. 6 mmol each of Na$^+$ and HCO$_3$$^-$), net price 56-cap pack = £10.12

Tablets, sodium bicarbonate 600 mg, net price 100 = £2.48

Important Oral solutions of sodium bicarbonate are required occasionally; these are available from 'special-order' manufacturers or specialist importing companies, see p. 969; the strength of sodium bicarbonate should be stated on the prescription

## POTASSIUM BICARBONATE

**Indications**   see notes above

**Cautions**   cardiac disease, renal impairment (avoid if severe; Appendix 3); **interactions:** Appendix 1 (potassium salts)

**Contra-indications**   hypochloraemia; plasma-potassium concentration above 5 mmol/litre

**Side-effects**   nausea and vomiting

**Dose**

- See notes above

**Potassium Tablets, Effervescent** (Non-proprietary)

Effervescent tablets, potassium bicarbonate 500 mg, potassium acid tartrate 300 mg, each tablet providing 6.5 mmol of K$^+$. To be dissolved in water before administration. Net price 56 = £29.76. Label: 13, 21

Note These tablets do not contain chloride; for effervescent tablets containing potassium and chloride, see under Potassium Chloride, section 9.2.1.1

## 9.2.2 Parenteral preparations for fluid and electrolyte imbalance

9.2.2.1 Electrolytes and water
9.2.2.2 Plasma and plasma substitutes

### 9.2.2.1 Electrolytes and water

Solutions of electrolytes are given intravenously, to meet normal fluid and electrolyte requirements or to replenish substantial deficits or continuing losses, when the patient is nauseated or vomiting and is unable to take adequate amounts by mouth. When intravenous administration is not possible, fluid (as sodium chloride 0.9% or glucose 5%) can also be given by subcutaneous infusion (hypodermoclysis).

The nature and severity of the electrolyte imbalance must be assessed from the history and clinical and biochemical investigations. Sodium, potassium, chloride, magnesium, phosphate, and water depletion can occur singly and in combination with or without disturbances of acid-base balance; for reference to the use of magnesium and phosphates, see section 9.5.

Isotonic solutions may be infused safely into a peripheral vein. Solutions more concentrated than plasma, e.g. 20% glucose, are best given through an indwelling catheter positioned in a large vein.

## Intravenous sodium

**Sodium chloride** in isotonic solution provides the most important extracellular ions in near physiological concentrations and is indicated in *sodium depletion*, which can arise from such conditions as gastro-enteritis, diabetic ketoacidosis, ileus, and ascites. In a severe deficit of 4 to 8 litres, 2 to 3 litres of isotonic sodium chloride may be given over 2 to 3 hours; thereafter the infusion can usually be at a slower rate. Excessive administration should be avoided; the jugular venous pressure should be assessed, the bases of the lungs should be examined for crepitations, and in elderly or seriously ill patients it is often helpful to monitor the right atrial (central) venous pressure.

Chronic hyponatraemia arising from inappropriate secretion of antidiuretic hormone should ideally be corrected by fluid restriction. However, if sodium chloride is required for acute or chronic hyponatraemia, regardless of the cause, the deficit should be corrected slowly to avoid the risk of osmotic demyelination syndrome and the rise in plasma-sodium concentration should not exceed 10 mmol/litre in 24 hours. In severe hyponatraemia, sodium chloride 1.8% may be used cautiously.

**Compound sodium lactate** (Hartmann's solution) can be used instead of isotonic sodium chloride solution during or after surgery, or in the initial management of the injured or wounded; it may avoid the risk of hyperchloraemic acidosis.

**Sodium chloride and glucose** solutions are indicated when there is combined *water and sodium depletion*. A 1:1 mixture of isotonic sodium chloride and 5% glucose allows some of the water (free of sodium) to enter body

cells which suffer most from dehydration while the sodium salt with a volume of water determined by the normal plasma $Na^+$ remains extracellular. Maintenance fluid should accurately reflect daily requirements and close monitoring is required to avoid fluid and electrolyte imbalance. Illness or injury increase the secretion of anti-diuretic hormone and therefore the ability to excrete excess water may be impaired. Injudicious use of hypotonic solutions such as sodium chloride 0.18% and glucose 4% may also cause dilutional hyponatraemia especially in children and the elderly; if necessary, guidance should be sought from a clinician experienced in the management of fluid and electrolytes.

Combined sodium, potassium, chloride, and water depletion may occur, for example, with severe diarrhoea or persistent vomiting; replacement is carried out with sodium chloride intravenous infusion 0.9% and glucose intravenous infusion 5% with potassium as appropriate.

## ■ SODIUM CHLORIDE

**Indications** electrolyte imbalance—see also section 9.2.1.2; nebuliser diluent (section 3.1.5); eye (section 11.8.1); oral hygiene (section 12.3.4); wound irrigation (section 13.11.1)

**Cautions** restrict intake in impaired renal function, cardiac failure, hypertension, peripheral and pulmonary oedema, toxaemia of pregnancy

**Side-effects** administration of large doses may give rise to sodium accumulation, oedema, and hyperchloraemic acidosis

**Dose**
• See notes above

**Sodium Chloride Intravenous Infusion** (Non-proprietary) PoM

Intravenous infusion, usual strength sodium chloride 0.9% (9 g, 150 mmol each of $Na^+$ and $Cl^-$/litre), this strength being supplied when normal saline for injection is requested. Net price 2-mL amp = 29p; 5-mL amp = 34p; 10-mL amp = 46p; 20-mL amp = £1.04; 50-mL amp = £2.01

In hospitals, 500- and 1000-mL packs, and sometimes other sizes, are available

Note The term 'normal saline' should **not** be used to describe sodium chloride intravenous infusion 0.9%; the term 'physiological saline' is acceptable but it is preferable to give the composition (i.e. sodium chloride intravenous infusion 0.9%).

### ◢With other ingredients

**Sodium Chloride and Glucose Intravenous Infusion** (Non-proprietary) PoM

Intravenous infusion, sodium chloride 0.18% ($Na^+$ and $Cl^-$ each 30 mmol/litre), glucose 4%

In hospitals, usually 500-mL packs and sometimes other sizes are available

Intravenous infusion, sodium chloride 0.45% ($Na^+$ and $Cl^-$ each 75 mmol/litre), glucose 2.5%

In hospitals, usually 500-mL packs and sometimes other sizes are available

Intravenous infusion, sodium chloride 0.45% ($Na^+$ and $Cl^-$ each 75 mmol/litre), glucose 5%

In hospitals, usually 500-mL packs and sometimes other sizes are available

Intravenous infusion, sodium chloride 0.9% ($Na^+$ and $Cl^-$ each 150 mmol/litre), glucose 5%

In hospitals, usually 500-mL packs and sometimes other sizes are available

Note See above for warning on hyponatraemia especially in children and elderly

9 Nutrition and blood

### Ringer's Solution for Injection [PoM]

Calcium chloride (dihydrate) 322 micrograms, potassium chloride 300 micrograms, sodium chloride 8.6 mg/mL, providing the following ions (in mmol/litre), $Ca^{2+}$ 2.2, $K^+$ 4, $Na^+$ 147, $Cl^-$ 156

In hospitals, 500- and 1000-mL packs, and sometimes other sizes, are available

### Sodium Lactate Intravenous Infusion, Compound (Non-proprietary) [PoM]

(Hartmann's Solution for Injection; Ringer-Lactate Solution for Injection)

Intravenous infusion, sodium chloride 0.6%, sodium lactate 0.32%, potassium chloride 0.04%, calcium chloride 0.027% (containing $Na^+$ 131 mmol, $K^+$ 5 mmol, $Ca^{2+}$ 2 mmol, $HCO_3^-$ (as lactate) 29 mmol, $Cl^-$ 111 mmol/litre)

In hospitals, 500- and 1000-mL packs, and sometimes other sizes, are available

## Intravenous glucose

**Glucose** solutions (5%) are used mainly to replace water deficit and should not be given alone except when there is no significant loss of electrolytes; prolonged administration of glucose solutions without electrolytes can lead to hyponatraemia and other electrolyte disturbances. Average water requirements in a healthy adult are 1.5 to 2.5 litres daily and this is needed to balance unavoidable losses of water through the skin and lungs and to provide sufficient for urinary excretion. Water depletion (dehydration) tends to occur when these losses are not matched by a comparable intake, as may occur in coma or dysphagia or in the elderly or apathetic who may not drink enough water on their own initiative.

Excessive loss of water without loss of electrolytes is uncommon, occurring in fevers, hyperthyroidism, and in uncommon water-losing renal states such as diabetes insipidus or hypercalcaemia. The volume of glucose solution needed to replace deficits varies with the severity of the disorder, but usually lies within the range of 2 to 6 litres.

Glucose solutions are also used to correct and prevent hypoglycaemia and to provide a source of energy in those too ill to be fed adequately by mouth; glucose solutions are a key component of parenteral nutrition (section 9.3).

Glucose solutions are given in regimens with calcium and insulin for the emergency management of *hyperkalaemia* (see p. 528). They are also given, after correction of hyperglycaemia, during treatment of diabetic ketoacidosis, when they must be accompanied by continuing insulin infusion.

### ▌ GLUCOSE

(Dextrose Monohydrate)

**Note** Glucose BP is the monohydrate but Glucose Intravenous Infusion BP is a sterile solution of anhydrous glucose or glucose monohydrate, potency being expressed in terms of anhydrous glucose

**Indications** fluid replacement (see notes above), provision of energy (section 9.3); hypoglycaemia (section 6.1.4)

**Side-effects** glucose injections especially if hypertonic may have a low pH and may cause venous irritation and thrombophlebitis

### Dose

- Water replacement, see notes above; energy source, 1–3 litres daily of 20–50% solution

### Glucose Intravenous Infusion (Non-proprietary) [PoM]

Intravenous infusion, glucose or anhydrous glucose (potency expressed in terms of anhydrous glucose), usual strength 5% (50 mg/mL) and 10% (100 mg/mL); 25% solution, net price 25-mL amp = £2.21; 50% solution,[1] 20-mL amp = 95p; 50-mL amp = £1.63

In hospitals, 500- and 1000-mL packs, and sometimes other sizes and strengths, are available; also available as *Minijet®* *Glucose*, 50% in 50-mL disposable syringe[1]

1. [PoM] restriction does not apply where administration is for saving life in emergency

## Intravenous potassium

**Potassium chloride and sodium chloride** intravenous infusion is the initial treatment for the correction of *severe hypokalaemia* and when sufficient potassium cannot be taken by mouth. Ready-mixed infusion solutions should be used when possible; alternatively, potassium chloride concentrate, as ampoules containing 1.5 g ($K^+$ 20 mmol) in 10 mL, is **thoroughly mixed** with 500 mL of sodium chloride 0.9% intravenous infusion and given slowly over 2 to 3 hours, with specialist advice and ECG monitoring in difficult cases. Higher concentrations of potassium chloride may be given in very severe depletion, but require specialist advice.

Repeated measurement of plasma-potassium concentration is necessary to determine whether further infusions are required and to avoid the development of hyperkalaemia, which is especially likely in renal impairment.

Initial potassium replacement therapy should **not** involve glucose infusions, because glucose may cause a further decrease in the plasma-potassium concentration.

### ▌ POTASSIUM CHLORIDE

**Indications** electrolyte imbalance; see also oral potassium supplements, section 9.2.1.1

**Cautions** for intravenous infusion the concentration of solution should not usually exceed 3 g (40 mmol)/litre; specialist advice and ECG monitoring (see notes above); renal impairment (avoid if severe; Appendix 3); **interactions**: Appendix 1 (potassium salts)

**Contra-indications** plasma-potassium concentration above 5 mmol/litre

**Side-effects** rapid infusion toxic to heart

### Dose

- By slow intravenous infusion, depending on the deficit or the daily maintenance requirements, see also notes above

### Potassium Chloride and Glucose Intravenous Infusion (Non-proprietary) [PoM]

Intravenous infusion, usual strength potassium chloride 0.3% (3 g, 40 mmol each of $K^+$ and $Cl^-$/litre) or 0.15% (1.5 g, 20 mmol each of $K^+$ and $Cl^-$/litre) with 5% of anhydrous glucose

In hospitals, 500- and 1000-mL packs, and sometimes other sizes, are available

9

Nutrition and blood

**Potassium Chloride and Sodium Chloride Intravenous Infusion** (Non-proprietary) PoM

Intravenous infusion, usual strength potassium chloride 0.15% (1.5 g/litre) with sodium chloride 0.9% (9 g/litre), containing K$^+$ 20 mmol, Na$^+$ 150 mmol, and Cl$^-$ 170 mmol/litre *or* potassium chloride 0.3% (3 g/litre) with sodium chloride 0.9% (9 g/litre), containing K$^+$ 40 mmol, Na$^+$ 150 mmol, and Cl$^-$ 190 mmol/litre

In hospitals, 500- and 1000-mL packs, and sometimes other sizes, are available

**Potassium Chloride, Sodium Chloride, and Glucose Intravenous Infusion** (Non-proprietary) PoM

Intravenous infusion, sodium chloride 0.45% (4.5 g, Na$^+$ 75 mmol/litre) with 5% of anhydrous glucose and usually sufficient potassium chloride to provide K$^+$ 10–40 mmol/litre (to be specified by the prescriber)

In hospitals, 500- and 1000-mL packs, and sometimes other sizes, are available

Intravenous infusion, sodium chloride 0.18% (1.8 g, Na$^+$ 30 mmol/litre) with 4% of anhydrous glucose and usually sufficient potassium chloride to provide K$^+$ 10–40 mmol/litre (to be specified by the prescriber)

In hospitals, 500- and 1000-mL packs, and sometimes other sizes, are available

**Potassium Chloride Concentrate, Sterile** (Non-proprietary) PoM

Sterile concentrate, potassium chloride 15% (150 mg, approximately 2 mmol each of K$^+$ and Cl$^-$/mL). Net price 10-mL amp = 48p

Important Must be diluted with **not less** than 50 times its volume of sodium chloride intravenous infusion 0.9% or other suitable diluent and **mixed well**

Solutions containing 10 and 20% of potassium chloride are also available in both 5- and 10-mL ampoules

## Bicarbonate and lactate

**Sodium bicarbonate** is used to control severe *metabolic acidosis* (pH < 7.1) particularly that caused by loss of bicarbonate (as in renal tubular acidosis or from excessive gastro-intestinal losses). Mild metabolic acidosis associated with volume depletion should first be managed by appropriate fluid replacement because acidosis usually resolves as tissue and renal perfusion are restored. In more severe metabolic acidosis or when the acidosis remains unresponsive to correction of anoxia or hypovolaemia, sodium bicarbonate (1.26%) can be infused over 3–4 hours with plasma-pH and electrolyte monitoring. In severe shock (section 2.7.1), for example in cardiac arrest, metabolic acidosis can develop without sodium or volume depletion; in these circumstances sodium bicarbonate is best given as a small volume of hypertonic solution, such as 50 mL of 8.4% solution intravenously; plasma-pH and electrolytes should be monitored.

**Sodium lactate** intravenous infusion is no longer used in metabolic acidosis because of the risk of producing lactic acidosis, particularly in seriously ill patients with poor tissue perfusion or impaired hepatic function.

For *chronic acidotic states*, sodium bicarbonate can be given by mouth (section 9.2.1.3).

## SODIUM BICARBONATE

**Indications** metabolic acidosis, see also notes above
**Dose**

• By slow intravenous injection, a strong solution (up to 8.4%), or by continuous intravenous infusion, a weaker solution (usually 1.26%), an amount appropriate to the body base deficit (see notes above)

**Sodium Bicarbonate Intravenous Infusion** PoM

Usual strength sodium bicarbonate 1.26% (12.6 g, 150 mmol each of Na$^+$ and HCO$_3^-$/litre); various other strengths available

In hospitals, 500- and 1000-mL packs, and sometimes other sizes, are available

**Minijet® Sodium Bicarbonate** (UCB Pharma) PoM

Intravenous injection, sodium bicarbonate in disposable syringe, net price 4.2%, 10 mL = £8.92; 8.4%, 10 mL = £9.95, 50 mL = £11.45

## SODIUM LACTATE

**Indications** see notes above

**Sodium Lactate** (Non-proprietary) PoM

Intravenous infusion, sodium lactate M/6, contains the following ions (in mmol/litre), Na$^+$ 167, HCO$_3^-$ (as lactate) 167

## Water

**Water for Injections** PoM

Net price 1-mL amp = 18p; 2-mL amp = 18p; 5-mL amp = 33p; 10-mL amp = 33p; 20-mL amp = 92p; 50-mL amp = £1.91; 100-mL vial = 23p

### 9.2.2.2 Plasma and plasma substitutes

Plasma and plasma substitutes ('colloids') contain large molecules that do not readily leave the intravascular space where they exert osmotic pressure to maintain circulatory volume. Compared to fluids containing electrolytes such as sodium chloride and glucose ('crystalloids'), a smaller volume of colloid is required to produce the same expansion of blood volume, thereby shifting salt and water from the extravascular space. If resuscitation requires a volume of fluid that exceeds the maximum dose of the colloid then crystalloids can be given; packed red cells may also be required.

**Albumin solutions**, prepared from whole blood, contain soluble proteins and electrolytes but no clotting factors, blood group antibodies, or plasma cholinesterases; they may be given without regard to the recipient's blood group.

Albumin is usually used after the acute phase of illness, to correct a plasma-volume deficit; hypoalbuminaemia itself is not an appropriate indication. The use of albumin solutions in acute plasma or blood loss may be wasteful; plasma substitutes are more appropriate. Concentrated albumin solutions (20%) can be used in patients with an intravascular fluid deficit and oedema because of interstitial fluid overload, to restore intravascular plasma volume without exacerbating the salt and water overload. Concentrated albumin solutions may also be used to obtain a diuresis in hypoalbuminaemic patients (e.g. in hepatic cirrhosis).

Recent evidence does not support the previous view that the use of albumin increases mortality.

Plasma and plasma substitutes are often used in very ill patients whose condition is unstable. Therefore, close monitoring is required and fluid and electrolyte therapy should be adjusted according to the patient's condition at all times.

## ALBUMIN SOLUTION
(Human Albumin Solution)

A solution containing protein derived from plasma, serum, or normal placentas; at least 95% of the protein is albumin. The solution may be isotonic (containing 3.5–5% protein) or concentrated (containing 15–25% protein).

**Indications** see under preparations, and also notes above

**Cautions** history of cardiac or circulatory disease (administer slowly to avoid rapid rise in blood pressure and cardiac failure, and monitor cardiovascular and respiratory function); increased capillary permeability; correct dehydration when administering concentrated solution

**Contra-indications** cardiac failure; severe anaemia

**Side-effects** hypersensitivity reactions (including anaphylaxis) with nausea, vomiting, increased salivation, fever, tachycardia, hypotension and chills reported

◢ Isotonic solutions

*Indications:* acute or sub-acute loss of plasma volume e.g. in burns, pancreatitis, trauma, and complications of surgery; plasma exchange

Available as: *Human Albumin Solution 4.5%* (50-, 100-, 250- and 400-mL bottles—Baxter); *Human Albumin Solution 5%* (250- and 500-mL bottles—Baxter); *Octalbin®* *5%* (100- and 250-mL bottles—Octapharm); *Zenalb®* *4.5%* (50-, 100-, 250-, and 500-mL bottles—BPL)

◢ Concentrated solutions (20%)

*Indications:* severe hypoalbuminaemia associated with low plasma volume and generalised oedema where salt and water restriction with plasma volume expansion are required; adjunct in the treatment of hyperbilirubinaemia by exchange transfusion in the newborn; paracentesis of large volume ascites associated with portal hypertension

Available as: *Human Albumin Solution 20%* (50- and 100-mL vials—Baxter); *Flexbumin®* 20% (50- and 100-mL bags—Baxter); *Octalbin®* *20%* (50- and 100-mL bottles—Octapharm); *Zenalb®* *20%* (50- and 100-mL bottles—BPL)

## Plasma substitutes

Dextran, gelatin, and the etherified starches (hetastarch, pentastarch, and tetrastarch) are macromolecular substances which are metabolised slowly; they may be used at the outset to expand and maintain blood volume in shock arising from conditions such as burns or septicaemia. Plasma substitutes may be used as an immediate short-term measure to treat haemorrhage until blood is available. They are rarely needed when shock is due to sodium and water depletion because, in these circumstances, the shock responds to water and electrolyte repletion; see also section 2.7.1 for the management of shock.

Plasma substitutes should **not** be used to maintain plasma volume in conditions such as burns or peritonitis where there is loss of plasma protein, water, and electrolytes over periods of several days or weeks. In these situations, plasma or plasma protein fractions containing large amounts of albumin should be given.

Large volumes of *some* plasma substitutes can increase the risk of bleeding through depletion of coagulation factors.

Dextran 70 by intravenous infusion is used for volume expansion. Dextran may interfere with blood group cross-matching or biochemical measurements, and these should be carried out before infusion is begun.

> Plasma and plasma substitutes are often used in very ill patients whose condition is unstable. Therefore, close monitoring is required and fluid and electrolyte therapy should be adjusted according to the patient's condition at all times.

**Cautions** Plasma substitutes should be used with caution in patients with cardiac disease, liver disease, or renal impairment; urine output should be monitored. Care should be taken to avoid haematocrit concentration from falling below 25–30% and the patient should be monitored for hypersensitivity reactions.

**Side-effects** Hypersensitivity reactions may occur including, rarely, severe anaphylactoid reactions. Transient increase in bleeding time may occur.

## DEXTRAN 70

Dextrans of weight average molecular weight about '70 000'

**Indications** short-term blood volume expansion

**Cautions** see notes above; can interfere with some laboratory tests (see also above); where possible, monitor central venous pressure; pregnancy (Appendix 4)

**Side-effects** see notes above

**Dose**

- See under preparation below

◢ Hypertonic solution

**RescueFlow®** (Vitaline) PoM

Intravenous infusion, dextran 70 intravenous infusion 6% in sodium chloride intravenous infusion 7.5%. Net price 250-mL bag = £28.50

Cautions see notes above; severe hyperglycaemia and hyperosmolality

Dose initial treatment of hypovolaemia with hypotension induced by traumatic injury, by intravenous infusion over 2–5 minutes, 250 mL, followed immediately by administration of isotonic fluids

## GELATIN

Note The gelatin is partially degraded

**Indications** low blood volume (but see notes above)

**Cautions** see notes above; pregnancy (Appendix 4)

**Side-effects** see notes above

**Dose**

- By intravenous infusion, initially 500–1000 mL of a 3.5–4% solution (see notes above)

**Gelofusine®** (Braun) PoM

Intravenous infusion, succinylated gelatin (modified fluid gelatin, average molecular weight 30 000) 40 g (4%), $Na^+$ 154 mmol, $Cl^-$ 120 mmol/litre, net price 500-mL *Ecobag®* = £4.70, 1-litre *Ecobag®* = £9.45

**Geloplasma®** (Fresenius Kabi) PoM

Intravenous infusion, partially hydrolysed and succinylated gelatin (modified liquid gelatin) (as anhy-

9

Nutrition and blood

drous gelatin) 30 g (3%), $Na^+$ 150 mmol, $K^+$ 5 mmol, $Mg^{2+}$ 1.5 mmol, $Cl^-$ 100 mmol, lactate 30 mmol/litre, net price 500-mL bag = £5.05

**Isoplex®** (IS Pharmaceuticals) [PoM]
Intravenous infusion, succinylated gelatin (modified fluid gelatin, average molecular weight 30 000) 40 g (4%), $Na^+$ 145 mmol, $K^+$ 4 mmol, $Mg^{2+}$ 0.9 mmol, $Cl^-$ 105 mmol, lactate 25 mmol/litre, net price 500-mL bag = £7.53, 1-litre bag = £14.54

**Volplex®** (IS Pharmaceuticals) [PoM]
Intravenous infusion, succinylated gelatin (modified fluid gelatin, average molecular weight 30 000) 40 g (4%), $Na^+$ 154 mmol, $Cl^-$ 125 mmol/litre, net price 500-mL bag = £4.70, 1-litre bag = £9.09

## ETHERIFIED STARCH

A starch composed of more than 90% of amylopectin that has been etherified with hydroxyethyl groups; the terms tetrastarch, pentastarch, and hetastarch reflect the degree of etherification

**Indications** low blood volume

**Cautions** see notes above; children

**Side-effects** see notes above; also pruritus, raised serum amylase

**Dose**
• See under preparations below

◀**Hetastarch**
**Hetastarch** (Non-proprietary) [PoM]
Intravenous infusion, hetastarch (weight average molecular weight 450 000) 6% in sodium chloride intravenous infusion 0.9%, net price 500-mL bag = £8.00
Dose by intravenous infusion, 500–1000 mL; usual daily max. 1500 mL (see notes above)

◀**Pentastarch**
**Pentastarch** (Non-proprietary) [PoM]
Intravenous infusion, pentastarch (weight average molecular weight 200 000), net price (in sodium chloride intravenous infusion 0.9%) 10%, 500-mL bag = £9.24
Dose by intravenous infusion, pentastarch 10%, 500 1000 mL; max. 1500 mL daily (see notes above)

**HAES-steril®** (Fresenius Kabi) [PoM]
Intravenous infusion, pentastarch (weight average molecular weight 200 000) 10% in sodium chloride intravenous infusion 0.9%, net price 500 mL = £16.50
Dose by intravenous infusion, up to 1500 mL daily (see notes above)

**Hemohes®** (Braun) [PoM]
Intravenous infusion, pentastarch (weight average molecular weight 200 000) 6% (both in sodium chloride intravenous infusion 0.9%) 500 mL = £12.50; 10%, 500 mL = £16.50
Cautions see notes above
Dose by intravenous infusion, pentastarch 6%, up to 2500 mL daily; pentastarch 10%, up to 1500 mL daily (see notes above)

◀**Tetrastarch**
**Tetraspan®** (Braun) [PoM]
Intravenous infusion, hydroxyethyl starch (weight average molecular weight 130 000) 6% in sodium chloride 0.625%, containing $Na^+$ 140 mmol, $K^+$ 4 mmol, $Mg^{2+}$ 1 mmol, $Cl^-$ 118 mmol, $Ca^{2+}$ 2.5 mmol,

acetate 24 mmol, malate 5 mmol/litre, net price 500-mL bag = £13.50
Dose by intravenous infusion, up to 50 mL/kg daily (see notes above)

Intravenous infusion, hydroxyethyl starch (weight average molecular weight 130 000) 10% in sodium chloride 0.625%, containing $Na^+$ 140 mmol, $K^+$ 4 mmol, $Mg^{2+}$ 1 mmol, $Cl^-$ 118 mmol, $Ca^{2+}$ 2.5 mmol, acetate 24 mmol, malate 5 mmol/litre, net price 500-mL bag = £17.50
Dose by intravenous infusion, up to 30 mL/kg daily (see notes above)

**Venofundin®** (Braun) [PoM]
Intravenous infusion, hydroxyethyl starch (weight average molecular weight 130 000) 6% in sodium chloride intravenous infusion 0.9%, net price 500-mL bag = £12.90
Dose by intravenous infusion, up to 50 mL/kg daily (see notes above)

**Volulyte®** (Fresenius Kabi) [PoM]
Intravenous infusion, hydroxyethyl starch (weight average molecular weight 130 000) 6% in sodium chloride intravenous infusion 0.6%, containing $Na^+$ 137 mmol, $K^+$ 4 mmol, $Mg^{2+}$ 1.5 mmol, $Cl^-$ 110 mmol, acetate 34 mmol/litre, net price 500-mL bag = £13.50
Dose by intravenous infusion, up to 50 mL/kg daily (see notes above)

**Voluven®** (Fresenius Kabi) [PoM]
Intravenous infusion, hydroxyethyl starch (weight average molecular weight 130 000) 6% in sodium chloride intravenous infusion 0.9%, net price 500-mL bag = £12.50
Dose by intravenous infusion, up to 50 mL/kg daily (see notes above)

◀**Hypertonic solution**
**HyperHAES®** (Fresenius Kabi) [PoM]
Intravenous infusion, hydroxyethyl starch (weight average molecular weight 200 000) 6% in sodium chloride intravenous infusion 7.2%, net price 250-mL bag = £28.00
Cautions see notes above; also diabetes
Dose by intravenous injection over 2–5 minutes, 4 mL/kg as a single dose, followed immediately by administration of appropriate replacement fluids

# 9.3 Intravenous nutrition

When adequate feeding through the alimentary tract is not possible, nutrients may be given by intravenous infusion. This may be in addition to ordinary oral or tube feeding—**supplemental parenteral nutrition**, or may be the sole source of nutrition—**total parenteral nutrition** (TPN). Indications for this method include preparation of undernourished patients for surgery, chemotherapy, or radiation therapy; severe or prolonged disorders of the gastro-intestinal tract; major surgery, trauma, or burns; prolonged coma or refusal to eat; and some patients with renal or hepatic failure. The composition of proprietary preparations available is given in the table Proprietary Infusion Fluids for Parenteral Feeding, p. 535.

Parenteral nutrition requires the use of a solution containing amino acids, glucose, fat, electrolytes, trace elements, and vitamins. This is now commonly provided by the pharmacy in the form of a 3-litre bag. A single dose of vitamin $B_{12}$, as hydroxocobalamin, is given by

## Proprietary Infusion Fluids for Parenteral Feeding

| Preparation | Nitrogen g/litre | [1,2]Energy kJ/litre | Electrolytes mmol/litre | | | | | Other components/litre |
|---|---|---|---|---|---|---|---|---|
| | | | K+ | Mg²⁺ | Na+ | Acet⁻ | Cl⁻ | |
| Aminoplasmal 5% E (Braun) Net price 500 mL = £9.02 | 8 | | 25 | 2.6 | 43 | 59 | 29 | dihydrogen phosphate 9 mmol, malic acid 1.01 g |
| Aminoplasmal 10% (Braun) Net price 500 mL = £17.06 | 16 | | | | | | 57 | |
| Aminoven 25 (Fresenius Kabi) Net price 500 mL = £23.20 | 25.7 | | | | | | | |
| Clinimix N9G20E (Baxter) Net price (dual compartment bag of amino acids with electrolytes 1000 mL and glucose 20% with calcium 1000 mL) = £29.00 | 4.6 | 1680 | 30 | 2.5 | 35 | 50 | 40 | Ca²⁺ 2.3 mmol, phosphate 15 mmol, anhydrous glucose 100 g |
| Clinimix N14G30E (Baxter) Net price (dual compartment bag of amino acids with electrolytes 1000 mL and glucose 30% with calcium 1000 mL) = £33.00 | 7 | 2520 | 30 | 2.5 | 35 | 70 | 40 | Ca²⁺ 2.3 mmol, phosphate 15 mmol, anhydrous glucose 150 g |
| ClinOleic 20% (Baxter) Net price 100 mL = £6.28; 250 mL = £10.08; 500 mL = £13.88 | | 8360 | | | | | | purified olive and soya oil 200 g, glycerol 22.5 g, egg phosphatides 12 g |
| Glamin (Fresenius Kabi) Net price 250 mL = £14.58; 500 mL = £27.20 | 22.4 | | | | 62 | | | |
| Hyperamine 30 (Braun) Net price 500 mL = £23.67 | 30 | | | | 5 | | | |
| Intralipid 10% (Fresenius Kabi) Net price 100 mL = £4.70; 500 mL = £10.30 | | 4600 | | | | | | soya oil 100 g, glycerol 22 g, purified egg phospholipids 12 g, phosphate 15 mmol |
| Intralipid 20% (Fresenius Kabi) Net price 100 mL = £7.05; 250 mL = £11.60; 500 mL = £15.45 | | 8400 | | | | | | soya oil 200 g, glycerol 22 g, purified egg phospholipids 12 g, phosphate 15 mmol |
| Intralipid 30% (Fresenius Kabi) Net price 333 mL = £17.30 | | 12600 | | | | | | soya oil 300 g, glycerol 16.7 g, purified egg phospholipids 12 g, phosphate 15 mmol |
| Kabiven (Fresenius Kabi) Net price (triple compartment bag of amino acids and electrolytes 300 mL, 450 mL, 600 mL, or 750 mL; glucose 526 mL, 790 mL, 1053 mL, or 1316 mL; lipid emulsion 200 mL, 300 mL, 400 mL, or 500 mL) 1026 mL = £35.00, 1540 mL = £50.00, 2053 mL = £67.00, 2566 mL = £70.00 | 5.3 | 3275 | 23 | 4 | 31 | 38 | 45 | Ca²⁺ 2 mmol, phosphate 9.7 mmol, anhydrous glucose 97 g, soya oil 39 g |
| Kabiven Peripheral (Fresenius Kabi) Net price (triple compartment bag of amino acids and electrolytes 300 mL, 400 mL, or 500 mL; glucose 885 mL, 1180 mL, or 1475 mL; lipid emulsion 255 mL, 340 mL, or 425 mL) 1440 mL = £35.00, 1920 mL = £50.00, 2400 mL = £64.00 | 3.75 | 2625 | 17 | 2.8 | 22 | 27 | 33 | Ca²⁺ 1.4 mmol, phosphate 7.5 mmol, anhydrous glucose 67.5 g, soya oil 35.4 g |
| Lipidem (Braun) Net price 100 mL = £18.00; 250 mL = £30.00; 500 mL = £38.00 | | 7900 | | | | | | omega-3-acid triglycerides 20 g, soya oil 80 g, medium-chain triglycerides 100 g |

9

Nutrition and blood

1. *Note.* 1000 kcal = 4200 kJ; 1000 kJ = 238.8 kcal. All entries are PoM
2. Excludes protein- or amino acid-derived energy

| Preparation | Nitrogen g/litre | [1,2]Energy kJ/litre | $K^+$ | $Mg^{2+}$ | $Na^+$ | Acet⁻ | Cl⁻ | Other components/litre |
|---|---|---|---|---|---|---|---|---|
| Lipofundin MCT/LCT 10% (Braun)<br>Net price 100 mL = £7.70; 500 mL = £12.90 | | 4430 | | | | | | soya oil 50 g, medium-chain triglycerides 50 g |
| Lipofundin MCT/LCT 20% (Braun)<br>Net price 100 mL = £12.51; 250 mL = £11.30; 500 mL = £19.18 | | 8000 | | | | | | soya oil 100 g, medium-chain triglycerides 100 g |
| Nutriflex basal (Braun)<br>Net price (dual compartment bag of amino acids 400 mL or 800 mL; glucose 600 mL or 1200 mL) 1000 mL = £24.99, 2000 mL = £27.50 | 4.6 | 2095 | 30 | 5.7 | 49.9 | 35 | 50 | $Ca^{2+}$ 3.6 mmol, acid phosphate 12.8 mmol, anhydrous glucose 125 g |
| Nutriflex peri (Braun)<br>Net price (dual compartment bag of amino acids 400 mL or 800 mL; glucose 600 mL or 1200 mL) 1000 mL = £26.00, 2000 mL = £28.70 | 5.7 | 1340 | 15 | 4 | 27 | 19.5 | 31.6 | $Ca^{2+}$ 2.5 mmol, acid phosphate 5.7 mmol, anhydrous glucose 80 g |
| Nutriflex plus (Braun)<br>Net price (dual compartment bag of amino acids 400 mL or 800 mL; glucose 600 mL or 1200 mL) 1000 mL = £27.15, 2000 mL = £31.10 | 6.8 | 2510 | 25 | 5.7 | 37.2 | 22.9 | 35.5 | $Ca^{2+}$ 3.6 mmol, acid phosphate 20 mmol, anhydrous glucose 150 g |
| Nutriflex special (Braun)<br>Net price (dual compartment bag of amino acids 500 mL or 750 mL; glucose 500 mL or 750 mL) 1000 mL = £28.65, 1500 mL = £31.26 | 10 | 4020 | 25.7 | 5 | 40.5 | 22 | 49.5 | $Ca^{2+}$ 4.1 mmol, acid phosphate 14.7 mmol, anhydrous glucose 240 g |
| NuTRIflex Lipid peri (Braun)<br>Net price (triple compartment bag of amino acids 500 mL or 1000 mL; glucose 500 mL or 1000 mL; lipid emulsion 20% 250 mL or 500 mL) 1250 mL = £43.38, 2500 mL = £65.05 | 4.56 | 2664 | 24 | 2.4 | 40 | 32 | 38.4 | $Ca^{2+}$ 2.4 mmol, $Zn^{2+}$ 24 micromol, phosphate 6 mmol, anhydrous glucose 64 g, soya oil 20 g, medium-chain triglycerides 20 g |
| NuTRIflex Lipid plus (Braun)<br>Net price (triple compartment bag of amino acids 500 mL, 750 mL or 1000 mL; glucose 500 mL, 750 mL or 1000 mL; lipid emulsion 20% 250 mL, 375 mL or 500 mL) 1250 mL = £47.17, 1875 mL = £60.23, 2500 mL = £69.27 | 5.44 | 3600 | 28 | 3.2 | 40 | 36 | 36 | $Ca^{2+}$ 3.2 mmol, $Zn^{2+}$ 24 micromol, phosphate 12 mmol, anhydrous glucose 120 g, soya oil 20 g, medium-chain triglycerides 20 g |
| NuTRIflex Lipid plus without Electrolytes (Braun)<br>Net price (triple compartment bag of amino acids 500 mL, 750 mL or 1000 mL; glucose 500 mL, 750 mL or 1000 mL; lipid emulsion 20% 250 mL, 375 mL or 500 mL) 1250 mL = £47.17, 1875 mL = £60.23, 2500 mL = £69.27 | 5.44 | 3600 | | | | | | anhydrous glucose 120 g, soya oil 20 g, medium-chain triglycerides 20 g |
| NuTRIflex Lipid special (Braun)<br>Net price (triple compartment bag of amino acids 500 mL, 750 mL or 1000 mL; glucose 500 mL, 750 mL or 1000 mL; lipid emulsion 20% 250 mL, 375 mL or 500 mL) 1250 mL = £57.69, 1875 mL = £75.58, 2500 mL = £89.21 | 8 | 4004 | 37.6 | 4.24 | 53.6 | 48 | 48 | $Ca^{2+}$ 4.24 mmol, $Zn^{2+}$ 32 micromol, phosphate 16 mmol, anhydrous glucose 144 g, soya oil 20 g, medium-chain triglycerides 20 g |

1. *Note.* 1000 kcal = 4200 kJ; 1000 kJ = 238.8 kcal. All entries are PoM
2. Excludes protein- or amino acid-derived energy

9 Nutrition and blood

| Preparation | Nitrogen g/litre | [1,2]Energy kJ/litre | K+ | Mg2+ | Na+ | Acet- | Cl- | Other components/litre |
|---|---|---|---|---|---|---|---|---|
| NuTRIflex Lipid special without Electrolytes (Braun)<br>Net price (triple compartment bag of amino acids 500 mL, 750 mL or 1000 mL; glucose 500 mL, 750 mL or 1000 mL; lipid emulsion 20% 250 mL, 375 mL or 500 mL) 1250 mL = £57.69, 1875 mL = £75.58, 2500 mL = £89.21 | 8 | 4004 | | | | | | anhydrous glucose 144 g, soya oil 20 g, medium-chain triglycerides 20 g |
| OliClinomel N4-550E (Baxter)<br>Net price (triple compartment bag of amino acids with electrolytes 1000 mL; glucose 20% 1000 mL; lipid emulsion 10% 500 mL) 2500 mL = £69.30 | 3.6 | 2184 | 16 | 2.2 | 21 | 30 | 33 | Ca2+ 2 mmol, phosphate 8.5 mmol, refined olive and soya oil 20 g, anhydrous glucose 80 g |
| OliClinomel N4-720E (Baxter)<br>Net price (triple compartment bag of amino acids with electrolytes 1000 mL; glucose 20% 1000 mL; lipid emulsion 20% 500 mL) 2500 mL = £69.30 | 3.64 | 3024 | 24 | 2 | 28 | 40 | 40 | Ca2+ 1.8 mmol, phosphate 8 mmol, refined olive and soya oil 40 g, anhydrous glucose 80 g |
| OliClinomel N5-800E (Baxter)<br>Net price (triple compartment bag of amino acids with electrolytes 800 mL or 1000 mL; glucose 25% 800 mL or 1000 mL; lipid emulsion 20% 400 mL or 500 mL) 2000 mL = £60.39, 2500 mL = £65.34 | 4.6 | 3360 | 24 | 2.2 | 32 | 49 | 44 | Ca2+ 2 mmol, phosphate 10 mmol, refined olive and soya oil 40 g, anhydrous glucose 100 g |
| OliClinomel N6-900E (Baxter)<br>Net price (triple compartment bag of amino acids with electrolytes 800 mL or 1000 mL; glucose 30% 800 mL or 1000 mL; lipid emulsion 20% 400 mL or 500 mL) 2000 mL = £70.40, 2500 mL = £75.90 | 5.6 | 3696 | 24 | 2.2 | 32 | 53 | 46 | Ca2+ 2 mmol, phosphate 10 mmol, refined olive and soya oil 40 g, anhydrous glucose 120 g |
| OliClinomel N7-1000 (Baxter)<br>Net price (triple compartment bag of amino acids 600 mL; glucose 40% 600 mL; lipid emulsion 20% 300 mL) 1500 mL = £43.70 | 6.6 | 4368 | | | | 37 | 16 | phosphate 3 mmol, refined olive and soya oil 40 g, anhydrous glucose 160 g |
| OliClinomel N7-1000E (Baxter)<br>Net price (triple compartment bag of amino acids with electrolytes 800 mL; glucose 40% 800 mL; lipid emulsion 20% 400 mL) 2000 mL = £66.33 | 6.6 | 4368 | 24 | 2.2 | 32 | 57 | 48 | Ca2+ 2 mmol, phosphate 10 mmol, refined olive and soya oil 40 g, anhydrous glucose 160 g |
| OliClinomel N8-800 (Baxter)<br>Net price (triple compartment bag of amino acids 800 mL; glucose 31.25% 800 mL; lipid emulsion 15% 400 mL) 2000 mL = £77.10 | 8.25 | 3360 | | | | 42.5 | 20 | phosphate 2.25 mmol, refined olive and soya oil 30 g, anhydrous glucose 125 g |
| Omegaven (Fresenius Kabi)<br>Net price 100 mL = £22.50 | | 4700 | | | | | | highly refined fish oil 100 g, glycerol 25 g, egg phosphatide 12 g |
| Plasma-Lyte 148 (water) (Baxter)<br>Net price 1000 mL = £1.59 | | | 5 | 1.5 | 140 | 27 | 98 | gluconate 23 mmol |
| Plasma-Lyte 148 (dextrose 5%) (Baxter)<br>Net price 1000 mL = £1.59 | | 840 | 5 | 1.5 | 140 | 27 | 98 | gluconate 23 mmol, anhydrous glucose 50 g |
| Plasma-Lyte M (dextrose 5%) (Baxter)<br>Net price 1000 mL = £1.33 | | 840 | 16 | 1.5 | 40 | 12 | 40 | Ca2+ 2.5 mmol, lactate 12 mmol, anhydrous glucose 50 g |
| [3]Primene 10% (Baxter)<br>Net price 100 mL = £5.78, 250 mL = £7.92 | 15 | | | | | | 19 | |

9 Nutrition and blood

1. *Note.* 1000 kcal = 4200 kJ; 1000 kJ = 238.8 kcal. All entries are [PoM]
2. Excludes protein- or amino acid-derived energy
3. For use in neonates and children only

| Preparation | Nitrogen g/litre | [1,2]Energy kJ/litre | Electrolytes mmol/litre | | | | | Other components/litre |
|---|---|---|---|---|---|---|---|---|
| | | | K$^+$ | Mg$^{2+}$ | Na$^+$ | Acet$^-$ | Cl$^-$ | |
| SMOFlipid (Fresenius Kabi)<br>Net price 500 mL = £20.50 | | 8400 | | | | | | fish oil 30 g, olive oil 50 g, soya oil 60 g, medium-chain triglycerides 60 g |
| StructoKabiven Electrolyte Free (Fresenius Kabi)<br>Net price (triple compartment bag of amino acids 500 mL, 750 mL or 1000 mL; glucose 42% 298 mL, 446 mL or 595 mL; lipid emulsion 188 mL, 281 mL or 375 mL) 986 mL = £66.50, 1477 mL = £69.00, 1970 mL = £74.00 | 8 | 3685 | | | | 74.5 | | phosphate 2.8 mmol, anhydrous glucose 127 g, glycerol 4.23 g, egg phospholipids 4.56 g, purified structured triglyceride 38.5 g (contains coconut oil, palm kernel oil and soya oil triglycerides) |
| Structolipid 20% (Fresenius Kabi)<br>Net price 500 mL = £16.09 | | 8200 | | | | | | purified structured triglyceride 200 g (contains coconut oil, palm kernel oil, and soya oil triglycerides) |
| Synthamin 9 (Baxter)<br>Net price 500 mL = £6.66; 1000 mL = £12.34 | 9.1 | | 60 | 5 | 70 | 100 | 70 | acid phosphate 30 mmol |
| Synthamin 9 EF (electrolyte-free) (Baxter)<br>Net price 500 mL = £6.66; 1000 mL = £12.34 | 9.1 | | | | | 44 | 22 | |
| Synthamin 14 (Baxter)<br>Net price 500 mL = £9.64; 1000 mL = £17.13; 3000 mL = £48.98 | 14 | | 60 | 5 | 70 | 140 | 70 | acid phosphate 30 mmol |
| Synthamin 14 EF (electrolyte-free) (Baxter)<br>Net price 500 mL = £9.87; 1000 mL = £17.51 | 14 | | | | | 68 | 34 | |
| Synthamin 17 (Baxter)<br>Net price 500 mL = £12.66; 1000 mL = £23.00 | 16.5 | | 60 | 5 | 70 | 150 | 70 | acid phosphate 30 mmol |
| Synthamin 17 EF (electrolyte-free) (Baxter)<br>Net price 500 mL = £12.66; 1000 mL = £23.00 | 16.5 | | | | | 82 | 40 | |
| Vamin 9 Glucose (Fresenius Kabi)<br>Net price 100 mL = £3.80; 500 mL = £7.70; 1000 mL = £13.40 | 9.4 | 1700 | 20 | 1.5 | 50 | | 50 | Ca$^{2+}$ 2.5 mmol, anhydrous glucose 100 g |
| Vamin 14 (Fresenius Kabi)<br>Net price 500 mL = £10.80; 1000 mL = £14.67 | 13.5 | | 50 | 8 | 100 | 135 | 100 | Ca$^{2+}$ 5 mmol, SO$_4$$^{2-}$ 8 mmol |
| Vamin 14 (Electrolyte-Free) (Fresenius Kabi)<br>Net price 500 mL = £10.80; 1000 mL = £18.30 | 13.5 | | | | | 90 | | |
| Vamin 18 (Electrolyte-Free) (Fresenius Kabi)<br>Net price 500 mL = £13.70; 1000 mL = £26.70 | 18 | | | | | 110 | | |
| Vaminolact (Fresenius Kabi)<br>Net price 100 mL = £4.35; 500 mL = £10.00 | 9.3 | | | | | | | |

1. *Note.* 1000 kcal = 4200 kJ; 1000 kJ = 238.8 kcal. All entries are [PoM]
2. Excludes protein- or amino acid-derived energy

**9** Nutrition and blood

intramuscular injection; regular vitamin B$_{12}$ injections are not usually required unless total parenteral nutrition continues for many months. Folic acid is given in a dose of 15 mg once or twice each week, usually in the nutrition solution. Other vitamins are usually given daily; they are generally introduced in the parenteral nutrition solution. Alternatively, if the patient is able to take small amounts by mouth, vitamins may be given orally.

The nutrition solution is infused through a central venous catheter inserted under full surgical precautions. Alternatively, infusion through a peripheral vein may be used for supplementary as well as total parenteral nutrition for periods of up to a month, depending on the availability of peripheral veins; factors prolonging cannula life and preventing thrombophlebitis include the use of soft polyurethane paediatric cannulas and use of feeds of low osmolality and neutral pH. Only nutritional fluids should be given by the dedicated intravenous line.

Before starting, the patient should be well oxygenated with a near normal circulating blood volume and attention should be given to renal function and acid-base status. Appropriate biochemical tests should have been carried out beforehand and serious deficits corrected. Nutritional and electrolyte status must be monitored throughout treatment.

Complications of long-term parenteral nutrition include gall bladder sludging, gall stones, cholestasis and abnormal liver function tests. For details of the prevention and management of parenteral nutrition complications, specialist literature should be consulted.

**Protein** is given as mixtures of essential and non-essential synthetic L-amino acids. Ideally, all essential amino acids should be included with a wide variety of non-essential ones to provide sufficient nitrogen together with electrolytes (see also section 9.2.2). Solutions vary in their composition of amino acids; they often contain an energy source (usually glucose) and electrolytes.

**Energy** is provided in a ratio of 0.6 to 1.1 megajoules (150–250 kcals) per gram of protein nitrogen. Energy requirements must be met if amino acids are to be utilised for tissue maintenance. A mixture of carbohydrate and fat energy sources (usually 30–50% as fat) gives better utilisation of amino acids than glucose alone.

**Glucose** is the preferred source of carbohydrate, but if more than 180 g is given per day frequent monitoring of blood glucose is required, and insulin may be necessary. Glucose in various strengths from 10 to 50% must be infused through a central venous catheter to avoid thrombosis.

In parenteral nutrition regimens, it is necessary to provide adequate **phosphate** in order to allow phosphorylation of glucose and to prevent hypophosphataemia; between 20 and 30 mmol of phosphate is required daily.

Fructose and sorbitol have been used in an attempt to avoid the problem of hyperosmolar hyperglycaemic non-ketotic acidosis but other metabolic problems may occur, as with xylitol and ethanol which are now rarely used.

**Fat** emulsions have the advantages of a high energy to fluid volume ratio, neutral pH, and iso-osmolarity with plasma, and provide essential fatty acids. Several days

of adaptation may be required to attain maximal utilisation. Reactions include occasional febrile episodes (usually only with 20% emulsions) and rare anaphylactic responses. Interference with biochemical measurements such as those for blood gases and calcium may occur if samples are taken before fat has been cleared. Daily checks are necessary to ensure complete clearance from the plasma in conditions where fat metabolism may be disturbed. **Additives should not be mixed with fat emulsions unless compatibility is known.**

> **Administration**
>
> Because of the complex requirements relating to parenteral nutrition full details relating to administration have been omitted. In all cases *product literature and other specialist literature should be consulted.*

## Supplementary preparations

> Compatibility with the infusion solution must be ascertained before adding supplementary preparations.

**Addiphos®** (Fresenius Kabi) PoM
Solution, sterile, phosphate 40 mmol, K$^+$ 30 mmol, Na$^+$ 30 mmol/20 mL. For addition to *Vamin®* solutions and glucose intravenous infusions. Net price 20-mL vial = £1.53

**Additrace®** (Fresenius Kabi) PoM
Solution, trace elements for addition to *Vamin®* solutions and glucose intravenous infusions, traces of Fe$^{3+}$, Zn$^{2+}$, Mn$^{2+}$, Cu$^{2+}$, Cr$^{3+}$, Se$^{4+}$, Mo$^{6+}$, F$^-$, I$^-$. For adults and children over 40 kg. Net price 10-mL amp = £2.31

**Cernevit®** (Baxter) PoM
Solution, *dl*-alpha tocopherol 11.2 units, ascorbic acid 125 mg, biotin 69 micrograms, colecalciferol 220 units, cyanocobalamin 6 micrograms, folic acid 414 micrograms, glycine 250 mg, nicotinamide 46 mg, pantothenic acid (as dexpanthenol) 17.25 mg, pyridoxine hydrochloride 5.5 mg, retinol (as palmitate) 3500 units, riboflavin (as dihydrated sodium phosphate) 4.14 mg, thiamine (as cocarboxylase tetrahydrate) 3.51 mg. Dissolve in 5 mL water for injections. Net price per vial = £3.32

**Decan®** (Baxter) PoM
Solution, trace elements for addition to infusion solutions, Fe$^{2+}$, Zn$^{2+}$, Cu$^{2+}$, Mn$^{2+}$, F$^-$, Co$^{2+}$, I$^-$, Se$^{4+}$, Mo$^{6+}$, Cr$^{3+}$. For adults over 40 kg. Net price 40-mL vial = £2.00

**Dipeptiven®** (Fresenius Kabi) PoM
Solution, *N*(2)-L-alanyl-L-glutamine 200 mg/mL (providing L-alanine 82 mg, L-glutamine 134.6 mg). For addition to infusion solutions containing amino acids. Net price 50 mL = £16.40, 100 mL = £30.50
Dose amino acid supplement for hypercatabolic or hypermetabolic states, 300–400 mg/kg daily; max. 400 mg/kg daily, dose not to exceed 20% of total amino acid intake

**Glycophos® Sterile Concentrate** (Fresenius Kabi) PoM
Solution, sterile, phosphate 20 mmol, Na$^+$ 40 mmol/20 mL. For addition to *Vamin®* and *Vaminolact®* solutions, and glucose intravenous infusions. Net price 20-mL vial = £4.60

9 Nutrition and blood

**Peditrace®** (Fresenius Kabi) PoM

Solution, trace elements for addition to *Vaminolact®*, *Vamin® 14 Electrolyte-Free* solutions and glucose intravenous infusions, traces of $Zn^{2+}$, $Cu^{2+}$, $Mn^{2+}$, $Se^{4+}$, $F^-$, $I^-$. For use in neonates (when kidney function established, usually second day of life), infants, and children. Net price 10-mL vial = £4.18

Cautions reduced biliary excretion especially in cholestatic liver disease or in markedly reduced urinary excretion (careful biochemical monitoring required); total parenteral nutrition exceeding 1 month (measure serum manganese concentration and check liver function before commencing treatment and regularly during treatment)—discontinue if manganese concentration raised or if cholestasis develops

**Solivito N®** (Fresenius Kabi) PoM

Solution, powder for reconstitution, biotin 60 micrograms, cyanocobalamin 5 micrograms, folic acid 400 micrograms, glycine 300 mg, nicotinamide 40 mg, pyridoxine hydrochloride 4.9 mg, riboflavin sodium phosphate 4.9 mg, sodium ascorbate 113 mg, sodium pantothenate 16.5 mg, thiamine mononitrate 3.1 mg. Dissolve in water for injections or glucose intravenous infusion for adding to glucose intravenous infusion or *Intralipid®*; dissolve in *Vitlipid N®* or *Intralipid®* for adding to *Intralipid®* only. Net price per vial = £2.32

**Vitlipid N®** (Fresenius Kabi) PoM

Emulsion, adult, vitamin A 330 units, ergocalciferol 20 units, *dl*-alpha tocopherol 1 unit, phytomenadione 15 micrograms/mL. For addition to *Intralipid®*. For adults and children over 11 years. Net price 10-mL amp = £2.32

Emulsion, infant, vitamin A 230 units, ergocalciferol 40 units, *dl*-alpha tocopherol 0.7 unit, phytomenadione 20 micrograms/mL. For addition to *Intralipid®*. Net price 10-mL amp = £2.32

## 9.4 Oral nutrition

9.4.1 Foods for special diets
9.4.2 Enteral nutrition

## 9.4.1 Foods for special diets

These are preparations that have been modified to eliminate a particular constituent from a food or that are nutrient mixtures formulated as food substitutes for patients who either cannot tolerate or cannot metabolise certain common constituents of food. In certain clinical conditions, some food preparations are regarded as drugs and can be prescribed within the NHS if they have been approved by the Advisory Committee on Borderline Substances (ACBS)—see Appendix 7.

**Phenylketonuria** Phenylketonuria (hyperphenylalaninaemia, PKU), which results from the inability to metabolise phenylalanine, is managed by restricting dietary intake of phenylalanine to a small amount sufficient for tissue building and repair.

**Sapropterin**, a synthetic form of tetrahydrobiopterin, is licensed as an adjunct to dietary restriction of phenylalanine in the management of patients with phenylketonuria and tetrahydrobiopterin deficiency.

**Aspartame** (used as a sweetener in some foods and medicines) contributes to the phenylalanine intake and may affect control of phenylketonuria. Where the presence of aspartame is specified in the product literature this is indicated in the BNF against the preparation; the patient should be informed of this.

**Coeliac disease** Intolerance to gluten in coeliac disease is managed by completely eliminating gluten from the diet. A range of gluten-free products is available for prescription—see Appendix 7, p. 903.

### ◼ SAPROPTERIN DIHYDROCHLORIDE

Note Sapropterin is a synthetic form of tetrahydrobiopterin

**Indications** see under Dose below

**Cautions** monitor blood-phenylalanine concentration before and after first week of treatment—if unsatisfactory response increase dose at weekly intervals to max. dose and monitor blood-phenylalanine concentration weekly; discontinue treatment if unsatisfactory response after 1 month; monitor blood-phenylalanine and tyrosine concentrations 1–2 weeks after dose adjustment and during treatment; history of convulsions; hepatic impairment; renal impairment; pregnancy (Appendix 4)

**Contra-indications** breast-feeding

**Side-effects** diarrhoea, vomiting, abdominal pain; nasal congestion, cough, pharyngolaryngeal pain; headache

**Dose**

* Phenylketonuria (specialist use only), by mouth, ADULT and CHILD over 4 years, initially 10 mg/kg once daily, preferably in the morning, adjusted according to response; usual dose 5–20 mg/kg daily

* Tetrahydrobiopterin deficiency (specialist use only), by mouth, ADULT and CHILD over 4 years, initially 2–5 mg/kg once daily, preferably in the morning, adjusted according to response; max. 20 mg/kg daily; total daily dose may alternatively be given in 2–3 divided doses

**Kuvan®** (Merck Serono) ▼ PoM

Dispersible tablets, sapropterin dihydrochloride 100 mg, net price 30-tab pack = £597.22, 120-tab pack = £2388.88. Label: 13, 21

Counselling Tablets should be dissolved in water and taken within 20 minutes

## 9.4.2 Enteral nutrition

The body's reserves of protein rapidly become exhausted in severely ill patients, especially during chronic illness or in those with severe burns, extensive trauma, pancreatitis, or intestinal fistula. Much can be achieved by frequent meals and by persuading the patient to take supplementary snacks of ordinary food between the meals.

However, extra calories, protein, other nutrients, and vitamins are often best given by supplementing ordinary meals with enteral sip or tube feeds (preparations, see Appendix 7).

When patients cannot feed normally, for example, patients with severe facial injury, oesophageal obstruction, or coma, a nutritionally complete diet of enteral feeds must be given. The advice of a dietitian should be sought to determine the protein and total energy requirement of the patient and the form and relative contribution of carbohydrate and fat to the energy requirements.

Most enteral feeds contain protein derived from cows' milk or soya. Elemental feeds containing protein hydrolysates or free amino acids can be used for patients who have diminished ability to break down protein, for example in inflammatory bowel disease or pancreatic insufficiency.

Even when nutritionally complete feeds are given, water and electrolyte balance should be monitored. Haematological and biochemical parameters should also be monitored, particularly in clinically unstable patients. Extra minerals (e.g. magnesium and zinc) may be needed in patients where gastro-intestinal secretions are being lost. Additional vitamins may also be needed. Feeds containing vitamin K may affect the INR in patients receiving warfarin—see **interactions**: Appendix 1 (vitamins).

**Children** Children have special requirements and in most situations liquid feeds prepared for adults are totally unsuitable—the advice of a paediatric dietitian should be sought; see also *BNF for Children*, section 9.4.2

◢**Preparations**
See Borderline Substances, Appendix 7.

# 9.5 Minerals

9.5.1 Calcium and magnesium
9.5.2 Phosphorus
9.5.3 Fluoride
9.5.4 Zinc
9.5.5 Selenium

See section 9.1.1 for iron salts.

# 9.5.1 Calcium and magnesium

9.5.1.1 Calcium supplements
9.5.1.2 Hypercalcaemia and hypercalciuria
9.5.1.3 Magnesium

## 9.5.1.1 Calcium supplements

Calcium supplements are usually only required where dietary calcium intake is deficient. This dietary requirement varies with age and is relatively greater in childhood, pregnancy, and lactation, due to an increased demand, and in old age, due to impaired absorption. In osteoporosis, a calcium intake which is double the recommended amount reduces the rate of bone loss. If the actual dietary intake is less than the recommended amount, a supplement of as much as 40 mmol is appropriate, see also Osteoporosis, p. 419 and Vitamin D, p. 549.

In severe acute hypocalcaemia or hypocalcaemic tetany, an initial slow intravenous injection of 10–20 mL of calcium gluconate injection 10% (providing approximately 2.25–4.5 mmol of calcium) should be

given, with plasma-calcium and ECG monitoring (risk of arrhythmias if given too rapidly), and either repeated as required or, if only temporary improvement, followed by a continuous intravenous infusion to prevent recurrence. For infusion, dilute 100 mL of calcium gluconate 10% in 1 litre of glucose 5% or sodium chloride 0.9% and give at an initial rate of 50 mL/hour adjusted according to response. Calcium chloride injection is also available, but is more irritant; care should be taken to prevent extravasation. Oral supplements of calcium and vitamin D may also be required in persistent hypocalcaemia (see also section 9.6.4). Concurrent hypomagnesaemia should be corrected with **magnesium sulphate** (section 9.5.1.3).

For the role of calcium gluconate in temporarily reducing the toxic effects of hyperkalaemia, see p. 528.

## ▮ CALCIUM SALTS

**Indications** see notes above; calcium deficiency

**Cautions** renal impairment; sarcoidosis; history of nephrolithiasis; avoid calcium chloride in respiratory acidosis or respiratory failure; **interactions**: Appendix 1 (antacids, calcium salts)

**Contra-indications** conditions associated with hypercalcaemia and hypercalciuria (e.g. some forms of malignant disease)

**Side-effects** gastro-intestinal disturbances; bradycardia, arrhythmias; *with injection*, peripheral vasodilatation, fall in blood pressure, injection-site reactions, severe tissue damage with extravasation

**Dose**
- By mouth, daily in divided doses, see notes above
- By slow intravenous injection, acute hypocalcaemia, calcium gluconate 1–2 g (Ca$^{2+}$ 2.25–4.5 mmol); CHILD see *BNF for Children*
- By continuous intravenous infusion, acute hypocalcaemia, see notes above

◢**Oral preparations**
**Calcium Gluconate** (Non-proprietary)
Tablets, calcium gluconate 600 mg (calcium 53.4 mg or Ca$^{2+}$ 1.35 mmol), net price 20 = £1.43. Label: 24
Effervescent tablets, calcium gluconate 1 g (calcium 89 mg or Ca$^{2+}$ 2.23 mmol), net price 28-tab pack = £10.66. Label: 13
Note Each tablet usually contains 4.46 mmol Na$^+$

**Calcium Lactate** (Non-proprietary)
Tablets, calcium lactate 300 mg (calcium 39 mg or Ca$^{2+}$ 1 mmol), net price 84 = £2.98

**Adcal®** (ProStrakan)
Chewable tablets, fruit flavour, calcium carbonate 1.5 g (calcium 600 mg or Ca$^{2+}$ 15 mmol), net price 100-tab pack = £7.25. Label: 24

**Cacit®** (Procter & Gamble Pharm.)
Tablets, effervescent, pink, calcium carbonate 1.25 g, providing calcium citrate when dispersed in water (calcium 500 mg or Ca$^{2+}$ 12.5 mmol), net price 76-tab pack = £12.05. Label: 13

**Calcichew®** (Shire)
Tablets (chewable), orange flavour, calcium carbonate 1.25 g (calcium 500 mg or Ca$^{2+}$ 12.5 mmol), net price 100-tab pack = £9.33. Label: 24

9

Nutrition and blood

Forte tablets (chewable), orange flavour, scored, calcium carbonate 2.5 g (calcium 1 g or Ca²⁺ 25 mmol), net price 60-tab pack = £13.16. Label: 24
Excipients include aspartame (section 9.4.1)

**Calcium-500** (Martindale)
Tablets, pink, f/c, calcium carbonate 1.25 g (calcium 500 mg or Ca²⁺ 12.5 mmol), net price 100-tab pack = £9.46. Label: 25

**Calcium-Sandoz®** (Alliance)
Syrup, orange flavour, calcium glubionate 1.09 g, calcium lactobionate 727 mg (calcium 108.3 mg or Ca²⁺ 2.7 mmol)/5 mL, net price 300 mL = £3.14

**Sandocal®** (Novartis Consumer Health)
Sandocal-400 tablets, effervescent, orange flavour, calcium lactate gluconate 930 mg, calcium carbonate 700 mg, anhydrous citric acid 1.189 g, providing calcium 400 mg (Ca²⁺ 10 mmol), net price 5 × 20-tab pack = £6.87. Label: 13
Excipients include aspartame (section 9.4.1)

Sandocal-1000 tablets, effervescent, orange flavour, calcium lactate gluconate 2.263 g, calcium carbonate 1.75 g, anhydrous citric acid 2.973 g providing 1 g calcium (Ca²⁺ 25 mmol), net price 3 × 10-tab pack = £6.17. Label: 13
Excipients include aspartame (section 9.4.1)

**◢Parenteral preparations**

**Calcium Gluconate** (Non-proprietary) [PoM]
Injection, calcium gluconate 10% (calcium 8.4 mg or Ca²⁺ 226 micromol/mL), net price 10-mL amp = 60p

**Calcium Chloride** (Non-proprietary) [PoM]
Injection, calcium chloride dihydrate 10% (calcium 27.3 mg or Ca²⁺ 680 micromol/mL), net price 10-mL disposable syringe = £5.10
Brands include *Minijet® Calcium Chloride 10%*

Injection, calcium chloride dihydrate 13.4% (calcium 36 mg or Ca²⁺ 910 micromol/mL), net price 10-mL amp = £14.94

**◢With vitamin D**
Section 9.6.4

**◢With disodium etidronate**
Section 6.6.2

**◢With risedronate sodium and colecalciferol**
Section 6.6.2

**9.5.1.2  Hypercalcaemia and hypercalciuria**

**Severe hypercalcaemia** Severe hypercalcaemia calls for urgent treatment before detailed investigation of the cause. Dehydration should be corrected first with intravenous infusion of **sodium chloride 0.9%**. Drugs (such as thiazides and vitamin D compounds) which promote hypercalcaemia, should be discontinued and dietary calcium should be restricted.

If *severe hypercalcaemia persists* drugs which inhibit mobilisation of calcium from the skeleton may be required. The **bisphosphonates** are useful and disodium pamidronate (section 6.6.2) is probably the most effective.

**Corticosteroids** (section 6.3) are widely given, but may only be useful where hypercalcaemia is due to sarcoi-

dosis or vitamin D intoxication; they often take several days to achieve the desired effect.

**Calcitonin** (section 6.6.1) is relatively non-toxic but its effect can wear off after a few days despite continued use; it is rarely effective where bisphosphonates have failed to reduce serum calcium adequately.

After treatment of severe hypercalcaemia the underlying cause must be established. *Further treatment* is governed by the same principles as for initial therapy. Salt and water depletion and drugs promoting hypercalcaemia should be avoided; oral administration of a bisphosphonate may be useful.

**Hyperparathyroidism** **Cinacalcet** is licensed for the treatment of secondary hyperparathyroidism in dialysis patients with end-stage renal disease (but see NICE guidance below), for primary hyperparathyroidism in patients where parathyroidectomy is inappropriate, and for the treatment of hypercalcaemia in parathyroid carcinoma. Cinacalcet reduces parathyroid hormone which leads to a decrease in serum calcium concentrations.

**Paricalcitol** (section 9.6.4) is also licensed for the prevention and treatment of secondary hyperparathyroidism associated with chronic renal failure.

Parathyroidectomy may be indicated for hyperparathyroidism.

---

**NICE guidance**
**Cinacalcet for the treatment of secondary hyperparathyroidism in patients with end-stage renal disease on maintenance dialysis therapy (January 2007)**
Cinacalcet is not recommended for the routine treatment of secondary hyperparathyroidism in patients with end-stage renal disease on maintenance dialysis therapy.
Cinacalcet is recommended for the treatment of refractory secondary hyperparathyroidism in patients with end-stage renal disease (including those with calciphylaxis) **only** in those:
• who have 'very uncontrolled' plasma concentration of intact parathyroid hormone (defined as greater than 85 picomol/litre) refractory to standard therapy, and a normal or high adjusted serum calcium concentration, **and**
• in whom surgical parathyroidectomy is contraindicated, in that the risks of surgery outweigh the benefits.
Response to treatment should be monitored regularly and treatment should be continued only if a reduction in the plasma concentration of intact parathyroid hormone of 30% or greater is seen within 4 months of treatment.

---

**Hypercalciuria** Hypercalciuria should be investigated for an underlying cause, which should be treated. Where a cause is not identified (idiopathic hypercalciuria), the condition is managed by increasing fluid intake and giving bendroflumethiazide in a dose of 2.5 mg daily (a higher dose is not usually necessary). Reducing dietary calcium intake may be beneficial but severe restriction of calcium intake has not proved beneficial and may even be harmful.

## ■ CINACALCET

**Indications** see under Dose and notes above

**Cautions** measure serum-calcium concentration before initiation of treatment and within 1 week after starting treatment or adjusting dose, then monthly for secondary hyperparathyroidism and every 2–3 months for primary hyperparathyroidism and parathyroid carcinoma; treatment should not be initiated in patients with hypocalcaemia; in secondary hyperparathyroidism measure parathyroid hormone concentration 1–4 weeks after starting treatment or adjusting dose, then every 1–3 months; dose adjustment may be necessary if smoking started or stopped during treatment; hepatic impairment (Appendix 2); pregnancy (Appendix 4); **interactions:** Appendix 1 (cinacalcet)

**Contra-indications** breast-feeding (Appendix 5)

**Side-effects** nausea, vomiting, anorexia; dizziness; paraesthesia, asthenia; reduced testosterone concentrations; myalgia; rash; *less commonly* dyspepsia, diarrhoea, and seizures; hypotension and heart failure also reported

**Dose**

- Secondary hyperparathyroidism in patients with end-stage renal disease on dialysis (but see notes above), ADULT over 18 years, initially 30 mg once daily, adjusted every 2–4 weeks to max. 180 mg daily
- Hypercalcaemia of primary hyperparathyroidism or parathyroid carcinoma, ADULT over 18 years, initially 30 mg twice daily, adjusted every 2–4 weeks according to response up to max. 90 mg 4 times daily

**Mimpara®** (Amgen) [PoM]
Tablets, green, f/c, cinacalcet (as hydrochloride) 30 mg, net price 28-tab pack = £121.36; 60 mg, 28-tab pack = £223.87; 90 mg, 28-tab pack = £335.81. Label: 21

### 9.5.1.3 Magnesium

Magnesium is an essential constituent of many enzyme systems, particularly those involved in energy generation; the largest stores are in the skeleton.

Magnesium salts are not well absorbed from the gastro-intestinal tract, which explains the use of magnesium sulphate (section 1.6.4) as an osmotic laxative.

Magnesium is excreted mainly by the kidneys and is therefore retained in renal failure, but significant *hypermagnesaemia* (causing muscle weakness and arrhythmias) is rare.

**Hypomagnesaemia** Since magnesium is secreted in large amounts in the gastro-intestinal fluid, excessive losses in diarrhoea, stoma or fistula are the most common causes of *hypomagnesaemia*; deficiency may also occur in alcoholism or as a result of treatment with certain drugs. Hypomagnesaemia often causes secondary hypocalcaemia, and also hypokalaemia and hyponatraemia.

Symptomatic *hypomagnesaemia* is associated with a deficit of 0.5–1 mmol/kg; up to 160 mmol $Mg^{2+}$ over up to 5 days may be required to replace the deficit (allowing for urinary losses). Magnesium is given initially by intravenous infusion or by intramuscular injection of **magnesium sulphate**; the intramuscular injection is painful. Plasma magnesium concentration should

be measured to determine the rate and duration of infusion and the dose should be reduced in renal impairment. To prevent *recurrence of the deficit*, magnesium may be given by mouth in a dose of 24 mmol $Mg^{2+}$ daily in divided doses; suitable preparations are magnesium glycerophosphate tablets or liquid [unlicensed], available from 'special-order' manufacturers or specialist importing companies, see p. 969. For maintenance (e.g. in intravenous nutrition), parenteral doses of magnesium are of the order of 10–20 mmol $Mg^{2+}$ daily (often about 12 mmol $Mg^{2+}$ daily).

**Arrhythmias** Magnesium sulphate has also been recommended for the emergency treatment of *serious arrhythmias*, especially in the presence of hypokalaemia (when hypomagnesaemia may also be present) and when salvos of rapid ventricular tachycardia show the characteristic twisting wave front known as *torsade de pointes* (see also section 2.3.1). The usual dose of magnesium sulphate by intravenous injection is 2 g (8 mmol $Mg^{2+}$) over 10–15 minutes (repeated once if necessary).

**Myocardial infarction** Limited evidence that magnesium sulphate prevents arrhythmias and reperfusion injury in patients with suspected myocardial infarction has not been confirmed by large studies. Routine use of magnesium sulphate for this purpose is not recommended. For the management of myocardial infarction, see section 2.10.1.

**Eclampsia and pre-eclampsia** Magnesium sulphate is the drug of choice for the prevention of recurrent seizures in *eclampsia*; see also Appendix 4. Regimens may vary between hospitals. Calcium gluconate injection is used for the management of magnesium toxicity.

Magnesium sulphate is also of benefit in women with *pre-eclampsia* in whom there is concern about developing eclampsia. The patient should be monitored carefully (see under Magnesium Sulphate).

## ■ MAGNESIUM SULPHATE

**Indications** see notes above; constipation (section 1.6.4); severe acute asthma (section 3.1); paste for boils (section 13.10.5)

**Cautions** see notes above; hepatic impairment (Appendix 2); renal impairment (Appendix 3); in severe hypomagnesaemia administer initially via controlled infusion device (preferably syringe pump); monitor blood pressure, respiratory rate, urinary output and for signs of overdosage (loss of patellar reflexes, weakness, nausea, sensation of warmth, flushing, drowsiness, double vision, and slurred speech); pregnancy (Appendix 4); **interactions:** Appendix 1 (magnesium, parenteral)

**Side-effects** generally associated with hypermagnesaemia, nausea, vomiting, thirst, flushing of skin, hypotension, arrhythmias, coma, respiratory depression, drowsiness, confusion, loss of tendon reflexes, muscle weakness; colic and diarrhoea following oral administration

**Dose**

- Hypomagnesaemia, see notes above
- Arrhythmias, see notes above
- Prevention of seizure recurrence in eclampsia, initially by intravenous injection over 5–15 minutes, 4 g, followed by intravenous infusion, 1 g/hour for at

least 24 hours after last seizure; if seizure recurs, additional dose by intravenous injection, 2 g (4 g if body-weight over 70 kg)

- Prevention of seizures in pre-eclampsia [unlicensed indication], initially by intravenous injection over 5–15 minutes, 4 g followed by intravenous infusion, 1 g/hour for 24 hours; if seizure occurs, additional dose by intravenous injection, 2 g

**Intravenous administration** For intravenous injection concentration of magnesium sulphate should not exceed 20% (dilute 1 part of magnesium sulphate injection 50% with at least 1.5 parts of water for injections)

**Note** Magnesium sulphate 1 g equivalent to $Mg^{2+}$ approx. 4 mmol

### Magnesium Sulphate (Non-proprietary) [PoM]

Injection, magnesium sulphate 20% ($Mg^{2+}$ approx. 0.8 mmol/mL), net price 20-mL (4-g) amp = £2.75; 50% ($Mg^{2+}$ approx. 2 mmol/mL), 2-mL (1-g) amp = £3.82, 4-mL (2-g) prefilled syringe = £7.39, 5-mL (2.5-g) amp = £3.00, 10-mL (5-g) amp = £3.35; 10-mL (5-g) prefilled syringe = £4.95
Brands include *Minijet® Magnesium Sulphate 50%*

## 9.5.2 Phosphorus

### 9.5.2.1 Phosphate supplements
### 9.5.2.2 Phosphate-binding agents

### 9.5.2.1 Phosphate supplements

Oral phosphate supplements may be required in addition to vitamin D in a small minority of patients with hypophosphataemic vitamin D-resistant rickets. Diarrhoea is a common side-effect and should prompt a reduction in dosage.

Phosphate infusion is occasionally needed in alcohol dependence or in phosphate deficiency arising from use of parenteral nutrition deficient in phosphate supplements; phosphate depletion also occurs in severe diabetic ketoacidosis. For *established hypophosphataemia*, monobasic potassium phosphate may be infused at a rate of 9 mmol every 12 hours. In critically ill patients, the dose of phosphate can be increased up to 500 micromol/kg (approx. 30 mmol in adults, max. 50 mmol), infused over 6–12 hours, according to severity. Excessive doses of phosphates may cause hypocalcaemia and metastatic calcification; it is **essential** to monitor closely plasma concentrations of calcium, phosphate, potassium, and other electrolytes.

For phosphate requirements in *total parenteral nutrition* regimens, see section 9.3.

### Phosphates (Fresenius Kabi) [PoM]

Intravenous infusion, phosphates (providing $PO_4^{3-}$ 100 mmol, $K^+$ 19 mmol, and $Na^+$ 162 mmol/litre), net price 500 mL (*Polyfusor®*) = £3.75.
For the treatment of moderate to severe hypophosphatemia

### Phosphate-Sandoz® (HK Pharma)

Tablets, effervescent, anhydrous sodium acid phosphate 1.936 g, sodium bicarbonate 350 mg, potassium bicarbonate 315 mg, equivalent to phosphorus 500 mg (phosphate 16.1 mmol), sodium 468.8 mg ($Na^+$ 20.4 mmol), potassium 123 mg ($K^+$ 3.1 mmol). Net price 20 = £3.29. Label: 13
**Dose** vitamin D-resistant hypophosphataemic osteomalacia, 4–6 tablets daily; CHILD under 5 years 2–3 tablets daily

### 9.5.2.2 Phosphate-binding agents

Calcium-containing preparations are used as phosphate-binding agents in the management of hyperphosphataemia complicating renal failure. Aluminium-containing preparations are rarely used as phosphate-binding agents and can cause aluminium accumulation.

**Sevelamer** is licensed for the treatment of hyperphosphataemia in patients on haemodialysis or peritoneal dialysis.

**Lanthanum** is licensed for the control of hyperphosphataemia in patients with chronic renal failure on haemodialysis or continuous ambulatory peritoneal dialysis (CAPD).

### ALUMINIUM HYDROXIDE

**Indications** hyperphosphataemia; dyspepsia (section 1.1)

**Cautions** hyperaluminaemia; see also notes above; renal impairment (Appendix 3); **interactions:** Appendix 1 (antacids)

**Side-effects** see section 1.1.1

**Alu-Cap®** (3M)
Capsules, green/red, dried aluminium hydroxide 475 mg (low $Na^+$). Net price 120-cap pack = £3.75
**Dose** phosphate-binding agent in renal failure, 4–20 capsules daily in divided doses with meals

### CALCIUM SALTS

**Indications** hyperphosphataemia

**Cautions** **interactions:** Appendix 1 (antacids, calcium salts)

**Contra-indications** hypercalcaemia, hypercalciuria

**Side-effects** hypercalcaemia

**Adcal®** section 9.5.1.1

**Calcichew®** section 9.5.1.1

**Calcium-500** section 9.5.1.1

**Phosex®** (Vitaline)
Tablets, yellow, calcium acetate 1 g (calcium 250 mg or $Ca^{2+}$ 6.2 mmol), net price 180-tab pack = £19.79. Label: 25, counselling, with meals
**Dose** phosphate-binding agent (with meals) in renal failure, according to the requirements of the patient

### LANTHANUM

**Indications** hyperphosphataemia in patients on haemodialysis or continuous ambulatory peritoneal dialysis (CAPD)

**Cautions** acute peptic ulcer; ulcerative colitis; Crohn's disease; bowel obstruction; hepatic impairment; breast-feeding (Appendix 5); **interactions:** Appendix 1 (lanthanum)

**Contra-indications** pregnancy (Appendix 4)

**Side-effects** gastro-intestinal disturbances; hypocalcaemia; *less commonly* anorexia, increased appetite, taste disturbances, dry mouth, thirst, stomatitis, chest pain, peripheral oedema, headache, dizziness, vertigo, asthenia, fatigue, malaise, hyperglycaemia, hyperparathyroidism, hypercalcaemia, hypophosphataemia, eosinophilia, arthralgia, myalgia, osteoporosis, sweating, alopecia, pruritus, and erythematous rash;

accumulation of lanthanum in bone, and transient changes in QT interval also reported

**Dose**

- ADULT over 18 years, initially 750 mg daily in divided doses chewed with or immediately after meals, adjusted according to plasma-phosphate concentration every 2–3 weeks (usual dose range 1.5–3 g daily in divided doses)

**Fosrenol®** (Shire) ▼ PoM
Tablets (chewable), lanthanum (as carbonate hydrate) 500 mg, net price 90-tab pack = £114.13; 750 mg, 90-tab pack = £152.17; 1 g, 90-tab pack = £161.33. Label: 21, counselling, to be chewed

## ▌ SEVELAMER

**Indications** hyperphosphataemia in patients on haemodialysis or peritoneal dialysis

**Cautions** gastro-intestinal disorders; pregnancy (Appendix 4); breast-feeding (Appendix 5); **interactions**: Appendix 1 (sevelamer)

**Contra-indications** bowel obstruction

**Side-effects** gastro-intestinal disturbances; *very rarely* intestinal obstruction

**Dose**

- ADULT over 18 years, initially 2.4–4.8 g daily in 3 divided doses with meals, then adjusted according to plasma-phosphate concentration (usual dose range 2.4–12 g daily in 3 divided doses)

**Renagel®** (Genzyme) PoM
Tablets, f/c, sevelamer 800 mg, net price 180-tab pack = £117.97. Label: 25, counselling, with meals

## 9.5.3 Fluoride

Availability of adequate fluoride confers significant resistance to dental caries. It is now considered that the topical action of fluoride on enamel and plaque is more important than the systemic effect.

When the fluoride content of drinking water is less than 700 micrograms per litre (0.7 parts per million), daily administration of fluoride tablets or drops provides suitable supplementation. Systemic fluoride supplements should not be prescribed without reference to the fluoride content of the local water supply. Infants need not receive fluoride supplements until the age of 6 months.

Dentifrices which incorporate sodium fluoride or monofluorophosphate are also a convenient source of fluoride.

Individuals who are either particularly caries prone or medically compromised may be given additional protection by use of fluoride rinses or by application of fluoride gels. Rinses may be used daily or weekly; daily use of a less concentrated rinse is more effective than weekly use of a more concentrated one. High-strength gels must be applied regularly under professional supervision; extreme caution is necessary to prevent children from swallowing any excess. Less concentrated gels are available for home use. Varnishes are also available and are particularly valuable for young or disabled children since they adhere to the teeth and set in the presence of moisture.

> Fluoride mouthwash, oral drops, tablets and toothpaste are prescribable on form FP10D (GP14 in Scotland, WP10D in Wales; for details see preparations, below).
> There are also arrangements for health authorities to supply fluoride tablets in the course of pre-school dental schemes, and they may also be supplied in school dental schemes.
> Fluoride gels are not prescribable on form FP10D (GP14 in Scotland, WP10D in Wales).

## ▌ FLUORIDES

**Note** Sodium fluoride 2.2 mg provides approx. 1 mg fluoride ion

**Indications** prophylaxis of dental caries—see notes above

**Contra-indications** not for areas where drinking water is fluoridated

**Side-effects** occasional white flecks on teeth with recommended doses; *rarely* yellowish-brown discoloration if recommended doses are exceeded

**Dose**

**Note** Dose expressed as fluoride ion ($F^-$)

- Water content less than $F^-$ 300 micrograms/litre (0.3 parts per million), CHILD up to 6 months none; 6 months–3 years $F^-$ 250 micrograms daily, 3–6 years $F^-$ 500 micrograms daily, over 6 years $F^-$ 1 mg daily
- Water content between $F^-$ 300 and 700 micrograms/litre (0.3–0.7 parts per million), CHILD up to 3 years none, 3–6 years $F^-$ 250 micrograms daily, over 6 years $F^-$ 500 micrograms daily
- Water content above $F^-$ 700 micrograms/litre (0.7 parts per million), supplements not advised

**Note** These doses reflect the recommendations of the British Dental Association, the British Society of Paediatric Dentistry and the British Association for the Study of Community Dentistry (*Br Dent J* 1997; **182**: 6–7)

**◢Tablets**
**Counselling** Tablets should be sucked or dissolved in the mouth and taken preferably in the evening

**En-De-Kay®** (Manx)
Fluotabs 3–6 years, orange-flavoured, scored, sodium fluoride 1.1 mg ($F^-$ 500 micrograms). Net price 200-tab pack = £2.38

Fluotabs 6+ years, orange-flavoured, scored, sodium fluoride 2.2 mg ($F^-$ 1 mg). Net price 200-tab pack = £2.38
**Dental prescribing on NHS** May be prescribed as Sodium Fluoride Tablets

**Fluor-a-day®** (Dental Health)
Tablets, buff, sodium fluoride 1.1 mg ($F^-$ 500 micrograms), net price 200-tab pack = £2.54; 2.2 mg ($F^-$ 1 mg), 200-tab pack = £2.54
**Dental prescribing on NHS** May be prescribed as Sodium Fluoride Tablets

**FluoriGard®** (Colgate-Palmolive)
Tablets 0.5, purple, grape-flavoured, scored, sodium fluoride 1.1 mg ($F^-$ 500 micrograms). Net price 200-tab pack = £1.91

Tablets 1.0, orange, orange-flavoured, scored, sodium fluoride 2.2 mg ($F^-$ 1 mg). Net price 200-tab pack = £1.91
**Dental prescribing on NHS** May be prescribed as Sodium Fluoride Tablets

**9** Nutrition and blood

**◢Oral drops**

**Note** Fluoride supplements not considered necessary below 6 months of age (see notes above)

**En-De-Kay®** (Manx)

Fluodrops® (= paediatric drops), sugar-free, sodium fluoride 550 micrograms (F⁻ 250 micrograms)/ 0.15 mL. Net price 60 mL = £2.38

Dental prescribing on NHS Corresponds to Sodium Fluoride Oral Drops DPF 0.37% equivalent to sodium fluoride 80 micrograms (F⁻ 36 micrograms)/drop

**◢Mouthwashes**

Rinse mouth for 1 minute and spit out

**Counselling** Avoid eating, drinking, or rinsing mouth for 15 minutes after use

**Duraphat®** (Colgate-Palmolive)

Weekly dental rinse (= mouthwash), blue, sodium fluoride 0.2%. Net price 150 mL = £2.37. Counselling, see above

Dose CHILD 6 years and over, for *weekly* use, rinse with 10 mL

Dental prescribing on NHS May be prescribed as Sodium Fluoride Mouthwash 0.2%

**En-De-Kay®** (Manx)

Daily fluoride mouthrinse (= mouthwash), blue, sodium fluoride 0.05%. Net price 250 mL = £1.51

Dose CHILD 6 years and over, for *daily* use, rinse with 10 mL

Dental prescribing on NHS May be prescribed as Sodium Fluoride Mouthwash 0.05%

Fluorinse (= mouthwash), red, sodium fluoride 2%. Net price 100 mL = £4.97. Counselling, see above

Dose CHILD 8 years and over, for *daily* use, dilute 5 drops to 10 mL of water; for *weekly* use, dilute 20 drops to 10 mL

Dental prescribing on NHS May be prescribed as Sodium Fluoride Mouthwash 2%

**FluoriGard®** (Colgate-Palmolive)

Daily dental rinse (= mouthwash), blue, sodium fluoride 0.05%. Net price 500 mL = £3.14. Counselling, see above

Dose CHILD 6 years and over, for *daily* use, rinse with 10 mL

Dental prescribing on NHS May be prescribed as Sodium Fluoride Mouthwash 0.05%

**◢Gels**

**FluoriGard®** (Colgate-Palmolive)

Gel-Kam (= gel), stannous fluoride 0.4% in glycerol basis. Net price 100 mL = £2.97. Counselling, see below

Dose ADULT and CHILD 3 years and over, for *daily* use, using a toothbrush, apply onto all tooth surfaces

**Counselling** Swish between teeth for 1 minute before spitting out. Avoid eating, drinking, or rinsing mouth for at least 30 minutes after use

**◢Toothpastes**

**Duraphat®** (Colgate-Palmolive) ℙₒₘ

*Duraphat®* '2800 ppm' toothpaste, sodium fluoride 0.619%. Net price 75 mL = £3.26, dual pack (2×75 mL) = £5.54. Counselling, see below

Dose ADULT and CHILD over 10 years, apply 1 cm twice daily using a toothbrush

**Counselling** Brush teeth for 1 minute before spitting out. Avoid drinking or rinsing mouth for 30 minutes after use

Dental prescribing on NHS May be prescribed as Sodium Fluoride Toothpaste 0.619%

*Duraphat®* '5000 ppm' toothpaste, sodium fluoride 1.1%. Net price 51 g = £4.45. Counselling, see below

Dose ADULT and ADOLESCENT over 16 years, apply 2 cm 3 times daily after meals using a toothbrush

**Counselling** Brush teeth for 3 minutes before spitting out

Dental prescribing on NHS May be prescribed as Sodium Fluoride Toothpaste 1.1%

## 9.5.4 Zinc

Zinc supplements should not be given unless there is good evidence of deficiency (hypoproteinaemia spuriously lowers plasma-zinc concentration) or in zinc-losing conditions. Zinc deficiency can occur as a result of inadequate diet or malabsorption; excessive loss of zinc can occur in trauma, burns, and protein-losing conditions. A zinc supplement is given until clinical improvement occurs, but it may need to be continued in severe malabsorption, metabolic disease (section 9.8.1), or in zinc-losing states.

Parenteral nutrition regimens usually include trace amounts of zinc (section 9.3). If necessary, further zinc can be added to intravenous feeding regimens. A suggested dose for intravenous nutrition is elemental zinc 6.5 mg (Zn²⁺ 100 micromol) daily.

### ZINC SULPHATE

**Indications** zinc deficiency or supplementation in zinc-losing conditions

**Cautions** acute renal failure (may accumulate); **interactions:** Appendix 1 (zinc)

**Side-effects** abdominal pain, dyspepsia, nausea, vomiting, diarrhoea, gastric irritation, gastritis; irritability, headache, lethargy

**Dose**

● See preparation below and notes above

**Zinc Sulphate** (Non-proprietary) ℙₒₘ

Injection, zinc sulphate 14.6 mg/mL (zinc 50 micromol/mL), net price 10 mL vial = £2.50

**Solvazinc®** (KoGEN)

Effervescent tablets, yellow-white, zinc sulphate monohydrate 125 mg (45 mg zinc), net price 30 = £4.32. Label: 13, 21

Dose ADULT and CHILD over 30 kg, 1 tablet in water 1–3 times daily after food; CHILD under 10 kg, ½ tablet daily; 10–30 kg, ½ tablet 1–3 times daily

## 9.5.5 Selenium

Selenium deficiency can occur as a result of inadequate diet or prolonged parenteral nutrition. A selenium supplement should not be given unless there is good evidence of deficiency.

### SELENIUM

**Indications** selenium deficiency

**Cautions** interactions: Appendix 1 (selenium)

**Dose**

● by mouth *or* by intramuscular injection *or* by intravenous injection, 100–500 micrograms daily

**Selenase®** (Oxford Nutrition) ℙₒₘ

Oral solution, selenium (as sodium selenite pentahydrate) 50 micrograms/mL, net price 2-mL amp = £1.03, 10-mL bottle = £3.75

Injection, selenium (as sodium selenite pentahydrate) 50 micrograms/mL, net price 2-mL amp = £1.50, 10-mL vial = £4.25

# 9.6 Vitamins

9.6.1 Vitamin A
9.6.2 Vitamin B group
9.6.3 Vitamin C
9.6.4 Vitamin D
9.6.5 Vitamin E
9.6.6 Vitamin K
9.6.7 Multivitamin preparations

Vitamins are used for the prevention and treatment of specific deficiency states or where the diet is known to be inadequate; they may be prescribed in the NHS to prevent or treat deficiency but not as dietary supplements.

Their use as general 'pick-me-ups' is of unproven value and, in the case of preparations containing vitamin A or D, may actually be harmful if patients take more than the prescribed dose. The 'fad' for mega-vitamin therapy with water-soluble vitamins, such as ascorbic acid and pyridoxine, is unscientific and can be harmful.

Dietary reference values for vitamins are available in the Department of Health publication:

Dietary Reference Values for Food Energy and Nutrients for the United Kingdom: Report of the Panel on Dietary Reference Values of the Committee on Medical Aspects of Food Policy. *Report on Health and Social Subjects 41.* London: HMSO, 1991

**Dental patients** It is unjustifiable to treat stomatitis or glossitis with mixtures of vitamin preparations; this delays diagnosis and correct treatment.

Most patients who develop a nutritional deficiency despite an adequate intake of vitamins have malabsorption and if this is suspected the patient should be referred to a medical practitioner.

## 9.6.1 Vitamin A

Deficiency of vitamin A (retinol) is associated with ocular defects (particularly xerophthalmia) and an increased susceptibility to infections, but deficiency is rare in the UK (even in disorders of fat absorption).

Massive overdose can cause rough skin, dry hair, an enlarged liver, and a raised erythrocyte sedimentation rate and raised serum calcium and serum alkaline phosphatase concentrations.

In view of evidence suggesting that high levels of vitamin A may cause birth defects, women who are (or may become) pregnant are advised not to take vitamin A supplements (including tablets and fish-liver oil drops), except on the advice of a doctor or an antenatal clinic; nor should they eat liver or products such as liver paté or liver sausage.

### VITAMIN A
(Retinol)

**Indications** see notes above

**Cautions** see notes above; **interactions:** Appendix 1 (vitamins)

**Side-effects** see notes above

**Dose**
- See notes above and under preparations

◢**Vitamins A and D**
**Halibut-liver Oil** (Non-proprietary)
Capsules, vitamin A 4000 units [also contains vitamin D], net price 100-cap pack = £1.05

**Vitamins A and D** (Non-proprietary)
Capsules, vitamin A 4000 units, vitamin D 400 units, net price 84-cap pack = £3.10
Note May be difficult to obtain

◢**Vitamins A, C and D**
**Healthy Start Children's Vitamin Drops** (Non-proprietary)
Oral drops, vitamin A 5000 units, vitamin D 2000 units, ascorbic acid 150 mg/mL
Available free of charge to children under 4 years through the Healthy Start Scheme; otherwise available direct to the public from maternity and child health clinics; community pharmacists may have difficulty obtaining supplies
Dose prevention of vitamin deficiency, CHILD 1 month–5 years, 5 drops daily (5 drops contain vitamin A approx. 700 units, vitamin D approx. 300 units, ascorbic acid approx. 20 mg)
Note *Healthy Start Vitamins for women* (containing ascorbic acid, vitamin D, and folic acid) are also available to women during pregnancy and until their baby is one year old, through the Healthy Start Scheme

## 9.6.2 Vitamin B group

Deficiency of the B vitamins, other than deficiency of vitamin $B_{12}$ (section 9.1.2), is rare in the UK and is usually treated by preparations containing thiamine ($B_1$), riboflavin ($B_2$), and nicotinamide, which is used in preference to nicotinic acid, as it does not cause vasodilatation. Other members (or substances traditionally classified as members) of the vitamin B complex such as aminobenzoic acid, biotin, choline, inositol, and pantothenic acid or panthenol may be included in vitamin B preparations but there is no evidence of their value.

The severe deficiency states Wernicke's encephalopathy and Korsakoff's psychosis, especially as seen in chronic alcoholism, are best treated initially by the parenteral administration of B vitamins (*Pabrinex*®), followed by oral administration of **thiamine** in the longer term. Anaphylaxis has been reported with parenteral B vitamins (see MHRA/CHM advice, below).

As with other vitamins of the B group, **pyridoxine** ($B_6$) deficiency is rare, but it may occur during isoniazid therapy (section 5.1.9) or penicillamine treatment in Wilson's disease (section 9.8.1) and is characterised by peripheral neuritis. High doses of pyridoxine are given in some metabolic disorders, such as hyperoxaluria, and it is also used in sideroblastic anaemia (section 9.1.3). There is evidence to suggest that pyridoxine in a dose not exceeding 100 mg daily may provide some benefit in premenstrual syndrome. It has been tried for a wide variety of other disorders, but there is little sound evidence to support the claims of efficacy, and overdosage induces toxic effects.

Nicotinic acid inhibits the synthesis of cholesterol and triglyceride (see section 2.12). Folic acid and vitamin $B_{12}$ are used in the treatment of megaloblastic anaemia (section 9.1.2). Folinic acid (available as calcium folinate) is used in association with cytotoxic therapy (section 8.1).

**9** Nutrition and blood

## RIBOFLAVIN
(Riboflavine, vitamin B₂)

**Indications** see notes above

◢ **Preparations**
Injections of vitamins B and C, see under Thiamine

◢ **Oral vitamin B complex preparations**
See below

## THIAMINE
(Vitamin B₁)

**MHRA/CHM advice (September 2007)**
Although potentially serious allergic adverse reactions may rarely occur during, or shortly after, parenteral administration, the CHM has recommended that:
1. This should not preclude the use of parenteral thiamine in patients where this route of administration is required, particularly in patients at risk of Wernicke-Korsakoff syndrome where treatment with thiamine is essential;
2. Intravenous administration should be by infusion over 30 minutes;
3. Facilities for treating anaphylaxis (including resuscitation facilities) should be available when parenteral thiamine is administered.

**Indications** see notes above
**Cautions** anaphylactic shock may occasionally follow injection (see MHRA/CHM advice above); breast-feeding (Appendix 5)
**Dose**
- Mild chronic deficiency, 10–25 mg daily; severe deficiency, 200–300 mg daily

**Thiamine** (Non-proprietary)
Tablets, thiamine hydrochloride 50 mg, net price 20 = 80p; 100 mg, 20 = £1.23
Brands include *Benerva®* ЈӉӅ

**Pabrinex®** (Link) Ⓟⓞⓜ
I/M High potency injection, for intramuscular use only, ascorbic acid 500 mg, nicotinamide 160 mg, pyridoxine hydrochloride 50 mg, riboflavin 4 mg, thiamine hydrochloride 250 mg/7 mL. Net price 7 mL (in 2 amps) = £2.35

I/V High potency injection, for intravenous use only, ascorbic acid 500 mg, anhydrous glucose 1 g, nicotinamide 160 mg, pyridoxine hydrochloride 50 mg, riboflavin 4 mg, thiamine hydrochloride 250 mg/10 mL. Net price 10 mL (in 2 amps) = £2.35
Parenteral vitamins B and C for rapid correction of severe depletion or malabsorption (e.g. in alcoholism, after acute infections, postoperatively, or in psychiatric states), maintenance of vitamins B and C in chronic intermittent haemodialysis
Dose see MHRA/CHM advice above
Coma or delirium from alcohol, from opioids, or from barbiturates, collapse following narcosis, by intravenous infusion of *I/V High potency*, 2–3 pairs every 8 hours
Psychosis following narcosis or electroconvulsive therapy, toxicity from acute infections, by intravenous infusion of *I/V High potency* or by deep intramuscular injection into the gluteal muscle of *I/M High potency*, 1 pair twice daily for up to 7 days
Haemodialysis, by intravenous infusion of *I/V High potency* in sodium chloride intravenous infusion 0.9%) 1 pair every 2 weeks

◢ **Oral vitamin B complex preparations**
See below

## PYRIDOXINE HYDROCHLORIDE
(Vitamin B₆)

**Indications** see under Dose
**Cautions** interactions: Appendix 1 (vitamins)
**Side-effects** sensory neuropathy reported with high doses given for extended periods
**Dose**
- Deficiency states, 20–50 mg up to 3 times daily
- Isoniazid-induced neuropathy, prophylaxis 10 mg daily [or 20 mg daily if suitable product not available]; treatment, 50 mg three times daily; CHILD under 18 years see *BNF for Children*
- Idiopathic sideroblastic anaemia, 100–400 mg daily in divided doses
- Penicillamine-induced neuropathy, prophylaxis in Wilson's disease [unlicensed use] (see also notes above), 20 mg daily; CHILD under 18 years see *BNF for Children*
- Premenstrual syndrome [unlicensed use], 50–100 mg daily (see notes above)

Prolonged use of pyridoxine in a dose of 10 mg daily is considered safe but the long-term use of pyridoxine in a dose of 200 mg or more daily has been associated with neuropathy. The safety of long-term pyridoxine supplementation with doses above 10 mg daily has not been established.

**Pyridoxine** (Non-proprietary)
Tablets, pyridoxine hydrochloride 10 mg, net price 20 = 34p; 20 mg, 20 = 34p; 50 mg, 28 = 76p

◢ **Injections of vitamins B and C**
See under Thiamine

## NICOTINAMIDE

**Indications** see notes above; acne vulgaris, see section 13.6.1

**Nicotinamide** (Non-proprietary)
Tablets, nicotinamide 50 mg. Net price 20 = £1.37

◢ **Injections of vitamins B and C**
See under Thiamine

## Oral vitamin B complex preparations
Note Other multivitamin preparations are in section 9.6.7.

**Vitamin B Tablets, Compound** ◪
Tablets, nicotinamide 15 mg, riboflavin 1 mg, thiamine hydrochloride 1 mg. Net price 20 = 7p
Dose prophylactic, 1–2 tablets daily

**Vitamin B Tablets, Compound, Strong** ◪
Tablets, brown, f/c or s/c, nicotinamide 20 mg, pyridoxine hydrochloride 2 mg, riboflavin 2 mg, thiamine hydrochloride 5 mg. Net price 28-tab pack = £2.07
Dose treatment of vitamin-B deficiency, 1–2 tablets 3 times daily

**Vigranon B®** (Wallace Mfg) ЈӉӅ ◪
Syrup, thiamine hydrochloride 5 mg, riboflavin 2 mg, nicotinamide 20 mg, pyridoxine hydrochloride 2 mg, panthenol 3 mg/5 mL. Net price 150 mL = £2.41

## Other compounds

**Potassium aminobenzoate** has been used in the treatment of various disorders associated with excessive fibrosis such as scleroderma but its therapeutic value is **doubtful**.

**Potaba®** (Glenwood) ◢

Capsules, potassium aminobenzoate 500 mg. Net price 20 = £1.59. Label: 21

Tablets, potassium aminobenzoate 500 mg. Net price 20 = £1.12. Label: 21

Envules® (= powder in sachets), potassium aminobenzoate 3 g. Net price 40 sachets = £17.21. Label: 13, 21

**Dose** Peyronie's disease, scleroderma, 12 g daily in divided doses after food

## 9.6.3 Vitamin C
### (Ascorbic acid)

Vitamin C therapy is essential in scurvy, but less florid manifestations of vitamin C deficiency are commonly found, especially in the elderly. It is rarely necessary to prescribe more than 100 mg daily except early in the treatment of scurvy.

Severe scurvy causes gingival swelling and bleeding margins as well as petechiae on the skin. This is, however, exceedingly rare and a patient with these signs is more likely to have leukaemia. Investigation should not be delayed by a trial period of vitamin treatment.

Claims that vitamin C ameliorates colds or promotes wound healing have not been proved.

### ASCORBIC ACID

**Indications** prevention and treatment of scurvy
**Cautions** interactions: Appendix 1 (vitamins)
**Dose**

- Prophylactic, 25–75 mg daily; therapeutic, not less than 250 mg daily in divided doses

**Ascorbic Acid** (Non-proprietary)

Tablets, ascorbic acid 50 mg, net price 28 = £1.21; 100 mg, 28 = £1.26; 200 mg, 28 = £1.27; 500 mg (label: 24), 28 = £3.23
Brands include *Redoxon®* (JHS)

Injection, ascorbic acid 100 mg/mL. Net price 5-mL amp = £2.51
Available from UCB Pharma

## 9.6.4 Vitamin D

**Note** The term Vitamin D is used for a range of compounds which possess the property of preventing or curing rickets. They include ergocalciferol (calciferol, vitamin D₂), colecalciferol (vitamin D₃), dihydrotachysterol, alfacalcidol (1α-hydroxycholecalciferol), and calcitriol (1,25-dihydroxycholecalciferol).

Simple vitamin D deficiency can be prevented by taking an oral supplement of only 10 micrograms (400 units) of **ergocalciferol** (calciferol, vitamin D₂) or **colecalciferol** (vitamin D₃) daily. Vitamin D deficiency can occur in people whose exposure to sunlight is limited and in those whose diet is deficient in vitamin D. In these individuals, ergocalciferol or colecalciferol in a dose of 20 micrograms (800 units) daily by mouth can prevent vitamin D deficiency. Since there is no plain tablet of this strength available, **calcium and ergocalciferol tablets** can be given (although the calcium is unnecessary).

Preparations containing calcium with colecalciferol are available for the management of combined calcium and vitamin D deficiency, or for those at high risk of deficiency (see also Osteoporosis, p. 419 and Calcium Supplements, p. 541).

Vitamin D deficiency caused by *intestinal malabsorption* or *chronic liver disease* usually requires vitamin D in pharmacological doses, such as **ergocalciferol tablets** up to 1 mg (40 000 units) daily; the hypocalcaemia of *hypoparathyroidism* often requires doses of up to 2.5 mg (100 000 units) daily in order to achieve normocalcaemia.

Vitamin D requires hydroxylation by the kidney to its active form, therefore the hydroxylated derivatives **alfacalcidol** or **calcitriol** should be prescribed if patients with *severe renal impairment* require vitamin D therapy. Calcitriol is also licensed for the management of postmenopausal osteoporosis.

**Paricalcitol**, a synthetic vitamin D analogue, is licensed for the prevention and treatment of secondary hyperparathyroidism associated with chronic renal failure (section 9.5.1.2).

**Important.** All patients receiving pharmacological doses of vitamin D should have their plasma-calcium concentration checked at intervals (initially once or twice weekly) and whenever nausea or vomiting occur. Breast milk from women taking pharmacological doses of vitamin D can cause hypercalcaemia if given to an infant.

### ERGOCALCIFEROL
#### (Calciferol, Vitamin D₂)

**Indications** see notes above
**Cautions** take care to ensure correct dose in infants; monitor plasma-calcium concentration in patients receiving high doses and in renal impairment; pregnancy (Appendix 4); breast-feeding (Appendix 5); **interactions**: Appendix 1 (vitamins)
**Contra-indications** hypercalcaemia; metastatic calcification
**Side-effects** symptoms of overdosage include anorexia, lassitude, nausea and vomiting, diarrhoea, constipation, weight loss, polyuria, sweating, headache, thirst, vertigo, and raised concentrations of calcium and phosphate in plasma and urine

**Dose**

- See notes above

◁**Daily supplements**
**Note** There is no plain vitamin D tablet available for treating simple deficiency (see notes above). Alternatives include vitamins capsules (section 9.6.7), preparations of vitamins A and D (section 9.6.1), and calcium and ergocalciferol tablets (see below).

For cautions, contra-indications, and side-effects of calcium, see section 9.5.1.1

**Calcium and Ergocalciferol** (Non-proprietary)
**(Calcium and Vitamin D)**

Tablets, calcium lactate 300 mg, calcium phosphate 150 mg (calcium 97 mg or Ca²⁺ 2.4 mmol), ergocalci-

**9**

**Nutrition and blood**

ferol 10 micrograms (400 units). Net price 28-tab pack = £2.88. Counselling, crush before administration or may be chewed

◢Pharmacological strengths (see notes above)
Note The BP directs that when calciferol is prescribed or demanded, colecalciferol or ergocalciferol should be dispensed or supplied

**Ergocalciferol** (Non-proprietary)
Tablets, ergocalciferol 250 micrograms (10 000 units), net price 100 = £21.99; 1.25 mg (50 000 units), 100 = £30.34
Note May be difficult to obtain
Important When the strength of the tablets ordered or prescribed is not clear, the intention of the prescriber with respect to the strength (expressed in micrograms or milligrams per tablet) should be ascertained.

Injection, for intramuscular use only, ergocalciferol, 7.5 mg (300 000 units)/mL in oil, net price 1-mL amp = £7.45, 2-mL amp = £8.95

## ◼ ALFACALCIDOL
(1α-Hydroxycholecalciferol)

**Indications** see notes above
**Cautions** see notes above and under Ergocalciferol; also nephrolithiasis
**Contra-indications** see under Ergocalciferol
**Side-effects** see under Ergocalciferol; also *rarely* nephrocalcinosis, pruritus, rash, and urticaria
**Dose**
• By mouth *or* by intravenous injection over 30 seconds, ADULT and CHILD over 20 kg, initially 1 microgram daily (elderly 500 nanograms), adjusted to avoid hypercalcaemia; maintenance, usually 0.25–1 microgram daily; NEONATE and PRETERM NEONATE initially 50–100 nanograms/kg daily, CHILD under 20 kg initially 50 nanograms/kg daily

**Alfacalcidol** (Non-proprietary) [PoM]
Capsules, alfacalcidol 250 nanograms, net price 30-cap pack = £5.33; 500 nanograms 30-cap pack = £10.45; 1 microgram 30-cap pack = £14.26

**One-Alpha®** (LEO) [PoM]
Capsules, alfacalcidol 250 nanograms (white), net price 30-cap pack = £3.37; 500 nanograms (red), 30-cap pack = £6.27; 1 microgram (brown), 30-cap pack = £8.75
Excipients include sesame oil

Oral drops, sugar-free, alfacalcidol 2 micrograms/mL (1 drop contains approx. 100 nanograms), net price 10 mL = £22.49
Excipients include alcohol
Note The concentration of alfacalcidol in *One-Alpha®* drops is 10 times greater than that of the former presentation *One-Alpha®* solution.

Injection, alfacalcidol 2 micrograms/mL, net price 0.5-mL amp = £2.16, 1-mL amp = £4.11
Excipients include alcohol, propylene glycol (caution in small preterm neonates), see Excipients, p. 2
Note Shake ampoule for at least 5 seconds before use

## ◼ CALCITRIOL
(1,25-Dihydroxycholecalciferol)

**Indications** see notes above
**Cautions** see under Ergocalciferol; monitor plasma calcium, phosphate, and creatinine during dosage titration

**Contra-indications** see under Ergocalciferol
**Side-effects** see under Ergocalciferol
**Dose**
• By mouth, renal osteodystrophy, initially 250 nanograms daily, or on alternate days (in patients with normal or only slightly reduced plasma-calcium concentration), increased if necessary in steps of 250 nanograms at intervals of 2–4 weeks; usual dose 0.5–1 microgram daily; CHILD not established
Established postmenopausal osteoporosis, 250 nanograms twice daily (monitor plasma-calcium concentration and creatinine, consult product literature)
• By intravenous injection (or injection through catheter after haemodialysis), hypocalcaemia in dialysis patients with chronic renal failure, initially 500 nanograms (approx. 10 nanograms/kg) 3 times a week, increased if necessary in steps of 250–500 nanograms at intervals of 2–4 weeks; usual dose 0.5–3 micrograms 3 times a week; CHILD see *BNF for Children*
Moderate to severe secondary hyperparathyroidism in dialysis patients, initially 0.5–4 micrograms 3 times a week, increased if necessary in steps of 250–500 nanograms at intervals of 2–4 weeks; max. 8 micrograms 3 times a week

**Calcitriol** (Non-proprietary) [PoM]
Capsules, calcitriol 250 nanograms, net price 30-cap pack = £5.87, 100-cap pack = £19.15; 500 nanograms, 30-cap pack = £10.50, 100-cap pack = £32.90

**Rocaltrol®** (Roche) [PoM]
Capsules, calcitriol 250 nanograms (red/white), net price 20 = £3.68; 500 nanograms (red), 20 = £6.58

**Calcijex®** (Abbott) [PoM]
Injection, calcitriol 1 microgram/mL, net price 1-mL amp = £5.14; 2 micrograms/mL, 1-mL amp = £10.28

## ◼ COLECALCIFEROL
(Cholecalciferol, vitamin D₃)

**Indications** see notes above
**Cautions** see under Ergocalciferol
**Contra-indications** see under Ergocalciferol
**Side-effects** see under Ergocalciferol
**Dose**
• see notes above

◢With calcium
For cautions, contra-indications, and side-effects of calcium, see section 9.5.1.1

**Adcal-D₃®** (ProStrakan)
Tablets (chewable) (lemon or tutti-frutti flavour), calcium carbonate 1.5 g (calcium 600 mg or Ca²⁺ 15 mmol), colecalciferol 10 micrograms (400 units), net price 56-tab pack = £3.89, 112-tab pack = £7.78. Label: 24

Dissolve (effervescent tablets), lemon flavour, calcium carbonate 1.5 g (calcium 600 mg or Ca²⁺ 15 mmol), colecalciferol 10 micrograms (400 units), net price 56-tab pack = £4.99. Label: 13

**Cacit® D3** (Procter & Gamble Pharm.)
Granules, effervescent, lemon flavour, calcium carbonate 1.25 g (calcium 500 mg or Ca²⁺ 12.5 mmol), colecalciferol 11 micrograms (440 units)/sachet, net price 30-sachet pack = £4.14. Label: 13

◼ **9** Nutrition and blood

**Calceos®** (Galen)
Tablets (chewable), lemon flavour, calcium carbonate 1.25 g (calcium 500 mg or $Ca^{2+}$ 12.5 mmol), colecalciferol 10 micrograms (400 units), net price 60-tab pack = £3.69. Label: 24

**Calcichew-D₃®** (Shire)
Tablets (chewable), orange flavour, calcium carbonate 1.25 g (calcium 500 mg or $Ca^{2+}$ 12.5 mmol), colecalciferol 5 micrograms (200 units), net price 100-tab pack = £14.43. Label: 24
Excipients include aspartame (section 9.4.1)

**Calcichew-D₃® Forte** (Shire)
Tablets (chewable), lemon flavour, calcium carbonate 1.25 g (calcium 500 mg or $Ca^{2+}$ 12.5 mmol), colecalciferol 10 micrograms (400 units), net price 60-tab pack = £4.32, 100-tab pack = £7.21. Label: 24
Excipients include aspartame (section 9.4.1)

**Calfovit D3®** (Menarini)
Powder, lemon flavour, calcium phosphate 3.1 g (calcium 1.2 g or $Ca^{2+}$ 30 mmol), colecalciferol 20 micrograms (800 units), net price 30-sachet pack = £4.32. Label: 13, 21

**Natecal D3®** (Chiesi)
Tablets, (aniseed, peppermint, and molasses flavour), calcium carbonate 1.5 g (calcium 600 mg or $Ca^{2+}$ 15 mmol), colecalciferol 10 micrograms (400 units), net price 60-tab pack = £3.70. Label: 24
Excipients include aspartame (section 9.4.1)

**Sandocal®+D 600** (Novartis Consumer Health)
Tablets, effervescent, orange flavour, calcium lactate gluconate 1.36 g, calcium carbonate 1.05 g, providing calcium 600 mg ($Ca^{2+}$ 15 mmol), colecalciferol concentrate 4 mg, providing colecalciferol 10 micrograms (400 units), net price 60-tab pack = £5.35, 100-tab pack = £8.75. Label: 13
Excipients include aspartame (section 9.4.1)

◢With alendronic acid
Section 6.6.2

◢With risedronate sodium and calcium
Section 6.6.2

## ▮ DIHYDROTACHYSTEROL

**Indications** see notes above
**Cautions** see under Ergocalciferol
**Contra-indications** see under Ergocalciferol
**Side-effects** see under Ergocalciferol

**AT 10®** (Intrapharm)
Oral solution, dihydrotachysterol 250 micrograms/mL. Net price 15-mL dropper bottle = £22.87
Excipients include arachis (peanut) oil
Dose acute, chronic, and latent forms of hypocalcaemic tetany due to hypoparathyroidism, consult product literature

## ▮ PARICALCITOL

**Indications** see under preparations below
**Cautions** monitor plasma calcium and phosphate during dose titration and at least monthly when stabilised; monitor parathyroid hormone concentration; pregnancy (Appendix 4); breast-feeding (Appendix 5); **interactions**: Appendix 1 (vitamins)
**Contra-indications** see under Ergocalciferol

**Side-effects** see under Ergocalciferol; also dyspepsia, taste disturbance, breast tenderness, acne, pruritus, and rash
**Dose**
● Consult product literature

**Zemplar®** (Abbott) ▼ PoM
Capsules, paricalcitol 1 microgram (grey), net price 28-cap pack = £69.44; 2 micrograms (orange-brown), 28-cap pack = £138.88; 4 micrograms (gold), 28-cap pack = £277.76
For prevention and treatment of secondary hyperparathyroidism associated with chronic renal failure

Injection, paricalcitol 5 micrograms/mL, net price 5 × 1-mL amp = £62.00, 5 × 2-mL amp = £124.00. For injection via haemodialysis access
Excipients include propylene glycol, see Excipients, p. 2
For prevention and treatment of secondary hyperparathyroidism associated with chronic renal failure in patients on haemodialysis

## ▮ 9.6.5 Vitamin E
(Tocopherols)

The daily requirement of vitamin E has not been well defined but is probably about 3 to 15 mg daily. There is little evidence that oral supplements of vitamin E are essential in adults, even where there is fat malabsorption secondary to cholestasis. In young children with congenital cholestasis, abnormally low vitamin E concentrations may be found in association with neuromuscular abnormalities, which usually respond only to the parenteral administration of vitamin E.

Vitamin E has been tried for various other conditions but there is little scientific evidence of its value.

## ▮ ALPHA TOCOPHERYL ACETATE
(Vitamin E)

**Indications** see notes above
**Cautions** predisposition to thrombosis; increased risk of necrotising enterocolitis in neonate weighing less than 1.5 kg; **interactions**: Appendix 1 (vitamins)
**Side-effects** diarrhoea and abdominal pain with doses more than 1 g daily

**Vitamin E Suspension** (Cambridge)
Suspension, alpha tocopheryl acetate 500 mg/5 mL. Net price 100 mL = £27.59
Dose malabsorption in cystic fibrosis, 100–200 mg daily; CHILD 1 month–1 year 50 mg daily; 1–12 years, 100 mg daily
Malabsorption in abetalipoproteinaemia, ADULT and CHILD 50–100 mg/kg daily
Malabsorption in chronic cholestasis and severe liver disease, CHILD see BNF for Children
Note Tablets containing tocopheryl acetate are available from 'special-order' manufacturers or specialist importing companies, see p. 969

## ▮ 9.6.6 Vitamin K

Vitamin K is necessary for the production of blood clotting factors and proteins necessary for the normal calcification of bone.

Because vitamin K is fat soluble, patients with fat malabsorption, especially in biliary obstruction or hepatic disease, may become deficient. **Menadiol sodium** phosphate is a water-soluble synthetic vitamin K derivative that can be given orally to prevent vitamin K deficiency in malabsorption syndromes.

Oral coumarin anticoagulants act by interfering with vitamin K metabolism in the hepatic cells and their effects can be antagonised by giving vitamin K; for British Society for Haematology Guidelines, see section 2.8.2.

**Vitamin K deficiency bleeding** Neonates are relatively deficient in vitamin K and those who do not receive supplements of vitamin K are at risk of serious bleeding including intracranial bleeding. The Chief Medical Officer and the Chief Nursing Officer have recommended that all newborn babies should receive vitamin K to prevent vitamin K deficiency bleeding (haemorrhagic disease of the newborn). An appropriate regimen should be selected after discussion with parents in the antenatal period.

Vitamin K (as **phytomenadione**) 1 mg may be given by a single intramuscular injection at birth; this prevents vitamin K deficiency bleeding in virtually all babies. For preterm neonates, see *BNF for Children*

Alternatively, vitamin K may be given by mouth, and arrangements must be in place to ensure the appropriate regimen is followed. Two doses of a colloidal (mixed micelle) preparation of phytomenadione 2 mg should be given in the first week. For exclusively breast-fed babies, a third dose of phytomenadione 2 mg is given at 1 month of age; the third dose is omitted in formula-fed babies because formula feeds contain vitamin K.

◀ **MENADIOL SODIUM PHOSPHATE**

**Indications** see notes above

**Cautions** G6PD deficiency (section 9.1.5) and vitamin E deficiency (risk of haemolysis); **interactions:** Appendix 1 (vitamins)

**Contra-indications** neonates and infants, late pregnancy

**Dose**

- 10–40 mg daily, adjusted as necessary; CHILD 1–12 years, 5–10 mg daily, adjusted as necessary, 12–18 years, 10–20 mg daily, adjusted as necessary

**Menadiol Phosphate** (Cambridge)
Tablets, menadiol sodium phosphate equivalent to 10 mg of menadiol phosphate. Net price 100-tab pack = £53.08

◀ **PHYTOMENADIONE**
(Vitamin K₁)

**Indications** see notes above

**Cautions** intravenous injections should be given very slowly (see also below); pregnancy (Appendix 4); **interactions:** Appendix 1 (vitamins)

**Dose**

- See notes above and section 2.8.2

**Konakion®** (Roche) [PoM]
Tablets, s/c, phytomenadione 10 mg, net price 10-tab pack = £1.59. To be chewed or allowed to dissolve slowly in the mouth (Label: 24)

◀ **Colloidal formulation**

**Konakion® MM** (Roche) [PoM]
Injection, phytomenadione 10 mg/mL in a mixed micelles vehicle, net price 1-mL amp = 39p
Excipients include glycocholic acid 54.6 mg/amp, lecithin
Cautions reduce dose in elderly; liver impairment (glycocholic acid may displace bilirubin); reports of anaphylactoid reactions
Note *Konakion® MM* may be administered by slow intravenous injection or by intravenous infusion in glucose 5% (see Appendix 6); **not** for intramuscular injection

**Konakion® MM Paediatric** (Roche) ▼ [PoM]
Injection, phytomenadione 10 mg/mL in a mixed micelles vehicle, net price 0.2-mL amp = 96p
Excipients include glycocholic acid 10.9 mg/amp, lecithin
Cautions parenteral administration in neonate of less than 2.5 kg (increased risk of kernicterus)
Note *Konakion® MM Paediatric* may be administered by mouth or by intramuscular injection or by intravenous injection

## 9.6.7 Multivitamin preparations

**Vitamins**
Capsules, ascorbic acid 15 mg, nicotinamide 7.5 mg, riboflavin 500 micrograms, thiamine hydrochloride 1 mg, vitamin A 2500 units, vitamin D 300 units, net price 20 = 22p

**Abidec®** (Chefaro UK)
Drops, vitamins A, B group, C, and D, net price 25 mL (with dropper) = £2.20
Excipients include arachis (peanut) oil
Note Contains 1333 units of vitamin A (as palmitate) per 0.6-mL dose

**Dalivit®** (LPC)
Oral drops, vitamins A, B group, C, and D, net price 25 mL = £2.98, 50 mL = £4.85
Note Contains 5000 units of vitamin A (as palmitate) per 0.6-mL dose

## Vitamin and mineral supplements and adjuncts to synthetic diets

**Forceval®** (Alliance)
Capsules, brown/red, vitamins (ascorbic acid 60 mg, biotin 100 micrograms, cyanocobalamin 3 micrograms, folic acid 400 micrograms, nicotinamide 18 mg, pantothenic acid 4 mg, pyridoxine 2 mg, riboflavin 1.6 mg, thiamine 1.2 mg, vitamin A 2500 units, vitamin D₂ 400 units, vitamin E 10 mg, minerals and trace elements (calcium 100 mg, chromium 200 micrograms, copper 2 mg, iodine 140 micrograms, iron 12 mg, magnesium 30 mg, manganese 3 mg, molybdenum 250 micrograms, phosphorus 77 mg, potassium 4 mg, selenium 50 micrograms, zinc 15 mg), net price 15-cap pack = £2.83, 30-cap pack = £5.19, 90-cap pack = £12.53. Label: 25
Dose vitamin and mineral deficiency and as adjunct in synthetic diets, ADULT 1 capsule daily one hour after a meal

Junior capsules, brown, vitamins (ascorbic acid 25 mg, biotin 50 micrograms, cyanocobalamin 2 micrograms, folic acid 100 micrograms, nicotinamide 7.5 mg, pantothenic acid 2 mg, pyridoxine 1 mg, riboflavin 1 mg, thiamine 1.5 mg, vitamin A 1250 units, vitamin D₂ 200 units, vitamin E 5 mg, vitamin K₁ 25 micrograms), minerals and trace elements (chromium 50 micrograms, copper 1 mg, iodine 75 micrograms, iron 5 mg, magnesium 1 mg, manganese 1.25 mg, molybdenum 50 micrograms, selenium 25 micrograms, zinc 5 mg), net price 30-cap pack = £3.52, 60-cap pack = £6.69

**Dose** vitamin and mineral deficiency and as adjunct in synthetic diets, CHILD over 5 years, 2 junior capsules daily

**Ketovite®** (Paines & Byrne)

Tablets PoM, yellow, ascorbic acid 16.6 mg, riboflavin 1 mg, thiamine hydrochloride 1 mg, pyridoxine hydrochloride 330 micrograms, nicotinamide 3.3 mg, calcium pantothenate 1.16 mg, alpha tocopheryl acetate 5 mg, inositol 50 mg, biotin 170 micrograms, folic acid 250 micrograms, acetomenaphthone 500 micrograms, net price 100-tab pack = £4.17

**Dose** prevention of vitamin deficiency in disorders of carbohydrate or amino-acid metabolism and adjunct in restricted, specialised, or synthetic diets, 1 tablet 3 times daily; use with *Ketovite® Liquid* for complete vitamin supplementation

Liquid, pink, sugar-free, vitamin A 2500 units, ergocalciferol 400 units, choline chloride 150 mg, cyanocobalamin 12.5 micrograms/5 mL, net price 150-mL pack = £2.70

**Dose** prevention of vitamin deficiency in disorders of carbohydrate or amino-acid metabolism and adjunct in restricted, specialised, or synthetic diets, 5 mL daily; use with *Ketovite® Tablets* for complete vitamin supplementation

## 9.7 Bitters and tonics

Mixtures containing simple and aromatic bitters are traditional remedies for loss of appetite; there is no evidence to support their use.

## 9.8 Metabolic disorders

**9.8.1 Drugs used in metabolic disorders**
**9.8.2 Acute porphyrias**

This section covers drugs used in metabolic disorders and not readily classified elsewhere.

## 9.8.1 Drugs used in metabolic disorders

### Wilson's disease

**Penicillamine** (see also section 10.1.3) is used in Wilson's disease (hepatolenticular degeneration) to aid the elimination of copper ions. See below for other indications.

**Trientine** is used for the treatment of Wilson's disease only in patients intolerant of penicillamine; it is **not** an alternative to penicillamine for rheumatoid arthritis or cystinuria. Penicillamine-induced systemic lupus erythematosus may not resolve on transfer to trientine.

**Zinc** prevents the absorption of copper in Wilson's disease. Symptomatic patients should be treated initially with a chelating agent because zinc has a slow onset of action. When transferring from chelating treatment to zinc maintenance therapy, chelating treatment should be co-administered for 2–3 weeks until zinc produces its maximal effect.

## PENICILLAMINE

**Indications** see under Dose below

**Cautions** see section 10.1.3; also neurological involvement in Wilson's disease

**Contra-indications** see section 10.1.3

**Side-effects** see section 10.1.3; also neuropathy (especially if previous neurological involvement in Wilson's disease—prophylactic pyridoxine recommended, see section 9.6.2)

**Dose**

- Wilson's disease, 1.5–2 g daily in divided doses before food; max. 2 g daily for 1 year; maintenance 0.75–1 g daily; ELDERLY 20 mg/kg daily in divided doses, adjusted according to response; CHILD under 12 years see *BNF for Children*
- Autoimmune hepatitis (used rarely; after disease controlled with corticosteroids), initially 500 mg daily in divided doses increased slowly over 3 months; usual maintenance dose 1.25 g daily; ELDERLY not recommended
- Cystinuria, therapeutic, 1–3 g daily in divided doses before food, adjusted to maintain urinary cystine below 200 mg/litre; prophylactic (maintain urinary cystine below 300 mg/litre) 0.5–1 g at bedtime; maintain adequate fluid intake (at least 3 litres daily); CHILD and ELDERLY minimum dose to maintain urinary cystine below 200 mg/litre
- Severe active rheumatoid arthritis, section 10.1.3

◢ **Preparations**
Section 10.1.3

## TRIENTINE DIHYDROCHLORIDE

**Indications** Wilson's disease in patients intolerant of penicillamine

**Cautions** see notes above; pregnancy (Appendix 4); **interactions:** Appendix 1 (trientine)

**Side-effects** nausea, rash; *very rarely* anaemia; duodenitis and colitis also reported

**Dose**

- ADULT and CHILD over 12 years, 1.2–2.4 g daily in 2–4 divided doses before food; CHILD 2–12 years, initially 0.6–1.5 g daily in 2–4 divided doses before food, adjusted according to response

**Trientine Dihydrochloride** (Univar) PoM
Capsules, trientine dihydrochloride 300 mg. Label: 6, 22

## ZINC ACETATE

**Indications** Wilson's disease (initiated under specialist supervision)

**Cautions** portal hypertension (risk of hepatic decompensation when switching from chelating agent); monitor full blood count and serum cholesterol; pregnancy (Appendix 4); **interactions:** Appendix 1 (zinc)

**Contra-indications** breast-feeding

**Side-effects** gastric irritation (usually transient; may be reduced if first dose taken mid-morning or with a little protein); *less commonly* sideroblastic anaemia and leucopenia

**9**

**Nutrition and blood**

**Dose**

Note Dose expressed as elemental zinc

- Wilson's disease, 50 mg 3 times daily (max. 50 mg 5 times daily), adjusted according to response; CHILD 1–6 years, 25 mg twice daily; 6–16 years, body-weight under 57 kg, 25 mg 3 times daily, body-weight over 57 kg, 50 mg 3 times daily; ADOLESCENT 16–18 years, 50 mg 3 times daily

**Wilzin®** (Orphan Europe) ▼ PoM

Capsules, zinc (as acetate) 25 mg (blue), net price 250-cap pack = £132.00; 50 mg (orange), 250-cap pack = £242.00. Label: 23

## Carnitine deficiency

**Carnitine** is available for the management of primary carnitine deficiency due to inborn errors of metabolism or of secondary deficiency in haemodialysis patients.

### ▮ CARNITINE

**Indications** primary and secondary carnitine deficiency

**Cautions** diabetes mellitus; monitoring of free and acyl carnitine in blood and urine recommended; renal impairment (Appendix 3); pregnancy (Appendix 4)

**Side-effects** nausea, vomiting, abdominal pain, diarrhoea, body odour; side-effects may be dose-related—monitor tolerance during first week and after any dose increase

**Dose**

- Primary deficiency, by mouth, up to 200 mg/kg daily in 2–4 divided doses; higher doses of up to 400 mg/kg daily occasionally required; by intravenous injection over 2–3 minutes, up to 100 mg/kg daily in 3–4 divided doses
- Secondary deficiency, by intravenous injection over 2–3 minutes, 20 mg/kg after each dialysis session (dosage adjusted according to plasma-carnitine concentration); maintenance (if benefit gained from first intravenous course), by mouth, 1 g daily

**Carnitor®** (Sigma-Tau) PoM

Oral liquid, L-carnitine 100 mg/mL (10%), net price 10 × 10-mL (1-g) single-dose bottle = £35.00

Paediatric solution, L-carnitine 300 mg/mL (30%), net price 20 mL = £21.00

Injection, L-carnitine 200 mg/mL. Net price 5-mL amp = £11.90

## Fabry's disease

**Agalsidase alfa** and **agalsidase beta**, enzymes produced by recombinant DNA technology, are licensed for long-term enzyme replacement therapy in Fabry's disease (a lysosomal storage disorder caused by deficiency of alpha-galactosidase A).

### ▮ AGALSIDASE ALFA and BETA

**Indications** Fabry's disease (specialist use only)

**Cautions** pregnancy (Appendix 4); breast-feeding (Appendix 5); **interactions:** Appendix 1 (agalsidase alfa and beta)

Infusion-related reactions Infusion-related reactions very common; manage by slowing the infusion rate or interrupt-ing the infusion, or minimise by pre-treatment with an anti-histamine, antipyretic, or corticosteroid—consult product literature

**Side-effects** gastro-intestinal disturbances, taste disturbances; tachycardia, bradycardia, palpitation, hypertension, hypotension, chest pain, oedema, flushing; dyspnoea, cough, wheezing, hoarseness, rhinorrhoea; headache, fatigue, dizziness, asthenia, paraesthesia, syncope, neuropathic pain, tremor, sleep disturbances; influenza-like symptoms, naso-pharyngitis; pain in extremities; eye irritation; tinnitus, vertigo; hypersensitivity reactions, pruritus, urticaria, rash, acne; *less commonly* bronchospasm, angioedema, cold extremities, parosmia, ear pain and swelling, skin discoloration, and injection-site reactions

**Fabrazyme®** (Genzyme) PoM

Intravenous infusion, powder for reconstitution, agalsidase beta, net price 5-mg vial = £325.50; 35-mg vial = £2269.20

**Dose** By intravenous infusion, ADULT and CHILD over 8 years 1 mg/kg every 2 weeks

**Replagal®** (Shire) PoM

Concentrate for intravenous infusion, agalsidase alfa 1 mg/mL, net price 1-mL vial = £356.85; 3.5-mL vial = £1068.64

**Dose** By intravenous infusion, ADULT and CHILD over 7 years 200 micrograms/kg every 2 weeks

## Gaucher's disease

**Imiglucerase**, an enzyme produced by recombinant DNA technology, is administered as enzyme replacement therapy for non-neurological manifestations of type I or type III Gaucher's disease, a familial disorder affecting principally the liver, spleen, bone marrow, and lymph nodes.

**Miglustat**, an inhibitor of glucosylceramide synthase, is licensed for the treatment of mild to moderate type I Gaucher's disease in patients for whom imiglucerase is unsuitable; it is given by mouth; see p. 557.

### ▮ IMIGLUCERASE

**Indications** (specialist use only) non-neurological manifestations of type I or type III Gaucher's disease

**Cautions** pregnancy (Appendix 4); breast-feeding (Appendix 5); monitor for imiglucerase antibodies; when stabilised, monitor all parameters and response to treatment at intervals of 6–12 months

**Side-effects** hypersensitivity reactions (including urticaria, angioedema, hypotension, flushing, tachycardia); less commonly nausea, vomiting, diarrhoea, abdominal cramps, headache, dizziness, paraesthesia, fatigue, fever, arthralgia, injection-site reactions

**Dose**

- By intravenous infusion, initially 60 units/kg once every 2 weeks (2.5 units/kg 3 times a week or 15 units/kg once every 2 weeks may improve haematological parameters and organomegaly, but not bone parameters); maintenance, adjust dose according to response

**Cerezyme®** (Genzyme) PoM

Intravenous infusion, powder for reconstitution, imiglucerase, net price 200-unit vial = £553.35; 400-unit vial = £1106.70

Electrolytes Na$^+$ 0.62 mmol/200-unit vial, 1.24 mmol/400-unit vial

*9 Nutrition and blood*

## Mucopolysaccharidosis

**Laronidase**, an enzyme produced by recombinant DNA technology, is licensed for long-term replacement therapy in the treatment of non-neurological manifestations of mucopolysaccharidosis I, a lysosomal storage disorder caused by deficiency of alpha-L-iduronidase.

**Idursulfase**, an enzyme produced by recombinant DNA technology, is licensed for long-term replacement therapy in mucopolysaccharidosis II (Hunter syndrome), a lysosomal storage disorder caused by deficiency of iduronate-2-sulfatase.

**Galsulfase**, a recombinant form of human N-acetylgalactosamine-4-sulfatase, is licensed for long-term replacement therapy in mucopolysaccharidosis VI (Maroteaux-Lamy syndrome).

Infusion-related reactions often occur with administration of laronidase, idursulfase, and galsulfase; they can be managed by slowing the infusion rate or interrupting the infusion, and can be minimised by pre-treatment with an antihistamine and an antipyretic. Recurrent infusion-related reactions may require pre-treatment with a corticosteroid—consult product literature for details.

### ▍ GALSULFASE

**Indications** (specialist use only) mucopolysaccharidosis VI

**Cautions** respiratory disease; acute febrile or respiratory illness (consider delaying treatment); pregnancy (Appendix 4)

Infusion-related reactions See notes above

**Contra-indications** breast-feeding (Appendix 5)

**Side-effects** abdominal pain, umbilical hernia, gastroenteritis; chest pain, hypertension; dyspnoea, apnoea, nasal congestion; rigors, malaise, areflexia; pharyngitis; conjunctivitis, corneal opacity; ear pain; facial oedema

**Dose**
● By intravenous infusion, ADULT and CHILD over 5 years, 1 mg/kg once weekly

**Naglazyme®** (BioMarin) ▼ PoM
Concentrate for intravenous infusion, galsulfase 1 mg/mL, net price 5-mL vial = £982.00

### ▍ IDURSULFASE

**Indications** (specialist use only) mucopolysaccharidosis II

**Cautions** severe respiratory disease; acute febrile respiratory illness (consider delaying treatment); breast-feeding (Appendix 5)

Infusion-related reactions See notes above

**Contra-indications** women of child-bearing potential (see Pregnancy—Appendix 4)

**Side-effects** gastro-intestinal disturbances, swollen tongue; arrhythmia, chest pain, cyanosis, peripheral oedema, hypertension, hypotension, flushing, pulmonary embolism; bronchospasm, cough, wheezing, tachypnoea, dyspnoea; headache, dizziness, tremor; pyrexia; arthralgia; increased lacrimation; facial oedema, urticaria, pruritus, rash, infusion-site swelling, erythema, and eczema; anaphylaxis also reported

**Dose**
● By intravenous infusion, ADULT and CHILD over 5 years, 500 micrograms/kg once weekly

**Elaprase®** (Shire) ▼ PoM
Concentrate for intravenous infusion, idursulfase 2 mg/mL, net price 3-mL vial = £1985.00

### ▍ LARONIDASE

**Indications** (specialist use only) non-neurological manifestations of mucopolysaccharidosis I

**Cautions** monitor immunoglobulin G (IgG) antibody concentration; pregnancy (Appendix 4); breast-feeding (Appendix 5); **interactions:** Appendix 1 (laronidase)

Infusion-related reactions See notes above

**Side-effects** nausea, vomiting, diarrhoea, abdominal pain; cold extremities, pallor, flushing, tachycardia, blood pressure changes; dyspnoea, cough, angioedema, anaphylaxis; headache, paraesthesia, dizziness, fatigue, restlessness; influenza-like symptoms; musculoskeletal pain, pain in extremities; rash, pruritus, urticaria, alopecia, infusion-site reactions; bronchospasm and respiratory arrest also reported

**Dose**
● By intravenous infusion, 100 units/kg once weekly; CHILD see *BNF for Children*

**Aldurazyme®** (Genzyme) ▼ PoM
Concentrate for intravenous infusion, laronidase 100 units/mL, net price 5-mL vial = £460.35
Electrolytes Na+ 1.29 mmol/5-mL vial

## Nephropathic cystinosis

**Mercaptamine** (cysteamine) is available for the treatment of nephropathic cystinosis.

### ▍ MERCAPTAMINE
(Cysteamine)

**Indications** (specialist use only) nephropathic cystinosis

**Cautions** leucocyte-cystine concentration and haematological monitoring required—consult product literature; dose of phosphate supplement may need to be adjusted

**Contra-indications** pregnancy and breast-feeding; hypersensitivity to mercaptamine or penicillamine

**Side-effects** breath and body odour, nausea, vomiting, diarrhoea, anorexia, lethargy, fever, rash; also reported dehydration, hypertension, abdominal discomfort, gastroenteritis, drowsiness, encephalopathy, headache, nervousness, depression; anaemia, leucopenia; *rarely* gastro-intestinal ulceration and bleeding, seizures, hallucinations, urticaria, interstitial nephritis

**Dose**
● Initial doses should be one-sixth to one-quarter of the expected maintenance dose, increased gradually over 4–6 weeks
● Maintenance, ADULT and CHILD over 50 kg bodyweight, 2 g daily in 4 divided doses
CHILD up to 12 years, 1.3 g/m² (approx. 50 mg/kg) daily in 4 divided doses

**9**

**Nutrition and blood**

**Cystagon®** (Orphan Europe) [PoM]
　Capsules, mercaptamine (as bitartrate) 50 mg, net price 100-cap pack = £59.00; 150 mg, 100-cap pack = £162.00
　Note CHILD under 6 years at risk of aspiration, capsules can be opened and contents sprinkled on food (at a temperature suitable for eating); avoid adding to acidic drinks (e.g. orange juice)

## Pompe disease

**Alglucosidase alfa**, an enzyme produced by recombinant DNA technology, is licensed for long-term replacement therapy in Pompe disease, a lysosomal storage disorder caused by deficiency of acid alpha-glucosidase.

### ■ ALGLUCOSIDASE ALFA

**Indications** (specialist use only) Pompe disease

**Cautions** cardiac and respiratory dysfunction—monitor closely; monitor immunoglobulin G (IgG) antibody concentration; pregnancy (Appendix 4)
　Infusion-related reactions Infusion-related reactions very common, calling for use of antihistamine, antipyretic or corticosteroid; consult product literature for details

**Contra-indications** breast-feeding (Appendix 5)

**Side-effects** nausea, vomiting; flushing, tachycardia, blood pressure changes, cold extremities, cyanosis, facial oedema; cough, tachypnoea, bronchospasm; headache, agitation, tremor, irritability, restlessness, paraesthesia, dizziness; pyrexia; antibody formation; sweating, rash, pruritus, and urticaria; anaphylaxis

**Dose**
● By intravenous infusion, ADULT and CHILD 20 mg/kg every 2 weeks

**Myozyme®** (Genzyme) ▼ [PoM]
　Intravenous infusion, powder for reconstitution, alglucosidase alfa, net price 50-mg vial = £368.59

## Tyrosinaemia type I

Nitisinone is licensed for the treatment of hereditary tyrosinaemia type I in combination with dietary restriction of tyrosine and phenylalanine.

### ■ NITISINONE
(NTBC)

**Indications** hereditary tyrosinaemia type I (specialist use only)

**Cautions** slit-lamp examination of eyes recommended before treatment; monitor liver function regularly; monitor platelet and white blood cell count every 6 months; pregnancy (Appendix 4)

**Contra-indications** breast-feeding (Appendix 5)

**Side-effects** thrombocytopenia, leucopenia, granulocytopenia; conjunctivitis, photophobia, corneal opacity, keratitis, eye pain; less commonly leucocytosis, blepharitis, pruritus, exfoliative dermatitis, and erythematous rash

**Dose**
● ADULT and CHILD initially 500 micrograms/kg twice daily, adjusted according to response; max. 2 mg/kg daily
　Note Capsules can be opened and the contents suspended in a small amount of water or formula diet and taken immediately

**Orfadin®** (Swedish Orphan) [PoM]
　Capsules, nitisinone 2 mg, net price 60-cap pack = £564.00; 5 mg, 60-cap pack = £1127.00; 10 mg, 60-cap pack = £2062.00

## Urea cycle disorders

**Sodium phenylbutyrate** is used in the management of urea cycle disorders. It is indicated as adjunctive therapy in all patients with neonatal-onset disease and in those with late-onset disease who have a history of hyperammonaemic encephalopathy.

**Carglumic acid** is licensed for the treatment of hyperammonaemia due to N-acetylglutamate synthase deficiency.

### ■ CARGLUMIC ACID

**Indications** hyperammonaemia due to N-acetylglutamate synthase deficiency (initiated under specialist supervision)

**Cautions** pregnancy (Appendix 4)

**Contra-indications** breast-feeding (Appendix 5)

**Side-effects** sweating

**Dose**
● ADULT and CHILD initially 100–250 mg/kg daily in 2–4 divided doses immediately before food, adjusted according to plasma–ammonia concentration; maintenance 10–100 mg/kg daily in 2–4 divided doses

**Carbaglu®** (Orphan Europe) [PoM]
　Dispersible tablets, carglumic acid 200 mg, net price 5-tab pack = £243.00, 60-tab pack = £2914.00. Label: 13

### ■ SODIUM PHENYLBUTYRATE

**Indications** adjunct in long-term treatment of urea cycle disorders (under specialist supervision)

**Cautions** congestive heart failure; hepatic and renal impairment; **interactions:** Appendix 1 (sodium phenylbutyrate)

**Contra-indications** pregnancy (Appendix 4); breast-feeding (Appendix 5)

**Side-effects** gastro-intestinal disturbances, weight gain, taste disturbance, decreased appetite; syncope, oedema; headache, depression, irritability; renal tubular acidosis, menstrual disorders; blood disorders, metabolic acidosis, alkalosis; rash, body odour; less commonly rectal bleeding, peptic ulcer, pancreatitis, and arrhythmias

**Dose**
● ADULT and CHILD body-weight over 20 kg, 9.9–13 g/m² daily in divided doses with meals (max. 20 g daily); CHILD body-weight less than 20 kg, 450–600 mg/kg daily in divided doses with meals

**Ammonaps®** (Swedish Orphan) [PoM]
　Tablets, sodium phenylbutyrate 500 mg. Contains Na⁺ 2.7 mmol/tablet. Net price 250-tab pack = £493.00

　Granules, sodium phenylbutyrate 940 mg/g. Contains Na⁺ 5.4 mmol/g. Net price 266-g pack = £860.00
　Note Granules should be mixed with food before taking

**9** Nutrition and blood

## Homocystinuria

**Betaine** is licensed for the adjunctive treatment of homocystinuria involving deficiencies or defects in cystathionine beta-synthase, 5,10-methylene-tetrahydrofolate reductase, or cobalamin cofactor metabolism. Betaine should be used in conjunction with dietary restrictions and may be given with supplements of Vitamin $B_{12}$, pyridoxine, and folate under specialist advice.

The *Scottish Medicines Consortium* (p. 3) has advised (February 2009) that betaine anhydrous oral powder (*Cystadane®*) is **not** recommended for use within NHS Scotland as adjunctive treatment of homocystinuria.

### ▊ BETAINE

**Indications**  (specialist use only) adjunctive treatment of homocystinuria

**Cautions**  monitor plasma-methionine concentration before and during treatment—interrupt treatment if symptoms of cerebral oedema occur; pregnancy (Appendix 4); breast-feeding (Appendix 5)

**Side-effects**  *less commonly* gastro-intestinal disorders, anorexia, reversible cerebral oedema (see Cautions), agitation, depression, personality disorder, sleep disturbances, urinary incontinence, alopecia, and urticaria

**Dose**

* ADULT and CHILD over 10 years, 3 g twice daily, adjusted according to response; max. 20 g/day; CHILD under 10 years 50 mg/kg twice daily, dose and frequency adjusted according to response; max. 75 mg/kg twice daily

**Cystadane®** (Orphan Europe) ℞

Powder, betaine (anhydrous), net price 180 g = £314.00

Note Powder should be mixed with water, juice, milk, formula, or food until completely dissolved and taken immediately; measuring spoons are provided to measure 1 g, 150 mg, and 100 mg of powder

## Other metabolic disorders

**Miglustat** is available for the treatment of progressive neurological manifestations of Niemann-Pick type C disease, a neurodegenerative disorder characterised by impaired intracellular lipid trafficking; it is also licensed for the treatment of mild to moderate type 1 Gaucher's disease for whom imiglucerase is unsuitable, see also p. 554.

### ▊ MIGLUSTAT

**Indications**  mild to moderate type I Gaucher's disease (specialist supervision only); Niemann-Pick type C disease (specialist supervision only)

**Cautions**  hepatic impairment; renal impairment (avoid if eGFR less than 30 mL/minute/1.73 m²; Appendix 3); monitor cognitive and neurological function; monitor growth and platelet count in Niemann-Pick type C disease

**Contra-indications**  pregnancy (Appendix 4); men should not father a child during or within 3 months of treatment; breast-feeding (Appendix 5)

**Side-effects**  diarrhoea, flatulence, abdominal pain, dyspepsia, constipation, nausea, vomiting, anorexia, weight changes; tremor, dizziness, headache, peripheral neuropathy, ataxia, hypoaesthesia, paraesthesia,

insomnia, fatigue, asthenia; decreased libido; thrombocytopenia; muscle spasm

**Dose**

* Gaucher's disease, ADULT over 18 years, 100 mg 3 times daily; reduced if not tolerated to 100 mg 1–2 times daily
* Niemann-Pick type C disease, ADULT and CHILD over 12 years, 200 mg 3 times daily; CHILD 4–12 years, body surface area less than 0.47 m², 100 mg once daily; body surface area 0.47–0.73 m², 100 mg twice daily; body surface area 0.73–0.88 m², 100 mg three times daily; body surface area 0.88–1.25 m², 200 mg twice daily; body surface area greater than 1.25 m², adult dose

**Zavesca®** (Actelion) ℞

Capsules, miglustat 100 mg, net price 84-cap pack = £3890.13 (hospital only)

## 9.8.2 Acute porphyrias

The acute porphyrias (acute intermittent porphyria, variegate porphyria, hereditary coproporphyria, and 5-aminolaevulinic acid dehydratase deficiency porphyria) are hereditary disorders of haem biosynthesis; they have a prevalence of about 1 in 10 000 of the population.

Great care must be taken when prescribing for patients with acute porphyria, since certain drugs can induce acute porphyric crises. Since acute porphyrias are hereditary, relatives of affected individuals should be screened and advised about the potential danger of certain drugs.

Treatment of serious or life-threatening conditions should not be withheld from patients with acute porphyria. When there is no safe alternative, urinary porphobilinogen excretion should be measured regularly; if it increases or symptoms occur, the drug can be withdrawn and the acute attack treated. If an acute attack of porphyria occurs during pregnancy, contact an expert porphyria service for further advice.

**Haem arginate** is administered by short intravenous infusion as haem replacement in moderate, severe, or unremitting acute porphyria crises.

Supplies of haem arginate may be obtained outside office hours from the on-call pharmacist at:

St Thomas' Hospital, London              (020) 7188 7188

### ▊ HAEM ARGINATE
(Human hemin)

**Indications**  acute porphyrias (acute intermittent porphyria, porphyria variegata, hereditary coproporphyria)

**Cautions**  pregnancy (Appendix 4); breast feeding (Appendix 5)

**Side-effects**  rarely hypersensitivity reactions and fever; pain and thrombophlebitis at injection site

**Dose**

* By intravenous infusion, ADULT and CHILD 3 mg/kg once daily (max. 250 mg daily) for 4 days; if response inadequate, repeat 4-day course with close biochemical monitoring

**Normosang®** (Orphan Europe) ▼ ℞

Concentrate for intravenous infusion, haem arginate 25 mg/mL, net price 10-mL amp = £338.50

**9**

**Nutrition and blood**

## Drugs unsafe for use in acute porphyrias

The following list contains drugs on the UK market that have been classified as 'unsafe' in porphyria because they have been shown to be porphyrinogenic in animals or *in vitro*, or have been associated with acute attacks in patients. Absence of a drug from the following lists does not necessarily imply that the drug is safe. For many drugs no information about porphyria is available.

An up-to-date list of drugs considered **safe** in acute porphyrias is available at www.wmic.wales.nhs.uk/porphyria_info.php

Further information may be obtained from:
www.porphyria-europe.org

and also from:

Welsh Medicines Information Centre
University Hospital of Wales
Cardiff, CF14 4XW
Tel: (029) 2074 2979/3877
**Note** Quite modest changes in chemical structure can lead to changes in porphyrinogenicity but where possible general statements have been made about groups of drugs; these should be checked first.

### Unsafe Drug Groups (check first)

| | | | |
|---|---|---|---|
| Alkylating drugs[1] | Calcium channel blockers[5] | Imidazole antifungals[8] | Sulphonamides[10] |
| Amphetamines | Contraceptives, hormonal[6] | Non-nucleoside reverse tran- | Sulphonylureas[11] |
| Anabolic steroids | Ergot derivatives[7] | scriptase inhibitors[1] | Taxanes[1] |
| Antidepressants[2] | Gold salts | Progestogens[6] | Tetracyclines |
| Antihistamines[3] | Hormone replacement | Protease inhibitors[1] | Thiazolidinediones[1] |
| Barbiturates[4] | therapy[6] | Statins[9] | Triazole antifungals[8] |

### Unsafe Drugs (check groups above first)

| | | | |
|---|---|---|---|
| Aceclofenac | Diclofenac | Metronidazole[16] | Risperidone |
| Alcohol | Erythromycin | Metyrapone | Spironolactone |
| Amiodarone | Etamsylate | Mifepristone | Sulfinpyrazone |
| Azapropazone | Ethosuximide | Minoxidil[16] | Sulpiride |
| Bosentan | Etomidate | Nalidixic acid | Tamoxifen |
| Bromocriptine | Fenfluramine | Nitrazepam | Telithromycin |
| Buspirone | Flupentixol | Nitrofurantoin | Temoporfin |
| Cabergoline | Griseofulvin | Orphenadrine | Theophylline[19] |
| Carbamazepine | Halothane | Oxcarbazepine | Tiagabine |
| Carisoprodol | Hydralazine | Oxybutynin | Tinidazole |
| Chloral hydrate[12] | Indapamide | Oxycodone[17] | Topiramate |
| Chloramphenicol | Isometheptene mucate | Pentazocine[17] | Toremifene |
| Chloroform[13] | Isoniazid | Pentoxifylline (oxpenti- | Tramadol[17] |
| Clindamycin | Ketamine | fylline) | Triclofos[12] |
| Clonidine | Ketorolac | Phenoxybenzamine | Trimethoprim |
| Cocaine | Lidocaine (lignocaine)[15] | Phenytoin | Valproate[14] |
| Colistin | Mebeverine | Pivmecillinam | Xipamide |
| Cycloserine | Mefenamic acid[16] | Porfimer | Zidovudine[1] |
| Danazol | Meprobamate | Probenecid | Zuclopenthixol |
| Dapsone | Methyldopa | Pyrazinamide | |
| Dexfenfluramine | Metoclopramide[16] | Rifabutin[18] | |
| Diazepam[14] | Metolazone | Rifampicin[18] | |

1. Contact Welsh Medicines Information Centre for further advice.
2. Includes tricyclic (and related) antidepressants and MAOIs; fluoxetine and mianserin thought to be safe.
3. Alimemazine (trimeprazine), chlorphenamine, desloratadine, fexofenadine, ketotifen, loratadine, and promethazine thought to be safe.
4. Includes primidone and thiopental.
5. Diltiazem may be used with caution if safer alternative not available
6. Progestogens are more porphyrinogenic than oestrogens; oestrogens may be safe at least in replacement doses. Progestogens should be avoided whenever possible by all women susceptible to acute porphyria; however, when non-hormonal contraception is inappropriate, progestogens may be used with extreme caution if the potential benefit outweighs risk. The risk of an acute attack is greatest in women who have had a previous attack or are aged under 30 years. Long-acting progestogen preparations should **never** be used in those at risk of acute porphyria.
7. Includes ergometrine (oxytocin probably safe) and pergolide.
8. Applies to oral and intravenous use; topical antifungals are thought to be safe due to low systemic exposure.
9. Rosuvastatin is thought to be safe.
10. Includes co-trimoxazole and sulfasalazine.
11. Glipizide is thought to be safe.
12. Although evidence of hazard is uncertain, manufacturer advises avoid.
13. Small amounts in medicines probably safe.
14. Status epilepticus has been treated successfully with intravenous diazepam.
15. When used for local anaesthesia, bupivacaine, lidocaine (lignocaine), prilocaine, and tetracaine are thought to be safe.
16. May be used with caution if safer alternative not available.
17. Buprenorphine, codeine, diamorphine, dihydrocodeine, fentanyl, methadone, morphine, and pethidine are thought to be safe.
18. Rifamycins have been used in a few patients without evidence of harm—use with caution if safer alternative not available.
19. Includes aminophylline.

# 10 Musculoskeletal and joint diseases

**10.1 Drugs used in rheumatic diseases and gout** 559

10.1.1 Non-steroidal anti-inflammatory drugs 560

10.1.2 Corticosteroids 569

10.1.2.1 Systemic corticosteroids 569

10.1.2.2 Local corticosteroid injections 569

10.1.3 Drugs that suppress the rheumatic disease process 570

10.1.4 Gout and cytotoxic-induced hyperuricaemia 581

10.1.5 Other drugs for rheumatic diseases 583

**10.2 Drugs used in neuromuscular disorders** 583

10.2.1 Drugs that enhance neuromuscular transmission 583

10.2.2 Skeletal muscle relaxants 585

**10.3 Drugs for the relief of soft-tissue inflammation** 587

10.3.1 Enzymes 588

10.3.2 Rubefacients and other topical antirheumatics 588

This chapter also includes advice on the drug management of the following:
dental and orofacial pain, p. 561
extravasation, p. 587
myasthenia gravis, p. 583
osteoarthritis and soft-tissue disorders, below
rheumatoid arthritis and other inflammatory disorders, below

For treatment of septic arthritis see Table 1, section 5.1.

## 10.1 Drugs used in rheumatic diseases and gout

10.1.1 Non-steroidal anti-inflammatory drugs

10.1.2 Corticosteroids

10.1.3 Drugs that suppress the rheumatic disease process

10.1.4 Gout and cytotoxic-induced hyperuricaemia

10.1.5 Other drugs for rheumatic diseases

### Rheumatoid arthritis and other inflammatory disorders

A **non-steroidal anti-inflammatory drug** (NSAID) or a **selective inhibitor of cyclo-oxygenase-2** is indicated for pain and stiffness resulting from inflammatory rheumatic disease. Analgesics such as **paracetamol** or **codeine** can also be used.

Drugs are also used to influence the rheumatic disease process itself (section 10.1.3). For *rheumatoid arthritis* these **disease-modifying antirheumatic drugs** (DMARDs) include methotrexate, cytokine modulators, azathioprine, ciclosporin, cyclophosphamide, leflunomide, penicillamine, gold salts, antimalarials (chloroquine and hydroxychloroquine), and sulfasalazine. **Corticosteroids** also have a significant role in the management of rheumatoid arthritis (section 10.1.2.1).

Drugs which may affect the disease process in *psoriatic arthritis* include sulfasalazine, gold salts, azathioprine, methotrexate, and etanercept (section 10.1.3).

For long-term control of *gout*, uricosuric drugs and allopurinol (section 10.1.4) can be used.

### Osteoarthritis and soft-tissue disorders

For pain relief in osteoarthritis and soft-tissue disorders, **paracetamol** (section 4.7.1) should be used first and may need to be taken regularly. A **topical NSAID** (section 10.3.2) or topical **capsaicin** 0.025% (section 10.3.2) should also be considered, particularly in knee or hand osteoarthritis. An **oral NSAID** (section 10.1.1), or a **selective inhibitor of cyclo-oxygenase-2** can be substituted for, or used in addition to, paracetamol. If further pain relief is required, then the addition of an **opioid** (section 4.7.2) should be considered; however, an opioid should be considered before a NSAID or selective inhibitor of cyclo-oxygenase-2 in patients taking low-dose aspirin.

10 Musculoskeletal and joint diseases

Intra-articular **corticosteroid** injections (section 10.1.2.2) may produce temporary benefit in osteoarthritis, especially if associated with soft-tissue inflammation.

Non-drug measures, such as weight reduction and exercise, should also be encouraged.

**Glucosamine** (section 10.1.5) and **rubefacients** (section 10.3.2) are not recommended for the treatment of osteoarthritis.

**Hyaluronic acid** and it's derivatives are available for osteoarthritis of the knee, but are not recommended. Sodium hyaluronate (*Durolane®*, *Euflexxa®*, *Fermathron®*, *Hyalgan®* ⟪JHS⟫ *Orthovisc®*, *Ostenil®*, *Suplasyn®*, *Synocrom®*) or hylan G-F 20 (*Synvisc®*) is injected intra-articularly to supplement natural hyaluronic acid in the synovial fluid. These injections may reduce pain over 1–6 months, but are associated with a short-term increase in knee inflammation.

## 10.1.1 Non-steroidal anti-inflammatory drugs

In *single doses* non-steroidal anti-inflammatory drugs (NSAIDs) have analgesic activity comparable to that of paracetamol (section 4.7.1), but paracetamol is preferred, particularly in the elderly (see also Prescribing for the Elderly, p. 20).

In regular *full dosage* NSAIDs have both a lasting analgesic and an anti-inflammatory effect which makes them particularly useful for the treatment of continuous or regular pain associated with inflammation. Therefore, although paracetamol often gives adequate pain control in osteoarthritis, NSAIDs are more appropriate than paracetamol or the opioid analgesics in the *inflammatory arthritides* (e.g. rheumatoid arthritis) and in some cases of *advanced osteoarthritis*. NSAIDs can also be of benefit in the less well defined conditions of *back pain* and *soft-tissue disorders*.

**Choice** Differences in anti-inflammatory activity between NSAIDs are small, but there is considerable variation in individuals' tolerance to these drugs and their response to them. About 60% of patients will respond to any NSAID; of the others, those who do not respond to one may well respond to another. Pain relief starts soon after taking the first dose and a full analgesic effect should normally be obtained within a week, whereas an anti-inflammatory effect may not be achieved (or may not be clinically assessable) for up to 3 weeks. If appropriate responses are not obtained within these times, another NSAID should be tried.

NSAIDs reduce the production of prostaglandins by inhibiting the enzyme cyclo-oxygenase. They vary in their selectivity for inhibiting different types of cyclo-oxygenase; selective inhibition of cyclo-oxygenase-2 is associated with less gastro-intestinal intolerance. Several other factors also influence susceptibility to gastro-intestinal effects, and a NSAID should be chosen on the basis of the incidence of gastro-intestinal and other side-effects.

**Ibuprofen** is a propionic acid derivative with anti-inflammatory, analgesic, and antipyretic properties. It has fewer side-effects than other non-selective NSAIDs but its anti-inflammatory properties are weaker. Doses of 1.6 to 2.4 g daily are needed for rheumatoid arthritis and it is unsuitable for conditions where inflammation is prominent, such as acute gout. **Dexibuprofen** is the active enantiomer of ibuprofen. It has similar properties to ibuprofen and is licensed for the relief of mild to moderate pain and inflammation.

Other propionic acid derivatives:

**Naproxen** is one of the first choices because it combines good efficacy with a low incidence of side-effects (but more than ibuprofen, see CSM comment below).

**Fenbufen** is claimed to be associated with less gastro-intestinal bleeding, but there is a high risk of rash (see p. 565).

**Fenoprofen** is as effective as naproxen, and **flurbiprofen** may be slightly more effective. Both are associated with slightly more gastro-intestinal side-effects than ibuprofen.

**Ketoprofen** has anti-inflammatory properties similar to ibuprofen and has more side-effects (see also CSM advice below). **Dexketoprofen**, an isomer of ketoprofen, has been introduced for the short-term relief of mild to moderate pain.

**Tiaprofenic acid** is as effective as naproxen; it has more side-effects than ibuprofen (**important**: reports of severe cystitis, see CSM advice on p. 569).

Drugs with properties similar to those of propionic acid derivatives:

**Azapropazone** is similar in effect to naproxen; it has a tendency to cause rashes and is associated with an increased risk of severe gastro-intestinal toxicity (**important**: see CSM restrictions on p. 562).

**Diclofenac** and **aceclofenac** have actions and side-effects similar to those of naproxen.

**Etodolac** is comparable in efficacy to naproxen; it is licensed for symptomatic relief of osteoarthritis and rheumatoid arthritis.

**Indometacin** (indomethacin) has an action equal to or superior to that of naproxen, but with a high incidence of side-effects including headache, dizziness, and gastro-intestinal disturbances (see also CSM advice below).

**Mefenamic acid** has minor anti-inflammatory properties. It has occasionally been associated with diarrhoea and haemolytic anaemia which require discontinuation of treatment.

**Meloxicam** is licensed for the short-term relief of pain in osteoarthritis and for long-term treatment of rheumatoid arthritis and ankylosing spondylitis.

**Nabumetone** is comparable in effect to naproxen.

**Piroxicam** is as effective as naproxen and has a long duration of action which permits once-daily administration. However, it has more gastro-intestinal side-effects than most other NSAIDs, and is associated with more frequent serious skin reactions (**important**: see CHMP advice, p. 568).

**Sulindac** is similar in tolerance to naproxen.

*10 Musculoskeletal and joint diseases*

**Tenoxicam** is similar in activity and tolerance to naproxen. Its long duration of action allows once-daily administration.

**Tolfenamic acid** is licensed for the treatment of migraine (section 4.7.4.1).

**Ketorolac** and the selective inhibitor of cyclo-oxygenase-2, **parecoxib**, are licensed for the short-term management of postoperative pain (section 15.1.4.2).

The selective inhibitors of cyclo-oxygenase-2, **etoricoxib** and **celecoxib**, are as effective as non-selective NSAIDs such as diclofenac and naproxen. Short-term data indicate that the risk of serious upper gastro-intestinal events is lower with selective inhibitors compared to non-selective NSAIDs; this advantage may be lost in patients who require concomitant low-dose aspirin. There are concerns about the cardiovascular safety of cyclo-oxygenase-2 selective inhibitors (see below).

**Celecoxib** and **etoricoxib** are licensed for the relief of pain in osteoarthritis, rheumatoid arthritis, and ankylosing spondylitis; etoricoxib is also licensed for the relief of pain from acute gout.

**Dental and orofacial pain**  Most mild to moderate dental pain and inflammation is effectively relieved by NSAIDs. Those used for dental pain include **ibuprofen** and **diclofenac**.

In an appraisal of the relative safety of 7 non-selective NSAIDs, the CSM assessed ibuprofen to have the lowest risk of serious gastro-intestinal side-effects (see p. 562).

For further information on the management of dental and orofacial pain, see p. 232.

**Cautions and contra-indications**  NSAIDs should be used with caution in the elderly (risk of serious side-effects and fatalities, see also Prescribing for the Elderly p. 20), in allergic disorders (they are **contra-indicated** in patients with a history of hypersensitivity to aspirin or any other NSAID—which includes those in whom attacks of asthma, angioedema, urticaria or rhinitis have been precipitated by aspirin or any other NSAID), during pregnancy and breast-feeding (see Appendix 4 and Appendix 5), and in coagulation defects. Long-term use of some NSAIDs is associated with reduced female fertility, which is reversible on stopping treatment.

In patients with renal or cardiac impairment, caution is required since NSAIDs may impair renal function (see also under Side-effects, below and Appendix 3); the dose should be kept as **low as possible** for the **shortest possible duration**, and renal function should be **monitored**. NSAIDs should be avoided if possible in renal impairment and used with caution in hepatic impairment (see also under side-effects, below and Appendix 2).

All NSAIDs are contra-indicated in severe heart failure. The selective inhibitors of cyclo-oxygenase-2 (celecoxib, etoricoxib, and parecoxib) are **contra-indicated** in ischaemic heart disease, cerebrovascular disease, peripheral arterial disease, and moderate or severe heart failure. The selective inhibitors of cyclo-oxygenase-2 should be used with caution in patients with a history of cardiac failure, left ventricular dysfunction, hypertension, in patients with oedema for any other reason, and in patients with risk factors for heart disease.

---

**NSAIDs and cardiovascular events**

Cyclo-oxygenase-2 selective inhibitors are associated with an increased risk of thrombotic events (e.g. myocardial infarction and stroke) and should not be used in preference to non-selective NSAIDs except when specifically indicated (i.e. for patients at a particularly high risk of developing gastroduodenal ulceration or bleeding) *and* after assessing their cardiovascular risk.

Non-selective NSAIDs are also associated with a small increased risk of thrombotic events even when used short-term in those with no cardiovascular risk factors. **Diclofenac** (150 mg daily) and **ibuprofen** (2.4 g daily) are associated with an increased risk of thrombotic events. The increased risk for diclofenac is similar to that of licensed doses of **etoricoxib**. **Naproxen** (1 g daily) is associated with a lower thrombotic risk, and low doses of ibuprofen (1.2 g daily or less) have not been associated with an increased risk of myocardial infarction.

The lowest effective dose of NSAID or cyclo-oxygenase-2 selective inhibitor should be prescribed for the shortest period to control symptoms and that the need for long-term treatment should be reviewed periodically.

---

The CSM has advised that non-selective NSAIDs are contra-indicated in patients with previous or active peptic ulceration and that selective inhibitors of cyclo-oxygenase-2 are contra-indicated in active peptic ulceration (see also **CSM advice** below). While it is preferable to avoid NSAIDs in patients with active or previous gastro-intestinal ulceration or bleeding, and to withdraw them if gastro-intestinal lesions develop, nevertheless patients with serious rheumatic diseases (e.g. rheumatoid arthritis) are usually dependent on NSAIDs for effective relief of pain and stiffness. For advice on the prophylaxis and treatment of NSAID-associated peptic ulcers, see section 1.3.

For **interactions** of NSAIDs, see Appendix 1 (NSAIDs).

**Side-effects**  Gastro-intestinal discomfort, nausea, diarrhoea, and occasionally bleeding and ulceration occur (see also CSM advice below). Systemic as well as local effects of NSAIDs contribute to gastro-intestinal damage; taking oral formulations with milk or food, or using enteric-coated formulations, or changing the route of administration may only partially reduce symptoms such as dyspepsia. Those at risk of duodenal or gastric ulceration (including the elderly) who need to continue NSAID treatment should receive either a selective inhibitor of cyclo-oxygenase-2 alone, or a non-selective NSAID with gastroprotective treatment (section 1.3).

Other side-effects include hypersensitivity reactions (particularly rashes, angioedema, and bronchospasm—see CSM advice below), headache, dizziness, nervousness, depression, drowsiness, insomnia, vertigo, hearing disturbances such as tinnitus, photosensitivity, and haematuria. Blood disorders have also occurred. Fluid retention may occur (rarely precipitating congestive heart failure); blood pressure may be raised.

Renal failure may be provoked by NSAIDs, especially in patients with renal impairment (**important**, see also under Cautions above). Rarely, papillary necrosis or interstitial fibrosis associated with NSAIDs can lead to renal failure.

**10**

**Musculoskeletal and joint diseases**

Hepatic damage, alveolitis, pulmonary eosinophilia, pancreatitis, eye changes, Stevens-Johnson syndrome and toxic epidermal necrolysis are other rare side-effects. Induction of or exacerbation of colitis has been reported. Aseptic meningitis has been reported rarely with NSAIDs; patients with connective-tissue disorders such as systemic lupus erythematosus may be especially susceptible.

**Overdosage:** see Emergency Treatment of Poisoning, p. 29.

> **CSM advice (gastro-intestinal side-effects)**
>
> All NSAIDs are associated with serious gastro-intestinal toxicity; the risk is higher in the elderly. Evidence on the relative safety of 7 **non-selective** NSAIDs indicates differences in the risks of serious upper gastro-intestinal side-effects. **Azapropazone** is associated with the *highest risk* (**important:** see also CSM restrictions, below) and **ibuprofen** with the *lowest*; **piroxicam, ketoprofen, indometacin, naproxen** and **diclofenac** are associated with *intermediate risks* (possibly higher in the case of piroxicam, see CHMP advice, p. 568). **Selective inhibitors of cyclo-oxygenase-2** are associated with a *lower risk* of serious upper gastro-intestinal side-effects than non-selective NSAIDs.
>
> Recommendations are that NSAIDs associated with a low risk e.g. ibuprofen are *generally preferred*, to start at the *lowest recommended dose*, not to use more than one oral NSAID at a time, and to remember that all NSAIDs (including selective inhibitors of cyclo-oxygenase-2) are *contra-indicated* in patients with active peptic ulceration. The CSM also contra-indicates non-selective NSAIDs in patients with a history of peptic ulceration.
>
> The combination of a NSAID and low-dose aspirin can increase the risk of gastro-intestinal side-effects; this combination should be used only if absolutely necessary and the patient should be monitored closely.

> **CSM warning (asthma)**
>
> Any degree of worsening of asthma may be related to the ingestion of NSAIDs, either prescribed or (in the case of ibuprofen and others) purchased over the counter.

## ACECLOFENAC

**Indications** pain and inflammation in rheumatoid arthritis, osteoarthritis and ankylosing spondylitis

**Cautions** see notes above; avoid in acute porphyria (section 9.8.2)

**Contra-indications** see notes above

**Side-effects** see notes above

**Dose**

- 100 mg twice daily; CHILD not recommended

**Preservex®** (Movianto) ℞

Tablets, f/c, aceclofenac 100 mg, net price 60-tab pack = £9.45. Label: 21

## ACEMETACIN

(Glycolic acid ester of indometacin)

**Indications** pain and inflammation in rheumatic disease and other musculoskeletal disorders; postoperative analgesia

**Cautions** see under Indometacin and notes above

Driving Dizziness may affect performance of skilled tasks (e.g. driving)

**Contra-indications** see notes above

**Side-effects** see under Indometacin and notes above

**Dose**

- 120 mg daily in divided doses with food, increased if necessary to 180 mg daily; CHILD not recommended

**Emflex®** (Merck) ℞

Capsules, yellow/orange, acemetacin 60 mg, net price 90-cap pack = £28.20. Label: 21, counselling, driving

## AZAPROPAZONE

**Indications** see under CSM restrictions

CSM restrictions CSM *has restricted* azapropazone to use in rheumatoid arthritis, ankylosing spondylitis, and acute gout only when other NSAIDs have been tried and failed, *has* contra-indicated it in patients with a history of peptic ulceration, and *has reduced* the maximum daily dose to 600 mg for rheumatoid arthritis and ankylosing spondylitis in patients over 60 years, and those with impaired renal function

**Cautions** see notes above

**Contra-indications** see notes above; also acute porphyria (section 9.8.2); history of inflammatory bowel disease or blood disorder

**Side-effects** see notes above; also see CSM advice below

Photosensitivity CSM has reminded of the need to advise patients taking azapropazone to avoid direct exposure to sunlight (or to use sunscreen preparations)

**Dose**

- Rheumatoid arthritis and ankylosing spondylitis, 1.2 g daily in 2 or 4 divided doses; ELDERLY over 60 years, 300 mg twice daily; CHILD not recommended

- Acute gout, 1.8 g daily in divided doses until acute symptoms subside (usually by day 4) *then* 1.2 g daily in divided doses until symptoms resolve—consider alternative therapy if symptoms persist; ELDERLY over 60 years, 1.8 g daily in divided doses for the first 24 hours *then* 1.2 g daily in divided doses, reduced to 600 mg daily in divided doses as soon as possible (preferably by day 4) until acute symptoms resolve—consider alternative therapy if symptoms persist; CHILD not recommended

**Rheumox®** (Goldshield) ℞ ◪

Capsules, orange, azapropazone 300 mg, net price 100-cap pack = £15.50. Label: 11, 21, counselling, photosensitivity (see above)

## CELECOXIB

**Indications** pain and inflammation in osteoarthritis, rheumatoid arthritis, and ankylosing spondylitis

**Cautions** see notes above; monitor blood pressure before treatment and during treatment

**Contra-indications** see notes above; sulphonamide sensitivity; inflammatory bowel disease

**Side-effects** see notes above; *less commonly* stomatitis, palpitation, cerebral infarction, fatigue, paraesthesia, muscle cramps; *rarely* taste disturbance, alopecia; *very rarely* seizures

**Dose**

- Osteoarthritis, 200 mg daily in 1–2 divided doses, increased if necessary to max. 200 mg twice daily; CHILD not recommended

- Rheumatoid arthritis, 100 mg twice daily, increased if necessary to 200 mg twice daily; CHILD not recommended

- Ankylosing spondylitis, 200 mg daily in 1–2 divided doses, increased if necessary to max. 400 mg daily in 1–2 divided doses; CHILD not recommended

**Note** Discontinue if no improvement after 2 weeks on max. dose

**Celebrex®** (Pharmacia) PoM

Capsules, celecoxib 100 mg (white/blue), net price 60-cap pack = £21.55; 200 mg (white/gold), 30-cap pack = £21.55

### ■ DEXIBUPROFEN

**Indications** pain and inflammation associated with osteoarthritis and other musculoskeletal disorders; mild to moderate pain and inflammation including dysmenorrhoea and dental pain

**Cautions** see notes above; systemic lupus erythematosus and other connective tissue disorders

**Contra-indications** see notes above

**Side-effects** see notes above

**Dose**

- 600–900 mg daily in up to 3 divided doses; increased if necessary to max. 1.2 g daily (900 mg daily for dysmenorrhoea); max. single dose 400 mg (300 mg for dysmenorrhoea); CHILD not recommended

**Seractil®** (Genus) ▼ PoM

Tablets, f/c, dexibuprofen 300 mg, net price 60–tab pack = £9.47; 400 mg (scored) 60–tab pack = £9.47. Label: 21

### ■ DEXKETOPROFEN

**Indications** short-term treatment of mild to moderate pain including dysmenorrhoea

**Cautions** see notes above

**Contra-indications** see notes above

**Side-effects** see notes above

**Dose**

- 12.5 mg every 4–6 hours *or* 25 mg every 8 hours; max. 75 mg daily; ELDERLY initially max. 50 mg daily; CHILD not recommended

**Keral®** (Menarini) PoM

Tablets, f/c, scored, dexketoprofen (as trometamol) 25 mg, net price 20-tab pack = £3.67, 50-tab pack = £9.18. Label: 22

### ■ DICLOFENAC SODIUM

**Indications** pain and inflammation in rheumatic disease (including juvenile idiopathic arthritis) and other musculoskeletal disorders; acute gout; postoperative pain

**Cautions** see notes above

**Contra-indications** see notes above; acute porphyria (section 9.8.2); avoid injections containing benzyl alcohol in neonates (see preparations below)

**Intravenous use** Additional contra-indications include concomitant NSAID or anticoagulant use (including low-dose heparin), history of haemorrhagic diathesis, history of confirmed or suspected cerebrovascular bleeding, operations with high risk of haemorrhage, history of asthma, moderate or severe renal impairment, hypovolaemia, dehydration

**Side-effects** see notes above; suppositories may cause rectal irritation; injection site reactions

**Dose**

- By mouth, 75–150 mg daily in 2–3 divided doses

- By rectum in suppositories, 75–150 mg daily in divided doses

- Juvenile idiopathic arthritis, CHILD 6 months–18 years, see *BNF for Children*

- CHILD 6–12 years, postoperative pain, by rectum, 1–2 mg/kg (max. 150 mg) daily in divided doses (12.5 mg and 25 mg suppositories only) for max. 4 days

**Diclofenac Sodium** (Non-proprietary) PoM

Tablets, e/c, diclofenac sodium 25 mg, net price 84-tab pack = £1.20; 50 mg, 84-tab pack = £1.37. Label: 5, 25

Brands include *Defenac®*, *Dicloflex®*, *Diclozip®*, *Fenactol®*, *Flamrase®*

**Dental prescribing on NHS** Diclofenac Sodium Tablets may be prescribed

Suppositories, diclofenac sodium 100 mg, net price 10 = £3.06

Brands include *Econac®*

**Dyloject®** (Javelin) PoM

Injection, diclofenac sodium 37.5 mg/mL, net price 2-mL vial = £4.80

**Dose** by deep intramuscular injection into the gluteal muscle, acute exacerbations of pain and postoperative pain, 75 mg once daily (twice daily in severe cases) for max. 2 days

Ureteric colic, 75 mg then a further 75 mg after 30 minutes if necessary

By intravenous injection (in supervised settings), acute postoperative pain, 75 mg repeated after 4–6 hours if necessary; max. 150 mg in 24 hours for 2 days

Prevention of postoperative pain, 25–50 mg after surgery; further doses given after 4–6 hours if necessary; max. 150 mg in 24 hours for 2 days

**Note** The *Scottish Medicines Consortium* (p. 3) has advised (Feb 2008) that *Dyloject®* is accepted for restricted use within NHS Scotland for the treatment or prevention of postoperative pain by intravenous injection in supervised healthcare settings

**Voltarol®** (Novartis) PoM

Tablets, e/c, diclofenac sodium 25 mg (yellow), net price 84-tab pack = £2.94; 50 mg (brown), 84-tab pack = £4.57. Label: 5, 25

Dispersible tablets, sugar-free, pink, diclofenac, equivalent to diclofenac sodium 50 mg, net price 21-tab pack = £6.19. Label: 13, 21

**Note** Voltarol Dispersible tablets are more suitable for **short-term** use in acute conditions for which treatment required for no more than 3 months (no information on use beyond 3 months)

Injection, diclofenac sodium 25 mg/mL, net price 3-mL amp = 83p

**Excipients** include benzyl alcohol (avoid in neonates unless there is no safer alternative, see Excipients, p. 2), propylene glycol

**Dose** by deep intramuscular injection into the gluteal muscle, acute exacerbations of pain and postoperative pain, 75 mg once daily (twice daily in severe cases) for max. 2 days; CHILD 2–18 years, see *BNF for Children*

Ureteric colic, 75 mg then a further 75 mg after 30 minutes if necessary

By intravenous infusion (in hospital setting), acute postoperative pain, 75 mg repeated if necessary after 4–6 hours; max. 150 mg in 24 hours for 2 days; CHILD 2–18 years, see *BNF for Children*

Prevention of postoperative pain, initially after surgery 25–50 mg over 15–60 minutes then 5 mg/hour; max. 150 mg in 24 hours for 2 days

Suppositories, diclofenac sodium 12.5 mg, net price 10 = 58p; 25 mg, 10 = £1.03; 50 mg, 10 = £1.70; 100 mg, 10 = £3.03

◢**Diclofenac potassium**
[1]**Voltarol® Rapid** (Novartis) [PoM]
Tablets, s/c, diclofenac potassium 25 mg (red), net
price 30-tab pack = £4.33; 50 mg (brown), 30-tab pack
= £8.28
> **Dose** rheumatic disease, musculoskeletal disorders, acute gout,
> postoperative pain, 75–150 mg daily in 2–3 divided doses; CHILD
> over 14 years, 75–100 mg daily in 2–3 divided doses
>
> Migraine, 50 mg at onset, repeated after 2 hours if necessary then
> after 4–6 hours; max. 200 mg in 24 hours; CHILD not
> recommended

1. 12.5 mg tablets can be sold to the public for the treatment of
headache, dental pain, period pain, rheumatic and muscular
pain, backache and the symptoms of cold and flu (including
fever), in patients aged over 14 years subject to max. single
dose of 25 mg, max. daily dose of 75 mg for max. 3 days, and
max. pack size of 18 × 12.5 mg

◢**Modified release**
**Diclomax SR®** (Provalis) [PoM]
Capsules, m/r, yellow, diclofenac sodium 75 mg, net
price 56-cap pack = £11.63. Label: 21, 25
> **Dose** 1 capsule 1–2 times daily *or* 2 capsules once daily, pre-
> ferably with food; CHILD not recommended

**Diclomax Retard®** (Provalis) [PoM]
Capsules, m/r, diclofenac sodium 100 mg, net price
28-cap pack = £8.36. Label: 21, 25
> **Dose** 1 capsule daily preferably with food; CHILD not recom-
> mended

**Motifene® 75 mg** (Daiichi Sankyo) [PoM]
Capsules, e/c, m/r, diclofenac sodium 75 mg
(enclosing e/c pellets containing diclofenac sodium
25 mg and m/r pellets containing diclofenac sodium
50 mg), net price 56-cap pack = £8.00. Label: 25
> **Dose** 1 capsule 1–2 times daily; CHILD not recommended

**Voltarol® 75 mg SR** (Novartis) [PoM]
Tablets, m/r, f/c, pink, diclofenac sodium 75 mg, net
price 28-tab pack = £6.46; 56-tab pack = £12.92.
Label: 21, 25
> **Dose** 75 mg 1–2 times daily preferably with food; CHILD not
> recommended
>
> **Note** Other brands of modified-release tablets containing diclo-
> fenac sodium 75 mg include *Defenac® SR, Dexomon® 75 SR,
> Dicloflex® 75 SR, Fenactol® 75 mg SR, Flamatak® 75 MR, Flamrase®
> SR, Flexotard® MR 75, Rheumatac® Retard 75, Rhumalgan® CR,
> Slofenac® SR, Volsaid® Retard 75*

**Voltarol® Retard** (Novartis) [PoM]
Tablets, m/r, f/c, red, diclofenac sodium 100 mg. Net
price 28-tab pack = £9.47. Label: 21, 25
> **Dose** 1 tablet daily preferably with food; CHILD not recom-
> mended
>
> **Note** Other brands of modified-release tablets containing diclo-
> fenac sodium 100 mg include *Defenac® Retard, Dexomon® Retard
> 100, Dicloflex® Retard, Fenactol® Retard 100 mg, Flamatak® 100
> MR, Flamrase® SR, Rhumalgan® CR, Slofenac® SR, Volsaid® Retard
> 100*

◢**With misoprostol**
For **cautions, contra-indications**, and **side-effects** of
misoprostol, see section 1.3.4

**Arthrotec®** (Pharmacia) [PoM]
Arthrotec® 50 tablets, diclofenac sodium (in e/c
core) 50 mg, misoprostol 200 micrograms, net price
60-tab pack = £11.98; Label: 21, 25
> **Dose** prophylaxis against NSAID-induced gastroduodenal
> ulceration in patients requiring diclofenac for rheumatoid arthritis
> or osteoarthritis, 1 tablet 2–3 times daily with food; CHILD not
> recommended

Arthrotec® 75 tablets, diclofenac sodium (in e/c
core) 75 mg, misoprostol 200 micrograms, net price
60-tab pack = £15.83. Label: 21, 25
> **Dose** prophylaxis against NSAID-induced gastroduodenal
> ulceration in patients requiring diclofenac for rheumatoid arthritis
> or osteoarthritis, 1 tablet twice daily with food; CHILD not
> recommended

◢**Topical preparations**
Section 10.3.2

## ETODOLAC

**Indications** pain and inflammation in rheumatoid
arthritis and osteoarthritis
**Cautions** see notes above
**Contra-indications** see notes above
**Side-effects** see notes above; also stomatitis, vascu-
litis, palpitation, dyspnoea, confusion, fatigue,
paraesthesia, tremor, urinary frequency, dysuria,
pyrexia, and pruritus
**Dose**
- ADULT over 18 years, 600 mg daily in 1–2 divided doses

**Etodolac** (Non-proprietary) [PoM]
Capsules, etodolac 300 mg, net price 60-cap pack =
£8.14
> Brands include *Eccoxolac®*

◢**Modified release**
**Etopan XL®** (Taro) [PoM]
Tablets, m/r, f/c, grey, etodolac 600 mg, net price 30-
tab pack = £14.90. Label: 25
> **Dose** 1 tablet daily; CHILD not recommended

**Lodine SR®** (Almirall) [PoM]
Tablets, m/r, f/c, light-grey, etodolac 600 mg, net
price 30-tab pack = £15.50. Label: 25
> **Dose** 1 tablet daily; CHILD not recommended

## ETORICOXIB

**Indications** pain and inflammation in osteoarthritis,
rheumatoid arthritis, and ankylosing spondylitis;
acute gout
**Cautions** see notes above; also dehydration; monitor
blood pressure before treatment, 2 weeks after
initiation and periodically during treatment
**Contra-indications** see notes above; inflammatory
bowel disease; uncontrolled hypertension (persistently above 140/90 mmHg)
**Side-effects** see notes above; also palpitation, fatigue,
influenza-like symptoms, ecchymosis; *less commonly*
dry mouth, taste disturbance, mouth ulcer, appetite
and weight change, atrial fibrillation, transient
ischaemic attack, chest pain, flushing, cough, dyspnoea, epistaxis, anxiety, mental acuity impaired,
paraesthesia, electrolyte disturbance, myalgia and
arthralgia; *very rarely* confusion and hallucinations
**Dose**
- Osteoarthritis, ADULT and CHILD over 16 years, 30 mg
once daily, increased if necessary to 60 mg once daily
- Rheumatoid arthritis and ankylosing spondylitis,
ADULT and CHILD over 16 years, 90 mg once daily
- Acute gout, ADULT and CHILD over 16 years, 120 mg
once daily for max. 8 days

**Arcoxia®** (MSD) ▼ [PoM]
Tablets, f/c, etoricoxib 30 mg (blue-green), net price
28-tab pack = £13.99; 60 mg (dark green), 28-tab pack
= £20.11; 90 mg (white), 28-tab pack = £22.96; 120 mg
(pale green), 7-tab pack = £5.74

## FENBUFEN

**Indications** pain and inflammation in rheumatic disease and other musculoskeletal disorders

**Cautions** see notes above

**Contra-indications** see notes above

**Side-effects** see notes above, but also high risk of rashes especially in seronegative rheumatoid arthritis, psoriatic arthritis and in women (discontinue immediately); erythema multiforme and Stevens-Johnson syndrome reported; also allergic interstitial lung disorders (may follow rashes)

**Dose**

- 300 mg in the morning and 600 mg at bed-time *or* 450 mg twice daily; CHILD under 14 years not recommended

**Fenbufen** (Non-proprietary) (PoM)

Capsules, fenbufen 300 mg, net price 84-cap pack = £20.71. Label: 21

Tablets, fenbufen 300 mg, net price 84-tab pack = £6.00; 450 mg, 56-tab pack = £24.97. Label: 21

**Lederfen®** (Goldshield) (PoM)

Capsules, dark blue, fenbufen 300 mg. Net price 84-cap pack = £20.71. Label: 21

Tablets, both light blue, f/c, fenbufen 300 mg, net price 84-tab pack = £6.00; 450 mg, 56-tab pack = £6.49. Label: 21

## FENOPROFEN

**Indications** pain and inflammation in rheumatic disease and other musculoskeletal disorders; mild to moderate pain

**Cautions** see notes above

**Contra-indications** see notes above

**Side-effects** see notes above; upper respiratory-tract infection, nasopharyngitis, and cystitis also reported

**Dose**

- 300–600 mg 3–4 times daily with food; max. 3 g daily; CHILD not recommended

**Fenopron®** (Typharm) (PoM)

Tablets, both orange, fenoprofen (as calcium salt) 300 mg (*Fenopron®* 300), net price 100-tab pack = £9.45; 600 mg (*Fenopron®* 600, scored), 100-tab pack = £18.29. Label: 21

## FLURBIPROFEN

**Indications** pain and inflammation in rheumatic disease and other musculoskeletal disorders; mild to moderate pain including dysmenorrhoea; migraine; postoperative analgesia; sore throat (section 12.3.1)

**Cautions** see notes above

**Contra-indications** see notes above

**Side-effects** see notes above; also stomatitis; *less commonly* paraesthesia, confusion, hallucinations, and fatigue

**Dose**

- ADULT and CHILD over 12 years, 150–200 mg daily in 2–4 divided doses, increased in acute conditions to 300 mg daily

- Dysmenorrhoea, ADULT and CHILD over 12 years, initially 100 mg, then 50–100 mg every 4–6 hours; max. 300 mg daily

**Flurbiprofen** (Non-proprietary) (PoM)

Tablets, flurbiprofen 50 mg, net price 20 = £2.59; 100 mg, 20 = £5.23. Label: 21

**Froben®** (Abbott) (PoM)

Tablets, yellow, s/c, flurbiprofen 50 mg, net price 20 = £2.09; 100 mg, 20 = £3.97. Label: 21

◀**Modified release**

**Froben SR®** (Abbott) (PoM)

Capsules, m/r, yellow, flurbiprofen 200 mg, net price 30-cap pack = £7.53. Label: 21, 25

Dose ADULT and CHILD over 12 years, 1 capsule daily, preferably in the evening

## IBUPROFEN

**Indications** pain and inflammation in rheumatic disease (including juvenile idiopathic arthritis) and other musculoskeletal disorders; mild to moderate pain including dysmenorrhoea; postoperative analgesia; migraine; dental pain; fever with discomfort and pain in children; post-immunisation pyrexia (section 14.1)

**Cautions** see notes above

**Contra-indications** see notes above

**Side-effects** see notes above; **overdosage:** see Emergency Treatment of Poisoning, p. 29

**Dose**

- ADULT and CHILD over 12 years, initially 300–400 mg 3–4 times daily; increased if necessary to max. 2.4 g daily; maintenance dose of 0.6–1.2 g daily may be adequate

- Pain and fever in children, CHILD 1–3 months, see *BNF for Children*; CHILD 3–6 months (body-weight over 5 kg), 50 mg 3 times daily (max. 30 mg/kg daily in 3–4 divided doses); CHILD 6 months–1 year, 50 mg 3–4 times daily (max. 30 mg/kg daily in 3–4 divided doses); CHILD 1–4 years, 100 mg 3 times daily (max. 30 mg/kg daily in 3–4 divided doses); CHILD 4–7 years, 150 mg 3 times daily (max. 30 mg/kg daily in 3–4 divided doses); CHILD 7–10 years, 200 mg 3 times daily (up to 30 mg/kg daily (max. 2.4 g) in 3–4 divided doses); CHILD 10–12 years, 300 mg 3 times daily (up to 30 mg/kg daily (max. 2.4 g) in 3–4 divided doses)

- Rheumatic disease in children (including juvenile idiopathic arthritis), CHILD 3 months–18 years (body-weight over 5 kg), 30–40 mg/kg (max. 2.4 g) daily in 3–4 divided doses; in systemic juvenile idiopathic arthritis up to 60 mg/kg (max. 2.4 g) daily [unlicensed] in 4–6 divided doses

[1] **Ibuprofen** (Non-proprietary) (PoM)

Tablets, coated, ibuprofen 200 mg, net price 84-tab pack = £2.03; 400 mg, 84-tab pack = £2.38; 600 mg, 84-tab pack = £3.73. Label: 21
Brands include *Arthrofen®*, *Ebufac®*, *Rimafen®*

Oral suspension, ibuprofen 100 mg/5 mL, net price 100 mL = £1.47, 150 mL = £2.71, 500 mL = £8.53. Label: 21

**Note** Sugar-free versions are available and can be ordered by specifying 'sugar-free' on the prescription
Brands include *Calprofen®*, *Fenpaed®*, *Feverfen®*, *Nurofen® for Children*, *Orbifen®* for Children

**Dental prescribing on NHS** Ibuprofen Tablets and Ibuprofen Oral Suspension Sugar-free may be prescribed

1. Can be sold to the public in certain circumstances; for exemptions see *Medicines, Ethics and Practice*, No. 33, London, Pharmaceutical Press, 2009 (and subsequent editions as available)

**Brufen®** (Abbott) (PoM)

Tablets, f/c, ibuprofen 200 mg, net price 100-tab pack = £3.92; 400 mg, 100-tab pack = £8.16; 600 mg, 100-tab pack = £12.24. Label: 21

Syrup, orange, ibuprofen 100 mg/5 mL, net price 500 mL (orange-flavoured) = £8.88. Label: 21

Granules, effervescent, ibuprofen 600 mg/sachet, net price 20-sachet pack = £6.53. Label: 13, 21
Electrolytes Na+ approx. 9 mmol/sachet

◄**Modified release**
**Brufen Retard®** (Abbott) (PoM)

Tablets, m/r, ibuprofen 800 mg, net price 56-tab pack = £6.48. Label: 25, 27
Dose ADULT and CHILD over 12 years, 2 tablets daily as a single dose, preferably in the early evening, increased in severe cases to 3 tablets daily in 2 divided doses

**Fenbid®** (Goldshield) (PoM)

Spansule® (= capsule m/r), maroon/pink, enclosing off-white pellets, ibuprofen 300 mg, net price 120-cap pack = £9.64. Label: 25
Dose ADULT and CHILD over 12 years, initially 2 capsules twice daily, increased in severe cases to 3 capsules twice daily; then 1–2 capsules twice daily

◄**Topical preparations**
Section 10.3.2

## INDOMETACIN
(Indomethacin)

**Indications** pain and moderate to severe inflammation in rheumatic disease and other acute musculoskeletal disorders; acute gout; dysmenorrhoea; closure of ductus arteriosus (section 7.1.1.1); premature labour (section 7.1.3)

**Cautions** see notes above; also epilepsy, parkinsonism, psychiatric disturbances; during prolonged therapy ophthalmic and blood examinations particularly advisable; avoid rectal administration in proctitis and haemorrhoids
Driving Dizziness may affect performance of skilled tasks (e.g. driving)

**Contra-indications** see notes above

**Side-effects** see notes above; *rarely*, confusion, convulsions, psychiatric disturbances, depression, syncope, blood disorders (particularly thrombocytopenia), hyperglycaemia, blurred vision, corneal deposits, peripheral neuropathy, and intestinal strictures; suppositories may cause rectal irritation and occasional bleeding

**Dose**
• By mouth, rheumatic disease, 50–200 mg daily in divided doses; CHILD see *BNF for Children*
Acute gout, 150–200 mg daily in divided doses
Dysmenorrhoea, up to 75 mg daily
• By rectum in suppositories, 100 mg at night and in the morning if required; CHILD not recommended
Combined oral and rectal treatment, max. total daily dose 150–200 mg

**Indometacin** (Non-proprietary) (PoM)

Capsules, indometacin 25 mg, net price 28-cap pack = £1.46; 50 mg, 28-cap pack = £1.76. Label: 21, counselling, driving, see above
Brands include *Rimacid®*

Suppositories, indometacin 100 mg, net price 10 = £15.04. Counselling, driving, see above

◄**Modified release**
**Indometacin m/r preparations** (PoM)

Capsules, m/r, indometacin 75 mg. Label: 21, 25, counselling, driving, see above
Brands include *Indolar SR®*, *Pardelprin®*,
Dose 1 capsule 1–2 times daily; CHILD not recommended

## KETOPROFEN

**Indications** pain and mild inflammation in rheumatic disease and other musculoskeletal disorders, and after orthopaedic surgery; acute gout; dysmenorrhoea

**Cautions** see notes above

**Contra-indications** see notes above

**Side-effects** see notes above; pain may occur at injection site (occasionally tissue damage); suppositories may cause rectal irritation

**Dose**
• By mouth, rheumatic disease, 100–200 mg daily in 2–4 divided doses; CHILD not recommended
Pain and dysmenorrhoea, 50 mg up to 3 times daily; CHILD not recommended
• By rectum in suppositories, rheumatic disease, 100 mg at bedtime; CHILD not recommended
Combined oral and rectal treatment, max. total daily dose 200 mg
• By deep intramuscular injection into the gluteal muscle, 50–100 mg every 4 hours (max. 200 mg in 24 hours) for up to 3 days; CHILD not recommended

**Ketoprofen** (Non-proprietary) (PoM)

Capsules, ketoprofen 50 mg, net price 28-cap pack = £9.32; 100 mg, 56-cap pack = £6.66. Label: 21

**Orudis®** (Sanofi-Aventis) (PoM)

Capsules, ketoprofen 50 mg (green/purple), net price 112-cap pack = £15.44; 100 mg (pink), 56-cap pack = £15.49. Label: 21

Suppositories, ketoprofen 100 mg. Net price 10 = £6.65

**Oruvail®** (Sanofi-Aventis) (PoM)

Injection, ketoprofen 50 mg/mL. Net price 2-mL amp = £1.07

◄**Modified release**
**Oruvail®** (Sanofi-Aventis) (PoM)

Capsules, all m/r, enclosing white pellets, ketoprofen 100 mg (pink/purple), net price 56-cap pack = £23.93; 150 mg (pink), 28-cap pack = £13.66; 200 mg (pink/white), 28-cap pack = £23.85. Label: 21, 25
Dose 100–200 mg once daily with food; CHILD not recommended
Note Other brands of modified-release capsules containing ketoprofen 100 mg and 200 mg include *Ketocid®* 200 mg, *Ketovail®*, *Tiloket®* CR

◄**Topical preparations**
Section 10.3.2

## MEFENAMIC ACID

**Indications** pain and inflammation in rheumatoid arthritis and osteoarthritis; postoperative pain; mild to moderate pain; dysmenorrhoea and menorrhagia

**Cautions** see notes above; epilepsy; acute porphyria (section 9.8.2)

**Contra-indications** see notes above; inflammatory bowel disease

**Side-effects** see notes above; also diarrhoea or rashes (withdraw treatment), stomatitis; *less commonly* paraesthesia and fatigue; *rarely* hypotension, palpitation, glucose intolerance, thrombocytopenia, haemolytic anaemia (positive Coombs' test), and aplastic anaemia reported

**Dose**

- ADULT over 18 years, 500 mg 3 times daily
- CHILD 12–18 years, acute pain including dysmenorrhoea, menorrhagia, 500 mg 3 times daily
- CHILD under 12 years not recommended

**Mefenamic Acid** (Non-proprietary) PoM

Capsules, mefenamic acid 250 mg, net price 100-cap pack = £3.72. Label: 21

Tablets, mefenamic acid 500 mg, net price 28-tab pack = £1.93. Label: 21

Suspension, mefenamic acid 50 mg/5 mL, net price 125 mL = £79.99. Label: 21
Excipients include ethanol

**Ponstan®** (Chemidex) PoM

Capsules, blue/ivory, mefenamic acid 250 mg, net price 100-cap pack = £8.17. Label: 21

Forte tablets, yellow, mefenamic acid 500 mg, net price 100-tab pack = £15.72. Label: 21

## ▌ MELOXICAM

**Indications** pain and inflammation in rheumatic disease; exacerbation of osteoarthritis (short-term); ankylosing spondylitis

**Cautions** see notes above; avoid rectal administration in proctitis or haemorrhoids

**Contra-indications** see notes above; severe heart failure

**Side-effects** see notes above

**Dose**

- By mouth, osteoarthritis, 7.5 mg daily, increased if necessary to max. 15 mg once daily
  Rheumatoid arthritis, ankylosing spondylitis, 15 mg once daily, may be reduced to 7.5 mg daily; ELDERLY 7.5 mg daily
- By rectum, in suppositories, osteoarthritis, 7.5 mg daily, increased if necessary to max. 15 mg once daily
  Rheumatoid arthritis, ankylosing spondylitis, 15 mg once daily, may be reduced to 7.5 mg daily; ELDERLY 7.5 mg daily
- CHILD under 15 years not recommended

**Meloxicam** (Non-proprietary) PoM

Tablets, meloxicam 7.5 mg, net price 30-tab pack = £2.65; 15 mg, 30-tab pack = £3.15. Label: 21

**Mobic®** (Boehringer Ingelheim) PoM

Tablets, yellow, scored, meloxicam 7.5 mg, net price 30-tab pack = £9.30; 15 mg, 30-tab pack = £12.93. Label: 21
Note Tablets may be dispersed in water

Suppositories, meloxicam 7.5 mg, net price 12 = £3.72; 15 mg, 12 = £5.58

## ▌ NABUMETONE

**Indications** pain and inflammation in osteoarthritis and rheumatoid arthritis

**Cautions** see notes above

**Contra-indications** see notes above

**Side-effects** see notes above

**Dose**

- 1 g at night; severe or persistent symptoms 0.5–1 g in morning and 1 g at night; ELDERLY 0.5–1 g daily; CHILD not recommended

**Nabumetone** (Non-proprietary) PoM

Tablets, nabumetone 500 mg, net price 56-tab pack = £6.80. Label: 21

**Relifex®** (Meda) PoM

Tablets, red, f/c, nabumetone 500 mg. Net price 56-tab pack = £5.18. Label: 21

Suspension, sugar-free, nabumetone 500 mg/5 mL. Net price 300-mL pack = £24.08. Label: 21

## ▌ NAPROXEN

**Indications** pain and inflammation in rheumatic disease (including juvenile idiopathic arthritis) and other musculoskeletal disorders; dysmenorrhoea; acute gout

**Cautions** see notes above

**Contra-indications** see notes above

**Side-effects** see notes above

**Dose**

- Rheumatic disease, 0.5–1 g daily in 1–2 divided doses; CHILD 2–18 years, juvenile idiopathic arthritis, see *BNF for Children*
- Acute musculoskeletal disorders and dysmenorrhoea, 500 mg initially, then 250 mg every 6–8 hours as required; max. dose after first day 1.25 g daily; CHILD under 18 years, see *BNF for Children*
- Acute gout, 750 mg initially, then 250 mg every 8 hours until attack has passed; CHILD under 16 years not recommended

[1]**Naproxen** (Non-proprietary) PoM

Tablets, naproxen 250 mg, net price 28-tab pack = £1.33; 500 mg, 28-tab pack = £1.78. Label: 21
Brands include *Arthroxen®*

Tablets, e/c, naproxen 250 mg, net price 56-tab pack = £5.67; 375 mg, 56-tab pack = £16.82; 500 mg, 56-tab pack = £8.11. Label: 5, 25

1. Can be sold to the public for the treatment of primary dysmenorrhoea in women aged 15–50 years subject to max. single dose of 500 mg, max. daily dose of 750 mg for max. 3 days, and a max. pack size of 9 × 250 mg tablets

**Naprosyn®** (Roche) PoM

Tablets, yellow, scored, naproxen 250 mg, net price 56-tab pack = £4.37; 500 mg, 56-tab pack = £8.74. Label: 21

Tablets, e/c, (*Naprosyn EC®*), naproxen 250 mg, net price 56-tab pack = £4.37; 375 mg, 56-tab pack = £6.55; 500 mg, 56-tab pack = £8.74. Label: 5, 25

**Synflex®** (Roche) PoM

Tablets, blue, naproxen sodium 275 mg, net price 60-tab pack = £7.25. Label: 21
Note 275 mg naproxen sodium ≡ 250 mg naproxen
Dose musculoskeletal disorders, postoperative analgesia, 550 mg twice daily when necessary, preferably after food; max. 1.1 g daily; CHILD under 16 years not recommended
Dysmenorrhoea and acute gout, initially 550 mg then 275 mg every 6–8 hours as required; max. of 1.375 g on first day and 1.1 g daily thereafter; CHILD under 16 years not recommended
Migraine, 825 mg at onset, then 275–550 mg at least 30 minutes after initial dose; max. 1.375 g in 24 hours; CHILD under 16 years not recommended

**10**

**Musculoskeletal and joint diseases**

**◄With misoprostol**

For **cautions**, **contra-indications**, and **side-effects** of misoprostol, see section 1.3.4

**Napratec®** (Pharmacia) ℗ℴ𝗠

Combination pack, 56 yellow scored tablets, naproxen 500 mg; 56 white scored tablets, misoprostol 200 micrograms. Net price = £23.76. Label: 21

Dose patients requiring naproxen for rheumatoid arthritis, osteoarthritis, or ankylosing spondylitis, with prophylaxis against NSAID-induced gastroduodenal ulceration, 1 naproxen 500-mg tablet and 1 misoprostol 200-microgram tablet taken together twice daily with food; CHILD not recommended

## ◼ PIROXICAM ▱

**Indications** pain and inflammation in rheumatic disease (including juvenile idiopathic arthritis) and other musculoskeletal disorders; acute gout

**Cautions** see notes above and CHMP advice below

**Contra-indications** see notes above

**Side-effects** see notes above; pain at injection site (occasionally tissue damage)

**Dose**

- By mouth, rheumatic disease, initially 20 mg daily, increased if necessary to 30 mg daily in single or divided doses; CHILD (6–18 years), juvenile idiopathic arthritis, under 15 kg, 5 mg daily; 16–25 kg, 10 mg; 26–45 kg, 15 mg; over 46 kg, 20 mg (but see CHMP advice below)

Acute musculoskeletal disorders, 40 mg daily in single or divided doses for 2 days, then 20 mg daily for 7–14 days (but see CHMP advice below); CHILD not recommended

Acute gout, 40 mg initially, then 40 mg daily in single or divided doses for 4–6 days (but see CHMP advice below); CHILD not recommended

> **CHMP advice**
> **Piroxicam (June 2007)**
> The CHMP has recommended restrictions on the use of piroxicam because of the increased risk of gastrointestinal side effects and serious skin reactions. The CHMP has advised that:
> - piroxicam should be initiated only by physicians experienced in treating inflammatory or degenerative rheumatic diseases
> - piroxicam should not be used as first-line treatment
> - in adults, use of piroxicam should be limited to the symptomatic relief of osteoarthritis, rheumatoid arthritis, and ankylosing spondylitis
> - piroxicam dose should not exceed 20 mg daily
> - piroxicam should no longer be used for the treatment of acute painful and inflammatory conditions
> - treatment should be reviewed 2 weeks after initiating piroxicam, and periodically thereafter
> - concomitant administration of a gastro-protective agent (section 1.3) should be considered
>
> **Note** Topical preparations containing piroxicam are not affected by these restrictions

**Piroxicam** (Non-proprietary) ℗ℴ𝗠 ▱

Capsules, piroxicam 10 mg, net price 56-cap pack = £1.96; 20 mg, 28-cap pack = £1.96. Label: 21

Dispersible tablets, piroxicam 10 mg, net price 56-tab pack = £9.96; 20 mg, 28-tab pack = £33.25. Label: 13, 21

**Brexidol®** (Chiesi) ℗ℴ𝗠 ▱

Tablets, yellow, scored, piroxicam (as betadex) 20 mg, net price 30-tab pack = £14.09. Label: 21

Dose osteoarthritis, rheumatic disease and acute musculoskeletal disorders, 1 tablet daily (may be halved in elderly); CHILD not recommended

**Feldene®** (Pfizer) ℗ℴ𝗠 ▱

Capsules, piroxicam 10 mg (red/blue), net price 56-cap pack = £7.20; 20 mg (white), 28-cap pack = £7.20. Label: 21

Tablets, (*Feldene Melt*), piroxicam 20 mg, net price 28-tab pack = £9.83. Label: 10, patient information leaflet, 21

Excipients include aspartame equivalent to phenylalanine 140 micrograms/tablet (section 9.4.1)

Note *Feldene Melt®* tablets can be taken by placing on tongue or by swallowing

**◄Topical preparations**

Section 10.3.2

## ◼ SULINDAC

**Indications** pain and inflammation in rheumatic disease and other musculoskeletal disorders; acute gout

**Cautions** see notes above; also history of renal stones and ensure adequate hydration

**Contra-indications** see notes above

**Side-effects** see notes above; jaundice with fever, cholestasis, hepatitis, hepatic failure; also urine discoloration occasionally reported

**Dose**

- 200 mg twice daily (may be reduced according to response); max. 400 mg daily; acute gout should respond within 7 days; limit treatment of peri-articular disorders to 7–10 days; CHILD not recommended

**Sulindac** (Non-proprietary) ℗ℴ𝗠

Tablets, sulindac 100 mg, net price 56-tab pack = £17.12; 200 mg, 56-tab pack = £34.60. Label: 21

## ◼ TENOXICAM

**Indications** pain and inflammation in rheumatic disease and other musculoskeletal disorders

**Cautions** see notes above

**Contra-indications** see notes above

**Side-effects** see notes above

**Dose**

- By mouth, rheumatic disease, 20 mg daily; CHILD not recommended

Acute musculoskeletal disorders, 20 mg daily for 7 days; max. duration of treatment 14 days (including treatment by intravenous or intramuscular injection); CHILD not recommended

- By intravenous *or* intramuscular injection, initial treatment for 1–2 days if oral administration not possible, 20 mg once daily; CHILD not recommended

**Tenoxicam** (Non-proprietary) ℗ℴ𝗠

Tablets, f/c, tenoxicam 20 mg, net price 28-tab pack = £12.76. Label: 21

Injection, powder for reconstitution, tenoxicam, net price 20-mg vial = £3.98

**Mobiflex®** (Roche) ℗ℴ𝗠

Tablets, yellow, f/c, tenoxicam 20 mg, net price 30-tab pack = £12.92. Label: 21

## TIAPROFENIC ACID

**Indications** pain and inflammation in rheumatic disease and other musculoskeletal disorders

**Cautions** see notes above

**Contra-indications** see notes above; also active bladder or prostate disease (or symptoms) and history of recurrent urinary-tract disorders—if urinary symptoms develop discontinue immediately and perform urine tests and culture; see also CSM advice below

> **CSM advice**
> Following reports of **severe cystitis** the CSM has recommended that tiaprofenic acid should not be given to patients with urinary-tract disorders and should be stopped if urinary symptoms develop. Patients should be advised to stop taking tiaprofenic acid and to report to their doctor promptly if they develop urinary-tract symptoms (such as increased frequency, nocturia, urgency, pain on urinating, or blood in urine)

**Side-effects** see notes above

**Dose**

- 300 mg twice daily; CHILD not recommended

**Surgam®** (Sanofi-Aventis) PoM
Tablets, tiaprofenic acid 300 mg, net price 56-tab pack = £14.95. Label: 21

---

## Aspirin

Aspirin (section 4.7.1) has been used in high doses to treat rheumatoid arthritis, but other NSAIDs are now preferred.

## 10.1.2 Corticosteroids

### 10.1.2.1 Systemic corticosteroids

The general actions, uses, and cautions of corticosteroids are described in section 6.3. Short-term treatment with corticosteroids can help to rapidly improve symptoms of rheumatoid arthritis. Long-term treatment in rheumatoid arthritis should be considered only after evaluating the risks and all other treatment options have been considered. Corticosteroids can induce osteoporosis, and prophylaxis should be considered on long-term treatment (section 6.6).

In severe, possibly life-threatening, situations a high initial dose of corticosteroid is given to induce remission and the dose is then reduced gradually and discontinued altogether. Relapse may occur as the dose of corticosteroid is reduced, particularly if the reduction is too rapid. The tendency is therefore to increase the maintenance dose and consequently the patient becomes dependent on corticosteroids. For this reason pulse doses of corticosteroids (e.g. methylprednisolone up to 1 g intravenously on 3 consecutive days) are used to suppress highly active inflammatory disease while longer-term treatment with a disease-modifying drug is commenced.

**Prednisolone** 7.5 mg daily may reduce the rate of joint destruction in moderate to severe *rheumatoid arthritis* of less than 2 years' duration. The reduction in joint destruction must be distinguished from mere symptomatic improvement (which lasts only 6 to 12 months at this dose) and care should be taken to avoid increasing the dose above 7.5 mg daily. Evidence supports maintenance of this anti-erosive dose for 2–4 years only after which treatment should be tapered off to reduce long-term adverse effects.

*Polymyalgia rheumatica* and *giant cell (temporal) arteritis* are always treated with corticosteroids. The usual initial dose of prednisolone in polymyalgia rheumatica is 10–15 mg daily and in giant cell arteritis 40–60 mg daily (the higher dose being used if visual symptoms occur). Treatment should be continued until remission of disease activity and doses are then reduced gradually to about 7.5–10 mg daily for maintenance. Relapse is common if therapy is stopped prematurely. Many patients require treatment for at least 2 years and in some patients it may be necessary to continue long-term low-dose corticosteroid treatment.

*Polyarteritis nodosa* and *polymyositis* are usually treated with corticosteroids. An initial dose of 60 mg of prednisolone daily is often used and reduced to a maintenance dose of 10–15 mg daily.

*Systemic lupus erythematosus* is treated with corticosteroids when necessary using a similar dosage regimen to that for polyarteritis nodosa and polymyositis (above). Patients with pleurisy, pericarditis, or other systemic manifestations will respond to corticosteroids. It may then be possible to reduce the dosage; alternate-day treatment is sometimes adequate, and the drug may be gradually withdrawn. In some mild cases corticosteroid treatment may be stopped after a few months. Many mild cases of systemic lupus erythematosus do not require corticosteroid treatment. Alternative treatment with anti-inflammatory analgesics, and possibly chloroquine or hydroxychloroquine, should be considered.

*Ankylosing spondylitis* should not be treated with long-term corticosteroids; rarely, pulse doses may be needed and may be useful in extremely active disease that does not respond to conventional treatment.

### 10.1.2.2 Local corticosteroid injections

Corticosteroids are injected locally for an anti-inflammatory effect. In inflammatory conditions of the joints, particularly in rheumatoid arthritis, they are given by *intra-articular injection* to relieve pain, increase mobility, and reduce deformity in one or a few joints. Full aseptic precautions are essential; infected areas should be avoided. Occasionally an acute inflammatory reaction develops after an intra-articular or soft-tissue injection of a corticosteroid. This may be a reaction to the microcrystalline suspension of the corticosteroid used, but must be distinguished from sepsis introduced into the injection site.

Smaller amounts of corticosteroids may also be injected directly into soft tissues for the relief of inflammation in conditions such as *tennis* or *golfer's elbow* or *compression neuropathies*. In *tendinitis*, injections should be made into the tendon sheath and not directly into the tendon (due to the absence of a true tendon sheath and a high risk of rupture, the Achilles tendon should not be injected).

Hydrocortisone acetate or one of the synthetic analogues is generally used for local injection. Intra-articular corticosteroid injections can cause flushing and may affect the hyaline cartilage. Each joint should usually be treated no more than 3 times in one year.

Corticosteroid injections are also injected into soft tissues for the treatment of skin lesions (see section 13.4).

## ■ LOCAL CORTICOSTEROID INJECTIONS

**Indications**  local inflammation of joints and soft tissues (for details, consult product literature)

**Cautions**  see notes above and consult product literature; see also section 6.3.2

**Contra-indications**  see notes above and consult product literature; avoid injections containing benzyl alcohol in neonates (see preparations below)

**Side-effects**  see notes above and consult product literature

**Dose**
• See under preparations

### ◢Betamethasone
**Betnesol®** (UCB Pharma) [PoM]
Injection, betamethasone (as sodium phosphate) 4 mg/mL, net price 1-mL amp = £1.17.

### ◢Dose calculated as dexamethasone
**Dexamethasone** (Organon) [PoM]
Injection, dexamethasone 4 mg/mL (as sodium phosphate) (≡ dexamethasone sodium phosphate 5.2 mg/mL ≡ dexamethasone phosphate 4.8 mg/mL), net price 1-mL amp = 83p; 2-mL vial = £1.27
Dose  by intra-articular or intrasynovial injection (for details consult product literature), 0.3–3 mg (calculated as dexamethasone) according to size; where appropriate may be repeated at intervals of 3–21 days according to response

### ◢Dose calculated as dexamethasone phosphate
**Dexamethasone** (Hospira) [PoM]
Injection, dexamethasone phosphate 4 mg/mL (as sodium phosphate) (≡ dexamethasone 3.3 mg/mL ≡ dexamethasone sodium phosphate 4.4 mg/mL), net price 1-mL amp = £1.00; 2-mL vial = £1.98
Dose  by intra-articular or intrasynovial injection (for details consult product literature), 0.4–4 mg (calculated as dexamethasone phosphate) according to size (by soft-tissue infiltration 2–6 mg); where appropriate may be repeated at intervals of 3–21 days

### ◢Hydrocortisone acetate
**Hydrocortistab®** (Sovereign) [PoM]
Injection (aqueous suspension), hydrocortisone acetate 25 mg/mL, net price 1-mL amp = £5.72
Dose  by intra-articular or intrasynovial injection (for details consult product literature), 5–50 mg according to size; where appropriate may be repeated at intervals of 21 days; not more than 3 joints should be treated on any one day; CHILD 5–30 mg (divided)

### ◢Methylprednisolone acetate
**Depo-Medrone®** (Pharmacia) [PoM]
Injection (aqueous suspension), methylprednisolone acetate 40 mg/mL, net price 1-mL vial = £2.87; 2-mL vial = £5.15; 3-mL vial = £7.47
Dose  by intra-articular or intrasynovial injection (for details consult product literature), 4–80 mg, according to size; where appropriate may be repeated at intervals of 7–35 days; also for intralesional injection

**Depo-Medrone® with Lidocaine** (Pharmacia) [PoM]
Injection (aqueous suspension), methylprednisolone acetate 40 mg, lidocaine hydrochloride 10 mg/mL, net price 1-mL vial = £3.28; 2-mL vial = £5.88
Dose  by intra-articular or intrasynovial injection (for details consult product literature), 4–80 mg, according to size; where appropriate may be repeated at intervals of 7–35 days

### ◢Prednisolone acetate
**Deltastab®** (Sovereign) [PoM]
Injection (aqueous suspension), prednisolone acetate 25 mg/mL, net price 1-mL amp = £5.73
Dose  by intra-articular or intrasynovial injection (for details consult product literature), 5–25 mg according to size; not more than 3 joints should be treated on any one day; where appropriate may be repeated when relapse occurs
For intramuscular injection, see section 6.3.2

### ◢Triamcinolone acetonide
**Adcortyl® Intra-articular/Intradermal** (Squibb) [PoM]
Injection (aqueous suspension), triamcinolone acetonide 10 mg/mL, net price 1-mL amp = 91p; 5-mL vial = £3.70
Excipients include benzyl alcohol (avoid in neonates, see Excipients, p. 2)
Dose  by intra-articular injection or intrasynovial injection (for details consult product literature), 2.5–15 mg according to size (for larger doses use Kenalog®); where appropriate may be repeated when relapse occurs
By intradermal injection, (for details consult product literature): 2–3 mg; max. 5 mg at any one site (total max. 30 mg); where appropriate may be repeated at intervals of 1–2 weeks
CHILD under 6 years not recommended

**Kenalog® Intra-articular/Intramuscular** (Squibb) [PoM]
Injection (aqueous suspension), triamcinolone acetonide 40 mg/mL, net price 1-mL vial = £1.52; 1-mL prefilled syringe = £1.88
Note Intramuscular needle with prefilled syringe should be replaced for intra-articular injection
Dose  by intra-articular or intrasynovial injection (for details consult product literature), 5–40 mg according to size; total max. 80 mg (for doses below 5 mg use Adcortyl® Intra-articular/Intradermal); where appropriate may be repeated when relapse occurs; CHILD under 18 years see BNF for Children
For intramuscular injection, see section 6.3.2

## 10.1.3 Drugs that suppress the rheumatic disease process

Certain drugs such as those affecting the immune response can suppress the disease process in *rheumatoid arthritis* and *psoriatic arthritis*; gold, penicillamine, hydroxychloroquine, chloroquine, and sulfasalazine can also suppress the disease process in *rheumatoid arthritis* while sulfasalazine and possibly gold can suppress the disease process in *psoriatic arthritis*. Unlike NSAIDs, disease-modifying anti-rheumatic drugs (DMARDs) can affect the progression of disease but may require 2–6 months of treatment for a full therapeutic response. Since in the first few months of treatment, the course of rheumatoid arthritis is unpredictable and the diagnosis uncertain, it is usual to start treatment with an NSAID alone. However, disease-modifying anti-rheumatic drugs should be initiated by specialists as soon as diagnosis, progression, and severity of the disease have been confirmed. Response to a disease-modifying anti-rheumatic drug may allow the dose of the NSAID to be reduced.

Disease-modifying antirheumatic drugs can improve not only the symptoms of inflammatory joint disease but also extra-articular manifestations such as vasculitis. They reduce the erythrocyte sedimentation rate, C-reactive protein, and sometimes the titre of rheumatoid factor; some also retard erosive damage as judged radiologically.

**Choice** The choice of a disease-modifying anti-rheumatic drug should take into account co-morbidity and patient preference. Methotrexate, sulfasalazine, intramuscular gold and penicillamine are similar in efficacy. However, **methotrexate** or **sulfasalazine** may be better tolerated.

A combination of **DMARDs** (including methotrexate and at least one other DMARD) and a short-term **corticosteroid** (section 10.1.2), should be given to patients with newly diagnosed active rheumatoid arthritis, ideally within 3 months of the onset of persistent symptoms. If the use of particular DMARDs is contra-indicated and combination therapy is not possible, monotherapy with a suitable DMARD should be given and the dose rapidly increased until clinically effective. In patients with established and stable rheumatoid arthritis, cautiously reduce drug doses to the lowest that are clinically effective. Response to drug treatment often produces a striking reduction in requirements of both corticosteroids and other drugs.

**Gold** and **penicillamine** are effective in *palindromic rheumatism*. *Systemic* and *discoid lupus erythematosus* are sometimes treated with **chloroquine** or **hydroxychloroquine**.

If a disease-modifying anti-rheumatic drug does not lead to an objective benefit within 6 months, it should be replaced by a different one.

**Juvenile idiopathic arthritis** Many children with *juvenile idiopathic arthritis* (juvenile chronic arthritis) do not require disease-modifying antirheumatic drugs. Methotrexate is effective [unlicensed indication]; sulfasalazine is an alternative [unlicensed indication] but it should be avoided in *systemic-onset juvenile idiopathic arthritis*. Gold and penicillamine are no longer used. For the role of adalimumab and etanercept in *polyarticular juvenile idiopathic arthritis*, see p. 576

## Gold

**Gold** can be given by intramuscular injection as sodium aurothiomalate or by mouth as auranofin.

**Sodium aurothiomalate** must be given by deep intramuscular injection and the area gently massaged. A test dose of 10 mg must be given followed by doses of 50 mg at weekly intervals until there is definite evidence of remission. Benefit is not to be expected until about 300–500 mg has been given. It should be discontinued if there is no remission after 1 g has been given. In patients who do respond, the interval between injections is then gradually increased to 4 weeks and treatment is continued for up to 5 years after complete remission. If relapse occurs the dosage frequency may be immediately increased to 50 mg weekly and only once control has been obtained again should the dosage frequency be decreased; if no response is seen within 2 months,

alternative treatment should be sought. It is important to avoid complete relapse since second courses of gold are not usually effective. Children can be given 1 mg/kg weekly to a maximum of 50 mg weekly, the intervals being gradually increased to 4 weeks according to response; an initial test dose is given corresponding to one-tenth to one-fifth of the calculated dose.

**Auranofin** is given by mouth. If there is no response after 6 months treatment should be discontinued. Auranofin is less effective than parenteral gold.

Gold therapy should be discontinued in the presence of blood disorders, gastro-intestinal bleeding (associated with ulcerative enterocolitis), or unexplained proteinuria (associated with immune complex nephritis) which is repeatedly above 300 mg/litre. Urine tests and full blood counts (including total and differential white cell and platelet counts) must therefore be performed before starting treatment with gold and before each intramuscular injection; in the case of oral treatment the urine and blood tests should be carried out monthly. Rashes with pruritus often occur after 2 to 6 months of intramuscular treatment and may necessitate discontinuation of treatment; the most common side-effect of oral therapy, diarrhoea with or without nausea or abdominal pain, may respond to bulking agents (such as bran) or temporary reduction in dosage.

### AURANOFIN

**Indications**  active progressive rheumatoid arthritis

**Cautions**  see under Sodium Aurothiomalate; inflammatory bowel disease; pregnancy (Appendix 4); breast-feeding (Appendix 5)

**Blood counts**  Withdraw if platelet count falls below 100 000/$mm^3$ or if signs and symptoms suggestive of thrombocytopenia occur, see also notes above

**Counselling**  Patients should be advised to seek prompt medical attention if diarrhoea, rectal bleeding, sore throat, fever, infection, non-specific illness, unexplained bleeding and bruising, purpura, mouth ulcers, metallic taste, rash, breathlessness, or cough develop

**Contra-indications**  see under Sodium Aurothiomalate

**Side-effects**  see under Sodium Aurothiomalate; headache and dizziness

**Dose**

● Administered on expert advice, 6 mg daily (initially in 2 divided doses then if tolerated as single dose), if response inadequate after 6 months, increase to 9 mg daily (in 3 divided doses), discontinue if no response after a further 3 months; CHILD not recommended

**Ridaura®** (Astellas) [PoM]
Tablets, yellow, f/c, auranofin 3 mg, net price 60-tab pack = £25.20. Label: 11, 21, counselling, blood disorder symptoms (see above)

### SODIUM AUROTHIOMALATE

**Indications**  active progressive rheumatoid arthritis, juvenile idiopathic arthritis

**Cautions**  see notes above; elderly, history of urticaria, eczema, colitis; monitor for pulmonary fibrosis with annual chest X-ray; hepatic impairment (avoid if severe); renal impairment (avoid if severe); pregnancy (Appendix 4); breast-feeding (Appendix 5); **interactions:** Appendix 1 (gold)

**Counselling**  Patients should be advised to seek prompt medical attention if diarrhoea, sore throat, fever, infection, non-specific illness, unexplained bleeding and bruising,

**10**

**Musculoskeletal and joint diseases**

purpura, mouth ulcers, metallic taste, rash, breathlessness, or cough develop

**Contra-indications** history of blood disorders or bone marrow aplasia, exfoliative dermatitis, systemic lupus erythematosus, necrotising enterocolitis, pulmonary fibrosis; acute porphyria (section 9.8.2)

**Side-effects** see notes above; also severe anaphylactic reactions; stomatitis, taste disturbances, colitis, hepatotoxicity with cholestatic jaundice, pulmonary fibrosis, peripheral neuropathy, mouth ulcers, proteinuria, blood disorders (sometimes sudden and fatal), nephrotic syndrome, gold deposits in eye, alopecia, and skin reactions (including, on prolonged parenteral treatment, irreversible pigmentation in sun-exposed areas)

**Dose**

● By deep intramuscular injection, administered on expert advice, see notes above

**Myocrisin®** (Sanofi-Aventis) [PoM]
Injection, sodium aurothiomalate 20 mg/mL, net price 0.5-mL (10-mg) amp = £3.80; 100 mg/mL, 0.5-mL (50-mg) amp = £11.23. Label: 11, counselling, blood disorder symptoms

---

## Penicillamine

Penicillamine has a similar action to gold. More patients are able to continue treatment than with gold but side-effects are common.

Patients should be warned not to expect improvement for at least 6 to 12 weeks after treatment is initiated. Penicillamine should be discontinued if there is no improvement within 1 year.

Blood counts, including platelets, and urine examinations should be carried out before starting treatment and then every 1 or 2 weeks for the first 2 months then every 4 weeks to detect blood disorders and proteinuria (they should also be carried out in the week after any dose increase). A reduction in platelet count calls for discontinuation with subsequent re-introduction at a lower dosage and then, if possible, gradual increase. Proteinuria, associated with immune complex nephritis, occurs in up to 30% of patients, but may resolve despite continuation of treatment; treatment may be continued provided that renal function tests remain normal, oedema is absent, and the 24-hour urinary excretion of protein does not exceed 2 g.

Nausea may occur but is not usually a problem provided that penicillamine is taken before food or on retiring and that low initial doses are used and only gradually increased. Loss of taste can occur about 6 weeks after treatment is started but usually returns 6 weeks later irrespective of whether treatment is discontinued; mineral supplements are not recommended. Rashes are a common side-effect. Those that occur in the first few months of treatment disappear when the drug is stopped and treatment may then be re-introduced at a lower dose level and gradually increased. Late rashes are more resistant and often necessitate discontinuation of treatment.

Patients who are hypersensitive to penicillin may react rarely to penicillamine.

## ▌ PENICILLAMINE

**Indications** see notes above and under Dose

**Cautions** see notes above; concomitant nephrotoxic drugs (increased risk of toxicity); gold treatment (avoid concomitant use if adverse reactions to gold); renal impairment (Appendix 3); pregnancy (Appendix 4); **interactions:** Appendix 1 (penicillamine)

**Blood counts and urine tests** See notes above. Longer intervals may be adequate in cystinuria and Wilson's disease. Consider withdrawal if platelet count falls below 120 000/ mm³ or white blood cells below 2500/mm³ or if 3 successive falls within reference range (can restart at reduced dose when counts return to within reference range but permanent withdrawal necessary if recurrence of leucopenia or thrombocytopenia)

**Counselling** Warn patient to tell doctor promptly if sore throat, fever, infection, non-specific illness, unexplained bleeding and bruising, purpura, mouth ulcers, or rashes develop

**Contra-indications** lupus erythematosus

**Side-effects** (see also notes above) initially nausea, anorexia, fever, and skin reactions; taste loss (mineral supplements not recommended); blood disorders including thrombocytopenia, leucopenia, agranulocytosis and aplastic anaemia; proteinuria, rarely haematuria (withdraw immediately); haemolytic anaemia, pancreatitis, cholestatic jaundice, nephrotic syndrome, lupus erythematosus-like syndrome, myasthenia gravis-like syndrome, neuropathy, polymyositis (rarely with cardiac involvement), dermatomyositis, mouth ulcers, stomatitis, alopecia, bronchiolitis and pneumonitis, pemphigus, Goodpasture's syndrome, neuropathy, and Stevens-Johnson syndrome also reported; male and female breast enlargement reported; in non-rheumatoid conditions rheumatoid arthritis-like syndrome also reported; late rashes (consider withdrawing treatment)

**Dose**

● Severe active rheumatoid arthritis, administered on expert advice, ADULT initially 125–250 mg daily for 1 month increased by similar amounts at intervals of not less than 4 weeks to usual maintenance of 500–750 mg daily in divided doses; max. 1.5 g daily; if remission sustained for 6 months, reduction of daily dose by 125–250 mg every 12 weeks may be attempted; ELDERLY initially up to 125 mg daily for 1 month increased by similar amounts at intervals of not less than 4 weeks; max. 1 g daily; CHILD maintenance of 15–20 mg/kg daily (initial dose lower and increased at intervals of 4 weeks over a period of 3–6 months)

● Wilson's disease, autoimmune hepatitis, and cystinuria, section 9.8.1

**Penicillamine** (Non-proprietary) [PoM]
Tablets, penicillamine 125 mg, net price 56-tab pack = £13.80; 250 mg, 56-tab pack = £20.82. Label: 6, 22, counselling, blood disorder symptoms (see above)

**Distamine®** (Alliance) [PoM]
Tablets, f/c, penicillamine 125 mg, net price 100-tab pack = £10.34; 250 mg, 100-tab pack= £17.78. Label: 6, 22, counselling, blood disorder symptoms (see above)

---

## Antimalarials

The antimalarial **hydroxychloroquine** is used to treat rheumatoid arthritis of moderate inflammatory activity; **chloroquine** is also licensed for treating inflammatory disorders but is used much less frequently and is generally reserved for use if other drugs have failed. Chloroquine and hydroxychloroquine are effective for mild systemic lupus erythematosus, particularly involving the skin and joints. These drugs should not be used for psoriatic arthritis.

Chloroquine and hydroxychloroquine are better tolerated than gold or penicillamine. Retinopathy (see below) rarely occurs provided that the recommended doses are not exceeded; in the elderly it is difficult to distinguish drug-induced retinopathy from changes of ageing.

**Mepacrine** (section 5.4.4) is sometimes used in discoid lupus erythematosus [unlicensed].

**Cautions**  Chloroquine and hydroxychloroquine should be used with caution in moderate to severe hepatic impairment and in renal impairment (Appendix 3). Manufacturers recommend regular ophthalmological examination but the evidence of practical value is unsatisfactory (see advice of the Royal College of Ophthalmologists, below). It is not necessary to withdraw an antimalarial drug during pregnancy (Appendix 4) if the rheumatic disease is well controlled. Chloroquine and hydroxychloroquine are present in breast milk and breast-feeding (Appendix 5) should be avoided when they are used to treat rheumatic disease; chloroquine can, however, be used for malaria during pregnancy and breast-feeding (section 5.4.1). Both should be used with caution in neurological disorders (especially in those with a history of epilepsy), in severe gastro-intestinal disorders, in G6PD deficiency (section 9.1.5), in acute porphyria, and in the elderly (see also above). Chloroquine and hydroxychloroquine may exacerbate psoriasis and aggravate myasthenia gravis. Concurrent use of hepatotoxic drugs should be avoided; other **interactions**: Appendix 1 (chloroquine and hydroxychloroquine).

**Screening for ocular toxicity**
A review group convened by the Royal College of Ophthalmologists has updated guidelines for screening to prevent ocular toxicity on long-term treatment with chloroquine, hydroxychloroquine, and mepacrine (*Ocular toxicity with hydroxychloroquine: guidelines for screening 2004*). Chloroquine should be considered (for treating chronic inflammatory conditions) **only** if other drugs have failed. All patients taking chloroquine should receive ocular examination according to a protocol arranged locally between the prescriber and the ophthalmologist. Mepacrine has negligible ocular toxicity. The following recommendations relate to hydroxychloroquine, which is only rarely associated with toxicity.

*Before treatment:*

● Assess renal and liver function (adjust dose if impaired)

● Ask patient about visual impairment (not corrected by glasses). If impairment or eye disease present, assessment by an optometrist is advised and any abnormality should be referred to an ophthalmologist

● Record near visual acuity of each eye (with glasses where appropriate) using a standard reading chart

● Initiate hydroxychloroquine treatment if no abnormality detected (at a dose not exceeding hydroxychloroquine sulphate 6.5 mg/kg daily)

*During treatment:*

● Ask patient about visual symptoms and monitor visual acuity annually using the standard reading chart

● Refer to ophthalmologist if visual acuity changes or if vision blurred and warn patient to stop treatment and seek prescribing doctor's advice

● A child treated for juvenile idiopathic arthritis should receive slit-lamp examination routinely to check for uveitis

● If long-term treatment is required (more than 5 years), individual arrangement should be agreed with the local ophthalmologist

Note  To avoid excessive dosage in obese patients, the doses of hydroxychloroquine and chloroquine should be calculated on the basis of lean body weight. Ocular toxicity is unlikely if the dose of chloroquine phosphate does not exceed 4 mg/kg daily (equivalent to chloroquine base approx. 2.5 mg/kg daily)

**Side-effects**  The side-effects of chloroquine and hydroxychloroquine include gastro-intestinal disturbances, headache and skin reactions (rashes, pruritus); those occurring less frequently include ECG changes, convulsions, visual changes, retinal damage (see above), keratopathy, ototoxicity, hair depigmentation, hair loss, and discoloration of skin, nails, and mucous membranes. Side-effects that occur rarely include blood disorders (including thrombocytopenia, agranulocytosis, and aplastic anaemia), mental changes (including emotional disturbances and psychosis), myopathy (including cardiomyopathy and neuromyopathy), acute generalised exanthematous pustulosis, exfoliative dermatitis, Stevens-Johnson syndrome, photosensitivity, and hepatic damage; angioedema has also been reported. **Important**: very toxic in overdosage—immediate advice from poisons centres essential (see also p. 32).

## CHLOROQUINE

**Indications**  active rheumatoid arthritis (including juvenile idiopathic arthritis), systemic and discoid lupus erythematosus; malaria (section 5.4.1)

**Cautions**  see notes above

**Side-effects**  see notes above

**Dose**

● Administered on expert advice, by mouth, chloroquine (base) 150 mg daily; max. 2.5 mg/kg daily, see recommendations above; CHILD up to 3 mg/kg daily
Note  Chloroquine base 150 mg ≡ chloroquine sulphate 200 mg ≡ chloroquine phosphate 250 mg (approx.).

◢**Preparations**
Section 5.4.1

## HYDROXYCHLOROQUINE SULPHATE

**Indications**  active rheumatoid arthritis (including juvenile idiopathic arthritis), systemic and discoid lupus erythematosus; dermatological conditions caused or aggravated by sunlight

**Cautions**  see notes above

**Side-effects**  see notes above; also reported bronchospasm

**Dose**

- Administered on expert advice, initially 400 mg daily in divided doses; maintenance 200–400 mg daily; max. 6.5 mg/kg daily (but not exceeding 400 mg daily), see recommendations above; CHILD up to 6.5 mg/kg daily (max. 400 mg daily)

**Plaquenil®** (Sanofi-Synthelabo) ᴘᴏᴹ
Tablets, f/c, hydroxychloroquine sulphate 200 mg, net price 60-tab pack = £5.25. Label: 5, 21

## Drugs affecting the immune response

**Methotrexate** is a disease-modifying antirheumatic drug suitable for moderate to severe rheumatoid arthritis. **Azathioprine, ciclosporin, cyclophosphamide, leflunomide**, and the **cytokine modulators** (adalimumab, anakinra, etanercept, and infliximab) are considered more toxic and they are used in cases that have not responded to other disease-modifying drugs.

**Methotrexate** is usually given in an initial dose of 7.5 mg by mouth once a week, adjusted according to response to a maximum of 15 mg once a week (occasionally 20 mg once a week). Regular full blood counts (including differential white cell count and platelet count), renal and liver function tests are required. In patients who experience mucosal or gastro-intestinal side-effects with methotrexate, folic acid 5 mg every week may help to reduce the frequency of such side-effects.

**Azathioprine** is usually given in a dose of 1.5 to 2.5 mg/kg daily in divided doses. Blood counts are needed to detect possible neutropenia or thrombocytopenia (usually resolved by reducing the dose). Nausea, vomiting, and diarrhoea may occur, usually starting early during the course of treatment, and may necessitate withdrawal of the drug; herpes zoster infection may also occur.

**Leflunomide** acts on the immune system as a disease-modifying antirheumatic drug. Its therapeutic effect starts after 4–6 weeks and improvement may continue for a further 4–6 months. Leflunomide, which is similar in efficacy to sulfasalazine and methotrexate, may be chosen when these drugs cannot be used. The active metabolite of leflunomide persists for a long period; active procedures to wash the drug out are required in case of serious adverse effects, or before starting treatment with another disease-modifying antirheumatic drug, or, in men or women, before conception. Side-effects of leflunomide include bone-marrow toxicity; its immunosuppressive effects increase the risk of infection and malignancy.

**Ciclosporin** (cyclosporin) is licensed for severe active rheumatoid arthritis when conventional second-line therapy is inappropriate or ineffective. There is some evidence that ciclosporin may retard the rate of erosive progression and improve symptom control in those who respond only partially to methotrexate.

**Cyclophosphamide** (section 8.1.1) may be used at a dose of 1 to 1.5 mg/kg daily by mouth for rheumatoid arthritis with severe systemic manifestations [unlicensed indication]; it is toxic and regular blood counts (including platelet counts) should be carried out. Cyclophosphamide can also be given intravenously in a dose of 0.5 to 1 g (with prophylactic mesna) for *severe systemic rheumatoid arthritis* and for other connective tissue dis-

eases (especially with active vasculitis), repeated initially at fortnightly then at monthly intervals (according to clinical response and haematological monitoring).

Drugs that affect the immune response are also used in the management of severe cases of *systemic lupus erythematosus* and other connective tissue disorders. They are often given in conjunction with corticosteroids for patients with severe or progressive renal disease. They may be used in cases of *polymyositis* that are resistant to corticosteroids. They are used for their corticosteroid-sparing effect in patients whose corticosteroid requirements are excessive. **Azathioprine** is usually used.

Azathioprine and methotrexate are used in the treatment of *psoriatic arthropathy* [unlicensed indication] for severe or progressive cases that are not controlled with anti-inflammatory drugs.

### ▌ AZATHIOPRINE

**Indications** see notes above; inflammatory bowel disease [unlicensed indication] (section 1.5.3); transplantation rejection, see section 8.2.1

**Cautions** see section 8.2.1

**Contra-indications** see section 8.2.1

**Side-effects** see section 8.2.1

**Dose**

- By mouth, initially, rarely more than 3 mg/kg daily, reduced according to response; maintenance 1–3 mg/kg daily; consider withdrawal if no improvement within 3 months

◢**Preparations**
Section 8.2.1

### ▌ CICLOSPORIN
(Cyclosporin)

**Indications** severe active rheumatoid arthritis when conventional second-line therapy inappropriate or ineffective; severe acute ulcerative colitis [unlicensed indication] (section 1.5.3); graft-versus-host disease (section 8.2.2); atopic dermatitis and psoriasis (section 13.5.3).

**Cautions** see section 8.2.2
Additional cautions in rheumatoid arthritis  *Contra-indicated* in abnormal renal function, uncontrolled hypertension (see also below), uncontrolled infections, and malignancy. Measure serum creatinine at least twice before treatment and monitor every 2 weeks for first 3 months, then every 4 weeks (or more frequently if dose increased or concomitant NSAIDs introduced or increased (see also *interactions*: Appendix 1 (ciclosporin)), reduce dose if serum creatinine increases more than 30% above baseline in more than 1 measurement; if above 50%, reduce dose by 50% (even if within normal range) and discontinue if reduction not successful within 1 month; monitor blood pressure (discontinue if hypertension develops that cannot be controlled by antihypertensive therapy); monitor hepatic function if concomitant NSAIDs given.

**Side-effects** see section 8.2.2

**Dose**

- By mouth, administered in accordance with expert advice, initially 2.5 mg/kg daily in 2 divided doses, if necessary increased gradually after 6 weeks; max. 4 mg/kg daily (discontinue if response insufficient after 3 months); dose adjusted according to response for maintenance and treatment reviewed after 6 months (continue only if benefits outweigh risks); CHILD and under 18 years, not recommended **Important** For preparations and counselling and for advice on conversion between the preparations, see section 8.2.2

◀**Preparations**
Section 8.2.2

---

# LEFLUNOMIDE

**Indications** (specialist use only) moderate to severe active rheumatoid arthritis; active psoriatic arthritis

**Cautions** renal impairment (avoid if moderate or severe; Appendix 3); impaired bone-marrow function including anaemia, leucopenia or thrombocytopenia (avoid if significant and due to causes other than rheumatoid arthritis); recent treatment with other hepatotoxic or myelotoxic disease-modifying anti-rheumatic drugs; washout procedures recommended for serious adverse effects or before switching to other disease-modifying antirheumatic drugs (consult product literature and see Washout Procedure, below); history of tuberculosis; exclude pregnancy before treatment; effective contraception **essential** during treatment and for at least 2 years after treatment in women and at least 3 months after treatment in men (plasma concentration monitoring required; waiting time before conception may be reduced with washout procedure—consult product literature and see Washout Procedure, below); monitor full blood count (including differential white cell count and platelet count) before treatment and every 2 weeks for 6 months then every 8 weeks; monitor liver function—see Hepatotoxicity, below; monitor blood pressure; **interactions:** Appendix 1 (leflunomide)

**Hepatotoxicity** Potentially life-threatening hepatotoxicity reported usually in the first 6 months; monitor liver function before treatment and every 2 weeks for first 6 months then every 8 weeks. Discontinue treatment (and institute washout procedure—consult product literature and see Washout Procedure below) or reduce dose according to liver-function abnormality; if liver-function abnormality persists after dose reduction, discontinue treatment and institute washout procedure

**Washout procedure** To aid drug elimination in case of serious adverse effect, or before starting another disease-modifying antirheumatic drug, or before conception (see also Appendix 4), stop treatment and give *either* colestyramine 8 g 3 times daily for 11 days *or* activated charcoal 50 g 4 times daily for 11 days; the concentration of the active metabolite after washout should be less than 20 micrograms/litre (measured on 2 occasions 14 days apart) in men or women before conception—consult product literature. Procedure may be repeated as necessary

**Contra-indications** severe immunodeficiency; severe hypoproteinaemia; serious infection; hepatic impairment (Appendix 2); pregnancy (**important terato-genic risk:** see Cautions and Appendix 4); breast-feeding (Appendix 5)

**Side-effects** diarrhoea, nausea, vomiting, anorexia, oral mucosal disorders, abdominal pain; increased blood pressure; headache, dizziness, asthenia, paraesthesia; leucopenia; tenosynovitis; alopecia; rash, dry skin, pruritus; *less commonly* taste disturbance, anxiety, hyperlipidaemia, hypokalaemia, hypophosphataemia, anaemia, thrombocytopenia, and tendon rupture; *rarely* hepatitis, jaundice (see Hepatotoxicity, above), interstitial lung disease, severe infection, eosinophilia, and pancytopenia; *very rarely* pancreatitis, hepatic failure (see Hepatotoxicity, above), peripheral neuropathy, vasculitis, Stevens-

Johnson syndrome, and toxic epidermal necrolysis; hypouricaemia, reduced sperm count, and renal failure also reported; **important:** discontinue treatment and institute washout procedure (see Washout Procedure under Cautions) in case of serious side-effect

**Dose**
- Rheumatoid arthritis, ADULT over 18 years, initially 100 mg once daily for 3 days, then 10–20 mg once daily
- Psoriatic arthritis, ADULT over 18 years, initially 100 mg once daily for 3 days, then 20 mg once daily

**Arava®** (Sanofi-Aventis) [PoM]
Tablets, f/c, leflunomide 10 mg (white), net price 30-tab pack = £51.13; 20 mg (yellow), 30-tab pack = £51.13; 100 mg (white), 3-tab pack = £25.56. Label: 4

---

# METHOTREXATE

**Indications** moderate to severe active rheumatoid arthritis; Crohn's disease [unlicensed indication] (section 1.5.3); malignant disease (section 8.1.3); psoriasis (section 13.5.3)

**Cautions** section 8.1; see CSM advice below (blood count, liver and pulmonary toxicity); extreme caution in blood disorders (avoid if severe); peptic ulceration, ulcerative colitis, diarrhoea and ulcerative stomatitis (withdraw if stomatitis develops—may be first sign of gastro-intestinal toxicity); risk of accumulation in pleural effusion or ascites—drain before treatment; acute porphyria (section 9.8.2); renal impairment (avoid in severe renal impairment; Appendix 3); **interactions:** see below and Appendix 1 (methotrexate)

> ### CSM advice
> In view of reports of blood dyscrasias (including fatalities) and liver cirrhosis with low-dose methotrexate, the CSM has advised:
> - full blood count and renal and liver function tests before starting treatment and repeated weekly until therapy stabilised, thereafter patients should be monitored every 2–3 months
> - that patients should be advised to report all symptoms and signs suggestive of infection, especially sore throat
>
> Treatment with folinic acid (as calcium folinate, section 8.1) may be required in acute toxicity

**Blood count** Bone marrow suppression can occur abruptly; factors likely to increase toxicity include advanced age, renal impairment, and concomitant use with another anti-folate drug. A clinically significant drop in white cell count or platelet count calls for immediate withdrawal of methotrexate and introduction of supportive therapy

**Liver toxicity** Liver cirrhosis reported. Treatment should not be started or should be discontinued if any abnormality of liver function tests or liver biopsy is present or develops during therapy. Abnormalities can return to normal within 2 weeks after which treatment may be recommenced if judged appropriate

**Pulmonary toxicity** Pulmonary toxicity may be a special problem in rheumatoid arthritis (patient to seek medical attention if dyspnoea, cough or fever); monitor for symptoms at each visit—discontinue if pneumonitis suspected.

**Aspirin and other NSAIDs** If aspirin or other NSAIDs are given concurrently the dose of methotrexate should be carefully monitored. Patients should be advised to avoid self-medication with over-the-counter aspirin or ibuprofen

**Contra-indications** see Cautions above; hepatic impairment (Appendix 2), pregnancy (following administration to a woman or a man, avoid conception for **at least 3 months** after stopping—Appendix 4), breast-feeding (Appendix 5), active infection and immunodeficiency syndromes

**10**

**Musculoskeletal and joint diseases**

**Side-effects** section 8.1; also anorexia, abdominal discomfort, dyspepsia, gastro-intestinal ulceration and bleeding, diarrhoea, toxic megacolon, hepatotoxicity (see Cautions above); hypotension, pericarditis, pericardial tamponade; pulmonary oedema, pleuritic pain, pulmonary fibrosis, interstitial pneumonitis (see also Pulmonary Toxicity above); anaphylactic reactions, urticaria; dizziness, fatigue, chills, fever, drowsiness, malaise, headache, mood changes, neurotoxicity, confusion, paraesthesia; precipitation of diabetes; menstrual disturbances, vaginitis, cystitis, reduced libido, impotence; blood disorders; haematuria, dysuria, renal failure; osteoporosis, arthralgia, myalgia, vasculitis; conjunctivitis, visual disturbance; rash, pruritus, Stevens-Johnson syndrome, toxic epidermal necrolysis, photosensitivity, changes in nail and skin pigmentation, telangiectasia, acne, furunclosis, ecchymosis; injection-site reactions

**Dose**

• Moderate to severe active rheumatoid arthritis, by mouth, 7.5 mg once weekly, adjusted according to response; max. weekly dose 20 mg

• Severe active rheumatoid arthritis, by subcutaneous *or* by intramuscular *or* by intravenous injection, 7.5 mg once weekly, increased according to response by 2.5 mg weekly; max. weekly dose 25 mg

> **Important**
>
> Note that the above dose is a **weekly** dose. To avoid error with low-dose methotrexate, it is recommended that:
>
> • the patient is carefully advised of the **dose** and **frequency** and the reason for taking methotrexate and any other prescribed medicine (e.g. folic acid);
>
> • only one strength of methotrexate tablet (usually 2.5 mg) is prescribed and dispensed;
>
> • the prescription and the dispensing label clearly show the dose and frequency of methotrexate administration;
>
> • the patient is warned to report immediately the onset of any feature of blood disorders (e.g. sore throat, bruising, and mouth ulcers), liver toxicity (e.g. nausea, vomiting, abdominal discomfort, and dark urine), and respiratory effects (e.g. shortness of breath).

**Methotrexate** (Non-proprietary) ▒PoM▒
Tablets, yellow, methotrexate 2.5 mg, net price 28-tab pack = £3.27. Counselling, dose, NSAIDs
Brands include *Maxtrex*®

Tablets, yellow, methotrexate 10 mg, net price 100-tab pack = £55.39. Counselling, dose, NSAIDs

◢**Parenteral preparations**
See also section 8.1.3

**Metoject**® (Medac) ▒PoM▒
Injection, prefilled syringe, methotrexate (as disodium salt) 10 mg/mL, net price 0.75 mL (7.5 mg) = £14.85, 1 mL (10 mg) = £15.29, 1.5 mL (15 mg) = £16.57, 2 mL (20 mg) = £17.84, 2.5 mL (25 mg) = £18.48

# Cytokine modulators

Cytokine modulators should be used under specialist supervision.

Adalimumab, etanercept, and infliximab inhibit the activity of tumour necrosis factor alpha (TNF-α).

**Adalimumab** is licensed for moderate to severe active *rheumatoid arthritis* when response to other disease-modifying antirheumatic drugs (including methotrexate) has been inadequate (see also NICE guidance, p. 577); it can also be used for severe, active, and progressive disease in adults not previously treated with methotrexate. It is also licensed for active *polyarticular juvenile idiopathic arthritis* in adolescents who have not responded adequately to one or more disease-modifying antirheumatic drugs. In the treatment of rheumatoid arthritis and polyarticular juvenile idiopathic arthritis, adalimumab should be used in combination with methotrexate, but it can be given alone if methotrexate is inappropriate. Adalimumab is also licensed for the treatment of active and progressive *psoriatic arthritis* (see also NICE guidance, below) and severe active *ankylosing spondylitis* (see also NICE guidance, p. 577) that have not responded adequately to other disease-modifying antirheumatic drugs. For the role of adalimumab in Crohn's disease, see section 1.5.3. For the role of adalimumab in plaque psoriasis, see section 13.5.3.

> **NICE guidance**
> **Adalimumab for the treatment of psoriatic arthritis (August 2007)**
> Adalimumab is an option for the treatment of active and progressive psoriatic arthritis in adults with at least 3 tender joints and at least 3 swollen joints, who have not responded adequately to at least 2 standard disease-modifying antirheumatic drugs (used alone or in combination). Adalimumab should be used under specialist supervision and should be discontinued if there is an inadequate response after 12 weeks.

**Etanercept** is licensed for the treatment of moderate to severe active *rheumatoid arthritis* either alone or in combination with methotrexate when the response to other disease-modifying antirheumatic drugs is inadequate (see also NICE guidance, p. 577). It is also licensed for the treatment of *active polyarticular juvenile idiopathic arthritis* in children who have not responded adequately to or are intolerant of methotrexate (see also NICE guidance, p. 577), active and progressive *psoriatic arthritis* inadequately responsive to other disease-modifying antirheumatic drugs (see also NICE guidance, p. 578), and for severe *ankylosing spondylitis* inadequately responsive to conventional therapy (see also NICE guidance, p. 577). For the role of etanercept in plaque psoriasis, see section 13.5.3.

**Infliximab** is licensed for the treatment of active *rheumatoid arthritis* in combination with methotrexate when the response to other disease-modifying antirheumatic drugs, including methotrexate, is inadequate (see also NICE guidance, p. 577); it is also licensed in combination with methotrexate for patients not previously treated with methotrexate or other DMARDs who have severe, active, and progressive rheumatoid arthritis. Infliximab is also licensed for the treatment of *ankylosing spondylitis*, in patients with severe axial symptoms who have not responded adequately to conventional therapy (see also NICE guidance, p. 577) and in combination with methotrexate (or alone if methotrexate is not tolerated or is contra-indicated) for the treatment of active and progressive *psoriatic arthritis* which has not responded adequately to disease-modifying antirheumatic drugs (see also NICE guidance, p. 578).

**Rituximab** is licensed in combination with metho-trexate for the treatment of severe active *rheumatoid arthritis* in patients whose condition has not responded adequately to other disease-modifying antirheumatic drugs (including one or more tumour necrosis factor inhibitors) or who are intolerant of them (see also NICE guidance, below). For the role of rituximab in malignant disease, see section 8.2.3.

> **NICE guidance**
> **Rituximab for the treatment of rheumatoid arthritis (August 2007)**
> Rituximab, in combination with methotrexate, is an option for the treatment of severe active rheumatoid arthritis in adults who have not had an adequate response to, or are intolerant of, other disease-mod-ifying antirheumatic drugs (DMARDs), including treatment with at least 1 tumour necrosis factor alpha (TNF-α) inhibitor.
> Treatment with rituximab plus methotrexate should be continued only if there is an adequate response to therapy; repeat courses should be given no more frequently than every 6 months.

**Side-effects** Adalimumab, etanercept, infliximab, and rituximab have been associated with infections, some-times severe, including tuberculosis, septicaemia, and hepatitis B reactivation. Other side-effects include nausea, abdominal pain, worsening heart failure, hyper-sensitivity reactions, fever, headache, depression, anti-body formation (including lupus erythematosus-like syndrome), pruritus, injection-site reactions, and blood disorders (including anaemia, leucopenia, thrombocyto-penia, pancytopenia, and aplastic anaemia).

> **NICE guidance**
> **Adalimumab, etanercept, and infliximab for the treatment of rheumatoid arthritis (October 2007)**
> The tumour necrosis factor alpha (TNF-α) inhibitors adalimumab, etanercept, and infliximab are options for the treatment of adults with active rheumatoid arthritis who have failed to respond to at least 2 disease-modifying antirheumatic drugs (DMARDs), including methotrexate (unless contra-indicated). TNF-α inhibitors should be given in combination with methotrexate; however, when methotrexate cannot be used because of intolerance or contra-indications, adalimumab or etanercept can be given as monotherapy.
>
> Adalimumab, etanercept, and infliximab should be withdrawn if response is not adequate within 6 months. Response to treatment should be monitored at least every 6 months in patients who respond initially; treatment should be withdrawn if response is not maintained. An alternative TNF-α inhibitor may be considered for patients in whom treatment is withdrawn because of intolerance before the initial 6-month assessment of efficacy.
>
> Use of TNF-α inhibitors for the treatment of severe, active, and progressive rheumatoid arthritis in adults not previously treated with methotrexate or other DMARDs is not recommended.

> **NICE guidance**
> **Adalimumab, etanercept, and infliximab for the treatment of ankylosing spondylitis (May 2008)**
> Adalimumab or etanercept are recommended as treatment options for adults with severe active anky-losing spondylitis whose disease satisfies specific criteria for diagnosis where there is confirmation of sustained active spinal disease, and where treatment with two or more NSAIDs taken sequentially at maximum tolerated or recommended doses for 4 weeks has failed to control symptoms.
> Response to adalimumab or etanercept treatment should be assessed at 12-week intervals and con-tinued only if response is adequate. If response to treatment is not maintained, a repeat assessment should be made after a further 6 weeks and treat-ment discontinued if there is an inadequate response. Patients who are intolerant of adalimumab or etanercept during the initial 12 weeks may receive the alternative TNF-α inhibitor (adalimumab or eta-nercept). However an alternative TNF-α inhibitor is not recommended in patients who fail to respond initially or fail to maintain an adequate response.
> Infliximab is not recommended for the treatment of ankylosing spondylitis. Patients who are already receiving infliximab for the treatment of ankylosing spondylitis can continue treatment until they and their specialist consider it appropriate to stop.
> See full NICE guidance for specific criteria to diag-nose severe active ankylosing spondylitis, confirm sustained active spinal disease, and assess response to treatment.

> **NICE guidance**
> **Etanercept for the treatment of juvenile idiopathic arthritis (March 2002)**
> Etanercept is recommended in children aged 4–17 years with active polyarticular-course juvenile idio-pathic arthritis who have not responded adequately to methotrexate or who are intolerant of it. Etaner-cept should be used under specialist supervision according to the guidelines of the British Society for Paediatric and Adolescent Rheumatology [pre-viously the British Paediatric Rheumatology Group].
>
> Etanercept should be withdrawn if severe side-effects develop or if there is no response after 6 months or if the initial response is not maintained. There is no evidence to support treatment for longer than 2 years; a decision to continue therapy should be based on disease activity and clinical effective-ness in individual cases.
>
> Prescribers of etanercept should register consenting patients with the Biologics Registry of the British Society for Paediatric and Adolescent Rheumatol-ogy.

**10**

**Musculoskeletal and joint diseases**

### NICE guidance
### Etanercept and infliximab for the treatment of psoriatic arthritis (July 2006)

Etanercept is recommended for severe active psoriatic arthritis in adults with at least 3 tender joints and at least 3 swollen joints, and who have not responded adequately to 2 other disease-modifying antirheumatic drugs (used alone or in combination); infliximab [in combination with methotrexate, unless contra-indicated or not tolerated] is recommended for those intolerant of etanercept.

Etanercept or infliximab should be used under specialist supervision and should be withdrawn if inadequate response after 12 weeks.

**Abatacept** prevents the full activation of T-lymphocytes. It is licensed for moderate to severe active *rheumatoid arthritis* in combination with methotrexate, in patients unresponsive or intolerant to other disease-modifying antirheumatic drugs (including at least one tumour necrosis factor (TNF) inhibitor). Abatacept is not recommended for use in combination with TNF inhibitors.

The *Scottish Medicines Consortium* (p. 3) has advised (August 2007) that abatacept is **not** recommended for the treatment of moderate to severe active rheumatoid arthritis within NHS Scotland.

### NICE guidance
### Abatacept for the treatment of rheumatoid arthritis (April 2008)

Abatacept is **not** recommended for the treatment of rheumatoid arthritis. Patients who are already receiving abatacept for rheumatoid arthritis can continue treatment until they and their specialist consider it appropriate to stop.

**Anakinra** inhibits the activity of interleukin-1. Anakinra (in combination with methotrexate) is licensed for the treatment of *rheumatoid arthritis* which has not responded to methotrexate alone; it is not, however, recommended for routine management of *rheumatoid arthritis*, see NICE guidance below.

The *Scottish Medicines Consortium* (p. 3) has advised (July 2002) that anakinra is **not** recommended for the treatment of rheumatoid arthritis within NHS Scotland.

### NICE guidance
### Anakinra for the treatment of rheumatoid arthritis (February 2009)

Anakinra is **not** recommended for the treatment of rheumatoid arthritis except when used in a controlled long-term clinical study. Patients who are already receiving anakinra for rheumatoid arthritis should continue treatment until they and their specialist consider it appropriate to stop.

## ◼ ABATACEPT

**Indications** see under Cytokine Modulators, above

**Cautions** predisposition to infection (screen for latent tuberculosis and viral hepatitis); do not initiate until active infections are controlled; elderly (increased risk of side-effects); **interactions:** Appendix 1 (abatacept)

**Contra-indications** severe infection (see also Cautions); pregnancy (Appendix 4); breast-feeding (Appendix 5)

**Side-effects** abdominal pain, diarrhoea, dyspepsia, nausea; flushing, hypertension; cough; dizziness, fatigue, headache; infection, rhinitis; rash; *less commonly* gastritis, stomatitis, tachycardia, bradycardia, palpitation, hypotension, dyspnoea, paraesthesia, weight gain, depression, anxiety, amenorrhoea, basal cell carcinoma, thrombocytopenia, leucopenia, arthralgia, pain in extremities, conjunctivitis, visual disturbance, vertigo, bruising, alopecia, and dry skin

**Dose**
- By intravenous infusion, ADULT over 18 years, body-weight less than 60 kg, 500 mg, repeated 2 weeks and 4 weeks after initial infusion, then every 4 weeks; body-weight 60–100 kg, 750 mg repeated 2 weeks and 4 weeks after initial infusion, then every 4 weeks; body-weight over 100 kg, 1 g repeated 2 weeks and 4 weeks after initial infusion, then every 4 weeks

**Note** Discontinue if no response within 6 months

**Orencia®** (Bristol-Myers Squibb) ▼ PoM
Intravenous infusion, powder for reconstitution, abatacept, net price 250-mg vial = £242.17
Electrolytes Na⁺<0.5 mmol/vial

## ◼ ADALIMUMAB

**Indications** see under Cytokine Modulators above; Crohn's disease (section 1.5.3); psoriasis (section 13.5.3)

**Cautions** predisposition to infection; monitor for infections before, during, and for 5 months after treatment (see also Tuberculosis below); do not initiate until active infections are controlled; discontinue if new serious infection develops; hepatitis B virus—monitor for active infection; children should be brought up to date with current immunisation schedule (section 14.1) before initiating therapy; mild heart failure (discontinue if symptoms develop or worsen—avoid in moderate or severe heart failure); demyelinating CNS disorders (risk of exacerbation); history of malignancy; monitor for non-melanoma skin cancer before and during treatment, especially in patients with a history of PUVA treatment for psoriasis or extensive immunosuppressant therapy; **interactions:** Appendix 1 (adalimumab)

**Tuberculosis** Patients should be evaluated for tuberculosis before treatment. Active tuberculosis should be treated with standard treatment (section 5.1.9) for at least 2 months before starting adalimumab. Patients who have previously received adequate treatment for tuberculosis can start adalimumab but should be monitored every 3 months for possible recurrence. In patients without active tuberculosis but who were previously not treated adequately, chemoprophylaxis should ideally be completed before starting adalimumab. In patients at high risk of tuberculosis who cannot be assessed by tuberculin skin test, chemoprophylaxis can be given concurrently with adalimumab. Patients should be advised to seek medical attention if symptoms suggestive of tuberculosis (e.g. persistent cough, weight loss, and fever) develop

**Contra-indications** pregnancy (Appendix 4); breast-feeding (Appendix 5); severe infection (see also Cautions)

**Side-effects** see under Cytokine Modulators (p. 577) and Cautions above; also mouth ulceration, stomatitis, diarrhoea, cough, dizziness, fatigue, paraesthesia, musculoskeletal pain, rash and pruritus; *less commonly* vomiting, dyspepsia, constipation, rectal bleeding, arrhythmias, syncope, chest pain, hyperlipidaemia, hypertension, flushing, dyspnoea, dysphonia, appetite disorders, anxiety, tremor, sleep disturbances, influenza-like symptoms, menstrual disorders, electrolyte disturbances, haematuria, renal impairment, hyperuricaemia, eye disorders, skin papilloma, and alopecia; *rarely* pancreatitis, colitis, oesophagitis, gastritis, hepatitis, cholelithiasis, palpitation, myocardial infarction, vascular occlusion, pleural effusion, demyelinating disorders, facial palsy, thyroid disorders, malignancy, rhabdomyolysis, hearing loss, tinnitus, and erythema multiforme; also reported intestinal perforation, vasculitis, and interstitial lung disease

**Dose**

- By subcutaneous injection, rheumatoid arthritis, ADULT over 18 years, 40 mg on alternate weeks; if necessary increased to 40 mg weekly in patients receiving adalimumab alone; review treatment if no response within 12 weeks

Polyarticular juvenile idiopathic arthritis, CHILD 13–17 years, 40 mg on alternate weeks; review treatment if no response within 12 weeks

Psoriatic arthritis, ankylosing spondylitis, ADULT over 18 years, 40 mg on alternate weeks; discontinue treatment if no response within 12 weeks

**Humira®** (Abbott) ▼ PoM
Injection, adalimumab, net price 40-mg prefilled pen or prefilled syringe = £357.50. Counselling, tuberculosis

### ANAKINRA

**Indications**   see under Cytokine Modulators above

**Cautions**   predisposition to infections; history of asthma (risk of serious infection); renal impairment (avoid if eGFR less than 30 mL/minute/1.73 m²; Appendix 3); **interactions:** Appendix 1 (anakinra)
**Blood disorders** Neutropenia reported commonly. Monitor neutrophil count before treatment, then every month for 6 months, then every 3 months—discontinue if neutropenia develops. Patients should be instructed to seek medical advice if symptoms suggestive of neutropenia (such as fever, sore throat, infection) develop

**Contra-indications**   pregnancy (Appendix 4); breast-feeding (Appendix 5); neutropenia

**Side-effects**   injection-site reactions; headache; infections, neutropenia (see also Cautions), and antibody formation; *also reported* malignancy

**Dose**

- By subcutaneous injection, ADULT over 18 years, 100 mg once daily

**Kineret®** (Amgen) PoM
Injection, anakinra, net price 100-mg prefilled syringe = £19.03. Counselling, blood disorder symptoms

### ETANERCEPT

**Indications**   see under Cytokine Modulators above; severe, active and progressive rheumatoid arthritis in patients not previously treated with methotrexate; psoriasis (section 13.5.3)

**Cautions**   predisposition to infection (avoid if predisposition to septicaemia); significant exposure to herpes zoster virus—interrupt treatment and consider varicella–zoster immunoglobulin; hepatitis B virus—monitor for active infection; heart failure (risk of exacerbation); demyelinating CNS disorders (risk of

exacerbation); history of blood disorders; **interactions:** Appendix 1 (etanercept)
**Tuberculosis** Patients should be evaluated for tuberculosis before treatment. Active tuberculosis should be treated with standard treatment (section 5.1.9) for at least 2 months before starting etanercept. Patients who have previously received adequate treatment for tuberculosis can start etanercept but should be monitored every 3 months for possible recurrence. In patients without active tuberculosis but who were previously not treated adequately, chemoprophylaxis should ideally be completed before starting etanercept. In patients at high risk of tuberculosis who cannot be assessed by tuberculin skin test, chemoprophylaxis can be given concurrently with etanercept. Patients should be advised to seek medical attention if symptoms suggestive of tuberculosis (e.g. persistent cough, weight loss, and fever) develop
**Blood disorders** Patients should be advised to seek medical attention if symptoms suggestive of blood disorders (such as fever, sore throat, bruising, or bleeding) develop

**Contra-indications**   active infection; avoid injections containing benzyl alcohol in neonates (see preparations below); pregnancy (Appendix 4); breast-feeding (Appendix 5)

**Side-effects**   see under Cytokine Modulators (p. 577); also *less commonly* interstitial lung disease, rash; *rarely* demyelinating disorders, seizures, Stevens-Johnson syndrome, and cutaneous vasculitis; *very rarely* toxic epidermal necrolysis; *also reported* appendicitis, cholecystitis, gastritis, gastro-intestinal haemorrhage, intestinal obstruction, liver damage, oesophagitis, pancreatitis, ulcerative colitis, vomiting, cerebral ischaemia, hypertension, hypotension, myocardial infarction, thrombophlebitis, thromboembolism, asthma, dyspnoea, aseptic meningitis, confusion, paresis, paraesthesia, vertigo, lymphadenopathy, diabetes mellitus, haematuria, malignancy, renal calculi, renal impairment, bone fracture, bursitis, polymyositis, scleritis, and cutaneous ulcer

**Dose**

- By subcutaneous injection, rheumatoid arthritis, psoriatic arthritis, ankylosing spondylitis, ADULT over 18 years, 25 mg twice weekly *or* 50 mg once weekly

Polyarticular-course juvenile idiopathic arthritis, CHILD 4–17 years, 400 micrograms/kg (max. 25 mg) twice weekly, with an interval of 3–4 days between doses

**Enbrel®** (Wyeth) ▼ PoM
Injection, powder for reconstitution, etanercept, net price 25-mg vial (with solvent) = £89.38. Label: 10, alert card, counselling, tuberculosis and blood disorders

Paediatric injection, powder for reconstitution, etanercept, net price 25-mg vial (with solvent) = £89.38. Label: 10, alert card, counselling, tuberculosis and blood disorders
Excipients include benzyl alcohol (avoid in neonates, see Excipients, p. 2)

Injection, etanercept, net price 25-mg prefilled syringe = £89.38; 50-mg prefilled syringe = £178.75. Label: 10, alert card, counselling, tuberculosis and blood disorders

### INFLIXIMAB

**Indications**   see under Cytokine Modulators above; inflammatory bowel disease (section 1.5.3); psoriasis (section 13.5.3)

**Cautions**   predisposition to infection; monitor for infections before, during, and for 6 months after treatment (see also Tuberculosis below); discontinue if new serious infection develops; hepatitis B virus—monitor for active infection; heart failure (discontinue

**10**

**Musculoskeletal and joint diseases**

if symptoms develop or worsen; avoid in moderate or severe heart failure; demyelinating CNS disorders (risk of exacerbation); history of malignancy (consider discontinuing treatment if malignancy develops); history of prolonged immunosuppressant or PUVA treatment in patients with psoriasis; **interactions:** Appendix 1 (infliximab)

**Tuberculosis** Patients should be evaluated for tuberculosis before treatment. Active tuberculosis should be treated with standard treatment (section 5.1.9) for at least 2 months before starting infliximab. Patients who have previously received adequate treatment for tuberculosis can start infliximab but should be monitored every 3 months for possible recurrence. In patients without active tuberculosis but who were previously not treated adequately, chemoprophylaxis should ideally be completed before starting infliximab. In patients at high risk of tuberculosis who cannot be assessed by tuberculin skin test, chemoprophylaxis can be given concurrently with infliximab. Patients should be advised to seek medical attention if symptoms suggestive of tuberculosis (e.g. persistent cough, weight loss, and fever) develop

**Hypersensitivity reactions** Hypersensitivity reactions (including fever, chest pain, hypotension, hypertension, dyspnoea, pruritus, urticaria, serum sickness-like reactions, angioedema, anaphylaxis) reported during or within 1–2 hours after infusion (risk greatest during first or second infusion or in patients who discontinue other immunosuppressants). All patients should be observed carefully for 1–2 hours after infusion and resuscitation equipment should be available for immediate use. Prophylactic antipyretics, antihistamines, or hydrocortisone may be administered. Monitor for symptoms of delayed hypersensitivity if readministered after a prolonged period. Patients should be advised to keep Alert card with them at all times and seek medical advice if symptoms of delayed hypersensitivity develop

**Contra-indications** severe infections (see also under Cautions); pregnancy (Appendix 4); breast-feeding (Appendix 5)

**Side-effects** see under Cytokine Modulators (p. 577) and under Cautions above; also diarrhoea, dyspepsia, hepatic impairment; flushing, chest pain; dyspnoea; dizziness, fatigue; sinusitis; rash, sweating, dry skin; *less commonly* constipation, gastro-oesophageal reflux, diverticulitis, cholecystitis, palpitation, arrhythmia, hypertension, hypotension, vasospasm, cyanosis, bradycardia, syncope, oedema, thrombophlebitis, epistaxis, bronchospasm, pleurisy, confusion, agitation, nervousness, amnesia, sleep disturbances, vaginitis, demyelinating disorders, antibody formation, pyelonephritis, myalgia, arthralgia, eye disorders, abnormal skin pigmentation, ecchymosis, cheilitis, and alopecia; *rarely* hepatitis, intestinal stenosis, intestinal perforation, gastro-intestinal haemorrhage, and circulatory failure, meningitis, seizure, and pancreatitis; *very rarely* pericardial and pleural effusion, and skin reactions (including Stevens-Johnson syndrome, toxic epidermal necrolysis); neuropathy, paraesthesia, lymphoma, and transverse myelitis; interstitial lung disease also reported

**Dose**
- By intravenous infusion, rheumatoid arthritis (in combination with methotrexate), ADULT over 18 years, 3 mg/kg, repeated 2 weeks and 6 weeks after initial infusion, then every 8 weeks; if response inadequate after 12 weeks, dose may be increased in steps of 1.5 mg/kg every 8 weeks, up to max. 7.5 mg/kg every 8 weeks; alternatively, 3 mg/kg may be given every 4 weeks; discontinue if no response by 12 weeks of initial infusion or after dose adjustment

Ankylosing spondylitis, ADULT over 18 years, 5 mg/kg, repeated 2 weeks and 6 weeks after initial infusion,

then every 6–8 weeks; discontinue if no response by 6 weeks of initial infusion

Psoriatic arthritis (in combination with methotrexate), ADULT over 18 years, 5 mg/kg, repeated 2 weeks and 6 weeks after initial infusion, then every 8 weeks

**Remicade®** (Schering-Plough) ▼ PoM
Intravenous infusion, powder for reconstitution, infliximab, net price 100-mg vial = £419.62. Label: 10, alert card, counselling, tuberculosis and hypersensitivity reactions

## ▮ RITUXIMAB

**Indications** see under Cytokine Modulators above; malignant disease (section 8.2.3)

**Cautions** section 8.2.3; predisposition to infection; hepatitis B virus—monitor for active infection

**Contra-indications** section 8.2.3; severe infection

**Side-effects** section 8.2.3 and under Cytokine Modulators (p. 577); *also* dyspepsia; hypertension, hypotension; rhinitis, sore throat; asthenia, paraesthesia, migraine; arthralgia, muscle spasm; urticaria

**Dose**
- By intravenous infusion, rheumatoid arthritis (in combination with methotrexate), 1 g, repeated 2 weeks after initial infusion; CHILD not recommended

◢**Preparations**
Section 8.2.3

---

# Sulfasalazine

**Sulfasalazine** (sulphasalazine) has a beneficial effect in suppressing the inflammatory activity of rheumatoid arthritis. Side-effects include rashes, gastro-intestinal intolerance and, especially in patients with rheumatoid arthritis, occasional leucopenia, neutropenia, and thrombocytopenia. These haematological abnormalities occur usually in the first 3 to 6 months of treatment and are reversible on cessation of treatment. Close monitoring of full blood counts (including differential white cell count and platelet count) is necessary initially, and at monthly intervals during the first 3 months (liver function tests also being performed at monthly intervals for the first 3 months). Although the manufacturer recommends renal function tests, evidence of practical value is unsatisfactory.

## ▮ SULFASALAZINE
(Sulphasalazine)

**Indications** active rheumatoid arthritis; inflammatory bowel disease, see section 1.5.1 and notes above

**Cautions** see section 1.5.1 and notes above
The CSM has recommended that patients should be advised to report any unexplained bleeding, bruising, purpura, sore throat, fever or malaise. A blood count should be performed and the drug stopped immediately if there is suspicion of a blood dyscrasia.

**Contra-indications** see section 1.5.1 and notes above

**Side-effects** see section 1.5.1 and notes above

**Dose**
- By mouth, administered on expert advice, as enteric-coated tablets, initially 500 mg daily, increased by 500 mg at intervals of 1 week to a max. of 2–3 g daily in divided doses

**Sulfasalazine** (Non-proprietary) [PoM]

Tablets, e/c, sulfasalazine 500 mg. Net price 112-tab pack = £16.15. Label: 5, 14, 25, counselling, blood disorder symptoms (see CSM recommendation above), contact lenses may be stained
Brands include *Sulazine EC®*

**Salazopyrin EN-Tabs®** (Pharmacia) [PoM]

Tablets, e/c, yellow, f/c, sulfasalazine 500 mg. Net price 112-tab pack = £8.43. Label: 5, 14, 25, counselling, blood disorder symptoms (see CSM recommendation above), contact lenses may be stained

## 10.1.4  Gout and cytotoxic-induced hyperuricaemia

It is important to distinguish drugs used for the treatment of acute attacks of gout from those used in the long-term control of the disease. The latter exacerbate and prolong the acute manifestations if started during an attack.

## Acute attacks of gout

Acute attacks of gout are usually treated with high doses of **NSAIDs** such as diclofenac, etoricoxib, indometacin, ketoprofen, naproxen, or sulindac (section 10.1.1). **Colchicine** is an alternative in patients in whom NSAIDs are contra-indicated. Aspirin is *not* indicated in gout. Allopurinol and uricosurics are not effective in treating an acute attack and may prolong it indefinitely if started during the acute episode.

The use of colchicine is limited by the development of toxicity at higher doses, but it is of value in patients with heart failure since, unlike NSAIDs, it does not induce fluid retention; moreover, it can be given to patients receiving anticoagulants.

Oral or parenteral **corticosteroids** are an effective alternative in those who cannot tolerate NSAIDs or who are resistant to other treatments. Intra-articular injection of a corticosteroid can be used in acute monoarticular gout [unlicensed indication]. A corticosteroid by intramuscular injection can be effective in podagra.

### ▌ COLCHICINE

**Indications** acute gout; short-term prophylaxis during initial therapy with allopurinol and uricosuric drugs; prophylaxis of familial Mediterranean fever (recurrent polyserositis)

**Cautions** elderly; gastro-intestinal disease; cardiac disease; hepatic impairment; renal impairment (avoid if eGFR less than 10 mL/minute/1.73 m²; Appendix 3); breast-feeding (Appendix 5); **interactions:** Appendix 1 (colchicine)

**Contra-indications** pregnancy (Appendix 4)

**Side-effects** nausea, vomiting, and abdominal pain; excessive doses may cause profuse diarrhoea, gastro-intestinal haemorrhage, rash, renal and hepatic damage; *rarely* peripheral neuritis, inhibition of spermatogenesis, myopathy, alopecia, and with prolonged treatment blood disorders

**Dose**

- Acute gout, 500 micrograms 2–4 times daily until symptoms relieved, max. 6 mg per course; course not to be repeated within 3 days

- Prevention of gout attacks during initial treatment with allopurinol or uricosuric drugs, 500 micrograms twice daily
- Prophylaxis of familial Mediterranean fever [unlicensed], 0.5–2 mg once daily

Note BNF doses may differ from those in the product literature

**Colchicine** (Non-proprietary) [PoM]

Tablets, colchicine 500 micrograms, net price 20 = £5.05

## Long-term control of gout

Frequent recurrence of acute attacks of gout, the presence of tophi, or signs of chronic gouty arthritis may call for the initiation of long-term ('interval') treatment. For long-term control of gout the formation of uric acid from purines may be reduced with the xanthine-oxidase inhibitor allopurinol, or the uricosuric drug sulfinpyrazone may be used to increase the excretion of uric acid in the urine. Treatment should be continued indefinitely to prevent further attacks of gout by correcting the hyperuricaemia. These drugs should never be started during an acute attack; they are usually started 1–2 weeks after the attack has settled. The initiation of treatment may precipitate an acute attack, and therefore an anti-inflammatory analgesic or colchicine should be used as a prophylactic and continued for at least one month after the hyperuricaemia has been corrected. However, if an acute attack develops during treatment, then the treatment should continue at the same dosage and the acute attack treated in its own right.

**Allopurinol** is widely used and is especially useful in patients with renal impairment or urate stones when uricosuric drugs cannot be used; it is *not* indicated for the treatment of asymptomatic hyperuricaemia. It can cause rashes.

**Sulfinpyrazone** (sulphinpyrazone) can be used instead of allopurinol, or in conjunction with it in cases that are resistant to treatment.

**Probenecid** (available from 'special-order' manufacturers or specialist importing companies, see p. 969) is a uricosuric drug used to prevent nephrotoxicity associated with cidofovir (section 5.3.2.2).

**Benzbromarone** (available from 'special-order' manufacturers or specialist importing companies, see p. 969) is a uricosuric drug that can be used in patients with mild renal impairment.

Crystallisation of urate in the urine can occur with the uricosuric drugs and it is important to ensure an adequate urine output especially in the first few weeks of treatment. As an additional precaution the urine may be rendered alkaline.

Aspirin and other salicylates antagonise the uricosuric drugs; they do not antagonise allopurinol but are nevertheless *not* indicated in gout.

### ▌ ALLOPURINOL

**Indications** prophylaxis of gout and of uric acid and calcium oxalate renal stones; prophylaxis of hyperuricaemia associated with cancer chemotherapy

**Cautions** administer prophylactic NSAID (*not* aspirin or salicylates) or colchicine until at least 1 month after hyperuricaemia corrected (usually for first 3 months) to avoid precipitating an acute attack; ensure adequate fluid intake (2–3 litres/day); for hyperuricaemia associated with cancer therapy, allopurinol treatment should be started before cancer therapy; hepatic impairment (Appendix 2); renal impairment (Appendix 3); pregnancy (Appendix 4); breast-feeding (Appendix 5); **interactions:** Appendix 1 (allopurinol)

**Contra-indications** not a treatment for acute gout but continue if attack develops when already receiving allopurinol, and treat attack separately (see notes above)

**Side-effects** rashes (**withdraw** therapy; if rash mild re-introduce cautiously but **discontinue** promptly if recurrence—hypersensitivity reactions occur rarely and include exfoliation, fever, lymphadenopathy, arthralgia, and eosinophilia resembling Stevens-Johnson syndrome or toxic epidermal necrolysis, vasculitis, hepatitis, renal impairment, and very rarely seizures); gastro-intestinal disorders; rarely malaise, headache, vertigo, drowsiness, visual and taste disturbances, hypertension, alopecia, hepatotoxicity, paraesthesia and neuropathy, gynaecomastia, blood disorders (including leucopenia, thrombocytopenia, haemolytic anaemia and aplastic anaemia)

**Dose**
- Initially 100 mg daily, preferably after food, then adjusted according to plasma or urinary uric acid concentration; usual maintenance dose in mild conditions 100–200 mg daily, in moderately severe conditions 300–600 mg daily, in severe conditions 700–900 mg daily; doses over 300 mg daily given in divided doses; CHILD under 15 years, (in neoplastic conditions, enzyme disorders) 10–20 mg/kg daily (max. 400 mg daily)

**Allopurinol** (Non-proprietary) PoM
Tablets, allopurinol 100 mg, net price 28-tab pack = £1.01; 300 mg, 28-tab pack = £1.20. Label: 8, 21, 27
Brands include *Caplenal®*, *Cosuric®*, *Rimapurinol®*

**Zyloric®** (GSK) PoM
Tablets, allopurinol 100 mg, net price 100-tab pack = £10.19; 300 mg, 28-tab pack = £7.31. Label: 8, 21, 27

## ▌ PROBENECID

**Indications** prevention of nephrotoxicity associated with cidofovir (section 5.3.2.2)

**Cautions** ensure adequate fluid intake (about 2–3 litres daily) and render urine alkaline if uric acid overload is high; peptic ulceration; transient false-positive Benedict's test; G6PD-deficiency (section 9.1.5); **interactions:** Appendix 1 (probenecid)

**Contra-indications** history of blood disorders, nephrolithiasis, acute porphyria (section 9.8.2), acute gout attack; avoid aspirin and salicylates; renal impairment (avoid if eGFR less than 30 mL/minute/1.73 m²; Appendix 3)

**Side-effects** gastro-intestinal disturbances; *less commonly* sore gums, flushing, headache, dizziness, urinary frequency, anaemia, alopecia; hepatic necrosis, hypersensitivity reactions (including anaphylaxis, pruritus, urticaria, fever, and Stevens-Johnson syndrome), nephrotic syndrome, haemolytic anaemia, leucopenia, and aplastic anaemia also reported

**Dose**
- Used with cidofovir, see section 5.3.2.2

**Probenecid** (Non-proprietary) PoM
Tablets, probenecid 500 mg. Label: 12, 21, 27
Available from 'special-order' manufacturers or specialist importing companies, see p. 969

## ▌ SULFINPYRAZONE
(Sulphinpyrazone)

**Indications** gout prophylaxis, hyperuricaemia

**Cautions** see under Probenecid; regular blood counts advisable; cardiac disease (may cause salt and water retention); renal impairment (avoid if severe; Appendix 3); **interactions:** Appendix 1 (sulfinpyrazone)

**Contra-indications** see under Probenecid; avoid in hypersensitivity to NSAIDs

**Side-effects** gastro-intestinal disturbances, occasionally allergic skin reactions, salt and water retention; rarely blood disorders, gastro-intestinal ulceration and bleeding, acute renal failure, raised liver enzymes, jaundice and hepatitis

**Dose**
- Initially 100–200 mg daily with food (or milk) increasing over 2–3 weeks to 600 mg daily (rarely 800 mg daily), continued until serum uric acid concentration normal then reduced for maintenance (maintenance dose may be as low as 200 mg daily)

**Anturan®** (Amdipharm) PoM
Tablets, both yellow, s/c, sulfinpyrazone 100 mg, net price 84-tab pack = £5.66; 200 mg, 84-tab pack = £11.25. Label: 12, 21

## Hyperuricaemia associated with cytotoxic drugs

**Allopurinol** is used to prevent hyperuricaemia associated with cytotoxic drugs—see section 8.1 (Hyperuricaemia) and Allopurinol above.

**Rasburicase** is licensed for the prophylaxis and treatment of acute hyperuricaemia, before and during initiation of chemotherapy, in patients with haematological malignancy and a high tumour burden at risk of rapid lysis.

## ▌ RASBURICASE

**Indications** prophylaxis and treatment of acute hyperuricaemia with initial chemotherapy for haematological malignancy

**Cautions** monitor closely for hypersensitivity; atopic allergies; may interfere with test for uric acid—consult product literature

**Contra-indications** G6PD deficiency (section 9.1.5); pregnancy (Appendix 4); breast-feeding (Appendix 5)

**Side-effects** fever; *less commonly* nausea, vomiting, diarrhoea, headache, hypersensitivity reactions (including rash, bronchospasm and anaphylaxis); haemolytic anaemia, methaemoglobinaemia

**Dose**
- By intravenous infusion, 200 micrograms/kg once daily for up to 7 days according to plasma-uric acid concentration

**Fasturtec®** (Sanofi-Aventis) PoM
Intravenous infusion, powder for reconstitution, rasburicase, net price 1.5-mg vial (with solvent) = £57.88; 7.5-mg vial (with solvent) = £241.20

Musculoskeletal and joint diseases    10

## 10.1.5 Other drugs for rheumatic diseases

### Glucosamine

Glucosamine is a natural substance found in mucopolysaccharides, mucoproteins, and chitin. It is licensed for symptomatic relief of mild to moderate osteoarthritis of the knee, but is not recommended. The mechanism of action is not understood and there is limited evidence to show it is effective.

The *Scottish Medicines Consortium* (p. 3) has advised (May 2008) that glucosamine (*Alateris®*) is **not** recommended for use within NHS Scotland for the symptomatic relief of mild to moderate osteoarthritis of the knee.

### ▌ GLUCOSAMINE ◢

**Indications** symptomatic relief of mild to moderate osteoarthritis of the knee

**Cautions** impaired glucose tolerance (monitor blood-glucose concentration before treatment and periodically thereafter); predisposition to cardiovascular disease (monitor cholesterol); asthma; **interactions**: Appendix 1 (glucosamine)

**Contra-indications** shellfish allergy; pregnancy (Appendix 4); breast-feeding (Appendix 5)

**Side-effects** nausea, abdominal pain, indigestion, diarrhoea, constipation; headache, fatigue; *less commonly* flushing, rash, pruritus; hypercholesterolaemia also reported

**Dose**
- ADULT over 18 years, 1.25 g once daily; review treatment if no benefit after 2–3 months

**Alateris®** (Dee) ▼ PoM ◢
Tablets, glucosamine (as hydrochloride) 625 mg, net price 60-tab pack = £18.40

## 10.2 Drugs used in neuromuscular disorders

### 10.2.1 Drugs that enhance neuromuscular transmission

### 10.2.2 Skeletal muscle relaxants

## 10.2.1 Drugs that enhance neuromuscular transmission

Anticholinesterases are used as first-line treatment in *ocular myasthenia gravis* and as an adjunct to immunosuppressant therapy for *generalised myasthenia gravis*.

Corticosteroids are used when anticholinesterases do not control symptoms completely. A second-line immunosuppressant such as azathioprine is frequently used to reduce the dose of corticosteroid.

Plasmapheresis or infusion of intravenous immunoglobulin [unlicensed indication] may induce temporary remission in severe relapses, particularly where bulbar or respiratory function is compromised or before thymectomy.

### Anticholinesterases

Anticholinesterase drugs enhance neuromuscular transmission in voluntary and involuntary muscle in myasthenia gravis. They prolong the action of acetylcholine by inhibiting the action of the enzyme acetylcholinesterase. Excessive dosage of these drugs can impair neuromuscular transmission and precipitate cholinergic crises by causing a depolarising block. This may be difficult to distinguish from a worsening myasthenic state.

Muscarinic side-effects of anticholinesterases include increased sweating, increased salivary and gastric secretions, increased gastro-intestinal and uterine motility, and bradycardia. These parasympathomimetic effects are antagonised by atropine.

**Edrophonium** has a very brief action and it is therefore used mainly for the diagnosis of myasthenia gravis. However, such testing should be performed only by those experienced in its use; other means of establishing the diagnosis are available. A single test-dose usually causes substantial improvement in muscle power (lasting about 5 minutes) in patients with the disease (if respiration already impaired, *only* in conjunction with someone skilled at intubation).

Edrophonium can also be used to determine whether a patient with myasthenia is receiving inadequate or excessive treatment with cholinergic drugs. If treatment is excessive an injection of edrophonium will either have no effect or will intensify symptoms (if respiration already impaired, give *only* in conjunction with someone skilled at intubation). Conversely, transient improvement may be seen if the patient is being inadequately treated. The test is best performed just before the next dose of anticholinesterase.

**Neostigmine** produces a therapeutic effect for up to 4 hours. Its pronounced muscarinic action is a disadvantage, and simultaneous administration of an antimuscarinic drug such as atropine or propantheline may be required to prevent colic, excessive salivation, or diarrhoea. In severe disease neostigmine can be given every 2 hours. The maximum that most patients can tolerate is 180 mg daily.

**Pyridostigmine** is less powerful and slower in action than neostigmine but it has a longer duration of action. It is preferable to neostigmine because of its smoother action and the need for less frequent dosage. It is particularly preferred in patients whose muscles are weak on waking. It has a comparatively mild gastro-intestinal effect but an antimuscarinic drug may still be required. It is inadvisable to exceed a total daily dose of 450 mg in order to avoid acetylcholine receptor down-regulation. Immunosuppressant therapy is usually considered if the dose of pyridostigmine exceeds 360 mg daily.

**Distigmine** has the longest action but the danger of a cholinergic crisis caused by accumulation of the drug is greater than with shorter-acting drugs; it is rarely used in the management of myasthenia gravis.

10

Musculoskeletal and joint diseases

Neostigmine and edrophonium are also used to reverse the actions of the non-depolarising neuromuscular blocking drugs (see section 15.1.6).

## NEOSTIGMINE

**Indications** myasthenia gravis; other indications (section 15.1.6)

**Cautions** asthma (*extreme* caution), bradycardia, arrhythmias, recent myocardial infarction, epilepsy, hypotension, parkinsonism, vagotonia, peptic ulceration, hyperthyroidism; atropine or other antidote to muscarinic effects may be necessary (particularly when neostigmine is given by injection), but not given routinely because it may mask signs of overdosage; renal impairment (Appendix 3), pregnancy (Appendix 4), breast-feeding (Appendix 5); **interactions:** Appendix 1 (parasympathomimetics)

**Contra-indications** intestinal or urinary obstruction

**Side-effects** nausea, vomiting, increased salivation, diarrhoea, abdominal cramps (more marked with higher doses); signs of overdosage include broncho-constriction, increased bronchial secretions, lacrimation, excessive sweating, involuntary defaecation and micturition, miosis, nystagmus, bradycardia, heart block, arrhythmias, hypotension, agitation, excessive dreaming, and weakness eventually leading to fasciculation and paralysis

**Dose**

- By mouth, neostigmine bromide 15–30 mg at suitable intervals throughout day, total daily dose 75–300 mg (but see also notes above); NEONATE 1–5 mg every 4 hours, half an hour before feeds; CHILD up to 6 years initially 7.5 mg, 6–12 years initially 15 mg, usual total daily dose 15–90 mg
- By subcutaneous *or* intramuscular injection, ADULT and CHILD over 12 years, neostigmine metilsulfate 1–2.5 mg at suitable intervals throughout day (usual total daily dose 5–20 mg); NEONATE 150 micrograms/kg every 6–8 hours 30 minutes before feeds, increased to max. 300 micrograms/kg every 4 hours, if necessary [unlicensed]; CHILD 1 month–12 years 200–500 micrograms as required

**Neostigmine** (Non-proprietary) ▣PoM▣
Tablets, scored, neostigmine bromide 15 mg, net price 20 = £8.01

Injection, neostigmine metilsulfate 2.5 mg/mL, net price 1-mL amp = 57p

## DISTIGMINE BROMIDE

**Indications** myasthenia gravis (but rarely used); urinary retention and other indications (section 7.4.1)

**Cautions** see section 7.4.1

**Contra-indications** see section 7.4.1

**Side-effects** see section 7.4.1

**Dose**

- Initially 5 mg daily half an hour before breakfast, increased at intervals of 3–4 days if necessary to a max. of 20 mg daily; CHILD up to 10 mg daily according to age

◢**Preparations**
Section 7.4.1

## EDROPHONIUM CHLORIDE

**Indications** see under Dose and notes above; reversal of non-depolarising neuromuscular blockade and diagnosis of dual block (section 15.1.6)

**Cautions** see under Neostigmine; have resuscitation facilities; *extreme* caution in respiratory distress (see notes above) and in asthma

Note Severe cholinergic reactions can be counteracted by injection of atropine sulphate (which should always be available)

**Contra-indications** see under Neostigmine

**Side-effects** see under Neostigmine

**Dose**

- Diagnosis of myasthenia gravis, by intravenous injection, 2 mg followed after 30 seconds (if no adverse reaction has occurred) by 8 mg; in adults without suitable veins, by intramuscular injection, 10 mg
- Detection of overdosage or underdosage of cholinergic drugs, by intravenous injection, 2 mg (preferably just before next dose of anticholinesterase, see notes above)
- CHILD by intravenous injection, 20 micrograms/kg followed after 30 seconds (if no adverse reaction has occurred) by 80 micrograms/kg

**Edrophonium** (Cambridge) ▣PoM▣
Injection, edrophonium chloride 10 mg/mL, net price 1-mL amp = £8.65

## PYRIDOSTIGMINE BROMIDE

**Indications** myasthenia gravis

**Cautions** see under Neostigmine; weaker muscarinic action

**Contra-indications** see under Neostigmine

**Side-effects** see under Neostigmine

**Dose**

- By mouth, 30–120 mg at suitable intervals throughout day, total daily dose 0.3–1.2 g (but see also notes above); CHILD under 12 years, see *BNF for Children*

**Mestinon®** (Valeant) ▣PoM▣
Tablets, scored, pyridostigmine (as bromide) 60 mg, net price 20 = £4.81

---

## Immunosuppressant therapy

**Corticosteroids** (section 6.3) are established as treatment for myasthenia gravis; although they are commonly given on alternate days there is little evidence of benefit over daily administration. Corticosteroid treatment is usually initiated under in-patient supervision and all patients should receive osteoporosis prophylaxis (section 6.6).

In *generalised myasthenia gravis* small initial doses of prednisolone (10 mg on alternate days) are increased in steps of 10 mg on alternate days to 1–1.5 mg/kg (max. 100 mg) on alternate days. When given daily, prednisolone is started at 5 mg daily and then increased in steps of 5 mg daily to 60 mg daily or occasionally up to 80 mg daily (0.75–1 mg/kg daily). About 10% of patients experience a transient but very serious worsening of symptoms in the first 2–3 weeks, especially if the corticosteroid is started at a high dose. However, ventilated patients may be started on 1.5 mg/kg (max. 100 mg) on alternate days. Smaller doses of corticosteroid are usually required in *ocular myasthenia*. Once clinical remission has occurred (usually after 2–6 months), the dose of prednisolone should be reduced slowly to the minimum effective dose (usually 10–40 mg on alternate days).

In generalised myasthenia gravis **azathioprine** (section 8.2.1) is usually started at the same time as the corticosteroid and it allows a lower maintenance dose of the corticosteroid to be used; azathioprine is initiated at a low dose, which is increased over 3–4 weeks to 2–2.5 mg/kg daily. Ciclosporin (section 8.2.2), **methotrexate** (section 8.1.3), or **mycophenolate mofetil** (section 8.2.1) can be used in patients unresponsive or intolerant to other treatments [unlicensed indications].

## 10.2.2 Skeletal muscle relaxants

The drugs described below are used for the relief of chronic muscle spasm or spasticity associated with multiple sclerosis or other neurological damage; they are not indicated for spasm associated with minor injuries. They act principally on the central nervous system with the exception of dantrolene, which has a peripheral site of action. They differ in action from the muscle relaxants used in anaesthesia (section 15.1.5), which block transmission at the neuromuscular junction.

The underlying cause of spasticity should be treated and any aggravating factors (e.g. pressure sores, infection) remedied. Skeletal muscle relaxants are effective in most forms of spasticity except the rare alpha variety. The major disadvantage of treatment with these drugs is that reduction in muscle tone can cause a loss of splinting action of the spastic leg and trunk muscles and sometimes lead to an increase in disability.

**Dantrolene** acts directly on skeletal muscle and produces fewer central adverse effects making it a drug of choice. The dose should be increased slowly.

**Baclofen** inhibits transmission at spinal level and also depresses the central nervous system. The dose should be increased slowly to avoid the major side-effects of sedation and muscular hypotonia (other adverse events are uncommon).

**Diazepam** can also be used. Sedation and occasionally extensor hypotonus are disadvantages. Other benzodiazepines also have muscle-relaxant properties. Muscle-relaxant doses of benzodiazepines are similar to anxiolytic doses (section 4.1.2).

**Tizanidine** is an alpha₂-adrenoceptor agonist indicated for spasticity associated with multiple sclerosis or spinal cord injury.

## ▌BACLOFEN

**Indications**  chronic severe spasticity resulting from disorders such as multiple sclerosis or traumatic partial section of spinal cord

**Cautions**  psychiatric illness, Parkinson's disease, cerebrovascular disease, elderly; respiratory impairment; epilepsy; history of peptic ulcer (avoid oral route in active peptic ulceration); diabetes; hypertonic bladder sphincter; avoid abrupt withdrawal (risk of

hyperactive state, may exacerbate spasticity, and precipitate autonomic dysfunction including hyperthermia, psychiatric reactions and convulsions, see also under Withdrawal below); renal impairment (Appendix 3); pregnancy (Appendix 4); **interactions:** Appendix 1 (muscle relaxants)

  **Withdrawal** CSM has advised that serious side-effects can occur on abrupt withdrawal; to minimise risk, discontinue by gradual dose reduction over at least 1–2 weeks (longer if symptoms occur)

  **Driving** Drowsiness may affect performance of skilled tasks (e.g. driving); effects of alcohol enhanced

**Side-effects**  gastro-intestinal disturbances, dry mouth; hypotension, respiratory or cardiovascular depression; sedation, drowsiness, confusion, dizziness, ataxia, hallucinations, nightmares, headache, euphoria, insomnia, depression, anxiety, agitation, tremor; seizure; urinary disturbances; myalgia; visual disorders; rash, hyperhidrosis; *rarely* taste disturbances, abdominal pain, paraesthesia, erectile dysfunction, dysarthria; *very rarely* hypothermia

**Dose**

- By mouth, 5 mg 3 times daily, preferably with or after food, gradually increased; max. 100 mg daily (discontinue if no benefit within 6 weeks); CHILD 0.75–2 mg/kg daily (over 10 years, max. 2.5 mg/kg daily) *or* 2.5 mg 4 times daily increased gradually according to age to maintenance: 1–2 years 10–20 mg daily, 2–6 years 20–30 mg daily, 6–10 years 30–60 mg daily

- By intrathecal injection, see preparation below

**Baclofen** (Non-proprietary) ▣PoM

  Tablets, baclofen 10 mg, net price 84-tab pack = £1.62. Label: 2, 8

  Oral solution, baclofen 5 mg/5 mL, net price 300 mL = £8.95. Label: 2, 8
  Brands include *Lyflex*® (sugar-free)

**Lioresal®** (Novartis) ▣PoM

  Tablets, scored, baclofen 10 mg, net price 84-tab pack = £10.84. Label: 2, 8
  Excipients include gluten

  Liquid, sugar-free, raspberry-flavoured, baclofen 5 mg/5 mL, net price 300 mL = £8.95. Label: 2, 8

### ◢By intrathecal injection

**Lioresal®** (Novartis) ▣PoM

  Intrathecal injection, baclofen, 50 micrograms/mL, net price 1-mL amp (for test dose) = £2.74; 500 micrograms/mL, 20-mL amp (for use with implantable pump) = £60.77; 2 mg/mL, 5-mL amp (for use with implantable pump) = £60.77

  **Important** Consult product literature for details on test dose and titration—important to monitor patients closely in appropriately equipped and staffed environment during screening and immediately after pump implantation. Resuscitation equipment must be available for immediate use

  **Dose**  by intrathecal injection, specialist use only, severe chronic spasticity unresponsive to oral antispastic drugs (or where side-effects of oral therapy unacceptable) *or* as alternative to ablative neurosurgical procedures, initial *test dose* 25–50 micrograms over at least 1 minute via catheter or lumbar puncture, increased in 25-microgram steps (not more often than every 24 hours) to max. 100 micrograms to determine appropriate dose *then dose-titration phase*, most often using infusion pump (implanted into chest wall or abdominal wall tissues) to establish *maintenance dose* (ranging from 12 micrograms to 2 mg daily for spasticity of spinal origin *or* 22 micrograms to 1.4 mg daily for spasticity of cerebral origin) retaining some spasticity to avoid sensation of paralysis; CHILD 4–18 years (spasticity of cerebral origin only), initial *test dose* 25 micrograms then titrated as for ADULT to *maintenance dose* (ranging from 24 micrograms to 1.2 mg daily in children under 12 years)

**10**

**Musculoskeletal and joint diseases**

# DANTROLENE SODIUM

**Indications** chronic severe spasticity of voluntary muscle; malignant hyperthermia (section 15.1.8)

**Cautions** impaired cardiac and pulmonary function; therapeutic effect may take a few weeks to develop—discontinue if no response within 45 days; **interactions**: Appendix 1 (muscle relaxants).
Hepatotoxicity Potentially life-threatening hepatotoxicity reported, usually if doses greater than 400 mg daily used, in females, patients over 30 years, if history of liver disorders, or concomitant use of hepatotoxic drugs; test liver function before and at intervals during therapy—discontinue if abnormal liver function tests or symptoms of liver disorder (counselling, see below); re-introduce only if complete reversal of hepatotoxicity
Counselling Patients should be told how to recognise signs of liver disorder and advised to seek prompt medical attention if symptoms such as anorexia, nausea, vomiting, fatigue, abdominal pain, dark urine, or pruritus develop
Driving Drowsiness may affect performance of skilled tasks (e.g. driving); effects of alcohol enhanced

**Contra-indications** hepatic impairment (may cause severe liver damage); acute muscle spasm; avoid when spasticity is useful, for example, locomotion; pregnancy (Appendix 4); breast-feeding (Appendix 5)

**Side-effects** diarrhoea (withdraw if severe, discontinue treatment if recurs on re-introduction), nausea, vomiting, anorexia, hepatotoxicity (see above), abdominal pain; pericarditis; pleural effusion, respiratory depression; headache, drowsiness, dizziness, asthenia, fatigue, seizures, fever, chills; speech and visual disturbances; rash; *less commonly* dysphagia, constipation, exacerbation of cardiac insufficiency, tachycardia, erratic blood pressure, dyspnoea, depression, confusion, nervousness, insomnia, increased urinary frequency, urinary incontinence or retention, haematuria, crystalluria, and increased sweating

**Dose**

- Initially 25 mg daily, may be increased at weekly intervals to max. 100 mg 4 times daily; usual dose 75 mg 3 times daily; CHILD 5–18 years see *BNF for Children*

**Dantrium®** (SpePharm) (PoM)
Capsules, orange/brown, dantrolene sodium 25 mg, net price 20 = £3.37; 100 mg, 20 = £8.61. Label: 2, counselling, driving, hepatotoxicity

# DIAZEPAM

**Indications** muscle spasm of varied aetiology, including tetanus; other indications (section 4.1.2, section 4.8, section 15.1.4.1)

**Cautions** see section 4.1.2; special precautions for intravenous injection (section 4.8.2)

**Contra-indications** see section 4.1.2

**Side-effects** see section 4.1.2; also hypotonia

**Dose**

- Muscle spasm, by mouth, 2–15 mg daily in divided doses, increased if necessary in spastic conditions to 60 mg daily according to response
Cerebral spasticity in selected cases, CHILD 2–40 mg daily in divided doses

By intramuscular *or* by slow intravenous injection (into a large vein at a rate of not more than

5 mg/minute), in acute muscle spasm, 10 mg repeated if necessary after 4 hours
Note Only use intramuscular route when oral and intravenous routes not possible; special precautions for intravenous injection see section 4.8.2

- Tetanus, ADULT and CHILD, by intravenous injection, 100–300 micrograms/kg repeated every 1–4 hours; by intravenous infusion (*or* by nasoduodenal tube), 3–10 mg/kg over 24 hours, adjusted according to response

◢**Preparations**
Section 4.1.2

# TIZANIDINE

**Indications** spasticity associated with multiple sclerosis or spinal cord injury or disease

**Cautions** elderly; monitor liver function monthly for first 4 months and in those who develop unexplained nausea, anorexia or fatigue; concomitant administration of drugs that prolong QT interval; renal impairment (Appendix 3), pregnancy (Appendix 4), breast-feeding (Appendix 5); **interactions**: Appendix 1 (muscle relaxants)
Driving Drowsiness may affect performance of skilled tasks (e.g. driving); effects of alcohol enhanced

**Contra-indications** severe hepatic impairment

**Side-effects** drowsiness, fatigue, dizziness, dry mouth, nausea, gastro-intestinal disturbances, hypotension; also reported, bradycardia, insomnia, hallucinations and altered liver enzymes (discontinue if persistently raised—consult product literature); rarely acute hepatitis

**Dose**

- ADULT over 18 years, initially 2 mg daily as a single dose increased according to response at intervals of at least 3–4 days in steps of 2 mg daily (and given in divided doses) usually up to 24 mg daily in 3–4 divided doses; max. 36 mg daily

**Tizanidine** (Non-proprietary) (PoM)
Tablets, tizanidine (as hydrochloride) 2 mg net price 120-tab pack = £14.19; 4 mg, 120-tab pack = £18.51. Label: 2

**Zanaflex®** (Cephalon) (PoM)
Tablets, scored, tizanidine (as hydrochloride) 2 mg, net price 120-tab pack = £63.00; 4 mg, 120-tab pack = £80.00. Label: 2

# Other muscle relaxants

The clinical efficacy of methocarbamol and meprobamate (section 4.1.2) as muscle relaxants is **not** well established, although they have been included in compound analgesic preparations.

# METHOCARBAMOL

**Indications** short-term symptomatic relief of muscle spasm (but see notes above)

**Cautions** hepatic impairment (Appendix 2); renal impairment (Appendix 3); pregnancy (Appendix 4); breast-feeding (Appendix 5); **interactions**: Appendix 1 (muscle relaxants)
Driving Drowsiness may affect performance of skilled tasks (e.g. driving); effects of alcohol enhanced

**Contra-indications** coma or pre-coma, brain damage, epilepsy, myasthenia gravis

**Side-effects** nausea, vomiting, dyspepsia; hypersensitivity reactions (including urticaria, angioedema, anaphylaxis); fever, headache, drowsiness, dizziness, confusion, amnesia, restlessness, anxiety, tremor, seizures; blurred vision, nasal congestion; rash, pruritus; leucopenia, cholestatic jaundice

**Dose**

• 1.5 g 4 times daily; may be reduced to 750 mg 3 times daily; ELDERLY up to 750 mg 4 times daily may be sufficient; CHILD not recommended

**Robaxin®** (Shire) [PoM] ◢

750 Tablets, f/c, scored, methocarbamol 750 mg, net price 20 = £2.53. Label: 2

## Nocturnal leg cramps

**Quinine** salts (section 5.4.1) 200–300 mg at bedtime are effective in reducing the frequency of nocturnal leg cramps by about 25% in ambulatory patients. It may take up to 4 weeks for improvement to become apparent; if there is benefit, quinine treatment can be continued. Patients should be monitored closely during the early stages for adverse effects as well as for benefit. Treatment should be interrupted at intervals of approximately 3 months to assess the need for further quinine treatment. Quinine is toxic in overdosage and accidental fatalities have occurred in children (see also below).

■ **QUININE**

**Indications** see notes above; malaria (section 5.4.1)

**Cautions** see section 5.4.1 and notes above

**Contra-indications** see section 5.4.1

**Side-effects** see section 5.4.1; **important: very toxic in overdosage**—immediate advice from poison centres essential (see also p. 32)

**Dose**

• See notes above

◢**Preparations**

Section 5.4.1

## 10.3  Drugs for the relief of soft-tissue inflammation

**10.3.1** Enzymes

**10.3.2** Rubefacients and other topical antirheumatics

## Extravasation

Local guidelines for the management of extravasation should be followed where they exist or specialist advice sought.

Extravasation injury follows leakage of drugs or intravenous fluids from the veins or inadvertent administration into the subcutaneous or subdermal tissue. It must be dealt with **promptly** to prevent tissue necrosis.

Acidic or alkaline preparations and those with an osmolarity greater than that of plasma can cause extravasation injury; excipients including alcohol and polyethylene glycol have also been implicated. Cytotoxic drugs commonly cause extravasation injury. In addition, certain patients such as the very young and the elderly are at increased risk. Those receiving anticoagulants are more likely to lose blood into surrounding tissues if extravasation occurs, while those receiving sedatives or analgesics may not notice the early signs or symptoms of extravasation.

**Prevention of extravasation** Precautions should be taken to avoid extravasation; ideally, drugs likely to cause extravasation injury should be given through a central line and patients receiving repeated doses of hazardous drugs peripherally should have the cannula resited at regular intervals. Attention should be paid to the manufacturers' recommendations for administration. Placing a glyceryl trinitrate patch (section 2.6.1) distal to the cannula may improve the patency of the vessel in patients with small veins or in those whose veins are prone to collapse.

Patients should be asked to report any pain or burning at the site of injection immediately.

**Management of extravasation** If extravasation is suspected the infusion should be stopped immediately but the cannula should not be removed until after an attempt has been made to aspirate the area (through the cannula) in order to remove as much of the drug as possible. Aspiration is sometimes possible if the extravasation presents with a raised bleb or blister at the injection site and is surrounded by hardened tissue, but it is often unsuccessful if the tissue is soft or soggy. **Corticosteroids** are usually given to treat inflammation, although there is little evidence to support their use in extravasation. Hydrocortisone or dexamethasone (section 6.3.2) can be given either locally by subcutaneous injection or intravenously at a site distant from the injury. **Antihistamines** (section 3.4.1) and **analgesics** (section 4.7) may be required for symptom relief.

The management of extravasation beyond these measures is not well standardised and calls for specialist advice. Treatment depends on the nature of the offending substance; one approach is to localise and neutralise the substance whereas another is to spread and dilute it. The first method may be appropriate following extravasation of vesicant drugs and involves administration of an antidote (if available) and the application of cold compresses 3–4 times a day (consult specialist literature for details of specific antidotes). Spreading and diluting the offending substance involves infiltrating the area with physiological saline, applying warm compresses, elevating the affected limb, and administering **hyaluronidase** (section 10.3.1). A saline flush-out technique (involving flushing the subcutaneous tissue with physiological saline) may be effective but requires specialist advice. Hyaluronidase should **not** be administered following extravasation of vesicant drugs (unless it is either specifically indicated or used in the saline flush-out technique). **Dexrazoxane** (section 8.1) is licensed for the treatment of anthracycline-induced extravasation.

**10**

**Musculoskeletal and joint diseases**

## 10.3.1 Enzymes

**Hyaluronidase** is used to render the tissues more readily permeable to injected fluids, e.g. for introduction of fluids by subcutaneous infusion (termed hypodermoclysis).

### ■ HYALURONIDASE

**Indications** enhance permeation of subcutaneous or intramuscular injections, local anaesthetics and subcutaneous infusions; promote resorption of excess fluids and blood

**Cautions** infants or elderly (control speed and total volume and avoid overhydration especially in renal impairment)

**Contra-indications** do not apply direct to cornea; avoid sites where infection or malignancy; not for anaesthesia in unexplained premature labour; not to be used to reduce swelling of bites or stings; not for intravenous administration

**Side-effects** oedema; *rarely* local irritation, infection, bleeding, bruising; occasional severe allergy (including anaphylaxis)

**Dose**
* With subcutaneous or intramuscular injection, 1500 units dissolved directly in solution to be injected (ensure compatibility)
* With local anaesthetics, 1500 units mixed with local anaesthetic solution (ophthalmology, 15 units/mL)
* Hypodermoclysis, 1500 units dissolved in 1 mL water for injections or 0.9% sodium chloride injection, administered before start of 500–1000 mL infusion fluid
* Extravasation (see notes above) or haematoma, 1500 units dissolved in 1 mL water for injections or 0.9% sodium chloride injection, infiltrated into affected area (as soon as possible after extravasation)

**Hyalase®** (CP) [PoM]
Injection, powder for reconstitution, hyaluronidase (ovine). Net price 1500-unit amp = £7.60

## 10.3.2 Rubefacients and other topical antirheumatics

**Rubefacients** act by counter-irritation. Pain, whether superficial or deep-seated, is relieved by any method which itself produces irritation of the skin. Counter-irritation is comforting in painful lesions of the muscles, tendons, and joints, and in non-articular rheumatism. Rubefacients probably all act through the same essential mechanism and differ mainly in intensity and duration of action.

The use of a NSAID by mouth is effective for relieving musculoskeletal pain. **Topical NSAIDs** (e.g. felbinac, ibuprofen, ketoprofen, and piroxicam) may provide some relief of pain in musculoskeletal conditions; they can be considered as an adjunctive treatment in knee or hand osteoarthritis (see section 10.1).

A preparation containing **capsaicin** 0.025% can also be considered as an adjunct in hand or knee osteoarthritis (see section 10.1). It may need to be used for 1–2 weeks before pain is relieved. A higher strength of capsaicin

0.075% cream is licensed for the symptomatic relief of postherpetic neuralgia (section 4.7.3) after lesions have healed, and for the relief of painful diabetic neuropathy (section 6.1.5).

---

### Topical NSAIDs and counter-irritants

**Cautions** Apply with gentle massage only. Avoid contact with eyes, mucous membranes, and inflamed or broken skin; discontinue if rash develops. Hands should be washed immediately after use. Not for use with occlusive dressings. Topical application of large amounts can result in systemic effects (see section 10.1.1), including hypersensitivity and asthma (renal disease has also been reported). Not generally suitable for children. Patient packs carry a **warning** to avoid during **pregnancy** or **breast-feeding**.

**Hypersensitivity** For NSAID hypersensitivity and asthma warning, see p. 561 and p. 562

**Photosensitivity** Patients should be advised against excessive exposure to sunlight of area treated in order to avoid possibility of photosensitivity

### ◢Non-proprietary preparations
**Ibuprofen** (Non-proprietary)
Gel, ibuprofen 5%, net price 30 g = £2.10, 50 g = £2.40, 100 g = £5.31
**Dose** apply up to 3 times daily

**Ketoprofen** (Non-proprietary) [PoM]
Gel, ketoprofen 2.5%, net price 30 g = £2.42, 50 g = £3.06, 100 g = £2.80
**Dose** apply 2–4 times daily for up to 7 days (usual max. 15 g daily)

**Piroxicam** (Non-proprietary) [PoM]
Gel, piroxicam 0.5%, net price 60 g = £1.79; 112 g = £2.73
**Dose** apply 3–4 times daily

### ◢Proprietary preparations
**Feldene®** (Pfizer) [PoM]
Gel, piroxicam 0.5%, net price 60 g = £6.00; 112 g = £9.41 (also 7.5 g starter pack, hosp. only)
Excipients include benzyl alcohol, propylene glycol
**Dose** apply 3–4 times daily; therapy should be reviewed after 4 weeks

**¹Fenbid® Forte Gel** (Goldshield) [PoM]
Gel, ibuprofen 10%, net price 100 g = £6.50
Excipients include benzyl alcohol
**Dose** apply up to 4 times daily; therapy should be reviewed after 14 days
1. Smaller pack sizes available on sale to the public

**Ibugel® Forte** (Dermal) [PoM]
Forte gel, ibuprofen 10%, net price 100 g = £5.87
Excipients none as listed in section 13.1.3
**Dose** apply up to 3 times daily

**¹Oruvail®** (Rhône-Poulenc Rorer) [PoM]
Gel, ketoprofen 2.5%, net price 100 g = £6.84
Excipients include fragrance
**Dose** apply 2–4 times daily for up to 7 days (usual recommended dose 15 g daily)
1. Smaller pack sizes available on sale to the public

**Pennsaid®** (Dimethaid) [PoM]
Cutaneous solution, diclofenac sodium 16 mg/mL in dimethyl sulfoxide, net price 60 mL = £16.00
Excipients include propylene glycol
Dose  pain in osteoarthritis of superficial joints, apply 0.5–1 mL 4 times daily

**Powergel®** (Menarini) [PoM]
Gel, ketoprofen 2.5%, net price 50 g = £3.06; 100 g = £5.89
Excipients include fragrance
Dose  apply 2–3 times daily for up to max. 10 days

**Traxam®** (Goldshield) [PoM]
Foam, felbinac 3.17%. Net price 100 g = £7.30. Label: 15
Excipients include cetostearyl alcohol

Gel, felbinac 3%. Net price 100 g = £7.00
Excipients none as listed in section 13.1.3
Dose  apply 2–4 times daily; max. 25 g daily; therapy should be reviewed after 14 days
Note Felbinac is an active metabolite of the NSAID fenbufen

**¹Voltarol Emulgel®** (Novartis) [PoM]
Gel, diclofenac diethylammonium salt 1.16% (equivalent to diclofenac sodium 1%), net price 20 g (hosp. only) = £1.55; 100 g = £7.00
Excipients include propylene glycol, fragrance
Dose  apply 3–4 times daily; therapy should be reviewed after 14 days (or after 28 days for osteoarthritis)
1. Smaller pack sizes available on sale to the public

**Voltarol Gel Patch®** (Novartis) [PoM]
Gel patch, diclofenac epolamine (equivalent to 140 mg diclofenac sodium per patch), net price 10-patch pack = £14.09
Excipients include hydroxybenzoates (parabens), propylene glycol
Dose  ADULT and CHILD over 15 years, ankle sprain, apply 1 patch daily for up to 3 days; epicondylitis, apply 1 patch twice daily for up to 14 days

## Capsaicin

**Cautions**  Avoid contact with eyes, and inflamed or broken skin. Hands should be washed immediately after use. Not for use under tight bandages. Avoid taking a hot shower or bath just before or after applying capsaicin—burning sensation enhanced.

**Side-effects**  Transient burning sensation can occur during initial treatment, particularly if too much cream is used, or if the frequency of administration is less than 3–4 times daily. Coughing, sneezing, and eye irritation rarely reported.

**Zacin®** (Cephalon) [PoM]
Cream, capsaicin 0.025%. net price 45 g = £18.05.
Excipients include benzyl alcohol, cetyl alcohol
Dose  symptomatic relief in osteoarthritis, apply sparingly 4 times daily (not more often than every 4 hours)

**Axsain®** (Cephalon) [PoM]
Cream, capsaicin 0.075%. net price 45 g = £14.58.
Excipients include benzyl alcohol, cetyl alcohol
Dose  post-herpetic neuralgia (**important: after** lesions have healed), apply sparingly up to 3–4 times daily (not more often than every 4 hours)

Painful diabetic neuropathy, under specialist supervision, apply sparingly 3–4 times daily (not more often than every 4 hours) for 8 weeks then review

## Poultices

**Kaolin Poultice** ◿
Poultice, heavy kaolin 52.7%, thymol 0.05%, boric acid 4.5%, peppermint oil 0.05%, methyl salicylate 0.2%, glycerol 42.5%. Net price 200 g = £2.44
Dose  warm and apply directly or between layers of muslin; avoid application of overheated poultice

**Kaolin Poultice K/L Pack®** (K/L) ◿
Kaolin poultice Net price 4 × 100-g pouches = £6.40

# 11 Eye

11.1 Administration of drugs to the eye 590

11.2 Control of microbial contamination 591

11.3 Anti-infective eye preparations 591

11.3.1 Antibacterials 591

11.3.2 Antifungals 593

11.3.3 Antivirals 593

11.4 Corticosteroids and other anti-inflammatory preparations 593

11.4.1 Corticosteroids 593

11.4.2 Other anti-inflammatory preparations 595

11.5 Mydriatics and cycloplegics 596

11.6 Treatment of glaucoma 597

11.7 Local anaesthetics 602

11.8 Miscellaneous ophthalmic preparations 603

11.8.1 Tear deficiency, ocular lubricants, and astringents 603

11.8.2 Ocular diagnostic and perioperative preparations and photodynamic treatment 604

11.9 Contact lenses 607

11 Eye

## 11.1 Administration of drugs to the eye

Drugs are most commonly administered to the eye by topical application as eye drops or eye ointments. When a higher drug concentration is required within the eye, a local injection may be necessary.

Eye-drop dispenser devices are available to aid the instillation of eye drops from plastic bottles; they are particularly useful for the elderly, visually impaired, arthritic, or otherwise physically limited patients.

**Eye drops and eye ointments** Eye drops are generally instilled into the pocket formed by gently pulling down the lower eyelid and keeping the eye closed for as long as possible after application; one drop is all that is needed. A small amount of eye ointment is applied similarly; the ointment melts rapidly and blinking helps to spread it.

When two different eye-drop preparations are used at the same time of day, dilution and overflow may occur when one immediately follows the other. The patient should therefore leave an interval of at least 5 minutes between the two.

Systemic effects may arise from absorption of drugs into the general circulation from conjunctival vessels or from the nasal mucosa after the excess preparation has drained down through the tear ducts. The extent of systemic absorption following ocular administration is highly variable; nasal drainage of drugs is associated with eye drops much more often than with eye ointments. Pressure on the lacrimal punctum for at least a minute after applying eye drops reduces nasolacrimal drainage and therefore decreases systemic absorption from the nasal mucosa.

For warnings relating to eye drops and contact lenses, see section 11.9.

**Eye lotions** These are solutions for the irrigation of the conjunctival sac. They act mechanically to flush out irritants or foreign bodies as a first-aid treatment. Sterile sodium chloride 0.9% solution (section 11.8.1) is usually used. Clean water will suffice in an emergency.

**Other preparations** Subconjunctival injection may be used to administer anti-infective drugs, mydriatics, or corticosteroids for conditions not responding to topical therapy. The drug diffuses through the cornea and sclera to the anterior and posterior chambers and vitreous humour. However, because the dose-volume is limited (usually not more than 1 mL), this route is suitable only for drugs which are readily soluble.

Drugs such as antimicrobials and corticosteroids may be administered systemically to treat susceptible eye conditions.

**Preservatives and sensitisers** Information on preservatives and on substances identified as skin sensitisers (see section 13.1.3) is provided under preparation entries.

# 11.2 Control of microbial contamination

Preparations for the eye should be sterile when issued. Eye drops in multiple-application containers include a preservative but care should nevertheless be taken to avoid contamination of the contents during use.

Eye drops in multiple-application containers for *domiciliary use* should not be used for more than 4 weeks after first opening (unless otherwise stated).

Eye drops for use in *hospital wards* are normally discarded 1 week after first opening. Individual containers should be provided for each patient. A separate bottle should be supplied for each eye only if there are special concerns about contamination. Containers used before an operation should be discarded at the time of the operation and fresh containers supplied. A fresh supply should also be provided upon discharge from hospital; in specialist ophthalmology units, it may be acceptable to issue eye-drop bottles that have been dispensed to the patient on the day of discharge.

In *out-patient departments* single-application packs should preferably be used; if multiple-application packs are used, they should be discarded at the end of each day. In clinics for eye diseases and in accident and emergency departments, where the dangers of infection are high, single-application packs should be used; if a multiple-application pack is used, it should be discarded after single use.

Diagnostic dyes (e.g. fluorescein) should be used only from single-application packs.

In *eye surgery* single-application containers should be used if possible; if a multiple-application pack is used, it should be discarded after single use. Preparations used during intra-ocular procedures and others that may penetrate into the anterior chamber must be isotonic and without preservatives and buffered if necessary to a neutral pH. Specially formulated fluids should be used for intra-ocular surgery; intravenous infusion preparations are not suitable for this purpose. For all surgical procedures, a previously unopened container is used for each patient.

# 11.3 Anti-infective eye preparations

11.3.1   **Antibacterials**

11.3.2   **Antifungals**

11.3.3   **Antivirals**

**Eye infections** Most acute superficial eye infections can be treated topically. Blepharitis and conjunctivitis are often caused by staphylococci; keratitis and endophthalmitis may be bacterial, viral, or fungal.

Bacterial *blepharitis* is treated by application of an antibacterial eye ointment to the conjunctival sac or to the lid margins. Systemic treatment may occasionally be required and is usually undertaken after culturing organisms from the lid margin and determining their antimicrobial sensitivity; antibiotics such as the tetracyclines given for 3 months or longer may be appropriate.

Most cases of acute bacterial conjunctivitis are self-limiting; where treatment is appropriate, antibacterial eye drops or an eye ointment are used. A poor response might indicate viral or allergic conjunctivitis. *Gonococcal conjunctivitis* is treated with systemic and topical antibacterials.

*Corneal ulcer* and *keratitis* require specialist treatment and may call for hospital admission for intensive therapy.

*Endophthalmitis* is a medical emergency which also calls for specialist management and often requires parenteral, subconjunctival, or intra-ocular administration of antimicrobials.

# 11.3.1 Antibacterials

Bacterial infections are generally treated topically with eye drops and eye ointments. Systemic administration is sometimes appropriate in blepharitis.

**Chloramphenicol** has a broad spectrum of activity and is the drug of choice for *superficial eye infections*. Chloramphenicol eye drops are well tolerated and the recommendation that chloramphenicol eye drops should be avoided because of an increased risk of aplastic anaemia is not well founded.

Other antibacterials with a broad spectrum of activity include the quinolones, **ciprofloxacin**, **levofloxacin**, and **ofloxacin**; the aminoglycosides, **gentamicin** and **neomycin** [unlicensed] are also active against a wide variety of bacteria. Gentamicin, quinolones, and **polymyxin B** are effective for infections caused by *Pseudomonas aeruginosa*.

**Ciprofloxacin** eye drops are licensed for *corneal ulcers*; intensive application (especially in the first 2 days) is required throughout the day and night.

*Trachoma* which results from chronic infection with *Chlamydia trachomatis* can be treated with **azithromycin** by mouth [unlicensed indication].

**Fusidic acid** is useful for staphylococcal infections.

**Propamidine isetionate** is of little value in bacterial infections but is specific for the rare but potentially devastating condition of *acanthamoeba keratitis* (see also section 11.9).

**With corticosteroids** Many antibacterial preparations also incorporate a corticosteroid but such mixtures should **not** be used unless a patient is under close specialist supervision. In particular they should not be prescribed for undiagnosed 'red eye' which is sometimes caused by the herpes simplex virus and may be difficult to diagnose (section 11.4).

**Administration** Frequency of application depends on the severity of the infection and the potential for irreversible ocular damage; antibacterial eye preparations are usually administered as follows:

**Eye drops** Apply 1 drop at least every 2 hours then reduce frequency as infection is controlled and continue for 48 hours after healing.

**Eye ointment** Apply *either* at night (if eye drops used during the day) *or* 3–4 times daily (if eye ointment used alone).

11

Eye

## CHLORAMPHENICOL

**Indications** see notes above

**Side-effects** transient stinging; see also notes above

**Dose**

- See Administration in notes above

### [1] Chloramphenicol (Non-proprietary) PoM

Eye drops, chloramphenicol 0.5%. Net price 10 mL = £2.31

Eye ointment, chloramphenicol 1%. Net price 4 g = £3.10

1. Chloramphenicol 0.5% eye drops (in max. pack size 10 mL) and 1% eye ointment (in max. pack size 4 g) can be sold to the public for treatment of acute bacterial conjunctivitis in adults and children over 2 years; max. duration of treatment 5 days

### Chloromycetin® (Goldshield) PoM

Redidrops (= eye drops), chloramphenicol 0.5%. Net price 5 mL = £1.65; 10 mL = 90p
Excipients include phenylmercuric acetate

Ophthalmic ointment (= eye ointment), chloramphenicol 1%. Net price 4 g = £1.08

#### ◢ Single use

**Minims® Chloramphenicol** (Chauvin) PoM

Eye drops, chloramphenicol 0.5%. Net price 20 × 0.5 mL = £8.61

## CIPROFLOXACIN

**Indications** superficial bacterial infections, see notes above; corneal ulcers

**Cautions** not recommended for children under 1 year; pregnancy (Appendix 4); breast-feeding (Appendix 5)

**Side-effects** local burning and itching; lid margin crusting; hyperaemia; taste disturbances; corneal staining, keratitis, lid oedema, lacrimation, photophobia, corneal infiltrates; nausea and visual disturbances reported

**Dose**

- Superficial bacterial infection, see Administration in notes above
- Corneal ulcer, apply *eye drops* throughout day and night, day 1 apply every 15 minutes for 6 hours then every 30 minutes, day 2 apply every hour, days 3–14 apply every 4 hours (max. duration of treatment 21 days)

  Apply *eye ointment* throughout day and night; apply 1.25 cm ointment every 1–2 hours for 2 days then every 4 hours for next 12 days

### Ciloxan® (Alcon) PoM

Ophthalmic solution (= eye drops), ciprofloxacin (as hydrochloride) 0.3%. Net price 5 mL = £4.79
Excipients include benzalkonium chloride

Eye ointment, ciprofloxacin (as hydrochloride) 0.3%. Net price 3.5 g = £5.32

## FUSIDIC ACID

**Indications** see notes above

**Dose**

- See under preparation below

### Fucithalmic® (LEO) PoM

Eye drops, m/r, fusidic acid 1% in gel basis (liquifies on contact with eye). Net price 5 g = £2.00
Excipients include benzalkonium chloride, disodium edetate
Dose apply twice daily

## GENTAMICIN

**Indications** see notes above

**Dose**

- See Administration in notes above

### Genticin® (Roche) PoM

Drops (for ear or eye), gentamicin 0.3% (as sulphate). Net price 10 mL = £2.13
Excipients include benzalkonium chloride

## LEVOFLOXACIN

**Indications** see notes above

**Cautions** not recommended for children under 1 year; pregnancy (Appendix 4); breast-feeding (Appendix 5)

**Side-effects** transient ocular irritation, visual disturbances, lid margin crusting, lid or conjunctival oedema, hyperaemia, conjunctival follicles, photophobia, headache, rhinitis

**Dose**

- See Administration in notes above

### Oftaquix® (Kestrel Ophthalmics) ▼ PoM

Eye drops, levofloxacin 0.5%, net price 5 mL = £6.95
Excipients include benzalkonium chloride

Eye drops, levofloxacin 0.5%, net price 30 × 0.5-mL single use units = £17.95

## NEOMYCIN SULPHATE

**Indications** see notes above

**Dose**

- See Administration in notes above

### Neomycin (Non-proprietary) PoM

Eye drops, neomycin sulphate 0.5% (3500 units/mL). Net price 10 mL = £3.11
Available from specialist importing companies, p. 969

Eye ointment, neomycin sulphate 0.5% (3500 units/g). Net price 3 g = £2.44
Available from specialist importing companies, p. 969

#### ◢ With other antibacterials

**Neosporin®** (TEVA UK) PoM

Eye drops, gramicidin 25 units, neomycin sulphate 1700 units, polymyxin B sulphate 5000 units/mL. Net price 5 mL = £4.86
Excipients include thiomersal
Dose apply 2–4 times daily or more frequently if required

## OFLOXACIN

**Indications** see notes above

**Cautions** pregnancy (Appendix 4); breast-feeding (Appendix 5)

**Side-effects** local irritation including photophobia; dizziness, numbness, nausea and headache reported

11 Eye

**Dose**

- Apply every 2–4 hours for the first 2 days then reduce frequency to 4 times daily (max. 10 days treatment)

**Exocin®** (Allergan) PoM
Ophthalmic solution (= eye drops), ofloxacin 0.3%. Net price 5 mL = £2.17
Excipients include benzalkonium chloride

## POLYMYXIN B SULPHATE

**Indications** see notes above
**Side-effects** local irritation and dermatitis
**Dose**

- See Administration in notes above

◀With other antibacterials
**Polyfax®** (TEVA UK) PoM
Eye ointment, polymyxin B sulphate 10 000 units, bacitracin zinc 500 units/g. Net price 4 g = £3.26

## PROPAMIDINE ISETIONATE

**Indications** local treatment of infections (but see notes above)
**Dose**

- See preparations

**Brolene®** (Aventis Pharma)
Eye drops, propamidine isetionate 0.1%. Net price 10 mL = £2.80
Excipients include benzalkonium chloride
Dose apply 4 times daily
Note Eye drops containing propamidine isetionate 0.1% also available from Typharm (*Golden Eye Drops*)

Eye ointment, dibromopropamidine isetionate 0.15%. Net price 5 g = £2.92
Dose apply 1–2 times daily
Note Eye ointment containing dibromopropamidine isetionate 0.15% also available from Typharm (*Golden Eye Ointment*)

## 11.3.2 Antifungals

Fungal infections of the cornea are rare but can occur after agricultural injuries, especially in hot and humid climates. Orbital mycosis is rarer, and when it occurs it is usually because of a direct spread of infection from the paranasal sinuses. Increasing age, debility, or immunosuppression may encourage fungal proliferation. The spread of infection through blood occasionally produces a metastatic endophthalmitis.

Many different fungi are capable of producing ocular infection; they may be identified by appropriate laboratory procedures.

Antifungal preparations for the eye are not generally available. Treatment will normally be carried out at specialist centres, but requests for information about supplies of preparations not available commercially should be addressed to the Strategic Health Authority (or equivalent), or to the nearest hospital ophthalmology unit, or to Moorfields Eye Hospital, 162 City Road, London EC1V 2PD (tel. (020) 7253 3411).

## 11.3.3 Antivirals

Herpes simplex infections producing, for example, dendritic corneal ulcers can be treated with **aciclovir** or **ganciclovir**.

Slow-release ocular implants containing **ganciclovir** (available on a named-patient basis from specialist importing companies, see p. 969) may be inserted surgically to treat immediate sight-threatening CMV retinitis. Local treatments do not protect against systemic infection or infection in the other eye. For systemic treatment of CMV retinitis, see section 5.3.2.2.

## ACICLOVIR
(Acyclovir)

**Indications** local treatment of herpes simplex infections
**Side-effects** local irritation and inflammation, superficial punctate keratopathy; *rarely* blepharitis; *very rarely* hypersensitivity reactions including angioedema
**Dose**

- Apply 5 times daily (continue for at least 3 days after complete healing)

**Zovirax®** (GSK) PoM
Eye ointment, aciclovir 3%. Net price 4.5 g = £9.53

## GANCICLOVIR

**Indications** local treatment of herpes simplex infections
**Side-effects** burning sensation, tingling, superficial punctate keratitis
**Dose**

- Apply 5 times daily until healing complete, then apply 3 times daily for a further 7 days

**Virgan®** (Spectrum) PoM
Ophthalmic gel, ganciclovir 0.15%, net price 5 g = £19.99

## 11.4 Corticosteroids and other anti-inflammatory preparations

11.4.1 Corticosteroids
11.4.2 Other anti-inflammatory preparations

## 11.4.1 Corticosteroids

Corticosteroids administered locally to the eye or given by mouth are effective for treating anterior segment inflammation, including that which results from surgery.

*Topical corticosteroids* are applied frequently for the first 24–48 hours; once inflammation is controlled, the frequency of application is reduced. They should normally only be used under expert supervision; three main dangers are associated with their use:

- a 'red eye', where the diagnosis is unconfirmed, may be due to herpes simplex virus, and a corticosteroid may aggravate the condition, leading to corneal ulceration, with possible damage to vision and even loss of the eye. Bacterial, fungal and amoebic infections pose a similar hazard;

- 'steroid glaucoma' may follow the use of corticosteroid eye preparations in susceptible individuals;

- a 'steroid cataract' may follow prolonged use.

Other side-effects of ocular corticosteroids include thinning of the cornea and sclera.

Combination products containing a corticosteroid with an anti-infective drug are sometimes used after ocular surgery to reduce inflammation and prevent infection; use of combination products is otherwise rarely justified.

*Systemic corticosteroids* (section 6.3.2) may be useful for ocular conditions. The risk of producing a 'steroid cataract' increases with the dose and duration of corticosteroid use.

The *Scottish Medicines Consortium* (p. 3) has advised (May 2008) that loteprednol etabonate 0.5% eye drops (*Lotemax®*) are **not** recommended for use within NHS Scotland.

## ■ BETAMETHASONE

**Indications** local treatment of inflammation (short-term)

**Cautions** see notes above

**Side-effects** see notes above

**Dose**

- Apply eye drops every 1–2 hours until controlled then reduce frequency; apply eye ointment 2–4 times daily *or* at night when used with eye drops

**Betnesol®** (UCB Pharma) PoM

Drops (for ear, eye, or nose), betamethasone sodium phosphate 0.1%. Net price 10 mL = £2.23
Excipients include benzalkonium chloride, disodium edetate

Eye ointment, betamethasone sodium phosphate 0.1%. Net price 3 g = £1.36

**Vistamethasone®** (Martindale) PoM

Drops (for ear, eye, or nose), betamethasone sodium phosphate 0.1%. Net price 5 mL = £1.02; 10 mL = £1.16
Excipients include benzalkonium chloride

◢With neomycin

**Betnesol-N®** (UCB Pharma) PoM

Drops (for ear, eye, or nose), see section 12.1.1
Dose apply up to 6 times daily

Eye ointment, betamethasone sodium phosphate 0.1%, neomycin sulphate 0.5%. Net price 3 g = £1.28

**Vistamethasone N®** (Martindale) PoM

Drops (for ear, eye, or nose), see section 12.1.1

## ■ DEXAMETHASONE

**Indications** local treatment of inflammation (short-term)

**Cautions** see notes above

**Side-effects** see notes above

**Dose**

- Apply eye drops every 30–60 minutes until controlled then reduce frequency to 4–6 times daily

**Maxidex®** (Alcon) PoM

Eye drops, dexamethasone 0.1%, hypromellose 0.5%. Net price 5 mL = £1.44; 10 mL = £2.86
Excipients include benzalkonium chloride, disodium edetate, polysorbate 80

◢Single use

**Minims® Dexamethasone** (Chauvin) PoM

Eye drops, dexamethasone sodium phosphate 0.1%. Net price 20 × 0.5 mL = £9.04
Excipients include disodium edetate

◢With antibacterials

**Maxitrol®** (Alcon) PoM

Eye drops, dexamethasone 0.1%, neomycin 0.35% (as sulphate), polymyxin B sulphate 6000 units/mL. Net price 5 mL = £1.72
Excipients include benzalkonium chloride, polysorbate 20

Eye ointment, dexamethasone 0.1%, neomycin 0.35% (as sulphate), polymyxin B sulphate 6000 units/g. Net price 3.5 g = £1.47
Excipients include hydroxybenzoates (parabens), wool fat
Dose apply 3–4 times daily *or* at night when used with eye drops

**Sofradex®** (Sanofi-Aventis) PoM

Drops (for ear or eye), see section 12.1.1

**Tobradex®** (Alcon) PoM

Eye drops, dexamethasone 0.1%, tobramycin 0.3%. Net price 5 mL = £5.47
Excipients include benzalkonium chloride, disodium edetate

## ■ FLUOROMETHOLONE

**Indications** local treatment of inflammation (short-term)

**Cautions** see notes above

**Side-effects** see notes above

**Dose**

- Apply every hour for 24–48 hours then reduce frequency to 2–4 times daily

**FML®** (Allergan) PoM

Ophthalmic suspension (= eye drops), fluorometholone 0.1%, polyvinyl alcohol (*Liquifilm®*) 1.4%. Net price 5 mL = £1.71; 10 mL = £2.95
Excipients include benzalkonium chloride, disodium edetate, polysorbate 80

## ■ HYDROCORTISONE ACETATE

**Indications** local treatment of inflammation (short-term)

**Cautions** see notes above

**Side-effects** see notes above

**Dose**

- Apply eye drops every 30–60 minutes until controlled then reduce frequency to every 4 hours

**Hydrocortisone** (Non-proprietary) PoM

Eye drops, hydrocortisone acetate 1%. Net price 10 mL = £3.21

Eye ointment, hydrocortisone acetate 0.5%, net price 3 g = £2.88; 1%, 3 g = £6.71; 2.5%, 3 g = £7.86

## ■ LOTEPREDNOL ETABONATE

**Indications**  treatment of post-operative inflammation following ocular surgery

**Cautions**  see notes above

**Side-effects**  see notes above

**Dose**

- Apply 4 times daily starting 24 hours after surgery; max. duration of treatment 14 days

**Lotemax®** (Bausch & Lomb) ▼ PoM
Opthalmic suspension (= eye drops), loteprednol etabonate 0.5%, net price 5 mL = £4.95
Excipients include benzalkonium chloride, disodium edetate

## ■ PREDNISOLONE

**Indications**  local treatment of inflammation (short-term)

**Cautions**  see notes above

**Side-effects**  see notes above

**Dose**

- Apply every 1–2 hours until controlled then reduce frequency

**Predsol®** (UCB Pharma) PoM
Drops (for ear or eye), prednisolone sodium phosphate 0.5%. Net price 10 mL = £1.92
Excipients include benzalkonium chloride, disodium edetate

**Pred Forte®** (Allergan) PoM
Eye drops, prednisolone acetate 1%. Net price 5 mL = £1.52; 10 mL = £3.05
Excipients include benzalkonium chloride, disodium edetate, polysorbate 80

◢Single use
**Minims® Prednisolone Sodium Phosphate** (Chauvin) PoM
Eye drops, prednisolone sodium phosphate 0.5%. Net price 20 × 0.5 mL = £9.78
Excipients include disodium edetate

◢With neomycin
**Predsol-N®** (UCB Pharma) PoM ◢
Drops (for ear or eye), see section 12.1.1
Dose apply up to 6 times daily

## ■ RIMEXOLONE

**Indications**  local treatment of inflammation (short-term)

**Cautions**  see notes above

**Side-effects**  see notes above

**Dose**

- Postoperative inflammation, apply 4 times daily for 2 weeks, beginning 24 hours after surgery
- Steroid-responsive inflammation, apply at least 4 times daily for up to 4 weeks
- Uveitis, apply every hour during daytime in week 1, then every 2 hours in week 2, then 4 times daily in week 3, then twice daily for first 4 days of week 4, then once daily for remaining 3 days of week 4

**Vexol®** (Alcon) PoM
Eye drops, rimexolone 1%, net price 5 mL = £5.77
Excipients include benzalkonium chloride, disodium edetate, polysorbate 80

## 11.4.2 Other anti-inflammatory preparations

Other preparations used for the topical treatment of inflammation and allergic conjunctivitis include antihistamines, lodoxamide, and sodium cromoglicate.

Eye drops of antihistamines, such as **antazoline** (with xylometazoline as *Otrivine-Antistin®*), **azelastine**, **epinastine**, **ketotifen**, and **olopatadine**, can be used for allergic conjunctivitis.

**Sodium cromoglicate** (sodium cromoglycate) and **nedocromil sodium** eye drops can be useful for vernal keratoconjunctivitis and other allergic forms of conjunctivitis.

**Lodoxamide** eye drops are used for allergic conjunctival conditions including seasonal allergic conjunctivitis.

**Diclofenac** eye drops (section 11.8.2) and **emedastine** eye drops are also licensed for seasonal allergic conjunctivitis.

## ■ ANTAZOLINE SULPHATE

**Indications**  allergic conjunctivitis

**Otrivine-Antistin®** (Novartis Consumer Health)
Eye drops, antazoline sulphate 0.5%, xylometazoline hydrochloride 0.05%. Net price 10 mL = £2.35
Excipients include benzalkonium chloride, disodium edetate
Dose ADULT and CHILD over 12 years apply 2–3 times daily (max. 7 days)
Note Xylometazoline is a sympathomimetic; it should be used with caution in patients susceptible to angle-closure glaucoma; absorption of antazoline and xylometazoline may result in systemic side-effects and the possibility of interaction with other drugs

## ■ AZELASTINE HYDROCHLORIDE

**Indications**  allergic conjunctivitis

**Side-effects**  mild transient irritation; bitter taste reported

**Dose**

- Seasonal allergic conjunctivitis, ADULT and CHILD over 4 years, apply twice daily, increased if necessary to 4 times daily
- Perennial conjunctivitis, ADULT and ADOLESCENT over 12 years, apply twice daily, increased if necessary to 4 times daily; max. duration of treatment 6 weeks

**Optilast®** (Viatris) PoM
Eye drops, azelastine hydrochloride 0.05%. Net price 8 mL = £6.40
Excipients include benzalkonium chloride, disodium edetate

## ■ EMEDASTINE

**Indications**  seasonal allergic conjunctivitis

**Side-effects**  transient burning or stinging; blurred vision, local oedema, keratitis, irritation, dry eye, lacrimation, corneal infiltrates (discontinue) and staining; photophobia; headache, and rhinitis occasionally reported

**Dose**

- ADULT and CHILD over 3 years, apply twice daily

**11
Eye**

**Emadine®** (Alcon) [PoM]
Eye drops, emedastine 0.05% (as difumarate), net price 5 mL = £7.45
Excipients include benzalkonium chloride

## EPINASTINE HYDROCHLORIDE

**Indications** seasonal allergic conjunctivitis

**Side-effects** burning; *less commonly* dry mouth, taste disturbance; nasal irritation, rhinitis; headache, blepharoptosis, conjunctival oedema and hyperaemia, dry eye, local irritation, photophobia, visual disturbance; pruritus

**Dose**
● ADULT and ADOLESCENT over 12 years, apply twice daily; max. duration of treatment 8 weeks

**Relestat®** (Allergan) [PoM]
Eye drops, epinastine hydrochloride 500 micrograms/mL, net price 5 mL = £9.90
Excipients include benzalkonium chloride, disodium edetate

## KETOTIFEN

**Indications** seasonal allergic conjunctivitis

**Side-effects** burning or stinging, punctate corneal epithelial erosion; *less commonly* dry eye, subconjunctival haemorrhage, photophobia; headache, drowsiness, skin reactions, and dry mouth also reported

**Dose**
● ADULT and CHILD over 3 years, apply twice daily

**Zaditen®** (Novartis) [PoM]
Eye drops, ketotifen (as fumarate) 250 micrograms/mL, net price 5 mL = £9.75
Excipients include benzalkonium chloride

## LODOXAMIDE

**Indications** allergic conjunctivitis

**Side-effects** burning, stinging, itching, and lacrimation; flushing and dizziness reported

**Dose**
● ADULT and CHILD over 4 years, apply 4 times daily

**Alomide®** (Alcon) [PoM]
Ophthalmic solution (= eye drops), lodoxamide 0.1% (as trometamol). Net price 10 mL = £5.31
Excipients include benzalkonium chloride, disodium edetate
Note Lodoxamide 0.1% eye drops can be sold to the public for treatment of allergic conjunctivitis in adults and children over 4 years

## NEDOCROMIL SODIUM

**Indications** allergic conjunctivitis; seasonal keratoconjunctivitis

**Side-effects** burning and stinging; distinctive taste reported

**Dose**
● Seasonal and perennial conjunctivitis, ADULT and CHILD over 6 years, apply twice daily increased if necessary to 4 times daily; max. 12 weeks treatment for seasonal allergic conjunctivitis
● Seasonal keratoconjunctivitis, ADULT and CHILD over 6 years, apply 4 times daily

**Rapitil®** (Aventis Pharma) [PoM]
Eye drops, nedocromil sodium 2%. Net price 5 mL = £4.92
Excipients include benzalkonium chloride, disodium edetate

## OLOPATADINE

**Indications** seasonal allergic conjunctivitis

**Side-effects** local irritation; less commonly keratitis, dry eye, local oedema, photophobia; headache, asthenia, dizziness; dry nose also reported

**Dose**
● ADULT and CHILD over 3 years, apply twice daily; max. duration of treatment 4 months

**Opatanol®** (Alcon) [PoM]
Eye drops, olopatadine (as hydrochloride) 1 mg/mL, net price 5 mL = £3.98
Excipients include benzalkonium chloride

## SODIUM CROMOGLICATE
### (Sodium cromoglycate)

**Indications** allergic conjunctivitis; seasonal keratoconjunctivitis

**Side-effects** burning and stinging

**Dose**
● ADULT and CHILD apply eye drops 4 times daily

[1]**Sodium Cromoglicate** (Non-proprietary) [PoM]
Eye drops, sodium cromoglicate 2%. Net price 13.5 mL = £1.55
Brands include *Hay-Crom® Aqueous, Opticrom® Aqueous, Vividrin®*)

1. Sodium cromoglicate 2% eye drops can be sold to the public (in max. pack size of 10 mL) for treatment of acute seasonal and perennial allergic conjunctivitis

# 11.5 Mydriatics and cycloplegics

Antimuscarinics dilate the pupil and paralyse the ciliary muscle; they vary in potency and duration of action.

Short-acting, relatively weak mydriatics, such as **tropicamide** 0.5% (action lasts for 4–6 hours), facilitate the examination of the fundus of the eye. **Cyclopentolate** 1% (action up to 24 hours) or **atropine** (action up to 7 days) are preferable for producing cycloplegia for refraction in young children. Atropine ointment 1% is sometimes preferred for children aged under 5 years because the ointment formulation reduces systemic absorption

Mydriatics and cycloplegics are used in the treatment of anterior uveitis, usually as an adjunct to corticosteroids (section 11.4.1). Atropine is used in anterior uveitis mainly to prevent posterior synechiae and to relieve ciliary spasm, often in combination with phenylephrine eye drops; cyclopentolate or **homatropine** (action up to 3 days) can also be used and may be preferred because they have a shorter duration of action.

**Phenylephrine** is used for mydriasis in diagnostic or therapeutic procedures; mydriasis occurs within 60–90 minutes and lasts up to 5–7 hours. Phenylephrine 10% drops are contra-indicated in children and the elderly owing to the risk of systemic effects.

**Cautions** Darkly pigmented iris is more resistant to pupillary dilatation and caution should be exercised to avoid overdosage. Mydriasis can precipitate acute angle-closure glaucoma in a few patients, usually aged over 60 years and hypermetropic (long-sighted), who are predisposed to the condition because of a shallow anterior chamber. Phenylephrine may interact with systemically administered monoamine-oxidase inhibitors; other **interactions**: Appendix 1 (sympathomimetics).

**Driving** Patients should be warned not to drive for 1–2 hours after mydriasis.

**Side-effects** Ocular side-effects of mydriatics and cycloplegics include transient stinging and raised intra-ocular pressure; on prolonged administration, local irritation, hyperaemia, oedema and conjunctivitis can occur. Contact dermatitis can occur with the antimuscarinic mydriatic drugs, especially atropine.

Systemic side-effects of atropine and cyclopentolate can occur, particularly in children and the elderly; see section 1.2 for systemic side-effects of antimuscarinic drugs.

## Antimuscarinics

### ATROPINE SULPHATE

**Indications** see notes above
**Cautions** risk of systemic effects with eye drops in infants under 3 months—eye ointment preferred; see also notes above
**Side-effects** see notes above

**Atropine** (Non-proprietary) (PoM)
Eye drops, atropine sulphate 0.5%, net price 10 mL = £2.78; 1%, 10 mL = £1.12

Eye ointment, atropine sulphate 1%. Net price 3 g = £2.97

◢Single use
**Minims® Atropine Sulphate** (Chauvin) (PoM)
Eye drops, atropine sulphate 1%. Net price 20 × 0.5 mL = £9.59

### CYCLOPENTOLATE HYDROCHLORIDE

**Indications** see notes above
**Cautions** see notes above
**Side-effects** see notes above

**Mydrilate®** (Intrapharm) (PoM)
Eye drops, cyclopentolate hydrochloride 0.5%, net price 5 mL = 97p; 1%, 5 mL = £1.19
Excipients include benzalkonium chloride

◢Single use
**Minims® Cyclopentolate Hydrochloride** (Chauvin) (PoM)
Eye drops, cyclopentolate hydrochloride 0.5% and 1%. Net price 20 × 0.5 mL (both) = £9.35

### HOMATROPINE HYDROBROMIDE

**Indications** see notes above
**Cautions** see notes above
**Side-effects** see notes above

**Homatropine** (Non-proprietary) (PoM)
Eye drops, homatropine hydrobromide 1%, net price 10 mL = £2.47; 2%, 10 mL = £2.60

### TROPICAMIDE

**Indications** see notes above
**Cautions** see notes above
**Side-effects** see notes above

**Mydriacyl®** (Alcon) (PoM)
Eye drops, tropicamide 0.5%, net price 5 mL = £1.32; 1%, 5 mL = £1.63
Excipients include benzalkonium chloride, disodium edetate

◢Single use
**Minims® Tropicamide** (Chauvin) (PoM)
Eye drops, tropicamide 0.5% and 1%. Net price 20 × 0.5 mL (both) = £8.63

## Sympathomimetics

### PHENYLEPHRINE HYDROCHLORIDE

**Indications** mydriasis; see also notes above
**Cautions** children and elderly (avoid 10% strength); cardiovascular disease (avoid or use 2.5% strength only); tachycardia; hyperthyroidism; diabetes; see also notes above
**Side-effects** eye pain and stinging; blurred vision, photophobia; systemic effects include palpitations, arrhythmias, hypertension, coronary artery spasm; *very rarely* angle-closure glaucoma

**Phenylephrine** (Non-proprietary)
Eye drops, phenylephrine hydrochloride 10%. Net price 10 mL = £3.89

◢Single use
**Minims® Phenylephrine Hydrochloride** (Chauvin)
Eye drops, phenylephrine hydrochloride 2.5%, net price 20 × 0.5 mL = £9.20; 10%, 20 × 0.5 mL = £9.20
Excipients include disodium edetate, sodium metabisulphite

## 11.6 Treatment of glaucoma

Glaucoma describes a group of disorders characterised by a loss of visual field associated with cupping of the optic disc and optic nerve damage. While glaucoma is generally associated with raised intra-ocular pressure, it can occur when the intra-ocular pressure is within the normal range.

The commonest form of glaucoma is *primary open-angle glaucoma* (chronic simple glaucoma; wide-angle glaucoma), where the obstruction is in the trabecular meshwork. The condition is often asymptomatic and the patient may present with significant loss of visual-field. *Primary angle-closure glaucoma* (acute closed-angle glaucoma, narrow-angle glaucoma) results from blockage of aqueous humour flow into the anterior chamber and is a medical emergency.

Drugs that reduce intra-ocular pressure by different mechanisms are available for managing glaucoma. A topical beta-blocker or a prostaglandin analogue is usually the drug of first choice. It may be necessary to

**11**
**Eye**

combine these drugs or add others, such as miotics, sympathomimetics, or carbonic anhydrase inhibitors, to control intra-ocular pressure.

For urgent reduction of intra-ocular pressure and before surgery, mannitol 20% (up to 500 mL) is given by slow intravenous infusion until the intra-ocular pressure has been satisfactorily reduced. Acetazolamide by intravenous injection can also be used for the emergency management of raised intra-ocular pressure.

Standard antiglaucoma therapy is used if supplementary treatment is required after iridotomy, iridectomy, or a drainage operation in either primary open-angle or primary angle-closure glaucoma.

## Beta-blockers

Topical application of a beta-blocker to the eye reduces intra-ocular pressure effectively in *primary open-angle glaucoma*, probably by reducing the rate of production of aqueous humour. Administration by mouth also reduces intra-ocular pressure but this route is not used since side-effects may be troublesome.

Beta-blockers used as eye drops include **betaxolol**, **carteolol**, **levobunolol**, **metipranolol**, and **timolol**.

**Cautions, contra-indications and side-effects** Systemic absorption may follow topical application to the eyes; therefore, eye drops containing a beta-blocker are contra-indicated in patients with bradycardia, heart block, or uncontrolled heart failure. **Important:** for a warning to avoid in asthma see CSM advice below. Consider also other cautions, contra-indications and side-effects of beta-blockers (p. 86). Local side-effects of eye drops include ocular stinging, burning, pain, itching, erythema, dry eyes and allergic reactions including anaphylaxis and blepharoconjunctivitis; occasionally corneal disorders have been reported.
**CSM advice** The CSM has advised that beta-blockers, even those with apparent cardioselectivity, should not be used in patients with asthma or a history of obstructive airways disease, unless no alternative treatment is available. In such cases the risk of inducing bronchospasm should be appreciated and appropriate precautions taken.

**Interactions** Since systemic absorption may follow topical application the possibility of interactions, in particular, with drugs such as verapamil should be borne in mind. See also Appendix 1 (beta-blockers).

### ■ BETAXOLOL HYDROCHLORIDE

**Indications** see notes above
**Cautions** see notes above
**Contra-indications** see notes above
**Side-effects** see notes above
**Dose**
- Apply twice daily

**Betoptic®** (Alcon) [PoM]
Ophthalmic solution (= eye drops), betaxolol (as hydrochloride) 0.5%, net price 5 mL = £1.94
Excipients include benzalkonium chloride, disodium edetate

Ophthalmic suspension (= eye drops), m/r, betaxolol (as hydrochloride) 0.25%, net price 5 mL = £2.71
Excipients include benzalkonium chloride, disodium edetate

Unit dose eye drop suspension, m/r, betaxolol (as hydrochloride) 0.25%, net price 50 × 0.25 mL = £14.04

### ■ CARTEOLOL HYDROCHLORIDE

**Indications** see notes above
**Cautions** see notes above
**Contra-indications** see notes above
**Side-effects** see notes above
**Dose**
- Apply twice daily

**Teoptic®** (Novartis) [PoM]
Eye drops, carteolol hydrochloride 1%, net price 5 mL = £4.60; 2%, 5 mL = £5.40
Excipients include benzalkonium chloride

### ■ LEVOBUNOLOL HYDROCHLORIDE

**Indications** see notes above
**Cautions** see notes above
**Contra-indications** see notes above
**Side-effects** see notes above; anterior uveitis occasionally reported
**Dose**
- Apply once or twice daily

**Levobunolol** (Non-proprietary) [PoM]
Eye drops, levobunolol hydrochloride 0.5%. Net price 5 mL = £2.77

**Betagan®** (Allergan) [PoM]
Eye drops, levobunolol hydrochloride 0.5%, polyvinyl alcohol (*Liquifilm®*) 1.4%. Net price 5-mL = £1.85
Excipients include benzalkonium chloride, disodium edetate, sodium metabisulphite

Unit dose eye drops, levobunolol hydrochloride 0.5%, polyvinyl alcohol (*Liquifilm®*) 1.4%. Net price 30 × 0.4 mL = £9.98
Excipients include disodium edetate

### ■ METIPRANOLOL

**Indications** see notes above but in chronic open-angle glaucoma **restricted** to patients allergic to preservatives or to those wearing soft contact lenses (in whom benzalkonium chloride should be avoided)
**Cautions** see notes above
**Contra-indications** see notes above
**Side-effects** see notes above; granulomatous anterior uveitis reported (discontinue treatment)
**Dose**
- Apply twice daily

**Minims® Metipranolol** (Chauvin) [PoM]
Eye drops, metipranolol 0.1%, net price 20 × 0.5 mL = £11.21

### ■ TIMOLOL MALEATE

**Indications** see notes above
**Cautions** see notes above
**Contra-indications** see notes above
**Side-effects** see notes above
**Dose**
- Apply twice daily; long-acting preparations, see under preparations below

**Timolol** (Non-proprietary) [PoM]
Eye drops, timolol (as maleate) 0.25%, net price 5 mL = £2.21; 0.5%, 5 mL = £2.04

**Timoptol®** (MSD) PoM

Eye drops, in *Ocumeter®* metered-dose unit, timolol (as maleate) 0.25%, net price 5 mL = £3.12; 0.5%, 5 mL = £3.12
Excipients include benzalkonium chloride

Unit dose eye drops, timolol (as maleate) 0.25%, net price 30 × 0.2 mL = £8.45; 0.5%, 30 × 0.2 mL = £9.65

◢**Once-daily preparations**

**Nyogel®** (Novartis) PoM

Eye gel (= eye drops), timolol (as maleate) 0.1%, net price 5 g = £2.85
Excipients include benzalkonium chloride

**Dose** apply once daily

**Timoptol®-LA** (MSD) PoM

Ophthalmic gel-forming solution (= eye drops), timolol (as maleate) 0.25%, net price 2.5 mL = £3.12; 0.5%, 2.5 mL = £3.12
Excipients include benzododecinium bromide

**Dose** apply once daily

◢**With bimatoprost**
See under Bimatoprost

◢**With brimonidine**
See under Brimonidine

◢**With brinzolomide**
See under Brinzolomide

◢**With dorzolamide**
See under Dorzolamide

◢**With latanoprost**
See under Latanoprost

◢**With travoprost**
See under Travoprost

## Prostaglandin analogues

**Latanoprost** and **travoprost** are prostaglandin analogues which increase uveoscleral outflow; **bimatoprost** is a related drug. They are used to reduce intra-ocular pressure in ocular hypertension or in open-angle glaucoma. Patients receiving prostaglandin analogues should be monitored for any changes to eye coloration since an increase in the brown pigment in the iris may occur; particular care is required in those with mixed coloured irides and those receiving treatment to one eye only.

### ▋ BIMATOPROST

**Indications** raised intra-ocular pressure in open-angle glaucoma; ocular hypertension

**Cautions** see under Latanoprost and notes above

**Side-effects** see under Latanoprost; also ocular pruritus, allergic conjunctivitis, cataract, conjunctival oedema, eye discharge, photophobia, superficial punctate keratitis, headache; hypertension

**Dose**

• Apply once daily, preferably in the evening; CHILD under 18 years, not recommended

**Lumigan®** (Allergan) PoM

Eye drops, bimatoprost 300 micrograms/mL, net price 3 mL = £10.30, triple pack (3 × 3 mL) = £30.90
Excipients include benzalkonium chloride

◢**With timolol**

For cautions, contra-indications, and side-effects of timolol, see section 11.6, Beta-blockers

**Ganfort®** (Allergan) ▼ PoM

Eye drops, bimatoprost 300 micrograms/mL, timolol (as maleate) 5 mg/mL, net price 3-mL = £13.95
Excipients include benzalkonium chloride

**Dose** for raised intra-ocular pressure in patients with open-angle glaucoma or ocular hypertension when beta-blocker or prostaglandin analogue alone not adequate; apply once daily, preferably in the morning

### ▋ LATANOPROST

**Indications** raised intra-ocular pressure in open-angle glaucoma; ocular hypertension

**Cautions** before initiating treatment, advise patients of possible change in eye colour; monitor for eye colour change (see also notes above); aphakia, or pseudo-phakia with torn posterior lens capsule or anterior chamber lenses; risk factors for iritis, uveitis, and cystoid macular oedema; brittle or severe asthma; not to be used within 5 minutes of use of thiomersal-containing preparations; pregnancy (Appendix 4); breast-feeding (Appendix 5)

**Side-effects** brown pigmentation particularly in those with mixed-colour irides; blepharitis, ocular irritation and pain; darkening, thickening and lengthening of eye lashes; conjunctival hyperaemia; transient punctate epithelial erosion; skin rash; *less commonly* eyelid oedema and rash; *rarely* dyspnoea, exacerbation of asthma, iritis, uveitis, local oedema, darkening of palpebral skin; *very rarely* chest pain, exacerbation of angina

**Dose**

• Apply once daily, preferably in the evening; CHILD not recommended

**Xalatan®** (Pharmacia) PoM

Eye drops, latanoprost 50 micrograms/mL, net price 2.5 mL = £12.48
Excipients include benzalkonium chloride

◢**With timolol**

For cautions, contra-indications, and side-effects of timolol, see section 11.6, Beta-blockers

**Xalacom®** (Pharmacia) PoM

Eye drops, latanoprost 50 micrograms, timolol (as maleate) 5 mg/mL, net price 2.5 mL = £14.32
Excipients include benzalkonium chloride

**Dose** for raised intra-ocular pressure in patients with open-angle glaucoma and ocular hypertension when beta-blocker alone not adequate; apply once daily

### ▋ TRAVOPROST

**Indications** raised intra-ocular pressure in open-angle glaucoma; ocular hypertension

**Cautions** see under Latanoprost and notes above

**Side-effects** see under Latanoprost; also headache, ocular pruritus, photophobia, and keratitis reported; rarely, hypotension, bradycardia, conjunctivitis, browache

**Dose**

• Apply once daily, preferably in the evening; CHILD under 18 years, not recommended

**11**

**Eye**

**Travatan®** (Alcon) PoM
Eye drops, travoprost 40 micrograms/mL, net price 2.5 mL = £10.17
Excipients include benzalkonium chloride

◀**With timolol**
For cautions, contra-indications, and side-effects of timolol, see section 11.6, Beta-blockers

**DuoTrav®** (Alcon) PoM
Eye drops, travoprost 40 micrograms, timolol (as maleate) 5 mg/mL, net price 2.5 mL = £12.79
Excipients include benzalkonium chloride, disodium edetate
Dose for raised intra-ocular pressure in patients with open-angle glaucoma or ocular hypertension when beta-blocker or prostaglandin analogue alone not adequate; apply once daily; CHILD and ADOLESCENT under 18 years, not recommended

## Sympathomimetics

**Dipivefrine** is a pro-drug of adrenaline (epinephrine). It is claimed to pass more rapidly than adrenaline through the cornea and is then converted to the active form.

Adrenaline probably acts both by reducing the rate of production of aqueous humour and by increasing the outflow through the trabecular meshwork. Because it is a mydriatic, adrenaline should be used with caution in patients susceptible to angle-closure glaucoma, unless an iridectomy has been carried out. Side-effects include severe smarting and redness of the eye; adrenaline should be used with caution in patients with hypertension and heart disease.

**Brimonidine**, a selective alpha₂-adrenoceptor agonist, is licensed for the reduction of intra-ocular pressure in open-angle glaucoma or ocular hypertension in patients for whom beta-blockers are inappropriate; it may also be used as adjunctive therapy when intra-ocular pressure is inadequately controlled by other antiglaucoma therapy.

**Apraclonidine** (section 11.8.2) is another alpha₂-adrenoceptor agonist. Eye drops containing apraclonidine 0.5% are used for a short term to delay laser treatment or surgery for glaucoma in patients not adequately controlled by another drug; eye drops containing 1% are used for control of intra-ocular pressure after anterior segment laser surgery.

### ▌ BRIMONIDINE TARTRATE

**Indications** raised intra-ocular pressure, see notes above
**Cautions** severe cardiovascular disease; cerebral or coronary insufficiency, Raynaud's syndrome, postural hypotension, depression, hepatic or renal impairment; pregnancy, breast-feeding; **interactions:** Appendix 1 (brimonidine)
Driving Drowsiness may affect performance of skilled tasks (e.g. driving)
**Side-effects** ocular reactions including conjunctival hyperaemia, stinging, pruritus, allergy, and conjunctival folliculosis, visual disturbances, blepharitis, epiphora, corneal erosion, superficial punctuate keratitis, eye pain, discharge, dryness, and irritation, eyelid inflammation, oedema, pruritus conjunctivitis, photophobia; also, hypertension, headache, depression, dry mouth, fatigue, drowsiness; *less commonly*, taste disturbances, palpitation, dizziness, syncope, rhinitis, nasal dryness

**Dose**
● Apply twice daily

**Alphagan®** (Allergan) PoM
Eye drops, brimonidine tartrate 0.2%, net price 5 mL = £6.85
Excipients include benzalkonium chloride

◀**With timolol**
For cautions, contra-indications, and side-effects of timolol, see section 11.6, Beta-blockers

**Combigan®** (Allergan) PoM
Eye drops, brimonidine tartrate 0.2%, timolol (as maleate) 0.5%, net price 5-mL = £10.00
Excipients include benzalkonium chloride
Dose for raised intra-ocular pressure in open-angle glaucoma and for ocular hypertension when beta-blocker alone not adequate, apply twice daily

### ▌ DIPIVEFRINE HYDROCHLORIDE

**Indications** see notes above
**Contra-indications** see notes above
**Side-effects** see notes above
**Dose**
● Apply twice daily

**Propine®** (Allergan) PoM
Eye drops, dipivefrine hydrochloride 0.1%, net price 5 mL = £3.81, 10 mL = £4.77
Excipients include benzalkonium chloride, disodium edetate

## Carbonic anhydrase inhibitors and systemic drugs

The **carbonic anhydrase inhibitors**, acetazolamide, brinzolamide, and dorzolamide, reduce intra-ocular pressure by reducing aqueous humour production. Systemic use also produces weak diuresis.

**Acetazolamide** is given by mouth or by intravenous injection (intramuscular injections are painful because of the alkaline pH of the solution). It is used as an adjunct to other treatment for reducing intra-ocular pressure. Acetazolamide is a sulphonamide; blood disorders, rashes, and other sulphonamide-related side-effects occur occasionally. It is not generally recommended for long-term use; electrolyte disturbances and metabolic acidosis that occur may be corrected by administering potassium bicarbonate (as effervescent potassium tablets, section 9.2.1.3).

**Dorzolamide** and **brinzolamide** are topical carbonic anhydrase inhibitors. They are licensed for use in patients resistant to beta-blockers or those in whom beta-blockers are contra-indicated. They are used alone or as an adjunct to a topical beta-blocker. Systemic absorption may rarely give rise to sulphonamide-like side-effects and may require discontinuation if severe.

The osmotic diuretics, intravenous hypertonic **mannitol** (section 2.2.5), or **glycerol** by mouth, are useful short-term ocular hypotensive drugs.

### ▌ ACETAZOLAMIDE

**Indications** reduction of intra-ocular pressure in open-angle glaucoma, secondary glaucoma, and perioperatively in angle-closure glaucoma; diuresis (section 2.2.7); epilepsy

**Cautions** not generally recommended for prolonged use but if given monitor blood count and plasma electrolyte concentration; pulmonary obstruction (risk of acidosis); elderly; pregnancy (Appendix 4); avoid extravasation at injection site (risk of necrosis); **interactions:** Appendix 1 (diuretics)

**Contra-indications** hypokalaemia, hyponatraemia, hyperchloraemic acidosis; severe hepatic impairment; renal impairment (Appendix 3); sulphonamide hypersensitivity

**Side-effects** nausea, vomiting, diarrhoea, taste disturbance; loss of appetite, paraesthesia, flushing, headache, dizziness, fatigue, irritability, depression; thirst, polyuria; reduced libido; metabolic acidosis and electrolyte disturbances on long-term therapy; occasionally, drowsiness, confusion, hearing disturbances, urticaria, melaena, glycosuria, haematuria, abnormal liver function, renal calculi, blood disorders including agranulocytosis and thrombocytopenia, rashes including Stevens-Johnson syndrome and toxic epidermal necrolysis; rarely, photosensitivity, liver damage, flaccid paralysis, convulsions; transient myopia reported

**Dose**

- Glaucoma, by mouth *or* by intravenous injection, 0.25–1 g daily in divided doses

- Epilepsy, by mouth *or* by intravenous injection, 0.25–1 g daily in divided doses; CHILD 8–30 mg/kg daily, max. 750 mg daily

**Note** Dose by intramuscular injection, as for intravenous injection but preferably avoided because of alkalinity

**Diamox®** (Goldshield) [PoM]

Tablets, acetazolamide 250 mg. Net price 112-tab pack = £12.68. Label: 3

Sodium Parenteral (= injection), powder for reconstitution, acetazolamide (as sodium salt). Net price 500-mg vial = £14.76

◢**Modified release**

**Diamox® SR** (Goldshield) [PoM]

Capsules, m/r, orange, enclosing orange f/c pellets, acetazolamide 250 mg. Net price 30-cap pack = £13.88. Label: 3, 25

Dose glaucoma, 1–2 capsules daily

▌ **BRINZOLAMIDE**

**Indications** adjunct to beta-blockers or used alone in raised intra-ocular pressure in ocular hypertension and in open-angle glaucoma if beta-blocker alone inadequate or inappropriate

**Cautions** systemic absorption follows topical application; hepatic impairment; pregnancy (Appendix 4); **interactions:** Appendix 1 (brinzolamide)

**Contra-indications** renal impairment; (avoid if eGFR less than 30 mL/minute/1.73 m²); hyperchloraemic acidosis; breast-feeding

**Side-effects** local irritation, taste disturbance; less commonly nausea, dyspepsia, dry mouth, chest pain, epistaxis, haemoptysis, dyspnoea, rhinitis, pharyngitis, bronchitis, paraesthesia, depression, dizziness, headache, dermatitis, alopecia, corneal erosion

**Dose**

- Apply twice daily increased to 3 times daily if necessary

**Azopt®** (Alcon) [PoM]

Eye drops, brinzolamide 10 mg/mL, net price 5 mL = £6.69

Excipients include benzalkonium chloride, disodium edetate

◢**With timolol**

For cautions, contra-indications, and side-effects of timolol, see section 11.6, Beta blockers

**Azarga®** (Alcon) ▼ [PoM]

Ophthalmic suspension ( = eye drops), brinzolamide 10 mg, timolol (as maleate) 5 mg/mL, net price 5 mL = £11.05

Excipients include benzalkonium chloride, disodium edetate

Dose for raised intra-ocular pressure in open-angle glaucoma or ocular hypertension when beta-blocker alone not adequate, ADULT over 18 years apply twice daily

▌ **DORZOLAMIDE**

**Indications** raised intra-ocular pressure in ocular hypertension, open-angle glaucoma, pseudo-exfoliative glaucoma *either* as adjunct to beta-blocker *or* used alone in patients unresponsive to beta-blockers or if beta-blockers contra-indicated

**Cautions** systemic absorption follows topical application; hepatic impairment; history of renal calculi; chronic corneal defects, history of intra-ocular surgery; **interactions:** Appendix 1 (dorzolamide)

**Contra-indications** renal impairment (avoid if eGFR less than 30 mL/minute/1.73 m²); hyperchloraemic acidosis; pregnancy and breast-feeding

**Side-effects** nausea, bitter taste, dry mouth; headache, asthenia; ocular irritation, blurred vision, lacrimation, conjunctivitis, superficial punctuate keratitis, eyelid inflammation; *less commonly* iridocyclitis; *rarely* hypersensitivity reactions (including urticaria, angioedema, bronchospasm), dizziness, paraesthesia, urolithiasis, eyelid crusting, transient myopia, corneal oedema, epistaxis, throat irritation

**Dose**

- Used alone, apply 3 times daily

- With topical beta-blocker, apply twice daily

**Trusopt®** (MSD) [PoM]

Ophthalmic solution (= eye drops), in *Ocumeter® Plus* metered-dose unit, dorzolamide (as hydrochloride) 2%, net price 5 mL = £6.33

Excipients include benzalkonium chloride

Unit dose eye drops, dorzolamide (as hydrochloride) 2%, net price 60 × 0.2 mL = £24.18

◢**With timolol**

For cautions, contra-indications, and side-effects of timolol, see section 11.6, Beta-blockers

**Cosopt®** (MSD) [PoM]

Ophthalmic solution (= eye drops), dorzolamide (as hydrochloride) 2%, timolol (as maleate) 0.5%, net price 5 mL = £10.05

Excipients include benzalkonium chloride

Unit dose eye drops, dorzolamide (as hydrochloride) 2%, timolol (as maleate) 0.5%, net price 60 × 0.2 mL = £28.59

## Miotics

The small pupil is an unfortunate side-effect of these drugs (except when pilocarpine is used temporarily before an operation for *angle-closure glaucoma*). They act by opening up the inefficient drainage channels in the trabecular meshwork resulting from contraction or spasm of the ciliary muscle.

Miotics used in the management of raised intra-ocular pressure include pilocarpine.

**Cautions** A darkly pigmented iris may require higher concentration of the miotic or more frequent administration and care should be taken to avoid overdosage. Retinal detachment has occurred in susceptible individuals and those with retinal disease; therefore fundus examination is advised before starting treatment with a miotic. Care is also required in conjunctival or corneal damage. Intra-ocular pressure and visual fields should be monitored in those with chronic simple glaucoma and those receiving long-term treatment with a miotic. Miotics should be used with caution in cardiac disease, hypertension, asthma, peptic ulceration, urinary-tract obstruction, and Parkinson's disease.
**Counselling** Blurred vision may affect performance of skilled tasks (e.g. driving) particularly at night or in reduced lighting

**Contra-indications** Miotics are contra-indicated in conditions where pupillary constriction is undesirable such as acute iritis, anterior uveitis and some forms of secondary glaucoma. They should be avoided in acute inflammatory disease of the anterior segment.

**Side-effects** Ciliary spasm leads to headache and browache which may be more severe in the initial 2–4 weeks of treatment (a particular disadvantage in patients under 40 years of age). Ocular side-effects include burning, itching, smarting, blurred vision, conjunctival vascular congestion, myopia, lens changes with chronic use, vitreous haemorrhage, and pupillary block. Systemic side-effects (see under Parasympathomimetics, section 7.4.1) are rare following application to the eye.

### PILOCARPINE

**Indications** see notes above; dry mouth (section 12.3.5)

**Cautions** see notes above

**Contra-indications** see notes above

**Side-effects** see notes above

**Dose**

- Apply up to 4 times daily; long-acting preparations, see under preparations below

**Pilocarpine Hydrochloride** (Non-proprietary) [PoM]
Eye drops, pilocarpine hydrochloride 0.5%, net price 10 mL = £1.60; 1%, 10 mL = £2.71; 2%, 10 mL = £2.59; 3%, 10 mL = £1.94; 4%, 10 mL = £3.46

◢Single use
**Minims® Pilocarpine Nitrate** (Chauvin) [PoM]
Eye drops, pilocarpine nitrate 2%, net price 20 × 0.5 mL = £9.84

◢Long acting
**Pilogel®** (Alcon) [PoM]
Ophthalmic gel, pilocarpine hydrochloride 4%, net price 5 g = £6.65
Excipients include benzalkonium chloride, disodium edetate
**Dose** apply 1–1.5 cm gel once daily at bedtime

## 11.7 Local anaesthetics

Oxybuprocaine and tetracaine (amethocaine) are probably the most widely used topical local anaesthetics. Proxymetacaine causes less initial stinging and is useful for children. Oxybuprocaine or a combined preparation of lidocaine (lignocaine) and fluorescein is used for tonometry. Tetracaine produces a more profound anaesthesia and is suitable for use before minor surgical procedures, such as the removal of corneal sutures. It has a temporary disruptive effect on the corneal epithelium. Lidocaine, with or without adrenaline (epinephrine), is injected into the eyelids for minor surgery, while retrobulbar or peribulbar injections are used for surgery of the globe itself. Local anaesthetics should never be used for the management of ocular symptoms.

Local anaesthetic eye drops should be avoided in preterm neonates because of the immaturity of the metabolising enzyme system.

### LIDOCAINE HYDROCHLORIDE
(Lignocaine hydrochloride)

**Indications** local anaesthetic

**Minims® Lignocaine and Fluorescein** (Chauvin) [PoM]
Eye drops, lidocaine hydrochloride 4%, fluorescein sodium 0.25%. Net price 20 × 0.5 mL = £10.40

### OXYBUPROCAINE HYDROCHLORIDE
(Benoxinate hydrochloride)

**Indications** local anaesthetic

**Minims® Oxybuprocaine Hydrochloride** (Chauvin)
[PoM]
Eye drops, oxybuprocaine hydrochloride 0.4%. Net price 20 × 0.5 mL = £8.61

### PROXYMETACAINE HYDROCHLORIDE

**Indications** local anaesthetic

**Minims® Proxymetacaine** (Chauvin) [PoM]
Eye drops, proxymetacaine hydrochloride 0.5%. Net price 20 × 0.5 mL = £9.04

◢With fluorescein
**Minims® Proxymetacaine and Fluorescein** (Chauvin)
[PoM]
Eye drops, proxymetacaine hydrochloride 0.5%, fluorescein sodium 0.25%. Net price 20 × 0.5 mL = £10.34

### TETRACAINE HYDROCHLORIDE
(Amethocaine hydrochloride)

**Indications** local anaesthetic

**Minims® Amethocaine Hydrochloride** (Chauvin) [PoM]
Eye drops, tetracaine hydrochloride 0.5% and 1%. Net price 20 × 0.5 mL (both) = £8.63

**11 Eye**

# 11.8 Miscellaneous ophthalmic preparations

**11.8.1** Tear deficiency, ocular lubricants, and astringents

**11.8.2** Ocular diagnostic and peri-operative preparations and photodynamic treatment

Certain eye drops, e.g. amphotericin, ceftazidime, cefuroxime, colistin, desferrioxamine, dexamethasone, gentamicin and vancomycin may be prepared aseptically from material supplied for injection.

# 11.8.1 Tear deficiency, ocular lubricants, and astringents

Chronic soreness of the eyes associated with reduced or abnormal tear secretion (e.g. in Sjögren's syndrome) often responds to tear replacement therapy or pilocarpine given by mouth (section 12.3.5). The severity of the condition and patient preference will often guide the choice of preparation.

**Hypromellose** is the traditional choice of treatment for tear deficiency. It may need to be instilled frequently (e.g. hourly) for adequate relief. Ocular surface mucin is often abnormal in tear deficiency and the combination of hypromellose with a mucolytic such as **acetylcysteine** can be helpful.

The ability of **carbomers** to cling to the eye surface may help reduce frequency of application to 4 times daily.

**Polyvinyl alcohol** increases the persistence of the tear film and is useful when the ocular surface mucin is reduced.

**Povidone** and **sodium hyaluronate** eye drops are also used in the management of tear deficiency.

**Sodium chloride 0.9%** drops are sometimes useful in tear deficiency, and can be used as 'comfort drops' by contact lens wearers, and to facilitate lens removal. Special presentations of sodium chloride 0.9% and other irrigation solutions are used routinely for intraocular surgery.

Eye ointments containing a **paraffin** may be used to lubricate the eye surface, especially in cases of recurrent corneal epithelial erosion. They may cause temporary visual disturbance and are best suited for application before sleep. Ointments should not be used during contact lens wear.

**Zinc sulphate** is a traditional astringent that is now little used.

## ACETYLCYSTEINE

**Indications** tear deficiency, impaired or abnormal mucus production

**Dose**
• Apply 3–4 times daily

**Ilube®** (Alcon) PoM
Eye drops, acetylcysteine 5%, hypromellose 0.35%. Net price 10 mL = £4.49
Excipients include benzalkonium chloride, disodium edetate

## CARBOMERS
(Polyacrylic acid)
**Note** Synthetic high molecular weight polymers of acrylic acid cross-linked with either allyl ethers of sucrose or allyl ethers of pentaerithrityl

**Indications** dry eyes including keratoconjunctivitis sicca, unstable tear film

**Dose**
• Apply 3–4 times daily or as required

**GelTears®** (Chauvin)
Gel (= eye drops), carbomer 980 (polyacrylic acid) 0.2%, net price 10 g = £2.80
Excipients include benzalkonium chloride

**Liposic®** (Bausch & Lomb)
Gel (= eye drops), carbomer 980 (polyacrylic acid) 0.2%, net price 10 g = £2.96
Excipients include cetrimide

**Liquivisc®** (Allergan)
Gel (= eye drops), carbomer 974P (polyacrylic acid) 0.25%, net price 10 g = £1.99
Excipients include benzalkonium chloride
**Note** May be difficult to obtain

**Viscotears®** (Novartis)
Liquid gel (= eye drops), carbomer 980 (polyacrylic acid) 0.2%, net price 10 g = £3.00
Excipients include cetrimide

Liquid gel (= eye drops), carbomer 980 (polyacrylic acid) 0.2%, net price 30 × 0.6-mL single-dose units = £5.53

## CARMELLOSE SODIUM

**Indications** dry eye conditions
**Dose**
• Apply as required

**Optive®** (Allergan)
Eye drops, carmellose sodium 0.5%, glycerol, net price 10 mL = £7.49

◄**Single use**
**Celluvisc®** (Allergan)
Eye drops, carmellose sodium 0.5%, net price 30 × 0.4 mL = £5.75, 90 × 0.4 mL = £15.53; 1%, 30 × 0.4 mL = £3.00, 60 × 0.4 mL = £10.99

## HYDROXYETHYLCELLULOSE

**Indications** tear deficiency

**Minims® Artificial Tears** (Chauvin)
Eye drops, hydroxyethylcellulose 0.44%, sodium chloride 0.35%. Net price 20 × 0.5 mL = £7.48

## HYPROMELLOSE

**Indications** tear deficiency
**Note** The Royal Pharmaceutical Society of Great Britain has stated that where it is not possible to ascertain the strength of

**11**
**Eye**

hypromellose prescribed, the prescriber should be contacted to clarify the strength intended.

**Hypromellose** (Non-proprietary)
Eye drops, hypromellose 0.3%, net price 10 mL = £2.02
Brands include *Artelac*®

**Isopto Alkaline**® (Alcon)
Eye drops, hypromellose 1%, net price 10 mL = 96p
Excipients include benzalkonium chloride

**Isopto Plain**® (Alcon)
Eye drops, hypromellose 0.5%, net price 10 mL = 82p
Excipients include benzalkonium chloride

**Tears Naturale**® (Alcon)
Eye drops, dextran '70' 0.1%, hypromellose 0.3%, net price 15 mL = £1.63
Excipients include benzalkonium chloride, disodium edetate

◢**Single use**
**Hypromellose** (Non-proprietary)
Eye drops, hypromellose 0.3%, net price 30 × 0.4 mL = £5.75

**Artelac**® **SDU** (Pharma-Global)
Eye drops, hypromellose 0.32%, net price 30 × 0.5 mL = £16.95

### LIQUID PARAFFIN

**Indications** dry eye conditions

**Lacri-Lube**® (Allergan)
Eye ointment, white soft paraffin 57.3%, liquid paraffin 42.5%, wool alcohols 0.2%. Net price 3.5 g = £2.28, 5 g = £3.32

**Lubri-Tears**® (Alcon)
Eye ointment, white soft paraffin 60%, liquid paraffin 30%, wool fat 10%. Net price 5 g = £2.22

### PARAFFIN, YELLOW, SOFT

**Indications** see notes above

**Simple Eye Ointment**
Ointment, liquid paraffin 10%, wool fat 10%, in yellow soft paraffin. Net price 4 g = £3.01

### POLYVINYL ALCOHOL

**Indications** tear deficiency

**Liquifilm Tears**® (Allergan)
Ophthalmic solution (= eye drops), polyvinyl alcohol 1.4%. Net price 15 mL = £1.93
Excipients include benzalkonium chloride, disodium edetate

Ophthalmic solution (= eye drops), polyvinyl alcohol 1.4%, povidone 0.6%. Net price 30 × 0.4 mL = £5.35

**Sno Tears**® (Chauvin)
Eye drops, polyvinyl alcohol 1.4%. Net price 10 mL = £1.06
Excipients include benzalkonium chloride, disodium edetate

### POVIDONE

**Indications** dry eye conditions
**Dose**
● Apply 4 times daily or as required

**Oculotect**® (Novartis)
Eye drops, povidone 5%. Net price 20 × 0.4 mL = £3.40

### SODIUM CHLORIDE

**Indications** irrigation, including first-aid removal of harmful substances

**Sodium Chloride 0.9% Solutions**
See section 13.11.1

**Balanced Salt Solution**
Solution (sterile), sodium chloride 0.64%, sodium acetate 0.39%, sodium citrate 0.17%, calcium chloride 0.048%, magnesium chloride 0.03%, potassium chloride 0.075%
For intra-ocular or topical irrigation during surgical procedures
Brands include *Iocare*®

◢**Single use**
**Minims**® **Saline** (Chauvin)
Eye drops, sodium chloride 0.9%. Net price 20 × 0.5 mL = £6.40

### SODIUM HYALURONATE

**Indications** dry eye conditions
**Dose**
● Apply as required

**Oxyal**® (Kestrel Ophthalmics)
Eye drops, sodium hyaluronate 0.15%, net price 10 mL = £4.15

**Vismed**® **Multi** (TRB Chemedica)
Eye drops, sodium hyaluronate 0.18%, net price 10 mL = £6.81

◢**Single use**
**Clinitas**® (Altacor)
Eye drops, sodium hyaluronate 0.4%, net price 30 × 0.5 mL = £5.70

**Ocusan**® (Agepha)
Eye drops, sodium hyaluronate 0.2%, net price 20 × 0.5 mL = £5.25

**Vismed**® (TRB Chemedica)
Eye drops, sodium hyaluronate 0.18%, net price 20 × 0.3 mL = £5.10

### ZINC SULPHATE

**Indications** see notes above

**Zinc Sulphate** (Non-proprietary)
Eye drops, zinc sulphate 0.25%. Net price 10 mL = £3.63

## 11.8.2 Ocular diagnostic and peri-operative preparations and photodynamic treatment

### Ocular diagnostic preparations

**Fluorescein sodium** is used in diagnostic procedures and for locating damaged areas of the cornea due to injury or disease.

## ■ FLUORESCEIN SODIUM

**Indications** detection of lesions and foreign bodies

**Minims® Fluorescein Sodium** (Chauvin)
Eye drops, fluorescein sodium 1% or 2%. Net price 20 × 0.5 mL (both) = £7.38

◢**With local anaesthetic**
Section 11.7

## Ocular peri-operative drugs

Drugs used to prepare the eye for surgery, drugs that are injected into the anterior chamber at the time of surgery, and those used after eye surgery, are included here.

Non-steroidal anti-inflammatory eye drops such as **diclofenac**, **flurbiprofen**, **ketorolac**, and **nepafenac**, are used for the prophylaxis and treatment of inflammation, pain, and other symptoms associated with ocular surgery or laser treatment of the eye. Diclofenac and flurbiprofen are also used to prevent miosis during ocular surgery.

**Apraclonidine**, an alpha$_1$-adrenoreceptor agonist, reduces intra-ocular pressure possibly by reducing the production of aqueous humour. It is used to control increases in intra-ocular pressure associated with ocular surgery and as short-term treatment to reduce intra-ocular pressure prior to surgery.

**Acetylcholine**, instilled into the anterior chamber of the eye during surgery, rapidly produces miosis which lasts approximately 20 minutes. If prolonged miosis is required, it can be applied again.

Intra-ocular **sodium hyaluronate** and balanced salt solution (section 11.8.1) are used during surgical procedures on the eye.

## ■ ACETYLCHOLINE CHLORIDE

**Indications** cataract surgery, penetrating keratoplasty, iridectomy, and other anterior segment surgery requiring rapid complete miosis
**Contra-indications** pregnancy; breast-feeding
**Side-effects** *rarely* bradycardia, hypotension, breathing difficulty, sweating, flushing

**Miochol-E®** (Novartis) PoM
Intra-ocular irrigation, powder for reconstitution, acetylcholine chloride 10 mg/mL (1%) when reconstituted, net price 20-mg vial (with solvent) = £9.10

## ■ APRACLONIDINE

**Note** Apraclonidine is a derivative of clonidine

**Indications** control of intra-ocular pressure
**Cautions** history of angina, severe coronary insufficiency, recent myocardial infarction, heart failure, cerebrovascular disease, vasovagal attack, chronic renal failure; depression; pregnancy and breast-feeding; monitor intra-ocular pressure and visual fields; loss of effect may occur over time; suspend treatment if reduction in vision occurs in end-stage glaucoma; monitor for excessive reduction in intra-ocular pressure following peri-operative use; **interactions:** Appendix 1 (apraclonidine)
**Driving** Drowsiness may affect performance of skilled tasks (e.g. driving)

**Contra-indications** history of severe or unstable and uncontrolled cardiovascular disease
**Side-effects** dry mouth, taste disturbance; hyperaemia, ocular pruritus, discomfort and lacrimation (withdraw if ocular intolerance including oedema of lids and conjunctiva); headache, asthenia, dry nose; lid retraction, conjunctival blanching and mydriasis reported after peri-operative use; since absorption may follow topical application systemic effects (see Clonidine Hydrochloride, section 2.5.2) may occur
**Dose**
● See under preparations below

**Iopidine®** (Alcon) PoM
Ophthalmic solution (= eye drops), apraclonidine 1% (as hydrochloride), net price 12 × 2 single use 0.25-mL units = £79.36
**Dose** control or prevention of postoperative elevation of intra-ocular pressure after anterior segment laser surgery, apply 1 drop 1 hour before laser procedure then 1 drop immediately after completion of procedure; CHILD not recommended

**Iopidine 0.5% ophthalmic solution** (= eye drops), apraclonidine 0.5% (as hydrochloride), net price 5 mL = £11.10
**Excipients** include benzalkonium chloride
**Dose** short-term adjunctive treatment of chronic glaucoma in patients not adequately controlled by another drug (see note below), apply 1 drop 3 times daily usually for max. 1 month; CHILD not recommended
**Note** May not provide additional benefit if patient already using two drugs that suppress the production of aqueous humour

## ■ DICLOFENAC SODIUM

**Indications** inhibition of intra-operative miosis during cataract surgery (but does not possess intrinsic mydriatic properties); postoperative inflammation in cataract surgery, strabismus surgery or argon laser trabeculoplasty; pain in corneal epithelial defects after photorefractive keratectomy, radial keratotomy or accidental trauma; seasonal allergic conjunctivitis (section 11.4.2)

**Voltarol® Ophtha Multidose** (Novartis) PoM
Eye drops, diclofenac sodium 0.1%, net price 5 mL = £6.68
**Excipients** include benzalkonium chloride, disodium edetate, propylene glycol

◢**Single use**
**Voltarol® Ophtha** (Novartis) PoM
Eye drops, diclofenac sodium 0.1%, net price pack of 5 single-dose units = £4.00, 40 single-dose units = £32.00

## ■ FLURBIPROFEN SODIUM

**Indications** inhibition of intra-operative miosis (but does not possess intrinsic mydriatic properties); anterior segment inflammation following postoperative and post-laser trabeculoplasty when corticosteroids contra-indicated

**Ocufen®** (Allergan) PoM
Ophthalmic solution (= eye drops), flurbiprofen sodium 0.03%, polyvinyl alcohol (*Liquifilm®*) 1.4%, net price 40 × 0.4 mL = £37.15

11
Eye

**KETOROLAC TROMETAMOL**

**Indications** prophylaxis and reduction of inflammation and associated symptoms following ocular surgery

**Acular®** (Allergan) PoM
Eye drops, ketorolac trometamol 0.5%, net price 5 mL = £3.00
Excipients include benzalkonium chloride, disodium edetate

**NEPAFENAC**

**Indications** prophylaxis and treatment of postoperative pain and inflammation associated with cataract surgery
**Cautions** avoid sunlight; discontinue immediately if evidence of corneal epithelial breakdown
**Side-effects** headache; punctuate keratitis, blurred vision, eye pruritus, dry eye; *less commonly* nausea, dry mouth; iritis; keratitis, corneal deposits, choroidal effusion, allergic conjunctivitis, increased lacrimation, photophobia, conjunctival hyperaemia

**Nevanac®** (Alcon) ▼ PoM
Ophthalmic suspension (= eye drops), nepafenac 1 mg/mL, net price 5 mL= £14.92
Excipients include benzalkonium chloride, disodium edetate

## Subfoveal choroidal neovascularisation

**Pegaptanib** and **ranibizumab** are vascular endothelial growth factor inhibitors licensed for the treatment of neovascular (wet) age-related macular degeneration; they are given by intravitreal injection by specialists experienced in the management of this condition.

---

NICE guidance
**Ranibizumab and pegaptanib for the treatment of wet age-related macular degeneration (August 2008)**
Ranibizumab is recommended for the treatment of wet age-related macular degeneration if all of the following apply:
- the best corrected visual acuity is between 6/12 and 6/96;
- there is no permanent structural damage to the central fovea;
- the lesion size is less than or equal to 12 disc areas in greatest linear dimension;
- there is evidence of recent disease progression;
- the cost of ranibizumab beyond 14 injections is met by the manufacturer.

Ranibizumab should only be continued in patients who maintain adequate response to therapy.
Pegaptanib is not recommended for the treatment of wet age-related macular degeneration; patients currently receiving pegaptanib for any lesion type can continue therapy until they and their specialist consider it appropriate to stop.

---

**Verteporfin** is licensed for use in the photodynamic treatment of age-related macular degeneration associated with predominantly classic subfoveal choroidal neovascularisation *or* with pathological myopia (see NICE guidance below). Following intravenous infusion, verteporfin is activated by local irradiation using non-thermal red light to produce cytotoxic derivatives. Only specialists experienced in the management of these conditions should use it.

---

NICE guidance
**Photodynamic therapy for wet age-related macular degeneration (September 2003)**
Photodynamic therapy is recommended for wet age-related macular degeneration with a confirmed diagnosis of classic (no occult) subfoveal choroidal neovascularisation and best-corrected visual acuity of 6/60 or better.
Photodynamic therapy is **not** recommended for wet age-related macular degeneration with predominantly classic but partly occult subfoveal choroidal neovascularisation *except* in clinical studies.

---

**PEGAPTANIB SODIUM**

**Indications** see notes above—specialist use only
**Cautions** monitor intra-ocular pressure following injection; pregnancy (Appendix 4); breast-feeding (Appendix 5)
**Contra-indications** ocular or periocular infection
**Side-effects** rhinorrhoea; headache; eye pain, anterior chamber inflammation, raised intra-ocular pressure, punctuate keratitis, vitreous floaters, cataract, conjunctival and retinal haemorrhage, local oedema, conjunctivitis, corneal dystrophy, dry eye, endophthalmitis, eye discharge, eye irritation, macular degeneration, mydriasis, periorbital haematoma, photophobia, flashing lights, vitreous disorders; *less commonly* vomiting, dyspepsia, palpitation, chest pain, hypertension, aortic aneurysm, influenza-like symptoms, nightmares, depression, back pain, asthenopia, blepharitis, corneal deposits, vitreous haemorrhage, chalazion, retinal exudates, eyelid ptosis, decreased intra-ocular pressure, injection-site reactions, retinal detachment, occlusion of retinal blood vessels, ectropion, eye movement disorder, pupillary disorder, iritis, optic nerve cupping, nasopharyngitis, deafness, vertigo, eczema, changes in hair colour, rash, pruritus, night sweats

**Dose**
- By intravitreal injection, 300 micrograms once every 6 weeks into the affected eye

Note For further information on administration, consult product literature

**Macugen®** (Pfizer) PoM
Solution for intravitreal injection, pegaptanib (as sodium salt), net price 300-microgram vial = £514.00

---

**RANIBIZUMAB**

**Indications** see notes above—specialist use only
**Cautions** monitor intra-ocular pressure and for signs of ocular infection following injection; pregnancy (Appendix 4); breast-feeding (Appendix 5)
**Contra-indications** ocular or periocular infection; severe intra-ocular inflammation
**Side-effects** nausea; headache; nasopharyngitis, cough; anxiety; anaemia; arthralgia; raised intra-ocular pressure, visual disturbance, conjunctival retinal and vitreous disorders, eye inflammation and irritation, eye haemorrhage; allergic skin reactions; *less commonly* atrial fibrillation, blindness, corneal disorders, iris adhesion, injection site reactions

**Dose**

- By intravitreal injection, initially 500 micrograms once a month for 3 months into the affected eye, thereafter monitor visual acuity once a month; if necessary subsequent doses may be given at least 1 month apart

  **Note** For further information on administration, consult product literature

  Antimicrobial eye drops should be administered into the affected eye for 3 days before and 3 days after each injection

**Lucentis®** (Novartis) ▼ PoM
Solution for intravitreal injection, ranibizumab 10 mg/mL, net price 0.23-mL vial = £761.20

---

## ▊ VERTEPORFIN

**Indications**  see notes above—specialist use only

**Cautions**  photosensitivity—avoid exposure of unprotected skin and eyes to bright light during infusion and for 48 hours afterwards; hepatic impairment (avoid if severe), biliary obstruction; avoid extravasation; pregnancy (Appendix 4)

**Contra-indications**  acute porphyria; breast-feeding (Appendix 5)

**Side-effects**  visual disturbances (including blurred vision, flashing lights, visual-field defects), nausea, back pain, asthenia, pruritus, hypercholesterolaemia, fever; *rarely* lacrimation disorder, subretinal or vitreous haemorrhage, hypersensitivity reactions (including chest pain, syncope, headache, dizziness, dyspnoea, urticaria, sweating, changes in blood pressure and in heart rate); injection-site reactions including pain, oedema, inflammation, haemorrhage, discoloration and blistering

**Dose**

- By intravenous infusion over 10 minutes, 6 mg/m$^2$

  **Note** For information on administration and light activation, consult product literature

**Visudyne®** (Novartis) PoM
Injection, powder for reconstitution, verteporfin, net price 15-mg vial = £850.00

---

## ▊ 11.9 Contact lenses

**Note** Some recommendations in this section involve non-licensed indications.

For cosmetic reasons many people prefer to wear contact lenses rather than spectacles; contact lenses are also sometimes required for medical indications. Visual defects are corrected by either rigid ('hard' or gas permeable) lenses or soft (hydrogel or silicone hydrogel) lenses; soft lenses are the most popular type, because they are the most comfortable, but they may not give the best vision. Lenses should usually be worn for a specified number of hours each day. Continuous (extended) wear involves much greater risks to eye health and is not recommended except where medically indicated.

Contact lenses require meticulous care. Poor compliance with directions for use, and with daily cleaning and disinfection, can result in complications including ulcerative keratitis and conjunctival problems (such as purulent or papillary conjunctivitis). One-day disposable lenses, which are worn only once and therefore require

no maintenance or storage, are becoming increasingly popular.

*Acanthamoeba keratitis*, a sight-threatening condition, is associated with ineffective lens cleaning and disinfection or the use of contaminated lens cases. The condition is especially associated with the use of soft lenses (including frequently replaced lenses). *Acanthamoeba keratitis* is treated, by specialists, with intensive use of polihexanide (polyhexamethylene biguanide), propamidine isetionate (section 11.3.1), chlorhexidine, and neomycin (section 11.3.1) drops, sometimes used in combination.

**Contact lenses and drug treatment**  Special care is required in prescribing eye preparations for contact lens users. Some drugs and preservatives in eye preparations can accumulate in hydrogel lenses and may induce toxic reactions. Therefore, unless medically indicated, the lenses should be removed before instillation and not worn during the period of treatment. Alternatively, unpreserved drops can be used. Eye drops may, however, be instilled over rigid corneal contact lenses. Ointment preparations should never be used in conjunction with contact lens wear; oily eye drops should also be avoided.

Many drugs given systemically can also have adverse effects on contact lens wear. These include oral contraceptives (particularly those with a higher oestrogen content), drugs which reduce blink rate (e.g. anxiolytics, hypnotics, antihistamines, and muscle relaxants), drugs which reduce lacrimation (e.g. antihistamines, antimuscarinics, phenothiazines and related drugs, some beta-blockers, diuretics, and tricyclic antidepressants), and drugs which increase lacrimation (including ephedrine and hydralazine). Other drugs that may affect contact lens wear are isotretinoin (can cause conjunctival inflammation), aspirin (salicylic acid appears in tears and can be absorbed by contact lenses—leading to irritation), and rifampicin and sulfasalazine (can discolour lenses).

# 12 Ear, nose, and oropharynx

12.1 Drugs acting on the ear                608
12.1.1 Otitis externa                       608
12.1.2 Otitis media                         611
12.1.3 Removal of ear wax                   611

12.2 Drugs acting on the nose               612
12.2.1 Drugs used in nasal allergy          612
12.2.2 Topical nasal decongestants          614
12.2.3 Nasal preparations for infection     615

12.3 Drugs acting on the oro-
pharynx                                     616
12.3.1 Drugs for oral ulceration and
inflammation                                616
12.3.2 Oropharyngeal anti-infective
drugs                                       618
12.3.3 Lozenges and sprays                  620
12.3.4 Mouthwashes, gargles, and
dentifrices                                 620
12.3.5 Treatment of dry mouth               621

This chapter also includes advice on the drug management of the following:
allergic rhinitis, p. 612
nasal polyps, p. 612
oropharyngeal infections, p. 618
periodontitis, p. 617

## 12.1 Drugs acting on the ear

12.1.1 Otitis externa
12.1.2 Otitis media
12.1.3 Removal of ear wax

### 12.1.1 Otitis externa

Otitis externa is an inflammatory reaction of the meatal skin. It is important to exclude an underlying chronic otitis media before treatment is commenced. Many cases recover after thorough cleansing of the external ear canal by suction or dry mopping. A frequent problem in resistant cases is the difficulty in applying lotions and ointments satisfactorily to the relatively inaccessible affected skin. The most effective method is to introduce a ribbon gauze dressing or sponge wick soaked with **corticosteroid** ear drops or with an astringent such as **aluminium acetate** solution. When this is not practical, the ear should be gently cleansed with a probe covered in cotton wool and the patient encouraged to lie with the affected ear uppermost for ten minutes after the canal has been filled with a liberal quantity of the appropriate solution.

If infection is present, a topical anti-infective which is not used systemically (such as **neomycin** or **clioquinol**) may be used, but for only about a week as excessive use may result in fungal infections; these may be difficult to treat and require expert advice. Sensitivity to the anti-infective or solvent may occur and resistance to anti-bacterials is a possibility with prolonged use. Aluminium acetate ear drops are also effective against bacterial infection and inflammation of the ear. **Chloramphenicol** may be used but the ear drops contain propylene glycol and cause hypersensitivity reactions in about 10% of patients. Solutions containing an anti-infective and a corticosteroid (such as *Locorten-Vioform®*) are used for treating cases where infection is present with inflammation and eczema.

In view of reports of ototoxicity in patients with a perforated tympanic membrane (eardrum), the CSM has stated that treatment with a topical aminoglycoside antibiotic is contra-indicated in those with a tympanic perforation. However, many specialists do use these drops cautiously in the presence of a perforation in patients with otitis media (section 12.1.2) and when other measures have failed for otitis externa.

A solution of **acetic acid** 2% acts as an antifungal and antibacterial in the external ear canal. It may be used to treat mild otitis externa but in severe cases an anti-inflammatory preparation with or without an anti-infective drug is required. A proprietary preparation containing acetic acid 2% (*EarCalm®* spray) is on sale to the public.

For severe pain associated with otitis externa, a simple analgesic, such as **paracetamol** (section 4.7.1) or **ibuprofen** (section 10.1.1), can be used. A systemic antibacterial (Table 1, section 5.1) can be used if there is spreading cellulitis or if the patient is systemically unwell. When a resistant staphylococcal infection (a boil) is present in the external auditory meatus, **flucloxacillin** is the drug of choice; **ciprofloxacin** (or an aminoglycoside) may be needed in pseudomonal infections which may occur if the patient has diabetes or is immunocompromised.

The skin of the pinna adjacent to the ear canal is often affected by eczema. Topical corticosteroid creams and ointments (section 13.4) are then required, but prolonged use should be avoided.

## Astringent preparations

### ▮ ALUMINIUM ACETATE

**Indications** inflammation in otitis externa (see notes above)

**Dose**
- Insert into meatus or apply on a ribbon gauze dressing or sponge wick which should be kept saturated with the ear drops

**Aluminium Acetate** (Non-proprietary)
Ear drops 13%, aluminium sulphate 2.25 g, calcium carbonate 1 g, tartaric acid 450 mg, acetic acid (33%) 2.5 mL, purified water 7.5 mL
Available from manufacturers of 'special order' products

Ear drops 8%, dilute 8 parts aluminium acetate ear drops (13%) with 5 parts purified water. Must be freshly prepared

## Anti-inflammatory preparations

### Corticosteroids

Topical corticosteroids are used to treat inflammation and eczema in otitis externa.

**Cautions** Prolonged use of topical corticosteroid ear preparations should be avoided.

**Contra-indications** Corticosteroid ear preparations should be avoided in the presence of an untreated ear infection. If infection is present, the corticosteroid should be used in combination with a suitable anti-infective (see notes above).

**Side-effects** Local sensitivity reactions may occur.

### ▮ BETAMETHASONE SODIUM PHOSPHATE

**Indications** eczematous inflammation in otitis externa (see notes above)
**Cautions** see notes above
**Contra-indications** see notes above
**Side-effects** see notes above

**Betnesol®** (UCB Pharma) (PoM)
Drops (for ear, eye, or nose), betamethasone sodium phosphate 0.1%. Net price 10 mL = £2.23
Excipients include benzalkonium chloride, disodium edetate
Dose ear, apply 2–3 drops every 2–3 hours; reduce frequency when relief obtained; eye, section 11.4.1; nose, section 12.2.1

**Vistamethasone®** (Martindale) (PoM)
Drops (for ear, eye, or nose), betamethasone sodium phosphate 0.1%. Net price 5 mL = £1.02; 10 mL = £1.16
Excipients include benzalkonium chloride, disodium edetate
Dose ear, apply 2–3 drops every 3–4 hours; reduce frequency when relief obtained; eye, section 11.4.1; nose, section 12.2.1

◢**With antibacterial**
**Betnesol-N®** (UCB Pharma) (PoM)
Drops (for ear, eye, or nose), betamethasone sodium phosphate 0.1%, neomycin sulphate 0.5%. Net price 10 mL = £2.30
Excipients include benzalkonium chloride, disodium edetate
Dose ear, apply 2–3 drops 3–4 times daily; eye, section 11.4.1; nose, section 12.2.3

**Vistamethasone N®** (Martindale) (PoM)
Drops (for ear, eye, or nose), betamethasone sodium phosphate 0.1%, neomycin sulphate 0.5%. Net price 5 mL = £1.09; 10 mL = £1.20
Excipients include thiomersal
Dose ear, apply 2–3 drops every 3–4 hours; reduce frequency when relief obtained; eye, section 11.4.1; nose, section 12.2.3

### ▮ DEXAMETHASONE

**Indications** eczematous inflammation in otitis externa (see notes above)
**Cautions** see notes above
**Contra-indications** see notes above
**Side-effects** see notes above

◢**With antibacterial**
**Otomize®** (GSK Consumer Healthcare) (PoM)
Ear spray, dexamethasone 0.1%, neomycin sulphate 3250 units/mL, glacial acetic acid 2%. Net price 5-mL pump-action aerosol unit = £3.79
Excipients include hydroxybenzoates (parabens)
Dose ear, apply 1 metered spray 3 times daily

**Sofradex®** (Sanofi-Aventis) (PoM) ◢
Drops (for ear or eye), dexamethasone (as sodium metasulphobenzoate) 0.05%, framycetin sulphate 0.5%, gramicidin 0.005%. Net price 10 mL = £6.25
Excipients include polysorbate 80
Dose ear, apply 2–3 drops 3–4 times daily; eye, section 11.4.1

### ▮ FLUMETASONE PIVALATE
(Flumethasone Pivalate)

**Indications** eczematous inflammation in otitis externa (see notes above)
**Cautions** see notes above
**Contra-indications** see notes above
**Side-effects** see notes above

◢**With antibacterial**
**Locorten-Vioform®** (Amdipharm) (PoM)
Ear drops, flumetasone pivalate 0.02%, clioquinol 1%. Net price 7.5 mL = £1.76
Contra-indications iodine sensitivity
Dose ADULT and CHILD over 2 years apply 2–3 drops into the ear twice daily for 7–10 days
Note Clioquinol stains skin and clothing

**12**

**Ear, nose, and oropharynx**

## HYDROCORTISONE

**Indications** eczematous inflammation in otitis externa (see notes above)

**Cautions** see notes above

**Contra-indications** see notes above

**Side-effects** see notes above

◢With antibacterial

**Gentisone® HC** (Amdipharm) PoM
Ear drops, hydrocortisone acetate 1%, gentamicin 0.3% (as sulphate). Net price 10 mL = £3.69
Excipients include benzalkonium chloride, disodium edetate
Dose ear, apply 2–4 drops 3–4 times daily and at night

**Otosporin®** (GSK) PoM ◢
Ear drops, hydrocortisone 1%, neomycin sulphate 3400 units, polymyxin B sulphate 10 000 units/mL. Net price 5 mL = £2.00; 10 mL = £4.00
Excipients include cetostearyl alcohol, hydroxybenzoates (parabens), polysorbate 20
Dose ADULT and CHILD over 3 years, ear, apply 3 drops 3–4 times daily

## PREDNISOLONE SODIUM PHOSPHATE

**Indications** eczematous inflammation in otitis externa (see notes above)

**Cautions** see notes above

**Contra-indications** see notes above

**Side-effects** see notes above

**Predsol®** (UCB Pharma) PoM
Drops (for ear or eye), prednisolone sodium phosphate 0.5%. Net price 10 mL = £1.92
Excipients include benzalkonium chloride, disodium edetate
Dose ear, apply 2–3 drops every 2–3 hours; reduce frequency when relief obtained; eye, section 11.4.1

◢With antibacterial

**Predsol-N®** (UCB Pharma) PoM
Drops (for ear or eye), prednisolone sodium phosphate 0.5%, neomycin sulphate 0.5%. Net price 10 mL = £2.27
Excipients include benzalkonium chloride, disodium edetate
Dose ear, apply 2–3 drops 3–4 times daily; eye, section 11.4.1

## Anti-infective preparations

### CHLORAMPHENICOL ◢

**Indications** bacterial infection in otitis externa (but see notes above)

**Cautions** avoid prolonged use (see notes above)

**Side-effects** high incidence of sensitivity reactions to vehicle

**Chloramphenicol** (Non-proprietary) PoM ◢
Ear drops, chloramphenicol in propylene glycol, net price 5%, 10 mL = £1.79; 10%, 10 mL = £5.62
Dose ear, apply 2–3 drops 2–3 times daily

### CLIOQUINOL ◢

**Indications** mild bacterial or fungal infections in otitis externa (see notes above)

**Cautions** avoid prolonged use (see notes above); manufacturer advises avoid in perforated tympanic membrane (but used by specialists for short periods)

**Side-effects** local sensitivity; stains skin and clothing

◢With corticosteroid
**Locorten-Vioform®** see Flumetasone, p. 609

### CLOTRIMAZOLE

**Indications** fungal infection in otitis externa (see notes above)

**Side-effects** occasional local irritation or sensitivity

**Canesten®** (Bayer Consumer Care)
Solution, clotrimazole 1% in polyethylene glycol 400 (macrogol 400). Net price 20 mL = £2.43
Dose ear, apply 2–3 times daily continuing for at least 14 days after disappearance of infection; skin, section 13.10.2

### FRAMYCETIN SULPHATE

**Indications** bacterial infection in otitis externa (see notes above)

**Cautions** avoid prolonged use (see notes above)

**Contra-indications** perforated tympanic membrane (see p. 608)

**Side-effects** local sensitivity

◢With corticosteroid
**Sofradex®** see Dexamethasone, p. 609

### GENTAMICIN

**Indications** bacterial infection in otitis externa (see notes above)

**Cautions** avoid prolonged use (see notes above)

**Contra-indications** perforated tympanic membrane (but see also p. 608 and section 12.1.2)

**Side-effects** local sensitivity

**Genticin®** (Amdipharm) PoM
Drops (for ear or eye), gentamicin 0.3% (as sulphate). Net price 10 mL = £2.13
Excipients include benzalkonium chloride
Dose ear, apply 2–3 drops 3–4 times daily and at night; eye, section 11.3.1

◢With corticosteroid
**Gentisone® HC** see Hydrocortisone, above

### NEOMYCIN SULPHATE

**Indications** bacterial infection in otitis externa (see notes above)

**Cautions** avoid prolonged use (see notes above)

**Contra-indications** perforated tympanic membrane (see p. 608)

**Side-effects** local sensitivity

◀**With corticosteroid**

**Betnesol-N®** see Betamethasone, p. 609

**Otomize®** see Dexamethasone, p. 609

**Otosporin®** see Hydrocortisone, p. 610

**Predsol-N®** see Prednisolone, p. 610

**Vistamethasone N®** see Betamethasone, p. 609

## 12.1.2 Otitis media

**Acute otitis media** Acute otitis media is the commonest cause of severe aural pain in small children. Many infections, especially those accompanying coryza, are caused by viruses. Most uncomplicated cases resolve without antibacterial treatment and a **simple analgesic**, such as paracetamol, may be sufficient. In children without systemic features, a **systemic antibacterial** (Table 1, section 5.1) may be started after 72 hours if there is no improvement, or earlier if there is deterioration, if the patient is systemically unwell, if the patient is at high risk of serious complications (e.g. in immunosuppression, cystic fibrosis), if mastoiditis is present, or in children under 2 years of age with bilateral otitis media. Perforation of the tympanic membrane in patients with *acute otitis media* usually heals spontaneously without treatment; if there is no improvement, e.g. pain or discharge persists, a systemic antibacterial (Table 1, section 5.1) can be given. Topical treatment of acute otitis media is ineffective and there is no place for drops containing a local anaesthetic.

**Otitis media with effusion** Otitis media with effusion ('glue ear') occurs in about 10% of children and in 90% of children with cleft palates. Systemic antibacterials are not usually required. If 'glue ear' persists for more than a month or two, the child should be referred for assessment and follow up because of the risk of long-term hearing impairment which can delay language development. Untreated or resistant glue ear may be responsible for some types of *chronic otitis media*.

**Chronic otitis media** Opportunistic organisms are often present in the debris, keratin, and necrotic bone of the middle ear and mastoid in patients with chronic otitis media. The mainstay of treatment is thorough cleansing with aural microsuction which may completely resolve long-standing infection. Local cleansing of the meatal and middle ear may be followed by treatment with a sponge wick or ribbon gauze dressing soaked with corticosteroid ear drops or with an astringent such as aluminium acetate solution; this is particularly beneficial for discharging ears or infections of the mastoid cavity. An antibacterial ear ointment may also be used. Acute exacerbations of chronic infection may also require systemic treatment with amoxicillin (or erythromycin if penicillin-allergic); treatment is adjusted according to the results of sensitivity testing. Parenteral antibacterials are required if *Pseudomonas aeruginosa* and *Proteus* spp. are present.

The CSM has stated that topical treatment with ototoxic antibacterials is contra-indicated in the presence of a perforation (section 12.1.1). However, many specialists use ear drops containing **aminoglycosides** (e.g. neomycin) or **polymyxins** if the otitis media has failed to settle with systemic antibacterials; it is considered that the pus in the middle ear associated with otitis media carries a higher risk of ototoxicity than the drops themselves. Ciprofloxacin or ofloxacin ear drops [both unlicensed; available on named-patient basis from a specialist importing company] or eye drops used in the ear [unlicensed indication] are an effective alternative to aminoglycoside ear drops for chronic otitis media in patients with perforation of the tympanic membrane.

## 12.1.3 Removal of ear wax

Wax is a normal bodily secretion which provides a protective film on the meatal skin and need only be removed if it causes deafness or interferes with a proper view of the ear drum. Ear irrigation is generally best avoided in young children, in patients with a history of recurrent otitis externa, a history of ear-drum perforation, or previous ear surgery. A person who has hearing in one ear only should not have that ear irrigated because even a very slight risk of damage is unacceptable in this situation.

Wax may be removed by irrigation with water (warmed to body temperature). If necessary, wax can be softened using simple remedies such as **olive oil** ear drops or **almond oil** ear drops; **sodium bicarbonate** ear drops are also effective but may cause dryness of the ear canal. If the wax is hard and impacted, the drops may be used twice daily for a few days before irrigation; otherwise the wax may be softened on the day of irrigation. The patient should lie with the affected ear uppermost for 5 to 10 minutes after a generous amount of the softening remedy has been introduced into the ear. Some proprietary preparations containing organic solvents can irritate the meatal skin, and in most cases the simple remedies indicated above are just as effective and less likely to cause irritation. Docusate sodium or urea–hydrogen peroxide are ingredients in a number of proprietary preparations for softening ear wax.

**Almond Oil** (Non-proprietary)
Ear drops, almond oil in a suitable container
Allow to warm to room temperature before use

**Olive Oil** (Non-proprietary)
Ear drops, olive oil in a suitable container
Allow to warm to room temperature before use

**Sodium Bicarbonate** (Non-proprietary)
Ear drops, sodium bicarbonate 5%, net price 10 mL = £1.25

**Cerumol®** (Thornton & Ross) ◪
Ear drops, chlorobutanol 5%, arachis (peanut) oil 57.3%. Net price 11 mL = £1.76

**Exterol®** (Dermal) ◪
Ear drops, urea–hydrogen peroxide complex 5% in glycerol. Net price 8 mL = £1.77

**Molcer®** (Wallace Mfg) ◪
Ear drops, docusate sodium 5%. Net price 15 mL = £5.60
Excipients include propylene glycol

**Otex®** (DDD) ◪
Ear drops, urea–hydrogen peroxide 5%. Net price 8 mL = £2.64

**Waxsol®** (Norgine) ◪
Ear drops, docusate sodium 0.5%. Net price 10 mL = £1.21

**12**

**Ear, nose, and oropharynx**

# 12.2 Drugs acting on the nose

**12.2.1** Drugs used in nasal allergy
**12.2.2** Topical nasal decongestants
**12.2.3** Nasal preparations for infection

Rhinitis is often self-limiting but bacterial sinusitis may require treatment with antibacterials (Table 1, section 5.1). There are few indications for nasal sprays and drops except in allergic rhinitis and perennial rhinitis (section 12.2.1). Many nasal preparations contain sympathomimetic drugs which may damage the nasal cilia (section 12.2.2). **Sodium chloride 0.9%** solution may be used as a douche or 'sniff' following endonasal surgery.

**Nasal polyps** Short-term use of corticosteroid nasal drops helps to shrink nasal polyps; to be effective, the drops must be administered with the patient in the 'head down' position. A short course of a systemic corticosteroid (section 6.3.2) may be required initially to shrink large polyps. A corticosteroid nasal spray can be used to maintain the reduction in swelling and also for the initial treatment of small polyps.

## 12.2.1 Drugs used in nasal allergy

Mild allergic rhinitis is controlled by **antihistamines** (see also section 3.4.1) or topical **nasal corticosteroids**; systemic nasal decongestants are of doubtful value (section 3.10). Topical nasal decongestants can be used for a short period to relieve congestion and allow penetration of a topical nasal corticosteroid.

More persistent symptoms and nasal congestion can be relieved by topical nasal **corticosteroids**; **cromoglicate** (cromoglycate) is an alternative, but may be less effective. The topical antihistamine **azelastine** is useful for controlling breakthrough symptoms in allergic rhinitis. Topical antihistamines are considered less effective than topical corticosteroids but probably more effective than cromoglicate. In seasonal allergic rhinitis (e.g. hay fever), treatment should begin 2 to 3 weeks before the season commences and may have to be continued for several months; continuous treatment may be required for years in perennial rhinitis.

**Montelukast** (section 3.3.2) can be used in patients with seasonal allergic rhinitis and concomitant asthma; montelukast is less effective than topical nasal corticosteroids.

Sometimes allergic rhinitis is accompanied by vasomotor rhinitis. In this situation, the addition of topical nasal ipratropium bromide (section 12.2.2) can reduce watery rhinorrhoea.

Very disabling symptoms occasionally justify the use of **systemic corticosteroids** for short periods (section 6.3), for example, in students taking important examinations. They may also be used at the beginning of a course of treatment with a corticosteroid spray to relieve severe mucosal oedema and allow the spray to penetrate the nasal cavity.

**Pregnancy** If a pregnant woman cannot tolerate the symptoms of allergic rhinitis, treatment with nasal beclometasone, budesonide, fluticasone, or sodium cromoglicate may be considered.

## Antihistamines

### ▌AZELASTINE HYDROCHLORIDE

**Indications** allergic rhinitis

**Side-effects** irritation of nasal mucosa; bitter taste (if applied incorrectly)

**Rhinolast®** (Viatris) ℗ℴ𝕄
Nasal spray, azelastine hydrochloride 140 micrograms (0.14 mL)/metered spray. Net price 22 mL (with metered pump) = £8.57
Excipients include sodium edetate
**Dose** ADULT and CHILD over 5 years, 140 micrograms (1 spray) into each nostril twice daily
Note Preparations of azelastine hydrochloride can be sold to the public for nasal administration in aqueous form (other than by aerosol) if supplied for the treatment of seasonal allergic rhinitis or perennial allergic rhinitis in adults and children over 5 years, subject to max. single dose of 140 micrograms per nostril, max. daily dose of 280 micrograms per nostril, and a pack size limit of 36 doses

## Corticosteroids

Nasal preparations containing corticosteroids (beclometasone, betamethasone, budesonide, flunisolide, fluticasone, mometasone, and triamcinolone) have a useful role in the prophylaxis and treatment of allergic rhinitis (see notes above).

**Cautions** Corticosteroid nasal preparations should be avoided in the presence of untreated nasal infections, and also after nasal surgery (until healing has occurred); they should also be avoided in pulmonary tuberculosis. Patients transferred from systemic corticosteroids may experience exacerbation of some symptoms. Systemic absorption may follow nasal administration particularly if high doses are used or if treatment is prolonged; for cautions and side-effects of systemic corticosteroids, see section 6.3.2. The risk of systemic effects may be greater with nasal drops than with nasal sprays; drops are administered incorrectly more often than sprays. The CSM recommends that the height of children receiving prolonged treatment with nasal corticosteroids is monitored; if growth is slowed, referral to a paediatrician should be considered.

**Side-effects** Local side-effects include dryness, irritation of nose and throat, and epistaxis. Nasal ulceration has been reported, but occurs commonly with nasal preparations containing fluticasone furoate or mometasone furoate. Nasal septal perforation (usually following nasal surgery) occurs very rarely. Raised intra-ocular pressure or glaucoma may occur rarely. Headache, smell and taste disturbances may also occur. Hypersensitivity reactions, including bronchospasm, have been reported.

## BECLOMETASONE DIPROPIONATE
### (Beclomethasone Dipropionate)

**Indications** prophylaxis and treatment of allergic and vasomotor rhinitis

**Cautions** see notes above

**Side-effects** see notes above

**Dose**

- ADULT and CHILD over 6 years, 100 micrograms (2 sprays) into each nostril twice daily; max. total 400 micrograms (8 sprays) daily; when symptoms controlled, dose reduced to 50 micrograms (1 spray) into each nostril twice daily

¹**Beclometasone** (Non-proprietary) (PoM)

Nasal spray, beclometasone dipropionate 50 micrograms/metered spray. Net price 200-spray unit = £2.79

Brands include *Nasobec Aqueous®*

1. Can be sold to the public for nasal administration (other than by aerosol) if supplied for the prevention and treatment of allergic rhinitis in adults over 18 years subject to max. single dose of 100 micrograms per nostril, max. daily dose of 200 micrograms per nostril for max. 3 months, and a pack size of 20 mg

**Beconase®** (A&H) (PoM)

Nasal spray (aqueous suspension), beclometasone dipropionate 50 micrograms/metered spray. Net price 200-spray unit with applicator = £2.19

Excipients include benzalkonium chloride, polysorbate 80

## BETAMETHASONE SODIUM PHOSPHATE

**Indications** non-infected inflammatory conditions of nose

**Cautions** see notes above

**Side-effects** see notes above

**Betnesol®** (UCB Pharma) (PoM)

Drops (for ear, eye, or nose), betamethasone sodium phosphate 0.1%, net price 10 mL = £2.23

Excipients include benzalkonium chloride, disodium edetate

Dose nose, 2–3 drops into each nostril 2–3 times daily; ear, section 12.1.1; eye, section 11.4.1

**Vistamethasone®** (Martindale) (PoM)

Drops (for ear, eye, or nose), betamethasone sodium phosphate 0.1%. Net price 5 mL = £1.02, 10 mL = £1.16

Excipients include benzalkonium chloride, disodium edetate

Dose nose, 2–3 drops into each nostril twice daily; ear, section 12.1.1; eye, section 11.4.1

## BUDESONIDE

**Indications** prophylaxis and treatment of allergic and vasomotor rhinitis; nasal polyps

**Cautions** see notes above; **interactions:** Appendix 1 (corticosteroids)

**Side-effects** see notes above

**Dose**

- See preparations

¹**Budesonide** (Non-proprietary) (PoM)

Nasal spray, budesonide 100 micrograms/metered spray, net price 100-spray unit = £5.90

Dose rhinitis, ADULT and CHILD over 12 years, 200 micrograms (2 sprays) into each nostril once daily in the morning *or* 100 micrograms (1 spray) into each nostril twice daily; when control

achieved reduce to 100 micrograms (1 spray) into each nostril once daily

Nasal polyps, ADULT and CHILD over 12 years, 100 micrograms (1 spray) into each nostril twice daily for up to 3 months

1. Can be sold to the public for nasal administration (other than by aerosol) if supplied for the prevention and treatment of seasonal allergic rhinitis in adults over 18 years subject to max. single dose of 200 micrograms per nostril, max. daily dose of 200 micrograms per nostril for max. period of 3 months, and a pack size of 10 mg

**Rhinocort Aqua®** (AstraZeneca) (PoM)

Nasal spray, budesonide 64 micrograms/metered spray. Net price 120-spray unit = £4.49

Excipients include disodium edetate, polysorbate 80, potassium sorbate

Dose rhinitis, ADULT and CHILD over 12 years, 128 micrograms (2 sprays) into each nostril once daily in the morning *or* 64 micrograms (1 spray) into each nostril twice daily; when control achieved reduce to 64 micrograms (1 spray) into each nostril once daily; max. duration of treatment 3 months

Nasal polyps, ADULT and CHILD over 12 years, 64 micrograms (1 spray) into each nostril twice daily for up to 3 months

## FLUNISOLIDE

**Indications** prophylaxis and treatment of allergic rhinitis

**Cautions** see notes above

**Side-effects** see notes above

**Syntaris®** (IVAX) (PoM)

Aqueous nasal spray, flunisolide 25 micrograms/metered spray. Net price 240-spray unit with pump and applicator = £5.05

Excipients include benzalkonium chloride, butylated hydroxytoluene, disodium edetate, polysorbate 20, propylene glycol

Dose ADULT, 50 micrograms (2 sprays) into each nostril twice daily, increased if necessary to max. 3 times daily then reduced for maintenance; CHILD 5–14 years initially 25 micrograms (1 spray) into each nostril up to 3 times daily

## FLUTICASONE PROPIONATE

**Indications** prophylaxis and treatment of allergic rhinitis and perennial rhinitis; nasal polyps

**Cautions** see notes above; **interactions:** Appendix 1 (corticosteroids)

**Side-effects** see notes above

**Dose**

- Rhinitis, 100 micrograms (2 sprays) into each nostril once daily, preferably in the morning, increased to max. twice daily if required; when control achieved reduce to 50 micrograms (1 spray) into each nostril once daily; CHILD 4–11 years, 50 micrograms (1 spray) into each nostril once daily, preferably in the morning, increased to max. twice daily if required

- Nasal polyps, see *Flixonase Nasule®* below

**Flixonase®** (A&H) (PoM)

Aqueous nasal spray, fluticasone propionate 50 micrograms/metered spray. Net price 150-spray unit with applicator = £11.23

Excipients include benzalkonium chloride, polysorbate 80

**Note** Preparations of fluticasone propionate can be sold to the public for nasal administration (other than by pressurised nasal spray) if supplied for the prevention and treatment of allergic rhinitis in adults over 18 years, subject to max. single dose of 100 micrograms per nostril, max. daily dose of 200 micrograms per nostril for max. 3 months, and a pack size of 3 mg

**12**

**Ear, nose, and oropharynx**

**Flixonase Nasule®** (A&H) [PoM]
Nasal drops, fluticasone propionate 400 micrograms/unit dose, net price 28 × 0.4-mL units = £13.25
Excipients include polysorbate 20

Dose nasal polyps, ADULT and ADOLESCENT over 16 years, 200 micrograms (approx. 6 drops) into each nostril once or twice daily; consider alternative treatment if no improvement after 4–6 weeks

**Nasofan®** (IVAX) [PoM]
Aqueous nasal spray fluticasone propionate 50 micrograms/metered spray. Net price 150-spray unit = £8.41
Excipients include benzalkonium chloride, polysorbate 80

◢Fluticasone furoate
**Avamys®** (GSK) ▼ [PoM]
Nasal spray, fluticasone furoate 27.5 micrograms/metered spray, net price 120-spray unit = £6.44
Excipients include benzalkonium chloride, disodium edetate, polysorbate 80

Dose prophylaxis and treatment of allergic rhinitis, ADULT and CHILD over 12 years, 55 micrograms (2 sprays) into each nostril once daily; when control achieved reduce to 27.5 micrograms (1 spray) into each nostril once daily; CHILD 6–12 years, 27.5 micrograms (1 spray) into each nostril once daily, increased if necessary to 55 micrograms (2 sprays) into each nostril once daily; when control achieved reduce to 27.5 micrograms (1 spray) into each nostril once daily

## ■ MOMETASONE FUROATE

**Indications** see preparations
**Cautions** see notes above
**Side-effects** see notes above

**Nasonex®** (Schering-Plough) [PoM]
Nasal spray, mometasone furoate 50 micrograms/metered spray. Net price 140-spray unit = £7.68
Excipients include benzalkonium chloride, polysorbate 80

Dose prophylaxis and treatment of allergic rhinitis, ADULT and CHILD over 12 years, 100 micrograms (2 sprays) into each nostril once daily, increased if necessary to max. 200 micrograms (4 sprays) into each nostril once daily; when control achieved reduce to 50 micrograms (1 spray) into each nostril once daily; CHILD 6–11 years, 50 micrograms (1 spray) into each nostril once daily
Nasal polyps, ADULT over 18 years, 100 micrograms (2 sprays) into each nostril once daily, increased if necessary after 5–6 weeks to 100 micrograms (2 sprays) into each nostril twice daily (consider alternative treatment if no improvement after further 5–6 weeks); reduce to the lowest effective dose when control achieved

## ■ TRIAMCINOLONE ACETONIDE

**Indications** prophylaxis and treatment of allergic rhinitis
**Cautions** see notes above
**Side-effects** see notes above

**Nasacort®** (Aventis Pharma) [PoM]
Aqueous nasal spray, triamcinolone acetonide 55 micrograms/metered spray. Net price 120-spray unit = £7.39
Excipients include benzalkonium chloride, disodium edetate, polysorbate 80

Dose ADULT and CHILD over 12 years 110 micrograms (2 sprays) into each nostril once daily; when control achieved, reduce to 55 micrograms (1 spray) into each nostril once daily; CHILD 6–12 years, 55 micrograms (1 spray) into each nostril once daily
Note Preparations of triamcinolone acetonide can be sold to the public for nasal administration as a non-pressurised nasal spray if supplied for the symptomatic treatment of seasonal allergic rhinitis in adults over 18 years, subject to max. daily dose of 110 micrograms per nostril for max. 3 months, and a pack size of 3.575 mg

## Cromoglicate

## ■ SODIUM CROMOGLICATE
(Sodium Cromoglycate)

**Indications** prophylaxis of allergic rhinitis
**Side-effects** local irritation; rarely transient bronchospasm

**Rynacrom®** (Sanofi-Aventis)
4% aqueous nasal spray, sodium cromoglicate 4% (5.2 mg/spray). Net price 22 mL with pump = £17.07
Excipients include benzalkonium chloride, disodium edetate
Dose ADULT and CHILD, 1 spray into each nostril 2–4 times daily

**Vividrin®** (Pharma-Global)
Nasal spray, sodium cromoglicate 2%. Net price 15 mL = £11.60
Excipients include benzalkonium chloride, edetic acid, polysorbate 80
Dose ADULT and CHILD, 1 spray into each nostril 4–6 times daily

## 12.2.2 Topical nasal decongestants

The nasal mucosa is sensitive to changes in atmospheric temperature and humidity and these alone may cause slight nasal congestion. The nose and nasal sinuses produce a litre of mucus in 24 hours and much of this finds its way silently into the stomach via the nasopharynx. Slight changes in the nasal airway, accompanied by an awareness of mucus passing along the nasopharynx causes some patients to be inaccurately diagnosed as suffering from chronic sinusitis. These symptoms are particularly noticeable in the later stages of the common cold. **Sodium chloride** 0.9% given as nasal drops may relieve nasal congestion by helping to liquefy mucous secretions.

Inhalation of **warm moist air** is useful in the treatment of symptoms of acute infective conditions. The addition of volatile substances such as menthol and eucalyptus may encourage the use of warm moist air (section 3.8).

Symptoms of nasal congestion associated with vasomotor rhinitis and the common cold can be relieved by the short-term use (usually not longer than 7 days) of decongestant nasal drops and sprays. These all contain sympathomimetic drugs which exert their effect by vasoconstriction of the mucosal blood vessels which in turn reduces oedema of the nasal mucosa. They are of limited value because they can give rise to a rebound congestion (rhinitis medicamentosa) on withdrawal, due to a secondary vasodilatation with a subsequent temporary increase in nasal congestion. This in turn tempts the further use of the decongestant, leading to a vicious cycle of events. **Ephedrine nasal drops** is the safest sympathomimetic preparation and can give relief for several hours. The more potent sympathomimetic drugs oxymetazoline and xylometazoline are more likely to cause a rebound effect. Sympathomimetics may cause a hypertensive crisis if used during treatment with a monoamine-oxidase inhibitor including moclobemide.

The CHM/MHRA has stated that non-prescription cough and cold medicines containing ephedrine, oxymetazoline, or xylometazoline can be considered in children aged 6–12 years after basic principles of best care have been tried; these medicines should not be used in children under 6 years of age (section 3.9.1).

**12** Ear, nose, and oropharynx

However, in special circumstances, some specialists prescribe nasal drops containing ephedrine or xylometazoline to children under 6 years of age for the short-term treatment of severe nasal obstruction that has not responded to sodium chloride 0.9% nose drops and inhalation of warm moist air.

Non-allergic watery rhinorrhoea often responds well to treatment with the antimuscarinic **ipratropium bromide**.

Systemic nasal decongestants—see section 3.10.

**Sinusitis and oral pain** Sinusitis affecting the maxillary antrum can cause pain in the upper jaw. Where this is associated with blockage of the opening from the sinus into the nasal cavity, it may be helpful to relieve the congestion with inhalation of warm moist air (section 3.8) or with **ephedrine nasal drops** (see above). For antibacterial treatment of sinusitis, see Table 1, section 5.1.

## Sympathomimetics

### ■ EPHEDRINE HYDROCHLORIDE

**Indications** nasal congestion

**Cautions** see notes above; also avoid excessive or prolonged use; caution in infants under 3 months (no good evidence of value—if irritation occurs might narrow nasal passage); **interactions:** Appendix 1 (sympathomimetics)

**Side-effects** local irritation, nausea, headache; after excessive use tolerance with diminished effect, rebound congestion; cardiovascular effects also reported

**Dose**
● See below

¹**Ephedrine** (Non-proprietary)
Nasal drops, ephedrine hydrochloride 0.5%, net price 10 mL = £1.25; 1%, 10 mL = £1.35
Note The BP directs that if no strength is specified 0.5% drops should be supplied
Dose 1–2 drops into each nostril up to 3 or 4 times daily when required, max. duration 7 days; CHILD 3 months–12 years (on a specialist's advice only for CHILD 3 months–6 years), 1–2 drops of 0.5% solution into each nostril 3–4 times daily when required, max. duration 5 days
Dental prescribing on NHS Ephedrine nasal drops may be prescribed

1. Can be sold to the public provided no more than 180 mg of ephedrine base (or salts) are supplied at one time, and pseudoephedrine salts are not supplied at the same time; for details see *Medicines, Ethics and Practice*, No. 33, London Pharmaceutical Press, 2009 (and subsequent editions as available)

### ■ XYLOMETAZOLINE HYDROCHLORIDE

**Indications** nasal congestion

**Cautions** see under Ephedrine Hydrochloride and notes above

**Side-effects** see under Ephedrine Hydrochloride and notes above

**Dose**
● See below

**Xylometazoline** (Non-proprietary)
Nasal drops, xylometazoline hydrochloride 0.1%, net price 10 mL = £1.91
Dose 2–3 drops into each nostril 2–3 times daily when required; max. duration 7 days; not recommended for children under 12 years
Brands include *Otradrops®*, *Otrivine®* ⁅NHS⁆

Paediatric nasal drops, xylometazoline hydrochloride 0.05%, net price 10 mL = £1.59
Dose CHILD 2–12 years 1–2 drops into each nostril 1–2 times daily when required (on a specialist's advice only for CHILD 3 months–6 years); max. duration 5 days
Brands include *Otradrops®*, *Otrivine®* ⁅NHS⁆, *Tixycolds®*

Nasal spray, xylometazoline hydrochloride 0.1%, net price 10 mL = £1.91
Dose 1 spray into each nostril 2–3 times daily when required; max. duration 7 days; not recommended for children under 12 years
Brands include *Otraspray®*, *Otrivine®* ⁅NHS⁆

## Antimuscarinic

### ■ IPRATROPIUM BROMIDE

**Indications** rhinorrhoea associated with allergic and non-allergic rhinitis

**Cautions** see section 3.1.2; avoid spraying near eyes

**Side-effects** epistaxis, nasal dryness, and irritation; less frequently nausea, headache, and pharyngitis; *very rarely* antimuscarinic effects such as gastrointestinal motility disturbances, palpitations, and urinary retention

**Dose**
● ADULT and CHILD over 12 years, 42 micrograms (2 sprays) into each nostril 2–3 times daily

**Rinatec®** (Boehringer Ingelheim) ⁅PoM⁆
Nasal spray 0.03%, ipratropium bromide 21 micrograms/metered spray. Net price 180-dose unit = £3.99
Excipients include benzalkonium chloride, disodium edetate

## 12.2.3 Nasal preparations for infection

There is **no** evidence that topical anti-infective nasal preparations have any therapeutic value in rhinitis or sinusitis; for elimination of nasal staphylococci, see below.

Systemic treatment of sinusitis—see Table 1 section 5.1

**Betnesol-N®** (UCB Pharma) ⁅PoM⁆ ◪
Drops (for ear, eye, or nose), betamethasone sodium phosphate 0.1%, neomycin sulphate 0.5%. Net price 10 mL = £2.30
Excipients include benzalkonium chloride, disodium edetate
Dose nose, 2–3 drops into each nostril 2–3 times daily; eye, section 11.4.1; ear, section 12.1.1

**Vistamethasone N®** (Martindale) ⁅PoM⁆ ◪
Drops (for ear, eye, or nose), betamethasone sodium phosphate 0.1%, neomycin sulphate 0.5%. Net price 5 mL = £1.09, 10 mL = £1.20
Excipients include thiomersal
Dose nose, 2–3 drops into each nostril twice daily; eye, section 11.4.1; ear, section 12.1.1

**12**

**Ear, nose, and oropharynx**

## Nasal staphylococci

Elimination of organisms such as staphylococci from the nasal vestibule can be achieved by the use of a cream containing **chlorhexidine and neomycin** (*Naseptin*®), but re-colonisation frequently occurs. Coagulase-positive staphylococci are present in the noses of 40% of the population.

A nasal ointment containing **mupirocin** is also available; it should probably be held in reserve for resistant cases. In hospital or in care establishments, mupirocin nasal ointment should be reserved for the eradication (in both patients and staff) of nasal carriage of meticillin-resistant *Staphylococcus aureus* (MRSA). The ointment should be applied 3 times daily for 5 days and a sample taken 2 days after treatment to confirm eradication. The course may be repeated if the sample is positive (and the throat is not colonised). To avoid the development of resistance, the treatment course should not exceed 7 days and the course should not be repeated on more than one occasion. If the MRSA strain is mupirocin-resistant or does not respond after 2 courses, consider alternative products such as chlorhexidine and neomycin cream.

### Bactroban Nasal® (GSK) [PoM]
Nasal ointment, mupirocin 2% (as calcium salt) in white soft paraffin basis. Net price 3 g = £5.80

**Dose** for eradication of nasal carriage of staphylococci, including meticillin-resistant *Staphylococcus aureus* (MRSA), apply 2–3 times daily to the inner surface of each nostril

### Naseptin® (Alliance) [PoM]
Cream, chlorhexidine hydrochloride 0.1%, neomycin sulphate 0.5%, net price 15 g = £1.90

**Excipients** include arachis (peanut) oil, cetostearyl alcohol

**Dose** for eradication of nasal carriage of staphylococci, apply to nostrils 4 times daily for 10 days; for preventing nasal carriage of staphylococci apply to nostrils twice daily

## 12.3 Drugs acting on the oropharynx

12.3.1 Drugs for oral ulceration and inflammation
12.3.2 Oropharyngeal anti-infective drugs
12.3.3 Lozenges and sprays
12.3.4 Mouthwashes, gargles, and dentifrices
12.3.5 Treatment of dry mouth

## 12.3.1 Drugs for oral ulceration and inflammation

Ulceration of the oral mucosa may be caused by trauma (physical or chemical), recurrent aphthae, infections, carcinoma, dermatological disorders, nutritional deficiencies, gastro-intestinal disease, haematopoietic disorders, and drug therapy (see also Chemotherapy-induced mucositis and myelosuppression, section 8.1). It is important to establish the diagnosis in each case as the majority of these lesions require specific management in addition to local treatment. Local treatment aims to protect the ulcerated area, to relieve pain, to reduce inflammation, or to control secondary infection.

Patients with an unexplained mouth ulcer of more than 3 weeks' duration require urgent referral to hospital to exclude oral cancer.

**Simple mouthwashes** A **saline** mouthwash (section 12.3.4) may relieve the pain of traumatic ulceration. The mouthwash is made up with warm water and used at frequent intervals until the discomfort and swelling subsides.

**Antiseptic mouthwashes** Secondary bacterial infection may be a feature of any mucosal ulceration; it can increase discomfort and delay healing. Use of **chlorhexidine** mouthwash (section 12.3.4) is often beneficial and may accelerate healing of recurrent aphthae.

**Mechanical protection** **Carmellose gelatin paste** may relieve some discomfort arising from ulceration by protecting the ulcer site. As the paste adheres to dry mucosa, it is difficult to apply it effectively to the tongue and oropharynx.

**Corticosteroids** Topical corticosteroid therapy may be used for some forms of oral ulceration. In the case of aphthous ulcers it is most effective if applied in the 'prodromal' phase.

Thrush or other types of candidiasis are recognised complications of corticosteroid treatment.

**Hydrocortisone oromucosal tablets** are allowed to dissolve next to an ulcer and are useful in recurrent aphthae and erosive lichenoid lesions.

**Triamcinolone dental paste** is designed to keep the corticosteroid in contact with the mucosa for long enough to permit penetration of the lesion. As the paste adheres to dry mucosa, it is difficult to apply it effectively to the tongue and oropharynx.

**Beclometasone dipropionate** inhaler 50–100 micrograms sprayed twice daily on the oral mucosa is used to manage oral ulceration [unlicensed indication]. Alternatively, **betamethasone** soluble tablets dissolved in water can be used as a mouthwash to treat oral ulceration [unlicensed indication].

Systemic corticosteroid therapy (section 6.3.2) is reserved for severe conditions such as pemphigus vulgaris.

**Local analgesics** Local analgesics have a limited role in the management of oral ulceration. When applied topically their action is of a relatively short duration so that analgesia cannot be maintained continuously throughout the day. The main indication for a topical local analgesic is to relieve the pain of otherwise intractable oral ulceration particularly when it is due to major aphthae. For this purpose lidocaine (lignocaine) 5% ointment or lozenges containing a local anaesthetic are applied to the ulcer. Lidocaine 10% solution as spray (section 15.2) can be applied thinly to the ulcer [unlicensed indication] using a cotton bud. When local anaesthetics are used in the mouth care must be taken not to produce anaesthesia of the pharynx before meals as this might lead to choking.

**Benzydamine** mouthwash or spray may be useful in reducing the discomfort associated with a variety of ulcerative conditions. It has also been found to be effective in reducing the discomfort of post-irradiation mucositis. Some patients find the full-strength

*Ear, nose, and oropharynx*

*12*

mouthwash causes some stinging and, for them, it should be diluted with an equal volume of water.

**Flurbiprofen** lozenges are licensed for the relief of sore throat.

**Choline salicylate** dental gel has some analgesic action and may provide relief for recurrent aphthae, but excessive application or confinement under a denture irritates the mucosa and can itself cause ulceration.

**Other preparations** Doxycycline rinsed in the mouth may be of value for recurrent aphthous ulceration.

**Periodontitis** Low-dose doxycycline (*Periostat®*) is licensed as an adjunct to scaling and root planing for the treatment of periodontitis; a low dose of doxycycline reduces collagenase activity without inhibiting bacteria associated with periodontitis. For anti-infectives used in the treatment of destructive (refractory) forms of periodontal disease, see section 12.3.2 and Table 1, section 5.1. For mouthwashes used for oral hygiene and plaque inhibition, see section 12.3.4.

## ■ BENZYDAMINE HYDROCHLORIDE

**Indications** painful inflammatory conditions of oropharynx

**Side-effects** occasional numbness or stinging; rarely hypersensitivity reactions

### Difflam® (3M)
Oral rinse, green, benzydamine hydrochloride 0.15%, net price 200 mL (*Difflam® Sore Throat Rinse*) = £2.50; 300 mL = £3.81

Dose ADULT and ADOLESCENT over 12 years, rinse or gargle, using 15 mL (dilute with an equal volume of water if stinging occurs) every 1½–3 hours as required, usually for not more than 7 days

Dental prescribing on NHS May be prescribed as Benzydamine Mouthwash 0.15%

Spray, benzydamine hydrochloride 0.15%. Net price 30-mL unit = £3.01

Dose ADULT, 4–8 sprays onto affected area every 1½–3 hours; CHILD under 6 years 1 spray per 4 kg body-weight to max. 4 sprays every 1½–3 hours; 6–12 years 4 sprays every 1½–3 hours

Dental prescribing on NHS May be prescribed as Benzydamine Oromucosal Spray 0.15%

## ■ CARMELLOSE SODIUM

**Indications** mechanical protection of oral and perioral lesions

### Orabase® (ConvaTec)
Protective paste (= oral paste), carmellose sodium 16.7%, pectin 16.7%, gelatin 16.7%, in *Plastibase®*. Net price 30 g = £2.02; 100 g = £4.48

Dose apply a thin layer when necessary after meals

Dental prescribing on NHS May be prescribed as Carmellose Gelatin Paste

### Orahesive® (ConvaTec)
Powder, carmellose sodium, pectin, gelatin, equal parts. Net price 25 g = £2.33

Dose sprinkle on the affected area

## ■ CORTICOSTEROIDS

**Indications** oral and perioral lesions

**Contra-indications** untreated oral infection; manufacturer of triamcinolone contra-indicates use on tuberculous and viral lesions

**Side-effects** occasional exacerbation of local infection; thrush or other candidal infections

### Adcortyl in Orabase® (Squibb)
Oral paste, triamcinolone acetonide 0.1% in adhesive basis. Net price 5 g = £2.25

Dose ADULT and CHILD, apply a thin layer 2–4 times daily; do not rub in; use limited to 5 days for children and short-term use also advised for elderly

Dental prescribing on NHS May be prescribed as Triamcinolone Dental Paste

Note A 5-g tube is on sale to the public for the treatment of common mouth ulcers for max. 5 days

### Betnesol® (UCB Pharma) [PoM]
Soluble tablets, pink, scored, betamethasone 500 micrograms (as sodium phosphate), net price 100-tab pack = £4.97. Label: 10, steroid card, 13, 21

Dose oral ulceration, [unlicensed indication] ADULT and CHILD over 12 years, 500 micrograms dissolved in 20 ml water and rinsed around the mouth 4 times daily; not to be swallowed

Dental prescribing on the NHS May be prescribed as Betamethasone Soluble Tablets 500 micrograms

### Corlan® (UCB Pharma)
Pellets (= oromucosal tablets), hydrocortisone 2.5 mg (as sodium succinate). Net price 20 = £2.03

Dose ADULT and CHILD over 12 years, 1 lozenge 4 times daily, allowed to dissolve slowly in the mouth in contact with the ulcer; CHILD under 12 years, only on medical advice

Dental prescribing on NHS May be prescribed as Hydrocortisone Oromucosal Tablets

## ■ DOXYCYCLINE

**Indications** see preparations; oral herpes (section 12.3.2); other indications (section 5.1.3)

**Cautions** section 5.1.3; monitor for superficial fungal infection, particularly, if predisposition to oral candidiasis

**Contra-indications** section 5.1.3

**Side-effects** section 5.1.3; fungal superinfection

**Dose**
- See preparations

Note Doxycycline stains teeth; avoid in children under 12 years of age

### Periostat® (Alliance) [PoM]
Tablets, f/c, doxycycline (as hyclate) 20 mg, net price 56-tab pack = £16.50. Label: 6, 11, 27, counselling, posture

Dose periodontitis (as an adjunct to gingival scaling and root planing), 20 mg twice daily for 3 months; CHILD under 12 years not recommended

Counselling Tablets should be swallowed whole with plenty of fluid (at least 100 mL), while sitting or standing

Dental prescribing on NHS May be prescribed as Doxycycline Tablets 20 mg

### ◢ Local application
For recurrent aphthous ulceration, the contents of a 100 mg doxycycline capsule can be stirred into a small amount of water then rinsed around the mouth for 2–3 minutes 4 times daily usually for 3 days; it should preferably not be swallowed [unlicensed indication].

## ■ FLURBIPROFEN

**Indications** relief of sore throat

**Cautions** see section 10.1.1

**Contra-indications** see section 10.1.1

**Side-effects** taste disturbance, mouth ulcers (move lozenge around mouth); see also section 10.1.1

**Strefen®** (Crookes)
Lozenges, flurbiprofen 8.75 mg, net price 16 = £2.24
Dose ADULT and CHILD over 12 years, allow 1 lozenge to dissolve slowly in the mouth every 3–6 hours, max. 5 lozenges in 24 hours, for max. 3 days

## ▐ LOCAL ANAESTHETICS

**Indications** relief of pain in oral lesions

**Cautions** avoid prolonged use; hypersensitivity; pregnancy (Appendix 4); avoid anaesthesia of the pharynx before meals—risk of choking

**Lidocaine** (Non-proprietary)
Ointment, lidocaine 5% in a water-miscible basis, net price 15 g = 80p
Dose rub sparingly and gently on affected areas
Dental prescribing on NHS Lidocaine 5% Ointment may be prescribed

**Xylocaine®** (AstraZeneca)
Spray (= pump spray), lidocaine 10% (100 mg/g) supplying 10 mg lidocaine/spray; 500 spray doses per container. Net price 50-mL bottle = £3.13
Dose apply thinly to the ulcer [unlicensed indication] using a cotton bud
Dental prescribing on NHS May be prescribed as Lidocaine Spray 10%

◢Preparations on sale to the public
Many mouth ulcer preparations, throat lozenges, and throat sprays on sale to the public contain a **local anaesthetic**. To identify the active ingredients in such preparations, consult the product literature of the manufacturer.
Note The correct proprietary name should be ascertained—many products have very similar names but different active ingredients

## ▐ SALICYLATES

**Indications** mild oral and perioral lesions

**Cautions** not to be applied to dentures—leave at least 30 minutes before re-insertion of dentures; frequent application, especially in children, may give rise to salicylate poisoning

**Contra-indications** children under 16 years
Reyes syndrome The CHM has advised that topical oral pain relief products containing salicylate salts should not be used in children under 16 years, as a cautionary measure due to the theoretical risk of Reye's syndrome

◢Choline salicylate
**Choline Salicylate Dental Gel, BP**
Oral gel, choline salicylate 8.7% in a flavoured gel basis, net price 15 g = £1.89
Brands include Bonjela® (sugar-free)
Dose ADULT and CHILD over 16 years, apply ½-inch of gel with gentle massage not more often than every 3 hours
Dental prescribing on NHS Choline Salicylate Dental Gel may be prescribed

◢Salicylic acid
**Pyralvex®** (Norgine)
Oral paint, brown, rhubarb extract (anthraquinone glycosides 0.5%), salicylic acid 1%. Net price 10 mL with brush = £3.25
Dose ADULT and CHILD over 16 years, apply 3–4 times daily

## 12.3.2 Oropharyngeal anti-infective drugs

The most common cause of a sore throat is a viral infection which does not benefit from anti-infective treatment. Streptococcal sore throats require systemic **penicillin** therapy (Table 1, section 5.1). Acute ulcerative gingivitis (Vincent's infection) responds to systemic **metronidazole** (section 5.1.11).

Preparations administered in the dental surgery for the local treatment of periodontal disease include gels of metronidazole (*Elyzol®*, Colgate-Palmolive) and of minocycline (*Dentomycin®*, Blackwell).

## Oropharyngeal fungal infections

Fungal infections of the mouth are usually caused by *Candida* spp. (candidiasis or candidosis). Different types of oropharyngeal candidiasis are managed as follows:

**Thrush** Acute pseudomembranous candidiasis (thrush), is usually an acute infection but it may persist for months in patients receiving inhaled corticosteroids, cytotoxics or broad-spectrum antibacterials. Thrush also occurs in patients with serious systemic disease associated with reduced immunity such as leukaemia, other malignancies, and HIV infection. Any predisposing condition should be managed appropriately. When thrush is associated with corticosteroid inhalers, rinsing the mouth with water (or cleaning a child's teeth) immediately after using the inhaler may avoid the problem. Treatment with **nystatin**, **amphotericin**, or **miconazole** may be needed. **Fluconazole** (section 5.2) is effective for unresponsive infections or if a topical antifungal drug cannot be used or if the patient has dry mouth. Topical therapy may not be adequate in immunocompromised patients and an oral triazole antifungal is preferred (section 5.2).

**Acute erythematous candidiasis** Acute erythematous (atrophic) candidiasis is a relatively uncommon condition associated with corticosteroid and broad-spectrum antibacterial use and with HIV disease. It is usually treated with **fluconazole** (section 5.2).

**Denture stomatitis** Patients with denture stomatitis (chronic atrophic candidiasis), should cleanse their dentures thoroughly and leave them out as often as possible during the treatment period. To prevent recurrence of the problem, dentures should not normally be worn at night. New dentures may be required if these measures fail despite good compliance.

**Miconazole** oral gel can be applied to the fitting surface of the denture before insertion (for short periods only). Alternatively, **amphotericin** lozenges can be allowed to dissolve slowly in the mouth but they are less effective at resolving the stomatitis. Denture stomatitis is not always associated with candidiasis and other factors such as mechanical or chemical irritation, bacterial infection, or rarely allergy to the dental base material, may be the cause.

**Chronic hyperplastic candidiasis** Chronic hyperplastic candidiasis (candidal leucoplakia) carries an increased risk of malignancy; biopsy is essential—this type of candidiasis may be associated with varying degrees of dysplasia, with oral cancer present in a high proportion of cases. Chronic hyperplastic candidiasis is treated with a systemic antifungal such as **fluconazole** (section 5.2) to eliminate candidal overlay. Patients should avoid the use of tobacco.

**Angular cheilitis** Angular cheilitis (angular stomatitis) is characterised by soreness, erythema and fissuring at the angles of the mouth. It is commonly associated with denture stomatitis but may represent a nutritional deficiency or it may be related to orofacial granulomatosis or HIV infection. Both yeasts (*Candida* spp.) and bacteria (*Staphylococcus aureus* and beta-haemolytic streptococci) are commonly involved as interacting, infective factors. A reduction in facial height related to ageing and tooth loss with maceration in the deep occlusive folds that may subsequently arise, predisposes to such infection. While the underlying cause is being identified and treated, it is often helpful to apply **miconazole** and **hydrocortisone** cream or ointment (see p. 631), **miconazole** cream (see p. 659), or **sodium fusidate** ointment (see p. 658).

**Immunocompromised patients** For advice on prevention of fungal infections in immunocompromised patients see p. 333.

**Drugs used in oropharyngeal candidiasis** Amphotericin and nystatin are not absorbed from the gastro-intestinal tract and are applied locally (as lozenges or suspension) to the mouth for treating local fungal infections. Miconazole is applied locally (as an oral gel) in the mouth but it is absorbed to the extent that potential interactions need to be considered. Miconazole also has some activity against Gram-positive bacteria including streptococci and staphylococci. **Fluconazole** (section 5.2) is given by mouth for infections that do not respond to topical therapy or when topical therapy cannot be used. It is reliably absorbed and effective. **Itraconazole** (section 5.2) can be used for fluconazole-resistant infections.

If candidal infection fails to respond to 1 to 2 weeks of treatment with antifungal drugs the patient should be sent for investigation to eliminate the possibility of underlying disease. Persistent infection may also be caused by reinfection from the genito-urinary or gastro-intestinal tract. Infection can be eliminated from these sources by appropriate anticandidal therapy; the patient's partner may also require treatment to prevent reinfection.

For the role of antiseptic mouthwashes in the prevention of oral candidiasis in immunocompromised patients and treatment of denture stomatitis, see section 12.3.4.

## ■ AMPHOTERICIN

**Indications** oral and perioral fungal infections

**Side-effects** mild gastro-intestinal disturbances reported

**Fungilin®** (Squibb) ℞
Lozenges, yellow, amphotericin 10 mg. Net price 60-lozenge pack = £3.53. Label: 9, 24, counselling, after food

**Dose** allow 1 lozenge to dissolve slowly in the mouth 4 times daily for 10–15 days (continued for 48 hours after lesions have resolved); increase to 8 daily if infection severe

**Dental prescribing on NHS** May be prescribed as Amphotericin Lozenges

## ■ MICONAZOLE

**Indications** see preparations

**Cautions** pregnancy (Appendix 4); breast-feeding; avoid in acute porphyria (section 9.8.2); **interactions**: Appendix 1 (antifungals, imidazole)

**Contra-indications** hepatic impairment; *with oral gel*, impaired swallowing reflex in infants, first 5–6 months of life of an infant born preterm

**Side-effects** nausea, vomiting; rash; *with buccal tablets*, abdominal pain, taste disturbance, burning sensation at application site, pruritus, and oedema; *with oral gel, very rarely* diarrhoea (usually on long-term treatment), hepatitis, toxic epidermal necrolysis, and Stevens-Johnson syndrome

**Dose**
● see preparations

**¹Daktarin®** (Janssen-Cilag) ℞
Oral gel, sugar-free, orange-flavoured, miconazole 24 mg/mL (20 mg/g). Net price 15-g tube = £2.84, 80-g tube = £4.47. Label: 9, counselling, hold in mouth, after food

**Dose** prevention and treatment of oral and intestinal fungal infections, 5–10 mL in the mouth after food 4 times daily, retained near oral lesions before swallowing; CHILD 4 months–2 years 2.5 mL twice daily, smeared around the mouth; 2–6 years 5 mL twice daily, retained near lesions before swallowing; over 6 years 5 mL 4 times daily, retained near lesions before swallowing

**Note** Treatment should be continued for 48 hours after lesions have healed

Localised lesions, smear small amount on affected area with clean finger 4 times daily for 5–7 days (dental prostheses should be removed at night and brushed with gel); treatment continued for 48 hours after lesions have healed

**Dental prescribing on NHS** May be prescribed as Miconazole Oromucosal Gel

1. 15-g tube can be sold to the public

**◢Buccal preparation**
**Loramyc®** (SpePharm) ▼ ℞
Mucoadhesive buccal tablets, white-yellow, miconazole 50 mg, net price 14-tab pack = £52.12. Label: 10, counselling, administration

**Dose** oropharyngeal candidiasis in immunocompromised ADULT, 50 mg daily preferably taken in the morning for 7 days; if no improvement, continue treatment for a further 7 days

**Counselling** Place rounded side of tablet on upper gum above an incisor tooth and hold upper lip firmly over the gum for 30 seconds using a finger. If tablet detaches within 6 hours, replace with a new tablet. With each dose, use alternate sides of the gum

**Note** The Scottish Medicines Consortium (p. 3) has advised (November 2008) that miconazole mucoadhesive buccal tablets (Loramyc®) are not recommended for use within NHS Scotland.

## ■ NYSTATIN

**Indications** oral and perioral fungal infections

**Side-effects** oral irritation and sensitisation, nausea reported; see also p. 338

**Dose**
● Treatment, ADULT and CHILD, 100 000 units 4 times daily after food, usually for 7 days (continued for 48 hours after lesions have resolved)

**Note** Unlicensed for treating candidiasis in NEONATE

**Nystan®** (Squibb) ℞
Oral suspension, yellow, nystatin 100 000 units/mL. Net price 30 mL with pipette = £1.91. Label: 9, counselling, use of pipette, hold in mouth, after food

**Dental prescribing on NHS** Nystatin Oral Suspension may be prescribed

## Oropharyngeal viral infections

The management of primary herpetic gingivostomatitis is a soft diet, adequate fluid intake, and analgesics as required, including local use of **benzydamine** (section 12.3.1). The use of chlorhexidine mouthwash (section 12.3.4) will control plaque accumulation if toothbrushing is painful and will also help to control secondary infection in general.

In the case of severe herpetic stomatitis, a systemic antiviral such as aciclovir is required (section 5.3.2.1). Valaciclovir and famciclovir are suitable alternatives for oral lesions associated with herpes zoster. Aciclovir and valaciclovir are also used for the prevention of frequently recurring herpes simplex lesions of the mouth, particularly when implicated in the initiation of erythema multiforme. See section 13.10.3 for the treatment of labial herpes simplex infections.

Herpes infections of the mouth may also respond to rinsing the mouth with **doxycycline**, see p. 617.

## 12.3.3 Lozenges and sprays

There is no convincing evidence that antiseptic lozenges and sprays have a beneficial action and they sometimes irritate and cause sore tongue and sore lips. Some of these preparations also contain local anaesthetics which relieve pain but may cause sensitisation.

## 12.3.4 Mouthwashes, gargles, and dentifrices

Superficial infections of the mouth are often helped by warm mouthwashes which have a mechanical cleansing effect and cause some local hyperaemia. However, to be effective, they must be used frequently and vigorously. A warm saline mouthwash is ideal and can be prepared either by dissolving half a teaspoonful of salt in a glassful of warm water or by diluting **compound sodium chloride mouthwash** with an equal volume of warm water. **Mouthwash solution-tablets** are used to remove unpleasant tastes.

Mouthwashes containing an oxidising agent, such as **hydrogen peroxide**, may be useful in the treatment of acute ulcerative gingivitis (Vincent's infection) since the organisms involved are anaerobes. It also has a mechanical cleansing effect arising from frothing when in contact with oral debris.

**Chlorhexidine** is an effective antiseptic which has the advantage of inhibiting plaque formation on the teeth. It does not, however, completely control plaque deposition and is not a substitute for effective toothbrushing. Moreover, chlorhexidine preparations do not penetrate significantly into stagnation areas and are therefore of little value in the control of dental caries or of periodontal disease once pocketing has developed. Chlorhexidine mouthwash is used in the treatment of denture stomatitis. It is also used in the prevention of oral candidiasis in immunocompromised patients. Chlorhexidine mouthwash reduces the incidence of alveolar osteitis following tooth extraction. Chlorhexidine mouthwash should not be used for the prevention of endocarditis in patients undergoing dental procedures.

Chlorhexidine can be used as a mouthwash, spray or gel for secondary infection in mucosal ulceration and for controlling gingivitis, as an adjunct to other oral hygiene measures. These preparations may also be used instead of toothbrushing where there is a painful periodontal condition (e.g. primary herpetic stomatitis) or if the patient has a haemorrhagic disorder, or is disabled. Chlorhexidine preparations are of little value in the control of acute necrotising ulcerative gingivitis.

There is no convincing evidence that gargles are effective.

---

### ▌ CHLORHEXIDINE GLUCONATE

**Indications** see under preparations below

**Side-effects** mucosal irritation (if desquamation occurs, discontinue treatment or dilute mouthwash with an equal volume of water); taste disturbance; reversible brown staining of teeth, and of silicate or composite restorations; tongue discoloration; parotid gland swelling reported

Note Chlorhexidine gluconate may be incompatible with some ingredients in toothpaste; leave an interval of at least 30 minutes between using mouthwash and toothpaste

**Chlorhexidine** (Non-proprietary)

Mouthwash, chlorhexidine gluconate 0.2%, net price 300 mL = £1.97

Dose oral hygiene and plaque inhibition, oral candidiasis, gingivitis, and management of aphthous ulcers, rinse mouth with 10 mL for about 1 minute twice daily

Denture stomatitis, cleanse and soak dentures in mouthwash solution for 15 minutes twice daily

Dental prescribing on NHS Chlorhexidine Mouthwash may be prescribed

**Chlorohex®** (Colgate-Palmolive)

Chlorohex 1200® mouthwash, chlorhexidine gluconate 0.12% (mint-flavoured). Net price 300 mL = £2.00

Dose oral hygiene and plaque inhibition, rinse mouth with 15 mL for about 30 seconds twice daily

**Corsodyl®** (GSK Consumer Healthcare)

Dental gel, chlorhexidine gluconate 1%. Net price 50 g = £1.21

Dose oral hygiene and plaque inhibition and gingivitis, brush on the teeth once or twice daily

Oral candidiasis and management of aphthous ulcers, apply to affected areas once or twice daily

Dental prescribing on NHS May be prescribed as Chlorhexidine Gluconate Gel

Mouthwash, chlorhexidine gluconate 0.2%. Net price 300 mL (original or mint) = £1.93, 600 mL (mint) = £3.85

Dose oral hygiene and plaque inhibition, oral candidiasis, gingivitis, and management of aphthous ulcers, rinse mouth with 10 mL for about 1 minute twice daily

Denture stomatitis, cleanse and soak dentures in mouthwash solution for 15 minutes twice daily

Oral spray, chlorhexidine gluconate 0.2% (mint-flavoured). Net price 60 mL = £4.10

Dose oral hygiene and plaque inhibition, oral candidiasis, gingivitis, and management of aphthous ulcers, apply as required to tooth, gingival, or ulcer surfaces using up to 12 actuations (approx. 0.14 mL/actuation) twice daily

Dental prescribing on NHS May be prescribed as Chlorhexidine Oral Spray

**Periogard®** (Colgate-Palmolive)
Oromucosal solution, alcohol-free, chlorhexidine gluconate 0.2%, net price 300 mL = £1.97

Dose short-term treatment of inflammation of gingival and oral mucosa, ADULT and CHILD over 6 years, rinse mouth with 10 mL for about 1 minute twice daily, usually for up to 7 days

Dental prescribing on NHS May be prescribed as Chlorhexidine Oromucosal Solution, Alcohol-free, 0.2%

◢With chlorobutanol
**Eludril®** (Fabre)
Mouthwash or *gargle*, chlorhexidine gluconate 0.1%, chlorobutanol 0.5% (mint-flavoured), net price 90 mL = £1.36, 250 mL = £2.83, 500 mL = £5.06

Dose oral hygiene and plaque inhibition, use 10–15 mL (diluted with warm water in measuring cup provided) 2–3 times daily

Denture disinfection, soak previously cleansed dentures in mouthwash (diluted with 2 volumes of water) for 60 minutes

### ▮ HEXETIDINE

**Indications** oral hygiene

**Side-effects** local irritation; *very rarely* taste disturbance and transient anaesthesia

**Oraldene®** (McNeil)
Mouthwash or *gargle*, red or blue-green (mint-flavoured), hexetidine 0.1%. Net price 100 mL = £1.31; 200 mL = £2.02

Dose ADULT and CHILD over 6 years, use 15 mL undiluted 2–3 times daily

### ▮ HYDROGEN PEROXIDE

**Indications** oral hygiene, see notes above

**Side-effects** hypertrophy of papillae of tongue on prolonged used

**Hydrogen Peroxide Mouthwash, BP**
Mouthwash, consists of Hydrogen Peroxide Solution 6% (= approx. 20 volume) BP

Dose rinse the mouth for 2–3 minutes with 15 mL diluted in half a tumblerful of warm water 2–3 times daily

Dental prescribing on NHS Hydrogen Peroxide Mouthwash may be prescribed

**Peroxyl®** (Colgate-Palmolive)
Mouthwash, hydrogen peroxide 1.5%, net price 300 mL = £2.95

Dose rinse the mouth with 10 mL for about 1 minute up to 4 times daily (after meals and at bedtime)

### ▮ SODIUM CHLORIDE

**Indications** oral hygiene, see notes above

**Sodium Chloride Mouthwash, Compound, BP**
Mouthwash, sodium bicarbonate 1%, sodium chloride 1.5% in a suitable vehicle with a peppermint flavour.

Dose extemporaneous preparations should be prepared according to the following formula: sodium chloride 1.5 g, sodium bicarbonate 1 g, concentrated peppermint emulsion 2.5 mL, double-strength chloroform water 50 mL, water to 100 mL

To be diluted with an equal volume of warm water

Dental prescribing on NHS Compound Sodium Chloride Mouthwash may be prescribed

### ▮ THYMOL

**Indications** oral hygiene, see notes above

**Mouthwash Solution-tablets**
Consist of tablets which may contain antimicrobial, colouring, and flavouring agents in a suitable soluble effervescent basis to make a mouthwash suitable for dental purposes. Net price 100-tab pack = £15.02

Dose dissolve 1 tablet in a tumblerful of warm water

Note Mouthwash solution tablets may contain ingredients such as thymol

Dental prescribing on NHS Mouthwash Solution-tablets may be prescribed

## 12.3.5 Treatment of dry mouth

Dry mouth (xerostomia) may be caused by drugs with antimuscarinic (anticholinergic) side-effects (e.g. antispasmodics, tricyclic antidepressants, and some antipsychotics), by diuretics, by irradiation of the head and neck region or by damage to or disease of the salivary glands. Patients with a persistently dry mouth may develop a burning or scalded sensation and have poor oral hygiene; they may develop increased dental caries, periodontal disease, intolerance of dentures, and oral infections (particularly candidiasis). Dry mouth may be relieved in many patients by simple measures such as frequent sips of cool drinks or sucking pieces of ice or sugar-free fruit pastilles. Sugar-free chewing gum stimulates salivation in patients with residual salivary function.

**Artificial saliva** can provide useful relief of dry mouth. A properly balanced artificial saliva should be of a neutral pH and contain electrolytes (including fluoride) to correspond approximately to the composition of saliva. The acidic pH of some artificial saliva products may be inappropriate. Of the proprietary preparations, *Luborant®* is licensed for any condition giving rise to a dry mouth; *Biotène Oralbalance®*, *BioXtra®*, *Glandosane®*, *Saliva Orthana®*, and *Saliveze®*, have ACBS approval for dry mouth associated only with radiotherapy or sicca syndrome. *Salivix®* pastilles, which act locally as salivary stimulants, are also available and have similar ACBS approval. *SST* tablets may be prescribed for dry mouth in patients with salivary gland impairment (and patent salivary ducts). *Salinum®* may also be prescribed for relief of symptoms of dry mouth.

**Pilocarpine** tablets are licensed for the treatment of xerostomia following irradiation for head and neck cancer and for dry mouth and dry eyes (xerophthalmia) in Sjögren's syndrome. They are effective only in patients who have some residual salivary gland function, and therefore should be withdrawn if there is no response.

### Local treatment

**AS Saliva Orthana®** (AS Pharma)
Oral spray, gastric mucin (porcine) 3.5%, xylitol 2%, sodium fluoride 4.2 mg/litre, with preservatives and flavouring agents, pH neutral. Net price 50-mL bottle = £4.92; 450-mL refill = £34.27

Dose ACBS: patients suffering from dry mouth as a result of having (or having undergone) radiotherapy, or sicca syndrome, spray 2–3 times onto oral and pharyngeal mucosa, when required

**12**

**Ear, nose, and oropharynx**

Lozenges, mucin 65 mg, xylitol 59 mg, in a sorbitol basis, pH neutral. Net price 30-lozenge pack = £3.50

**Dose** ACBS: patients suffering from dry mouth as a result of having (or having undergone) radiotherapy, or sicca syndrome

**Note** *AS Saliva Orthana®* lozenges do not contain fluoride

**Dental prescribing on NHS** *AS Saliva Orthana®* Oral Spray and Lozenges may be prescribed

### Biotène Oralbalance® (Anglian)

Saliva replacement gel, lactoperoxidase, lactoferrin, lysozyme, glucose oxidase, xylitol in a gel basis, net price 50-g tube = £4.10, 24 × 12.4-mL tube = £30.40 (for hospital use)

**Dose** ACBS: patients suffering from dry mouth as a result of having (or having undergone) radiotherapy, or sicca syndrome, apply to gums and tongue as required

**Note** Avoid use with toothpastes containing detergents (including foaming agents)

**Dental prescribing on NHS** *Biotène Oralbalance®* Saliva Replacement Gel may be prescribed

### BioXtra® (RIS Products)

Gel, lactoperoxidase, lactoferrin, lysozyme, whey colostrum, xylitol and other ingredients, net price 40-mL tube = £3.94, 50-mL spray = £3.94

**Dose** ACBS: patients suffering from dry mouth as a result of having (or having undergone) radiotherapy, or sicca syndrome, apply to oral mucosa as required

**Dental prescribing on NHS** *BioXtra®* Gel may be prescribed

### Glandosane® (Fresenius Kabi)

Aerosol spray, carmellose sodium 500 mg, sorbitol 1.5 g, potassium chloride 60 mg, sodium chloride 42.2 mg, magnesium chloride 2.6 mg, calcium chloride 7.3 mg, and dipotassium hydrogen phosphate 17.1 mg/50 g, pH 5.75. Net price 50-mL unit (neutral, lemon or peppermint flavoured) = £4.70

**Dose** ACBS: patients suffering from dry mouth as a result of having (or having undergone) radiotherapy, or sicca syndrome, spray onto oral and pharyngeal mucosa as required

**Dental prescribing on NHS** *Glandosane®* Aerosol Spray may be prescribed

### Luborant® (Goldshield)

Oral spray, pink, sorbitol 1.8 g, carmellose sodium (sodium carboxymethylcellulose) 390 mg, dibasic potassium phosphate 48.23 mg, potassium chloride 37.5 mg, monobasic potassium phosphate 21.97 mg, calcium chloride 9.972 mg, magnesium chloride 3.528 mg, sodium fluoride 258 micrograms/60 mL, with preservatives and colouring agents. Net price 60-mL unit = £3.96

**Dose** saliva deficiency, 2–3 sprays onto oral mucosa up to 4 times daily, or as directed

**Note** May be difficult to obtain

**Dental prescribing on NHS** *Luborant®* Oral Spray may be prescribed as Artificial Saliva Oral Spray

### Salinum® (Crawford)

Liquid, sugar-free, linseed extract (containing polysaccharides) with dipotassium phosphate buffer and preservatives, pH 6–7, net price 300-mL bottle = £13.50

**Dose** symptomatic treatment of dry mouth, approx. 2 mL rinsed around the mouth and then swallowed, when required

**Dental prescribing on NHS** *Salinum®* liquid may be prescribed as Artificial Saliva Liquid

### Saliveze® (Wyvern)

Oral spray, carmellose sodium (sodium carboxymethylcellulose), calcium chloride, magnesium chloride, potassium chloride, sodium chloride, and dibasic sodium phosphate, pH neutral. Net price 50-mL bottle (mint-flavoured) = £3.50

**Dose** ACBS: patients suffering from dry mouth as a result of having (or having undergone) radiotherapy, or sicca syndrome, 1 spray onto oral mucosa as required

**Dental prescribing on NHS** *Saliveze®* Oral Spray may be prescribed

### Salivix® (KoGEN)

Pastilles, sugar-free, reddish-amber, acacia, malic acid and other ingredients. Net price 50-pastille pack = £3.50

**Dose** ACBS: patients suffering from dry mouth as a result of having (or having undergone) radiotherapy, or sicca syndrome, suck 1 pastille when required

**Dental prescribing on NHS** *Salivix®* Pastilles may be prescribed

### SST (Medac)

Tablets, sugar-free, citric acid, malic acid and other ingredients in a sorbitol base, net price 100-tab pack = £4.86

**Dose** symptomatic treatment of dry mouth in patients with impaired salivary gland function and patent salivary ducts, allow 1 tablet to dissolve slowly in the mouth when required

**Dental prescribing on NHS** May be prescribed as Saliva Stimulating Tablets

### Xerotin® (SpePharm)

Oral spray, sugar-free, water, sorbitol, carmellose (carboxymethylcellulose), potassium chloride, sodium chloride, potassium phosphate, magnesium chloride, calcium chloride and other ingredients, pH neutral. Net price 100-mL unit = £6.86

**Dose** symptomatic treatment of dry mouth, spray as required

## Systemic treatment

### PILOCARPINE HYDROCHLORIDE

**Indications** xerostomia following irradiation for head and neck cancer (see also notes above); dry mouth and dry eyes in Sjögren's syndrome

**Cautions** asthma and chronic obstructive pulmonary disease (avoid if uncontrolled, see Contra-indications), cardiovascular disease (avoid if uncontrolled); cholelithiasis or biliary-tract disease, peptic ulcer, hepatic impairment (Appendix 2), renal impairment; risk of increased urethral smooth muscle tone and renal colic; maintain adequate fluid intake to avoid dehydration associated with excessive sweating; cognitive or psychiatric disturbances; susceptibility to angle-closure glaucoma; **interactions:** Appendix 1 (parasympathomimetics)

**Counselling** Blurred vision or dizziness may affect performance of skilled tasks (e.g. driving) particularly at night or in reduced lighting

**Contra-indications** uncontrolled asthma and chronic obstructive pulmonary disease (increased bronchial secretions and increased airways resistance); uncontrolled cardiorenal disease; acute iritis; pregnancy (Appendix 4); breast-feeding (Appendix 5)

**Side-effects** dyspepsia, diarrhoea, abdominal pain, nausea, vomiting, constipation; flushing, hypertension, palpitation, headache, dizziness, asthenia, influenza-like symptoms, sweating; increased urinary frequency; visual disturbances, lacrimation, ocular pain, conjunctivitis; rhinitis; rash, pruritus; *less commonly* flatulence, urinary urgency

## Dose

- Xerostomia following irradiation for head and neck cancer, 5 mg 3 times daily with or immediately after meals (last dose always with evening meal); if tolerated but response insufficient after 4 weeks, may be increased to max. 30 mg daily in divided doses; max. therapeutic effect normally within 4–8 weeks; discontinue if no improvement after 2–3 months; CHILD not recommended

- Dry mouth and dry eyes in Sjögren's syndrome, 5 mg 4 times daily (with meals and at bedtime); if tolerated but response insufficient, may be increased to max. 30 mg daily in divided doses; discontinue if no improvement after 2–3 months; CHILD not recommended

**Salagen®** (Novartis) PoM
Tablets, f/c, pilocarpine hydrochloride 5 mg. Net price 84-tab pack = £51.43. Label: 21, 27, counselling, driving

# 13 Skin

**13.1 Management of skin conditions** **624**

13.1.1 Vehicles 624

13.1.2 Suitable quantities for prescribing 625

13.1.3 Excipients and sensitisation 625

**13.2 Emollient and barrier preparations** **625**

13.2.1 Emollients 625

13.2.1.1 Emollient bath additives 628

13.2.2 Barrier preparations 629

**13.3 Topical local anaesthetics and antipruritics** **630**

**13.4 Topical corticosteroids** **630**

**13.5 Preparations for eczema and psoriasis** **637**

13.5.1 Preparations for eczema 637

13.5.2 Preparations for psoriasis 639

13.5.3 Drugs affecting the immune response 643

**13.6 Acne and rosacea** **646**

13.6.1 Topical preparations for acne 647

13.6.2 Oral preparations for acne 649

**13.7 Preparations for warts and calluses** **651**

**13.8 Sunscreens and camouflagers** **653**

13.8.1 Sunscreen preparations 653

13.8.2 Camouflagers 654

**13.9 Shampoos and other preparations for scalp and hair conditions** **655**

**13.10 Anti-infective skin preparations** **656**

13.10.1 Antibacterial preparations 656

13.10.1.1 Antibacterial preparations only used topically 657

13.10.1.2 Antibacterial preparations also used systemically 658

13.10.2 Antifungal preparations 659

13.10.3 Antiviral preparations 661

13.10.4 Parasiticidal preparations 662

13.10.5 Preparations for minor cuts and abrasions 664

**13.11 Skin cleansers and antiseptics** **665**

13.11.1 Alcohols and saline 665

13.11.2 Chlorhexidine salts 666

13.11.3 Cationic surfactants and soaps 667

13.11.4 Iodine 667

13.11.5 Phenolics 667

13.11.6 Oxidisers and dyes 667

13.11.7 Preparations for promotion of wound healing 667

**13.12 Antiperspirants** **668**

**13.13 Topical circulatory preparations** **668**

This chapter also includes advice on the drug management of the following:

candidiasis, p. 659
crab lice, p. 663
dermatophytoses, p. 659
head lice, p. 663
hirsutism, p. 656
nappy rash, p. 629
photodamage, p. 654
pityriasis versicolor, p. 659
scabies, p. 662

For further information on wound management products and elastic hosiery see Appendix 8, p. 911

The British Association of Dermatologists list of preferred unlicensed dermatological preparations (specials) is available at http://88.208.244.6/BAD/site/495/default.aspx

## 13.1 Management of skin conditions

### 13.1.1 Vehicles

Both vehicle and active ingredients are important in the treatment of skin conditions; the vehicle alone may have more than a mere placebo effect. The vehicle affects the degree of hydration of the skin, has a mild anti-inflammatory effect, and aids the penetration of active drug.

**Applications** are usually viscous solutions, emulsions, or suspensions for application to the skin (including the scalp) or nails.

**Collodions** are painted on the skin and allowed to dry to leave a flexible film over the site of application.

**Creams** are emulsions of oil and water and are generally well absorbed into the skin. They may contain an antimicrobial preservative unless the active ingredient or basis is intrinsically bactericidal and fungicidal. Generally, creams are cosmetically more acceptable than ointments because they are less greasy and easier to apply.

Gels consist of active ingredients in suitable hydrophilic or hydrophobic bases; they generally have a high water content. Gels are particularly suitable for application to the face and scalp.

Lotions have a cooling effect and may be preferred to ointments or creams for application over a hairy area. Lotions in alcoholic basis can sting if used on broken skin. *Shake lotions* (such as calamine lotion) contain insoluble powders which leave a deposit on the skin surface.

Ointments are greasy preparations which are normally anhydrous and insoluble in water, and are more occlusive than creams. They are particularly suitable for chronic, dry lesions. The most commonly used ointment bases consist of soft paraffin or a combination of soft, liquid and hard paraffin. Some ointment bases have both *hydrophilic and lipophilic* properties; they may have occlusive properties on the skin surface, encourage hydration, and also be miscible with water; they often have a mild anti-inflammatory effect. *Water-soluble ointments* contain macrogols which are freely soluble in water and are therefore readily washed off; they have a limited but useful role where ready removal is desirable.

Pastes are stiff preparations containing a high proportion of finely powdered solids such as zinc oxide and starch suspended in an ointment. They are used for circumscribed lesions such as those which occur in lichen simplex, chronic eczema, or psoriasis. They are less occlusive than ointments and can be used to protect inflamed, lichenified, or excoriated skin.

Dusting powders are used only rarely. They reduce friction between opposing skin surfaces. Dusting powders should not be applied to moist areas because they can cake and abrade the skin. Talc is a lubricant but it does not absorb moisture; it can cause respiratory irritation. Starch is less lubricant but absorbs water.

Dilution    The BP directs that creams and ointments should **not** normally be diluted but that should dilution be necessary care should be taken, in particular, to prevent microbial contamination. The appropriate diluent should be used and heating should be avoided during mixing; excessive dilution may affect the stability of some creams. Diluted creams should normally be used within 2 weeks of preparation.

## 13.1.2 Suitable quantities for prescribing

**Suitable quantities of dermatological preparations to be prescribed for specific areas of the body**

|  | Creams and Ointments | Lotions |
|---|---|---|
| Face | 15–30 g | 100 mL |
| Both hands | 25–50 g | 200 mL |
| Scalp | 50–100 g | 200 mL |
| Both arms or both legs | 100–200 g | 200 mL |
| Trunk | 400 g | 500 mL |
| Groins and genitalia | 15–25 g | 100 mL |

These amounts are usually suitable for an adult for twice daily application for 1 week. The recommendations do **not** apply to corticosteroid preparations—for suitable quantities of corticosteroid preparations see section 13.4.

## 13.1.3 Excipients and sensitisation

Excipients in topical products rarely cause problems. If a patch test indicates allergy to an excipient, products containing the substance should be avoided (see also Anaphylaxis, p. 176). The following excipients in topical preparations are rarely associated with sensitisation; the presence of these excipients is indicated in the entries for topical products. See also Excipients, under General Guidance, p. 2.

| | |
|---|---|
| Beeswax | Imidurea |
| Benzyl alcohol | Isopropyl palmitate |
| Butylated hydroxyanisole | *N*-(3-Chloroallyl)hexami- |
| Butylated hydroxytoluene | nium chloride (quater- |
| Cetostearyl alcohol (includ- | nium 15) |
| ing cetyl and stearyl | Polysorbates |
| alcohol) | Propylene glycol |
| Chlorocresol | Sodium metabisulphite |
| Edetic acid (EDTA) | Sorbic acid |
| Ethylenediamine | Wool fat and related sub- |
| Fragrances | stances including |
| Hydroxybenzoates (para- | lanolin[1] |
| bens) | |

1. Purified versions of wool fat have reduced the problem

## 13.2 Emollient and barrier preparations

### 13.2.1 Emollients
### 13.2.2 Barrier preparations

**Borderline substances**    The preparations marked 'ACBS' are regarded as drugs when prescribed in accordance with the advice of the Advisory Committee on Borderline Substances for the clinical conditions listed. Prescriptions issued in accordance with this advice and endorsed 'ACBS' will normally not be investigated. See Appendix 7 for listing by clinical condition.

## 13.2.1 Emollients

Emollients soothe, smooth and hydrate the skin and are indicated for all dry or scaling disorders. Their effects are short-lived and they should be applied frequently even after improvement occurs. They are useful in dry and eczematous disorders, and to a lesser extent in psoriasis (section 13.5.2). Light emollients such as **aqueous cream** are suitable for many patients with dry skin but a wide range of more greasy preparations, including **white soft paraffin**, **emulsifying ointment**, and **liquid and white soft paraffin ointment**, are available; the severity of the condition, patient preference and site of application will often guide the choice of

13

Skin

emollient; emollients should be applied in the direction of hair growth. Ointments may exacerbate acne and folliculitis. Some ingredients rarely cause sensitisation (section 13.1.3) and this should be suspected if an eczematous reaction occurs.

> ### Fire hazard with paraffin-based emollients
> Emulsifying ointment *or* 50% Liquid Paraffin and 50% White Soft Paraffin Ointment in contact with dressings and clothing is easily ignited by a naked flame. The risk is greater when these preparations are applied to large areas of the body, and clothing or dressings become soaked with the ointment. Patients should be told to keep away from fire or flames, and not to smoke when using these preparations. The risk of fire should be considered when using large quantities of any paraffin-based emollient.

Preparations such as **aqueous cream** and **emulsifying ointment** can be used as soap substitutes for hand washing and in the bath; the preparation is rubbed on the skin before rinsing off completely. The addition of a bath oil (section 13.2.1.1) may also be helpful.

Preparations containing an antibacterial (section 13.10) should be avoided unless infection is present or is a frequent complication.

**Urea** is a hydrating agent used in the treatment of dry, scaling conditions (including ichthyosis) and may be useful in elderly patients. It is occasionally used with other topical agents such as corticosteroids to enhance penetration of the skin.

#### ◀Non-proprietary emollient preparations

**Aqueous Cream, BP**

Cream, emulsifying ointment 30%, [1]phenoxyethanol 1% in freshly boiled and cooled purified water, net price 100 g = 70p, 500 g = £1.70
Excipients include cetostearyl alcohol

1. The BP permits use of alternative antimicrobials provided their identity and concentration are stated on the label

**Emulsifying Ointment, BP**

Ointment, emulsifying wax 30%, white soft paraffin 50%, liquid paraffin 20%, net price 500 g = £2.15
Excipients include cetostearyl alcohol

**Hydrous Ointment, BP**

Ointment, (oily cream), dried magnesium sulphate 0.5%, phenoxyethanol 1%, wool alcohols ointment 50%, in freshly boiled and cooled purified water, net price 500 g = £2.18

**Liquid and White Soft Paraffin Ointment, NPF**

Ointment, liquid paraffin 50%, white soft paraffin 50%, net price 500 g = £3.94

**Paraffin, White Soft, BP**

White petroleum jelly, net price 100 g = 46p

**Paraffin, Yellow Soft, BP**

Yellow petroleum jelly, net price 100 g = 38p

#### ◀Proprietary emollient preparations

**Aveeno®** (J&J)

Cream, colloidal oatmeal in emollient basis, net price 100 mL = £3.78, 300-mL pump pack = £6.80
Excipients include benzyl alcohol, cetyl alcohol, isopropyl palmitate
ACBS: For endogenous and exogenous eczema, xeroderma, ichthyosis, and senile pruritus (pruritus of the elderly) associated with dry skin

Lotion, colloidal oatmeal in emollient basis, net price 400 mL = £6.42
Excipients include benzyl alcohol, cetyl alcohol, isopropyl palmitate
ACBS: as for *Aveeno®* Cream

**Cetraben®** (Genus)

Emollient cream, white soft paraffin 13.2%, light liquid paraffin 10.5%, net price 50-g pump pack = £1.17, 150-g pump pack = £2.88, 500-g pump pack = £5.39, 1.05-kg pump pack = £11.11
Excipients include cetostearyl alcohol, hydroxybenzoates (parabens)
For inflamed, damaged, dry or chapped skin including eczema

**Dermamist®** (Alliance)

Spray application, white soft paraffin 10% in a basis containing liquid paraffin, fractionated coconut oil, net price 250-mL pressurised aerosol unit = £6.45
Excipients none as listed in section 13.1.3
For dry skin conditions including eczema, ichthyosis, pruritus of the elderly
Note Flammable

**Diprobase®** (Schering-Plough)

Cream, cetomacrogol 2.25%, cetostearyl alcohol 7.2%, liquid paraffin 6%, white soft paraffin 15%, water-miscible basis used for *Diprosone®* cream, net price 50 g = £1.30; 500-g pump pack = £6.58
Excipients include cetostearyl alcohol, chlorocresol
For dry skin conditions

Ointment, liquid paraffin 5%, white soft paraffin 95%, basis used for *Diprosone®* ointment, net price 50 g = £1.30
Excipients none as listed in section 13.1.3
For dry skin conditions

**Doublebase®** (Dermal)

Gel, isopropyl myristate 15%, liquid paraffin 15%, net price 100 g = £2.69, 500 g = £5.92
Excipients none as listed in section 13.1.3
For dry, chapped, or itchy skin conditions

Emollient shower gel, isopropyl myristate 15%, liquid paraffin 15%, net price 200 g = £5.29
Excipients none as listed in section 13.1.3
For dry, chapped, or itchy skin conditions
Note Also available as *Doublebase® Emollient Wash Gel*

**E45®** (Crookes)

Cream, light liquid paraffin 12.6%, white soft paraffin 14.5%, hypoallergenic anhydrous wool fat (hypoallergenic lanolin) 1% in self-emulsifying monostearin, net price 50 g = £1.40, 125 g = £2.55, 350 g = £4.46, 500-g pump pack = £5.39
Excipients include cetyl alcohol, hydroxybenzoates (parabens)
For dry skin conditions

Emollient Wash Cream, soap substitute, zinc oxide 5% in an emollient basis, net price 250-mL pump pack = £3.19
Excipients none as listed in section 13.1.3
ACBS: For endogenous and exogenous eczema, xeroderma, ichthyosis and senile pruritus (pruritus of the elderly) associated with dry skin

Lotion, light liquid paraffin 4%, cetomacrogol, white soft paraffin 10%, hypoallergenic anhydrous wool fat (hypoallergenic lanolin) 1% in glyceryl monostearate, net price 200 mL = £2.40, 500-mL pump pack = £4.50
Excipients include isopropyl palmitate, hydroxybenzoates (parabens), benzyl alcohol
ACBS: for symptomatic relief of dry skin conditions, such as those associated with atopic eczema and contact dermatitis

**13 Skin**

**Emollin®** (C D Medical)

Spray, liquid paraffin 50%, white soft paraffin 50% in aerosol basis, net price 150 mL = £3.74, 240 mL = £5.98

Excipients none as listed in section 13.1.3

For dry skin conditions

**Epaderm®** (Mölnlycke)

Ointment, emulsifying wax 30%, yellow soft paraffin 30%, liquid paraffin 40%, net price 125 g = £3.62, 500 g = £6.14, 1 kg = £11.44

Excipients include cetostearyl alcohol

For use as an emollient or soap substitute

**Hewletts®** (Kestrel)

Cream, hydrous wool fat 4%, zinc oxide 8%, arachis (peanut) oil, oleic acid, white soft paraffin, net price 35 g = £1.43, 400 g = £6.69

Excipients include fragrance

For nursing hygiene and care of skin, and chapped hands

**Hydromol®** (Alliance)

Cream, sodium pidolate 2.5%, liquid paraffin 13.8%, net price 50 g = £2.04, 100 g = £3.80, 500 g = £11.09

Excipients include cetostearyl alcohol, hydroxybenzoates (parabens)

For dry skin conditions

Ointment, yellow soft paraffin 30%, emulsifying wax 30%, liquid paraffin 40%, net price 125 g = £2.79, 500 g = £4.74

Excipients include cetostearyl alcohol

For use as an emollient, bath additive, or soap substitute

**Linola® Gamma** (Linderma)

Cream, evening primrose oil 20%, net price 50 g = £2.83, 250 g = £8.20

Excipients include beeswax, hydroxybenzoates (parabens), propylene glycol

Cautions epilepsy (but hazard unlikely with topical preparations)

For dry skin conditions

**Lipobase®** (Astellas)

Cream, fatty cream basis used for *Locoid Lipocream®*, net price 50 g = £2.08

Excipients include cetostearyl alcohol, hydroxybenzoates (parabens)

For dry skin conditions, also for use during treatment with topical corticosteroid and as diluent for *Locoid Lipocream®*

**Oilatum®** (Stiefel)

Cream, light liquid paraffin 6%, white soft paraffin 15%, net price 40 g = £1.30, 150 g = £2.46, 500-mL pump pack = £4.99, 1.05-litre pump pack = £9.98; *Oilatum® Junior* 150 g = £3.38, 350 mL = £4.65, 500 mL = £4.99, 1.05-litre pump pack = £9.98

Excipients include benzyl alcohol, cetostearyl alcohol

For dry skin conditions

Shower emollient (gel), light liquid paraffin 70%, net price 150 g = £5.15

Excipients include fragrance

For dry skin conditions including dermatitis

**QV®** (Crawford)

Cream, glycerol 10%, light liquid paraffin 10%, white soft paraffin 5%, net price 100 g = £1.95, 500 g = £5.60

Excipients include cetostearyl alcohol, hydroxybenzoates (parabens)

For dry skin conditions including eczema, psoriasis, ichthyosis, pruritus

Lotion, white soft paraffin 5%, net price 250 mL = £3.00

Excipients include cetostearyl alcohol, hydroxybenzoates (parabens)

For dry skin conditions including eczema, psoriasis, ichthyosis, pruritus

Wash, glycerol 10%, net price 200 mL = £2.50

Excipients include hydroxybenzoates (parabens)

For dry skin conditions including eczema, psoriasis, ichthyosis, and pruritus, use as soap substitute

**Ultrabase®** (Valeant)

Cream, water-miscible, containing liquid paraffin and white soft paraffin, net price 50 g = 89p, 500-g pump pack = £6.44

Excipients include fragrance, hydroxybenzoates (parabens), disodium edetate, stearyl alcohol

For dry skin conditions

**Unguentum M®** (Almirall)

Cream, containing saturated neutral oil, liquid paraffin, white soft paraffin, net price 50 g = £1.41, 100 g = £2.78, 200-mL pump pack = £5.50, 500 g = £8.48

Excipients include cetostearyl alcohol, polysorbate 40, propylene glycol, sorbic acid

For dry skin conditions and nappy rash

**Zerobase®** (Zeroderma)

Cream, liquid paraffin 11%, net price 500-g pump pack = £5.99

Excipients include cetostearyl alcohol, chlorocresol

For dry skin conditions

◀**Preparations containing urea**

**Aquadrate®** (Alliance)

Cream, urea 10%, net price 100 g = £4.37

Excipients none as listed in section 13.1.3

Dose for dry, scaling and itching skin, apply thinly and rub into area when required

**Balneum® Plus** (Almirall)

Cream, urea 5%, lauromacrogols 3%, net price 100 g = £3.29, 175-g pump pack = £8.33, 500-g pump pack = £17.09

Excipients include benzyl alcohol, polysorbates

Dose for dry, scaling and itching skin, apply twice daily

**Calmurid®** (Galderma)

Cream, urea 10%, lactic acid 5%, net price 100 g = £5.70, 500-g pump pack = £27.42

Excipients none as listed in section 13.1.3

Dose for dry, scaling and itching skin, apply a thick layer for 3–5 minutes, massage into area, and remove excess, usually twice daily. Use half-strength cream for 1 week if stinging occurs

Note Can be diluted with aqueous cream (life of diluted cream 14 days)

**E45® Itch Relief Cream** (Crookes)

Cream, urea 5%, macrogol lauryl ether 3%, net price 50 g = £2.55, 100 g = £3.47, 500-g pump pack = £16.42

Excipients include benzyl alcohol, polysorbates

Dose for dry, scaling, and itching skin, apply twice a day

**Eucerin® Intensive** (Beiersdorf)

Cream, urea 10%, net price 100 mL = £7.59

Excipients include benzyl alcohol, isopropyl palmitate, wool fat

Dose for dry skin conditions including eczema, ichthyosis, xeroderma, hyperkeratosis, apply thinly and rub into area twice daily

Lotion, urea 10%, net price 250 mL = £7.93

Excipients include benzyl alcohol, isopropyl palmitate

Dose for dry skin conditions including eczema, ichthyosis, xeroderma, hyperkeratosis, apply sparingly and rub into area twice daily

**Nutraplus®** (Galderma)

Cream, urea 10%, net price 100 g = £4.37

Excipients include hydroxybenzoates (parabens), propylene glycol

Dose for dry, scaling and itching skin, apply 2–3 times daily

◀**With antimicrobials**

**Dermol®** (Dermal)

Cream, benzalkonium chloride 0.1%, chlorhexidine hydrochloride 0.1%, isopropyl myristate 10%, liquid paraffin 10%, net price 100-g tube = £2.90, 500-g pump pack = £6.72

Excipients include cetostearyl alcohol

Dose for dry and pruritic skin conditions including eczema and dermatitis, apply to skin or use as soap substitute

**13**

**Skin**

Dermol® 500 Lotion, benzalkonium chloride 0.1%, chlorhexidine hydrochloride 0.1%, liquid paraffin 2.5%, isopropyl myristate 2.5%, net price 500-mL pump pack = £6.13
Excipients include cetostearyl alcohol

**Dose** for dry and pruritic skin conditions including eczema and dermatitis, apply to skin or use as soap substitute

Dermol® 200 Shower Emollient, benzalkonium chloride 0.1%, chlorhexidine hydrochloride 0.1%, liquid paraffin 2.5%, isopropyl myristate 2.5%, net price 200 mL = £3.61
Excipients include cetostearyl alcohol

**Dose** for dry and pruritic skin conditions including eczema and dermatitis, apply to skin or use as soap substitute

### 13.2.1.1 Emollient bath additives

Emollient bath additives should be added to bath water; hydration can be improved by soaking in the bath for 10–20 minutes. Some bath emollients can be applied to wet skin undiluted and rinsed off. In dry skin conditions soap should be avoided (see section 13.2.1 for soap substitutes). The quantities of bath additives recommended for adults are suitable for an adult-size bath. Proportionately less should be used for a child-size bath or a washbasin; recommended bath additive quantities for children reflect this.

> These preparations make skin and surfaces slippery—particular care is needed when bathing

**Alpha Keri Bath®** (Novartis Consumer Health)
Bath oil, liquid paraffin 91.7%, oil-soluble fraction of wool fat 3%, net price 240 mL = £3.45, 480 mL = £6.43
Excipients include fragrance

**Dose** for dry skin conditions including ichthyosis and pruritus of the elderly, add 10–20 mL/bath (INFANT 5 mL) or apply to wet skin and rinse

**Aveeno®** (J&J)
Aveeno® Bath oil, colloidal oatmeal, white oat fraction in emollient basis, net price 250 mL = £4.28
Excipients include beeswax, fragrance

**Dose** ACBS: for endogenous and exogenous eczema, xeroderma, ichthyosis, and senile pruritus (pruritus of the elderly) associated with dry skin, add 20–30 mL/bath or apply to wet skin and rinse

Aveeno Colloidal® Bath additive, oatmeal, white oat fraction in emollient basis, net price 10 × 50-g sachets = £7.33; *Baby Bath Additive*, 10 × 15-g sachets = £4.39
Excipients none as listed in section 13.1.3

**Dose** ACBS: as for *Aveeno®* Bath oil; add 50 g/bath (INFANT and CHILD under 12 years, 15 g)

**Balneum®** (Almirall)
Balneum® bath oil, soya oil 84.75%, net price 200 mL = £2.48, 500 mL = £5.38, 1 litre = £10.39
Excipients include butylated hydroxytoluene, propylene glycol, fragrance

**Dose** for dry skin conditions including those associated with dermatitis and eczema; add 20–60 mL/bath (INFANT 5–15 mL); do not use undiluted

Balneum Plus® bath oil, soya oil 82.95%, mixed lauromacrogols 15%, net price 500 mL = £6.66
Excipients include butylated hydroxytoluene, propylene glycol, fragrance

**Dose** for dry skin conditions including those associated with dermatitis and eczema where pruritus also experienced; add 20 mL/bath (INFANT 5 mL) or apply to wet skin and rinse

**Cetraben®** (Genus)
Emollient bath additive, light liquid paraffin 82.8%, net price 500 mL = £5.25

**Dose** for dry skin conditions, including eczema, add 1–2 capfuls/bath (CHILD ½–1 capful) or apply to wet skin and rinse

**Dermalo®** (Dermal)
Bath emollient, acetylated wool alcohols 5%, liquid paraffin 65%, net price 500 mL = £3.50
Excipients none as listed in section 13.1.3

**Dose** for dermatitis, dry skin conditions including ichthyosis and pruritus of the elderly; add 15–20 mL/bath (INFANT and CHILD 5–10 mL) or apply to wet skin and rinse

**Diprobath®** (Schering-Plough)
Bath additive, isopropyl myristate 39%, light liquid paraffin 46%, net price 500 mL = £6.84
Excipients none as listed in section 13.1.3

**Dose** for dry skin conditions including dermatitis and eczema; add 25–50 mL/bath (INFANT 10 mL); do not use undiluted

**Doublebase®** (Dermal)
Emollient bath additive, liquid paraffin 65%, net price 500 mL = £5.54
Excipients include cetostearyl alcohol

**Dose** for dry skin conditions including dermatitis, ichthyosis, and pruritus of the elderly; add 15–20 mL/bath, (INFANT and CHILD 5–10 mL)

**E45®** (Crookes)
Emollient bath oil, cetyl dimeticone 5%, liquid paraffin 91%, net price 250 mL = £3.19, 500 mL = £5.11
Excipients none as listed in section 13.1.3

**Dose** ACBS: for endogenous and exogenous eczema, xeroderma, ichthyosis, and senile pruritus (pruritus of the elderly) associated with dry skin; add 15 mL/bath (CHILD 5–10 mL) or apply to wet skin and rinse

**Hydromol®** (Alliance)
Bath and Shower Emollient, isopropyl myristate 13%, light liquid paraffin 37.8%, net price 350 mL = £3.61, 500 mL = £4.11, 1 litre = £8.19
Excipients none as listed in section 13.1.3

**Dose** for dry skin conditions including eczema, ichthyosis and pruritus of the elderly; add 1–3 capfuls/bath (INFANT ½–2 capfuls) or apply to wet skin and rinse

**Imuderm®** (Goldshield)
Bath oil, almond oil 30%, light liquid paraffin 69.6%, net price 250 mL = £3.75
Excipients include butylated hydroxyanisole

**Dose** for dry skin conditions including dermatitis, eczema, pruritus of the elderly, and ichthyosis, add 15–30 mL/bath (INFANT and CHILD 7.5–15 mL) or rub into dry skin until absorbed

**Oilatum®** (Stiefel)
Emollient bath additive (emulsion), acetylated wool alcohols 5%, liquid paraffin 63.4%, net price 250 mL = £2.75, 500 mL = £4.57
Excipients include isopropyl palmitate, fragrance

**Dose** for dry skin conditions including dermatitis, pruritus of the elderly and ichthyosis; add 1–3 capfuls/bath (INFANT 0.5–2 capfuls) or apply to wet skin and rinse

Junior Emollient bath additive, light liquid paraffin 63.4%, net price 150 mL = £2.82, 250 mL = £3.25, 300 mL = £5.10, 500 mL = £5.75
Excipients include wool fat, isopropyl palmitate

**Dose** for dry skin conditions including dermatitis, pruritus of the elderly and ichthyosis; add 1–3 capfuls/bath (INFANT 0.5–2 capfuls) or apply to wet skin and rinse

**QV®** (Crawford)
Bath oil, light liquid paraffin 85.09%, net price 200 mL = £2.20, 500 mL = £4.50
Excipients include hydroxybenzoates (parabens)

**Dose** for dry skin conditions including eczema, ichthyosis, and pruritus of the elderly, add 10 mL/bath (CHILD 7 mL, INFANT 4 mL) or apply to wet skin and rinse

**13 Skin**

◀**With antimicrobials**

**Dermol® 600** (Dermal)

Bath Emollient, benzalkonium chloride 0.5%, liquid paraffin 25%, isopropyl myristate 25%, net price 600 mL = £7.67

Excipients include polysorbate 60

**Dose** for dry and pruritic skin conditions including eczema and dermatitis, add up to 30 mL/bath (INFANT up to 15 mL); do not use undiluted

**Emulsiderm®** (Dermal)

Liquid emulsion, liquid paraffin 25%, isopropyl myristate 25%, benzalkonium chloride 0.5%, net price 300 mL (with 15-mL measure) = £3.92, 1 litre (with 30-mL measure) = £12.18

Excipients include polysorbate 60

**Dose** for dry skin conditions including eczema and ichthyosis; add 7–30 mL/bath or rub into dry skin until absorbed

**Oilatum® Plus** (Stiefel)

Bath additive, benzalkonium chloride 6%, triclosan 2%, light liquid paraffin 52.5%, net price 500 mL = £6.98

Excipients include wool fat, isopropyl palmitate

**Dose** for topical treatment of eczema including eczema at risk from infection; add 1–2 capfuls/bath (CHILD over 6 months 1 mL); do not use undiluted

◀**With tar**

Section 13.5.2

## 13.2.2 Barrier preparations

Barrier preparations often contain water-repellent substances such as **dimeticone** (dimethicone) or other silicones. They are used on the skin around stomas, bedsores, and pressure areas in the elderly where the skin is intact. Where the skin has broken down, barrier preparations have a limited role in protecting adjacent skin. They are no substitute for adequate nursing care and it is doubtful if they are any more effective than **zinc ointments**.

**Nappy rash** Barrier creams and ointments are used for protection against nappy rash which is usually a local dermatitis. The first line of treatment is to ensure that nappies are changed frequently and that tightly fitting water-proof pants are avoided. The rash may clear when left exposed to the air and a barrier preparation can be helpful. If the rash is associated with a fungal infection, an antifungal cream such as clotrimazole cream (section 13.10.2) is useful. A mild corticosteroid such as hydrocortisone 1% is useful in moderate to severe inflammation, but it should be avoided in neonates. The barrier preparation is applied after the corticosteroid preparation to prevent further damage. Hydrocortisone can be used in combination with antifungal and antibacterial drugs (section 13.4) if there is considerable inflammation, erosion, and infection. Preparations containing hydrocortisone should be applied for no more than a week; the hydrocortisone should be discontinued as soon as the inflammation subsides. The occlusive effect of nappies and water-proof pants may increase absorption (for cautions, see p. 631).

◀**Non-proprietary barrier preparations**

**Zinc Cream, BP**

Cream, zinc oxide 32%, arachis (peanut) oil 32%, calcium hydroxide 0.045%, oleic acid 0.5%, wool fat

8%, in freshly boiled and cooled purified water, net price 50 g = 50p

For nappy and urinary rash and eczematous conditions

**Zinc Ointment, BP**

Ointment, zinc oxide 15%, in Simple Ointment BP 1988 (which contains wool fat 5%, hard paraffin 5%, cetostearyl alcohol 5%, white soft paraffin 85%), net price 25 g = 22p

For nappy and urinary rash and eczematous conditions

**Zinc and Castor Oil Ointment, BP**

Ointment, zinc oxide 7.5%, castor oil 50%, arachis (peanut) oil 30.5%, white beeswax 10%, cetostearyl alcohol 2%, net price 100 g = 70p

For nappy and urinary rash

◀**Proprietary barrier preparations**

**Conotrane®** (Astellas)

Cream, benzalkonium chloride 0.1%, dimeticone '350' 22%, net price 100 g = 88p, 500 g = £3.51

Excipients include cetostearyl alcohol, fragrance

For nappy and urinary rash and pressure sores

**Drapolene®** (Chefaro UK)

Cream, benzalkonium chloride 0.01%, cetrimide 0.2% in a basis containing white soft paraffin, cetyl alcohol and wool fat, net price 100 g = £1.54, 200 g = £2.50, 350 g = £3.75

Excipients include cetyl alcohol, chlorocresol, wool fat

For nappy and urinary rash; minor wounds

**Medicaid®** (LPC)

Cream, cetrimide 0.5% in a basis containing light liquid paraffin, white soft paraffin, cetostearyl alcohol, glyceryl monostearate, net price 50 g = £1.69

Excipients include cetostearyl alcohol, fragrance, hydroxybenzoates (parabens), wool fat

For nappy rash, minor burns and abrasions

**Metanium®** (Ransom)

Ointment, titanium dioxide 20%, titanium peroxide 5%, titanium salicylate 3% in a basis containing dimeticone, light liquid paraffin, white soft paraffin, and benzoin tincture, net price 30 g = £2.01

Excipients none as listed in section 13.1.3

For nappy rash

**Morhulin®** (Actavis)

Ointment, cod-liver oil 11.4%, zinc oxide 38%, in a basis containing liquid paraffin and yellow soft paraffin, net price 50 g = £1.72

Excipients include wool fat derivative

For minor wounds, varicose ulcers, pressure sores, eczema and nappy rash

**Siopel®** (Centrapharm)

Barrier cream, dimeticone '1000' 10%, cetrimide 0.3%, arachis (peanut) oil, net price 50 g = £2.15

Excipients include butylated hydroxytoluene, cetostearyl alcohol, hydroxybenzoates (parabens)

For protection against water-soluble irritants

**Sprilon®** (Ayrton Saunders)

Spray application, dimeticone 1.04%, zinc oxide 12.5%, in a basis containing wool alcohols, cetostearyl alcohol, dextran, white soft paraffin, liquid paraffin, propellants, net price 115-g pressurised aerosol unit = £3.54

Excipients include cetostearyl alcohol, hydroxybenzoates (parabens), wool fat

For urinary rash, pressure sores, leg ulcers, moist eczema, fissures, fistulae and ileostomy care

**Note** Flammable

**13**

**Skin**

**Sudocrem®** (Forest)

Cream, benzyl alcohol 0.39%, benzyl benzoate 1.01%, benzyl cinnamate 0.15%, hydrous wool fat (hypoallergenic lanolin) 4%, zinc oxide 15.25%, net price 30 g = £1.13, 60 g = £1.25, 125 g = £1.84, 250 g = £3.09, 400 g = £4.34

Excipients include beeswax (synthetic), propylene glycol, fragrance

For nappy rash and pressure sores

**Vasogen®** (Forest)

Barrier cream, dimeticone 20%, calamine 1.5%, zinc oxide 7.5%, net price 50 g = 80p, 100 g = £1.36

Excipients include hydroxybenzoates (parabens), wool fat

For nappy rash, pressure sores, ileostomy and colostomy care

## 13.3 Topical local anaesthetics and antipruritics

*Pruritus* may be caused by systemic disease (such as drug hypersensitivity, obstructive jaundice, endocrine disease, and certain malignant diseases), skin disease (e.g. psoriasis, eczema, urticaria, and scabies) or as a side-effect of opioid analgesics. Where possible the underlying causes should be treated. An **emollient** (section 13.2.1) may be of value where the pruritus is associated with dry skin. Pruritus that occurs in otherwise healthy elderly people can also be treated with an emollient. For advice on the treatment of pruritus in palliative care, see p. 17.

Preparations containing **crotamiton** are sometimes used but are of uncertain value. Preparations containing **calamine** are often ineffective.

A topical preparation containing **doxepin** 5% is licensed for the relief of pruritus in eczema; it can cause drowsiness and there may be a risk of sensitisation.

Pruritus is common in biliary obstruction, especially in primary biliary cirrhosis and drug-induced cholestasis. Oral administration of **colestyramine** (cholestyramine) is the treatment of choice (section 1.9.2).

Topical antihistamines and local anaesthetics are only marginally effective and occasionally cause sensitisation. For *insect stings* and *insect bites*, a short course of a topical corticosteroid is appropriate. Short-term treatment with a **sedating antihistamine** (section 3.4.1) may help in insect stings and in intractable pruritus where sedation is desirable. Calamine preparations are of little value for the treatment of insect stings or bites.

For preparations used in *pruritus ani*, see section 1.7.1.

### CALAMINE

**Indications** pruritus

**Calamine** (Non-proprietary)

Aqueous cream, calamine 4%, zinc oxide 3%, liquid paraffin 20%, self-emulsifying glyceryl monostearate 5%, cetomacrogol emulsifying wax 5%, phenoxyethanol 0.5%, freshly boiled and cooled purified water 62.5%, net price 100 mL = 84p

Lotion (= cutaneous suspension), calamine 15%, zinc oxide 5%, glycerol 5%, bentonite 3%, sodium citrate 0.5%, liquefied phenol 0.5%, in freshly boiled and cooled purified water, net price 200 mL = 63p

Oily lotion (BP 1980), calamine 5%, arachis (peanut) oil 50%, oleic acid 0.5%, wool fat 1%, in calcium hydroxide solution, net price 200 mL = £1.57

### CROTAMITON

**Indications** pruritus (including pruritus after scabies—section 13.10.4); see notes above

**Cautions** avoid use near eyes and broken skin; use on doctor's advice for children under 3 years

**Contra-indications** acute exudative dermatoses

**Dose**

- Pruritus, apply 2–3 times daily; CHILD below 3 years, apply once daily

**Eurax®** (Novartis Consumer Health)

Cream, crotamiton 10%, net price 30 g = £2.27, 100 g = £3.95

Excipients include beeswax, fragrance, hydroxybenzoates (parabens), stearyl alcohol

Lotion, crotamiton 10%, net price 100 mL = £2.99

Excipients include cetyl alcohol, fragrance, propylene glycol, sorbic acid, stearyl alcohol

### DOXEPIN HYDROCHLORIDE

**Indications** pruritus in eczema; depressive illness (section 4.3.1)

**Cautions** susceptibility to angle-closure glaucoma, urinary retention, severe liver impairment, mania; avoid application to large areas; pregnancy and breast-feeding; **interactions:** Appendix 1 (antidepressants, tricyclic)

Driving Drowsiness may affect performance of skilled tasks (e.g. driving); effects of alcohol enhanced

**Side-effects** drowsiness; local burning, stinging, irritation, tingling and rash; systemic side-effects such as antimuscarinic effects, headache, fever, dizziness, gastro-intestinal disturbances also reported

**Dose**

- ADULT and CHILD over 12 years, apply thinly 3–4 times daily; usual max. 3 g per application; usual total max. 12 g daily; coverage should be less than 10% of body surface area

**Xepin®** (CHS) PoM

Cream, doxepin hydrochloride 5%, net price 30 g = £11.70. Label: 2, 10, patient information leaflet

Excipients include benzyl alcohol

### TOPICAL LOCAL ANAESTHETICS

**Indications** relief of local pain, see notes above. See section 15.2 for use in surface anaesthesia

**Cautions** occasionally cause hypersensitivity

Note Topical local anaesthetic preparations may be absorbed, especially through mucosal surfaces, therefore excessive application should be avoided and they should preferably not be used for more than about 3 days; not generally suitable for young children

### TOPICAL ANTIHISTAMINES

**Indications** see notes above

**Cautions** may cause hypersensitivity; avoid in eczema; photosensitivity (diphenhydramine); not recommended for longer than 3 days

## 13.4 Topical corticosteroids

Topical corticosteroids are used for the treatment of inflammatory conditions of the skin (other than those arising from an infection), in particular eczema (section

13.5.1), contact dermatitis, insect stings (p. 36), and eczema of scabies (section 13.10.4). Corticosteroids suppress the inflammatory reaction during use; they are not curative and on discontinuation a rebound exacerbation of the condition may occur. They are generally used to relieve symptoms and suppress signs of the disorder when other measures such as emollients are ineffective.

Topical corticosteroids are of no value in the treatment of urticaria and they are **contra-indicated** in rosacea; they may worsen ulcerated or secondarily infected lesions. They should not be used indiscriminately in pruritus (where they will only benefit if inflammation is causing the itch) and are **not** recommended for acne vulgaris.

Systemic or potent topical corticosteroids should be avoided or given only under specialist supervision in *psoriasis* because, although they may suppress the psoriasis in the short term, relapse or vigorous rebound occurs on withdrawal (sometimes precipitating severe pustular psoriasis). Topical use of potent corticosteroids on widespread psoriasis can lead to systemic as well as to local side-effects. It is reasonable, however, to prescribe a mild to moderate topical corticosteroid for a short period (2–4 weeks) for *flexural* and *facial* psoriasis and to use a more potent corticosteroid such as betamethasone or fluocinonide for psoriasis of the *scalp, palms,* or *soles* (see below for cautions in psoriasis).

In general, the most potent topical corticosteroids should be reserved for recalcitrant dermatoses such as *chronic discoid lupus erythematosus, lichen simplex chronicus, hypertrophic lichen planus,* and *palmoplantar pustulosis.* Potent corticosteroids should generally be avoided on the face and skin flexures, but specialists occasionally prescribe them for use on these areas in certain circumstances.

When topical treatment has failed, intralesional corticosteroid injections (section 10.1.2.2) may be used. These are more effective than the very potent topical corticosteroid preparations and should be reserved for severe cases where there are localised lesions such as *keloid scars, hypertrophic lichen planus,* or *localised alopecia areata.*

**Perioral lesions** Hydrocortisone cream 1% can be used for up to 7 days to treat uninfected inflammatory lesions on the lips and on the skin surrounding the mouth. **Hydrocortisone and miconazole** cream or ointment is useful where infection by susceptible organisms and inflammation co-exist, particularly for initial treatment (up to 7 days) e.g. in angular cheilitis (see also p. 619). Organisms susceptible to miconazole include *Candida* spp. and many Gram-positive bacteria including streptococci and staphylococci.

**Children** Children, especially infants, are particularly susceptible to side-effects. However, concern about the safety of topical corticosteroids in children should not result in the child being undertreated. The aim is to control the condition as well as possible; inadequate treatment will perpetuate the condition. A mild corticosteroid such as hydrocortisone 1% ointment or cream is useful for treating nappy rash (section 13.2.2) and for atopic eczema in childhood (section 13.5.1). A moderately potent or potent corticosteroid may be appropriate for severe atopic eczema on the limbs, for 1–2 weeks only, switching to a less potent preparation as the condition improves. In an acute flare-up of atopic eczema, it may be appropriate to use more potent formulations of topical corticosteroids for a short period to regain control of the condition. A very potent corticosteroid should be initiated under the supervision of a specialist. Continuous daily application of a mild corticosteroid such as hydrocortisone 1% is equivalent to a potent corticosteroid such as betamethasone 0.1% applied intermittently. Carers of young children should be advised that treatment should **not** necessarily be reserved to 'treat only the worst areas' and they may need to be advised that patient information leaflets may contain inappropriate advice for the patient's condition.

**Choice of formulation** Water-miscible corticosteroid *creams* are suitable for moist or weeping lesions whereas *ointments* are generally chosen for dry, lichenified or scaly lesions or where a more occlusive effect is required. *Lotions* may be useful when minimal application to a large or hair-bearing area is required or for the treatment of exudative lesions. *Occlusive polythene or hydrocolloid dressings* increase absorption, but also increase the risk of side-effects; they are therefore used only under supervision on a short-term basis for areas of very thick skin (such as the palms and soles). The inclusion of urea or salicylic acid also increases the penetration of the corticosteroid.

In the BNF topical corticosteroids for the skin are categorised as 'mild', 'moderately potent', 'potent' or 'very potent' (see p. 632); the **least potent** preparation which is effective should be chosen but dilution should be avoided whenever possible.

**Cautions** Avoid prolonged use of a topical corticosteroid on the face (and keep away from eyes). In children avoid prolonged use and use potent or very potent corticosteroids under specialist supervision; extreme caution is required in dermatoses of infancy including nappy rash—treatment should be limited to 5–7 days.

**Psoriasis** The use of potent or very potent corticosteroids in psoriasis can result in rebound relapse, development of generalised pustular psoriasis, and local and systemic toxicity.

**Contra-indications** Topical corticosteroids are contra-indicated in untreated bacterial, fungal, or viral skin lesions, in rosacea, and in perioral dermatitis; potent corticosteroids are contra-indicated in widespread plaque psoriasis (see notes above).

**Side-effects** *Mild* and *moderately potent* topical corticosteroids are associated with few side-effects but care is required in the use of *potent* and *very potent* corticosteroids. Absorption through the skin can rarely cause adrenal suppression and even Cushing's syndrome (section 6.3.2), depending on the area of the body being treated and the duration of treatment. Absorption is greatest where the skin is thin or raw, and from intertriginous areas; it is increased by occlusion. Local side-effects include:

- spread and worsening of untreated infection;
- thinning of the skin which may be restored over a period after stopping treatment but the original structure may never return;
- irreversible striae atrophicae and telangiectasia;
- contact dermatitis;
- perioral dermatitis;

**13 Skin**

- acne, or worsening of acne or rosacea;
- mild depigmentation which may be reversible;
- hypertrichosis also reported.

> In order to minimise the side-effects of a topical corticosteroid, it is important to apply it **thinly** to affected areas **only**, no more frequently than **twice daily**, and to use the least potent formulation which is fully effective.

**Application** Topical corticosteroid preparations should be applied no more frequently than twice daily; once daily is often sufficient.

Topical corticosteroids are spread thinly on the skin; the length of cream or ointment expelled from a tube may be used to specify the quantity to be applied to a given area of skin. This length can be measured in terms of a *fingertip unit* (the distance from the tip of the adult index finger to the first crease). One fingertip unit (approximately 500 mg) is sufficient to cover an area that is twice that of the flat adult palm.

### Suitable quantities of corticosteroid preparations to be prescribed for specific areas of the body

|  | Creams and Ointments |
|---|---|
| Face and neck | 15 to 30 g |
| Both hands | 15 to 30 g |
| Scalp | 15 to 30 g |
| Both arms | 30 to 60 g |
| Both legs | 100 g |
| Trunk | 100 g |
| Groins and genitalia | 15 to 30 g |

These amounts are usually suitable for an adult for a single daily application for 2 weeks

If a patient is using topical corticosteroids of different potencies, the patient should be told when to use each corticosteroid. The potency of each topical corticosteroid (see Topical Corticosteroid Preparation Potencies, below) should be included on the label with the directions for use. The label should be attached to the container (for example, the tube) rather than the outer packaging.

Mixing topical preparations on the skin should be avoided where possible; several minutes should elapse between application of different preparations.

**Compound preparations** The advantages of including other substances (such as antibacterials or antifungals) with corticosteroids in topical preparations are uncertain, but such combinations may have a place where inflammatory skin conditions are associated with bacterial or fungal infection, such as infected eczema. In these cases the antimicrobial drug should be chosen according to the sensitivity of the infecting organism and used regularly for a short period (typically twice daily for 1 week). Longer use increases the likelihood of resistance and of sensitisation.

## Topical corticosteroid preparation potencies

Potency of a topical corticosteroid preparation is a result of the formulation as well as the corticosteroid. Therefore, proprietary names are shown below.

### Mild

Hydrocortisone 0.1–2.5%, *Dioderm, Mildison, Synalar 1 in 10 dilution*

- Mild with antimicrobials: *Canesten HC, Daktacort, Econacort, Fucidin H, Nystaform-HC, Timodine*
- Mild with crotamiton: *Eurax-Hydrocortisone*

### Moderate

*Betnovate-RD, Eumovate, Haelan, Modrasone, Synalar 1 in 4 Dilution, Ultralanum Plain*

- Moderate with antimicrobials: *Trimovate*
- Moderate with urea: *Alphaderm, Calmurid HC*

### Potent

Betamethasone valerate 0.1%, *Betacap, Bettamousse, Betnovate, Cutivate, Diprosone, Elocon,* Hydrocortisone butyrate, *Locoid, Locoid Crelo, Metosyn, Nerisone, Synalar*

- Potent with antimicrobials: *Aureocort, Betnovate-C, Betnovate-N, Fucibet, Lotriderm, Synalar C, Synalar N*
- Potent with salicylic acid: *Diprosalic*

### Very potent

*Clarelux, Dermovate, Etrivex, Nerisone Forte*

## ■ HYDROCORTISONE

**Indications** mild inflammatory skin disorders such as eczemas (but for over-the-counter preparations, see below); nappy rash, see notes above and section 13.2.2

**Cautions** see notes above

**Contra-indications** see notes above

**Side-effects** see notes above

**Dose**
- Apply thinly 1–2 times daily

**Hydrocortisone** (Non-proprietary) ℗oM
Cream, hydrocortisone 0.5%, net price, 15 g = £2.75; 30 g = £5.19; 1%, 15 g = £2.19, 30 g = £2.79, 50 g = £14.12; 2.5%, 15 g = £19.03. Label: 28, counselling, application, see above. Potency: mild
**Dental prescribing on NHS** Hydrocortisone Cream 1% 15 g may be prescribed

Ointment, hydrocortisone 0.5%, net price 15 g = £2.65, 30 g = £5.23; 1%, 15 g = £2.59, 30 g = £2.84, 50 g = £17.50; 2.5%, 15 g = £22.53. Label: 28, counselling, application, see above. Potency: mild
When hydrocortisone cream or ointment is prescribed and no strength is stated, the 1% strength should be supplied

◀ **Over-the-counter hydrocortisone preparations**
Skin creams and ointments containing hydrocortisone (alone or with other ingredients) can be sold to the public for the treatment of allergic contact dermatitis, irritant dermatitis, insect bite reactions and mild to moderate eczema, to be applied sparingly over the affected area 1–2 times daily for max. 1 week. Over-

the-counter hydrocortisone preparations should not be sold without medical advice for children under 10 years or for pregnant women; they should **not** be sold for application to the face, anogenital region, broken or infected skin (including cold sores, acne, and athlete's foot).

### ◢ Proprietary hydrocortisone preparations

**Dioderm®** (Dermal) [PoM]

Cream, hydrocortisone 0.1%, net price 30 g = £2.43. Label: 28, counselling, application, see p. 632. Potency: mild
Excipients include cetostearyl alcohol, propylene glycol
Note Although this contains only 0.1% hydrocortisone, the formulation is designed to provide a clinical activity comparable to that of Hydrocortisone Cream 1% BP

**Mildison®** (Astellas) [PoM]

Lipocream, hydrocortisone 1%, net price 30 g = £2.45. Label: 28, counselling, application, see p. 632. Potency: mild
Excipients include cetostearyl alcohol, hydroxybenzoates (parabens)

### ◢ Compound preparations

Compound preparations with coal tar see section 13.5.2

**Alphaderm®** (Alliance) [PoM]

Cream, hydrocortisone 1%, urea 10%, net price 30 g = £2.38; 100 g = £7.03. Label: 28, counselling, application, see p. 632. Potency: moderate
Excipients none as listed in section 13.1.3

**Calmurid HC®** (Galderma) [PoM]

Cream, hydrocortisone 1%, urea 10%, lactic acid 5%, net price 30 g = £2.80, 50 g = £4.67. Label: 28, counselling, application, see p. 632. Potency: moderate
Excipients none as listed in section 13.1.3
Note Manufacturer advises dilute to half-strength with aqueous cream for 1 week if stinging occurs then transfer to undiluted preparation (but see section 13.1.1 for advice to avoid dilution where possible)

[1]**Eurax-Hydrocortisone®** (Novartis Consumer Health) [PoM]

Cream, hydrocortisone 0.25%, crotamiton 10%, net price 30 g = 87p. Label: 28, counselling, application, see p. 632. Potency: mild
Excipients include fragrance, hydroxybenzoates (parabens), propylene glycol, stearyl alcohol

1. A 15-g tube is on sale to the public for treatment of contact dermatitis and insect bites

### ◢ With antimicrobials

See notes above for comment on compound preparations

[1]**Canesten HC®** (Bayer Consumer Care) [PoM]

Cream, hydrocortisone 1%, clotrimazole 1%, net price 30 g = £2.42. Label: 28, counselling, application, see p. 632. Potency: mild
Excipients include benzyl alcohol, cetostearyl alcohol

1. A 15-g tube is on sale to the public for the treatment of athlete's foot and fungal infection of skin folds with associated inflammation

**Daktacort®** (Janssen-Cilag) [PoM]

Cream, hydrocortisone 1%, miconazole nitrate 2%, net price 30 g = £1.83. Label: 28, counselling, application, see p. 632. Potency: mild
Excipients include butylated hydroxyanisole, disodium edetate
Note A 15-g tube is on sale to the public for the treatment of athlete's foot and candidal intertrigo

Ointment, hydrocortisone 1%, miconazole nitrate 2%, net price 30 g = £2.01. Label: 28, counselling, application, see p. 632. Potency: mild
Excipients none as listed in section 13.1.3
Dental prescribing on NHS May be prescribed as Miconazole and Hydrocortisone Cream or Ointment for max. 7 days

**Econacort®** (Squibb) [PoM]

Cream, hydrocortisone 1%, econazole nitrate 1%, net price 30 g = £2.25. Label: 28, counselling, application, see p. 632. Potency: mild
Excipients include butylated hydroxyanisole

**Fucidin H®** (LEO) [PoM]

Cream, hydrocortisone acetate 1%, fusidic acid 2%, net price 30 g = £5.09, 60 g = £10.18. Label: 28, counselling, application, see p. 632. Potency: mild
Excipients include butylated hydroxyanisole, cetyl alcohol, polysorbate 60, potassium sorbate

Ointment, hydrocortisone acetate 1%, sodium fusidate 2%, net price 30 g = £3.26, 60 g = £6.53. Label: 28, counselling, application, see p. 632. Potency: mild
Excipients include cetyl alcohol, wool fat

**Nystaform-HC®** (Typharm) [PoM]

Cream, hydrocortisone 0.5%, nystatin 100 000 units/g, chlorhexidine hydrochloride 1%, net price 30 g = £2.66. Label: 28, counselling, application, see p. 632. Potency: mild
Excipients include benzyl alcohol, cetostearyl alcohol, polysorbate '60'

Ointment, hydrocortisone 1%, nystatin 100 000 units/g, chlorhexidine acetate 1%, net price 30 g = £2.66. Label: 28, counselling, application, see p. 632. Potency: mild
Excipients none as listed in section 13.1.3

**Timodine®** (R&C) [PoM]

Cream, hydrocortisone 0.5%, nystatin 100 000 units/g, benzalkonium chloride solution 0.2%, dimeticone '350' 10%, net price 30 g = £2.03. Label: 28, counselling, application, see p. 632. Potency: mild
Excipients include butylated hydroxyanisole, cetostearyl alcohol, hydroxybenzoates (parabens), sodium metabisulphite, sorbic acid

### ■ HYDROCORTISONE BUTYRATE

**Indications** severe inflammatory skin disorders such as eczemas unresponsive to less potent corticosteroids; psoriasis, see notes above

**Cautions** see notes above

**Contra-indications** see notes above

**Side-effects** see notes above

**Dose**

• Apply thinly 1–2 times daily

**Locoid®** (Astellas) [PoM]

Cream, hydrocortisone butyrate 0.1%, net price 30 g = £2.29, 100 g = £7.05. Label: 28, counselling, application, see p. 632. Potency: potent
Excipients include cetostearyl alcohol, hydroxybenzoates (parabens)

Lipocream, hydrocortisone butyrate 0.1%, net price 30 g = £2.41, 100 g = £7.38. Label: 28, counselling, application, see p. 632. Potency: potent
Excipients include benzyl alcohol, cetostearyl alcohol, hydroxybenzoates (parabens)
Note For bland cream basis see *Lipobase®*, section 13.2.1

Ointment, hydrocortisone butyrate 0.1%, net price 30 g = £2.29, 100 g = £7.05. Label: 28, counselling, application, see p. 632. Potency: potent
Excipients none as listed in section 13.1.3

Scalp lotion, hydrocortisone butyrate 0.1%, in an aqueous isopropyl alcohol basis, net price 100 mL =

£9.76. Label: 15, 28, counselling, application, see p. 632. Potency: potent
Excipients none as listed in section 13.1.3

**Locoid Crelo®** (Astellas) [PoM]
Lotion (topical emulsion), hydrocortisone butyrate 0.1% in a water-miscible basis, net price 100 g (with applicator nozzle) = £8.44. Label: 28, counselling, application, see p. 632. Potency: potent
Excipients include butylated hydroxytoluene, cetostearyl alcohol, hydroxybenzoates (parabens), propylene glycol

## ◼ ALCLOMETASONE DIPROPIONATE

**Indications** inflammatory skin disorders such as eczemas
**Cautions** see notes above
**Contra-indications** see notes above
**Side-effects** see notes above
**Dose**
• Apply thinly 1–2 times daily

**Modrasone®** (TEVA UK) [PoM]
Cream, alclometasone dipropionate 0.05%, net price 50 g = £2.68. Label: 28, counselling, application, see p. 632. Potency: moderate
Excipients include cetostearyl alcohol, chlorocresol, propylene glycol

Ointment, alclometasone dipropionate 0.05%, net price 50 g = £2.68. Label: 28, counselling, application, see p. 632. Potency: moderate
Excipients include beeswax, propylene glycol

## ◼ BETAMETHASONE ESTERS

**Indications** severe inflammatory skin disorders such as eczemas unresponsive to less potent corticosteroids; psoriasis, see notes above
**Cautions** see notes above; use of more than 100 g per week of 0.1% preparation likely to cause adrenal suppression
**Contra-indications** see notes above
**Side-effects** see notes above
**Dose**
• Apply thinly 1–2 times daily

**Betamethasone Valerate** (Non-proprietary) [PoM]
Cream, betamethasone (as valerate) 0.1%, net price 30 g = £1.58, 100 g = £4.30. Label: 28, counselling, application, see p. 632. Potency: potent

Ointment, betamethasone (as valerate) 0.1%, net price 30 g = £1.69, 100 g = £4.21. Label: 28, counselling, application, see p. 632. Potency: potent

**Betacap®** (Dermal) [PoM]
Scalp application, betamethasone (as valerate) 0.1% in a water-miscible basis containing coconut oil derivative, net price 100 mL = £3.81. Label: 15, 28, counselling, application, see p. 632. Potency: potent
Excipients none as listed in section 13.1.3

**Betnovate®** (GSK) [PoM]
Cream, betamethasone (as valerate) 0.1% in a water-miscible basis, net price 30 g = £1.43, 100 g = £4.05. Label: 28, counselling, application, see p. 632. Potency: potent
Excipients include cetostearyl alcohol, chlorocresol

Ointment, betamethasone (as valerate) 0.1% in an anhydrous paraffin basis, net price 30 g = £1.43, 100 g = £4.05. Label: 28, counselling, application, see p. 632. Potency: potent
Excipients none as listed in section 13.1.3

Lotion, betamethasone (as valerate) 0.1%, net price 100 mL = £4.67. Label: 28, counselling, application, see p. 632. Potency: potent
Excipients include cetostearyl alcohol, hydroxybenzoates (parabens)

Scalp application, betamethasone (as valerate) 0.1% in a water-miscible basis, net price 100 mL = £5.09. Label: 15, 28, counselling, application, see p. 632. Potency: potent
Excipients none as listed in section 13.1.3

**Betnovate-RD®** (GSK) [PoM]
Cream, betamethasone (as valerate) 0.025% in a water-miscible basis (1 in 4 dilution of *Betnovate®* cream), net price 100 g = £3.21. Label: 28, counselling, application, see p. 632. Potency: moderate
Excipients include cetostearyl alcohol, chlorocresol

Ointment, betamethasone (as valerate) 0.025% in an anhydrous paraffin basis (1 in 4 dilution of *Betnovate®* ointment), net price 100 g = £3.21. Label: 28, counselling, application, see p. 632. Potency: moderate
Excipients none as listed in section 13.1.3

**Bettamousse®** (UCB Pharma) [PoM]
Foam (= scalp application), betamethasone valerate 0.12% (≡ betamethasone 0.1%), net price 100 g = £9.37. Label: 28, counselling, application, see p. 632. Potency: potent
Excipients include cetyl alcohol, polysorbate 60, propylene glycol, stearyl alcohol
Note Flammable

**Diprosone®** (Schering-Plough) [PoM]
Cream, betamethasone (as dipropionate) 0.05%, net price 30 g = £2.20, 100 g = £6.24. Label: 28, counselling, application, see p. 632. Potency: potent
Excipients include cetostearyl alcohol, chlorocresol

Ointment, betamethasone (as dipropionate) 0.05%, net price 30 g = £2.20, 100 g = £6.24. Label: 28, counselling, application, see p. 632. Potency: potent
Excipients none as listed in section 13.1.3

Lotion, betamethasone (as dipropionate) 0.05%, net price 30 mL = £2.78, 100 mL = £7.95. Label: 28, counselling, application, see p. 632. Potency: potent
Excipients none as listed in section 13.1.3

### ◢ With salicylic acid
See notes above for comment on compound preparations

**Diprosalic®** (Schering-Plough) [PoM]
Ointment, betamethasone (as dipropionate) 0.05%, salicylic acid 3%, net price 30 g = £3.24, 100 g = £9.32. Label: 28, counselling, application, see p. 632. Potency: potent
Excipients none as listed in section 13.1.3
Dose apply thinly 1–2 times daily; max. 60 g per week

Scalp application, betamethasone (as dipropionate) 0.05%, salicylic acid 2%, in an alcoholic basis, net price 100 mL = £10.30. Label: 28, counselling, application, see p. 632. Potency: potent
Excipients include disodium edetate
Dose apply a few drops 1–2 times daily

### ◢ With antimicrobials
See notes above for comment on compound preparations

**Betnovate-C®** (Chemidex) [PoM]
Cream, betamethasone (as valerate) 0.1%, clioquinol 3%, net price 30 g = £1.76. Label: 28, counselling, application, see p. 632. Potency: potent
Excipients include cetostearyl alcohol, chlorocresol
Note Stains clothing

Ointment, betamethasone (as valerate) 0.1%, clioquinol 3%, net price 30 g = £1.76. Label: 28, counselling, application, see p. 632. Potency: potent
Excipients none as listed in section 13.1.3
Note Stains clothing

**Betnovate-N®** (Chemidex) PoM
Cream, betamethasone (as valerate) 0.1%, neomycin sulphate 0.5%, net price 30 g = £1.76, 100 g = £4.88. Label: 28, counselling, application, see p. 632. Potency: potent
Excipients include cetostearyl alcohol, chlorocresol

Ointment, betamethasone (as valerate) 0.1%, neomycin sulphate 0.5%, net price 30 g = £1.76, 100 g = £4.88. Label: 28, counselling, application, see p. 632. Potency: potent
Excipients none as listed in section 13.1.3

**Fucibet®** (LEO) PoM
Cream, betamethasone (as valerate) 0.1%, fusidic acid 2%, net price 30 g = £5.40, 60 g = £10.79. Label: 28, counselling, application, see p. 632. Potency: potent
Excipients include cetostearyl alcohol, chlorocresol

Lipid cream, betamethasone (as valerate) 0.1%, fusidic acid 2%, net price 30 g = £5.62. Label: 28, counselling, application, see p. 632. Potency: potent
Excipients include cetostearyl alcohol, hydroxybenzoates (parabens)

**Lotriderm®** (TEVA UK) PoM
Cream, betamethasone dipropionate 0.064% (≡ betamethasone 0.05%), clotrimazole 1%, net price 30 g = £6.34. Label: 28, counselling, application, see p. 632. Potency: potent
Excipients include benzyl alcohol, cetostearyl alcohol, propylene glycol

## ■ CLOBETASOL PROPIONATE

**Indications** short-term treatment only of severe resistant inflammatory skin disorders such as recalcitrant eczemas unresponsive to less potent corticosteroids; psoriasis, see notes above

**Cautions** see notes above

**Contra-indications** see notes above

**Side-effects** see notes above

**Dose**

• Apply thinly 1–2 times daily for up to 4 weeks; max. 50 g of 0.05% preparation per week

**Clarelux®** (Fabre) PoM
Foam (= scalp application), clobetasol propionate 0.05%, net price 100 g = £11.06. Label: 15, 28, counselling, application, see p. 632. Potency: very potent
Excipients include cetyl alcohol, polysorbate 60, propylene glycol, stearyl alcohol
Caution flammable
Note Apply directly to scalp lesions (foam begins to subside immediately on contact with skin)

**Dermovate®** (GSK) PoM
Cream, clobetasol propionate 0.05%, net price 30 g = £2.75, 100 g = £8.06. Label: 28, counselling, application, see p. 632. Potency: very potent
Excipients include beeswax (or beeswax substitute), cetostearyl alcohol, chlorocresol, propylene glycol

Ointment, clobetasol propionate 0.05%, net price 30 g = £2.75, 100 g = £8.06. Label: 28, counselling, application, see p. 632. Potency: very potent
Excipients include propylene glycol

Scalp application, clobetasol propionate 0.05%, in a thickened alcoholic basis, net price 30 mL = £3.13, 100 mL = £10.63. Label: 15, 28, counselling, application, see p. 632. Potency: very potent
Excipients none as listed in section 13.1.3

**Etrivex®** (Galderma) PoM
Shampoo, clobetasol propionate 0.05%, net price 125 mL = £15.43. Label: 28, counselling, application, see p. 632. Potency: very potent
Excipients none as listed in section 13.1.3
Dose moderate scalp psoriasis, ADULT over 18 years, apply thinly once daily, rinse off after 15 minutes; reduce frequency of application after clinical improvement; max. duration of treatment 4 weeks

## ■ CLOBETASONE BUTYRATE

**Indications** eczemas and dermatitis of all types; maintenance between courses of more potent corticosteroids

**Cautions** see notes above

**Contra-indications** see notes above

**Side-effects** see notes above

**Dose**

• Apply thinly 1–2 times daily

**¹Eumovate®** (GSK) PoM
Cream, clobetasone butyrate 0.05%, net price 30 g = £1.89, 100 g = £5.54. Label: 28, counselling, application, see p. 632. Potency: moderate
Excipients include beeswax substitute, cetostearyl alcohol, chlorocresol

Ointment, clobetasone butyrate 0.05%, net price 30 g = £1.89, 100 g = £5.54. Label: 28, counselling, application, see p. 632. Potency: moderate
Excipients none as listed in section 13.1.3

1. Cream can be sold to the public for short-term symptomatic treatment and control of patches of eczema and dermatitis (but not seborrhoeic dermatitis) in adults and children over 12 years provided pack does not contain more than 15 g

## ◢With antimicrobials

See notes above for comment on compound preparations

**Trimovate®** (GSK) PoM
Cream, clobetasone butyrate 0.05%, oxytetracycline 3% (as calcium salt), nystatin 100 000 units/g, net price 30 g = £3.35. Label: 28, counselling, application, see p. 632. Potency: moderate
Excipients include cetostearyl alcohol, chlorocresol, sodium metabisulphite
Note Stains clothing

## ■ DIFLUCORTOLONE VALERATE

**Indications** severe inflammatory skin disorders such as eczemas unresponsive to less potent corticosteroids; high strength (0.3%), short-term treatment of severe exacerbations; psoriasis, see notes above

**Cautions** see notes above

**Contra-indications** see notes above

**Side-effects** see notes above

**Dose**

• Apply thinly 1–2 times daily for up to 4 weeks (0.1% preparations) or 2 weeks (0.3% preparations), reducing strength as condition responds; max. 60 g of 0.3% per week

**Nerisone®** (Meadow) PoM
Cream, diflucortolone valerate 0.1%, net price 30 g = £1.59. Label: 28, counselling, application, see p. 632. Potency: potent
Excipients include disodium edetate, hydroxybenzoates (parabens), stearyl alcohol

Oily cream, diflucortolone valerate 0.1%, net price 30 g = £2.56. Label: 28, counselling, application, see p. 632. Potency: potent
Excipients include beeswax

Ointment, diflucortolone valerate 0.1%, net price 30 g = £1.59. Label: 28, counselling, application, see p. 632. Potency: potent
Excipients none as listed in section 13.1.3

**Nerisone Forte®** (Meadow) [PoM]
Oily cream, diflucortolone valerate 0.3%, net price 15 g = £2.09. Label: 28, counselling, application, see p. 632. Potency: very potent
Excipients include beeswax

Ointment, diflucortolone valerate 0.3%, net price 15 g = £2.09. Label: 28, counselling, application, see p. 632. Potency: very potent
Excipients none as listed in section 13.1.3

## ▌ FLUDROXYCORTIDE
(Flurandrenolone)

**Indications** inflammatory skin disorders such as eczemas

**Cautions** see notes above

**Contra-indications** see notes above

**Side-effects** see notes above

**Dose**
● Apply thinly 1–2 times daily

**Haelan®** (Typharm) [PoM]
Cream, fludroxycortide 0.0125%, net price 60 g = £3.26. Label: 28, counselling, application, see p. 632. Potency: moderate
Excipients include cetyl alcohol, propylene glycol

Ointment, fludroxycortide 0.0125%, net price 60 g = £3.26. Label: 28, counselling, application, see p. 632. Potency: moderate
Excipients include beeswax, cetyl alcohol, polysorbate

Tape, polythene adhesive film impregnated with fludroxycortide 4 micrograms /cm², net price 7.5 cm × 50 cm = £9.27, 7.5 cm × 200 cm = £24.95
Dose for chronic localised recalcitrant dermatoses (but not acute or weeping), cut tape to fit lesion, apply to clean, dry skin shorn of hair, usually for 12 hours daily

## ▌ FLUOCINOLONE ACETONIDE

**Indications** inflammatory skin disorders such as eczemas, psoriasis, see notes above

**Cautions** see notes above

**Contra-indications** see notes above

**Side-effects** see notes above

**Dose**
● Apply thinly 1–2 times daily, reducing strength as condition responds

**Synalar®** (GP Pharma) [PoM]
Cream, fluocinolone acetonide 0.025%, net price 30 g = £3.76, 100 g = £10.68. Label: 28, counselling, application, see p. 632. Potency: potent
Excipients include benzyl alcohol, cetostearyl alcohol, polysorbates, propylene glycol

Gel, fluocinolone acetonide 0.025%, net price 30 g = £5.56, 60 g = £10.02. For use on scalp and other hairy areas. Label: 28, counselling, application, see p. 632. Potency: potent
Excipients include hydroxybenzoates (parabens), propylene glycol

Ointment, fluocinolone acetonide 0.025%, net price 30 g = £3.76, 100 g = £10.68. Label: 28, counselling, application, see p. 632. Potency: potent
Excipients include propylene glycol, wool fat

**Synalar 1 in 4 Dilution®** (GP Pharma) [PoM]
Cream, fluocinolone acetonide 0.00625%, net price 50 g = £4.40. Label: 28, counselling, application, see p. 632. Potency: moderate
Excipients include benzyl alcohol, cetostearyl alcohol, polysorbates, propylene glycol

Ointment, fluocinolone acetonide 0.00625%, net price 50 g = £4.40. Label: 28, counselling, application, see p. 632. Potency: moderate
Excipients include propylene glycol, wool fat

**Synalar 1 in 10 Dilution®** (GP Pharma) [PoM]
Cream, fluocinolone acetonide 0.0025%, net price 50 g = £4.16. Label: 28, counselling, application, see p. 632. Potency: mild
Excipients include benzyl alcohol, cetostearyl alcohol, polysorbates, propylene glycol

◢With antibacterials
See notes above for comment on compound preparations

**Synalar C®** (GP Pharma) [PoM]
Cream, fluocinolone acetonide 0.025%, clioquinol 3%, net price 15 g = £2.42. Label: 28, counselling, application, see p. 632. Potency: potent
Excipients include cetostearyl alcohol, disodium edetate, hydroxybenzoates (parabens), polysorbates, propylene glycol

Ointment, fluocinolone acetonide 0.025%, clioquinol 3%, net price 15 g = £2.42. Label: 28, counselling, application, see p. 632. Potency: potent.
Note stains clothing
Excipients include propylene glycol, wool fat

**Synalar N®** (GP Pharma) [PoM]
Cream, fluocinolone acetonide 0.025%, neomycin sulphate 0.5%, net price 30 g = £3.96. Label: 28, counselling, application, see p. 632. Potency: potent
Excipients include cetostearyl alcohol, hydroxybenzoates (parabens), polysorbates, propylene glycol

Ointment, fluocinolone acetonide 0.025%, neomycin sulphate 0.5%, in a greasy basis, net price 30 g = £3.96. Label: 28, counselling, application, see p. 632. Potency: potent
Excipients include propylene glycol, wool fat

## ▌ FLUOCINONIDE

**Indications** severe inflammatory skin disorders such as eczemas unresponsive to less potent corticosteroids; psoriasis, see notes above

**Cautions** see notes above

**Contra-indications** see notes above

**Side-effects** see notes above

**Dose**
● Apply thinly 1–2 times daily

**Metosyn®** (GP Pharma) [PoM]
FAPG cream, fluocinonide 0.05%, net price 25 g = £3.30, 100 g = £11.12. Label: 28, counselling, application, see p. 632. Potency: potent
Excipients include propylene glycol

Ointment, fluocinonide 0.05%, net price 25 g = £2.92, 100 g = £10.96. Label: 28, counselling, application, see p. 632. Potency: potent
Excipients include propylene glycol, wool fat

## ▌ FLUOCORTOLONE

**Indications** severe inflammatory skin disorders such as eczemas unresponsive to less potent corticosteroids; psoriasis, see notes above

**Cautions** see notes above

**13 Skin**

**Contra-indications** see notes above

**Side-effects** see notes above

**Dose**

- Apply thinly 1–2 times daily, reducing strength as condition responds

**Ultralanum Plain®** (Meadow) ⟨PoM⟩

Cream, fluocortolone caproate 0.25%, fluocortolone pivalate 0.25%, net price 50 g = £2.95. Label: 28, counselling, application, see p. 632. Potency: moderate

Excipients include disodium edetate, fragrance, hydroxybenzoates (parabens), stearyl alcohol

Ointment, fluocortolone 0.25%, fluocortolone caproate 0.25%, net price 50 g = £2.95. Label: 28, counselling, application, see p. 632. Potency: moderate

Excipients include wool fat, fragrance

## ■ FLUTICASONE PROPIONATE

**Indications** inflammatory skin disorders such as dermatitis and eczemas unresponsive to less potent corticosteroids

**Cautions** see notes above

**Contra-indications** see notes above

**Side-effects** see notes above

**Dose**

- Apply thinly 1–2 times daily

**Cutivate®** (GSK) ⟨PoM⟩

Cream, fluticasone propionate 0.05%, net price 15 g = £2.32, 30 g = £4.50. Label: 28, counselling, application, see p. 632. Potency: potent

Excipients include cetostearyl alcohol, imidurea, propylene glycol

Ointment, fluticasone propionate 0.005%, net price 15 g = £2.32, 30 g = £4.50. Label: 28, counselling, application, see p. 632. Potency: potent

Excipients include propylene glycol

## ■ MOMETASONE FUROATE

**Indications** severe inflammatory skin disorders such as eczemas unresponsive to less potent corticosteroids; psoriasis, see notes above

**Cautions** see notes above

**Contra-indications** see notes above

**Side-effects** see notes above

**Dose**

- Apply thinly once daily (to scalp in case of lotion)

**Elocon®** (Schering-Plough) ⟨PoM⟩

Cream, mometasone furoate 0.1%, net price 30 g = £4.45, 100 g = £12.82. Label: 28, counselling, application, see p. 632. Potency: potent

Excipients include propylene glycol, stearyl alcohol

Ointment, mometasone furoate 0.1%, net price 30 g = £4.45, 100 g = £12.82. Label: 28, counselling, application, see p. 632. Potency: potent

Excipients include propylene glycol

Scalp lotion, mometasone furoate 0.1% in an aqueous isopropyl alcohol basis, net price 30 mL = £4.45. Label: 28, counselling, application, see p. 632. Potency: potent

Excipients include propylene glycol

## ■ TRIAMCINOLONE ACETONIDE

**Indications** severe inflammatory skin disorders such as eczemas unresponsive to less potent corticosteroids; psoriasis, see notes above

**Cautions** see notes above

**Contra-indications** see notes above

**Side-effects** see notes above

**Dose**

- Apply thinly 1–2 times daily

**◢With antimicrobials**

See notes above for comment on compound preparations

**Aureocort®** (Goldshield) ⟨PoM⟩

Ointment, triamcinolone acetonide 0.1%, chlortetracycline hydrochloride 3%, in an anhydrous greasy basis containing wool fat and white soft paraffin, net price 15 g = £2.70. Label: 28, counselling, application, see p. 632. Potency: potent

Excipients include wool fat

Note Stains clothing

## 13.5 Preparations for eczema and psoriasis

13.5.1 Preparations for eczema

13.5.2 Preparations for psoriasis

13.5.3 Drugs affecting the immune response

## 13.5.1 Preparations for eczema

Eczema (dermatitis) has several causes, which may influence treatment. The main types of eczema are irritant, allergic contact, atopic, venous and discoid; different types may co-exist. Lichenification, due to scratching and rubbing, may complicate any chronic eczema. *Atopic eczema* is the most common type and it usually involves dry skin as well as infection and lichenification.

Management of eczema involves the removal or treatment of contributory factors including occupational and domestic irritants. Known or suspected contact allergens should be avoided. Rarely, ingredients in topical medicinal products may sensitise the skin; the BNF lists active ingredients together with excipients that have been associated with skin sensitisation.

Skin dryness and the consequent irritant eczema requires **emollients** (section 13.2.1) applied regularly and liberally to the affected area; this can be supplemented with bath or shower emollients. The use of emollients should continue even if the eczema improves or if other treatment is being used.

**Topical corticosteroids** (section 13.4) are also required in the management of eczema; the potency of the corticosteroid should be appropriate to the severity and site of the condition. Mild corticosteroids are generally used on the face and on flexures; potent corticosteroids are generally required for use on adults with discoid or lichenified eczema or with eczema on the scalp, limbs, and trunk. Treatment should be reviewed regularly, especially if a potent corticosteroid is required. Bandages (including those containing **zinc** and **ichthammol**) are sometimes applied over topical corticosteroids or emollients to treat eczema of the limbs.

**13** Skin

For the role of topical **pimecrolimus** and **tacrolimus** in atopic eczema see section 13.5.3.

**Infection** Bacterial infection (commonly with *Staphylococcus aureus* and occasionally with *Streptococcus pyogenes*) can exacerbate eczema and requires treatment with topical or systemic **antibacterial drugs** (section 13.10.1 and section 5.1). Antibacterial drugs, particularly fusidic acid, should be used in short courses (typically 1 week) to reduce the risk of drug resistance or skin sensitisation. Associated eczema is treated simultaneously with a topical corticosteroid usually of moderate or high potency.

Eczema involving widespread or recurrent infection requires the use of a systemic antibacterial that is active against the infecting organism. Products that combine an antiseptic with an emollient application (section 13.2.1) and with a bath emollient (section 13.2.1.1) can also be used; antiseptic shampoos (section 13.9) can be used on the scalp.

Intertriginous eczema commonly involves candida and bacteria; it is best treated with a mild or moderately potent topical corticosteroid and a suitable antimicrobial drug.

Widespread herpes simplex infection may complicate atopic eczema and treatment with a systemic antiviral drug (section 5.3.2.1) is indicated.

The management of *seborrhoeic dermatitis* is described below.

**Management of other features of eczema** *Lichenification*, which results from repeated scratching is treated initially with a potent corticosteroid. Bandages containing **ichthammol paste** (to reduce pruritus) and other substances such as **zinc oxide** can be applied over the corticosteroid or emollient. **Coal tar** (section 13.5.2) and **ichthammol** can be useful in some cases of *chronic eczema*.

A *non-sedating* **antihistamine** (section 3.4.1) may be of some value in relieving severe itching or urticaria associated with eczema. A *sedating* antihistamine (section 3.4.1) can be used if itching causes sleep disturbance.

*Exudative ('weeping') eczema* requires a potent corticosteroid initially; infection may also be present and require specific treatment (see above). **Potassium permanganate** solution (1 in 10 000) can be used in exudating eczema for its antiseptic and astringent effects; treatment should be stopped when exudation stops.

**Severe refractory eczema** *Severe refractory eczema* is best managed under specialist supervision; it may require phototherapy or drugs that act on the immune system (section 13.5.3). **Alitretinoin** (see below) is licensed for the treatment of severe chronic hand eczema refractory to potent topical corticosteroids; patients with hyperkeratotic features are more likely to respond to alitretinoin than those with pompholyx.

**Seborrhoeic dermatitis** *Seborrhoeic dermatitis* (*seborrhoeic eczema*) is associated with species of the yeast *Malassezia* and affects the scalp, paranasal areas, and eyebrows. Shampoos active against the yeast (including those containing ketoconazole and coal tar, section 13.9) and combinations of mild corticosteroids with suitable antimicrobials (section 13.4) are used.

## Topical preparations for eczema

### ICHTHAMMOL

**Indications** chronic lichenified eczema
**Side-effects** skin irritation
**Dose**
• Apply 1–3 times daily

**Ichthammol Ointment, BP 1980**
Ointment, ichthammol 10%, yellow soft paraffin 45%, wool fat 45%

**Zinc and Ichthammol Cream, BP**
Cream, ichthammol 5%, cetostearyl alcohol 3%, wool fat 10%, in zinc cream

**Zinc Paste and Ichthammol Bandage, BP 1993**
See Appendix 8 (section A8.2.9)

## Oral retinoid for eczema

The retinoid, **alitretinoin**, is licensed for the treatment of severe chronic hand eczema refractory to potent topical corticosteroids; patients with hyperkeratotic features are more likely to respond to alitretinoin than those with pompholyx.

Alitretinoin should be prescribed **only** by, or under the supervision of, a consultant dermatologist.

Alitretinoin is **teratogenic** and must **not** be given to women of child-bearing potential unless they practise effective contraception and then only after detailed assessment and explanation by the physician. See also Pregnancy Prevention under Cautions, below.

### ALITRETINOIN

**Indications** severe chronic hand eczema refractory to potent topical corticosteroids
**Cautions** avoid blood donation during treatment and for at least 1 month after stopping treatment; monitor serum lipids (more frequently in those with diabetes, history of hyperlipidaemia, or risk factors for cardiovascular disease)—discontinue if uncontrolled hyperlipidaemia; history of depression; dry eye syndrome; **interactions:** Appendix 1 (retinoids)
**Pregnancy prevention** In women of child-bearing potential, exclude pregnancy 1 month before treatment, up to 5 days before treatment, every month during treatment (unless there are compelling reasons to indicate that there is no risk of pregnancy), and 5 weeks after stopping treatment—perform pregnancy test in the first 3 days of the menstrual cycle. Women must practise effective contraception for at least 1 month before starting treatment, during treatment, and for at least 1 month after stopping treatment. Women should be advised to use at least 1 method of contraception but ideally they should use 2 methods of contraception. Oral progestogen-only contraceptives are not considered effective. Barrier methods should not be used alone but can be used in conjunction with other contraceptive methods. Each prescription for alitretinoin should be limited to a supply of up to 30 days' treatment and dispensed within 7 days of the date stated on the prescription. Women should be advised to discontinue treatment and to seek prompt medical attention if they become pregnant during treatment or within 1 month of stopping treatment
**Contra-indications** hepatic impairment; severe renal impairment (Appendix 3); uncontrolled hyperlipidaemia; uncontrolled hypothyroidism; hypervitaminosis A; pregnancy (**important teratogenic risk:** see Pregnancy Prevention, above); breast-feeding

**Side-effects**  raised serum concentration of tri-glycerides and of cholesterol (risk of pancreatitis if triglycerides above 9 mmol/litre), flushing; headache; changes in thyroid function tests; anaemia; myalgia, raised creatine kinase, arthralgia; conjunctivitis, dry eyes (may respond to lubricating eye ointment or tear replacement therapy)—sometimes decreased toler-ance to contact lenses, eye irritation; dryness of skin and lips, cheilitis, erythema, alopecia; *less commonly* epistaxis, hyperostosis, ankylosing spondylitis, blurred vision, cataracts, pruritus, and asteototic eczema; *rarely* benign intracranial hypertension (dis-continue if severe headache, nausea, vomiting, papill-oedema, or visual disturbances occur) and vasculitis; also reported keratitis and impaired night vision

**Dose**

- ADULT over 18 years, 30 mg once daily, reduced to 10 mg once daily if not tolerated; patients with dia-betes, history of hyperlipidaemia, or risk factors for cardiovascular disease, initially 10 mg once daily, increased if necessary up to max. 30 mg daily

  Note Duration of treatment 12–24 weeks; discontinue if no response after 12 weeks. Course may be repeated in those who relapse. See also Pregnancy Prevention, above

**Toctino®** (Basilea) ▼ PoM

Capsules, alitretinoin 10 mg (brown), net price 30-cap pack = £411.43; 30 mg (red-brown), 30-cap pack = £411.43. Label: 10, patient information leaflet, 11, 21

## 13.5.2  Preparations for psoriasis

Psoriasis is characterised by epidermal thickening and scaling. It commonly affects extensor surfaces and the scalp. For mild psoriasis, reassurance and treatment with an emollient may be all that is necessary.

Occasionally psoriasis is provoked or exacerbated by drugs such as lithium, chloroquine and hydroxychloro-quine, beta-blockers, non-steroidal anti-inflammatory drugs, and ACE inhibitors. Psoriasis may not be seen until the drug has been taken for weeks or months.

**Emollients** (section 13.2.1), in addition to their effects on dryness, scaling and cracking, may have an anti-proliferative effect in psoriasis. They are particularly useful in *inflammatory psoriasis* and in *plaque psoriasis of palms and soles*, in which irritant factors can perpe-tuate the condition. Emollients are useful adjuncts to other more specific treatment.

More specific topical treatment for *chronic stable plaque psoriasis* on extensor surfaces of trunk and limbs involves the use of **vitamin D analogues**, **coal tar**, **dithranol**, and the retinoid **tazarotene**. However, they can irritate the skin and they are not suitable for the more inflammatory forms of psoriasis; their use should be suspended during an inflammatory phase of psor-iasis. The efficacy and the irritancy of each substance varies between patients. If a substance irritates signifi-cantly, it should be stopped or the concentration reduced; if it is tolerated, its effects should be assessed after 4 to 6 weeks and treatment continued if it is effective.

Widespread *unstable psoriasis* of erythrodermic or gen-eralised pustular type requires urgent specialist assess-ment. Initial topical treatment should be limited to using emollients frequently and generously; emollients should be prescribed in quantities of 1 kg or more. More loca-lised acute or subacute *inflammatory psoriasis* with hot, spreading or itchy lesions, should be treated topically with emollients or with a corticosteroid of moderate potency.

**Calcipotriol** and **tacalcitol** are analogues of vitamin D that affect cell division and differentiation. **Calcitriol** is an active form of vitamin D. Vitamin D and its analogues are used as first-line treatment for plaque psoriasis; they do not smell or stain and they may be more acceptable than tar or dithranol products. Of the vitamin D analo-gues, tacalcitol and calcitriol are less likely to irritate.

**Coal tar** has anti-inflammatory properties that are use-ful in chronic plaque psoriasis; it also has antiscaling properties. Crude coal tar (coal tar, BP) is the most effective form, typically in a concentration of 1 to 10% in a soft paraffin base, but few outpatients tolerate the smell and mess. Cleaner extracts of coal tar included in proprietary preparations, are more practicable for home use but they are less effective and improvement takes longer. Contact of coal tar products with normal skin is not normally harmful and they can be used for wide-spread small lesions; however, irritation, contact allergy, and sterile folliculitis can occur. The milder tar extracts can be used on the face and flexures. Tar baths and tar shampoos are also helpful.

**Dithranol** is effective for chronic plaque psoriasis. Its major disadvantages are irritation (for which individual susceptibility varies) and staining of skin and of clothing. It should be applied to chronic extensor plaques only, carefully avoiding normal skin. Dithranol is not gener-ally suitable for widespread small lesions nor should it be used in the flexures or on the face. Treatment should be started with a low concentration such as dithranol 0.1%, and the strength increased gradually every few days up to 3%, according to tolerance. Proprietary preparations are more suitable for home use; they are usually washed off after 5 to 60 minutes ('short con-tact'). Specialist nurses may apply intensive treatment with dithranol paste which is covered by stockinette dressings and usually retained overnight. Dithranol should be discontinued if even a low concentration causes acute inflammation; continued use can result in the psoriasis becoming unstable. When applying dith-ranol, hands should be protected by gloves or they should be washed thoroughly afterwards.

**Tazarotene**, a retinoid, seems to be less effective than calcipotriol with a greater incidence of irritation. Although irritation is common, it is minimised by apply-ing tazarotene sparingly to the plaques and avoiding normal skin. Tazarotene is clean and odourless.

A topical **corticosteroid** (section 13.4) is not generally suitable as the sole treatment of extensive chronic plaque psoriasis; any early improvement is not usually maintained and there is a risk of the condition deterior-ating or of precipitating an unstable form of psoriasis (e.g. erythrodermic psoriasis or generalised pustular psoriasis). However, it may be appropriate to treat psor-iasis in specific sites, such as the face and flexures, usually with a mild corticosteroid, and psoriasis of the scalp, palms, and soles with a potent corticosteroid.

Combining the use of a corticosteroid with another specific topical treatment may be beneficial in chronic plaque psoriasis; the drugs may be used separately at different times of the day or used together in a single

**13**

**Skin**

formulation. *Eczema* co-existing with psoriasis may be treated with a corticosteroid, or coal tar, or both.

*Scalp psoriasis* is usually scaly, and the scale may be thick and adherent. This requires softening with an emollient ointment, cream, or oil and usually combined with **salicylic acid** as a keratolytic.

Some preparations prescribed for psoriasis affecting the scalp combine salicylic acid with coal tar or **sulphur**. Preparations containing salicylic acid, sulphur, and coal tar are available as proprietary products. The product should be applied generously and an adequate quantity should be prescribed. It should be left on for at least an hour, often more conveniently overnight, before washing it off. If a corticosteroid lotion or gel is required (e.g. for itch), it can be used in the morning.

**Phototherapy** Phototherapy is available in specialist centres under the supervision of a dermatologist. **Ultra-violet B** (UVB) radiation is usually effective for *chronic stable psoriasis* and for *guttate psoriasis*. It may be considered for patients with moderately severe psoriasis in whom topical treatment has failed, but it may irritate inflammatory psoriasis.

**Photochemotherapy** combining long-wave ultraviolet A radiation with a psoralen (PUVA) is available in specialist centres under the supervision of a dermatologist. The psoralen, which enhances the effect of irradiation, is administered either by mouth or topically. PUVA is effective in most forms of psoriasis, including *localised palmoplantar pustular psoriasis*. Early adverse effects include phototoxicity and pruritus. Higher cumulative doses exaggerate skin ageing, increase the risk of dysplastic and neoplastic skin lesions, especially squamous cancer, and pose a theoretical risk of cataracts.

Phototherapy combined with coal tar, dithranol, tazarotene, topical vitamin D or vitamin D analogues, or oral acitretin, allows reduction of the cumulative dose of phototherapy required to treat psoriasis.

**Systemic treatment** Systemic treatment is required for severe, resistant, unstable or complicated forms of psoriasis, and it should be initiated only under specialist supervision. Systemic drugs for psoriasis include acitretin (see below) and drugs that affect the immune response (such as ciclosporin and methotrexate, section 13.5.3).

Systemic corticosteroids should be used only rarely in psoriasis because rebound deterioration may occur on reducing the dose.

**Acitretin**, a metabolite of etretinate, is a retinoid (vitamin A derivative); it is prescribed by specialists. The main indication for acitretin is *psoriasis*, but it is also used in disorders of keratinisation such as severe *Darier's disease* (keratosis follicularis), and some forms of *ichthyosis*. Although a minority of cases of psoriasis respond well to acitretin alone, it is only moderately effective in many cases and it is combined with other treatments. A therapeutic effect occurs after 2 to 4 weeks and the maximum benefit after 4 to 6 weeks or longer. The manufacturers of acitretin do not recommend continuous treatment for longer than 6 months. However, some patients may benefit from longer treatment, provided that the lowest effective dose is used, patients are monitored carefully for adverse effects, and the need for treatment is reviewed regularly.

Apart from teratogenicity, which remains a risk for 3 years after stopping, acitretin is the least toxic systemic treatment for psoriasis; in women with a potential for child-bearing, the possibility of pregnancy must be excluded before treatment and effective contraception must be used during treatment and for at least 3 years afterwards (oral progestogen-only contraceptives not considered effective). Common side-effects derive from its widespread but reversible effects on epithelia, such as dry and cracking lips, dry skin and mucosal surfaces, hair thinning, paronychia, and soft and sticky palms and soles. Liver function and blood lipid concentration should be monitored.

# Topical preparations for psoriasis

## Vitamin D and analogues

**Calcipotriol, calcitriol,** and **tacalcitol** are used for the management of *plaque psoriasis*. They should be avoided by those with calcium metabolism disorders, and used with caution in *generalised pustular* or *erythrodermic exfoliative psoriasis* (enhanced risk of hypercalcaemia). Local skin reactions (itching, erythema, burning, paraesthesia, dermatitis) are common. Hands should be washed thoroughly after application to avoid inadvertent transfer to other body areas. Aggravation of psoriasis has also been reported.

## ▌ CALCIPOTRIOL

**Indications** plaque psoriasis

**Cautions** see notes above; avoid use on face; avoid excessive exposure to sunlight and sunlamps; pregnancy (Appendix 4); breast-feeding (Appendix 5)

**Contra-indications** see notes above

**Side-effects** see notes above; also photosensitivity; rarely facial or perioral dermatitis, skin atrophy

**Dose**

- *Cream* or *ointment* apply once or twice daily; max. 100 g weekly (less with *scalp solution*, see below); CHILD over 6 years, apply twice daily; 6–12 years max. 50 g weekly; over 12 years max. 75 g weekly
  Note Patient information leaflet for *Dovonex®* cream advises liberal application (but note max. recommended weekly dose, above)

**Calcipotriol** (Non-proprietary) PoM
  Ointment, calcipotriol 50 micrograms/g, net price 120 g = £24.65
  Note Not licensed for use in children under 18 years

**Dovonex®** (LEO) PoM
  Cream, calcipotriol 50 micrograms/g, net price 60 g = £11.55, 120 g = £23.10
  Excipients include cetostearyl alcohol, disodium edetate

  Scalp solution, calcipotriol 50 micrograms/mL, net price 60 mL = £12.53, 120 mL = £26.07
  Excipients include propylene glycol

  Dose scalp psoriasis, apply to scalp twice daily; max. 60 mL weekly (less with cream or ointment, see below); CHILD under 18 years, see *BNF for Children*
  Note When preparations used together max. total calcipotriol 5 mg in any one week (e.g. scalp solution 60 mL with cream or ointment 30 g *or* cream or ointment 60 g with scalp solution 30 mL)

**13 Skin**

◀With betamethasone
For cautions, contra-indications, side-effects, and for comment on the limited role of corticosteroids in psoriasis, see section 13.4.

**Dovobet®** (LEO) PoM
Ointment, betamethasone 0.05% (as dipropionate), calcipotriol 50 micrograms/g, net price 60 g = £33.63, 120 g = £62.46. Label: 28
Excipients none as listed in section 13.1.3
Dose initial treatment of stable plaque psoriasis, apply once daily to max. 30% of body surface (max. 15 g daily, max. 100 g weekly) for 4 weeks; if necessary, subsequent courses repeated after an interval of at least 4 weeks; CHILD under 18 years see *BNF for Children*
Note When different preparations containing calcipotriol used together, max. total calcipotriol 5 mg in any one week

**Xamiol®** (LEO) PoM
Scalp gel, betamethasone 0.05% (as dipropionate), calcipotriol 50 micrograms/g, net price 60 g = £36.50. Label: 28
Excipients include butylated hydroxytoluene
Dose scalp psoriasis, ADULT over 18 years, apply 1–4 g to scalp once daily, shampoo off after leaving on scalp overnight or during day; usual duration of therapy, 4 weeks
Note When different preparations containing calcipotriol used together, max. total calcipotriol 5 mg in any one week

## ■ CALCITRIOL
**(1,25-Dihydroxycholecalciferol)**

**Indications** mild to moderate plaque psoriasis
**Cautions** see notes above; liver impairment (Appendix 2); pregnancy (Appendix 4)
**Contra-indications** see notes above; do not apply under occlusion; renal impairment (Appendix 3); breast-feeding (Appendix 5)
**Side-effects** see notes above
**Dose**
● ADULT and CHILD over 12 years, apply twice daily; not more than 35% of body surface to be treated daily, max. 30 g daily

**Silkis®** (Galderma) PoM
Ointment, calcitriol 3 micrograms/g, net price 100 g = £13.87
Excipients none as listed in section 13.1.3

## ■ TACALCITOL

**Indications** plaque psoriasis
**Cautions** see notes above; pregnancy (Appendix 4), breast-feeding (Appendix 5); avoid eyes; monitor plasma calcium if risk of hypercalcaemia or in renal impairment; if used in conjunction with UV treatment, UV radiation should be given in the morning and tacalcitol applied at bedtime
**Contra-indications** see notes above
**Side-effects** see notes above
**Dose**
● ADULT and CHILD over 12 years, apply once daily preferably at bedtime; max. 10 g *ointment* or 10 mL *lotion* daily
Note When lotion and ointment used together, max. total tacalcitol 280 micrograms in any one week (e.g. lotion 30 mL with ointment 40 g)

**Curatoderm®** (Almirall) PoM
Lotion, tacalcitol (as monohydrate) 4 micrograms/g, net price 30 mL = £12.73
Excipients include disodium edetate, propylene glycol

Ointment, tacalcitol (as monohydrate) 4 micrograms/ g, net price 30 g = £13.40, 60 g = £23.14, 100 g = £30.86
Excipients none as listed in section 13.1.3

**Tazarotene**

## ■ TAZAROTENE

**Indications** mild to moderate plaque psoriasis affecting up to 10% of skin area
**Cautions** wash hands immediately after use, avoid contact with eyes, face, intertriginous areas, hair-covered scalp, eczematous or inflamed skin; avoid excessive exposure to UV light (including sunlight, solariums, PUVA or UVB treatment); do not apply emollients or cosmetics within 1 hour of application
**Contra-indications** pregnancy—women of child-bearing potential must use effective contraception (Appendix 4); breast-feeding (Appendix 5)
**Side-effects** local irritation (more common with higher concentration and may require discontinuation), pruritus, burning, erythema, desquamation, non-specific rash, contact dermatitis, and worsening of psoriasis; rarely stinging and inflamed, dry or painful skin
**Dose**
● Apply once daily in the evening usually for up to 12 weeks; CHILD under 18 years not recommended

**Zorac®** (Allergan) PoM
Gel, tazarotene 0.05%, net price 30 g = £14.09; 0.1%, 30 g = £14.80
Excipients include benzyl alcohol, butylated hydroxyanisole, butylated hydroxytoluene, disodium edetate, polysorbate 40

**Tars**

## ■ TARS

**Indications** psoriasis and occasionally chronic atopic eczema
**Cautions** avoid eyes, mucosa, genital or rectal areas, and broken or inflamed skin; use suitable chemical protection gloves for extemporaneous preparation
**Contra-indications** not for use in sore, acute, or pustular psoriasis or in presence of infection
**Side-effects** skin irritation and acne-like eruptions, photosensitivity; stains skin, hair, and fabric
**Dose**
● Apply 1–3 times daily starting with low-strength preparations
Note For shampoo preparations see section 13.9; impregnated dressings see Appendix 8 (section A8.2.9)

◀Non-proprietary preparations
May be difficult to obtain. Patients may find newer proprietary preparations more acceptable

**Calamine and Coal Tar Ointment, BP**
Ointment, calamine 12.5 g, strong coal tar solution 2.5 g, zinc oxide 12.5 g, hydrous wool fat 25 g, white soft paraffin 47.5 g
Excipients include wool fat
Dose apply 1–2 times daily

**Coal Tar and Salicylic Acid Ointment, BP**
Ointment, coal tar 2 g, salicylic acid 2 g, emulsifying wax 11.4 g, white soft paraffin 19 g, coconut oil 54 g, polysorbate '80' 4 g, liquid paraffin 7.6 g
Excipients include cetostearyl alcohol
Dose apply 1–2 times daily

## Coal Tar Paste, BP

Paste, strong coal tar solution 7.5%, in compound zinc paste
Dose apply 1–2 times daily

## Zinc and Coal Tar Paste, BP

Paste, zinc oxide 6%, coal tar 6%, emulsifying wax 5%, starch 38%, yellow soft paraffin 45%
Excipients include cetostearyl alcohol
Dose apply 1–2 times daily

### ◢Proprietary preparations

**Carbo-Dome®** (Sandoz)
Cream, coal tar solution 10%, in a water-miscible basis, net price 30 g = £4.77, 100 g = £16.38
Excipients include beeswax, hydroxybenzoates (parabens)
Dose psoriasis, apply to skin 2–3 times daily

**Clinitar®** (CHS)
Cream, coal tar extract 1%, net price 100 g = £10.99
Excipients include cetostearyl alcohol, isopropyl palmitate, propylene glycol
Dose psoriasis and eczema, apply to skin 1–2 times daily

**Cocois®** (UCB Pharma)
Scalp ointment, coal tar solution 12%, salicylic acid 2%, precipitated sulphur 4%, in a coconut oil emollient basis, net price 40 g (with applicator nozzle) = £5.98, 100 g = £11.23
Excipients include cetostearyl alcohol
Dose scaly scalp disorders including psoriasis, eczema, seborrhoeic dermatitis and dandruff, apply to scalp once weekly as necessary (if severe use daily for first 3–7 days), shampoo off after 1 hour; CHILD 6–12 years, medical supervision required (not recommended under 6 years)

**Exorex®** (Forest)
Lotion, prepared coal tar 1% in an emollient basis, net price 100 mL = £8.11, 250 mL = £16.24
Excipients include hydroxybenzoates (parabens), polysorbate 80
Dose psoriasis, apply to skin or scalp 2–3 times daily; CHILD under 12 years and ELDERLY, lotion can be diluted with a few drops of water before applying

**Psoriderm®** (Dermal)
Cream, coal tar 6%, lecithin 0.4%, net price 225 mL = £9.57
Excipients include isopropyl palmitate, propylene glycol
Dose psoriasis, apply to skin or scalp 1–2 times daily

Scalp lotion—section 13.9

**Sebco®** (Centrapharm)
Scalp ointment, coal tar solution 12%, salicylic acid 2%, precipitated sulphur 4%, in a coconut oil emollient basis, net price 40 g = £4.54, 100 g = £8.52
Excipients include cetostearyl alcohol
Dose scaly scalp disorders including psoriasis, eczema, seborrhoeic dermatitis and dandruff, apply to scalp as necessary (if severe use daily for first 3–7 days), shampoo off after 1 hour; CHILD 6–12 years, medical supervision required (not recommended under 6 years)

### ◢Bath preparations

**Coal Tar Solution, BP**
Solution, coal tar 20%, polysorbate '80' 5%, in alcohol (96%), net price 500 mL = £7.25
Excipients include polysorbates
Dose use 100 mL in a bath
Note Strong Coal Tar Solution BP contains coal tar 40%

**Pinetarsol®** (Crawford)
Bath oil, tar 2.3% in a light liquid paraffin basis, net price 200 mL = £4.75, 500 mL = £7.95
Excipients include fragrance
Dose eczema and psoriasis, use 15–30 mL in a bath or apply directly to wet skin and rinse after a few minutes; can be used as soap substitute

Gel, tar 1.6%, net price 100 g = £4.95
Dose eczema and psoriasis, apply directly to wet skin and rinse after a few minutes; can be used as soap substitute

Solution, tar 2.3%, net price 200 mL = £4.45, 500 mL = £7.45
Dose eczema and psoriasis, use 15–30 mL in a bath or dilute 15 mL with 3 litres of water and apply to affected areas or apply solution directly to wet skin and rinse after a few minutes; can be used as soap substitute

**Polytar Emollient®** (Stiefel)
Bath additive, coal tar solution 2.5%, arachis (peanut) oil extract of coal tar 7.5%, tar 7.5%, cade oil 7.5%, liquid paraffin 35%, net price 500 mL = £5.78
Excipients include isopropyl palmitate
Dose psoriasis, eczema, atopic and pruritic dermatoses, use 2–4 capfuls (15–30 mL) in bath and soak for 20 minutes

**Psoriderm®** (Dermal)
Bath emulsion, coal tar 40%, net price 200 mL = £2.79
Excipients include polysorbate 20
Dose psoriasis, use 30 mL in a bath and soak for 5 minutes

### ◢With corticosteroids

**Alphosyl HC®** (GSK Consumer Healthcare) [PoM]
Cream, alcoholic coal tar extract 5%, hydrocortisone 0.5%, allantoin 2%, net price 100 g = £3.16. Label: 28. Potency: mild
Excipients include beeswax, cetyl alcohol, hydroxybenzoates (parabens), isopropyl palmitate, wool fat
Dose ADULT and CHILD over 5 years, psoriasis, apply thinly twice daily

## Dithranol

---

### ▌DITHRANOL
### (Anthralin)

**Indications** subacute and chronic psoriasis, see notes above

**Cautions** avoid use near eyes and sensitive areas of skin; see also notes above

**Contra-indications** hypersensitivity; acute and pustular psoriasis

**Side-effects** local burning sensation and irritation; stains skin, hair, and fabrics

**Dose**

- See notes above and under preparations
Note Some of these dithranol preparations also contain coal tar or salicylic acid—for cautions, contra-indications, and side-effects see under Tars (above) or under Salicylic Acid

### ◢Non-proprietary preparations

**¹Dithranol Ointment, BP** [PoM]
Ointment, dithranol, in yellow soft paraffin; usual strengths 0.1–2%. Part of basis may be replaced by hard paraffin if a stiffer preparation is required. Label: 28

1. [PoM] if dithranol content more than 1%, otherwise may be sold to the public

**Dithranol Paste, BP**
Paste, dithranol in zinc and salicylic acid (Lassar's) paste. Usual strengths 0.1–1% of dithranol. Label: 28

### ◢Proprietary preparations

**Dithrocream®** (Dermal)
Cream, dithranol 0.1%, net price 50 g = £3.83; 0.25%, 50 g = £4.10; 0.5%, 50 g = £4.73; 1%, 50 g = £5.51; [PoM] 2%, 50 g = £6.89. Label: 28
Excipients include cetostearyl alcohol, chlorocresol
Dose for application to skin or scalp; 0.1–0.5% cream suitable for overnight treatment, 1–2% cream for max. 1 hour

**Micanol®** (GP Pharma)

Cream, dithranol 1% in a lipid-stabilised basis, net price 50 g = £13.48; PoM 3%, 50 g = £16.79. Label: 28

Excipients none as listed in section 13.1.3

**Dose** for application to skin or scalp, apply 1% cream for up to 30 minutes once daily, if necessary 3% cream can be used under medical supervision

**Note** At the end of contact time, use plenty of lukewarm (not hot) water to rinse off cream; soap may be used *after* the cream has been rinsed off; use shampoo before applying cream to scalp and if necessary after cream has been rinsed off

**Psorin®** (LPC)

Ointment, dithranol 0.11%, coal tar 1%, salicylic acid 1.6%, net price 50 g = £9.22, 100 g = £18.44. Label: 28

Excipients include beeswax, wool fat

**Dose** for application to skin up to twice daily

Scalp gel, dithranol 0.25%, salicylic acid 1.6% in gel basis containing methyl salicylate, net price 50 g = £7.03. Label: 28

Excipients none as listed in section 13.1.3

**Dose** for application to scalp, initially apply on alternate days for 10–20 minutes; may be increased to daily application for max. 1 hour and then wash off

## Salicylic acid

### ▌ SALICYLIC ACID

For coal tar preparations containing salicylic acid, see under Tars, p. 641; for dithranol preparations containing salicylic acid see under Dithranol, p. 642

**Indications** hyperkeratotic skin disorders; acne (section 13.6.1); warts and calluses (section 13.7); scalp conditions (section 13.9); fungal nail infections (section 13.10.2)

**Cautions** see notes above; avoid broken or inflamed skin

**Salicylate toxicity** If large areas of skin are treated, salicylate toxicity may occur

**Side-effects** sensitivity, excessive drying, irritation, systemic effects after widespread use (see under Cautions)

**Dose**

● See preparations

**Zinc and Salicylic Acid Paste, BP**

Paste, (Lassar's Paste), zinc oxide 24%, salicylic acid 2%, starch 24%, white soft paraffin 50%, net price 25 g = 17p

**Dose** apply twice daily

## Oral retinoids for psoriasis

### ▌ ACITRETIN

**Note** Acitretin is a metabolite of etretinate

**Indications** severe extensive psoriasis resistant to other forms of therapy; palmoplantar pustular psoriasis; severe congenital ichthyosis; severe Darier's disease (keratosis follicularis)

**Cautions** exclude pregnancy before starting (test for pregnancy within 2 weeks before treatment and monthly thereafter; start treatment on day 2 or 3 of menstrual cycle)—women (including those with history of infertility) should avoid pregnancy for at least 1 month before, during, and for at least 3 years after treatment; patients should avoid concomitant tetracycline or methotrexate, high doses of vitamin A (more than 4000–5000 units daily) and use of keratolytics, and should not donate blood during or for at least 1 year after stopping therapy (teratogenic risk); check liver function at start, then every 1–2 weeks for

2 months, then every 3 months; monitor plasma lipids; diabetes (can alter glucose tolerance—initial frequent blood glucose checks); radiographic assessment on long-term treatment; investigate atypical musculoskeletal symptoms; in children use only in exceptional circumstances (premature epiphyseal closure reported); avoid excessive exposure to sunlight and unsupervised use of sunlamps; **interactions:** Appendix 1 (retinoids)

**Contra-indications** hepatic impairment (Appendix 2); renal impairment (Appendix 3); hyperlipidaemia, pregnancy (**important teratogenic risk:** see Cautions and Appendix 4); breast-feeding

**Side-effects** dryness of mucous membranes (sometimes erosion), of skin (sometimes scaling, thinning, erythema especially of face, and pruritus), and of conjunctiva (sometimes conjunctivitis and decreased tolerance of contact lenses); sticky skin, dermatitis; other side-effects reported include palmoplantar exfoliation, epistaxis, epidermal and nail fragility, oedema, paronychia, granulomatous lesions, bullous eruptions, reversible hair thinning and alopecia, myalgia and arthralgia, occasional nausea, headache, malaise, drowsiness, rhinitis, sweating, taste disturbance, and gingivitis; benign intracranial hypertension (discontinue if severe headache, vomiting, diarrhoea, abdominal pain, and visual disturbance occur; **avoid** concomitant tetracyclines); photosensitivity, corneal ulceration, raised liver enzymes, rarely jaundice and hepatitis (**avoid** concomitant methotrexate); raised serum triglycerides or cholesterol; decreased night vision reported; skeletal hyperostosis and extra-osseous calcification reported following long-term administration of etretinate (and premature epiphyseal closure in children, see Cautions)

**Dose**

● Under expert supervision, initially 25–30 mg daily (Darier's disease 10 mg daily) for 2–4 weeks, then adjusted according to response, usual range 25–50 mg daily; up to 75 mg daily for short periods in psoriasis and ichthyosis; CHILD (**important:** exceptional circumstances only, see Cautions), 500 micrograms/kg daily (occasionally up to 1 mg/kg daily to max. 35 mg daily) with careful monitoring of musculoskeletal development (see p. 640)

**Neotigason®** (Actavis) PoM

Capsules, acitretin 10 mg (brown/white), net price 60-cap pack = £24.27; 25 mg (brown/yellow), 60-cap pack = £56.30. Label: 10, patient information leaflet, 21

## ▌13.5.3▐ Drugs affecting the immune response

Drugs affecting the immune response are used for eczema or psoriasis. Systemic drugs acting on the immune system are used under specialist supervision.

**Pimecrolimus** by topical application is licensed for *mild to moderate atopic eczema.* **Tacrolimus** is licensed for topical use in *moderate to severe atopic eczema.* Both are drugs whose long-term safety is still being evaluated and they should not usually be considered first-line treatments unless there is a specific reason to avoid or reduce the use of topical corticosteroids. Treatment with topical pimecrolimus or topical tacrolimus should be initiated only by prescribers experienced in treating atopic eczema

> **NICE guidance**
> **Tacrolimus and pimecrolimus for atopic eczema (August 2004)**
> Topical pimecrolimus and tacrolimus are options for atopic eczema not controlled by maximal topical corticosteroid treatment or if there is a risk of important corticosteroid side-effects (particularly skin atrophy).
> Topical pimecrolimus is recommended for moderate atopic eczema on the face and neck of children aged 2–16 years and topical tacrolimus is recommended for moderate to severe atopic eczema in adults and children over 2 years. Pimecrolimus and tacrolimus should be used within their licensed indications.

For the role of topical corticosteroids in eczema, see section 13.5.1, and for comment on their limited role in psoriasis, see section 13.4. A short course of a systemic corticosteroid (section 6.3.2) can be given for eczema flares that have not improved despite appropriate topical treatment.

**Ciclosporin** (cyclosporin) by mouth can be used for *severe psoriasis* and for *severe eczema*. **Azathioprine** (section 8.2.1) or **mycophenolate mofetil** (section 8.2.1) are used for severe refractory eczema [unlicensed indication]. **Hydroxycarbamide** (hydroxyurea) (section 8.1.5) is used by mouth for severe psoriasis [unlicensed indication].

**Methotrexate** can be used for *severe psoriasis*, the dose being adjusted according to severity of the condition and haematological and biochemical measurements. Folic acid 5 mg (section 9.1.2) can be given once weekly to reduce the possibility of side-effects associated with methotrexate; alternative regimens of folic acid may be used in some settings.

**Etanercept**, **adalimumab**, and **infliximab** inhibit the activity of tumour necrosis factor (TNFα); they are used for *severe plaque psoriasis* either refractory to at least 2 standard systemic treatments and photochemotherapy, or when standard treatments cannot be used because of intolerance or contra-indications. **Ustekinumab** (a monoclonal antibody that inhibits interleukins 12 and 23) can be used for *severe plaque psoriasis* that has not responded to etanercept, adalimumab, or infliximab, or when these drugs cannot be used because of intolerance or contra-indications. Adalimumab, etanercept, and infliximab are also licensed for psoriatic arthritis (section 10.1.3).

> **NICE guidance[1]**
> **Adalimumab for plaque psoriasis in adults (June 2008)**
> Adalimumab is recommended for the treatment of severe plaque psoriasis which has failed to respond to standard systemic treatments (including ciclosporin and methotrexate) and photochemotherapy, or when standard treatments cannot be used because of intolerance or contra-indications. Adalimumab should be withdrawn if the response is not adequate after 16 weeks.

1. The *Scottish Medicines Consortium* issued similar advice in May 2008.

> **NICE guidance**
> **Etanercept and efalizumab for plaque psoriasis in adults (July 2006)**
> Etanercept is recommended for severe plaque psoriasis which has failed to respond to standard systemic treatments (including ciclosporin and methotrexate) and to photochemotherapy, or when standard treatments cannot be used because of intolerance or contra-indications. Etanercept should be withdrawn if the response is not adequate after 12 weeks.
> Following suspension of the marketing authorisation for efalizumab, NICE has temporarily withdrawn its guidance on the use of efalizumab for plaque psoriasis.

> **NICE guidance**
> **Infliximab for plaque psoriasis in adults (January 2008)**
> Infliximab is recommended for the treatment of very severe plaque psoriasis which has failed to respond to standard systemic treatments (including ciclosporin and methotrexate) or to photochemotherapy, or when standard treatments cannot be used because of intolerance or contra-indications. Infliximab should be withdrawn if the response is not adequate after 10 weeks.

> **Efalizumab**
> The marketing authorisation for **efalizumab** has been suspended following a review by the CHMP. The CHMP concluded that the benefits of efalizumab do not outweigh the risks. Efalizumab should not be prescribed for patients who are not already taking it. Treatment for patients who are taking efalizumab should be reviewed.

## CICLOSPORIN
(Cyclosporin)

**Indications** see under Dose; severe acute ulcerative colitis (section 1.5.3); transplantation and graft-versus-host disease (section 8.2.2)

**Cautions** see section 8.2.2
Additional cautions in atopic dermatitis and psoriasis *Contra-indicated* in abnormal renal function, uncontrolled hypertension (see also below), infections not under control, and malignancy (see also below). Dermatological and physical examination, including blood pressure and renal function measurements required at least twice before starting. During treatment, monitor serum creatinine every 2 weeks for first 3 months then every month; reduce dose by 25–50% if serum creatinine increases more than 30% above baseline (even if within normal range) and discontinue if reduction not successful within 1 month. Discontinue if hypertension develops that cannot be controlled by dose reduction or antihypertensive therapy. Avoid excessive exposure to sunlight and avoid use of UVB or PUVA. *In atopic dermatitis*, also allow herpes simplex infections to clear before starting (if they occur during treatment withdraw if severe); *Staphylococcus aureus* skin infections not absolute contra-indication providing controlled (but avoid erythromycin unless no other alternative—see also **interactions**: Appendix 1 (ciclosporin)); investigate lymphadenopathy that persists despite improvement in atopic dermatitis. *In psoriasis*, also exclude malignancies (including those of skin and cervix) before starting (biopsy any lesions not typical of psoriasis) and treat patients with malignant or pre-malignant conditions of skin only after appropriate treatment (and if no other option); discontinue if lymphoproliferative disorder develops

**Side-effects** see section 8.2.2

**Dose**

- Short-term treatment (usually for max. 8 weeks but can be longer under specialists) of severe atopic dermatitis where conventional therapy ineffective or inappropriate, administered in accordance with expert advice, by mouth, ADULT and CHILD over 16 years, initially 2.5 mg/kg daily in 2 divided doses, if good initial response not achieved within 2 weeks, increase rapidly to max. 5 mg/kg daily; initial dose of 5 mg/kg daily in 2 divided doses if very severe; CHILD under 16 years, see *BNF for Children*

- Severe psoriasis where conventional therapy ineffective or inappropriate, administered in accordance with expert advice, by mouth, ADULT and CHILD over 16 years, initially 2.5 mg/kg daily in 2 divided doses, increased gradually to max. 5 mg/kg daily if no improvement within 1 month (discontinue if response still insufficient after 6 weeks); initial dose of 5 mg/kg daily justified if rapid control required; CHILD under 16 years, see *BNF for Children*

**Important** For preparations and counselling and for advice on conversion between the preparations, see section 8.2.2

◢**Preparations**
Section 8.2.2

## ▌ METHOTREXATE

**Indications** severe psoriasis unresponsive to conventional therapy (specialist use only); Crohn's disease (section 1.5.3); malignant disease (section 8.1.3); rheumatoid arthritis (section 10.1.3)

**Cautions** section 10.1.3; also photosensitivity—psoriasis lesions aggravated by UV radiation (skin ulceration reported)

**Contra-indications** section 10.1.3

**Side-effects** section 10.1.3

**Dose**

- By mouth *or* by intramuscular *or* intravenous injection, 2.5–10 mg once weekly, increased according to response; max. weekly dose 30 mg; ELDERLY consider dose reduction (extreme caution); CHILD 12–18 years see *BNF for Children*

| Important |
|---|
| Note that the above dose is a **weekly** dose. To avoid error with low dose methotrexate, it is recommended that: |
| • the patient is carefully advised of the **dose** and **frequency** and the reason for taking methotrexate and any other prescribed medicine (e.g. folic acid); |
| • only one **strength** of methotrexate tablet (usually 2.5 mg) is prescribed and dispensed; |
| • the prescription and the dispensing label clearly show the dose and frequency of methotrexate administration; |
| • the patient is warned to report immediately the onset of any feature of blood disorders (e.g. sore throat, bruising, and mouth ulcers), liver toxicity (e.g. nausea, vomiting, abdominal discomfort and dark urine), and respiratory effects (e.g. shortness of breath). |

◢**Preparations**
Section 8.1.3 (parenteral) and section 10.1.3 (oral)

## ▌ PIMECROLIMUS

**Indications** short-term treatment of mild to moderate atopic eczema (including flares) when topical corticosteroids cannot be used; see also notes above

**Cautions** UV light (avoid excessive exposure to sunlight and sunlamps), avoid other topical treatments except emollients at treatment site; alcohol consumption (risk of facial flushing and skin irritation)

**Contra-indications** contact with eyes and mucous membranes, application under occlusion, infection at treatment site; congenital epidermal barrier defects; generalised erythroderma; immunodeficiency; concomitant use with drugs that cause immunosuppression (may be prescribed in exceptional circumstances by specialists); application to malignant or potentially malignant skin lesions

**Side-effects** burning sensation, pruritus, erythema, skin infections (including folliculitis and *less commonly* impetigo, herpes simplex and zoster, molluscum contagiosum); *rarely* papilloma, skin discoloration, local reactions including pain, paraesthesia, peeling, dryness, oedema, and worsening of eczema; skin malignancy reported

**Dose**

- Short-term treatment, apply twice daily until symptoms resolve (stop treatment if eczema worsens or no response after 6 weeks); CHILD under 2 years not recommended

**Elidel®** (Novartis) [PoM]
Cream, pimecrolimus 1%, net price 30 g = £19.69, 60 g = £37.41, 100 g = £59.07. Label: 4, 28
**Excipients** include benzyl alcohol, cetyl alcohol, propylene glycol, stearyl alcohol

## ▌ TACROLIMUS

**Indications** short-term treatment of moderate to severe atopic eczema (including flares) either unresponsive to, or in patients intolerant of conventional therapy; prevention of flares in patients with moderate to severe atopic eczema and 4 or more flares a year who have responded to initial treatment with topical tacrolimus; see also notes above; other indications section 8.2.2

**Cautions** infection at treatment site, UV light (avoid excessive exposure to sunlight and sunlamps); alcohol consumption (risk of facial flushing and skin irritation); pregnancy

**Contra-indications** congenital epidermal barrier defects; generalised erythroderma; immunodeficiency; concomitant use with drugs that cause immunosuppression (may be prescribed in exceptional circumstances by specialists); application to malignant or potentially malignant skin lesions; avoid contact with eyes and mucous membranes; application under occlusion; breast-feeding (Appendix 5)

**Side-effects** application-site reactions including rash, irritation, pain and paraesthesia; herpes simplex infection, Kaposi's varicelliform eruption; application-site infections (with preventative therapy); *less commonly* acne; rosacea and skin malignancy also reported

**Dose**

- Short-term treatment, ADULT and CHILD over 16 years initially apply 0.1% ointment thinly twice daily until lesion clears (consider other treatment if eczema worsens or no improvement after 2 weeks); reduce to once daily or switch to 0.03% ointment if condition allows; CHILD 2–16 years, initially apply 0.03% ointment thinly twice daily for up to 3 weeks (consider other treatment if eczema worsens or if no improvement after 2 weeks) then reduce to once daily until lesion clears

- Prevention of flares, ADULT and CHILD over 16 years, apply 0.1% ointment thinly twice weekly; use short-term treatment regimen during an acute flare; review need for preventative therapy after 1 year; CHILD 2–16 years, apply 0.03% ointment thinly twice weekly; use short-term treatment regimen during an acute flare; interrupt preventative therapy after 1 year to reassess condition

**Protopic®** (Astellas) [PoM]
Ointment, tacrolimus (as monohydrate) 0.03%, net price 30 g = £19.44, 60 g = £36.94; 0.1%, 30 g = £21.60, 60 g = £41.04. Label: 4, 11, 28
Excipients include beeswax

## Cytokine modulators

### ▌ ADALIMUMAB

**Indications** see notes above; Crohn's disease (section 1.5.3); ankylosing spondylitis, polyarticular juvenile idiopathic arthritis, psoriatic arthritis, rheumatoid arthritis (section 10.1.3)
**Cautions** section 10.1.3; monitor for non-melanoma skin cancer before and during treatment
**Contra-indications** section 10.1.3
**Side-effects** section 10.1.3
**Dose**

- By subcutaneous injection, plaque psoriasis, ADULT over 18 years, initially 80 mg, then 40 mg on alternate weeks starting 1 week after initial dose; discontinue treatment if no response within 16 weeks

◢**Preparations**
Section 10.1.3

### ▌ ETANERCEPT

**Indications** see notes above; ankylosing spondylitis, psoriatic arthritis, polyarticular course juvenile idiopathic arthritis, rheumatoid arthritis (section 10.1.3)
**Cautions** section 10.1.3; monitor for non-melanoma skin cancer before and during treatment
**Contra-indications** section 10.1.3
**Side-effects** section 10.1.3
**Dose**

- By subcutaneous injection, plaque psoriasis, 25 mg twice weekly or 50 mg once weekly; max. treatment duration 24 weeks; discontinue if no response after 12 weeks; CHILD 8–18 years, 800 micrograms/kg (max. 50 mg) once weekly; max. treatment duration 24 weeks; discontinue if no response after 12 weeks

◢**Preparations**
Section 10.1.3

### ▌ INFLIXIMAB

**Indications** see notes above; inflammatory bowel disease (section 1.5.3); ankylosing spondylitis, psoriatic arthritis, rheumatoid arthritis (section 10.1.3)
**Cautions** section 10.1.3; monitor for non-melanoma skin cancer before and during treatment
**Contra-indications** section 10.1.3

**Side-effects** section 10.1.3
**Dose**

- By intravenous infusion, plaque psoriasis, ADULT over 18 years, 5 mg/kg, repeated 2 weeks and 6 weeks after initial infusion, then every 8 weeks; discontinue if no response within 14 weeks of initial infusion

◢**Preparations**
Section 10.1.3

### ▌ USTEKINUMAB

**Indications** see notes above
**Cautions** predisposition to infection; history of malignancy; elderly; **interactions:** Appendix 1 (ustekinumab)

Tuberculosis Patients should be evaluated for tuberculosis before treatment. Active tuberculosis should be treated with standard treatment (section 5.1.9) for at least 2 months before starting ustekinumab. Patients who have previously received adequate treatment for tuberculosis can start ustekinumab but should be monitored every 3 months for possible recurrence. In patients without active tuberculosis but who were previously not treated adequately, chemoprophylaxis should ideally be completed before starting ustekinumab. In patients at high risk of tuberculosis who cannot be assessed by tuberculin skin test, chemoprophylaxis can be given concurrently with ustekinumab. Patients should be advised to seek medical attention if symptoms suggestive of tuberculosis (e.g. persistent cough, weight loss, and fever) develop

**Contra-indications** active infection; pregnancy (Appendix 4); breast-feeding (Appendix 5)
**Side-effects** infections (sometimes severe); diarrhoea; hypersensitivity reactions, pain in pharynx and larynx; headache, fatigue, dizziness, depression; arthralgia; myalgia; nasal congestion; pruritus, injection-site reactions
**Dose**

- By subcutaneous injection, plaque psoriasis, ADULT over 18 years, body-weight under 100 kg, initially 45 mg, then 45 mg 4 weeks after initial dose, then 45 mg every 12 weeks; body-weight over 100 kg, initially 45–90 mg, then 45–90 mg 4 weeks after initial dose, then 45–90 mg every 12 weeks
Note Discontinue if no response within 28 weeks

**Stelara®** (Janssen-Cilag) ▼ [PoM]
Injection, ustekinumab 90 mg/mL, net price 0.5-mL (45-mg) vial = £2147.00. Label: 10, counselling, tuberculosis

## 13.6 Acne and rosacea

**13.6.1** Topical preparations for acne
**13.6.2** Oral preparations for acne

**Acne** Treatment of acne should be commenced early to prevent scarring. Patients should be counselled that an improvement may not be seen for at least a couple of months. The choice of treatment depends on whether the acne is predominantly inflammatory or comedonal and its severity.

*Mild to moderate acne* is generally treated with topical preparations (section 13.6.1). Systemic treatment (section 13.6.2) with oral antibacterials is generally used for *moderate to severe acne* or where topical preparations are not tolerated or are ineffective or where application to the site is difficult. Another oral preparation used for acne is the hormone treatment co-cyprindiol (cyproterone acetate with ethinylestradiol); it is for women only.

*Severe acne*, acne unresponsive to prolonged courses of oral antibacterials, scarring, or acne associated with psychological problems calls for early referral to a consultant dermatologist who may prescribe isotretinoin for administration by mouth.

**Rosacea** Rosacea is not comedonal (but may exist with acne which may be comedonal). The pustules and papules of rosacea respond to topical metronidazole (section 13.10.1.2) or to topical azelaic acid (section 13.6.1). Alternatively, oral administration of oxytetracycline or tetracycline 500 mg twice daily (section 5.1.3) or of erythromycin 500 mg twice daily (section 5.1.5) can be used; courses usually last 6–12 weeks and are repeated intermittently. Doxycycline (section 5.1.3) 100 mg once daily can be used [unlicensed indication] if oxytetracycline or tetracycline is inappropriate (e.g. in renal impairment). Isotretinoin is occasionally given in refractory cases [unlicensed indication]. Camouflagers (section 13.8.2) may be required for the redness.

## 13.6.1 Topical preparations for acne

In mild to moderate acne, comedones and inflamed lesions respond well to benzoyl peroxide (see below) or to a topical retinoid (see p. 648). Alternatively, topical application of an antibacterial such as erythromycin or clindamycin may be effective for inflammatory acne. If topical preparations prove inadequate, oral preparations may be needed (section 13.6.2).

### Benzoyl peroxide and azelaic acid

**Benzoyl peroxide** is effective in mild to moderate acne. Both comedones and inflamed lesions respond well to benzoyl peroxide. The lower concentrations seem to be as effective as higher concentrations in reducing inflammation. It is usual to start with a lower strength and to increase the concentration of benzoyl peroxide gradually. Adverse effects include local skin irritation, particularly when therapy is initiated, but the scaling and redness often subside with treatment continued at a reduced frequency of application. If the acne does not respond after 2 months then use of a topical antibacterial should be considered.

**Azelaic acid** has antimicrobial and anticomedonal properties. It may be an alternative to benzoyl peroxide or to a topical retinoid for treating mild to moderate comedonal acne, particularly of the face. Some patients prefer azelaic acid because it is less likely to cause local irritation than benzoyl peroxide.

### ▌ BENZOYL PEROXIDE

**Indications** acne vulgaris

**Cautions** avoid contact with eyes, mouth, and mucous membranes; may bleach fabrics and hair; avoid excessive exposure to sunlight

**Side-effects** skin irritation (reduce frequency or suspend use until irritation subsides and re-introduce at reduced frequency)

**Dose**
- Apply 1–2 times daily preferably after washing with soap and water, start treatment with lower-strength preparations
Note May bleach clothing

**Acnecide®** (Galderma)
Gel, benzoyl peroxide 5% in an aqueous gel basis, net price 60 g = £4.17
Excipients include propylene glycol

**Brevoxyl®** (Stiefel)
Cream, benzoyl peroxide 4% in an aqueous basis, net price 40 g = £3.30
Excipients include cetyl alcohol, fragrance, stearyl alcohol

**PanOxyl®** (Stiefel)
Aquagel (= aqueous gel), benzoyl peroxide 2.5%, net price 40 g = £1.76; 5%, 40 g = £1.92; 10%, 40 g = £2.13
Excipients include propylene glycol

Cream, benzoyl peroxide 5% in a non-greasy basis, net price 40 g = £1.89
Excipients include isopropyl palmitate, propylene glycol

Gel, benzoyl peroxide 5% in an aqueous alcoholic basis, net price 40 g = £1.51; 10%, 40 g = £1.69
Excipients include fragrance

Wash, benzoyl peroxide 10% in a detergent basis, net price 150 mL = £4.00
Excipients include imidurea

#### ◢ With antimicrobials
**Duac® Once Daily** (Stiefel) PoM
Gel, benzoyl peroxide 5%, clindamycin 1% (as phosphate) in an aqueous basis, net price 25 g = £9.95, 50 g = £19.90
Excipients include disodium edetate
Dose apply once daily in the evening

**Quinoderm®** (Ferndale)
Cream, benzoyl peroxide 5%, potassium hydroxyquinoline sulphate 0.5%, in an astringent vanishing-cream basis, net price 50 g = £2.21
Excipients include cetostearyl alcohol, edetic acid (EDTA)

Cream, benzoyl peroxide 10%, potassium hydroxyquinoline sulphate 0.5%, in an astringent vanishing-cream basis, net price 25 g = £1.30, 50 g = £2.49
Excipients include cetostearyl alcohol, edetic acid (EDTA)

### ▌ AZELAIC ACID

**Indications** see preparations

**Cautions** avoid contact with eyes, mouth, and mucous membranes

**Side-effects** local irritation (reduce frequency or discontinue temporarily); *less commonly* skin discoloration; *very rarely* photosensitisation

**Finacea®** (Valeant) PoM
Gel, azelaic acid 15%, net price 30 g = £7.48
Excipients include disodium edetate, polysorbate 80, propylene glycol
Dose facial acne vulgaris, ADULT and CHILD over 14 years, apply twice daily; discontinue if no improvement after 1 month
Papulopustular rosacea, ADULT over 18 years, apply twice daily

**Skinoren®** (Valeant) PoM
Cream, azelaic acid 20%, net price 30 g = £3.74
Excipients include propylene glycol
Dose acne vulgaris, apply twice daily (sensitive skin, once daily for first week). Extended treatment may be required but manufacturer advises period of treatment should not exceed 6 months

13
Skin

## Topical antibacterials for acne

For many patients with mild to moderate inflammatory acne, topical antibacterials may be no more effective than topical benzoyl peroxide or tretinoin. Topical antibacterials are probably best reserved for patients who wish to avoid oral antibacterials or who cannot tolerate them. Topical preparations of **erythromycin** and **clindamycin** are effective for inflammatory acne. Topical antibacterials can produce mild irritation of the skin, and on rare occasions cause sensitisation.

Antibacterial resistance of *Propionibacterium acnes* is increasing; there is cross-resistance between erythromycin and clindamycin. To avoid development of resistance:

- when possible use non-antibiotic antimicrobials (such as benzoyl peroxide or azelaic acid);

- avoid concomitant treatment with different oral and topical antibacterials;

- if a particular antibacterial is effective, use it for repeat courses if needed (short intervening courses of benzoyl peroxide or azelaic acid may eliminate any resistant propionibacteria);

- do not continue treatment for longer than necessary (however, treatment with a topical preparation should be continued for at least 6 months).

### ◢ ANTIBACTERIALS

**Indications** acne vulgaris

**Cautions** some manufacturers advise preparations containing alcohol are not suitable for use with benzoyl peroxide

**Dalacin T®** (Pharmacia) PoM
Topical solution, clindamycin 1% (as phosphate), in an aqueous alcoholic basis, net price (both with applicator) 30 mL = £4.34, 50 mL = £7.23
Excipients include propylene glycol
**Dose** apply twice daily

Lotion, clindamycin 1% (as phosphate) in an aqueous basis, net price 30 mL = £5.08, 50 mL = £8.47
Excipients include cetostearyl alcohol, hydroxybenzoates (parabens)
**Dose** apply twice daily

**Stiemycin®** (Stiefel) PoM
Solution, erythromycin 2% in an alcoholic basis, net price 50 mL = £7.69
Excipients include propylene glycol
**Dose** apply twice daily

**Zindaclin®** (Crawford) PoM
Gel, clindamycin 1% (as phosphate), net price 30 g = £8.66
Excipients include propylene glycol
**Dose** apply once daily

**Zineryt®** (Astellas) PoM
Topical solution, powder for reconstitution, erythromycin 40 mg, zinc acetate 12 mg/mL when reconstituted with solvent containing ethanol, net price per pack of powder and solvent to provide 30 mL = £7.71, 90 mL = £22.24
Excipients none as listed in section 13.1.3
**Dose** apply twice daily

## Topical retinoids and related preparations for acne

Topical **tretinoin** and its isomer **isotretinoin** are useful for treating comedones and inflammatory lesions in mild to moderate acne. Patients should be warned that some redness and skin peeling may occur initially but settles with time. Several months of treatment may be needed to achieve an optimal response and the treatment should be continued until no new lesions develop.

Isotretinoin is given by mouth in severe acne; see section 13.6.2 for **warnings** relating to use by mouth.

**Adapalene**, a retinoid-like drug, is licensed for mild to moderate acne. It is less irritant than topical retinoids.

**Cautions** Topical retinoids should be avoided in severe acne involving large areas. Contact with eyes, nostrils, mouth and mucous membranes, eczematous, broken or sunburned skin should be avoided. These drugs should be used with caution in sensitive areas such as the neck, and accumulation in angles of the nose should be avoided. Exposure to UV light (including sunlight, solariums) should be avoided; if sun exposure is unavoidable, an appropriate sunscreen or protective clothing should be used. Use of retinoids with abrasive cleaners, comedogenic or astringent cosmetics should be avoided. Allow peeling (e.g. resulting from use of benzoyl peroxide) to subside before using a topical retinoid; alternating a preparation that causes peeling with a topical retinoid may give rise to contact dermatitis (reduce frequency of retinoid application).

**Contra-indications** Topical retinoids are contra-indicated in pregnancy (Appendix 4); women of child-bearing age must use effective contraception (oral progestogen-only contraceptives not considered effective). Tretinoin is contra-indicated in personal or familial history of cutaneous epithelioma.

**Side-effects** Local reactions include burning, erythema, stinging, pruritus, dry or peeling skin (discontinue if severe). Increased sensitivity to UVB light or sunlight occurs. Temporary changes of skin pigmentation have been reported. Eye irritation and oedema, and blistering or crusting of skin have been reported rarely.

### ◢ ADAPALENE

**Indications** mild to moderate acne
**Cautions** see notes above
**Contra-indications** see notes above
**Side-effects** see notes above
**Dose**
- Apply thinly once daily before retiring

**Differin®** (Galderma) PoM
Cream, adapalene 0.1%, net price 45 g = £11.40
Excipients include disodium edetate, hydroxybenzoates (parabens)

Gel, adapalene 0.1%, net price 45 g = £11.40
Excipients include disodium edetate, hydroxybenzoates (parabens), propylene glycol

### ◢ TRETINOIN

**Note** Tretinoin is the acid form of vitamin A

**Indications** see preparations; malignant disease (section 8.1.5)
**Cautions** see notes above

**Contra-indications** see notes above
**Side-effects** see notes above
**Dose**

- See preparations

**Retin-A®** (Janssen-Cilag) PoM
Gel, tretinoin 0.01%, net price 60 g = £5.39; 0.025%, 60 g = £5.39
Excipients include butylated hydroxytoluene
Dose acne vulgaris, apply thinly 1–2 times daily

◢With antibacterial
**Aknemycin® Plus** (Almirall) PoM
Solution, tretinoin 0.025%, erythromycin 4% in an alcoholic basis, net price 25 mL = £7.05
Excipients none as listed in section 13.1.3
Dose acne, apply thinly 1–2 times daily

### ISOTRETINOIN

Note Isotretinoin is an isomer of tretinoin
Important For **indications, cautions, contra-indications** and **side-effects** of isotretinoin **when given by mouth**, see p. 650

**Indications** see notes above; oral treatment (see section 13.6.2)
**Cautions** (*topical application* only) see notes above
**Contra-indications** (*topical application* only) see notes above
**Dose**

- Apply thinly 1–2 times daily

**Isotrex®** (Stiefel) PoM
Gel, isotretinoin 0.05%, net price 30 g = £5.94
Excipients include butylated hydroxytoluene

◢With antibacterial
**Isotrexin®** (Stiefel) PoM
Gel, isotretinoin 0.05%, erythromycin 2% in ethanolic basis, net price 30 g = £7.47
Excipients include butylated hydroxytoluene

---

## Other topical preparations for acne

**Salicylic acid** is available in various preparations for sale direct to the public for the treatment of mild acne. Other products are more suitable for acne; salicylic acid is used mainly for its keratolytic effect.

Preparations containing **sulphur** and **abrasive agents** are not considered beneficial in acne.

Topical **corticosteroids** should **not** be used in acne.

A topical preparation of **nicotinamide** is available for inflammatory acne.

### ABRASIVE AGENTS ◢

**Indications** acne vulgaris (but see notes above)
**Cautions** avoid contact with eyes; discontinue use temporarily if skin becomes irritated
**Contra-indications** superficial venules, telangiectasia

**Brasivol®** (Stiefel) ◢
Paste No. 1, aluminium oxide 38.09% in fine particles, in a soap-detergent basis, net price 75 g = £2.21
Excipients include fragrance, N-(3-Chloroallyl)hexaminium chloride (quaternium 15)
Dose use instead of soap 1–3 times daily

### CORTICOSTEROIDS ◢

**Indications** use in acne not recommended (see notes above)
**Cautions** see section 13.4 and notes above
**Contra-indications** see section 13.4 and notes above

**Side-effects** see section 13.4 and notes above

**Actinac®** (Peckforton) PoM ◢
Lotion (powder for reconstitution with solvent), chloramphenicol 40 mg, hydrocortisone acetate 40 mg, allantoin 24 mg, butoxyethyl nicotinate 24 mg, precipitated sulphur 320 mg/g. Discard 21 days after reconstitution, net price 2 × 6.25-g bottles powder with 2 × 20-mL bottles solvent = £16.28. Label: 28. Potency: mild
Excipients none as listed in section 13.1.3

### NICOTINAMIDE

**Indications** see under preparation
**Cautions** avoid contact with eyes and mucous membranes (including nose and mouth); reduce frequency of application if excessive dryness, irritation or peeling
**Side-effects** dryness of skin; also pruritus, erythema, burning and irritation

**Nicam®** (Dermal)
Gel, nicotinamide 4%, net price 60 g = £7.20
Excipients none as listed in section 13.1.3
Dose inflammatory acne vulgaris, apply twice daily; reduce to once daily or on alternate days if irritation occurs

### SALICYLIC ACID ◢

**Indications** acne; psoriasis (section 13.5.2); warts and calluses (section 13.7); fungal nail infections (section 13.10.2)
**Cautions** avoid contact with mouth, eyes, mucous membranes; systemic effects after excessive use (see section 4.7.1)
**Side-effects** local irritation

**Acnisal®** (Alliance) ◢
Topical solution, salicylic acid 2% in a detergent and emollient basis, net price 177 mL = £3.39.
Excipients include benzyl alcohol
Dose use up to 3 times daily

---

## 13.6.2 Oral preparations for acne

### Oral antibacterials for acne

Systemic antibacterial treatment is useful for inflammatory acne if topical treatment is not adequately effective or if it is inappropriate. Anticomedonal treatment (e.g. with topical benzoyl peroxide) may also be required.

Either **oxytetracycline** or **tetracycline** (section 5.1.3) is usually given for acne in a dose of 500 mg twice daily. If there is no improvement after the first 3 months another oral antibacterial should be used. Maximum improvement usually occurs after 4 to 6 months but in more severe cases treatment may need to be continued for 2 years or longer.

**Doxycycline** and **lymecycline** (section 5.1.3) are alternatives to tetracycline. Doxycycline can be used in a dose of 100 mg daily. Lymecycline is given in a dose of 408 mg daily.

Although **minocycline** is as effective as other tetracyclines for acne, it is associated with a greater risk of lupus erythematosus-like syndrome. Minocycline sometimes causes irreversible pigmentation; it is given in a dose of 100 mg once daily *or* 50 mg twice daily.

**13**
Skin

**Erythromycin** (section 5.1.5) in a dose of 500 mg twice daily is an alternative for the management of acne but propionibacteria strains resistant to erythromycin are becoming widespread and this may explain poor response.

**Trimethoprim** (section 5.1.8) in a dose of 300 mg twice daily may be used for acne resistant to other antibacterials [unlicensed indication]. Prolonged treatment with trimethoprim may depress haematopoiesis; it should generally be initiated by specialists.

Concomitant use of different topical and systemic antibacterials is undesirable owing to the increased likelihood of the development of bacterial resistance.

## Hormone treatment for acne

**Co-cyprindiol** (cyproterone acetate with ethinylestradiol) contains an anti-androgen. It is no more effective than an oral broad-spectrum antibacterial but is useful in women who also wish to receive oral contraception.

Improvement of acne with co-cyprindiol probably occurs because of decreased sebum secretion which is under androgen control. Some women with moderately severe hirsutism may also benefit because hair growth is also androgen-dependent. Contra-indications of co-cyprindiol include pregnancy and a predisposition to thrombosis.

> **CSM advice**
> Venous thromboembolism occurs more frequently in women taking co-cyprindiol than those taking a low-dose combined oral contraceptive. The CSM has reminded prescribers that co-cyprindiol is licensed for use in women with severe acne which has not responded to oral antibacterials and for moderately severe hirsutism; it should not be used solely for contraception. It is contra-indicated in those with a personal or close family history of venous thromboembolism. Women with severe acne or hirsutism may have an inherently increased risk of cardiovascular disease.

### ■ CO-CYPRINDIOL

A mixture of cyproterone acetate and ethinylestradiol in the mass proportions 2000 parts to 35 parts, respectively

**Indications** severe acne in women refractory to prolonged oral antibacterial therapy (but see notes above); moderately severe hirsutism

**Cautions** see under Combined Hormonal Contraceptives, section 7.3.1

**Contra-indications** see under Combined Hormonal Contraceptives, section 7.3.1

**Side-effects** see under Combined Hormonal Contraceptives, section 7.3.1

**Dose**
* 1 tablet daily for 21 days starting on day 1 of menstrual cycle and repeated after a 7-day interval, usually for several months; withdraw 3–4 months after acne or hirsutism completely resolved (repeat courses may be given if recurrence); long-term treatment may be necessary for severe symptoms

**Co-cyprindiol** (Non-proprietary) ▸PoM◂
Tablets, co-cyprindiol 2000/35 (cyproterone acetate 2 mg, ethinylestradiol 35 micrograms), net price 21-tab pack = £3.64
Brands include *Acnocin*®, *Cicafem*®, *Clairette*®, *Diva*®

**Dianette**® (Schering Health) ▸PoM◂
Tablets, beige, s/c, co-cyprindiol 2000/35 (cyproterone acetate 2 mg, ethinylestradiol 35 micrograms), net price 21-tab pack = £2.92

## Oral retinoid for acne

The retinoid **isotretinoin** reduces sebum secretion. It is used for the systemic treatment of nodulo-cystic and conglobate acne, severe acne, scarring, acne which has not responded to an adequate course of a systemic antibacterial, or acne which is associated with psychological problems. It is also useful in women who develop acne in the third or fourth decades of life, since late onset acne is frequently unresponsive to antibacterials.

Isotretinoin is a toxic drug that should be prescribed **only** by, or under the supervision of, a consultant dermatologist. It is given for at least 16 weeks; repeat courses are not normally required.

Side-effects of isotretinoin include severe dryness of the skin and mucous membranes, nose bleeds, and joint pains. The drug is **teratogenic** and must **not** be given to women of child-bearing age unless they practise effective contraception (oral progestogen-only contraceptives not considered effective) and then only after detailed assessment and explanation by the physician. Women must also be registered with a pregnancy prevention programme (see under Cautions below).

Although a causal link between isotretinoin use and psychiatric changes (including suicidal ideation) has not been established, the possibility should be considered before initiating treatment; if psychiatric changes occur during treatment, isotretinoin should be stopped, the prescriber informed, and specialist psychiatric advice should be sought.

### ■ ISOTRETINOIN

**Note** Isotretinoin is an isomer of tretinoin

**Indications** see notes above

**Cautions** avoid blood donation during treatment and for at least 1 month after treatment; history of depression; measure hepatic function and serum lipids before treatment, 1 month after starting and then every 3 months (reduce dose or discontinue if transaminase or serum lipids persistently raised); discontinue if uncontrolled hypertriglyceridaemia or pancreatitis; dry eye syndrome (associated with risk of keratitis); avoid keratolytics; renal impairment (Appendix 3) **interactions:** Appendix 1 (retinoids)

**Pregnancy prevention** In women of child-bearing potential, exclude pregnancy up to 3 days before treatment (start treatment on day 2 or 3 of menstrual cycle), every month during treatment (unless there are compelling reasons to indicate that there is no risk of pregnancy), and 5 weeks after stopping treatment—perform pregnancy test in the first 3 days of the menstrual cycle. Women must practise effective contraception for at least 1 month before starting treatment, during treatment, and for at least 1 month after stopping treatment. Women should be advised to use at least 1 method of contraception, but ideally they should use 2 methods of contraception. Oral progestogen-only contraceptives are not considered effective. Barrier methods should not be used alone, but can be used in conjunction with other contraceptive methods. Each prescription for isotretinoin should be limited to a supply of up to 30 days' treatment and dispensed within 7 days of the date stated on the prescription. Women should be advised to discontinue treatment and to seek prompt medical attention if they become pregnant during treatment or within 1 month of stopping treatment.

**Counselling** Warn patient to avoid wax epilation (risk of epidermal stripping), dermabrasion, and laser skin treatments (risk of scarring) during treatment and for at least 6 months after stopping; patient should avoid exposure to UV light (including sunlight) and use sunscreen and emollient (including lip balm) preparations from the start of treatment.

**Contra-indications** pregnancy (**important teratogenic risk:** see Cautions above and Appendix 4); breast-feeding; hepatic impairment (Appendix 2); hypervitaminosis A, hyperlipidaemia

**Side-effects** dryness of skin (with dermatitis, scaling, thinning, erythema, pruritus); epidermal fragility (trauma may cause blistering), dryness of lips (sometimes cheilitis), dryness of eyes (with blepharitis and conjunctivitis), dryness of pharyngeal mucosa (with hoarseness), dryness of nasal mucosa (with epistaxis), headache, myalgia and arthralgia, raised plasma concentration of triglycerides, of glucose, of serum transaminases, and of cholesterol (risk of pancreatitis if triglycerides above 9 mmol/litre), haematuria and proteinuria, thrombocytopenia, thrombocytosis, neutropenia and anaemia; *rarely* mood changes (depression, suicidal ideation, aggressive behaviour, anxiety)—expert referral required, exacerbation of acne, acne fulminans, allergic skin reactions, and hypersensitivity, alopecia; *very rarely* nausea, inflammatory bowel disease, diarrhoea (discontinue if severe), benign intracranial hypertension (avoid concomitant tetracyclines), convulsions, malaise, drowsiness, dizziness, lymphadenopathy, increased sweating, hyperuricaemia, raised serum creatinine concentration and glomerulonephritis, hepatitis, tendinitis, bone changes (including reduced bone density, early epiphyseal closure, and skeletal hyperostosis following long-term administration), visual disturbances (papilloedema, corneal opacities, cataracts, decreased night vision, photophobia, blurred vision, colour blindness)—expert referral required and consider withdrawal, decreased tolerance to contact lenses and keratitis, impaired hearing, Grampositive infections of skin and mucous membranes, allergic vasculitis and granulomatous lesions, paronychia, hirsutism, nail dystrophy, skin hyperpigmentation, photosensitivity

**Dose**
- ADULT and CHILD over 12 years, 500 micrograms/kg daily increased if necessary to 1 mg/kg (in 1–2 divided doses) for 16–24 weeks (repeat treatment course after a period of at least 8 weeks if failure or relapse after first course); max. cumulative dose 150 mg/kg per course

**Isotretinoin** (Non-proprietary) ⓅⓄⓂ
Capsules, isotretinoin 5 mg, net price 56-cap pack = £14.99; 20 mg, 56-cap pack = £39.99. Label: 10, patient information leaflet, 11, 21

**Roaccutane®** (Roche) ⓅⓄⓂ
Capsules, isotretinoin 10 mg (brown-red), net price 30-cap pack = £17.46; 20 mg (brown-red/white), 30-

cap pack = £24.04. Label: 10, patient information card, 11, 21
Excipients may include arachis (peanut) oil in *Roaccutane®* 20 mg capsules; *Roaccutane®* 5 mg capsules are discontinued, but those in circulation contain arachis (peanut) oil

## 13.7 Preparations for warts and calluses

Warts (verrucas) are caused by a human papillomavirus, which most frequently affects the hands, feet (plantar warts), and the anogenital region (see below); treatment usually relies on local tissue destruction. Warts may regress on their own and treatment is required only if the warts are painful, unsightly, persistent, or cause distress.

Preparations of **salicylic acid, formaldehyde, gluteraldehyde** or **silver nitrate** are available for purchase by the public; they are suitable for the removal of warts on hands and feet. **Salicylic acid** is a useful keratolytic which may be considered first; it is also suitable for the removal of *corns and calluses*. Preparations of salicylic acid in a collodion basis are available but some patients may develop an allergy to colophony in the formulation. An ointment combining **salicylic acid** with **podophyllum resin** (*Posalfilin®*) is available for treating plantar warts. Cryotherapy causes pain, swelling, and blistering and may be no more effective than topical salicylic acid in the treatment of warts.

### SALICYLIC ACID

**Indications** see under preparations; psoriasis (section 13.5.2); acne (section 13.6.1); fungal nail infections (section 13.10.2)

**Cautions** significant peripheral neuropathy, patients with diabetes at risk of neuropathic ulcers; protect surrounding skin and avoid broken skin; not suitable for application to face, anogenital region, or large areas

**Side-effects** skin irritation, see notes above

**Dose**
- See under preparations; advise patient to apply carefully to wart and to protect surrounding skin (e.g. with soft paraffin or specially designed plaster); rub wart surface gently with file or pumice stone once weekly; treatment may need to be continued for up to 3 months

**Cuplex®** (Crawford)
Gel, salicylic acid 11%, lactic acid 4%, in a collodion basis, net price 5 g = £2.23. Label: 15
Dose for plantar and mosaic warts, corns, and calluses, apply twice daily
Note Contains colophony (see notes above)

**Duofilm®** (Stiefel)
Paint, salicylic acid 16.7%, lactic acid 16.7%, in flexible collodion, net price 15 mL (with applicator) = £2.25. Label: 15
Dose for plantar and mosaic warts, apply daily

**Occlusal®** (Alliance)
Cutaneous solution, salicylic acid 26% in polyacrylic solution, net price 10 mL (with applicator) = £3.56. Label: 15
Dose for common and plantar warts, apply daily

**13**

**Skin**

**Salactol®** (Dermal)

Paint, salicylic acid 16.7%, lactic acid 16.7%, in flexible collodion, net price 10 mL (with applicator) = £1.74. Label: 15

Dose for warts, particularly plantar warts, verrucas, corns, and calluses, apply daily

Note Contains colophony (see notes above)

**Salatac®** (Dermal)

Gel, salicylic acid 12%, lactic acid 4% in a collodion basis, net price 8 g (with applicator) = £3.03. Label: 15

Dose for warts, verrucas, corns, and calluses, apply daily

**Verrugon®** (Ransom)

Ointment, salicylic acid 50% in a paraffin basis, net price 6 g = £2.83

Dose for plantar warts, apply daily

◢**With podophyllum**

**Posalfilin®** (Norgine)

Ointment, podophyllum resin 20%, salicylic acid 25%, net price 10 g = £3.37

Dose for plantar warts apply daily

Note Owing to the salicylic acid content, not suitable for anogenital warts; owing to the podophyllum content also contra-indicated in pregnancy and breast-feeding

### ▌FORMALDEHYDE

**Indications** see under preparations

**Cautions** see under Salicylic Acid

**Side-effects** see under Salicylic Acid

**Veracur®** (Typharm)

Gel, formaldehyde 0.75% in a water-miscible gel basis, net price 15 g = £2.41.

Dose for warts, particularly plantar warts, apply twice daily

### ▌GLUTARALDEHYDE

**Indications** warts, particularly plantar warts

**Cautions** protect surrounding skin; not for application to face, mucosa, or anogenital areas

**Side-effects** rashes, skin irritation (discontinue if severe); stains skin brown

**Dose**

• Apply twice daily (see also under Salicylic acid)

**Glutarol®** (Dermal)

Solution (= application), glutaraldehyde 10%, net price 10 mL (with applicator) = £2.10

### ▌SILVER NITRATE

**Indications** warts, verrucas, umbilical granulomas, over-granulating tissue, cauterisation

**Cautions** protect surrounding skin and avoid broken skin; not suitable for application to face, ano-genital region, or large areas

**Side-effects** chemical burns on surrounding skin; stains skin and fabric

**Dose**

• Common warts and verrucas, apply moistened caustic pencil tip for 1–2 minutes; repeat after 24 hours up to max. 3 applications for warts *or* max. 6 applications for verrucas

Note Instructions in proprietary packs generally incorporate advice to remove dead skin before use by gentle filing and to cover with adhesive dressing after application

• Umbilical granulomas, apply moistened caustic pencil tip (usually containing silver nitrate 40%) for 1–2

minutes while protecting surrounding skin with soft paraffin

**Silver nitrate** (Non-proprietary)

Caustic pencil, tip containing silver nitrate 40%, potassium nitrate 60%, net price = 93p

**AVOCA®** (Bray)

Caustic pencil, tip containing silver nitrate 95%, potassium nitrate 5%, net price, treatment pack (including emery file, 6 adhesive dressings and protector pads) = £1.94.

## Anogenital warts

The treatment of anogenital warts (condylomata acuminata) should be accompanied by screening for other sexually transmitted diseases. **Podophyllotoxin** (the major active ingredient of podophyllum) may be used for *soft, non-keratinised* external anogenital warts. Patients with a limited number of external warts or *keratinised* lesions may be better treated with cryotherapy or other forms of physical ablation.

**Imiquimod** cream is licensed for the treatment of external anogenital warts; it may be used for both keratinised and non-keratinised lesions. It is also licensed for the treatment of superficial basal cell carcinoma and actinic keratosis (section 13.8.1).

**Inosine pranobex** (section 5.3.2.1) is licensed for adjunctive treatment of genital warts but it has been superseded by more effective drugs.

### ▌IMIQUIMOD

**Indications** see under Dose

**Cautions** avoid normal or broken skin, and open wounds; not suitable for internal genital warts; uncircumcised males (risk of phimosis or stricture of foreskin); autoimmune disease; immunosuppressed patients; pregnancy (Appendix 4)

**Side-effects** local reactions (including itching, burning sensation, erythema, erosion, oedema, excoriation, and scabbing); headache; influenza-like symptoms; myalgia; *less commonly* local ulceration and alopecia; *rarely* Stevens-Johnson syndrome and cutaneous lupus erythematosus-like effect; *very rarely* dysuria in women; permanent hypopigmentation or hyperpigmentation reported

**Dose**

• Warts (external genital and perianal), apply thinly 3 times a week at night until lesions resolve (max. 16 weeks)

• Superficial basal cell carcinoma, apply to lesion (and 1 cm beyond it) on 5 days each week for 6 weeks; assess response 12 weeks after completing treatment

• Actinic keratosis, apply to lesion 3 times a week for 4 weeks; assess response after a 4 week treatment-free interval; repeat 4-week course if lesions persist; max. 2 courses

• CHILD under 18 years, see *BNF for Children*

Important Should be rubbed in and allowed to stay on the treated area for 6–10 hours for warts or for 8 hours for basal cell carcinoma and actinic keratosis, then washed off with mild soap and water (uncircumcised males treating warts under foreskin should wash the area daily). The cream should be washed off before sexual contact

**Aldara®** (3M) [PoM]

Cream, imiquimod 5%, net price 12-sachet pack = £51.32. Label: 10, patient information leaflet

Excipients include benzyl alcohol, cetyl alcohol, hydroxybenzoates (parabens), polysorbate 60, stearyl alcohol

Condoms may damage latex condoms and diaphragms

## ▌ PODOPHYLLOTOXIN

**Indications** see under preparations

**Cautions** avoid normal skin and open wounds; keep away from face; very irritant to eyes

**Contra-indications** pregnancy and breast-feeding; children

**Side-effects** local irritation

**Condyline®** (Ardern) [PoM]

Solution, podophyllotoxin 0.5% in alcoholic basis, net price 3.5 mL (with applicators) = £14.49. Label: 15

**Dose** condylomata acuminata affecting the penis or the female external genitalia, apply twice daily for 3 consecutive days; treatment may be repeated at weekly intervals if necessary for a total of five 3-day treatment courses; direct medical supervision for lesions in the female and for lesions greater than 4 cm² in the male; max. 50 single applications ('loops') per session (consult product literature)

**Warticon®** (Stiefel) [PoM]

Cream, podophyllotoxin 0.15%, net price 5 g (with mirror) = £14.86

Excipients include butylated hydroxyanisole, cetyl alcohol, hydroxybenzoates (parabens), sorbic acid, stearyl alcohol

**Dose** condylomata acuminata affecting the penis or the female external genitalia, apply twice daily for 3 consecutive days; treatment may be repeated at weekly intervals if necessary for a total of four 3-day treatment courses; direct medical supervision for lesions greater than 4 cm²

Solution, blue, podophyllotoxin 0.5% in alcoholic basis, net price 3 mL (with applicators—*Warticon®* [for men]; with applicators and mirror—*Warticon Fem®* [for women]) = £12.38. Label: 15

**Dose** condylomata acuminata affecting the penis or the female external genitalia, apply twice daily for 3 consecutive days; treatment may be repeated at weekly intervals if necessary for a total of four 3-day treatment courses; direct medical supervision for lesions greater than 4 cm²; max. 50 single applications ('loops') per session (consult product literature)

## ▌13.8 ▌ Sunscreens and camouflagers

**13.8.1** Sunscreen preparations

**13.8.2** Camouflagers

## ▌13.8.1 ▌ Sunscreen preparations

Solar ultraviolet irradiation can be harmful to the skin. It is responsible for disorders such as *polymorphic light eruption, solar urticaria,* and it provokes the various *cutaneous porphyrias.* It also provokes (or at least aggravates) skin lesions of *lupus erythematosus* and may aggravate *rosacea* and some other *dermatoses.* Certain drugs, such as *demeclocycline, phenothiazines,* or *amiodarone,* can cause photosensitivity. All these conditions (as well as *sunburn*) may occur after relatively short periods of exposure to the sun. Solar ultraviolet irradiation may provoke attacks of recurrent herpes labialis (but it is not known whether the effect of sunlight exposure is local or systemic).

The effects of exposure over longer periods include *ageing changes* and more importantly the initiation of *skin cancer.*

Solar ultraviolet radiation is approximately 200–400 nm in wavelength. The medium wavelengths (290–320 nm, known as UVB) cause *sunburn.* The long wavelengths (320–400 nm, known as UVA) are responsible for many *photosensitivity reactions* and *photodermatoses.* Both UVA and UVB contribute to long-term *photodamage* and to the changes responsible for *skin cancer* and ageing.

Sunscreen preparations contain substances that protect the skin against UVA and UVB radiation, but they are no substitute for covering the skin and avoiding sunlight. The sun protection factor (SPF, usually indicated in the preparation title) provides guidance on the degree of protection offered against UVB; it indicates the multiples of protection provided against burning, compared with unprotected skin; for example, an SPF of 8 should enable a person to remain 8 times longer in the sun without burning. However, in practice, users do not apply sufficient sunscreen product and the protection is lower than that found in experimental studies.

Some manufacturers use a star rating system to indicate the protection against UVA relative to protection against UVB for sunscreen products. However, the usefulness of the star rating system remains controversial. The EU Commission (September 2006) has recommended that the UVA protection factor for a sunscreen should be at least one-third of the sun protection factor (SPF); products that achieve this requirement will be labelled with a UVA logo alongside the SPF classification. Preparations that also contain reflective substances, such as titanium dioxide, provide the most effective protection against UVA.

Sunscreen preparations may rarely cause allergic reactions.

> For optimum photoprotection, sunscreen preparations should be applied **thickly** and **frequently** (approximately 2 hourly). In photodermatoses, they should be used from spring to autumn. As maximum protection from sunlight is desirable, preparations with the highest SPF should be prescribed.

**Borderline substances** The preparations marked 'ACBS' are regarded as drugs when prescribed for skin protection against ultraviolet radiation in abnormal cutaneous photosensitivity resulting from genetic disorders or photodermatoses, including vitiligo and those resulting from radiotherapy; chronic or recurrent herpes simplex labialis. Preparations with SPF less than 30 should not normally be prescribed. See also Appendix 7.

**Delph®** (Fenton)

Lotion, (UVA and UVB protection; UVB-SPF 30), avobenzone 4%, octinoxate 4.8%, oxybenzone 1.5%, titanium dioxide 2.5%, net price 200 mL = £3.53. ACBS

Excipients include cetostearyl alcohol, fragrance, hydroxybenzoates (parabens), imidurea

**E45 Sun®** (Crookes)

Reflective Sunscreen (UVA and UVB protection; UVB-SPF 50), waterproof, titanium dioxide 6.4%, zinc oxide 16%, net price 150 mL = £7.09. ACBS

Excipients include hydroxybenzoates (parabens), isopropyl palmitate

**SpectraBan®** (Stiefel)

Ultra lotion (UVA and UVB protection; UVB-SPF 28), water resistant, avobenzone 2%, oxybenzone 3%, padimate-O 8%, titanium dioxide 2%, net price 150 mL = £6.54. ACBS

Excipients include benzyl alcohol, disodium edetate, sorbic acid, fragrance

**Sunsense® Ultra** (Crawford)
    Lotion (UVA and UVB protection; UVB-SPF 60), octinoxate
    7.5% oxybenzone 3%, titanium dioxide 3.5%, net price 50-
    mL bottle with roll-on applicator = £3.11, 125 mL = £5.10.
    ACBS
    Excipients include butylated hydroxytoluene, cetyl alcohol, fragrance,
    hydroxybenzoates (parabens), propylene glycol

**Uvistat®** (LPC)
    Cream (UVA and UVB protection; UVB-SPF 30), avoben-
    zone 5%, bisoctrizole 1.5%, octinoxate 7.5%, octrocrilene
    4%, titanium dioxide 5.2%, net price 125 mL = £7.45. ACBS
    Excipients include disodium edetate, hydroxybenzoates (parabens),
    propylene glycol

    Cream (UVA and UVB protection; UVB-SPF 50), amiloxate
    2%, avobenzone 5%, bisoctrizole 6%, octinoxate 10%,
    octrocrilene 4%, titanium dioxide 4.8%, net price 125 mL =
    £8.45. ACBS
    Excipients include disodium edetate, polysorbate 60, propylene glycol

    Lipscreen (UVA and UVB protection; UVB-SPF 50), avo-
    benzone 5%, bemotrizinol 3%, octinoxate 10%, octocrilene
    4%, titanium dioxide 3%, net price 5 g = £2.99. ACBS
    Excipients include butylated hydroxytoluene, hydroxybenzoates (para-
    bens)

---

## Photodamage

Patients should be advised to use a high-SPF sunscreen
and to minimise exposure of the skin to direct sunlight
or sun lamps.

Topical treatments are used for non-hypertrophic *actinic
keratosis*. An **emollient** may be sufficient for mild
lesions. **Diclofenac** gel is suitable for the treatment of
superficial lesions in mild disease. **Fluorouracil** cream is
effective against most types of non-hypertrophic actinic
keratosis. **Imiquimod** (section 13.7) is used for lesions
on the face and scalp when cryotherapy or other topical
treatments cannot be used. Fluorouracil and imiquimod
produce a more marked inflammatory reaction than
diclofenac but lesions resolve faster. **Photodynamic
therapy** in combination with methyl-5-aminolevulinate
cream (*Metvix®*, available from Galderma) is used in
specialist centres for treating superficial and confluent,
non-hypertrophic actinic keratosis when other treatments are inadequate or unsuitable; it is particularly
suitable for multiple lesions, for periorbital lesions, or for
lesions located at sites of poor healing.

Imiquimod or topical fluorouracil is used for treating
superficial *basal cell carcinomas*. Photodynamic therapy
in combination with methyl-5-aminolevulinate cream is
used in specialist centres for treating superficial, nodular
basal cell carcinomas when other treatments are unsuitable.

---

### ■ DICLOFENAC SODIUM

**Indications**   actinic keratosis
**Cautions**   as for topical NSAIDs, see section 10.3.2
**Contra-indications**   as for topical NSAIDs, see section
    10.3.2
**Side-effects**   as for topical NSAIDs, see section 10.3.2;
    also paraesthesia; application of large amounts may
    result in systemic effects, see section 10.1
**Dose**
• Apply thinly twice daily for 60–90 days; max. 8 g daily

**Solaraze®** (Almirall) [PoM]
    Gel, diclofenac sodium 3% in a sodium hyaluronate
    basis, net price 50 g = £33.30
    Excipients include benzyl alcohol

---

### ■ FLUOROURACIL

**Indications**   superficial malignant and pre-malignant
    skin lesions; other malignant disease (section 8.1.3)
**Cautions**   avoid contact with mucous membranes;
    caution in handling—irritant to tissues
**Contra-indications**   pregnancy (Appendix 4); breast-
    feeding
**Side-effects**   local irritation (use a topical cortico-
    steroid for severe discomfort associated with
    inflammatory reactions), photosensitivity; *rarely*
    erythema multiforme
**Dose**
• Apply thinly to the affected area once or twice daily; if
    possible, cover malignant lesions with occlusive
    dressing; max. area of skin treated at one time,
    500 cm²; usual duration of initial therapy, 3–4 weeks
    Note Alternative regimens may be in use in some settings

**Efudix®** (Valeant) [PoM]
    Cream, fluorouracil 5%, net price 40 g = £34.74
    Excipients include hydroxybenzoates (parabens), polysorbate 60, pro-
    pylene glycol, stearyl alcohol

---

### **13.8.2** Camouflagers

Disfigurement of the skin can be very distressing to
patients and may have a marked psychological effect. In
skilled hands, or with experience, camouflage cosmetics
can be very effective in concealing scars and birthmarks. The depigmented patches in vitiligo are also
very disfiguring and camouflage creams are of great
cosmetic value.

**Borderline substances**   The preparations marked
'ACBS' are regarded as drugs when prescribed for postoperative scars and other deformities and as an adjunctive therapy in the relief of emotional disturbances due
to disfiguring skin disease, such as vitiligo. See also
Appendix 7.

**Covermark®** (Skin Camouflage Co.)
    Classic foundation (masking cream), net price 15 mL (10
    shades) = £11.32. ACBS
    Excipients include beeswax, hydroxybenzoates (parabens), fragrance
    Finishing powder, net price 25 g = £11.32. ACBS
    Excipients include beeswax, hydroxybenzoates (parabens), fragrance

**Dermacolor®** (Fox)
    Camouflage creme, (100 shades), net price 25 g = £9.05.
    ACBS
    Excipients include beeswax, butylated hydroxytoluene, fragrance, pro-
    pylene glycol, stearyl alcohol, wool fat
    Fixing powder, (7 shades), net price 60 g = £7.68. ACBS
    Excipients include fragrance

**Keromask®** (Lornamead)
    Masking cream, (2 shades), net price 15 mL = £5.67. ACBS
    Excipients include butylated hydroxyanisole, hydroxybenzoates (para-
    bens), wool fat, propylene glycol
    Finishing powder, net price 20 g = £5.67. ACBS
    Excipients include butylated hydroxytoluene, hydroxybenzoates (para-
    bens)

**Veil®** (Blake)
    Cover cream, (40 shades), net price 19 g = £19.65, 44 g =
    £29.22, 70 g = £36.90. ACBS
    Excipients include hydroxybenzoates (parabens), wool fat derivative
    Finishing powder, translucent, net price 35 g = £21.55. ACBS
    Excipients include butylated hydroxyanisole, hydroxybenzoates (para-
    bens)

## 13.9 Shampoos and other preparations for scalp and hair conditions

*Dandruff* is considered to be a mild form of seborrhoeic dermatitis (see also section 13.5.1). Shampoos containing antimicrobial agents such as **pyrithione zinc** (which are widely available) and **selenium sulphide** may have beneficial effects. Shampoos containing **tar** extracts may be useful and they are also used in *psoriasis*. **Ketoconazole** shampoo should be considered for more persistent or severe dandruff or for seborrhoeic dermatitis of the scalp.

**Corticosteroid** gels and lotions (section 13.4) can also be used.

Shampoos containing **coal tar** and **salicylic acid** may also be useful. A cream or an ointment containing coal tar and salicylic acid is very helpful in *psoriasis* that affects the scalp (section 13.5.2). Patients who do not respond to these treatments may need to be referred to exclude the possibility of other skin conditions.

*Cradle cap* in infants may be treated with **coconut oil** or **olive oil** applications followed by shampooing.

See below for male-pattern baldness and also section 13.5 (psoriasis and eczema), section 13.10.4 (lice), and section 13.10.2 (ringworm).

◢**Shampoos**
[1]**Ketoconazole** (Non-proprietary) (PoM)
Cream—section 13.10.2

Shampoo, ketoconazole 2%, net price 120 mL = £3.70
Excipients include imidurea
Brands include *Dandrazol® 2% Shampoo, Nizoral®*
Dose  treatment of seborrhoeic dermatitis and dandruff apply twice weekly for 2–4 weeks (prophylaxis apply once every 1–2 weeks); treatment of pityriasis versicolor apply once daily for max. 5 days (prophylaxis apply once daily for up to 3 days before sun exposure); leave preparation on for 3–5 minutes before rinsing

1. Can be sold to the public for the prevention and treatment of dandruff and seborrhoeic dermatitis of the scalp as a shampoo formulation containing ketoconazole max. 2%, in a pack containing max. 120 mL and labelled to show a max. frequency of application of once every 3 days

**Alphosyl 2 in 1®** (GSK Consumer Healthcare)
Shampoo, alcoholic coal tar extract 5%, net price 125 mL = £1.81, 250 mL = £3.43
Excipients include hydroxybenzoates (parabens), fragrance
Dose  dandruff, use once or twice weekly as necessary; psoriasis, seborrhoeic dermatitis, scaling and itching, use every 2–3 days

**Capasal®** (Dermal)
Shampoo, coal tar 1%, coconut oil 1%, salicylic acid 0.5%, net price 250 mL = £4.78
Excipients none as listed in section 13.1.3
Dose  scaly scalp disorders including psoriasis, seborrhoeic dermatitis, dandruff, and cradle cap, apply daily as necessary

**Ceanel Concentrate®** (Ferndale)
Shampoo, cetrimide 10%, undecenoic acid 1%, phenylethyl alcohol 7.5%, net price 150 mL = £3.40, 500 mL = £9.80
Excipients none as listed in section 13.1.3
Dose  scaly scalp disorders, seborrhoeic dermatitis, dandruff, apply 3 times in first week then twice weekly

**Clinitar®** (CHS)
Shampoo, coal tar extract 2%, net price 100 g = £2.50
Excipients include polysorbates, fragrance
Dose  scalp psoriasis, seborrhoeic dermatitis, and dandruff, apply up to 3 times weekly

**Dermax®** (Dermal)
Shampoo, benzalkonium chloride 0.5%, net price 250 mL = £5.78
Excipients none as listed in section 13.1.3
Dose  seborrhoeic scalp conditions associated with dandruff and scaling, apply as necessary

**Meted®** (Alliance)
Shampoo, salicylic acid 3%, sulphur 5%, net price 120 mL = £3.80
Excipients include fragrance
Dose  scaly scalp disorders including psoriasis, seborrhoeic dermatitis, and dandruff, apply at least twice weekly

**Pentrax®** (Alliance)
Shampoo, coal tar 4.3%, net price 120 mL = £3.80
Excipients none as listed in section 13.1.3
Dose  scaly scalp disorders including psoriasis, seborrhoeic dermatitis, and dandruff, apply at least twice weekly

**Polytar AF®** (Stiefel)
Shampoo, arachis (peanut) oil extract of coal tar 0.3%, cade oil 0.3%, coal tar solution 0.1%, pine tar 0.3%, pyrithione zinc 1%, net price 250 mL = £6.52
Excipients include fragrance, imidurea
Dose  scaly scalp disorders including psoriasis, seborrhoeic dermatitis, and dandruff, apply 2–3 times weekly for at least 3 weeks

**Psoriderm®** (Dermal)
Scalp lotion (= shampoo), coal tar 2.5%, lecithin 0.3%, net price 250 mL = £4.81
Excipients include disodium edetate
Dose  scalp psoriasis, use as necessary

**Selsun®** (Chattem UK)
Shampoo, selenium sulphide 2.5%, net price 50 mL = £1.44, 100 mL = £1.96, 150 mL = £2.75
Excipients include fragrance
Cautions  avoid using 48 hours before or after applying hair colouring, straightening or waving preparations
Dose  seborrhoeic dermatitis and dandruff, apply twice weekly for 2 weeks then once weekly for 2 weeks and then as necessary; CHILD under 5 years not recommended; pityriasis versicolor, section 13.10.2 [unlicensed indication]

**T/Gel®** (J&J)
Shampoo, coal tar extract 2%, net price 125 mL = £3.18, 250 mL = £4.78
Excipients include fragrance, hydroxybenzoates (parabens), imidurea, tetrasodium edetate
Dose  scalp psoriasis, seborrhoeic dermatitis, dandruff, apply as necessary

◢**Other scalp preparations**
**Cocois®**
Section 13.5.2

**Etrivex®**
Section 13.4

**Polytar®** (Stiefel)
Liquid, arachis (peanut) oil extract of coal tar 0.3%, cade oil 0.3%, coal tar solution 0.1%, oleyl alcohol 1%, tar 0.3%, net price 250 mL = £2.23
Excipients include fragrance, imidurea, polysorbate 80
Dose  scalp disorders including psoriasis, seborrhoea, eczema, pruritus, and dandruff, apply 1–2 times weekly

**13**

**Skin**

**Polytar Plus®** (Stiefel)
Liquid, ingredients as *Polytar®* liquid with hydrolysed animal protein 3%, net price 500 mL = £3.91
Excipients include fragrance, imidurea, polysorbate 80
Dose scalp disorders including psoriasis, seborrhoea, eczema, pruritus, and dandruff, apply 1–2 times weekly

## Hirsutism

Hirsutism may result from hormonal disorders or as a side-effect of drugs such as minoxidil, corticosteroids, anabolic steroids, androgens, danazol, and progestogens.

Weight loss can reduce hirsutism in obese women.

Women should be advised about local methods of hair removal, and in the mildest cases this may be all that is required.

**Eflornithine**, an antiprotozoal drug, inhibits the enzyme ornithine decarboxylase in hair follicles. Topical eflornithine can be used as an adjunct to laser therapy for facial hirsutism in women. Eflornithine should be discontinued in the absence of improvement after treatment for 4 months.

**Co-cyprindiol** (section 13.6.2) may be effective for moderately severe hirsutism. **Metformin** (section 6.1.2.2) is an alternative in women with polycystic ovary syndrome [unlicensed indication]. Systemic treatment is required for 6–12 months before benefit is seen.

### ▉ EFLORNITHINE

**Indications** see notes above
**Contra-indications** pregnancy (Appendix 4); breast-feeding (Appendix 5)
**Side-effects** acne, application site reactions including burning and stinging sensation, rash; *less commonly* abnormal hair texture and growth
**Dose**
• Apply thinly twice daily; CHILD under 12 years not recommended
Note Preparation must be rubbed in thoroughly; cosmetics may be applied over treated area 5 minutes after eflornithine; do not wash treated area for 4 hours after application

**Vaniqa®** (Almirall) ⒫ⓄⓂ
Cream, eflornithine (as hydrochloride) 11.5%, net price 60 g = £52.08
Excipients include cetostearyl alcohol, hydroxybenzoates, stearyl alcohol
Note The *Scottish Medicines Consortium* has advised (September 2005) that eflornithine for facial hirsutism be restricted for use in women in whom alternative drug treatment cannot be used

## Androgenetic alopecia

**Finasteride** is licensed for the treatment of androgenetic alopecia in men. Continuous use for 3–6 months is required before benefit is seen, and effects are reversed 6–12 months after treatment is discontinued.

Topical application of **minoxidil** may stimulate limited hair growth in a small proportion of adults but only for as long as it is used.

### ▉ FINASTERIDE

**Indications** androgenetic alopecia in men
**Cautions** see section 6.4.2
**Side-effects** see section 6.4.2
**Dose**
• By mouth 1 mg daily

**Propecia®** (MSD) ⒫ⓄⓂ ⓃⒽⓈ
Tablets, f/c, beige, finasteride 1 mg, net price 28-tab pack = £26.99, 84-tab pack = £81.55

### ▉ MINOXIDIL

**Indications** androgenetic alopecia (men and women)
**Cautions** section 2.5.1 (only about 1.4–1.7% absorbed); avoid contact with eyes, mouth and mucous membranes, broken, infected, shaved, or inflamed skin; avoid inhalation of spray mist; avoid occlusive dressings and topical drugs which enhance absorption
**Contra-indications** section 2.5.1
**Side-effects** section 2.5.1; irritant dermatitis, allergic contact dermatitis, changes in hair colour or texture, discontinue if increased hair loss persists for more than 2 weeks
**Dose**
• Apply 1 mL twice daily to dry hair and scalp (discontinue if no improvement after 1 year); 5% strength licensed for use in men only

**Regaine®** (McNeil) ⓃⒽⓈ
Regaine® Regular Strength topical solution, minoxidil 2% in an aqueous alcoholic basis, net price 60-mL bottle with applicators = £14.16
Excipients include propylene glycol
Cautions flammable; wash hands after application

Regaine® Extra Strength topical solution, minoxidil 5% in an aqueous alcoholic basis, net price 60-mL bottle with applicators = £17.00, 3 × 60-mL bottles = £34.03
Excipients include propylene glycol
Cautions flammable; wash hands after application

## 13.10 Anti-infective skin preparations

13.10.1 **Antibacterial preparations**
13.10.2 **Antifungal preparations**
13.10.3 **Antiviral preparations**
13.10.4 **Parasiticidal preparations**
13.10.5 **Preparations for minor cuts and abrasions**

## 13.10.1 Antibacterial preparations

13.10.1.1 **Antibacterial preparations only used topically**
13.10.1.2 **Antibacterial preparations also used systemically**

*Cellulitis*, a rapidly spreading deeply seated inflammation of the skin and subcutaneous tissue, requires systemic antibacterial treatment (see Table 1, section 5.1); it often involves staphylococcal infection. Lower leg infections or infections spreading around wounds are almost always cellulitis. *Erysipelas*, a superficial infection with clearly defined edges (and often affecting the face), is also treated with a systemic antibacterial (see Table 1, section 5.1); it usually involves streptococcal infection.

In the community acute *impetigo* on small areas of the skin may be treated by short-term topical application of **fusidic acid**; **mupirocin** should be used only to treat methicillin-resistant *Staphylococcus aureus*. If the impetigo is extensive or longstanding, an oral antibacterial such as **flucloxacillin** (or **erythromycin** in penicillin-allergy) (Table 1, section 5.1) should be used. Mild antiseptics such as **povidone–iodine** (section 13.11.4) are used to soften crusts and exudate.

Although many antibacterial drugs are available in topical preparations, some are potentially hazardous and frequently their use is not necessary if adequate hygienic measures can be taken. Moreover, not all skin conditions that are oozing, crusted, or characterised by pustules are actually infected. Topical antibacterials should be **avoided** on *leg ulcers* unless used in short courses for defined infections; treatment of bacterial colonisation is generally inappropriate.

To minimise the development of resistant organisms it is advisable to limit the choice of antibacterials applied topically to those not used systemically. Unfortunately some of these, for example neomycin, may cause sensitisation, and there is cross-sensitivity with other aminoglycoside antibiotics, such as gentamicin. If *large areas of skin* are being treated, ototoxicity may also be a hazard with aminoglycoside antibiotics (and also with polymyxins), particularly in children, in the elderly, and in those with renal impairment. *Resistant organisms* are more common in hospitals, and whenever possible swabs should be taken for bacteriological examination before beginning treatment.

**Mupirocin** is not related to any other antibacterial in use; it is effective for skin infections, particularly those due to Gram-positive organisms but it is not indicated for pseudomonal infection. Although *Staphylococcus aureus* strains with low-level resistance to mupirocin are emerging, it is generally useful in infections resistant to other antibacterials. To avoid the development of resistance, mupirocin or fusidic acid should not be used for longer than 10 days and local microbiology advice should be sought before using it in hospital. In the presence of mupirocin-resistant MRSA infection, a topical antiseptic such as povidone–iodine, chlorhexidine, or alcohol can be used; their use should be discussed with the local microbiologist.

**Retapamulin** can be used for impetigo and other superficial bacterial skin infections caused by *Staphylococcus aureus* and *Streptococcus pyogenes* that are resistant to first-line topical antibacterials. However, it is not effective against MRSA. The *Scottish Medicines Consortium* (p. 3) has advised (March 2008) that retapamulin (*Altargo®*) is **not** recommended for use within NHS Scotland for the treatment of superficial skin infections.

**Silver sulfadiazine** (silver sulphadiazine) is used in the treatment of infected burns.

## 13.10.1.1 Antibacterial preparations only used topically

### ■ MUPIROCIN

**Indications** bacterial skin infections (see also notes above)

**Side-effects** local reactions including urticaria, pruritus, burning sensation, rash

**Dose**
- ADULT and CHILD over 1 year, apply up to 3 times daily for up to 10 days; CHILD under 1 year see *BNF for Children*

**Bactroban®** (GSK) (PoM)
Cream, mupirocin (as mupirocin calcium) 2%, net price 15 g = £4.38
Excipients include benzyl alcohol, cetyl alcohol, stearyl alcohol

Ointment, mupirocin 2%, net price 15 g = £4.38
Excipients none as listed in section 13.1.3
Note Contains macrogol and manufacturer advises caution in renal impairment; may sting

Nasal ointment—section 12.2.3

### ■ NEOMYCIN SULPHATE

**Indications** bacterial skin infections

**Cautions** large areas, see below
Large areas If large areas of skin are being treated ototoxicity may be a hazard, particularly in children, in the elderly, and in those with renal impairment

**Contra-indications** neonates

**Side-effects** sensitisation (see also notes above)

**Neomycin Cream BPC** (PoM)
Cream, neomycin sulphate 0.5%, cetomacrogol emulsifying ointment 30%, chlorocresol 0.1%, disodium edetate 0.01%, in freshly boiled and cooled purified water, net price 15 g = £2.17
Excipients include cetostearyl alcohol, edetic acid (EDTA)
Dose apply up to 3 times daily (short-term use)

### ■ POLYMYXINS

**Indications** bacterial skin infections

**Cautions** large areas, see below
Large areas If large areas of skin are being treated nephrotoxicity and neurotoxicity may be a hazard, particularly in children, in the elderly, and in those with renal impairment

**Side-effects** sensitisation (see also notes above)

**Polyfax®** (TEVA UK) (PoM)
Ointment, polymyxin B sulphate 10 000 units, bacitracin zinc 500 units/g, net price 4 g = £3.26, 20 g = £4.62
Excipients none as listed in section 13.1.3
Dose apply twice daily or more frequently if required

### ■ RETAPAMULIN

**Indications** superficial bacterial skin infections (see also notes above)

**Contra-indications** contact with eyes and mucous membranes

**Side-effects** local reactions including irritation, erythema, pain, and pruritus

13

Skin

**Dose**

- ADULT and CHILD over 9 months, apply thinly twice daily for 5 days; review treatment if no response within 2–3 days

**Altargo®** (GSK) ▼ PoM
Ointment, retapamulin 1%, net price 5 g = £7.89. Label: 28
Excipients include butylated hydroxytoluene

## SILVER SULFADIAZINE
(Silver sulphadiazine)

**Indications** prophylaxis and treatment of infection in burn wounds; as an adjunct to short-term treatment of infection in leg ulcers and pressure sores; as an adjunct to prophylaxis of infection in skin graft donor sites and extensive abrasions; for conservative management of finger-tip injuries

**Cautions** hepatic impairment; renal impairment; G6PD deficiency; pregnancy and breast-feeding (avoid in late pregnancy and in neonate—see also Appendix 4); may inactivate enzymatic debriding agents—concomitant use may be inappropriate; for large amounts see also **interactions:** Appendix 1 (sulphonamides)

Large areas Plasma-sulfadiazine concentrations may approach therapeutic levels with *side-effects* and *interactions* as for sulphonamides (see section 5.1.8) if large areas of skin are treated. Owing to the association of sulphonamides with severe blood and skin disorders treatment should be stopped immediately if blood disorders or rashes develop—but leucopenia developing 2–3 days after starting treatment of burns patients is reported usually to be self-limiting and silver sulfadiazine need not usually be discontinued provided blood counts are monitored carefully to ensure return to normality within a few days. Argyria may also occur if large areas of skin are treated (or if application is prolonged).

**Contra-indications** pregnancy (Appendix 4) and breast-feeding (Appendix 5); sensitivity to sulphonamides; not recommended for neonates (see also Appendix 4)

**Side-effects** allergic reactions including burning, itching and rashes; argyria reported following prolonged use; leucopenia reported (monitor blood levels)

**Flamazine®** (S&N Hlth.) PoM
Cream, silver sulfadiazine 1%, net price 20 g = £2.91, 50 g = £3.85, 250 g = £10.32, 500 g = £18.27
Excipients include cetyl alcohol, polysorbates, propylene glycol
Dose burns, apply daily or more frequently if very exudative; leg ulcers or pressure sores, apply daily or on alternate days (not recommended if ulcer very exudative); finger-tip injuries, apply every 2–3 days; consult product literature for details
Note Apply with sterile applicator

### 13.10.1.2 Antibacterial preparations also used systemically

**Sodium fusidate** is a narrow-spectrum antibacterial used for staphylococcal infections. For the role of sodium fusidate in the treatment of impetigo see p. 657.

**Metronidazole** is used topically for rosacea and to reduce the odour associated with anaerobic infections; oral metronidazole (section 5.1.11) is used to treat wounds infected with anaerobic bacteria.

**Angular cheilitis** An ointment containing sodium fusidate is used in the fissures of angular cheilitis when associated with staphylococcal infection. For

further information on angular cheilitis, see section 12.3.2.

## FUSIDIC ACID

**Indications** staphylococcal skin infections; penicillin-resistant staphylococcal infections (section 5.1.7); staphylococcal eye infections (section 11.3.1)
**Cautions** see notes above; avoid contact with eyes
**Side-effects** rarely hypersensitivity reactions
**Dose**

- Apply 3–4 times daily

**Fucidin®** (LEO) PoM
Cream, fusidic acid 2%, net price 15 g = £1.92, 30 g = £3.64
Excipients include butylated hydroxyanisole, cetyl alcohol

Ointment, sodium fusidate 2%, net price 15 g = £2.23, 30 g = £3.79
Excipients include cetyl alcohol, wool fat
Dental prescribing on NHS May be prescribed as Sodium Fusidate ointment

## METRONIDAZOLE

**Indications** see preparations; rosacea (see also section 13.6); *Helicobacter pylori* eradication (section 1.3); anaerobic infections (section 5.1.11 and section 7.2.2); protozoal infections (section 5.4.2)
**Cautions** avoid exposure to strong sunlight or UV light
**Side-effects** skin irritation
**Dose**

- See preparations

**Acea®** (Ferndale) PoM
Gel, metronidazole 0.75%, net price 40 g = £9.95
Excipients include disodium edetate, hydroxybenzoates (parabens)
Dose acute inflammatory exacerbation of rosacea, apply thinly twice daily for 8 weeks

**Anabact®** (CHS) PoM
Gel, metronidazole 0.75%, net price 15 g = £4.47, 30 g = £7.89
Excipients include hydroxybenzoates (parabens), propylene glycol
Dose malodorous fungating tumours and malodorous decubitus ulcers, apply to clean wound 1–2 times daily and cover with non-adherent dressing

**Metrogel®** (Galderma) PoM
Gel, metronidazole 0.75%, net price 40 g = £9.95
Excipients include hydroxybenzoates (parabens), propylene glycol
Dose acute inflammatory exacerbation of rosacea, apply thinly twice daily for 8–9 weeks
Malodorous fungating tumours, apply to clean wound 1–2 times daily and cover with non-adherent dressing

**Metrosa®** (Linderma) PoM
Gel, metronidazole 0.75%, net price 40 g = £19.90
Excipients include propylene glycol
Dose acute exacerbation of rosacea, apply thinly twice daily for up to 8 weeks

**Metrotop®** (Medlock) PoM
Gel, metronidazole 0.8%, net price 15 g = £4.59
Excipients none as listed in section 13.1.3
Dose malodorous fungating tumours and malodorous gravitational and decubitus ulcers, apply to clean wound 1–2 times daily and cover (flat wounds, apply liberally; cavities, smear on paraffin gauze and pack loosely)

**Rosiced®** (Fabre) PoM
Cream, metronidazole 0.75%, net price 30 g = £7.50
Excipients include propylene glycol
Dose inflammatory papules and pustules of rosacea, apply twice daily for 6 weeks (longer if necessary)

**Rozex®** (Galderma) [PoM]

  Cream, metronidazole 0.75%, net price 40 g = £9.95
  Excipients include benzyl alcohol, isopropyl palmitate

  Gel, metronidazole 0.75%, net price 40 g = £9.95
  Excipients include disodium edetate, hydroxybenzoates (parabens), propylene glycol
  **Dose** inflammatory papules, pustules and erythema of rosacea, apply twice daily for 3–4 months

**Zyomet®** (Goldshield) [PoM]

  Gel, metronidazole 0.75%, net price 30 g = £12.00
  Excipients include benzyl alcohol, disodium edetate, propylene glycol
  **Dose** acute inflammatory exacerbation of rosacea, apply thinly twice daily for 8–9 weeks

## 13.10.2 Antifungal preparations

Most localised fungal infections are treated with topical preparations. To prevent relapse, local antifungal treatment should be continued for 1–2 weeks after the disappearance of all signs of infection. Systemic therapy (section 5.2) is necessary for nail or scalp infection or if the skin infection is widespread, disseminated, or intractable. Skin scrapings should be examined if systemic therapy is being considered or where there is doubt about the diagnosis.

**Dermatophytoses** Ringworm infection can affect the scalp (tinea capitis), body (tinea corporis), groin (tinea cruris), hand (tinea manuum), foot (tinea pedis, athlete's foot), or nail (tinea unguium). Scalp infection requires systemic treatment (section 5.2); additional application of a topical antifungal, during the early stages of treatment, may reduce the risk of transmission. A topical antifungal can also be used to treat asymptomatic carriers of scalp ringworm. Most other local ringworm infections can be treated adequately with topical antifungal preparations (including shampoos, section 13.9). The imidazole antifungals **clotrimazole, econazole, ketoconazole, miconazole,** and **sulconazole** are all effective. **Terbinafine** cream is also effective but it is more expensive. Other topical antifungals include **amorolfine, griseofulvin,** and the **undecenoates**. **Compound benzoic acid ointment** (Whitfield's ointment) has been used for ringworm infections but it is cosmetically less acceptable than proprietary preparations. Topical preparations for athlete's foot containing **tolnaftate** are on sale to the public.

Antifungal dusting powders are of little therapeutic value in the treatment of fungal skin infections and may cause skin irritation; they may have some role in preventing re-infection.

Antifungal treatment may not be necessary in asymptomatic patients with tinea infection of the nails. If treatment is necessary, a systemic antifungal (section 5.2) is more effective than topical therapy. However, topical application of **amorolfine** or **tioconazole** may be useful for treating early onychomycosis when involvement is limited to mild distal disease in up to 2 nails, or for superficial white onychomycosis, or where there are contra-indications to systemic therapy.

**Pityriasis versicolor** Pityriasis (tinea) versicolor can be treated with **ketoconazole** shampoo (section 13.9). Alternatively, **selenium sulphide** shampoo [unlicensed indication] (section 13.9) can be used as a lotion (diluted with water to reduce irritation) and left on for at least 30 minutes or overnight; it is applied 2–7 times over a fortnight and the course repeated if necessary.

Topical imidazole antifungals **clotrimazole, econazole, ketoconazole, miconazole,** and **sulconazole,** and topical **terbinafine** are alternatives, but large quantities may be required.

If topical therapy fails, or if the infection is widespread, pityriasis versicolor is treated systemically with a triazole antifungal (section 5.2). Relapse is common, especially in the immunocompromised.

**Candidiasis** Candidal skin infections can be treated with a topical imidazole antifungal, such as **clotrimazole, econazole, ketoconazole, miconazole,** or **sulconazole**; topical terbinafine is an alternative. Topical application of **nystatin** is also effective for candidiasis but it is ineffective against dermatophytosis. Refractory candidiasis requires systemic treatment (section 5.2) generally with a triazole such as fluconazole; systemic treatment with terbinafine is **not appropriate** for refractory candidiasis.

**Angular cheilitis** Miconazole cream is used in the fissures of angular cheilitis when associated with *Candida*. For further information on angular cheilitis, see p. 619.

**Compound topical preparations** Combination of an imidazole and a mild corticosteroid (such as hydrocortisone 1%) (section 13.4) may be of value in the treatment of eczematous intertrigo and, in the first few days only, of a severely inflamed patch of ringworm. Combination of a mild corticosteroid with either an imidazole or nystatin may be of use in the treatment of intertrigo associated with candida.

**Cautions** Contact with eyes and mucous membranes should be avoided.

**Side-effects** Occasional local irritation and hypersensitivity reactions include mild burning sensation, erythema, and itching. Treatment should be discontinued if these are severe.

---

## ▌ AMOROLFINE

**Indications** see under preparations
**Cautions** see notes above; also avoid contact with ears; pregnancy and breast-feeding
**Side-effects** see notes above

**Loceryl®** (Galderma) [PoM]

Cream, amorolfine (as hydrochloride) 0.25%, net price 20 g = £3.52. Label: 10, patient information leaflet
Excipients include cetostearyl alcohol, disodium edetate
**Dose** fungal skin infections, apply once daily after cleansing in the evening for at least 2–3 weeks (up to 6 weeks for foot infection) continuing for 3–5 days after lesions have healed

Nail lacquer, amorolfine (as hydrochloride) 5%, net price 5-mL pack (with nail files, spatulas and cleansing swabs) = £18.17. Label: 10, patient information leaflet
Excipients none as listed in section 13.1.3
**Dose** fungal nail infections, apply to infected nails 1–2 times weekly after filing and cleansing; allow to dry (approx. 3 minutes); treat finger nails for 6 months, toe nails for 9–12 months (review at intervals of 3 months); avoid nail varnish or artificial nails during treatment
**Note** Amorolfine nail lacquer can be sold to the public if supplied for the treatment of mild cases of distal and lateral subungual onychomycoses caused by dermatophytes, yeasts and moulds; subject to treatment of max. 2 nails, max. strength of nail lacquer amorolfine 5% and a pack size of 3 mL

**13**

**Skin**

## BENZOIC ACID

**Indications** ringworm (tinea), but see notes above

**Benzoic Acid Ointment, Compound, BP (Whitfield's ointment)**
Ointment, benzoic acid 6%, salicylic acid 3%, in emulsifying ointment
Excipients include cetostearyl alcohol
Dose apply twice daily

## CLOTRIMAZOLE

**Indications** fungal skin infections; vaginal candidiasis (section 7.2.2); otitis externa (section 12.1.1)
**Cautions** see notes above
**Side-effects** see notes above
**Dose**
- Apply 2–3 times daily

**Clotrimazole** (Non-proprietary)
Cream, clotrimazole 1%, net price 20 g = £1.84

**Canesten®** (Bayer Consumer Care)
Cream, clotrimazole 1%, net price 20 g = £2.14, 50 g = £3.50
Excipients include benzyl alcohol, cetostearyl alcohol, polysorbate 60

Powder, clotrimazole 1%, net price 30 g = £1.52
Excipients none as listed in section 13.1.3

Solution, clotrimazole 1% in macrogol 400 (polyethylene glycol 400), net price 20 mL = £2.43. For hairy areas
Excipients none as listed in section 13.1.3

Spray, clotrimazole 1%, in 30% isopropyl alcohol, net price 40-mL atomiser = £4.99. Label: 15. For large or hairy areas
Excipients include propylene glycol

## ECONAZOLE NITRATE

**Indications** fungal skin infections; vaginal candidiasis (section 7.2.2)
**Cautions** see notes above
**Side-effects** see notes above
**Dose**
- Skin infections apply twice daily; nail infections, apply once daily under occlusive dressing

**Ecostatin®** (Squibb)
Cream, econazole nitrate 1%, net price 15 g = £1.49; 30 g = £2.75
Excipients include butylated hydroxyanisole, fragrance

**Pevaryl®** (Janssen-Cilag)
Cream, econazole nitrate 1%, net price 30 g = £2.65
Excipients include butylated hydroxyanisole, fragrance

## GRISEOFULVIN

**Indications** tinea pedis; resistant fungal infections (section 5.2)
**Cautions** see notes above
**Side-effects** see notes above
**Dose**
- Apply 400 micrograms (1 spray) to an area approx. 13 cm² once daily, increased to 1.2 mg (3 sprays, allowing each spray to dry between applications) once daily if necessary; max. treatment duration 4 weeks

**Grisol AF®** (Transdermal)
Spray, griseofulvin 400 micrograms/metered spray, net price 20-mL (400-dose) spray = £4.00. Label: 15
Excipients include benzyl alcohol

## KETOCONAZOLE

**Indications** fungal skin infections; systemic or resistant fungal infections (section 5.2); vulval candidiasis (section 7.2.2)
**Cautions** see notes above; do **not** use within 2 weeks of a topical corticosteroid for seborrhoeic dermatitis—risk of skin sensitisation
**Side-effects** see notes above
**Dose**
- Tinea pedis, apply twice daily; other fungal infections, apply 1–2 times daily

**Nizoral®** (Janssen-Cilag) [PoM]
¹Cream, ketoconazole 2%, net price 30 g = £3.40
Excipients include cetyl alcohol, polysorbates, propylene glycol, stearyl alcohol
Note A 15-g tube is available for sale to the public for the treatment of tinea pedis, tinea cruris, and candidal intertrigo

Shampoo—section 13.9

1. [NHS] except for seborrhoeic dermatitis and pityriasis versicolor and endorsed 'SLS'

## MICONAZOLE NITRATE

**Indications** fungal skin infections; oral and intestinal fungal infections (section 12.3.2); vaginal candidiasis (section 7.2.2)
**Cautions** see notes above
**Side-effects** see notes above
**Dose**
- Apply twice daily continuing for 10 days after lesions have healed; nail infections, apply 1–2 times daily

**Miconazole** (Non-proprietary)
Cream, miconazole nitrate 2%, net price 20 g = £2.05, 45 g = £1.97
**Dental prescribing on NHS** Miconazole cream may be prescribed

**Daktarin®** (Janssen-Cilag)
Cream, miconazole nitrate 2%, net price 30 g = £1.85
Excipients include butylated hydroxyanisole
Note A 15-g tube [NHS] is on sale to the public

Powder[NHS], miconazole nitrate 2%, net price 20 g = £2.27
Excipients none as listed in section 13.1.3

Dual Action Spray powder, miconazole nitrate 0.16%, in an aerosol basis, net price 100 g = £2.27
Excipients none as listed in section 13.1.3

## NYSTATIN

**Indications** skin infections due to *Candida* spp.; intestinal candidiasis (section 5.2); oral fungal infections (section 12.3.2)
**Cautions** see notes above
**Side-effects** see notes above

**Nystaform®** (Typharm) [PoM]
Cream, nystatin 100 000 units/g, chlorhexidine hydrochloride 1%, net price 30 g = £2.62
Excipients include benzyl alcohol, cetostearyl alcohol, polysorbate 60
Dose apply 2–3 times daily continuing for 7 days after lesions have healed.

13 Skin

**Tinaderm-M®** (Schering-Plough) [PoM]
Cream, nystatin 100 000 units/g, tolnaftate 1%, net
price 20 g = £1.83
Excipients include butylated hydroxytoluene, cetostearyl alcohol,
hydroxybenzoates (parabens), fragrance
Dose apply 2–3 times daily

## SALICYLIC ACID

**Indications** fungal nail infections, particularly tinea;
hyperkeratotic skin disorders (section 13.5.2); acne
vulgaris (section 13.6.1); warts and calluses (section
13.7)
**Cautions** avoid broken or inflamed skin
**Salicylate toxicity** Salicylate toxicity can occur particularly if
applied on large areas of skin
**Contra-indications** pregnancy
**Side-effects** see notes above
**Dose**

• ADULT and CHILD over 5 years, apply twice daily and
after washing

**Phytex®** (Wynlit) ▱
Paint, salicylic acid 1.46% (total combined), tannic
acid 4.89% and boric acid 3.12% (as borotannic
complex), in a vehicle containing alcohol and ethyl
acetate, net price 25 mL (with brush) = £2.81
Excipients none as listed in section 13.1.3
Note Flammable

## SULCONAZOLE NITRATE

**Indications** fungal skin infections
**Cautions** see notes above
**Side-effects** see notes above; also blistering
**Dose**

• Apply 1–2 times daily continuing for 2–3 weeks after
lesions have healed

**Exelderm®** (Centrapharm)
Cream, sulconazole nitrate 1%, net price 30 g = £3.90
Excipients include cetyl alcohol, polysorbates, propylene glycol, stearyl
alcohol

## TERBINAFINE

**Indications** fungal skin infections
**Cautions** pregnancy, breast-feeding; avoid contact
with eyes
**Side-effects** see notes above
**Dose**

• Apply thinly 1–2 times daily for up to 1 week in tinea
pedis, 1–2 weeks in tinea corporis and tinea cruris, 2
weeks in cutaneous candidiasis and pityriasis versicolor; review after 2 weeks; CHILD see *BNF for Children*

[1]**Terbinafine** (Non-proprietary) [PoM]
Cream, terbinafine hydrochloride 1%, net price 15 g =
£4.86, 30 g = £8.76

1. Preparations of terbinafine hydrochloride (max. 1%) can be
sold to the public for external use for the treatment of tinea
pedis as a cutaneous solution in a pack containing max. 15 g,
*or* for the treatment of tinea pedis and cruris as a cream in a
pack containing max. 15 g, *or* for the treatment of tinea
pedis, cruris, and corporis as a spray in a pack containing
max. 30 mL spray or as a gel in a pack containing max. 30 g
gel

**Lamisil®** (Novartis Consumer Health) [PoM]
Cream, terbinafine hydrochloride 1%, net price 15 g =
£4.86, 30 g = £8.76
Excipients include benzyl alcohol, cetyl alcohol, polysorbate 60, stearyl
alcohol

Tablets—section 5.2

## TIOCONAZOLE

**Indications** fungal nail infections
**Cautions** see notes above
**Contra-indications** pregnancy
**Side-effects** see notes above; also local oedema, dry
skin, nail discoloration, periungual inflammation, nail
pain, rash, exfoliation
**Dose**

• Apply to nails and surrounding skin twice daily usually
for up to 6 months (may be extended to 12 months)

**Trosyl®** (Pfizer) [PoM]
Cutaneous solution, tioconazole 28%, net price
12 mL (with applicator brush) = £27.38
Excipients none as listed in section 13.1.3

## UNDECENOATES

**Indications** see under preparations below
**Side-effects** see notes above
**Dose**

• See under preparations below

**Mycota®** (Thornton & Ross)
Cream, zinc undecenoate 20%, undecenoic acid 5%,
net price 25 g = £1.49
Excipients include fragrance
Dose treatment of athlete's foot, apply twice daily continuing for
7 days after lesions have healed
Prevention of athlete's foot, apply once daily

Powder, zinc undecenoate 20%, undecenoic acid 2%,
net price 70 g = £2.07
Excipients include fragrance
Dose treatment of athlete's foot, apply twice daily continuing for
7 days after lesions have healed
Prevention of athlete's foot, apply once daily

Spray application, undecenoic acid 3.9%, dichloro-
phen 0.4% (pressurised aerosol pack), net price
100 mL = £2.34
Excipients include fragrance
Dose treatment of athlete's foot, apply twice daily continuing for
7 days after lesions have healed
Prevention of athlete's foot, apply once daily

## 13.10.3 Antiviral preparations

**Aciclovir** cream is licensed for the treatment of initial
and recurrent labial and genital *herpes simplex infections*;
treatment should begin as early as possible. Systemic
treatment is necessary for buccal or vaginal infections
and for *herpes zoster (shingles)* (for details of systemic use
see section 5.3.2.1).

**Idoxuridine** solution (5% in dimethyl sulfoxide) is of
little value.

**Herpes labialis** Aciclovir cream can be used for the
treatment of initial and recurrent labial herpes simplex
infections (cold sores). It is best applied at the earliest
possible stage, usually when prodromal changes of
sensation are felt in the lip and before vesicles appear.

13 Skin

Penciclovir cream is also licensed for the treatment of herpes labialis; it needs to be applied more frequently than aciclovir cream. These creams should not be used in the mouth.

Systemic treatment is necessary if cold sores recur frequently or for infections in the mouth (see p. 348).

## ACICLOVIR
(Acyclovir)

**Indications** see notes above; herpes simplex and varicella–zoster infections (section 5.3.2.1); eye infections (section 11.3.3)

**Cautions** avoid contact with eyes and mucous membranes

**Side-effects** transient stinging or burning; occasionally erythema, itching or drying of the skin

**Dose**
- Apply to lesions every 4 hours (5 times daily) for 5–10 days, starting at first sign of attack

¹**Aciclovir** (Non-proprietary) PoM
Cream, aciclovir 5%, net price 2 g = £1.22, 10 g = £2.13
Excipients include propylene glycol
Brands include *Zuvogen®* (*excipients* also include cetyl alcohol, propylene glycol)
Dental prescribing on NHS Aciclovir Cream may be prescribed

1. A 2-g tube and a pump pack are on sale to the public for the treatment of cold sores

**Zovirax®** (GSK) PoM
Cream, aciclovir 5%, net price 2 g = £4.73, 10 g = £14.24
Excipients include cetostearyl alcohol, propylene glycol
Eye ointment—section 11.3.3
Tablets—section 5.3.2.1

## PENCICLOVIR

**Indications** see notes above

**Cautions** avoid contact with eyes and mucous membranes

**Side-effects** transient stinging, burning, numbness; hypersensitivity reactions also reported

**Vectavir®** (Novartis Consumer Health) PoM
Cream, penciclovir 1%, net price 2 g = £4.20
Excipients include cetostearyl alcohol, propylene glycol
Dose herpes labialis, apply to lesions every 2 hours during waking hours for 4 days, starting at first sign of attack; CHILD under 12 years, not recommended
Dental prescribing on NHS May be prescribed as Penciclovir Cream

## IDOXURIDINE IN DIMETHYL SULFOXIDE

**Indications** herpes simplex and herpes zoster infection but of little value

**Cautions** avoid contact with the eyes, mucous membranes, and textiles; breast-feeding (Appendix 5); **interactions:** Appendix 1 (dimethyl sulfoxide)

**Contra-indications** pregnancy (Appendix 4); **not** to be used in mouth

**Side-effects** stinging on application, changes in taste; overuse may cause maceration

**Herpid®** (Astellas) PoM
Application, idoxuridine 5% in dimethyl sulfoxide, net price 5 mL (with applicator) = £6.33
Dose apply to lesions 4 times daily for 4 days, starting at first sign of attack; CHILD under 12 years, not recommended

## 13.10.4 Parasiticidal preparations

### Suitable quantities of parasiticidal preparations

| | Skin creams | Lotions | Cream rinses |
|---|---|---|---|
| Scalp (head lice) | — | 50–100 mL | 50–100 mL |
| Body (scabies) | 30–60 g | 100 mL | — |
| Body (crab lice) | 30–60 g | 100 mL | — |

These amounts are usually suitable for an adult for single application.

## Scabies

**Permethrin** is used for the treatment of *scabies* (*Sarcoptes scabiei*); **malathion** can be used if permethrin is inappropriate.

Aqueous preparations are preferable to alcoholic lotions, which are not recommended owing to irritation of excoriated skin and the genitalia.

**Benzyl benzoate** is an irritant and should be avoided in children; it is less effective than malathion and permethrin.

**Ivermectin** (available on a named patient basis from 'special-order' manufacturers or specialist importing companies, see p. 969) in a single dose of 200 micrograms/kg by mouth has been used, in combination with topical drugs, for the treatment of hyperkeratotic (crusted or 'Norwegian') scabies that does not respond to topical treatment alone.

**Application** Although acaricides have traditionally been applied after a hot bath, this is **not** necessary and there is even evidence that a hot bath may increase absorption into the blood, removing them from their site of action on the skin.

All members of the affected household should be treated simultaneously. Treatment should be applied to the whole body including the scalp, neck, face, and ears. Particular attention should be paid to the webs of the fingers and toes and lotion brushed under the ends of nails. It is now recommended that malathion and permethrin should be applied twice, one week apart; in the case of benzyl benzoate up to 3 applications on consecutive days may be needed. It is important to warn users to reapply treatment to the hands if they are washed. Patients with hyperkeratotic scabies may require 2 or 3 applications of acaricide on consecutive days to ensure that enough penetrates the skin crusts to kill all the mites.

**Itching** The *itch* and *eczema* of scabies persists for some weeks after the infestation has been eliminated and treatment for pruritus and eczema (section 13.5.1) may be required. Application of **crotamiton** can be used to control itching after treatment with more effective acaricides. A topical corticosteroid may help to reduce itch and inflammation after scabies has been treated successfully; however, persistent symptoms suggest that scabies eradication was not successful. Oral administration of a **sedating antihistamine** (section 3.4.1) at night may also be useful.

## Head lice

**Malathion** and the **pyrethroid** (phenothrin) can be used against head lice (*Pediculus humanus capitis*) but lice in some districts have developed resistance; resistance to two or more parasiticidal preparations has also been reported. Careful application of **dimeticone**, which acts on the surface of head lice, is also effective. Benzyl benzoate is licensed for the treatment of head lice but it is less effective than other drugs.

Head lice infestation (pediculosis) should be treated using lotion or liquid formulations. Shampoos are diluted too much in use to be effective. Alcoholic formulations are effective but aqueous formulations are preferred in severe eczema, for patients with asthma, and small children. A contact time of 12 hours or overnight treatment is recommended for lotions and liquids; a 2-hour treatment is not sufficient to kill eggs.

In general, a course of treatment for head lice should be 2 applications of product 7 days apart to prevent lice emerging from any eggs that survive the first application.

The policy of rotating insecticides on a district-wide basis is now considered outmoded. To overcome the development of resistance, a mosaic strategy is required whereby, if a course of treatment fails to cure, a different insecticide is used for the next course. If a course of treatment with phenothrin fails, then a non-pyrethroid parasiticidal product should be used for the next course.

**Wet combing methods** Head lice can be mechanically removed by combing wet hair meticulously with a plastic detection comb (probably for at least 30 minutes each time) over the whole scalp at 4-day intervals for a minimum of 2 weeks; hair conditioner or vegetable oil can be used to facilitate the process. Several products are available and some are prescribable on the NHS.

## Crab lice

**Permethrin** and **malathion** are used to eliminate *crab lice* (*Pthirus pubis*). An aqueous preparation should be applied, allowed to dry naturally and washed off after 12 hours; a second treatment is needed after 7 days to kill lice emerging from surviving eggs. All surfaces of the body should be treated, including the scalp, neck, and face (paying particular attention to the eyebrows and other facial hair). A different insecticide should be used if a course of treatment fails. Alcoholic lotions are not recommended (owing to irritation of excoriated skin and the genitalia).

## Benzyl benzoate

**Benzyl benzoate** is effective for *scabies* but is not a first-choice for *scabies* (see notes above).

### ▌ BENZYL BENZOATE ◪

**Indications** scabies (but see notes above)

**Cautions** children (not recommended, see also under Dose, below), avoid contact with eyes and mucous membranes; do not use on broken or secondarily infected skin; breast-feeding (suspend feeding until product has been washed off)

**Side-effects** skin irritation, burning sensation especially on genitalia and excoriations, occasionally rashes

**Dose**
- Apply over the whole body; repeat without bathing on the following day and wash off 24 hours later; a third application may be required in some cases
  **Note** Not recommended for children—dilution to reduce irritant effect also reduces efficacy. Some manufacturers recommend application to the body but to exclude the head and neck. However, application should be extended to the scalp, neck, face, and ears

**Benzyl Benzoate Application, BP** (Non-proprietary) ◪

Application, benzyl benzoate 25% in an emulsion basis, net price 500 mL = £2.50
Brands include *Ascabiol®* (*excipients: include* triethanolamine)

## Dimeticone

**Dimeticone** coats head lice and interferes with water balance in lice by preventing the excretion of water; it is less active against eggs and treatment should be repeated after 7 days.

### ▌ DIMETICONE

**Indications** head lice

**Cautions** avoid contact with eyes; children under 6 months, medical supervision required

**Side-effects** skin irritation

**Dose**
- Rub into dry hair and scalp, allow to dry naturally, shampoo after minimum 8 hours (or overnight); repeat application after 7 days

**Hedrin®** (Thornton & Ross)
Lotion, dimeticone 4%, net price 50 mL = £2.98, 120 mL spray pack = £7.13, 150 mL = £6.83
**Note** Patients should be told to keep hair away from fire and flames during treatment

## Malathion

**Malathion** is recommended for *scabies*, *head lice* and *crab lice* (for details see notes above).

The risk of systemic effects associated with 1–2 applications of malathion is considered to be very low; however, applications of lotion repeated at intervals of less than 1 week *or* application for more than 3 consecutive weeks should be **avoided** since the likelihood of eradication of lice is not increased.

**13**

**Skin**

## MALATHION

**Indications** see notes above and under preparations

**Cautions** avoid contact with eyes; do not use on broken or secondarily infected skin; children under 6 months, medical supervision required

**Side-effects** skin irritation and hypersensitivity reactions; chemical burns also reported

**Dose**

* Head lice, rub 0.5% preparation into dry hair and scalp, allow to dry naturally, remove by washing after 12 hours (see also notes above); repeat application after 7 days

* Crab lice, apply 0.5% aqueous preparation over whole body, allow to dry naturally, wash off after 12 hours or overnight; repeat application after 7 days

* Scabies, apply 0.5% preparation over whole body, and wash off after 24 hours; if hands are washed with soap within 24 hours, they should be retreated; see also notes above; repeat application after 7 days

  Note For scabies, manufacturer recommends application to the body but not necessarily to the head and neck. However, application should be extended to the scalp, neck, face, and ears

**Derbac-M®** (SSL)

Liquid, malathion 0.5% in an aqueous basis, net price 50 mL = £2.27, 200 mL = £5.70

Excipients include cetostearyl alcohol, fragrance, hydroxybenzoates (parabens)

For crab lice, head lice, and scabies

**Prioderm®** (SSL)

Cream shampoo (NHS) malathion 1%, net price 40 g = £2.77

Excipients include cetostearyl alcohol, fragrance, hydroxybenzoates (parabens), sodium edetate, wool fat

Dose head and crab lice, not recommended, therefore no dose stated (product too diluted in use and insufficient contact time)

**Quellada M®** (GSK Consumer Healthcare)

Liquid, malathion 0.5% in an aqueous basis, net price 50 mL = £1.85, 200 mL = £4.62

Excipients include cetostearyl alcohol, fragrance, hydroxybenzoates (parabens)

For crab lice, head lice, and scabies

Cream shampoo malathion 1%, net price 40 g = £2.18

Excipients include cetostearyl alcohol, fragrance, hydroxybenzoates (parabens), sodium edetate, wool fat

Dose head and crab lice, not recommended, therefore no dose stated (product too diluted in use and insufficient contact time)

## Permethrin

**Permethrin** is effective for *scabies* and *crab lice* (for details see notes above). Permethrin is active against *head lice* but the formulation and licensed methods of application of the current products make them unsuitable for the treatment of head lice.

## PERMETHRIN

**Indications** see notes above and under Dose

**Cautions** avoid contact with eyes; do not use on broken or secondarily infected skin; children under 6 months, medical supervision required for cream rinse (head lice); children aged 2 months–2 years, medical supervision required for dermal cream (scabies)

**Side-effects** pruritus, erythema, and stinging; rarely rashes and oedema

**Dose**

* Scabies, apply 5% preparation over whole body and wash off after 8–12 hours; CHILD (see also Cautions, above) apply over whole body including face, neck, scalp and ears; if hands washed with soap within 8 hours of application, they should be treated again with cream (see notes above); repeat application after 7 days

  Note Manufacturer recommends application to the body but to exclude head and neck. However, application should be extended to the scalp, neck, face, and ears

  Larger patients may require up to two 30-g packs for adequate treatment

* Crab lice, ADULT over 18 years, apply 5% cream over whole body, allow to dry naturally and wash off after 12 hours or after leaving on overnight; repeat application after 7 days

**Permethrin** (Non-proprietary)

Cream, permethrin 5%, net price 30 g = £5.52

**Lyclear® Creme Rinse** (Chefaro UK)

Cream rinse, permethrin 1% in basis containing isopropyl alcohol 20%, net price 59 mL = £2.38, 2 × 59-mL pack = £4.32

Excipients include cetyl alcohol

Dose head lice, not recommended, therefore no dose stated (insufficient contact time)

**Lyclear® Dermal Cream** (Chefaro UK)

Dermal cream, permethrin 5%, net price 30 g = £5.71. Label: 10, patient information leaflet

Excipients include butylated hydroxytoluene, wool fat derivative

## Phenothrin

**Phenothrin** is recommended for *head lice* (for details see notes above).

## PHENOTHRIN

**Indications** see notes above and under preparations

**Cautions** avoid contact with eyes; do not use on broken or secondarily infected skin; do not use more than once a week for 3 weeks at a time; children under 6 months, medical supervision required

**Side-effects** skin irritation

**Dose**

* See under preparations

**Full Marks®** (SSL)

Liquid, phenothrin 0.5% in an aqueous basis, net price 200 mL = £6.27

Excipients include cetostearyl alcohol, fragrance, hydroxybenzoates (parabens)

Dose head lice, apply to dry hair, allow to dry naturally; shampoo after 12 hours or next day, comb wet hair; repeat application after 7 days [unlicensed use]

## 13.10.5 Preparations for minor cuts and abrasions

Some of the preparations listed are used in minor burns, and abrasions. They are applied as necessary but should not be used on large wounds or for prolonged periods because of the possibility of hypersensitivity. The effervescent effect of hydrogen peroxide (section 13.11.6) is used to clean minor cuts and abrasions. Preparations containing camphor and sulphonamides should be **avoided**. Preparations such as magnesium sulphate paste are also listed but are now rarely used to treat carbuncles and boils as these are best treated with antibiotics (section 5.1.1.2).

### Cetrimide Cream, BP

Cream, cetrimide 0.5% in a suitable water-miscible basis such as cetostearyl alcohol 5%, liquid paraffin 50% in freshly boiled and cooled purified water, net price 50 g = £1.11

### Proflavine Cream, BPC

Cream, proflavine hemisulphate 0.1%, yellow beeswax 2.5%, chlorocresol 0.1%, liquid paraffin 67.3%, freshly boiled and cooled purified water 25%, wool fat 5%, net price 100 mL = 68p
**Excipients** include beeswax, wool fat
**Note** Stains clothing

◢**Preparations for boils**
### Magnesium Sulphate Paste, BP

Paste, dried magnesium sulphate 45 g, glycerol 55 g, phenol 500 mg, net price 25 g = 70p, 50 g = 81p
**Note** Should be stirred before use
**Dose** apply under dressing

## Collodion

**Flexible collodion** may be used to seal minor cuts and wounds that have partially healed.

### Collodion, Flexible, BP

Collodion, castor oil 2.5%, colophony 2.5% in a collodion basis, prepared by dissolving pyroxylin (10%) in a mixture of 3 volumes of ether and 1 volume of alcohol (90%), net price 10 mL = 25p. Label: 15
**Contra-indications** allergy to colophony in elastic adhesive plasters and tape

## Skin tissue adhesive

Tissue adhesives are used for closure of minor skin wounds and for additional suture support. They should be applied by an appropriately trained healthcare professional. Skin tissue adhesives may cause skin sensitisation.

### Dermabond ProPen® (Ethicon)

Topical Skin Adhesive, sterile, octyl 2-cyanoacrylate, net price 0.5 mL = £18.38

### Epiglu® (Schuco)

Tissue adhesive, sterile, ethyl-2-cyanoacrylate 954.5 mg/g, polymethylmethacrylate, net price 4 × 3-g vials = £149.50 (with dispensing pipettes and pallete)

### Histoacryl® (Braun)

Tissue adhesive, sterile, enbucrilate, net price 5 × 200-mg unit (blue) = £32.00, 10 × 200-mg unit (blue) = £67.20, 5 × 500-mg unit (clear or blue) = £34.65, 10 × 500-mg unit (blue) = £69.30

### LiquiBand® (MedLogic)

Tissue adhesive, sterile, enbucrilate, net price 0.5-g amp = £5.50

## 13.11 Skin cleansers and antiseptics

13.11.1 Alcohols and saline
13.11.2 Chlorhexidine salts
13.11.3 Cationic surfactants and soaps
13.11.4 Iodine
13.11.5 Phenolics
13.11.6 Oxidisers and dyes
13.11.7 Preparations for promotion of wound healing

Soap or detergent is used with water to cleanse intact skin; emollient preparations such as aqueous cream or emulsifying ointment (section 13.2.1) that do not irritate the skin are best used in place of soap or detergent for cleansing dry skin.

An antiseptic is used for skin that is infected or that is susceptible to recurrent infection. Detergent preparations containing **chlorhexidine** or **povidone–iodine**, which should be thoroughly rinsed off, are used. Emollients may also contain antiseptics (section 13.2.1).

Antiseptics such as **chlorhexidine** or **povidone–iodine** are used on intact skin before surgical procedures; their antiseptic effect is enhanced by an alcoholic solvent. Antiseptic solutions containing **cetrimide** can be used if a detergent effect is also required.

For irrigating ulcers or wounds, lukewarm sterile sodium chloride 0.9% solution is used, but tap water is often appropriate.

**Potassium permanganate** solution 1 in 10 000, a mild antiseptic with astringent properties, can be used for exudative eczematous areas; treatment should be stopped when the skin becomes dry. It can stain skin and nails especially with prolonged use.

## 13.11.1 Alcohols and saline

### ALCOHOL

**Indications** skin preparation before injection
**Cautions** flammable; avoid broken skin; patients have suffered severe burns when diathermy has been preceded by application of alcoholic skin disinfectants

### Industrial Methylated Spirit, BP

Solution, 19 volumes of ethanol and 1 volume approved wood naphtha, net price '66 OP' (containing 95% by volume alcohol) 100 mL = 39p; '74 OP' (containing 99% by volume alcohol) 100 mL = 39p. Label: 15

### Surgical Spirit, BP

Spirit, methyl salicylate 0.5 mL, diethyl phthalate 2%, castor oil 2.5%, in industrial methylated spirit, net price 100 mL = 20p. Label: 15

### SODIUM CHLORIDE

**Indications** see notes above; nebuliser diluent (section 3.1.5); sodium depletion (section 9.2.1.2); electrolyte imbalance (section 9.2.2.1); eye (section 11.8.1); oral hygiene (section 12.3.4)

**13**

**Skin**

**Sodium Chloride** (Non-proprietary)
Solution (sterile), sodium chloride 0.9%, net price 25 × 20-mL unit = £5.50, 200-mL can = £2.65, 1 litre = 97p

**Flowfusor®** (Fresenius Kabi)
Solution (sterile), sodium chloride 0.9%, net price 120-mL Bellows Pack = £1.53

**Irriclens®** (ConvaTec)
Solution in aerosol can (sterile), sodium chloride 0.9%, net price 240-mL can = £3.24

**Irripod®** (C D Medical)
Solution (sterile), sodium chloride 0.9%, net price 25 × 20-mL sachet = £5.50

**Miniversol®** (Aguettant)
Solution (sterile), sodium chloride 0.9%, net price 30 × 45-mL unit = £13.20; 30 × 100-mL unit = £19.50

**Normasol®** (Medlock)
Solution (sterile), sodium chloride 0.9%, net price 25 × 25-mL sachet = £5.98; 10 × 100-mL sachet = £7.27

**Stericlens®** (C D Medical)
Solution in aerosol can (sterile), sodium chloride 0.9%, net price 100-mL can = £1.94, 240-mL can = £2.95

**Steripod® Sodium Chloride** (Medlock)
Solution (sterile), sodium chloride 0.9%, net price 25 × 20-mL sachet = £7.36

## 13.11.2 Chlorhexidine salts

### CHLORHEXIDINE

**Indications** see under preparations; bladder irrigation and catheter patency solutions (see section 7.4.4)
**Cautions** avoid contact with eyes, brain, meninges and middle ear; not for use in body cavities; alcoholic solutions not suitable before diathermy
**Side-effects** occasional sensitivity

**Chlorhexidine 0.05%** (Baxter)
2000 Solution (sterile), pink, chlorhexidine acetate 0.05%, net price 500 mL = 72p, 1000 mL = 77p
For cleansing and disinfecting wounds and burns

**Cepton®** (LPC)
Skin wash (= solution), red, chlorhexidine gluconate 1%, net price 150 mL = £2.48
For use as skin wash in acne

Lotion, blue, chlorhexidine gluconate 0.1%, net price 150 mL = £2.48
For skin disinfection in acne

**ChloraPrep®** (Enturia)
Cutaneous solution, sterile, chlorhexidine gluconate 2% in isopropyl alcohol 70%, net price (single applicator) 0.67 mL = 30p, 1.5 mL = 55p, 3 mL = 85p, 10.5 mL = £2.92, 26 mL = £6.50
For skin disinfection before invasive procedures; CHILD under 2 months, not recommended
Note Flammable

**CX Antiseptic Dusting Powder®** (Ecolab)
Dusting powder, sterile, chlorhexidine acetate 1%, net price 15 g = £2.68
For skin disinfection

**Hibiscrub®** (Regent Medical)
Cleansing solution, red, chlorhexidine gluconate 4%, perfumed, in a surfactant solution, net price 250 mL = £4.25, 500 mL = £5.25, 5 litres = £16.20
Excipients include fragrance
Use instead of soap for pre-operative hand and skin preparation and for general hand and skin disinfection

**Hibitane Obstetric®** (Centrapharm)
Cream, chlorhexidine gluconate solution 5% (≡ 1% chlorhexidine gluconate), in a pourable water-miscible basis, net price 250 mL = £4.44
For use in obstetrics and gynaecology as an antiseptic and lubricant (for application to skin around vulva and perineum and to hands of midwife or doctor)

**Hydrex®** (Ecolab)
Solution, chlorhexidine gluconate solution 2.5% (≡ chlorhexidine gluconate 0.5%), in an alcoholic solution, net price 600 mL (clear) = £2.06; 600 mL (pink) = £2.06, 200-mL spray = £1.77, 500-mL spray = £3.01; 600 mL (blue) = £2.26
For pre-operative skin disinfection
Note Flammable

Surgical scrub, chlorhexidine gluconate 4% in a surfactant solution, net price 250 mL = £1.93, 500 mL = £2.05
For pre-operative hand and skin preparation and for general hand disinfection

**Unisept®** (Medlock)
Solution (sterile), pink, chlorhexidine gluconate 0.05%, net price 25 × 25-mL sachet = £5.40; 10 × 100-mL sachet = £6.67
For cleansing and disinfecting wounds and burns and swabbing in obstetrics

### With cetrimide
**Tisept®** (Medlock)
Solution (sterile), yellow, chlorhexidine gluconate 0.015%, cetrimide 0.15%, net price 25 × 25-mL sachet = £5.20; 10 × 100-mL sachet = £6.68
To be used undiluted for general skin disinfection and wound cleansing

**Travasept 100®** (Baxter)
Solution (sterile), yellow, chlorhexidine acetate 0.015%, cetrimide 0.15%, net price 500 mL = 72p, 1 litre = 77p
To be used undiluted in skin disinfection such as wound cleansing and obstetrics

### Concentrates
**Hibitane 5% Concentrate®** (Regent Medical)
Solution, red, chlorhexidine gluconate 5%, in a perfumed aqueous solution, net price 5 litres = £14.50
Dose to be used diluted 1 in 10 (0.5%) with alcohol 70% for pre-operative skin preparation, or 1 in 100 (0.05%) with water for general skin disinfection
Note Alcoholic solutions not suitable before diathermy (see Alcohol, p. 665)

13 Skin

## 13.11.3 Cationic surfactants and soaps

### CETRIMIDE

**Indications** skin disinfection

**Cautions** avoid contact with eyes; avoid use in body cavities

**Side-effects** skin irritation and occasionally sensitisation

◢**Preparations**

Ingredient of *Tisept®* and *Travasept® 100*, see above

## 13.11.4 Iodine

### POVIDONE–IODINE

**Indications** skin disinfection

**Cautions** pregnancy (Appendix 4), breast-feeding (Appendix 5); broken skin (see below); renal impairment (Appendix 3)

**Large open wounds** The application of povidone–iodine to large wounds or severe burns may produce systemic adverse effects such as metabolic acidosis, hypernatraemia and impairment of renal function.

**Contra-indications** preterm neonate gestational age under 32 weeks; avoid regular use in patients with thyroid disorders or those receiving lithium therapy

**Side-effects** rarely sensitivity; may interfere with thyroid function tests

**Betadine®** (Mölnlycke)

Dry powder spray, povidone–iodine 2.5% in a pressurised aerosol unit, net price 150-g unit = £2.63
For skin disinfection, particularly minor wounds and infections; CHILD under 2 years not recommended
Note Not for use in serous cavities

Ointment, povidone–iodine 10%, in a water-miscible basis, net price 20 g = £1.33, 80 g = £2.66
Excipients none as listed in section 13.1.3
For skin disinfection, particularly minor wounds and infections; CHILD under 2 years not recommended

**Savlon® Dry** (Novartis Consumer Health)

Powder spray, povidone–iodine 1.14% in a pressurised aerosol unit, net price 50-mL unit = £2.39
For minor wounds

**Videne®** (Ecolab)

Alcoholic tincture, povidone–iodine 10%, net price 500 mL = £2.50
To be applied undiluted in pre-operative skin disinfection

Antiseptic solution, povidone–iodine 10% in aqueous solution, net price 500 mL = £2.50
To be applied undiluted in pre-operative skin disinfection and general antisepsis

Surgical scrub, povidone–iodine 7.5% in aqueous solution, net price 500 mL = £2.50
To be used as a pre-operative scrub for hand and skin disinfection

## 13.11.5 Phenolics

Triclosan has been used for disinfection of the hands and wounds, and for disinfection of the skin before surgery.

## 13.11.6 Oxidisers and dyes

### HYDROGEN PEROXIDE

**Indications** see under preparations below

**Cautions** large or deep wounds; avoid on healthy skin and eyes; bleaches fabric; incompatible with products containing iodine or potassium permanganate

**Hydrogen Peroxide Solution, BP**

Solution 6% (20 vols), net price 200 mL = 43p

Solution 3% (10 vols), net price 200 mL = 42p
For skin disinfection, particularly cleansing and deodorising wounds and ulcers
Note The BP directs that when hydrogen peroxide is prescribed, hydrogen peroxide solution 6% (20 vols) should be dispensed.
Important Strong solutions of hydrogen peroxide which contain 27% (90 vols) and 30% (100 vols) are only for the preparation of weaker solutions

**Crystacide®** (GP Pharma)

Cream, hydrogen peroxide 1%, net price 10 g = £4.82, 25 g = £8.07, 40 g = £11.62
Dose superficial bacterial skin infection, apply 2–3 times daily for up to 3 weeks
Excipients include edetic acid (EDTA), propylene glycol

### POTASSIUM PERMANGANATE

**Indications** cleansing and deodorising suppurating eczematous reactions and wounds

**Cautions** irritant to mucous membranes

**Dose**

- Wet dressings or baths, approx. 0.01% solution
  Note Stains skin and clothing

**Potassium Permanganate Solution**

Solution, potassium permanganate 0.1% (1 in 1000) in water
Dose to be diluted 1 in 10 to provide a 0.01% (1 in 10 000) solution

**Permitabs®** (Alliance)

Solution tablets, for preparation of topical solution, potassium permanganate 400 mg, net price 30-tab pack = £9.85
Note 1 tablet dissolved in 4 litres of water provides a 0.01% (1 in 10 000) solution

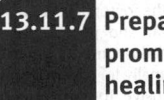

## 13.11.7 Preparations for promotion of wound healing

### Desloughing agents

Alginate, hydrogel and hydrocolloid dressings (Appendix 8) are effective at wound debridement. Sterile larvae (maggots) (*LarvE®*, Zoobiotic) are also used for managing sloughing wounds and are prescribable on the NHS.

Desloughing solutions and creams are of little clinical value. Substances applied to an open area are easily absorbed and perilesional skin is easily sensitised; gravitational dermatitis may be complicated by superimposed contact sensitivity to substances such as neomycin or lanolin.

For further information on wound management products see Appendix 8, p. 911.

## Growth factor

A topical preparation of **becaplermin** (recombinant human platelet-derived growth factor) is licensed as an adjunct treatment of full-thickness, neuropathic, diabetic ulcers. It enhances the formation of granulation tissue, thereby promoting wound healing.

### ▋ BECAPLERMIN
(Recombinant human platelet-derived growth factor)

**Indications** see notes above

**Cautions** malignant disease; avoid on sites with infection, malignancy, or peripheral arteriopathy

**Side-effects** pain; infections including cellulitis and osteomyelitis; local reactions including erythema; *rarely* bullous eruption, oedema, and hypertrophic granulation

**Dose**

- Full-thickness, neuropathic, diabetic ulcers (no larger than 5 cm²), apply thin layer daily and cover with gauze dressing moistened with physiological saline; max. duration of treatment 20 weeks (reassess if no healing after first 10 weeks); CHILD under 18 years, see *BNF for Children*

**Regranex®** (Janssen-Cilag) PoM
Gel, becaplermin (recombinant human platelet-derived growth factor) 0.01%, net price 15 g = £245.78
Excipients include hydroxybenzoates (parabens)

### ▋13.12 Antiperspirants

**Aluminium chloride** is a potent antiperspirant used in the treatment of hyperhidrosis. Aluminium salts are also incorporated in preparations for minor fungal skin infections associated with hyperhidrosis.

In more severe cases specialists use **glycopyrronium bromide** as a 0.05% solution in the iontophoretic treatment of hyperhidrosis of plantar and palmar areas. **Botulinum A toxin-haemagglutinin complex** (section 4.9.3) is licensed for use intradermally for severe hyperhidrosis of the axillae unresponsive to topical antiperspirant or other antihidrotic treatment.

### ▋ ALUMINIUM SALTS

**Indications** see under Dose below

**Cautions** avoid contact with eyes or mucous membranes; avoid use on broken or irritated skin; do not shave axillae or use depilatories within 12 hours of application; avoid contact with clothing

**Side-effects** skin irritation

**Dose**

- Hyperhidrosis affecting axillae, hands or feet, apply liquid formulation at night to dry skin, wash off the

following morning, initially daily then reduce frequency as condition improves—do not bathe immediately before use

- Hyperhidrosis, bromidrosis, intertrigo, and prevention of tinea pedis and related conditions, apply powder to dry skin

**Anhydrol® Forte** (Dermal)
Solution (= application), aluminium chloride hexahydrate 20% in an alcoholic basis, net price 60-mL bottle with roll-on applicator = £2.54. Label: 15
Excipients none as listed in section 13.1.3

¹**Driclor®** (Stiefel)
Application, aluminium chloride hexahydrate 20% in an alcoholic basis, net price 60-mL bottle with roll-on applicator = £2.82. Label: 15
Excipients none as listed in section 13.1.3

1. A 30-mL pack is on sale to the public

**ZeaSORB®** (Stiefel)
Dusting powder, aldioxa 0.22%, chloroxylenol 0.5%, net price 50 g = £2.61
Excipients include fragrance

### ▋ GLYCOPYRRONIUM BROMIDE

**Indications** iontophoretic treatment of hyperhidrosis; other indications section 15.1.3

**Cautions** see section 15.1.3 (but poorly absorbed and systemic effects unlikely)

**Contra-indications** see section 15.1.3 (but poorly absorbed and systemic effects unlikely), infections affecting the treatment site

**Side-effects** see section 15.1.3 (but poorly absorbed and systemic effects unlikely), tingling at administration site

**Dose**

- Consult product literature; only 1 site to be treated at a time, max. 2 sites treated in any 24 hours, treatment not to be repeated within 7 days

**Robinul®** (Antigen) PoM
Powder, glycopyrronium bromide, net price 3 g = £110.00

### ▋13.13 Topical circulatory preparations

These preparations are used to improve circulation in conditions such as bruising, superficial thrombophlebitis, chilblains and varicose veins but are of little value. Chilblains are best managed by avoidance of exposure to cold; neither systemic nor topical vasodilator therapy is established as being effective. Sclerotherapy of varicose veins is described in section 2.13.

Rubefacients are described in section 10.3.2.

**Hirudoid®** (Genus) ◢
Cream, heparinoid 0.3% in a vanishing-cream basis, net price 50 g = £3.99
Excipients include cetostearyl alcohol, hydroxybenzoates (parabens)

Gel, heparinoid 0.3%, net price 50 g = £3.99
Excipients include propylene glycol, fragrance

**Dose** apply up to 4 times daily in superficial soft-tissue injuries and superficial thrombophlebitis

13 Skin

# 14 Immunological products and vaccines

| | | |
|---|---|---|
| **14.1** | Active immunity | **669** |
| **14.2** | Passive immunity | **672** |
| **14.3** | Storage and use | **672** |
| **14.4** | Vaccines and antisera | **672** |
| **14.5** | Immunoglobulins | **690** |
| 14.5.1 | Normal immunoglobulin | 690 |
| 14.5.2 | Disease-specific immunoglobulins | 692 |
| 14.5.3 | Anti-D (Rh$_0$) immunoglobulin | 693 |
| **14.6** | International travel | **695** |

## 14.1 Active immunity

Active immunity can be acquired by natural disease or by vaccination. **Vaccines** stimulate production of antibodies and other components of the immune mechanism; they consist of either:

1. a *live attenuated* form of a virus (e.g. measles, mumps and rubella vaccine) or bacteria (e.g. BCG vaccine), or

2. *inactivated* preparations of the virus (e.g. influenza vaccine) or bacteria, or

3. *extracts of* or *detoxified exotoxins* produced by a micro-organism (e.g. tetanus vaccine).

**Live attenuated vaccines** usually produce a durable immunity, but not always as long-lasting as that resulting from natural infection.

**Inactivated vaccines** may require a primary series of injections of vaccine to produce an adequate antibody response, and in most cases booster (reinforcing) injections are required; the duration of immunity varies from months to many years. Some inactivated vaccines are adsorbed onto an adjuvant (such as aluminium hydroxide) to enhance the antibody response.

> Advice in this chapter reflects that in the handbook *Immunisation against Infectious Disease* (2006), which in turn reflects the guidance of the Joint Committee on Vaccination and Immunisation (JCVI).
> Chapters from the handbook are available at www.dh.gov.uk
> The advice in this chapter also incorporates changes announced by the Chief Medical Officer and Health Department Updates.

**Cautions** Most individuals can safely receive the majority of vaccines. Vaccination may be postponed if the individual is suffering from an acute illness; however, it is not necessary to postpone immunisation in patients with minor illnesses without fever or systemic upset. See also Predisposition to Neurological Problems, below. For individuals with bleeding disorders, see Route of administration, below. If alcohol or disinfectant is used for cleansing the skin it should be allowed to

evaporate before vaccination to prevent possible inactivation of live vaccines.

When two live virus vaccines are required (and are not available as a combined preparation) they should be given either simultaneously at different sites or separated by an interval of at least 4 weeks. For **interactions** see Appendix 1 (vaccines).

*See also* Cautions under individual vaccines

**Contra-indications** Vaccines are contra-indicated in those who have a confirmed anaphylactic reaction to a preceding dose of a vaccine containing the same antigens or vaccine component (such as antibacterials in viral vaccines). The presence of the following excipients in vaccines and immunological products has been noted under the relevant entries:

| | | |
|---|---|---|
| Gelatin | Neomycin | Streptomycin |
| Gentamicin | Penicillins | Thiomersal |
| Kanamycin | Polymyxin B | |

*Hypersensitivity to egg* with evidence of previous anaphylactic reaction, contra-indicates influenza vaccine, tick-borne encephalitis vaccine, and yellow fever vaccine. See also Cautions under MMR vaccine.

See also Vaccines and HIV infection, below.

Live vaccines may be contra-indicated temporarily in individuals who are:

- immunosuppressed (see Impaired immune response, below);

- pregnant (see Pregnancy and breast-feeding, below).

*See also* Contra-indications under individual vaccines.

**Impaired immune response** Immune response to vaccines may be reduced in immunosuppressed patients and there is a risk of generalised infection with live vaccines. Severely immunosuppressed patients should not be given live vaccines (including those with severe primary immunodeficiency). Specialist advice should be sought for those being treated with high doses of corticosteroids (dose equivalents of prednisolone: **adults**, at least 40 mg daily for more than 1 week; **children**, 2 mg/kg daily for at least 1 week or 1 mg/kg daily for 1 month), or other immunosuppressive drugs[1], and those being treated for malignant conditions with chemotherapy or generalised radiotherapy[1,2]. For special reference to *HIV infection*, see below.

The Royal College of Paediatrics and Child Health has produced a statement, *Immunisation of the Immunocompromised Child (2002)* (available at www.rcpch.ac.uk).

1. Live vaccines should be postponed until at least 3 months after stopping high-dose systemic corticosteroids and at least 6 months after stopping other immunosuppressive drugs or generalised radiotherapy (at least 12 months after discontinuing immunosuppressants following bone-marrow transplantation).
2. Use of normal immunoglobulin should be considered after exposure to measles (see p. 691) and varicella–zoster immunoglobulin considered after exposure to chickenpox or herpes zoster (see p. 693).

**Pregnancy and breast-feeding** Live vaccines should not be administered routinely to *pregnant women* because of the theoretical risk of fetal infection but where there is a significant risk of exposure to disease (e.g. to yellow fever), the need for vaccination usually outweighs any possible risk to the fetus. Termination of pregnancy following inadvertent immunisation is not recommended. Although there is a theoretical risk of live vaccine being present in breast milk, vaccination is not contra-indicated for women who are breast-feeding when there is significant risk of exposure to disease. There is no evidence of risk from vaccinating pregnant women, or those who are breast-feeding, with inactivated viral or bacterial vaccines or toxoids. For use of specific vaccines during pregnancy or breast-feeding, see under individual vaccines.

**Side-effects** Injection of a vaccine may be followed by local reactions such as pain, inflammation, redness, and lymphangitis. An induration or sterile abscess may develop at the injection site. Gastro-intestinal disturbances, fever, headache, irritability, loss of appetite, fatigue, myalgia, and malaise are among the most commonly reported side-effects. Other side-effects include influenza-like symptoms, dizziness, paraesthesia, asthenia, drowsiness, arthralgia, rash, and lymphadenopathy. Hypersensitivity reactions, such as bronchospasm, angioedema, urticaria, and anaphylaxis, are very rare but can be fatal (see section 3.4.3 for management of allergic emergencies).

**Oral** vaccines such as cholera, live poliomyelitis, rotavirus, and live typhoid can also cause gastro-intestinal disturbances such as nausea, vomiting, abdominal pain and cramps, and diarrhoea.

*See also* Predisposition to neurological problems, below.

Some vaccines (e.g. poliomyelitis) produce very few reactions, while others (e.g. measles, mumps and rubella) may cause a very mild form of the disease. Occasionally more serious adverse reactions can occur—these should always be reported to the CHM (see Adverse Reactions to Drugs, p. 11).

There is no evidence that premature babies are at increased risk of adverse reactions from vaccines, see also Prematurity, below.

---

**Predisposition to neurological problems**

When there is a personal or family history of *febrile* convulsions, there is an increased risk of these occurring during fever from any cause including immunisation, but this is not a contra-indication to immunisation. In children who have had a seizure associated with fever without neurological deterioration, immunisation is *recommended*; advice on the *prevention of fever* (see Post-immunisation pyrexia in infants, above) should be given before immunisation. When a child has had a convulsion not associated with fever, and the neurological condition is not deteriorating, immunisation is *recommended*.

Children with stable neurological disorders (e.g. spina bifida, congenital brain abnormality, and perinatal hypoxic-ischaemic encephalopathy) should be immunised according to the recommended schedule. Where there is a *still evolving neurological problem*, including poorly controlled epilepsy, immunisation should be *deferred* and the child referred to a specialist. Immunisation is recommended if a cause for the neurological disorder is identified. If a cause is not identified, immunisation should be deferred until the condition is stable.

---

**Post-immunisation pyrexia in infants**

The parent should be advised that if pyrexia develops after childhood immunisation, the infant can be given a dose of paracetamol and, if necessary, a second dose given 6 hours later; ibuprofen may be used if paracetamol is unsuitable. The parent should be warned to seek medical advice if the pyrexia persists.

For post-immunisation pyrexia in an infant aged 2–3 months, the dose of paracetamol is 60 mg; the dose of ibuprofen is 50 mg (on doctor's advice). An oral syringe can be obtained from any pharmacy to give the small volume required.

---

Further information on adverse effects associated with specific vaccines can be found under individual vaccines.

**Vaccines and HIV infection** HIV-positive individuals with or without symptoms can receive the following live vaccines:

MMR (but avoid if immunity significantly impaired), varicella-zoster (but avoid if immunity significantly impaired—consult product literature);[1,2]

and the following inactivated vaccines:

anthrax, cholera (oral), diphtheria, haemophilus influenzae type b, hepatitis A, hepatitis B, human papilloma virus, influenza, meningococcal, pertussis, pneumococcal, poliomyelitis, rabies, tetanus, tick-borne encephalitis, typhoid (injection).

HIV-positive individuals should **not** receive:

BCG, typhoid (oral), yellow fever[3]

**Note** The above advice differs from that for other immunocompromised patients; *Immunisation Guidelines for HIV-infected Adults* issued by *British HIV Association* (BHIVA) are available at www.bhiva.org and, *Immunisation of HIV-infected Children* issued by *Children's HIV Association* (CHIVA) are available at www.chiva.org.uk

**Vaccines and asplenia** The following vaccines are recommended for asplenic patients or those with splenic dysfunction:

haemophilus influenzae type b, influenza, meningococcal group C, pneumococcal.

For antibiotic prophylaxis in asplenia see p. 293.

**Route of administration** Vaccines should not be given intravenously. Most vaccines are given by the intramuscular route; some vaccines are given by others routes—the intradermal route for BCG vaccine, deep subcutaneous route for Japanese encephalitis, and varicella vaccine, and the oral route for cholera, live poliomyelitis, rotavirus, and live typhoid vaccines. The intramuscular route should not be used in patients with **bleeding disorders** such as haemophilia or thrombocytopenia. Vaccines usually given by the intramuscular route should be given by deep subcutaneous injection instead.

**Note** The Department of Health has advised *against the use of jet guns* for vaccination owing to the risk of transmitting blood-borne infections, such as HIV.

---

1. Use of normal immunoglobulin should be considered after exposure to measles (see p. 691) and varicella–zoster immunoglobulin considered after exposure to chickenpox or herpes zoster (see p. 693).
2. The Royal College of Paediatrics and Child Health recommends that MMR is not given to a child with HIV infection whilst severely immunosuppressed.
3. If yellow fever risk is unavoidable, specialist advice should be sought.

14 Immunological products and vaccines

# Immunisation schedule

Vaccines for the childhood immunisation schedule should be obtained from **local health organisations** or **direct from Movianto**—not to be prescribed on FP10 (HS21 in Northern Ireland; GP10 in Scotland; WP10 in Wales).

## Prematurity

Children born prematurely should receive all routine immunisations based on the actual date of birth. There is no evidence that premature infants are at increased risk of adverse reactions directly related to vaccines. However, for those in neonatal units with cardiorespiratory problems, and those infants who have had one or more apnoeic attacks in the 24 hours prior to immunisation, it may be appropriate to monitor for apnoea for 48 hours after immunistaion. Seroconversion may be unreliable in babies born earlier than 28 weeks' gestation or in babies treated with corticosteroids for chronic lung disease; consideration should be given to testing for antibodies against *Haemophilus influenzae* (type b), meningococcal C, and hepatitis B after primary immunisation.

| When to immunise (for premature infants—see note above) | Vaccine given and dose schedule (for details of dose, see under individual vaccines) |
|---|---|
| Neonates at risk only | • **BCG Vaccine**<br>See section 14.4, BCG Vaccines<br>• **Hepatitis B Vaccine**<br>See section 14.4, Hepatitis B Vaccine |
| 2 months | • **Diptheria, Tetanus, Pertussis (Acellular, Component), Poliomyelitis (Inactivated), and Haemophilus Type b Conjugate Vaccine (Adsorbed)**<br>First dose<br>• **Pneumococcal Polysaccharide Conjugate Vaccine (Adsorbed)**<br>First dose |
| 3 months | • **Diptheria, Tetanus, Pertussis (Acellular, Component), Poliomyelitis (Inactivated), and Haemophilus Type b Conjugate Vaccine (Adsorbed)**<br>Second dose<br>• **Meningococcal Group C Conjugate Vaccine**<br>First dose |
| 4 months | • **Diphtheria, Tetanus, Pertussis (Acellular, Component), Poliomyelitis (Inactivated), and Haemophilus Type b Conjugate Vaccine (Adsorbed)**<br>Third dose<br>• **Meningococcal Group C Conjugate Vaccine**<br>Second dose<br>• **Pneumococcal Polysaccharide Conjugate Vaccine (Adsorbed)**<br>Second dose |
| 12 months | • **Haemophilus Type b Conjugate Vaccine and Meningococcal Group C Conjugate Vaccine**<br>Single booster dose |
| 13 months | • **Measles, Mumps and Rubella Vaccine, Live (MMR)**<br>First dose<br>• **Pneumococcal Polysaccharide Conjugate Vaccine (Adsorbed)**<br>Single booster dose |
| Between 3 years and 4 months, and 5 years | • **Adsorbed Diphtheria [low dose], Tetanus, Pertussis (Acellular, Component) and Poliomyelitis (Inactivated) Vaccine**<br>*or*<br>**Adsorbed Diphtheria, Tetanus, Pertussis (Acellular, Component) and Poliomyelitis (Inactivated) Vaccine**<br>*or*<br>**Diphtheria, Tetanus, Pertussis (Acellular, Component) Poliomyelitis (Inactivated) and Haemophilus Type b Conjugate Vaccine (Adsorbed)**<br>Single booster dose<br>**Note:** Preferably allow interval of at least 3 years after completing primary course; can be given at same session as MMR Vaccine but use separate syringe and needle, and give in different limb<br>• **Measles, Mumps and Rubella Vaccine, Live (MMR)**<br>Second dose |
| 12–13 years (females only) | • **Human Papilloma Virus Vaccine**<br>3 doses; second dose 1–2 months, and third dose 6 months after first dose[1,2] |
| 13–18 years | • **Adsorbed Diphtheria [low dose], Tetanus, and Poliomyelitis (Inactivated) Vaccine**<br>Single booster dose |
| During adult life<br>Women of child-bearing age susceptible to rubella | • **Measles, Mumps and Rubella Vaccine, Live (MMR)**<br>Women of child-bearing age who have not received 2 doses of a rubella-containing vaccine or who do not have a positive antibody test for rubella should be offered rubella immunisation (using the MMR vaccine)—exclude pregnancy before immunisation, but see also section 14.4, Measles, Mumps and Rubella Vaccine |
| During adult life<br>If not previously immunised | • **Adsorbed Diphtheria [low dose], Tetanus, and Poliomyelitis (Inactivated) Vaccine**<br>3 doses at intervals of 1 month<br>Booster dose at least 1 year after primary course and again 5–10 years later |

1. The two human papilloma virus vaccines are not interchangeable and one vaccine product should be used for the entire course; however for individuals with previous incomplete vaccination with *Gardasil*® who are eligible for HPV vaccination under the national programme, *Cervarix*® can be used to complete the vaccination course if necessary; the individual must be informed that *Cervarix*® does not protect against genital warts.
2. For females aged 14 to under 18 years, see 'Catch-Up' Programme, p. 679.

14

Immunological products and vaccines

## High-risk groups

For information on high-risk groups, see section 14.4 under individual vaccines

BCG Vaccines

Hepatitis A Vaccine

Hepatitis B Vaccine

Influenza Vaccine

Pneumococcal Vaccines

Tetanus Vaccines

## 14.2 Passive immunity

Immunity with immediate protection against certain infective organisms can be obtained by injecting preparations made from the plasma of immune individuals with adequate levels of antibody to the disease for which protection is sought (see under Immunoglobulins, section 14.5). The duration of this passive immunity varies according to the dose and the type of immunoglobulin. Passive immunity may last only a few weeks; when necessary, passive immunisation can be repeated.

Antibodies of human origin are usually termed *immunoglobulins*. The term *antiserum* is applied to material prepared in animals. Because of serum sickness and other allergic-type reactions that may follow injections of antisera, this therapy has been replaced wherever possible by the use of immunoglobulins. Reactions are theoretically possible after injection of human immunoglobulins but reports of such reactions are very rare.

## 14.3 Storage and use

Care must be taken to store all vaccines and other immunological products under the conditions recommended in the product literature, otherwise the preparation may become ineffective. **Refrigerated storage** is usually necessary; many vaccines and immunoglobulins need to be stored at 2–8°C and not allowed to freeze. Vaccines and immunoglobulins should be protected from light. Reconstituted vaccines and opened multidose vials must be used within the period recommended in the product literature. Unused vaccines should be disposed of by incineration at a registered disposal contractor.

Particular attention must be paid to instructions on the use of diluents. Vaccines which are liquid suspensions or are reconstituted before use should be adequately mixed to ensure uniformity of the material to be injected.

## 14.4 Vaccines and antisera

**Availability** Anthrax and yellow fever vaccines, botulism antitoxin, diphtheria antitoxin, and snake and spider venom antitoxins are available from local designated holding centres.

For antivenom, see Emergency Treatment of Poisoning, p. 36.

Enquiries for vaccines not available commercially can also be made to:

Immunisation Policy, Monitoring and Surveillance
Department of Health
Wellington House
133–155 Waterloo Road
London, SE1 8UG
Tel: (020) 7972 4047

In Scotland information about availability of vaccines can be obtained from a Specialist in Pharmaceutical Public Health. In Wales enquiries for vaccines not available commercially should be directed to:

Welsh Medicines Information Centre
University Hospital of Wales
Cardiff, CF14 4XW
Tel: (029) 2074 2979

and in Northern Ireland:

Regional Pharmacist (procurement co-ordination)-
United Hospitals Trust Pharmacy Dept
Whiteabbey Hospital
Doagh Road
Newtownabbey, BT37 9RH
Tel: (028) 9086 5181 ext 2386

For further details of availability, see under individual vaccines.

## Anthrax vaccine

Anthrax vaccine is made from antigens from *B. anthracis*. Anthrax immunisation is indicated for individuals who handle infected animals, for those exposed to imported infected animal products, and for laboratory staff who work with *Bacillus anthracis*. A 4-dose regimen is used for primary immunisation; booster doses should be given annually to workers at continued risk of exposure to anthrax.

In the event of possible contact with *B. anthracis*, post-exposure immunisation may be indicated, in addition to antimicrobial prophylaxis (section 5.1.12). Advice on the use of anthrax vaccine for post-exposure prophylaxis must be obtained from the Centre for Infections, Health Protection Agency (tel. 020 8200 4400).

### ■ ANTHRAX VACCINE

**Indications** pre-exposure immunisation against anthrax; post-exposure immunisation (see notes above)

**Cautions** see section 14.1

**Contra-indications** see section 14.1

**Side-effects** see section 14.1

**Dose**

- By intramuscular injection in deltoid region, initial course 3 doses of 0.5 mL at intervals of 3 weeks followed by a fourth dose after an interval of 6 months; booster, 0.5 mL every 12 months

**Anthrax Vaccine** (PoM)

Injection, suspension of anthrax antigens (not less than 0.125 mL/0.5 mL dose), sterile filtrate, adsorbed on to aluminium potassium sulphate
Excipients include thiomersal
Available from the Health Protection Agency's Centre for Emergency Preparedness and Response (Porton Down)

# BCG vaccines

BCG (Bacillus Calmette-Guérin) is a live attenuated strain derived from *Mycobacterium bovis* which stimulates the development of hypersensitivity to *M. tuberculosis*. BCG vaccine should be given intradermally by operators skilled in the technique (see below).

The expected reaction to successful BCG vaccination is induration at the site of injection followed by a local lesion which starts as a papule 2 or more weeks after vaccination; the lesion may ulcerate then subside over several weeks or months, leaving a small, flat scar. A dry dressing may be used if the ulcer discharges, but air should **not** be excluded.

Apart from children under 6 years, any person being considered for BCG immunisation must first be given a skin test for hypersensitivity to tuberculoprotein (see under Diagnostic Agents, below). A skin test is not necessary for a child under 6 years provided that the child has not stayed for longer than 3 months in a country with an incidence of tuberculosis greater than 40 per 100 000, the child has not had contact with a person with tuberculosis, and there is no family history of tuberculosis within the last 5 years.

BCG is recommended for the following groups if BCG immunisation has not previously been carried out:

- all neonates and infants (0–12 months) born in areas where the incidence[1] of tuberculosis is greater than 40 per 100 000;

- neonates, infants, and children under 16 years with a parent or grandparent born in a country with an incidence[1] of tuberculosis greater than 40 per 100 000;

- new immigrants aged under 16 years who were born in, or lived for more than 3 months in a country with an incidence[1] of tuberculosis greater than 40 per 100 000;

- new immigrants aged 16–35 years from Sub-Saharan Africa or a country with an incidence[1] of tuberculosis greater than 500 per 100 000

- contacts aged under 36 years of those with active respiratory tuberculosis (for healthcare or laboratory workers who have had contact with clinical materials or patients with tuberculosis, age limit does not apply);

- healthcare workers and laboratory staff (irrespective of age) who are likely to have contact with patients, clinical materials, or derived isolates; other individuals under 35 years[2] at occupational risk including veterinary and other staff who handle animal species susceptible to tuberculosis, and staff working directly with prisoners, in care homes for the elderly, or in hostels or facilities for the homeless or refugees;

- individuals under 16 years intending to live with local people for more than 3 months in a country with an incidence[1] of tuberculosis greater than 40 per 100 000 (section 14.6).

BCG vaccine can be given simultaneously with another live vaccine (see also section 14.1), but if they are not given at the same time an interval of 4 weeks should normally be allowed. When BCG is given to infants, there is no need to delay routine primary immunisa-

tions. No further vaccination should be given in the arm used for BCG vaccination for at least 3 months because of the risk of regional lymphadenitis.

Bladder instillations of BCG are licensed for the management of bladder carcinoma (section 8.2.4).

For advice on chemoprophylaxis against tuberculosis, see section 5.1.9; for the treatment of infection following vaccination, seek expert advice.

## ▊ BACILLUS CALMETTE-GUÉRIN VACCINE
### BCG Vaccine

**Indications** immunisation against tuberculosis

**Cautions** see section 14.1; **interactions:** Appendix 1 (vaccines)

**Contra-indications** see section 14.1; *also* neonate in household contact with known or suspected case of active tuberculosis; generalised septic skin conditions (for patients with eczema, lesion-free site should be used)

**Side-effects** see section 14.1 and notes above; *also* at the injection site, subcutaneous abscess, prolonged ulceration; *rarely* disseminated complications such as osteitis or osteomyelitis

**Dose**

- By intradermal injection ADULT and CHILD over 1 year, 0.1 mL; NEONATE and CHILD under 1 year, 0.05 mL
  **Intradermal injection technique** Skin is stretched between thumb and forefinger and needle (size 25G or 26G) inserted (bevel upwards) for about 3 mm into superficial layers of dermis (almost parallel with surface). Needle should be short with short bevel (can usually be seen through epidermis during insertion). Tense raised blanched bleb showing tips of hair follicles is sign of correct injection; 7 mm bleb ≡ 0.1 mL injection, 3 mm bleb ≡ 0.05 mL injection; if considerable resistance not felt, needle too deep and should be removed and reinserted before giving more vaccine.
  To be injected at insertion of deltoid muscle onto humerus (keloid formation more likely with sites higher on arm); tip of shoulder should be **avoided**.

▐ Intradermal
**Bacillus Calmette-Guérin Vaccine** [PoM]
BCG Vaccine, Dried/Tub/BCG
  Injection (powder for suspension), freeze-dried preparation of live bacteria of a strain derived from the bacillus of Calmette and Guérin.
  Available from health organisations or direct from Movianto (SSI brand, multidose vial with diluent)

## Diagnostic agents

The *Mantoux test* is recommended for tuberculin skin testing, but no licensed preparation is currently available. Guidance for healthcare professionals is available at www.immunisation.nhs.uk.

In the Mantoux test, the diagnostic dose is administered by intradermal injection of Tuberculin Purified Protein Derivative (PPD).

The *Heaf test* (involving the use of multiple-puncture apparatus) is no longer available.

**Note** Response to tuberculin may be suppressed by live viral vaccines, viral infection, sarcoidosis, corticosteroid therapy, or immunosuppression due to disease or treatment. Tuberculin testing should not be carried out within 4 weeks of receiving a live viral vaccine.

---

1. List of countries or primary care trusts where the incidence of tuberculosis is greater than 40 cases per 100 000 is available at www.hpa.org.uk

2. There is inadequate evidence of protection by BCG vaccine in adults aged over 35 years; however, vaccination is recommended for healthcare workers irrespective of age because of the increased risk to them or their patients

Two interferon gamma release assay (IGRA) tests are also available as an aid in the diagnosis of tuberculosis infection: QuanitFERON® TB Gold and T-SPOT®.TB. Both tests measure T-cell mediated immune response to synthetic antigens. For further information on the use of interferon gamma release assay tests for tuberculosis, see www.hpa.org.uk.

### Tuberculin Purified Protein Derivative [PoM]
(Tuberculin PPD)

Injection, heat-treated products of growth and lysis of appropriate *Mycobacterium* spp. 20 units/mL (2 units/0.1-mL dose) (for routine use), 1.5-mL vial; 100 units/mL (10 units/0.1-mL dose), 1.5-mL vial

**Dose** by intradermal injection, for Mantoux test, 2 units (0.1 mL of 20 units/mL strength) for routine Mantoux test; if first test is negative and a further test is considered appropriate 10 units (0.1 mL of 100 units/mL strength)

Available from Movianto (SSI brand)

**Note** The strength of tuberculin PPD in this product may be different to the strengths of products used previously for the Mantoux test; care is required to select the correct strength

## Botulism antitoxin

A polyvalent botulism antitoxin is available for the post-exposure prophylaxis of botulism and for the treatment of persons thought to be suffering from botulism. It specifically neutralises the toxins produced by *Clostridium botulinum* types A, B, and E. It is not effective against infantile botulism as the toxin (type A) is seldom, if ever, found in the blood in this type of infection.

Hypersensitivity reactions are a problem. It is essential to read the contra-indications, warnings, and details of sensitivity tests on the package insert. Prior to treatment checks should be made regarding previous administration of any antitoxin and history of any allergic condition, e.g. asthma, hay fever, etc. All patients should be tested for sensitivity (diluting the antitoxin if history of allergy).

### Botulism Antitoxin [PoM]
A preparation containing the specific antitoxic globulins that have the power of neutralising the toxins formed by types A, B, and E of *Clostridium botulinum*.

**Note** The BP title Botulinum Antitoxin is not used because the preparation currently in use may have a different specification.

**Dose** prophylaxis, consult product literature

Available from local designated centres, for details see TOXBASE (requires registration) www.toxbase.org. For supplies outside working hours apply to other designated centres or to the duty doctor at the Health Protection Agency (Tel (020) 8200 6868). For major incidents, obtain supplies from the local blood bank

## Cholera vaccine

**Cholera vaccine** (oral) contains inactivated Inaba (including El-Tor biotype) and Ogawa strains of *Vibrio cholerae*, serotype O1 together with recombinant B-subunit of the cholera toxin produced in Inaba strains of *V.cholerae*, serotype O1.

Oral cholera vaccine is licensed for travellers to endemic or epidemic areas on the basis of current recommendations (see also section 14.6). Immunisation should be completed at least 1 week before potential exposure. However, there is no requirement for cholera vaccination for international travel.

Immunisation with cholera vaccine does not provide complete protection and all travellers to a country where cholera exists should be warned that scrupulous attention to food, water, and personal hygiene is **essential**.

*Injectable cholera vaccine provides unreliable protection and is no longer available in the UK.*

### ▍ CHOLERA VACCINE

**Indications** see notes above

**Cautions** see section 14.1 and notes above

**Contra-indications** see section 14.1

**Side-effects** see section 14.1; also *rarely* respiratory symptoms such as rhinitis and cough; *very rarely* sore throat, insomnia

**Dose**

- ADULT and CHILD over 6 years 2 doses separated by an interval of 1–6 weeks; CHILD 2–6 years 3 doses each separated by an interval of 1–6 weeks

  **Note** If more than 6 weeks have elapsed between doses, the primary course should be restarted

- A single booster dose can be given 2 years after primary course for adults and children over 6 years, and 6 months after primary course for children 2–6 years. If more than 2 years have elapsed since the last vaccination, the primary course should be repeated

  **Counselling** Dissolve effervescent sodium bicarbonate granules in a glassful of water (approximately 150 mL). For adults and children over 6 years, add vaccine suspension to make one dose. For child 2–6 years, discard half (approximately 75 mL) of the solution, then add vaccine suspension to make one dose. Drink within 2 hours. Food, drink, and other oral medicines should be avoided for 1 hour before and after vaccination

**Dukoral®** (Novartis Vaccines) [PoM]
Oral suspension, for dilution with solution of effervescent sodium bicarbonate granules, heat- and formaldehyde-inactivated Inaba (including El-Tor biotype) and Ogawa strains of *Vibrio cholerae* bacteria and recombinant cholera toxin B-subunit produced in *V. cholerae*, net price 2-dose pack = £23.42. Counselling, administration

## Diphtheria vaccines

Diphtheria vaccines are prepared from the toxin of *Corynebacterium diphtheriae* and adsorption on aluminium hydroxide or aluminium phosphate improves antigenicity. The vaccine stimulates the production of the protective antitoxin. The quantity of diphtheria toxoid in a preparation determines whether the vaccine is defined as 'high dose' or 'low dose'. Vaccines containing the higher dose of diphtheria toxoid are used for primary immunisation of children under 10 years of age. Vaccines containing the lower dose of diphtheria toxoid are used for primary immunisation in adults and children over 10 years. Single-antigen diphtheria vaccine is not available and adsorbed diphtheria vaccine is given as a combination product containing other vaccines.

For primary immunisation *of children aged between 2 months and 10 years* vaccination is recommended usually in the form of 3 doses (separated by 1-month intervals) of **diphtheria, tetanus, pertussis (acellular, component), poliomyelitis (inactivated) and haemophilus type b conjugate vaccine (adsorbed)** (see Immunisation schedule, section 14.1). In unimmunised individuals aged *over 10 years* the primary course comprises of 3 doses of **adsorbed diphtheria** [low dose], **tetanus and poliomyelitis (inactivated) vaccine**.

A booster dose should be given 3 years after the primary course (this interval can be reduced to a minimum of 1 year if the primary course was delayed). Children *under 10 years* should receive *either* adsorbed diphtheria, tetanus, pertussis (acellular, component) and poliomyelitis (inactivated) vaccine *or* adsorbed diphtheria [low dose], tetanus, pertussis (acellular, component) and poliomyelitis (inactivated) vaccine. Individuals aged *over 10 years* should receive adsorbed diphtheria [low dose], tetanus, and poliomyelitis (inactivated) vaccine.

A second booster dose, of adsorbed diphtheria [low dose], tetanus and poliomyelitis (inactivated) vaccine, should be given 10 years after the previous booster dose (this interval can be reduced to a minimum of 5 years if previous doses were delayed).

**Travel** Those intending to travel to areas with a risk of diphtheria infection should be fully immunised according to the UK schedule (see also section 14.6). If more than 10 years have lapsed since completion of the UK schedule, a dose of **adsorbed diphtheria** [low dose], **tetanus and poliomyelitis (inactivated) vaccine** should be administered.

**Contacts** Staff in contact with diphtheria patients or with potentially pathogenic clinical specimens or working directly with *C. diphtheriae* or *C. ulcerans* should receive a booster dose if fully immunised (with 5 doses of diphtheria-containing vaccine given at appropriate intervals); further doses should be given at 10-year intervals if risk persists. Individuals at risk who are not fully immunised should complete the primary course; a booster dose should be given after 5 years and then at 10-year intervals. **Adsorbed diphtheria** [low dose], **tetanus and poliomyelitis (inactivated) vaccine** is used for this purpose; immunity should be checked by antibody testing at least 3 months after completion of immunisation.

Advice on the management of cases, carriers, contacts and outbreaks must be sought from health protection units. The immunisation history of infected individuals and their contacts should be determined; those who have been incompletely immunised should complete their immunisation and fully immunised individuals should receive a reinforcing dose. For advice on antibacterial treatment to prevent a secondary case of diphtheria in a non-immune individual, see Table 2, section 5.1.

---

### ◢ DIPHTHERIA-CONTAINING VACCINES

**Indications** see notes above

**Cautions** see section 14.1 and see also individual components of vaccines

**Contra-indications** see section 14.1 and see also individual components of vaccines

**Side-effects** see section 14.1; also restlessness, sleep disturbances, and unusual crying in infants

**Dose**
- See under preparations

### ◢Diphtheria-containing vaccines for children under 10 years

**Important** Not recommended for persons *aged 10 years or over* (see Diphtheria-containing Vaccines for Children over 10 years and Adults, below)

### Diphtheria, Tetanus, Pertussis (Acellular, Component), Poliomyelitis (Inactivated) and Haemophilus Type b Conjugate Vaccine (Adsorbed) [PoM]

Injection, suspension of diphtheria toxoid, tetanus toxoid, acellular pertussis, inactivated poliomyelitis and *Haemophilus influenzae* type b (conjugated to tetanus protein), net price 0.5-mL vial = £19.94
**Excipients** may include neomycin, polymyxin B and streptomycin
**Dose** by intramuscular injection, CHILD 2 months–10 years, primary immunisation, 3 doses each of 0.5 mL separated by intervals of 1 month; see also notes on booster doses, above
Brands include *Infanrix-IPV+Hib*®, *Pediacel*®; available as part of childhood immunisation schedule, from health organisations or Movianto

### Adsorbed Diphtheria, Tetanus, Pertussis (Acellular, Component) and Poliomyelitis (Inactivated) Vaccine [PoM]

Injection, suspension of diphtheria toxoid, tetanus toxoid, acellular pertussis and inactivated poliomyelitis vaccine components adsorbed on a mineral carrier, net price 0.5-mL prefilled syringe = £17.56
**Excipients** may include neomycin and polymyxin B
**Dose** by intramuscular injection, CHILD 3–10 years, first booster dose 3 years after primary immunisation, 0.5 mL; *see also* notes on booster doses, above
Brands include *Infanrix-IPV*®; available as part of childhood immunisation schedule, from health organisations or Movianto

### Adsorbed Diphtheria [low dose], Tetanus, Pertussis (Acellular, Component) and Poliomyelitis (Inactivated) Vaccine [PoM]

Injection, suspension of diphtheria toxoid [low dose], tetanus toxoid, acellular pertussis and inactivated poliomyelitis vaccine components adsorbed on a mineral carrier, net price 0.5-mL prefilled syringe = £11.98
**Excipients** may include neomycin, polymyxin B and streptomycin
**Dose** by intramuscular injection, CHILD 3–10 years, first booster dose 3 years after primary immunisation, 0.5 mL; *see also* notes on booster doses, above
Brands include *Repevax*®; available as part of childhood immunisation schedule, from health organisations or Movianto

### ◢Diphtheria-containing vaccines for children over 10 years and adults

A **low dose** of diphtheria toxoid is sufficient to recall immunity in individuals previously immunised against diphtheria but whose immunity may have diminished with time; it is insufficient to cause serious reactions in an individual who is already immune. Preparations containing low dose diphtheria should be used for adults and children *over 10 years*, for both primary immunisation and booster doses.

### Adsorbed Diphtheria [low dose], Tetanus and Poliomyelitis (Inactivated) Vaccine [PoM]

Injection, suspension of diphtheria toxoid [low dose], tetanus toxoid and inactivated poliomyelitis vaccine components adsorbed on a mineral carrier, net price 0.5-mL prefilled syringe = £6.48
**Excipients** may include neomycin, polymyxin B and streptomycin
**Dose** by intramuscular injection, ADULT and CHILD over 10 years, primary immunisation, 3 doses each of 0.5 mL separated by intervals of 1 month; second booster dose, 0.5 mL given 10 years after first booster dose (may also be used as first booster dose in those over 10 years who have received only 3 previous doses of a diphtheria-containing vaccine); see also notes on booster doses and contacts, above
Brands include *Revaxis*®; available as part of immunisation schedule, from health organisations or Movianto

**14**

**Immunological products and vaccines**

◢Diphtheria antitoxin

**Diphtheria antitoxin** is used for passive immunisation in suspected cases of diphtheria only (without waiting for bacteriological confirmation); tests for hypersensitivity should be first carried out. It is derived from horse serum, and reactions are common after administration; resuscitation facilities should be available immediately.

It is no longer used for prophylaxis because of the risk of hypersensitivity; unimmunised contacts should be promptly investigated and given antibacterial prophylaxis (section 5.1, table 2) and vaccine (see Contacts above).

**Diphtheria Antitoxin** PoM
Dip/Ser

**Dose** prophylaxis, not recommended therefore no dose stated (see notes above)

Treatment, consult product literature

Available from Centre for Infections (Tel (020) 8200 6868) or in Northern Ireland from Public Health Laboratory, Belfast City Hospital (Tel (028) 9032 9241)

---

## Haemophilus type B conjugate vaccine

**Haemophilus influenzae type b (Hib) vaccine** is made from capsular polysaccharide; it is conjugated with a protein such as tetanus toxoid to increase immunogenicity, especially in young children. Haemophilus influenzae type b vaccine immunisation is given in combination with diptheria, tetanus, pertussis (acellular, component) and poliomyelitis (inactivated) vaccine, as a component of the primary course of childhood immunisation (see Immunisation schedule, section 14.1) (see under Diphtheria-containing Vaccines). For infants under 1 year, the course consists of 3 doses of a vaccine containing haemophilus influenzae type b component with an interval of 1 month between doses. A booster dose of haemophilus influenzae type b vaccine (combined with meningococcal group C conjugate vaccine) should be given at around 12 months of age.

Children 1–10 years who have not been immunised against *Haemophilus influenzae* type b need to receive only 1 dose of Haemophilus influenzae type b vaccine (combined with meningococcal group C conjuate vaccine). However, if a primary course of immunisation has not been completed, these children should be given 3 doses of diphtheria, tetanus, pertussis (acellular, component), poliomyelitis (inactivated) and haemophilus type b conjugate vaccine (adsorbed). The risk of infection falls sharply in older children and the vaccine is not normally required for children over 10 years.

Haemophilus influenzae type b vaccine may be given to those over 10 years who are considered to be at increased risk of invasive *H. influenzae* type b disease (such as those with sickle-cell disease and those receiving treatment for malignancy).

For use of Rifampicin in the prevention of secondary cases of *Haemophilus influenzae type b* disease, see Table 2, section 5.1.

**Asplenia or splenic dysfunction**   Haemophilus influenzae type b vaccine is recommended for patients with asplenia or splenic dysfunction. Immunised adults and children over 1 year, who develop splenic dysfunction, should be given 1 additional dose of haemophilus influenzae type b vaccine (combined with meningococcal group C conjugate vaccine). For elective splenec-

tomy, the vaccine should ideally be given at least 2 weeks before surgery. Adults and children over 1 year, who are not immunised against haemophilus influenzae type b, should be given 2 doses of haemophilus influenzae type b vaccine (combined with meningococcal group C conjugate vaccine) with an interval of 2 months between doses. However, children under 10 years, who are not immunised against diphtheria, tetanus, pertussis, poliomyelitis, and haemophilus influenzae type b should be given 3 doses (with an interval of 1 month between doses) of combined diphtheria, tetanus, pertussis (acellular component), poliomyelitis (inactivated) and haemophilus type b conjugate vaccine.

## ◼ HAEMOPHILUS TYPE B CONJUGATE VACCINE

**Indications** see notes above

**Cautions** see section 14.1

**Contra-indications** see section 14.1

**Side-effects** see section 14.1; also atopic dermatitis and hypotonia

**Dose**

- Primary immunisation, see under Diphtheria
- Booster dose, see notes above and under preparation below

**Menitorix®** (GSK) PoM

Injection, powder for reconstitution, capsular polysaccharide of *Haemophilus influenzae* type b and capsular polysaccharide of *Neisseria meningitidis* group C (both conjugated to tetanus protein), net price single-dose vial (with syringe containing 0.5 mL diluent) = £39.87

**Dose** by intramuscular injection, CHILD 1–10 years, 0.5 mL
ADULT and CHILD over 1 year, with asplenia or splenic dysfunction (see notes above), 0.5 mL

Available as part of the childhood immunisation schedule from Movianto

◢Combined vaccines

See also under Diphtheria-containing Vaccines

---

## Hepatitis A vaccine

**Hepatitis A vaccine** is prepared from formaldehyde-inactivated hepatitis A virus grown in human diploid cells.

Immunisation is recommended for:

- laboratory staff who work directly with the virus;
- staff and residents of homes for those with severe learning difficulties;
- workers at risk of exposure to untreated sewage;
- individuals who work with primates;
- patients with haemophilia treated with plasma-derived clotting factors;
- patients with severe liver disease;
- travellers to high-risk areas (see p. 695);
- individuals who are at risk due to their sexual behaviour;
- parenteral drug abusers.

Immunisation should be considered for :

- patients with chronic liver disease including chronic hepatitis B or chronic hepatitis C;

*Immunological products and vaccines*

**14**

- prevention of secondary cases in close contacts of confirmed cases of hepatitis A, within 7 days of onset of disease in the primary case.

A booster dose is usually given 6–12 months after the initial dose. A second booster dose can be given 20 years after the previous booster dose to those who continue to be at risk. Specialist advice should be sought on re-immunisation of immunocompromised individuals.

For rapid protection against hepatitis A after exposure or during an outbreak, in adults a single dose of a monovalent vaccine is recommended; for children under 16 years, a single dose of the combined vaccine *Ambirix®* can also be used.

Intramuscular **normal immunoglobulin** (section 14.5.1) is recommended for use in addition to Hepatitis A vaccine, for contacts of patients with delayed confirmation of hepatitis A infection, or for individuals at high-risk of severe disease.

## ◼ HEPATITIS A VACCINE

**Indications** immunisation against hepatitis A infection
**Cautions** see section 14.1
**Contra-indications** see section 14.1
**Side-effects** see section 14.1; for combination vaccines, see also Typhoid vaccine, p. 688
**Dose**
- See under preparations

### ◢ Single component

**Avaxim®** (Sanofi Pasteur) PoM
Injection, suspension of formaldehyde-inactivated hepatitis A virus (GBM grown in human diploid cells) 320 antigen units/mL adsorbed onto aluminium hydroxide, net price 0.5-mL prefilled syringe = £18.44
Excipients include neomycin
Dose by intramuscular injection (see note below), ADULT and CHILD over 16 years, 0.5 mL as a single dose; booster dose 0.5 mL 6–12 months after initial dose
Note Booster dose may be delayed by up to 3 years if not given after recommended interval following primary dose with *Avaxim®*. The deltoid region is the preferred site of injection. The subcutaneous route may be used for patients with bleeding disorders; not to be injected into the buttock (vaccine efficacy reduced)

**Epaxal®** (MASTA) PoM
Injection, suspension of formaldehyde-inactivated hepatitis A virus (RG-SB grown in human diploid cells) at least 48 units/mL, net price 0.5-mL prefilled syringe = £23.81
Dose by intramuscular injection (see note below), ADULT and CHILD over 1 year, 0.5 mL as a single dose; booster dose 0.5 mL 6–12 months after initial dose (1–6 months if splenectomised)
Note Booster dose may be delayed by up to 4 years in adults if not given after recommended interval following primary dose. The deltoid region is the preferred site of injection. The subcutaneous route may be used for patients with bleeding disorders
Important *Epaxal®* contains influenza virus haemagglutinin grown in the allantoic cavity of chick embryos, therefore contra-indicated in those hypersensitive to eggs or chicken protein.

**Havrix Monodose®** (GSK) PoM
Injection, suspension of formaldehyde-inactivated hepatitis A virus (HM 175 grown in human diploid cells) 1440 ELISA units/mL adsorbed onto aluminium hydroxide, net price 1-mL prefilled syringe = £22.14, 0.5-mL (720 ELISA units) prefilled syringe (*Havrix Junior Monodose®*) = £16.77
Excipients include neomycin
Dose by intramuscular injection (see note below), ADULT and CHILD over 16 years, 1 mL as a single dose; booster dose, 1 mL 6–

12 months after initial dose; CHILD 1–15 years 0.5 mL; booster dose, 0.5 mL 6–12 months after initial dose
Note Booster dose may be delayed by up to 3 years if not given after recommended interval following primary dose with *Havrix Monodose®*. The deltoid region is the preferred site of injection. The subcutaneous route may be used for patients with bleeding disorders

**Vaqta® Paediatric** (Sanofi Pasteur) PoM
Injection, suspension of formaldehyde-inactivated hepatitis A virus (grown in human diploid cells) 50 antigen units/mL adsorbed onto aluminium hydroxyphosphate sulphate, net price 0.5-mL prefilled syringe = £15.04
Excipients include neomycin
Dose by intramuscular injection (see note below) CHILD 1–17 years, 0.5 mL as a single dose; booster dose 0.5 mL 6–18 months after initial dose; under 1 year, not recommended
Note The deltoid region is the preferred site of injection. The subcutaneous route may be used for patients with bleeding disorders (but immune response may be reduced)

### ◢ With hepatitis B vaccine

**Ambirix®** (GSK) ▼ PoM
Injection, suspension of inactivated hepatitis A virus (grown in human diploid cells) 720 ELISA units/mL adsorbed onto aluminium hydroxide, and recombinant (DNA) hepatitis B surface antigen (grown in yeast cells) 20 micrograms/mL adsorbed onto aluminium phosphate, net price 1-mL prefilled syringe = £31.18
Excipients include neomycin and traces of thiomersal
Dose CHILD 1–15 years, by intramuscular injection (see note below); primary course, 2 doses of 1 mL, the second 6–12 months after initial dose
Note Primary course should be completed with *Ambirix®* (single component vaccines given at appropriate intervals may be used for booster dose); the deltoid region is the preferred site of injection in older children; anterolateral thigh is the preferred site in infants; not to be injected into the buttock (vaccine efficacy reduced); subcutaneous route used for patients with bleeding disorders (but immune response may be reduced)
Important *Ambirix®* is **not** recommended for post-exposure prophylaxis following percutaneous (needle-stick), ocular, or mucous membrane exposure to hepatitis B virus

**Twinrix®** (GSK) PoM
Injection, inactivated hepatitis A virus (grown in human diploid cells) 720 ELISA units/mL adsorbed onto aluminium hydroxide and recombinant (DNA) hepatitis B surface antigen (grown in yeast cells) 20 micrograms/mL adsorbed onto aluminium phosphate, net price 1-mL prefilled syringe (*Twinrix® Adult*) = £27.76, 0.5-mL prefilled syringe (*Twinrix® Paediatric*) = £20.79
Excipients include neomycin and traces of thiomersal
Dose by intramuscular injection (see note below); ADULT and CHILD over 16 years, primary course of 3 doses of 1 mL, the second 1 month and the third 6 months after the first dose; CHILD 1–15 years, 3 doses of 0.5 mL
Accelerated schedule (e.g. for travellers departing within 1 month), ADULT, second dose 7 days after first dose, third dose after further 14 days and a fourth dose 12 months after the first dose
Note Primary course should be completed with *Twinrix®* (single component vaccines given at appropriate intervals may be used for booster dose); the deltoid region is the preferred site of injection in adults and older children; anterolateral thigh is preferred site in infants; not to be injected into the buttock (vaccine efficacy reduced); subcutaneous route used for patients with bleeding disorders (but immune response may be reduced).
Important *Twinrix®* **not** recommended for post-exposure prophylaxis following percutaneous (needle-stick), ocular or mucous membrane exposure to hepatitis B virus.

### ◢ With typhoid vaccine

**Hepatyrix®** (GSK) PoM
Injection, suspension of inactivated hepatitis A virus (grown in human diploid cells) 1440 ELISA units/mL adsorbed onto aluminium hydroxide, combined with typhoid vaccine containing 25 micrograms/mL viru-

**14**

**Immunological products and vaccines**

lence polysaccharide antigen of *Salmonella typhi*, net price 1-mL prefilled syringe = £32.08
Excipients include neomycin

**Dose** by intramuscular injection (see note below), ADULT and CHILD over 15 years, 1 mL as a single dose; booster doses, see under single component hepatitis A vaccine (above) and under polysaccharide typhoid vaccine, p. 688

**Note** The deltoid region is the preferred site of injection. The subcutaneous route may be used for patients with bleeding disorders; not to be injected into the buttock (vaccine efficacy reduced)

**ViATIM®** (Sanofi Pasteur) PoM

Injection, suspension of inactivated hepatitis A virus (grown in human diploid cells) 160 antigen units/mL adsorbed onto aluminium hydroxide, combined with typhoid vaccine containing 25 micrograms/mL virulence polysaccharide antigen of *Salmonella typhi*, net price 1-mL prefilled syringe = £29.04
Excipients include neomycin

**Dose** by intramuscular injection (see note below), ADULT and CHILD over 16 years, 1 mL as a single dose; booster doses, see under single component hepatitis A vaccine (above) and under polysaccharide typhoid vaccine, p. 688

**Note** The deltoid region is the preferred site of injection. The subcutaneous route may be used for patients with bleeding disorders; not to be injected into the buttock (vaccine efficacy reduced)

## Hepatitis B vaccine

**Hepatitis B vaccine** contains inactivated hepatitis B virus surface antigen (HBsAg) adsorbed onto aluminium hydroxide adjuvant. It is made biosynthetically using recombinant DNA technology. The vaccine is used in individuals at high risk of contracting hepatitis B.

In the UK, groups at high-risk of hepatitis B include:

- parenteral drug misusers, their sexual partners, and household contacts; other drug misusers who are likely to 'progress' to injecting;

- individuals who change sexual partners frequently;

- close family contacts of a case or individual with chronic hepatitis B infection;

- babies whose mothers have had acute hepatitis B during pregnancy *or* are positive for hepatitis B surface antigen (regardless of e-antigen markers); hepatitis B vaccination is started immediately on delivery and *hepatitis B immunoglobulin* (see p. 692) given at the same time (but preferably at a different site). Babies whose mothers are positive for hepatitis B surface antigen and for e-antigen antibody should receive the vaccine only (but babies weighing 1.5 kg or less should also receive the immunoglobulin regardless of the mother's e-antigen antibody status);

- individuals with haemophilia, those receiving regular blood transfusions or blood products, and carers responsible for the administration of such products;

- patients with chronic renal failure including those on haemodialysis. Haemodialysis patients should be monitored for antibodies annually and re-immunised if necessary. Home carers (of dialysis patients) should be vaccinated;

- individuals with chronic liver disease;

- healthcare personnel (including trainees) who have direct contact with blood or blood-stained body fluids or with patients' tissues;

- laboratory staff who handle material that may contain the virus;

- other occupational risk groups such as morticians and embalmers;

- staff and patients of day-care or residential accommodation for those with severe learning difficulties;

- staff and inmates of custodial institutions;

- those travelling to areas of high or intermediate prevalence who are at increased risk or who plan to remain there for lengthy periods (see p. 695);

- families adopting children from countries with a high or intermediate prevalence of hepatitis B;

- foster carers and their families.

Different immunisation schedules for hepatitis B vaccine are recommended for specific circumstances (see under individual preparations). Generally, three or four doses are required for primary immunisation; an 'accelerated schedule' is recommended for pre-exposure prophylaxis in high-risk groups where rapid protection is required, and for post-exposure prophylaxis (see below).

Immunisation may take up to 6 months to confer adequate protection; the duration of immunity is not known precisely, but a single booster 5 years after the primary course may be sufficient to maintain immunity for those who continue to be at risk.

Immunisation does not eliminate the need for common-sense precautions for avoiding the risk of infection from known carriers by the routes of infection which have been clearly established, consult *Guidance for Clinical Health Care Workers: Protection against Infection with Blood-borne Viruses* (available at www.dh.gov.uk). Accidental inoculation of hepatitis B virus-infected blood into a wound, incision, needle-prick, or abrasion may lead to infection, whereas it is unlikely that indirect exposure to a carrier will do so.

Following significant exposure to hepatitis B, an accelerated schedule, with the second dose given 1 month, and the third dose 2 months after the first dose, is recommended. For those at continued risk, a fourth dose should be given 12 months after the first dose. More detailed guidance is given in the handbook *Immunisation against Infectious Disease* see p. 669

Specific **hepatitis B immunoglobulin** ('HBIG') is available for use with the vaccine in those accidentally inoculated and in neonates at special risk of infection (section 14.5.2).

A combined hepatitis A and hepatitis B vaccine is also available.

## ▌ HEPATITIS B VACCINE

**Indications** immunisation against hepatitis B infection
**Cautions** see section 14.1
**Contra-indications** see section 14.1
**Side-effects** see section 14.1
**Dose**
- See under preparations

◢**Single component**
**Engerix B®** (GSK) PoM

Injection, suspension of hepatitis B surface antigen (prepared from yeast cells by recombinant DNA technique) 20 micrograms/mL adsorbed onto alu-

minium hydroxide, net price 0.5-mL (paediatric) pre-filled syringe = £9.67, 1-mL vial = £12.34, 1-mL prefilled syringe = £12.99
Excipients include traces of thiomersal

**Dose** by intramuscular injection (see note below), ADULT and CHILD over 16 years, 3 doses of 20 micrograms, the second 1 month and the third 6 months after the first dose; NEONATE (except if born to hepatitis B surface antigen positive mother, see below) and CHILD 1 month–16 years, 3 doses of 10 micrograms

Accelerated schedule (all ages), second dose 1 month after first dose, third dose 2 months after first dose and fourth dose 12 months after first dose; *exceptionally* (e.g. for travellers departing within 1 month), ADULT over 18 years, second dose 7 days after first dose, third dose 21 days after first dose, and fourth dose 12 months after first dose

Alternative schedule for CHILD 11–15 years, 2 doses of 20 micrograms, the second dose 6 months after the first dose (this schedule not suitable if high risk of infection between doses or if compliance with second dose uncertain)

NEONATE born to hepatitis B surface antigen-positive mother (see also notes above), 4 doses of 10 micrograms, first dose at birth with hepatitis B immunoglobulin injection (separate site) the second 1 month, the third 2 months and the fourth 12 months after the first dose

Renal insufficiency (including haemodialysis patients), by intramuscular injection (see note below), ADULT and CHILD over 16 years, 4 doses of 40 micrograms, the second 1 month, the third 2 months and the fourth 6 months after the first dose; immunisation schedule and booster doses may need to be adjusted in those with low antibody concentration; NEONATE (except if born to hepatitis B surface antigen positive mother, see above) and CHILD 1 month–16 years 3 doses of 10 micrograms, second dose 1 month and third dose 6 months after first dose *or* accelerated schedule, 4 doses of 10 micrograms, second dose 1 month, third dose 2 months and fourth dose 12 months after first dose; immunisation schedule and booster doses may need to be adjusted in those with low antibody concentration

**Note** Deltoid muscle is preferred site of injection in adults and older children; anterolateral thigh is preferred site in neonates, infants and young children; not to be injected into the buttock (vaccine efficacy reduced)

**Fendrix®** (GSK) ▨[PoM]

Injection, suspension of hepatitis B surface antigen (prepared from yeast cells by recombinant DNA technique) 40 micrograms/mL adsorbed onto aluminium phosphate, net price 0.5-mL prefilled syringe = £38.10
Excipients include traces of thiomersal

**Dose** ADULT and CHILD over 15 years with renal insufficiency (including pre-haemodialysis and haemodialysis patients), by intramuscular injection (see note below) 4 doses of 20 micrograms, the second 1 month, the third 2 months and the fourth 6 months after the first dose; immunisation schedule and booster doses may need to be adjusted in those with low antibody concentration

**Note** Deltoid muscle is preferred site of injection; not to be injected into the buttock (vaccine efficacy reduced)

**HBvaxPRO®** (Sanofi Pasteur) ▨[PoM]

Injection, suspension of hepatitis B surface antigen (prepared from yeast cells by recombinant DNA technique) 10 micrograms/mL adsorbed onto aluminium hydroxyphosphate sulphate, net price 0.5-mL (5-microgram) prefilled syringe = £9.13, 1-mL (10-microgram) prefilled syringe = £12.44; 40 micrograms/mL, 1-mL (40-microgram) vial = £28.16

**Dose** by intramuscular injection (see note below), ADULT and CHILD over 16 years, 3 doses of 10 micrograms, the second 1 month and the third 6 months after the first dose; CHILD under 16 years, 3 doses of 5 micrograms

Accelerated schedule (all ages), second dose 1 month after first dose, third dose 2 months after first dose with fourth dose at 12 months

Booster doses may be required in immunocompromised patients with low antibody concentration

NEONATE born to hepatitis B surface antigen-positive mother (see also notes above), 5 micrograms, first dose at birth with hepatitis B immunoglobulin injection (separate site), the second 1 month, the third 2 months and the fourth 12 months after the first dose

Chronic haemodialysis patients, by intramuscular injection (see note below) 3 doses of 40 micrograms, the second 1 month and the third 6 months after the first dose; booster doses may be required in those with low antibody concentration

**Note** Deltoid muscle is preferred site of injection in adults and older children; anterolateral thigh is preferred site in neonates and infants; not to be injected into the buttock (vaccine efficacy reduced)

◢**With hepatitis A vaccine**
See Hepatitis A Vaccine

## Human papilloma virus vaccines

**Human papilloma virus vaccine** is available as a bivalent vaccine (*Cervarix®*) or a quadrivalent vaccine (*Gardasil®*). *Cervarix®* is licensed for use in females for the prevention of cervical cancer and other pre-cancerous lesions caused by human papilloma virus types 16 and 18. *Gardasil®* is licensed for use in females for the prevention of cervical cancer, genital warts and pre-cancerous lesions caused by human papilloma virus types 6, 11, 16, and 18. The two vaccines are not interchangeable and one vaccine product should be used for an entire course. However, the Department of Health (November 2008) states that for individuals with previous incomplete vaccination with *Gardasil®*, who are eligible for HPV vaccination under the national programme, *Cervarix®* can be used to complete the vaccination course if necessary; the individual must be informed that *Cervarix®* does not protect against genital warts.

Human papilloma virus vaccine will be most effective if given before sexual activity starts. The first dose is given to females aged 12 to 13 years, the second and third doses are given 1–2 and 6 months after the first dose (see Immunisation schedule, section 14.1); all 3 doses should be given within a 12-month period. If the course is interrupted, it should be resumed but not repeated, allowing the appropriate interval between the remaining doses. Where there are significant challenges in scheduling vaccinations, or a high likelihood that the third dose will not be given, the third dose of *Cervarix®* can be given 3 months after the second dose. Where appropriate, immunisation with human papilloma virus vaccine should be offered to females coming into the UK as they may not have been offered protection in their country of origin. The duration of protection has not been established, but current studies suggest that protection is maintained for at least 6 years after completion of the primary course.

As the vaccines do not protect against all strains of human papilloma virus, routine cervical screening should continue.

> **Human papilloma virus vaccine 'Catch-up' programme for England, Wales, and Northern Ireland**
> A 'catch-up' programme will be offered as follows:
> - from September 2008 [January 2009 in Wales] to all females born between 1 September 1990 and 31 August 1991 (aged 17–18 years)
> - from September 2009 to all females born between 1 September 1991 and 31 August 1995 (aged 14–18 years)

**Human papilloma virus vaccine 'Catch-up' programme for Scotland**

The 'catch-up' programme in Scotland will be offered as follows:

- from 1 September 2008 to all females aged 16–17 years
- from September 2009 to all females aged 14–16 years

# HUMAN PAPILLOMA VIRUS VACCINES

**Indications**  see notes above and under preparations

**Cautions**  see section 14.1

**Contra-indications**  see section 14.1

**Side-effects**  see section 14.1

**Dose**

- see notes above and under preparations
  Note  To avoid confusion, prescribers should specify the brand to be dispensed

**Cervarix®** (GSK) ▼ PoM
Injection, suspension of virus-like particles of human papilloma virus type 16 (40 micrograms/mL), type 18 (40 micrograms/mL) capsid protein (prepared by recombinant DNA technique using a Baculovirus expression system) in monophosphoryl lipid A adjuvant adsorbed onto aluminium hydroxide, net price 0.5-mL prefilled syringe = £80.50
Dose  prevention of premalignant genital lesions and cervical cancer, by intramuscular injection into deltoid region, ADULT and CHILD 10–25 years, 3 doses of 0.5 mL, the second 1 month and the third 6 months after the first dose

**Gardasil®** (Sanofi Pasteur) ▼ PoM
Injection, suspension of virus-like particles of human papilloma virus type 6 (40 micrograms/mL), type 11 (80 micrograms/mL), type 16 (80 micrograms/mL), type 18 (40 micrograms/mL) capsid protein (prepared from yeast cells by recombinant DNA technique) adsorbed onto aluminium hydroxyphosphate sulphate, net price 0.5-mL prefilled syringe = £77.36
Dose  prevention of premalignant genital lesions, cervical cancer and genital warts, by intramuscular injection preferably into deltoid region or higher anterolateral thigh, ADULT and CHILD 9–26 years, 3 doses of 0.5 mL, the second 2 months and the third 6 months after the first dose
Alternative schedule for ADULT and CHILD 9–26 years, 3 doses of 0.5 mL, the second at least 1 month, and the third at least 4 months after the first dose; schedule should be completed within 12 months

# Influenza vaccines

While most viruses are antigenically stable, the influenza viruses A and B (especially A) are constantly altering their antigenic structure as indicated by changes in the haemagglutinins (H) and neuraminidases (N) on the surface of the viruses. It is essential that influenza vaccines in use contain the H and N components of the prevalent strain or strains as recommended each year by the World Health Organization.

**Influenza vaccines** will not control epidemics—immunisation is recommended *only for persons at high risk*. Annual immunisation is strongly recommended for

individuals aged over 6 months with the following conditions:

- chronic respiratory disease (includes asthma treated with continuous or repeated use of inhaled or systemic corticosteroids or asthma with previous exacerbations requiring hospital admission);
- chronic heart disease;
- chronic liver disease;
- chronic renal disease;
- chronic neurological disease
- diabetes mellitus
- immunosuppression because of disease (including asplenia or splenic dysfunction) or treatment (including chemotherapy and prolonged corticosteroid treatment);
- HIV infection (regardless of immune status).

Influenza immunisation is also recommended for all persons aged over 65 years, for residents of nursing or residential homes for the elderly and other long-stay facilities, and for carers of persons whose welfare may be at risk if the carer falls ill. Influenza immunisation should also be considered for household contacts of immunocompromised individuals.

As part of winter planning, NHS employers should offer vaccination to healthcare workers who are directly involved in patient care. Employers of social care workers should consider similar action.

Where possible, pregnant women and children should receive a thiomersal-free influenza vaccine; if this is not available, a thiomersal containing influenza vaccine should be given.

For people who work in close contact with poultry on a regular basis, influenza immunisation is recommended as a precautionary public health measure. Seasonal human influenza vaccine does not protect against avian influenza, but it reduces the risk of poultry workers contracting both human and avian influenza simultaneously, and therefore also reduces the risk of a new influenza virus emerging.

Information on pandemic influenza and avian influenza may be found at www.dh.gov.uk/pandemicflu and at www.hpa.org.uk.

# INFLUENZA VACCINE

**Indications**  annual immunisation against influenza

**Cautions**  see section 14.1 **interactions:** Appendix 1 (vaccines)

**Contra-indications**  see section 14.1

**Side-effects**  see section 14.1; also reported febrile convulsions and transient thrombocytopenia

**Dose**

- By intramuscular injection ADULT and CHILD over 13 years, 0.5 mL as a single dose; CHILD 6 months–3 years, 0.25–0.5 mL; 3–13 years 0.5 mL; for children 6 months to 13 years who have not been previously vaccinated repeat after 4–6 weeks
- By intradermal injection, see under *Intanza®* below

◢**For intramuscular use**

**Inactivated Influenza Vaccine (Split Virion)** PoM
Flu
Injection, suspension of formaldehyde-inactivated influenza virus (split virion grown in fertilised hens' egg's), net price 0.25-mL prefilled syringe = £6.29; 0.5-mL prefilled syringe = £6.29
Excipients  may include neomycin and polymyxin
Available from Sanofi Pasteur

## Inactivated Influenza Vaccine (Surface Antigen)
PoM

**Flu or Flu(adj)**
Injection, suspension of propiolactone-inactivated influenza virus (surface antigen, grown in fertilised hens' eggs), net price 0.5-mL prefilled syringe = £4.40
Excipients may include neomycin and polymyxin B, and traces of thiomersal
Available from Novartis Vaccines
Note Not licensed for children under 4 years

**Agrippal®** (Novartis Vaccines) PoM
Injection, suspension of formaldehyde-inactivated influenza virus (surface antigen, grown in fertilised hens' eggs), net price 0.5-mL prefilled syringe = £5.85
Excipients include kanamycin and neomycin

**Begrivac®** (Novartis Vaccines) PoM
Injection, suspension of formaldehyde-inactivated influenza virus (split virion, grown in fertilised hens' eggs), net price 0.5-mL prefilled syringe = £5.85
Excipients include polymyxin B

**Enzira®** (Wyeth) PoM
Injection, suspension of inactivated influenza virus (split virion, grown in fertilised hens' eggs), net price 0.5-mL prefilled syringe = £6.33
Excipients include neomycin and polymyxin B

**Fluarix®** (GSK) PoM
Injection, suspension of formaldehyde-inactivated influenza virus (split virion, grown in fertilised hens' eggs), net price 0.5-mL prefilled syringe = £4.49
Excipients include gentamicin

**Fluvirin®** (Novartis Vaccines) PoM
Injection, suspension of formaldehyde-inactivated influenza virus (surface antigen, grown in fertilised hens' eggs), net price 0.5-mL prefilled syringe = £5.55
Excipients include neomycin, polymyxin B, and traces of thiomersal
Note Not licensed for use in children under 4 years

**Imuvac®** (Solvay) PoM
Injection, suspension of inactivated influenza virus (surface antigen, grown in fertilised hens' eggs), net price 0.5-mL prefilled syringe = £6.59
Excipients include gentamicin

**Influvac Sub-unit®** (Solvay) PoM
Injection, suspension of inactivated influenza virus (surface antigen, grown in fertilised hens' eggs), net price 0.5-mL prefilled syringe = £5.22
Excipients include gentamicin

**Mastaflu®** (MASTA) PoM
Injection, suspension of formaldehyde-inactivated influenza virus (surface antigen, grown in fertilised hens' eggs), net price 0.5-mL prefilled syringe = £6.50
Excipients include gentamicin

**Viroflu®** (Sanofi Pasteur) PoM
Injection, suspension of inactivated influenza virus (surface antigen, virosome, grown in fertilised hens' eggs), net price 0.5-mL prefilled syringe = £6.33
Excipients include neomycin and polymyxin B

◢**For intradermal use**
**Intanza®** (Sanofi Pasteur) ▼ PoM
Injection, suspension of formaldehyde-inactivated influenza virus (split virion, grown in fertilised hens' eggs), net price prefilled syringe, 9 micrograms (0.1 mL) = £9.05; prefilled syringe, 15 micrograms (0.1 mL) = £9.05
Excipients include neomycin
Dose by intradermal injection into deltoid region, ADULT 18–60 years, 9 micrograms as a single dose; ADULT over 60 years, 15 micrograms as a single dose

## Japanese encephalitis vaccine

Japanese encephalitis vaccine is indicated for travellers to areas in Asia and the Far East where infection is endemic and for laboratory staff at risk of exposure to the virus. The primary immunisation course of 2 doses should be completed at least one week before potential exposure to Japanese encephalitis virus. The duration of protection has not been established and the recommended schedule for booster doses is uncertain.

Up-to-date information on the risk of Japanese encephalitis in specific countries can be obtained from the National Travel Health Network and Centre (www.nathnac.org)

### ◼ JAPANESE ENCEPHALITIS VACCINE

**Indications** immunisation against Japanese encephalitis
**Cautions** see section 14.1
**Contra-indications** see section 14.1; hypersensitivity reaction after first dose—do not give the second dose
**Side-effects** see section 14.1; also *less commonly* migraine, vertigo, pharyngolaryngeal pain
**Dose**
● see under preparation

[1]**Ixiaro®** (Novartis Vaccines) ▼ PoM ⒿⒽⓈ
Injection, suspension, inactivated Japanese encephalitis virus (produced in Vero cells), adsorbed onto aluminium hydroxide, net price 0.5-mL (6 micrograms) prefilled syringe = £48.00
Dose by intramuscular injection in deltoid region, ADULT over 18 years 2 doses of 0.5 mL separated by interval of 28 days
Note *Ixiaro®* doses differ from the other previously available unlicensed Japanese encephalitis vaccines

## Measles vaccine

Measles vaccine has been replaced by a combined live measles, mumps and rubella vaccine (MMR vaccine).
MMR vaccine may be used in the control of outbreaks of measles (see under MMR Vaccine).

◢**Single antigen vaccine**
No longer available in the UK

◢**Combined vaccines**
See MMR vaccine

## Measles, Mumps and Rubella (MMR) vaccine

A combined live **measles, mumps, and rubella vaccine** (MMR vaccine) aims to eliminate measles, mumps, and rubella (and congenital rubella syndrome). Every child should receive two doses of MMR vaccine by entry to primary school, unless there is a valid contra-indication (see section 14.1). MMR vaccine should be given irrespective of previous measles, mumps, or rubella infection or vaccination.

The first dose of MMR vaccine is given to children aged 13 months. A second dose is given before starting school at 3–5 years of age (see Immunisation Schedule, section 14.1

1. Japanese encephalitis vaccine not prescribable on the NHS; health authorities may investigate circumstances under which vaccine prescribed

**14**

Immunological products and vaccines

When protection against measles is required urgently (e.g. during a measles outbreak), the second dose of MMR vaccine can be given 1 month after the first dose; if the second dose is given before 18 months of age, then children should still receive the routine dose before starting school at 3–5 years of age.

Children presenting for pre-school booster who have not received the first dose of MMR vaccine should be given a dose of MMR vaccine followed 3 months later by a second dose. At school-leaving age or at entry into further education, MMR immunisation should be offered to individuals of both sexes who have not received 2 doses during childhood. In a young adult who has received only a single dose of MMR in childhood, a second dose is recommended to achieve full protection. If 2 doses of MMR vaccine are required, the second dose should be given one month after initial dose.

MMR vaccine should be used to protect against rubella in *seronegative women of child-bearing age* (see Immunisation Schedule, section 14.1); unimmunised healthcare workers who might put pregnant women and other vulnerable groups at risk of rubella (or measles) should be vaccinated. MMR vaccine may also be offered to previously *unimmunised and seronegative post-partum women*—vaccination a few days after delivery is important because about 60% of congenital abnormalities from rubella infection occur in babies of women who have borne more than one child. Immigrants arriving after the age of school immunisation are particularly likely to require immunisation.

**Contacts** MMR vaccine may also be used in the control of outbreaks of measles and should be offered to susceptible children aged over 6 months who are contacts of a case, within 3 days of exposure to infection; these children should still receive routine MMR vaccinations at the recommended ages. Children aged under 9 months for whom avoidance of measles infection is particularly important (such as those with history of recent severe illness) can be given normal immunoglobulin (section 14.5.1) after exposure to measles; routine MMR immunisation should then be given after at least 3 months at the appropriate age.

MMR vaccine is **not suitable** for prophylaxis following exposure to mumps or rubella since the antibody response to the mumps and rubella components is too slow for effective prophylaxis.

Children and adults with impaired immune response should not receive live vaccines (for advice on HIV see section 14.1). If they have been exposed to measles infection they should be given normal immunoglobulin (section 14.5.1).

**Travel** Unimmunised travellers, including children over 6 months, to areas where measles is endemic or epidemic should receive MMR vaccine. Children immunised before 12 months of age should still receive two doses of MMR at the recommended ages. If one dose of MMR has already been given to a child, then the second dose should be brought forward to at least one month after the first, to ensure complete protection. If the child is under 18 months of age and the second dose is given within 3 months of the first, then the routine dose before starting school at 3–5 years should still be given.

**Side-effects** See section 14.1; also malaise, fever, or a rash can occur after the first dose of MMR vaccine, most commonly about a week after vaccination and lasting about 2 to 3 days. Leaflets are available for parents on advice for reducing fever (including the use of paracetamol). Febrile seizures occur less commonly 6 to 11 days after MMR vaccination; the incidence of febrile seizures is lower than that following measles infection. Parotid swelling occurs occasionally, usually in the third week, and rarely, arthropathy 2 to 3 weeks after immunisation. Adverse reactions are considerably less frequent after the second dose of MMR vaccine than after the first dose.

Hypersensitivity to egg— there is increasing evidence that MMR vaccine can be given safely even when the child has had an anaphylactic reaction to food containing egg (dislike of egg or refusal to eat eggs is not a contra-indication). For children with a confirmed anaphylactic reaction to egg-containing food, MMR vaccine should be administered in a hospital setting.

Idiopathic thrombocytopenic purpura has occurred rarely following MMR vaccination, usually within 6 weeks of the first dose. The risk of idiopathic thrombocytopenic purpura after MMR vaccine is much less than the risk after infection with wild measles or rubella virus. The CSM has recommended that children who develop idiopathic thrombocytopenic purpura within 6 weeks of the first dose of MMR should undergo serological testing before the second dose is due; if the results suggest incomplete immunity against measles, mumps or rubella then a second dose of MMR is recommended. The Specialist and Reference Microbiology Division, Health Protection Agency offers free serological testing for children who develop idiopathic thrombocytopenic purpura *within 6 weeks* of the first dose of MMR.

Post-vaccination aseptic meningitis was reported (rarely and with complete recovery) following vaccination with MMR vaccine containing Urabe mumps vaccine, which has now been discontinued; no cases have been confirmed in association with the currently used Jeryl Lynn mumps vaccine. Children with post-vaccination symptoms are not infectious.

> Reviews undertaken on behalf of the CSM, the Medical Research Council, and the Cochrane Collaboration, have not found any evidence of a link between MMR vaccination and bowel disease or autism. The Chief Medical Officers have advised that the MMR vaccine is the safest and best way to protect children against measles, mumps, and rubella. Information (including fact sheets and a list of references) may be obtained from:
> www.immunisation.nhs.uk/Vaccines/MMR

## ▌ MEASLES, MUMPS AND RUBELLA VACCINE, LIVE

**Indications** immunisation against measles, mumps, and rubella

**Cautions** see section 14.1; also, after immunoglobulin administration or blood transfusion, leave an interval of at least 3 months before MMR immunisation as antibody response to measles component may be reduced—see also p. 693; **interactions:** Appendix 1 (vaccines)

**Hypersensitivity to egg** There is increasing evidence that MMR vaccine can be given safely even when the child has had an anaphylactic reaction to food containing egg (dislike of egg or refusal to eat egg is not a contra-indication). For children with a confirmed anaphylactic reaction to egg-containing food, MMR vaccine should be administered in a hospital setting

**Contra-indications**   see section 14.1; also pregnancy (avoid pregnancy for at least 1 month after vaccination)

**Side-effects**   see section 14.1 and notes above; also *less commonly* sleep disturbances, unusual crying in infants; also reported peripheral and optic neuritis

**Dose**

- By intramuscular or deep subcutaneous injection, ADULT and CHILD over 9 months (but see also notes above), primary immunisation, 2 doses each of 0.5 mL, see Immunisation Schedule , section 14.1, p. 671; see also notes above for use in outbreaks, for contacts of cases, and for travel

◢**Combined vaccines**

**MMRvaxPro®** (Sanofi Pasteur) ▼ PoM

Injection, powder for reconstitution, live attenuated, measles virus (Enders' Edmonston strain) and mumps virus (Jeryl Lynn strain) prepared in chick embryo cells, and rubella virus (Wistar RA 27/3 strain); single-dose vial (with syringe containing solvent)
Excipients include gelatin and neomycin
Only available as part of childhood immunisation schedule from health organisations or Movianto

**Priorix®** (GSK) PoM

Injection, powder for reconstitution, live attenuated, measles virus (Schwarz strain) and mumps virus (RIT 4385 strain) prepared in chick embryo cells, and rubella virus (Wistar RA 27/3 strain); net price single-dose vial (with syringe containing solvent) = £6.37
Excipients include neomycin
Also available as part of childhood immunisation schedule from health organisations or Movianto

---

## Meningococcal vaccines

Almost all childhood meningococcal disease in the UK is caused by *Neisseria meningitidis* serogroups B and C. **Meningococcal group C conjugate vaccine** protects only against infection by serogroup C. The risk of meningococcal disease declines with age—immunisation is not generally recommended after the age of 25 years.

**Childhood immunisation** Meningococcal group C conjugate vaccine provides long-term protection against infection by serogroup C of *Neisseria meningitidis*. Immunisation consists of 2 doses given at 3 months and 4 months of age; a booster should be given at 12 months of age, usually combined with haemophilus influenzae type b vaccine. This routine booster dose should be given one month before the booster dose of pneumococcal conjugate vaccine (see Immunisation schedule, section 14.1, p. 671). It is recommended that meningococcal group C conjugate vaccine be given to anyone aged under 25 years who has not been vaccinated previously with this vaccine; those over 1 year receive a single dose.

A single dose of meningococcal group C conjugate vaccine is also recommended for unimmunised individuals attending university, irrespective of age.

**Meningococcal group C conjugate vaccine in patients with asplenia or splenic dysfunction**
Meningococcal group C conjugate vaccine is recommended for patients with asplenia or splenic dysfunc-

tion. Children under 1 year should be vaccinated according to the Immunisation Schedule (section 14.1). Unimmunised adults and children over 1 year should be given 2 doses of meningococcal group C conjugate vaccine (usually combined with haemophilus influenzae type b vaccine) with an interval of 2 months between doses. Immunised adults and children who develop splenic dysfunction should be given 1 additional dose of meningococcal group C conjugate vaccine (usually combined with haemophilus influenzae type b vaccine).

**Travel** Individuals travelling to countries of risk (see below) should be immunised with a meningococcal polysaccharide vaccine that covers serotypes A, C, W135, and Y, even if they have previously received meningitis C conjugate vaccine. If an individual has recently received meningococcal group C conjugate vaccine, an interval of at least 2 weeks should be allowed before administration of the tetravalent (A, C, W135, and Y) vaccine. The antibody response to serotype C in unconjugated meningococcal polysaccharide vaccines in children under 18 months may be suboptimal.

Vaccination is particularly important for those living or working with local people or visiting an area of risk during outbreaks.

Immunisation recommendations and requirements for visa entry for individual countries should be checked before travelling, particularly to countries in Sub-Saharan Africa, Asia, and the Indian sub-continent where epidemics of meningococcal outbreaks and infection are reported. Country-by-country information is available from the National Travel Health Network and Centre (www.nathnac.org).

Proof of vaccination with the tetravalent (A, C, W135, and Y) meningococcal vaccine is required for those travelling to Saudi Arabia during the Hajj and Umrah pilgrimages (where outbreaks of the W135 strain have occurred).

**Contacts** For advice on the immunisation of *laboratory workers and close contacts* of cases of meningococcal disease in the UK and on the role of the vaccine in the control of *local outbreaks*, consult Guidance for Public Health Management of Meningococcal Disease in the UK at www.hpa.org.uk. See Table 2, section 5.1 for antibacterial prophylaxis for prevention of secondary cases of meningococcal meningitis.

The need for immunisation of laboratory staff who work directly with *Neisseria meningitidis* should be considered.

---

◼ **MENINGOCOCCAL VACCINES**

**Indications**   immunisation against *Neisseria meningitidis*

**Cautions**   see section 14.1

**Contra-indications**   see section 14.1

**Side-effects**   see section 14.1; also *rarely* symptoms of meningitis reported (but no evidence that the vaccine causes meningococcal C meningitis)

**Dose**

- See under preparations

◢**Meningococcal group C conjugate vaccine**
**Meningitec®** (Wyeth) PoM

Injection, suspension of capsular polysaccharide antigen of *Neisseria meningitidis* group C (conjugated to *Corynebacterium diphtheriae* protein), adsorbed onto aluminium phosphate, net price 0.5-mL prefilled syringe = £7.50

**Dose** by intramuscular injection, ADULT and CHILD over 1 year 0.5 mL as a single dose; for routine immunisation in CHILD 2 months–1 year, 0.5 mL, see notes above and Immunisation schedule, section 14.1

Available as part of childhood immunisation schedule from Movianto

**Menjugate Kit®** (Sanofi Pasteur) PoM
Injection, powder for reconstitution, capsular poly-saccharide antigen of *Neisseria meningitidis* group C (conjugated to *Corynebacterium diphtheriae* protein), adsorbed onto aluminium hydroxide, single-dose vial with diluent

**Dose** by intramuscular injection, ADULT and CHILD over 1 year 0.5 mL as a single dose; for routine immunisation in CHILD 2 months–1 year, 0.5 mL, see notes above and Immunisation schedule, section 14.1

**NeisVac-C®** (Baxter) PoM
Injection, suspension of polysaccharide antigen of *Neisseria meningitidis* group C (conjugated to tetanus toxoid protein), adsorbed onto aluminium hydroxide, 0.5-mL prefilled syringe

**Dose** by intramuscular injection, ADULT and CHILD over 1 year 0.5 mL as a single dose; for routine immunisation in CHILD 3 months–1 year, 0.5 mL, see notes above and Immunisation schedule, section 14.1

◢Meningococcal Group C conjugate vaccine with Haemophilus Influenzae type B vaccine
See Haemophilus Influenzae type B vaccine

◢Meningococcal polysaccharide A, C, W135 and Y vaccine

**ACWY Vax®** (GSK) ▼ PoM
Injection, powder for reconstitution, capsular poly-saccharide antigens of *Neisseria meningitidis* groups A, C, W135, and Y, net price single-dose vial (with syringe containing diluent) = £16.73

**Dose** by deep subcutaneous injection, ADULT and CHILD over 2 years 0.5 mL as a single dose; booster dose for those at continued risk, 0.5 mL 5 years after initial dose (children who were under 5 years of age when first vaccinated, should be given a booster dose after 2–3 years)

**Note** Two doses of 0.5 mL separated by an interval of 3 months can be given to CHILD 3 months–2 years [unlicensed] but antibody response may be suboptimal

---

## Mumps vaccine

◢Single antigen vaccine
No longer available in the UK

◢Combined vaccines
See MMR Vaccine

---

## Pertussis vaccine

**Pertussis vaccine** is given as a combination preparation containing other vaccines (see Diphtheria containing Vaccines). Acellular vaccines are derived from highly purified components of *Bordetella pertussis*. Primary immunisation against pertussis (whooping cough) requires 3 doses of an acellular pertussis-containing vaccine (see Immunisation schedule, section 14.1), given at intervals of 1 month from the age of 2 months.

A booster dose of an acellular pertussis-containing vaccine should be given 3 years after the primary course.

All children up to the age of 10 years should receive primary immunisation with diphtheria, tetanus, pertussis (acellular, component), poliomyelitis (inactivated) and haemophilus type b conjugate vaccine (adsorbed).

Children aged 1–10 years who have not received a *pertussis-containing* vaccine as part of their primary immunisation should be offered 1 dose of a suitable pertussis-containing vaccine; after an interval of at least 1 year, a booster dose of a suitable pertussis-containing vaccine should be given. Immunisation against pertussis is not currently recommended in individuals over 10 years of age.

**Cautions** Section 14.1.

**Contra-indications** Section 14.1.

**Side-effects** See also section 14.1. The incidence of local and systemic effects is generally lower with vaccines containing acellular pertussis components than with the whole-cell pertussis vaccine used previously. However, compared with primary vaccination, booster doses with vaccines containing acellular pertussis are reported to increase the risk of injection-site reactions (some of which affect the entire limb); local reactions do not contra-indicate further doses (see below).

The vaccine should not be withheld from children with a history to a preceding dose of:

- fever, irrespective of severity;
- persistent crying or screaming for more than 3 hours;
- severe local reaction, irrespective of extent.

These side-effects were associated with whole-cell pertussis vaccine.

◢Combined vaccines
Combined vaccines, see under Diphtheria-containing vaccines

---

## Pneumococcal vaccines

Pneumococcal vaccines protect against infection with *Streptococcus pneumoniae* (pneumococcus); the vaccines contain polysaccharide from capsular pneumococci. **Pneumococcal polysaccharide vaccine** contains purified polysaccharide from 23 capsular types of pneumococci whereas **pneumococcal polysaccharide conjugate vaccine (adsorbed)** contains polysaccharide from 7 capsular types, the polysaccharide being conjugated to protein.

The conjugate vaccine is used for childhood immunisation schedule. The recommended schedule consists of 3 doses, the first at 2 months of age, the second at 4 months, and the third at 13 months (see Immunisation Schedule, section 14.1).

Pneumococcal vaccination is recommended for individuals at increased risk of pneumococcal infection as follows:

- age over 65 years;
- asplenia or splenic dysfunction (including homozygous sickle cell disease and coeliac disease which could lead to splenic dysfunction);
- chronic respiratory disease (includes asthma treated with continuous or frequent use of a systemic corticosteroid);

- chronic heart disease;
- chronic renal disease;
- chronic liver disease;
- diabetes mellitus requiring insulin or oral hypogly-caemic drugs;
- immune deficiency because of disease (e.g. HIV infection) or treatment (including prolonged systemic corticosteroid treatment);
- presence of cochlear implant;
- conditions where leakage of cerebrospinal fluid may occur;
- child under 5 years with a history of invasive pneumococcal disease.

Where possible, the vaccine should be given at least 2 weeks before splenectomy, cochlear implant surgery, and chemotherapy; patients should be given advice about increased risk of pneumococcal infection. Prophylactic antibacterial therapy against pneumococcal infection (Table 2, section 5.1) should not be stopped after immunisation. A patient card and information leaflet for patients with asplenia are available from the Department of Health or in Scotland from the Scottish Executive, Public Health Division 1 (Tel (0131) 244 2501).

**Choice of vaccine**  Children under 2 years at increased risk of pneumococcal infection (see list above) should receive pneumococcal polysaccharide conjugate vaccine (adsorbed) at the recommended ages, followed by a single dose of the 23-valent pneumococcal polysaccharide vaccine after their second birthday (see below). Children at increased risk of pneumococcal infection presenting late for vaccination should receive 2 doses (separated by at least 1 month) of pneumococcal polysaccharide conjugate vaccine (adsorbed) before the age of 12 months, and a third dose at 13 months. Children over 12 months and under 5 years (who have not been vaccinated or not completed the primary course) should receive a single dose of pneumococcal polysaccharide conjugate vaccine (adsorbed) (2 doses separated by an interval of 2 months in the immunocompromised or those with asplenia or splenic dysfunction). All children under 5 years at increased risk of pneumococcal infection should receive a single dose of the 23-valent pneumococcal polysaccharide vaccine after their second birthday and at least 2 months after the final dose of the 7-valent pneumococcal polysaccharide conjugate vaccine (adsorbed).

Children over 5 years and adults who are at increased risk of pneumococcal disease should receive a single dose of the 23-valent unconjugated pneumococcal polysaccharide vaccine.

**Revaccination**  In individuals with higher concentrations of antibodies to pneumococcal polysaccharides, revaccination with the 23-valent pneumococcal polysaccharide vaccine more commonly produces adverse reactions. Revaccination is therefore not recommended, except every 5 years in individuals in whom the antibody concentration is likely to decline rapidly (e.g. asplenia, splenic dysfunction and nephrotic syndrome). If there is doubt, the need for revaccination should be discussed with a haematologist, immunologist, or microbiologist.

## ■ PNEUMOCOCCAL VACCINE

**Indications**  immunisation against pneumococcal infection
**Cautions**  see section 14.1
**Contra-indications**  see section 14.1
**Side-effects**  see section 14.1; *also* Revaccination, above
**Dose**
- See under preparations

▲**Pneumococcal polysaccharide vaccine**
**Pneumovax® II** (Sanofi Pasteur) PoM
Injection, polysaccharide from each of 23 capsular types of pneumococcus, net price 0.5-mL vial = £8.49
**Dose** by intramuscular or subcutaneous injection, ADULT and CHILD over 2 years, 0.5 mL; revaccination, see notes above

▲**Pneumococcal polysaccharide conjugate vaccine (adsorbed)**
**Prevenar®** (Wyeth) PoM
Injection, polysaccharide from each of 7 capsular types of pneumococcus (conjugated to diphtheria toxoid) adsorbed onto aluminium phosphate, net price 0.5-mL prefilled syringe = £34.50
**Dose** by intramuscular injection, CHILD 2 months–5 years, 0.5 mL (see notes above and Immunisation schedule, section 14.1)
**Note** Deltoid muscle is preferred site of injection in young children; anterolateral thigh is preferred site in infants
The dose in the BNF may differ from that in product literature

## Poliomyelitis vaccines

Two types of poliomyelitis vaccine (containing strains of poliovirus types 1, 2, and 3) are available, inactivated poliomyelitis vaccine (for injection) and live (oral) poliomyelitis vaccine. **Inactivated poliomyelitis vaccine**, only available in combined preparation (see under Diptheria Vaccines), is recommended for routine immunisation.

A course of primary immunisation consists of 3 doses of a combined preparation containing inactivated poliomyelitis vaccine, starting at 2 months of age with intervals of 1 month between doses (see Immunisation schedule, section 14.1). A course of 3 doses should also be given to all unimmunised adults; no adult should remain unimmunised against poliomyelitis.

Two booster doses of a preparation containing inactivated poliomyelitis vaccine are recommended, the first before school entry and the second before leaving school (see Immunisation schedule, section 14.1). Further booster doses are only necessary for adults at special risk, such as travellers to endemic areas, or laboratory staff likely to be exposed to the viruses, or healthcare workers in possible contact with cases; booster doses should be given to such individuals every 10 years.

Preparations containing inactivated poliomyelitis vaccine can be used to complete an immunisation course initiated with the live (oral) poliomyelitis vaccine. **Live (oral) poliomyelitis vaccine** is available only for use during outbreaks. The live (oral) vaccine poses a very rare risk of vaccine-associated paralytic polio because the attenuated strain of the virus can revert to a virulent form. For this reason the live (oral) vaccine must **not** be used for immunosuppressed individuals or their household contacts. The use of inactivated poliomyelitis vaccine removes the risk of vaccine-associated paralytic polio altogether.

**14**

**Immunological products and vaccines**

**Travel** Unimmunised travellers to areas with a high incidence of poliomyelitis should receive a full 3-dose course of a preparation containing inactivated poliomyelitis vaccine. Those who have not been vaccinated in the last 10 years should receive a booster dose of **adsorbed diphtheria [low dose], tetanus and poliomyelitis (inactivated) vaccine**. Information about countries with a high incidence of poliomyelitis can be obtained from www.travax.nhs.uk or from the National Travel Health Network and Centre (www.nathnac.org).

## POLIOMYELITIS VACCINES

**Indications** immunisation against poliomyelitis

**Cautions** see section 14.1; *also for live vaccine*, **interactions:** Appendix 1 (vaccines)

**Contra-indications** see notes above and section 14.1

**Side-effects** see notes above and section 14.1

**Dose**

- See under preparations

◢**Combined vaccines**

See under Diphtheria-containing Vaccines

◢**Inactivated (Salk) vaccine**

See under Diptheria-containing vaccines

◢**Live (oral) (Sabin) vaccine**

**Poliomyelitis Vaccine, Live (Oral)** (GSK) [PoM]

OPV

A suspension of suitable live attenuated strains of poliomyelitis virus, types 1, 2, and 3. Available in single-dose and 10-dose containers

Excipients include neomycin and polymyxin B

**Dose** control of outbreaks, 3 drops; may be given on a lump of sugar; not to be given with foods which contain preservatives

**Note** Live poliomyelitis vaccine loses potency once the container has been opened—any vaccine remaining at the end of an immunisation session should be discarded; whenever possible sessions should be arranged to avoid undue wastage.

## Rabies vaccine

Rabies vaccine contains inactivated rabies virus cultivated in either human diploid cells or purified chick embryo cells; vaccines are used for pre- and post-exposure prophylaxis.

**Pre-exposure prophylaxis** Immunisation should be offered to those at high risk of exposure to rabies—laboratory staff who handle the rabies virus, those working in quarantine stations, animal handlers, veterinary surgeons and field workers who are likely to be bitten by infected wild animals, certain port officials, and bat handlers. Transmission of rabies by humans has not been recorded but it is advised that those caring for patients with the disease should be vaccinated.

Immunisation against rabies is also recommended where there is limited access to prompt medical care for those living in areas where rabies is enzootic, for those travelling to such areas for longer than 1 month, and for those on shorter visits who may be exposed to unusual risk.

Immunisation against rabies is indicated during pregnancy if there is substantial risk of exposure to rabies and rapid access to post-exposure prophylaxis is likely to be limited.

Up-to-date country-by-country information on the incidence of rabies can be obtained from the National Travel Health Network and Centre (www.nathnac.org) and, in Scotland, from Health Protection Scotland (www.hps.scot.nhs.uk).

Immunisation against rabies requires 3 doses of rabies vaccine, with further booster doses for those who remain at continued risk . To ensure continued protection in persons at high risk (e.g. laboratory workers), the concentration of antirabies antibodies in plasma is used to determine the intervals between doses.

**Post-exposure management** Following potential exposure to rabies, the wound or site of exposure (e.g. mucous membrane) should be cleansed under running water and washed for several minutes with soapy water as soon as possible after exposure. Disinfectant and a simple dressing can be applied, but suturing should be delayed because it may increase the risk of introducing rabies virus into the nerves.

Post-exposure prophylaxis against rabies depends on the level of risk in the country, the nature of exposure, and the individual's immunity. In each case, expert risk assessment and advice on appropriate management should be obtained from the Health Protection Agency Virus Reference Department, Colindale, London (tel. (020) 8200 4400) or the Centre for Infections (tel. (020) 8200 6868), in Scotland from Health Protection Scotland (tel. (0141) 300 1100), in Northern Ireland from the Public Health Laboratory, Belfast City Hospital (tel. (028) 9032 9241).

There are no specific contra-indications to the use of rabies vaccine for post-exposure prophylaxis and its use should be considered whenever a patient has been attacked by an animal in a country where rabies is enzootic, even if there is no direct evidence of rabies in the attacking animal. Because of the potential consequences of untreated rabies exposure and because rabies vaccination has not been associated with fetal abnormalities, pregnancy is not considered a contra-indication to post-exposure prophylaxis.

For post-exposure prophylaxis of *fully immunised* individuals (who have previously received pre-exposure or post-exposure prophylaxis with cell-derived rabies vaccine), 2 doses of cell-derived vaccine, given on day 0 and day 3, are likely to be sufficient. Rabies immunoglobulin is not necessary in such cases.

Post-exposure treatment for *unimmunised individuals* (or those whose prophylaxis is possibly incomplete) comprises 5 doses of rabies vaccine given over 1 month (on days 0, 3, 7, 14, and 30); also, depending on the level of risk (determined by factors such as the nature of the bite and the country where it was sustained), rabies immunoglobulin (section 14.5.2) is given on day 0. The immunisation course can be discontinued if it is proved that the individual was not at risk.

## RABIES VACCINE

**Indications** immunisation against rabies

**Cautions** see section 14.1

**Contra-indications** see section 14.1; but see also Post-exposure Management in notes above

**Side-effects** see section 14.1; also reported paresis

*Immunological products and vaccines*

**14**

**Dose**

- Pre-exposure prophylaxis, by intramuscular injection in deltoid region or anterolateral thigh in infants, 1 mL on days 0, 7, and 21 or 28; for those at continued risk give a single reinforcing dose 1 year after the primary course is completed and booster doses every 3–5 years; for those at intermittent risk give booster doses every 2–5 years
- Post-exposure prophylaxis, by intramuscular injection in deltoid region or anterolateral thigh in infants, 1 mL (see notes above)

**Rabies Vaccine** (Sanofi Pasteur) ℗ₒₘ
**Rab**
Injection, powder for reconstitution, freeze-dried inactivated Wistar rabies virus strain PM/WI 38 1503-3M cultivated in human diploid cells, net price single-dose vial with syringe containing diluent = £24.40
Excipients include neomycin

**Rabipur®** (Novartis Vaccines) ℗ₒₘ
Injection, powder for reconstitution, freeze-dried inactivated Flury LEP rabies virus strain cultivated in chick embryo cells, net price single-dose vial = £24.40
Excipients include neomycin

## Rotavirus vaccine

Rotavirus vaccine a live, oral vaccine is licensed for immunisation of infants over 6 weeks of age for protection against gastro-enteritis caused by rotavirus infection.

The rotavirus vaccine virus is excreted in the stool and may be transmitted to close contacts; the vaccine should be used with caution in those with *immunosuppressed* close contacts. Carers of a recently vaccinated baby should be advised of the need to wash their hands after changing the baby's nappies.

### ▌ ROTAVIRUS VACCINE

**Indications** immunisation against gastro-enteritis caused by rotavirus
**Cautions** see section 14.1; *also* diarrhoea or vomiting (postpone vaccination); immunosuppressed close contacts (see notes above); **interactions:** Appendix 1 (vaccines)
**Contra-indications** see section 14.1; *also* predisposition to, or history of, intussusception
**Side-effects** see section 14.1
**Dose**

- By mouth, CHILD over 6 weeks, 2 doses of 1 mL separated by an interval of at least 4 weeks; course should be completed before 24 weeks of age (preferably before 16 weeks)

**Rotarix®** (GSK) ▼ ℗ₒₘ
Oral suspension, powder for reconstitution, live attenuated rotavirus (RIX4414 strain), net price single-dose vial (with oral syringe containing diluent) = £41.38

## Rubella vaccine

A combined measles, mumps and rubella vaccine (MMR vaccine) aims to eliminate rubella (German measles) and congenital rubella syndrome. MMR vaccine is used for childhood vaccination as well as for vaccinating adults (including women of child-bearing age) who do

not have immunity against rubella (see MMR vaccine, p. 681)

◀**Single antigen vaccine**
No longer available in the UK; the combined live measles, mumps and rubella vaccine is a suitable alternative

◀**Combined vaccines**
see MMR vaccine

## Smallpox vaccine

Limited supplies of **smallpox vaccine** are held at the Specialist and Reference Microbiology Division, Health Protection Agency (Tel. (020) 8200 4400) for the exclusive use of workers in laboratories where pox viruses (such as vaccinia) are handled.

If a wider use of the vaccine is being considered, *Guidelines for smallpox response and management in the post-eradication era* should be consulted at www.dh.gov.uk

## Tetanus Vaccines

**Tetanus vaccine** contains a cell-free purified toxin of *Clostridium tetani* adsorbed on aluminium hydroxide or aluminium phosphate to improve antigenicity.

Primary immunisation for children under 10 years consists of 3 doses of a combined preparation containing adsorbed tetanus vaccine (see Diphtheria-containing Vaccines), with an interval of 1 month between doses. Following routine childhood vaccination, 2 booster doses of a preparation containing adsorbed tetanus vaccine are recommended, the first before school entry and the second before leaving school (see Immunisation schedule, section 14.1).

The recommended schedule of tetanus vaccination not only gives protection against tetanus in childhood but also gives the basic immunity for subsequent booster doses. In most circumstances, a total of 5 doses of tetanus vaccine is considered sufficient for long term protection.

For primary immunisation of adults and children over 10 years previously unimmunised against tetanus, 3 doses of **adsorbed diphtheria [low dose], tetanus and poliomyelitis (inactivated) vaccine** are given with an interval of 1 month between doses (see Diphtheria-containing Vaccines).

**Cautions** See also section 14.1. When an individual presents for a booster dose but has been vaccinated following a tetanus-prone wound, the vaccine preparation administered at the time of injury should be determined. If this is not possible, the booster should still be given to ensure adequate protection against all antigens in the booster vaccine.

Very rarely, tetanus has developed after abdominal surgery; patients awaiting elective surgery should be asked about tetanus immunisation and immunised if necessary.

Parenteral drug abuse is also associated with tetanus; those abusing drugs by injection should be vaccinated if unimmunised—booster doses should be given if there is any doubt about their immunisation status.

All laboratory staff should be offered a primary course if unimmunised.

Travel recommendations see section 14.6.

**14**

*Immunological products and vaccines*

**Contra-indications** See section 14.1.

**Side effects** See section 14.1.

**Wounds** Wounds are considered to be tetanus-prone if they are sustained more than 6 hours before surgical treatment *or* at any interval after injury and are puncture-type (particularly if contaminated with soil or manure) *or* show much devitalised tissue *or* are septic *or* are compound fractures *or* contain foreign bodies. All wounds should receive thorough cleansing.

- For *clean wounds*: fully immunised individuals (those who have received a total of 5 doses of a tetanus-containing vaccine at appropriate intervals) and those whose primary immunisation is complete (with boosters up to date), do not require tetanus vaccine; individuals whose primary immunisation is incomplete or whose boosters are not up to date require a reinforcing dose of a tetanus-containing vaccine (followed by further doses as required to complete the schedule); non-immunised individuals (or those whose immunisation status is not known or who have been fully immunised but are now immunocompromised) should be given a dose of the appropriate tetanus-containing vaccine immediately (followed by completion of the full course of the vaccine if records confirm the need).

- For *tetanus-prone wounds*: management is as for clean wounds with the addition of a dose of tetanus immunoglobulin (section 14.5.2) given at a different site; in fully immunised individuals and those whose primary immunisation is complete (with boosters up to date) the immunoglobulin is needed only if the risk of infection is especially high (e.g. contamination with manure). Antibacterial prophylaxis (with benzylpenicillin, co-amoxiclav, or metronidazole) may also be required for tetanus-prone wounds.

◢**Combined vaccines**

See Diphtheria-containing Vaccines

---

## Tick-borne encephalitis vaccine

Tick-borne encephalitis vaccine contains inactivated tick-borne encephalitis virus cultivated in chick embryo cells. It is recommended for immunisation of those working in, or visiting, high-risk areas (see International Travel, section 14.6). Those working, walking or camping in warm forested areas of Central and Eastern Europe and Scandinavia, particularly from April to October when ticks are most prevalent, are at greatest risk of tick-borne encephalitis. For full protection, 3 doses of the vaccine are required; booster doses are required every 3–5 years for those still at risk. Ideally, immunisation should be completed at least one month before travel.

### ■ TICK-BORNE ENCEPHALITIS VACCINE, INACTIVATED

**Indications** immunisation against tick-borne encephalitis

**Cautions** see section 14.1

**Contra-indications** see section 14.1

**Side-effects** see section 14.1

**Dose**

- Initial immunisation, by intramuscular injection in deltoid region or anterolateral thigh in infants, ADULT and CHILD over 16 years, 3 doses each of 0.5 mL, second dose after 1–3 months and third dose after further 5–12 months; CHILD 1–16 years 3 doses of 0.25 mL, second dose after 1–3 months and third dose after further 5–12 months; ELDERLY over 60 years and immunocompromised (including those receiving immunosuppressants), antibody concentration may be measured 4 weeks after second dose and dose repeated if protective levels not achieved Note To achieve more rapid protection, second dose may be given 14 days after first dose

- Booster doses, give first dose within 3 years after initial course completed, then every 3–5 years

**TicoVac®** (MASTA) ℞

Injection, suspension, formaldehyde-inactivated Neudörfl tick-borne encephalitis virus strain (cultivated in chick embryo cells) adsorbed onto hydrated aluminium hydroxide, net price 0.25-mL prefilled syringe (*TicoVac Junior®*) = £28.00, 0.5-mL prefilled syringe = £32.00
Excipients include gentamicin and neomycin

---

## Typhoid vaccines

Typhoid vaccine is available as Vi capsular polysaccharide (from *Salmonella typhi*) vaccine for injection and as live attenuated *Salmonella typhi* for oral use.

Typhoid immunisation is advised for

- travellers to areas where typhoid is endemic, especially if staying with or visiting local people

- travellers to endemic areas where frequent or prolonged exposure to poor sanitation and poor food hygiene is likely

- laboratory personnel who, in the course of their work, may be exposed to *Salmonella typhi*

Typhoid vaccination is not a substitute for scrupulous personal hygiene (see p. 695).

Capsular **polysaccharide typhoid vaccine** is usually given by *intramuscular injection*. Children under 2 years may respond suboptimally to the vaccine, but children aged between 1–2 years should be immunised if the risk of typhoid fever is considered high (immunisation is not recommended for infants under 12 months). Booster doses are needed every 3 years on continued exposure.

**Oral typhoid vaccine** is a **live attenuated** vaccine contained in an enteric-coated capsule. One capsule taken on alternate days for a total of 3 doses, provides protection 7–10 days after the last dose. Protection may persist for up to 3 years in those constantly (or repeatedly) exposed to *Salmonella typhi*, but occasional travellers require further courses at intervals of 1 year.

**Interactions** Oral typhoid vaccine is inactivated by concomitant administration of antibacterials or antimalarials:

- Antibacterials should be avoided for 3 days before and after oral typhoid vaccination;

- *Mefloquine* should be avoided for at least 12 hours before or after oral typhoid; vaccination with oral typhoid should preferably be completed at least 3 days before the first dose of mefloquine;

- For other antimalarials vaccination with oral typhoid vaccine should be completed at least 3 days before the first dose of the antimalarial (except proguanil hydrochloride with atovaquone, which may be given concomitantly).

### ■ TYPHOID VACCINE

**Indications** immunisation against typhoid fever
**Cautions** section 14.1; **interactions:** see above and Appendix 1 (vaccines)
**Contra-indications** section 14.1; also for *oral* vaccine, acute gastro-intestinal illness
**Side-effects** section 14.1
**Dose**
- See under preparations

◢**Typhoid polysaccharide vaccine for injection**
**Typherix®** (GSK) [PoM]
Injection, Vi capsular polysaccharide typhoid vaccine, 50 micrograms/mL virulence polysaccharide antigen of *Salmonella typhi*, net price 0.5-mL prefilled syringe = £9.93
Dose by intramuscular injection, 0.5 mL at least 2 weeks before potential exposure to typhoid infection; CHILD under 2 years (see notes above)

**Typhim Vi®** (Sanofi Pasteur) [PoM]
Injection, Vi capsular polysaccharide typhoid vaccine, 50 micrograms/mL virulence polysaccharide antigen of formaldehyde-inactivated *Salmonella typhi*, net price 0.5-mL prefilled syringe = £9.12
Dose by intramuscular injection, 0.5 mL at least 2 weeks before potential exposure to typhoid infection CHILD under 2 years (see notes above)

◢**Polysaccharide vaccine with hepatitis A vaccine**
See Hepatitis A Vaccine

◢**Typhoid vaccine, live (oral)**
**Vivotif®** (MASTA) [PoM]
Capsules, e/c, live attenuated *Salmonella typhi* (Ty21a), net price 3-cap pack = £14.77. Label: 23, 25, counselling, administration
Dose ADULT and CHILD over 6 years, 1 capsule on days 1, 3, and 5
Counselling Swallow as soon as possible after placing in mouth with a cold or lukewarm drink; it is important to store capsules in a refrigerator

## Varicella–zoster vaccine

Varicella–zoster vaccine (live) is licensed for immunisation against varicella in seronegative individuals. It is not recommended for routine use in children but can be given to seronegative healthy children over 1 year who come into close contact with individuals at high risk of severe varicella infections. The Department of Health recommends varicella–zoster vaccine for seronegative healthcare workers who come into direct contact with patients. Those with a history of chickenpox or shingles can be considered immune, but healthcare workers with a negative or uncertain history should be tested.

Rarely, the varicella–zoster vaccine virus has been transmitted from the vaccinated individual to close contacts. Therefore, contact with the following should be avoided if a vaccine-related cutaneous rash develops within 4–6 weeks of the first or second dose:

- varicella-susceptible pregnant women;
- individuals at high risk of severe varicella, including those with immunodeficiency or those receiving immunosuppressive therapy.

Healthcare workers who develop a generalised papular or vesicular rash on vaccination should avoid contact with patients until the lesions have crusted. Those who develop a localised rash after vaccination should cover the lesions and be allowed to continue working unless in contact with patients at high risk of severe varicella.

**Varicella–zoster immunoglobulin** is used to protect susceptible individuals at increased risk of varicella infection, see p. 693.

### ■ VARICELLA-ZOSTER VACCINE

**Indications** immunisation against varicella infection (see notes above)
**Cautions** see section 14.1; *also* post-vaccination close-contact with susceptible individuals (see notes above); **interactions:** Appendix 1 (vaccines)
**Contra-indications** see section 14.1; *also* pregnancy (avoid pregnancy for 3 months after vaccination)
**Side-effects** see section 14.1; also varicella-like rash; *rarely* thrombocytopenia
**Dose**
- See under preparations

**Varilrix®** (GSK) ▼ [PoM]
Injection, powder for reconstitution, live attenuated varicella–zoster virus (Oka strain) propagated in human diploid cells, net price 0.5-mL vial (with diluent) = £27.31
Excipients include neomycin
Dose by subcutaneous injection preferably into deltoid region, ADULT and CHILD over 1 year (see notes above), 2 doses of 0.5 mL separated by an interval of at least 6 weeks (minimum 4 weeks)

**Varivax®** (Sanofi Pasteur) ▼ [PoM]
Injection powder for reconstitution, live attenuated varicella-zoster virus (Oka/Merck strain) propagated in human diploid cells, net price 0.5-mL vial (with diluent) = £30.89
Excipients include gelatin and neomycin
Dose by intramuscular or subcutaneous injection into deltoid region (or higher anterolateral thigh in children), ADULT and CHILD over 13 years (see notes above), 2 doses of 0.5 mL separated by 4–8 weeks; CHILD 1–13 years (see notes above) 2 doses of 0.5 mL separated by an interval of at least 4 weeks (two doses separated by 12 weeks in children with asymptomatic HIV infection)

## Yellow fever vaccine

Live yellow fever vaccine is indicated for those travelling or living in areas where infection is endemic (see p. 695) and for laboratory staff who handle the virus or who handle clinical material from suspected cases. Infants under 6 months of age should not be vaccinated because there is a small risk of encephalitis; infants 6–9 months should be vaccinated only if the risk of yellow fever is high and unavoidable (seek expert advice). The immunity which probably lasts for life is officially accepted for 10 years starting from 10 days after primary immunisation and for a further 10 years immediately after revaccination.

Very rare, vaccine-associated adverse effects have been reported, such as viscerotropic disease (yellow fever vaccine-associated viscerotropic disease, YEL-AVD), a syndrome which may include metabolic acidosis, muscle and liver cytolysis, and multi-organ failure. Neurological disorders (yellow fever vaccine-associated neurotropic disease, YEL-AND) such as encephalitis have also been reported. These *very rare* adverse effects usually have occurred after the first dose of yellow fever vaccine in those with no previous immunity.

**Pregnancy and breast-feeding** Live yellow fever vaccine should not be given during pregnancy but if a significant risk of exposure cannot be avoided then vaccination should be delayed to the third trimester if possible (but the need for immunisation usually outweighs risk to the fetus). Vaccination should be considered in breast-feeding women when there is a real risk to the mother from yellow fever disease.

### ■ YELLOW FEVER VACCINE, LIVE

**Indications** immunisation against yellow fever

**Cautions** see section 14.1; *also* individuals over 60 years—greater risk of vaccine-associated adverse effects, see notes above; pregnancy and breast-feeding, see notes above; **interactions:** Appendix 1 (vaccines)

**Contra-indications** see section 14.1 and notes above; *also* children under 6 months; history of thymus dysfunction

**Side-effects** see section 14.1; also reported neurotropic disease and viscerotropic disease (see notes above)

**Dose**

• By deep subcutaneous injection, ADULT and CHILD over 9 months, 0.5 mL (see also notes above)

**Yellow Fever Vaccine, Live** PoM
Yel(live)
Injection, powder for reconstitution, live, attenuated 17D-204 strain of yellow fever virus, cultivated in chick embryos; single dose vial with syringe containing 0.5 mL diluent
Available (only to designated Yellow Fever Vaccination centres) as *Stamaril®*

### 14.5 Immunoglobulins

14.5.1    Normal immunoglobulin
14.5.2    Disease-specific immunoglobulins
14.5.3    Anti-D (Rh₀) immunoglobulin

Two types of human immunoglobulin preparation are available, **normal immunoglobulin** and **disease-specific immunoglobulins.**

Human immunoglobulin is a sterile preparation of concentrated antibodies (immune globulins) recovered from pooled human plasma or serum obtained from outside the UK, tested and found non-reactive for hepatitis B surface antigen and for antibodies against hepatitis C virus and human immunodeficiency virus (types 1 and 2). A global shortage of human immunoglobulin and the rapidly increasing range of clinical indications for treatment with immunoglobulins has resulted in the need for a Demand Management programme in the UK (for further information consult www.ivig.nhs.uk and Clinical Guidelines for Immunoglobulin Use, www.dh.gov.uk).

Immunoglobulins of animal origin (antisera were frequently associated with hypersensitivity reactions and are no longer used.

Further information on the use of immunoglobulins is included in the Health Protection Agency's *Immunoglobulin Handbook* www.hpa.org.uk, and in the Department of Health's publication, *Immunisation against Infectious Disease*, www.dh.gov.uk.

**Availability** Normal immunoglobulin for intramuscular administration is available from some regional Health Protection Agencies and microbiology laboratories for protection of contacts and the control of outbreaks of hepatitis A, measles and rubella, only. For other indications, subcutaneous or intravenous normal immunoglobulin should be purchased from the manufacturer.

**Disease-specific immunoglobulins** (section 14.5.2) are available from some regional Health Protection Agencies and microbiology laboratories, with the exception of **tetanus immunoglobulin** which is available from BPL, hospital pharmacies, or blood transfusion departments. **Rabies immunoglobulin** is available from the Specialist and Reference Microbiology Division, Health Protection Agency. **Hepatitis B immunoglobulin** required by transplant centres should be obtained commercially.

In Scotland all immunoglobulins are available from the *Blood Transfusion Service.*

### 14.5.1 Normal immunoglobulin

Human **normal immunoglobulin** ('HNIG') is prepared from pools of at least 1000 donations of human plasma; it contains immunoglobulin G (IgG) and antibodies to hepatitis A, measles, mumps, rubella, varicella, and other viruses that are currently prevalent in the general population.

Normal immunoglobulin may **interfere with the immune response to live virus vaccines** which should therefore only be given **at least 3 weeks before or 3 months after** an injection of normal immunoglobulin (this does not apply to yellow fever vaccine since normal immunoglobulin does not contain antibody to this virus).

**Uses** Normal immunoglobulin (containing 10%–18%) is administered by *intramuscular injection* for the protection of susceptible contacts against **hepatitis A** virus (infectious hepatitis), **measles** and, to a lesser extent, **rubella.** Injection of immunoglobulin produces immediate protection lasting several weeks.

Normal immunoglobulin (containing 3%–12% protein) for *intravenous administration* is used as *replacement therapy* for patients with congenital agammaglobulinaemia and hypogammaglobulinaemia, and for the short-term treatment of idiopathic thrombocytopenic purpura and Kawasaki syndrome; it is also used for the prophylaxis of infection following bone-marrow transplantation and in children with symptomatic HIV infection who have recurrent bacterial infections. Normal immunoglobulin for replacement therapy may also be given intramuscularly or subcutaneously, but intravenous formulations are normally preferred.Intravenous immunoglobulin is also used in the treatment of Guillain-Barré syndrome as an alternative to plasma exchange.

For guidance on the use of intravenous normal immunoglobulins and alternative therapies for certain conditions, consult *Clinical Guidelines for Immunoglobulin Use* (www.dh.gov.uk).

**Hepatitis A** Hepatitis A vaccine is preferred for individuals at risk of infection (see p. 676) including those visiting areas where the disease is highly endemic (all countries excluding Northern and Western Europe, North America, Japan, Australia, and New Zealand). In unimmunised individuals, transmission of hepatitis A is reduced by good hygiene. Intramuscular normal immunoglobulin is no longer recommended for routine prophylaxis in travellers but it may be indicated for immunocompromised patients if their antibody response to vaccine is unlikely to be adequate.

Intramuscular normal immunoglobulin is of value in the prevention of infection in close contacts of confirmed cases of hepatitis A where there has been a delay of more than 7 days in identifying contacts, or for close contacts at high risk of severe disease. Hepatitis A vaccine may be given at the same time, but it should be given at a separate injection site.

**Measles** Intramuscular normal immunoglobulin may be given to prevent or attenuate an attack of measles in individuals who do not have adequate immunity. Children and adults with compromised immunity who have come into contact with measles should receive intramuscular normal immunoglobulin as soon as possible after exposure. It is most effective if given within 72 hours but can be effective if given within 6 days. For individuals receiving intravenous immunoglobulin, 100 mg/kg given within 3 weeks before measles exposure should prevent measles. Intramuscular normal immunoglobulin should also be considered for the following individuals if they have been in contact with a confirmed case of measles or with a person associated with a local outbreak:

- non-immune pregnant women;
- infants under 9 months.

Further advice should be sought from the Centre for Infections, Health Protection Agency (tel. (020) 8200 6868).

Individuals with normal immunity who are not in the above categories and who have not been fully immunised against measles, can be given MMR vaccine (section 14.4) for prophylaxis following exposure to measles.

**Rubella** Intramuscular immunoglobulin after exposure to rubella does **not** prevent infection in non-immune contacts and is **not** recommended for protection of pregnant women exposed to rubella. It may, however, reduce the likelihood of a clinical attack which may possibly reduce the risk to the fetus. Risk of intrauterine transmission is greatest in the first 11 weeks of pregnancy, between 16 and 20 weeks there is minimal risk of deafness only, after 20 weeks there is no increased risk. Intramuscular normal immunoglobulin should be used only if termination of pregnancy would be unacceptable to the pregnant woman—it should be given as soon as possible after exposure. Serological follow-up of recipients is essential to determine if the woman has become infected despite receiving immunoglobulin.

For routine prophylaxis against Rubella, see MMR vaccine (p. 681).

## ■ NORMAL IMMUNOGLOBULIN

**Indications**  see notes above

**Cautions**  hypo- or agammaglobulinaemia with or without IgA deficiency; interference with live virus vaccines—see p. 690
**Intravenous use** thrombophilic disorders, or risk factors for arterial or venous thromboembolic events; obesity; ensure adequate hydration, renal insufficiency— monitor for acute renal failure (intravenous preparations with added sucrose have been associated with cases of renal dysfunction and acute renal failure)

**Contra-indications**  patients with selective IgA deficiency who have known antibody against IgA

**Side-effects**  nausea, chills, fever, headache, arthralgia, low back pain *rarely*; hypotension; anaphylaxis, cutaneous skin reactions; aseptic meningitis, acute renal failure, also reported with *intravenous use* haemolytic anaemia, thromboembolic events including myocardial infarction, stroke, pulmonary embolism, and deep vein thrombosis,
**Note** Adverse reactions are more likely to occur in patients receiving normal immunoglobulin for the first time, or following a prolonged period between treatments, or when a different brand of normal immunoglobulin is administered.

**Dose**
- See under preparations
**Note** Antibody titres can vary widely between normal immunoglobulin preparations from different manufacturers—formulations are **not interchangeable**; patients should be maintained on the same formulation throughout long-term treatment to avoid adverse effects

### ◢For intramuscular use
**Normal Immunoglobulin** ⓘPoM
Normal immunoglobulin injection. 250-mg vial; 750-mg vial
**Dose**  by deep intramuscular injection, to control outbreaks of hepatitis A (see notes above), 500 mg; CHILD under 10 years 250 mg
Measles prophylaxis, CHILD under 1 year 250 mg, 1–2 years 500 mg, 3 years and over 750 mg
Rubella in pregnancy, prevention of clinical attack, 750 mg
Available from the Centre for Infections and other regional Health Protection Agency offices (for contacts and control of outbreaks only, see above)

### ◢For subcutaneous use
**Subcuvia®** (Baxter) ⓘPoM
Normal immunoglobulin (protein 16%) injection, net price 5-mL vial = £32.56, 10-mL vial = £65.12
**Dose**  by subcutaneous injection, ADULT and CHILD over 12 years antibody deficiency syndromes, consult product literature
**Note** May be administered by intramuscular injection (if subcutaneous route not possible) but **not** for patients with thrombocytopenia or other bleeding disorders

**Subgam®** (BPL) ⓘPoM
Normal immunoglobulin (protein 14%-18%) injection, net price 250-mg vial = £11.20, 750-mg vial = £28.50, 1.5-g vial = £57.00
**Dose**  by subcutaneous injection, antibody deficiency syndromes, consult product literature by intramuscular injection, Hepatitis A prophylaxis in outbreaks (see notes above), ADULT and CHILD over 10 years, 750 mg, CHILD under 10 years, 500 mg
Measles prophylaxis (see also notes above), ADULT and CHILD over 3 years, 750 mg, CHILD 1–3 years 500 mg, CHILD under 1 year, 250 mg
Rubella, in pregnancy, prevention of clinical attack (see also notes above), 750 mg
Tetanus prophylaxis (when tetanus immunoglobulin unavailable—see also p. 693), 250 units
**Note** Subgam® is not licensed for prophylactic use, but due to difficulty in obtaining suitable immunoglobulin products, the Health Protection Agency recommends intramuscular use for prophylaxis against Hepatitis A, measles, or rubella

**14**

**Immunological products and vaccines**

**Vivaglobin®** (CSL Behring) [PoM]
Normal immunoglobulin (protein 16%) injection, net price 3-mL vial = £17.76, 10-mL vial = £59.20, 20-mL vial = £118.40
Dose by subcutaneous injection, antibody deficiency syndromes, consult product literature

◀ **For intravenous use**
Note Dose recommendation for Kawasaki's syndrome, see *BNF for Children*; other indications—consult product literature for dosage regimens

**Flebogamma®** (Grifols) [PoM]
Intravenous infusion, human normal immunoglobulin (protein 5%), net price 0.5 g (10 mL) = £20.00, 2.5 g (50 mL) = £100.00, 5 g (100 mL) = £200.00, 10 g (200 mL) = £400.00

**Gammagard S/D®** (Baxter) [PoM]
Intravenous infusion, (providing protein 5% or 10%), net price 0.5 g (with diluent) = £20.05, 2.5 g (with diluent) = £100.25, 5 g (with diluent) = £200.50, 10 g (with diluent) = £401.00

**Intratect®** (Biotest UK) [PoM]
Intravenous infusion, human normal immunoglobulin (protein 5%), net price 1 g (20 mL) = £45.00, 2.5 g (50 mL) = £112.50, 5 g (100 mL) = £225.00, 10 g (200 mL) = £450.00,

**Octagam®** (Octapharma) ▼ [PoM]
Intravenous infusion, human normal immunoglobulin (protein 5%), net price 2.5 g (50 mL) = £120.00, 5 g (100 mL) = £240.00, 10 g (200 mL) = £480.00, (protein 10%), 5 g (50 mL) = £345.00, 10 g (100 mL) = £690.00,
Note Contains maltose (may cause falsely elevated results with blood glucose testing systems

**Privigen®** (CSL Behring) ▼ [PoM]
Intravenous infusion, human normal immunoglobulin (protein 10%), net price 2.5 g (25 mL) = £135.00, 5 g (50 mL) = £270.00, 10 g (100 mL) = £540.00, 20 g (200 mL) = £1080.00
Note Contains L-proline; contra-indicated in patients with hyperprolinaemia

**Vigam®** (BPL) [PoM]
Intravenous infusion, human normal immunoglobulin (protein 5%), net price 2.5 g (50 mL) = £95.00, 5 g (100 mL) = £190.00, 10 g (200 mL) = £380.00
Note Contains sucrose (see cautions, above)

## 14.5.2 Disease-specific immunoglobulins

Specific immunoglobulins are prepared by pooling the plasma of selected human donors with high levels of the specific antibody required. For further information, see Immunoglobulin Handbook (www.hpa.org.uk).

There are no specific immunoglobulins for hepatitis A, measles, or rubella—normal immunoglobulin, section 14.5.1 is used in certain circumstances. There is no specific immunoglobulin for mumps; neither normal immunoglobulin nor MMR vaccine is effective as post-exposure prophylaxis.

## Hepatitis B

Disease-specific **hepatitis B immunoglobulin** ('HBIG') is available for use in association with hepatitis B vaccine for the prevention of infection in laboratory and other personnel who have been accidentally inoculated with hepatitis B virus, and in infants born to mothers who have become infected with this virus in pregnancy or who are high-risk carriers (see Hepatitis B Vaccine, p. 678). Hepatitis B immunoglobulin will not inhibit the antibody response when given at the same time as hepatitis B vaccine but should be given in different sites.

## ◼ HEPATITIS B IMMUNOGLOBULIN

**Indications** prophylaxis against hepatitis B infection
**Cautions** IgA deficiency; interference with live virus vaccines see under Normal Immunoglobulin, p. 690.
**Side-effects** injection site swelling and pain, anthralgia; *rarely* anaphylaxis (for side-effects associated with *intravenous* immunoglobulins, see section 14.5.1) chest tightness and dyspnoea also reported
**Dose**
● see under preparations and see also notes above

**Hepatitis B Immunoglobulin** [PoM]
Injection, hepatitis B-specific immunoglobulin, 100 units/mL. Vials containing 200 units or 500 units, available from selected Health Protection Agency and NHS laboratories (except for Transplant Centres, see p. 690), also available from BPL
Dose by intramuscular injection (as soon as possible after exposure; ideally within 12–48 hours, but no later than 7 days after exposure), ADULT and CHILD over 10 years 500 units; CHILD under 5 years 200 units, 5–9 years 300 units; NEONATE 200 units
Prevention of transmitted infection at birth, NEONATE 200 units as soon as possible after birth; for full details consult *Immunisation against Infectious Disease* (www.dh.gov.uk)
Note Hepatitis B immunoglobulin for *intravenous use* is available from BPL on a named-patient basis

**Hepatect®CP** (Biotest UK) ▼ [PoM]
Intravenous infusion, hepatitis B-specific immunoglobulin 50 units/mL, net price 500 units (10 mL) = £300.00, 2000 units (40 mL) = £1100.00
Dose By intravenous infusion, after exposure to hepatitis B virus-contaminated material, (as soon as possible after exposure, but no later than 72 hours) ADULT and CHILD over 2 years, 8–10 units/kg; repeat dose after 2 months if necessary; infuse at initial rate of 0.1 mL/kg/hour for 10 minutes, then increase rate to max. 1 mL/kg/hour
Prevention of transmitted infection at birth, NEONATE, 20–50 units/kg (minimum dose 100 units) given at a rate of 2 mL over 5–15 minutes
Prophylaxis against re-infection of transplanted liver—consult product literature

## Rabies

Following exposure of an unimmunised individual to an animak in or from a country where the risk of rabies is high the site of the bite should be washed with soapy water and specific rabies immunoglobulin of human origin administered. As much of the dose as possible should be injected in and around the cleansed wound; the remainder should be given intramuscularly into the anterolateral thigh (remote from the site used for vaccination)

Rabies vaccine should also be given intramuscularly at a different site (for details see Rabies vaccine p. 686)

## ▬ RABIES IMMUNOGLOBULIN

**Indications**   post-exposure prophylaxis against rabies infection

**Cautions**   IgA deficiency; interference with live virus vaccines—see, p. 690 under Normal Immunoglobulin

**Side-effects**   injection site swelling and pain, arthralgia; *rarely* anaphylaxis; buccal ulceration, chest tightness, dyspnoea, and facial oedema also reported

**Dose**

• See under preparation

**Rabies Immunoglobulin** PoM
(Antirabies Immunoglobulin Injection)
See notes above

Dose   20 units/kg by infiltration in and around the cleansed wound; if wound not visible or healed or if infiltration of whole volume not possible, give remainder by intramuscular injection into anterolateral thigh (remote from vaccination site)

Note The potency of individual batches of rabies immunoglobulin from the same manufacturer may vary. The potency on individual vials indicates the volume needed to administer 500 units—it is necessary to calculate the specific volume required to provide the dose (units)

Available from Specialist and Reference Microbiology Division, Health Protection Agency (see section 14.5 under availability) (also from BPL)

## Tetanus

For the management of tetanus-prone wounds, **tetanus immunoglobulin** should be used in addition to wound cleansing and, where appropriate, antibacterial prophylaxis and a tetanus-containing vaccine (see diptheria containing vaccinessection 14.4). Tetanus immunoglobulin, together with metronidazole (section 5.1.11) and wound cleansing, should also be used for the treatment of established cases of tetanus.

Where intramuscular tetanus immunoglobulin is in short supply it should be reserved for treatment of tetanus. For tetanus-prone wounds in patients who are not fully immunised against tetanus, consider using intramuscular normal immunoglobulin (section 14.5.1); further details are available at www.hpa.org.uk

## ▬ TETANUS IMMUNOGLOBULIN

**Indications**   post-exposure prophylaxis and treatment of tetanus infection

**Cautions**   IgA deficiency; interference with live virus vaccines—see p. 690

**Side-effects**   injection site swelling and pain; *rarely* anaphylaxis

**Dose**

• Post-exposure prophylaxis, by intramuscular injection 250 units, increased to 500 units if more than 24 hours have elapsed or there is risk of heavy contamination or following burns

• Treatment of tetanus infection, by intramuscular injection 150 units/kg (multiple sites)

**Tetanus Immunoglobulin** PoM
(Antitetanus Immunoglobulin Injection)
Available from BPL
Note May be difficult to obtain

## Varicella–zoster

**Varicella–zoster immunoglobulin** (VZIG) is recommended for individuals who are at increased risk of severe varicella *and* who have no antibodies to varicella–zoster virus *and* who have significant exposure to chickenpox or herpes zoster. Those at increased risk include:

• neonates whose mothers develop chickenpox in the period 7 days before to 7 days after delivery;

• susceptible neonates exposed in the first 7 days of life;

• susceptible neonates or infants exposed whilst requiring intensive or prolonged special care nursing;

• susceptible women exposed at any stage of pregnancy (but when supplies of VZIG are short, may only be issued to those exposed in the first 20 weeks' gestation or to those near term) providing VZIG is given within 10 days of contact;

• immunocompromised individuals including those who have received corticosteroids in the previous 3 months at the following dose equivalents of prednisolone; *children* 2 mg/kg daily for at least 1 week or 1 mg/kg daily for 1 month; *adults* about 40 mg daily for more than 1 week.

**Important:** for full details consult *Immunisation against Infectious Disease*. **Varicella–zoster vaccine** is available—see section 14.4. For treatment of varicella–zoster infections, see section 5.3.2.1

## ▬ VARICELLA–ZOSTER IMMUNOGLOBULIN

**Indications**   prophylaxis against varicella infection

**Cautions**   IgA deficiency; interference with live virus vaccines—see p. 690

**Side-effects**   injection site swelling and pain; *rarely* anaphylaxis

**Dose**

• By intramuscular injection, prophylaxis (as soon as possible—not later than 10 days after exposure), ADULT and CHILD over 14 years, 1 g; NEONATE, INFANT and CHILD up to 5 years 250 mg, 5–10 years 500 mg, 10–14 years 750 mg; give second dose if further exposure occurs more than 3 weeks after first dose
Note No evidence that effective in treatment of severe disease. Normal immunoglobulin for intravenous use (section 14.5.1) may be used in those unable to receive intramuscular injections

**Varicella–Zoster Immunoglobulin** PoM
(Antivaricella–zoster Immunoglobulin)

Available from selected Health Protection Agency and NHS laboratories; (see section 14.5 under Availability) also from BPL

## 14.5.3 Anti-D (Rh$_0$) immunoglobulin

Anti-D (Rh$_0$) immunoglobulin is prepared from plasma taken from rhesus-negative donors who have been immunised against the anti-D-antigen. Anti-D (Rh$_0$) immunoglobulin is used to prevent a rhesus-negative mother from forming antibodies to fetal rhesus-positive cells which may pass into the maternal circulation. The objective is to protect any subsequent child from the hazard of haemolytic disease of the newborn.

Anti-D immunoglobulin should be administered to the mother following any sensitising episode (e.g. abortion, miscarriage and birth); it should be injected within 72 hours of the episode but even if a longer period has elapsed it may still give protection and should be administered. Anti-D (Rh₀) immunoglobulin is also given when significant feto-maternal haemorrhage occurs in rhesus-negative women during delivery. The dose of anti-D immunoglobulin is determined according to the level of exposure to rhesus-positive blood.

For routine antenatal prophylaxis NICE recommends that two doses of either 500 units *or* 1000–1650 units of anti-D immunoglobulin should be given, the first at 28 weeks' gestation and the second at 34 weeks; alternatively a single dose of 1500 units given between 28 and 30 weeks gestation can be used (see also NICE guidance below).

Use of routine *antenatal* anti-D prophylaxis should be given irrespective of previous anti-D prophylaxis for a sensitising event early in the same pregnancy. Similarly, *postpartum* anti-D prophylaxis should be given irrespective of previous routine antenatal anti-D prophylaxis or antenatal anti-D prophylaxis for a sensitising event in the same pregnancy.

---

**NICE guidance**

**Routine antenatal anti-D prophylaxis for rhesus-negative women (August 2008)**

Routine antenatal anti-D prophylaxis should be offered to all non-sensitised pregnant women who are rhesus negative.

---

**Note**

MMR vaccine may be given in the postpartum period with anti-D (Rh₀) immunoglobulin injection provided that separate syringes are used and the products are administered into different limbs. If blood is transfused, the antibody response to the vaccine may be inhibited—measure rubella antibodies after 6–8 weeks and revaccinate if necessary.

---

Anti-D (Rh₀) immunoglobulin is also given to women of child-bearing potential after the inadvertent transfusion of rhesus-incompatible blood components and is used for the treatment of idiopathic thrombocytopenia purpura.

## ■ ANTI-D (Rh₀) IMMUNOGLOBULIN

**Indications** see notes above

**Cautions** immunoglobulin A deficiency; possible interference with live virus vaccines, see under p. 690, but see notes above about administration with MMR vaccine

**Contra-indications** treatment of idiopathic thrombocytopenia purpura in rhesus negative or splenectomised patients

**Side-effects** nausea, vomiting, diarrhoea, abdominal pain; hypotension, hypertension, headache, fever, malaise, asthenia, drowsiness, dizziness, back pain, arthralgia, myalgia; pruritus, rash, sweating, injection site pain; *rarely* tachycardia, anaphylaxis, dyspnoea, hypotension, and urticaria; (for side-effects associated with *intravenous* immunoglobulins, see section 14.5.1

**Dose**
• See preparations below

**Anti-D (Rh₀) Immunoglobulin** PoM

Injection, anti-D (Rh₀) immunoglobulin, net price 250-unit vial = £19.00, 500-unit vial = £27.00, 1500-unit vial = £58.00, 2500-unit vial = £94.40

Dose by deep intramuscular injection, to rhesus-negative woman for prevention of Rh₀(D) sensitisation:

Following birth of rhesus-positive infant, 500 units immediately or within 72 hours; for transplacental bleed of over 4 mL fetal red cells, extra 100–125 units per mL fetal red cells

Following any potentially sensitising episode (e.g. stillbirth, abortion, amniocentesis) up to 20 weeks' gestation 250 units per episode (after 20 weeks, 500 units) immediately or within 72 hours

Antenatal prophylaxis, 500 units given at weeks 28 and 34 of pregnancy; if infant rhesus-positive, a further dose is still needed immediately or within 72 hours of delivery

Following Rh₀(D) incompatible blood transfusion, 100–125 units per mL transfused rhesus-positive red cells

Note Subcutaneous route used for patients with bleeding disorders

Available from Blood Centres and from BPL (*D-Gam®*)

**Partobulin SDF®** (Baxter) PoM

Injection, anti-D (Rh₀) immunoglobulin 1250 units/mL (250 micrograms/mL), net price 1-mL prefilled syringe = £35.00

Dose by intramuscular injection, to rhesus-negative woman for prevention of Rh₀ (D) sensitisation:

Following birth of rhesus-positive infant, 1000–1650 units immediately or within 72 hours; for large transplacental blood loss, 50–125 units per mL of fetal red cells

Antenatal prophylaxis, 1000–1650 units given at weeks 28 and 34 of pregnancy; if infant rhesus-positive, further dose is needed immediately or within 72 hours of delivery

Following abortion, ectopic pregnancy or hydatidiform mole up to 12 weeks' gestation, 600–750 units (after 12 weeks, 1250–1650 units) immediately or within 72 hours

Following amniocentesis or chorionic villous sampling, 1250–1650 units immediately or within 72 hours

Following Rh₀ (D) incompatible blood or red cell transfusion, 1250 units per 10 mL of transfused rhesus-positive red cells immediately or within 72 hours

Note Subcutaneous route recommended for patients with bleeding disorders.

**Rhophylac®** (CSL Behring) PoM

Injection, anti-D (Rh₀) immunoglobulin 750 units/mL (150 micrograms/mL), net price 2-mL (1500-unit) prefilled syringe = £46.50.

Dose by intramuscular *or* intravenous injection, to rhesus-negative woman for prevention of Rh₀(D) sensitisation:

Following birth of rhesus-positive infant, 1000–1500 units immediately or within 72 hours; for large transplacental bleed, extra 100 units per mL fetal red cells (preferably by intravenous injection)

Following any potentially sensitising episode (e.g. abortion, amniocentesis, chorionic villous sampling) up to 12 weeks' gestation 1000 units per episode (after 12 weeks, higher doses may be required) immediately or within 72 hours

Antenatal prophylaxis, 1500 units given between weeks 28–30 of pregnancy; if infant rhesus-positive, a further dose is still needed immediately or within 72 hours of delivery

Following Rh₀(D) incompatible blood transfusion, by intravenous injection, 50 units per mL transfused rhesus-positive blood (or 100 units per mL of erythrocyte concentrate)

Note Intravenous route recommended for patients with bleeding disorders.

**WinRho SDF®** (Baxter) PoM
Injection, anti-D (Rh₀) immunoglobulin, powder for reconstitution, net price 1500-unit (300-microgram) vial (with diluent) = £313.50, 5000-unit (1-mg) vial (with diluent) = £1045.00

**Dose** to rhesus-negative woman for prevention of Rh₀(D) sensitisation:

Following birth of rhesus-positive infant, by intramuscular injection, 1500 units or by intravenous injection, 600 units immediately or within 72 hours; for transplacental bleed of over 4 mL fetal blood, by intramuscular or intravenous injection, extra 100 units per mL fetal blood (further doses required for large bleed)

Following any potentially sensitising episode (e.g. abortion, amniocentesis, chorionic villous sampling) up to 12 weeks' gestation, by intramuscular or intravenous injection, 600 units per episode (after 12 weeks, 1500 units) immediately or within 72 hours

Antenatal prophylaxis, by intramuscular or intravenous injection, 1500 units given at week 28 of pregnancy; if infant rhesus positive; a further dose is still needed immediately or within 72 hours of delivery

Following Rh₀(D) incompatible blood transfusion, by intravenous injection, 50 units per mL transfused rhesus-positive blood (or 100 units per mL of erythrocyte concentrate); if intramuscular route used give in divided doses over several days

Following Rh₀(D) incompatible thrombocyte transfusion in rhesus-negative female child or woman of child-bearing age, by intravenous injection, 600 units

Autoimmune (idiopathic) thrombocytopenic purpura, consult product literature

**Note** Intravenous route recommended for patients with bleeding disorders

# 14.6 International travel

**Note** For advice on **malaria chemoprophylaxis**, see section 5.4.1.

No special immunisation is required for travellers to the United States, Europe, Australia, or New Zealand, although all travellers should have immunity to tetanus and poliomyelitis (and childhood immunisations should be up to date). Certain special precautions are required in non-European areas surrounding the Mediterranean, in Africa, the Middle East, Asia, and South America.

Travellers to areas that have a high incidence of **poliomyelitis** or **tuberculosis** should be immunised with the appropriate vaccine; in the case of poliomyelitis previously immunised adults may be given a booster dose of a preparation containing inactivated poliomyelitis vaccine (see p. 686). BCG immunisation (see p. 673) is recommended for travellers aged under 16 years[1] proposing to stay for longer than 3 months (or in close contact with the local population) in countries with an incidence of tuberculosis greater than 40 per 100 000[2]; it should preferably be given 3 months or more before departure.

**Yellow fever** immunisation (see p. 689) is recommended for travel to the endemic zones of Africa and South America. Many countries require an International Certificate of Vaccination from individuals arriving from, or who have been travelling through, endemic areas; other countries require a certificate from all entering travellers (consult the Department of Health handbook, *Health Information for Overseas Travel*, www.dh.gov.uk).

Immunisation against **meningococcal meningitis** is recommended for a number of areas of the world (for details, see p. 683).

Protection against **hepatitis A** is recommended for travellers to high-risk areas outside Northern and Western Europe, North America, Japan, Australia and New Zealand. Hepatitis A vaccine (see p. 676) is preferred and it is likely to be effective even if given shortly before departure; normal immunoglobulin is no longer given routinely but may be indicated in the immunocompromised (see p. 691). Special care must also be taken with food hygiene (see below).

**Hepatitis B** vaccine (see p. 678) is recommended for those travelling to areas of high or intermediate prevalence who intend to seek employment as healthcare workers or who plan to remain there for lengthy periods and who may therefore be at increased risk of acquiring infection as the result of medical or dental procedures carried out in those countries. Short-term tourists or business travellers are not generally at increased risk of infection but may put themselves at risk by their sexual behaviour when abroad.

Prophylactic immunisation against **rabies** (see p. 686) is recommended for travellers to enzootic areas on long journeys or to areas out of reach of immediate medical attention.

Travellers who have not had a **tetanus** booster in the last 10 years and are visiting areas where medical attention may not be accessible should receive a booster dose of adsorbed diphtheria [low dose], tetanus and poliomyelitis (inactivated) vaccine (see p. 674), even if they have received 5 doses of a tetanus-containing vaccine previously.

**Typhoid vaccine** (see p. 688) is indicated for travellers to countries where typhoid is endemic, but the vaccine is no substitute for personal precautions (see below).

There is no requirement for cholera vaccination as a condition for entry into any country, but **oral cholera vaccine** (see p. 674) should be considered for backpackers and those travelling to situations where the risk is greatest (e.g. refugee camps). Regardless of vaccination, travellers to areas where cholera is endemic should take special care with food hygiene (see below).

Advice on **diphtheria** (see p. 675), on **Japanese encephalitis**[3] (see p. 681) and on **tick-borne encephalitis** (see p. 688) is included in *Health Information for Overseas Travel*, see below.

**Food hygiene** In areas where sanitation is poor, good food hygiene is important to help prevent hepatitis A, typhoid, cholera, and other diarrhoeal diseases (including travellers' diarrhoea). Food should be freshly prepared and hot, and uncooked vegetables (including green salads) should be avoided; only fruits which can be peeled should be eaten. Only suitable bottled water, or tap water that has been boiled or treated with sterilising tablets, should be used for drinking.

---

1. There is inadequate evidence of protection by BCG vaccine in adults aged over 35 years; however, vaccination is recommended for healthcare workers irrespective of age because of the increased risk to them or their patients

2. List of countries where the incidence of tuberculosis is greater than 40 cases per 100 000 is available at www.hpa.org.uk

3. Japanese encephalitis vaccine not prescribable on the NHS; health authorities may investigate circumstances under which vaccine prescribed

**Information on health advice for travellers**
The Department of Health handbook, *Health Information for Overseas Travel* (2001), which draws together essential information *for healthcare professionals* regarding health advice for travellers, can be obtained from
The Stationery Office
PO Box 29, Norwich NR3 1GN
Telephone orders, 0870 600 5522
Fax: 0870 600 5533
www.tso.co.uk
Health professionals and travellers can find the latest information on immunisation requirements and precautions for avoiding disease while travelling from:
www.nathnac.org

Immunisation requirements change from time to time, and information on the current requirements for any particular country may be obtained from the embassy or legation of the appropriate country or from:

National Travel Health Network and Centre
Hospital for Tropical Diseases
Mortimer Market Centre
Capper Street, off Tottenham Court Road
London, WC1E 6AU
Tel: 0845 602 6712
(9 a.m.–noon, 2–4.30 p.m. weekdays for healthcare professionals **only**)
www.nathnac.org

Travel Medicine Team
Health Protection Scotland
Clifton House
Clifton Place
Glasgow, G3 7LN
Tel: (0141) 300 1100
(2 p.m.–4 p.m. weekdays)
www.travax.nhs.uk (registration required. Annual fee may be payable for users outside NHS Scotland)

Welsh Medicines Information Centre
University Hospital of Wales
Cardiff, CF14 4XW
Tel: (029) 2074 2979 (8.30 a.m.–5 p.m. weekdays for health professionals in Wales **only**)

Department of Health and Social Services
Castle Buildings
Stormont
Belfast, BT4 3PP
Tel: (028) 9052 0000

# 697

# 15 Anaesthesia

**15.1 General anaesthesia** 697

**15.1.1** Intravenous anaesthetics 698

**15.1.2** Inhalational anaesthetics 701

**15.1.3** Antimuscarinic drugs 703

**15.1.4** Sedative and analgesic peri-operative drugs 704

**15.1.4.1** Anxiolytics and neuroleptics 704

**15.1.4.2** Non-opioid analgesics 706

**15.1.4.3** Opioid analgesics 707

**15.1.5** Neuromuscular blocking drugs 708

**15.1.6** Drugs for reversal of neuro-muscular blockade 711

**15.1.7** Antagonists for central and respiratory depression 712

**15.1.8** Drugs for malignant hyper-thermia 713

**15.2 Local anaesthesia** 713

## 15.1 General anaesthesia

**15.1.1** Intravenous anaesthetics

**15.1.2** Inhalational anaesthetics

**15.1.3** Antimuscarinic drugs

**15.1.4** Sedative and analgesic peri-operative drugs

**15.1.5** Neuromuscular blocking drugs

**15.1.6** Drugs for reversal of neuromuscular blockade

**15.1.7** Antagonists for central and respiratory depression

**15.1.8** Drugs for malignant hyperthermia

> **Important** The drugs in section 15.1 should be used only by experienced personnel and where adequate resuscitation equipment is available.

Several different types of drug are given together during general anaesthesia. Anaesthesia is induced with either a volatile drug given by inhalation (section 15.1.2) or with an intravenously administered drug (section 15.1.1); anaesthesia is maintained with an intravenous or inhalational anaesthetic. Analgesics (section 15.1.4), usually short-acting opioids, are also used. The use of neuromuscular blocking drugs (section 15.1.5) necessitates intermittent positive-pressure ventilation. Following surgery, anticholinesterases (section 15.1.6) can be given to reverse the effects of neuromuscular blocking drugs; specific antagonists (section 15.1.7) can be used to reverse central and respiratory depression caused by some drugs used in surgery. A local anaesthetic (section 15.2) can be used to reduce pain at the injection site.

Individual requirements vary considerably and the recommended doses are only a guide. Smaller doses are indicated in ill, shocked, or debilitated patients and in significant hepatic impairment, while robust individuals may require larger doses. The required dose of induction agent may be less if the patient has been premedicated with a sedative agent or if an opioid analgesic has been used.

**Surgery and long-term medication** The risk of losing disease control on stopping long-term medication before surgery is often greater than the risk posed by continuing it during surgery. It is vital that the anaesthetist knows about **all** drugs that a patient is (or has been) taking.

Patients with adrenal atrophy resulting from long-term corticosteroid use (section 6.3.2) may suffer a precipitous fall in blood pressure unless corticosteroid cover is provided during anaesthesia and in the immediate postoperative period. Anaesthetists must therefore know whether a patient is, or has been, receiving corticosteroids (including high-dose inhaled corticosteroids).

Other drugs that should normally not be stopped before surgery include antiepileptics, antiparkinsonian drugs, antipsychotics, anxiolytics, bronchodilators, cardiovascular drugs (but see potassium-sparing diuretics, angiotensin-converting enzyme inhibitors, and angiotensin-II receptor antagonists below), glaucoma drugs, immunosuppressants, drugs of dependence, and thyroid or antithyroid drugs. Expert advice is required for patients receiving antivirals for HIV infection. For general advice on surgery in diabetic patients see section 6.1.1.

Patients taking antiplatelet medication or an oral anticoagulant present an increased risk for surgery. In these circumstances, the anaesthetist and surgeon should assess the relative risks and decide jointly whether the antiplatelet or anticoagulant should be stopped or replaced with heparin therapy.

Drugs that should be stopped before surgery include combined oral contraceptives (see Surgery, section 7.3.1 for details); for advice on hormone replacement therapy, see section 6.4.1.1. If antidepressants need to be stopped, they should be withdrawn gradually to avoid withdrawal symptoms. In view of their hazardous interactions MAOIs should normally be stopped 2 weeks before surgery. Tricyclic antidepressants need not be stopped, but there may be an increased risk of arrhythmias and hypotension (and dangerous interactions with vasopressor drugs); therefore, the anaesthetist should be informed if they are not stopped. Lithium should be stopped 24 hours before major surgery but the normal dose can be continued for minor surgery (with careful monitoring of fluids and electrolytes). Potassium-sparing diuretics may need to be withheld on the morning of surgery because hyperkalaemia may develop if renal perfusion is impaired or if there is tissue damage. Angiotensin-converting enzyme (ACE) inhibitors and angiotensin-II receptor antagonists can be associated with severe hypotension after induction of anaesthesia; these drugs may need to be discontinued 24 hours before surgery.

**Anaesthesia and driving**  Patients given sedatives and analgesics during minor outpatient procedures should be very carefully warned about the risk of driving afterwards. For intravenous benzodiazepines and for a short general anaesthetic the risk extends to **at least 24 hours** after administration. Responsible persons should be available to take patients home. The dangers of taking **alcohol** should also be emphasised.

**Prophylaxis of acid aspiration**  Regurgitation and aspiration of gastric contents (Mendelson's syndrome) is an important complication of general anaesthesia, particularly in obstetrics and during emergency surgery, and requires prophylaxis against acid aspiration. Prophylaxis is also needed in those with gastro-oesophageal reflux disease and in circumstances where gastric emptying may be delayed.

An **H$_2$-receptor antagonist** (section 1.3.1) or a **proton pump inhibitor** (section 1.3.5) such as omeprazole may be used before surgery to increase the pH and reduce the volume of gastric fluid. They do not affect the pH of fluid already in the stomach and this limits their value in emergency procedures; oral H$_2$-receptor antagonists can be given 1–2 hours before the procedure but omeprazole must be given at least 12 hours earlier. Antacids are frequently used to neutralise the acidity of the fluid already in the stomach; 'clear' (non-particulate) antacids such as sodium citrate are preferred. Sodium citrate 300 mmol/litre (88.2 mg/mL) oral solution is licensed for use before general anaesthesia for caesarean section (available from Viridian).

## Gas cylinders

Each gas cylinder bears a label with the name of the gas contained in the cylinder. The name or chemical symbol of the gas appears on the shoulder of the cylinder and is also clearly and indelibly stamped on the cylinder valve.

The colours on the valve end of the cylinder extend down to the shoulder; in the case of mixed gases the colours for the individual gases are applied in four segments, two for each colour.

Gas cylinders should be stored in a cool well-ventilated room, free from flammable materials.

**No lubricant of any description should be used on the cylinder valves.**

## Anaesthesia, sedation, and resuscitation in dental practice

For details see *A Conscious Decision: A review of the use of general anaesthesia and conscious sedation in primary dental care*; report by a group chaired by the Chief Medical Officer and Chief Dental Officer, July 2000 and associated documents. Further details can also be found in *Conscious Sedation in the Provision of Dental Care*; report of an Expert Group on Sedation for Dentistry (commissioned by the Department of Health), 2003. Both documents are available at www.dh.gov.uk.

Guidance is also included in *Standards for Dental Professionals*, London, General Dental Council, May 2005 (and as amended subsequently), and *Conscious Sedation in Dentistry: Dental Clinical Guidance*, Scottish Dental Effectiveness Programme, May 2006.

## 15.1.1 Intravenous anaesthetics

Intravenous anaesthetics may be used either to induce anaesthesia or for maintenance of anaesthesia throughout surgery. Intravenous anaesthetics nearly all produce their effect in one arm-brain circulation time and can cause apnoea and hypotension, and so adequate resuscitative facilities **must** be available. They are **contraindicated** if the anaesthetist is not confident of being able to maintain the airway (e.g. in the presence of a tumour in the pharynx or larynx). Extreme care is required in surgery of the mouth, pharynx, or larynx and in patients with acute circulatory failure (shock) or fixed cardiac output.

To facilitate tracheal intubation, induction is usually followed by a neuromuscular blocking drug (section 15.1.5) or short-acting opioid (section 15.1.4.3).

The dose of all intravenous anaesthetic drugs should be titrated to effect (except when using 'rapid sequence induction'). The dose and rate of administration should be lower in the elderly, and particularly in those with hypovolaemia or cardiovascular disease; lower doses may also be required in premedicated patients.

**Total intravenous anaesthesia** This is a technique in which major surgery is carried out with all drugs given intravenously. Respiration can be spontaneous, or controlled with oxygen-enriched air. Neuromuscular blocking drugs can be used to provide relaxation and prevent reflex muscle movements. The main problem to be overcome is the assessment of depth of anaesthesia. Target Controlled Infusion (TCI) systems can be used to titrate intravenous anaesthetic infusions to predicted plasma-drug concentrations in ventilated adult patients.

**Anaesthesia and driving** See section 15.1.

---

# Drugs used for intravenous anaesthesia

**Propofol**, the most widely used intravenous anaesthetic, can be used for induction or maintenance of anaesthesia in adults and children, but it is not recommended in neonates. Propofol is associated with rapid recovery and less hangover effect than other intravenous anaesthetics. It causes pain on intravenous injection, which can be reduced by intravenous lidocaine. Significant extraneous muscle movements may occur. Rarely, convulsions, anaphylaxis, and delayed recovery from anaesthesia can occur after propofol administration; since the onset of convulsions can be delayed, caution should be taken after day surgery. Propofol is associated with bradycardia, occasionally profound; intravenous administration of an antimuscarinic drug may prevent this. In adults, propofol can be used for sedation during diagnostic procedures or in intensive care. It is contraindicated in children under 17 years receiving intensive care because of the risk of potentially fatal effects including metabolic acidosis, cardiac failure, rhabdomyolysis, hyperlipidaemia, and hepatomegaly. When used for maintenance of anaesthesia in children, the maximum duration of administration should not exceed 60 minutes except in exceptional circumstances (e.g malignant hyperthermia where volatile agents must be avoided).

**Thiopental sodium** (thiopentone sodium) is a barbiturate that is used for induction of anaesthesia, but has no analgesic properties. Induction is generally smooth and rapid, but dose-related cardiovascular and respiratory depression can occur. Awakening from a moderate dose of thiopental is rapid because the drug redistributes into other tissues, particularly fat. However, metabolism is slow and sedative effects can persist for 24 hours. Repeated doses have a cumulative effect and recovery is much slower.

**Etomidate** is an intravenous agent associated with rapid recovery without a hangover effect. It causes less hypotension than thiopental and propofol during induction. Etomidate produces a high incidence of extraneous muscle movement, which can be minimised by an opioid analgesic or a short-acting benzodiazepine given just before induction. Pain on injection can be reduced by injecting into a larger vein or by giving an opioid analgesic just before induction. Etomidate can suppress adrenocortical function, particularly during continuous administration, and it should not be used for maintenance of anaesthesia.

**Ketamine** is used rarely. It has good analgesic properties at sub-anaesthetic dosage and is used under specialist supervision in palliative care for pain that is unresponsive to standard treatment. Ketamine causes

less hypotension than thiopental and propofol during induction. It is used mainly for paediatric anaesthesia, particularly when repeated administration is required (such as for serial burns dressings); recovery is relatively slow and there is a high incidence of extraneous muscle movements. The main disadvantage of ketamine is the high incidence of hallucinations, nightmares, and other transient psychotic effects; these can be reduced by a benzodiazepine such as diazepam or midazolam. Ketamine also has abuse potential and can itself cause dependence.

---

## ■ ETOMIDATE

**Indications** induction of anaesthesia

**Cautions** see under Intravenous Anaesthetics and notes above; hepatic impairment (Appendix 2); avoid in acute porphyria (section 9.8.2); pregnancy (Appendix 4); breast-feeding (Appendix 5); **interactions:** Appendix 1 (anaesthetics, general)

**Contra-indications** see under Intravenous Anaesthetics and notes above

**Side-effects** see notes above; also coughing, hiccups, shivering, allergic reaction (including bronchospasm and anaphylaxis); respiratory depression, arrhythmia, and convulsions also reported

**Dose**

● See under preparations

**Etomidate-Lipuro®** (Braun) PoM
Injection (emulsion), etomidate 2 mg/mL, net price 10-mL amp = £1.53
Dose ADULT and CHILD over 6 months, by slow intravenous injection, 150–300 micrograms/kg; CHILD under 10 years may need up to 400 micrograms/kg, ELDERLY 150–200 micrograms/kg

**Hypnomidate®** (Janssen-Cilag) PoM
Injection, etomidate 2 mg/mL, net price 10-mL amp = £1.41
Excipients include propylene glycol (see Excipients, p. 2)
Dose ADULT and CHILD, by slow intravenous injection, 300 micrograms/kg max.total dose 60 mg; ELDERLY 150–200 micrograms/kg; max. total dose 60 mg

---

## ■ KETAMINE

**Indications** induction and maintenance of anaesthesia (but rarely used)

**Cautions** see under Intravenous Anaesthetics and notes above; increased cerebrospinal fluid pressure; predisposition to hallucinations or nightmares; pregnancy (Appendix 4); **interactions:** Appendix 1 (anaesthetics, general)

**Contra-indications** see under Intravenous Anaesthetics; hypertension, pre-eclampsia or eclampsia, severe cardiac disease, stroke; raised intracranial pressure; head trauma; acute porphyria (section 9.8.2)

**Side-effects** see notes above; also tachycardia, hypertension, arrhythmias, hypotension, bradycardia; increased salivation, laryngospasm; anxiety, insomnia; diplopia, nystagmus, raised intra-ocular pressure; rashes, injection-site reactions; anaphylaxis also reported

**Dose**

● By intramuscular injection, short procedures, initially 6.5–13 mg/kg, adjusted according to response (10 mg/kg usually produces 12–25 minutes of surgical anaesthesia)

Diagnostic manoeuvres and procedures not involving intense pain, initially 4 mg/kg

**15**

**Anaesthesia**

- By intravenous injection over at least 60 seconds, short procedures, initially 1–4.5 mg/kg, adjusted according to response (2 mg/kg usually produces 5–10 minutes of surgical anaesthesia)
- By intravenous infusion of a solution containing 1 mg/mL, longer procedures, induction, total dose of 0.5–2 mg/kg; maintenance, 10–45 micrograms/kg/minute, rate adjusted according to response

**Ketalar®** (Pfizer) (PoM)
Injection, ketamine (as hydrochloride) 10 mg/mL, net price 20-mL vial = £5.06; 50 mg/mL, 10-mL vial = £8.77; 100 mg/mL, 10-mL vial = £16.10
Note For *intravenous injection*, dilute 100 mg/mL strength to a concentration of not more than 50 mg/mL with Glucose 5% *or* Sodium Chloride 0.9% *or* Water for Injections

## ▮ PROPOFOL

**Indications** see under dose

**Cautions** see under Intravenous Anaesthetics and notes above; cardiac impairment; respiratory impairment; elderly; hypovolaemia; epilepsy; hypotension; raised intracranial pressure; monitor blood-lipid concentration if risk of fat overload or if sedation longer than 3 days; hepatic impairment; renal impairment; pregnancy (Appendix 4); breast-feeding (Appendix 5); **interactions:** Appendix 1 (anaesthetics, general)

**Contra-indications** see notes above

**Side-effects** see notes above; also hypotension, tachycardia, flushing; transient apnoea, hyperventilation, coughing, and hiccup during induction; headache; *less commonly* thrombosis, phlebitis; *rarely* arrhythmia, headache, vertigo, shivering, euphoria; *very rarely* pancreatitis, pulmonary oedema, sexual disinhibition, and discoloration of urine; serious and sometimes fatal side-effects reported with prolonged infusion of doses exceeding 5 mg/kg/hour, including metabolic acidosis, rhabdomyolysis, hyperkalaemia, and cardiac failure, dystonia and dyskinesia also reported

**Dose**
- *1% injection*
- Induction of anaesthesia, by intravenous injection *or* infusion, 1.5–2.5 mg/kg (1–1.5 mg in those over 55 years) at a rate of 20–40 mg every 10 seconds until response; CHILD over 1 month, administer slowly until response (usual dose in child over 8 years 2.5 mg/kg, may need more in younger child e.g. 2.5–4 mg/kg)
- Maintenance of anaesthesia, by intravenous infusion, 4–12 mg/kg/hour *or* by intravenous injection, 25–50 mg repeated according to response; CHILD over 1 month, by intravenous infusion, 9–15 mg/kg/hour
- Sedation of ventilated patients in intensive care, by intravenous infusion, ADULT and CHILD over 17 years, 0.3–4 mg/kg/hour
- Sedation for surgical and diagnostic procedures, ADULT and CHILD over 17 years, initially by intravenous injection over 1–5 minutes, 0.5–1 mg/kg; maintenance, by intravenous infusion, 1.5–4.5 mg/kg/hour (additionally, if rapid increase in sedation required, by intravenous injection, 10–20 mg); patients over 55 years may require lower dose

- *2% injection*
- Induction of anaesthesia, by intravenous infusion, 1.5–2.5 mg/kg (1–1.5 mg in those over 55 years) at a rate of 20–40 mg every 10 seconds; CHILD over 3 years, administer slowly until response (usual dose in child over 8 years 2.5 mg/kg, may need more in younger child e.g. 2.5–4 mg/kg)
- Maintenance of anaesthesia, by intravenous infusion, 4–12 mg/kg/hour; CHILD over 3 years, by intravenous infusion, 9–15 mg/kg/hour
- Sedation in intensive care, by intravenous infusion, ADULT and CHILD over 17 years, 0.3–4 mg/kg/hour

**Propofol** (Non-proprietary) (PoM)
1% injection (emulsion), propofol 10 mg/mL, net price 20-mL amp = £2.33, 50-mL bottle = £5.82, 100-mL bottle = £11.64

2% injection (emulsion), propofol 20 mg/mL, net price 50-mL vial = £11.64
Brands include *Propofol-Lipuro®*, *Propoven*

**Diprivan®** (AstraZeneca) (PoM)
1% injection (emulsion), propofol 10 mg/mL, net price 20-mL amp = £1.07, 50-mL prefilled syringe (for use with *Diprifusor® TCI* system) = £4.72

2% injection (emulsion), propofol 20 mg/mL, net price 50-mL prefilled syringe (for use with *Diprifusor® TCI* system) = £5.27
Note *Diprifusor® TCI* ('target controlled infusion') system is licensed **only** for induction and maintenance of general anaesthesia in adults

## ▮ THIOPENTAL SODIUM
### (Thiopentone sodium)

**Indications** induction of general anaesthesia; anaesthesia of short duration; reduction of raised intracranial pressure if ventilation controlled; status epilepticus (see also section 4.8.2)

**Cautions** see notes above; cardiovascular disease; reconstituted solution is highly alkaline—extravasation causes tissue necrosis and severe pain; avoid intra-arterial injection; hepatic impairment (Appendix 2); pregnancy (Appendix 4); **interactions:** Appendix 1 (anaesthetics, general)

**Contra-indications** see notes above; acute porphyria (section 9.8.2); myotonic dystrophy; breast-feeding (Appendix 5)

**Side-effects** hypotension, arrhythmias, myocardial depression, laryngeal spasm, cough, sneezing, hypersensitivity reactions, rash, injection-site reactions; excessive doses associated with hypothermia and profound cerebral impairment

**Dose**
- Induction of general anaesthesia, by slow intravenous injection usually as a 2.5% (25 mg/mL) solution, ADULT over 18 years, fit and premedicated, initially 100–150 mg (reduced in elderly or debilitated) over 10–15 seconds (longer in elderly or debilitated), followed by further quantity if necessary according to response after 30–60 seconds; *or* up to 4 mg/kg (max. 500 mg); CHILD 1 month–18 years, initially up to 4 mg/kg, *then* 1 mg/kg repeated as necessary (max. total dose 7 mg/kg)
- Raised intracranial pressure, by slow intravenous injection, 1.5–3 mg/kg, repeated as required

- Status epilepticus (only if other measures fail, see section 4.8.2), by slow intravenous injection as a 2.5% (25 mg/mL) solution, ADULT over 18 years, 75–125 mg as a single dose; CHILD 1 month–18 years, initially up to 4 mg/kg by slow intravenous injection, *then* up to 8 mg/kg/hour by continuous intravenous infusion, adjusted according to response

**Thiopental** (Link) [PoM]

Injection, powder for reconstitution, thiopental sodium, net price 500-mg vial = £3.06

## 15.1.2 Inhalational anaesthetics

Inhalational anaesthetics may be gases or volatile liquids. *Gaseous anaesthetics* require suitable equipment for storage and administration. They may be supplied via hospital pipelines or from metal cylinders (section 15.1). *Volatile liquid anaesthetics* are administered using calibrated vaporisers, using air, oxygen, or nitrous oxide–oxygen mixtures as the carrier gas. To prevent hypoxia, the inspired gas mixture should contain a minimum of 25% oxygen at all times. Higher concentrations of oxygen (greater than 30%) are usually required during inhalational anaesthesia when nitrous oxide is being administered, see below.

**Anaesthesia and driving** See section 15.1.

## Volatile liquid anaesthetics

Volatile liquid anaesthetics can be used for induction and maintenance of anaesthesia, and following induction with an intravenous anaesthetic (section 15.1.1).

Volatile liquid anaesthetics can trigger malignant hyperthermia (section 15.1.8) and are contra-indicated in those susceptible to malignant hyperthermia. They can increase cerebrospinal pressure and should be used with caution in those with raised intracranial pressure. They may also cause hepatotoxicity in those sensitised to halogenated anaesthetics; halothane has been associated with *severe hepatotoxicity* (**important:** see CSM advice, below). In children with neuromuscular disease, inhalational anaesthetics are associated with very rare cases of hyperkalaemia resulting in cardiac arrhythmias and death. Cardiorespiratory depression, hypotension, and arrhythmias are common side-effects of volatile liquid anaesthetics.

**Isoflurane** is a volatile liquid anaesthetic. Heart rhythm is generally stable during isoflurane anaesthesia, but heart-rate can rise, particularly in younger patients. Systemic arterial pressure can fall and cardiac output can decrease, owing to a decrease in systemic vascular resistance. Muscle relaxation occurs and the effects of muscle relaxant drugs are potentiated. Isoflurane can irritate mucous membranes causing cough, breath-holding, and laryngospasm.

**Desflurane** is a rapid acting volatile liquid anaesthetic; it is reported to have about one-fifth the potency of isoflurane. Emergence and recovery from anaesthesia are particularly rapid because of its low solubility. Desflurane is not recommended for induction of anaesthesia as it is irritant to the upper respiratory tract; cough, breath-holding, apnoea, laryngospasm, and increased secretions can occur.

**Sevoflurane** is a rapid acting volatile liquid anaesthetic and is more potent than desflurane. Emergence and recovery are particularly rapid, but slower than desflurane. Sevoflurane is non-irritant and is therefore often used for inhalational induction of anaesthesia. Sevoflurane can interact with carbon dioxide absorbents to form compound A, a potentially nephrotoxic vinyl ether. However, in spite of extensive use, no cases of sevoflurane-induced permanent renal injury have been reported and the carbon dioxide absorbents used in the UK produce very low concentrations of compound A, even in low-flow anaesthetic systems.

**Halothane** is a volatile liquid anaesthetic that has largely been superseded by newer agents, but is occasionally used for inhalation induction of anaesthesia with careful monitoring for cardiorespiratory depression and arrhythmias. It is potent, induction is smooth, and the vapour is non-irritant and seldom induces coughing or breath holding. Halothane produces moderate muscle relaxation, but this may be inadequate for major abdominal surgery for which specific muscle relaxants should be used.

> **CSM advice (halothane hepatotoxicity)**
> *Severe hepatotoxicity* can follow halothane anaesthesia. The CSM has reported that this occurs more frequently after repeated exposure to halothane and has a high mortality. The risk of severe hepatotoxicity appears to be increased by repeated exposures within a short time interval, but even after a long interval (sometimes of several years), susceptible patients have been reported to develop jaundice. Since there is no reliable way of identifying susceptible patients, the CSM recommends the following precautions before the use of halothane:
> - a careful anaesthetic history should be taken to determine previous exposure and previous reactions to halothane;
> - repeated exposure to halothane within a period of **at least** 3 months should be **avoided** unless there are **overriding** clinical circumstances;
> - a history of unexplained jaundice or pyrexia in a patient following exposure to halothane is an absolute **contra-indication** to its future use in that patient.

## ▌ DESFLURANE

**Indications**   see notes above

**Cautions**   see notes above; pregnancy (Appendix 4); interactions: Appendix 1 (anaesthetics, general)

**Contra-indications**   see notes above; breast-feeding (Appendix 5)

**Side-effects**   see notes above

**Dose**

- Induction of anaesthesia (but not recommended), by inhalation through specifically calibrated vaporiser, ADULT 4–11%
- Maintenance of anaesthesia, by inhalation through specifically calibrated vaporiser, ADULT 2–6% in nitrous oxide; 2.5–8.5% in oxygen or oxygen-enriched air; CHILD see *BNF for Children*

**Suprane®** (Baxter) [PoM]

Desflurane, net price 240 mL = £63.31

15   Anaesthesia

## HALOTHANE

**Indications** see notes above

**Cautions** see notes above (**important**: CSM advice above); avoid for dental procedures in those under 18 years unless treated in hospital (high risk of arrhythmia); avoid in acute porphyria (section 9.8.2); hepatic impairment (Appendix 2); pregnancy (Appendix 4); **interactions**: Appendix 1 (anaesthetics, general)

**Contra-indications** see notes above; breast-feeding (Appendix 5)

**Side-effects** see notes above

**Dose**

• Induction of anaesthesia, using specifically calibrated vaporiser, in oxygen or nitrous oxide–oxygen, ADULT and CHILD over 1 month, initially 0.5% then increased gradually according to response to 2–4%

• Maintenance of anaesthesia, using specifically calibrated vaporiser, in oxygen or nitrous oxide–oxygen, ADULT and CHILD over 1 month, 0.5–2%

**Halothane** (Non-proprietary) [PoM]

Available from 'special-order' manufacturers or specialist importing companies, see p. 969

## ISOFLURANE

**Indications** see notes above

**Cautions** see notes above; pregnancy (Appendix 4); **interactions**: Appendix 1 (anaesthetics, general)

**Contra-indications** see notes above; breast-feeding (Appendix 5)

**Side-effects** see notes above

**Dose**

• Induction of anaesthesia, using specifically calibrated vaporiser, in oxygen or nitrous oxide–oxygen, increased gradually from 0.5% to 3%

• Maintenance of anaesthesia, using specifically calibrated vaporiser, 1–2.5% in nitrous oxide–oxygen; an additional 0.5–1% may be required when given with oxygen alone; caesarean section, 0.5–0.75% in nitrous oxide–oxygen

**Isoflurane** (Abbott)

Isoflurane, net price 250 mL = £47.50

**AErrane®** (Baxter)

Isoflurane, net price 250 mL = £27.00

## SEVOFLURANE

**Indications** see notes above

**Cautions** see notes above; obstetric use (risk of uterine haemorrhage); renal impairment (Appendix 3); pregnancy (Appendix 4); **interactions**: Appendix 1 (anaesthetics, general)

**Contra-indications** see notes above; breast-feeding (Appendix 5)

**Side-effects** see notes above; also urinary retention, leucopenia, agitation in children; dystonia, rash, and seizures also reported

**Dose**

• Induction of anaesthesia, using a specifically calibrated vaporiser, in oxygen or nitrous oxide–oxygen, adjusted according to response, ADULT and CHILD over 1 month initially 0.5–1% then increased gradually up to 8%

• Maintenance of anaesthesia, using a specifically calibrated vaporiser, in oxygen or nitrous oxide–oxygen, adjusted according to response, ADULT and CHILD over 1 month 0.5–3%

**Sevoflurane** (Non-proprietary) [PoM]

Sevoflurane, net price 250 mL = £123.00

# Nitrous oxide

**Nitrous oxide** is used for maintenance of anaesthesia and, in sub-anaesthetic concentrations, for analgesia. For *anaesthesia*, nitrous oxide is commonly used in a concentration of 50 to 66% in oxygen as part of a balanced technique in association with other inhalational or intravenous agents. Nitrous oxide is unsatisfactory as a sole anaesthetic owing to lack of potency, but is useful as part of a combination of drugs since it allows a significant reduction in dosage.

For *analgesia* (without loss of consciousness), a mixture of nitrous oxide and oxygen containing 50% of each gas (*Entonox®*, *Equanox®*) is used. Self-administration using a demand valve is popular in obstetric practice, for changing painful dressings, as an aid to postoperative physiotherapy, and in emergency ambulances.

Nitrous oxide may have a deleterious effect if used in patients with an air-containing closed space since nitrous oxide diffuses into such a space with a resulting increase in pressure. This effect may be dangerous in the presence of a pneumothorax, which may enlarge to compromise respiration, or in the presence of intracranial air after head injury.

Hypoxia can occur immediately following the administration of nitrous oxide; additional oxygen should always be given for several minutes after stopping the flow of nitrous oxide.

Exposure of patients to nitrous oxide for prolonged periods, either by continuous or by intermittent administration, may result in megaloblastic anaemia owing to interference with the action of vitamin $B_{12}$; neurological toxic effects can occur without preceding overt haematological changes. For the same reason, exposure of theatre staff to nitrous oxide should be minimised. Depression of white cell formation may also occur.

Assessment of plasma-vitamin $B_{12}$ concentration should be considered in those at risk of deficiency, including the elderly, those who have a poor or vegetarian diet, and those with a history of anaemia. Nitrous oxide should **not** be given continuously for longer than 24 hours or more frequently than every 4 days without close supervision and haematological monitoring.

## NITROUS OXIDE

**Indications** see notes above

**Cautions** see notes above; pregnancy (Appendix 4); **interactions**: Appendix 1 (anaesthetics, general)

**Contra-indications** susceptibility to malignant hyperthermia

**Side-effects** see notes above

**Dose**

• Maintenance of light anaesthesia (using suitable anaesthetic apparatus), up to 66% in oxygen

• Analgesia, up to 50% in oxygen, according to the patient's needs

## 15.1.3 Antimuscarinic drugs

Antimuscarinic drugs are used (less commonly nowadays) as premedicants to dry bronchial and salivary secretions which are increased by intubation, upper airway surgery, or some inhalational anaesthetics. They are also used before or with neostigmine (section 15.1.6) to prevent bradycardia, excessive salivation, and other muscarinic actions of neostigmine. They also prevent bradycardia and hypotension associated with drugs such as halothane, propofol, and suxamethonium.

**Atropine sulphate** is now rarely used for premedication but still has an emergency role in the treatment of vagotonic side-effects. For its role in acute arrhythmias after myocardial infarction, see section 2.3.1; see also cardiopulmonary resuscitation, section 2.7.3.

**Hyoscine hydrobromide** reduces secretions and also provides a degree of amnesia, sedation and anti-emesis. Unlike atropine it may produce bradycardia rather than tachycardia. In some patients, especially the elderly, hyoscine may cause the central anticholinergic syndrome (excitement, ataxia, hallucinations, behavioural abnormalities, and drowsiness).

**Glycopyrronium bromide** reduces salivary secretions. When given intravenously it produces less tachycardia than atropine. It is widely used with neostigmine for reversal of non-depolarising neuromuscular blocking drugs (section 15.1.5).

**Phenothiazines** do not effectively reduce secretions when used alone.

### ATROPINE SULPHATE

**Indications** drying secretions; reversal of excessive bradycardia; with anticholinesterases for reversal of non-depolarising neuromuscular block; antidote to organophosphorous poisoning (see Emergency Treatment of Poisoning p. 36), antispasmodic (section 1.2); bradycardia (section 2.3.1); cardiopulmonary resuscitation (section 2.7.3); cycloplegia, anterior uveitis (section 11.5)

**Cautions** section 1.2; also paralytic ileus; pyloric stenosis; cardiovascular disease; myasthenia gravis; prostatic enlargement; pregnancy (Appendix 4); breast-feeding (Appendix 5); **interactions:** Appendix 1 (antimuscarinics)

  **Duration of action** Since atropine has a shorter duration of action than neostigmine, late unopposed bradycardia may result; close monitoring of the patient is necessary

**Side-effects** section 1.2

**Dose**
• Premedication, by intravenous injection, 300–600 micrograms immediately before induction of anaesthesia; CHILD 20 micrograms/kg (max. 600 micrograms)

  By subcutaneous or intramuscular injection, 300–600 micrograms 30–60 minutes before induction; CHILD 20 micrograms/kg (max. 600 micrograms)

• Intra-operative bradycardia, by intravenous injection, 300–600 micrograms (larger doses in emergencies); CHILD [unlicensed indication] 1–12 years 10–20 micrograms/kg

• Control of muscarinic side-effects of neostigmine in reversal of competitive neuromuscular block, by intravenous injection, 0.6–1.2 mg; CHILD under 12 years 20 micrograms/kg (max. 600 micrograms)

• Control of muscarinic side-effects of edrophonium in reversal of competitive neuromuscular block, by intravenous injection, 600 micrograms; CHILD under 18 years 7 micrograms/kg (max. 600 micrograms) [unlicensed]

• Arrhythmias after myocardial infarction, see section 2.3.1 and 2.7.3; see also cardiopulmonary resuscitation algorithm, inside back cover

**¹Atropine** (Non-proprietary) ℗ℴ𝔐
Injection, atropine sulphate 600 micrograms/mL, net price 1-mL amp = 57p
**Note** Other strengths also available

Injection, prefilled disposable syringe, atropine sulphate 100 micrograms/mL, net price 5 mL = £4.58, 10 mL = £5.39, 30 mL = £8.95

Injection, prefilled disposable syringe, atropine sulphate 200 micrograms/mL, net price 5 mL = £5.90; 300 micrograms/mL, 10 mL = £5.91; 600 micrograms/mL, 1 mL = £5.91

1. ℗ℴ𝔐 restriction does not apply where administration is for saving life in emergency

**¹Minijet® Atropine** (UCB Pharma) ℗ℴ𝔐
Injection, atropine sulphate 100 micrograms/mL, net price 5 mL = £5.04, 10 mL = £5.93, 30 mL = £9.85

1. ℗ℴ𝔐 restriction does not apply where administration is for saving life in emergency

### GLYCOPYRRONIUM BROMIDE
(Glycopyrrolate)

**Indications** drying secretions (see Prescribing in Palliative Care, p. 17); reversal of excessive bradycardia; with neostigmine for reversal of non-depolarising neuromuscular block; hyperhidrosis (section 13.12)

**Cautions** section 1.2; also paralytic ileus, pyloric stenosis; cardiovascular disease; myasthenia gravis; prostatic enlargement; **interactions:** Appendix 1 (antimuscarinics)

**Side-effects** see section 1.2

**Dose**
• Premedication, by intramuscular *or* intravenous injection, 200–400 micrograms *or* 4–5 micrograms/kg (max. 400 micrograms); CHILD by intramuscular *or* by intravenous injection, 4–8 micrograms/kg (max. 200 micrograms)

• Intra-operative use, by intravenous injection, 200–400 micrograms *or* 4–5 micrograms/kg (max. 400 micrograms), repeated if necessary; CHILD under 18 years 4–8 micrograms/kg (max. 200 micrograms), repeated if necessary

• Control of muscarinic side-effects of neostigmine in reversal of non-depolarising neuromuscular block, by intravenous injection, 200 micrograms per 1 mg of neostigmine, *or* 10–15 micrograms/kg; CHILD 10 micrograms/kg (max. 500 micrograms)

**Glycopyrronium bromide** (Non-proprietary) ℗ℴ𝔐
Injection, glycopyrronium bromide 200 micrograms/mL, net price 1-mL amp = 54p; 3-mL amp = 91p

**Robinul®** (Anpharm) ℗ℴ𝔐
Injection, glycopyrronium bromide 200 micrograms/mL, net price 1-mL amp = 70p; 3-mL amp = £1.50
**Note** May be difficult to obtain

◢**With neostigmine metilsulphate**
Section 15.1.6

**15**

**Anaesthesia**

## ■ HYOSCINE HYDROBROMIDE
### (Scopolamine hydrobromide)

**Indications** premedication; motion sickness (section 4.6); hypersalivation associated with clozapine therapy (section 4.6); excessive respiratory secretions (see Prescribing in Palliative Care, p. 17)

**Cautions** see Antimuscarinics (section 1.2); also gastro-intestinal obstruction, paralytic ileus, myasthenia gravis, epilepsy, prostatic enlargement; avoid in the elderly (see notes above)

**Side-effects** see Antimuscarinics (section 1.2)

**Dose**

• Premedication, by subcutaneous *or* intramuscular injection, 200–600 micrograms 30–60 minutes before induction of anaesthesia; CHILD 15 micrograms/kg

**Hyoscine** (Non-proprietary) PoM
Injection, hyoscine hydrobromide 400 micrograms/mL, net price 1-mL amp = £2.80; 600 micrograms/mL, 1-mL amp = £2.67

◀With papaveretum
See under papaveretum (section 4.7.2)

## 15.1.4 Sedative and analgesic peri-operative drugs

15.1.4.1 Anxiolytics and neuroleptics
15.1.4.2 Non-opioid analgesics
15.1.4.3 Opioid analgesics

**Premedication** These drugs are given to allay fear and anxiety in the pre-operative period (including the night before an operation), to relieve pain and discomfort when present, and to augment the action of subsequent anaesthetic agents. A number of the drugs used also provide some degree of pre-operative amnesia. The choice will vary with the individual patient, the nature of the operative procedure, the anaesthetic to be used, and other prevailing circumstances such as outpatients, obstetrics, and recovery facilities. The choice also varies between elective and emergency operations.

**Premedication in children** Oral administration is preferred where possible; the rectal route should only be used in exceptional circumstances. For further details, consult *BNF for Children*.

Application of a local anaesthetic (section 15.2) to the injection site can help to prevent pain.

**Dental procedures** Anxiolytics diminish tension, anxiety and panic, and may benefit anxious patients. However, their use is no substitute for sympathy and reassurance.

Diazepam and temazepam are effective anxiolytics for dental treatment in adults, but they are less suitable for children. Diazepam has a longer duration of action than temazepam. When given at night diazepam is associated with more residual effects the following day; patients should be very carefully warned **not** to drive (**important**: for general advice on anaesthesia and driving see p. 698). For further information on hypnotics

and anxiolytics, see section 4.1. For further information on hypnotics used for dental procedures, see section 4.1.1.

**Anaesthesia and driving** See section 15.1.

### 15.1.4.1 Anxiolytics and neuroleptics

Anxiolytic benzodiazepines are widely used for premedication; neuroleptics such as **chlorpromazine** are rarely used.

## Benzodiazepines

Benzodiazepines possess useful properties for premedication including relief of anxiety, sedation, and amnesia; short-acting benzodiazepines taken by mouth are the most common premedicants. They have no analgesic effect so an opioid analgesic may sometimes be required for pain.

Benzodiazepines can alleviate anxiety at doses that do not necessarily cause excessive sedation and they are of particular value during short procedures or during operations under local anaesthesia (including dentistry). Amnesia reduces the likelihood of any unpleasant memories of the procedure (although benzodiazepines, particularly when used for more profound sedation, can sometimes induce sexual fantasies). Benzodiazepines are also used in intensive care units for sedation, particularly in those receiving assisted ventilation.

Benzodiazepines may occasionally cause marked respiratory depression and facilities for its treatment are essential; flumazenil (section 15.1.7) is used to antagonise the effects of benzodiazepines. They are best avoided in myasthenia gravis, especially peri-operatively.

**Diazepam** is used to produce mild sedation with amnesia. It is a long-acting drug with active metabolites and a second period of drowsiness can occur several hours after its administration. Peri-operative use of diazepam in children is not generally recommended; its effect and timing of response are unreliable and paradoxical effects may occur.

Diazepam is relatively insoluble in water and preparations formulated in organic solvents are painful on intravenous injection and give rise to a high incidence of venous thrombosis (which may not be noticed for several days after the injection). Intramuscular injection of diazepam is painful and absorption is erratic. An emulsion formulated for intravenous injection is less irritant and reduces the risk of venous thrombosis; it is not suitable for intramuscular injection. Diazepam is also available as a rectal solution but this preparation is not used for premedication or sedation.

**Temazepam** is given by mouth and has a shorter duration of action and a more rapid onset than diazepam given by mouth. It has been used as a premedicant in inpatient and day-case surgery; anxiolytic and sedative effects last about 90 minutes although there may be residual drowsiness.

**Lorazepam** produces more prolonged sedation than temazepam and it has marked amnesic effects. It is used as a premedicant the night before major surgery; a further, smaller dose may be required the following morning if any delay in starting surgery is anticipated.

Alternatively the first dose may be given early in the morning on the day of operation.

**Midazolam** is a water-soluble benzodiazepine that is often used in preference to intravenous diazepam; recovery is faster than from diazepam, but may be significantly longer in the elderly, in patients with a low cardiac output, or after repeated dosing. Midazolam is associated with profound sedation when high doses are given intravenously or when used with certain other drugs.

> There have been reports of overdosage when high strength midazolam has been used for conscious sedation. The use of high-strength midazolam (5 mg/mL in 2 mL and 10 mL ampoules, or 2 mg/mL in 5 mL ampoules) should be restricted to general anaesthesia, intensive care, palliative care, or other situations where the risk has been assessed. It is advised that flumazenil (section 15.1.7) is available when midazolam is used, to reverse the effects if necessary.

### DIAZEPAM

**Indications** premedication; sedation with amnesia, and in conjunction with local anaesthesia; short-term use in anxiety or insomnia, adjunct in acute alcohol withdrawal (section 4.1.2); status epilepticus (section 4.8.2); muscle spasms (section 10.2.2)

**Cautions** see notes above, section 4.1.2, and section 4.8.2

**Contra-indications** see notes above and section 4.1.2

**Side-effects** see notes above and section 4.1.2

**Dose**

- By mouth, 5–20 mg 1–2 hours before procedure *or* 5 mg on night before dental surgery then 5 mg 2 hours before procedure; ELDERLY (or debilitated), half adult dose; CHILD 1 month–18 years, see *BNF for Children*
- By intravenous injection into a large vein (emulsion preparation preferred), sedative cover for minor surgical and medical procedures, ADULT over 18 years, 10–20 mg over 2–4 minutes, immediately before procedure; premedication 100–200 micrograms/kg, CHILD under 18 years see *BNF for Children*
- By rectum, CHILD 1–18 years, see *BNF for Children*

◢**Preparations**
Section 4.1.2

### LORAZEPAM

**Indications** sedation with amnesia; premedication; short-term use in anxiety or insomnia (section 4.1.2); status epilepticus (section 4.8.2)

**Cautions** see notes above and section 4.1.2; **interactions:** Appendix 1 (anxiolytics and hypnotics)

**Contra-indications** see notes above and under Diazepam (section 4.1.2)

**Side-effects** see notes above and under Diazepam (section 4.1.2)

**Dose**

- By mouth, 2–3 mg the night before operation; 2–4 mg 1–2 hours before operation

- By slow intravenous injection, preferably diluted with an equal volume of sodium chloride intravenous infusion 0.9% or water for injections, 50 micrograms/kg 30–45 minutes before operation
- By intramuscular injection, diluted as above, 50 micrograms/kg 60–90 minutes before operation

◢**Preparations**
Section 4.1.2

### MIDAZOLAM

**Indications** conscious sedation; sedation in intensive care; sedation in anaesthesia; premedication; induction of anaesthesia; status epilepticus (section 4.8.2)

**Cautions** see notes above; cardiac disease; respiratory disease; myasthenia gravis; neonates; children (particularly if cardiovascular impairment); risk of airways obstruction and hypoventilation in children under 6 months (monitor respiratory rate and oxygen saturation); history of drug or alcohol abuse; reduce dose in elderly and debilitated; risk of severe hypotension in hypovolaemia, vasoconstriction, hypothermia; avoid prolonged use (and abrupt withdrawal thereafter); concentration of midazolam in children under 15 kg not to exceed 1 mg/mL; hepatic impairment (Appendix 2); renal impairment (Appendix 3); pregnancy (Appendix 4) and breast-feeding (Appendix 5); **interactions:** Appendix 1 (anxiolytics and hypnotics)

**Contra-indications** marked neuromuscular respiratory weakness including unstable myasthenia gravis; severe respiratory depression; acute pulmonary insufficiency

**Side-effects** see notes above; gastro-intestinal disturbances, increased appetite, jaundice; hypotension, cardiac arrest, heart rate changes, anaphylaxis, thrombosis; laryngospasm, bronchospasm, respiratory depression and respiratory arrest (particularly with high doses or on rapid injection); drowsiness, confusion, ataxia, amnesia, headache, euphoria, hallucinations, convulsions (more common in neonates), dizziness, vertigo, involuntary movements, paradoxical excitement and aggression (especially in children and elderly), dysarthria; urinary retention, incontinence, changes in libido; blood disorders; muscle weakness; visual disturbances; salivation changes; skin reactions; injection-site reactions

**Dose**

- Conscious sedation, by slow intravenous injection (approx. 2 mg/minute) 5–10 minutes before procedure, initially 2–2.5 mg (ELDERLY 0.5–1 mg), increased if necessary in steps of 1 mg (ELDERLY 0.5–1 mg); usual total dose 3.5–5 mg (max. 7.5 mg), ELDERLY max. 3.5 mg; CHILD 1 month–18 years, see *BNF for Children*

  By rectum, CHILD 6 months–18 years, see *BNF for Children*

  By mouth, CHILD 1 month–18 years, see *BNF for Children*

  By buccal administration, CHILD 6 months–18 years, see *BNF for Children*

- Conscious sedation in dental patients (specialist use only), by mouth, 20 mg 30–60 minutes before procedure with close monitoring [unlicensed]

- Sedative in combined anaesthesia, by intravenous injection, 30–100 micrograms/kg repeated as required or by continuous intravenous infusion, 30–100 micrograms/kg/hour (ELDERLY lower doses needed); CHILD not recommended
- Premedication, by deep intramuscular injection, 70–100 micrograms/kg (ELDERLY and debilitated 25–50 micrograms/kg) 20–60 minutes before induction

By intravenous injection, 1–2 mg repeated as required (ELDERLY and debilitated 0.5 mg, repeat dose slowly as required); CHILD 12–18 years, see *BNF for Children*

By rectum, CHILD 6 months–12 years, see *BNF for Children*

By mouth, CHILD 1 month–18 years, see *BNF for Children*

- Induction (but rarely used), by slow intravenous injection, 150–200 micrograms/kg (ELDERLY and debilitated 50–150 micrograms/kg) given in divided doses (max. 5 mg) at intervals of 2 minutes; max. total dose 600 micrograms/kg; CHILD 7–18 years initially 150 micrograms/kg (max. 7.5 mg) given in steps of 50 micrograms/kg (max. 2.5 mg) over 2–5 minutes; wait for 2–5 minutes then give additional doses of 50 micrograms/kg (max. 2.5 mg) every 2 minutes if necessary; max. total dose 500 micrograms/kg (not exceeding 25 mg)
- Sedation of patients receiving intensive care, by slow intravenous injection, initially 30–300 micrograms/kg given in steps of 1–2.5 mg every 2 minutes, then by slow intravenous injection *or* by continuous intravenous infusion, 30–200 micrograms/kg/hour; reduce dose (or reduce or omit initial dose) in hypovolaemia, vasoconstriction, or hypothermia; lower doses may be adequate if opioid analgesic also used; NEONATE under 32 weeks gestational age by continuous intravenous infusion, 30 micrograms/kg/hour, NEONATE over 32 weeks gestational age and CHILD under 6 months 60 micrograms/kg/hour, CHILD over 6 months by slow intravenous injection, initially 50–200 micrograms/kg, then by continuous intravenous infusion, 60–120 micrograms/kg/hour, adjusted according to response

**Midazolam** (Non-proprietary) ⓒᴅ
Oral liquid, midazolam 2.5 mg/mL, 100 mL
Available from 'special-order' manufacturers or specialist importing companies, see p. 969

Injection, midazolam (as hydrochloride) 1 mg/mL, net price 2-mL amp = 50p, 5-mL amp = 60p, 50-mL vial = £7.87; 2 mg/mL, 5-mL amp = 65p; 5 mg/mL, 2-mL amp = 58p, 10-mL amp = £2.50

**Hypnovel®** (Roche) ⓒᴅ
Injection, midazolam (as hydrochloride) 2 mg/mL, net price 5-mL amp = 86p; 5 mg/mL, 2-mL amp = 73p

## ▌ TEMAZEPAM

**Indications** premedication before surgery; anxiety before investigatory procedures; hypnotic (section 4.1.1)

**Cautions** see notes above and under Diazepam (section 4.1.2; **interactions:** Appendix 1 (anxiolytics and hypnotics)

**Contra-indications** see notes above and under Diazepam (section 4.1.2)

**Side-effects** see notes above and under Diazepam (section 4.1.2)

**Dose**
- By mouth, premedication, 20–40 mg (elderly, 10–20 mg) 1 hour before operation; CHILD 1 mg/kg (max. 30 mg)

◢**Preparations**
Section 4.1.1

## ▌15.1.4.2 Non-opioid analgesics

Since non-steroidal anti-inflammatory drugs (NSAIDs) do not depress respiration, do not impair gastro-intestinal motility, and do not cause dependence, they may be useful alternatives or adjuncts to opioids for the relief of postoperative pain. NSAIDs may be inadequate for the relief of severe pain.

**Acemetacin, diclofenac, flurbiprofen, ibuprofen, ketoprofen,** (section 10.1.1), **paracetamol** (section 4.7.1), **parecoxib,** and **ketorolac** are licensed for postoperative use. Diclofenac, ketoprofen, ketorolac, and paracetamol can be given by injection as well as by mouth. Diclofenac can be given by intravenous infusion for the treatment or prevention of postoperative pain. Intramuscular injections of diclofenac and ketoprofen are rarely used; they are given deep into the gluteal muscle to minimise pain and tissue damage. Ketorolac is less irritant on intramuscular injection but pain has been reported; it can also be given by intravenous injection.

Parecoxib (a selective inhibitor of cyclo-oxygenase-2) can be given by intramuscular or intravenous injection (but see also NSAIDs and Cardiovascular Events, section 10.1.1). The *Scottish Medicines Consortium* has advised (January 2003) that parecoxib should **not** be used because there is no evidence of a reduction in postoperative haemorrhagic or gastro-intestinal complications compared with non-selective NSAIDs.

Suppositories of diclofenac and ketoprofen may be effective alternatives to the parenteral use of these drugs. Flurbiprofen is also available as suppositories.

## ▌ KETOROLAC TROMETAMOL

**Indications** short-term management of moderate to severe acute postoperative pain **only**

**Cautions** section 10.1.1; avoid in acute porphyria (section 9.8.2); **interactions:** Appendix 1 (NSAIDs)

**Contra-indications** section 10.1.1; also complete or partial syndrome of nasal polyps; haemorrhagic diatheses (including coagulation disorders) and following operations with high risk of haemorrhage or incomplete haemostasis; confirmed or suspected cerebrovascular bleeding; hypovolaemia or dehydration

**Side-effects** section 10.1.1; also gastro-intestinal disturbances, taste disturbances, dry mouth; flushing, bradycardia, palpitation, chest pain, hypertension, pallor; dyspnoea, asthma; malaise, euphoria, psychosis, paraesthesia, convulsions, abnormal dreams, hyperkinesia, confusion, hallucinations; urinary frequency, thirst, sweating; hyponatraemia, hyperkalaemia, myalgia; visual disturbances (including optic neuritis); hearing disorders, purpura, pain at injection site

**Dose**

- ADULT and CHILD over 16 years, by mouth, 10 mg every 4–6 hours (ELDERLY every 6–8 hours) as required; max. 40 mg daily; max. duration of treatment 7 days
- ADULT and CHILD over 16 years, by intramuscular injection *or* by intravenous injection over at least 15 seconds, initially 10 mg, then 10–30 mg every 4–6 hours as required (up to every 2 hours during initial postoperative period); max. 90 mg daily (ELDERLY and patients weighing less than 50 kg max. 60 mg daily); max. duration of treatment 2 days; CHILD 6 months–16 years, see *BNF for Children*

**Note** When converting from parenteral to oral administration, total combined dose on the day of converting should not exceed 90 mg (60 mg in the elderly and patients weighing less than 50 kg) of which the oral component should not exceed 40 mg

**Ketorolac** (Non-proprietary) ▢PoM

Injection, ketorolac trometamol 30 mg/mL, net price 1-mL amp = £1.14

**Toradol®** (Roche) ▢PoM

Tablets, ivory, f/c, ketorolac trometamol 10 mg, net price 20-tab pack = £5.56. Label: 17, 21

Injection, ketorolac trometamol 10 mg/mL, net price 1-mL amp = 91p; 30 mg/mL, 1-mL amp = £1.09

## ▮ PARECOXIB

**Indications** short-term management of acute postoperative pain

**Cautions** section 10.1.1; dehydration; following coronary artery bypass graft surgery; **interactions:** Appendix 1 (NSAIDs)

**Contra-indications** section 10.1.1; also history of allergic drug reactions including sulphonamide hypersensitivity; inflammatory bowel disease

**Side-effects** section 10.1.1; also flatulence; hypertension, hypotension, peripheral oedema; pharyngitis; respiratory insufficiency; hypoaesthesia; alveolar osteitis; oliguria; postoperative anaemia, hypokalaemia; back pain; pruritus; *less commonly* bradycardia, cardiovascular events, increased blood urea nitrogen, ecchymosis, thrombocytopenia, *rarely* vomiting, tachycardia, rash (discontinue—risk of serious reactions including Stevens-Johnson syndrome and toxic epidermal necrolysis), anaphylaxis

**Dose**

- By deep intramuscular injection *or* by intravenous injection, initially 40 mg, then 20–40 mg every 6–12 hours when required for up to 3 days; max. 80 mg daily; ELDERLY weighing less than 50 kg, initially 20 mg, then max. 40 mg daily; CHILD under 18 years, not recommended

**Dynastat®** (Pharmacia) ▼ ▢PoM

Injection, powder for reconstitution, parecoxib (as sodium salt), net price 40-mg vial = £4.96, 40-mg vial (with solvent) = £5.67

### ▮ 15.1.4.3 Opioid analgesics

Opioid analgesics are now rarely used as premedicants; they are more likely to be administered at induction. Pre-operative use of opioid analgesics is generally limited to those patients who require control of existing pain. The main side-effects of opioid analgesics are respiratory depression, cardiovascular depression, nausea, and vomiting; for general notes on opioid analgesics and their use in postoperative pain, see section 4.7.2.

For the management of opioid-induced respiratory depression, see section 15.1.7.

**Intra-operative analgesia** Opioid analgesics given in small doses before or with induction reduce the dose requirement of some drugs used during anaesthesia.

**Alfentanil**, **fentanyl**, and **remifentanil** are particularly useful because they act within 1–2 minutes and have short durations of action. The initial doses of alfentanil or fentanyl are followed either by successive intravenous injections or by an intravenous infusion; prolonged infusions increase the duration of effect. Repeated intra-operative doses of alfentanil or fentanyl should be given with care since the resulting respiratory depression can persist postoperatively and occasionally it may become apparent for the first time postoperatively when monitoring of the patient might be less intensive. Alfentanil, fentanyl, and remifentanil can cause muscle rigidity, particularly of the chest wall or jaw; this can be managed by the use of neuromuscular blocking drugs.

In contrast to other opioids which are metabolised in the liver, remifentanil undergoes rapid metabolism by non-specific blood and tissue esterases; its short duration of action allows prolonged administration at high dosage, without accumulation, and with little risk of residual postoperative respiratory depression. Remifentanil should not be given by intravenous injection intraoperatively, but it is well suited to continuous infusion; a supplementary analgesic is given before stopping the infusion of remifentanil.

## ▮ ALFENTANIL

**Indications** analgesia especially during short operative procedure and outpatient surgery; enhancement of anaesthesia; analgesia and suppression of respiratory activity in patients receiving intensive care, with assisted ventilation, for up to 4 days

**Cautions** section 4.7.2 and notes above

**Contra-indications** section 4.7.2

**Side-effects** section 4.7.2 and notes above; also hypertension, myoclonic movements; *less commonly* arrhythmias, cough, hiccup, laryngospasm; also reported cardiac arrest, convulsions, and pyrexia

**Dose**

To avoid excessive dosage in obese patients, dose may need to be calculated on the basis of ideal body-weight

- By intravenous injection, spontaneous respiration, ADULT, initially up to 500 micrograms over 30 seconds; supplemental, 250 micrograms

  With assisted ventilation, ADULT over 18 years, initially 30–50 micrograms/kg; supplemental, 15 micrograms/kg; CHILD 1 month–18 years, initially 10–20 micrograms/kg; supplemental doses up to 10 micrograms/kg

- By intravenous infusion, with assisted ventilation, ADULT and CHILD, initially 50–100 micrograms/kg over 10 minutes *or* as a bolus, followed by maintenance of 0.5–1 micrograms/kg/minute

**15** **Anaesthesia**

Analgesia and suppression of respiratory activity during intensive care, with assisted ventilation, by intravenous infusion, initially 2 mg/hour subsequently adjusted according to response (usual range 0.5–10 mg/hour); more rapid initial control may be obtained with an intravenous dose of 5 mg given in divided portions over 10 minutes (slowing if hypotension or bradycardia occur); additional doses of 0.5–1 mg may be given by intravenous injection during short painful procedures

**Rapifen®** (Janssen-Cilag) ᴄᴅ
Injection, alfentanil (as hydrochloride) 500 micrograms/mL, net price 2-mL amp = 65p; 10-mL amp = £2.96
Intensive care injection, alfentanil (as hydrochloride) 5 mg/mL. To be diluted before use. Net price 1-mL amp = £2.37

### ■ FENTANYL

**Indications** analgesia during operation, enhancement of anaesthesia; respiratory depressant in assisted respiration; analgesia in other situations (section 4.7.2)

**Cautions** section 4.7.2 and notes above

**Contra-indications** section 4.7.2

**Side-effects** section 4.7.2 and notes above; also myoclonic movements; *less commonly* laryngospasm; *rarely* asystole, insomnia

**Dose**

> To avoid excessive dosage in obese patients, dose may need to be calculated on the basis of ideal body-weight

- By slow intravenous injection, with spontaneous respiration, ADULT and CHILD over 12 years, initially 50–100 micrograms (max. 200 micrograms on specialist advice), then 25–50 micrograms as required; CHILD 1 month–12 years see *BNF for Children*
  With assisted ventilation, ADULT and CHILD over 12 years, initially 0.3–3.5 mg, then 100–200 micrograms as required; CHILD 1 month–12 years see *BNF for Children*
- By intravenous infusion, with spontaneous respiration, ADULT, 50–80 nanograms/kg/minute adjusted according to response
  With assisted ventilation, ADULT, initially 10 micrograms/kg over 10 minutes then 100 nanograms/kg/minute adjusted according to response; may require up to 3 micrograms/kg/minute during cardiac surgery

**Fentanyl** (Non-proprietary) ᴄᴅ
Injection, fentanyl (as citrate) 50 micrograms/mL, net price 2-mL amp = 54p, 10-mL amp = £1.65

**Sublimaze®** (Janssen-Cilag) ᴄᴅ
Injection, fentanyl (as citrate) 50 micrograms/mL, net price 2-mL amp = 22p, 10-mL amp = £1.05

### ■ REMIFENTANIL

**Indications** supplementation of general anaesthesia during induction and analgesia during maintenance of anaesthesia (consult product literature for use in patients undergoing cardiac surgery); analgesia and sedation in ventilated, intensive care patients

**Cautions** section 4.7.2 (but no dose adjustment necessary in renal impairment) and notes above

**Contra-indications** section 4.7.2 and notes above; left ventricular dysfunction

**Side-effects** section 4.7.2 and notes above; also hypertension, hypoxia; *very rarely* asystole and anaphylaxis

**Dose**

> To avoid excessive dosage in obese patients, dose should be calculated on the basis of ideal body-weight

- Induction of anaesthesia, ADULT and CHILD over 12 years, by intravenous infusion, 0.5–1 micrograms/kg/minute, *with or without* an initial dose by intravenous injection of 0.25–1 microgram/kg over at least 30 seconds
  **Note** If patient to be intubated more than 8 minutes after start of intravenous infusion, initial intravenous injection dose is not necessary
- Maintenance of anaesthesia in ventilated patients, ADULT and CHILD over 12 years, by intravenous infusion, 0.05–2 micrograms/kg/minute (*with or without* an initial dose by intravenous injection of 0.25–1 micrograms/kg over at least 30 seconds) according to anaesthetic technique and adjusted according to response; in light anaesthesia supplemental doses by intravenous injection every 2–5 minutes
- Maintenance of anaesthesia with spontaneous respiration, ADULT and CHILD over 12 years, by intravenous infusion, initially 40 nanograms/kg/minute adjusted according to response, usual range 25–100 nanograms/kg/minute
- Maintenance of anaesthesia, CHILD 1–12 years, by intravenous infusion, 0.05–1.3 micrograms/kg/minute (*with or without* an initial dose by intravenous injection of 0.1–1 microgram/kg over at least 30 seconds) according to anaesthetic technique and adjusted according to response
- Analgesia and sedation in ventilated, intensive-care patients, by intravenous infusion, ADULT over 18 years, initially 100–150 nanograms/kg/minute adjusted according to response in steps of 25 nanograms/kg/minute (allow at least 5 minutes between dose adjustments); usual range 6–740 nanograms/kg/minute; if an infusion rate of 200 nanograms/kg/minute does not produce adequate sedation add another sedative (consult product literature for details)
- Additional analgesia during stimulating or painful procedures in ventilated, intensive-care patients, by intravenous infusion, ADULT over 18 years, maintain infusion rate of at least 100 nanograms/kg/minute for at least 5 minutes before procedure and adjust every 2–5 minutes according to requirements, usual range 250–750 nanograms/kg/minute
- Cardiac surgery, consult product literature
**Note** Remifentanil doses in BNF may differ from those in product literature

**Ultiva®** (GSK) ᴄᴅ
Injection, powder for reconstitution, remifentanil (as hydrochloride), net price 1-mg vial = £5.12; 2-mg vial = £10.23; 5-mg vial = £25.58

## 15.1.5 Neuromuscular blocking drugs

Neuromuscular blocking drugs used in anaesthesia are also known as **muscle relaxants**. By specific blockade of the neuromuscular junction they enable light anaesthesia to be used with adequate relaxation of the muscles of the abdomen and diaphragm. They also relax the vocal cords and allow the passage of a tracheal tube. Their action differs from the muscle relaxants used in musculoskeletal disorders (section 10.2.2) that act on the spinal cord or brain.

Patients who have received a neuromuscular blocking drug should **always** have their respiration assisted or controlled until the drug has been inactivated or antagonised (section 15.1.6). They should also receive sufficient concomitant inhalational or intravenous anaesthetic or sedative drugs to prevent awareness.

## Non-depolarising neuromuscular blocking drugs

Non-depolarising neuromuscular blocking drugs (also known as competitive muscle relaxants) compete with acetylcholine for receptor sites at the neuromuscular junction and their action can be reversed with anticholinesterases such as neostigmine (section 15.1.6). Non-depolarising neuromuscular blocking drugs can be divided into the **aminosteroid** group, comprising pancuronium, rocuronium, and vecuronium, and the **benzylisoquinolinium** group, comprising atracurium, cisatracurium, and mivacurium.

Non-depolarising neuromuscular blocking drugs have a slower onset of action than suxamethonium. These drugs can be classified by their duration of action as short-acting (15–30 minutes), intermediate-acting (30–40 minutes), and long-acting (60–120 minutes), although duration of action is dose-dependent. Drugs with a shorter or intermediate duration of action, such as atracurium and vecuronium, are more widely used than those with a longer duration of action, such as pancuronium.

Non-depolarising neuromuscular blocking drugs have no sedative or analgesic effects and are not considered to trigger malignant hyperthermia.

For patients receiving intensive care and who require tracheal intubation and mechanical ventilation, a non-depolarising neuromuscular blocking drug is chosen according to its onset of effect, duration of action, and side-effects. Rocuronium, with a rapid onset of effect, may facilitate intubation. Atracurium or cisatracurium may be suitable for long-term neuromuscular blockade since their duration of action is not dependent on elimination by the liver or the kidneys.

**Cautions** Allergic cross-reactivity between neuromuscular blocking drugs has been reported; caution is advised in cases of hypersensitivity to these drugs. Their activity is prolonged in patients with myasthenia gravis and in hypothermia, and lower doses are required. Non-depolarising neuromuscular blocking drugs should be used with great care in those with other neuromuscular disorders and those with fluid and electrolyte disturbances, as response is unpredictable. Resistance can develop in patients with burns, who may require increased doses; low plasma cholinesterase activity in these patients requires dose titration for mivacurium. **Interactions:** Appendix 1 (muscle relaxants).

**Side-effects** Benzylisoquinolinium non-depolarising neuromuscular blocking drugs (except cisatracurium) are associated with histamine release, which can cause skin flushing, hypotension, tachycardia, bronchospasm, and very rarely anaphylactoid reactions. Most aminosteroid neuromuscular blocking drugs produce minimal histamine release. Drugs with vagolytic activity can counteract any bradycardia that occurs during surgery. Acute myopathy has also been reported after prolonged use in intensive care.

**Atracurium**, a mixture of 10 isomers, is a benzylisoquinolinium neuromuscular blocking drug with an intermediate duration of action. It undergoes non-enzymatic metabolism which is independent of liver and kidney function, thus allowing its use in patients with hepatic or renal impairment. Cardiovascular effects are associated with significant histamine release.

**Cisatracurium** is a single isomer of atracurium. It is more potent and has a slightly longer duration of action than atracurium and provides greater cardiovascular stability because cisatracurium lacks histamine-releasing effects.

**Mivacurium**, a benzylisoquinolinium neuromuscular blocking drug, has a short duration of action. It is metabolised by plasma cholinesterase and muscle paralysis is prolonged in individuals deficient in this enzyme. It is not associated with vagolytic activity or ganglionic blockade although histamine release can occur, particularly with rapid injection.

**Pancuronium**, an aminosteroid neuromuscular blocking drug, has a long duration of action and is often used in patients receiving long-term mechanical ventilation in intensive care units. It lacks a histamine-releasing effect, but vagolytic and sympathomimetic effects can cause tachycardia and hypertension.

**Rocuronium** exerts an effect within 2 minutes and has the most rapid onset of any of the non-depolarising neuromuscular blocking drugs. It is an aminosteroid neuromuscular blocking drug with an intermediate duration of action. It is reported to have minimal cardiovascular effects; high doses produce mild vagolytic activity.

**Vecuronium**, an aminosteroid neuromuscular blocking drug, has an intermediate duration of action. It does not generally produce histamine release and lacks cardiovascular effects.

## ATRACURIUM BESILATE
(Atracurium besylate)

**Indications** neuromuscular blockade (short to intermediate duration) for surgery or during intensive care

**Cautions** see notes above; pregnancy (Appendix 4); breast-feeding (Appendix 5)

**Side-effects** see notes above; seizures also reported

**Dose**

> To avoid excessive dosage in obese patients, dose should be calculated on the basis of ideal body-weight

- Surgery or intubation, ADULT and CHILD over 1 month, by intravenous injection, initially 300–600 micrograms/kg, then 100–200 micrograms/kg as required *or* initially by intravenous injection, 200–600 micrograms/kg followed by intravenous infusion, 5–10 micrograms/kg/minute (300–600 micrograms/kg/hour)
- Intensive care, ADULT and CHILD over 1 month, by intravenous injection, initially 300–600 micrograms/kg (optional) then by intravenous infusion 4.5–29.5 micrograms/kg/minute (usual dose 11–13 micrograms/kg/minute)

**Atracurium** (Non-proprietary) PoM

Injection, atracurium besilate 10 mg/mL, net price 2.5-mL amp = £1.85; 5-mL amp = £3.37; 25-mL amp = £14.45

**Tracrium®** (GSK) PoM

Injection, atracurium besilate 10 mg/mL, net price 2.5-mL amp = £1.66; 5-mL amp = £3.00; 25-mL amp = £12.91

## CISATRACURIUM

**Indications** neuromuscular blockade (intermediate duration) for surgery or during intensive care

**Cautions** see notes above; pregnancy (Appendix 4); breast-feeding

**Side-effects** see notes above; also bradycardia

**Dose**

> To avoid excessive dosage in obese patients, dose should be calculated on the basis of ideal body-weight

- Intubation, by intravenous injection, ADULT and CHILD over 1 month, initially 150 micrograms/kg; maintenance, by intravenous injection, 30 micrograms/kg approx. every 20 minutes; CHILD 2–12 years, 20 micrograms/kg approx. every 9 minutes; or maintenance, by intravenous infusion, ADULT and CHILD over 2 years, initially, 3 micrograms/kg/minute, *then after stabilisation*, 1–2 micrograms/minute; dose reduced by up to 40% if used with isoflurane
- Intensive care, by intravenous infusion, ADULT 0.5–10.2 micrograms/kg/minute (usual dose 3 micrograms/kg/minute)
  Note Lower doses can be used for children over 2 years when *not* for intubation

**Nimbex®** (GSK) PoM

Injection, cisatracurium (as besilate) 2 mg/mL, net price 10-mL amp = £7.55

Forte injection, cisatracurium (as besilate) 5 mg/mL, net price 30-mL vial = £31.09

## MIVACURIUM

**Indications** neuromuscular blockade (short duration) for surgery

**Cautions** see notes above; low plasma cholinesterase activity; elderly; hepatic impairment (Appendix 2); renal impairment (Appendix 3); pregnancy (Appendix 4)

**Side-effects** see notes above

**Dose**

> To avoid excessive dosage in obese patients, dose should be calculated on the basis of ideal body-weight

- By intravenous injection, 70–250 micrograms/kg; maintenance 100 micrograms/kg every 15 minutes; CHILD 2–6 months initially 150 micrograms/kg, 7 months–12 years initially 200 micrograms/kg; maintenance (CHILD 2 months–12 years) 100 micrograms/kg every 6–9 minutes
  Note Doses up to 150 micrograms/kg may be given over 5–15 seconds, higher doses should be given over 30 seconds. In patients with asthma, cardiovascular disease or those who are sensitive to falls in arterial blood pressure give over 60 seconds

- By intravenous infusion, maintenance of block, 8–10 micrograms/kg/minute, adjusted if necessary every 3 minutes by 1 microgram/kg/minute to usual dose of 6–7 micrograms/kg/minute; CHILD 2 months–12 years, usual dose 11–14 micrograms/kg/minute

**Mivacron®** (GSK) PoM

Injection, mivacurium (as chloride) 2 mg/mL, net price 5-mL amp = £2.79; 10-mL amp = £4.51

## PANCURONIUM BROMIDE

**Indications** neuromuscular blockade (long duration) for surgery or during intensive care

**Cautions** see notes above; hepatic impairment (Appendix 2); renal impairment (Appendix 3); pregnancy (Appendix 4); breast-feeding (Appendix 5)

**Side-effects** see notes above

**Dose**

> To avoid excessive dosage in obese patients, dose should be calculated on the basis of ideal body-weight

- Intubation, by intravenous injection, initially 50–100 micrograms/kg then 10–20 micrograms/kg as required; NEONATE see BNF for Children; CHILD 1 month–18 years, initially 100 micrograms/kg, then 20 micrograms/kg
- Intensive care, by intravenous injection, 60 micrograms/kg every 60–90 minutes

**Pancuronium** (Non-proprietary) PoM

Injection, pancuronium bromide 2 mg/mL, net price 2-mL amp = £1.20

## ROCURONIUM BROMIDE

**Indications** neuromuscular blockade (intermediate duration) for surgery or during intensive care

**Cautions** see notes above; hepatic impairment (Appendix 2); renal impairment (Appendix 3); pregnancy (Appendix 4) and breast-feeding (Appendix 5)

**Side-effects** see notes above

**Dose**

> To avoid excessive dosage in obese patients, dose should be calculated on the basis of ideal body-weight

- Intubation, ADULT and CHILD over 1 month, by intravenous injection, initially 600 micrograms/kg; maintenance by intravenous injection, 150 micrograms/kg (ELDERLY 75–100 micrograms/kg) or maintenance by intravenous infusion, 300–600 micrograms/kg/hour (ELDERLY up to 400 micrograms/kg/hour) adjusted according to response
- Intensive care, by intravenous injection, ADULT initially 600 micrograms/kg; maintenance by intravenous infusion, 300–600 micrograms/kg/hour for first hour, then adjusted according to response

**Esmeron®** (Organon) PoM

Injection, rocuronium bromide 10 mg/mL, net price 5-mL vial = £2.95; 10-mL vial = £5.90

*15 Anaesthesia*

## ■ VECURONIUM BROMIDE

**Indications** neuromuscular blockade (intermediate duration) for surgery

**Cautions** see notes above; pregnancy (Appendix 4)

**Side-effects** see notes above

**Dose**

> To avoid excessive dosage in obese patients, dose should be calculated on the basis of ideal body-weight

- By intravenous injection, intubation, ADULT and CHILD, initially 80–100 micrograms/kg; maintenance 20–30 micrograms/kg adjusted according to response; NEONATE, see *BNF for Children*
- By intravenous infusion, 0.8–1.4 micrograms/kg/minute (after initial intravenous injection of 40–100 micrograms/kg)

**Norcuron®** (Organon) ▣ᴾᵒᴹ
Injection, powder for reconstitution, vecuronium bromide, net price 10-mg vial = £3.75 (with water for injections)

---

## Depolarising neuromuscular blocking drugs

**Suxamethonium** has the most rapid onset of action of any of the neuromuscular blocking drugs and is ideal if fast onset and brief duration of action are required, e.g. with tracheal intubation.

Suxamethonium acts by mimicking acetylcholine at the neuromuscular junction but hydrolysis is much slower than for acetylcholine; depolarisation is therefore prolonged, resulting in neuromuscular blockade. Unlike the non-depolarising neuromuscular blocking drugs, its action cannot be reversed and recovery is spontaneous; anticholinesterases such as neostigmine potentiate the neuromuscular block.

Suxamethonium should be given after anaesthetic induction because paralysis is usually preceded by painful muscle fasciculations. While tachycardia occurs with single use, bradycardia may occur with repeated doses in adults and with the first dose in children. Premedication with atropine reduces bradycardia as well as the excessive salivation associated with suxamethonium use.

Prolonged paralysis may occur in **dual block**, which occurs with high or repeated doses of suxamethonium and is caused by the development of a non-depolarising block following the initial depolarising block; edrophonium (section 15.1.6) may be used to confirm the diagnosis of dual block. Individuals with myasthenia gravis are resistant to suxamethonium but can develop dual block resulting in delayed recovery. Prolonged paralysis may also occur in those with low or atypical plasma cholinesterase. Assisted ventilation should be continued until muscle function is restored.

## ■ SUXAMETHONIUM CHLORIDE
(Succinylcholine chloride)

**Indications** neuromuscular blockade (short duration)

**Cautions** see notes above; hypersensitivity to other neuromuscular blocking drugs; patients with cardiac, respiratory or neuromuscular disease; raised intraocular pressure (avoid in penetrating eye injury); severe sepsis (risk of hyperkalaemia); pregnancy (Appendix 4); **interactions**: Appendix 1 (muscle relaxants)

**Contra-indications** family history of malignant hyperthermia, hyperkalaemia; major trauma, severe burns, neurological disease involving acute wasting of major muscle, prolonged immobilisation—risk of hyperkalaemia, personal or family history of congenital myotonic disease, Duchenne muscular dystrophy, low plasma-cholinesterase activity (including severe liver disease) (Appendix 2)

**Side-effects** see notes above; also increased gastric pressure; hyperkalaemia; postoperative muscle pain, myoglobinuria, myoglobinaemia; increased intraocular pressure; flushing, rash; *rarely* arrhythmias, cardiac arrest; bronchospasm, apnoea, prolonged respiratory depression; limited jaw mobility; *very rarely* anaphylactic reactions, malignant hyperthermia; *also reported* hypertension, hypotension, rhabdomyolysis

**Dose**

- By intravenous injection, initially 1 mg/kg; maintenance, usually 0.5–1 mg/kg at 5–10 minute intervals; max. 500 mg/hour; CHILD under 1 year, 2 mg/kg; CHILD over 1 year, 1 mg/kg
- By intravenous infusion of a solution containing 1–2 mg/mL (0.1–0.2%), 2.5–4 mg/minute; max. 500 mg/hour; CHILD reduce infusion rate according to body-weight
- By intramuscular injection, CHILD under 1 year, up to 4–5 mg/kg, CHILD over 1 year, up to 4 mg/kg; max. 150 mg

**Suxamethonium Chloride** (Non-proprietary) ᴾᵒᴹ
Injection, suxamethonium chloride 50 mg/mL, net price 2-mL amp = 64p, 2-mL prefilled syringe = £7.35

**Anectine®** (GSK) ᴾᵒᴹ
Injection, suxamethonium chloride 50 mg/mL, net price 2-mL amp = 71p

---

## 15.1.6 Drugs for reversal of neuromuscular blockade

---

## Anticholinesterases

Anticholinesterases reverse the effects of the non-depolarising (competitive) neuromuscular blocking drugs such as pancuronium but they prolong the action of the depolarising neuromuscular blocking drug suxamethonium.

**Edrophonium** has a transient action and may be used in the diagnosis of suspected dual block due to suxamethonium. Atropine (section 15.1.3) is given before or with edrophonium to prevent muscarinic effects when given for reversal of non-depolarising neuromuscular blockade.

**Neostigmine** has a longer duration of action than edrophonium and is used specifically for reversal of non-depolarising (competitive) blockade. It acts within one minute of intravenous injection and its effects last for 20 to 30 minutes; a second dose may then be necessary. Glycopyrronium or alternatively atropine (section

**15** Anaesthesia

15.1.3), given before or with neostigmine, prevent bradycardia, excessive salivation, and other muscarinic effects of neostigmine.

## EDROPHONIUM CHLORIDE

**Indications** see under Dose; myasthenia gravis (section 10.2.1)

**Cautions** section 10.2.1; atropine should also be given

**Contra-indications** section 10.2.1

**Side-effects** section 10.2.1

**Dose**

- Brief reversal of non-depolarising neuromuscular blockade, by intravenous injection over several minutes, 500–700 micrograms/kg (after or with atropine)

- Diagnosis of dual block, by intravenous injection, 10 mg

**Edrophonium** (Cambridge) [PoM]
Injection, edrophonium chloride 10 mg/mL, net price 1-mL amp = £8.65

## NEOSTIGMINE METILSULFATE
(Neostigmine methylsulphate)

**Indications** see under Dose

**Cautions** section 10.2.1 and notes above; glycopyrronium or atropine should also be given

**Contra-indications** section 10.2.1 and notes above

**Side-effects** section 10.2.1 and notes above

**Dose**

- Reversal of non-depolarising neuromuscular blockade, by intravenous injection over 1 minute, 50–70 micrograms/kg (max. 5 mg) after or with glycopyrronium or atropine

- Myasthenia gravis, see section 10.2.1

**Neostigmine** (Non-proprietary) [PoM]
Injection, neostigmine metilsulfate 2.5 mg/mL, net price 1-mL amp = 58p

◢With glycopyrronium
**Robinul-Neostigmine®** (Anpharm) [PoM]
Injection, neostigmine metilsulfate 2.5 mg, glycopyrronium bromide 500 micrograms/mL, net price 1-mL amp = £1.15
Dose reversal of non-depolarising neuromuscular blockade by intravenous injection over 10–30 seconds, 1–2 mL or 0.02 mL/kg, dose may be repeated if required (total max. 2 mL); CHILD 0.02 mL/kg (or 0.2 mL/kg of a 1 in 10 dilution using water for injections or sodium chloride injection 0.9%), dose may be repeated if required (total max. 2 mL)
Note May be difficult to obtain

## Other drugs for reversal of neuromuscular blockade

Sugammadex is a modified gamma cyclodextrin used for reversal of neuromuscular blockade induced by rocuronium or vecuronium (section 15.1.5).

## SUGAMMADEX

**Indications** reversal of neuromuscular blockade induced by rocuronium or vecuronium

**Cautions** recurrence of neuromuscular blockade—monitor respiratory function until fully recovered;

recovery may be delayed in cardiovascular disease and elderly; wait 24 hours before re-administering rocuronium or vecuronium; renal impairment (Appendix 3); pregnancy (Appendix 4); **interactions:** Appendix 1 (sugammadex)

**Side-effects** taste disturbances; *less commonly* allergic reactions; bronchospasm also reported

**Dose**

- Routine reversal of neuromuscular blockade induced by rocuronium or vecuronium, by intravenous injection, ADULT over 18 years, 2–4 mg/kg (consult product literature); a further dose of 4 mg/kg may be required if recurrence of neuromuscular blockade occurs

- Routine reversal of neuromuscular blockade induced by rocuronium, by intravenous injection, CHILD 2–18 years, 2 mg/kg (consult product literature)

- Immediate reversal of neuromuscular blockade induced by rocuronium, by intravenous injection, ADULT over 18 years, 16 mg/kg (consult product literature)

**Bridion®** (Schering-Plough) ▼ [PoM]
Injection, sugammadex (as sodium salt) 100 mg/mL, net price 2-mL amp = £59.64, 5-mL amp = £149.10
Electrolytes Na+ 0.42 mmol/mL

## 15.1.7 Antagonists for central and respiratory depression

Respiratory depression is a major concern with opioid analgesics and it may be treated by artificial ventilation or be reversed by **naloxone**. Naloxone will immediately reverse opioid-induced respiratory depression but the dose may have to be repeated because of the short duration of action of naloxone; however, naloxone will also antagonise the analgesic effect.

**Flumazenil** is a benzodiazepine antagonist for the reversal of the central sedative effects of benzodiazepines after anaesthetic and similar procedures. Flumazenil has a shorter half-life and duration of action than diazepam or midazolam so patients may become resedated.

**Doxapram** (section 3.5.1) is a central and respiratory stimulant but is of limited value in anaesthesia.

## FLUMAZENIL

**Indications** reversal of sedative effects of benzodiazepines in anaesthetic, intensive care, and diagnostic procedures

**Cautions** short-acting (repeat doses may be necessary—benzodiazepine effects may persist for at least 24 hours); benzodiazepine dependence (may precipitate withdrawal symptoms); prolonged benzodiazepine therapy for epilepsy (risk of convulsions); history of panic disorders (risk of recurrence); ensure neuromuscular blockade cleared before giving; avoid rapid injection in high-risk or anxious patients and following major surgery; head injury (rapid reversal of benzodiazepine sedation may cause convulsions); elderly;-

15 Anaesthesia

children; hepatic impairment (Appendix 2); pregnancy (Appendix 4); breast-feeding

**Contra-indications** life-threatening condition (e.g. raised intracranial pressure, status epilepticus) controlled by benzodiazepines

**Side-effects** nausea, vomiting, and flushing; if wakening too rapid, agitation, anxiety, and fear; transient increase in blood pressure and heart-rate in intensive care patients; *very rarely* convulsions (particularly in those with epilepsy), hypersensitivity reactions including anaphylaxis

**Dose**

- By intravenous injection, 200 micrograms over 15 seconds, then 100 micrograms at 60-second intervals if required; usual dose range, 300–600 micrograms; max. total dose 1 mg (2 mg in intensive care); question aetiology if no response to repeated doses
- By intravenous infusion, if drowsiness recurs after injection, 100–400 micrograms/hour, adjusted according to level of arousal

**Flumazenil** (Non-proprietary) PoM
Injection, flumazenil 100 micrograms/mL, net price 5-mL amp = £14.00

**Anexate®** (Roche) PoM
Injection, flumazenil 100 micrograms/mL, net price 5-mL amp = £13.93

▌ **NALOXONE HYDROCHLORIDE**

**Indications** reversal of opioid-induced respiratory depression; reversal of neonatal respiratory depression resulting from opioid administration to mother during labour; overdosage with opioids (see Emergency Treatment of Poisoning)

**Cautions** cardiovascular disease or those receiving cardiotoxic drugs (serious adverse cardiovascular effects reported); physical dependence on opioids (precipitates withdrawal); pain (see also under Titration of Dose, below); has short duration of action (repeated doses or infusion may be necessary to reverse effects of opioids with longer duration of action); pregnancy (Appendix 4)

**Titration of dose** In postoperative use, the dose should be titrated for each patient in order to obtain sufficient respiratory response; however, naloxone antagonises analgesia

**Side-effects** nausea, vomiting; hypotension, hypertension, ventricular tachycardia and fibrillation, cardiac arrest; hyperventilation, dyspnoea, pulmonary oedema; headache, dizziness; *less commonly* diarrhoea, dry mouth, agitation, excitement, paraesthesia, tremor, sweating; *very rarely* seizures, erythema multiforme, and hypersensitivity reactions including anaphylaxis

**Dose**

- ADULT and CHILD over 12 years, by intravenous injection, 100–200 micrograms (1.5–3 micrograms/kg); if response inadequate, give subsequent dose of 100 micrograms every 2 minutes; alternatively, subsequent doses can be given by intramuscular injection every 1–2 hours; CHILD 1 month–12 years by intravenous injection, 5–10 micrograms/kg; if response inadequate, give subsequent dose of 100 micrograms/kg (max. 2 mg); if intravenous route not possible, may be given in divided doses by intramuscular *or* subcutaneous injection

- NEONATE, reversal of respiratory and CNS depression resulting from opioid administration to mother during labour, by intramuscular injection, 200 micrograms (60 micrograms/kg) as a single dose at birth; alternatively by subcutaneous, intramuscular, *or* intravenous injection, 10 micrograms/kg, repeated every 2–3 minutes

**Note** Naloxone doses in BNF may differ from those in product literature

**Naloxone** PoM
See under Emergency Treatment of Poisoning p. 31

▌ **15.1.8 Drugs for malignant hyperthermia**

Malignant hyperthermia is a rare but potentially lethal complication of anaesthesia. It is characterised by a rapid rise in temperature, increased muscle rigidity, tachycardia, and acidosis. The most common triggers of malignant hyperthermia are the volatile anaesthetics. Suxamethonium has also been implicated, but malignant hyperthermia is more likely if it is given following a volatile anaesthetic. Volatile anaesthetics and suxamethonium should be avoided during anaesthesia in patients at high risk of malignant hyperthermia.

**Dantrolene** is used in the treatment of malignant hyperthermia. It acts on skeletal muscle cells by interfering with calcium efflux, thereby stopping the contractile process.

▌ **DANTROLENE SODIUM**

**Indications** malignant hyperthermia; chronic severe spasticity of voluntary muscle (section 10.2.2)

**Cautions** avoid extravasation (risk of tissue necrosis); pregnancy (Appendix 4); breast-feeding (Appendix 5); **interactions:** Appendix 1 (muscle relaxants)

**Side-effects** hepatotoxicity, pulmonary oedema, dizziness, weakness, and injection-site reactions including erythema, rash, swelling, and thrombophlebitis

**Dose**

- By rapid intravenous injection, initially 2–3 mg/kg, then 1 mg/kg repeated as required to a cumulative max. of 10 mg/kg

**Dantrium Intravenous®** (SpePharm) PoM
Injection, powder for reconstitution, dantrolene sodium, net price 20-mg vial = £51.00 (hosp. only)

▌ **15.2 Local anaesthesia**

The use of local anaesthetics by injection or by application to mucous membranes to produce local analgesia is discussed in this section.

See also section 1.7 (anus), section 11.7 (eye), section 12.3 (oropharynx), and section 13.3 (skin).

**Use of local anaesthetics** Local anaesthetic drugs act by causing a reversible block to conduction along nerve fibres. The drugs used vary widely in their potency, toxicity, duration of action, stability, solubility in water, and ability to penetrate mucous membranes. These variations determine their suitability for use by various routes, e.g. topical (surface), infiltration, periph-

15

Anaesthesia

eral nerve block, intravenous regional anaesthesia (Bier's block), plexus, epidural (extradural) or spinal block. Local anaesthetics may also be used for postoperative pain relief, thereby reducing the need for analgesics such as opioids.

**Administration** In estimating the safe dosage of these drugs it is important to take account of the rate at which they are absorbed and excreted as well as their potency. The patient's age, weight, physique, and clinical condition, the degree of vascularity of the area to which the drug is to be applied, and the duration of administration are other factors which must be taken into account.

Local anaesthetics do not rely on the circulation to transport them to their sites of action, but uptake into the systemic circulation is important in terminating their action and producing toxicity. Following most regional anaesthetic procedures, maximum arterial plasma concentrations of anaesthetic develop within about 10 to 25 minutes, so **careful surveillance** for toxic effects is necessary during the first 30 minutes after injection. Great care must be taken to avoid accidental intravascular injection. Local anaesthesia around the oral cavity may impair swallowing and therefore increase the risk of aspiration.

Epidural anaesthesia is commonly used during surgery, often combined with general anaesthesia, because of its protective effect against the stress response of surgery. It is often used when good postoperative pain relief is essential (e.g. major thoracic or intra-abdominal surgery).

**Toxicity** Toxic effects associated with local anaesthetics usually result from excessively high plasma concentrations; single application of topical lidocaine preparations does not generally cause systemic side-effects. Effects initially include a feeling of inebriation and lightheadedness followed by sedation, circumoral paraesthesia and twitching; convulsions can occur in severe reactions. On intravenous injection convulsions and cardiovascular collapse may occur very rapidly. Hypersensitivity reactions occur mainly with the ester-type local anaesthetics such as benzocaine, cocaine, and tetracaine (amethocaine); reactions are less frequent with the amide types such as lidocaine (lignocaine), bupivacaine, levobupivacaine, prilocaine, and ropivacaine. Cross-sensitivity reactions may be avoided by using the alternative chemical type. Local anaesthetics may be associated with methaemoglobinaemia; prilocaine and benzocaine have been implicated.

When prolonged analgesia is required, a long-acting local anaesthetic is preferred to minimise the likelihood of cumulative systemic toxicity. Local anaesthetic injections should be given slowly in order to detect inadvertent intravascular administration. Local anaesthetics should **not** be injected into inflamed or infected tissues nor should they be applied to the traumatised urethra. In such cases absorption into the blood may increase the possibility of systemic side-effects. The local anaesthetic effect may also be reduced by the altered local pH. Local anaesthetics can be ototoxic and should not be applied to the middle ear.

**Use of vasoconstrictors** Most local anaesthetics, with the exception of cocaine, cause dilation of blood vessels. The addition of a vasoconstrictor such as **adrenaline (epinephrine)** diminishes local blood flow, slows the rate of absorption of the local anaesthetic,

and prolongs its local effect. Adrenaline must be used in a low concentration (e.g. 1 in 200 000) for this purpose and it is not advisable to give adrenaline with a local anaesthetic injection in digits or appendages because of the risk of ischaemic necrosis.

When adrenaline is included the final concentration should be 1 in 200 000 (5 micrograms/mL), but see also Dental Anaesthesia below.

The total dose of adrenaline should **not** exceed 500 micrograms and it is essential not to exceed a concentration of 1 in 200 000 (5 micrograms/mL) if more than 50 mL of the mixture is to be injected. Care must also be taken to calculate a safe maximum dose of local anaesthetic when using combination products. For general cautions associated with the use of adrenaline, see section 2.7.3. For drug interactions, see Appendix 1 (sympathomimetics).

**Dental anaesthesia** Lidocaine (lignocaine) is widely used in dental procedures; it is most often used in combination with **adrenaline** (epinephrine). Lidocaine 2% combined with adrenaline 1 in 80 000 (12.5 micrograms/mL) is a safe and effective preparation; there is no justification for using higher concentrations of adrenaline.

The local anaesthetics **articaine** (carticaine) and **mepivacaine** are also used in dentistry; they are available in cartridges suitable for dental use. Mepivacaine is available with or without adrenaline (as *Scandonest®*) and articaine is available with adrenaline (as *Septanest®*).

In patients with severe hypertension or unstable cardiac rhythm, the use of adrenaline in a local anaesthetic may be hazardous. For these patients **prilocaine** with or without felypressin can be used but there is no evidence that it is any safer. Felypressin can cause coronary vasoconstriction when used at high doses; limit dose in patients with coronary artery disease.

Great care should be taken to avoid inadvertent intravenous administration of a preparation containing adrenaline.

---

## Lidocaine

Lidocaine (lignocaine) is effectively absorbed from mucous membranes and is a useful surface anaesthetic in concentrations up to 10%. Except for surface anaesthesia and dental anaesthesia, solutions should **not** usually exceed 1% in strength. The duration of the block (with adrenaline) is about 90 minutes.

### ▌LIDOCAINE HYDROCHLORIDE
(Lignocaine hydrochloride)

**Indications** see under Dose; also dental anaesthesia (see p. 715); ventricular arrhythmias (section 2.3.2)

**Cautions** see notes above; see section 2.3.2 for effects on heart; epilepsy, respiratory impairment, impaired cardiac conduction, bradycardia, severe shock; acute porphyria (section 9.8.2); myasthenia gravis; reduce dose in elderly or debilitated; resuscitative equipment should be available; hepatic impairment (Appendix 2); renal impairment (Appendix 3); pregnancy (Appendix 4); **interactions:** Appendix 1 (lidocaine)

**Contra-indications** see notes above; hypovolaemia, complete heart block; do not use solutions containing adrenaline for anaesthesia in appendages

**Side-effects** see notes above and section 2.3.2; also CNS effects include confusion, respiratory depression and convulsions; hypotension and bradycardia (may lead to cardiac arrest); *rarely* hypersensitivity reported

**Dose**

- Infiltration anaesthesia, by injection, according to patient's weight and nature of procedure, max. 200 mg (or 500 mg if given in solutions containing adrenaline)—see also Administration on p. 714 and see also **important** warning below
- Intravenous regional anaesthesia and nerve blocks, seek expert advice
- Surface anaesthesia, usual strengths 2–4%, see preparations below

> **Important**
> The licensed doses stated above may not be appropriate in some settings and expert advice should be sought

◢**Lidocaine hydrochloride injections**

**Lidocaine** (Non-proprietary) [PoM]

Injection 0.5%, lidocaine hydrochloride 5 mg/mL, net price 10-mL amp = 35p

Injection 1%, lidocaine hydrochloride 10 mg/mL, net price 2-mL amp = 21p; 5-mL amp = 26p; 10-mL amp = 38p; 10-mL prefilled syringe = £4.53; 20-mL amp = 78p

Injection 2%, lidocaine hydrochloride 20 mg/mL, net price 2-mL amp = 27p; 5-mL amp = 28p

**Xylocaine®** (AstraZeneca) [PoM]

Injection 1% with adrenaline 1 in 200 000, anhydrous lidocaine hydrochloride 10 mg/mL, adrenaline 1 in 200 000 (5 micrograms/mL), net price 20-mL vial = 99p

Injection 2% with adrenaline 1 in 200 000, anhydrous lidocaine hydrochloride 20 mg/mL, adrenaline 1 in 200 000 (5 micrograms/mL), net price 20-mL vial = £1.04

◢**Lidocaine injections for dental use**

**Note** Consult expert dental sources for specific advice in relation to dose of lidocaine for dental anaesthesia

A variety of lidocaine injections with adrenaline is available in dental cartridges; brands include *Lignospan Special®*, *Rexocaine®* and *Xylocaine®*

◢**Lidocaine for surface anaesthesia**

**Important**. Rapid and extensive absorption may result in systemic side-effects

**Lidocaine** (Non-proprietary)

Ointment, lidocaine hydrochloride 5%, net price 15 g = 88p

**Dose** dental practice, rub gently into dry gum

Sore nipples from breast-feeding, apply using gauze and wash off immediately before feed

Pain relief (in anal fissures, haemorrhoids, pruritus ani, pruritus vulvae, herpes zoster, or herpes labialis), 1–2 mL applied when necessary; avoid long-term use

Solution, lidocaine hydrochloride 4%, net price 25 mL = £1.35

**Dose** biopsy in mouth, 3–4 mL with suitable spray *or* swab (with adrenaline if necessary); max. 5 mL, ELDERLY lower max. dose, CHILD max. 3 mg/kg

Puncture of maxillary sinus or polypectomy, apply with swab for 2–3 minutes (with adrenaline); max. 5 mL, ELDERLY lower max. dose, CHILD max. 3 mg/kg

Bronchoscopy and bronchography, 2–3 mL with suitable spray; max. 5 mL, ELDERLY lower max. dose, CHILD max. 3 mg/kg

**EMLA®** (AstraZeneca)

Drug Tariff cream, lidocaine 2.5%, prilocaine 2.5%, net price 5-g tube = £1.73

Surgical pack cream, lidocaine 2.5%, prilocaine 2.5%, net price 30-g tube = £10.25

Premedication pack cream, lidocaine 2.5%, prilocaine 2.5%, net price 5 × 5-g tube with 12 occlusive dressings = £9.75

**Cautions** not for preterm neonates, children under 1 year receiving treatment with methaemoglobin-inducing agents, wounds, mucous membranes (except genital mucosa in adults), or atopic dermatitis; avoid use near eyes or middle ear; although systemic absorption low, caution in anaemia, in congenital or acquired methaemoglobinaemia or in G6PD deficiency (see also Prilocaine, p. 717)

**Side-effects** include administration site reactions such as transient paleness, redness, oedema, itching, burning sensation, and localised lesions

**Dose** ADULT and CHILD over 1 year, anaesthesia before minor skin procedures including venepuncture, apply thick layer under occlusive dressing 1–5 hours before procedure (2–5 hours before procedures on large areas e.g. split skin grafting); max. 2 doses in 24 hours for CHILD 1–12 years; CHILD under 3 months or body-weight less than 5 kg, apply max. 1 g under occlusive dressing for max. 1 hour before procedure; max. 1 dose in 24 hours, CHILD 3–12 months and body-weight over 5 kg, apply max. 2 g under occlusive dressing for max. 4 hours before procedure; max. 2 doses in 24 hours

**Note** Shorter application time of 15–30 minutes is recommended for children with atopic dermatitis

Anaesthesia on genital skin before injection of local anaesthetics in adult men, apply under occlusive dressing for 15 minutes

Anaesthesia before surgical treatment of lesions on genital mucosa in adults, apply up to 10 g 5–10 minutes before procedure

**Instillagel®** (CliniMed)

Gel, lidocaine hydrochloride 2%, chlorhexidine gluconate solution 0.25%, in a sterile lubricant basis in disposable syringe, net price 6-mL syringe = £1.41, 11-mL syringe = £1.58

**Excipients** include hydroxybenzoates (parabens)

**Dose** 6–11 mL into urethra

**Laryngojet®** (UCB Pharma) [PoM]

Jet spray 4% (disposable kit for laryngotracheal anaesthesia), lidocaine hydrochloride 40 mg/mL, net price per unit (4-mL vial and disposable sterile cannula with cover and vial injector) = £5.10

**Cautions** may be rapidly and almost completely absorbed from respiratory tract and systemic side-effects may occur; extreme caution if mucosa has been traumatised or if sepsis present

**Dose** usually 160 mg (4 mL) as a single dose instilled as jet spray to larynx and trachea or applied with a swab (reduce dose according to size, age and condition of patient); max. 200 mg (5 mL); CHILD up to 3 mg/kg

**LMX 4®** (Ferndale)

Cream lidocaine 4%, net price 5-g tube = £2.98; 5 × 5-g tube with 10 occlusive dressings = £16.90

**Excipients** include benzyl alcohol and propylene glycol

**Cautions** not for wounds, mucous membranes, or atopic dermatitis; avoid use near eyes or middle ear; although systemic absorption low, caution in severe hepatic impairment, acutely ill, debilitated, or elderly patients

**Side-effects** irritation and rash

**Dose** ADULT and CHILD over 1 month, anaesthesia before venous cannulation or venepuncture, apply thick layer (1–2.5 g; CHILD under 1 year max. 1 g) to small area (2.5 cm × 2.5 cm) of non-irritated skin at least 30 minutes before procedure (max. 60 minutes); remove cream with gauze and perform procedure after approximately 5 minutes

**15**

**Anaesthesia**

**Rapydan®** (EUSA Pharma) [PoM]

Medicated plasters, lidocaine 70 mg, tetracaine 70 mg, net price 25 = £98.00
Excipients include hydroxybenzoates (parabens)

**Dose** needle puncture or superficial surgical procedures, ADULT over 18 years, apply 1–4 plasters to intact skin 30 minutes before needle puncture or procedure; max. 4 plasters daily; CHILD 3–18 years, needle puncture, apply 1–2 plasters to intact skin 30 minutes before needle puncture; max. 2 plasters daily

The *Scottish Medicines Consortium* (p. 3) has advised (May 2008) that lidocaine 70 mg/tetracaine 70 mg (*Rapydan®* medicated plaster) is **not** recommended for use within NHS Scotland for surface anaesthesia of the skin in connection with needle puncture or for cases of superficial surgical procedures on normal skin in adults or children over 3 years.

**Versatis®** (Grünenthal) [PoM]

Medicated plasters, lidocaine 5% (700 mg/medicated plaster), net price 30 = £72.40
Excipients include hydroxybenzoates (parabens), propylene glycol

**Cautions** should not be applied to mucous membranes

**Side-effects** include administration site reactions such as skin lesions or injury

**Dose** postherpetic neuralgia, ADULT over 18 years, apply to intact, dry, non-hairy, non-irritated skin once daily for up to 12 hours, followed by a 12-hour plaster-free period; discontinue if no response after 4 weeks

**Note** Up to 3 plasters may be used to cover large areas; plasters may be cut

**Note** The *Scottish Medicines Consortium* (p. 3) has advised (July 2008) that *Versatis®* is accepted for restricted use within NHS Scotland for the treatment of postherpetic neuralgia in patients who are intolerant of first-line systemic therapies or when they have been ineffective

**Xylocaine®** (AstraZeneca)

Spray (= pump spray), lidocaine 10% (100 mg/g) supplying 10 mg lidocaine/dose; 500 spray doses per container. Net price 50-mL bottle = £3.13

**Dose** dental practice, 1–5 doses

Maxillary sinus puncture, 3 doses

During delivery in obstetrics, up to 20 doses

Bronchoscopy, laryngoscopy, oesophagoscopy, endotracheal intubation, up to 20 doses; CHILD up to 3 mg/kg

**Note** Lidocaine can damage plastic cuffs of endotracheal tubes

### ◢Lidocaine for ear, nose, and oropharyngeal use

For **cautions**, **contra-indications** and **side-effects** of phenylephrine, see section 2.7.2

**Lidocaine with Phenylephrine** (Non-proprietary)

Topical solution, lidocaine hydrochloride 5%, phenylephrine hydrochloride 0.5%, net price 2.5 mL (with nasal applicator) = £9.60.

## Bupivacaine

The advantage of bupivacaine over other local anaesthetics is its longer duration of action. It has a slow onset of action, taking up to 30 minutes for full effect. It is often used in lumbar epidural blockade and is particularly suitable for continuous epidural analgesia in labour, or for postoperative pain relief. It is the principal drug used for spinal anaesthesia.

### ◼ BUPIVACAINE HYDROCHLORIDE

**Indications** see under Dose

**Cautions** see under Lidocaine Hydrochloride and notes above; myocardial depression may be more

severe and more resistant to treatment; **interactions**: Appendix 1 (bupivacaine)

**Contra-indications** see under Lidocaine Hydrochloride and notes above; intravenous regional anaesthesia (Bier's block)

**Side-effects** see under Lidocaine Hydrochloride and notes above

**Dose**

**Note** Doses should be adjusted according to patient's physical status and nature of procedure—**important**: see also under Administration, p. 714

- Local infiltration, max. 60 mL, using a 2.5 mg/mL (0.25%) solution
- Peripheral nerve block, max. 60 mL, using a 2.5 mg/mL (0.25%) solution; max. 30 mL, using a 5 mg/mL (0.5%) solution
- Epidural block

  Surgery, *lumbar*, max. 20 mL, using a 5 mg/mL (0.5%) solution

  Surgery, *caudal*, max. 30 mL, using a 5 mg/mL (0.5%) solution; CHILD (up to 10 years) using a 2.5 mg/mL (0.25%) solution, up to lower-thoracic (T10) 0.3–0.4 mL/kg, up to mid-thoracic (T6) 0.4–0.8 mL/kg

  Labour, *lumbar*, max. 12 mL using a 2.5 mg/mL (0.25%) or 5 mg/mL (0.5%) solution; *caudal* (but rarely used) max. 20 mL using a 2.5 mg/mL (0.25%) or 5 mg/mL (0.5%) solution

- Sympathetic block, max. 50 mL, using a 2.5 mg/mL (0.25%) solution

- Intrathecal anaesthesia, see under preparations

> **Important**
> The licensed doses stated above may not be appropriate in some settings and expert advice should be sought

**Bupivacaine** (Non-proprietary) [PoM]

Injection, anhydrous bupivacaine hydrochloride 2.5 mg/mL (0.25%), net price 10 mL = 82p; 5 mg/mL (0.5%), 10 mL = 94p

**Note** Bupivacaine hydrochloride injection 0.25% and 0.5% are available in glass or plastic ampoules, and sterile-wrapped glass ampoules

Infusion, anhydrous bupivacaine hydrochloride 1 mg/mL (0.1%), net price 100 mL = £8.41, 250 mL = £10.59; 1.25 mg/mL (0.125%), 250 mL = £10.80

**Dose** Continuous lumbar epidural infusion during labour (once epidural block established), 10–15 mg/hour of 0.1% or 0.125% solution; max. 2 mg/kg over 4 hours and total of 400 mg in 24 hours

Continuous thoracic, upper abdominal, or lower abdominal epidural infusion for postoperative pain (once epidural block established), 4–15 mg/hour of 0.1% or 0.125% solution; max. 2 mg/kg over 4 hours and total of 400 mg in 24 hours; not recommended for use in children

**Marcain®** (AstraZeneca) [PoM]

Injection, anhydrous bupivacaine hydrochloride 2.5 mg/mL (*Marcain® 0.25%*), net price 10-mL *Polyamp®* = £1.06; 5 mg/mL (*Marcain® 0.5%*), 10-mL *Polyamp®* = £1.21

**Marcain Heavy®** (AstraZeneca) [PoM]

Injection, anhydrous bupivacaine hydrochloride 5 mg, glucose 80 mg/mL, net price 4-mL amp = £1.21

**Dose** intrathecal anaesthesia for surgery, 2–4 mL (dose may need to be reduced in elderly and in late pregnancy)

◢With adrenaline

For **cautions**, **contra-indications**, and **side-effects** of adrenaline, see section 3.4.3

**Bupivacaine and Adrenaline** (Non-proprietary) [PoM]

Injection, anhydrous bupivacaine hydrochloride 2.5 mg/mL (0.25%), adrenaline 1 in 200 000 (5 micrograms/mL), net price 10-mL amp = £1.23

Injection, anhydrous bupivacaine hydrochloride 5 mg/mL (0.5%), adrenaline 1 in 200 000 (5 micrograms/mL), net price 10-mL amp = £1.40

## Levobupivacaine

Levobupivacaine, an isomer of bupivacaine, has anaesthetic and analgesic properties similar to bupivacaine, but is thought to have fewer adverse effects.

### ▮ LEVOBUPIVACAINE

Note Levobupivacaine is an isomer of bupivacaine

**Indications** see under Dose

**Cautions** see under Lidocaine Hydrochloride and notes above; **interactions**: Appendix 1 (levobupivacaine)

**Contra-indications** see under Lidocaine Hydrochloride and notes above; intravenous regional anaesthesia (Bier's block); paracervical block in obstetrics; do not use 7.5 mg/mL strength in obstetrics

**Side-effects** see under Lidocaine Hydrochloride and notes above

**Dose**

Note Doses should be adjusted according to patient's physical status and nature of procedure—**important**: see also under Administration, p. 714

• Surgical anaesthesia

Lumbar epidural, 10–20 mL (50–150 mg) of 5 mg/mL or 7.5 mg/mL solution over 5 minutes; caesarean section, 15–30 mL (75–150 mg) of 5 mg/mL solution over 15–20 minutes

Intrathecal, 3 mL (15 mg) of 5 mg/mL solution

Peripheral nerve block, 1–40 mL of 2.5 mg/mL or 5 mg/mL solution (max. 150 mg); ilioinguinal/iliohypogastric block, CHILD under 12 years 0.25–0.5 mL/kg (0.625–2.5 mg/kg) of a 2.5 mg/mL or 5 mg/mL solution

Peribulbar block, 5–15 mL (37.5–112.5 mg) of 7.5 mg/mL solution

Local infiltration, 1–60 mL (max. 150 mg) of 2.5 mg/mL solution

• Acute pain

Lumbar epidural, labour pain, 6–10 mL (15–25 mg) of 2.5 mg/mL solution at intervals of at least 15 minutes or 5–12.5 mg/hour as a continuous epidural infusion, postoperative pain, 12.5–18.75 mg/hour as a continuous epidural infusion; max. 400 mg in 24 hours

> **Important**
> The licensed doses stated above may not be appropriate in some settings and expert advice should be sought

**Chirocaine®** (Abbott) [PoM]

Injection, levobupivacaine (as hydrochloride) 2.5 mg/mL, net price 10-mL amp = £1.66; 5 mg/mL, 10-mL amp = £1.90; 7.5 mg/mL, 10-mL amp = £2.85
Note For 1.25 mg/mL concentration dilute standard solutions with sodium chloride 0.9%

Infusion, levobupivacaine (as hydrochloride) 625 micrograms/mL, net price 100 mL = £7.80, 200 mL = £10.40; 1.25 mg/mL, net price 100 mL = £8.54, 200 mL = £12.20

## Prilocaine

Prilocaine is a local anaesthetic of low toxicity which is similar to lidocaine (lignocaine). If used in high doses, methaemoglobinaemia may occur which can be treated with intravenous injection of methylthioninium chloride (methylene blue) 1% using a dose of 1 mg/kg. Infants under 6 months are particularly susceptible to methaemoglobinaemia.

### ▮ PRILOCAINE HYDROCHLORIDE

**Indications** infiltration anaesthesia (higher strengths for dental use only), nerve block

**Cautions** see under Lidocaine Hydrochloride and notes above; severe or untreated hypertension, severe heart disease; concomitant drugs which cause methaemoglobinaemia; reduce dose in elderly or debilitated; pregnancy (Appendix 4); **interactions**: Appendix 1 (prilocaine)

**Contra-indications** see under Lidocaine Hydrochloride and notes above; anaemia or congenital or acquired methaemoglobinaemia

**Side-effects** see under Lidocaine Hydrochloride and notes above; ocular toxicity (including blindness) reported with excessively high strengths used for ophthalmic procedures

**Dose**

• See under preparations—**important**: see also under Administration, p. 714

**Citanest®** (AstraZeneca) [PoM]

Injection 1%, prilocaine hydrochloride 10 mg/mL, net price 50-mL multidose vial = £2.01
Dose adjusted according to site of administration and response, 100–200 mg/minute, or in incremental doses, to max. total dose 400 mg; CHILD over 6 months up to 5 mg/kg

◢With lidocaine

**EMLA®** see Lidocaine, p. 715

◢For dental use

Note Consult expert dental sources for specific advice in relation to dose of prilocaine for dental anaesthesia.

**Citanest®** (Dentsply) [PoM]

Injection 4%, prilocaine hydrochloride 40 mg/mL, net price 2.2-mL cartridge = 17p

**Citanest with Octapressin®** (Dentsply) [PoM]

Injection 3%, prilocaine hydrochloride 30 mg/mL, felypressin 0.03 unit/mL, net price 1.8-mL cartridge and self-aspirating cartridge (both) = 15p

**15**

**Anaesthesia**

## Ropivacaine

Ropivacaine is an amide-type local anaesthetic agent similar to bupivacaine. It is less cardiotoxic than bupivacaine, but also less potent.

### ▌ROPIVACAINE HYDROCHLORIDE

**Indications** see under Dose

**Cautions** see under Lidocaine Hydrochloride and notes above; also acute porphyria (section 9.8.2); **interactions**: Appendix 1 (ropivacaine)

**Contra-indications** see under Lidocaine Hydrochloride and notes above; intravenous regional anaesthesia (Bier's block); paracervical block in obstetrics

**Side-effects** see under Lidocaine Hydrochloride and notes above; also nausea, vomiting; hypertension, tachycardia; headache, rigors, impaired temperature regulation; urinary retention; back pain; *less commonly* syncope, dyspnoea, anxiety; *rarely* arrhythmia

**Dose**

Note Doses should be adjusted according to patient's physical status and nature of procedure—**important** see also under Administration on p. 714

* Surgical anaesthesia

Lumbar epidural, ADULT and CHILD over 12 years, 15–20 mL of 10 mg/mL solution *or* 15–25 mL of 7.5 mg/mL solution (max. total dose 200 mg); caesarean section, 15–20 mL of 7.5 mg/mL solution in incremental doses (max. total dose 150 mg)

Thoracic epidural (to establish block for postoperative pain), ADULT and CHILD over 12 years, 5–15 mL of 7.5 mg/mL solution

Major nerve block (brachial plexus block), ADULT and CHILD over 12 years, 30–40 mL of 7.5 mg/mL solution

Field block, ADULT and CHILD over 12 years, 1–30 mL of 7.5 mg/mL solution

* Acute pain

Lumbar epidural, ADULT and CHILD over 12 years, 10–20 mL of 2 mg/mL solution followed by 10–15 mL of 2 mg/mL solution at intervals of at least 30 minutes *or* 6–10 mL/hour of 2 mg/mL solution as a continuous epidural infusion for labour pain *or* 6–14 mL/hour of 2 mg/mL solution as a continuous epidural infusion for postoperative pain

Thoracic epidural, ADULT and CHILD over 12 years, 6–14 mL/hour of 2 mg/mL solution as a continuous infusion

Field block, ADULT and CHILD over 12 years, 1–100 mL of 2 mg/mL solution

Peripheral nerve block, ADULT and CHILD over 12 years, 5–10 mL/hour of 2 mg/mL solution as a continuous infusion *or* by intermittent injection

CHILD under 12 years, consult product literature

**Naropin®** (AstraZeneca) [PoM]

Injection, ropivacaine hydrochloride 2 mg/mL, net price 10-mL *Polyamp®* = £1.78; 7.5 mg/mL, 10-mL *Polyamp®* = £2.65; 10 mg/mL, 10-mL *Polyamp®* = £3.20
Electrolytes Na⁺<0.5 mmol/mL

Infusion, ropivacaine hydrochloride 2 mg/mL, net price 200-mL *Polybag®* = £14.45
Electrolytes Na⁺<0.5 mmol/mL

## Tetracaine

**Tetracaine** (amethocaine) is an effective local anaesthetic for topical application; a 4% gel is indicated for anaesthesia before venepuncture or venous cannulation. It is rapidly absorbed from mucous membranes and should **never** be applied to inflamed, traumatised, or highly vascular surfaces. It should **never** be used to provide anaesthesia for bronchoscopy or cystoscopy, as lidocaine (lignocaine) is a safer alternative. It is used in ophthalmology (section 11.7) and in skin preparations (section 13.3).

### ▌TETRACAINE
(Amethocaine)

**Indications** see under preparation below

**Cautions** see notes above

**Contra-indications** see notes above

**Side-effects** see notes above; also erythema, oedema and pruritus; *very rarely* blistering
**Important**. Rapid and extensive absorption may result in systemic side-effects (see also notes above)

**Ametop®** (S&N Hlth.)

Gel, tetracaine 4%, net price 1.5-g tube = £1.08
Dose ADULT and CHILD over 1 month, apply contents of tube to site of venepuncture or venous cannulation and cover with occlusive dressing; remove gel and dressing after 30 minutes for venepuncture and after 45 minutes for venous cannulation; NEONATE see *BNF for Children*
Note ADULT and CHILD over 5 years, contents of max. 5 tubes applied at separate sites at a single time; CHILD 1 month–5 years, contents of max. 1 tube applied at separate sites at a single time

◀With lidocaine
**Rapydan®** see Lidocaine, p. 716

## Other local anaesthetics

**Benzocaine** is a local anaesthetic of low potency and toxicity. It is used in concentrations of up to 20% for topical anaesthesia of the oral mucosa before injection. It is an ingredient of some proprietary topical preparations for musculoskeletal conditions (section 10.3.2), mouth-ulcer preparations (section 12.3.1), and throat lozenges (section 12.3.3). Benzocaine sprays used in the mouth and throat have been associated with methaemoglobinaemia.

**Cocaine** readily penetrates mucous membranes and is an effective surface anaesthetic with an intense vasoconstrictor action. However, apart from its use in otolaryngology (see below), it has now been replaced by less toxic alternatives. It has marked sympathomimetic activity and should **never** be given by injection because of its toxicity. As a result of its intense stimulant effect it is a drug of addiction. In otolaryngology cocaine is applied to the nasal mucosa in concentrations of 4 to 10% (40–100 mg/mL); an oromucosal solution and nasal spray both containing cocaine hydrochloride 10% are available (Aurum). In order to avoid systemic effects, the maximum dose recommended for application to the nasal mucosa in fit adults is a total of 1.5 mg/kg, which is equivalent to a total topical dose of approximately 100 mg for an adult male; this dose relates to direct application of cocaine (application on gauze may reduce systemic absorption). It should be used only by those skilled in the precautions needed to *minimise absorption* and the *consequent risk of arrhythmias*. Although cocaine interacts with other drugs liable to induce arrhythmias, including adrenaline, some otolaryngologists consider that combined use of topical cocaine with topical adrenaline (in the form of a paste or a solution) improves the operative field and may possibly reduce absorption. Cocaine is a mydriatic as well as a local anaesthetic but owing to corneal toxicity it is now little used in ophthalmology. Cocaine should be avoided in acute porphyria (section 9.8.2).

# A1 Interactions

Two or more drugs given at the same time may exert their effects independently or may interact. The interaction may be potentiation or antagonism of one drug by another, or occasionally some other effect. Adverse drug interactions should be reported to the CHM as for other adverse drug reactions.

Drug interactions may be **pharmacodynamic** or **pharmacokinetic**.

## Pharmacodynamic interactions

These are interactions between drugs which have similar or antagonistic pharmacological effects or side-effects. They may be due to competition at receptor sites, or occur between drugs acting on the same physiological system. They are usually predictable from a knowledge of the pharmacology of the interacting drugs; in general, those demonstrated with one drug are likely to occur with related drugs. They occur to a greater or lesser extent in most patients who receive the interacting drugs.

## Pharmacokinetic interactions

These occur when one drug alters the absorption, distribution, metabolism, or excretion of another, thus increasing or reducing the amount of drug available to produce its pharmacological effects. They are not easily predicted and many of them affect only a small proportion of patients taking the combination of drugs. Pharmacokinetic interactions occurring with one drug cannot be assumed to occur with related drugs unless their pharmacokinetic properties are known to be similar.

Pharmacokinetic interactions are of several types:

**Affecting absorption** The rate of absorption or the total amount absorbed can both be altered by drug interactions. Delayed absorption is rarely of clinical importance unless high peak plasma concentrations are required (e.g. when giving an analgesic). Reduction in the total amount absorbed, however, may result in ineffective therapy.

**Due to changes in protein binding** To a variable extent most drugs are loosely bound to plasma proteins. Protein-binding sites are non-specific and one drug can displace another thereby increasing its proportion free to diffuse from plasma to its site of action. This only produces a detectable increase in effect if it is an extensively bound (more than 90%) that is not widely distributed throughout the body. Even so displacement rarely produces more than transient potentiation because this increased concentration of free drug results in an increased rate of elimination.

Displacement from protein binding plays a part in the potentiation of warfarin by sulphonamides and tolbutamide but the importance of these interactions is due mainly to the fact that warfarin metabolism is also inhibited.

**Affecting metabolism** Many drugs are metabolised in the liver. Induction of the hepatic microsomal enzyme system by one drug can gradually increase the rate of metabolism of another, resulting in lower plasma concentrations and a reduced effect. On withdrawal of the inducer plasma concentrations increase and toxicity may occur. Barbiturates, griseofulvin, many antiepileptics, and rifampicin are the most important enzyme inducers. Drugs affected include warfarin and the oral contraceptives.

Conversely when one drug inhibits the metabolism of another higher plasma concentrations are produced, rapidly resulting in an increased effect with risk of toxicity. Some drugs which potentiate warfarin and phenytoin do so by this mechanism.

> Isoenzymes of the hepatic cytochrome P450 system interact with a wide range of drugs. Drugs may be substrates, inducers or inhibitors of the different isoenzymes. A great deal of *in-vitro* information is available on the effect of drugs on the isoenzymes; however, since drugs are eliminated by a number of different metabolic routes as well as renal excretion, the clinical effects of interactions cannot be predicted accurately from laboratory data on the cytochrome P450 isoenzymes. Except where a combination of drugs is specifically contra-indicated, the BNF presents only interactions that have been reported in clinical practice. In all cases the possibility of an interaction must be considered if toxic effects occur or if the activity of a drug diminishes.

**Affecting renal excretion** Drugs are eliminated through the kidney both by glomerular filtration and by active tubular secretion. Competition occurs between those which share active transport mechanisms in the proximal tubule. For example, salicylates and some other NSAIDs delay the excretion of methotrexate; serious methotrexate toxicity is possible.

## Relative importance of interactions

Many drug interactions are harmless and many of those which are potentially harmful only occur in a small proportion of patients; moreover, the severity of an interaction varies from one patient to another. Drugs with a small therapeutic ratio (e.g. phenytoin) and those which require careful control of dosage (e.g. anticoagulants, antihypertensives, and antidiabetics) are most often involved.

Patients at increased risk from drug interactions include the elderly and those with impaired renal or liver function.

**Hazardous interactions** The symbol • has been placed against interactions that are **potentially hazardous** and where combined administration of the drugs involved should be **avoided** (or only undertaken with caution and appropriate monitoring).

Interactions that have no symbol do not usually have serious consequences.

## List of drug interactions

The following is an alphabetical list of drugs and their interactions; to avoid excessive cross-referencing each drug or group is listed twice: in the alphabetical list and also against the drug or group with which it interacts; changes in the interactions lists since BNF No. 57 (March 2009) are underlined.

For explanation of symbol • see above

**Abacavir**

Analgesics: abacavir possibly reduces plasma concentration of methadone

Antibacterials: plasma concentration of abacavir possibly reduced by rifampicin

Antiepileptics: plasma concentration of abacavir possibly reduced by phenytoin

• Antivirals: plasma concentration of abacavir reduced by •tipranavir

Barbiturates: plasma concentration of abacavir possibly reduced by phenobarbital

**Abatacept**

Adalimumab: increased risk of side-effects when abatacept given with adalimumab

Etanercept: increased risk of side-effects when abatacept given with etanercept

Infliximab: increased risk of side-effects when abatacept given with infliximab

• Vaccines: avoid concomitant use of abatacept with live •vaccines (see p. 669)

**Acarbose** see Antidiabetics

**ACE Inhibitors**

Alcohol: enhanced hypotensive effect when ACE inhibitors given with alcohol

Aldesleukin: enhanced hypotensive effect when ACE inhibitors given with aldesleukin

Allopurinol: increased risk of leucopenia and hypersensitivity reactions when ACE inhibitors given with allopurinol especially in renal impairment

Alpha-blockers: enhanced hypotensive effect when ACE inhibitors given with alpha-blockers

Anaesthetics, General: enhanced hypotensive effect when ACE inhibitors given with general anaesthetics

Analgesics: increased risk of renal impairment when ACE inhibitors given with NSAIDs, also hypotensive effect antagonised

Angiotensin-II Receptor Antagonists: increased risk of hyperkalaemia when ACE inhibitors given with angiotensin-II receptor antagonists

Antacids: absorption of ACE inhibitors possibly reduced by antacids; absorption of captopril, enalapril and fosinopril reduced by antacids

Antibacterials: plasma concentration of active metabolite of imidapril reduced by rifampicin (reduced antihypertensive effect); quinapril tablets reduce absorption of tetracyclines (quinapril tablets contain magnesium carbonate)

Anticoagulants: increased risk of hyperkalaemia when ACE inhibitors given with heparins

Antidepressants: hypotensive effect of ACE inhibitors possibly enhanced by MAOIs

Antidiabetics: ACE inhibitors possibly enhance hypoglycaemic effect of insulin, metformin and sulphonylureas

Antipsychotics: enhanced hypotensive effect when ACE inhibitors given with antipsychotics

Anxiolytics and Hypnotics: enhanced hypotensive effect when ACE inhibitors given with anxiolytics and hypnotics

Azathioprine: increased risk of anaemia or leucopenia when captopril given with azathioprine especially in renal impairment; increased risk of anaemia when enalapril given with azathioprine especially in renal impairment

Beta-blockers: enhanced hypotensive effect when ACE inhibitors given with beta-blockers

Calcium-channel Blockers: enhanced hypotensive effect when ACE inhibitors given with calcium-channel blockers

**ACE Inhibitors** *(continued)*

Cardiac Glycosides: captopril possibly increases plasma concentration of digoxin

• Ciclosporin: increased risk of hyperkalaemia when ACE inhibitors given with •ciclosporin

Clonidine: enhanced hypotensive effect when ACE inhibitors given with clonidine; antihypertensive effect of captopril possibly delayed by previous treatment with clonidine

Corticosteroids: hypotensive effect of ACE inhibitors antagonised by corticosteroids

Diazoxide: enhanced hypotensive effect when ACE inhibitors given with diazoxide

• Diuretics: enhanced hypotensive effect when ACE inhibitors given with •diuretics; increased risk of severe hyperkalaemia when ACE inhibitors given with •potassium-sparing diuretics and aldosterone antagonists (monitor potassium concentration with low-dose spironolactone in heart failure)

Dopaminergics: enhanced hypotensive effect when ACE inhibitors given with levodopa

• Lithium: ACE inhibitors reduce excretion of •lithium (increased plasma concentration)

Methyldopa: enhanced hypotensive effect when ACE inhibitors given with methyldopa

Moxisylyte (thymoxamine): enhanced hypotensive effect when ACE inhibitors given with moxisylyte

Moxonidine: enhanced hypotensive effect when ACE inhibitors given with moxonidine

Muscle Relaxants: enhanced hypotensive effect when ACE inhibitors given with baclofen or tizanidine

Nitrates: enhanced hypotensive effect when ACE inhibitors given with nitrates

Oestrogens: hypotensive effect of ACE inhibitors antagonised by oestrogens

• Potassium Salts: increased risk of severe hyperkalaemia when ACE inhibitors given with •potassium salts

Probenecid: excretion of captopril reduced by probenecid

Prostaglandins: enhanced hypotensive effect when ACE inhibitors given with alprostadil

Vasodilator Antihypertensives: enhanced hypotensive effect when ACE inhibitors given with hydralazine, minoxidil or sodium nitroprusside

**Acebutolol** see Beta-blockers

**Aceclofenac** see NSAIDs

**Acemetacin** see NSAIDs

**Acenocoumarol (nicoumalone)** see Coumarins

**Acetazolamide** see Diuretics

**Aciclovir**

Note  Interactions do not apply to topical aciclovir preparations

Note  Valaciclovir interactions as for aciclovir

Ciclosporin: increased risk of nephrotoxicity when aciclovir given with ciclosporin

Mycophenolate: plasma concentration of aciclovir increased by mycophenolate, also plasma concentration of inactive metabolite of mycophenolate increased

Probenecid: excretion of aciclovir reduced by probenecid (increased plasma concentration)

Tacrolimus: possible increased risk of nephrotoxicity when aciclovir given with tacrolimus

**Acitretin** see Retinoids

**Adalimumab**

Abatacept: increased risk of side-effects when adalimumab given with abatacept

• Anakinra: avoid concomitant use of adalimumab with •anakinra

• Vaccines: avoid concomitant use of adalimumab with live •vaccines (see p. 669)

**Adefovir**

Antivirals: avoidance of adefovir advised by manufacturer of tenofovir

**Adenosine**

Note Possibility of interaction with drugs tending to impair myocardial conduction

Anaesthetics, Local: increased myocardial depression when anti-arrhythmics given with bupivacaine, levobupivacaine, prilocaine or ropivacaine

• Anti-arrhythmics: increased myocardial depression when anti-arrhythmics given with other ●anti-arrhythmics

• Antipsychotics: increased risk of ventricular arrhythmias when anti-arrhythmics that prolong the QT interval given with ●antipsychotics that prolong the QT interval

• Beta-blockers: increased myocardial depression when anti-arrhythmics given with ●beta-blockers

• Dipyridamole: effect of adenosine enhanced and extended by ●dipyridamole (important risk of toxicity)

Theophylline: anti-arrhythmic effect of adenosine antagonised by theophylline

**Adrenaline (epinephrine)** see Sympathomimetics

**Adrenergic Neurone Blockers**

Alcohol: enhanced hypotensive effect when adrenergic neurone blockers given with alcohol

Alpha-blockers: enhanced hypotensive effect when adrenergic neurone blockers given with alpha-blockers

• Anaesthetics, General: enhanced hypotensive effect when adrenergic neurone blockers given with ●general anaesthetics

Analgesics: hypotensive effect of adrenergic neurone blockers antagonised by NSAIDs

Angiotensin-II Receptor Antagonists: enhanced hypotensive effect when adrenergic neurone blockers given with angiotensin-II receptor antagonists

Antidepressants: enhanced hypotensive effect when adrenergic neurone blockers given with MAOIs; hypotensive effect of adrenergic neurone blockers antagonised by tricyclics

Antipsychotics: hypotensive effect of adrenergic neurone blockers antagonised by haloperidol; hypotensive effect of adrenergic neurone blockers antagonised by higher doses of chlorpromazine; enhanced hypotensive effect when adrenergic neurone blockers given with phenothiazines

Anxiolytics and Hypnotics: enhanced hypotensive effect when adrenergic neurone blockers given with anxiolytics and hypnotics

Beta-blockers: enhanced hypotensive effect when adrenergic neurone blockers given with beta-blockers

Calcium-channel Blockers: enhanced hypotensive effect when adrenergic neurone blockers given with calcium-channel blockers

Clonidine: enhanced hypotensive effect when adrenergic neurone blockers given with clonidine

Corticosteroids: hypotensive effect of adrenergic neurone blockers antagonised by corticosteroids

Diazoxide: enhanced hypotensive effect when adrenergic neurone blockers given with diazoxide

Diuretics: enhanced hypotensive effect when adrenergic neurone blockers given with diuretics

Dopaminergics: enhanced hypotensive effect when adrenergic neurone blockers given with levodopa

Methyldopa: enhanced hypotensive effect when adrenergic neurone blockers given with methyldopa

Moxisylyte (thymoxamine): enhanced hypotensive effect when adrenergic neurone blockers given with moxisylyte

Moxonidine: enhanced hypotensive effect when adrenergic neurone blockers given with moxonidine

Muscle Relaxants: enhanced hypotensive effect when adrenergic neurone blockers given with baclofen or tizanidine

Nitrates: enhanced hypotensive effect when adrenergic neurone blockers given with nitrates

Oestrogens: hypotensive effect of adrenergic neurone blockers antagonised by oestrogens

Pizotifen: hypotensive effect of adrenergic neurone blockers antagonised by pizotifen

**Adrenergic Neurone Blockers** *(continued)*

Prostaglandins: enhanced hypotensive effect when adrenergic neurone blockers given with alprostadil

• Sympathomimetics: hypotensive effect of guanethidine antagonised by ●dexamfetamine; hypotensive effect of adrenergic neurone blockers antagonised by ●ephedrine, ●isometheptene, ●metaraminol, ●methylphenidate, ●noradrenaline (norepinephrine), ●oxymetazoline, ●phenylephrine, ●pseudoephedrine or ●xylometazoline

Vasodilator Antihypertensives: enhanced hypotensive effect when adrenergic neurone blockers given with hydralazine, minoxidil or sodium nitroprusside

**Adsorbents** see Kaolin

**Agalsidase Alfa and Beta**

Anti-arrhythmics: effects of agalsidase alfa and beta possibly inhibited by amiodarone (manufacturers of agalsidase alfa and beta advise avoid concomitant use)

Antibacterials: effects of agalsidase alfa and beta possibly inhibited by gentamicin (manufacturers of agalsidase alfa and beta advise avoid concomitant use)

Antimalarials: effects of agalsidase alfa and beta possibly inhibited by chloroquine and hydroxychloroquine (manufacturers of agalsidase alfa and beta advise avoid concomitant use)

**Agomelatine**

• Antibacterials: manufacturer of agomelatine advises avoid concomitant use with ●ciprofloxacin

• Antidepressants: metabolism of agomelatine inhibited by ●fluvoxamine (increased plasma concentration)

• Antimalarials: avoidance of antidepressants advised by manufacturer of ●artemether/lumefantrine

Atomoxetine: possible increased risk of convulsions when antidepressants given with atomoxetine

**Alcohol**

ACE Inhibitors: enhanced hypotensive effect when alcohol given with ACE inhibitors

Adrenergic Neurone Blockers: enhanced hypotensive effect when alcohol given with adrenergic neurone blockers

Alpha-blockers: increased sedative effect when alcohol given with indoramin; enhanced hypotensive effect when alcohol given with alpha-blockers

Analgesics: enhanced hypotensive and sedative effects when alcohol given with opioid analgesics

Angiotensin-II Receptor Antagonists: enhanced hypotensive effect when alcohol given with angiotensin-II receptor antagonists

• Antibacterials: disulfiram-like reaction when alcohol given with metronidazole; possibility of disulfiram-like reaction when alcohol given with tinidazole; increased risk of convulsions when alcohol given with ●cycloserine

• Anticoagulants: major changes in consumption of alcohol may affect anticoagulant control with ●coumarins or ●phenindione

• Antidepressants: some beverages containing alcohol and some dealcoholised beverages contain tyramine which interacts with ●MAOIs (hypertensive crisis)—if no tyramine, enhanced hypotensive effect; sedative effects possibly increased when alcohol given with SSRIs; increased sedative effect when alcohol given with ●mirtazapine, ●tricyclic-related antidepressants or ●tricyclics

Antidiabetics: alcohol enhances hypoglycaemic effect of antidiabetics; increased risk of lactic acidosis when alcohol given with metformin; flushing, in susceptible subjects, when alcohol given with chlorpropamide

Antiepileptics: alcohol possibly increases CNS side-effects of carbamazepine; increased sedative effect when alcohol given with primidone

Antifungals: effects of alcohol possibly enhanced by griseofulvin

Antihistamines: increased sedative effect when alcohol given with antihistamines (possibly less effect with non-sedating antihistamines)

Alcohol *(continued)*

Antimuscarinics: increased sedative effect when alcohol given with hyoscine

Antipsychotics: increased sedative effect when alcohol given with antipsychotics

Anxiolytics and Hypnotics: increased sedative effect when alcohol given with anxiolytics and hypnotics

Barbiturates: increased sedative effect when alcohol given with barbiturates

Beta-blockers: enhanced hypotensive effect when alcohol given with beta-blockers

Calcium-channel Blockers: enhanced hypotensive effect when alcohol given with calcium-channel blockers; plasma concentration of alcohol possibly increased by verapamil

Clonidine: enhanced hypotensive effect when alcohol given with clonidine

Cytotoxics: disulfiram-like reaction when alcohol given with procarbazine

Diazoxide: enhanced hypotensive effect when alcohol given with diazoxide

Disulfiram: disulfiram reaction when alcohol given with disulfiram (see p. 280)

Diuretics: enhanced hypotensive effect when alcohol given with diuretics

Dopaminergics: alcohol reduces tolerance to bromo-criptine

Levamisole: possibility of disulfiram-like reaction when alcohol given with levamisole

Lofexidine: increased sedative effect when alcohol given with lofexidine

Methyldopa: enhanced hypotensive effect when alcohol given with methyldopa

Moxonidine: enhanced hypotensive effect when alcohol given with moxonidine

Muscle Relaxants: increased sedative effect when alcohol given with baclofen, methocarbamol or tizanidine

Nabilone: increased sedative effect when alcohol given with nabilone

Nicorandil: alcohol possibly enhances hypotensive effect of nicorandil

Nitrates: enhanced hypotensive effect when alcohol given with nitrates

• Paraldehyde: increased sedative effect when alcohol given with ●paraldehyde

• Retinoids: presence of alcohol causes etretinate to be formed from ●acitretin (increased risk of teratogenicity in women of child-bearing potential)

Sympathomimetics: alcohol possibly enhances effects of methylphenidate

Vasodilator Antihypertensives: enhanced hypotensive effect when alcohol given with hydralazine, minoxidil or sodium nitroprusside

Aldesleukin

ACE Inhibitors: enhanced hypotensive effect when aldesleukin given with ACE inhibitors

Alpha-blockers: enhanced hypotensive effect when aldesleukin given with alpha-blockers

Angiotensin-II Receptor Antagonists: enhanced hypotensive effect when aldesleukin given with angiotensin-II receptor antagonists

Beta-blockers: enhanced hypotensive effect when aldesleukin given with beta-blockers

Calcium-channel Blockers: enhanced hypotensive effect when aldesleukin given with calcium-channel blockers

Clonidine: enhanced hypotensive effect when aldesleukin given with clonidine

Diazoxide: enhanced hypotensive effect when aldesleukin given with diazoxide

Diuretics: enhanced hypotensive effect when aldesleukin given with diuretics

Methyldopa: enhanced hypotensive effect when aldesleukin given with methyldopa

Moxonidine: enhanced hypotensive effect when aldesleukin given with moxonidine

Nitrates: enhanced hypotensive effect when aldesleukin given with nitrates

Aldesleukin *(continued)*

Vasodilator Antihypertensives: enhanced hypotensive effect when aldesleukin given with hydralazine, minoxidil or sodium nitroprusside

**Alendronic Acid** *see* Bisphosphonates

**Alfentanil** *see* Opioid Analgesics

**Alfuzosin** *see* Alpha-blockers

**Alimemazine (trimeprazine)** *see* Antihistamines

**Aliskiren**

Angiotensin-II Receptor Antagonists: plasma concentration of aliskiren possibly reduced by irbesartan

Anticoagulants: increased risk of hyperkalaemia when aliskiren given with heparins

Antifungals: plasma concentration of aliskiren increased by ketoconazole

Calcium-channel Blockers: manufacturer of aliskiren advises avoid concomitant use with verapamil

• Ciclosporin: plasma concentration of aliskiren increased by ●ciclosporin—avoid concomitant use

Diuretics: aliskiren reduces plasma concentration of furosemide (frusemide); increased risk of hyperkalaemia when aliskiren given with potassium-sparing diuretics and aldosterone antagonists

Potassium Salts: increased risk of hyperkalaemia when aliskiren given with potassium salts

**Alitretinoin** *see* Retinoids

**Alkylating Drugs** *see* Busulfan, Carmustine, Cyclophosphamide, Estramustine, Ifosfamide, Lomustine, Melphalan, and Thiotepa

**Allopurinol**

ACE Inhibitors: increased risk of leucopenia and hypersensitivity reactions when allopurinol given with ACE inhibitors especially in renal impairment

Antibacterials: increased risk of rash when allopurinol given with amoxicillin or ampicillin

Anticoagulants: allopurinol possibly enhances anticoagulant effect of coumarins

• Antivirals: allopurinol increases plasma concentration of ●didanosine (risk of toxicity)—avoid concomitant use

• Azathioprine: allopurinol enhances effects and increases toxicity of ●azathioprine (reduce dose of azathioprine to one quarter of usual dose)

Ciclosporin: allopurinol possibly increases plasma concentration of ciclosporin (risk of nephrotoxicity)

• Cytotoxics: allopurinol enhances effects and increases toxicity of ●mercaptopurine (reduce dose of mercaptopurine to one quarter of usual dose); avoidance of allopurinol advised by manufacturer of ●capecitabine

Diuretics: increased risk of hypersensitivity when allopurinol given with thiazides and related diuretics especially in renal impairment

Theophylline: allopurinol possibly increases plasma concentration of theophylline

**Almotriptan** *see* 5HT$_1$ Agonists

**Alpha$_2$-adrenoceptor Stimulants** *see* Apraclonidine, Brimonidine, Clonidine and Methyldopa

**Alpha-blockers**

ACE Inhibitors: enhanced hypotensive effect when alpha-blockers given with ACE inhibitors

Adrenergic Neurone Blockers: enhanced hypotensive effect when alpha-blockers given with adrenergic neurone blockers

Alcohol: enhanced hypotensive effect when alpha-blockers given with alcohol; increased sedative effect when indoramin given with alcohol

Aldesleukin: enhanced hypotensive effect when alpha-blockers given with aldesleukin

• Anaesthetics, General: enhanced hypotensive effect when alpha-blockers given with ●general anaesthetics

Analgesics: hypotensive effect of alpha-blockers antagonised by NSAIDs

Angiotensin-II Receptor Antagonists: enhanced hypotensive effect when alpha-blockers given with angiotensin-II receptor antagonists

• Antidepressants: manufacturer of indoramin advises avoid concomitant use with ●MAOIs; enhanced

**Alpha-blockers**
- Antidepressants *(continued)*
  hypotensive effect when alpha-blockers given with MAOIs
  Antipsychotics: enhanced hypotensive effect when alpha-blockers given with antipsychotics
- Antivirals: plasma concentration of alfuzosin possibly increased by ●ritonavir—avoid concomitant use
  Anxiolytics and Hypnotics: enhanced hypotensive and sedative effects when alpha-blockers given with anxiolytics and hypnotics
- Beta-blockers: enhanced hypotensive effect when alpha-blockers given with ●beta-blockers, also increased risk of first-dose hypotension with post-synaptic alpha-blockers such as prazosin
- Calcium-channel Blockers: enhanced hypotensive effect when alpha-blockers given with ●calcium-channel blockers, also increased risk of first-dose hypotension with post-synaptic alpha-blockers such as prazosin
  Cardiac Glycosides: prazosin increases plasma concentration of digoxin
  Clonidine: enhanced hypotensive effect when alpha-blockers given with clonidine
  Corticosteroids: hypotensive effect of alpha-blockers antagonised by corticosteroids
  Diazoxide: enhanced hypotensive effect when alpha-blockers given with diazoxide
- Diuretics: enhanced hypotensive effect when alpha-blockers given with ●diuretics, also increased risk of first-dose hypotension with post-synaptic alpha-blockers such as prazosin
  Dopaminergics: enhanced hypotensive effect when alpha-blockers given with levodopa
  Methyldopa: enhanced hypotensive effect when alpha-blockers given with methyldopa
- Moxisylyte (thymoxamine): possible severe postural hypotension when alpha-blockers given with ●moxisylyte
  Moxonidine: enhanced hypotensive effect when alpha-blockers given with moxonidine
  Muscle Relaxants: enhanced hypotensive effect when alpha-blockers given with baclofen or tizanidine
  Nitrates: enhanced hypotensive effect when alpha-blockers given with nitrates
  Oestrogens: hypotensive effect of alpha-blockers antagonised by oestrogens
  Prostaglandins: enhanced hypotensive effect when alpha-blockers given with alprostadil
- Sildenafil: enhanced hypotensive effect when alpha-blockers given with ●sildenafil (avoid alpha-blockers for 4 hours after sildenafil)—see also p. 463
- Sympathomimetics: avoid concomitant use of tolazoline with ●adrenaline (epinephrine) or ●dopamine
- Tadalafil: enhanced hypotensive effect when alpha-blockers given with ●tadalafil—see also p. 463; enhanced hypotensive effect when doxazosin given with ●tadalafil—manufacturer of tadalafil advises avoid concomitant use
- Ulcer-healing Drugs: effects of tolazoline antagonised by ●cimetidine and ●ranitidine
- Vardenafil: enhanced hypotensive effect when alpha-blockers (excludes tamsulosin) given with ●vardenafil—separate doses by 6 hours—see also p. 463
  Vasodilator Antihypertensives: enhanced hypotensive effect when alpha-blockers given with hydralazine, minoxidil or sodium nitroprusside

**Alpha-blockers (post-synaptic)** *see* Alpha-blockers
**Alprazolam** *see* Anxiolytics and Hypnotics
**Alprostadil** *see* Prostaglandins
**Aluminium Hydroxide** *see* Antacids
**Amantadine**
  Antipsychotics: increased risk of extrapyramidal side-effects when amantadine given with antipsychotics
  Bupropion: increased risk of side-effects when amantadine given with bupropion
- Memantine: increased risk of CNS toxicity when amantadine given with ●memantine (manufacturer of

**Amantadine**
- Memantine *(continued)*
  memantine advises avoid concomitant use); effects of dopaminergics possibly enhanced by memantine
  Methyldopa: increased risk of extrapyramidal side-effects when amantadine given with methyldopa; antiparkinsonian effect of dopaminergics antagonised by methyldopa
  Tetrabenazine: increased risk of extrapyramidal side-effects when amantadine given with tetrabenazine

**Amikacin** *see* Aminoglycosides
**Amiloride** *see* Diuretics
**Aminoglycosides**
  Agalsidase Alfa and Beta: gentamicin possibly inhibits effects of agalsidase alfa and beta (manufacturers of agalsidase alfa and beta advise avoid concomitant use)
  Analgesics: plasma concentration of amikacin and gentamicin in neonates possibly increased by indometacin
  Antibacterials: neomycin reduces absorption of phenoxymethylpenicillin; increased risk of nephrotoxicity when aminoglycosides given with colistin or polymyxins; increased risk of nephrotoxicity and ototoxicity when aminoglycosides given with capreomycin, teicoplanin or vancomycin; possible increased risk of nephrotoxicity when aminoglycosides given with cephalosporins
- Anticoagulants: experience in anticoagulant clinics suggests that INR possibly altered when neomycin (given for local action on gut) is given with ●coumarins or ●phenindione
  Antidiabetics: neomycin possibly enhances hypoglycaemic effect of acarbose, also severity of gastro-intestinal effects increased
  Antifungals: increased risk of nephrotoxicity when aminoglycosides given with amphotericin
  Bisphosphonates: increased risk of hypocalcaemia when aminoglycosides given with bisphosphonates
  Cardiac Glycosides: neomycin reduces absorption of digoxin; gentamicin possibly increases plasma concentration of digoxin
- Ciclosporin: increased risk of nephrotoxicity when aminoglycosides given with ●ciclosporin
- Cytotoxics: neomycin possibly reduces absorption of methotrexate; increased risk of nephrotoxicity and possibly of ototoxicity when aminoglycosides given with ●platinum compounds
- Diuretics: increased risk of otoxicity when aminoglycosides given with ●loop diuretics
- Muscle Relaxants: aminoglycosides enhance effects of ●non-depolarising muscle relaxants and ●suxamethonium
  Oestrogens: antibacterials that do not induce liver enzymes possibly reduce contraceptive effect of oestrogens (risk probably small, see p. 445)
- Parasympathomimetics: aminoglycosides antagonise effects of ●neostigmine and ●pyridostigmine
- Tacrolimus: increased risk of nephrotoxicity when aminoglycosides given with ●tacrolimus
  Vaccines: antibacterials inactivate oral typhoid vaccine–see p. 688
  Vitamins: neomycin possibly reduces absorption of vitamin A

**Aminophylline** *see* Theophylline
**Aminosalicylates**
  Azathioprine: possible increased risk of leucopenia when aminosalicylates given with azathioprine
  Cardiac Glycosides: sulfasalazine possibly reduces absorption of digoxin
  Cytotoxics: possible increased risk of leucopenia when aminosalicylates given with mercaptopurine
  Folates: sulfasalazine possibly reduces absorption of folic acid

## Amiodarone

Note Amiodarone has a long half-life; there is a potential for drug interactions to occur for several weeks (or even months) after treatment with it has been stopped

Agalsidase Alfa and Beta: amiodarone possibly inhibits effects of agalsidase alfa and beta (manufacturers of agalsidase alfa and beta advise avoid concomitant use)

Anaesthetics, Local: increased myocardial depression when anti-arrhythmics given with bupivacaine, levo-bupivacaine, prilocaine or ropivacaine

- Anti-arrhythmics: increased myocardial depression when anti-arrhythmics given with other ●anti-arrhythmics; increased risk of ventricular arrhythmias when amiodarone given with ●disopyramide—avoid concomitant use; amiodarone increases plasma concentration of ●flecainide (halve dose of flecainide)
- Antibacterials: increased risk of ventricular arrhythmias when amiodarone given with parenteral ●erythromycin—avoid concomitant use; increased risk of ventricular arrhythmias when amiodarone given with ●levofloxacin or ●moxifloxacin—avoid concomitant use; increased risk of ventricular arrhythmias when amiodarone given with ●sulfamethoxazole and ●trimethoprim (as co-trimoxazole)—avoid concomitant use of co-trimoxazole
- Anticoagulants: amiodarone inhibits metabolism of ●coumarins and ●phenindione (enhanced anticoagulant effect); amiodarone increases plasma concentration of ●dabigatran etexilate (reduce dose of dabigatran etexilate)
- Antidepressants: increased risk of ventricular arrhythmias when amiodarone given with ●tricyclics—avoid concomitant use
- Antiepileptics: amiodarone inhibits metabolism of ●phenytoin (increased plasma concentration)
- Antihistamines: increased risk of ventricular arrhythmias when amiodarone given with ●mizolastine—avoid concomitant use
- Antimalarials: avoidance of amiodarone advised by manufacturer of ●artemether/lumefantrine (risk of ventricular arrhythmias); increased risk of ventricular arrhythmias when amiodarone given with ●chloroquine and hydroxychloroquine, ●mefloquine or ●quinine—avoid concomitant use
- Antimuscarinics: increased risk of ventricular arrhythmias when amiodarone given with ●tolterodine
- Antipsychotics: increased risk of ventricular arrhythmias when anti-arrhythmics that prolong the QT interval given with ●antipsychotics that prolong the QT interval; increased risk of ventricular arrhythmias when amiodarone given with ●benperidol—manufacturer of benperidol advises avoid concomitant use; increased risk of ventricular arrhythmias when amiodarone given with ●amisulpride, ●droperidol, ●haloperidol, ●phenothiazines, ●pimozide, ●sertindole or ●zuclopenthixol—avoid concomitant use; increased risk of ventricular arrhythmias when amiodarone given with ●sulpiride
- Antivirals: plasma concentration of amiodarone possibly increased by ●atazanavir; plasma concentration of amiodarone possibly increased by ●fosamprenavir (increased risk of ventricular arrhythmias—avoid concomitant use); plasma concentration of amiodarone possibly increased by ●indinavir—avoid concomitant use; increased risk of ventricular arrhythmias when amiodarone given with ●nelfinavir—avoid concomitant use; plasma concentration of amiodarone increased by ●ritonavir (increased risk of ventricular arrhythmias—avoid concomitant use)
- Atomoxetine: increased risk of ventricular arrhythmias when amiodarone given with ●atomoxetine
- Beta-blockers: increased risk of bradycardia, AV block and myocardial depression when amiodarone given with ●beta-blockers; increased myocardial depression when anti-arrhythmics given with ●beta-blockers; increased risk of ventricular arrhythmias when

## Amiodarone

- Beta-blockers *(continued)* amiodarone given with ●sotalol—avoid concomitant use
- Calcium-channel Blockers: increased risk of bradycardia, AV block and myocardial depression when amiodarone given with ●diltiazem or ●verapamil
- Cardiac Glycosides: amiodarone increases plasma concentration of ●digoxin (halve dose of digoxin)

Ciclosporin: amiodarone possibly increases plasma concentration of ciclosporin

Diuretics: increased cardiac toxicity with amiodarone if hypokalaemia occurs with acetazolamide, loop diuretics or thiazides and related diuretics; amiodarone increases plasma concentration of eplerenone (reduce dose of eplerenone)

Grapefruit Juice: plasma concentration of amiodarone increased by grapefruit juice

- 5HT₃ Antagonists: increased risk of ventricular arrhythmias when amiodarone given with ●dolasetron—avoid concomitant use
- Ivabradine: increased risk of ventricular arrhythmias when amiodarone given with ●ivabradine
- Lipid-regulating Drugs: increased risk of myopathy when amiodarone given with ●simvastatin
- Lithium: manufacturer of amiodarone advises avoid concomitant use with ●lithium (risk of ventricular arrhythmias)

Orlistat: plasma concentration of amiodarone possibly reduced by orlistat

- Pentamidine Isetionate: increased risk of ventricular arrhythmias when amiodarone given with ●pentamidine isetionate—avoid concomitant use

Thyroid Hormones: for concomitant use of amiodarone and thyroid hormones see p. 83

Ulcer-healing Drugs: plasma concentration of amiodarone increased by cimetidine

**Amisulpride** see Antipsychotics

**Amitriptyline** see Antidepressants, Tricyclic

**Amlodipine** see Calcium-channel Blockers

**Amobarbital** see Barbiturates

**Amoxicillin** see Penicillins

## Amphotericin

Note Close monitoring required with concomitant administration of nephrotoxic drugs or cytotoxics

Antibacterials: increased risk of nephrotoxicity when amphotericin given with aminoglycosides or polymyxins; possible increased risk of nephrotoxicity when amphotericin given with vancomycin

Antifungals: amphotericin reduces renal excretion and increases cellular uptake of flucytosine (toxicity possibly increased); effects of amphotericin possibly antagonised by imidazoles and triazoles

- Cardiac Glycosides: hypokalaemia caused by amphotericin increases cardiac toxicity with ●cardiac glycosides
- Ciclosporin: increased risk of nephrotoxicity when amphotericin given with ●ciclosporin
- Corticosteroids: increased risk of hypokalaemia when amphotericin given with ●corticosteroids—avoid concomitant use unless corticosteroids needed to control reactions

Diuretics: increased risk of hypokalaemia when amphotericin given with loop diuretics or thiazides and related diuretics

Pentamidine Isetionate: possible increased risk of nephrotoxicity when amphotericin given with pentamidine isetionate

- Tacrolimus: increased risk of nephrotoxicity when amphotericin given with ●tacrolimus

**Ampicillin** see Penicillins

## Anabolic Steroids

- Anticoagulants: anabolic steroids enhance anticoagulant effect of ●coumarins and ●phenindione

Antidiabetics: anabolic steroids possibly enhance hypoglycaemic effect of antidiabetics

## Anaesthetics, General

Note *See also* Surgery and Long-term Medication, p. 697

ACE Inhibitors: enhanced hypotensive effect when general anaesthetics given with ACE inhibitors

- Adrenergic Neurone Blockers: enhanced hypotensive effect when general anaesthetics given with •adrenergic neurone blockers

- Alpha-blockers: enhanced hypotensive effect when general anaesthetics given with •alpha-blockers

Angiotensin-II Receptor Antagonists: enhanced hypotensive effect when general anaesthetics given with angiotensin-II receptor antagonists

Antibacterials: general anaesthetics possibly potentiate hepatotoxicity of isoniazid; effects of thiopental enhanced by sulphonamides; hypersensitivity-like reactions can occur when general anaesthetics given with intravenous vancomycin

- Antidepressants: Because of hazardous interactions between general anaesthetics and •MAOIs, MAOIs should normally be stopped 2 weeks before surgery; increased risk of arrhythmias and hypotension when general anaesthetics given with tricyclics

- <u>Antipsychotics</u>: enhanced hypotensive effect when general anaesthetics given with •antipsychotics; effects of thiopental enhanced by droperidol

Anxiolytics and Hypnotics: increased sedative effect when general anaesthetics given with anxiolytics and hypnotics

Beta-blockers: enhanced hypotensive effect when general anaesthetics given with beta-blockers

- Calcium-channel Blockers: enhanced hypotensive effect when general anaesthetics or isoflurane given with calcium-channel blockers; general anaesthetics enhance hypotensive effect of •verapamil (also AV delay)

Clonidine: enhanced hypotensive effect when general anaesthetics given with clonidine

- Cytotoxics: nitrous oxide increases antifolate effect of •methotrexate—avoid concomitant use

Diazoxide: enhanced hypotensive effect when general anaesthetics given with diazoxide

Diuretics: enhanced hypotensive effect when general anaesthetics given with diuretics

- Dopaminergics: increased risk of arrhythmias when volatile liquid general anaesthetics given with •levodopa

Ergot Alkaloids: halothane reduces effects of ergometrine on the parturient uterus

- Memantine: increased risk of CNS toxicity when ketamine given with •memantine (manufacturer of memantine advises avoid concomitant use)

Methyldopa: enhanced hypotensive effect when general anaesthetics given with methyldopa

Moxonidine: enhanced hypotensive effect when general anaesthetics given with moxonidine

- <u>Muscle Relaxants</u>: increased risk of myocardial depression and bradycardia when propofol given with •suxamethonium; volatile liquid general anaesthetics enhance effects of non-depolarising muscle relaxants and suxamethonium; ketamine enhances effects of atracurium

Nitrates: enhanced hypotensive effect when general anaesthetics given with nitrates

Oxytocin: oxytocic effect possibly reduced, also enhanced hypotensive effect and risk of arrhythmias when volatile liquid general anaesthetics given with oxytocin

Probenecid: effects of thiopental possibly enhanced by probenecid

- Sympathomimetics: increased risk of arrhythmias when volatile liquid general anaesthetics given with •adrenaline (epinephrine); increased risk of hypertension when volatile liquid general anaesthetics given with •methylphenidate

Theophylline: increased risk of convulsions when ketamine given with theophylline; increased risk of arrhythmias when halothane given with theophylline

## Anaesthetics, General *(continued)*

Vasodilator Antihypertensives: enhanced hypotensive effect when general anaesthetics given with hydralazine, minoxidil or sodium nitroprusside

**Anaesthetics, General (intravenous)** *see* Anaesthetics, General

**Anaesthetics, General (volatile liquids)** *see* Anaesthetics, General

**Anaesthetics, Local** *see* Bupivacaine, Levobupivacaine, Lidocaine (lignocaine), Prilocaine, and Ropivacaine

## Anagrelide

- Cilostazol: manufacturer of anagrelide advises avoid concomitant use with •cilostazol

- Phosphodiesterase Inhibitors: manufacturer of anagrelide advises avoid concomitant use with •enoximone and •milrinone

## Anakinra

- Adalimumab: avoid concomitant use of anakinra with •adalimumab

- Etanercept: increased risk of side-effects when anakinra given with •etanercept—avoid concomitant use

- Infliximab: avoid concomitant use of anakinra with •infliximab

- Vaccines: avoid concomitant use of anakinra with live •vaccines (see p. 669)

**Analgesics** *see* Aspirin, Nefopam, NSAIDs, Opioid Analgesics, and Paracetamol

## Angiotensin-II Receptor Antagonists

ACE Inhibitors: increased risk of hyperkalaemia when angiotensin-II receptor antagonists given with ACE inhibitors

Adrenergic Neurone Blockers: enhanced hypotensive effect when angiotensin-II receptor antagonists given with adrenergic neurone blockers

Alcohol: enhanced hypotensive effect when angiotensin-II receptor antagonists given with alcohol

Aldesleukin: enhanced hypotensive effect when angiotensin-II receptor antagonists given with aldesleukin

Aliskiren: irbesartan possibly reduces plasma concentration of aliskiren

Alpha-blockers: enhanced hypotensive effect when angiotensin-II receptor antagonists given with alpha-blockers

Anaesthetics, General: enhanced hypotensive effect when angiotensin-II receptor antagonists given with general anaesthetics

Analgesics: increased risk of renal impairment when angiotensin-II receptor antagonists given with NSAIDs, also hypotensive effect antagonised

Anticoagulants: increased risk of hyperkalaemia when angiotensin-II receptor antagonists given with heparin

Antidepressants: hypotensive effect of angiotensin-II receptor antagonists possibly enhanced by MAOIs

Antipsychotics: enhanced hypotensive effect when angiotensin-II receptor antagonists given with antipsychotics

Anxiolytics and Hypnotics: enhanced hypotensive effect when angiotensin-II receptor antagonists given with anxiolytics and hypnotics

Beta-blockers: enhanced hypotensive effect when angiotensin-II receptor antagonists given with beta-blockers

Calcium-channel Blockers: enhanced hypotensive effect when angiotensin-II receptor antagonists given with calcium-channel blockers

- Ciclosporin: increased risk of hyperkalaemia when angiotensin-II receptor antagonists given with •ciclosporin

Clonidine: enhanced hypotensive effect when angiotensin-II receptor antagonists given with clonidine

Corticosteroids: hypotensive effect of angiotensin-II receptor antagonists antagonised by corticosteroids

Diazoxide: enhanced hypotensive effect when angiotensin-II receptor antagonists given with diazoxide

- Diuretics: enhanced hypotensive effect when angiotensin-II receptor antagonists given with •diuretics; increased risk of hyperkalaemia when angiotensin-II

**Angiotensin-II Receptor Antagonists**

- Diuretics *(continued)*
  receptor antagonists given with •potassium-sparing diuretics and aldosterone antagonists
  Dopaminergics: enhanced hypotensive effect when angiotensin-II receptor antagonists given with levodopa
- Lithium: angiotensin-II receptor antagonists reduce excretion of •lithium (increased plasma concentration)
  Methyldopa: enhanced hypotensive effect when angiotensin-II receptor antagonists given with methyldopa
  Moxisylyte (thymoxamine): enhanced hypotensive effect when angiotensin-II receptor antagonists given with moxisylyte
  Moxonidine: enhanced hypotensive effect when angiotensin-II receptor antagonists given with moxonidine
  Muscle Relaxants: enhanced hypotensive effect when angiotensin-II receptor antagonists given with baclofen or tizanidine
  Nitrates: enhanced hypotensive effect when angiotensin-II receptor antagonists given with nitrates
  Oestrogens: hypotensive effect of angiotensin-II receptor antagonists antagonised by oestrogens
- Potassium Salts: increased risk of hyperkalaemia when angiotensin-II receptor antagonists given with •potassium salts
  Prostaglandins: enhanced hypotensive effect when angiotensin-II receptor antagonists given with alprostadil
  Tacrolimus: increased risk of hyperkalaemia when angiotensin-II receptor antagonists given with tacrolimus
  Vasodilator Antihypertensives: enhanced hypotensive effect when angiotensin-II receptor antagonists given with hydralazine, minoxidil or sodium nitroprusside

**Antacids**

Note Antacids should preferably not be taken at the same time as other drugs since they may impair absorption

ACE Inhibitors: antacids possibly reduce absorption of ACE inhibitors; antacids reduce absorption of captopril, enalapril and fosinopril

Analgesics: alkaline urine due to some antacids increases excretion of aspirin

Antibacterials: antacids reduce absorption of azithromycin, cefaclor, cefpodoxime, ciprofloxacin, isoniazid, levofloxacin, moxifloxacin, norfloxacin, ofloxacin, rifampicin and tetracyclines; oral magnesium salts (as magnesium trisilicate) reduce absorption of nitrofurantoin

Antiepileptics: antacids reduce absorption of gabapentin and phenytoin

Antifungals: antacids reduce absorption of itraconazole and ketoconazole

Antihistamines: antacids reduce absorption of fexofenadine

Antimalarials: antacids reduce absorption of chloroquine and hydroxychloroquine; oral magnesium salts (as magnesium trisilicate) reduce absorption of proguanil

Antipsychotics: antacids reduce absorption of phenothiazines and sulpiride

Antivirals: antacids possibly reduce plasma concentration of atazanavir; antacids possibly reduce absorption of fosamprenavir; antacids reduce absorption of tipranavir

Bile Acids: antacids possibly reduce absorption of bile acids

Bisphosphonates: antacids reduce absorption of bisphosphonates

Cardiac Glycosides: antacids possibly reduce absorption of digoxin

Corticosteroids: antacids reduce absorption of deflazacort

Cytotoxics: avoidance of antacids advised by manufacturer of nilotinib

**Antacids** *(continued)*

Deferasirox: antacids containing aluminium possibly reduce absorption of deferasirox (manufacturer of deferasirox advises avoid concomitant use)

Dipyridamole: antacids possibly reduce absorption of dipyridamole

Iron: oral magnesium salts (as magnesium trisilicate) reduce absorption of *oral* iron

Lipid-regulating Drugs: antacids reduce absorption of rosuvastatin

Lithium: sodium bicarbonate increases excretion of lithium (reduced plasma concentration)

Mycophenolate: antacids reduce absorption of mycophenolate

Penicillamine: antacids reduce absorption of penicillamine

Thyroid Hormones: antacids possibly reduce absorption of levothyroxine (thyroxine)

Ulcer-healing Drugs: antacids possibly reduce absorption of lansoprazole

**Antazoline** *see* Antihistamines

**Anti-arrhythmics** *see* Adenosine, Amiodarone, Disopyramide, Flecainide, Lidocaine (lignocaine), and Propafenone

**Antibacterials** *see* individual drugs

**Antibiotics (cytotoxic)** *see* Bleomycin, Doxorubicin, Epirubicin, Mitomycin

**Anticoagulants** *see* Coumarins, Dabigatran etexilate, Heparins, Phenindione, and Rivaroxaban

**Antidepressants** *see* Agomelatine; Antidepressants, SSRI; Antidepressants, Tricyclic; Antidepressants, Tricyclic (related); MAOIs; Mirtazapine; Moclobemide; Reboxetine; St John's Wort; Tryptophan; Venlafaxine

**Antidepressants, Noradrenaline Re-uptake Inhibitors** *see* Reboxetine

**Antidepressants, SSRI**

Alcohol: sedative effects possibly increased when SSRIs given with alcohol

Anaesthetics, Local: fluvoxamine inhibits metabolism of ropivacaine—avoid prolonged administration of ropivacaine

- Analgesics: increased risk of bleeding when SSRIs given with •NSAIDs or •aspirin; fluoxetine, fluvoxamine, paroxetine and sertraline possibly increase plasma concentration of methadone; increased risk of CNS toxicity when SSRIs given with •tramadol
  Anti-arrhythmics: fluvoxamine increases plasma concentration of flecainide; paroxetine possibly inhibits metabolism of propafenone (increased risk of toxicity)
- Anticoagulants: SSRIs possibly enhance anticoagulant effect of •coumarins
- Antidepressants: avoidance of fluvoxamine advised by manufacturer of •reboxetine; possible increased serotonergic effects when SSRIs given with duloxetine; fluvoxamine inhibits metabolism of •duloxetine—avoid concomitant use; citalopram, escitalopram, fluvoxamine or paroxetine should not be started until 2 weeks after stopping •MAOIs, also MAOIs should not be started until at least 1 week after stopping citalopram, escitalopram, fluvoxamine or paroxetine; fluoxetine should not be started until 2 weeks after stopping •MAOIs, also MAOIs should not be started until at least 5 weeks after stopping fluoxetine; CNS effects of SSRIs increased by •MAOIs (risk of serious toxicity); sertraline should not be started until 2 weeks after stopping •MAOIs, also MAOIs should not be started until at least 2 weeks after stopping sertraline; increased risk of CNS toxicity when escitalopram given with •moclobemide, preferably avoid concomitant use; after stopping citalopram, fluvoxamine or paroxetine do not start •moclobemide for at least 1 week; after stopping fluoxetine do not start •moclobemide for 5 weeks; after stopping sertraline do not start •moclobemide for 2 weeks; increased serotonergic effects when SSRIs given with •St John's wort—avoid concomitant use; fluvoxamine inhibits metabolism of •agomelatine (increased plasma con-

**Antidepressants, SSRI**

- Antidepressants *(continued)*
centration); possible increased serotonergic effects when fluoxetine or fluvoxamine given with mirtazapine; SSRIs increase plasma concentration of some •tricyclics; agitation and nausea may occur when SSRIs given with •tryptophan
- Antiepileptics: SSRIs antagonise anticonvulsant effect of •antiepileptics (convulsive threshold lowered); fluoxetine and fluvoxamine increase plasma concentration of •carbamazepine; plasma concentration of paroxetine reduced by carbamazepine, phenytoin and primidone; fluoxetine and fluvoxamine increase plasma concentration of •phenytoin
Antihistamines: antidepressant effect of SSRIs possibly antagonised by cyproheptadine
- Antimalarials: avoidance of antidepressants advised by manufacturer of •artemether/lumefantrine
Antimuscarinics: paroxetine increases plasma concentration of darifenacin and procyclidine
- Antipsychotics: avoidance of fluoxetine, fluvoxamine or sertraline advised by manufacturer of •droperidol (risk of ventricular arrhythmias); fluoxetine increases plasma concentration of •clozapine, •haloperidol, risperidone, •sertindole and •zotepine; paroxetine inhibits metabolism of perphenazine (reduce dose of perphenazine); fluoxetine and paroxetine possibly inhibit metabolism of •aripiprazole (reduce dose of aripiprazole); fluvoxamine, paroxetine and sertraline increase plasma concentration of •clozapine; citalopram possibly increases plasma concentration of clozapine (increased risk of toxicity); fluvoxamine increases plasma concentration of olanzapine; SSRIs possibly increase plasma concentration of •pimozide (increased risk of ventricular arrhythmias—avoid concomitant use); paroxetine possibly increases plasma concentration of risperidone (increased risk of toxicity); paroxetine increases plasma concentration of •sertindole
- Antivirals: plasma concentration of paroxetine and sertraline possibly reduced by darunavir; plasma concentration of SSRIs possibly increased by •ritonavir; plasma concentration of paroxetine possibly reduced by ritonavir
- Anxiolytics and Hypnotics: fluvoxamine increases plasma concentration of some benzodiazepines; fluvoxamine increases plasma concentration of •melatonin—avoid concomitant use; sedative effects possibly increased when sertraline given with zolpidem
Atomoxetine: possible increased risk of convulsions when antidepressants given with atomoxetine; fluoxetine and paroxetine possibly inhibit metabolism of atomoxetine
Barbiturates: SSRIs antagonise anticonvulsant effect of barbiturates (convulsive threshold lowered); plasma concentration of paroxetine reduced by phenobarbital
Beta-blockers: citalopram and escitalopram increase plasma concentration of metoprolol; paroxetine possibly increases plasma concentration of metoprolol (enhanced effect); fluvoxamine increases plasma concentration of propranolol
Bupropion: plasma concentration of citalopram possibly increased by bupropion
Calcium-channel Blockers: fluoxetine possibly inhibits metabolism of nifedipine (increased plasma concentration)
- Dopaminergics: caution with paroxetine advised by manufacturer of entacapone; increased risk of CNS toxicity when SSRIs given with •rasagiline; fluvoxamine should not be started until 2 weeks after stopping •rasagiline; fluoxetine should not be started until 2 weeks after stopping •rasagiline, also rasagiline should not be started until at least 5 weeks after stopping fluoxetine; theoretical risk of serotonin syndrome if citalopram given with selegiline (espe-

**Antidepressants, SSRI**

- Dopaminergics *(continued)*
cially if dose of selegiline exceeds 10 mg daily); manufacturer of escitalopram advises caution with selegiline; increased risk of hypertension and CNS excitation when paroxetine or sertraline given with •selegiline (selegiline should not be started until 2 weeks after stopping paroxetine or sertraline, avoid paroxetine or sertraline for 2 weeks after stopping selegiline); increased risk of hypertension and CNS excitation when fluvoxamine given with •selegiline (selegiline should not be started until 1 week after stopping fluvoxamine, avoid fluvoxamine for 2 weeks after stopping selegiline); increased risk of hypertension and CNS excitation when fluoxetine given with •selegiline (selegiline should not be started until 5 weeks after stopping fluoxetine, avoid fluoxetine for 2 weeks after stopping selegiline)
- Hormone Antagonists: fluoxetine and paroxetine possibly inhibit metabolism of •tamoxifen to active metabolite (avoid concomitant use)
- $5HT_1$ Agonists: fluvoxamine inhibits the metabolism of frovatriptan; possible increased serotonergic effects when SSRIs given with frovatriptan; increased risk of CNS toxicity when sertraline given with •sumatriptan (manufacturer of sertraline advises avoid concomitant use); increased risk of CNS toxicity when citalopram, escitalopram, fluoxetine, fluvoxamine or paroxetine given with •sumatriptan; fluvoxamine possibly inhibits metabolism of zolmitriptan (reduce dose of zolmitriptan)
- Lithium: Increased risk of CNS effects when SSRIs given with •lithium (lithium toxicity reported)
- Muscle Relaxants: fluvoxamine increases plasma concentration of •tizanidine (increased risk of toxicity)—avoid concomitant use
Parasympathomimetics: paroxetine increases plasma concentration of galantamine
Ranolazine: paroxetine increases plasma concentration of ranolazine
- Sibutramine: increased risk of CNS toxicity when SSRIs given with •sibutramine (manufacturer of sibutramine advises avoid concomitant use)
Sympathomimetics: metabolism of SSRIs possibly inhibited by methylphenidate
- Theophylline: fluvoxamine increases plasma concentration of •theophylline (concomitant use should usually be avoided, but where not possible halve theophylline dose and monitor plasma-theophylline concentration)
Ulcer-healing Drugs: plasma concentration of citalopram, escitalopram and sertraline increased by cimetidine; fluvoxamine possibly increases plasma concentration of lansoprazole; plasma concentration of escitalopram increased by omeprazole

**Antidepressants, SSRI (related)** *see* Duloxetine and Venlafaxine

**Antidepressants, Tricyclic**

Adrenergic Neurone Blockers: tricyclics antagonise hypotensive effect of adrenergic neurone blockers
- Alcohol: increased sedative effect when tricyclics given with •alcohol
Alpha₂-adrenoceptor Stimulants: avoidance of tricyclics advised by manufacturer of apraclonidine and brimonidine
Anaesthetics, General: increased risk of arrhythmias and hypotension when tricyclics given with general anaesthetics
- Analgesics: increased risk of CNS toxicity when tricyclics given with •tramadol; side-effects possibly increased when tricyclics given with nefopam; sedative effects possibly increased when tricyclics given with opioid analgesics
- Anti-arrhythmics: increased risk of ventricular arrhythmias when tricyclics given with •amiodarone—

## Antidepressants, Tricyclic

- Anti-arrhythmics *(continued)*
  avoid concomitant use; increased risk of ventricular arrhythmias when tricyclics given with ●disopyramide or ●flecainide; increased risk of arrhythmias when tricyclics given with ●propafenone
- Antibacterials: increased risk of ventricular arrhythmias when tricyclics given with ●moxifloxacin—avoid concomitant use; plasma concentration of tricyclics possibly reduced by rifampicin
- Anticoagulants: tricyclics may enhance or reduce anticoagulant effect of ●coumarins
- Antidepressants: possible increased serotonergic effects when amitriptyline or clomipramine given with duloxetine; increased risk of hypertension and CNS excitation when tricyclics given with ●MAOIs, tricyclics should not be started until 2 weeks after stopping MAOIs (3 weeks if starting clomipramine or imipramine), also MAOIs should not be started for at least 1–2 weeks after stopping tricyclics (3 weeks in the case of clomipramine or imipramine); after stopping tricyclics do not start ●moclobemide for at least 1 week; plasma concentration of some tricyclics increased by ●SSRIs; plasma concentration of amitriptyline reduced by St John's wort
- Antiepileptics: tricyclics antagonise anticonvulsant effect of ●antiepileptics (convulsive threshold lowered); metabolism of tricyclics accelerated by ●carbamazepine (reduced plasma concentration and reduced effect); plasma concentration of tricyclics possibly reduced by ●phenytoin; tricyclics antagonises anticonvulsant effect of ●primidone (convulsive threshold lowered), also metabolism of tricyclics possibly accelerated (reduced plasma concentration)
  Antifungals: plasma concentration of imipramine and nortriptyline possibly increased by terbinafine
  Antihistamines: increased antimuscarinic and sedative effects when tricyclics given with antihistamines
- Antimalarials: avoidance of antidepressants advised by manufacturer of ●artemether/lumefantrine
  Antimuscarinics: increased risk of antimuscarinic side-effects when tricyclics given with antimuscarinics
- Antipsychotics: plasma concentration of tricyclics increased by ●antipsychotics—possibly increased risk of ventricular arrhythmias; avoidance of tricyclics advised by manufacturer of ●droperidol (risk of ventricular arrhythmias); possibly increased antimuscarinic side-effects when tricyclics given with clozapine; increased risk of antimuscarinic side-effects when tricyclics given with phenothiazines; increased risk of ventricular arrhythmias when tricyclics given with ●pimozide—avoid concomitant use
- Antivirals: side-effects of tricyclics possibly increased by fosamprenavir; plasma concentration of tricyclics possibly increased by ●ritonavir
  Anxiolytics and Hypnotics: increased sedative effect when tricyclics given with anxiolytics and hypnotics
- Atomoxetine: increased risk of ventricular arrhythmias when tricyclics given with ●atomoxetine; possible increased risk of convulsions when antidepressants given with atomoxetine
- Barbiturates: tricyclics antagonises anticonvulsant effect of ●barbiturates (convulsive threshold lowered), also metabolism of tricyclics possibly accelerated (reduced plasma concentration)
- Beta-blockers: plasma concentration of imipramine increased by labetalol and propranolol; increased risk of ventricular arrhythmias when tricyclics given with ●sotalol
  Calcium-channel Blockers: plasma concentration of tricyclics possibly increased by diltiazem and verapamil; plasma concentration of imipramine increased by diltiazem and verapamil
- Clonidine: tricyclics antagonise hypotensive effect of ●clonidine, also increased risk of hypertension on clonidine withdrawal

## Antidepressants, Tricyclic *(continued)*

Disulfiram: metabolism of tricyclics inhibited by disulfiram (increased plasma concentration); concomitant amitriptyline reported to increase disulfiram reaction with alcohol
Diuretics: increased risk of postural hypotension when tricyclics given with diuretics
- Dopaminergics: caution with tricyclics advised by manufacturer of entacapone; increased risk of CNS toxicity when tricyclics given with ●rasagiline; CNS toxicity reported when tricyclics given with ●selegiline
Lithium: risk of toxicity when tricyclics given with lithium
Muscle Relaxants: tricyclics enhance muscle relaxant effect of baclofen
Nicorandil: tricyclics possibly enhance hypotensive effect of nicorandil
Nitrates: tricyclics reduce effects of sublingual tablets of nitrates (failure to dissolve under tongue owing to dry mouth)
Oestrogens: antidepressant effect of tricyclics antagonised by oestrogens (but side-effects of tricyclics possibly increased due to increased plasma concentration)
- Pentamidine Isetionate: increased risk of ventricular arrhythmias when tricyclics given with ●pentamidine isetionate
- Sibutramine: increased risk of CNS toxicity when tricyclics given with ●sibutramine (manufacturer of sibutramine advises avoid concomitant use)
Sodium Oxybate: increased risk of side-effects when tricyclics given with sodium oxybate
- Sympathomimetics: increased risk of hypertension and arrhythmias when tricyclics given with ●adrenaline (epinephrine) (but local anaesthetics with adrenaline appear to be safe); metabolism of tricyclics possibly inhibited by methylphenidate; increased risk of hypertension and arrhythmias when tricyclics given with ●noradrenaline (norepinephrine)
Thyroid Hormones: effects of tricyclics possibly enhanced by thyroid hormones; effects of amitriptyline and imipramine enhanced by thyroid hormones
Ulcer-healing Drugs: plasma concentration of tricyclics possibly increased by cimetidine; metabolism of amitriptyline, doxepin, imipramine and nortriptyline inhibited by cimetidine (increased plasma concentration)

## Antidepressants, Tricyclic *(related)*

- Alcohol: increased sedative effect when tricyclic-related antidepressants given with ●alcohol
  Alpha$_2$-adrenoceptor Stimulants: avoidance of tricyclic-related antidepressants advised by manufacturer of apraclonidine and brimonidine
- Antidepressants: tricyclic-related antidepressants should not be started until 2 weeks after stopping ●MAOIs, also MAOIs should not be started until at least 1–2 weeks after stopping tricyclic-related antidepressants; after stopping tricyclic-related antidepressants do not start ●moclobemide for at least 1 week
- Antiepileptics: tricyclic-related antidepressants possibly antagonise anticonvulsant effect of ●antiepileptics (convulsive threshold lowered); plasma concentration of mianserin reduced by ●carbamazepine and ●phenytoin; metabolism of mianserin accelerated by ●primidone (reduced plasma concentration)
  Antihistamines: possible increased antimuscarinic and sedative effects when tricyclic-related antidepressants given with antihistamines
- Antimalarials: avoidance of antidepressants advised by manufacturer of ●artemether/lumefantrine
  Antimuscarinics: possibly increased antimuscarinic side-effects when tricyclic-related antidepressants given with antimuscarinics
  Antivirals: side-effects possibly increased when trazodone given with ritonavir

**Antidepressants, Tricyclic (related)** *(continued)*

Anxiolytics and Hypnotics: increased sedative effect when tricyclic-related antidepressants given with anxiolytics and hypnotics

Atomoxetine: possible increased risk of convulsions when antidepressants given with atomoxetine

● Barbiturates: tricyclic-related antidepressants possibly antagonise anticonvulsant effect of ●barbiturates (convulsive threshold lowered); metabolism of mianserin accelerated by ●phenobarbital (reduced plasma concentration)

Diazoxide: enhanced hypotensive effect when tricyclic-related antidepressants given with diazoxide

Nitrates: tricyclic-related antidepressants possibly reduce effects of sublingual tablets of nitrates (failure to dissolve under tongue owing to dry mouth)

● Sibutramine: increased risk of CNS toxicity when tricyclic-related antidepressants given with ●sibutramine (manufacturer of sibutramine advises avoid concomitant use)

Vasodilator Antihypertensives: enhanced hypotensive effect when tricyclic-related antidepressants given with hydralazine or sodium nitroprusside

**Antidiabetics**

Note  Other oral drugs may be taken at least 1 hour before or 4 hours after exenatide injection, or taken with a meal when exenatide is not administered, to minimise possible interference with absorption

ACE Inhibitors: hypoglycaemic effect of insulin, metformin and sulphonylureas possibly enhanced by ACE inhibitors

Alcohol: hypoglycaemic effect of antidiabetics enhanced by alcohol; increased risk of lactic acidosis when metformin given with alcohol; flushing, in susceptible subjects, when chlorpropamide given with alcohol

Anabolic Steroids: hypoglycaemic effect of antidiabetics possibly enhanced by anabolic steroids

● Analgesics: effects of sulphonylureas possibly enhanced by ●NSAIDs; effects of tolbutamide enhanced by ●azapropazone (avoid concomitant use)

Anti-arrhythmics: hypoglycaemic effect of gliclazide, insulin and metformin possibly enhanced by disopyramide

● Antibacterials: hypoglycaemic effect of acarbose possibly enhanced by neomycin, also severity of gastro-intestinal effects increased; effects of repaglinide enhanced by clarithromycin; effects of glibenclamide possibly enhanced by ciprofloxacin and norfloxacin; plasma concentration of nateglinide reduced by rifampicin; hypoglycaemic effect of repaglinide possibly antagonised by rifampicin; plasma concentration of rosiglitazone reduced by ●rifampicin—consider increasing dose of rosiglitazone; effects of sulphonylureas enhanced by ●chloramphenicol, metabolism of sulphonylureas possibly accelerated by ●rifamycins (reduced effect); metabolism of chlorpropamide and tolbutamide accelerated by ●rifamycins (reduced effect); effects of sulphonylureas rarely enhanced by sulphonamides and trimethoprim; hypoglycaemic effect of repaglinide possibly enhanced by trimethoprim—manufacturer advises avoid concomitant use

● Anticoagulants: exenatide possibly enhances anticoagulant effect of warfarin; hypoglycaemic effect of sulphonylureas possibly enhanced by ●coumarins, also possibly changes to anticoagulant effect

Antidepressants: hypoglycaemic effect of insulin, metformin and sulphonylureas enhanced by MAOIs; hypoglycaemic effect of antidiabetics possibly enhanced by MAOIs

Antiepileptics: tolbutamide transiently increases plasma concentration of phenytoin (possibility of toxicity); plasma concentration of glibenclamide possibly reduced by topiramate

● Antifungals: plasma concentration of sulphonylureas increased by ●fluconazole and ●miconazole; hypoglycaemic effect of gliclazide and glipizide enhanced by ●miconazole—avoid concomitant use; hypogly-

**Antidiabetics**

● Antifungals *(continued)*

caemic effect of nateglinide possibly enhanced by fluconazole; hypoglycaemic effect of repaglinide possibly enhanced by itraconazole; hypoglycaemic effect of glipizide possibly enhanced by posaconazole; plasma concentration of sulphonylureas possibly increased by voriconazole

Antihistamines: thrombocyte count depressed when metformin given with ketotifen (manufacturer of ketotifen advises avoid concomitant use)

Antipsychotics: hypoglycaemic effect of sulphonylureas possibly antagonised by phenothiazines

Antivirals: plasma concentration of tolbutamide possibly increased by ritonavir

Aprepitant: plasma concentration of tolbutamide reduced by aprepitant

Beta-blockers: warning signs of hypoglycaemia (such as tremor) with antidiabetics may be masked when given with beta-blockers; hypoglycaemic effect of insulin enhanced by beta-blockers

● Bosentan: increased risk of hepatotoxicity when glibenclamide given with ●bosentan—avoid concomitant use

Calcium-channel Blockers: glucose tolerance occasionally impaired when insulin given with nifedipine

Cardiac Glycosides: acarbose possibly reduces plasma concentration of digoxin; sitagliptin increases plasma concentration of digoxin

Ciclosporin: hypoglycaemic effect of repaglinide possibly enhanced by ciclosporin

Corticosteroids: hypoglycaemic effect of antidiabetics antagonised by corticosteroids

● Cytotoxics: avoidance of repaglinide advised by manufacturer of ●lapatinib; metabolism of rosiglitazone possibly inhibited by paclitaxel

Deferasirox: plasma concentration of repaglinide increased by deferasirox

Diazoxide: hypoglycaemic effect of antidiabetics antagonised by diazoxide

Diuretics: hypoglycaemic effect of antidiabetics antagonised by loop diuretics and thiazides and related diuretics; increased risk of hyponatraemia when chlorpropamide given with potassium-sparing diuretics and aldosterone antagonists plus thiazide; increased risk of hyponatraemia when chlorpropamide given with thiazides and related diuretics plus potassium-sparing diuretic

Hormone Antagonists: requirements for insulin, metformin, repaglinide and sulphonylureas possibly reduced by lanreotide; requirements for insulin, metformin, repaglinide and sulphonylureas possibly reduced by octreotide

Leflunomide: hypoglycaemic effect of tolbutamide possibly enhanced by leflunomide

● Lipid-regulating Drugs: hypoglycaemic effect of acarbose possibly enhanced by colestyramine; hypoglycaemic effect of nateglinide possibly enhanced by gemfibrozil; increased risk of severe hypoglycaemia when repaglinide given with ●gemfibrozil—avoid concomitant use; plasma concentration of rosiglitazone increased by ●gemfibrozil (consider reducing dose of rosiglitazone); plasma concentration of glibenclamide possibly increased by fluvastatin; may be improved glucose tolerance and an additive effect when insulin or sulphonylureas given with fibrates

Oestrogens: hypoglycaemic effect of antidiabetics antagonised by oestrogens

Orlistat: avoidance of acarbose advised by manufacturer of orlistat

Pancreatin: hypoglycaemic effect of acarbose antagonised by pancreatin

Probenecid: hypoglycaemic effect of chlorpropamide possibly enhanced by probenecid

Progestogens: hypoglycaemic effect of antidiabetics antagonised by progestogens

● Sulfinpyrazone: effects of sulphonylureas enhanced by ●sulfinpyrazone

**Antidiabetics** *(continued)*

Testosterone: hypoglycaemic effect of antidiabetics possibly enhanced by testosterone

Ulcer-healing Drugs: excretion of metformin reduced by cimetidine (increased plasma concentration); hypoglycaemic effect of sulphonylureas enhanced by cimetidine

**Antiepileptics** *see* Carbamazepine, Ethosuximide, Gabapentin, Lacosamide, Lamotrigine, Levetiracetam, Oxcarbazepine, Phenytoin, Primidone, Rufinamide, Stiripentol, Tiagabine, Topiramate, Valproate, Vigabatrin, and Zonisamide

**Antifungals** *see* Amphotericin; Antifungals, Imidazole; Antifungals, Triazole; Caspofungin; Flucytosine; Griseofulvin; Micafungin; Terbinafine

**Antifungals, Imidazole**

Aliskiren: ketoconazole increases plasma concentration of aliskiren

● Analgesics: ketoconazole inhibits metabolism of ●buprenorphine (reduce dose of buprenorphine)

Antacids: absorption of ketoconazole reduced by antacids

● Anti-arrhythmics: increased risk of ventricular arrhythmias when ketoconazole given with ●disopyramide—avoid concomitant use

● Antibacterials: metabolism of ketoconazole accelerated by ●rifampicin (reduced plasma concentration), also plasma concentration of rifampicin may be reduced by ketoconazole; plasma concentration of ketoconazole possibly reduced by isoniazid; avoidance of concomitant ketoconazole in severe renal and hepatic impairment advised by manufacturer of ●telithromycin

● Anticoagulants: miconazole enhances anticoagulant effect of ●coumarins (miconazole oral gel and possibly vaginal formulations absorbed); ketoconazole enhances anticoagulant effect of ●coumarins; ketoconazole increases plasma concentration of ●rivaroxaban—avoid concomitant use

● Antidepressants: avoidance of imidazoles advised by manufacturer of ●reboxetine; ketoconazole increases plasma concentration of mirtazapine

● Antidiabetics: miconazole enhances hypoglycaemic effect of ●gliclazide and ●glipizide—avoid concomitant use; miconazole increases plasma concentration of ●sulphonylureas

● Antiepileptics: ketoconazole and miconazole possibly increase plasma concentration of carbamazepine; miconazole enhances anticonvulsant effect of ●phenytoin (plasma concentration of phenytoin increased); plasma concentration of ketoconazole reduced by ●phenytoin

Antifungals: imidazoles possibly antagonise effects of amphotericin

● Antihistamines: manufacturer of loratadine advises ketoconazole possibly increases plasma concentration of loratadine; imidazoles possibly inhibit metabolism of ●mizolastine (avoid concomitant use); ketoconazole inhibits metabolism of ●mizolastine—avoid concomitant use

● Antimalarials: avoidance of imidazoles advised by manufacturer of ●artemether/lumefantrine

Antimuscarinics: absorption of ketoconazole reduced by antimuscarinics; ketoconazole increases plasma concentration of darifenacin—avoid concomitant use; manufacturer of fesoterodine advises dose reduction when ketoconazole given with fesoterodine—consult fesoterodine product literature; ketoconazole increases plasma concentration of solifenacin; avoidance of ketoconazole advised by manufacturer of tolterodine

● Antipsychotics: ketoconazole inhibits metabolism of ●aripiprazole (reduce dose of aripiprazole); increased risk of ventricular arrhythmias when imidazoles given with ●pimozide—avoid concomitant use; imidazoles possibly increase plasma concentration of quetiapine (reduce dose of quetiapine); possible increased risk of ventricular arrhythmias when imidazoles given with ●sertindole—avoid concomitant use; increased risk of

**Antifungals, Imidazole**

● Antipsychotics *(continued)*
ventricular arrhythmias when ketoconazole given with ●sertindole—avoid concomitant use

● Antivirals: plasma concentration of both drugs increased when ketoconazole given with darunavir; plasma concentration of ketoconazole increased by fosamprenavir; ketoconazole increases plasma concentration of ●indinavir and ●maraviroc (consider reducing dose of indinavir and maraviroc); plasma concentration of ketoconazole reduced by ●nevirapine—avoid concomitant use; combination of ketoconazole with ●ritonavir may increase plasma concentration of either drug (or both); imidazoles possibly increase plasma concentration of saquinavir; ketoconazole increases plasma concentration of saquinavir

● Anxiolytics and Hypnotics: ketoconazole increases plasma concentration of alprazolam; ketoconazole increases plasma concentration of ●midazolam (risk of prolonged sedation)

Aprepitant: ketoconazole increases plasma concentration of aprepitant

Bosentan: ketoconazole increases plasma concentration of bosentan

● Calcium-channel Blockers: ketoconazole inhibits metabolism of ●felodipine (increased plasma concentration); avoidance of ketoconazole advised by manufacturer of lercanidipine; ketoconazole possibly inhibits metabolism of dihydropyridines (increased plasma concentration)

● Ciclosporin: ketoconazole inhibits metabolism of ●ciclosporin (increased plasma concentration); miconazole possibly inhibits metabolism of ●ciclosporin (increased plasma concentration)

● Cilostazol: ketoconazole possibly increases plasma concentration of ●cilostazol—avoid concomitant use

Cinacalcet: ketoconazole inhibits metabolism of cinacalcet (increased plasma concentration)

Corticosteroids: ketoconazole possibly inhibits metabolism of corticosteroids; ketoconazole increases plasma concentration of inhaled and oral budesonide; ketoconazole increases plasma concentration of active metabolite of ciclesonide; ketoconazole inhibits the metabolism of methylprednisolone; ketoconazole increases plasma concentration of inhaled mometasone

● Cytotoxics: ketoconazole inhibits metabolism of erlotinib and sunitinib (increased plasma concentration); ketoconazole increases plasma concentration of bortezomib and imatinib; ketoconazole increases plasma concentration of ●lapatinib and ●nilotinib—avoid concomitant use; ketoconazole increases plasma concentration of active metabolite of ●temsirolimus—avoid concomitant use; *in vitro* studies suggest a possible interaction between ketoconazole and docetaxel (consult docetaxel product literature); ketoconazole reduces plasma concentration of ●irinotecan (but concentration of active metabolite of irinotecan increased)—avoid concomitant use

● Diuretics: ketoconazole increases plasma concentration of ●eplerenone—avoid concomitant use

● Domperidone: ketoconazole possibly increases risk of arrhythmias with ●domperidone

● Ergot Alkaloids: increased risk of ergotism when imidazoles given with ●ergotamine and methysergide—avoid concomitant use

● 5HT$_1$ Agonists: ketoconazole increases plasma concentration of almotriptan (increased risk of toxicity); ketoconazole increases plasma concentration of ●eletriptan (risk of toxicity)—avoid concomitant use

● Ivabradine: ketoconazole increases plasma concentration of ●ivabradine—avoid concomitant use

Lanthanum: absorption of ketoconazole possibly reduced by lanthanum (give at least 2 hours apart)

● Lipid-regulating Drugs: possible increased risk of myopathy when imidazoles given with atorvastatin or simvastatin; increased risk of myopathy when keto-

Appendix 1: Interactions

## Antifungals, Imidazole

- Lipid-regulating Drugs *(continued)*
  conazole given with •simvastatin (avoid concomitant use); possible increased risk of myopathy when miconazole given with •simvastatin—avoid concomitant use

  Oestrogens: anecdotal reports of contraceptive failure when imidazoles or ketoconazole given with oestrogens

  Parasympathomimetics: ketoconazole increases plasma concentration of galantamine
- Ranolazine: ketoconazole increases plasma concentration of •ranolazine—avoid concomitant use

  Retinoids: ketoconazole increases plasma concentration of alitretinoin

  Rimonabant: ketoconazole increases plasma concentration of rimonabant

  Sildenafil: ketoconazole increases plasma concentration of sildenafil—reduce initial dose of sildenafil
- Sirolimus: ketoconazole increases plasma concentration of •sirolimus—avoid concomitant use; miconazole increases plasma concentration of •sirolimus
- Tacrolimus: imidazoles possibly increase plasma concentration of •tacrolimus; ketoconazole increases plasma concentration of •tacrolimus

  Tadalafil: ketoconazole increases plasma concentration of tadalafil
- Theophylline: ketoconazole possibly increases plasma concentration of •theophylline

  Ulcer-healing Drugs: absorption of ketoconazole reduced by histamine H$_2$-antagonists, proton pump inhibitors and sucralfate
- Vardenafil: ketoconazole increases plasma concentration of •vardenafil—avoid concomitant use

  Vitamins: ketoconazole possibly increases plasma concentration of paricalcitol

## Antifungals, Polyene *see* Amphotericin

## Antifungals, Triazole

Note In general, fluconazole interactions relate to multiple-dose treatment

- Analgesics: fluconazole increases plasma concentration of celecoxib (halve dose of celecoxib); voriconazole increases plasma concentration of diclofenac and ibuprofen; fluconazole increases plasma concentration of parecoxib (reduce dose of parecoxib); voriconazole increases plasma concentration of •alfentanil and •methadone (consider reducing dose of alfentanil and methadone); fluconazole inhibits metabolism of alfentanil (risk of prolonged or delayed respiratory depression); itraconazole possibly inhibits metabolism of alfentanil; fluconazole and itraconazole possibly increase plasma concentration of fentanyl

  Antacids: absorption of itraconazole reduced by antacids
- Anti-arrhythmics: manufacturer of itraconazole advises avoid concomitant use with •disopyramide
- Antibacterials: plasma concentration of itraconazole increased by clarithromycin; triazoles possibly increase plasma concentration of •rifabutin (increased risk of uveitis—reduce rifabutin dose); posaconazole increases plasma concentration of •rifabutin (also plasma concentration of posaconazole reduced); voriconazole increases plasma concentration of •rifabutin, also rifabutin reduces plasma concentration of voriconazole (increase dose of voriconazole and also monitor for rifabutin toxicity); fluconazole increases plasma concentration of •rifabutin (increased risk of uveitis—reduce rifabutin dose); plasma concentration of itraconazole reduced by •rifabutin—avoid concomitant use; plasma concentration of posaconazole reduced by •rifampicin; plasma concentration of voriconazole reduced by •rifampicin—avoid concomitant use; metabolism of fluconazole and itraconazole accelerated by •rifampicin (reduced plasma concentration)
- Anticoagulants: fluconazole, itraconazole and voriconazole enhance anticoagulant effect of •coumarins;

## Antifungals, Triazole

- Anticoagulants *(continued)*
  avoidance of itraconazole, posaconazole and voriconazole advised by manufacturer of rivaroxaban
- Antidepressants: avoidance of triazoles advised by manufacturer of •reboxetine; plasma concentration of voriconazole reduced by •St John's wort—avoid concomitant use
- Antidiabetics: posaconazole possibly enhances hypoglycaemic effect of glipizide; fluconazole possibly enhances hypoglycaemic effect of nateglinide; itraconazole possibly enhances hypoglycaemic effect of repaglinide; fluconazole increases plasma concentration of •sulphonylureas; voriconazole possibly increases plasma concentration of sulphonylureas
- Antiepileptics: plasma concentration of itraconazole and posaconazole possibly reduced by •carbamazepine; fluconazole possibly increases plasma concentration of carbamazepine; plasma concentration of voriconazole possibly reduced by •carbamazepine and •primidone—avoid concomitant use; plasma concentration of itraconazole reduced by •phenytoin—avoid concomitant use; fluconazole increases plasma concentration of •phenytoin (consider reducing dose of phenytoin); voriconazole increases plasma concentration of •phenytoin, also phenytoin reduces plasma concentration of voriconazole (increase dose of voriconazole and also monitor for phenytoin toxicity); plasma concentration of posaconazole reduced by •phenytoin; plasma concentration of posaconazole possibly reduced by •primidone

  Antifungals: triazoles possibly antagonise effects of amphotericin; plasma concentration of itraconazole increased by micafungin (consider reducing dose of itraconazole)
- Antihistamines: itraconazole inhibits metabolism of •mizolastine—avoid concomitant use
- Antimalarials: avoidance of triazoles advised by manufacturer of •artemether/lumefantrine

  Antimuscarinics: avoidance of itraconazole advised by manufacturer of darifenacin and tolterodine; manufacturer of fesoterodine advises dose reduction when itraconazole given with fesoterodine—consult fesoterodine product literature; itraconazole increases plasma concentration of solifenacin
- Antipsychotics: itraconazole possibly inhibits metabolism of •aripiprazole (reduce dose of aripiprazole); increased risk of ventricular arrhythmias when triazoles given with •pimozide—avoid concomitant use; triazoles possibly increase plasma concentration of quetiapine (reduce dose of quetiapine); possible increased risk of ventricular arrhythmias when triazoles given with •sertindole—avoid concomitant use; increased risk of ventricular arrhythmias when itraconazole given with •sertindole—avoid concomitant use
- Antivirals: posaconazole increases plasma concentration of •atazanavir; plasma concentration of itraconazole and posaconazole reduced by •efavirenz; plasma concentration of voriconazole reduced by •efavirenz, also plasma concentration of efavirenz increased (increase voriconazole dose and reduce efavirenz dose); plasma concentration of itraconazole possibly increased by fosamprenavir; itraconazole increases plasma concentration of •indinavir (consider reducing dose of indinavir); fluconazole increases plasma concentration of •nevirapine, ritonavir and tipranavir; plasma concentration of itraconazole possibly reduced by nevirapine—consider increasing dose of itraconazole; plasma concentration of voriconazole reduced by •ritonavir—avoid concomitant use; combination of itraconazole with •ritonavir may increase plasma concentration of either drug (or both); triazoles possibly increase plasma concentration of saquinavir;

## Antifungals, Triazole
- <u>Antivirals</u> *(continued)*
  fluconazole increases plasma concentration of
  ●zidovudine (increased risk of toxicity)
- Anxiolytics and Hypnotics: itraconazole increases
  plasma concentration of alprazolam; posaconazole
  increases plasma concentration of ●midazolam;
  fluconazole and itraconazole increase plasma concentration of ●midazolam (risk of prolonged sedation); itraconazole increases plasma concentration of
  buspirone (reduce dose of buspirone)
- Barbiturates: plasma concentration of voriconazole
  possibly reduced by ●phenobarbital—avoid concomitant use; plasma concentration of itraconazole and
  posaconazole possibly reduced by ●phenobarbital
- Bosentan: fluconazole possibly increases plasma concentration of ●bosentan—avoid concomitant use;
  itraconazole possibly increases plasma concentration
  of bosentan
- Calcium-channel Blockers: negative inotropic effect
  possibly increased when itraconazole given with
  calcium-channel blockers; itraconazole inhibits
  metabolism of ●felodipine (increased plasma concentration); avoidance of itraconazole advised by
  manufacturer of lercanidipine; itraconazole possibly
  inhibits metabolism of dihydropyridines (increased
  plasma concentration)
- Cardiac Glycosides: itraconazole increases plasma
  concentration of ●digoxin
- Ciclosporin: fluconazole, itraconazole,
  posaconazole and voriconazole inhibit metabolism of
  ●ciclosporin (increased plasma concentration)
  Corticosteroids: itraconazole possibly inhibits metabolism of corticosteroids and methylprednisolone;
  itraconazole increases plasma concentration of
  inhaled budesonide
- Cytotoxics: itraconazole inhibits metabolism of busulfan (increased risk of toxicity); itraconazole possibly
  increases side-effects of cyclophosphamide; avoidance of itraconazole, posaconazole and voriconazole
  advised by manufacturer of ●lapatinib; avoidance of
  itraconazole and voriconazole advised by manufacturer of ●nilotinib; posaconazole possibly inhibits
  metabolism of ●vinblastine and ●vincristine
  (increased risk of neurotoxicity); itraconazole possibly inhibits metabolism of ●vincristine (increased risk
  of neurotoxicity)
- Diuretics: fluconazole increases plasma concentration
  of eplerenone (reduce dose of eplerenone); itraconazole increases plasma concentration of
  ●eplerenone—avoid concomitant use; plasma concentration of fluconazole increased by hydrochlorothiazide
- Ergot Alkaloids: increased risk of ergotism when
  triazoles given with ●ergotamine and methysergide—
  avoid concomitant use
- 5HT$_1$ Agonists: itraconazole increases plasma concentration of ●eletriptan (risk of toxicity)—avoid concomitant use
- Ivabradine: fluconazole increases plasma concentration of ivabradine—reduce initial dose of ivabradine;
  itraconazole possibly increases plasma concentration
  of ●ivabradine—avoid concomitant use
- Lipid-regulating Drugs: possible increased risk of
  myopathy when triazoles given with atorvastatin or
  simvastatin; increased risk of myopathy when
  itraconazole or posaconazole given with
  ●atorvastatin (avoid concomitant use); fluconazole
  increases plasma concentration of fluvastatin;
  increased risk of myopathy when itraconazole or
  posaconazole given with ●simvastatin (avoid concomitant use)
  Oestrogens: anecdotal reports of contraceptive failure
  when fluconazole or itraconazole given with oestrogens
- Ranolazine: itraconazole, posaconazole and voriconazole increase plasma concentration of
  ●ranolazine—manufacturer of ranolazine advises
  avoid concomitant use

## Antifungals, Triazole *(continued)*
  Sildenafil: itraconazole increases plasma concentration of sildenafil—reduce initial dose of sildenafil
- Sirolimus: posaconazole possibly increases plasma
  concentration of sirolimus; itraconazole and voriconazole increase plasma concentration of ●sirolimus—
  avoid concomitant use
- Tacrolimus: triazoles possibly increase plasma concentration of ●tacrolimus; posaconazole increases
  plasma concentration of ●tacrolimus (reduce dose of
  tacrolimus); fluconazole, itraconazole and voriconazole increase plasma concentration of ●tacrolimus
  Tadalafil: itraconazole possibly increases plasma concentration of tadalafil
- Theophylline: fluconazole possibly increases plasma
  concentration of ●theophylline
- Ulcer-healing Drugs: plasma concentration of posaconazole reduced by ●cimetidine; voriconazole possibly
  increases plasma concentration of esomeprazole;
  voriconazole increases plasma concentration of
  omeprazole (consider reducing dose of omeprazole);
  absorption of itraconazole reduced by histamine H$_2$-
  antagonists and proton pump inhibitors
- Vardenafil: itraconazole possibly increases plasma
  concentration of ●vardenafil—avoid concomitant use

## Antihistamines
Note Sedative interactions apply to a lesser extent to the
non-sedating antihistamines. Interactions do not generally
apply to antihistamines used for topical action (including
inhalation)
  Alcohol: increased sedative effect when antihistamines
  given with alcohol (possibly less effect with non-
  sedating antihistamines)
- Analgesics: sedative effects possibly increased when
  sedating antihistamines given with ●opioid analgesics
  Antacids: absorption of fexofenadine reduced by
  antacids
- Anti-arrhythmics: increased risk of ventricular arrhythmias when mizolastine given with ●amiodarone,
  ●disopyramide, ●flecainide or ●propafenone—avoid
  concomitant use
- Antibacterials: manufacturer of loratadine advises
  plasma concentration possibly increased by erythromycin; metabolism of mizolastine inhibited by
  ●erythromycin—avoid concomitant use; increased
  risk of ventricular arrhythmias when mizolastine
  given with ●moxifloxacin—avoid concomitant use;
  metabolism of mizolastine possibly inhibited by
  ●macrolides (avoid concomitant use)
  Antidepressants: increased antimuscarinic and sedative effects when antihistamines given with MAOIs or
  tricyclics; cyproheptadine possibly antagonises antidepressant effect of SSRIs; possible increased antimuscarinic and sedative effects when antihistamines
  given with tricyclic-related antidepressants
  Antidiabetics: thrombocyte count depressed when
  ketotifen given with metformin (manufacturer of
  ketotifen advises avoid concomitant use)
- Antifungals: manufacturer of loratadine advises plasma
  concentration possibly increased by ketoconazole;
  metabolism of mizolastine inhibited by
  ●itraconazole or ●ketoconazole—avoid concomitant
  use; metabolism of mizolastine possibly inhibited by
  ●imidazoles (avoid concomitant use)
  Antimuscarinics: increased risk of antimuscarinic side-
  effects when antihistamines given with antimuscarinics
  Antivirals: plasma concentration of loratadine possibly
  increased by fosamprenavir; plasma concentration of
  chlorphenamine (chlorpheniramine) possibly
  increased by lopinavir; plasma concentration of non-
  sedating antihistamines possibly increased by ritonavir
  Anxiolytics and Hypnotics: increased sedative effect
  when antihistamines given with anxiolytics and
  hypnotics
- Beta-blockers: increased risk of ventricular arrhythmias when mizolastine given with ●sotalol—avoid
  concomitant use

**Antihistamines** *(continued)*

Betahistine: antihistamines theoretically antagonise effect of betahistine

Ulcer-healing Drugs: manufacturer of loratadine advises plasma concentration possibly increased by cimetidine

**Antihistamines, Non-sedating** *see* Antihistamines

**Antihistamines, Sedating** *see* Antihistamines

**Antimalarials** *see* Artemether with Lumefantrine, Chloroquine and Hydroxychloroquine, Mefloquine, Primaquine, Proguanil, and Quinine

**Antimetabolites** *see* Cytarabine, Fludarabine, Fluorouracil, Gemcitabine, Mercaptopurine, Methotrexate, and Tioguanine

**Antimuscarinics**

Note Many drugs have antimuscarinic effects; concomitant use of two or more such drugs can increase side-effects such as dry mouth, urine retention, and constipation; concomitant use can also lead to confusion in the elderly. Interactions do not generally apply to antimuscarinics used by inhalation

Alcohol: increased sedative effect when hyoscine given with alcohol

Analgesics: increased risk of antimuscarinic side-effects when antimuscarinics given with nefopam

- Anti-arrhythmics: increased risk of ventricular arrhythmias when tolterodine given with ●amiodarone, ●disopyramide or ●flecainide; increased risk of antimuscarinic side-effects when antimuscarinics given with disopyramide

Antibacterials: manufacturer of fesoterodine advises dose reduction when fesoterodine given with clarithromycin and telithromycin—consult fesoterodine product literature; manufacturer of tolterodine advises avoid concomitant use with clarithromycin and erythromycin; plasma concentration of darifenacin possibly increased by erythromycin; plasma concentration of active metabolite of fesoterodine reduced by rifampicin

Antidepressants: plasma concentration of darifenacin and procyclidine increased by paroxetine; increased risk of antimuscarinic side-effects when antimuscarinics given with MAOIs or tricyclics; possibly increased antimuscarinic side-effects when antimuscarinics given with tricyclic-related antidepressants

Antifungals: antimuscarinics reduce absorption of ketoconazole; manufacturer of fesoterodine advises dose reduction when fesoterodine given with itraconazole and ketoconazole—consult fesoterodine product literature; plasma concentration of darifenacin increased by ketoconazole—avoid concomitant use; plasma concentration of solifenacin increased by itraconazole and ketoconazole; manufacturer of tolterodine advises avoid concomitant use with itraconazole and ketoconazole; manufacturer of darifenacin advises avoid concomitant use with itraconazole

Antihistamines: increased risk of antimuscarinic side-effects when antimuscarinics given with antihistamines

Antipsychotics: antimuscarinics possibly reduce effects of haloperidol; increased risk of antimuscarinic side-effects when antimuscarinics given with clozapine; antimuscarinics reduce plasma concentration of phenothiazines, but risk of antimuscarinic side-effects increased

Antivirals: manufacturer of fesoterodine advises dose reduction when fesoterodine given with atazanavir, indinavir, nelfinavir, ritonavir and saquinavir—consult fesoterodine product literature; manufacturer of darifenacin advises avoid concomitant use with atazanavir, fosamprenavir, indinavir, lopinavir, nelfinavir, ritonavir, saquinavir and tipranavir; manufacturer of tolterodine advises avoid concomitant use with fosamprenavir, indinavir, lopinavir, nelfinavir, ritonavir and saquinavir; plasma concentration of solifenacin increased by nelfinavir and ritonavir

- Beta-blockers: increased risk of ventricular arrhythmias when tolterodine given with ●sotalol

**Antimuscarinics** *(continued)*

Calcium-channel Blockers: manufacturer of darifenacin advises avoid concomitant use with verapamil

Cardiac Glycosides: darifenacin possibly increases plasma concentration of digoxin

Ciclosporin: manufacturer of darifenacin advises avoid concomitant use with ciclosporin

Domperidone: antimuscarinics antagonise effects of domperidone on gastro-intestinal activity

Dopaminergics: antimuscarinics possibly reduce absorption of levodopa

Memantine: effects of antimuscarinics possibly enhanced by memantine

Metoclopramide: antimuscarinics antagonise effects of metoclopramide on gastro-intestinal activity

Nitrates: antimuscarinics possibly reduce effects of sublingual tablets of nitrates (failure to dissolve under tongue owing to dry mouth)

Parasympathomimetics: antimuscarinics antagonise effects of parasympathomimetics

**Antipsychotics**

Note Increased risk of toxicity with myelosuppressive drugs

Note Avoid concomitant use of clozapine with drugs that have a substantial potential for causing agranulocytosis

ACE Inhibitors: enhanced hypotensive effect when antipsychotics given with ACE inhibitors

Adrenergic Neurone Blockers: enhanced hypotensive effect when phenothiazines given with adrenergic neurone blockers; higher doses of chlorpromazine antagonise hypotensive effect of adrenergic neurone blockers; haloperidol antagonises hypotensive effect of adrenergic neurone blockers

Adsorbents: absorption of phenothiazines possibly reduced by kaolin

Alcohol: increased sedative effect when antipsychotics given with alcohol

Alpha-blockers: enhanced hypotensive effect when antipsychotics given with alpha-blockers

- Anaesthetics, General: droperidol enhances effects of thiopental; enhanced hypotensive effect when antipsychotics given with ●general anaesthetics

- Analgesics: avoid concomitant use of clozapine with ●azapropazone (increased risk of agranulocytosis); possible severe drowsiness when haloperidol given with indometacin; increased risk of ventricular arrhythmias when antipsychotics that prolong the QT interval given with ●methadone; increased risk of ventricular arrhythmias when amisulpride given with ●methadone—avoid concomitant use; increased risk of convulsions when antipsychotics given with tramadol; enhanced hypotensive and sedative effects when antipsychotics given with opioid analgesics

Angiotensin-II Receptor Antagonists: enhanced hypotensive effect when antipsychotics given with angiotensin-II receptor antagonists

Antacids: absorption of phenothiazines and sulpiride reduced by antacids

- Anti-arrhythmics: increased risk of ventricular arrhythmias when antipsychotics that prolong the QT interval given with ●anti-arrhythmics that prolong the QT interval; increased risk of ventricular arrhythmias when benperidol given with ●amiodarone—manufacturer of benperidol advises avoid concomitant use; increased risk of ventricular arrhythmias when amisulpride, droperidol, haloperidol, phenothiazines, pimozide, sertindole or zuclopenthixol given with ●amiodarone—avoid concomitant use; increased risk of ventricular arrhythmias when sulpiride given with ●amiodarone or ●disopyramide; increased risk of ventricular arrhythmias when amisulpride, droperidol, pimozide, sertindole or zuclopenthixol given with ●disopyramide—avoid concomitant use; increased risk of ventricular arrhythmias when phenothiazines given with ●disopyramide; increased risk of arrhythmias when clozapine given with ●flecainide

- Antibacterials: increased risk of ventricular arrhythmias when pimozide given with ●clarithromycin, ●moxifloxacin or ●telithromycin—avoid concomitant use; increased risk of ventricular arrhythmias when

**Antipsychotics**

- <u>Antibacterials</u> *(continued)*

  sertindole given with ●erythromycin or ●moxifloxacin—avoid concomitant use; increased risk of ventricular arrhythmias when amisulpride or zuclopenthixol given with parenteral ●erythromycin—avoid concomitant use; plasma concentration of clozapine possibly increased by ●erythromycin (possible increased risk of convulsions); possible increased risk of ventricular arrhythmias when pimozide given with ●erythromycin—avoid concomitant use; increased risk of ventricular arrhythmias when sulpiride given with parenteral ●erythromycin; plasma concentration of clozapine increased by ciprofloxacin; plasma concentration of olanzapine possibly increased by ciprofloxacin; increased risk of ventricular arrhythmias when droperidol, haloperidol, phenothiazines or zuclopenthixol given with ●moxifloxacin—avoid concomitant use; increased risk of ventricular arrhythmias when benperidol given with ●moxifloxacin—manufacturer of benperidol advises avoid concomitant use; plasma concentration of aripiprazole possibly reduced by ●rifabutin and ●rifampicin—increase dose of aripiprazole; plasma concentration of clozapine possibly reduced by rifampicin; metabolism of haloperidol accelerated by ●rifampicin (reduced plasma concentration); avoid concomitant use of clozapine with ●chloramphenicol or ●sulphonamides (increased risk of agranulocytosis); possible increased risk of ventricular arrhythmias when sertindole given with ●macrolides—avoid concomitant use; manufacturer of droperidol advises avoid concomitant use with ●macrolides (risk of ventricular arrhythmias); plasma concentration of quetiapine possibly increased by macrolides (reduce dose of quetiapine)

- <u>Antidepressants</u>: plasma concentration of clozapine possibly increased by citalopram (increased risk of toxicity); metabolism of aripiprazole possibly inhibited by ●fluoxetine and ●paroxetine (reduce dose of aripiprazole); plasma concentration of clozapine, haloperidol, risperidone, sertindole and zotepine increased by ●fluoxetine; manufacturer of droperidol advises avoid concomitant use with ●fluoxetine, ●fluvoxamine, ●sertraline or ●tricyclics (risk of ventricular arrhythmias); plasma concentration of clozapine and olanzapine increased by ●fluvoxamine; plasma concentration of clozapine and sertindole increased by ●paroxetine; plasma concentration of risperidone possibly increased by paroxetine (increased risk of toxicity); metabolism of perphenazine inhibited by paroxetine (reduce dose of perphenazine); plasma concentration of clozapine increased by ●sertraline and ●venlafaxine; plasma concentration of haloperidol increased by venlafaxine; clozapine possibly increases CNS effects of ●MAOIs; plasma concentration of pimozide possibly increased by ●SSRIs (increased risk of ventricular arrhythmias—avoid concomitant use); plasma concentration of aripiprazole possibly reduced by ●St John's wort—increase dose of aripiprazole; possibly increased antimuscarinic side-effects when clozapine given with tricyclics; antipsychotics increase plasma concentration of ●tricyclics—possibly increased risk of ventricular arrhythmias; increased risk of antimuscarinic side-effects when phenothiazines given with tricyclics; increased risk of ventricular arrhythmias when pimozide given with ●tricyclics—avoid concomitant use

  Antidiabetics: phenothiazines possibly antagonise hypoglycaemic effect of sulphonylureas

- Antiepileptics: metabolism of haloperidol, olanzapine, quetiapine, risperidone and sertindole accelerated by

**Antipsychotics**

- Antiepileptics *(continued)*

  carbamazepine (reduced plasma concentration); metabolism of clozapine accelerated by ●carbamazepine (reduced plasma concentration), also avoid concomitant use of drugs with substantial potential for causing agranulocytosis; plasma concentration of aripiprazole reduced by ●carbamazepine—increase dose of aripiprazole; plasma concentration of paliperidone reduced by carbamazepine; antipsychotics antagonise anticonvulsant effect of ●carbamazepine, ●ethosuximide, ●oxcarbazepine, ●phenytoin, ●primidone and ●valproate (convulsive threshold lowered); metabolism of clozapine, quetiapine and sertindole accelerated by phenytoin (reduced plasma concentration); plasma concentration of aripiprazole possibly reduced by ●phenytoin and ●primidone—increase dose of aripiprazole; metabolism of haloperidol accelerated by primidone (reduced plasma concentration); increased risk of neutropenia when olanzapine given with ●valproate

- Antifungals: metabolism of aripiprazole inhibited by ●ketoconazole (reduce dose of aripiprazole); increased risk of ventricular arrhythmias when sertindole given with ●itraconazole or ●ketoconazole—avoid concomitant use; metabolism of aripiprazole possibly inhibited by ●itraconazole (reduce dose of aripiprazole); plasma concentration of quetiapine possibly increased by imidazoles and triazoles (reduce dose of quetiapine); increased risk of ventricular arrhythmias when pimozide given with ●imidazoles or ●triazoles—avoid concomitant use; possible increased risk of ventricular arrhythmias when sertindole given with ●imidazoles or ●triazoles—avoid concomitant use

- <u>Antimalarials</u>: avoidance of antipsychotics advised by manufacturer of ●artemether/lumefantrine; increased risk of ventricular arrhythmias when droperidol given with ●chloroquine and hydroxychloroquine or ●quinine—avoid concomitant use; increased risk of ventricular arrhythmias when pimozide given with ●mefloquine or ●quinine—avoid concomitant use

  Antimuscarinics: increased risk of antimuscarinic side-effects when clozapine given with antimuscarinics; plasma concentration of phenothiazines reduced by antimuscarinics, but risk of antimuscarinic side-effects increased; effects of haloperidol possibly reduced by antimuscarinics

- <u>Antipsychotics</u>: increased risk of ventricular arrhythmias when amisulpride, pimozide, sertindole or sulpiride given with ●droperidol—avoid concomitant use; increased risk of ventricular arrhythmias when phenothiazines that prolong the QT interval given with ●droperidol—avoid concomitant use; avoid concomitant use of clozapine with depot formulation of ●flupentixol, ●fluphenazine, ●haloperidol, ●pipotiazine, ●risperidone or ●zuclopenthixol as cannot be withdrawn quickly if neutropenia occurs; increased risk of ventricular arrhythmias when sulpiride given with ●haloperidol; increased risk of ventricular arrhythmias when droperidol given with ●haloperidol—avoid concomitant use; increased risk of ventricular arrhythmias when sertindole given with ●amisulpride—avoid concomitant use; increased risk of ventricular arrhythmias when pimozide given with ●phenothiazines—avoid concomitant use; increased risk of ventricular arrhythmias when pimozide given with ●sulpiride

- Antivirals: plasma concentration of pimozide possibly increased by ●atazanavir—avoid concomitant use; metabolism of aripiprazole possibly inhibited by ●atazanavir, ●fosamprenavir, ●indinavir, ●lopinavir, ●nelfinavir, ●ritonavir and ●saquinavir (reduce dose of aripiprazole); plasma concentration of aripiprazole possibly reduced by ●efavirenz and ●nevirapine—

**Antipsychotics**

- **Antivirals** *(continued)*
  increase dose of aripiprazole; plasma concentration of pimozide possibly increased by ●efavirenz, ●indinavir, ●nelfinavir and ●saquinavir (increased risk of ventricular arrhythmias—avoid concomitant use); plasma concentration of clozapine possibly increased by fosamprenavir; plasma concentration of pimozide and sertindole increased by ●fosamprenavir (increased risk of ventricular arrhythmias—avoid concomitant use); plasma concentration of sertindole increased by ●indinavir, ●lopinavir, ●nelfinavir, ●ritonavir and ●saquinavir (increased risk of ventricular arrhythmias—avoid concomitant use); plasma concentration of antipsychotics possibly increased by ●ritonavir; plasma concentration of pimozide increased by ●ritonavir (increased risk of ventricular arrhythmias—avoid concomitant use); plasma concentration of olanzapine reduced by ritonavir—consider increasing dose of olanzapine; plasma concentration of clozapine increased by ●ritonavir (increased risk of toxicity)—avoid concomitant use

- **Anxiolytics and Hypnotics:** increased sedative effect when antipsychotics given with anxiolytics and hypnotics; plasma concentration of zotepine increased by diazepam; increased risk of hypotension, bradycardia and respiratory depression when intramuscular olanzapine given with parenteral ●benzodiazepines; plasma concentration of haloperidol increased by buspirone

- **Aprepitant:** avoidance of pimozide advised by manufacturer of ●aprepitant

- **Atomoxetine:** increased risk of ventricular arrhythmias when antipsychotics that prolong the QT interval given with ●atomoxetine

- **Barbiturates:** antipsychotics antagonise anticonvulsant effect of ●barbiturates (convulsive threshold lowered); metabolism of haloperidol accelerated by phenobarbital (reduced plasma concentration); plasma concentration of both drugs reduced when chlorpromazine given with phenobarbital; plasma concentration of aripiprazole possibly reduced by ●phenobarbital—increase dose of aripiprazole

- <u>Beta-blockers:</u> enhanced hypotensive effect when phenothiazines given with beta-blockers; plasma concentration of both drugs may increase when chlorpromazine given with ●propranolol; increased risk of ventricular arrhythmias when amisulpride, phenothiazines, pimozide, sertindole or sulpiride given with ●sotalol; increased risk of ventricular arrhythmias when droperidol or zuclopenthixol given with ●sotalol—avoid concomitant use

  Calcium-channel Blockers: enhanced hypotensive effect when antipsychotics given with calcium-channel blockers

  Clonidine: enhanced hypotensive effect when phenothiazines given with clonidine

- **Cytotoxics:** avoid concomitant use of clozapine with ●cytotoxics (increased risk of agranulocytosis); avoidance of pimozide advised by manufacturer of ●lapatinib

  Desferrioxamine: manufacturer of levomepromazine (methotrimeprazine) advises avoid concomitant use with desferrioxamine; avoidance of prochlorperazine advised by manufacturer of desferrioxamine

  Diazoxide: enhanced hypotensive effect when phenothiazines given with diazoxide

- **Diuretics:** risk of ventricular arrhythmias with amisulpride or sertindole increased by hypokalaemia caused by ●diuretics; risk of ventricular arrhythmias with pimozide increased by hypokalaemia caused by ●diuretics (avoid concomitant use); enhanced hypotensive effect when phenothiazines given with diuretics

**Antipsychotics** *(continued)*

  Dopaminergics: increased risk of extrapyramidal side-effects when antipsychotics given with amantadine; antipsychotics antagonise effects of apomorphine, levodopa and pergolide; antipsychotics antagonise hypoprolactinaemic and antiparkinsonian effects of bromocriptine and cabergoline; manufacturer of amisulpride advises avoid concomitant use of levodopa (antagonism of effect); avoidance of antipsychotics advised by manufacturer of pramipexole, ropinirole and rotigotine (antagonism of effect)

- <u>Hormone Antagonists:</u> manufacturer of droperidol advises avoid concomitant use with ●tamoxifen (risk of ventricular arrhythmias)

- **Ivabradine:** increased risk of ventricular arrhythmias when pimozide or sertindole given with ●ivabradine

- **Lithium:** increased risk of ventricular arrhythmias when sertindole given with ●lithium—avoid concomitant use; increased risk of extrapyramidal side-effects and possibly neurotoxicity when clozapine, flupentixol, haloperidol, phenothiazines or zuclopenthixol given with lithium; increased risk of extrapyramidal side-effects when sulpiride given with lithium

  Memantine: effects of antipsychotics possibly reduced by memantine

  Methyldopa: enhanced hypotensive effect when antipsychotics given with methyldopa (also increased risk of extrapyramidal effects)

  Metoclopramide: increased risk of extrapyramidal side-effects when antipsychotics given with metoclopramide

  Moxonidine: enhanced hypotensive effect when phenothiazines given with moxonidine

  Muscle Relaxants: promazine possibly enhances effects of suxamethonium

  Nitrates: enhanced hypotensive effect when phenothiazines given with nitrates

- **Penicillamine:** avoid concomitant use of clozapine with ●penicillamine (increased risk of agranulocytosis)

- <u>Pentamidine Isetionate:</u> increased risk of ventricular arrhythmias when amisulpride or droperidol given with ●pentamidine isetionate—avoid concomitant use; increased risk of ventricular arrhythmias when phenothiazines given with ●pentamidine isetionate

- **Sibutramine:** increased risk of CNS toxicity when antipsychotics given with ●sibutramine (manufacturer of sibutramine advises avoid concomitant use)

  Sodium Benzoate: haloperidol possibly reduces effects of sodium benzoate

  Sodium Oxybate: antipsychotics possibly enhance effects of sodium oxybate

  Sodium Phenylbutyrate: haloperidol possibly reduces effects of sodium phenylbutyrate

  <u>Sympathomimetics:</u> antipsychotics antagonise hypertensive effect of sympathomimetics; antipsychotic effects of chlorpromazine possibly antagonised by dexamfetamine; side-effects of risperidone possibly increased by methylphenidate

- **Tacrolimus:** manufacturer of droperidol advises avoid concomitant use with ●tacrolimus (risk of ventricular arrhythmias)

  Tetrabenazine: increased risk of extrapyramidal side-effects when antipsychotics given with tetrabenazine

- **Ulcer-healing Drugs:** effects of antipsychotics, chlorpromazine and clozapine possibly enhanced by cimetidine; increased risk of ventricular arrhythmias when sertindole given with ●cimetidine—avoid concomitant use; plasma concentration of clozapine possibly reduced by omeprazole; absorption of sulpiride reduced by sucralfate

  Vasodilator Antihypertensives: enhanced hypotensive effect when phenothiazines given with hydralazine, minoxidil or sodium nitroprusside

**Antivirals** see Abacavir, Aciclovir, Adefovir, Atazanavir, Cidofovir, Darunavir, Didanosine, Efavirenz, Emtricitabine, Etravirine, Famciclovir, Fosamprenavir, Foscarnet, Ganciclovir, Indinavir, Lamivudine, Lopinavir, Maraviroc, Nelfinavir, Nevirapine, Raltegravir, Ribavirin, Ritonavir, Saquinavir, Stavudine, Telbivudine, Tenofovir, Tipranavir, Valaciclovir, and Zidovudine

**Anxiolytics and Hypnotics**

ACE Inhibitors: enhanced hypotensive effect when anxiolytics and hypnotics given with ACE inhibitors

Adrenergic Neurone Blockers: enhanced hypotensive effect when anxiolytics and hypnotics given with adrenergic neurone blockers

Alcohol: increased sedative effect when anxiolytics and hypnotics given with alcohol

Alpha-blockers: enhanced hypotensive and sedative effects when anxiolytics and hypnotics given with alpha-blockers

Anaesthetics, General: increased sedative effect when anxiolytics and hypnotics given with general anaesthetics

Analgesics: increased sedative effect when anxiolytics and hypnotics given with opioid analgesics

Angiotensin-II Receptor Antagonists: enhanced hypotensive effect when anxiolytics and hypnotics given with angiotensin-II receptor antagonists

• Antibacterials: metabolism of midazolam inhibited by •clarithromycin, •erythromycin, •quinupristin/ dalfopristin and •telithromycin (increased plasma concentration with increased sedation); plasma concentration of buspirone increased by erythromycin (reduce dose of buspirone); metabolism of zopiclone inhibited by erythromycin and quinupristin/dalfopristin; metabolism of benzodiazepines possibly accelerated by rifampicin (reduced plasma concentration); metabolism of diazepam accelerated by rifampicin (reduced plasma concentration); metabolism of buspirone and zaleplon possibly accelerated by rifampicin; metabolism of zolpidem accelerated by rifampicin (reduced plasma concentration and reduced effect); plasma concentration of zopiclone significantly reduced by rifampicin; metabolism of diazepam inhibited by isoniazid

Anticoagulants: chloral and triclofos may transiently enhance anticoagulant effect of coumarins

• Antidepressants: plasma concentration of melatonin increased by •fluvoxamine—avoid concomitant use; plasma concentration of some benzodiazepines increased by fluvoxamine; sedative effects possibly increased when zolpidem given with sertraline; manufacturer of buspirone advises avoid concomitant use with MAOIs; plasma concentration of oral midazolam possibly reduced by St John's wort; increased sedative effect when anxiolytics and hypnotics given with mirtazapine, tricyclic-related antidepressants or tricyclics

Antiepileptics: plasma concentration of midazolam reduced by carbamazepine; plasma concentration of clonazepam often reduced by carbamazepine, phenytoin and primidone; benzodiazepines possibly increase or decrease plasma concentration of phenytoin; diazepam increases or decreases plasma concentration of phenytoin; plasma concentration of clobazam increased by stiripentol; plasma concentration of diazepam and lorazepam possibly increased by valproate; increased risk of side-effects when clonazepam given with valproate; clobazam possibly increases plasma concentration of valproate

• Antifungals: plasma concentration of alprazolam increased by itraconazole and ketoconazole; plasma concentration of midazolam increased by •fluconazole, •itraconazole and •ketoconazole (risk of prolonged sedation); plasma concentration of buspirone increased by itraconazole (reduce dose of buspirone); plasma concentration of midazolam increased by •posaconazole

Antihistamines: increased sedative effect when anxiolytics and hypnotics given with antihistamines

• Antipsychotics: increased sedative effect when anxiolytics and hypnotics given with antipsychotics; buspirone increases plasma concentration of haloperidol; increased risk of hypotension, bradycardia and respiratory depression when parenteral benzo-

**Anxiolytics and Hypnotics**

• Antipsychotics *(continued)*
diazepines given with intramuscular •olanzapine; diazepam increases plasma concentration of zotepine

• Antivirals: plasma concentration of midazolam possibly increased by •atazanavir—avoid concomitant use of oral midazolam; increased risk of prolonged sedation when midazolam given with •efavirenz—avoid concomitant use; increased risk of prolonged sedation and respiratory depression when alprazolam, clonazepam, diazepam, flurazepam or midazolam given with •fosamprenavir; plasma concentration of midazolam possibly increased by •indinavir, •nelfinavir and •ritonavir (risk of prolonged sedation—avoid concomitant use of oral midazolam); increased risk of prolonged sedation when alprazolam given with •indinavir—avoid concomitant use; plasma concentration of alprazolam, diazepam, flurazepam and zolpidem possibly increased by •ritonavir (risk of extreme sedation and respiratory depression—avoid concomitant use); plasma concentration of anxiolytics and hypnotics possibly increased by •ritonavir; plasma concentration of buspirone increased by ritonavir (increased risk of toxicity); plasma concentration of midazolam increased by •saquinavir (risk of prolonged sedation—avoid concomitant use of oral midazolam)

Aprepitant: plasma concentration of midazolam increased by aprepitant (risk of prolonged sedation)

Barbiturates: plasma concentration of clonazepam often reduced by phenobarbital

Beta-blockers: enhanced hypotensive effect when anxiolytics and hypnotics given with beta-blockers

Calcium-channel Blockers: enhanced hypotensive effect when anxiolytics and hypnotics given with calcium-channel blockers; midazolam increases absorption of lercanidipine; metabolism of midazolam inhibited by diltiazem and verapamil (increased plasma concentration with increased sedation); plasma concentration of buspirone increased by diltiazem and verapamil (reduce dose of buspirone)

Cardiac Glycosides: alprazolam increases plasma concentration of digoxin (increased risk of toxicity)

Clonidine: enhanced hypotensive effect when anxiolytics and hypnotics given with clonidine

Cytotoxics: plasma concentration of midazolam increased by nilotinib

Deferasirox: plasma concentration of midazolam possibly reduced by deferasirox

Diazoxide: enhanced hypotensive effect when anxiolytics and hypnotics given with diazoxide

Disulfiram: metabolism of benzodiazepines inhibited by disulfiram (increased sedative effects); increased risk of temazepam toxicity when given with disulfiram

Diuretics: enhanced hypotensive effect when anxiolytics and hypnotics given with diuretics; administration of chloral or triclofos with parenteral furosemide (frusemide) may displace thyroid hormone from binding sites

Dopaminergics: benzodiazepines possibly antagonise effects of levodopa

Grapefruit Juice: plasma concentration of buspirone increased by grapefruit juice

Lofexidine: increased sedative effect when anxiolytics and hypnotics given with lofexidine

Methyldopa: enhanced hypotensive effect when anxiolytics and hypnotics given with methyldopa

Moxonidine: enhanced hypotensive effect when anxiolytics and hypnotics given with moxonidine; sedative effects possibly increased when benzodiazepines given with moxonidine

Muscle Relaxants: increased sedative effect when anxiolytics and hypnotics given with baclofen or tizanidine

**Anxiolytics and Hypnotics** *(continued)*

Nabilone: increased sedative effect when anxiolytics and hypnotics given with nabilone

Nitrates: enhanced hypotensive effect when anxiolytics and hypnotics given with nitrates

Oestrogens: plasma concentration of melatonin increased by oestrogens

Probenecid: excretion of lorazepam reduced by probenecid (increased plasma concentration); excretion of nitrazepam possibly reduced by probenecid (increased plasma concentration)

● Sodium Oxybate: benzodiazepines enhance effects of ●sodium oxybate (avoid concomitant use)

Theophylline: effects of benzodiazepines possibly reduced by theophylline

Ulcer-healing Drugs: plasma concentration of melatonin increased by cimetidine; metabolism of benzodiazepines, clomethiazole and zaleplon inhibited by cimetidine (increased plasma concentration); metabolism of diazepam possibly inhibited by esomeprazole and omeprazole (increased plasma concentration)

Vasodilator Antihypertensives: enhanced hypotensive effect when anxiolytics and hypnotics given with hydralazine, minoxidil or sodium nitroprusside

**Apomorphine**

Antipsychotics: effects of apomorphine antagonised by antipsychotics

Dopaminergics: effects of apomorphine possibly enhanced by entacapone

Memantine: effects of dopaminergics possibly enhanced by memantine

Methyldopa: antiparkinsonian effect of dopaminergics antagonised by methyldopa

**Apraclonidine**

Antidepressants: manufacturer of apraclonidine advises avoid concomitant use with MAOIs, tricyclic-related antidepressants and tricyclics

**Aprepitant**

Note  Fosaprepitant is a prodrug of aprepitant

Antibacterials: plasma concentration of aprepitant possibly increased by clarithromycin and telithromycin; plasma concentration of aprepitant reduced by rifampicin

Anticoagulants: aprepitant possibly reduces anticoagulant effect of warfarin

● Antidepressants: manufacturer of aprepitant advises avoid concomitant use with ●St John's wort

Antidiabetics: aprepitant reduces plasma concentration of tolbutamide

Antiepileptics: plasma concentration of aprepitant possibly reduced by carbamazepine and phenytoin

Antifungals: plasma concentration of aprepitant increased by ketoconazole

● Antipsychotics: manufacturer of aprepitant advises avoid concomitant use with ●pimozide

Antivirals: plasma concentration of aprepitant possibly increased by ritonavir

Anxiolytics and Hypnotics: aprepitant increases plasma concentration of midazolam (risk of prolonged sedation)

Barbiturates: plasma concentration of aprepitant possibly reduced by phenobarbital

Corticosteroids: aprepitant inhibits metabolism of dexamethasone and methylprednisolone (reduce dose of dexamethasone and methylprednisolone)

● Oestrogens: aprepitant possibly causes contraceptive failure of hormonal contraceptives containing ●oestrogens (alternative contraception recommended)

● Progestogens: aprepitant possibly causes contraceptive failure of hormonal contraceptives containing ●progestogens (alternative contraception recommended)

**Aripiprazole** *see* Antipsychotics

**Artemether with Lumefantrine**

● Anti-arrhythmics: manufacturer of artemether/lumefantrine advises avoid concomitant use with

**Artemether with Lumefantrine**

● Anti-arrhythmics *(continued)*

●amiodarone, ●disopyramide or ●flecainide (risk of ventricular arrhythmias)

● Antibacterials: manufacturer of artemether/lumefantrine advises avoid concomitant use with ●macrolides and ●quinolones

● Antidepressants: manufacturer of artemether/lumefantrine advises avoid concomitant use with ●antidepressants

● Antifungals: manufacturer of artemether/lumefantrine advises avoid concomitant use with ●imidazoles and ●triazoles

● Antimalarials: manufacturer of artemether/lumefantrine advises avoid concomitant use with ●antimalarials; increased risk of ventricular arrhythmias when artemether/lumefantrine given with ●quinine

● Antipsychotics: manufacturer of artemether/lumefantrine advises avoid concomitant use with ●antipsychotics

Antivirals: manufacturer of artemether/lumefantrine advises caution with atazanavir, darunavir, fosamprenavir, indinavir, lopinavir, nelfinavir, ritonavir, saquinavir and tipranavir

● Beta-blockers: manufacturer of artemether/lumefantrine advises avoid concomitant use with ●metoprolol and ●sotalol

Grapefruit Juice: plasma concentration of artemether/lumefantrine possibly increased by grapefruit juice

● Ulcer-healing Drugs: manufacturer of artemether/lumefantrine advises avoid concomitant use with ●cimetidine

Vaccines: antimalarials inactivate oral typhoid vaccine–see p. 688

**Ascorbic acid** *see* Vitamins

**Aspirin**

Adsorbents: absorption of aspirin possibly reduced by kaolin

● Analgesics: avoid concomitant use of aspirin with ●NSAIDs (increased side-effects); antiplatelet effect of aspirin possibly reduced by ibuprofen

Antacids: excretion of aspirin increased by alkaline urine due to some antacids

● Anticoagulants: increased risk of bleeding when aspirin given with ●coumarins or ●phenindione (due to antiplatelet effect); aspirin enhances anticoagulant effect of ●heparins

● Antidepressants: increased risk of bleeding when aspirin given with ●SSRIs or ●venlafaxine

Antiepileptics: aspirin enhances effects of phenytoin and valproate

Cilostazol: manufacturer of cilostazol recommends dose of aspirin should not exceed 80 mg daily when given with cilostazol

Clopidogrel: increased risk of bleeding when aspirin given with clopidogrel

Corticosteroids: increased risk of gastro-intestinal bleeding and ulceration when aspirin given with corticosteroids, also corticosteroids reduce plasma concentration of salicylate

● Cytotoxics: aspirin reduces excretion of ●methotrexate (increased risk of toxicity)—but for concomitant use in rheumatic disease see p. 575

Diuretics: aspirin antagonises diuretic effect of spironolactone; increased risk of toxicity when high-dose aspirin given with carbonic anhydrase inhibitors

Iloprost: increased risk of bleeding when aspirin given with iloprost

Leukotriene Receptor Antagonists: aspirin increases plasma concentration of zafirlukast

Metoclopramide: rate of absorption of aspirin increased by metoclopramide (enhanced effect)

Probenecid: aspirin antagonises effects of probenecid

Sibutramine: increased risk of bleeding when aspirin given with sibutramine

Sulfinpyrazone: aspirin antagonises effects of sulfinpyrazone

**Atazanavir**

Antacids: plasma concentration of atazanavir possibly reduced by antacids

- Anti-arrhythmics: atazanavir possibly increases plasma concentration of ●amiodarone and ●lidocaine (lignocaine)
- Antibacterials: plasma concentration of both drugs increased when atazanavir given with clarithromycin; atazanavir increases plasma concentration of ●rifabutin (reduce dose of rifabutin); plasma concentration of atazanavir reduced by ●rifampicin—avoid concomitant use; avoidance of concomitant atazanavir in severe renal and hepatic impairment advised by manufacturer of ●telithromycin

Anticoagulants: atazanavir may enhance or reduce anticoagulant effect of warfarin; avoidance of atazanavir advised by manufacturer of rivaroxaban

- Antidepressants: plasma concentration of atazanavir reduced by ●St John's wort—avoid concomitant use
- Antifungals: plasma concentration of atazanavir increased by ●posaconazole

Antimalarials: caution with atazanavir advised by manufacturer of artemether/lumefantrine

Antimuscarinics: avoidance of atazanavir advised by manufacturer of darifenacin; manufacturer of fesoterodine advises dose reduction when atazanavir given with fesoterodine—consult fesoterodine product literature

- Antipsychotics: atazanavir possibly inhibits metabolism of ●aripiprazole (reduce dose of aripiprazole); atazanavir possibly increases plasma concentration of ●pimozide—avoid concomitant use
- Antivirals: manufacturer of atazanavir advises avoid concomitant use with ●efavirenz (plasma concentration of atazanavir reduced); avoid concomitant use of atazanavir with ●indinavir; atazanavir increases plasma concentration of ●maraviroc (consider reducing dose of maraviroc); plasma concentration of atazanavir possibly reduced by ●nevirapine—avoid concomitant use; atazanavir increases plasma concentration of ●saquinavir; plasma concentration of atazanavir reduced by tenofovir, also plasma concentration of tenofovir possibly increased; atazanavir increases plasma concentration of ●tipranavir (also plasma concentration of atazanavir reduced)
- Anxiolytics and Hypnotics: atazanavir possibly increases plasma concentration of ●midazolam—avoid concomitant use of oral midazolam
- Calcium-channel Blockers: atazanavir increases plasma concentration of ●diltiazem (reduce dose of diltiazem); atazanavir possibly increases plasma concentration of verapamil
- Ciclosporin: atazanavir possibly increases plasma concentration of ●ciclosporin
- Cytotoxics: atazanavir possibly inhibits metabolism of ●irinotecan (increased risk of toxicity)
- Ergot Alkaloids: atazanavir possibly increases plasma concentration of ●ergot alkaloids—avoid concomitant use
- Lipid-regulating Drugs: possible increased risk of myopathy when atazanavir given with atorvastatin; possible increased risk of myopathy when atazanavir given with ●rosuvastatin—avoid concomitant use; increased risk of myopathy when atazanavir given with ●simvastatin (avoid concomitant use)
- Oestrogens: atazanavir increases plasma concentration of ●ethinylestradiol—avoid concomitant use
- Ranolazine: atazanavir possibly increases plasma concentration of ●ranolazine—manufacturer of ranolazine advises avoid concomitant use
- Sildenafil: atazanavir possibly increases side-effects of ●sildenafil
- Sirolimus: atazanavir possibly increases plasma concentration of ●sirolimus
- Tacrolimus: atazanavir possibly increases plasma concentration of ●tacrolimus
- Ulcer-healing Drugs: plasma concentration of atazanavir possibly reduced by histamine H$_2$-antagonists;

**Atazanavir**

- Ulcer-healing Drugs *(continued)*
  plasma concentration of atazanavir reduced by ●proton pump inhibitors

**Atenolol** *see* Beta-blockers

**Atomoxetine**

- Analgesics: increased risk of ventricular arrhythmias when atomoxetine given with ●methadone; possible increased risk of convulsions when atomoxetine given with tramadol
- Anti-arrhythmics: increased risk of ventricular arrhythmias when atomoxetine given with ●amiodarone or ●disopyramide
- Antibacterials: increased risk of ventricular arrhythmias when atomoxetine given with parenteral ●erythromycin; increased risk of ventricular arrhythmias when atomoxetine given with ●moxifloxacin
- Antidepressants: metabolism of atomoxetine possibly inhibited by fluoxetine and paroxetine; possible increased risk of convulsions when atomoxetine given with antidepressants; atomoxetine should not be started until 2 weeks after stopping ●MAOIs, also MAOIs should not be started until at least 2 weeks after stopping atomoxetine; increased risk of ventricular arrhythmias when atomoxetine given with ●tricyclics
- Antimalarials: increased risk of ventricular arrhythmias when atomoxetine given with ●mefloquine
- Antipsychotics: increased risk of ventricular arrhythmias when atomoxetine given with ●antipsychotics that prolong the QT interval
- Beta-blockers: increased risk of ventricular arrhythmias when atomoxetine given with ●sotalol

Bupropion: possible increased risk of convulsions when atomoxetine given with bupropion

- Diuretics: risk of ventricular arrhythmias with atomoxetine increased by hypokalaemia caused by ●diuretics

Sympathomimetics, Beta$_2$: Increased risk of cardiovascular side-effects when atomoxetine given with parenteral salbutamol

**Atorvastatin** *see* Statins

**Atovaquone**

- Antibacterials: plasma concentration of atovaquone reduced by ●rifabutin and ●rifampicin (possible therapeutic failure of atovaquone); plasma concentration of atovaquone reduced by tetracycline

Antivirals: atovaquone possibly reduces plasma concentration of indinavir; atovaquone possibly inhibits metabolism of zidovudine (increased plasma concentration)

Metoclopramide: plasma concentration of atovaquone reduced by metoclopramide

**Atracurium** *see* Muscle Relaxants

**Atropine** *see* Antimuscarinics

**Auranofin** *see* Gold

**Azapropazone** *see* NSAIDs

**Azathioprine**

ACE Inhibitors: increased risk of anaemia or leucopenia when azathioprine given with captopril especially in renal impairment; increased risk of anaemia when azathioprine given with enalapril especially in renal impairment

- Allopurinol: enhanced effects and increased toxicity of azathioprine when azathioprine given with ●allopurinol (reduce dose of azathioprine to one quarter of usual dose)

Aminosalicylates: possible increased risk of leucopenia when azathioprine given with aminosalicylates

- Antibacterials: increased risk of haematological toxicity when azathioprine given with ●sulfamethoxazole (as co-trimoxazole); increased risk of haematological toxicity when azathioprine given with ●trimethoprim (also with co-trimoxazole)
- Anticoagulants: azathioprine possibly reduces anticoagulant effect of ●coumarins

**Azithromycin** *see* Macrolides

**Aztreonam**

- Anticoagulants: aztreonam possibly enhances anticoagulant effect of ●coumarins

*Appendix 1: Interactions*

**Aztreonam** *(continued)*

Oestrogens: antibacterials that do not induce liver enzymes possibly reduce contraceptive effect of oestrogens (risk probably small, see p. 445)

Vaccines: antibacterials inactivate oral typhoid vaccine–see p. 688

**Baclofen** *see* Muscle Relaxants

**Balsalazide** *see* Aminosalicylates

**Bambuterol** *see* Sympathomimetics, Beta$_2$

**Barbiturates**

Alcohol: increased sedative effect when barbiturates given with alcohol

Analgesics: phenobarbital reduces plasma concentration of methadone; barbiturates possibly increase CNS effects of opioid analgesics

Anti-arrhythmics: barbiturates accelerate metabolism of disopyramide (reduced plasma concentration)

• Antibacterials: barbiturates accelerate metabolism of •chloramphenicol, doxycycline and metronidazole (reduced plasma concentration); phenobarbital possibly reduces plasma concentration of rifampicin; phenobarbital reduces plasma concentration of •telithromycin (avoid during and for 2 weeks after phenobarbital)

• Anticoagulants: barbiturates accelerate metabolism of •coumarins (reduced anticoagulant effect)

• Antidepressants: phenobarbital reduces plasma concentration of paroxetine; phenobarbital accelerates metabolism of •mianserin (reduced plasma concentration); anticonvulsant effect of barbiturates possibly antagonised by MAOIs and •tricyclic-related antidepressants (convulsive threshold lowered); anticonvulsant effect of barbiturates antagonised by SSRIs (convulsive threshold lowered); avoid concomitant use of phenobarbital with •St John's wort; anticonvulsant effect of barbiturates antagonised by •tricyclics (convulsive threshold lowered), also metabolism of tricyclics possibly accelerated (reduced plasma concentration)

• Antiepileptics: phenobarbital reduces plasma concentration of carbamazepine, lamotrigine, tiagabine and zonisamide; phenobarbital possibly reduces plasma concentration of ethosuximide; plasma concentration of phenobarbital increased by oxcarbazepine, also plasma concentration of an active metabolite of oxcarbazepine reduced; plasma concentration of phenobarbital often increased by phenytoin, plasma concentration of phenytoin often reduced but may be increased; increased sedative effect when barbiturates given with primidone; plasma concentration of phenobarbital increased by •stiripentol; plasma concentration of phenobarbital increased by valproate (also plasma concentration of valproate reduced); plasma concentration of phenobarbital possibly reduced by vigabatrin

• Antifungals: phenobarbital possibly reduces plasma concentration of itraconazole and •posaconazole; phenobarbital possibly reduces plasma concentration of •voriconazole—avoid concomitant use; phenobarbital reduces absorption of griseofulvin (reduced effect)

• Antipsychotics: anticonvulsant effect of barbiturates antagonised by •antipsychotics (convulsive threshold lowered); phenobarbital accelerates metabolism of haloperidol (reduced plasma concentration); plasma concentration of both drugs reduced when phenobarbital given with chlorpromazine; phenobarbital possibly reduces plasma concentration of •aripiprazole—increase dose of aripiprazole

• Antivirals: phenobarbital possibly reduces plasma concentration of abacavir, darunavir, fosamprenavir and •lopinavir; avoidance of phenobarbital advised by manufacturer of etravirine; phenobarbital possibly reduces plasma concentration of •indinavir, also plasma concentration of phenobarbital possibly increased; barbiturates possibly reduce plasma concentration of •indinavir, •nelfinavir and •saquinavir

**Barbiturates** *(continued)*

Anxiolytics and Hypnotics: phenobarbital often reduces plasma concentration of clonazepam

Aprepitant: phenobarbital possibly reduces plasma concentration of aprepitant

Beta-blockers: barbiturates reduce plasma concentration of metoprolol and timolol; barbiturates possibly reduce plasma concentration of propranolol

• Calcium-channel Blockers: barbiturates reduce effects of •felodipine and •isradipine; barbiturates probably reduce effects of •dihydropyridines, •diltiazem and •verapamil

Cardiac Glycosides: barbiturates accelerate metabolism of digitoxin (reduced effect)

• Ciclosporin: barbiturates accelerate metabolism of •ciclosporin (reduced effect)

• Corticosteroids: barbiturates accelerate metabolism of •corticosteroids (reduced effect)

Cytotoxics: phenobarbital possibly reduces plasma concentration of etoposide; phenobarbital reduces plasma concentration of irinotecan and its active metabolite

• Diuretics: phenobarbital reduces plasma concentration of •eplerenone—avoid concomitant use; increased risk of osteomalacia when phenobarbital given with carbonic anhydrase inhibitors

Folates: plasma concentration of phenobarbital possibly reduced by folates

Hormone Antagonists: barbiturates accelerate metabolism of gestrinone (reduced plasma concentration); barbiturates possibly accelerate metabolism of toremifene (reduced plasma concentration)

Leukotriene Receptor Antagonists: phenobarbital reduces plasma concentration of montelukast

Lofexidine: increased sedative effect when barbiturates given with lofexidine

Memantine: effects of barbiturates possibly reduced by memantine

• Oestrogens: barbiturates accelerate metabolism of •oestrogens (reduced contraceptive effect—see p. 445)

• Progestogens: barbiturates accelerate metabolism of •progestogens (reduced contraceptive effect—see p. 445)

• Sodium Oxybate: barbiturates enhance effects of •sodium oxybate (avoid concomitant use)

Sympathomimetics: plasma concentration of phenobarbital possibly increased by methylphenidate

• Tacrolimus: phenobarbital reduces plasma concentration of •tacrolimus

Theophylline: barbiturates accelerate metabolism of theophylline (reduced effect)

Thyroid Hormones: barbiturates accelerate metabolism of thyroid hormones (may increase requirements for thyroid hormones in hypothyroidism)

Tibolone: barbiturates accelerate metabolism of tibolone (reduced plasma concentration)

Vitamins: barbiturates possibly increase requirements for vitamin D

**Beclometasone** *see* Corticosteroids

**Bemiparin** *see* Heparins

**Bendroflumethiazide (bendrofluazide)** *see* Diuretics

**Benperidol** *see* Antipsychotics

**Benzodiazepines** *see* Anxiolytics and Hypnotics

**Benzthiazide** *see* Diuretics

**Benzylpenicillin** *see* Penicillins

**Beta-blockers**

Note Since systemic absorption may follow topical application of beta-blockers to the eye the possibility of interactions, in particular, with drugs such as verapamil should be borne in mind

ACE Inhibitors: enhanced hypotensive effect when beta-blockers given with ACE inhibitors

Adrenergic Neurone Blockers: enhanced hypotensive effect when beta-blockers given with adrenergic neurone blockers

Alcohol: enhanced hypotensive effect when beta-blockers given with alcohol

*Appendix 1: Interactions*

## Beta-blockers *(continued)*

Aldesleukin: enhanced hypotensive effect when beta-blockers given with aldesleukin

- Alpha-blockers: enhanced hypotensive effect when beta-blockers given with ●alpha-blockers, also increased risk of first-dose hypotension with post-synaptic alpha-blockers such as prazosin

Anaesthetics, General: enhanced hypotensive effect when beta-blockers given with general anaesthetics

- Anaesthetics, Local: propranolol increases risk of ●bupivacaine toxicity

Analgesics: hypotensive effect of beta-blockers antagonised by NSAIDs; plasma concentration of esmolol possibly increased by morphine

Angiotensin-II Receptor Antagonists: enhanced hypotensive effect when beta-blockers given with angiotensin-II receptor antagonists

- Anti-arrhythmics: increased myocardial depression when beta-blockers given with ●anti-arrhythmics; increased risk of ventricular arrhythmias when sotalol given with ●amiodarone or ●disopyramide—avoid concomitant use; increased risk of bradycardia, AV block and myocardial depression when beta-blockers given with ●amiodarone; increased risk of myocardial depression and bradycardia when beta-blockers given with ●flecainide; propranolol increases risk of ●lidocaine (lignocaine) toxicity; plasma concentration of metoprolol and propranolol increased by propafenone

- Antibacterials: increased risk of ventricular arrhythmias when sotalol given with ●moxifloxacin—avoid concomitant use; metabolism of bisoprolol and propranolol accelerated by rifampicin (plasma concentration significantly reduced); plasma concentration of carvedilol, celiprolol and metoprolol reduced by rifampicin

- Antidepressants: plasma concentration of metoprolol increased by citalopram and escitalopram; plasma concentration of propranolol increased by fluvoxamine; plasma concentration of metoprolol possibly increased by paroxetine (enhanced effect); labetalol and propranolol increase plasma concentration of imipramine; enhanced hypotensive effect when beta-blockers given with MAOIs; increased risk of ventricular arrhythmias when sotalol given with ●tricyclics

Antidiabetics: beta-blockers may mask warning signs of hypoglycaemia (such as tremor) with antidiabetics; beta-blockers enhance hypoglycaemic effect of insulin

- Antihistamines: increased risk of ventricular arrhythmias when sotalol given with ●mizolastine—avoid concomitant use

- Antimalarials: avoidance of metoprolol and sotalol advised by manufacturer of ●artemether/lumefantrine; increased risk of bradycardia when beta-blockers given with mefloquine

- Antimuscarinics: increased risk of ventricular arrhythmias when sotalol given with ●tolterodine

- Antipsychotics: increased risk of ventricular arrhythmias when sotalol given with ●droperidol or ●zuclopenthixol—avoid concomitant use; plasma concentration of both drugs may increase when propranolol given with ●chlorpromazine; increased risk of ventricular arrhythmias when sotalol given with ●amisulpride, ●phenothiazines, ●pimozide, ●sertindole or ●sulpiride; enhanced hypotensive effect when beta-blockers given with phenothiazines

- Antivirals: avoidance of metoprolol for heart failure advised by manufacturer of ●tipranavir

Anxiolytics and Hypnotics: enhanced hypotensive effect when beta-blockers given with anxiolytics and hypnotics

- Atomoxetine: increased risk of ventricular arrhythmias when sotalol given with ●atomoxetine

Barbiturates: plasma concentration of metoprolol and timolol reduced by barbiturates; plasma concentration of propranolol possibly reduced by barbiturates

## Beta-blockers *(continued)*

- Calcium-channel Blockers: enhanced hypotensive effect when beta-blockers given with calcium-channel blockers; possible severe hypotension and heart failure when beta-blockers given with ●nifedipine; increased risk of AV block and bradycardia when beta-blockers given with ●diltiazem; asystole, severe hypotension and heart failure when beta-blockers given with ●verapamil (see p. 119)

Cardiac Glycosides: increased risk of AV block and bradycardia when beta-blockers given with cardiac glycosides

- Ciclosporin: carvedilol increases plasma concentration of ●ciclosporin

- Clonidine: increased risk of withdrawal hypertension when beta-blockers given with ●clonidine (withdraw beta-blockers several days before slowly withdrawing clonidine)

Corticosteroids: hypotensive effect of beta-blockers antagonised by corticosteroids

Diazoxide: enhanced hypotensive effect when beta-blockers given with diazoxide

- Diuretics: enhanced hypotensive effect when beta-blockers given with diuretics; risk of ventricular arrhythmias with sotalol increased by hypokalaemia caused by ●loop diuretics or ●thiazides and related diuretics

Dopaminergics: enhanced hypotensive effect when beta-blockers given with levodopa

Ergot Alkaloids: increased peripheral vasoconstriction when beta-blockers given with ergotamine and methysergide

5HT₁ Agonists: propranolol increases plasma concentration of rizatriptan (manufacturer of rizatriptan advises halve dose and avoid within 2 hours of propranolol)

- 5HT₃ Antagonists: increased risk of ventricular arrhythmias when sotalol given with ●dolasetron—avoid concomitant use

- Ivabradine: increased risk of ventricular arrhythmias when sotalol given with ●ivabradine

Methyldopa: enhanced hypotensive effect when beta-blockers given with methyldopa

- Moxisylyte (thymoxamine): possible severe postural hypotension when beta-blockers given with ●moxisylyte

Moxonidine: enhanced hypotensive effect when beta-blockers given with moxonidine

Muscle Relaxants: propranolol enhances effects of muscle relaxants; enhanced hypotensive effect when beta-blockers given with baclofen; possible enhanced hypotensive effect and bradycardia when beta-blockers given with tizanidine

Nitrates: enhanced hypotensive effect when beta-blockers given with nitrates

Oestrogens: hypotensive effect of beta-blockers antagonised by oestrogens

Parasympathomimetics: propranolol antagonises effects of neostigmine and pyridostigmine; increased risk of arrhythmias when beta-blockers given with pilocarpine

Prostaglandins: enhanced hypotensive effect when beta-blockers given with alprostadil

- Ranolazine: avoidance of sotalol advised by manufacturer of ●ranolazine

- Sympathomimetics: increased risk of severe hypertension and bradycardia when non-cardioselective beta-blockers given with ●adrenaline (epinephrine), also reponse to adrenaline (epinephrine) may be reduced; increased risk of severe hypertension and bradycardia when non-cardioselective beta-blockers given with ●dobutamine; possible increased risk of severe hypertension and bradycardia when non-cardioselective beta-blockers given with ●noradrenaline (norepinephrine)

Thyroid Hormones: metabolism of propranolol accelerated by levothyroxine (thyroxine)

**Beta-blockers** (continued)

Ulcer-healing Drugs: plasma concentration of labetalol, metoprolol and propranolol increased by cimetidine

Vasodilator Antihypertensives: enhanced hypotensive effect when beta-blockers given with hydralazine, minoxidil or sodium nitroprusside

**Betahistine**

Antihistamines: effect of betahistine theoretically antagonised by antihistamines

**Betamethasone** see Corticosteroids

**Betaxolol** see Beta-blockers

**Bethanechol** see Parasympathomimetics

**Bexarotene**

Antiepileptics: cytotoxics possibly reduce absorption of phenytoin

● Antipsychotics: avoid concomitant use of cytotoxics with ●clozapine (increased risk of agranulocytosis)

Cardiac Glycosides: cytotoxics reduce absorption of digoxin tablets

● Lipid-regulating Drugs: plasma concentration of bexarotene increased by ●gemfibrozil—avoid concomitant use

**Bezafibrate** see Fibrates

**Bicalutamide**

Anticoagulants: bicalutamide possibly enhances anticoagulant effect of coumarins

**Biguanides** see Antidiabetics

**Bile Acid Sequestrants** see Colesevelam, Colestipol, and Colestyramine

**Bile Acids** see Ursodeoxycholic Acid

**Bisoprolol** see Beta-blockers

**Bisphosphonates**

Analgesics: bioavailability of tiludronic acid increased by indometacin

Antacids: absorption of bisphosphonates reduced by antacids

Antibacterials: increased risk of hypocalcaemia when bisphosphonates given with aminoglycosides

Calcium Salts: absorption of bisphosphonates reduced by calcium salts

● Cytotoxics: sodium clodronate increases plasma concentration of ●estramustine

Iron: absorption of bisphosphonates reduced by oral iron

**Bleomycin**

Antiepileptics: cytotoxics possibly reduce absorption of phenytoin

● Antipsychotics: avoid concomitant use of cytotoxics with ●clozapine (increased risk of agranulocytosis)

Cardiac Glycosides: cytotoxics reduce absorption of digoxin tablets

● Cytotoxics: increased pulmonary toxicity when bleomycin given with ●cisplatin

**Bortezomib**

Antiepileptics: cytotoxics possibly reduce absorption of phenytoin

Antifungals: plasma concentration of bortezomib increased by ketoconazole

● Antipsychotics: avoid concomitant use of cytotoxics with ●clozapine (increased risk of agranulocytosis)

Cardiac Glycosides: cytotoxics reduce absorption of digoxin tablets

**Bosentan**

● Antibacterials: plasma concentration of bosentan reduced by ●rifampicin—avoid concomitant use

Anticoagulants: manufacturer of bosentan recommends monitoring anticoagulant effect of coumarins

● Antidiabetics: increased risk of hepatotoxicity when bosentan given with ●glibenclamide—avoid concomitant use

● Antifungals: plasma concentration of bosentan increased by ketoconazole; plasma concentration of bosentan possibly increased by ●fluconazole—avoid concomitant use; plasma concentration of bosentan possibly increased by itraconazole

Antivirals: plasma concentration of bosentan possibly increased by ritonavir

**Bosentan** (continued)

● Ciclosporin: plasma concentration of bosentan increased by ●ciclosporin (also plasma concentration of ciclosporin reduced—avoid concomitant use)

Lipid-regulating Drugs: bosentan reduces plasma concentration of simvastatin

● Oestrogens: bosentan possibly causes contraceptive failure of hormonal contraceptives containing ●oestrogens (alternative contraception recommended)

● Progestogens: bosentan possibly causes contraceptive failure of hormonal contraceptives containing ●progestogens (alternative contraception recommended)

Sildenafil: bosentan reduces plasma concentration of sildenafil

**Brimonidine**

Antidepressants: manufacturer of brimonidine advises avoid concomitant use with MAOIs, tricyclic-related antidepressants and tricyclics

**Brinzolamide** see Diuretics

**Bromocriptine**

Alcohol: tolerance of bromocriptine reduced by alcohol

Antibacterials: plasma concentration of bromocriptine increased by erythromycin (increased risk of toxicity); plasma concentration of bromocriptine possibly increased by macrolides (increased risk of toxicity)

Antipsychotics: hypoprolactinaemic and antiparkinsonian effects of bromocriptine antagonised by antipsychotics

Domperidone: hypoprolactinaemic effect of bromocriptine possibly antagonised by domperidone

Hormone Antagonists: plasma concentration of bromocriptine increased by octreotide

Memantine: effects of dopaminergics possibly enhanced by memantine

Methyldopa: antiparkinsonian effect of dopaminergics antagonised by methyldopa

Metoclopramide: hypoprolactinaemic effect of bromocriptine antagonised by metoclopramide

● Sympathomimetics: risk of toxicity when bromocriptine given with ●isometheptene

**Buclizine** see Antihistamines

**Budesonide** see Corticosteroids

**Bumetanide** see Diuretics

**Bupivacaine**

Anti-arrhythmics: increased myocardial depression when bupivacaine given with anti-arrhythmics

● Beta-blockers: increased risk of bupivacaine toxicity when given with ●propranolol

**Buprenorphine** see Opioid Analgesics

**Bupropion**

Note Bupropion should be administered with extreme caution to patients receiving other medication known to lower the seizure threshold—see CSM advice p. 281 and Cautions, Contra-indications and Side-effects of individual drugs

● Antidepressants: bupropion possibly increases plasma concentration of citalopram; manufacturer of bupropion advises avoid for 2 weeks after stopping ●MAOIs; manufacturer of bupropion advises avoid concomitant use with ●moclobemide

Antiepileptics: plasma concentration of bupropion reduced by carbamazepine and phenytoin; metabolism of bupropion inhibited by valproate

● Antivirals: plasma concentration of bupropion increased or decreased by ●ritonavir

Atomoxetine: possible increased risk of convulsions when bupropion given with atomoxetine

Dopaminergics: increased risk of side-effects when bupropion given with amantadine or levodopa

● Hormone Antagonists: bupropion possibly inhibits metabolism of ●tamoxifen to active metabolite (avoid concomitant use)

**Buspirone** see Anxiolytics and Hypnotics

**Busulfan**

Analgesics: metabolism of intravenous busulfan possibly inhibited by paracetamol (manufacturer of intravenous busulfan advises caution within 72 hours of paracetamol)

**Busulfan** *(continued)*

- Antibacterials: plasma concentration of busulfan increased by •metronidazole (increased risk of toxicity)
  Antiepileptics: cytotoxics possibly reduce absorption of phenytoin; plasma concentration of busulfan possibly reduced by phenytoin
  Antifungals: metabolism of busulfan inhibited by itraconazole (increased risk of toxicity)
- Antipsychotics: avoid concomitant use of cytotoxics with •clozapine (increased risk of agranulocytosis)
  Cardiac Glycosides: cytotoxics reduce absorption of digoxin tablets
  Cytotoxics: increased risk of hepatotoxicity when busulfan given with tioguanine

**Butobarbital** *see* Barbiturates

**Butyrophenones** *see* Antipsychotics

**Cabergoline**

Antibacterials: plasma concentration of cabergoline increased by erythromycin (increased risk of toxicity); plasma concentration of cabergoline possibly increased by macrolides (increased risk of toxicity)
Antipsychotics: hypoprolactinaemic and antiparkinsonian effects of cabergoline antagonised by antipsychotics
Domperidone: hypoprolactinaemic effect of cabergoline possibly antagonised by domperidone
Memantine: effects of dopaminergics possibly enhanced by memantine
Methyldopa: antiparkinsonian effect of dopaminergics antagonised by methyldopa
Metoclopramide: hypoprolactinaemic effect of cabergoline antagonised by metoclopramide

**Calcium Salts**

Note *see also* Antacids
Antibacterials: calcium salts reduce absorption of ciprofloxacin and tetracycline
Bisphosphonates: calcium salts reduce absorption of bisphosphonates
Cardiac Glycosides: large intravenous doses of calcium salts can precipitate arrhythmias when given with cardiac glycosides
Corticosteroids: absorption of calcium salts reduced by corticosteroids
Diuretics: increased risk of hypercalcaemia when calcium salts given with thiazides and related diuretics
Fluorides: calcium salts reduce absorption of fluorides
Iron: calcium salts reduce absorption of *oral* iron
Thyroid Hormones: calcium salts reduce absorption of levothyroxine (thyroxine)
Zinc: calcium salts reduce absorption of zinc

**Calcium-channel Blockers**

Note Dihydropyridine calcium-channel blockers include amlodipine, felodipine, isradipine, lacidipine, lercanidipine, nicardipine, nifedipine, and nimodipine
ACE Inhibitors: enhanced hypotensive effect when calcium-channel blockers given with ACE inhibitors
Adrenergic Neurone Blockers: enhanced hypotensive effect when calcium-channel blockers given with adrenergic neurone blockers
Alcohol: enhanced hypotensive effect when calcium-channel blockers given with alcohol; verapamil possibly increases plasma concentration of alcohol
Aldesleukin: enhanced hypotensive effect when calcium-channel blockers given with aldesleukin
Aliskiren: avoidance of verapamil advised by manufacturer of aliskiren
- Alpha-blockers: enhanced hypotensive effect when calcium-channel blockers given with •alpha-blockers, also increased risk of first-dose hypotension with post-synaptic alpha-blockers such as prazosin
- Anaesthetics, General: enhanced hypotensive effect when calcium-channel blockers given with general anaesthetics or isoflurane; hypotensive effect of verapamil enhanced by •general anaesthetics (also AV delay)
  Analgesics: hypotensive effect of calcium-channel blockers antagonised by NSAIDs; diltiazem inhibits

**Calcium-channel Blockers**

Analgesics *(continued)*
metabolism of alfentanil (risk of prolonged or delayed respiratory depression)
Angiotensin-II Receptor Antagonists: enhanced hypotensive effect when calcium-channel blockers given with angiotensin-II receptor antagonists
- Anti-arrhythmics: increased risk of bradycardia, AV block and myocardial depression when diltiazem or verapamil given with •amiodarone; increased risk of myocardial depression and asystole when verapamil given with •disopyramide or •flecainide
- Antibacterials: metabolism of verapamil possibly inhibited by •clarithromycin and •erythromycin (increased risk of toxicity); metabolism of felodipine possibly inhibited by erythromycin (increased plasma concentration); manufacturer of lercanidipine advises avoid concomitant use with erythromycin; metabolism of diltiazem, nifedipine, nimodipine and verapamil accelerated by •rifampicin (plasma concentration significantly reduced); metabolism of isradipine and nicardipine possibly accelerated by •rifampicin (possible significantly reduced plasma concentration); plasma concentration of nifedipine increased by •quinupristin/dalfopristin
  Antidepressants: metabolism of nifedipine possibly inhibited by fluoxetine (increased plasma concentration); diltiazem and verapamil increase plasma concentration of imipramine; enhanced hypotensive effect when calcium-channel blockers given with MAOIs; plasma concentration of amlodipine possibly reduced by St John's wort; diltiazem and verapamil possibly increase plasma concentration of tricyclics
  Antidiabetics: glucose tolerance occasionally impaired when nifedipine given with insulin
- Antiepileptics: effects of felodipine and isradipine reduced by carbamazepine; effects of dihydropyridines, nicardipine and nifedipine probably reduced by carbamazepine; diltiazem and verapamil enhance effects of •carbamazepine; effects of felodipine, isradipine and verapamil reduced by phenytoin; effects of dihydropyridines, nicardipine and nifedipine probably reduced by •phenytoin; diltiazem increases plasma concentration of •phenytoin but also effect of diltiazem reduced; effects of dihydropyridines, diltiazem and verapamil probably reduced by •primidone; effects of felodipine and isradipine reduced by •primidone
- Antifungals: metabolism of dihydropyridines possibly inhibited by itraconazole and ketoconazole (increased plasma concentration); metabolism of felodipine inhibited by •itraconazole and •ketoconazole (increased plasma concentration); manufacturer of lercanidipine advises avoid concomitant use with itraconazole and ketoconazole; negative inotropic effect possibly increased when calcium-channel blockers given with itraconazole; plasma concentration of nifedipine increased by micafungin
  Antimalarials: possible increased risk of bradycardia when calcium-channel blockers given with mefloquine
  Antimuscarinics: avoidance of verapamil advised by manufacturer of darifenacin
  Antipsychotics: enhanced hypotensive effect when calcium-channel blockers given with antipsychotics
- Antivirals: plasma concentration of diltiazem increased by •atazanavir (reduce dose of diltiazem); plasma concentration of verapamil possibly increased by atazanavir; plasma concentration of diltiazem reduced by efavirenz; plasma concentration of calcium-channel blockers possibly increased by •ritonavir; manufacturer of lercanidipine advises avoid concomitant use with ritonavir
  Anxiolytics and Hypnotics: enhanced hypotensive effect when calcium-channel blockers given with anxiolytics and hypnotics; diltiazem and verapamil inhibit metabolism of midazolam (increased plasma concentration with increased sedation); absorption of

## Calcium-channel Blockers

**Anxiolytics and Hypnotics** (continued)
lercanidipine increased by midazolam; diltiazem and verapamil increase plasma concentration of buspirone (reduce dose of buspirone)

- **Barbiturates:** effects of dihydropyridines, diltiazem and verapamil probably reduced by ●barbiturates; effects of felodipine and isradipine reduced by ●barbiturates
- **Beta-blockers:** enhanced hypotensive effect when calcium-channel blockers given with beta-blockers; increased risk of AV block and bradycardia when diltiazem given with ●beta-blockers; asystole, severe hypotension and heart failure when verapamil given with ●beta-blockers (see p. 119); possible severe hypotension and heart failure when nifedipine given with ●beta-blockers

**Calcium-channel Blockers:** plasma concentration of both drugs may increase when diltiazem given with nifedipine

- **Cardiac Glycosides:** verapamil increases plasma concentration of ●digoxin, also increased risk of AV block and bradycardia; diltiazem, lercanidipine and nicardipine increase plasma concentration of ●digoxin; nifedipine possibly increases plasma concentration of ●digoxin
- **Ciclosporin:** diltiazem, nicardipine and verapamil increase plasma concentration of ●ciclosporin; combination of lercanidipine with ●ciclosporin may increase plasma concentration of either drug (or both)—avoid concomitant use; plasma concentration of nifedipine possibly increased by ciclosporin (increased risk of toxicity including gingival hyperplasia)
- **Cilostazol:** diltiazem increases plasma concentration of ●cilostazol—avoid concomitant use

**Clonidine:** enhanced hypotensive effect when calcium-channel blockers given with clonidine

**Corticosteroids:** hypotensive effect of calcium-channel blockers antagonised by corticosteroids

**Cytotoxics:** nifedipine possibly inhibits metabolism of vincristine

**Diazoxide:** enhanced hypotensive effect when calcium-channel blockers given with diazoxide

**Diuretics:** enhanced hypotensive effect when calcium-channel blockers given with diuretics; diltiazem and verapamil increase plasma concentration of eplerenone (reduce dose of eplerenone)

**Dopaminergics:** enhanced hypotensive effect when calcium-channel blockers given with levodopa

**Grapefruit Juice:** plasma concentration of felodipine, isradipine, lacidipine, lercanidipine, nicardipine, nifedipine, nimodipine and verapamil increased by grapefruit juice

**Hormone Antagonists:** diltiazem and verapamil increase plasma concentration of dutasteride

- **Ivabradine:** diltiazem and verapamil increase plasma concentration of ●ivabradine—avoid concomitant use
- **Lipid-regulating Drugs:** diltiazem increases plasma concentration of atorvastatin; possible increased risk of myopathy when diltiazem given with simvastatin; increased risk of myopathy when verapamil given with ●simvastatin

**Lithium:** neurotoxicity may occur when diltiazem or verapamil given with lithium without increased plasma concentration of lithium

- **Magnesium** (parenteral): profound hypotension reported with concomitant use of nifedipine and ●parenteral magnesium in pre-eclampsia

**Methyldopa:** enhanced hypotensive effect when calcium-channel blockers given with methyldopa

**Moxisylyte** (thymoxamine): enhanced hypotensive effect when calcium-channel blockers given with moxisylyte

**Moxonidine:** enhanced hypotensive effect when calcium-channel blockers given with moxonidine

## Calcium-channel Blockers (continued)

**Muscle Relaxants:** verapamil enhances effects of non-depolarising muscle relaxants and suxamethonium; enhanced hypotensive effect when calcium-channel blockers given with baclofen or tizanidine; risk of arrhythmias when diltiazem given with intravenous dantrolene; hypotension, myocardial depression, and hyperkalaemia when verapamil given with intravenous dantrolene; nifedipine enhances effects of non-depolarising muscle relaxants

**Nitrates:** enhanced hypotensive effect when calcium-channel blockers given with nitrates

**Oestrogens:** hypotensive effect of calcium-channel blockers antagonised by oestrogens

**Prostaglandins:** enhanced hypotensive effect when calcium-channel blockers given with alprostadil

**Ranolazine:** diltiazem and verapamil increase plasma concentration of ranolazine (consider reducing dose of ranolazine)

**Sildenafil:** enhanced hypotensive effect when amlodipine given with sildenafil

- **Sirolimus:** diltiazem increases plasma concentration of ●sirolimus; plasma concentration of both drugs increased when verapamil given with ●sirolimus
- **Tacrolimus:** diltiazem and nifedipine increase plasma concentration of ●tacrolimus; felodipine, nicardipine and verapamil possibly increase plasma concentration of tacrolimus
- **Theophylline:** calcium-channel blockers possibly increase plasma concentration of ●theophylline (enhanced effect); diltiazem increases plasma concentration of theophylline; verapamil increases plasma concentration of ●theophylline (enhanced effect)

**Ulcer-healing Drugs:** metabolism of calcium-channel blockers possibly inhibited by cimetidine (increased plasma concentration); plasma concentration of isradipine increased by cimetidine (halve dose of isradipine)

**Vardenafil:** enhanced hypotensive effect when nifedipine given with vardenafil

**Vasodilator Antihypertensives:** enhanced hypotensive effect when calcium-channel blockers given with hydralazine, minoxidil or sodium nitroprusside

**Calcium-channel Blockers (dihydropyridines)** *see* Calcium-channel Blockers

**Candesartan** *see* Angiotensin-II Receptor Antagonists

**Capecitabine** *see* Fluorouracil

## Capreomycin

**Antibacterials:** increased risk of nephrotoxicity when capreomycin given with colistin or polymyxins; increased risk of nephrotoxicity and ototoxicity when capreomycin given with aminoglycosides or vancomycin

**Cytotoxics:** increased risk of nephrotoxicity and ototoxicity when capreomycin given with platinum compounds

**Oestrogens:** antibacterials that do not induce liver enzymes possibly reduce contraceptive effect of oestrogens (risk probably small, see p. 445)

**Vaccines:** antibacterials inactivate oral typhoid vaccine–see p. 688

**Captopril** *see* ACE Inhibitors

## Carbamazepine

**Alcohol:** CNS side-effects of carbamazepine possibly increased by alcohol

- **Analgesics:** effects of carbamazepine enhanced by ●dextropropoxyphene; carbamazepine reduces plasma concentration of methadone; carbamazepine reduces effects of tramadol; carbamazepine possibly accelerates metabolism of paracetamol
- **Antibacterials:** plasma concentration of carbamazepine increased by ●clarithromycin and ●erythromycin; plasma concentration of carbamazepine reduced by ●rifabutin; carbamazepine accelerates metabolism of doxycycline (reduced effect); plasma concentration of carbamazepine increased by ●isoniazid (also possibly increased isoniazid hepatotoxicity); carbamazepine reduces plasma concentra-

Carbamazepine
- Antibacterials *(continued)*
  tion of ●telithromycin (avoid during and for 2 weeks after carbamazepine)
- Anticoagulants: carbamazepine accelerates metabolism of ●coumarins (reduced anticoagulant effect)
- Antidepressants: plasma concentration of carbamazepine increased by ●fluoxetine and ●fluvoxamine; carbamazepine reduces plasma concentration of ●mianserin, mirtazapine and paroxetine; manufacturer of carbamazepine advises avoid for 2 weeks after stopping ●MAOIs, also antagonism of anticonvulsant effect; anticonvulsant effect of antiepileptics possibly antagonised by MAOIs and ●tricyclic-related antidepressants (convulsive threshold lowered); anticonvulsant effect of antiepileptics antagonised by ●SSRIs and ●tricyclics (convulsive threshold lowered); avoid concomitant use of antiepileptics with ●St John's wort; carbamazepine accelerates metabolism of ●tricyclics (reduced plasma concentration and reduced effect)
- Antiepileptics: carbamazepine possibly reduces plasma concentration of ethosuximide; carbamazepine often reduces plasma concentration of lamotrigine, also plasma concentration of an active metabolite of carbamazepine sometimes raised (but evidence is conflicting); plasma concentration of carbamazepine sometimes reduced by oxcarbazepine (but concentration of an active metabolite of carbamazepine may be increased), also plasma concentration of an active metabolite of oxcarbazepine often reduced; plasma concentration of both drugs often reduced when carbamazepine given with phenytoin, also plasma concentration of phenytoin may be increased; plasma concentration of carbamazepine often reduced by primidone, also plasma concentration of primidone sometimes reduced (but concentration of an active metabolite of primidone often increased); plasma concentration of carbamazepine increased by ●stiripentol; carbamazepine reduces plasma concentration of tiagabine and zonisamide; carbamazepine often reduces plasma concentration of topiramate; carbamazepine reduces plasma concentration of valproate, also plasma concentration of active metabolite of carbamazepine increased
- Antifungals: plasma concentration of carbamazepine possibly increased by fluconazole, ketoconazole and miconazole; carbamazepine possibly reduces plasma concentration of itraconazole and ●posaconazole; carbamazepine possibly reduces plasma concentration of ●voriconazole—avoid concomitant use; carbamazepine possibly reduces plasma concentration of caspofungin—consider increasing dose of caspofungin
- Antimalarials: possible increased risk of convulsions when antiepileptics given with chloroquine and hydroxychloroquine; anticonvulsant effect of antiepileptics antagonised by ●mefloquine
- Antipsychotics: anticonvulsant effect of carbamazepine antagonised by ●antipsychotics (convulsive threshold lowered); carbamazepine accelerates metabolism of haloperidol, olanzapine, quetiapine, risperidone and sertindole (reduced plasma concentration); carbamazepine reduces plasma concentration of ●aripiprazole—increase dose of aripiprazole; carbamazepine accelerates metabolism of ●clozapine (reduced plasma concentration), also avoid concomitant use of drugs with substantial potential for causing agranulocytosis; carbamazepine reduces plasma concentration of paliperidone
- Antivirals: carbamazepine possibly reduces plasma concentration of darunavir, fosamprenavir, lopinavir, nelfinavir, saquinavir and tipranavir; plasma concentration of both drugs reduced when carbamazepine given with efavirenz; avoidance of carbamazepine advised by manufacturer of etravirine; carbamazepine possibly reduces plasma concentration of ●indinavir, also plasma concentration of carbamaze-

Carbamazepine
- Antivirals *(continued)*
  pine possibly increased; plasma concentration of carbamazepine possibly increased by ●ritonavir
  Anxiolytics and Hypnotics: carbamazepine often reduces plasma concentration of clonazepam; carbamazepine reduces plasma concentration of midazolam
  Aprepitant: carbamazepine possibly reduces plasma concentration of aprepitant
  Barbiturates: plasma concentration of carbamazepine reduced by phenobarbital
  Bupropion: carbamazepine reduces plasma concentration of bupropion
- Calcium-channel Blockers: carbamazepine reduces effects of felodipine and isradipine; carbamazepine probably reduces effects of dihydropyridines, nicardipine and nifedipine; effects of carbamazepine enhanced by ●diltiazem and ●verapamil
  Cardiac Glycosides: carbamazepine accelerates metabolism of digitoxin (reduced effect)
- Ciclosporin: carbamazepine accelerates metabolism of ●ciclosporin (reduced plasma concentration)
- Corticosteroids: carbamazepine accelerates metabolism of ●corticosteroids (reduced effect)
- Cytotoxics: carbamazepine reduces plasma concentration of ●imatinib and ●lapatinib—avoid concomitant use; carbamazepine reduces plasma concentration of irinotecan and its active metabolite
- Diuretics: increased risk of hyponatraemia when carbamazepine given with diuretics; plasma concentration of carbamazepine increased by ●acetazolamide; carbamazepine reduces plasma concentration of ●eplerenone—avoid concomitant use
- Hormone Antagonists: metabolism of carbamazepine inhibited by ●danazol (increased risk of toxicity); carbamazepine accelerates metabolism of gestrinone (reduced plasma concentration); carbamazepine possibly accelerates metabolism of toremifene (reduced plasma concentration)
  5HT$_3$ Antagonists: carbamazepine accelerates metabolism of ondansetron (reduced effect)
  Lithium: neurotoxicity may occur when carbamazepine given with lithium without increased plasma concentration of lithium
  Muscle Relaxants: carbamazepine antagonises muscle relaxant effect of non-depolarising muscle relaxants (accelerated recovery from neuromuscular blockade)
- Oestrogens: carbamazepine accelerates metabolism of ●oestrogens (reduced contraceptive effect—see p. 445)
- Progestogens: carbamazepine accelerates metabolism of ●progestogens (reduced contraceptive effect—see p. 445)
  Retinoids: plasma concentration of carbamazepine possibly reduced by isotretinoin
  Theophylline: carbamazepine accelerates metabolism of theophylline (reduced effect)
  Thyroid Hormones: carbamazepine accelerates metabolism of thyroid hormones (may increase requirements for thyroid hormones in hypothyroidism)
  Tibolone: carbamazepine accelerates metabolism of tibolone (reduced plasma concentration)
- Ulcer-healing Drugs: metabolism of carbamazepine inhibited by ●cimetidine (increased plasma concentration)
  Vitamins: carbamazepine possibly increases requirements for vitamin D
Carbapenems *see* Doripenem, Ertapenem, Imipenem with Cilastatin, and Meropenem
**Carbonic Anhydrase Inhibitors** *see* Diuretics
Carboplatin *see* Platinum Compounds
Carboprost *see* Prostaglandins
**Cardiac Glycosides**
  ACE Inhibitors: plasma concentration of digoxin possibly increased by captopril

**Appendix 1: Interactions**

**Cardiac Glycosides** *(continued)*

Alpha-blockers: plasma concentration of digoxin increased by prazosin

Aminosalicylates: absorption of digoxin possibly reduced by sulfasalazine

Analgesics: plasma concentration of cardiac glycosides possibly increased by NSAIDs, also possible exacerbation of heart failure and reduction of renal function

Antacids: absorption of digoxin possibly reduced by antacids

• Anti-arrhythmics: plasma concentration of digoxin increased by ●amiodarone and ●propafenone (halve dose of digoxin)

Antibacterials: plasma concentration of digoxin possibly increased by gentamicin, telithromycin and trimethoprim; absorption of digoxin reduced by neomycin; plasma concentration of digoxin possibly reduced by rifampicin; plasma concentration of digoxin increased by macrolides (increased risk of toxicity); metabolism of digitoxin accelerated by rifamycins (reduced effect)

• Antidepressants: plasma concentration of digoxin reduced by ●St John's wort—avoid concomitant use

Antidiabetics: plasma concentration of digoxin possibly reduced by acarbose; plasma concentration of digoxin increased by sitagliptin

Antiepileptics: metabolism of digitoxin accelerated by carbamazepine, phenytoin and primidone (reduced effect); plasma concentration of digoxin possibly reduced by phenytoin

• Antifungals: increased cardiac toxicity with cardiac glycosides if hypokalaemia occurs with ●amphotericin; plasma concentration of digoxin increased by ●itraconazole

• Antimalarials: plasma concentration of digoxin possibly increased by ●chloroquine and hydroxychloroquine; possible increased risk of bradycardia when digoxin given with mefloquine; plasma concentration of digoxin increased by ●quinine

Antimuscarinics: plasma concentration of digoxin possibly increased by darifenacin

Antivirals: plasma concentration of digoxin increased by etravirine; plasma concentration of digoxin possibly increased by ritonavir

Anxiolytics and Hypnotics: plasma concentration of digoxin increased by alprazolam (increased risk of toxicity)

Barbiturates: metabolism of digitoxin accelerated by barbiturates (reduced effect)

Beta-blockers: increased risk of AV block and bradycardia when cardiac glycosides given with beta-blockers

Calcium Salts: arrhythmias can be precipitated when cardiac glycosides given with large intravenous doses of calcium salts

• Calcium-channel Blockers: plasma concentration of digoxin increased by ●diltiazem, ●lercanidipine and ●nicardipine; plasma concentration of digoxin possibly increased by ●nifedipine; plasma concentration of digoxin increased by ●verapamil, also increased risk of AV block and bradycardia

• Ciclosporin: plasma concentration of digoxin increased by ●ciclosporin (increased risk of toxicity)

Corticosteroids: increased risk of hypokalaemia when cardiac glycosides given with corticosteroids

Cytotoxics: absorption of digoxin tablets reduced by cytotoxics

• Diuretics: increased cardiac toxicity with cardiac glycosides if hypokalaemia occurs with ●acetazolamide, ●loop diuretics or ●thiazides and related diuretics; plasma concentration of digoxin possibly increased by potassium canrenoate; plasma concentration of digitoxin possibly affected by spironolactone; plasma concentration of digoxin increased by ●spironolactone

Lenalidomide: plasma concentration of digoxin possibly increased by lenalidomide

Lipid-regulating Drugs: absorption of cardiac glycosides possibly reduced by colestipol and colestyr-

**Cardiac Glycosides**

Lipid-regulating Drugs *(continued)*

amine; plasma concentration of digoxin possibly increased by atorvastatin

Muscle Relaxants: risk of ventricular arrhythmias when cardiac glycosides given with suxamethonium; possible increased risk of bradycardia when cardiac glycosides given with tizanidine

Penicillamine: plasma concentration of digoxin possibly reduced by penicillamine

Ranolazine: plasma concentration of digoxin increased by ranolazine

Sympathomimetics, Beta$_2$: plasma concentration of digoxin possibly reduced by salbutamol

Ulcer-healing Drugs: plasma concentration of digoxin possibly slightly increased by proton pump inhibitors; absorption of cardiac glycosides possibly reduced by sucralfate

**Carmustine**

Antiepileptics: cytotoxics possibly reduce absorption of phenytoin

• Antipsychotics: avoid concomitant use of cytotoxics with ●clozapine (increased risk of agranulocytosis)

Cardiac Glycosides: cytotoxics reduce absorption of digoxin tablets

Ulcer-healing Drugs: myelosuppressive effects of carmustine possibly enhanced by cimetidine

**Carteolol** *see* Beta-blockers

**Carvedilol** *see* Beta-blockers

**Caspofungin**

Antibacterials: plasma concentration of caspofungin initially increased and then reduced by rifampicin (consider increasing dose of caspofungin)

Antiepileptics: plasma concentration of caspofungin possibly reduced by carbamazepine and phenytoin—consider increasing dose of caspofungin

Antivirals: plasma concentration of caspofungin possibly reduced by efavirenz and nevirapine—consider increasing dose of caspofungin

• Ciclosporin: plasma concentration of caspofungin increased by ●ciclosporin (manufacturer of caspofungin recommends monitoring liver enzymes)

Corticosteroids: plasma concentration of caspofungin possibly reduced by dexamethasone—consider increasing dose of caspofungin

• Tacrolimus: caspofungin reduces plasma concentration of ●tacrolimus

**Cefaclor** *see* Cephalosporins

**Cefadroxil** *see* Cephalosporins

**Cefalexin** *see* Cephalosporins

**Cefixime** *see* Cephalosporins

**Cefotaxime** *see* Cephalosporins

**Cefpodoxime** *see* Cephalosporins

**Cefradine** *see* Cephalosporins

**Ceftazidime** *see* Cephalosporins

**Ceftriaxone** *see* Cephalosporins

**Cefuroxime** *see* Cephalosporins

**Celecoxib** *see* NSAIDs

**Celiprolol** *see* Beta-blockers

**Cephalosporins**

Antacids: absorption of cefaclor and cefpodoxime reduced by antacids

Antibacterials: possible increased risk of nephrotoxicity when cephalosporins given with aminoglycosides

• Anticoagulants: cephalosporins possibly enhance anticoagulant effect of ●coumarins

Oestrogens: antibacterials that do not induce liver enzymes possibly reduce contraceptive effect of oestrogens (risk probably small, see p. 445)

Probenecid: excretion of cephalosporins reduced by probenecid (increased plasma concentration)

Ulcer-healing Drugs: absorption of cefpodoxime reduced by histamine H$_2$-antagonists

Vaccines: antibacterials inactivate oral typhoid vaccine–see p. 688

**Cetirizine** *see* Antihistamines

**Chloral** *see* Anxiolytics and Hypnotics

**Chloramphenicol**

Antibacterials: metabolism of chloramphenicol accelerated by rifampicin (reduced plasma concentration)

- Anticoagulants: chloramphenicol enhances anticoagulant effect of ●coumarins
- Antidiabetics: chloramphenicol enhances effects of ●sulphonylureas
- Antiepileptics: chloramphenicol increases plasma concentration of ●phenytoin (increased risk of toxicity); metabolism of chloramphenicol accelerated by ●primidone (reduced plasma concentration)
- Antipsychotics: avoid concomitant use of chloramphenicol with ●clozapine (increased risk of agranulocytosis)
- Barbiturates: metabolism of chloramphenicol accelerated by ●barbiturates (reduced plasma concentration)
- Ciclosporin: chloramphenicol possibly increases plasma concentration of ●ciclosporin

Hydroxocobalamin: chloramphenicol reduces response to hydroxocobalamin

Oestrogens: antibacterials that do not induce liver enzymes possibly reduce contraceptive effect of oestrogens (risk probably small, see p. 445)

- Tacrolimus: chloramphenicol possibly increases plasma concentration of ●tacrolimus

Vaccines: antibacterials inactivate oral typhoid vaccine–see p. 688

**Chlordiazepoxide** *see* Anxiolytics and Hypnotics

**Chloroquine and Hydroxychloroquine**

Adsorbents: absorption of chloroquine and hydroxychloroquine reduced by kaolin

Agalsidase Alfa and Beta: chloroquine and hydroxychloroquine possibly inhibit effects of agalsidase alfa and beta (manufacturers of agalsidase alfa and beta advise avoid concomitant use)

Antacids: absorption of chloroquine and hydroxychloroquine reduced by antacids

- Anti-arrhythmics: increased risk of ventricular arrhythmias when chloroquine and hydroxychloroquine given with ●amiodarone–avoid concomitant use
- Antibacterials: increased risk of ventricular arrhythmias when chloroquine and hydroxychloroquine given with ●moxifloxacin–avoid concomitant use

Antiepileptics: possible increased risk of convulsions when chloroquine and hydroxychloroquine given with antiepileptics

- Antimalarials: avoidance of antimalarials advised by manufacturer of ●artemether/lumefantrine; increased risk of convulsions when chloroquine and hydroxychloroquine given with ●mefloquine
- Antipsychotics: increased risk of ventricular arrhythmias when chloroquine and hydroxychloroquine given with ●droperidol–avoid concomitant use
- Cardiac Glycosides: chloroquine and hydroxychloroquine possibly increase plasma concentration of ●digoxin
- Ciclosporin: chloroquine and hydroxychloroquine increase plasma concentration of ●ciclosporin (increased risk of toxicity)

Lanthanum: absorption of chloroquine and hydroxychloroquine possibly reduced by lanthanum (give at least 2 hours apart)

Laronidase: chloroquine and hydroxychloroquine possibly inhibit effects of laronidase (manufacturer of laronidase advises avoid concomitant use)

Parasympathomimetics: chloroquine and hydroxychloroquine have potential to increase symptoms of myasthenia gravis and thus diminish effect of neostigmine and pyridostigmine

Ulcer-healing Drugs: metabolism of chloroquine and hydroxychloroquine inhibited by cimetidine (increased plasma concentration)

Vaccines: antimalarials inactivate oral typhoid vaccine–see p. 688

**Chlorothiazide** *see* Diuretics

**Chlorphenamine (chlorpheniramine)** *see* Antihistamines

**Chlorpromazine** *see* Antipsychotics

**Chlorpropamide** *see* Antidiabetics

**Chlortalidone** *see* Diuretics

**Ciclesonide** *see* Corticosteroids

**Ciclosporin**

- ACE Inhibitors: increased risk of hyperkalaemia when ciclosporin given with ●ACE inhibitors
- Aliskiren: ciclosporin increases plasma concentration of ●aliskiren—avoid concomitant use

Allopurinol: plasma concentration of ciclosporin possibly increased by allopurinol (risk of nephrotoxicity)

- Analgesics: increased risk of nephrotoxicity when ciclosporin given with ●NSAIDs; ciclosporin increases plasma concentration of ●diclofenac (halve dose of diclofenac)
- Angiotensin-II Receptor Antagonists: increased risk of hyperkalaemia when ciclosporin given with ●angiotensin-II receptor antagonists

Anti-arrhythmics: plasma concentration of ciclosporin possibly increased by amiodarone and propafenone

- Antibacterials: metabolism of ciclosporin inhibited by ●clarithromycin and ●erythromycin (increased plasma concentration); metabolism of ciclosporin accelerated by ●rifampicin (reduced plasma concentration); plasma concentration of ciclosporin possibly reduced by ●sulfadiazine; plasma concentration of ciclosporin possibly increased by ●chloramphenicol, ●doxycycline and ●telithromycin; increased risk of nephrotoxicity when ciclosporin given with ●aminoglycosides, ●polymyxins, ●quinolones, ●sulphonamides or ●vancomycin; increased risk of myopathy when ciclosporin given with ●daptomycin (preferably avoid concomitant use); metabolism of ciclosporin possibly inhibited by ●macrolides (increased plasma concentration); plasma concentration of ciclosporin increased by ●quinupristin/dalfopristin; increased risk of nephrotoxicity when ciclosporin given with ●trimethoprim, also plasma concentration of ciclosporin reduced by intravenous trimethoprim
- Antidepressants: plasma concentration of ciclosporin reduced by ●St John's wort—avoid concomitant use

Antidiabetics: ciclosporin possibly enhances hypoglycaemic effect of repaglinide

- Antiepileptics: metabolism of ciclosporin accelerated by ●carbamazepine and ●phenytoin (reduced plasma concentration); plasma concentration of ciclosporin possibly reduced by oxcarbazepine; metabolism of ciclosporin accelerated by ●primidone (reduced effect)
- Antifungals: metabolism of ciclosporin inhibited by ●fluconazole, ●itraconazole, ●ketoconazole, ●posaconazole and ●voriconazole (increased plasma concentration); metabolism of ciclosporin possibly inhibited by ●miconazole (increased plasma concentration); increased risk of nephrotoxicity when ciclosporin given with ●amphotericin; ciclosporin increases plasma concentration of ●caspofungin (manufacturer of caspofungin recommends monitoring liver enzymes); plasma concentration of ciclosporin possibly reduced by griseofulvin and terbinafine; plasma concentration of ciclosporin possibly increased by micafungin
- Antimalarials: plasma concentration of ciclosporin increased by ●chloroquine and hydroxychloroquine (increased risk of toxicity)

Antimuscarinics: avoidance of ciclosporin advised by manufacturer of darifenacin

- Antivirals: increased risk of nephrotoxicity when ciclosporin given with aciclovir; plasma concentration of ciclosporin possibly increased by ●atazanavir, ●nelfinavir and ●ritonavir; plasma concentration of ciclosporin possibly reduced by ●efavirenz; plasma concentration of ciclosporin increased by ●indinavir; plasma concentration of both drugs increased when ciclosporin given with ●saquinavir
- Barbiturates: metabolism of ciclosporin accelerated by ●barbiturates (reduced effect)
- Beta-blockers: plasma concentration of ciclosporin increased by ●carvedilol
- Bile Acids: absorption of ciclosporin increased by ●ursodeoxycholic acid

**Appendix 1: Interactions**

**Ciclosporin** *(continued)*
- Bosentan: ciclosporin increases plasma concentration of ●bosentan (also plasma concentration of ciclosporin reduced—avoid concomitant use)
- Calcium-channel Blockers: combination of ciclosporin with ●lercanidipine may increase plasma concentration of either drug (or both)—avoid concomitant use; plasma concentration of ciclosporin increased by ●diltiazem, ●nicardipine and ●verapamil; ciclosporin possibly increases plasma concentration of nifedipine (increased risk of toxicity including gingival hyperplasia)
- Cardiac Glycosides: ciclosporin increases plasma concentration of ●digoxin (increased risk of toxicity)
- Colchicine: possible increased risk of nephrotoxicity and myotoxicity when ciclosporin given with ●colchicine (increased plasma concentration of ciclosporin)
- Corticosteroids: plasma concentration of ciclosporin increased by high-dose ●methylprednisolone (risk of convulsions); ciclosporin increases plasma concentration of prednisolone
- Cytotoxics: increased risk of nephrotoxicity when ciclosporin given with ●melphalan; increased risk of neurotoxicity when ciclosporin given with ●doxorubicin; risk of toxicity when ciclosporin given with ●methotrexate; plasma concentration of ciclosporin possibly increased by imatinib; *in vitro* studies suggest a possible interaction between ciclosporin and docetaxel (consult docetaxel product literature); ciclosporin possibly increases plasma concentration of etoposide (increased risk of toxicity)
- Diuretics: increased risk of hyperkalaemia when ciclosporin given with ●potassium-sparing diuretics and aldosterone antagonists; increased risk of nephrotoxicity and possibly hypermagnesaemia when ciclosporin given with thiazides and related diuretics
- Grapefruit Juice: plasma concentration of ciclosporin increased by ●grapefruit juice (increased risk of toxicity)
- Hormone Antagonists: metabolism of ciclosporin inhibited by ●danazol (increased plasma concentration); plasma concentration of ciclosporin reduced by lanreotide and ●octreotide
- Lipid-regulating Drugs: increased risk of renal impairment when ciclosporin given with bezafibrate or fenofibrate; increased risk of myopathy when ciclosporin given with ●rosuvastatin (avoid concomitant use); plasma concentration of both drugs may increase when ciclosporin given with ●ezetimibe; increased risk of myopathy when ciclosporin given with ●statins
  Mannitol: possible increased risk of nephrotoxicity when ciclosporin given with mannitol
- Metoclopramide: plasma concentration of ciclosporin increased by ●metoclopramide
- Modafinil: plasma concentration of ciclosporin reduced by ●modafinil
  Oestrogens: plasma concentration of ciclosporin possibly increased by oestrogens
- Orlistat: absorption of ciclosporin possibly reduced by ●orlistat
- Potassium Salts: increased risk of hyperkalaemia when ciclosporin given with ●potassium salts
- Progestogens: metabolism of ciclosporin inhibited by ●progestogens (increased plasma concentration)
  Ranolazine: ciclosporin possibly increases plasma concentration of ranolazine
  Sevelamer: plasma concentration of ciclosporin possibly reduced by sevelamer
  Sirolimus: ciclosporin increases plasma concentration of sirolimus
- Sitaxentan: ciclosporin increases plasma concentration of ●sitaxentan—avoid concomitant use
- Sulfinpyrazone: plasma concentration of ciclosporin reduced by ●sulfinpyrazone

**Ciclosporin** *(continued)*
- Tacrolimus: plasma concentration of ciclosporin increased by ●tacrolimus (increased risk of nephrotoxicity)—avoid concomitant use
- Ulcer-healing Drugs: plasma concentration of ciclosporin possibly increased by ●cimetidine; plasma concentration of ciclosporin possibly affected by omeprazole

**Cidofovir**
  Antivirals: combination of cidofovir with tenofovir may increase plasma concentration of either drug (or both)

**Cilazapril** *see* ACE Inhibitors

**Cilostazol**
- Anagrelide: avoidance of cilostazol advised by manufacturer of ●anagrelide
  Analgesics: manufacturer of cilostazol recommends dose of concomitant aspirin should not exceed 80 mg daily
- Antibacterials: plasma concentration of cilostazol increased by ●erythromycin (also plasma concentration of erythromycin reduced)—avoid concomitant use
- Antifungals: plasma concentration of cilostazol possibly increased by ●ketoconazole—avoid concomitant use
- Antivirals: plasma concentration of cilostazol possibly increased by ●fosamprenavir, ●indinavir, ●lopinavir, ●nelfinavir, ●ritonavir and ●saquinavir—avoid concomitant use
- Calcium-channel Blockers: plasma concentration of cilostazol increased by ●diltiazem—avoid concomitant use
- Ulcer-healing Drugs: plasma concentration of cilostazol possibly increased by ●cimetidine and ●lansoprazole—avoid concomitant use; plasma concentration of cilostazol increased by ●omeprazole (risk of toxicity)—avoid concomitant use

**Cimetidine** *see* Histamine H₂-antagonists

**Cinacalcet**
  Antifungals: metabolism of cinacalcet inhibited by ketoconazole (increased plasma concentration)
  Tobacco: metabolism of cinacalcet increased by tobacco smoking (reduced plasma concentration)

**Cinnarizine** *see* Antihistamines
**Ciprofibrate** *see* Fibrates
**Ciprofloxacin** *see* Quinolones
**Cisatracurium** *see* Muscle Relaxants
**Cisplatin** *see* Platinum Compounds
**Citalopram** *see* Antidepressants, SSRI
**Clarithromycin** *see* Macrolides
**Clemastine** *see* Antihistamines

**Clindamycin**
- Muscle Relaxants: clindamycin enhances effects of ●non-depolarising muscle relaxants and ●suxamethonium
  Oestrogens: antibacterials that do not induce liver enzymes possibly reduce contraceptive effect of oestrogens (risk probably small, see p. 445)
  Parasympathomimetics: clindamycin antagonises effects of neostigmine and pyridostigmine
  Vaccines: antibacterials inactivate oral typhoid vaccine—see p. 688

**Clobazam** *see* Anxiolytics and Hypnotics
**Clomethiazole** *see* Anxiolytics and Hypnotics
**Clomipramine** *see* Antidepressants, Tricyclic
**Clonazepam** *see* Anxiolytics and Hypnotics

**Clonidine**
  ACE Inhibitors: enhanced hypotensive effect when clonidine given with ACE inhibitors; previous treatment with clonidine possibly delays antihypertensive effect of captopril
  Adrenergic Neurone Blockers: enhanced hypotensive effect when clonidine given with adrenergic neurone blockers
  Alcohol: enhanced hypotensive effect when clonidine given with alcohol
  Aldesleukin: enhanced hypotensive effect when clonidine given with aldesleukin

**Clonidine** *(continued)*

Alpha-blockers: enhanced hypotensive effect when clonidine given with alpha-blockers

Anaesthetics, General: enhanced hypotensive effect when clonidine given with general anaesthetics

Analgesics: hypotensive effect of clonidine antagonised by NSAIDs

Angiotensin-II Receptor Antagonists: enhanced hypotensive effect when clonidine given with angiotensin-II receptor antagonists

● Antidepressants: enhanced hypotensive effect when clonidine given with MAOIs; hypotensive effect of clonidine antagonised by ●tricyclics, also increased risk of hypertension on clonidine withdrawal

Antipsychotics: enhanced hypotensive effect when clonidine given with phenothiazines

Anxiolytics and Hypnotics: enhanced hypotensive effect when clonidine given with anxiolytics and hypnotics

● Beta-blockers: increased risk of withdrawal hypertension when clonidine given with ●beta-blockers (withdraw beta-blockers several days before slowly withdrawing clonidine)

Calcium-channel Blockers: enhanced hypotensive effect when clonidine given with calcium-channel blockers

Corticosteroids: hypotensive effect of clonidine antagonised by corticosteroids

Diazoxide: enhanced hypotensive effect when clonidine given with diazoxide

Diuretics: enhanced hypotensive effect when clonidine given with diuretics

Dopaminergics: enhanced hypotensive effect when clonidine given with levodopa

Methyldopa: enhanced hypotensive effect when clonidine given with methyldopa

Moxisylyte (thymoxamine): enhanced hypotensive effect when clonidine given with moxisylyte

Moxonidine: enhanced hypotensive effect when clonidine given with moxonidine

Muscle Relaxants: enhanced hypotensive effect when clonidine given with baclofen or tizanidine

Nitrates: enhanced hypotensive effect when clonidine given with nitrates

Oestrogens: hypotensive effect of clonidine antagonised by oestrogens

Prostaglandins: enhanced hypotensive effect when clonidine given with alprostadil

● Sympathomimetics: possible risk of hypertension when clonidine given with adrenaline (epinephrine) or noradrenaline (norepinephrine); serious adverse events reported with concomitant use of clonidine and ●methylphenidate (causality not established)

Vasodilator Antihypertensives: enhanced hypotensive effect when clonidine given with hydralazine, minoxidil or sodium nitroprusside

**Clopamide** *see* Diuretics

**Clopidogrel**

Analgesics: increased risk of bleeding when clopidogrel given with NSAIDs or aspirin

● Anticoagulants: manufacturer of clopidogrel advises avoid concomitant use with ●warfarin; antiplatelet action of clopidogrel enhances anticoagulant effect of ●coumarins and ●phenindione; increased risk of bleeding when clopidogrel given with heparins

Dipyridamole: increased risk of bleeding when clopidogrel given with dipyridamole

Iloprost: increased risk of bleeding when clopidogrel given with iloprost

Prasugrel: possible increased risk of bleeding when clopidogrel given with prasugrel

● Ulcer-healing Drugs: antiplatelet effect of clopidogrel possibly reduced by ●proton pump inhibitors—avoid concomitant use

**Clotrimazole** *see* Antifungals, Imidazole

**Clozapine** *see* Antipsychotics

**Co-amoxiclav** *see* Penicillins

**Co-beneldopa** *see* Levodopa

**Co-careldopa** *see* Levodopa

**Codeine** *see* Opioid Analgesics

**Co-fluampicil** *see* Penicillins

**Colchicine**

● Antibacterials: increased risk of colchicine toxicity when given with ●clarithromycin or ●erythromycin

● Ciclosporin: possible increased risk of nephrotoxicity and myotoxicity when colchicine given with ●ciclosporin (increased plasma concentration of ciclosporin)

● Lipid-regulating Drugs: possible increased risk of myopathy when colchicine given with ●statins

**Colesevelam**

Note Other drugs should be taken at least 1 hour before or 4 hours after colesevelam to reduce possible interference with absorption

**Colestipol**

Note Other drugs should be taken at least 1 hour before or 4-6 hours after colestipol to reduce possible interference with absorption

Antibacterials: colestipol possibly reduces absorption of tetracycline

Bile Acids: colestipol possibly reduces absorption of bile acids

Cardiac Glycosides: colestipol possibly reduces absorption of cardiac glycosides

Diuretics: colestipol reduces absorption of thiazides and related diuretics (give at least 2 hours apart)

Thyroid Hormones: colestipol reduces absorption of thyroid hormones

**Colestyramine**

Note Other drugs should be taken at least 1 hour before or 4-6 hours after colestyramine to reduce possible interference with absorption

Analgesics: colestyramine increases the excretion of meloxicam; colestyramine reduces absorption of paracetamol

Antibacterials: colestyramine possibly reduces absorption of tetracycline; colestyramine antagonises effects of oral vancomycin

● Anticoagulants: colestyramine may enhance or reduce anticoagulant effect of ●coumarins and ●phenindione

Antidiabetics: colestyramine possibly enhances hypoglycaemic effect of acarbose

Antiepileptics: colestyramine possibly reduces absorption of valproate

Bile Acids: colestyramine possibly reduces absorption of bile acids

Cardiac Glycosides: colestyramine possibly reduces absorption of cardiac glycosides

Diuretics: colestyramine reduces absorption of thiazides and related diuretics (give at least 2 hours apart)

Leflunomide: colestyramine significantly decreases effect of leflunomide (enhanced elimination)—avoid unless drug elimination desired

Mycophenolate: colestyramine reduces absorption of mycophenolate

Raloxifene: colestyramine reduces absorption of raloxifene (manufacturer of raloxifene advises avoid concomitant administration)

Thyroid Hormones: colestyramine reduces absorption of thyroid hormones

**Colistin** *see* Polymyxins

**Contraceptives, oral** *see* Oestrogens and Progestogens

**Corticosteroids**

Note Interactions do not generally apply to corticosteroids used for topical action (including inhalation) unless specified

ACE Inhibitors: corticosteroids antagonise hypotensive effect of ACE inhibitors

Adrenergic Neurone Blockers: corticosteroids antagonise hypotensive effect of adrenergic neurone blockers

Alpha-blockers: corticosteroids antagonise hypotensive effect of alpha-blockers

Analgesics: increased risk of gastro-intestinal bleeding and ulceration when corticosteroids given with NSAIDs; increased risk of gastro-intestinal bleeding and ulceration when corticosteroids given with

## Corticosteroids

**Analgesics** *(continued)*
aspirin, also corticosteroids reduce plasma concentration of salicylate

**Angiotensin-II Receptor Antagonists:** corticosteroids antagonise hypotensive effect of angiotensin-II receptor antagonists

**Antacids:** absorption of deflazacort reduced by antacids

- **Antibacterials:** plasma concentration of methylprednisolone possibly increased by clarithromycin; metabolism of corticosteroids possibly inhibited by erythromycin; metabolism of methylprednisolone inhibited by erythromycin; corticosteroids possibly reduce plasma concentration of isoniazid; metabolism of corticosteroids accelerated by ●rifamycins (reduced effect)

- **Anticoagulants:** corticosteroids may enhance or reduce anticoagulant effect of ●coumarins (high-dose corticosteroids enhance anticoagulant effect)

**Antidiabetics:** corticosteroids antagonise hypoglycaemic effect of antidiabetics

- **Antiepileptics:** metabolism of corticosteroids accelerated by ●carbamazepine, ●phenytoin and ●primidone (reduced effect)

- **Antifungals:** metabolism of corticosteroids possibly inhibited by itraconazole and ketoconazole; plasma concentration of active metabolite of ciclesonide increased by ketoconazole; plasma concentration of inhaled mometasone increased by ketoconazole; plasma concentration of inhaled and oral budesonide increased by ketoconazole; metabolism of methylprednisolone inhibited by ketoconazole; increased risk of hypokalaemia when corticosteroids given with ●amphotericin—avoid concomitant use unless corticosteroids needed to control reactions; plasma concentration of inhaled budesonide increased by itraconazole; metabolism of methylprednisolone possibly inhibited by itraconazole; dexamethasone possibly reduces plasma concentration of caspofungin—consider increasing dose of caspofungin

- **Antivirals:** dexamethasone possibly reduces plasma concentration of indinavir, lopinavir and saquinavir; plasma concentration of corticosteroids, dexamethasone and prednisolone possibly increased by ritonavir; plasma concentration of inhaled and intranasal budesonide and fluticasone increased by ●ritonavir

**Aprepitant:** metabolism of dexamethasone and methylprednisolone inhibited by aprepitant (reduce dose of dexamethasone and methylprednisolone)

- **Barbiturates:** metabolism of corticosteroids accelerated by ●barbiturates (reduced effect)

**Beta-blockers:** corticosteroids antagonise hypotensive effect of beta-blockers

**Calcium Salts:** corticosteroids reduce absorption of calcium salts

**Calcium-channel Blockers:** corticosteroids antagonise hypotensive effect of calcium-channel blockers

**Cardiac Glycosides:** increased risk of hypokalaemia when corticosteroids given with cardiac glycosides

- **Ciclosporin:** high-dose methylprednisolone increases plasma concentration of ●ciclosporin (risk of convulsions); plasma concentration of prednisolone increased by ciclosporin

**Clonidine:** corticosteroids antagonise hypotensive effect of clonidine

- **Cytotoxics:** increased risk of haematological toxicity when corticosteroids given with ●methotrexate

**Diazoxide:** corticosteroids antagonise hypotensive effect of diazoxide

**Diuretics:** corticosteroids antagonise diuretic effect of diuretics; increased risk of hypokalaemia when corticosteroids given with acetazolamide, loop diuretics or thiazides and related diuretics

**Methyldopa:** corticosteroids antagonise hypotensive effect of methyldopa

## Corticosteroids *(continued)*

**Mifepristone:** effect of corticosteroids (including inhaled corticosteroids) may be reduced for 3–4 days after mifepristone

**Moxonidine:** corticosteroids antagonise hypotensive effect of moxonidine

**Muscle Relaxants:** corticosteroids possibly antagonise effects of pancuronium and vecuronium

**Nitrates:** corticosteroids antagonise hypotensive effect of nitrates

**Oestrogens:** plasma concentration of corticosteroids increased by oral contraceptives containing oestrogens

**Sodium Benzoate:** corticosteroids possibly reduce effects of sodium benzoate

**Sodium Phenylbutyrate:** corticosteroids possibly reduce effects of sodium phenylbutyrate

**Somatropin:** corticosteroids may inhibit growth-promoting effect of somatropin

**Sympathomimetics:** metabolism of dexamethasone accelerated by ephedrine

**Sympathomimetics, Beta$_2$:** increased risk of hypokalaemia when corticosteroids given with high doses of beta$_2$ sympathomimetics—for CSM advice (hypokalaemia) see p. 155

**Theophylline:** increased risk of hypokalaemia when corticosteroids given with theophylline

- **Vaccines:** high doses of corticosteroids impair immune response to ●vaccines, avoid concomitant use with live vaccines (see p. 669)

**Vasodilator Antihypertensives:** corticosteroids antagonise hypotensive effect of hydralazine, minoxidil and sodium nitroprusside

**Cortisone** *see* Corticosteroids

**Co-trimoxazole** *see* Trimethoprim and Sulfamethoxazole

## Coumarins

Note Change in patient's clinical condition, particularly associated with liver disease, intercurrent illness, or drug administration, necessitates more frequent testing. Major changes in diet (especially involving salads and vegetables) and in alcohol consumption may also affect anticoagulant control

- **Alcohol:** anticoagulant control with coumarins may be affected by major changes in consumption of ●alcohol

**Allopurinol:** anticoagulant effect of coumarins possibly enhanced by allopurinol

- **Anabolic Steroids:** anticoagulant effect of coumarins enhanced by ●anabolic steroids

- **Analgesics:** anticoagulant effect of coumarins possibly enhanced by ●NSAIDs; anticoagulant effect of coumarins enhanced by ●azapropazone (avoid concomitant use); increased risk of haemorrhage when anticoagulants given with intravenous ●diclofenac (avoid concomitant use, including low-dose heparin); increased risk of haemorrhage when anticoagulants given with ●ketorolac (avoid concomitant use, including low-dose heparin); anticoagulant effect of coumarins enhanced by ●tramadol; increased risk of bleeding when coumarins given with ●aspirin (due to antiplatelet effect); anticoagulant effect of coumarins possibly enhanced by prolonged regular use of paracetamol

- **Anti-arrhythmics:** metabolism of coumarins inhibited by ●amiodarone (enhanced anticoagulant effect); anticoagulant effect of coumarins enhanced by ●propafenone

- **Antibacterials:** experience in anticoagulant clinics suggests that INR possibly altered when coumarins are given with ●neomycin (given for local action on gut); anticoagulant effect of coumarins possibly enhanced by ●azithromycin, ●aztreonam, ●cephalosporins, levofloxacin, ●tetracyclines, tigecycline and trimethoprim; anticoagulant effect of coumarins enhanced by ●chloramphenicol, ●ciprofloxacin, ●clarithromycin, ●erythromycin, ●metronidazole, ●nalidixic acid, ●norfloxacin, ●ofloxacin and ●sulphonamides; studies have failed to demonstrate an interaction with coumarins, but

Coumarins
- Antibacterials *(continued)*
  common experience in anticoagulant clinics is
  that INR can be altered by a course of broad-
  spectrum penicillins such as ampicillin; metabolism of coumarins accelerated by ●rifamycins
  (reduced anticoagulant effect)
- Antidepressants: anticoagulant effect of warfarin
  possibly enhanced by ●venlafaxine; anticoagulant
  effect of coumarins possibly enhanced by ●SSRIs;
  anticoagulant effect of coumarins reduced by ●St
  John's wort (avoid concomitant use); anticoagulant
  effect of warfarin enhanced by mirtazapine; anticoagulant effect of coumarins may be enhanced or
  reduced by ●tricyclics
- Antidiabetics: anticoagulant effect of warfarin possibly
  enhanced by exenatide; coumarins possibly enhance
  hypoglycaemic effect of ●sulphonylureas, also possible changes to anticoagulant effect
- Antiepileptics: metabolism of coumarins accelerated
  by ●carbamazepine and ●primidone (reduced anticoagulant effect); metabolism of coumarins accelerated by ●phenytoin (possibility of reduced
  anticoagulant effect, but enhancement also reported);
  anticoagulant effect of coumarins possibly enhanced
  by valproate
- Antifungals: anticoagulant effect of coumarins
  enhanced by ●fluconazole, ●itraconazole,
  ●ketoconazole and ●voriconazole; anticoagulant
  effect of coumarins enhanced by ●miconazole
  (miconazole oral gel and possibly vaginal formulations absorbed); anticoagulant effect of coumarins
  reduced by ●griseofulvin
  Antimalarials: isolated reports that anticoagulant effect
  of warfarin may be enhanced by proguanil
- Antivirals: anticoagulant effect of warfarin may be
  enhanced or reduced by atazanavir, ●nevirapine and
  ●ritonavir; anticoagulant effect of coumarins may be
  enhanced or reduced by fosamprenavir; anticoagulant effect of coumarins possibly enhanced by
  ●ritonavir; anticoagulant effect of warfarin possibly
  enhanced by saquinavir
  Anxiolytics and Hypnotics: anticoagulant effect of
  coumarins may transiently be enhanced by
  chloral and triclofos
  Aprepitant: anticoagulant effect of warfarin possibly
  reduced by aprepitant
- Azathioprine: anticoagulant effect of coumarins possibly reduced by ●azathioprine
- Barbiturates: metabolism of coumarins accelerated by
  ●barbiturates (reduced anticoagulant effect)
  Bosentan: monitoring anticoagulant effect of coumarins recommended by manufacturer of bosentan
- Clopidogrel: anticoagulant effect of coumarins
  enhanced due to antiplatelet action of ●clopidogrel;
  avoidance of warfarin advised by manufacturer of
  ●clopidogrel
- Corticosteroids: anticoagulant effect of coumarins may
  be enhanced or reduced by ●corticosteroids (high-
  dose corticosteroids enhance anticoagulant effect)
- Cranberry Juice: anticoagulant effect of coumarins
  possibly enhanced by ●cranberry juice—avoid concomitant use
- Cytotoxics: anticoagulant effect of coumarins possibly
  enhanced by ●etoposide, ●ifosfamide and ●sorafenib;
  anticoagulant effect of coumarins enhanced by
  ●fluorouracil; anticoagulant effect of warfarin possibly enhanced by gemcitabine; anticoagulant effect of
  coumarins possibly reduced by ●mercaptopurine and
  ●mitotane; increased risk of bleeding when coumarins given with ●erlotinib; replacement of warfarin
  with a heparin advised by manufacturer of imatinib
  (possibility of enhanced warfarin effect)
- Dipyridamole: anticoagulant effect of coumarins
  enhanced due to antiplatelet action of ●dipyridamole
- Disulfiram: anticoagulant effect of coumarins
  enhanced by ●disulfiram

Coumarins *(continued)*
- Dopaminergics: anticoagulant effect of warfarin
  enhanced by ●entacapone
- Enteral Foods: anticoagulant effect of coumarins
  antagonised by vitamin K (present in some ●enteral
  feeds )
- Glucosamine: anticoagulant effect of warfarin
  enhanced by ●glucosamine (avoid concomitant use)
- Hormone Antagonists: anticoagulant effect of coumarins possibly enhanced by bicalutamide and
  ●toremifene; metabolism of coumarins inhibited by
  ●danazol (enhanced anticoagulant effect); anticoagulant effect of coumarins enhanced by
  ●flutamide and ●tamoxifen
  Iloprost: anticoagulant effect of coumarins possibly
  enhanced by iloprost
  Lactulose: anticoagulant effect of coumarins possibly
  enhanced by lactulose
  Leflunomide: anticoagulant effect of warfarin possibly
  enhanced by leflunomide
  Leukotriene Receptor Antagonists: anticoagulant
  effect of warfarin enhanced by zafirlukast
- Levamisole: anticoagulant effect of warfarin possibly
  enhanced by ●levamisole
- Lipid-regulating Drugs: anticoagulant effect of coumarins may be enhanced or reduced by
  ●colestyramine; anticoagulant effect of warfarin may
  be transiently reduced by atorvastatin; anticoagulant
  effect of coumarins enhanced by ●fibrates,
  ●fluvastatin and simvastatin; anticoagulant effect of
  coumarins possibly enhanced by ezetimibe and
  ●rosuvastatin
  Memantine: anticoagulant effect of warfarin possibly
  enhanced by memantine
- Oestrogens: anticoagulant effect of coumarins may be
  enhanced or reduced by ●oestrogens
  Orlistat: monitoring anticoagulant effect of coumarins
  recommended by manufacturer of orlistat
  Prasugrel: possible increased risk of bleeding when
  coumarins given with prasugrel
- Progestogens: anticoagulant effect of coumarins may
  be enhanced or reduced by ●progestogens
  Raloxifene: anticoagulant effect of coumarins antagonised by raloxifene
- Retinoids: anticoagulant effect of coumarins possibly
  reduced by ●acitretin
  Sibutramine: increased risk of bleeding when anticoagulants given with sibutramine
- Sitaxentan: anticoagulant effect of coumarins
  enhanced by ●sitaxentan
- Sulfinpyrazone: anticoagulant effect of coumarins
  enhanced by ●sulfinpyrazone
- Sympathomimetics: anticoagulant effect of coumarins
  possibly enhanced by ●methylphenidate
  Terpene Mixture: anticoagulant effect of coumarins
  possibly reduced by Rowachol®
- Testolactone: anticoagulant effect of coumarins
  enhanced by ●testolactone
- Testosterone: anticoagulant effect of coumarins
  enhanced by ●testosterone
- Thyroid Hormones: anticoagulant effect of coumarins
  enhanced by ●thyroid hormones
  Ubidecarenone: anticoagulant effect of warfarin may
  be enhanced or reduced by ubidecarenone
- Ulcer-healing Drugs: metabolism of coumarins inhibited by ●cimetidine (enhanced anticoagulant effect);
  anticoagulant effect of coumarins possibly enhanced
  by ●esomeprazole, ●omeprazole and pantoprazole;
  absorption of coumarins possibly reduced by
  ●sucralfate (reduced anticoagulant effect)
  Vaccines: anticoagulant effect of warfarin possibly
  enhanced by influenza vaccine
- Vitamins: anticoagulant effect of coumarins antagonised by ●vitamin K
Cranberry Juice
- Anticoagulants: cranberry juice possibly enhances
  anticoagulant effect of ●coumarins—avoid concomitant use

Cyclizine *see* Antihistamines

Cyclopenthiazide *see* Diuretics

Cyclopentolate *see* Antimuscarinics

**Cyclophosphamide**

Antiepileptics: cytotoxics possibly reduce absorption of phenytoin

Antifungals: side-effects of cyclophosphamide possibly increased by itraconazole

• Antipsychotics: avoid concomitant use of cytotoxics with •clozapine (increased risk of agranulocytosis)

Cardiac Glycosides: cytotoxics reduce absorption of digoxin tablets

• Cytotoxics: increased toxicity when high-dose cyclophosphamide given with •pentostatin—avoid concomitant use

Muscle Relaxants: cyclophosphamide enhances effects of suxamethonium

**Cycloserine**

• Alcohol: increased risk of convulsions when cycloserine given with •alcohol

Antibacterials: increased risk of CNS toxicity when cycloserine given with isoniazid

Oestrogens: antibacterials that do not induce liver enzymes possibly reduce contraceptive effect of oestrogens (risk probably small, see p. 445)

Vaccines: antibacterials inactivate oral typhoid vaccine–see p. 688

Cyproheptadine *see* Antihistamines

**Cytarabine**

Antiepileptics: cytotoxics possibly reduce absorption of phenytoin

Antifungals: cytarabine possibly reduces plasma concentration of flucytosine

• Antipsychotics: avoid concomitant use of cytotoxics with •clozapine (increased risk of agranulocytosis)

Cardiac Glycosides: cytotoxics reduce absorption of digoxin tablets

Cytotoxics: intracellular concentration of cytarabine increased by fludarabine

Cytotoxics *see* individual drugs

**Dabigatran Etexilate**

• Analgesics: possible increased risk of bleeding when dabigatran etexilate given with •NSAIDs; increased risk of haemorrhage when anticoagulants given with intravenous •diclofenac (avoid concomitant use, including low-dose heparin); increased risk of haemorrhage when anticoagulants given with •ketorolac (avoid concomitant use, including low-dose heparin)

• Anti-arrhythmics: plasma concentration of dabigatran etexilate increased by •amiodarone (reduce dose of dabigatran etexilate)

Sibutramine: increased risk of bleeding when anticoagulants given with sibutramine

**Dairy Products**

Antibacterials: dairy products reduce absorption of ciprofloxacin and norfloxacin; dairy products reduce absorption of tetracyclines (except doxycycline and minocycline)

Dalteparin *see* Heparins

**Danazol**

• Anticoagulants: danazol inhibits metabolism of •coumarins (enhanced anticoagulant effect)

• Antiepileptics: danazol inhibits metabolism of •carbamazepine (increased risk of toxicity)

• Ciclosporin: danazol inhibits metabolism of •ciclosporin (increased plasma concentration)

• Lipid-regulating Drugs: possible increased risk of myopathy when danazol given with •simvastatin

Tacrolimus: danazol possibly increases plasma concentration of tacrolimus

Dantrolene *see* Muscle Relaxants

**Dapsone**

Antibacterials: plasma concentration of dapsone reduced by rifamycins; plasma concentration of both drugs may increase when dapsone given with trimethoprim

Antivirals: plasma concentration of dapsone possibly increased by fosamprenavir

**Dapsone** *(continued)*

Oestrogens: antibacterials that do not induce liver enzymes possibly reduce contraceptive effect of oestrogens (risk probably small, see p. 445)

Probenecid: excretion of dapsone reduced by probenecid (increased risk of side-effects)

Vaccines: antibacterials inactivate oral typhoid vaccine–see p. 688

**Daptomycin**

• Ciclosporin: increased risk of myopathy when daptomycin given with •ciclosporin (preferably avoid concomitant use)

• Lipid-regulating Drugs: increased risk of myopathy when daptomycin given with •fibrates or •statins (preferably avoid concomitant use)

Oestrogens: antibacterials that do not induce liver enzymes possibly reduce contraceptive effect of oestrogens (risk probably small, see p. 445)

Vaccines: antibacterials inactivate oral typhoid vaccine–see p. 688

Darifenacin *see* Antimuscarinics

**Darunavir**

Anti-arrhythmics: darunavir possibly increases plasma concentration of lidocaine (lignocaine)—avoid concomitant use

• Antibacterials: darunavir increases plasma concentration of •rifabutin (reduce dose of rifabutin); plasma concentration of darunavir significantly reduced by •rifampicin—avoid concomitant use

Anticoagulants: avoidance of darunavir advised by manufacturer of rivaroxaban

• Antidepressants: darunavir possibly reduces plasma concentration of paroxetine and sertraline; plasma concentration of darunavir reduced by •St John's wort—avoid concomitant use

Antiepileptics: plasma concentration of darunavir possibly reduced by carbamazepine and phenytoin

Antifungals: plasma concentration of both drugs increased when darunavir given with ketoconazole

Antimalarials: caution with darunavir advised by manufacturer of artemether/lumefantrine

• Antivirals: plasma concentration of darunavir reduced by efavirenz and saquinavir; plasma concentration of both drugs increased when darunavir given with indinavir; plasma concentration of darunavir reduced by •lopinavir, also plasma concentration of lopinavir increased (avoid concomitant use); darunavir increases plasma concentration of •maraviroc (consider reducing dose of maraviroc)

Barbiturates: plasma concentration of darunavir possibly reduced by phenobarbital

• Lipid-regulating Drugs: darunavir possibly increases plasma concentration of pravastatin; possible increased risk of myopathy when darunavir given with •rosuvastatin—avoid concomitant use

• Ranolazine: darunavir possibly increases plasma concentration of •ranolazine—manufacturer of ranolazine advises avoid concomitant use

**Dasatinib**

• Antibacterials: metabolism of dasatinib accelerated by •rifampicin (reduced plasma concentration—avoid concomitant use)

Antiepileptics: cytotoxics possibly reduce absorption of phenytoin

• Antipsychotics: avoid concomitant use of cytotoxics with •clozapine (increased risk of agranulocytosis)

Cardiac Glycosides: cytotoxics reduce absorption of digoxin tablets

Lipid-regulating Drugs: dasatinib possibly increases plasma concentration of simvastatin

Ulcer-healing Drugs: plasma concentration of dasatinib possibly reduced by famotidine

**Deferasirox**

Antacids: absorption of deferasirox possibly reduced by antacids containing aluminium (manufacturer of deferasirox advises avoid concomitant use)

Antibacterials: plasma concentration of deferasirox reduced by rifampicin

**Deferasirox** *(continued)*

Antidiabetics: deferasirox increases plasma concentration of repaglinide

Anxiolytics and Hypnotics: deferasirox possibly reduces plasma concentration of midazolam

**Deflazacort** *see* Corticosteroids

**Demeclocycline** *see* Tetracyclines

**Desferrioxamine**

Antipsychotics: avoidance of desferrioxamine advised by manufacturer of levomepromazine (methotrimeprazine); manufacturer of desferrioxamine advises avoid concomitant use with prochlorperazine

**Desflurane** *see* Anaesthetics, General

**Desloratadine** *see* Antihistamines

**Desmopressin**

Analgesics: effects of desmopressin enhanced by indometacin

Loperamide: plasma concentration of *oral* desmopressin increased by loperamide

**Desogestrel** *see* Progestogens

**Dexamethasone** *see* Corticosteroids

**Dexamfetamine** *see* Sympathomimetics

**Dexibuprofen** *see* NSAIDs

**Dexketoprofen** *see* NSAIDs

**Dextromethorphan** *see* Opioid Analgesics

**Dextropropoxyphene** *see* Opioid Analgesics

**Diamorphine** *see* Opioid Analgesics

**Diazepam** *see* Anxiolytics and Hypnotics

**Diazoxide**

ACE Inhibitors: enhanced hypotensive effect when diazoxide given with ACE inhibitors

Adrenergic Neurone Blockers: enhanced hypotensive effect when diazoxide given with adrenergic neurone blockers

Alcohol: enhanced hypotensive effect when diazoxide given with alcohol

Aldesleukin: enhanced hypotensive effect when diazoxide given with aldesleukin

Alpha-blockers: enhanced hypotensive effect when diazoxide given with alpha-blockers

Anaesthetics, General: enhanced hypotensive effect when diazoxide given with general anaesthetics

Analgesics: hypotensive effect of diazoxide antagonised by NSAIDs

Angiotensin-II Receptor Antagonists: enhanced hypotensive effect when diazoxide given with angiotensin-II receptor antagonists

Antidepressants: enhanced hypotensive effect when diazoxide given with MAOIs or tricyclic-related antidepressants

Antidiabetics: diazoxide antagonises hypoglycaemic effect of antidiabetics

Antiepileptics: diazoxide reduces plasma concentration of phenytoin, also effect of diazoxide may be reduced

Antipsychotics: enhanced hypotensive effect when diazoxide given with phenothiazines

Anxiolytics and Hypnotics: enhanced hypotensive effect when diazoxide given with anxiolytics and hypnotics

Beta-blockers: enhanced hypotensive effect when diazoxide given with beta-blockers

Calcium-channel Blockers: enhanced hypotensive effect when diazoxide given with calcium-channel blockers

Clonidine: enhanced hypotensive effect when diazoxide given with clonidine

Corticosteroids: hypotensive effect of diazoxide antagonised by corticosteroids

Diuretics: enhanced hypotensive and hyperglycaemic effects when diazoxide given with diuretics

Dopaminergics: enhanced hypotensive effect when diazoxide given with levodopa

Methyldopa: enhanced hypotensive effect when diazoxide given with methyldopa

Moxisylyte (thymoxamine): enhanced hypotensive effect when diazoxide given with moxisylyte

Moxonidine: enhanced hypotensive effect when diazoxide given with moxonidine

**Diazoxide** *(continued)*

Muscle Relaxants: enhanced hypotensive effect when diazoxide given with baclofen or tizanidine

Nitrates: enhanced hypotensive effect when diazoxide given with nitrates

Oestrogens: hypotensive effect of diazoxide antagonised by oestrogens

Prostaglandins: enhanced hypotensive effect when diazoxide given with alprostadil

Vasodilator Antihypertensives: enhanced hypotensive effect when diazoxide given with hydralazine, minoxidil or sodium nitroprusside

**Diclofenac** *see* NSAIDs

**Dicycloverine (dicyclomine)** *see* Antimuscarinics

**Didanosine**

Note Antacids in tablet formulation may affect absorption of other drugs

● Allopurinol: plasma concentration of didanosine increased by ●allopurinol (risk of toxicity)—avoid concomitant use

● Antivirals: plasma concentration of didanosine possibly increased by ganciclovir; increased risk of side-effects when didanosine given with ●ribavirin—avoid concomitant use; increased risk of side-effects when didanosine given with ●stavudine; plasma concentration of didanosine increased by ●tenofovir (increased risk of toxicity)—avoid concomitant use; plasma concentration of didanosine reduced by ●tipranavir

● Cytotoxics: increased risk of toxicity when didanosine given with ●hydroxycarbamide—avoid concomitant use

**Digitoxin** *see* Cardiac Glycosides

**Digoxin** *see* Cardiac Glycosides

**Dihydrocodeine** *see* Opioid Analgesics

**Diltiazem** *see* Calcium-channel Blockers

**Dimercaprol**

● Iron: avoid concomitant use of dimercaprol with ●iron

**Dimethyl sulfoxide**

● Analgesics: avoid concomitant use of dimethyl sulfoxide with ●sulindac

**Dinoprostone** *see* Prostaglandins

**Diphenoxylate** *see* Opioid Analgesics

**Dipipanone** *see* Opioid Analgesics

**Dipivefrine** *see* Sympathomimetics

**Dipyridamole**

Antacids: absorption of dipyridamole possibly reduced by antacids

● Anti-arrhythmics: dipyridamole enhances and extends the effects of ●adenosine (important risk of toxicity)

● Anticoagulants: antiplatelet action of dipyridamole enhances anticoagulant effect of ●coumarins and ●phenindione; dipyridamole enhances anticoagulant effect of heparins

Clopidogrel: increased risk of bleeding when dipyridamole given with clopidogrel

Cytotoxics: dipyridamole possibly reduces effects of fludarabine

**Disodium Etidronate** *see* Bisphosphonates

**Disodium Pamidronate** *see* Bisphosphonates

**Disopyramide**

Anaesthetics, Local: increased myocardial depression when anti-arrhythmics given with bupivacaine, levobupivacaine, prilocaine or ropivacaine

● Anti-arrhythmics: increased myocardial depression when anti-arrhythmics given with other ●anti-arrhythmics; increased risk of ventricular arrhythmias when disopyramide given with ●amiodarone—avoid concomitant use

● Antibacterials: plasma concentration of disopyramide possibly increased by ●clarithromycin (increased risk of toxicity); plasma concentration of disopyramide increased by ●erythromycin (increased risk of toxicity); increased risk of ventricular arrhythmias when disopyramide given with ●moxifloxacin or ●quinupristin/dalfopristin—avoid concomitant use; metabolism of disopyramide accelerated by ●rifamycins (reduced plasma concentration)

Appendix 1: Interactions

**Disopyramide** *(continued)*
- Antidepressants: increased risk of ventricular arrhythmias when disopyramide given with ●tricyclics
  Antidiabetics: disopyramide possibly enhances hypoglycaemic effect of gliclazide, insulin and metformin
  Antiepileptics: plasma concentration of disopyramide reduced by phenytoin; metabolism of disopyramide accelerated by primidone (reduced plasma concentration)
- Antifungals: increased risk of ventricular arrhythmias when disopyramide given with ●ketoconazole—avoid concomitant use; avoidance of disopyramide advised by manufacturer of ●itraconazole
- Antihistamines: increased risk of ventricular arrhythmias when disopyramide given with ●mizolastine—avoid concomitant use
- Antimalarials: avoidance of disopyramide advised by manufacturer of ●artemether/lumefantrine (risk of ventricular arrhythmias)
- Antimuscarinics: increased risk of antimuscarinic side-effects when disopyramide given with antimuscarinics; increased risk of ventricular arrhythmias when disopyramide given with ●tolterodine
- Antipsychotics: increased risk of ventricular arrhythmias when anti-arrhythmics that prolong the QT interval given with ●antipsychotics that prolong the QT interval; increased risk of ventricular arrhythmias when disopyramide given with ●amisulpride, ●droperidol, ●pimozide, ●sertindole or ●zuclopenthixol—avoid concomitant use; increased risk of ventricular arrhythmias when disopyramide given with ●phenothiazines or ●sulpiride
- Antivirals: plasma concentration of disopyramide possibly increased by ●ritonavir (increased risk of toxicity)
- Atomoxetine: increased risk of ventricular arrhythmias when disopyramide given with ●atomoxetine
  Barbiturates: metabolism of disopyramide accelerated by barbiturates (reduced plasma concentration)
- Beta-blockers: increased myocardial depression when anti-arrhythmics given with ●beta-blockers; increased risk of ventricular arrhythmias when disopyramide given with ●sotalol—avoid concomitant use
- Calcium-channel Blockers: increased risk of myocardial depression and asystole when disopyramide given with ●verapamil
- Diuretics: increased cardiac toxicity with disopyramide if hypokalaemia occurs with ●acetazolamide, ●loop diuretics or ●thiazides and related diuretics
- 5HT₃ Antagonists: increased risk of ventricular arrhythmias when disopyramide given with ●dolasetron—avoid concomitant use
- Ivabradine: increased risk of ventricular arrhythmias when disopyramide given with ●ivabradine
  Nitrates: disopyramide reduces effects of sublingual tablets of nitrates (failure to dissolve under tongue owing to dry mouth)
- Ranolazine: avoidance of disopyramide advised by manufacturer of ●ranolazine

**Distigmine** *see* Parasympathomimetics

**Disulfiram**
  Alcohol: disulfiram reaction when disulfiram given with alcohol (see p. 280)
  Antibacterials: psychotic reaction reported when disulfiram given with metronidazole
- Anticoagulants: disulfiram enhances anticoagulant effect of ●coumarins
  Antidepressants: increased disulfiram reaction with alcohol reported with concomitant amitriptyline; disulfiram inhibits metabolism of tricyclics (increased plasma concentration)
- Antiepileptics: disulfiram inhibits metabolism of ●phenytoin (increased risk of toxicity)
  Anxiolytics and Hypnotics: disulfiram increases risk of temazepam toxicity; disulfiram inhibits metabolism of benzodiazepines (increased sedative effects)

**Disulfiram** *(continued)*
- Paraldehyde: risk of toxicity when disulfiram given with ●paraldehyde
  Theophylline: disulfiram inhibits metabolism of theophylline (increased risk of toxicity)

**Diuretics**
  Note Since systemic absorption may follow topical application of brinzolamide to the eye, the possibility of interactions should be borne in mind
  Note Since systemic absorption may follow topical application of dorzolamide to the eye, the possibility of interactions should be borne in mind
- ACE Inhibitors: enhanced hypotensive effect when diuretics given with ●ACE inhibitors; increased risk of severe hyperkalaemia when potassium-sparing diuretics and aldosterone antagonists given with ●ACE inhibitors (monitor potassium concentration with low-dose spironolactone in heart failure)
  Adrenergic Neurone Blockers: enhanced hypotensive effect when diuretics given with adrenergic neurone blockers
  Alcohol: enhanced hypotensive effect when diuretics given with alcohol
  Aldesleukin: enhanced hypotensive effect when diuretics given with aldesleukin
  Aliskiren: plasma concentration of furosemide (frusemide) reduced by aliskiren; increased risk of hyperkalaemia when potassium-sparing diuretics and aldosterone antagonists given with aliskiren
  Allopurinol: increased risk of hypersensitivity when thiazides and related diuretics given with allopurinol especially in renal impairment
- Alpha-blockers: enhanced hypotensive effect when diuretics given with ●alpha-blockers, also increased risk of first-dose hypotension with post-synaptic alpha-blockers such as prazosin
  Anaesthetics, General: enhanced hypotensive effect when diuretics given with general anaesthetics
- Analgesics: Diuretic effect of potassium canrenoate possibly antagonised by NSAIDs; possibly increased risk of hyperkalaemia when potassium-sparing diuretics and aldosterone antagonists given with NSAIDs; diuretics increase risk of nephrotoxicity of NSAIDs, also antagonism of diuretic effect; effects of diuretics antagonised by indometacin and ketorolac; increased risk of hyperkalaemia when potassium-sparing diuretics and aldosterone antagonists given with indometacin; occasional reports of reduced renal function when triamterene given with ●indometacin—avoid concomitant use; increased risk of toxicity when carbonic anhydrase inhibitors given with high-dose aspirin; diuretic effect of spironolactone antagonised by aspirin
- Angiotensin-II Receptor Antagonists: enhanced hypotensive effect when diuretics given with ●angiotensin-II receptor antagonists; increased risk of hyperkalaemia when potassium-sparing diuretics and aldosterone antagonists given with ●angiotensin-II receptor antagonists
- Anti-arrhythmics: plasma concentration of eplerenone increased by amiodarone (reduce dose of eplerenone); hypokalaemia caused by acetazolamide, loop diuretics or thiazides and related diuretics increases cardiac toxicity with amiodarone; hypokalaemia caused by acetazolamide, loop diuretics or thiazides and related diuretics increases cardiac toxicity with ●disopyramide; hypokalaemia caused by acetazolamide, loop diuretics or thiazides and related diuretics increases cardiac toxicity with ●flecainide; hypokalaemia caused by acetazolamide, loop diuretics or thiazides and related diuretics antagonises action of ●lidocaine (lignocaine)
- Antibacterials: plasma concentration of eplerenone increased by clarithromycin and ●telithromycin—avoid concomitant use; plasma concentration of eplerenone increased by erythromycin (reduce dose of eplerenone); plasma concentration of eplerenone reduced by ●rifampicin—avoid concomitant use; avoidance of diuretics advised by manufacturer of

**Diuretics**
- Antibacterials *(continued)*
  lymecycline; increased risk of otoxicity when loop diuretics given with ●aminoglycosides, ●polymyxins or ●vancomycin; acetazolamide antagonises effects of ●methenamine; increased risk of hyperkalaemia when eplerenone given with trimethoprim
- Antidepressants: possible increased risk of hypokalaemia when loop diuretics or thiazides and related diuretics given with reboxetine; enhanced hypotensive effect when diuretics given with MAOIs; plasma concentration of eplerenone reduced by ●St John's wort—avoid concomitant use; increased risk of postural hypotension when diuretics given with tricyclics

  Antidiabetics: loop diuretics and thiazides and related diuretics antagonise hypoglycaemic effect of antidiabetics; increased risk of hyponatraemia when thiazides and related diuretics plus potassium-sparing diuretic given with chlorpropamide; increased risk of hyponatraemia when potassium-sparing diuretics and aldosterone antagonists plus thiazide given with chlorpropamide
- Antiepileptics: plasma concentration of eplerenone reduced by ●carbamazepine and ●phenytoin—avoid concomitant use; increased risk of hyponatraemia when diuretics given with carbamazepine; acetazolamide increases plasma concentration of ●carbamazepine; effects of furosemide (frusemide) antagonised by phenytoin; increased risk of osteomalacia when carbonic anhydrase inhibitors given with phenytoin or primidone; acetazolamide possibly reduces plasma concentration of primidone
- Antifungals: plasma concentration of eplerenone increased by ●itraconazole and ●ketoconazole—avoid concomitant use; increased risk of hypokalaemia when loop diuretics or thiazides and related diuretics given with amphotericin; hydrochlorothiazide increases plasma concentration of fluconazole; plasma concentration of eplerenone increased by fluconazole (reduce dose of eplerenone)
- Antipsychotics: hypokalaemia caused by diuretics increases risk of ventricular arrhythmias with ●amisulpride or ●sertindole; enhanced hypotensive effect when diuretics given with phenothiazines; hypokalaemia caused by diuretics increases risk of ventricular arrhythmias with ●pimozide (avoid concomitant use)
- Antivirals: plasma concentration of eplerenone increased by ●nelfinavir and ●ritonavir—avoid concomitant use; plasma concentration of eplerenone increased by saquinavir (reduce dose of eplerenone)

  Anxiolytics and Hypnotics: enhanced hypotensive effect when diuretics given with anxiolytics and hypnotics; administration of parenteral furosemide (frusemide) with chloral or triclofos may displace thyroid hormone from binding sites
- Atomoxetine: hypokalaemia caused by diuretics increases risk of ventricular arrhythmias with ●atomoxetine
- Barbiturates: increased risk of osteomalacia when carbonic anhydrase inhibitors given with phenobarbital; plasma concentration of eplerenone reduced by ●phenobarbital—avoid concomitant use
- Beta-blockers: enhanced hypotensive effect when diuretics given with beta-blockers; hypokalaemia caused by loop diuretics or thiazides and related diuretics increases risk of ventricular arrhythmias with ●sotalol

  Calcium Salts: increased risk of hypercalcaemia when thiazides and related diuretics given with calcium salts

  Calcium-channel Blockers: enhanced hypotensive effect when diuretics given with calcium-channel blockers; plasma concentration of eplerenone increased by diltiazem and verapamil (reduce dose of eplerenone)

**Diuretics** *(continued)*
- Cardiac Glycosides: hypokalaemia caused by acetazolamide, loop diuretics or thiazides and related diuretics increases cardiac toxicity with ●cardiac glycosides; spironolactone possibly affects plasma concentration of digitoxin; spironolactone increases plasma concentration of ●digoxin; potassium canrenoate possibly increases plasma concentration of digoxin
- Ciclosporin: increased risk of nephrotoxicity and possibly hypermagnesaemia when thiazides and related diuretics given with ciclosporin; increased risk of hyperkalaemia when potassium-sparing diuretics and aldosterone antagonists given with ●ciclosporin

  Clonidine: enhanced hypotensive effect when diuretics given with clonidine

  Corticosteroids: diuretic effect of diuretics antagonised by corticosteroids; increased risk of hypokalaemia when acetazolamide, loop diuretics or thiazides and related diuretics given with corticosteroids

  Cytotoxics: avoidance of spironolactone advised by manufacturer of mitotane (antagonism of effect); increased risk of nephrotoxicity and ototoxicity when diuretics given with platinum compounds

  Diazoxide: enhanced hypotensive and hyperglycaemic effects when diuretics given with diazoxide

  Diuretics: increased risk of hypokalaemia when loop diuretics or thiazides and related diuretics given with acetazolamide; profound diuresis possible when metolazone given with furosemide (frusemide); increased risk of hypokalaemia when thiazides and related diuretics given with loop diuretics

  Dopaminergics: enhanced hypotensive effect when diuretics given with levodopa

  Hormone Antagonists: increased risk of hypercalcaemia when thiazides and related diuretics given with toremifene; increased risk of hyperkalaemia when potassium-sparing diuretics and aldosterone antagonists given with trilostane

  Lipid-regulating Drugs: absorption of thiazides and related diuretics reduced by colestipol and colestyramine (give at least 2 hours apart)
- Lithium: loop diuretics and thiazides and related diuretics reduce excretion of ●lithium (increased plasma concentration and risk of toxicity)—loop diuretics safer than thiazides; potassium-sparing diuretics and aldosterone antagonists reduce excretion of ●lithium (increased plasma concentration and risk of toxicity); acetazolamide increases the excretion of ●lithium

  Methyldopa: enhanced hypotensive effect when diuretics given with methyldopa

  Moxisylyte (thymoxamine): enhanced hypotensive effect when diuretics given with moxisylyte

  Moxonidine: enhanced hypotensive effect when diuretics given with moxonidine

  Muscle Relaxants: enhanced hypotensive effect when diuretics given with baclofen or tizanidine

  Nitrates: enhanced hypotensive effect when diuretics given with nitrates

  Oestrogens: diuretic effect of diuretics antagonised by oestrogens
- Potassium Salts: increased risk of hyperkalaemia when potassium-sparing diuretics and aldosterone antagonists given with ●potassium salts

  Progestogens: risk of hyperkalaemia when potassium-sparing diuretics and aldosterone antagonists given with drospirenone (monitor serum potassium during first cycle)

  Prostaglandins: enhanced hypotensive effect when diuretics given with alprostadil

  Sympathomimetics, Beta$_2$: increased risk of hypokalaemia when acetazolamide, loop diuretics or thiazides and related diuretics given with high doses of beta$_2$ sympathomimetics—for CSM advice (hypokalaemia) see p. 155
- Tacrolimus: increased risk of hyperkalaemia when potassium-sparing diuretics and aldosterone antagonists given with ●tacrolimus

**Diuretics** (continued)

Theophylline: increased risk of hypokalaemia when acetazolamide, loop diuretics or thiazides and related diuretics given with theophylline

Vasodilator Antihypertensives: enhanced hypotensive effect when diuretics given with hydralazine, minoxidil or sodium nitroprusside

Vitamins: increased risk of hypercalcaemia when thiazides and related diuretics given with vitamin D

**Diuretics, Loop** see Diuretics

**Diuretics, Potassium-sparing and Aldosterone Antagonists** see Diuretics

**Diuretics, Thiazide and related** see Diuretics

**Dobutamine** see Sympathomimetics

**Docetaxel**

Antibacterials: in vitro studies suggest a possible interaction between docetaxel and erythromycin (consult docetaxel product literature)

Antiepileptics: cytotoxics possibly reduce absorption of phenytoin

Antifungals: in vitro studies suggest a possible interaction between docetaxel and ketoconazole (consult docetaxel product literature)

● Antipsychotics: avoid concomitant use of cytotoxics with ●clozapine (increased risk of agranulocytosis)

Cardiac Glycosides: cytotoxics reduce absorption of digoxin tablets

Ciclosporin: in vitro studies suggest a possible interaction between docetaxel and ciclosporin (consult docetaxel product literature)

Cytotoxics: plasma concentration of docetaxel increased by sorafenib

**Dolasetron** see 5HT$_3$ Antagonists

**Domperidone**

Analgesics: effects of domperidone on gastro-intestinal activity antagonised by opioid analgesics

● Antifungals: risk of arrhythmias with domperidone possibly increased by ●ketoconazole

Antimuscarinics: effects of domperidone on gastro-intestinal activity antagonised by antimuscarinics

Dopaminergics: domperidone possibly antagonises hypoprolactinaemic effects of bromocriptine and cabergoline

**Donepezil** see Parasympathomimetics

**Dopamine** see Sympathomimetics

**Dopaminergics** see Amantadine, Apomorphine, Bromocriptine, Cabergoline, Entacapone, Levodopa, Pergolide, Pramipexole, Quinagolide, Rasagiline, Ropinirole, Rotigotine, Selegiline, and Tolcapone

**Dopexamine** see Sympathomimetics

**Doripenem**

Antiepileptics: doripenem possibly reduces plasma concentration of valproate

Oestrogens: antibacterials that do not induce liver enzymes possibly reduce contraceptive effect of oestrogens (risk probably small, see p. 445)

Probenecid: excretion of doripenem reduced by probenecid (manufacturers of doripenem advise avoid concomitant use)

Vaccines: antibacterials inactivate oral typhoid vaccine–see p. 688

**Dorzolamide** see Diuretics

**Dosulepin (dothiepin)** see Antidepressants, Tricyclic

**Doxapram**

Antidepressants: effects of doxapram enhanced by MAOIs

Sympathomimetics: increased risk of hypertension when doxapram given with sympathomimetics

Theophylline: increased CNS stimulation when doxapram given with theophylline

**Doxazosin** see Alpha-blockers

**Doxepin** see Antidepressants, Tricyclic

**Doxorubicin**

Antiepileptics: cytotoxics possibly reduce absorption of phenytoin

● Antipsychotics: avoid concomitant use of cytotoxics with ●clozapine (increased risk of agranulocytosis)

Antivirals: doxorubicin possibly inhibits effects of stavudine

**Doxorubicin** (continued)

Cardiac Glycosides: cytotoxics reduce absorption of digoxin tablets

● Ciclosporin: increased risk of neurotoxicity when doxorubicin given with ●ciclosporin

Cytotoxics: plasma concentration of doxorubicin possibly increased by sorafenib

**Doxycycline** see Tetracyclines

**Droperidol** see Antipsychotics

**Drospirenone** see Progestogens

**Drotrecogin Alfa**

● Anticoagulants: manufacturer of drotrecogin alfa advises avoid concomitant use with high doses of ●heparin—consult product literature

**Duloxetine**

Analgesics: possible increased serotonergic effects when duloxetine given with pethidine or tramadol

● Antibacterials: metabolism of duloxetine inhibited by ●ciprofloxacin—avoid concomitant use

● Antidepressants: metabolism of duloxetine inhibited by ●fluvoxamine—avoid concomitant use; possible increased serotonergic effects when duloxetine given with SSRIs, St John's wort, amitriptyline, clomipramine, ●moclobemide, tryptophan or venlafaxine; duloxetine should not be started until 2 weeks after stopping ●MAOIs, also MAOIs should not be started until at least 5 days after stopping duloxetine; after stopping SSRI-related antidepressants do not start ●moclobemide for at least 1 week

● Antimalarials: avoidance of antidepressants advised by manufacturer of ●artemether/lumefantrine

Atomoxetine: possible increased risk of convulsions when antidepressants given with atomoxetine

● Hormone Antagonists: duloxetine possibly inhibits metabolism of ●tamoxifen to active metabolite (avoid concomitant use)

5HT$_1$ Agonists: possible increased serotonergic effects when duloxetine given with 5HT$_1$ agonists

● Sibutramine: increased risk of CNS toxicity when SSRI-related antidepressants given with ●sibutramine (manufacturer of sibutramine advises avoid concomitant use)

**Dutasteride**

Calcium-channel Blockers: plasma concentration of dutasteride increased by diltiazem and verapamil

**Dydrogesterone** see Progestogens

**Edrophonium** see Parasympathomimetics

**Efavirenz**

Analgesics: efavirenz reduces plasma concentration of methadone

Antibacterials: increased risk of rash when efavirenz given with clarithromycin; efavirenz reduces plasma concentration of rifabutin—increase dose of rifabutin; plasma concentration of efavirenz reduced by rifampicin—increase dose of efavirenz

● Antidepressants: plasma concentration of efavirenz reduced by ●St John's wort—avoid concomitant use

Antiepileptics: plasma concentration of both drugs reduced when efavirenz given with carbamazepine

● Antifungals: efavirenz reduces plasma concentration of itraconazole and ●posaconazole; efavirenz reduces plasma concentration of ●voriconazole, also plasma concentration of efavirenz increased (increase voriconazole dose and reduce efavirenz dose); efavirenz possibly reduces plasma concentration of caspofungin—consider increasing dose of caspofungin

● Antipsychotics: efavirenz possibly reduces plasma concentration of ●aripiprazole—increase dose of aripiprazole; efavirenz possibly increases plasma concentration of ●pimozide (increased risk of ventricular arrhythmias—avoid concomitant use)

● Antivirals: avoidance of efavirenz advised by manufacturer of ●atazanavir (plasma concentration of atazanavir reduced); efavirenz reduces plasma concentration of darunavir, fosamprenavir and indinavir; efavirenz possibly reduces plasma concentration of ●etravirine—avoid concomitant use; efavirenz reduces plasma concentration of ●lopinavir—consider increasing dose of lopinavir; efavirenz possibly

**Efavirenz**
- Antivirals *(continued)*
  reduces plasma concentration of ●maraviroc—consider increasing dose of maraviroc; plasma concentration of efavirenz reduced by nevirapine; toxicity of efavirenz increased by ritonavir, monitor liver function tests; efavirenz significantly reduces plasma concentration of saquinavir
- Anxiolytics and Hypnotics: increased risk of prolonged sedation when efavirenz given with ●midazolam—avoid concomitant use
  Calcium-channel Blockers: efavirenz reduces plasma concentration of diltiazem
- Ciclosporin: efavirenz possibly reduces plasma concentration of ●ciclosporin
- Ergot Alkaloids: increased risk of ergotism when efavirenz given with ●ergot alkaloids—avoid concomitant use
  Grapefruit Juice: plasma concentration of efavirenz possibly increased by grapefruit juice
  Lipid-regulating Drugs: efavirenz reduces plasma concentration of atorvastatin, pravastatin and simvastatin
  Oestrogens: efavirenz possibly reduces contraceptive effect of oestrogens
- Tacrolimus: efavirenz possibly affects plasma concentration of ●tacrolimus

**Eletriptan** *see* 5HT₁ Agonists

**Emtricitabine**
  Antivirals: manufacturer of emtricitabine advises avoid concomitant use with lamivudine

**Enalapril** *see* ACE Inhibitors

**Enoxaparin** *see* Heparins

**Enoximone** *see* Phosphodiesterase Inhibitors

**Entacapone**
- Anticoagulants: entacapone enhances anticoagulant effect of ●warfarin
- Antidepressants: manufacturer of entacapone advises caution with moclobemide, paroxetine, tricyclics and venlafaxine; avoid concomitant use of entacapone with non-selective ●MAOIs
  Dopaminergics: entacapone possibly enhances effects of apomorphine; entacapone possibly reduces plasma concentration of rasagiline; manufacturer of entacapone advises max. dose of 10 mg selegiline if used concomitantly
  Iron: absorption of entacapone reduced by *oral* iron
  Memantine: effects of dopaminergics possibly enhanced by memantine
  Methyldopa: entacapone possibly enhances effects of methyldopa; antiparkinsonian effect of dopaminergics antagonised by methyldopa
  Sympathomimetics: entacapone possibly enhances effects of adrenaline (epinephrine), dobutamine, dopamine and noradrenaline (norepinephrine)

**Enteral Foods**
- Anticoagulants: the presence of vitamin K in some enteral feeds can antagonise the anticoagulant effect of ●coumarins and ●phenindione
  Antiepileptics: enteral feeds possibly reduce absorption of phenytoin

**Ephedrine** *see* Sympathomimetics

**Epinephrine (adrenaline)** *see* Sympathomimetics

**Epirubicin**
  Antiepileptics: cytotoxics possibly reduce absorption of phenytoin
- Antipsychotics: avoid concomitant use of cytotoxics with ●clozapine (increased risk of agranulocytosis)
  Cardiac Glycosides: cytotoxics reduce absorption of digoxin tablets
- Ulcer-healing Drugs: plasma concentration of epirubicin increased by ●cimetidine

**Eplerenone** *see* Diuretics

**Eprosartan** *see* Angiotensin-II Receptor Antagonists

**Eptifibatide**
  Iloprost: increased risk of bleeding when eptifibatide given with iloprost

**Ergometrine** *see* Ergot Alkaloids

**Ergot Alkaloids**
  Anaesthetics, General: effects of ergometrine on the parturient uterus reduced by halothane
- Antibacterials: increased risk of ergotism when ergotamine and methysergide given with ●macrolides or ●telithromycin—avoid concomitant use; avoidance of ergotamine and methysergide advised by manufacturer of ●quinupristin/dalfopristin; increased risk of ergotism when ergotamine and methysergide given with tetracyclines
  Antidepressants: possible risk of hypertension when ergotamine and methysergide given with reboxetine
- Antifungals: increased risk of ergotism when ergotamine and methysergide given with ●imidazoles or ●triazoles—avoid concomitant use
- Antivirals: plasma concentration of ergot alkaloids possibly increased by ●atazanavir—avoid concomitant use; increased risk of ergotism when ergot alkaloids given with ●efavirenz—avoid concomitant use; increased risk of ergotism when ergotamine and methysergide given with ●fosamprenavir, ●indinavir, ●nelfinavir, ●ritonavir or ●saquinavir—avoid concomitant use
  Beta-blockers: increased peripheral vasoconstriction when ergotamine and methysergide given with beta-blockers
- 5HT₁ Agonists: increased risk of vasospasm when ergotamine and methysergide given with ●almotriptan, ●rizatriptan, ●sumatriptan or ●zolmitriptan (avoid ergotamine and methysergide for 6 hours after almotriptan, rizatriptan, sumatriptan or zolmitriptan, avoid almotriptan, rizatriptan, sumatriptan or zolmitriptan for 24 hours after ergotamine and methysergide); increased risk of vasospasm when ergotamine and methysergide given with ●eletriptan or ●frovatriptan (avoid ergotamine and methysergide for 24 hours after eletriptan or frovatriptan, avoid eletriptan or frovatriptan for 24 hours after ergotamine and methysergide); avoid concomitant use of ergotamine and methysergide with ●naratriptan
  Sympathomimetics: increased risk of ergotism when ergotamine and methysergide given with sympathomimetics
- Ulcer-healing Drugs: increased risk of ergotism when ergotamine and methysergide given with ●cimetidine—avoid concomitant use

**Ergotamine and Methysergide** *see* Ergot Alkaloids

**Erlotinib**
- Analgesics: increased risk of bleeding when erlotinib given with ●NSAIDs
  Antibacterials: metabolism of erlotinib accelerated by rifampicin (reduced plasma concentration)
- Anticoagulants: increased risk of bleeding when erlotinib given with ●coumarins
  Antiepileptics: cytotoxics possibly reduce absorption of phenytoin
  Antifungals: metabolism of erlotinib inhibited by ketoconazole (increased plasma concentration)
- Antipsychotics: avoid concomitant use of cytotoxics with ●clozapine (increased risk of agranulocytosis)
  Cardiac Glycosides: cytotoxics reduce absorption of digoxin tablets
  Cytotoxics: plasma concentration of erlotinib possibly increased by capecitabine
  Tobacco: plasma concentration of erlotinib reduced by tobacco smoking

**Ertapenem**
  Antiepileptics: ertapenem possibly reduces plasma concentration of valproate
  Oestrogens: antibacterials that do not induce liver enzymes possibly reduce contraceptive effect of oestrogens (risk probably small, see p. 445)
  Vaccines: antibacterials inactivate oral typhoid vaccine—see p. 688

**Erythromycin** *see* Macrolides

**Escitalopram** *see* Antidepressants, SSRI

**Esmolol** *see* Beta-blockers

**Esomeprazole** *see* Proton Pump Inhibitors

Estradiol *see* Oestrogens

Estramustine

Antiepileptics: cytotoxics possibly reduce absorption of phenytoin
- Antipsychotics: avoid concomitant use of cytotoxics with ●clozapine (increased risk of agranulocytosis)
- Bisphosphonates: plasma concentration of estramustine increased by ●sodium clodronate

Cardiac Glycosides: cytotoxics reduce absorption of digoxin tablets

Estriol *see* Oestrogens

Estrone *see* Oestrogens

Estropipate *see* Oestrogens

Etanercept

Abatacept: increased risk of side-effects when etanercept given with abatacept
- Anakinra: increased risk of side-effects when etanercept given with ●anakinra—avoid concomitant use
- Vaccines: avoid concomitant use of etanercept with live ●vaccines (see p. 669)

Ethinylestradiol *see* Oestrogens

Ethosuximide
- Antibacterials: metabolism of ethosuximide inhibited by ●isoniazid (increased plasma concentration and risk of toxicity)
- Antidepressants: anticonvulsant effect of antiepileptics possibly antagonised by MAOIs and ●tricyclic-related antidepressants (convulsive threshold lowered); anticonvulsant effect of antiepileptics antagonised by ●SSRIs and ●tricyclics (convulsive threshold lowered); avoid concomitant use of antiepileptics with ●St John's wort
- Antiepileptics: plasma concentration of ethosuximide possibly reduced by carbamazepine and primidone; plasma concentration of ethosuximide possibly reduced by ●phenytoin, also plasma concentration of phenytoin possibly increased; plasma concentration of ethosuximide possibly increased by valproate
- Antimalarials: possible increased risk of convulsions when antiepileptics given with chloroquine and hydroxychloroquine; anticonvulsant effect of antiepileptics antagonised by ●mefloquine
- Antipsychotics: anticonvulsant effect of ethosuximide antagonised by ●antipsychotics (convulsive threshold lowered)

Barbiturates: plasma concentration of ethosuximide possibly reduced by phenobarbital

Etodolac *see* NSAIDs

Etomidate *see* Anaesthetics, General

Etonogestrel *see* Progestogens

Etoposide
- Anticoagulant: etoposide possibly enhances anticoagulant effect of ●coumarins

Antiepileptics: plasma concentration of etoposide possibly reduced by phenytoin; cytotoxics possibly reduce absorption of phenytoin
- Antipsychotics: avoid concomitant use of cytotoxics with ●clozapine (increased risk of agranulocytosis)

Barbiturates: plasma concentration of etoposide possibly reduced by phenobarbital

Cardiac Glycosides: cytotoxics reduce absorption of digoxin tablets

Ciclosporin: plasma concentration of etoposide possibly increased by ciclosporin (increased risk of toxicity)

Etoricoxib *see* NSAIDs

Etravirine
- Antibacterials: plasma concentration of etravirine increased by ●clarithromycin, also plasma concentration of clarithromycin reduced; plasma concentration of both drugs reduced when etravirine given with ●rifabutin; manufacturer of etravirine advises avoid concomitant use with rifampicin

Antidepressants: manufacturer of etravirine advises avoid concomitant use with St John's wort

Antiepileptics: manufacturer of etravirine advises avoid concomitant use with carbamazepine and phenytoin

Etravirine *(continued)*
- Antivirals: plasma concentration of etravirine possibly reduced by ●efavirenz and ●nevirapine—avoid concomitant use; etravirine increases plasma concentration of ●fosamprenavir (consider reducing dose of fosamprenavir); etravirine possibly reduces plasma concentration of ●indinavir—avoid concomitant use; etravirine possibly reduces plasma concentration of maraviroc; etravirine possibly increases plasma concentration of nelfinavir—avoid concomitant use; plasma concentration of etravirine reduced by ●tipranavir, also plasma concentration of tipranavir increased (avoid concomitant use)

Barbiturates: manufacturer of etravirine advises avoid concomitant use with phenobarbital

Cardiac Glycosides: etravirine increases plasma concentration of digoxin

Lipid-regulating Drugs: etravirine possibly reduces plasma concentration of atorvastatin

Sildenafil: etravirine reduces plasma concentration of sildenafil

Etynodiol *see* Progestogens

Exemestane

Antibacterials: plasma concentration of exemestane possibly reduced by rifampicin

Ezetimibe

Anticoagulants: ezetimibe possibly enhances anticoagulant effect of coumarins
- Ciclosporin: plasma concentration of both drugs may increase when ezetimibe given with ●ciclosporin

Lipid-regulating Drugs: increased risk of cholelithiasis and gallbladder disease when ezetimibe given with fibrates—discontinue if suspected

Famciclovir

Probenecid: excretion of famciclovir possibly reduced by probenecid (increased plasma concentration)

Famotidine *see* Histamine H₂-antagonists

Felodipine *see* Calcium-channel Blockers

Fenbufen *see* NSAIDs

Fenofibrate *see* Fibrates

Fenoprofen *see* NSAIDs

Fenoterol *see* Sympathomimetics, Beta₂

Fentanyl *see* Opioid Analgesics

Ferrous Salts *see* Iron

Fesoterodine *see* Antimuscarinics

Fexofenadine *see* Antihistamines

Fibrates
- Antibacterials: increased risk of myopathy when fibrates given with ●daptomycin (preferably avoid concomitant use)
- Anticoagulants: fibrates enhance anticoagulant effect of ●coumarins and ●phenindione
- Antidiabetics: gemfibrozil increases plasma concentration of ●rosiglitazone (consider reducing dose of rosiglitazone); fibrates may improve glucose tolerance and have an additive effect with insulin or sulphonylureas; gemfibrozil possibly enhances hypoglycaemic effect of nateglinide; increased risk of severe hypoglycaemia when gemfibrozil given with ●repaglinide—avoid concomitant use

Ciclosporin: increased risk of renal impairment when bezafibrate or fenofibrate given with ciclosporin
- Cytotoxics: gemfibrozil increases plasma concentration of ●bexarotene—avoid concomitant use
- Lipid-regulating Drugs: increased risk of cholelithiasis and gallbladder disaese when fibrates given with ezetimibe—discontinue if suspected; increased risk of myopathy when fibrates given with ●statins; increased risk of myopathy when gemfibrozil given with ●statins (preferably avoid concomitant use)

Filgrastim

Note Pegfilgrastim interactions as for filgrastim

Cytotoxics: neutropenia possibly exacerbated when filgrastim given with fluorouracil

Flavoxate *see* Antimuscarinics

Flecainide

Anaesthetics, Local: increased myocardial depression when anti-arrhythmics given with bupivacaine, levo-bupivacaine, prilocaine or ropivacaine

**Flecainide** *(continued)*

- Anti-arrhythmics: increased myocardial depression when anti-arrhythmics given with other ●anti-arrhythmics; plasma concentration of flecainide increased by ●amiodarone (halve dose of flecainide)
- Antidepressants: plasma concentration of flecainide increased by fluoxetine; increased risk of ventricular arrhythmias when flecainide given with ●tricyclics
- Antihistamines: increased risk of ventricular arrhythmias when flecainide given with ●mizolastine—avoid concomitant use
- Antimalarials: avoidance of flecainide advised by manufacturer of ●artemether/lumefantrine (risk of ventricular arrhythmias); plasma concentration of flecainide increased by ●quinine
- Antimuscarinics: increased risk of ventricular arrhythmias when flecainide given with ●tolterodine
- Antipsychotics: increased risk of ventricular arrhythmias when anti-arrhythmics that prolong the QT interval given with ●antipsychotics that prolong the QT interval; increased risk of arrhythmias when flecainide given with ●clozapine
- Antivirals: plasma concentration of flecainide possibly increased by ●fosamprenavir, ●indinavir, ●lopinavir and ●ritonavir (increased risk of ventricular arrhythmias—avoid concomitant use)
- Beta-blockers: increased risk of myocardial depression and bradycardia when flecainide given with ●beta-blockers; increased myocardial depression when anti-arrhythmics given with ●beta-blockers
- Calcium-channel Blockers: increased risk of myocardial depression and asystole when flecainide given with ●verapamil
- Diuretics: increased cardiac toxicity with flecainide if hypokalaemia occurs with ●acetazolamide, ●loop diuretics or ●thiazides and related diuretics
- 5HT₃ Antagonists: increased risk of ventricular arrhythmias when flecainide given with ●dolasetron—avoid concomitant use

   Ulcer-healing Drugs: metabolism of flecainide inhibited by cimetidine (increased plasma concentration)

**Flucloxacillin** *see* Penicillins

**Fluconazole** *see* Antifungals, Triazole

**Flucytosine**

   Antifungals: renal excretion of flucytosine decreased and cellular uptake increased by amphotericin (toxicity possibly increased)

   Cytotoxics: plasma concentration of flucytosine possibly reduced by cytarabine

**Fludarabine**

   Antiepileptics: cytotoxics possibly reduce absorption of phenytoin

- Antipsychotics: avoid concomitant use of cytotoxics with ●clozapine (increased risk of agranulocytosis)

   Cardiac Glycosides: cytotoxics reduce absorption of digoxin tablets

- Cytotoxics: fludarabine increases intracellular concentration of cytarabine; increased pulmonary toxicity when fludarabine given with ●pentostatin (unacceptably high incidence of fatalities)

   Dipyridamole: effects of fludarabine possibly reduced by dipyridamole

**Fludrocortisone** *see* Corticosteroids

**Flunisolide** *see* Corticosteroids

**Fluorides**

   Calcium Salts: absorption of fluorides reduced by calcium salts

**Fluorouracil**

   Note  Capecitabine is a prodrug of fluorouracil

   Note  Tegafur is a prodrug of fluorouracil

- Allopurinol: manufacturer of capecitabine advises avoid concomitant use with ●allopurinol

   Antibacterials: metabolism of fluorouracil inhibited by metronidazole (increased toxicity)

- Anticoagulants: fluorouracil enhances anticoagulant effect of ●coumarins

   Antiepileptics: fluorouracil possibly inhibits metabolism of phenytoin (increased risk of toxicity); cytotoxics possibly reduce absorption of phenytoin

**Fluorouracil** *(continued)*

- Antipsychotics: avoid concomitant use of cytotoxics with ●clozapine (increased risk of agranulocytosis)

   Cardiac Glycosides: cytotoxics reduce absorption of digoxin tablets

   Cytotoxics: capecitabine possibly increases plasma concentration of erlotinib

   Filgrastim: neutropenia possibly exacerbated when fluorouracil given with filgrastim

- Temoporfin: increased skin photosensitivity when topical fluorouracil used with ●temoporfin

   Ulcer-healing Drugs: metabolism of fluorouracil inhibited by cimetidine (increased plasma concentration)

**Fluoxetine** *see* Antidepressants, SSRI

**Flupentixol** *see* Antipsychotics

**Fluphenazine** *see* Antipsychotics

**Flurazepam** *see* Anxiolytics and Hypnotics

**Flurbiprofen** *see* NSAIDs

**Flutamide**

- Anticoagulants: flutamide enhances anticoagulant effect of ●coumarins

**Fluticasone** *see* Corticosteroids

**Fluvastatin** *see* Statins

**Fluvoxamine** *see* Antidepressants, SSRI

**Folates**

   Aminosalicylates: absorption of folic acid possibly reduced by sulfasalazine

   Antiepileptics: folates possibly reduce plasma concentration of phenytoin and primidone

   Barbiturates: folates possibly reduce plasma concentration of phenobarbital

**Folic Acid** *see* Folates

**Folinic Acid** *see* Folates

**Formoterol (eformoterol)** *see* Sympathomimetics, Beta₂

**Fosamprenavir**

   Note  Fosamprenavir is a prodrug of amprenavir

   Analgesics: fosamprenavir reduces plasma concentration of methadone

   Antacids: absorption of fosamprenavir possibly reduced by antacids

- Anti-arrhythmics: fosamprenavir possibly increases plasma concentration of ●amiodarone, ●flecainide and ●propafenone (increased risk of ventricular arrhythmias—avoid concomitant use); fosamprenavir possibly increases plasma concentration of ●lidocaine (lignocaine)—avoid concomitant use

- Antibacterials: plasma concentration of both drugs increased when fosamprenavir given with erythromycin; fosamprenavir increases plasma concentration of ●rifabutin (reduce dose of rifabutin); plasma concentration of fosamprenavir significantly reduced by ●rifampicin—avoid concomitant use; fosamprenavir possibly increases plasma concentration of dapsone; avoidance of concomitant fosamprenavir in severe renal and hepatic impairment advised by manufacturer of ●telithromycin

   Anticoagulants: fosamprenavir may enhance or reduce anticoagulant effect of coumarins; avoidance of fosamprenavir advised by manufacturer of rivaroxaban

- Antidepressants: plasma concentration of fosamprenavir reduced by ●St John's wort—avoid concomitant use; fosamprenavir possibly increases side-effects of tricyclics

   Antiepileptics: plasma concentration of fosamprenavir possibly reduced by carbamazepine and phenytoin

   Antifungals: fosamprenavir increases plasma concentration of ketoconazole; fosamprenavir possibly increases plasma concentration of itraconazole

   Antihistamines: fosamprenavir possibly increases plasma concentration of loratadine

   Antimalarials: caution with fosamprenavir advised by manufacturer of artemether/lumefantrine

   Antimuscarinics: avoidance of fosamprenavir advised by manufacturer of darifenacin and tolterodine

- Antipsychotics: fosamprenavir possibly inhibits metabolism of ●aripiprazole (reduce dose of aripi-

**Fosamprenavir**
- Antipsychotics *(continued)*
  prazole); fosamprenavir possibly increases
  plasma concentration of clozapine; fosamprenavir increases plasma concentration of
  ●pimozide and ●sertindole (increased risk of
  ventricular arrhythmias—avoid concomitant use)
- Antivirals: plasma concentration of fosamprenavir
  reduced by efavirenz and ●tipranavir; plasma concentration of fosamprenavir increased by ●etravirine
  (consider reducing dose of fosamprenavir); plasma
  concentration of fosamprenavir reduced by lopinavir,
  effect on lopinavir plasma concentration not predictable—avoid concomitant use; plasma concentration of fosamprenavir possibly reduced by nevirapine
- Anxiolytics and Hypnotics: increased risk of prolonged
  sedation and respiratory depression when fosamprenavir given with ●alprazolam, clonazepam,
  ●diazepam, ●flurazepam or ●midazolam
  Barbiturates: plasma concentration of fosamprenavir
  possibly reduced by phenobarbital
- Cilostazol: fosamprenavir possibly increases plasma
  concentration of ●cilostazol—avoid concomitant use
- Ergot Alkaloids: increased risk of ergotism when
  fosamprenavir given with ●ergotamine and methysergide—avoid concomitant use
- Lipid-regulating Drugs: possible increased risk of
  myopathy when fosamprenavir given with atorvastatin; possible increased risk of myopathy when
  fosamprenavir given with ●rosuvastatin or
  ●simvastatin—avoid concomitant use
  Oestrogens: fosamprenavir increases plasma concentration of oestrogens, also plasma concentration of
  fosamprenavir reduced—alternative contraception
  recommended
  Progestogens: fosamprenavir increases plasma concentration of progestogens, also plasma concentration of fosamprenavir reduced—alternative
  contraception recommended
- Ranolazine: fosamprenavir possibly increases plasma
  concentration of ●ranolazine—manufacturer of
  ranolazine advises avoid concomitant use
  Sildenafil: fosamprenavir possibly increases plasma
  concentration of sildenafil—reduce initial dose of
  sildenafil
  Tadalafil: fosamprenavir possibly increases plasma
  concentration of tadalafil
  Ulcer-healing Drugs: fosamprenavir possibly increases
  plasma concentration of cimetidine
  Vardenafil: fosamprenavir possibly increases plasma
  concentration of vardenafil
**Fosaprepitant** *see* Aprepitant
**Foscarnet**
  Antivirals: avoidance of foscarnet advised by manu-
  facturer of lamivudine
**Fosinopril** *see* ACE Inhibitors
**Fosphenytoin** *see* Phenytoin
**Framycetin** *see* Aminoglycosides
**Frovatriptan** *see* 5HT$_1$ Agonists
**Furosemide (frusemide)** *see* Diuretics
**Fusidic Acid**
- Antivirals: plasma concentration of both drugs
  increased when fusidic acid given with ●ritonavir—
  avoid concomitant use
- Lipid-regulating Drugs: possible increased risk of
  myopathy when fusidic acid given with atorvastatin;
  increased risk of myopathy when fusidic acid given
  with ●simvastatin
  Oestrogens: antibacterials that do not induce liver
  enzymes possibly reduce contraceptive effect of
  oestrogens (risk probably small, see p. 445)
  Sugammadex: fusidic acid possibly reduces response
  to sugammadex
  Vaccines: antibacterials inactivate oral typhoid
  vaccine—see p. 688
**Gabapentin**
  Analgesics: bioavailability of gabapentin increased by
  morphine

**Gabapentin** *(continued)*
  Antacids: absorption of gabapentin reduced by
  antacids
- Antidepressants: anticonvulsant effect of antiepileptics
  possibly antagonised by MAOIs and ●tricyclic-related
  antidepressants (convulsive threshold lowered); anticonvulsant effect of antiepileptics antagonised by
  ●SSRIs and ●tricyclics (convulsive threshold
  lowered); avoid concomitant use of antiepileptics
  with ●St John's wort
- Antimalarials: possible increased risk of convulsions
  when antiepileptics given with chloroquine and
  hydroxychloroquine; anticonvulsant effect of antiepileptics antagonised by ●mefloquine
**Galantamine** *see* Parasympathomimetics
**Ganciclovir**
  Note Increased risk of myelosuppression with other myelosuppressive drugs—consult product literature
  Note Valganciclovir interactions as for ganciclovir
- Antibacterials: increased risk of convulsions when
  ganciclovir given with ●imipenem with cilastatin
- Antivirals: ganciclovir possibly increases plasma concentration of didanosine; avoidance of intravenous
  ganciclovir advised by manufacturer of lamivudine;
  profound myelosuppression when ganciclovir given
  with ●zidovudine (if possible avoid concomitant
  administration, particularly during initial ganciclovir
  therapy)
  Mycophenolate: plasma concentration of ganciclovir
  possibly increased by mycophenolate, also plasma
  concentration of inactive metabolite of mycophenolate possibly increased
  Probenecid: excretion of ganciclovir reduced by probenecid (increased plasma concentration and risk of
  toxicity)
  Tacrolimus: possible increased risk of nephrotoxicity
  when ganciclovir given with tacrolimus
**Gemcitabine**
  Anticoagulants: gemcitabine possibly enhances anti-
  coagulant effect of warfarin
  Antiepileptics: cytotoxics possibly reduce absorption
  of phenytoin
- Antipsychotics: avoid concomitant use of cytotoxics
  with ●clozapine (increased risk of agranulocytosis)
  Cardiac Glycosides: cytotoxics reduce absorption of
  digoxin tablets
**Gemeprost** *see* Prostaglandins
**Gemfibrozil** *see* Fibrates
**Gentamicin** *see* Aminoglycosides
**Gestodene** *see* Progestogens
**Gestrinone**
  Antibacterials: metabolism of gestrinone accelerated
  by rifampicin (reduced plasma concentration)
  Antiepileptics: metabolism of gestrinone accelerated
  by carbamazepine, phenytoin and primidone
  (reduced plasma concentration)
  Barbiturates: metabolism of gestrinone accelerated by
  barbiturates (reduced plasma concentration)
**Glibenclamide** *see* Antidiabetics
**Gliclazide** *see* Antidiabetics
**Glimepiride** *see* Antidiabetics
**Glipizide** *see* Antidiabetics
**Glucosamine**
- Anticoagulants: glucosamine enhances anticoagulant
  effect of ●warfarin (avoid concomitant use)
**Glyceryl Trinitrate** *see* Nitrates
**Glycopyrronium** *see* Antimuscarinics
**Gold**
  Penicillamine: avoidance of gold advised by manu-
  facturer of penicillamine (increased risk of toxicity)
**Grapefruit Juice**
  Anti-arrhythmics: grapefruit juice increases plasma
  concentration of amiodarone
  Antimalarials: grapefruit juice possibly increases
  plasma concentration of artemether/lumefantrine
  Antivirals: grapefruit juice possibly increases plasma
  concentration of efavirenz
  Anxiolytics and Hypnotics: grapefruit juice increases
  plasma concentration of buspirone

**Grapefruit Juice** *(continued)*

Calcium-channel Blockers: grapefruit juice increases plasma concentration of felodipine, isradipine, lacidipine, lercanidipine, nicardipine, nifedipine, nimodipine and verapamil

- Ciclosporin: grapefruit juice increases plasma concentration of ●ciclosporin (increased risk of toxicity)
- Cytotoxics: avoidance of grapefruit juice advised by manufacturer of ●lapatinib and ●nilotinib

Ivabradine: grapefruit juice increases plasma concentration of ivabradine

- Lipid-regulating Drugs: grapefruit juice possibly increases plasma concentration of atorvastatin; grapefruit juice increases plasma concentration of ●simvastatin—avoid concomitant use
- Ranolazine: grapefruit juice possibly increases plasma concentration of ●ranolazine—manufacturer of ranolazine advises avoid concomitant use

Sildenafil: grapefruit juice possibly increases plasma concentration of sildenafil

- Sirolimus: grapefruit juice increases plasma concentration of ●sirolimus—avoid concomitant use
- Tacrolimus: grapefruit juice increases plasma concentration of ●tacrolimus

Tadalafil: grapefruit juice possibly increases plasma concentration of tadalafil

- Vardenafil: grapefruit juice possibly increases plasma concentration of ●vardenafil—avoid concomitant use

**Griseofulvin**

Alcohol: griseofulvin possibly enhances effects of alcohol

- Anticoagulants: griseofulvin reduces anticoagulant effect of ●coumarins

Antiepileptics: absorption of griseofulvin reduced by primidone (reduced effect)

Barbiturates: absorption of griseofulvin reduced by phenobarbital (reduced effect)

Ciclosporin: griseofulvin possibly reduces plasma concentration of ciclosporin

- Oestrogens: griseofulvin accelerates metabolism of ●oestrogens (reduced contraceptive effect—see p. 445)
- Progestogens: griseofulvin accelerates metabolism of ●progestogens (reduced contraceptive effect—see p. 445)

**Guanethidine** *see* Adrenergic Neurone Blockers

**Haloperidol** *see* Antipsychotics

**Halothane** *see* Anaesthetics, General

**Heparin** *see* Heparins

**Heparins**

ACE Inhibitors: increased risk of hyperkalaemia when heparins given with ACE inhibitors

Aliskiren: increased risk of hyperkalaemia when heparins given with aliskiren

- Analgesics: possible increased risk of bleeding when heparins given with NSAIDs; increased risk of haemorrhage when anticoagulants given with intravenous ●diclofenac (avoid concomitant use, including low-dose heparin); increased risk of haemorrhage when anticoagulants given with ●ketorolac (avoid concomitant use, including low-dose heparin); anticoagulant effect of heparins enhanced by ●aspirin

Angiotensin-II Receptor Antagonists: increased risk of hyperkalaemia when heparin given with angiotensin-II receptor antagonists

Clopidogrel: increased risk of bleeding when heparins given with clopidogrel

Dipyridamole: anticoagulant effect of heparins enhanced by dipyridamole

- Drotrecogin Alfa: avoidance of concomitant use of high doses of heparin with drotrecogin alfa advised by manufacturer of ●drotrecogin alfa—consult product literature

Iloprost: anticoagulant effect of heparins possibly enhanced by iloprost

- Nitrates: anticoagulant effect of heparins reduced by infusion of ●glyceryl trinitrate

Sibutramine: increased risk of bleeding when anticoagulants given with sibutramine

**Histamine H₂-antagonists**

- Alpha-blockers: cimetidine and ranitidine antagonise effects of ●tolazoline

Analgesics: cimetidine possibly increases plasma concentration of azapropazone; cimetidine inhibits metabolism of opioid analgesics (increased plasma concentration)

- Anti-arrhythmics: cimetidine increases plasma concentration of amiodarone and ●propafenone; cimetidine inhibits metabolism of flecainide (increased plasma concentration); cimetidine increases plasma concentration of ●lidocaine (lignocaine) (increased risk of toxicity)

Antibacterials: histamine H₂-antagonists reduce absorption of cefpodoxime; cimetidine increases plasma concentration of erythromycin (increased risk of toxicity, including deafness); cimetidine inhibits metabolism of metronidazole (increased plasma concentration); metabolism of cimetidine accelerated by rifampicin (reduced plasma concentration)

- Anticoagulants: cimetidine inhibits metabolism of ●coumarins (enhanced anticoagulant effect)

Antidepressants: cimetidine increases plasma concentration of citalopram, escitalopram, mirtazapine and sertraline; cimetidine inhibits metabolism of amitriptyline, doxepin, imipramine and nortriptyline (increased plasma concentration); cimetidine increases plasma concentration of moclobemide (halve dose of moclobemide); cimetidine possibly increases plasma concentration of tricyclics

Antidiabetics: cimetidine reduces excretion of metformin (increased plasma concentration); cimetidine enhances hypoglycaemic effect of sulphonylureas

- Antiepileptics: cimetidine inhibits metabolism of ●carbamazepine, ●phenytoin and ●valproate (increased plasma concentration)
- Antifungals: histamine H₂-antagonists reduce absorption of itraconazole and ketoconazole; cimetidine reduces plasma concentration of ●posaconazole; cimetidine increases plasma concentration of terbinafine

Antihistamines: manufacturer of loratadine advises cimetidine possibly increases plasma concentration of loratadine

- Antimalarials: avoidance of cimetidine advised by manufacturer of ●artemether/lumefantrine; cimetidine inhibits metabolism of chloroquine and hydroxychloroquine and quinine (increased plasma concentration)
- Antipsychotics: cimetidine possibly enhances effects of antipsychotics, chlorpromazine and clozapine; increased risk of ventricular arrhythmias when cimetidine given with ●sertindole—avoid concomitant use
- Antivirals: histamine H₂-antagonists possibly reduce plasma concentration of atazanavir; plasma concentration of cimetidine possibly increased by fosamprenavir; histamine H₂-antagonists possibly increase plasma concentration of raltegravir—manufacturer of raltegravir advises avoid concomitant use; cimetidine possibly increases plasma concentration of saquinavir

Anxiolytics and Hypnotics: cimetidine inhibits metabolism of benzodiazepines, clomethiazole and zaleplon (increased plasma concentration); cimetidine increases plasma concentration of melatonin

Beta-blockers: cimetidine increases plasma concentration of labetalol, metoprolol and propranolol

Calcium-channel Blockers: cimetidine possibly inhibits metabolism of calcium-channel blockers (increased plasma concentration); cimetidine increases plasma concentration of isradipine (halve dose of isradipine)

- Ciclosporin: cimetidine possibly increases plasma concentration of ●ciclosporin
- Cilostazol: cimetidine possibly increases plasma concentration of ●cilostazol—avoid concomitant use
- Cytotoxics: cimetidine possibly enhances myelosuppressive effects of carmustine and lomustine; cime-

**Histamine H₂-antagonists**
● <u>Cytotoxics</u> *(continued)*
tidine increases plasma concentration of
●epirubicin; cimetidine inhibits metabolism of
fluorouracil (increased plasma concentration);
famotidine possibly reduces plasma concentration of dasatinib; histamine H₂-antagonists possibly reduce absorption of lapatinib; avoidance of
histamine H₂-antagonists advised by manufacturer of nilotinib
Dopaminergics: cimetidine reduces excretion of pramipexole (increased plasma concentration)
● Ergot Alkaloids: increased risk of ergotism when
cimetidine given with ●ergotamine and methysergide—avoid concomitant use
Hormone Antagonists: absorption of cimetidine possibly delayed by octreotide
5HT₁ Agonists: cimetidine inhibits metabolism of
zolmitriptan (reduce dose of zolmitriptan)
Mebendazole: cimetidine possibly inhibits metabolism
of mebendazole (increased plasma concentration)
Sildenafil: cimetidine increases plasma concentration
of sildenafil (reduce initial dose of sildenafil)
● Theophylline: cimetidine inhibits metabolism of
●theophylline (increased plasma concentration)
Thyroid Hormones: cimetidine reduces absorption of
levothyroxine (thyroxine)
**Homatropine** *see* Antimuscarinics
**Hormone Antagonists** *see* Bicalutamide, Danazol, Dutasteride, Exemestane, Flutamide, Gestrinone, Lanreotide,
Octreotide, Tamoxifen, Toremifene, and Trilostane
**5HT₁ Agonists**
● Antibacterials: plasma concentration of eletriptan
increased by ●clarithromycin and ●erythromycin (risk
of toxicity)—avoid concomitant use; metabolism of
zolmitriptan possibly inhibited by quinolones (reduce
dose of zolmitriptan)
● Antidepressants: increased risk of CNS toxicity when
sumatriptan given with ●citalopram, ●escitalopram,
●fluoxetine, ●fluvoxamine or ●paroxetine; metabolism of frovatriptan inhibited by fluvoxamine;
metabolism of zolmitriptan possibly inhibited by
fluvoxamine (reduce dose of zolmitriptan); increased
risk of CNS toxicity when sumatriptan given with
●sertraline (manufacturer of sertraline advises avoid
concomitant use); possible increased serotonergic
effects when 5HT₁ agonists given with duloxetine;
risk of CNS toxicity when rizatriptan or sumatriptan
given with ●MAOIs (avoid rizatriptan or sumatriptan
for 2 weeks after MAOIs); increased risk of CNS
toxicity when zolmitriptan given with ●MAOIs; risk of
CNS toxicity when rizatriptan or sumatriptan given
with ●moclobemide (avoid rizatriptan or sumatriptan
for 2 weeks after moclobemide); risk of CNS toxicity
when zolmitriptan given with ●moclobemide (reduce
dose of zolmitriptan); possible increased serotonergic
effects when frovatriptan given with SSRIs; increased
serotonergic effects when 5HT₁ agonists given with
●St John's wort—avoid concomitant use
● Antifungals: plasma concentration of eletriptan
increased by ●itraconazole and ●ketoconazole (risk of
toxicity)—avoid concomitant use; plasma concentration of almotriptan increased by ketoconazole
(increased risk of toxicity)
● Antivirals: plasma concentration of eletriptan increased
by ●indinavir, ●nelfinavir and ●ritonavir (risk of
toxicity)—avoid concomitant use
Beta-blockers: plasma concentration of rizatriptan
increased by propranolol (manufacturer of rizatriptan
advises halve dose and avoid within 2 hours of
propranolol)
● <u>Ergot Alkaloids</u>: increased risk of vasospasm when
almotriptan, rizatriptan, sumatriptan or zolmitriptan
given with ●ergotamine and methysergide (avoid
ergotamine and methysergide for 6 hours after
almotriptan, rizatriptan, sumatriptan or zolmitriptan,
avoid almotriptan, rizatriptan, sumatriptan or zolmitriptan for 24 hours after ergotamine and methy-

**5HT₁ Agonists**
● <u>Ergot Alkaloids</u> *(continued)*
sergide); avoid concomitant use of naratriptan
with ●ergotamine and methysergide; increased
risk of vasospasm when eletriptan or frovatriptan
given with ●ergotamine and methysergide (avoid
ergotamine and methysergide for 24 hours after
eletriptan or frovatriptan, avoid eletriptan or
frovatriptan for 24 hours after ergotamine and
methysergide)
Ulcer-healing Drugs: metabolism of zolmitriptan
inhibited by cimetidine (reduce dose of zolmitriptan)
**5HT₃ Antagonists**
Analgesics: ondansetron possibly antagonises effects
of tramadol
● Anti-arrhythmics: increased risk of ventricular arrhythmias when dolasetron given with ●amiodarone,
●disopyramide, ●flecainide, ●lidocaine (lignocaine) or
●propafenone—avoid concomitant use
Antibacterials: metabolism of ondansetron accelerated
by rifampicin (reduced effect)
Antiepileptics: metabolism of ondansetron accelerated
by carbamazepine and phenytoin (reduced effect)
● Beta-blockers: increased risk of ventricular arrhyth-
mias when dolasetron given with ●sotalol—avoid
concomitant use
**Hydralazine** *see* Vasodilator Antihypertensives
**Hydrochlorothiazide** *see* Diuretics
**Hydrocortisone** *see* Corticosteroids
**Hydroflumethiazide** *see* Diuretics
**Hydromorphone** *see* Opioid Analgesics
**Hydrotalcite** *see* Antacids
**Hydroxocobalamin**
Antibacterials: response to hydroxocobalamin reduced
by chloramphenicol
**Hydroxycarbamide**
Antiepileptics: cytotoxics possibly reduce absorption
of phenytoin
● Antipsychotics: avoid concomitant use of cytotoxics
with ●clozapine (increased risk of agranulocytosis)
● Antivirals: increased risk of toxicity when hydroxycar-
bamide given with ●didanosine and ●stavudine—
avoid concomitant use
Cardiac Glycosides: cytotoxics reduce absorption of
digoxin tablets
**Hydroxychloroquine** *see* Chloroquine and Hydroxychloro-
quine
**Hydroxyzine** *see* Antihistamines
**Hyoscine** *see* Antimuscarinics
**Ibandronic Acid** *see* Bisphosphonates
**Ibuprofen** *see* NSAIDs
**Ifosfamide**
● Anticoagulants: ifosfamide possibly enhances anti-
coagulant effect of ●coumarins
Antiepileptics: cytotoxics possibly reduce absorption
of phenytoin
● Antipsychotics: avoid concomitant use of cytotoxics
with ●clozapine (increased risk of agranulocytosis)
Cardiac Glycosides: cytotoxics reduce absorption of
digoxin tablets
**Iloprost**
Analgesics: increased risk of bleeding when iloprost
given with NSAIDs or aspirin
Anticoagulants: iloprost possibly enhances anti-
coagulant effect of coumarins and heparins;
increased risk of bleeding when iloprost given with
phenindione
Clopidogrel: increased risk of bleeding when iloprost
given with clopidogrel
Eptifibatide: increased risk of bleeding when iloprost
given with eptifibatide
Tirofiban: increased risk of bleeding when iloprost
given with tirofiban
**Imatinib**
● Antibacterials: plasma concentration of imatinib
reduced by ●rifampicin—avoid concomitant use

**Imatinib** *(continued)*

Anticoagulants: manufacturer of imatinib advises replacement of warfarin with a heparin (possibility of enhanced warfarin effect)

● Antidepressants: plasma concentration of imatinib reduced by ●St John's wort—avoid concomitant use

● Antiepileptics: plasma concentration of imatinib reduced by ●carbamazepine, ●oxcarbazepine and ●phenytoin—avoid concomitant use; cytotoxics possibly reduce absorption of phenytoin

Antifungals: plasma concentration of imatinib increased by ketoconazole

● Antipsychotics: avoid concomitant use of cytotoxics with ●clozapine (increased risk of agranulocytosis)

Cardiac Glycosides: cytotoxics reduce absorption of digoxin tablets

Ciclosporin: imatinib possibly increases plasma concentration of ciclosporin

Lipid-regulating Drugs: imatinib increases plasma concentration of simvastatin

Thyroid Hormones: imatinib possibly reduces plasma concentration of levothyroxine (thyroxine)

**Imidapril** *see* ACE Inhibitors

**Imipenem with Cilastatin**

Antiepileptics: imipenem with cilastatin reduces plasma concentration of valproate

● Antivirals: increased risk of convulsions when imipenem with cilastatin given with ●ganciclovir

Oestrogens: antibacterials that do not induce liver enzymes possibly reduce contraceptive effect of oestrogens (risk probably small, see p. 445)

Vaccines: antibacterials inactivate oral typhoid vaccine–see p. 688

**Imipramine** *see* Antidepressants, Tricyclic

**Immunoglobulins**

Note For advice on immunoglobulins and live virus vaccines, see under Normal Immunoglobulin, p. 690

**Indapamide** *see* Diuretics

**Indinavir**

● Anti-arrhythmics: indinavir possibly increases plasma concentration of ●amiodarone—avoid concomitant use; indinavir possibly increases plasma concentration of ●flecainide (increased risk of ventricular arrhythmias—avoid concomitant use)

● Antibacterials: indinavir increases plasma concentration of ●rifabutin—avoid concomitant use; metabolism of indinavir accelerated by ●rifampicin (reduced plasma concentration—avoid concomitant use); avoidance of concomitant indinavir in severe renal and hepatic impairment advised by manufacturer of ●telithromycin

Anticoagulants: avoidance of indinavir advised by manufacturer of rivaroxaban

● Antidepressants: plasma concentration of indinavir reduced by ●St John's wort—avoid concomitant use

● Antiepileptics: plasma concentration of indinavir possibly reduced by ●carbamazepine and ●phenytoin, also plasma concentration of carbamazepine and phenytoin possibly increased; plasma concentration of indinavir possibly reduced by ●primidone

● Antifungals: plasma concentration of indinavir increased by ●itraconazole and ●ketoconazole (consider reducing dose of indinavir)

Antimalarials: caution with indinavir advised by manufacturer of artemether/lumefantrine

Antimuscarinics: avoidance of indinavir advised by manufacturer of darifenacin and tolterodine; manufacturer of fesoterodine advises dose reduction when indinavir given with fesoterodine—consult fesoterodine product literature

● Antipsychotics: indinavir possibly inhibits metabolism of ●aripiprazole (reduce dose of aripiprazole); indinavir possibly increases plasma concentration of ●pimozide (increased risk of ventricular arrhythmias—avoid concomitant use); indinavir increases plasma concentration of ●sertindole (increased risk of ventricular arrhythmias—avoid concomitant use)

● Antivirals: avoid concomitant use of indinavir with ●atazanavir; plasma concentration of both drugs

**Indinavir**

● Antivirals *(continued)*
increased when indinavir given with darunavir; plasma concentration of indinavir reduced by efavirenz and nevirapine; plasma concentration of indinavir possibly reduced by ●etravirine— avoid concomitant use; indinavir increases plasma concentration of ●maraviroc (consider reducing dose of maraviroc); combination of indinavir with nelfinavir may increase plasma concentration of either drug (or both); plasma concentration of indinavir increased by ritonavir; indinavir increases plasma concentration of saquinavir

● Anxiolytics and Hypnotics: increased risk of prolonged sedation when indinavir given with ●alprazolam— avoid concomitant use; indinavir possibly increases plasma concentration of ●midazolam (risk of prolonged sedation—avoid concomitant use of oral midazolam)

Atovaquone: plasma concentration of indinavir possibly reduced by atovaquone

● Barbiturates: plasma concentration of indinavir possibly reduced by ●barbiturates; plasma concentration of indinavir possibly reduced by ●phenobarbital, also plasma concentration of phenobarbital possibly increased

● Ciclosporin: indinavir increases plasma concentration of ●ciclosporin

● Cilostazol: indinavir possibly increases plasma concentration of ●cilostazol—avoid concomitant use

Corticosteroids: plasma concentration of indinavir possibly reduced by dexamethasone

● Ergot Alkaloids: increased risk of ergotism when indinavir given with ●ergotamine and methysergide—avoid concomitant use

● 5HT₁ Agonists: indinavir increases plasma concentration of ●eletriptan (risk of toxicity)—avoid concomitant use

● Lipid-regulating Drugs: possible increased risk of myopathy when indinavir given with atorvastatin; possible increased risk of myopathy when indinavir given with ●rosuvastatin—avoid concomitant use; increased risk of myopathy when indinavir given with ●simvastatin (avoid concomitant use)

● Ranolazine: indinavir possibly increases plasma concentration of ●ranolazine—manufacturer of ranolazine advises avoid concomitant use

● Sildenafil: indinavir increases plasma concentration of ●sildenafil—reduce initial dose of sildenafil

Tadalafil: indinavir possibly increases plasma concentration of tadalafil

● Vardenafil: indinavir increases plasma concentration of ●vardenafil—avoid concomitant use

**Indometacin** *see* NSAIDs

**Indoramin** *see* Alpha-blockers

**Infliximab**

Abatacept: increased risk of side-effects when infliximab given with abatacept

● Anakinra: avoid concomitant use of infliximab with ●anakinra

● Vaccines: avoid concomitant use of infliximab with live ●vaccines (see p. 669)

**Influenza Vaccine** *see* Vaccines

**Insulin** *see* Antidiabetics

**Interferon Alfa** *see* Interferons

**Interferon Gamma** *see* Interferons

**Interferons**

Note Peginterferon alfa interactions as for interferon alfa

● Antivirals: increased risk of peripheral neuropathy when interferon alfa given with ●telbivudine

Theophylline: interferon alfa inhibits metabolism of theophylline (increased plasma concentration)

Vaccines: manufacturer of interferon gamma advises avoid concomitant use with vaccines

**Ipratropium** *see* Antimuscarinics

**Irbesartan** *see* Angiotensin-II Receptor Antagonists

**Irinotecan**
- Antidepressants: metabolism of irinotecan accelerated by ●St John's wort (reduced plasma concentration—avoid concomitant use)

  Antiepileptics: plasma concentration of irinotecan and its active metabolite reduced by carbamazepine and phenytoin; cytotoxics possibly reduce absorption of phenytoin
- Antifungals: plasma concentration of irinotecan reduced by ●ketoconazole (but concentration of active metabolite of irinotecan increased)—avoid concomitant use
- Antipsychotics: avoid concomitant use of cytotoxics with ●clozapine (increased risk of agranulocytosis)
- Antivirals: metabolism of irinotecan possibly inhibited by ●atazanavir (increased risk of toxicity)

  Barbiturates: plasma concentration of irinotecan and its active metabolite reduced by phenobarbital

  Cardiac Glycosides: cytotoxics reduce absorption of digoxin tablets

  Cytotoxics: plasma concentration of irinotecan possibly increased by sorafenib

**Iron**
  Antacids: absorption of *oral* iron reduced by oral magnesium salts (as magnesium trisilicate)

  Antibacterials: *oral* iron reduces absorption of ciprofloxacin, levofloxacin, moxifloxacin, norfloxacin and ofloxacin; *oral* iron reduces absorption of tetracyclines, also absorption of *oral* iron reduced by tetracyclines

  Bisphosphonates: *oral* iron reduces absorption of bisphosphonates

  Calcium Salts: absorption of *oral* iron reduced by calcium salts
- Dimercaprol: avoid concomitant use of iron with ●dimercaprol

  Dopaminergics: *oral* iron reduces absorption of entacapone; *oral* iron possibly reduces absorption of levodopa

  Methyldopa: *oral* iron antagonises hypotensive effect of methyldopa

  Mycophenolate: *oral* iron reduces absorption of mycophenolate

  Penicillamine: *oral* iron reduces absorption of penicillamine

  Thyroid Hormones: *oral* iron reduces absorption of levothyroxine (thyroxine) (give at least 2 hours apart)

  Trientine: absorption of *oral* iron reduced by trientine

  Zinc: *oral* iron reduces absorption of zinc, also absorption of *oral* iron reduced by zinc

**Isocarboxazid** see MAOIs
**Isoflurane** see Anaesthetics, General
**Isometheptene** see Sympathomimetics
**Isoniazid**
  Anaesthetics, General: hepatotoxicity of isoniazid possibly potentiated by general anaesthetics

  Antacids: absorption of isoniazid reduced by antacids

  Antibacterials: increased risk of CNS toxicity when isoniazid given with cycloserine
- Antiepileptics: isoniazid increases plasma concentration of ●carbamazepine (also possibly increased isoniazid hepatotoxicity); isoniazid inhibits metabolism of ●ethosuximide (increased plasma concentration and risk of toxicity); isoniazid inhibits metabolism of ●phenytoin (increased plasma concentration)

  Antifungals: isoniazid possibly reduces plasma concentration of ketoconazole

  Anxiolytics and Hypnotics: isoniazid inhibits the metabolism of diazepam

  Corticosteroids: plasma concentration of isoniazid possibly reduced by corticosteroids

  Oestrogens: antibacterials that do not induce liver enzymes possibly reduce contraceptive effect of oestrogens (risk probably small, see p. 445)

  Theophylline: isoniazid possibly increases plasma concentration of theophylline

  Vaccines: antibacterials inactivate oral typhoid vaccine—see p. 688

**Isosorbide Dinitrate** see Nitrates
**Isosorbide Mononitrate** see Nitrates
**Isotretinoin** see Retinoids
**Isradipine** see Calcium-channel Blockers
**Itraconazole** see Antifungals, Triazole
**Ivabradine**
- Anti-arrhythmics: increased risk of ventricular arrhythmias when ivabradine given with ●amiodarone or ●disopyramide
- Antibacterials: plasma concentration of ivabradine possibly increased by ●clarithromycin and ●telithromycin—avoid concomitant use; increased risk of ventricular arrhythmias when ivabradine given with ●erythromycin—avoid concomitant use

  Antidepressants: plasma concentration of ivabradine reduced by St John's wort—avoid concomitant use
- Antifungals: plasma concentration of ivabradine increased by ●ketoconazole—avoid concomitant use; plasma concentration of ivabradine increased by fluconazole—reduce initial dose of ivabradine; plasma concentration of ivabradine possibly increased by ●itraconazole—avoid concomitant use
- Antimalarials: increased risk of ventricular arrhythmias when ivabradine given with ●mefloquine
- Antipsychotics: increased risk of ventricular arrhythmias when ivabradine given with ●pimozide or ●sertindole
- Antivirals: plasma concentration of ivabradine possibly increased by ●nelfinavir and ●ritonavir—avoid concomitant use
- Beta-blockers: increased risk of ventricular arrhythmias when ivabradine given with ●sotalol
- Calcium-channel Blockers: plasma concentration of ivabradine increased by ●diltiazem and ●verapamil—avoid concomitant use

  Grapefruit Juice: plasma concentration of ivabradine increased by grapefruit juice
- Pentamidine Isetionate: increased risk of ventricular arrhythmias when ivabradine given with ●pentamidine isetionate

**Kaolin**
  Analgesics: kaolin possibly reduces absorption of aspirin

  Antibacterials: kaolin possibly reduces absorption of tetracyclines

  Antimalarials: kaolin reduces absorption of chloroquine and hydroxychloroquine

  Antipsychotics: kaolin possibly reduces absorption of phenothiazines

**Ketamine** see Anaesthetics, General
**Ketoconazole** see Antifungals, Imidazole
**Ketoprofen** see NSAIDs
**Ketorolac** see NSAIDs
**Ketotifen** see Antihistamines
**Labetalol** see Beta-blockers
**Lacidipine** see Calcium-channel Blockers
**Lacosamide**
- Antidepressants: anticonvulsant effect of antiepileptics possibly antagonised by MAOIs and ●tricyclic-related antidepressants (convulsive threshold lowered); anticonvulsant effect of antiepileptics antagonised by ●SSRIs and ●tricyclics (convulsive threshold lowered); avoid concomitant use of antiepileptics with ●St John's wort
- Antimalarials: possible increased risk of convulsions when antiepileptics given with chloroquine and hydroxychloroquine; anticonvulsant effect of antiepileptics antagonised by ●mefloquine

**Lactulose**
  Anticoagulants: lactulose possibly enhances anticoagulant effect of coumarins

**Lamivudine**
  Antibacterials: plasma concentration of lamivudine increased by trimethoprim (as co-trimoxazole)—avoid concomitant use of high-dose co-trimoxazole

  Antivirals: avoidance of lamivudine advised by manufacturer of emtricitabine; manufacturer of lamivudine advises avoid concomitant use with foscarnet;

Lamivudine
  Antivirals *(continued)*
    manufacturer of lamivudine advises avoid concomitant use of intravenous ganciclovir
Lamotrigine
  • Antibacterials: plasma concentration of lamotrigine reduced by •rifampicin
  • Antidepressants: anticonvulsant effect of antiepileptics possibly antagonised by MAOIs and •tricyclic-related antidepressants (convulsive threshold lowered); anticonvulsant effect of antiepileptics antagonised by •SSRIs and •tricyclics (convulsive threshold lowered); avoid concomitant use of antiepileptics with •St John's wort
    Antiepileptics: plasma concentration of lamotrigine often reduced by carbamazepine, also plasma concentration of an active metabolite of carbamazepine sometimes raised (but evidence is conflicting); plasma concentration of lamotrigine reduced by phenytoin and primidone; plasma concentration of lamotrigine increased by valproate
  • Antimalarials: possible increased risk of convulsions when antiepileptics given with chloroquine and hydroxychloroquine; anticonvulsant effect of antiepileptics antagonised by •mefloquine
    Barbiturates: plasma concentration of lamotrigine reduced by phenobarbital
  • Oestrogens: plasma concentration of lamotrigine reduced by •oestrogens
  • Progestogens: plasma concentration of lamotrigine reduced by •progestogens
Lanreotide
  Antidiabetics: lanreotide possibly reduces requirements for insulin, metformin, repaglinide and sulphonylureas
  Ciclosporin: lanreotide reduces plasma concentration of ciclosporin
Lansoprazole *see* Proton Pump Inhibitors
Lanthanum
  Antifungals: lanthanum possibly reduces absorption of ketoconazole (give at least 2 hours apart)
  Antimalarials: lanthanum possibly reduces absorption of chloroquine and hydroxychloroquine (give at least 2 hours apart)
Lapatinib
  • Antibacterials: manufacturer of lapatinib advises avoid concomitant use with •rifabutin, •rifampicin and •telithromycin
  • Antidepressants: manufacturer of lapatinib advises avoid concomitant use with •St John's wort
  • Antidiabetics: manufacturer of lapatinib advises avoid concomitant use with •repaglinide
  • Antiepileptics: plasma concentration of lapatinib reduced by •carbamazepine—avoid concomitant use; cytotoxics possibly reduce absorption of phenytoin; manufacturer of lapatinib advises avoid concomitant use with •phenytoin
  • Antifungals: plasma concentration of lapatinib increased by •ketoconazole—avoid concomitant use; manufacturer of lapatinib advises avoid concomitant use with •itraconazole, •posaconazole and •voriconazole
  • Antipsychotics: avoid concomitant use of cytotoxics with •clozapine (increased risk of agranulocytosis); manufacturer of lapatinib advises avoid concomitant use with •pimozide
  • Antivirals: manufacturer of lapatinib advises avoid concomitant use with •ritonavir and •saquinavir
    Cardiac Glycosides: cytotoxics reduce absorption of digoxin tablets
  • Grapefruit Juice: manufacturer of lapatinib advises avoid concomitant use with •grapefruit juice
    Ulcer-healing Drugs: absorption of lapatinib possibly reduced by histamine $H_2$-antagonists and proton pump inhibitors
Laronidase
  Antimalarials: effects of laronidase possibly inhibited by chloroquine and hydroxychloroquine (manufacturer of laronidase advises avoid concomitant use)

Leflunomide
  Note Increased risk of toxicity with other haematotoxic and hepatotoxic drugs
    Antibacterials: plasma concentration of active metabolite of leflunomide possibly increased by rifampicin
    Anticoagulants: leflunomide possibly enhances anticoagulant effect of warfarin
    Antidiabetics: leflunomide possibly enhances hypoglycaemic effect of tolbutamide
    Antiepileptics: leflunomide possibly increases plasma concentration of phenytoin
  • Cytotoxics: risk of toxicity when leflunomide given with •methotrexate
    Lipid-regulating Drugs: the effect of leflunomide is significantly decreased by colestyramine (enhanced elimination)—avoid unless drug elimination desired
  • Vaccines: avoid concomitant use of leflunomide with live •vaccines (see p. 669)
Lenalidomide
  Cardiac Glycosides: lenalidomide possibly increases plasma concentration of digoxin
Lercanidipine *see* Calcium-channel Blockers
Leukotriene Receptor Antagonists
  Analgesics: plasma concentration of zafirlukast increased by aspirin
  Antibacterials: plasma concentration of zafirlukast reduced by erythromycin
  Anticoagulants: zafirlukast enhances anticoagulant effect of warfarin
  Antiepileptics: plasma concentration of montelukast reduced by primidone
  Barbiturates: plasma concentration of montelukast reduced by phenobarbital
  Theophylline: zafirlukast possibly increases plasma concentration of theophylline, also plasma concentration of zafirlukast reduced
Levamisole
  Alcohol: possibility of disulfiram-like reaction when levamisole given with alcohol
  • Anticoagulants: levamisole possibly enhances anticoagulant effect of •warfarin
    Antiepileptics: levamisole possibly increases plasma concentration of phenytoin
Levetiracetam
  • Antidepressants: anticonvulsant effect of antiepileptics possibly antagonised by MAOIs and •tricyclic-related antidepressants (convulsive threshold lowered); anticonvulsant effect of antiepileptics antagonised by •SSRIs and •tricyclics (convulsive threshold lowered); avoid concomitant use of antiepileptics with •St John's wort
  • Antimalarials: possible increased risk of convulsions when antiepileptics given with chloroquine and hydroxychloroquine; anticonvulsant effect of antiepileptics antagonised by •mefloquine
Levobunolol *see* Beta-blockers
Levobupivacaine
  Anti-arrhythmics: increased myocardial depression when levobupivacaine given with anti-arrhythmics
Levocetirizine *see* Antihistamines
Levodopa
  ACE Inhibitors: enhanced hypotensive effect when levodopa given with ACE inhibitors
  Adrenergic Neurone Blockers: enhanced hypotensive effect when levodopa given with adrenergic neurone blockers
  Alpha-blockers: enhanced hypotensive effect when levodopa given with alpha-blockers
  • Anaesthetics, General: increased risk of arrhythmias when levodopa given with •volatile liquid general anaesthetics
  Angiotensin-II Receptor Antagonists: enhanced hypotensive effect when levodopa given with angiotensin-II receptor antagonists
  • Antidepressants: risk of hypertensive crisis when levodopa given with •MAOIs, avoid levodopa for at least 2 weeks after stopping MAOIs; increased risk of side-effects when levodopa given with moclobemide

**Levodopa** *(continued)*

Antiepileptics: effects of levodopa possibly reduced by phenytoin

Antimuscarinics: absorption of levodopa possibly reduced by antimuscarinics

Antipsychotics: effects of levodopa antagonised by antipsychotics; avoidance of levodopa advised by manufacturer of amisulpride (antagonism of effect)

Anxiolytics and Hypnotics: effects of levodopa possibly antagonised by benzodiazepines

Beta-blockers: enhanced hypotensive effect when levodopa given with beta-blockers

Bupropion: increased risk of side-effects when levodopa given with bupropion

Calcium-channel Blockers: enhanced hypotensive effect when levodopa given with calcium-channel blockers

Clonidine: enhanced hypotensive effect when levodopa given with clonidine

Diazoxide: enhanced hypotensive effect when levodopa given with diazoxide

Diuretics: enhanced hypotensive effect when levodopa given with diuretics

Dopaminergics: enhanced effects and increased toxicity of levodopa when given with selegiline (reduce dose of levodopa)

Iron: absorption of levodopa possibly reduced by *oral* iron

Memantine: effects of dopaminergics possibly enhanced by memantine

Methyldopa: enhanced hypotensive effect when levodopa given with methyldopa; antiparkinsonian effect of dopaminergics antagonised by methyldopa

Moxonidine: enhanced hypotensive effect when levodopa given with moxonidine

Muscle Relaxants: possible agitation, confusion and hallucinations when levodopa given with baclofen

Nitrates: enhanced hypotensive effect when levodopa given with nitrates

Vasodilator Antihypertensives: enhanced hypotensive effect when levodopa given with hydralazine, minoxidil or sodium nitroprusside

Vitamins: effects of levodopa reduced by pyridoxine when given without dopa-decarboxylase inhibitor

**Levofloxacin** *see* Quinolones

**Levomepromazine (methotrimeprazine)** *see* Antipsychotics

**Levonorgestrel** *see* Progestogens

**Levothyroxine (thyroxine)** *see* Thyroid Hormones

**Lidocaine (lignocaine)**

Note Interactions less likely when lidocaine used topically

Anaesthetics, Local: increased myocardial depression when anti-arrhythmics given with bupivacaine, levobupivacaine, prilocaine or ropivacaine

● Anti-arrhythmics: increased myocardial depression when anti-arrhythmics given with other ●anti-arrhythmics

● Antibacterials: increased risk of ventricular arrhythmias when lidocaine (lignocaine) given with ●quinupristin/dalfopristin—avoid concomitant use

● Antipsychotics: increased risk of ventricular arrhythmias when anti-arrhythmics that prolong the QT interval given with ●antipsychotics that prolong the QT interval

● Antivirals: plasma concentration of lidocaine (lignocaine) possibly increased by ●atazanavir and lopinavir; plasma concentration of lidocaine (lignocaine) possibly increased by darunavir and ●fosamprenavir—avoid concomitant use

● Beta-blockers: increased myocardial depression when anti-arrhythmics given with ●beta-blockers; increased risk of lidocaine (lignocaine) toxicity when given with ●propranolol

● Diuretics: action of lidocaine (lignocaine) antagonised by hypokalaemia caused by ●acetazolamide, ●loop diuretics or ●thiazides and related diuretics

● 5HT₃ Antagonists: increased risk of ventricular arrhythmias when lidocaine (lignocaine) given with ●dolasetron—avoid concomitant use

**Lidocaine (lignocaine)** *(continued)*

Muscle Relaxants: neuromuscular blockade enhanced and prolonged when lidocaine (lignocaine) given with suxamethonium

● Ulcer-healing Drugs: plasma concentration of lidocaine (lignocaine) increased by ●cimetidine (increased risk of toxicity)

**Linezolid**

Note Linezolid is a reversible, non-selective MAO inhibitor—see interactions of MAOIs

Oestrogens: antibacterials that do not induce liver enzymes possibly reduce contraceptive effect of oestrogens (risk probably small, see p. 445)

Vaccines: antibacterials inactivate oral typhoid vaccine–see p. 688

**Liothyronine** *see* Thyroid Hormones

**Lipid-regulating Drugs** *see* Colestipol, Colestyramine, Ezetimibe, Fibrates, Nicotinic Acid, and Statins

**Lisinopril** *see* ACE Inhibitors

**Lithium**

● ACE Inhibitors: excretion of lithium reduced by ●ACE inhibitors (increased plasma concentration)

● Analgesics: excretion of lithium reduced by ●NSAIDs (increased risk of toxicity); excretion of lithium reduced by ●ketorolac (increased risk of toxicity)—avoid concomitant use

● Angiotensin-II Receptor Antagonists: excretion of lithium reduced by ●angiotensin-II receptor antagonists (increased plasma concentration)

Antacids: excretion of lithium increased by sodium bicarbonate (reduced plasma concentration)

● Anti-arrhythmics: avoidance of lithium advised by manufacturer of ●amiodarone (risk of ventricular arrhythmias)

Antibacterials: increased risk of lithium toxicity when given with metronidazole

● Antidepressants: possible increased serotonergic effects when lithium given with venlafaxine; increased risk of CNS effects when lithium given with ●SSRIs (lithium toxicity reported); risk of toxicity when lithium given with tricyclics

Antiepileptics: neurotoxicity may occur when lithium given with carbamazepine or phenytoin without increased plasma concentration of lithium; plasma concentration of lithium possibly affected by topiramate

● Antipsychotics: increased risk of extrapyramidal side-effects and possibly neurotoxicity when lithium given with clozapine, flupentixol, haloperidol, phenothiazines or zuclopenthixol; increased risk of ventricular arrhythmias when lithium given with ●sertindole—avoid concomitant use; increased risk of extrapyramidal side-effects when lithium given with sulpiride

Calcium-channel Blockers: neurotoxicity may occur when lithium given with diltiazem or verapamil without increased plasma concentration of lithium

● Diuretics: excretion of lithium increased by ●acetazolamide; excretion of lithium reduced by ●loop diuretics and ●thiazides and related diuretics (increased plasma concentration and risk of toxicity)—loop diuretics safer than thiazides; excretion of lithium reduced by ●potassium-sparing diuretics and aldosterone antagonists (increased plasma concentration and risk of toxicity)

● Methyldopa: neurotoxicity may occur when lithium given with ●methyldopa without increased plasma concentration of lithium

Muscle Relaxants: lithium enhances effects of muscle relaxants; hyperkinesis caused by lithium possibly aggravated by baclofen

Parasympathomimetics: lithium antagonises effects of neostigmine and pyridostigmine

Theophylline: excretion of lithium increased by theophylline (reduced plasma concentration)

**Lofepramine** *see* Antidepressants, Tricyclic

**Lofexidine**

Alcohol: increased sedative effect when lofexidine given with alcohol

**Lofexidine** *(continued)*

Anxiolytics and Hypnotics: increased sedative effect when lofexidine given with anxiolytics and hypnotics

Barbiturates: increased sedative effect when lofexidine given with barbiturates

**Lomustine**

Antiepileptics: cytotoxics possibly reduce absorption of phenytoin

● Antipsychotics: avoid concomitant use of cytotoxics with ●clozapine (increased risk of agranulocytosis)

Cardiac Glycosides: cytotoxics reduce absorption of digoxin tablets

Ulcer-healing Drugs: myelosuppressive effects of lomustine possibly enhanced by cimetidine

**Loperamide**

Desmopressin: loperamide increases plasma concentration of *oral* desmopressin

**Lopinavir**

Note In combination with ritonavir as *Kaletra*® (ritonavir is present to inhibit lopinavir metabolism and increase plasma-lopinavir concentration)—see also Ritonavir

● Anti-arrhythmics: lopinavir possibly increases plasma concentration of ●flecainide (increased risk of ventricular arrhythmias—avoid concomitant use); lopinavir possibly increases plasma concentration of lidocaine (lignocaine)

● Antibacterials: plasma concentration of lopinavir reduced by ●rifampicin—avoid concomitant use; avoidance of concomitant lopinavir in severe renal and hepatic impairment advised by manufacturer of ●telithromycin

Anticoagulants: avoidance of lopinavir advised by manufacturer of rivaroxaban

● Antidepressants: plasma concentration of lopinavir reduced by ●St John's wort—avoid concomitant use

● Antiepileptics: plasma concentration of lopinavir possibly reduced by carbamazepine, phenytoin and ●primidone

Antihistamines: lopinavir possibly increases plasma concentration of chlorphenamine (chlorpheniramine)

Antimalarials: caution with lopinavir advised by manufacturer of artemether/lumefantrine

Antimuscarinics: avoidance of lopinavir advised by manufacturer of darifenacin and tolterodine

● Antipsychotics: lopinavir possibly inhibits metabolism of ●aripiprazole (reduce dose of aripiprazole); lopinavir increases plasma concentration of ●sertindole (increased risk of ventricular arrhythmias—avoid concomitant use)

● Antivirals: lopinavir reduces plasma concentration of ●darunavir, also plasma concentration of lopinavir increased (avoid concomitant use); plasma concentration of lopinavir reduced by ●efavirenz—consider increasing dose of lopinavir; lopinavir reduces plasma concentration of fosamprenavir, effect on lopinavir plasma concentration not predictable—avoid concomitant use; lopinavir increases plasma concentration of ●maraviroc (consider reducing dose of maraviroc); plasma concentration of lopinavir reduced by nelfinavir, also plasma concentration of active metabolite of nelfinavir increased; plasma concentration of lopinavir possibly reduced by ●nevirapine—consider increasing dose of lopinavir; lopinavir increases plasma concentration of saquinavir and tenofovir; plasma concentration of lopinavir reduced by ●tipranavir

● Barbiturates: plasma concentration of lopinavir possibly reduced by ●phenobarbital

● Cilostazol: lopinavir possibly increases plasma concentration of ●cilostazol—avoid concomitant use

Corticosteroids: plasma concentration of lopinavir possibly reduced by dexamethasone

● Lipid-regulating Drugs: possible increased risk of myopathy when lopinavir given with atorvastatin; possible increased risk of myopathy when lopinavir given with ●rosuvastatin or ●simvastatin—avoid concomitant use

**Lopinavir** *(continued)*

● Ranolazine: lopinavir possibly increases plasma concentration of ●ranolazine—manufacturer of ranolazine advises avoid concomitant use

Sirolimus: lopinavir possibly increases plasma concentration of sirolimus

**Loprazolam** *see* Anxiolytics and Hypnotics

**Loratadine** *see* Antihistamines

**Lorazepam** *see* Anxiolytics and Hypnotics

**Lormetazepam** *see* Anxiolytics and Hypnotics

**Losartan** *see* Angiotensin-II Receptor Antagonists

**Lumefantrine** *see* Artemether with Lumefantrine

**Lymecycline** *see* Tetracyclines

**Macrolides**

Note *See also* Telithromycin

Note Interactions do not apply to small amounts of erythromycin used topically

Analgesics: erythromycin increases plasma concentration of alfentanil

Antacids: absorption of azithromycin reduced by antacids

● Anti-arrhythmics: increased risk of ventricular arrhythmias when parenteral erythromycin given with ●amiodarone—avoid concomitant use; erythromycin increases plasma concentration of ●disopyramide (increased risk of toxicity); clarithromycin possibly increases plasma concentration of ●disopyramide (increased risk of toxicity)

● Antibacterials: increased risk of ventricular arrhythmias when parenteral erythromycin given with ●moxifloxacin—avoid concomitant use; macrolides possibly increase plasma concentration of ●rifabutin (increased risk of uveitis—reduce rifabutin dose); clarithromycin increases plasma concentration of ●rifabutin (increased risk of uveitis—reduce rifabutin dose); plasma concentration of clarithromycin reduced by rifamycins

● Anticoagulants: clarithromycin and erythromycin enhance anticoagulant effect of ●coumarins; azithromycin possibly enhances anticoagulant effect of ●coumarins

● Antidepressants: avoidance of macrolides advised by manufacturer of ●reboxetine

Antidiabetics: clarithromycin enhances effects of repaglinide

● Antiepileptics: clarithromycin and erythromycin increase plasma concentration of ●carbamazepine; clarithromycin inhibits metabolism of phenytoin (increased plasma concentration); erythromycin possibly inhibits metabolism of valproate (increased plasma concentration)

Antifungals: clarithromycin increases plasma concentration of itraconazole

● Antihistamines: manufacturer of loratadine advises erythromycin possibly increases plasma concentration of loratadine; macrolides possibly inhibit metabolism of ●mizolastine (avoid concomitant use); erythromycin inhibits metabolism of ●mizolastine—avoid concomitant use

● Antimalarials: avoidance of macrolides advised by manufacturer of ●artemether/lumefantrine

Antimuscarinics: erythromycin possibly increases plasma concentration of darifenacin; manufacturer of fesoterodine advises dose reduction when clarithromycin given with fesoterodine—consult fesoterodine product literature; avoidance of clarithromycin and erythromycin advised by manufacturer of tolterodine

● Antipsychotics: avoidance of macrolides advised by manufacturer of ●droperidol (risk of ventricular arrhythmias); increased risk of ventricular arrhythmias when parenteral erythromycin given with ●amisulpride or ●zuclopenthixol—avoid concomitant use; erythromycin possibly increases plasma concentration of ●clozapine (possible increased risk of convulsions); increased risk of ventricular arrhythmias when clarithromycin given with ●pimozide—avoid concomitant use; possible increased risk of ventricular arrhythmias when erythromycin given with ●pimozide—avoid concomitant use; macrolides

**Macrolides**

- Antipsychotics (continued)
  possibly increase plasma concentration of quetiapine (reduce dose of quetiapine); possible increased risk of ventricular arrhythmias when macrolides given with ●sertindole—avoid concomitant use; increased risk of ventricular arrhythmias when erythromycin given with ●sertindole—avoid concomitant use; increased risk of ventricular arrhythmias when parenteral erythromycin given with ●sulpiride
- Antivirals: plasma concentration of both drugs increased when clarithromycin given with atazanavir; increased risk of rash when clarithromycin given with efavirenz; clarithromycin increases plasma concentration of ●etravirine, also plasma concentration of clarithromycin reduced; plasma concentration of both drugs increased when erythromycin given with fosamprenavir; clarithromycin possibly increases plasma concentration of ●maraviroc (consider reducing dose of maraviroc); plasma concentration of azithromycin and erythromycin possibly increased by ritonavir; plasma concentration of clarithromycin increased by ●ritonavir (reduce dose of clarithromycin in renal impairment); plasma concentration of clarithromycin increased by ●tipranavir (reduce dose of clarithromycin in renal impairment), also clarithromycin increases plasma concentration of tipranavir; clarithromycin tablets reduce absorption of zidovudine (give at least 2 hours apart)
- Anxiolytics and Hypnotics: clarithromycin and erythromycin inhibit metabolism of ●midazolam (increased plasma concentration with increased sedation); erythromycin increases plasma concentration of buspirone (reduce dose of buspirone); erythromycin inhibits the metabolism of zopiclone
  Aprepitant: clarithromycin possibly increases plasma concentration of aprepitant
- Atomoxetine: increased risk of ventricular arrhythmias when parenteral erythromycin given with ●atomoxetine
- Calcium-channel Blockers: erythromycin possibly inhibits metabolism of felodipine (increased plasma concentration); avoidance of erythromycin advised by manufacturer of lercanidipine; clarithromycin and erythromycin possibly inhibit metabolism of ●verapamil (increased risk of toxicity)
  Cardiac Glycosides: macrolides increase plasma concentration of digoxin (increased risk of toxicity)
- Ciclosporin: macrolides possibly inhibit metabolism of ●ciclosporin (increased plasma concentration); clarithromycin and erythromycin inhibit metabolism of ●ciclosporin (increased plasma concentration)
- Cilostazol: erythromycin increases plasma concentration of ●cilostazol (also plasma concentration of erythromycin reduced)—avoid concomitant use
- Colchicine: clarithromycin or erythromycin increase risk of ●colchicine toxicity
  Corticosteroids: erythromycin possibly inhibits metabolism of corticosteroids; clarithromycin possibly increases plasma concentration of methylprednisolone; erythromycin inhibits the metabolism of methylprednisolone
- Cytotoxics: avoidance of clarithromycin advised by manufacturer of ●nilotinib; in vitro studies suggest a possible interaction between erythromycin and docetaxel (consult docetaxel product literature); erythromycin increases toxicity of ●vinblastine—avoid concomitant use
- Diuretics: clarithromycin increases plasma concentration of ●eplerenone—avoid concomitant use; erythromycin increases plasma concentration of eplerenone (reduce dose of eplerenone)
  Dopaminergics: macrolides possibly increase plasma concentration of bromocriptine and cabergoline (increased risk of toxicity); erythromycin increases plasma concentration of bromocriptine and cabergoline (increased risk of toxicity)

**Macrolides** (continued)

- Ergot Alkaloids: increased risk of ergotism when macrolides given with ●ergotamine and methysergide—avoid concomitant use
- 5HT₁ Agonists: clarithromycin and erythromycin increase plasma concentration of ●eletriptan (risk of toxicity)—avoid concomitant use
- Ivabradine: clarithromycin possibly increases plasma concentration of ●ivabradine—avoid concomitant use; increased risk of ventricular arrhythmias when erythromycin given with ●ivabradine—avoid concomitant use
  Leukotriene Receptor Antagonists: erythromycin reduces plasma concentration of zafirlukast
- Lipid-regulating Drugs: clarithromycin increases plasma concentration of ●atorvastatin and pravastatin; possible increased risk of myopathy when erythromycin given with atorvastatin; erythromycin increases plasma concentration of pravastatin; erythromycin reduces plasma concentration of rosuvastatin; increased risk of myopathy when clarithromycin or erythromycin given with ●simvastatin (avoid concomitant use)
  Oestrogens: antibacterials that do not induce liver enzymes possibly reduce contraceptive effect of oestrogens (risk probably small, see p. 445)
  Parasympathomimetics: erythromycin increases plasma concentration of galantamine
- Pentamidine Isetionate: increased risk of ventricular arrhythmias when parenteral erythromycin given with ●pentamidine isetionate
- Ranolazine: clarithromycin possibly increases plasma concentration of ●ranolazine—manufacturer of ranolazine advises avoid concomitant use
  Sildenafil: clarithromycin possibly increases plasma concentration of sildenafil—reduce initial dose of sildenafil; erythromycin increases plasma concentration of sildenafil—reduce initial dose of sildenafil
- Sirolimus: clarithromycin increases plasma concentration of ●sirolimus—avoid concomitant use; plasma concentration of both drugs increased when erythromycin given with ●sirolimus
- Tacrolimus: clarithromycin and erythromycin increase plasma concentration of ●tacrolimus
  Tadalafil: clarithromycin and erythromycin possibly increase plasma concentration of tadalafil
- Theophylline: azithromycin possibly increases plasma concentration of theophylline; clarithromycin inhibits metabolism of ●theophylline (increased plasma concentration); erythromycin inhibits metabolism of ●theophylline (increased plasma concentration), if erythromycin given by mouth, also decreased plasma-erythromycin concentration
  Ulcer-healing Drugs: plasma concentration of erythromycin increased by cimetidine (increased risk of toxicity, including deafness); plasma concentration of both drugs increased when clarithromycin given with omeprazole
  Vaccines: antibacterials inactivate oral typhoid vaccine—see p. 688
  Vardenafil: erythromycin increases plasma concentration of vardenafil (reduce dose of vardenafil)

**Magnesium (parenteral)**

- Calcium-channel Blockers: profound hypotension reported with concomitant use of parenteral magnesium and ●nifedipine in pre-eclampsia
  Muscle Relaxants: parenteral magnesium enhances effects of non-depolarising muscle relaxants and suxamethonium

**Magnesium Salts (oral)** see Antacids

**Mannitol**

  Ciclosporin: possible increased risk of nephrotoxicity when mannitol given with ciclosporin

## MAOIs

Note For interactions of reversible MAO-A inhibitors (RIMAs) see Moclobemide, and for interactions of MAO-B inhibitors see Rasagiline and Selegiline; the antibacterial Linezolid is a reversible, non-selective MAO inhibitor

**ACE Inhibitors:** MAOIs possibly enhance hypotensive effect of ACE inhibitors

**Adrenergic Neurone Blockers:** enhanced hypotensive effect when MAOIs given with adrenergic neurone blockers

- **Alcohol:** MAOIs interact with tyramine found in some beverages containing ●alcohol and some dealcoholised beverages (hypertensive crisis)—if no tyramine, enhanced hypotensive effect

**Alpha$_2$-adrenoceptor Stimulants:** avoidance of MAOIs advised by manufacturer of apraclonidine and brimonidine

- **Alpha-blockers:** avoidance of MAOIs advised by manufacturer of ●indoramin; enhanced hypotensive effect when MAOIs given with alpha-blockers

- **Anaesthetics, General:** Because of hazardous interactions between MAOIs and ●general anaesthetics, MAOIs should normally be stopped 2 weeks before surgery

- **Analgesics:** CNS excitation or depression (hypertension or hypotension) when MAOIs given with ●pethidine—avoid concomitant use and for 2 weeks after stopping MAOIs; avoidance of MAOIs advised by manufacturer of ●nefopam; possible CNS excitation or depression (hypertension or hypotension) when MAOIs given with ●opioid analgesics—avoid concomitant use and for 2 weeks after stopping MAOIs

**Angiotensin-II Receptor Antagonists:** MAOIs possibly enhance hypotensive effect of angiotensin-II receptor antagonists

- **Antidepressants:** increased risk of hypertension and CNS excitation when MAOIs given with ●reboxetine (MAOIs should not be started until 1 week after stopping reboxetine, avoid reboxetine for 2 weeks after stopping MAOIs); after stopping MAOIs do not start ●citalopram, ●escitalopram, ●fluvoxamine or ●paroxetine for 2 weeks, also MAOIs should not be started until at least 1 week after stopping citalopram, escitalopram, fluvoxamine or paroxetine; after stopping MAOIs do not start ●fluoxetine for 2 weeks, also MAOIs should not be started until at least 5 weeks after stopping fluoxetine; after stopping MAOIs do not start ●mirtazapine or ●sertraline for 2 weeks, also MAOIs should not be started until at least 2 weeks after stopping mirtazapine or sertraline; after stopping MAOIs do not start ●duloxetine for 2 weeks, also MAOIs should not be started until at least 5 days after stopping duloxetine; enhanced CNS effects and toxicity when MAOIs given with ●venlafaxine (venlafaxine should not be started until 2 weeks after stopping MAOIs, avoid MAOIs for 1 week after stopping venlafaxine); increased risk of hypertension and CNS excitation when MAOIs given with other ●MAOIs (avoid for at least 2 weeks after stopping previous MAOIs and then start at a reduced dose); after stopping MAOIs do not start ●moclobemide for at least 1 week; MAOIs increase CNS effects of ●SSRIs (risk of serious toxicity); after stopping MAOIs do not start ●tricyclic-related antidepressants for 2 weeks, also MAOIs should not be started until at least 1–2 weeks after stopping tricyclic-related antidepressants; increased risk of hypertension and CNS excitation when MAOIs given with ●tricyclics, tricyclics should not be started until 2 weeks after stopping MAOIs (3 weeks if starting clomipramine or imipramine), also MAOIs should not be started for at least 1–2 weeks after stopping tricyclics (3 weeks in the case of clomipramine or imipramine); CNS excitation and confusion when MAOIs given with ●tryptophan (reduce dose of tryptophan)

**Antidiabetics:** MAOIs possibly enhance hypoglycaemic effect of antidiabetics; MAOIs enhance hypo-

## MAOIs

**Antidiabetics** (continued)
glycaemic effect of insulin, metformin and sulphonylureas

- **Antiepileptics:** MAOIs possibly antagonise anticonvulsant effect of antiepileptics (convulsive threshold lowered); avoidance for 2 weeks after stopping MAOIs advised by manufacturer of ●carbamazepine, also antagonism of anticonvulsant effect

**Antihistamines:** increased antimuscarinic and sedative effects when MAOIs given with antihistamines

- **Antimalarials:** avoidance of antidepressants advised by manufacturer of ●artemether/lumefantrine

**Antimuscarinics:** increased risk of antimuscarinic side-effects when MAOIs given with antimuscarinics

- **Antipsychotics:** CNS effects of MAOIs possibly increased by ●clozapine

**Anxiolytics and Hypnotics:** avoidance of MAOIs advised by manufacturer of buspirone

- **Atomoxetine:** after stopping MAOIs do not start ●atomoxetine for 2 weeks, also MAOIs should not be started until at least 2 weeks after stopping atomoxetine; possible increased risk of convulsions when antidepressants given with atomoxetine

**Barbiturates:** MAOIs possibly antagonise anticonvulsant effect of barbiturates (convulsive threshold lowered)

**Beta-blockers:** enhanced hypotensive effect when MAOIs given with beta-blockers

- **Bupropion:** avoidance of bupropion for 2 weeks after stopping MAOIs advised by manufacturer of ●bupropion

**Calcium-channel Blockers:** enhanced hypotensive effect when MAOIs given with calcium-channel blockers

**Clonidine:** enhanced hypotensive effect when MAOIs given with clonidine

**Diazoxide:** enhanced hypotensive effect when MAOIs given with diazoxide

**Diuretics:** enhanced hypotensive effect when MAOIs given with diuretics

- **Dopaminergics:** avoid concomitant use of non-selective MAOIs with ●entacapone; risk of hypertensive crisis when MAOIs given with ●levodopa, avoid levodopa for at least 2 weeks after stopping MAOIs; risk of hypertensive crisis when MAOIs given with ●rasagiline, avoid MAOIs for at least 2 weeks after stopping rasagiline; enhanced hypotensive effect when MAOIs given with selegiline; avoid concomitant use of MAOIs with tolcapone

**Doxapram:** MAOIs enhance effects of doxapram

- **5HT$_1$ Agonists:** risk of CNS toxicity when MAOIs given with ●rizatriptan or ●sumatriptan (avoid rizatriptan or sumatriptan for 2 weeks after MAOIs); increased risk of CNS toxicity when MAOIs given with ●zolmitriptan

- **Methyldopa:** avoidance of MAOIs advised by manufacturer of ●methyldopa

**Moxonidine:** enhanced hypotensive effect when MAOIs given with moxonidine

**Muscle Relaxants:** phenelzine enhances effects of suxamethonium

**Nicorandil:** enhanced hypotensive effect when MAOIs given with nicorandil

**Nitrates:** enhanced hypotensive effect when MAOIs given with nitrates

- **Sibutramine:** increased CNS toxicity when MAOIs given with ●sibutramine (manufacturer of sibutramine advises avoid concomitant use), also avoid sibutramine for 2 weeks after stopping MAOIs

- **Sympathomimetics:** risk of hypertensive crisis when MAOIs given with ●sympathomimetics; risk of hypertensive crisis when MAOIs given with ●methylphenidate, some manufacturers advise avoid methylphenidate for at least 2 weeks after stopping MAOIs

- **Tetrabenazine:** risk of CNS excitation and hypertension when MAOIs given with ●tetrabenazine

**MAOIs** *(continued)*
Vasodilator Antihypertensives: enhanced hypotensive effect when MAOIs given with hydralazine, minoxidil or sodium nitroprusside
**MAOIs, reversible** *see* Moclobemide
**Maraviroc**
● Antibacterials: plasma concentration of maraviroc possibly increased by ●clarithromycin and ●telithromycin (consider reducing dose of maraviroc); plasma concentration of maraviroc reduced by ●rifampicin—consider increasing dose of maraviroc
● Antidepressants: plasma concentration of maraviroc possibly reduced by ●St John's wort—avoid concomitant use
● Antifungals: plasma concentration of maraviroc increased by ●ketoconazole (consider reducing dose of maraviroc)
● Antivirals: plasma concentration of maraviroc increased by ●atazanavir, ●darunavir, ●indinavir, ●lopinavir and ●saquinavir (consider reducing dose of maraviroc); plasma concentration of maraviroc possibly reduced by ●efavirenz—consider increasing dose of maraviroc; plasma concentration of maraviroc possibly reduced by etravirine; plasma concentration of maraviroc possibly increased by ●nelfinavir (consider reducing dose of maraviroc)
**Mebendazole**
Ulcer-healing Drugs: metabolism of mebendazole possibly inhibited by cimetidine (increased plasma concentration)
**Medroxyprogesterone** *see* Progestogens
**Mefenamic Acid** *see* NSAIDs
**Mefloquine**
● Anti-arrhythmics: increased risk of ventricular arrhythmias when mefloquine given with ●amiodarone—avoid concomitant use
● Antibacterials: increased risk of ventricular arrhythmias when mefloquine given with ●moxifloxacin—avoid concomitant use; plasma concentration of mefloquine reduced by ●rifampicin—avoid concomitant use
● Antiepileptics: mefloquine antagonises anticonvulsant effect of ●antiepileptics
● Antimalarials: avoidance of antimalarials advised by manufacturer of ●artemether/lumefantrine; increased risk of convulsions when mefloquine given with ●chloroquine and hydroxychloroquine; increased risk of convulsions when mefloquine given with ●quinine (but should not prevent the use of intravenous quinine in severe cases)
● Antipsychotics: increased risk of ventricular arrhythmias when mefloquine given with ●pimozide—avoid concomitant use
● Atomoxetine: increased risk of ventricular arrhythmias when mefloquine given with ●atomoxetine
Beta-blockers: increased risk of bradycardia when mefloquine given with beta-blockers
Calcium-channel Blockers: possible increased risk of bradycardia when mefloquine given with calcium-channel blockers
Cardiac Glycosides: possible increased risk of bradycardia when mefloquine given with digoxin
● Ivabradine: increased risk of ventricular arrhythmias when mefloquine given with ●ivabradine
Vaccines: antimalarials inactivate oral typhoid vaccine–see p. 688
**Megestrol** *see* Progestogens
**Melatonin** *see* Anxiolytics and Hypnotics
**Meloxicam** *see* NSAIDs
**Melphalan**
Antibacterials: increased risk of melphalan toxicity when given with nalidixic acid
Antiepileptics: cytotoxics possibly reduce absorption of phenytoin
● Antipsychotics: avoid concomitant use of cytotoxics with ●clozapine (increased risk of agranulocytosis)
Cardiac Glycosides: cytotoxics reduce absorption of digoxin tablets

**Melphalan** *(continued)*
● Ciclosporin: increased risk of nephrotoxicity when melphalan given with ●ciclosporin
**Memantine**
● Anaesthetics, General: increased risk of CNS toxicity when memantine given with ●ketamine (manufacturer of memantine advises avoid concomitant use)
● Analgesics: increased risk of CNS toxicity when memantine given with ●dextromethorphan (manufacturer of memantine advises avoid concomitant use)
Anticoagulants: memantine possibly enhances anticoagulant effect of warfarin
Antiepileptics: memantine possibly reduces effects of primidone
Antimuscarinics: memantine possibly enhances effects of antimuscarinics
Antipsychotics: memantine possibly reduces effects of antipsychotics
Barbiturates: memantine possibly reduces effects of barbiturates
● Dopaminergics: memantine possibly enhances effects of dopaminergics and selegiline; increased risk of CNS toxicity when memantine given with ●amantadine (manufacturer of memantine advises avoid concomitant use)
Muscle Relaxants: memantine possibly modifies effects of baclofen and dantrolene
**Mepacrine**
Antimalarials: mepacrine increases plasma concentration of primaquine (increased risk of toxicity)
**Meprobamate** *see* Anxiolytics and Hypnotics
**Meptazinol** *see* Opioid Analgesics
**Mercaptopurine**
● Allopurinol: enhanced effects and increased toxicity of mercaptopurine when given with ●allopurinol (reduce dose of mercaptopurine to one quarter of usual dose)
Aminosalicylates: possible increased risk of leucopenia when mercaptopurine given with aminosalicylates
● Antibacterials: increased risk of haematological toxicity when mercaptopurine given with ●sulfamethoxazole (as co-trimoxazole); increased risk of haematological toxicity when mercaptopurine given with ●trimethoprim (also with co-trimoxazole)
● Anticoagulants: mercaptopurine possibly reduces anticoagulant effect of ●coumarins
Antiepileptics: cytotoxics possibly reduce absorption of phenytoin
● Antipsychotics: avoid concomitant use of cytotoxics with ●clozapine (increased risk of agranulocytosis)
Cardiac Glycosides: cytotoxics reduce absorption of digoxin tablets
**Meropenem**
Antiepileptics: meropenem reduces plasma concentration of valproate
Oestrogens: antibacterials that do not induce liver enzymes possibly reduce contraceptive effect of oestrogens (risk probably small, see p. 445)
Probenecid: excretion of meropenem reduced by probenecid (manufacturers of meropenem advise avoid concomitant use)
Vaccines: antibacterials inactivate oral typhoid vaccine–see p. 688
**Mesalazine** *see* Aminosalicylates
**Mestranol** *see* Oestrogens
**Metaraminol** *see* Sympathomimetics
**Metformin** *see* Antidiabetics
**Methadone** *see* Opioid Analgesics
**Methenamine**
● Antibacterials: increased risk of crystalluria when methenamine given with ●sulphonamides
● Diuretics: effects of methenamine antagonised by ●acetazolamide
Oestrogens: antibacterials that do not induce liver enzymes possibly reduce contraceptive effect of oestrogens (risk probably small, see p. 445)

**Methenamine** *(continued)*

Potassium Salts: avoid concomitant use of methenamine with potassium citrate

Vaccines: antibacterials inactivate oral typhoid vaccine–see p. 688

**Methocarbamol** *see* Muscle Relaxants

**Methotrexate**

● Anaesthetics, General: antifolate effect of methotrexate increased by ●nitrous oxide—avoid concomitant use

● Analgesics: excretion of methotrexate probably reduced by ●NSAIDs (increased risk of toxicity)—but for concomitant use in rheumatic disease see p. 575; excretion of methotrexate reduced by ●azapropazone (avoid concomitant use); excretion of methotrexate reduced by ●aspirin, ●diclofenac, ●ibuprofen, ●indometacin, ●ketoprofen, ●meloxicam and ●naproxen (increased risk of toxicity)—but for concomitant use in rheumatic disease see p. 575

● Antibacterials: absorption of methotrexate possibly reduced by neomycin; excretion of methotrexate possibly reduced by ciprofloxacin (increased risk of toxicity); increased risk of haematological toxicity when methotrexate given with ●sulfamethoxazole (as co-trimoxazole); increased risk of methotrexate toxicity when given with doxycycline, sulphonamides or tetracycline; excretion of methotrexate reduced by penicillins (increased risk of toxicity); increased risk of haematological toxicity when methotrexate given with ●trimethoprim (also with co-trimoxazole)

Antiepileptics: cytotoxics possibly reduce absorption of phenytoin; antifolate effect of methotrexate increased by phenytoin

● Antimalarials: antifolate effect of methotrexate increased by ●pyrimethamine

● Antipsychotics: avoid concomitant use of cytotoxics with ●clozapine (increased risk of agranulocytosis)

Cardiac Glycosides: cytotoxics reduce absorption of digoxin tablets

● Ciclosporin: risk of toxicity when methotrexate given with ●ciclosporin

● Corticosteroids: increased risk of haematological toxicity when methotrexate given with ●corticosteroids

● Cytotoxics: increased pulmonary toxicity when methotrexate given with ●cisplatin

● Leflunomide: risk of toxicity when methotrexate given with ●leflunomide

● Probenecid: excretion of methotrexate reduced by ●probenecid (increased risk of toxicity)

● Retinoids: plasma concentration of methotrexate increased by ●acitretin (also increased risk of hepatotoxicity)—avoid concomitant use

Theophylline: methotrexate possibly increases plasma concentration of theophylline

Ulcer-healing Drugs: excretion of methotrexate possibly reduced by omeprazole (increased risk of toxicity)

**Methoxamine** *see* Sympathomimetics

**Methyldopa**

ACE Inhibitors: enhanced hypotensive effect when methyldopa given with ACE inhibitors

Adrenergic Neurone Blockers: enhanced hypotensive effect when methyldopa given with adrenergic neurone blockers

Alcohol: enhanced hypotensive effect when methyldopa given with alcohol

Aldesleukin: enhanced hypotensive effect when methyldopa given with aldesleukin

Alpha-blockers: enhanced hypotensive effect when methyldopa given with alpha-blockers

Anaesthetics, General: enhanced hypotensive effect when methyldopa given with general anaesthetics

Analgesics: hypotensive effect of methyldopa antagonised by NSAIDs

Angiotensin-II Receptor Antagonists: enhanced hypotensive effect when methyldopa given with angiotensin-II receptor antagonists

**Methyldopa** *(continued)*

● Antidepressants: manufacturer of methyldopa advises avoid concomitant use with ●MAOIs

Antipsychotics: enhanced hypotensive effect when methyldopa given with antipsychotics (also increased risk of extrapyramidal effects)

Anxiolytics and Hypnotics: enhanced hypotensive effect when methyldopa given with anxiolytics and hypnotics

Beta-blockers: enhanced hypotensive effect when methyldopa given with beta-blockers

Calcium-channel Blockers: enhanced hypotensive effect when methyldopa given with calcium-channel blockers

Clonidine: enhanced hypotensive effect when methyldopa given with clonidine

Corticosteroids: hypotensive effect of methyldopa antagonised by corticosteroids

Diazoxide: enhanced hypotensive effect when methyldopa given with diazoxide

Diuretics: enhanced hypotensive effect when methyldopa given with diuretics

Dopaminergics: methyldopa antagonises antiparkinsonian effect of dopaminergics; increased risk of extrapyramidal side-effects when methyldopa given with amantadine; effects of methyldopa possibly enhanced by entacapone; enhanced hypotensive effect when methyldopa given with levodopa

Iron: hypotensive effect of methyldopa antagonised by *oral* iron

● Lithium: neurotoxicity may occur when methyldopa given with ●lithium without increased plasma concentration of lithium

Moxisylyte (thymoxamine): enhanced hypotensive effect when methyldopa given with moxisylyte

Moxonidine: enhanced hypotensive effect when methyldopa given with moxonidine

Muscle Relaxants: enhanced hypotensive effect when methyldopa given with baclofen or tizanidine

Nitrates: enhanced hypotensive effect when methyldopa given with nitrates

Oestrogens: hypotensive effect of methyldopa antagonised by oestrogens

Prostaglandins: enhanced hypotensive effect when methyldopa given with alprostadil

● Sympathomimetics, Beta$_2$: acute hypotension reported when methyldopa given with infusion of ●salbutamol

Vasodilator Antihypertensives: enhanced hypotensive effect when methyldopa given with hydralazine, minoxidil or sodium nitroprusside

**Methylphenidate** *see* Sympathomimetics

**Methylprednisolone** *see* Corticosteroids

**Methysergide** *see* Ergot Alkaloids

**Metipranolol** *see* Beta-blockers

**Metoclopramide**

Analgesics: metoclopramide increases rate of absorption of aspirin (enhanced effect); effects of metoclopramide on gastro-intestinal activity antagonised by opioid analgesics; metoclopramide increases rate of absorption of paracetamol

Antimuscarinics: effects of metoclopramide on gastro-intestinal activity antagonised by antimuscarinics

Antipsychotics: increased risk of extrapyramidal side-effects when metoclopramide given with antipsychotics

Atovaquone: metoclopramide reduces plasma concentration of atovaquone

● Ciclosporin: metoclopramide increases plasma concentration of ●ciclosporin

Dopaminergics: metoclopramide antagonises hypoprolactinaemic effects of bromocriptine and cabergoline; metoclopramide antagonises antiparkinsonian effect of pergolide; avoidance of metoclopramide advised by manufacturer of ropinirole and rotigotine (antagonism of effect)

Muscle Relaxants: metoclopramide enhances effects of suxamethonium

**Metoclopramide** *(continued)*
Tetrabenazine: increased risk of extrapyramidal side-effects when metoclopramide given with tetrabenazine

**Metolazone** *see* Diuretics

**Metoprolol** *see* Beta-blockers

**Metronidazole**
Note Interactions do not apply to topical metronidazole preparations
Alcohol: disulfiram-like reaction when metronidazole given with alcohol
- Anticoagulants: metronidazole enhances anticoagulant effect of ●coumarins
- Antiepileptics: metronidazole inhibits metabolism of ●phenytoin (increased plasma concentration); metabolism of metronidazole accelerated by primidone (reduced plasma concentration)
Barbiturates: metabolism of metronidazole accelerated by barbiturates (reduced plasma concentration)
- Cytotoxics: metronidazole increases plasma concentration of ●busulfan (increased risk of toxicity); metronidazole inhibits metabolism of fluorouracil (increased toxicity)
Disulfiram: psychotic reaction reported when metronidazole given with disulfiram
Lithium: metronidazole increases risk of lithium toxicity
Mycophenolate: metronidazole possibly reduces bioavailability of mycophenolate
Oestrogens: antibacterials that do not induce liver enzymes possibly reduce contraceptive effect of oestrogens (risk probably small, see p. 445)
Ulcer-healing Drugs: metabolism of metronidazole inhibited by cimetidine (increased plasma concentration)
Vaccines: antibacterials inactivate oral typhoid vaccine–see p. 688

**Mianserin** *see* Antidepressants, Tricyclic (related)

**Micafungin**
Antifungals: micafungin increases plasma concentration of itraconazole (consider reducing dose of itraconazole)
Calcium-channel Blockers: micafungin increases plasma concentration of nifedipine
Ciclosporin: micafungin possibly increases plasma concentration of ciclosporin
Sirolimus: micafungin increases plasma concentration of sirolimus

**Miconazole** *see* Antifungals, Imidazole

**Midazolam** *see* Anxiolytics and Hypnotics

**Mifepristone**
Corticosteroids: mifepristone may reduce effect of corticosteroids (including inhaled corticosteroids) for 3–4 days

**Milrinone** *see* Phosphodiesterase Inhibitors

**Minocycline** *see* Tetracyclines

**Minoxidil** *see* Vasodilator Antihypertensives

**Mirtazapine**
- Alcohol: increased sedative effect when mirtazapine given with ●alcohol
Analgesics: possible increased serotonergic effects when mirtazapine given with tramadol
Anticoagulants: mirtazapine enhances anticoagulant effect of warfarin
- Antidepressants: possible increased serotonergic effects when mirtazapine given with fluoxetine, fluvoxamine or venlafaxine; mirtazapine should not be started until 2 weeks after stopping ●MAOIs, also MAOIs should not be started until at least 2 weeks after stopping mirtazapine; after stopping mirtazapine do not start ●moclobemide for at least 1 week
Antiepileptics: plasma concentration of mirtazapine reduced by carbamazepine and phenytoin
Antifungals: plasma concentration of mirtazapine increased by ketoconazole
- Antimalarials: avoidance of antidepressants advised by manufacturer of ●artemether/lumefantrine

**Mirtazapine** *(continued)*
Anxiolytics and Hypnotics: increased sedative effect when mirtazapine given with anxiolytics and hypnotics
Atomoxetine: possible increased risk of convulsions when antidepressants given with atomoxetine
- Sibutramine: increased risk of CNS toxicity when mirtazapine given with ●sibutramine (manufacturer of sibutramine advises avoid concomitant use)
Ulcer-healing Drugs: plasma concentration of mirtazapine increased by cimetidine

**Mitomycin**
Antiepileptics: cytotoxics possibly reduce absorption of phenytoin
- Antipsychotics: avoid concomitant use of cytotoxics with ●clozapine (increased risk of agranulocytosis)
Cardiac Glycosides: cytotoxics reduce absorption of digoxin tablets

**Mitotane**
- Anticoagulants: mitotane possibly reduces anticoagulant effect of ●coumarins
Antiepileptics: cytotoxics possibly reduce absorption of phenytoin
- Antipsychotics: avoid concomitant use of cytotoxics with ●clozapine (increased risk of agranulocytosis)
Cardiac Glycosides: cytotoxics reduce absorption of digoxin tablets
Diuretics: manufacturer of mitotane advises avoid concomitant use of spironolactone (antagonism of effect)

**Mivacurium** *see* Muscle Relaxants

**Mizolastine** *see* Antihistamines

**Moclobemide**
- Analgesics: possible CNS excitation or depression (hypertension or hypotension) when moclobemide given with ●dextromethorphan or ●pethidine—avoid concomitant use; possible CNS excitation or depression (hypertension or hypotension) when moclobemide given with ●opioid analgesics
- Antidepressants: moclobemide should not be started for at least 1 week after stopping ●MAOIs, ●SSRI-related antidepressants, ●citalopram, ●fluvoxamine, ●mirtazapine, ●paroxetine, ●tricyclic-related antidepressants or ●tricyclics; increased risk of CNS toxicity when moclobemide given with ●escitalopram, preferably avoid concomitant use; moclobemide should not be started until 5 weeks after stopping ●fluoxetine; moclobemide should not be started until 2 weeks after stopping ●sertraline; possible increased serotonergic effects when moclobemide given with ●duloxetine
- Antimalarials: avoidance of antidepressants advised by manufacturer of ●artemether/lumefantrine
Atomoxetine: possible increased risk of convulsions when antidepressants given with atomoxetine
- Bupropion: avoidance of moclobemide advised by manufacturer of ●bupropion
- Dopaminergics: caution with moclobemide advised by manufacturer of entacapone; increased risk of side-effects when moclobemide given with levodopa; avoid concomitant use of moclobemide with ●selegiline
- 5HT₁ Agonists: risk of CNS toxicity when moclobemide given with ●rizatriptan or ●sumatriptan (avoid rizatriptan or sumatriptan for 2 weeks after moclobemide); risk of CNS toxicity when moclobemide given with ●zolmitriptan (reduce dose of zolmitriptan)
- Sibutramine: increased CNS toxicity when moclobemide given with ●sibutramine (manufacturer of sibutramine advises avoid concomitant use), also avoid sibutramine for 2 weeks after stopping moclobemide
- Sympathomimetics: risk of hypertensive crisis when moclobemide given with ●sympathomimetics
Ulcer-healing Drugs: plasma concentration of moclobemide increased by cimetidine (halve dose of moclobemide)

**Modafinil**

Antiepileptics: modafinil possibly increases plasma concentration of phenytoin

● Ciclosporin: modafinil reduces plasma concentration of ●ciclosporin

● Oestrogens: modafinil accelerates metabolism of ●oestrogens (reduced contraceptive effect—see p. 445)

**Moexipril** *see* ACE Inhibitors

**Mometasone** *see* Corticosteroids

**Monobactams** *see* Aztreonam

**Montelukast** *see* Leukotriene Receptor Antagonists

**Morphine** *see* Opioid Analgesics

**Moxifloxacin** *see* Quinolones

**Moxisylyte (thymoxamine)**

ACE Inhibitors: enhanced hypotensive effect when moxisylyte given with ACE inhibitors

Adrenergic Neurone Blockers: enhanced hypotensive effect when moxisylyte given with adrenergic neurone blockers

● Alpha-blockers: possible severe postural hypotension when moxisylyte given with ●alpha-blockers

Angiotensin-II Receptor Antagonists: enhanced hypotensive effect when moxisylyte given with angiotensin-II receptor antagonists

● Beta-blockers: possible severe postural hypotension when moxisylyte given with ●beta-blockers

Calcium-channel Blockers: enhanced hypotensive effect when moxisylyte given with calcium-channel blockers

Clonidine: enhanced hypotensive effect when moxisylyte given with clonidine

Diazoxide: enhanced hypotensive effect when moxisylyte given with diazoxide

Diuretics: enhanced hypotensive effect when moxisylyte given with diuretics

Methyldopa: enhanced hypotensive effect when moxisylyte given with methyldopa

Moxonidine: enhanced hypotensive effect when moxisylyte given with moxonidine

Nitrates: enhanced hypotensive effect when moxisylyte given with nitrates

Vasodilator Antihypertensives: enhanced hypotensive effect when moxisylyte given with hydralazine, minoxidil or sodium nitroprusside

**Moxonidine**

ACE Inhibitors: enhanced hypotensive effect when moxonidine given with ACE inhibitors

Adrenergic Neurone Blockers: enhanced hypotensive effect when moxonidine given with adrenergic neurone blockers

Alcohol: enhanced hypotensive effect when moxonidine given with alcohol

Aldesleukin: enhanced hypotensive effect when moxonidine given with aldesleukin

Alpha-blockers: enhanced hypotensive effect when moxonidine given with alpha-blockers

Anaesthetics, General: enhanced hypotensive effect when moxonidine given with general anaesthetics

Analgesics: hypotensive effect of moxonidine antagonised by NSAIDs

Angiotensin-II Receptor Antagonists: enhanced hypotensive effect when moxonidine given with angiotensin-II receptor antagonists

Antidepressants: enhanced hypotensive effect when moxonidine given with MAOIs

Antipsychotics: enhanced hypotensive effect when moxonidine given with phenothiazines

Anxiolytics and Hypnotics: enhanced hypotensive effect when moxonidine given with anxiolytics and hypnotics; sedative effects possibly increased when moxonidine given with benzodiazepines

Beta-blockers: enhanced hypotensive effect when moxonidine given with beta-blockers

Calcium-channel Blockers: enhanced hypotensive effect when moxonidine given with calcium-channel blockers

Clonidine: enhanced hypotensive effect when moxonidine given with clonidine

**Moxonidine** *(continued)*

Corticosteroids: hypotensive effect of moxonidine antagonised by corticosteroids

Diazoxide: enhanced hypotensive effect when moxonidine given with diazoxide

Diuretics: enhanced hypotensive effect when moxonidine given with diuretics

Dopaminergics: enhanced hypotensive effect when moxonidine given with levodopa

Methyldopa: enhanced hypotensive effect when moxonidine given with methyldopa

Moxisylyte (thymoxamine): enhanced hypotensive effect when moxonidine given with moxisylyte

Muscle Relaxants: enhanced hypotensive effect when moxonidine given with baclofen or tizanidine

Nitrates: enhanced hypotensive effect when moxonidine given with nitrates

Oestrogens: hypotensive effect of moxonidine antagonised by oestrogens

Prostaglandins: enhanced hypotensive effect when moxonidine given with alprostadil

Vasodilator Antihypertensives: enhanced hypotensive effect when moxonidine given with hydralazine, minoxidil or sodium nitroprusside

**Muscle Relaxants**

ACE Inhibitors: enhanced hypotensive effect when baclofen or tizanidine given with ACE inhibitors

Adrenergic Neurone Blockers: enhanced hypotensive effect when baclofen or tizanidine given with adrenergic neurone blockers

Alcohol: increased sedative effect when baclofen, methocarbamol or tizanidine given with alcohol

Alpha-blockers: enhanced hypotensive effect when baclofen or tizanidine given with alpha-blockers

● Anaesthetics, General: effects of atracurium enhanced by ketamine; increased risk of myocardial depression and bradycardia when suxamethonium given with ●propofol; effects of non-depolarising muscle relaxants and suxamethonium enhanced by volatile liquid general anaesthetics

Analgesics: excretion of baclofen possibly reduced by NSAIDs (increased risk of toxicity); excretion of baclofen reduced by ibuprofen (increased risk of toxicity)

Angiotensin-II Receptor Antagonists: enhanced hypotensive effect when baclofen or tizanidine given with angiotensin-II receptor antagonists

Anti-arrhythmics: neuromuscular blockade enhanced and prolonged when suxamethonium given with lidocaine (lignocaine)

● Antibacterials: effects of non-depolarising muscle relaxants and suxamethonium enhanced by piperacillin; plasma concentration of tizanidine increased by ●ciprofloxacin (increased risk of toxicity)—avoid concomitant use; plasma concentration of tizanidine possibly increased by norfloxacin (increased risk of toxicity); effects of non-depolarising muscle relaxants and suxamethonium enhanced by ●aminoglycosides; effects of non-depolarising muscle relaxants and suxamethonium enhanced by ●clindamycin; effects of non-depolarising muscle relaxants and suxamethonium enhanced by ●polymyxins; effects of suxamethonium enhanced by ●vancomycin

● Antidepressants: plasma concentration of tizanidine increased by ●fluvoxamine (increased risk of toxicity)—avoid concomitant use; effects of suxamethonium enhanced by phenelzine; muscle relaxant effect of baclofen enhanced by tricyclics

Antiepileptics: muscle relaxant effect of non-depolarising muscle relaxants antagonised by carbamazepine and phenytoin (accelerated recovery from neuromuscular blockade)

Antimalarials: effects of suxamethonium possibly enhanced by quinine

Antipsychotics: effects of suxamethonium possibly enhanced by promazine

**Muscle Relaxants** *(continued)*

Anxiolytics and Hypnotics: increased sedative effect when baclofen or tizanidine given with anxiolytics and hypnotics

Beta-blockers: enhanced hypotensive effect when baclofen given with beta-blockers; possible enhanced hypotensive effect and bradycardia when tizanidine given with beta-blockers; effects of muscle relaxants enhanced by propranolol

Calcium-channel Blockers: enhanced hypotensive effect when baclofen or tizanidine given with calcium-channel blockers; effects of non-depolarising muscle relaxants enhanced by nifedipine and verapamil; risk of arrhythmias when intravenous dantrolene given with diltiazem; hypotension, myocardial depression, and hyperkalaemia when intravenous dantrolene given with verapamil; effects of suxamethonium enhanced by verapamil

Cardiac Glycosides: possible increased risk of bradycardia when tizanidine given with cardiac glycosides; risk of ventricular arrhythmias when suxamethonium given with cardiac glycosides

Clonidine: enhanced hypotensive effect when baclofen or tizanidine given with clonidine

Corticosteroids: effects of pancuronium and vecuronium possibly antagonised by corticosteroids

Cytotoxics: effects of suxamethonium enhanced by cyclophosphamide and thiotepa

Diazoxide: enhanced hypotensive effect when baclofen or tizanidine given with diazoxide

Diuretics: enhanced hypotensive effect when baclofen or tizanidine given with diuretics

Dopaminergics: possible agitation, confusion and hallucinations when baclofen given with levodopa

Lithium: effects of muscle relaxants enhanced by lithium; baclofen possibly aggravates hyperkinesis caused by lithium

Magnesium (parenteral): effects of non-depolarising muscle relaxants and suxamethonium enhanced by parenteral magnesium

Memantine: effects of baclofen and dantrolene possibly modified by memantine

Methyldopa: enhanced hypotensive effect when baclofen or tizanidine given with methyldopa

Metoclopramide: effects of suxamethonium enhanced by metoclopramide

Moxonidine: enhanced hypotensive effect when baclofen or tizanidine given with moxonidine

Nitrates: enhanced hypotensive effect when baclofen or tizanidine given with nitrates

Oestrogens: plasma concentration of tizanidine possibly increased by oestrogens (increased risk of toxicity)

Parasympathomimetics: effects of non-depolarising muscle relaxants possibly antagonised by donepezil; effects of suxamethonium possibly enhanced by donepezil; effects of non-depolarising muscle relaxants antagonised by edrophonium, neostigmine, pyridostigmine and rivastigmine; effects of suxamethonium enhanced by edrophonium, galantamine, neostigmine, pyridostigmine and rivastigmine

Progestogens: plasma concentration of tizanidine possibly increased by progestogens (increased risk of toxicity)

Sympathomimetics, Beta$_2$: effects of suxamethonium enhanced by bambuterol

Vasodilator Antihypertensives: enhanced hypotensive effect when baclofen or tizanidine given with hydralazine; enhanced hypotensive effect when baclofen or tizanidine given with minoxidil; enhanced hypotensive effect when baclofen or tizanidine given with sodium nitroprusside

**Muscle Relaxants, depolarising** *see* Muscle Relaxants

**Muscle Relaxants, non-depolarising** *see* Muscle Relaxants

**Mycophenolate**

Antacids: absorption of mycophenolate reduced by antacids

**Mycophenolate** *(continued)*

● Antibacterials: bioavailability of mycophenolate possibly reduced by metronidazole and norfloxacin; plasma concentration of active metabolite of mycophenolate reduced by ●rifampicin

Antivirals: mycophenolate increases plasma concentration of aciclovir, also plasma concentration of inactive metabolite of mycophenolate increased; mycophenolate possibly increases plasma concentration of ganciclovir, also plasma concentration of inactive metabolite of mycophenolate possibly increased

Iron: absorption of mycophenolate reduced by *oral* iron

Lipid-regulating Drugs: absorption of mycophenolate reduced by colestyramine

Sevelamer: plasma concentration of mycophenolate possibly reduced by sevelamer

**Mycophenolate Mofetil** *see* Mycophenolate

**Mycophenolate Sodium** *see* Mycophenolate

**Mycophenolic Acid** *see* Mycophenolate

**Nabilone**

Alcohol: increased sedative effect when nabilone given with alcohol

Anxiolytics and Hypnotics: increased sedative effect when nabilone given with anxiolytics and hypnotics

**Nabumetone** *see* NSAIDs

**Nadolol** *see* Beta-blockers

**Nalidixic Acid** *see* Quinolones

**Nandrolone** *see* Anabolic Steroids

**Naproxen** *see* NSAIDs

**Naratriptan** *see* 5HT$_1$ Agonists

**Nateglinide** *see* Antidiabetics

**Nebivolol** *see* Beta-blockers

**Nefopam**

● Antidepressants: manufacturer of nefopam advises avoid concomitant use with ●MAOIs; side-effects possibly increased when nefopam given with tricyclics

Antimuscarinics: increased risk of antimuscarinic side-effects when nefopam given with antimuscarinics

**Nelfinavir**

Analgesics: nelfinavir reduces plasma concentration of methadone

● Anti-arrhythmics: increased risk of ventricular arrhythmias when nelfinavir given with ●amiodarone—avoid concomitant use

● Antibacterials: nelfinavir increases plasma concentration of ●rifabutin (halve dose of rifabutin); plasma concentration of nelfinavir significantly reduced by ●rifampicin—avoid concomitant use; avoidance of concomitant nelfinavir in severe renal and hepatic impairment advised by manufacturer of ●telithromycin

Anticoagulants: avoidance of nelfinavir advised by manufacturer of rivaroxaban

● Antidepressants: plasma concentration of nelfinavir reduced by ●St John's wort—avoid concomitant use

● Antiepileptics: plasma concentration of nelfinavir possibly reduced by carbamazepine and ●primidone; nelfinavir reduces plasma concentration of phenytoin

Antimalarials: caution with nelfinavir advised by manufacturer of artemether/lumefantrine

Antimuscarinics: avoidance of nelfinavir advised by manufacturer of darifenacin and tolterodine; manufacturer of fesoterodine advises dose reduction when nelfinavir given with fesoterodine—consult fesoterodine product literature; nelfinavir increases plasma concentration of solifenacin

● Antipsychotics: nelfinavir possibly inhibits metabolism of ●aripiprazole (reduce dose of aripiprazole); nelfinavir possibly increases plasma concentration of ●pimozide (increased risk of ventricular arrhythmias—avoid concomitant use); nelfinavir increases plasma concentration of ●sertindole (increased risk of ventricular arrhythmias—avoid concomitant use)

● Antivirals: plasma concentration of nelfinavir possibly increased by etravirine—avoid concomitant use; combination of nelfinavir with indinavir, ritonavir or saquinavir may increase plasma concentration of

**Nelfinavir**
- Antivirals *(continued)*
  either drug (or both); nelfinavir reduces plasma concentration of lopinavir, also plasma concentration of active metabolite of nelfinavir increased; nelfinavir possibly increases plasma concentration of ●maraviroc (consider reducing dose of maraviroc)
- Anxiolytics and Hypnotics: nelfinavir possibly increases plasma concentration of ●midazolam (risk of prolonged sedation—avoid concomitant use of oral midazolam)
- Barbiturates: plasma concentration of nelfinavir possibly reduced by ●barbiturates
- Ciclosporin: nelfinavir possibly increases plasma concentration of ●ciclosporin
- Cilostazol: nelfinavir possibly increases plasma concentration of ●cilostazol—avoid concomitant use
  Cytotoxics: nelfinavir increases plasma concentration of paclitaxel
- Diuretics: nelfinavir increases plasma concentration of ●eplerenone—avoid concomitant use
- Ergot Alkaloids: increased risk of ergotism when nelfinavir given with ●ergotamine and methysergide—avoid concomitant use
- 5HT₁ Agonists: nelfinavir increases plasma concentration of ●eletriptan (risk of toxicity)—avoid concomitant use
- Ivabradine: nelfinavir possibly increases plasma concentration of ●ivabradine—avoid concomitant use
- Lipid-regulating Drugs: possible increased risk of myopathy when nelfinavir given with atorvastatin; possible increased risk of myopathy when nelfinavir given with ●rosuvastatin—avoid concomitant use; increased risk of myopathy when nelfinavir given with ●simvastatin (avoid concomitant use)
- Oestrogens: nelfinavir accelerates metabolism of ●oestrogens (reduced contraceptive effect—see p. 445)
  Progestogens: nelfinavir possibly reduces contraceptive effect of progestogens
- Ranolazine: nelfinavir possibly increases plasma concentration of ●ranolazine—manufacturer of ranolazine advises avoid concomitant use
  Sildenafil: nelfinavir possibly increases plasma concentration of sildenafil—reduce initial dose of sildenafil
- Tacrolimus: nelfinavir possibly increases plasma concentration of ●tacrolimus
- Ulcer-healing Drugs: plasma concentration of nelfinavir reduced by ●omeprazole—avoid concomitant use

**Neomycin** *see* Aminoglycosides
**Neostigmine** *see* Parasympathomimetics
**Nevirapine**
  Analgesics: nevirapine possibly reduces plasma concentration of methadone
- Antibacterials: nevirapine possibly increases plasma concentration of rifabutin; plasma concentration of nevirapine reduced by ●rifampicin—avoid concomitant use
- Anticoagulants: nevirapine may enhance or reduce anticoagulant effect of ●warfarin
- Antidepressants: plasma concentration of nevirapine reduced by ●St John's wort—avoid concomitant use
- Antifungals: nevirapine reduces plasma concentration of ●ketoconazole—avoid concomitant use; plasma concentration of nevirapine increased by ●fluconazole; nevirapine possibly reduces plasma concentration of caspofungin and itraconazole—consider increasing dose of caspofungin and itraconazole
- Antipsychotics: nevirapine possibly reduces plasma concentration of ●aripiprazole—increase dose of aripiprazole
- Antivirals: nevirapine possibly reduces plasma concentration of ●atazanavir and ●etravirine—avoid concomitant use; nevirapine reduces plasma concentration of efavirenz and indinavir; nevirapine

**Nevirapine**
- Antivirals *(continued)*
  possibly reduces plasma concentration of fosamprenavir; nevirapine possibly reduces plasma concentration of ●lopinavir—consider increasing dose of lopinavir
- Oestrogens: nevirapine accelerates metabolism of ●oestrogens (reduced contraceptive effect—see p. 445)
- Progestogens: nevirapine accelerates metabolism of ●progestogens (reduced contraceptive effect—see p. 445)

**Nicardipine** *see* Calcium-channel Blockers
**Nicorandil**
  Alcohol: hypotensive effect of nicorandil possibly enhanced by alcohol
  Antidepressants: enhanced hypotensive effect when nicorandil given with MAOIs; hypotensive effect of nicorandil possibly enhanced by tricyclics
- Sildenafil: hypotensive effect of nicorandil significantly enhanced by ●sildenafil (avoid concomitant use)
- Tadalafil: hypotensive effect of nicorandil significantly enhanced by ●tadalafil (avoid concomitant use)
- Vardenafil: possible increased hypotensive effect when nicorandil given with ●vardenafil—avoid concomitant use
  Vasodilator Antihypertensives: possible enhanced hypotensive effect when nicorandil given with hydralazine, minoxidil or sodium nitroprusside

**Nicotinic Acid**
  Note Interactions apply to lipid-regulating doses of nicotinic acid
- Lipid-regulating Drugs: increased risk of myopathy when nicotinic acid given with ●statins (applies to lipid regulating doses of nicotinic acid)

**Nifedipine** *see* Calcium-channel Blockers
**Nilotinib**
  Antacids: manufacturer of nilotinib advises avoid concomitant use with antacids
- Antibacterials: manufacturer of nilotinib advises avoid concomitant use with ●clarithromycin, ●moxifloxacin and ●telithromycin; plasma concentration of nilotinib reduced by ●rifampicin—avoid concomitant use
  Antiepileptics: cytotoxics possibly reduce absorption of phenytoin
- Antifungals: plasma concentration of nilotinib increased by ●ketoconazole—avoid concomitant use; manufacturer of nilotinib advises avoid concomitant use with ●itraconazole and ●voriconazole
- Antipsychotics: avoid concomitant use of cytotoxics with ●clozapine (increased risk of agranulocytosis)
- Antivirals: manufacturer of nilotinib advises avoid concomitant use with ●ritonavir
  Anxiolytics and Hypnotics: nilotinib increases plasma concentration of midazolam
  Cardiac Glycosides: cytotoxics reduce absorption of digoxin tablets
- Grapefruit Juice: manufacturer of nilotinib advises avoid concomitant use with ●grapefruit juice
  Ulcer-healing Drugs: manufacturer of nilotinib advises avoid concomitant use with histamine H₂-antagonists and proton pump inhibitors

**Nimodipine** *see* Calcium-channel Blockers
**Nitrates**
  ACE Inhibitors: enhanced hypotensive effect when nitrates given with ACE inhibitors
  Adrenergic Neurone Blockers: enhanced hypotensive effect when nitrates given with adrenergic neurone blockers
  Alcohol: enhanced hypotensive effect when nitrates given with alcohol
  Aldesleukin: enhanced hypotensive effect when nitrates given with aldesleukin
  Alpha-blockers: enhanced hypotensive effect when nitrates given with alpha-blockers
  Anaesthetics, General: enhanced hypotensive effect when nitrates given with general anaesthetics

**Nitrates** *(continued)*

Analgesics: hypotensive effect of nitrates antagonised by NSAIDs

Angiotensin-II Receptor Antagonists: enhanced hypotensive effect when nitrates given with angiotensin-II receptor antagonists

Anti-arrhythmics: effects of sublingual tablets of nitrates reduced by disopyramide (failure to dissolve under tongue owing to dry mouth)

- Anticoagulants: infusion of glyceryl trinitrate reduces anticoagulant effect of ●heparins

Antidepressants: enhanced hypotensive effect when nitrates given with MAOIs; effects of sublingual tablets of nitrates possibly reduced by tricyclic-related antidepressants (failure to dissolve under tongue owing to dry mouth); effects of sublingual tablets of nitrates reduced by tricyclics (failure to dissolve under tongue owing to dry mouth)

Antimuscarinics: effects of sublingual tablets of nitrates possibly reduced by antimuscarinics (failure to dissolve under tongue owing to dry mouth)

Antipsychotics: enhanced hypotensive effect when nitrates given with phenothiazines

Anxiolytics and Hypnotics: enhanced hypotensive effect when nitrates given with anxiolytics and hypnotics

Beta-blockers: enhanced hypotensive effect when nitrates given with beta-blockers

Calcium-channel Blockers: enhanced hypotensive effect when nitrates given with calcium-channel blockers

Clonidine: enhanced hypotensive effect when nitrates given with clonidine

Corticosteroids: hypotensive effect of nitrates antagonised by corticosteroids

Diazoxide: enhanced hypotensive effect when nitrates given with diazoxide

Diuretics: enhanced hypotensive effect when nitrates given with diuretics

Dopaminergics: enhanced hypotensive effect when nitrates given with levodopa

Methyldopa: enhanced hypotensive effect when nitrates given with methyldopa

Moxisylyte (thymoxamine): enhanced hypotensive effect when nitrates given with moxisylyte

Moxonidine: enhanced hypotensive effect when nitrates given with moxonidine

Muscle Relaxants: enhanced hypotensive effect when nitrates given with baclofen or tizanidine

Oestrogens: hypotensive effect of nitrates antagonised by oestrogens

Prostaglandins: enhanced hypotensive effect when nitrates given with alprostadil

- Sildenafil: hypotensive effect of nitrates significantly enhanced by ●sildenafil (avoid concomitant use)
- Tadalafil: hypotensive effect of nitrates significantly enhanced by ●tadalafil (avoid concomitant use)
- Vardenafil: possible increased hypotensive effect when nitrates given with ●vardenafil—avoid concomitant use

Vasodilator Antihypertensives: enhanced hypotensive effect when nitrates given with hydralazine, minoxidil or sodium nitroprusside

**Nitrazepam** *see* Anxiolytics and Hypnotics

**Nitrofurantoin**

Antacids: absorption of nitrofurantoin reduced by oral magnesium salts (as magnesium trisilicate)

Oestrogens: antibacterials that do not induce liver enzymes possibly reduce contraceptive effect of oestrogens (risk probably small, see p. 445)

Probenecid: excretion of nitrofurantoin reduced by probenecid (increased risk of side-effects)

Sulfinpyrazone: excretion of nitrofurantoin reduced by sulfinpyrazone (increased risk of toxicity)

Vaccines: antibacterials inactivate oral typhoid vaccine—see p. 688

**Nitroimidazoles** *see* Metronidazole and Tinidazole

**Nitrous Oxide** *see* Anaesthetics, General

**Nizatidine** *see* Histamine H$_2$-antagonists

**Noradrenaline (norepinephrine)** *see* Sympathomimetics

**Norelgestromin** *see* Progestogens

**Norepinephrine (noradrenaline)** *see* Sympathomimetics

**Norethisterone** *see* Progestogens

**Norfloxacin** *see* Quinolones

**Norgestimate** *see* Progestogens

**Norgestrel** *see* Progestogens

**Nortriptyline** *see* Antidepressants, Tricyclic

**NSAIDs**

Note *See also* Aspirin. Interactions do not generally apply to topical NSAIDs

ACE Inhibitors: increased risk of renal impairment when NSAIDs given with ACE inhibitors, also hypotensive effect antagonised

Adrenergic Neurone Blockers: NSAIDs antagonise hypotensive effect of adrenergic neurone blockers

Alpha-blockers: NSAIDs antagonise hypotensive effect of alpha-blockers

- Analgesics: avoid concomitant use of NSAIDs with ●NSAIDs or ●aspirin (increased side-effects); avoid concomitant use of NSAIDs with ●ketorolac (increased side-effects and haemorrhage); ibuprofen possibly reduces antiplatelet effect of aspirin

Angiotensin-II Receptor Antagonists: increased risk of renal impairment when NSAIDs given with angiotensin-II receptor antagonists, also hypotensive effect antagonised

- Antibacterials: indometacin possibly increases plasma concentration of amikacin and gentamicin in neonates; plasma concentration of etoricoxib reduced by rifampicin; possible increased risk of convulsions when NSAIDs given with ●quinolones

- Anticoagulants: increased risk of haemorrhage when intravenous diclofenac given with ●anticoagulants (avoid concomitant use, including low-dose heparin); increased risk of haemorrhage when ketorolac given with ●anticoagulants (avoid concomitant use, including low-dose heparin); NSAIDs possibly enhance anticoagulant effect of ●coumarins and ●phenindione; azapropazone enhances anticoagulant effect of ●coumarins (avoid concomitant use); possible increased risk of bleeding when NSAIDs given with ●dabigatran etexilate or heparins

- Antidepressants: increased risk of bleeding when NSAIDs given with ●SSRIs or ●venlafaxine

- Antidiabetics: azapropazone enhances effects of ●tolbutamide (avoid concomitant use); NSAIDs possibly enhance effects of ●sulphonylureas

- Antiepileptics: NSAIDs possibly enhance effects of ●phenytoin; azapropazone significantly increases plasma concentration of ●phenytoin—avoid concomitant use

Antifungals: plasma concentration of parecoxib increased by fluconazole (reduce dose of parecoxib); plasma concentration of celecoxib increased by fluconazole (halve dose of celecoxib); plasma concentration of diclofenac and ibuprofen increased by voriconazole

- Antipsychotics: possible severe drowsiness when indometacin given with haloperidol; avoid concomitant use of azapropazone with ●clozapine (increased risk of agranulocytosis)

- Antivirals: plasma concentration of piroxicam increased by ●ritonavir (risk of toxicity)—avoid concomitant use; plasma concentration of NSAIDs possibly increased by ritonavir; increased risk of haematological toxicity when NSAIDs given with zidovudine

Beta-blockers: NSAIDs antagonise hypotensive effect of beta-blockers

Bisphosphonates: indometacin increases bioavailability of tiludronic acid

Calcium-channel Blockers: NSAIDs antagonise hypotensive effect of calcium-channel blockers

Cardiac Glycosides: NSAIDs possibly increase plasma concentration of cardiac glycosides, also possible exacerbation of heart failure and reduction of renal function

**NSAIDs** *(continued)*

- Ciclosporin: increased risk of nephrotoxicity when NSAIDs given with ●ciclosporin; plasma concentration of diclofenac increased by ●ciclosporin (halve dose of diclofenac)

  Clonidine: NSAIDs antagonise hypotensive effect of clonidine

  Clopidogrel: increased risk of bleeding when NSAIDs given with clopidogrel

  Corticosteroids: increased risk of gastro-intestinal bleeding and ulceration when NSAIDs given with corticosteroids

- Cytotoxics: NSAIDs probably reduce excretion of ●methotrexate (increased risk of toxicity)—but for concomitant use in rheumatic disease see p. 575; azapropazone reduces excretion of ●methotrexate (avoid concomitant use); diclofenac, ibuprofen, indometacin, ketoprofen, meloxicam and naproxen reduce excretion of ●methotrexate (increased risk of toxicity)—but for concomitant use in rheumatic disease see p. 575; increased risk of bleeding when NSAIDs given with ●erlotinib

  Desmopressin: indometacin enhances effects of desmopressin

  Diazoxide: NSAIDs antagonise hypotensive effect of diazoxide

- Dimethyl sulfoxide: avoid concomitant use of sulindac with ●dimethyl sulfoxide

- Diuretics: risk of nephrotoxicity of NSAIDs increased by diuretics, also antagonism of diuretic effect; indometacin and ketorolac antagonise effects of diuretics; NSAIDs possibly antagonise diuretic effect of potassium canrenoate; occasional reports of reduced renal function when indometacin given with ●triamterene—avoid concomitant use; possibly increased risk of hyperkalaemia when NSAIDs given with potassium-sparing diuretics and aldosterone antagonists; increased risk of hyperkalaemia when indometacin given with potassium-sparing diuretics and aldosterone antagonists

  Iloprost: increased risk of bleeding when NSAIDs given with iloprost

  Lipid-regulating Drugs: excretion of meloxicam increased by colestyramine

- Lithium: NSAIDs reduce excretion of ●lithium (increased risk of toxicity); ketorolac reduces excretion of ●lithium (increased risk of toxicity)—avoid concomitant use

  Methyldopa: NSAIDs antagonise hypotensive effect of methyldopa

  Moxonidine: NSAIDs antagonise hypotensive effect of moxonidine

  Muscle Relaxants: ibuprofen reduces excretion of baclofen (increased risk of toxicity); NSAIDs possibly reduce excretion of baclofen (increased risk of toxicity)

  Nitrates: NSAIDs antagonise hypotensive effect of nitrates

  Oestrogens: etoricoxib increases plasma concentration of ethinylestradiol

  Penicillamine: possible increased risk of nephrotoxicity when NSAIDs given with penicillamine

- Pentoxifylline (oxpentifylline): possible increased risk of bleeding when NSAIDs given with pentoxifylline (oxpentifylline); increased risk of bleeding when ketorolac given with ●pentoxifylline (oxpentifylline) (avoid concomitant use)

  Prasugrel: possible increased risk of bleeding when NSAIDs given with prasugrel

- Probenecid: excretion of dexketoprofen, indometacin, ketoprofen and naproxen reduced by ●probenecid (increased plasma concentration); excretion of ketorolac reduced by ●probenecid (increased plasma concentration)—avoid concomitant use

  Sibutramine: increased risk of bleeding when NSAIDs given with sibutramine

- Tacrolimus: possible increased risk of nephrotoxicity when NSAIDs given with tacrolimus; increased risk of

**NSAIDs**

- Tacrolimus *(continued)*
  nephrotoxicity when ibuprofen given with ●tacrolimus

  Ulcer-healing Drugs: plasma concentration of azapropazone possibly increased by cimetidine

  Vasodilator Antihypertensives: NSAIDs antagonise hypotensive effect of hydralazine, minoxidil and sodium nitroprusside

**Octreotide**

  Antidiabetics: octreotide possibly reduces requirements for insulin, metformin, repaglinide and sulphonylureas

- Ciclosporin: octreotide reduces plasma concentration of ●ciclosporin

  Dopaminergics: octreotide increases plasma concentration of bromocriptine

  Ulcer-healing Drugs: octreotide possibly delays absorption of cimetidine

**Oestrogens**

  Note  Interactions of combined oral contraceptives may also apply to combined contraceptive patches and vaginal rings

  ACE Inhibitors: oestrogens antagonise hypotensive effect of ACE inhibitors

  Adrenergic Neurone Blockers: oestrogens antagonise hypotensive effect of adrenergic neurone blockers

  Alpha-blockers: oestrogens antagonise hypotensive effect of alpha-blockers

  Analgesics: plasma concentration of ethinylestradiol increased by etoricoxib

  Angiotensin-II Receptor Antagonists: oestrogens antagonise hypotensive effect of angiotensin-II receptor antagonists

- Antibacterials: contraceptive effect of oestrogens possibly reduced by antibacterials that do not induce liver enzymes (risk probably small, see p. 445); metabolism of oestrogens accelerated by ●rifamycins (reduced contraceptive effect—see p. 445)

- Anticoagulants: oestrogens may enhance or reduce anticoagulant effect of ●coumarins; oestrogens antagonise anticoagulant effect of ●phenindione

- Antidepressants: contraceptive effect of oestrogens reduced by ●St John's wort (avoid concomitant use); oestrogens antagonise antidepressant effect of tricyclics (but side-effects of tricyclics possibly increased due to increased plasma concentration)

  Antidiabetics: oestrogens antagonise hypoglycaemic effect of antidiabetics

- Antiepileptics: metabolism of oestrogens accelerated by ●carbamazepine, ●oxcarbazepine, ●phenytoin, ●primidone, ●rufinamide and ●topiramate (reduced contraceptive effect—see p. 445); oestrogens reduce plasma concentration of ●lamotrigine

- Antifungals: anecdotal reports of contraceptive failure when oestrogens given with fluconazole, imidazoles, itraconazole or ketoconazole; metabolism of oestrogens accelerated by ●griseofulvin (reduced contraceptive effect—see p. 445); occasional reports of breakthrough bleeding when oestrogens (used for contraception) given with terbinafine

- Antivirals: plasma concentration of ethinylestradiol increased by ●atazanavir—avoid concomitant use; contraceptive effect of oestrogens possibly reduced by efavirenz; plasma concentration of oestrogens increased by fosamprenavir, also plasma concentration of fosamprenavir reduced—alternative contraception recommended; metabolism of oestrogens accelerated by ●nelfinavir, ●nevirapine and ●ritonavir (reduced contraceptive effect—see p. 445)

  Anxiolytics and Hypnotics: oestrogens increase plasma concentration of melatonin

- Aprepitant: possible contraceptive failure of hormonal contraceptives containing oestrogens when given with ●aprepitant (alternative contraception recommended)

- Barbiturates: metabolism of oestrogens accelerated by ●barbiturates (reduced contraceptive effect—see p. 445)

**Appendix 1: Interactions**

**Oestrogens** (continued)

Beta-blockers: oestrogens antagonise hypotensive effect of beta-blockers

Bile Acids: elimination of cholesterol in bile increased when oestrogens given with bile acids

• Bosentan: possible contraceptive failure of hormonal contraceptives containing oestrogens when given with •bosentan (alternative contraception recommended)

Calcium-channel Blockers: oestrogens antagonise hypotensive effect of calcium-channel blockers

Ciclosporin: oestrogens possibly increase plasma concentration of ciclosporin

Clonidine: oestrogens antagonise hypotensive effect of clonidine

Corticosteroids: oral contraceptives containing oestrogens increase plasma concentration of corticosteroids

Diazoxide: oestrogens antagonise hypotensive effect of diazoxide

Diuretics: oestrogens antagonise diuretic effect of diuretics

Dopaminergics: oestrogens increase plasma concentration of ropinirole; oestrogens increase plasma concentration of selegiline (increased risk of toxicity)

Lipid-regulating Drugs: plasma concentration of ethinylestradiol increased by atorvastatin and rosuvastatin

Methyldopa: oestrogens antagonise hypotensive effect of methyldopa

• Modafinil: metabolism of oestrogens accelerated by •modafinil (reduced contraceptive effect—see p. 445)

Moxonidine: oestrogens antagonise hypotensive effect of moxonidine

Muscle Relaxants: oestrogens possibly increase plasma concentration of tizanidine (increased risk of toxicity)

Nitrates: oestrogens antagonise hypotensive effect of nitrates

Sitaxentan: plasma concentration of oestrogens increased by sitaxentan

Somatropin: oestrogens (when used as oral replacement therapy) may increase dose requirements of somatropin

Sugammadex: plasma concentration of oestrogens possibly reduced by sugammadex

Tacrolimus: metabolism of oestrogens possibly inhibited by tacrolimus; ethinylestradiol possibly increases plasma concentration of tacrolimus

Theophylline: oestrogens reduce excretion of theophylline (increased plasma concentration)

Thyroid Hormones: oestrogens may increase requirements for thyroid hormones in hypothyroidism

Vasodilator Antihypertensives: oestrogens antagonise hypotensive effect of hydralazine, minoxidil and sodium nitroprusside

**Oestrogens, conjugated** see Oestrogens

**Ofloxacin** see Quinolones

**Olanzapine** see Antipsychotics

**Olmesartan** see Angiotensin-II Receptor Antagonists

**Olsalazine** see Aminosalicylates

**Omeprazole** see Proton Pump Inhibitors

**Ondansetron** see 5HT$_3$ Antagonists

**Opioid Analgesics**

Alcohol: enhanced hypotensive and sedative effects when opioid analgesics given with alcohol

Antibacterials: plasma concentration of alfentanil increased by erythromycin; avoidance of premedication with opioid analgesics advised by manufacturer of ciprofloxacin (reduced plasma concentration of ciprofloxacin) when ciprofloxacin used for surgical prophylaxis; metabolism of methadone accelerated by rifampicin (reduced effect)

• Anticoagulants: tramadol enhances anticoagulant effect of •coumarins

• Antidepressants: plasma concentration of methadone possibly increased by fluoxetine, fluvoxamine, paroxetine and sertraline; possible increased seroto-

**Opioid Analgesics**

• Antidepressants (continued)

nergic effects when pethidine or tramadol given with duloxetine; CNS excitation or depression (hypertension or hypotension) when pethidine given with •MAOIs—avoid concomitant use and for 2 weeks after stopping MAOIs; possible CNS excitation or depression (hypertension or hypotension) when opioid analgesics given with •MAOIs—avoid concomitant use and for 2 weeks after stopping MAOIs; possible CNS excitation or depression (hypertension or hypotension) when opioid analgesics given with •moclobemide; possible CNS excitation or depression (hypertension or hypotension) when dextromethorphan or pethidine given with •moclobemide—avoid concomitant use; increased risk of CNS toxicity when tramadol given with •SSRIs or •tricyclics; possible increased serotonergic effects when tramadol given with mirtazapine; sedative effects possibly increased when opioid analgesics given with tricyclics

• Antiepileptics: plasma concentration of methadone reduced by carbamazepine; dextropropoxyphene enhances effects of •carbamazepine; effects of tramadol reduced by carbamazepine; morphine increases bioavailability of gabapentin; metabolism of methadone accelerated by phenytoin (reduced effect and risk of withdrawal effects); plasma concentration of methadone possibly reduced by primidone

• Antifungals: metabolism of buprenorphine inhibited by •ketoconazole (reduce dose of buprenorphine); metabolism of alfentanil inhibited by fluconazole (risk of prolonged or delayed respiratory depression); plasma concentration of fentanyl possibly increased by fluconazole and itraconazole; metabolism of alfentanil possibly inhibited by itraconazole; plasma concentration of alfentanil and methadone increased by •voriconazole (consider reducing dose of alfentanil and methadone)

• Antihistamines: sedative effects possibly increased when opioid analgesics given with •sedating antihistamines

• Antipsychotics: enhanced hypotensive and sedative effects when opioid analgesics given with antipsychotics; increased risk of ventricular arrhythmias when methadone given with •antipsychotics that prolong the QT interval; increased risk of convulsions when tramadol given with antipsychotics; increased risk of ventricular arrhythmias when methadone given with •amisulpride—avoid concomitant use

• Antivirals: plasma concentration of methadone possibly reduced by abacavir and nevirapine; plasma concentration of methadone reduced by efavirenz, fosamprenavir, nelfinavir and ritonavir; plasma concentration of alfentanil and fentanyl increased by •ritonavir; plasma concentration of pethidine reduced by •ritonavir, but plasma concentration of toxic pethidine metabolite increased (avoid concomitant use); plasma concentration of morphine possibly reduced by ritonavir; plasma concentration of dextropropoxyphene increased by •ritonavir (risk of toxicity)—avoid concomitant use; plasma concentration of buprenorphine possibly increased by ritonavir; methadone possibly increases plasma concentration of zidovudine

Anxiolytics and Hypnotics: increased sedative effect when opioid analgesics given with anxiolytics and hypnotics

• Atomoxetine: increased risk of ventricular arrhythmias when methadone given with •atomoxetine; possible increased risk of convulsions when tramadol given with atomoxetine

Barbiturates: CNS effects of opioid analgesics possibly increased by barbiturates; plasma concentration of methadone reduced by phenobarbital

**Opioid Analgesics** *(continued)*

Beta-blockers: morphine possibly increases plasma concentration of esmolol

Calcium-channel Blockers: metabolism of alfentanil inhibited by diltiazem (risk of prolonged or delayed respiratory depression)

Domperidone: opioid analgesics antagonise effects of domperidone on gastro-intestinal activity

● Dopaminergics: avoid concomitant use of dextromethorphan with ●rasagiline; risk of CNS toxicity when pethidine given with ●rasagiline (avoid pethidine for 2 weeks after rasagiline); hyperpyrexia and CNS toxicity reported when pethidine given with ●selegiline (avoid concomitant use); caution with tramadol advised by manufacturer of selegiline

5HT$_3$ Antagonists: effects of tramadol possibly antagonised by ondansetron

● Memantine: increased risk of CNS toxicity when dextromethorphan given with ●memantine (manufacturer of memantine advises avoid concomitant use)

Metoclopramide: opioid analgesics antagonise effects of metoclopramide on gastro-intestinal activity

● Sodium Oxybate: opioid analgesics enhance effects of ●sodium oxybate (avoid concomitant use)

Ulcer-healing Drugs: metabolism of opioid analgesics inhibited by cimetidine (increased plasma concentration)

**Orciprenaline** *see* Sympathomimetics

**Orlistat**

Anti-arrhythmics: orlistat possibly reduces plasma concentration of amiodarone

Anticoagulants: manufacturer of orlistat recommends monitoring anticoagulant effect of coumarins

Antidiabetics: manufacturer of orlistat advises avoid concomitant use with acarbose

● Ciclosporin: orlistat possibly reduces absorption of ●ciclosporin

**Orphenadrine** *see* Antimuscarinics

**Oxaliplatin** *see* Platinum Compounds

**Oxandrolone** *see* Anabolic Steroids

**Oxazepam** *see* Anxiolytics and Hypnotics

**Oxcarbazepine**

● Antidepressants: anticonvulsant effect of antiepileptics possibly antagonised by MAOIs and ●tricyclic-related antidepressants (convulsive threshold lowered); anticonvulsant effect of antiepileptics antagonised by ●SSRIs and ●tricyclics (convulsive threshold lowered); avoid concomitant use of antiepileptics with ●St John's wort

Antiepileptics: oxcarbazepine sometimes reduces plasma concentration of carbamazepine (but concentration of an active metabolite of carbamazepine may be increased), also plasma concentration of an active metabolite of oxcarbazepine often reduced; oxcarbazepine increases plasma concentration of phenytoin, also plasma concentration of an active metabolite of oxcarbazepine reduced; plasma concentration of an active metabolite of oxcarbazepine sometimes reduced by valproate

● Antimalarials: possible increased risk of convulsions when antiepileptics given with chloroquine and hydroxychloroquine; anticonvulsant effect of antiepileptics antagonised by ●mefloquine

● Antipsychotics: anticonvulsant effect of oxcarbazepine antagonised by ●antipsychotics (convulsive threshold lowered)

Barbiturates: oxcarbazepine increases plasma concentration of phenobarbital, also plasma concentration of an active metabolite of oxcarbazepine reduced

Ciclosporin: oxcarbazepine possibly reduces plasma concentration of ciclosporin

● Cytotoxics: oxcarbazepine reduces plasma concentration of ●imatinib—avoid concomitant use

● Oestrogens: oxcarbazepine accelerates metabolism of ●oestrogens (reduced contraceptive effect—see p. 445)

**Oxcarbazepine** *(continued)*

● Progestogens: oxcarbazepine accelerates metabolism of ●progestogens (reduced contraceptive effect—see p. 445)

**Oxprenolol** *see* Beta-blockers

**Oxybutynin** *see* Antimuscarinics

**Oxycodone** *see* Opioid Analgesics

**Oxymetazoline** *see* Sympathomimetics

**Oxytetracycline** *see* Tetracyclines

**Oxytocin**

Anaesthetics, General: oxytocic effect possibly reduced, also enhanced hypotensive effect and risk of arrhythmias when oxytocin given with volatile liquid general anaesthetics

Prostaglandins: uterotonic effect of oxytocin potentiated by prostaglandins

Sympathomimetics: risk of hypertension when oxytocin given with vasoconstrictor sympathomimetics (due to enhanced vasopressor effect)

**Paclitaxel**

Antidiabetics: paclitaxel possibly inhibits metabolism of rosiglitazone

Antiepileptics: cytotoxics possibly reduce absorption of phenytoin

● Antipsychotics: avoid concomitant use of cytotoxics with ●clozapine (increased risk of agranulocytosis)

Antivirals: plasma concentration of paclitaxel increased by nelfinavir and ritonavir

Cardiac Glycosides: cytotoxics reduce absorption of digoxin tablets

**Paliperidone** *see* Antipsychotics

**Pancreatin**

Antidiabetics: pancreatin antagonises hypoglycaemic effect of acarbose

**Pancuronium** *see* Muscle Relaxants

**Pantoprazole** *see* Proton Pump Inhibitors

**Papaveretum** *see* Opioid Analgesics

**Paracetamol**

Anticoagulants: prolonged regular use of paracetamol possibly enhances anticoagulant effect of coumarins

Antiepileptics: metabolism of paracetamol possibly accelerated by carbamazepine

Cytotoxics: paracetamol possibly inhibits metabolism of *intravenous* busulfan (manufacturer of *intravenous* busulfan advises caution within 72 hours of paracetamol)

Lipid-regulating Drugs: absorption of paracetamol reduced by colestyramine

Metoclopramide: rate of absorption of paracetamol increased by metoclopramide

**Paraldehyde**

● Alcohol: increased sedative effect when paraldehyde given with ●alcohol

● Disulfiram: risk of toxicity when paraldehyde given with ●disulfiram

**Parasympathomimetics**

Anti-arrhythmics: effects of neostigmine and pyridostigmine possibly antagonised by propafenone

● Antibacterials: plasma concentration of galantamine increased by erythromycin; effects of neostigmine and pyridostigmine antagonised by ●aminoglycosides; effects of neostigmine and pyridostigmine antagonised by clindamycin; effects of neostigmine and pyridostigmine antagonised by ●polymyxins

Antidepressants: plasma concentration of galantamine increased by paroxetine

Antifungals: plasma concentration of galantamine increased by ketoconazole

Antimalarials: effects of neostigmine and pyridostigmine may be diminished because of potential for chloroquine and hydroxychloroquine to increase symptoms of myasthenia gravis

Antimuscarinics: effects of parasympathomimetics antagonised by antimuscarinics

Beta-blockers: increased risk of arrhythmias when pilocarpine given with beta-blockers; effects of neostigmine and pyridostigmine antagonised by propranolol

**Parasympathomimetics** *(continued)*
Lithium: effects of neostigmine and pyridostigmine antagonised by lithium
Muscle Relaxants: donepezil possibly enhances effects of suxamethonium; edrophonium, galantamine, neostigmine, pyridostigmine and rivastigmine enhance effects of suxamethonium; donepezil possibly antagonises effects of non-depolarising muscle relaxants; edrophonium, neostigmine, pyridostigmine and rivastigmine antagonise effects of non-depolarising muscle relaxants

**Parecoxib** *see* NSAIDs
**Paricalcitol** *see* Vitamins
**Paroxetine** *see* Antidepressants, SSRI
**Pegfilgrastim** *see* Filgrastim
**Peginterferon Alfa** *see* Interferons
**Penicillamine**
Analgesics: possible increased risk of nephrotoxicity when penicillamine given with NSAIDs
Antacids: absorption of penicillamine reduced by antacids
● Antipsychotics: avoid concomitant use of penicillamine with ●clozapine (increased risk of agranulocytosis)
Cardiac Glycosides: penicillamine possibly reduces plasma concentration of digoxin
Gold: manufacturer of penicillamine advises avoid concomitant use with gold (increased risk of toxicity)
Iron: absorption of penicillamine reduced by *oral* iron
Zinc: penicillamine reduces absorption of zinc, also absorption of penicillamine reduced by zinc
**Penicillins**
Allopurinol: increased risk of rash when amoxicillin or ampicillin given with allopurinol
Antibacterials: absorption of phenoxymethylpenicillin reduced by neomycin
Anticoagulants: common experience in anticoagulant clinics is that INR can be altered by a course of broad-spectrum penicillins such as ampicillin, although studies have failed to demonstrate an interaction with coumarins or phenindione
Cytotoxics: penicillins reduce excretion of methotrexate (increased risk of toxicity)
Muscle Relaxants: piperacillin enhances effects of non-depolarising muscle relaxants and suxamethonium
Oestrogens: antibacterials that do not induce liver enzymes possibly reduce contraceptive effect of oestrogens (risk probably small, see p. 445)
Probenecid: excretion of penicillins reduced by probenecid (increased plasma concentration)
Sugammadex: flucloxacillin possibly reduces response to sugammadex
Sulfinpyrazone: excretion of penicillins reduced by sulfinpyrazone
Vaccines: antibacterials inactivate oral typhoid vaccine–see p. 688
**Pentamidine Isetionate**
● Anti-arrhythmics: increased risk of ventricular arrhythmias when pentamidine isetionate given with ●amiodarone–avoid concomitant use
● Antibacterials: increased risk of ventricular arrhythmias when pentamidine isetionate given with parenteral ●erythromycin; increased risk of ventricular arrhythmias when pentamidine isetionate given with ●moxifloxacin–avoid concomitant use
● Antidepressants: increased risk of ventricular arrhythmias when pentamidine isetionate given with ●tricyclics
Antifungals: possible increased risk of nephrotoxicity when pentamidine isetionate given with amphotericin
● Antipsychotics: increased risk of ventricular arrhythmias when pentamidine isetionate given with ●amisulpride or ●droperidol–avoid concomitant use; increased risk of ventricular arrhythmias when pentamidine isetionate given with ●phenothiazines
● Ivabradine: increased risk of ventricular arrhythmias when pentamidine isetionate given with ●ivabradine

**Pentazocine** *see* Opioid Analgesics
**Pentostatin**
Antiepileptics: cytotoxics possibly reduce absorption of phenytoin
● Antipsychotics: avoid concomitant use of cytotoxics with ●clozapine (increased risk of agranulocytosis)
Cardiac Glycosides: cytotoxics reduce absorption of digoxin tablets
● Cytotoxics: increased toxicity when pentostatin given with high-dose ●cyclophosphamide—avoid concomitant use; increased pulmonary toxicity when pentostatin given with ●fludarabine (unacceptably high incidence of fatalities)
**Pentoxifylline (oxpentifylline)**
● Analgesics: possible increased risk of bleeding when pentoxifylline (oxpentifylline) given with NSAIDs; increased risk of bleeding when pentoxifylline (oxpentifylline) given with ●ketorolac (avoid concomitant use)
Theophylline: pentoxifylline (oxpentifylline) increases plasma concentration of theophylline
**Pergolide**
Antipsychotics: effects of pergolide antagonised by antipsychotics
Memantine: effects of dopaminergics possibly enhanced by memantine
Methyldopa: antiparkinsonian effect of dopaminergics antagonised by methyldopa
Metoclopramide: antiparkinsonian effect of pergolide antagonised by metoclopramide
**Pericyazine** *see* Antipsychotics
**Perindopril** *see* ACE Inhibitors
**Perphenazine** *see* Antipsychotics
**Pethidine** *see* Opioid Analgesics
**Phenazocine** *see* Opioid Analgesics
**Phenelzine** *see* MAOIs
**Phenindione**
Note Change in patient's clinical condition particularly associated with liver disease, intercurrent illness, or drug administration, necessitates more frequent testing. Major changes in diet (especially involving salads and vegetables) and in alcohol consumption may also affect anticoagulant control
● Alcohol: anticoagulant control with phenindione may be affected by major changes in consumption of ●alcohol
● Anabolic Steroids: anticoagulant effect of phenindione enhanced by ●anabolic steroids
● Analgesics: anticoagulant effect of phenindione possibly enhanced by ●NSAIDs; increased risk of haemorrhage when anticoagulants given with intravenous ●diclofenac (avoid concomitant use, including low-dose heparin); increased risk of haemorrhage when anticoagulants given with ●ketorolac (avoid concomitant use, including low-dose heparin); increased risk of bleeding when phenindione given with ●aspirin (due to antiplatelet effect)
● Anti-arrhythmics: metabolism of phenindione inhibited by ●amiodarone (enhanced anticoagulant effect)
● Antibacterials: experience in anticoagulant clinics suggests that INR possibly altered when phenindione is given with ●neomycin (given for local action on gut); anticoagulant effect of phenindione possibly enhanced by levofloxacin and ●tetracyclines; studies have failed to demonstrate an interaction with phenindione, but common experience in anticoagulant clinics is that INR can be altered by a course of broad-spectrum penicillins such as ampicillin
● Antivirals: anticoagulant effect of phenindione possibly enhanced by ●ritonavir
● Clopidogrel: anticoagulant effect of phenindione enhanced due to antiplatelet action of ●clopidogrel
● Dipyridamole: anticoagulant effect of phenindione enhanced due to antiplatelet action of ●dipyridamole
● Enteral Foods: anticoagulant effect of phenindione antagonised by vitamin K (present in some ●enteral feeds)

**Phenindione** *(continued)*

Iloprost: increased risk of bleeding when phenindione given with iloprost

- Lipid-regulating Drugs: anticoagulant effect of phenindione may be enhanced or reduced by ●colestyramine; anticoagulant effect of phenindione possibly enhanced by ●rosuvastatin; anticoagulant effect of phenindione enhanced by ●fibrates
- Oestrogens: anticoagulant effect of phenindione antagonised by ●oestrogens

Prasugrel: possible increased risk of bleeding when phenindione given with prasugrel

- Progestogens: anticoagulant effect of phenindione antagonised by ●progestogens

Sibutramine: increased risk of bleeding when anticoagulants given with sibutramine

- Testolactone: anticoagulant effect of phenindione enhanced by ●testolactone
- Testosterone: anticoagulant effect of phenindione enhanced by ●testosterone
- Thyroid Hormones: anticoagulant effect of phenindione enhanced by ●thyroid hormones
- Vitamins: anticoagulant effect of phenindione antagonised by ●vitamin K

**Phenobarbital** *see* Barbiturates

**Phenothiazines** *see* Antipsychotics

**Phenoxybenzamine** *see* Alpha-blockers

**Phenoxymethylpenicillin** *see* Penicillins

**Phentolamine** *see* Alpha-blockers

**Phenylephrine** *see* Sympathomimetics

**Phenytoin**

Note Fosphenytoin interactions as for phenytoin

- Analgesics: effects of phenytoin possibly enhanced by ●NSAIDs; plasma concentration of phenytoin significantly increased by ●azapropazone—avoid concomitant use; phenytoin accelerates metabolism of methadone (reduced effect and risk of withdrawal effects); effects of phenytoin enhanced by aspirin

Antacids: absorption of phenytoin reduced by antacids

- Anti-arrhythmics: metabolism of phenytoin inhibited by ●amiodarone (increased plasma concentration); phenytoin reduces plasma concentration of disopyramide
- Antibacterials: metabolism of phenytoin inhibited by clarithromycin, ●isoniazid and ●metronidazole (increased plasma concentration); plasma concentration of phenytoin increased or decreased by ciprofloxacin; phenytoin accelerates metabolism of doxycycline (reduced plasma concentration); plasma concentration of phenytoin increased by ●chloramphenicol (increased risk of toxicity); metabolism of phenytoin accelerated by ●rifamycins (reduced plasma concentration); plasma concentration of phenytoin possibly increased by sulphonamides; phenytoin reduces plasma concentration of ●telithromycin (avoid during and for 2 weeks after phenytoin); plasma concentration of phenytoin increased by ●trimethoprim (also increased antifolate effect)
- Anticoagulants: phenytoin accelerates metabolism of ●coumarins (possibility of reduced anticoagulant effect, but enhancement also reported)
- Antidepressants: plasma concentration of phenytoin increased by ●fluoxetine and ●fluvoxamine; phenytoin reduces plasma concentration of ●mianserin, mirtazapine and paroxetine; anticonvulsant effect of antiepileptics possibly antagonised by MAOIs and ●tricyclic-related antidepressants (convulsive threshold lowered); anticonvulsant effect of antiepileptics antagonised by ●SSRIs and ●tricyclics (convulsive threshold lowered); avoid concomitant use of antiepileptics with ●St John's wort; phenytoin possibly reduces plasma concentration of ●tricyclics

Antidiabetics: plasma concentration of phenytoin transiently increased by tolbutamide (possibility of toxicity)

- Antiepileptics: plasma concentration of both drugs often reduced when phenytoin given with carbamazepine, also plasma concentration of phenytoin

**Phenytoin**

- Antiepileptics *(continued)*

may be increased; plasma concentration of phenytoin possibly increased by ●ethosuximide, also plasma concentration of ethosuximide possibly reduced; phenytoin reduces plasma concentration of lamotrigine, tiagabine and zonisamide; plasma concentration of phenytoin increased by oxcarbazepine, also plasma concentration of an active metabolite of oxcarbazepine reduced; phenytoin possibly reduces plasma concentration of primidone (but concentration of an active metabolite increased), plasma concentration of phenytoin often reduced but may be increased; plasma concentration of phenytoin possibly increased by rufinamide; plasma concentration of phenytoin increased by ●stiripentol; plasma concentration of phenytoin increased by ●topiramate (also plasma concentration of topiramate reduced); plasma concentration of phenytoin increased or possibly reduced when given with valproate, also plasma concentration of valproate reduced; plasma concentration of phenytoin reduced by vigabatrin

- Antifungals: phenytoin reduces plasma concentration of ●ketoconazole and ●posaconazole; anticonvulsant effect of phenytoin enhanced by ●miconazole (plasma concentration of phenytoin increased); plasma concentration of phenytoin increased by ●fluconazole (consider reducing dose of phenytoin); phenytoin reduces plasma concentration of ●itraconazole—avoid concomitant use; plasma concentration of phenytoin increased by ●voriconazole, also phenytoin reduces plasma concentration of voriconazole (increase dose of voriconazole and also monitor for phenytoin toxicity); phenytoin possibly reduces plasma concentration of caspofungin—consider increasing dose of caspofungin
- Antimalarials: possible increased risk of convulsions when antiepileptics given with chloroquine and hydroxychloroquine; anticonvulsant effect of antiepileptics antagonised by ●mefloquine; anticonvulsant effect of phenytoin antagonised by ●pyrimethamine, also increased antifolate effect
- Antipsychotics: anticonvulsant effect of phenytoin antagonised by ●antipsychotics (convulsive threshold lowered); phenytoin possibly reduces plasma concentration of ●aripiprazole—increase dose of aripiprazole; phenytoin accelerates metabolism of clozapine, quetiapine and sertindole (reduced plasma concentration)
- Antivirals: phenytoin possibly reduces plasma concentration of abacavir, darunavir, fosamprenavir, lopinavir and saquinavir; avoidance of phenytoin advised by manufacturer of etravirine; phenytoin possibly reduces plasma concentration of ●indinavir, also plasma concentration of phenytoin possibly increased; plasma concentration of phenytoin reduced by nelfinavir; phenytoin possibly reduces plasma concentration of ritonavir, also plasma concentration of phenytoin possibly affected; plasma concentration of phenytoin increased or decreased by zidovudine

Anxiolytics and Hypnotics: phenytoin often reduces plasma concentration of clonazepam; plasma concentration of phenytoin increased or decreased by diazepam; plasma concentration of phenytoin possibly increased or decreased by benzodiazepines

Aprepitant: phenytoin possibly reduces plasma concentration of aprepitant

Barbiturates: phenytoin often increases plasma concentration of phenobarbital, plasma concentration of phenytoin often reduced but may be increased

Bupropion: phenytoin reduces plasma concentration of bupropion

- Calcium-channel Blockers: phenytoin reduces effects of felodipine, isradipine and verapamil; phenytoin

**Phenytoin**
- Calcium-channel Blockers *(continued)*
  probably reduces effects of dihydropyridines, nicardipine and ●nifedipine; plasma concentration of phenytoin increased by ●diltiazem but also effect of diltiazem reduced

  Cardiac Glycosides: phenytoin accelerates metabolism of digitoxin (reduced effect); phenytoin possibly reduces plasma concentration of digoxin
- Ciclosporin: phenytoin accelerates metabolism of ●ciclosporin (reduced plasma concentration)
- Corticosteroids: phenytoin accelerates metabolism of ●corticosteroids (reduced effect)
- Cytotoxics: phenytoin possibly reduces plasma concentration of busulfan and etoposide; metabolism of phenytoin possibly inhibited by fluorouracil (increased risk of toxicity); phenytoin increases antifolate effect of methotrexate; absorption of phenytoin possibly reduced by cytotoxics; phenytoin reduces plasma concentration of ●imatinib—avoid concomitant use; avoidance of phenytoin advised by manufacturer of ●lapatinib; phenytoin reduces plasma concentration of irinotecan and its active metabolite

  Diazoxide: plasma concentration of phenytoin reduced by diazoxide, also effect of diazoxide may be reduced
- Disulfiram: metabolism of phenytoin inhibited by ●disulfiram (increased risk of toxicity)
- Diuretics: phenytoin antagonises effects of furosemide (frusemide); phenytoin reduces plasma concentration of ●eplerenone—avoid concomitant use; increased risk of osteomalacia when phenytoin given with carbonic anhydrase inhibitors

  Dopaminergics: phenytoin possibly reduces effects of levodopa

  Enteral Foods: absorption of phenytoin possibly reduced by enteral feeds

  Folates: plasma concentration of phenytoin possibly reduced by folates

  Hormone Antagonists: phenytoin accelerates metabolism of gestrinone (reduced plasma concentration); phenytoin possibly accelerates metabolism of toremifene

  5HT₃ Antagonists: phenytoin accelerates metabolism of ondansetron (reduced effect)

  Leflunomide: plasma concentration of phenytoin possibly increased by leflunomide

  Levamisole: plasma concentration of phenytoin possibly increased by levamisole

  Lipid-regulating Drugs: combination of phenytoin with fluvastatin may increase plasma concentration of either drug (or both)

  Lithium: neurotoxicity may occur when phenytoin given with lithium without increased plasma concentration of lithium

  Modafinil: plasma concentration of phenytoin possibly increased by modafinil

  Muscle Relaxants: phenytoin antagonises muscle relaxant effect of non-depolarising muscle relaxants (accelerated recovery from neuromuscular blockade)
- Oestrogens: phenytoin accelerates metabolism of ●oestrogens (reduced contraceptive effect—see p. 445)
- Progestogens: phenytoin accelerates metabolism of ●progestogens (reduced contraceptive effect—see p. 445)
- Sulfinpyrazone: plasma concentration of phenytoin increased by ●sulfinpyrazone

  Sympathomimetics: plasma concentration of phenytoin increased by methylphenidate

  Tacrolimus: phenytoin reduces plasma concentration of tacrolimus, also plasma concentration of phenytoin possibly increased
- Theophylline: plasma concentration of both drugs reduced when phenytoin given with ●theophylline

  Thyroid Hormones: phenytoin accelerates metabolism of thyroid hormones (may increase requirements in hypothyroidism), also plasma concentration of phenytoin possibly increased

**Phenytoin** *(continued)*
  Tibolone: phenytoin accelerates metabolism of tibolone
- Ulcer-healing Drugs: metabolism of phenytoin inhibited by ●cimetidine (increased plasma concentration); effects of phenytoin enhanced by ●esomeprazole; effects of phenytoin possibly enhanced by omeprazole; absorption of phenytoin reduced by ●sucralfate

  Vaccines: effects of phenytoin enhanced by influenza vaccine

  Vitamins: phenytoin possibly increases requirements for vitamin D

**Phosphodiesterase Inhibitors**
- Anagrelide: avoidance of enoximone and milrinone advised by manufacturer of ●anagrelide

**Physostigmine** *see* Parasympathomimetics
**Pilocarpine** *see* Parasympathomimetics
**Pimozide** *see* Antipsychotics
**Pindolol** *see* Beta-blockers
**Pioglitazone** *see* Antidiabetics
**Piperacillin** *see* Penicillins
**Pipotiazine** *see* Antipsychotics
**Piroxicam** *see* NSAIDs
**Pivmecillinam** *see* Penicillins

**Pizotifen**
  Adrenergic Neurone Blockers: pizotifen antagonises hypotensive effect of adrenergic neurone blockers

**Platinum Compounds**
- Antibacterials: increased risk of nephrotoxicity and possibly of ototoxicity when platinum compounds given with ●aminoglycosides or ●polymyxins; increased risk of nephrotoxicity and ototoxicity when platinum compounds given with capreomycin; increased risk of nephrotoxicity and possibly of ototoxicity when cisplatin given with vancomycin

  Antiepileptics: cytotoxics possibly reduce absorption of phenytoin
- Antipsychotics: avoid concomitant use of cytotoxics with ●clozapine (increased risk of agranulocytosis)

  Cardiac Glycosides: cytotoxics reduce absorption of digoxin tablets
- Cytotoxics: increased pulmonary toxicity when cisplatin given with ●bleomycin and ●methotrexate

  Diuretics: increased risk of nephrotoxicity and ototoxicity when platinum compounds given with diuretics

**Polymyxin B** *see* Polymyxins

**Polymyxins**
  Antibacterials: increased risk of nephrotoxicity when colistin or polymyxins given with aminoglycosides; increased risk of nephrotoxicity when colistin or polymyxins given with capreomycin; increased risk of nephrotoxicity and ototoxicity when colistin given with teicoplanin or vancomycin; increased risk of nephrotoxicity when polymyxins given with vancomycin

  Antifungals: increased risk of nephrotoxicity when polymyxins given with amphotericin
- Ciclosporin: increased risk of nephrotoxicity when polymyxins given with ●ciclosporin
- Cytotoxics: increased risk of nephrotoxicity and possibly of ototoxicity when polymyxins given with ●platinum compounds
- Diuretics: increased risk of ototoxicity when polymyxins given with ●loop diuretics
- Muscle Relaxants: polymyxins enhance effects of ●non-depolarising muscle relaxants and ●suxamethonium

  Oestrogens: antibacterials that do not induce liver enzymes possibly reduce contraceptive effect of oestrogens (risk probably small, see p. 445)
- Parasympathomimetics: polymyxins antagonise effects of ●neostigmine and ●pyridostigmine

  Vaccines: antibacterials inactivate oral typhoid vaccine—see p. 688

**Polystyrene Sulphonate Resins**
  Thyroid Hormones: polystyrene sulphonate resins reduce absorption of levothyroxine (thyroxine)

Posaconazole *see* Antifungals, Triazole
Potassium Canrenoate *see* Diuretics
Potassium Aminobenzoate
   Antibacterials: potassium aminobenzoate inhibits
     effects of sulphonamides
Potassium Bicarbonate *see* Potassium Salts
Potassium Chloride *see* Potassium Salts
Potassium Citrate *see* Potassium Salts
Potassium Salts
   Note  Includes salt substitutes
• ACE Inhibitors: increased risk of severe hyperkalaemia
   when potassium salts given with •ACE inhibitors
   Aliskiren: increased risk of hyperkalaemia when
     potassium salts given with aliskiren
• Angiotensin-II Receptor Antagonists: increased risk of
   hyperkalaemia when potassium salts given with
   •angiotensin-II receptor antagonists
   Antibacterials: avoid concomitant use of potassium
     citrate with methenamine
• Ciclosporin: increased risk of hyperkalaemia when
   potassium salts given with •ciclosporin
• Diuretics: increased risk of hyperkalaemia when
   potassium salts given with •potassium-sparing diur-
   etics and aldosterone antagonists
• Tacrolimus: increased risk of hyperkalaemia when
   potassium salts given with •tacrolimus
Pramipexole
   Antipsychotics: manufacturer of pramipexole advises
     avoid concomitant use of antipsychotics (antagonism
     of effect)
   Memantine: effects of dopaminergics possibly
     enhanced by memantine
   Methyldopa: antiparkinsonian effect of dopaminergics
     antagonised by methyldopa
   Ulcer-healing Drugs: excretion of pramipexole reduced
     by cimetidine (increased plasma concentration)
Prasugrel
   <u>Analgesics</u>: possible increased risk of bleeding when
     prasugrel given with NSAIDs
   <u>Anticoagulants</u>: possible increased risk of bleeding
     when prasugrel given with coumarins or phenindione
   <u>Clopidogrel</u>: possible increased risk of bleeding when
     prasugrel given with clopidogrel
Pravastatin *see* Statins
Prazosin *see* Alpha-blockers
Prednisolone *see* Corticosteroids
Prilocaine
   Anti-arrhythmics: increased myocardial depression
     when prilocaine given with anti-arrhythmics
   Antibacterials: increased risk of methaemoglobin-
     aemia when prilocaine given with sulphonamides
Primaquine
• Antimalarials: avoidance of antimalarials advised by
   manufacturer of •artemether/lumefantrine
   Mepacrine: plasma concentration of primaquine
     increased by mepacrine (increased risk of toxicity)
   Vaccines: antimalarials inactivate oral typhoid
     vaccine–see p. 688
Primidone
   Alcohol: increased sedative effect when primidone
     given with alcohol
   <u>Analgesics</u>: primidone possibly reduces plasma con-
     centration of methadone
   Anti-arrhythmics: primidone accelerates metabolism of
     disopyramide (reduced plasma concentration)
• Antibacterials: primidone accelerates metabolism of
   •chloramphenicol, doxycycline and metronidazole
   (reduced plasma concentration); primidone reduces
   plasma concentration of •telithromycin (avoid during
   and for 2 weeks after primidone)
• Anticoagulants: primidone accelerates metabolism of
   •coumarins (reduced anticoagulant effect)
• Antidepressants: primidone reduces plasma concentration of paroxetine; primidone accelerates metabolism of •mianserin (reduced plasma concentration);
   anticonvulsant effect of antiepileptics possibly
   antagonised by MAOIs and •tricyclic-related antidepressants (convulsive threshold lowered); anticonvulsant effect of antiepileptics antagonised by

Primidone
• Antidepressants *(continued)*
    •SSRIs and •tricyclics (convulsive threshold
    lowered); avoid concomitant use of antiepileptics
    with •St John's wort; anticonvulsant effect of
    primidone antagonised by •tricyclics (convulsive
    threshold lowered), also metabolism of tricyclics
    possibly accelerated (reduced plasma concentration)
• Antiepileptics: primidone often reduces plasma concentration of carbamazepine, also plasma concentration of primidone sometimes reduced (but
   concentration of an active metabolite of primidone
   often increased); primidone possibly reduces plasma
   concentration of ethosuximide; primidone reduces
   plasma concentration of lamotrigine and tiagabine;
   plasma concentration of primidone possibly reduced
   by phenytoin (but concentration of an active metabolite increased), plasma concentration of phenytoin
   often reduced but may be increased; plasma concentration of primidone possibly increased by
   •valproate (plasma concentration of active metabolite of primidone increased), also plasma concentration of valproate reduced; plasma concentration of
   primidone possibly reduced by vigabatrin
• Antifungals: primidone possibly reduces plasma concentration of •posaconazole; primidone possibly
   reduces plasma concentration of •voriconazole—
   avoid concomitant use; primidone reduces absorption of griseofulvin (reduced effect)
• Antimalarials: possible increased risk of convulsions
   when antiepileptics given with chloroquine and
   hydroxychloroquine; anticonvulsant effect of antiepileptics antagonised by •mefloquine
• Antipsychotics: anticonvulsant effect of primidone
   antagonised by •antipsychotics (convulsive threshold
   lowered); primidone accelerates metabolism of haloperidol (reduced plasma concentration); primidone
   possibly reduces plasma concentration of
   •aripiprazole—increase dose of aripiprazole
• Antivirals: primidone possibly reduces plasma concentration of •indinavir, •lopinavir, •nelfinavir and
   •saquinavir
   Anxiolytics and Hypnotics: primidone often reduces
     plasma concentration of clonazepam
   Barbiturates: increased sedative effect when primid-
     one given with barbiturates
• Calcium-channel Blockers: primidone reduces effects
   of •felodipine and •isradipine; primidone probably
   reduces effects of •dihydropyridines, •diltiazem and
   •verapamil
   Cardiac Glycosides: primidone accelerates metabolism
     of digitoxin (reduced effect)
• Ciclosporin: primidone accelerates metabolism of
   •ciclosporin (reduced effect)
• Corticosteroids: primidone accelerates metabolism of
   •corticosteroids (reduced effect)
   Diuretics: plasma concentration of primidone possibly
     reduced by acetazolamide; increased risk of osteo-
     malacia when primidone given with carbonic
     anhydrase inhibitors
   Folates: plasma concentration of primidone possibly
     reduced by folates
   Hormone Antagonists: primidone accelerates metab-
     olism of gestrinone and toremifene (reduced plasma
     concentration)
   Leukotriene Receptor Antagonists: primidone reduces
     plasma concentration of montelukast
   Memantine: effects of primidone possibly reduced by
     memantine
• Oestrogens: primidone accelerates metabolism of
   •oestrogens (reduced contraceptive effect—see
   p. 445)
• Progestogens: primidone accelerates metabolism of
   •progestogens (reduced contraceptive effect—see
   p. 445)
   Sympathomimetics: plasma concentration of primid-
     one possibly increased by methylphenidate
   Theophylline: primidone accelerates metabolism of
     theophylline (reduced effect)

Appendix 1: Interactions

**Primidone** *(continued)*

Thyroid Hormones: primidone accelerates metabolism of thyroid hormones (may increase requirements for thyroid hormones in hypothyroidism)

Tibolone: primidone accelerates metabolism of tibolone (reduced plasma concentration)

Vitamins: primidone possibly increases requirements for vitamin D

**Probenecid**

ACE Inhibitors: probenecid reduces excretion of captopril

Anaesthetics, General: probenecid possibly enhances effects of thiopental

• Analgesics: probenecid reduces excretion of ●dexketoprofen, ●indometacin, ●ketoprofen and ●naproxen (increased plasma concentration); probenecid reduces excretion of ●ketorolac (increased plasma concentration)—avoid concomitant use; effects of probenecid antagonised by aspirin

Antibacterials: probenecid reduces excretion of doripenem and meropenem (manufacturers of doripenem and meropenem advise avoid concomitant use); probenecid reduces excretion of cephalosporins, ciprofloxacin, nalidixic acid, norfloxacin and penicillins (increased plasma concentration); probenecid reduces excretion of dapsone and nitrofurantoin (increased risk of side-effects); effects of probenecid antagonised by pyrazinamide

Antidiabetics: probenecid possibly enhances hypoglycaemic effect of chlorpropamide

• Antivirals: probenecid reduces excretion of aciclovir (increased plasma concentration); probenecid possibly reduces excretion of famciclovir (increased plasma concentration); probenecid reduces excretion of ganciclovir and ●zidovudine (increased plasma concentration and risk of toxicity)

Anxiolytics and Hypnotics: probenecid reduces excretion of lorazepam (increased plasma concentration); probenecid possibly reduces excretion of nitrazepam (increased plasma concentration)

• Cytotoxics: probenecid reduces excretion of ●methotrexate (increased risk of toxicity)

Sodium Benzoate: probenecid possibly reduces excretion of conjugate formed by sodium benzoate

Sodium Phenylbutyrate: probenecid possibly reduces excretion of conjugate formed by sodium phenylbutyrate

**Procarbazine**

Alcohol: disulfiram-like reaction when procarbazine given with alcohol

Antiepileptics: cytotoxics possibly reduce absorption of phenytoin

• Antipsychotics: avoid concomitant use of cytotoxics with ●clozapine (increased risk of agranulocytosis)

Cardiac Glycosides: cytotoxics reduce absorption of digoxin tablets

**Prochlorperazine** *see* Antipsychotics

**Procyclidine** *see* Antimuscarinics

**Progesterone** *see* Progestogens

**Progestogens**

Note Interactions of combined oral contraceptives may also apply to combined contraceptive patches and vaginal rings

• Antibacterials: metabolism of progestogens accelerated by ●rifamycins (reduced contraceptive effect—see p. 445)

• Anticoagulants: progestogens may enhance or reduce anticoagulant effect of ●coumarins; progestogens antagonise anticoagulant effect of ●phenindione

• Antidepressants: contraceptive effect of progestogens reduced by ●St John's wort (avoid concomitant use)

Antidiabetics: progestogens antagonise hypoglycaemic effect of antidiabetics

• Antiepileptics: metabolism of progestogens accelerated by ●carbamazepine, ●oxcarbazepine, ●phenytoin, ●primidone, ●rufinamide and ●topiramate (reduced contraceptive effect—see p. 445); progestogens reduce plasma concentration of ●lamotrigine

**Progestogens** *(continued)*

• Antifungals: metabolism of progestogens accelerated by ●griseofulvin (reduced contraceptive effect—see p. 445); occasional reports of breakthrough bleeding when progestogens (used for contraception) given with terbinafine

• Antivirals: plasma concentration of progestogens increased by fosamprenavir, also plasma concentration of fosamprenavir reduced—alternative contraception recommended; contraceptive effect of progestogens possibly reduced by nelfinavir; metabolism of progestogens accelerated by ●nevirapine (reduced contraceptive effect—see p. 445)

• Aprepitant: possible contraceptive failure of hormonal contraceptives containing progestogens when given with ●aprepitant (alternative contraception recommended)

• Barbiturates: metabolism of progestogens accelerated by ●barbiturates (reduced contraceptive effect—see p. 445)

• Bosentan: possible contraceptive failure of hormonal contraceptives containing progestogens when given with ●bosentan (alternative contraception recommended)

• Ciclosporin: progestogens inhibit metabolism of ●ciclosporin (increased plasma concentration)

Diuretics: risk of hyperkalaemia when drospirenone given with potassium-sparing diuretics and aldosterone antagonists (monitor serum potassium during first cycle)

Dopaminergics: progestogens increase plasma concentration of selegiline (increased risk of toxicity)

Lipid-regulating Drugs: plasma concentration of norethisterone increased by atorvastatin; plasma concentration of norgestrel increased by rosuvastatin

Muscle Relaxants: progestogens possibly increase plasma concentration of tizanidine (increased risk of toxicity)

Sitaxentan: plasma concentration of progestogens increased by sitaxentan

Sugammadex: plasma concentration of progestogens possibly reduced by sugammadex

Tacrolimus: metabolism of progestogens possibly inhibited by tacrolimus

**Proguanil**

Antacids: absorption of proguanil reduced by oral magnesium salts (as magnesium trisilicate)

Anticoagulants: isolated reports that proguanil may enhance anticoagulant effect of warfarin

• Antimalarials: avoidance of antimalarials advised by manufacturer of ●artemether/lumefantrine; increased antifolate effect when proguanil given with pyrimethamine

Vaccines: antimalarials inactivate oral typhoid vaccine—see p. 688

**Promazine** *see* Antipsychotics

**Promethazine** *see* Antihistamines

**Propafenone**

Anaesthetics, Local: increased myocardial depression when anti-arrhythmics given with bupivacaine, levobupivacaine, prilocaine or ropivacaine

• Anti-arrhythmics: increased myocardial depression when anti-arrhythmics given with other ●anti-arrhythmics

• Antibacterials: metabolism of propafenone accelerated by ●rifampicin (reduced effect)

• Anticoagulants: propafenone enhances anticoagulant effect of ●coumarins

• Antidepressants: metabolism of propafenone possibly inhibited by paroxetine (increased risk of toxicity); increased risk of arrhythmias when propafenone given with ●tricyclics

• Antihistamines: increased risk of ventricular arrhythmias when propafenone given with ●mizolastine—avoid concomitant use

• Antipsychotics: increased risk of ventricular arrhythmias when anti-arrhythmics that prolong the QT interval given with ●antipsychotics that prolong the QT interval

**Propafenone** *(continued)*
- Antivirals: plasma concentration of propafenone possibly increased by ●fosamprenavir (increased risk of ventricular arrhythmias—avoid concomitant use); plasma concentration of propafenone increased by ●ritonavir (increased risk of ventricular arrhythmias—avoid concomitant use)
- Beta-blockers: increased myocardial depression when anti-arrhythmics given with ●beta-blockers; propafenone increases plasma concentration of metoprolol and propranolol
- Cardiac Glycosides: propafenone increases plasma concentration of ●digoxin (halve dose of digoxin)
Ciclosporin: propafenone possibly increases plasma concentration of ciclosporin
- 5HT₃ Antagonists: increased risk of ventricular arrhythmias when propafenone given with ●dolasetron—avoid concomitant use
Parasympathomimetics: propafenone possibly antagonises effects of neostigmine and pyridostigmine
Theophylline: propafenone increases plasma concentration of theophylline
- Ulcer-healing Drugs: plasma concentration of propafenone increased by ●cimetidine

**Propantheline** *see* Antimuscarinics
**Propiverine** *see* Antimuscarinics
**Propofol** *see* Anaesthetics, General
**Propranolol** *see* Beta-blockers
**Prostaglandins**
ACE Inhibitors: enhanced hypotensive effect when alprostadil given with ACE inhibitors
Adrenergic Neurone Blockers: enhanced hypotensive effect when alprostadil given with adrenergic neurone blockers
Alpha-blockers: enhanced hypotensive effect when alprostadil given with alpha-blockers
Angiotensin-II Receptor Antagonists: enhanced hypotensive effect when alprostadil given with angiotensin-II receptor antagonists
Beta-blockers: enhanced hypotensive effect when alprostadil given with beta-blockers
Calcium-channel Blockers: enhanced hypotensive effect when alprostadil given with calcium-channel blockers
Clonidine: enhanced hypotensive effect when alprostadil given with clonidine
Diazoxide: enhanced hypotensive effect when alprostadil given with diazoxide
Diuretics: enhanced hypotensive effect when alprostadil given with diuretics
Methyldopa: enhanced hypotensive effect when alprostadil given with methyldopa
Moxonidine: enhanced hypotensive effect when alprostadil given with moxonidine
Nitrates: enhanced hypotensive effect when alprostadil given with nitrates
Oxytocin: prostaglandins potentiate uterotonic effect of oxytocin
Vasodilator Antihypertensives: enhanced hypotensive effect when alprostadil given with hydralazine, minoxidil or sodium nitroprusside
**Protein Kinase Inhibitors** *see* Dasatinib, Erlotinib, Imatinib, Lapatinib, Nilotinib, Sorafenib, Sunitinib, and Temsirolimus
**Proton Pump Inhibitors**
Antacids: absorption of lansoprazole possibly reduced by antacids
Antibacterials: plasma concentration of both drugs increased when omeprazole given with clarithromycin
- Anticoagulants: esomeprazole, omeprazole and pantoprazole possibly enhance anticoagulant effect of ●coumarins
Antidepressants: omeprazole increases plasma concentration of escitalopram; plasma concentration of lansoprazole possibly increased by fluvoxamine
- Antiepileptics: esomeprazole enhances effects of ●phenytoin; omeprazole possibly enhances effects of phenytoin

**Proton Pump Inhibitors** *(continued)*
Antifungals: proton pump inhibitors reduce absorption of itraconazole and ketoconazole; plasma concentration of esomeprazole possibly increased by voriconazole; plasma concentration of omeprazole increased by voriconazole (consider reducing dose of omeprazole)
Antipsychotics: omeprazole possibly reduces plasma concentration of clozapine
- Antivirals: proton pump inhibitors reduce plasma concentration of ●atazanavir; omeprazole reduces plasma concentration of ●nelfinavir—avoid concomitant use; proton pump inhibitors possibly increase plasma concentration of raltegravir—manufacturer of raltegravir advises avoid concomitant use; omeprazole increases plasma concentration of ●raltegravir—avoid concomitant use; omeprazole increases plasma concentration of saquinavir; plasma concentration of esomeprazole and omeprazole reduced by ●tipranavir
Anxiolytics and Hypnotics: esomeprazole and omeprazole possibly inhibit metabolism of diazepam (increased plasma concentration)
Cardiac Glycosides: proton pump inhibitors possibly slightly increase plasma concentration of digoxin
Ciclosporin: omeprazole possibly affects plasma concentration of ciclosporin
- Cilostazol: omeprazole increases plasma concentration of ●cilostazol (risk of toxicity)—avoid concomitant use; lansoprazole possibly increases plasma concentration of ●cilostazol—avoid concomitant use
- Clopidogrel: proton pump inhibitors possibly reduce antiplatelet effect of ●clopidogrel—avoid concomitant use
Cytotoxics: omeprazole possibly reduces excretion of methotrexate (increased risk of toxicity); proton pump inhibitors possibly reduce absorption of lapatinib; avoidance of proton pump inhibitors advised by manufacturer of nilotinib
Tacrolimus: omeprazole possibly increases plasma concentration of tacrolimus
Ulcer-healing Drugs: absorption of lansoprazole possibly reduced by sucralfate
**Pseudoephedrine** *see* Sympathomimetics
**Pyrazinamide**
Oestrogens: antibacterials that do not induce liver enzymes possibly reduce contraceptive effect of oestrogens (risk probably small, see p. 445)
Probenecid: pyrazinamide antagonises effects of probenecid
Sulfinpyrazone: pyrazinamide antagonises effects of sulfinpyrazone
Vaccines: antibacterials inactivate oral typhoid vaccine—see p. 688
**Pyridostigmine** *see* Parasympathomimetics
**Pyridoxine** *see* Vitamins
**Pyrimethamine**
- Antibacterials: increased antifolate effect when pyrimethamine given with ●sulphonamides or ●trimethoprim
- Antiepileptics: pyrimethamine antagonises anticonvulsant effect of ●phenytoin, also increased antifolate effect
- Antimalarials: avoidance of antimalarials advised by manufacturer of ●artemether/lumefantrine; increased antifolate effect when pyrimethamine given with proguanil
Antivirals: increased antifolate effect when pyrimethamine given with zidovudine
- Cytotoxics: pyrimethamine increases antifolate effect of ●methotrexate
Vaccines: antimalarials inactivate oral typhoid vaccine—see p. 688
**Quetiapine** *see* Antipsychotics
**Quinagolide**
Memantine: effects of dopaminergics possibly enhanced by memantine
Methyldopa: antiparkinsonian effect of dopaminergics antagonised by methyldopa

Quinapril *see* ACE Inhibitors

Quinine
- Anti-arrhythmics: increased risk of ventricular arrhythmias when quinine given with ●amiodarone—avoid concomitant use; quinine increases plasma concentration of ●flecainide
- Antibacterials: increased risk of ventricular arrhythmias when quinine given with ●moxifloxacin—avoid concomitant use
- Antimalarials: increased risk of ventricular arrhythmias when quinine given with ●artemether/lumefantrine; avoidance of antimalarials advised by manufacturer of ●artemether/lumefantrine; increased risk of convulsions when quinine given with ●mefloquine (but should not prevent the use of intravenous quinine in severe cases)
- Antipsychotics: increased risk of ventricular arrhythmias when quinine given with ●droperidol or ●pimozide—avoid concomitant use
- Cardiac Glycosides: quinine increases plasma concentration of ●digoxin
  Muscle Relaxants: quinine possibly enhances effects of suxamethonium
  Ulcer-healing Drugs: metabolism of quinine inhibited by cimetidine (increased plasma concentration)
  Vaccines: antimalarials inactivate oral typhoid vaccine–see p. 688

Quinolones
- Analgesics: possible increased risk of convulsions when quinolones given with ●NSAIDs; manufacturer of ciprofloxacin advises avoid premedication with opioid analgesics (reduced plasma concentration of ciprofloxacin) when ciprofloxacin used for surgical prophylaxis
  Antacids: absorption of ciprofloxacin, levofloxacin, moxifloxacin, norfloxacin and ofloxacin reduced by antacids
- Anti-arrhythmics: increased risk of ventricular arrhythmias when levofloxacin or moxifloxacin given with ●amiodarone—avoid concomitant use; increased risk of ventricular arrhythmias when moxifloxacin given with ●disopyramide—avoid concomitant use
- Antibacterials: increased risk of ventricular arrhythmias when moxifloxacin given with parenteral ●erythromycin—avoid concomitant use
- Anticoagulants: ciprofloxacin, nalidixic acid, norfloxacin and ofloxacin enhance anticoagulant effect of ●coumarins; levofloxacin possibly enhances anticoagulant effect of coumarins and phenindione
- Antidepressants: ciprofloxacin inhibits metabolism of ●duloxetine—avoid concomitant use; avoidance of ciprofloxacin advised by manufacturer of ●agomelatine; increased risk of ventricular arrhythmias when moxifloxacin given with ●tricyclics—avoid concomitant use
  Antidiabetics: ciprofloxacin and norfloxacin possibly enhance effects of glibenclamide
  Antiepileptics: ciprofloxacin increases or decreases plasma concentration of phenytoin
- Antihistamines: increased risk of ventricular arrhythmias when moxifloxacin given with ●mizolastine—avoid concomitant use
- Antimalarials: avoidance of quinolones advised by manufacturer of ●artemether/lumefantrine; increased risk of ventricular arrhythmias when moxifloxacin given with ●chloroquine and hydroxychloroquine, ●mefloquine or ●quinine—avoid concomitant use
- Antipsychotics: increased risk of ventricular arrhythmias when moxifloxacin given with ●benperidol—manufacturer of benperidol advises avoid concomitant use; increased risk of ventricular arrhythmias when moxifloxacin given with ●droperidol, ●haloperidol, ●phenothiazines, ●pimozide, ●sertindole or ●zuclopenthixol—avoid concomitant use; ciprofloxacin increases plasma concentration of clozapine; ciprofloxacin possibly increases plasma concentration of olanzapine

Quinolones *(continued)*
- Atomoxetine: increased risk of ventricular arrhythmias when moxifloxacin given with ●atomoxetine
- Beta-blockers: increased risk of ventricular arrhythmias when moxifloxacin given with ●sotalol—avoid concomitant use
  Calcium Salts: absorption of ciprofloxacin reduced by calcium salts
- Ciclosporin: increased risk of nephrotoxicity when quinolones given with ●ciclosporin
- Cytotoxics: nalidixic acid increases risk of melphalan toxicity; ciprofloxacin possibly reduces excretion of methotrexate (increased risk of toxicity); avoidance of moxifloxacin advised by manufacturer of ●nilotinib
  Dairy Products: absorption of ciprofloxacin and norfloxacin reduced by dairy products
  Dopaminergics: ciprofloxacin inhibits metabolism of ropinirole (increased plasma concentration)
  5HT$_1$ Agonists: quinolones possibly inhibit metabolism of zolmitriptan (reduce dose of zolmitriptan)
  Iron: absorption of ciprofloxacin, levofloxacin, moxifloxacin, norfloxacin and ofloxacin reduced by *oral* iron
- Muscle Relaxants: ciprofloxacin increases plasma concentration of ●tizanidine (increased risk of toxicity)—avoid concomitant use; norfloxacin possibly increases plasma concentration of tizanidine (increased risk of toxicity)
  Mycophenolate: norfloxacin possibly reduces bioavailability of mycophenolate
  Oestrogens: antibacterials that do not induce liver enzymes possibly reduce contraceptive effect of oestrogens (risk probably small, see p. 445)
- Pentamidine Isetionate: increased risk of ventricular arrhythmias when moxifloxacin given with ●pentamidine isetionate—avoid concomitant use
  Probenecid: excretion of ciprofloxacin, nalidixic acid and norfloxacin reduced by probenecid (increased plasma concentration)
  Sevelamer: bioavailability of ciprofloxacin reduced by sevelamer
  Strontium Ranelate: absorption of quinolones reduced by strontium ranelate (manufacturer of strontium ranelate advises avoid concomitant use)
- Theophylline: possible increased risk of convulsions when quinolones given with ●theophylline; ciprofloxacin and norfloxacin increase plasma concentration of ●theophylline
  Ulcer-healing Drugs: absorption of ciprofloxacin, levofloxacin, moxifloxacin, norfloxacin and ofloxacin reduced by sucralfate
  Vaccines: antibacterials inactivate oral typhoid vaccine–see p. 688
  Zinc: absorption of ciprofloxacin, levofloxacin, moxifloxacin, norfloxacin and ofloxacin reduced by zinc

Quinupristin with Dalfopristin
- Anti-arrhythmics: increased risk of ventricular arrhythmias when quinupristin/dalfopristin given with ●disopyramide or ●lidocaine (lignocaine)—avoid concomitant use
  Antibacterials: manufacturer of quinupristin/dalfopristin recommends monitoring liver function when given with rifampicin
  Antivirals: quinupristin/dalfopristin possibly increases plasma concentration of saquinavir
- Anxiolytics and Hypnotics: quinupristin/dalfopristin inhibits metabolism of ●midazolam (increased plasma concentration with increased sedation); quinupristin/dalfopristin inhibits the metabolism of zopiclone
- Calcium-channel Blockers: quinupristin/dalfopristin increases plasma concentration of ●nifedipine
- Ciclosporin: quinupristin/dalfopristin increases plasma concentration of ●ciclosporin
- Ergot Alkaloids: manufacturer of quinupristin/dalfopristin advises avoid concomitant use with ●ergotamine and methysergide

**Quinupristin with Dalfopristin** *(continued)*

Oestrogens: antibacterials that do not induce liver enzymes possibly reduce contraceptive effect of oestrogens (risk probably small, see p. 445)

● Tacrolimus: quinupristin/dalfopristin increases plasma concentration of ●tacrolimus

Vaccines: antibacterials inactivate oral typhoid vaccine–see p. 688

**Rabeprazole** *see* Proton Pump Inhibitors

**Raloxifene**

Anticoagulants: raloxifene antagonises anticoagulant effect of coumarins

Lipid-regulating Drugs: absorption of raloxifene reduced by colestyramine (manufacturer of raloxifene advises avoid concomitant administration)

**Raltegravir**

● Antibacterials: plasma concentration of raltegravir reduced by ●rifampicin—consider increasing dose of raltegravir

● Ulcer-healing Drugs: plasma concentration of raltegravir increased by ●omeprazole—avoid concomitant use; plasma concentration of raltegravir possibly increased by histamine H$_2$-antagonists and proton pump inhibitors—manufacturer of raltegravir advises avoid concomitant use

**Ramipril** *see* ACE Inhibitors

**Ranitidine** *see* Histamine H$_2$-antagonists

**Ranolazine**

● <u>Anti-arrhythmics</u>: manufacturer of ranolazine advises avoid concomitant use with ●disopyramide

● <u>Antibacterials</u>: plasma concentration of ranolazine possibly increased by ●clarithromycin and ●telithromycin—manufacturer of ranolazine advises avoid concomitant use; plasma concentration of ranolazine reduced by ●rifampicin—manufacturer of ranolazine advises avoid concomitant use

<u>Antidepressants</u>: plasma concentration of ranolazine increased by paroxetine

● <u>Antifungals</u>: plasma concentration of ranolazine increased by ●ketoconazole—avoid concomitant use; plasma concentration of ranolazine possibly increased by ●itraconazole, ●posaconazole and ●voriconazole—manufacturer of ranolazine advises avoid concomitant use

● <u>Antivirals</u>: plasma concentration of ranolazine possibly increased by ●atazanavir, ●darunavir, ●fosamprenavir, ●indinavir, ●lopinavir, ●nelfinavir, ●ritonavir, ●saquinavir and ●tipranavir—manufacturer of ranolazine advises avoid concomitant use

● <u>Beta-blockers</u>: manufacturer of ranolazine advises avoid concomitant use with ●sotalol

<u>Calcium channel Blockers</u>: plasma concentration of ranolazine increased by diltiazem and verapamil (consider reducing dose of ranolazine)

<u>Cardiac Glycosides</u>: ranolazine increases plasma concentration of digoxin

<u>Ciclosporin</u>: plasma concentration of ranolazine possibly increased by ciclosporin

● <u>Grapefruit Juice</u>: plasma concentration of ranolazine possibly increased by ●grapefruit juice—manufacturer of ranolazine advises avoid concomitant use

<u>Lipid-regulating Drugs</u>: ranolazine increases plasma concentration of simvastatin (consider reducing dose of simvastatin)

**Rasagiline**

Note Rasagiline is a MAO-B inhibitor

● Analgesics: avoid concomitant use of rasagiline with ●dextromethorphan; risk of CNS toxicity when rasagiline given with ●pethidine (avoid pethidine for 2 weeks after rasagiline)

● Antidepressants: after stopping rasagiline do not start ●fluoxetine for 2 weeks, also rasagiline should not be started until at least 5 weeks after stopping fluoxetine; after stopping rasagiline do not start ●fluvoxamine for 2 weeks; risk of hypertensive crisis when rasagiline given with ●MAOIs, avoid MAOIs for at least 2 weeks after stopping rasagiline; increased risk of CNS toxicity when rasagiline given with ●SSRIs or ●tricyclics

**Rasagiline** *(continued)*

Dopaminergics: plasma concentration of rasagiline possibly reduced by entacapone

Memantine: effects of dopaminergics possibly enhanced by memantine

Methyldopa: antiparkinsonian effect of dopaminergics antagonised by methyldopa

● Sympathomimetics: avoid concomitant use of rasagiline with ●sympathomimetics

**Reboxetine**

● Antibacterials: manufacturer of reboxetine advises avoid concomitant use with ●macrolides

● Antidepressants: manufacturer of reboxetine advises avoid concomitant use with ●fluvoxamine; increased risk of hypertension and CNS excitation when reboxetine given with ●MAOIs (MAOIs should not be started until 1 week after stopping reboxetine, avoid reboxetine for 2 weeks after stopping MAOIs)

● Antifungals: manufacturer of reboxetine advises avoid concomitant use with ●imidazoles and ●triazoles

● Antimalarials: avoidance of antidepressants advised by manufacturer of ●artemether/lumefantrine

Atomoxetine: possible increased risk of convulsions when antidepressants given with atomoxetine

Diuretics: possible increased risk of hypokalaemia when reboxetine given with loop diuretics or thiazides and related diuretics

Ergot Alkaloids: possible risk of hypertension when reboxetine given with ergotamine and methysergide

● Sibutramine: increased risk of CNS toxicity when noradrenaline re-uptake inhibitors given with ●sibutramine (manufacturer of sibutramine advises avoid concomitant use)

**Remifentanil** *see* Opioid Analgesics

**Repaglinide** *see* Antidiabetics

**Retinoids**

● Alcohol: etretinate formed from acitretin in presence of ●alcohol (increased risk of teratogenicity in women of child-bearing potential)

● Antibacterials: possible increased risk of benign intracranial hypertension when retinoids given with ●tetracyclines (avoid concomitant use)

● Anticoagulants: acitretin possibly reduces anticoagulant effect of ●coumarins

Antiepileptics: isotretinoin possibly reduces plasma concentration of carbamazepine

Antifungals: plasma concentration of alitretinoin increased by ketoconazole

● Cytotoxics: acitretin increases plasma concentration of ●methotrexate (also increased risk of hepatotoxicity)—avoid concomitant use

Lipid-regulating Drugs: alitretinoin reduces plasma concentration of simvastatin

Vitamins: risk of hypervitaminosis A when retinoids given with vitamin A

**Ribavirin**

● Antivirals: increased risk of side-effects when ribavirin given with ●didanosine—avoid concomitant use; ribavirin possibly inhibits effects of ●stavudine; increased risk of anaemia when ribavirin given with ●zidovudine—avoid concomitant use

**Rifabutin** *see* Rifamycins

**Rifampicin** *see* Rifamycins

**Rifamycins**

ACE Inhibitors: rifampicin reduces plasma concentration of active metabolite of imidapril (reduced antihypertensive effect)

Analgesics: rifampicin reduces plasma concentration of etoricoxib; rifampicin accelerates metabolism of methadone (reduced effect)

Antacids: absorption of rifampicin reduced by antacids

● Anti-arrhythmics: rifamycins accelerate metabolism of ●disopyramide (reduced plasma concentration); rifampicin accelerates metabolism of ●propafenone (reduced effect)

● Antibacterials: rifamycins reduce plasma concentration of clarithromycin and dapsone; plasma concentration of rifabutin increased by ●clarithromycin (increased risk of uveitis—reduce rifabutin dose);

**Rifamycins**

- **Antibacterials** *(continued)*

  rifampicin accelerates metabolism of chloramphenicol (reduced plasma concentration); plasma concentration of rifabutin possibly increased by ●macrolides (increased risk of uveitis—reduce rifabutin dose); monitoring of liver function with rifampicin recommended by manufacturer of quinupristin/dalfopristin; rifampicin reduces plasma concentration of ●telithromycin (avoid during and for 2 weeks after rifampicin); rifampicin possibly reduces plasma concentration of trimethoprim

- **Anticoagulants:** rifamycins accelerate metabolism of ●coumarins (reduced anticoagulant effect); rifampicin reduces plasma concentration of rivaroxaban

  **Antidepressants:** rifampicin possibly reduces plasma concentration of tricyclics

- **Antidiabetics:** rifamycins accelerate metabolism of ●chlorpropamide and ●tolbutamide (reduced effect); rifampicin reduces plasma concentration of ●rosiglitazone—consider increasing dose of rosiglitazone; rifampicin reduces plasma concentration of nateglinide; rifampicin possibly antagonises hypoglycaemic effect of repaglinide; rifamycins possibly accelerate metabolism of ●sulphonylureas (reduced effect)

- **Antiepileptics:** rifabutin reduces plasma concentration of ●carbamazepine; rifampicin reduces concentration of ●lamotrigine; rifamycins accelerate metabolism of ●phenytoin (reduced plasma concentration)

- <u>**Antifungals:**</u> rifampicin accelerates metabolism of ●ketoconazole (reduced plasma concentration), also plasma concentration of rifampicin may be reduced by ketoconazole; plasma concentration of rifabutin increased by ●fluconazole (increased risk of uveitis—reduce rifabutin dose); rifampicin accelerates metabolism of ●fluconazole and ●itraconazole (reduced plasma concentration); rifabutin reduces plasma concentration of ●itraconazole—avoid concomitant use; plasma concentration of rifabutin increased by ●posaconazole (also plasma concentration of posaconazole reduced); rifampicin reduces plasma concentration of ●posaconazole and ●terbinafine; plasma concentration of rifabutin increased by ●voriconazole, also rifabutin reduces plasma concentration of voriconazole (increase dose of voriconazole and also monitor for rifabutin toxicity); rifampicin reduces plasma concentration of ●voriconazole—avoid concomitant use; rifampicin initially increases and then reduces plasma concentration of caspofungin (consider increasing dose of caspofungin); plasma concentration of rifabutin possibly increased by ●triazoles (increased risk of uveitis—reduce rifabutin dose)

- **Antimalarials:** rifampicin reduces plasma concentration of ●mefloquine—avoid concomitant use

  **Antimuscarinics:** rifampicin reduces plasma concentration of active metabolite of fesoterodine

- **Antipsychotics:** rifampicin accelerates metabolism of ●haloperidol (reduced plasma concentration); rifabutin and rifampicin possibly reduce plasma concentration of ●aripiprazole—increase dose of aripiprazole; rifampicin possibly reduces plasma concentration of clozapine

- **Antivirals:** rifampicin possibly reduces plasma concentration of abacavir and ritonavir; plasma concentration of rifabutin increased by ●atazanavir, ●darunavir, ●fosamprenavir and ●tipranavir (reduce dose of rifabutin); rifampicin reduces plasma concentration of ●atazanavir, ●lopinavir and ●nevirapine—avoid concomitant use; rifampicin significantly reduces plasma concentration of ●darunavir, ●fosamprenavir and ●nelfinavir—avoid concomitant use; rifampicin reduces plasma concentration of efavirenz—increase dose of efavirenz; plasma concentration of rifabutin reduced by efavir-

**Rifamycins**

- **Antivirals** *(continued)*

  enz—increase dose of rifabutin; avoidance of rifampicin advised by manufacturer of etravirine and zidovudine; plasma concentration of both drugs reduced when rifabutin given with ●etravirine; rifampicin accelerates metabolism of ●indinavir (reduced plasma concentration—avoid concomitant use); plasma concentration of rifabutin increased by ●indinavir—avoid concomitant use; rifampicin reduces plasma concentration of ●maraviroc and ●raltegravir—consider increasing dose of maraviroc and raltegravir; plasma concentration of rifabutin increased by ●nelfinavir (halve dose of rifabutin); plasma concentration of rifabutin possibly increased by nevirapine; plasma concentration of rifabutin increased by ●ritonavir (increased risk of toxicity); rifampicin significantly reduces plasma concentration of ●saquinavir, also risk of hepatotoxicity—avoid concomitant use; rifabutin reduces plasma concentration of ●saquinavir; rifampicin possibly reduces plasma concentration of ●tipranavir—avoid concomitant use

  **Anxiolytics and Hypnotics:** rifampicin accelerates metabolism of diazepam (reduced plasma concentration); rifampicin possibly accelerates metabolism of benzodiazepines (reduced plasma concentration); rifampicin possibly accelerates metabolism of buspirone and zaleplon; rifampicin accelerates metabolism of zolpidem (reduced plasma concentration and reduced effect); rifampicin significantly reduces plasma concentration of zopiclone

  **Aprepitant:** rifampicin reduces plasma concentration of aprepitant

- **Atovaquone:** rifabutin and rifampicin reduce plasma concentration of ●atovaquone (possible therapeutic failure of atovaquone)

  **Barbiturates:** plasma concentration of rifampicin possibly reduced by phenobarbital

  **Beta-blockers:** rifampicin accelerates metabolism of bisoprolol and propranolol (plasma concentration significantly reduced); rifampicin reduces plasma concentration of carvedilol, celiprolol and metoprolol

- **Bosentan:** rifampicin reduces plasma concentration of ●bosentan—avoid concomitant use

- **Calcium-channel Blockers:** rifampicin possibly accelerates metabolism of ●isradipine and ●nicardipine (possible significantly reduced plasma concentration); rifampicin accelerates metabolism of ●diltiazem, ●nifedipine, ●nimodipine and ●verapamil (plasma concentration significantly reduced)

  **Cardiac Glycosides:** rifamycins accelerate metabolism of digitoxin (reduced effect); rifampicin possibly reduces plasma concentration of digoxin

- **Ciclosporin:** rifampicin accelerates metabolism of ●ciclosporin (reduced plasma concentration)

- **Corticosteroids:** rifamycins accelerate metabolism of ●corticosteroids (reduced effect)

- <u>**Cytotoxics:**</u> rifampicin accelerates metabolism of ●dasatinib (reduced plasma concentration—avoid concomitant use); rifampicin accelerates metabolism of erlotinib and sunitinib (reduced plasma concentration); rifampicin reduces plasma concentration of ●imatinib and ●nilotinib—avoid concomitant use; avoidance of rifabutin and rifampicin advised by manufacturer of ●lapatinib; rifampicin reduces plasma concentration of sorafenib; rifampicin reduces plasma concentration of active metabolite of ●temsirolimus—avoid concomitant use

- <u>**Deferasirox:**</u> rifampicin reduces plasma concentration of deferasirox

- **Diuretics:** rifampicin reduces plasma concentration of ●eplerenone—avoid concomitant use

  <u>**Hormone Antagonists:**</u> rifampicin possibly reduces plasma concentration of exemestane; rifampicin

Rifamycins

Hormone Antagonists *(continued)*
accelerates metabolism of gestrinone and tamoxifen (reduced plasma concentration)

5HT₃ Antagonists: rifampicin accelerates metabolism of ondansetron (reduced effect)

Leflunomide: rifampicin possibly increases plasma concentration of active metabolite of leflunomide

Lipid-regulating Drugs: rifampicin possibly reduces plasma concentration of atorvastatin and simvastatin; rifampicin accelerates metabolism of fluvastatin (reduced effect)

● Mycophenolate: rifampicin reduces plasma concentration of active metabolite of ●mycophenolate

● Oestrogens: rifamycins accelerate metabolism of ●oestrogens (reduced contraceptive effect—see p. 445); antibacterials that do not induce liver enzymes possibly reduce contraceptive effect of oestrogens (risk probably small, see p. 445)

● Progestogens: rifamycins accelerate metabolism of ●progestogens (reduced contraceptive effect—see p. 445)

● Ranolazine: rifampicin reduces plasma concentration of ●ranolazine—manufacturer of ranolazine advises avoid concomitant use

● Sirolimus: rifabutin and rifampicin reduce plasma concentration of ●sirolimus—avoid concomitant use

● Tacrolimus: rifampicin reduces plasma concentration of ●tacrolimus

Tadalafil: rifampicin reduces plasma concentration of tadalafil

Theophylline: rifampicin accelerates metabolism of theophylline (reduced plasma concentration)

Thyroid Hormones: rifampicin accelerates metabolism of levothyroxine (thyroxine) (may increase requirements for levothyroxine (thyroxine) in hypothyroidism)

Tibolone: rifampicin accelerates metabolism of tibolone (reduced plasma concentration)

Ulcer-healing Drugs: rifampicin accelerates metabolism of cimetidine (reduced plasma concentration)

Vaccines: antibacterials inactivate oral typhoid vaccine—see p. 688

Rimonabant
Antifungals: plasma concentration of rimonabant increased by ketoconazole

Risedronate Sodium *see* Bisphosphonates

Risperidone *see* Antipsychotics

Ritodrine *see* Sympathomimetics, Beta₂

Ritonavir

● Alpha-blockers: ritonavir possibly increases plasma concentration of ●alfuzosin—avoid concomitant use

● Analgesics: ritonavir possibly increases plasma concentration of NSAIDs and buprenorphine; ritonavir increases plasma concentration of ●dextropropoxyphene and ●piroxicam (risk of toxicity)—avoid concomitant use; ritonavir increases plasma concentration of ●alfentanil and ●fentanyl; ritonavir reduces plasma concentration of methadone; ritonavir possibly reduces plasma concentration of morphine; ritonavir reduces plasma concentration of ●pethidine, but increases plasma concentration of toxic metabolite of pethidine (avoid concomitant use)

● Anti-arrhythmics: ritonavir increases plasma concentration of ●amiodarone and ●propafenone (increased risk of ventricular arrhythmias—avoid concomitant use); ritonavir possibly increases plasma concentration of ●disopyramide (increased risk of toxicity); ritonavir possibly increases plasma concentration of ●flecainide (increased risk of ventricular arrhythmias—avoid concomitant use)

● Antibacterials: ritonavir possibly increases plasma concentration of azithromycin and erythromycin; ritonavir increases plasma concentration of ●clarithromycin (reduce dose of clarithromycin in renal impairment); ritonavir increases plasma concentration of ●rifabutin (increased risk of toxicity); plasma concentration of ritonavir possibly reduced

Ritonavir

● Antibacterials *(continued)*
by rifampicin; plasma concentration of both drugs increased when ritonavir given with ●fusidic acid—avoid concomitant use; avoidance of concomitant ritonavir in severe renal and hepatic impairment advised by manufacturer of ●telithromycin

● Anticoagulants: ritonavir may enhance or reduce anticoagulant effect of ●warfarin; ritonavir possibly enhances anticoagulant effect of ●coumarins and ●phenindione; ritonavir increases plasma concentration of ●rivaroxaban—manufacturer of rivaroxaban advises avoid concomitant use

● Antidepressants: ritonavir possibly reduces plasma concentration of paroxetine; side-effects possibly increased when ritonavir given with trazodone; ritonavir possibly increases plasma concentration of ●SSRIs and ●tricyclics; plasma concentration of ritonavir reduced by ●St John's wort—avoid concomitant use

Antidiabetics: ritonavir possibly increases plasma concentration of tolbutamide

● Antiepileptics: ritonavir possibly increases plasma concentration of ●carbamazepine; plasma concentration of ritonavir possibly reduced by phenytoin, also plasma concentration of phenytoin possibly affected

● Antifungals: combination of ritonavir with ●itraconazole or ●ketoconazole may increase plasma concentration of either drug (or both); plasma concentration of ritonavir increased by fluconazole; ritonavir reduces plasma concentration of ●voriconazole—avoid concomitant use

Antihistamines: ritonavir possibly increases plasma concentration of non-sedating antihistamines

Antimalarials: caution with ritonavir advised by manufacturer of artemether/lumefantrine

Antimuscarinics: avoidance of ritonavir advised by manufacturer of darifenacin and tolterodine; manufacturer of fesoterodine advises dose reduction when ritonavir given with fesoterodine—consult fesoterodine product literature; ritonavir increases plasma concentration of solifenacin

● Antipsychotics: ritonavir possibly increases plasma concentration of ●antipsychotics; ritonavir possibly inhibits metabolism of ●aripiprazole (reduce dose of aripiprazole); ritonavir increases plasma concentration of ●clozapine (increased risk of toxicity)—avoid concomitant use; ritonavir reduces plasma concentration of olanzapine—consider increasing dose of olanzapine; ritonavir increases plasma concentration of ●pimozide and ●sertindole (increased risk of ventricular arrhythmias—avoid concomitant use)

● Antivirals: ritonavir increases toxicity of efavirenz, monitor liver function tests; ritonavir increases plasma concentration of indinavir and ●saquinavir; combination of ritonavir with nelfinavir may increase plasma concentration of either drug (or both)

● Anxiolytics and Hypnotics: ritonavir possibly increases plasma concentration of ●anxiolytics and hypnotics; ritonavir possibly increases plasma concentration of ●alprazolam, ●diazepam, ●flurazepam and ●zolpidem (risk of extreme sedation and respiratory depression—avoid concomitant use); ritonavir possibly increases plasma concentration of ●midazolam (risk of prolonged sedation—avoid concomitant use of oral midazolam); ritonavir increases plasma concentration of buspirone (increased risk of toxicity)

Aprepitant: ritonavir possibly increases plasma concentration of aprepitant

Bosentan: ritonavir possibly increases plasma concentration of bosentan

● Bupropion: ritonavir increases or decreases plasma concentration of ●bupropion

● Calcium-channel Blockers: ritonavir possibly increases plasma concentration of ●calcium-channel blockers;

**Ritonavir**

- Calcium-channel Blockers (continued)
  avoidance of ritonavir advised by manufacturer of lercanidipine
  Cardiac Glycosides: ritonavir possibly increases plasma concentration of digoxin
- Ciclosporin: ritonavir possibly increases plasma concentration of ●ciclosporin
- Cilostazol: ritonavir possibly increases plasma concentration of ●cilostazol—avoid concomitant use
- Corticosteroids: ritonavir possibly increases plasma concentration of corticosteroids, dexamethasone and prednisolone; ritonavir increases plasma concentration of inhaled and intranasal budesonide and ●fluticasone
- Cytotoxics: avoidance of ritonavir advised by manufacturer of ●lapatinib and ●nilotinib; ritonavir increases plasma concentration of paclitaxel
- Diuretics: ritonavir increases plasma concentration of ●eplerenone—avoid concomitant use
- Ergot Alkaloids: increased risk of ergotism when ritonavir given with ●ergotamine and methysergide—avoid concomitant use
- 5HT₁ Agonists: ritonavir increases plasma concentration of ●eletriptan (risk of toxicity)—avoid concomitant use
- Ivabradine: ritonavir possibly increases plasma concentration of ●ivabradine—avoid concomitant use
- Lipid-regulating Drugs: possible increased risk of myopathy when ritonavir given with atorvastatin; possible increased risk of myopathy when ritonavir given with ●rosuvastatin—avoid concomitant use; increased risk of myopathy when ritonavir given with ●simvastatin (avoid concomitant use)
- Oestrogens: ritonavir accelerates metabolism of ●oestrogens (reduced contraceptive effect—see p. 445)
- <u>Ranolazine</u>: ritonavir possibly increases plasma concentration of ●ranolazine—manufacturer of ranolazine advises avoid concomitant use
- Sildenafil: ritonavir significantly increases plasma concentration of ●sildenafil—avoid concomitant use
  Sympathomimetics: ritonavir possibly increases plasma concentration of dexamfetamine
- Tacrolimus: ritonavir possibly increases plasma concentration of ●tacrolimus
  Tadalafil: ritonavir increases plasma concentration of tadalafil
- Theophylline: ritonavir accelerates metabolism of ●theophylline (reduced plasma concentration)
- Vardenafil: ritonavir possibly increases plasma concentration of ●vardenafil—avoid concomitant use

**Rivaroxaban**

- <u>Analgesics</u>: increased risk of haemorrhage when anticoagulants given with intravenous ●diclofenac (avoid concomitant use, including low-dose heparin); increased risk of haemorrhage when anticoagulants given with ●ketorolac (avoid concomitant use, including low-dose heparin)
  Antibacterials: plasma concentration of rivaroxaban reduced by rifampicin
- Antifungals: plasma concentration of rivaroxaban increased by ●ketoconazole—avoid concomitant use; manufacturer of rivaroxaban advises avoid concomitant use with itraconazole, posaconazole and voriconazole
- Antivirals: manufacturer of rivaroxaban advises avoid concomitant use with atazanavir, darunavir, fosamprenavir, indinavir, lopinavir, nelfinavir, saquinavir and tipranavir; plasma concentration of rivaroxaban increased by ●ritonavir—manufacturer of rivaroxaban advises avoid concomitant use
  Sibutramine: increased risk of bleeding when anticoagulants given with sibutramine

**Rivastigmine** see Parasympathomimetics
**Rizatriptan** see 5HT₁ Agonists
**Rocuronium** see Muscle Relaxants

**Ropinirole**

  Antibacterials: metabolism of ropinirole inhibited by ciprofloxacin (increased plasma concentration)
  Antipsychotics: manufacturer of ropinirole advises avoid concomitant use of antipsychotics (antagonism of effect)
  Memantine: effects of dopaminergics possibly enhanced by memantine
  Methyldopa: antiparkinsonian effect of dopaminergics antagonised by methyldopa
  Metoclopramide: manufacturer of ropinirole advises avoid concomitant use of metoclopramide (antagonism of effect)
  Oestrogens: plasma concentration of ropinirole increased by oestrogens

**Ropivacaine**

  Anti-arrhythmics: increased myocardial depression when ropivacaine given with anti-arrhythmics
  Antidepressants: metabolism of ropivacaine inhibited by fluvoxamine—avoid prolonged administration of ropivacaine

**Rosiglitazone** see Antidiabetics
**Rosuvastatin** see Statins

**Rotigotine**

  Antipsychotics: manufacturer of rotigotine advises avoid concomitant use of antipsychotics (antagonism of effect)
  Memantine: effects of dopaminergics possibly enhanced by memantine
  Methyldopa: antiparkinsonian effect of dopaminergics antagonised by methyldopa
  Metoclopramide: manufacturer of rotigotine advises avoid concomitant use of metoclopramide (antagonism of effect)

**Rowachol®**

  Anticoagulants: Rowachol® possibly reduces anticoagulant effect of coumarins

**Rufinamide**

- Antidepressants: anticonvulsant effect of antiepileptics possibly antagonised by MAOIs and ●tricyclic-related antidepressants (convulsive threshold lowered); anticonvulsant effect of antiepileptics antagonised by ●SSRIs and ●tricyclics (convulsive threshold lowered); avoid concomitant use of antiepileptics with ●St John's wort
  Antiepileptics: rufinamide possibly increases plasma concentration of phenytoin; plasma concentration of rufinamide possibly increased by valproate (reduce dose of rufinamide)
- Antimalarials: possible increased risk of convulsions when antiepileptics given with chloroquine and hydroxychloroquine; anticonvulsant effect of antiepileptics antagonised by ●mefloquine
- Oestrogens: rufinamide accelerates metabolism of ●oestrogens (reduced contraceptive effect—see p. 445)
- Progestogens: rufinamide accelerates metabolism of ●progestogens (reduced contraceptive effect—see p. 445)

**St John's Wort**

- Antibacterials: St John's wort reduces plasma concentration of ●telithromycin (avoid during and for 2 weeks after St John's wort)
- Anticoagulants: St John's wort reduces anticoagulant effect of ●coumarins (avoid concomitant use)
- Antidepressants: possible increased serotonergic effects when St John's wort given with duloxetine; St John's wort reduces plasma concentration of amitriptyline; increased serotonergic effects when St John's wort given with ●SSRIs—avoid concomitant use
- Antiepileptics: avoid concomitant use of St John's wort with ●antiepileptics
- Antifungals: St John's wort reduces plasma concentration of ●voriconazole—avoid concomitant use
- Antimalarials: avoidance of antidepressants advised by manufacturer of ●artemether/lumefantrine

**St John's Wort** *(continued)*

- Antipsychotics: St John's wort possibly reduces plasma concentration of ●aripiprazole—increase dose of aripiprazole
- Antivirals: St John's wort reduces plasma concentration of ●atazanavir, ●darunavir, ●efavirenz, ●fosamprenavir, ●indinavir, ●lopinavir, ●nelfinavir, ●nevirapine, ●ritonavir and ●saquinavir—avoid concomitant use; avoidance of St John's wort advised by manufacturer of etravirine; St John's wort possibly reduces plasma concentration of ●maraviroc and ●tipranavir—avoid concomitant use

  Anxiolytics and Hypnotics: St John's wort possibly reduces plasma concentration of oral midazolam
- Aprepitant: avoidance of St John's wort advised by manufacturer of ●aprepitant

  Atomoxetine: possible increased risk of convulsions when antidepressants given with atomoxetine
- Barbiturates: avoid concomitant use of St John's wort with ●phenobarbital

  Calcium-channel Blockers: St John's wort possibly reduces plasma concentration of amlodipine
- Cardiac Glycosides: St John's wort reduces plasma concentration of ●digoxin—avoid concomitant use
- Ciclosporin: St John's wort reduces plasma concentration of ●ciclosporin—avoid concomitant use
- Cytotoxics: St John's wort reduces plasma concentration of ●imatinib—avoid concomitant use; avoidance of St John's wort advised by manufacturer of ●lapatinib; St John's wort accelerates metabolism of ●irinotecan (reduced plasma concentration—avoid concomitant use)
- Diuretics: St John's wort reduces plasma concentration of ●eplerenone—avoid concomitant use
- 5HT$_1$ Agonists: increased serotonergic effects when St John's wort given with ●5HT$_1$ agonists—avoid concomitant use

  Ivabradine: St John's wort reduces plasma concentration of ivabradine—avoid concomitant use

  Lipid-regulating Drugs: St John's wort reduces plasma concentration of simvastatin
- Oestrogens: St John's wort reduces contraceptive effect of ●oestrogens (avoid concomitant use)
- Progestogens: St John's wort reduces contraceptive effect of ●progestogens (avoid concomitant use)
- Tacrolimus: St John's wort reduces plasma concentration of ●tacrolimus—avoid concomitant use
- Theophylline: St John's wort reduces plasma concentration of ●theophylline—avoid concomitant use

**Salbutamol** *see* Sympathomimetics, Beta$_2$

**Salmeterol** *see* Sympathomimetics, Beta$_2$

**Saquinavir**

- Antibacterials: plasma concentration of saquinavir reduced by ●rifabutin; plasma concentration of saquinavir significantly reduced by ●rifampicin, also risk of hepatotoxicity—avoid concomitant use; plasma concentration of saquinavir possibly increased by quinupristin/dalfopristin; avoidance of concomitant saquinavir in severe renal and hepatic impairment advised by manufacturer of ●telithromycin

  Anticoagulants: saquinavir possibly enhances anticoagulant effect of warfarin; avoidance of saquinavir advised by manufacturer of rivaroxaban
- Antidepressants: plasma concentration of saquinavir reduced by ●St John's wort—avoid concomitant use
- Antiepileptics: plasma concentration of saquinavir possibly reduced by carbamazepine, phenytoin and ●primidone

  Antifungals: plasma concentration of saquinavir increased by ketoconazole; plasma concentration of saquinavir possibly increased by imidazoles and triazoles

  Antimalarials: caution with saquinavir advised by manufacturer of artemether/lumefantrine

  Antimuscarinics: avoidance of saquinavir advised by manufacturer of darifenacin and tolterodine; manufacturer of fesoterodine advises dose reduction when

**Saquinavir**

Antimuscarinics *(continued)*

  saquinavir given with fesoterodine—consult fesoterodine product literature
- Antipsychotics: saquinavir possibly inhibits metabolism of ●aripiprazole (reduce dose of aripiprazole); saquinavir possibly increases plasma concentration of ●pimozide (increased risk of ventricular arrhythmias—avoid concomitant use); saquinavir increases plasma concentration of ●sertindole (increased risk of ventricular arrhythmias—avoid concomitant use)
- Antivirals: plasma concentration of saquinavir increased by atazanavir, indinavir, lopinavir and ●ritonavir; saquinavir reduces plasma concentration of darunavir; plasma concentration of saquinavir significantly reduced by efavirenz; saquinavir increases plasma concentration of ●maraviroc (consider reducing dose of maraviroc); combination of saquinavir with nelfinavir may increase plasma concentration of either drug (or both); plasma concentration of saquinavir reduced by ●tipranavir
- Anxiolytics and Hypnotics: saquinavir increases plasma concentration of ●midazolam (risk of prolonged sedation—avoid concomitant use of oral midazolam)
- Barbiturates: plasma concentration of saquinavir possibly reduced by ●barbiturates
- Ciclosporin: plasma concentration of both drugs increased when saquinavir given with ●ciclosporin
- Cilostazol: saquinavir possibly increases plasma concentration of ●cilostazol—avoid concomitant use

  Corticosteroids: plasma concentration of saquinavir possibly reduced by dexamethasone
- Cytotoxics: avoidance of saquinavir advised by manufacturer of ●lapatinib

  Diuretics: saquinavir increases plasma concentration of eplerenone (reduce dose of eplerenone)
- Ergot Alkaloids: increased risk of ergotism when saquinavir given with ●ergotamine and methysergide—avoid concomitant use
- Lipid-regulating Drugs: possible increased risk of myopathy when saquinavir given with atorvastatin; possible increased risk of myopathy when saquinavir given with ●rosuvastatin—avoid concomitant use; increased risk of myopathy when saquinavir given with ●simvastatin (avoid concomitant use)
- Ranolazine: saquinavir possibly increases plasma concentration of ●ranolazine—manufacturer of ranolazine advises avoid concomitant use

  Sildenafil: saquinavir possibly increases plasma concentration of sildenafil—reduce initial dose of sildenafil
- Tacrolimus: saquinavir increases plasma concentration of ●tacrolimus (consider reducing dose of tacrolimus)

  Tadalafil: saquinavir possibly increases plasma concentration of tadalafil—reduce initial dose of tadalafil

  Ulcer-healing Drugs: plasma concentration of saquinavir possibly increased by cimetidine; plasma concentration of saquinavir increased by omeprazole

  Vardenafil: saquinavir possibly increases plasma concentration of vardenafil—reduce initial dose of vardenafil

**Secobarbital** *see* Barbiturates

**Selegiline**

Note  Selegiline is a MAO-B inhibitor

- Analgesics: hyperpyrexia and CNS toxicity reported when selegiline given with ●pethidine (avoid concomitant use); manufacturer of selegiline advises caution with tramadol
- Antidepressants: theoretical risk of serotonin syndrome if selegiline given with citalopram (especially if dose of selegiline exceeds 10 mg daily); caution with selegiline advised by manufacturer of escitalopram; increased risk of hypertension and CNS excitation when selegiline given with ●fluoxetine (selegiline should not be started until 5 weeks after stopping fluoxetine, avoid fluoxetine for 2 weeks after stopping selegiline); increased risk of hypertension and CNS excitation when selegiline given with

**Selegiline**
- Antidepressants *(continued)*
  - •fluvoxamine or •venlafaxine (selegiline should not be started until 1 week after stopping fluvoxamine or venlafaxine, avoid fluvoxamine or venlafaxine for 2 weeks after stopping selegiline); increased risk of hypertension and CNS excitation when selegiline given with •paroxetine or •sertraline (selegiline should not be started until 2 weeks after stopping paroxetine or sertraline, avoid paroxetine or sertraline for 2 weeks after stopping selegiline); enhanced hypotensive effect when selegiline given with MAOIs; avoid concomitant use of selegiline with •moclobemide; CNS toxicity reported when selegiline given with •tricyclics

Dopaminergics: max. dose of 10 mg selegiline advised by manufacturer of entacapone if used concomitantly; selegiline enhances effects and increases toxicity of levodopa (reduce dose of levodopa)

Memantine: effects of dopaminergics and selegiline possibly enhanced by memantine

Methyldopa: antiparkinsonian effect of dopaminergics antagonised by methyldopa

Oestrogens: plasma concentration of selegiline increased by oestrogens (increased risk of toxicity)

Progestogens: plasma concentration of selegiline increased by progestogens (increased risk of toxicity)
- Sympathomimetics: risk of hypertensive crisis when selegiline given with •dopamine

**Selenium**
Vitamins: absorption of selenium possibly reduced by ascorbic acid (give at least 4 hours apart)

**Sertindole** *see* Antipsychotics

**Sertraline** *see* Antidepressants, SSRI

**Sevelamer**
Antibacterials: sevelamer reduces bioavailability of ciprofloxacin

Ciclosporin: sevelamer possibly reduces plasma concentration of ciclosporin

Mycophenolate: sevelamer possibly reduces plasma concentration of mycophenolate

Tacrolimus: sevelamer possibly reduces plasma concentration of tacrolimus

**Sevoflurane** *see* Anaesthetics, General

**Sibutramine**
Analgesics: increased risk of bleeding when sibutramine given with NSAIDs or aspirin

Anticoagulants: increased risk of bleeding when sibutramine given with anticoagulants
- Antidepressants: increased CNS toxicity when sibutramine given with •MAOIs or •moclobemide (manufacturer of sibutramine advises avoid concomitant use), also avoid sibutramine for 2 weeks after stopping MAOIs or moclobemide; increased risk of CNS toxicity when sibutramine given with •SSRI-related antidepressants, •SSRIs, •mirtazapine, •noradrenaline re-uptake inhibitors, •tricyclic-related antidepressants, •tricyclics or •tryptophan (manufacturer of sibutramine advises avoid concomitant use)
- Antipsychotics: increased risk of CNS toxicity when sibutramine given with •antipsychotics (manufacturer of sibutramine advises avoid concomitant use)

**Sildenafil**
- Alpha-blockers: enhanced hypotensive effect when sildenafil given with •alpha-blockers (avoid alpha-blockers for 4 hours after sildenafil)—see also p. 463

Antibacterials: plasma concentration of sildenafil possibly increased by clarithromycin and telithromycin—reduce initial dose of sildenafil; plasma concentration of sildenafil increased by erythromycin—reduce initial dose of sildenafil

Antifungals: plasma concentration of sildenafil increased by itraconazole and ketoconazole—reduce initial dose of sildenafil
- Antivirals: side-effects of sildenafil possibly increased by •atazanavir; plasma concentration of sildenafil reduced by etravirine; plasma concentration of sildenafil possibly increased by fosamprenavir,

**Sildenafil**
- Antivirals *(continued)*
  nelfinavir and saquinavir—reduce initial dose of sildenafil; plasma concentration of sildenafil increased by •indinavir—reduce initial dose of sildenafil; plasma concentration of sildenafil significantly increased by •ritonavir—avoid concomitant use

Bosentan: plasma concentration of sildenafil reduced by bosentan

Calcium-channel Blockers: enhanced hypotensive effect when sildenafil given with amlodipine

Grapefruit Juice: plasma concentration of sildenafil possibly increased by grapefruit juice
- Nicorandil: sildenafil significantly enhances hypotensive effect of •nicorandil (avoid concomitant use)
- Nitrates: sildenafil significantly enhances hypotensive effect of •nitrates (avoid concomitant use)

Ulcer-healing Drugs: plasma concentration of sildenafil increased by cimetidine (reduce initial dose of sildenafil)

**Simvastatin** *see* Statins

**Sirolimus**
- Antibacterials: plasma concentration of sirolimus increased by •clarithromycin and •telithromycin—avoid concomitant use; plasma concentration of both drugs increased when sirolimus given with •erythromycin; plasma concentration of sirolimus reduced by •rifabutin and •rifampicin—avoid concomitant use
- Antifungals: plasma concentration of sirolimus increased by •itraconazole, •ketoconazole and •voriconazole—avoid concomitant use; plasma concentration of sirolimus increased by micafungin and •miconazole; plasma concentration of sirolimus possibly increased by posaconazole
- Antivirals: plasma concentration of sirolimus possibly increased by •atazanavir and lopinavir
- Calcium-channel Blockers: plasma concentration of sirolimus increased by •diltiazem; plasma concentration of both drugs increased when sirolimus given with •verapamil

Ciclosporin: plasma concentration of sirolimus increased by ciclosporin
- Grapefruit Juice: plasma concentration of sirolimus increased by •grapefruit juice—avoid concomitant use

**Sitaxentan**
- Anticoagulants: sitaxentan enhances anticoagulant effect of •coumarins
- Ciclosporin: plasma concentration of sitaxentan increased by •ciclosporin—avoid concomitant use

Oestrogens: sitaxentan increases plasma concentration of oestrogens

Progestogens: sitaxentan increases plasma concentration of progestogens

**Sodium Aurothiomalate** *see* Gold

**Sodium Benzoate**
Antiepileptics: effects of sodium benzoate possibly reduced by valproate

Antipsychotics: effects of sodium benzoate possibly reduced by haloperidol

Corticosteroids: effects of sodium benzoate possibly reduced by corticosteroids

Probenecid: excretion of conjugate formed by sodium benzoate possibly reduced by probenecid

**Sodium Bicarbonate** *see* Antacids

**Sodium Clodronate** *see* Bisphosphonates

**Sodium Nitroprusside** *see* Vasodilator Antihypertensives

**Sodium Oxybate**
- Analgesics: effects of sodium oxybate enhanced by •opioid analgesics (avoid concomitant use)

Antidepressants: increased risk of side-effects when sodium oxybate given with tricyclics

Antipsychotics: effects of sodium oxybate possibly enhanced by antipsychotics

**Sodium Oxybate** *(continued)*
- Anxiolytics and Hypnotics: effects of sodium oxybate enhanced by ●benzodiazepines (avoid concomitant use)
- Barbiturates: effects of sodium oxybate enhanced by ●barbiturates (avoid concomitant use)

**Sodium Phenylbutyrate**
Antiepileptics: effects of sodium phenylbutyrate possibly reduced by valproate
Antipsychotics: effects of sodium phenylbutyrate possibly reduced by haloperidol
Corticosteroids: effects of sodium phenylbutyrate possibly reduced by corticosteroids
Probenecid: excretion of conjugate formed by sodium phenylbutyrate possibly reduced by probenecid

**Sodium Valproate** *see* Valproate

**Solifenacin** *see* Antimuscarinics

**Somatropin**
Corticosteroids: growth-promoting effect of somatropin may be inhibited by corticosteroids
Oestrogens: increased doses of somatropin may be needed when given with oestrogens (when used as oral replacement therapy)

**Sorafenib**
Antibacterials: plasma concentration of sorafenib reduced by rifampicin
- Anticoagulants: sorafenib possibly enhances anticoagulant effect of ●coumarins
Antiepileptics: cytotoxics possibly reduce absorption of phenytoin
- Antipsychotics: avoid concomitant use of cytotoxics with ●clozapine (increased risk of agranulocytosis)
Cardiac Glycosides: cytotoxics reduce absorption of digoxin tablets
Cytotoxics: sorafenib possibly increases plasma concentration of doxorubicin and irinotecan; sorafenib increases plasma concentration of docetaxel

**Sotalol** *see* Beta-blockers

**Spironolactone** *see* Diuretics

**Statins**
Antacids: absorption of rosuvastatin reduced by antacids
- Anti-arrhythmics: increased risk of myopathy when simvastatin given with ●amiodarone
- Antibacterials: plasma concentration of atorvastatin and pravastatin increased by ●clarithromycin; increased risk of myopathy when simvastatin given with ●clarithromycin, ●erythromycin or ●telithromycin (avoid concomitant use); plasma concentration of rosuvastatin reduced by erythromycin; possible increased risk of myopathy when atorvastatin given with erythromycin or fusidic acid; plasma concentration of pravastatin increased by erythromycin; plasma concentration of atorvastatin and simvastatin possibly reduced by rifampicin; metabolism of fluvastatin accelerated by rifampicin (reduced effect); increased risk of myopathy when statins given with ●daptomycin (preferably avoid concomitant use); increased risk of myopathy when simvastatin given with ●fusidic acid; increased risk of myopathy when atorvastatin given with ●telithromycin (avoid concomitant use)
- Anticoagulants: atorvastatin may transiently reduce anticoagulant effect of warfarin; fluvastatin and simvastatin enhance anticoagulant effect of ●coumarins; rosuvastatin possibly enhances anticoagulant effect of ●coumarins and ●phenindione
Antidepressants: plasma concentration of simvastatin reduced by St John's wort
Antidiabetics: fluvastatin possibly increases plasma concentration of glibenclamide
Antiepileptics: combination of fluvastatin with phenytoin may increase plasma concentration of either drug (or both)
- Antifungals: increased risk of myopathy when simvastatin given with ●itraconazole, ●ketoconazole or ●posaconazole (avoid concomitant use); possible increased risk of myopathy when simvastatin given with ●miconazole—avoid concomitant use; plasma

**Statins**
- Antifungals *(continued)*
concentration of fluvastatin increased by fluconazole; increased risk of myopathy when atorvastatin given with ●itraconazole or ●posaconazole (avoid concomitant use); possible increased risk of myopathy when atorvastatin or simvastatin given with imidazoles; possible increased risk of myopathy when atorvastatin or simvastatin given with triazoles
- Antivirals: increased risk of myopathy when simvastatin given with ●atazanavir, ●indinavir, ●nelfinavir, ●ritonavir or ●saquinavir (avoid concomitant use); possible increased risk of myopathy when atorvastatin given with atazanavir, fosamprenavir, indinavir, lopinavir, nelfinavir, ritonavir or saquinavir; possible increased risk of myopathy when rosuvastatin given with ●atazanavir, ●darunavir, ●fosamprenavir, ●indinavir, ●lopinavir, ●nelfinavir, ●ritonavir, ●saquinavir or ●tipranavir—avoid concomitant use; plasma concentration of pravastatin possibly increased by darunavir; plasma concentration of atorvastatin, pravastatin and simvastatin reduced by efavirenz; plasma concentration of atorvastatin possibly reduced by etravirine; possible increased risk of myopathy when simvastatin given with ●fosamprenavir or ●lopinavir—avoid concomitant use
Bosentan: plasma concentration of simvastatin reduced by bosentan
- Calcium-channel Blockers: possible increased risk of myopathy when simvastatin given with diltiazem; plasma concentration of atorvastatin increased by diltiazem; increased risk of myopathy when simvastatin given with ●verapamil
Cardiac Glycosides: atorvastatin possibly increases plasma concentration of digoxin
- Ciclosporin: increased risk of myopathy when statins given with ●ciclosporin; increased risk of myopathy when rosuvastatin given with ●ciclosporin (avoid concomitant use)
- Colchicine: possible increased risk of myopathy when statins given with ●colchicine
Cytotoxics: plasma concentration of simvastatin possibly increased by dasatinib; plasma concentration of simvastatin increased by imatinib
- Grapefruit Juice: plasma concentration of atorvastatin possibly increased by grapefruit juice; plasma concentration of simvastatin increased by ●grapefruit juice—avoid concomitant use
- Hormone Antagonists: possible increased risk of myopathy when simvastatin given with ●danazol
- Lipid-regulating Drugs: increased risk of myopathy when statins given with ●gemfibrozil (preferably avoid concomitant use); increased risk of myopathy when statins given with ●fibrates; increased risk of myopathy when statins given with ●nicotinic acid (applies to lipid regulating doses of nicotinic acid)
Oestrogens: atorvastatin and rosuvastatin increase plasma concentration of ethinylestradiol
Progestogens: atorvastatin increases plasma concentration of norethisterone; rosuvastatin increases plasma concentration of norgestrel
Ranolazine: plasma concentration of simvastatin increased by ranolazine (consider reducing dose of simvastatin)
Retinoids: plasma concentration of simvastatin reduced by alitretinoin

**Stavudine**
- Antivirals: increased risk of side-effects when stavudine given with ●didanosine; effects of stavudine possibly inhibited by ●ribavirin; effects of stavudine possibly inhibited by ●zidovudine (manufacturers advise avoid concomitant use)
- Cytotoxics: effects of stavudine possibly inhibited by doxorubicin; increased risk of toxicity when stavudine given with ●hydroxycarbamide—avoid concomitant use

**Stiripentol**
- Antidepressants: anticonvulsant effect of antiepileptics possibly antagonised by MAOIs and ●tricyclic-related antidepressants (convulsive threshold lowered); anticonvulsant effect of antiepileptics antagonised by ●SSRIs and ●tricyclics (convulsive threshold lowered); avoid concomitant use of antiepileptics with ●St John's wort
- <u>Antiepileptics</u>: stiripentol increases plasma concentration of ●carbamazepine and ●phenytoin
- Antimalarials: possible increased risk of convulsions when antiepileptics given with chloroquine and hydroxychloroquine; anticonvulsant effect of antiepileptics antagonised by ●mefloquine
  <u>Anxiolytics and Hypnotics</u>: stiripentol increases plasma concentration of clobazam
- <u>Barbiturates</u>: stiripentol increases plasma concentration of ●phenobarbital

**Streptomycin** *see* Aminoglycosides

**Strontium Ranelate**
  Antibacterials: strontium ranelate reduces absorption of quinolones and tetracyclines (manufacturer of strontium ranelate advises avoid concomitant use)

**Sucralfate**
  Antibacterials: sucralfate reduces absorption of ciprofloxacin, levofloxacin, moxifloxacin, norfloxacin, ofloxacin and tetracyclines
- Anticoagulants: sucralfate possibly reduces absorption of ●coumarins (reduced anticoagulant effect)
- Antiepileptics: sucralfate reduces absorption of ●phenytoin
  Antifungals: sucralfate reduces absorption of ketoconazole
  Antipsychotics: sucralfate reduces absorption of sulpiride
  Cardiac Glycosides: sucralfate possibly reduces absorption of cardiac glycosides
  Theophylline: sucralfate possibly reduces absorption of theophylline (give at least 2 hours apart)
  Thyroid Hormones: sucralfate reduces absorption of levothyroxine (thyroxine)
  Ulcer-healing Drugs: sucralfate possibly reduces absorption of lansoprazole

**Sugammadex**
  Antibacterials: response to sugammadex possibly reduced by flucloxacillin and fusidic acid
  Hormone Antagonists: response to sugammadex possibly reduced by toremifene
  Oestrogens: sugammadex possibly reduces plasma concentration of oestrogens
  Progestogens: sugammadex possibly reduces plasma concentration of progestogens

**Sulfadiazine** *see* Sulphonamides
**Sulfadoxine** *see* Sulphonamides
**Sulfamethoxazole** *see* Sulphonamides
**Sulfasalazine** *see* Aminosalicylates

**Sulfinpyrazone**
  Analgesics: effects of sulfinpyrazone antagonised by aspirin
  Antibacterials: sulfinpyrazone reduces excretion of nitrofurantoin (increased risk of toxicity); sulfinpyrazone reduces excretion of penicillins; effects of sulfinpyrazone antagonised by pyrazinamide
- Anticoagulants: sulfinpyrazone enhances anticoagulant effect of ●coumarins
- Antidiabetics: sulfinpyrazone enhances effects of ●sulphonylureas
- Antiepileptics: sulfinpyrazone increases plasma concentration of ●phenytoin
- Ciclosporin: sulfinpyrazone reduces plasma concentration of ●ciclosporin
  Theophylline: sulfinpyrazone reduces plasma concentration of theophylline

**Sulindac** *see* NSAIDs

**Sulphonamides**
  Anaesthetics, General: sulphonamides enhance effects of thiopental

**Sulphonamides** *(continued)*
  Anaesthetics, Local: increased risk of methaemoglobinaemia when sulphonamides given with prilocaine
- Anti-arrhythmics: increased risk of ventricular arrhythmias when sulfamethoxazole (as co-trimoxazole) given with ●amiodarone—avoid concomitant use of co-trimoxazole
- Antibacterials: increased risk of crystalluria when sulphonamides given with ●methenamine
- Anticoagulants: sulphonamides enhance anticoagulant effect of ●coumarins
  Antidiabetics: sulphonamides rarely enhance the effects of sulphonylureas
  Antiepileptics: sulphonamides possibly increase plasma concentration of phenytoin
- Antimalarials: increased antifolate effect when sulphonamides given with ●pyrimethamine
- Antipsychotics: avoid concomitant use of sulphonamides with ●clozapine (increased risk of agranulocytosis)
- Azathioprine: increased risk of haematological toxicity when sulfamethoxazole (as co-trimoxazole) given with ●azathioprine
- Ciclosporin: increased risk of nephrotoxicity when sulphonamides given with ●ciclosporin; sulfadiazine possibly reduces plasma concentration of ●ciclosporin
- Cytotoxics: increased risk of haematological toxicity when sulfamethoxazole (as co-trimoxazole) given with ●mercaptopurine or ●methotrexate; sulphonamides increase risk of methotrexate toxicity
  Oestrogens: antibacterials that do not induce liver enzymes possibly reduce contraceptive effect of oestrogens (risk probably small, see p. 445)
  Potassium Aminobenzoate: effects of sulphonamides inhibited by potassium aminobenzoate
  Vaccines: antibacterials inactivate oral typhoid vaccine–see p. 688

**Sulphonylureas** *see* Antidiabetics
**Sulpiride** *see* Antipsychotics
**Sumatriptan** *see* 5HT$_1$ Agonists

**Sunitinib**
  Antibacterials: metabolism of sunitinib accelerated by rifampicin (reduced plasma concentration)
  Antiepileptics: cytotoxics possibly reduce absorption of phenytoin
  Antifungals: metabolism of sunitinib inhibited by ketoconazole (increased plasma concentration)
- Antipsychotics: avoid concomitant use of cytotoxics with ●clozapine (increased risk of agranulocytosis)
  Cardiac Glycosides: cytotoxics reduce absorption of digoxin tablets

**Suxamethonium** *see* Muscle Relaxants

**Sympathomimetics**
- <u>Adrenergic Neurone Blockers</u>: ephedrine, isometheptene, metaraminol, methylphenidate, noradrenaline (norepinephrine), oxymetazoline, phenylephrine, pseudoephedrine and xylometazoline antagonise hypotensive effect of ●adrenergic neurone blockers; dexamfetamine antagonises hypotensive effect of ●guanethidine
  <u>Alcohol</u>: effects of methylphenidate possibly enhanced by alcohol
- Alpha-blockers: avoid concomitant use of adrenaline (epinephrine) or dopamine with ●tolazoline
- Anaesthetics, General: increased risk of hypertension when methylphenidate given with ●volatile liquid general anaesthetics; increased risk of arrhythmias when adrenaline (epinephrine) given with ●volatile liquid general anaesthetics
- Anticoagulants: methylphenidate possibly enhances anticoagulant effect of ●coumarins
- Antidepressants: risk of hypertensive crisis when methylphenidate given with ●MAOIs, some manufacturers advise avoid methylphenidate for at least 2 weeks after stopping MAOIs; risk of hypertensive crisis when sympathomimetics given with ●MAOIs or ●moclobemide; methylphenidate possibly inhibits

**Sympathomimetics**

● Antidepressants *(continued)*
metabolism of SSRIs and tricyclics; increased risk
of hypertension and arrhythmias when
noradrenaline (norepinephrine) given with
●tricyclics; increased risk of hypertension and
arrhythmias when adrenaline (epinephrine) given
with ●tricyclics (but local anaesthetics with adrenaline appear to be safe)

Antiepileptics: methylphenidate increases plasma
concentration of phenytoin; methylphenidate possibly increases plasma concentration of primidone

Antipsychotics: hypertensive effect of sympathomimetics antagonised by antipsychotics; dexamfetamine possibly antagonises antipsychotic effects of
chlorpromazine; methylphenidate possibly increases
side-effects of risperidone

Antivirals: plasma concentration of dexamfetamine
possibly increased by ritonavir

Barbiturates: methylphenidate possibly increases
plasma concentration of phenobarbital

● Beta-blockers: increased risk of severe hypertension
and bradycardia when adrenaline (epinephrine) given
with non-cardioselective ●beta-blockers, also
response to adrenaline (epinephrine) may be
reduced; increased risk of severe hypertension and
bradycardia when dobutamine given with non-
cardioselective ●beta-blockers; possible increased
risk of severe hypertension and bradycardia when
noradrenaline (norepinephrine) given with non-cardioselective ●beta-blockers

● Clonidine: possible risk of hypertension when adrenaline (epinephrine) or noradrenaline (norepinephrine)
given with clonidine; serious adverse events reported
with concomitant use of methylphenidate and
●clonidine (causality not established)

Corticosteroids: ephedrine accelerates metabolism of
dexamethasone

● Dopaminergics: risk of toxicity when isometheptene
given with ●bromocriptine; effects of adrenaline
(epinephrine), dobutamine, dopamine and noradrenaline (norepinephrine) possibly enhanced by entacapone; avoid concomitant use of sympathomimetics
with ●rasagiline; risk of hypertensive crisis when
dopamine given with ●selegiline

Doxapram: increased risk of hypertension when
sympathomimetics given with doxapram

Ergot Alkaloids: increased risk of ergotism when
sympathomimetics given with ergotamine and
methysergide

Oxytocin: risk of hypertension when vasoconstrictor
sympathomimetics given with oxytocin (due to
enhanced vasopressor effect)

● Sympathomimetics: effects of adrenaline (epinephrine)
possibly enhanced by ●dopexamine; dopexamine
possibly enhances effects of ●noradrenaline (norepinephrine)

Theophylline: avoidance of ephedrine in children
advised by manufacturer of theophylline

**Sympathomimetics, Beta₂**

Atomoxetine: Increased risk of cardiovascular side-
effects when parenteral salbutamol given with
atomoxetine

Cardiac Glycosides: salbutamol possibly reduces
plasma concentration of digoxin

Corticosteroids: increased risk of hypokalaemia when
high doses of beta₂ sympathomimetics given with
corticosteroids—for CSM advice (hypokalaemia) see
p. 155

Diuretics: increased risk of hypokalaemia when high
doses of beta₂ sympathomimetics given with acetazolamide, loop diuretics or thiazides and related
diuretics—for CSM advice (hypokalaemia) see p. 155

● Methyldopa: acute hypotension reported when infusion of salbutamol given with ●methyldopa

Muscle Relaxants: bambuterol enhances effects of
suxamethonium

**Sympathomimetics, Beta₂** *(continued)*

Theophylline: increased risk of hypokalaemia when
high doses of beta₂ sympathomimetics given with
theophylline—for CSM advice (hypokalaemia) see
p. 155

**Tacrolimus**

Note Interactions do not generally apply to tacrolimus used
topically; risk of facial flushing and skin irritation with
alcohol consumption (p. 645) does not apply to tacrolimus
taken systemically

● Analgesics: possible increased risk of nephrotoxicity
when tacrolimus given with NSAIDs; increased risk of
nephrotoxicity when tacrolimus given with
●ibuprofen

Angiotensin-II Receptor Antagonists: increased risk of
hyperkalaemia when tacrolimus given with angiotensin-II receptor antagonists

● Antibacterials: plasma concentration of tacrolimus
increased by ●clarithromycin, ●erythromycin and
●quinupristin/dalfopristin; plasma concentration of
tacrolimus reduced by ●rifampicin; increased risk of
nephrotoxicity when tacrolimus given with
●aminoglycosides; plasma concentration of tacrolimus possibly increased by ●chloramphenicol and
●telithromycin; possible increased risk of nephrotoxicity when tacrolimus given with vancomycin

● Antidepressants: plasma concentration of tacrolimus
reduced by ●St John's wort—avoid concomitant use

Antiepileptics: plasma concentration of tacrolimus
reduced by phenytoin, also plasma concentration of
phenytoin possibly increased

● Antifungals: plasma concentration of tacrolimus
increased by ●fluconazole, ●itraconazole,
●ketoconazole and ●voriconazole; increased risk of
nephrotoxicity when tacrolimus given with
●amphotericin; plasma concentration of tacrolimus
increased by ●posaconazole (reduce dose of tacrolimus); plasma concentration of tacrolimus reduced by
●caspofungin; plasma concentration of tacrolimus
possibly increased by ●imidazoles and ●triazoles

● Antipsychotics: avoidance of tacrolimus advised by
manufacturer of ●droperidol (risk of ventricular
arrhythmias)

● Antivirals: possible increased risk of nephrotoxicity
when tacrolimus given with aciclovir or ganciclovir;
plasma concentration of tacrolimus possibly
increased by ●atazanavir, ●nelfinavir and ●ritonavir;
plasma concentration of tacrolimus possibly affected
by ●efavirenz; plasma concentration of tacrolimus
increased by ●saquinavir (consider reducing dose of
tacrolimus)

● Barbiturates: plasma concentration of tacrolimus
reduced by ●phenobarbital

● Calcium-channel Blockers: plasma concentration of
tacrolimus possibly increased by felodipine,
nicardipine and verapamil; plasma concentration of
tacrolimus increased by ●diltiazem and ●nifedipine

● Ciclosporin: tacrolimus increases plasma concentration
of ●ciclosporin (increased risk of nephrotoxicity)—
avoid concomitant use

● Diuretics: increased risk of hyperkalaemia when
tacrolimus given with ●potassium-sparing diuretics
and aldosterone antagonists

● Grapefruit Juice: plasma concentration of tacrolimus
increased by ●grapefruit juice

Hormone Antagonists: plasma concentration of
tacrolimus possibly increased by danazol

Oestrogens: tacrolimus possibly inhibits metabolism of
oestrogens; plasma concentration of tacrolimus
possibly increased by ethinylestradiol

● Potassium Salts: increased risk of hyperkalaemia
when tacrolimus given with ●potassium salts

Progestogens: tacrolimus possibly inhibits metabolism
of progestogens

Sevelamer: plasma concentration of tacrolimus possibly reduced by sevelamer

Ulcer-healing Drugs: plasma concentration of tacrolimus possibly increased by omeprazole

**Tadalafil**
- Alpha-blockers: enhanced hypotensive effect when tadalafil given with ●doxazosin—manufacturer of tadalafil advises avoid concomitant use; enhanced hypotensive effect when tadalafil given with ●alpha-blockers—see also p. 463

  Antibacterials: plasma concentration of tadalafil possibly increased by clarithromycin and erythromycin; plasma concentration of tadalafil reduced by rifampicin

  Antifungals: plasma concentration of tadalafil increased by ketoconazole; plasma concentration of tadalafil possibly increased by itraconazole

  Antivirals: plasma concentration of tadalafil possibly increased by fosamprenavir and indinavir; plasma concentration of tadalafil increased by ritonavir; plasma concentration of tadalafil possibly increased by saquinavir—reduce initial dose of tadalafil

  Grapefruit Juice: plasma concentration of tadalafil possibly increased by grapefruit juice
- Nicorandil: tadalafil significantly enhances hypotensive effect of ●nicorandil (avoid concomitant use)
- Nitrates: tadalafil significantly enhances hypotensive effect of ●nitrates (avoid concomitant use)

**Tamoxifen**
- Antibacterials: metabolism of tamoxifen accelerated by rifampicin (reduced plasma concentration)
- Anticoagulants: tamoxifen enhances anticoagulant effect of ●coumarins
- Antidepressants: metabolism of tamoxifen to active metabolite possibly inhibited by ●duloxetine, ●fluoxetine and ●paroxetine (avoid concomitant use)
- Antipsychotics: avoidance of tamoxifen advised by manufacturer of ●droperidol (risk of ventricular arrhythmias)
- Bupropion: metabolism of tamoxifen to active metabolite possibly inhibited by ●bupropion (avoid concomitant use)

**Tamsulosin** see Alpha-blockers
**Taxanes** see Docetaxel and Paclitaxel
**Tegafur with uracil** see Fluorouracil
**Teicoplanin**
  Antibacterials: increased risk of nephrotoxicity and ototoxicity when teicoplanin given with aminoglycosides or colistin

  Oestrogens: antibacterials that do not induce liver enzymes possibly reduce contraceptive effect of oestrogens (risk probably small, see p. 445)

  Vaccines: antibacterials inactivate oral typhoid vaccine–see p. 688

**Telbivudine**
- Interferons: increased risk of peripheral neuropathy when telbivudine given with ●interferon alfa

**Telithromycin**
- Antibacterials: plasma concentration of telithromycin reduced by ●rifampicin (avoid during and for 2 weeks after rifampicin)
- Antidepressants: plasma concentration of telithromycin reduced by ●St John's wort (avoid during and for 2 weeks after St John's wort)
- Antiepileptics: plasma concentration of telithromycin reduced by ●carbamazepine, ●phenytoin and ●primidone (avoid during and for 2 weeks after carbamazepine, phenytoin and primidone)
- Antifungals: manufacturer of telithromycin advises avoid concomitant use with ●ketoconazole in severe renal and hepatic impairment

  Antimuscarinics: manufacturer of fesoterodine advises dose reduction when telithromycin given with fesoterodine—consult fesoterodine product literature
- Antipsychotics: increased risk of ventricular arrhythmias when telithromycin given with ●pimozide—avoid concomitant use
- Antivirals: manufacturer of telithromycin advises avoid concomitant use with ●atazanavir, ●fosamprenavir, ●indinavir, ●lopinavir, ●nelfinavir, ●ritonavir, ●saquinavir and ●tipranavir in severe renal and hepatic impairment; telithromycin possibly increases

**Telithromycin**
- Antivirals (continued)

  plasma concentration of ●maraviroc (consider reducing dose of maraviroc)
- Anxiolytics and Hypnotics: telithromycin inhibits metabolism of ●midazolam (increased plasma concentration with increased sedation)

  Aprepitant: telithromycin possibly increases plasma concentration of aprepitant
- Barbiturates: plasma concentration of telithromycin reduced by ●phenobarbital (avoid during and for 2 weeks after phenobarbital)

  Cardiac Glycosides: telithromycin possibly increases plasma concentration of digoxin
- Ciclosporin: telithromycin possibly increases plasma concentration of ●ciclosporin
- Cytotoxics: avoidance of telithromycin advised by manufacturer of ●lapatinib and ●nilotinib
- Diuretics: telithromycin increases plasma concentration of ●eplerenone—avoid concomitant use
- Ergot Alkaloids: increased risk of ergotism when telithromycin given with ●ergotamine and methysergide—avoid concomitant use
- Ivabradine: telithromycin possibly increases plasma concentration of ●ivabradine—avoid concomitant use
- Lipid-regulating Drugs: increased risk of myopathy when telithromycin given with ●atorvastatin or ●simvastatin (avoid concomitant use)

  Oestrogens: antibacterials that do not induce liver enzymes possibly reduce contraceptive effect of oestrogens (risk probably small, see p. 445)
- Ranolazine: telithromycin possibly increases plasma concentration of ●ranolazine—manufacturer of ranolazine advises avoid concomitant use

  Sildenafil: telithromycin possibly increases plasma concentration of sildenafil—reduce initial dose of sildenafil
- Sirolimus: telithromycin increases plasma concentration of ●sirolimus—avoid concomitant use
- Tacrolimus: telithromycin possibly increases plasma concentration of ●tacrolimus

  Vaccines: antibacterials inactivate oral typhoid vaccine–see p. 688

**Telmisartan** see Angiotensin-II Receptor Antagonists
**Temazepam** see Anxiolytics and Hypnotics
**Temocillin** see Penicillins
**Temoporfin**
- Cytotoxics: increased skin photosensitivity when temoporfin given with topical ●fluorouracil

**Temozolomide**
  Antiepileptics: cytotoxics possibly reduce absorption of phenytoin; plasma concentration of temozolomide increased by valproate
- Antipsychotics: avoid concomitant use of cytotoxics with ●clozapine (increased risk of agranulocytosis)

  Cardiac Glycosides: cytotoxics reduce absorption of digoxin tablets

**Temsirolimus**
  Note The main active metabolite of temsirolimus is sirolimus—see also interactions of sirolimus and consult product literature
- Antibacterials: plasma concentration of active metabolite of temsirolimus reduced by ●rifampicin—avoid concomitant use

  Antiepileptics: cytotoxics possibly reduce absorption of phenytoin
- Antifungals: plasma concentration of active metabolite of temsirolimus increased by ●ketoconazole—avoid concomitant use
- Antipsychotics: avoid concomitant use of cytotoxics with ●clozapine (increased risk of agranulocytosis)

  Cardiac Glycosides: cytotoxics reduce absorption of digoxin tablets

**Tenofovir**
- Antivirals: manufacturer of tenofovir advises avoid concomitant use with adefovir; tenofovir reduces plasma concentration of atazanavir, also plasma concentration of tenofovir possibly increased;

**Tenofovir**

● Antivirals *(continued)*
combination of tenofovir with cidofovir may increase plasma concentration of either drug (or both); tenofovir increases plasma concentration of ●didanosine (increased risk of toxicity)—avoid concomitant use; plasma concentration of tenofovir increased by lopinavir

**Tenoxicam** *see* NSAIDs

**Terazosin** *see* Alpha-blockers

**Terbinafine**

● <u>Antibacterials</u>: plasma concentration of terbinafine reduced by ●rifampicin

Antidepressants: terbinafine possibly increases plasma concentration of imipramine and nortriptyline

<u>Ciclosporin</u>: terbinafine possibly reduces plasma concentration of ciclosporin

Oestrogens: occasional reports of breakthrough bleeding when terbinafine given with oestrogens (when used for contraception)

Progestogens: occasional reports of breakthrough bleeding when terbinafine given with progestogens (when used for contraception)

Ulcer-healing Drugs: plasma concentration of terbinafine increased by cimetidine

**Terbutaline** *see* Sympathomimetics, Beta$_2$

**Terpene Mixture** *see* Rowachol®

**Testolactone**

● Anticoagulants: testolactone enhances anticoagulant effect of ●coumarins and ●phenindione

**Testosterone**

● Anticoagulants: testosterone enhances anticoagulant effect of ●coumarins and ●phenindione

Antidiabetics: testosterone possibly enhances hypoglycaemic effect of antidiabetics

**Tetrabenazine**

● Antidepressants: risk of CNS excitation and hypertension when tetrabenazine given with ●MAOIs

Antipsychotics: increased risk of extrapyramidal side-effects when tetrabenazine given with antipsychotics

Dopaminergics: increased risk of extrapyramidal side-effects when tetrabenazine given with amantadine

Metoclopramide: increased risk of extrapyramidal side-effects when tetrabenazine given with metoclopramide

**Tetracosactide** *see* Corticosteroids

**Tetracycline** *see* Tetracyclines

**Tetracyclines**

ACE Inhibitors: absorption of tetracyclines reduced by quinapril tablets (quinapril tablets contain magnesium carbonate)

Adsorbents: absorption of tetracyclines possibly reduced by kaolin

Antacids: absorption of tetracyclines reduced by antacids

● Anticoagulants: tetracyclines possibly enhance anticoagulant effect of ●coumarins and ●phenindione

Antiepileptics: metabolism of doxycycline accelerated by carbamazepine (reduced effect); metabolism of doxycycline accelerated by phenytoin and primidone (reduced plasma concentration)

Atovaquone: tetracycline reduces plasma concentration of atovaquone

Barbiturates: metabolism of doxycycline accelerated by barbiturates (reduced plasma concentration)

Calcium Salts: absorption of tetracycline reduced by calcium salts

● Ciclosporin: doxycycline possibly increases plasma concentration of ●ciclosporin

Cytotoxics: doxycycline or tetracycline increase risk of methotrexate toxicity

Dairy Products: absorption of tetracyclines (except doxycycline and minocycline) reduced by dairy products

Diuretics: manufacturer of lymecycline advises avoid concomitant use with diuretics

**Tetracyclines** *(continued)*

Ergot Alkaloids: increased risk of ergotism when tetracyclines given with ergotamine and methysergide

Iron: absorption of tetracyclines reduced by *oral* iron, also absorption of *oral* iron reduced by tetracyclines

Lipid-regulating Drugs: absorption of tetracycline possibly reduced by colestipol and colestyramine

Oestrogens: antibacterials that do not induce liver enzymes possibly reduce contraceptive effect of oestrogens (risk probably small, see p. 445)

● Retinoids: possible increased risk of benign intracranial hypertension when tetracyclines given with ●retinoids (avoid concomitant use)

Strontium Ranelate: absorption of tetracyclines reduced by strontium ranelate (manufacturer of strontium ranelate advises avoid concomitant use)

Ulcer-healing Drugs: absorption of tetracyclines reduced by sucralfate and tripotassium dicitratobismuthate

Vaccines: antibacterials inactivate oral typhoid vaccine–see p. 688

Zinc: absorption of tetracyclines reduced by zinc, also absorption of zinc reduced by tetracyclines

**Theophylline**

Allopurinol: plasma concentration of theophylline possibly increased by allopurinol

Anaesthetics, General: increased risk of convulsions when theophylline given with ketamine; increased risk of arrhythmias when theophylline given with halothane

Anti-arrhythmics: theophylline antagonises anti-arrhythmic effect of adenosine; plasma concentration of theophylline increased by propafenone

● Antibacterials: plasma concentration of theophylline possibly increased by azithromycin and isoniazid; metabolism of theophylline inhibited by ●clarithromycin (increased plasma concentration); metabolism of theophylline inhibited by ●erythromycin (increased plasma concentration), if erythromycin given by mouth, also decreased plasma-erythromycin concentration; plasma concentration of theophylline increased by ●ciprofloxacin and ●norfloxacin; metabolism of theophylline accelerated by rifampicin (reduced plasma concentration); possible increased risk of convulsions when theophylline given with ●quinolones

● Antidepressants: plasma concentration of theophylline increased by ●fluvoxamine (concomitant use should usually be avoided, but where not possible halve theophylline dose and monitor plasma-theophylline concentration); plasma concentration of theophylline reduced by ●St John's wort—avoid concomitant use

● Antiepileptics: metabolism of theophylline accelerated by carbamazepine and primidone (reduced effect); plasma concentration of both drugs reduced when theophylline given with ●phenytoin

● Antifungals: plasma concentration of theophylline possibly increased by ●fluconazole and ●ketoconazole

● Antivirals: metabolism of theophylline accelerated by ●ritonavir (reduced plasma concentration)

Anxiolytics and Hypnotics: theophylline possibly reduces effects of benzodiazepines

Barbiturates: metabolism of theophylline accelerated by barbiturates (reduced effect)

● Calcium-channel Blockers: plasma concentration of theophylline possibly increased by ●calcium-channel blockers (enhanced effect); plasma concentration of theophylline increased by diltiazem; plasma concentration of theophylline increased by ●verapamil (enhanced effect)

Corticosteroids: increased risk of hypokalaemia when theophylline given with corticosteroids

Cytotoxics: plasma concentration of theophylline possibly increased by methotrexate

Disulfiram: metabolism of theophylline inhibited by disulfiram (increased risk of toxicity)

**Theophylline** *(continued)*

Diuretics: increased risk of hypokalaemia when theophylline given with acetazolamide, loop diuretics or thiazides and related diuretics

Doxapram: increased CNS stimulation when theophylline given with doxapram

Interferons: metabolism of theophylline inhibited by interferon alfa (increased plasma concentration)

Leukotriene Receptor Antagonists: plasma concentration of theophylline possibly increased by zafirlukast, also plasma concentration of zafirlukast reduced

Lithium: theophylline increases excretion of lithium (reduced plasma concentration)

Oestrogens: excretion of theophylline reduced by oestrogens (increased plasma concentration)

Pentoxifylline (oxpentifylline): plasma concentration of theophylline increased by pentoxifylline (oxpentifylline)

Sulfinpyrazone: plasma concentration of theophylline reduced by sulfinpyrazone

Sympathomimetics: manufacturer of theophylline advises avoid concomitant use with ephedrine in children

Sympathomimetics, Beta$_2$: increased risk of hypokalaemia when theophylline given with high doses of beta$_2$ sympathomimetics—for CSM advice (hypokalaemia) see p. 155

Tobacco: metabolism of theophylline increased by tobacco smoking (reduced plasma concentration)

• Ulcer-healing Drugs: metabolism of theophylline inhibited by ●cimetidine (increased plasma concentration); absorption of theophylline possibly reduced by sucralfate (give at least 2 hours apart)

Vaccines: plasma concentration of theophylline possibly increased by influenza vaccine

**Thiazolidinediones** *see* Antidiabetics

**Thiopental** *see* Anaesthetics, General

**Thiotepa**

Antiepileptics: cytotoxics possibly reduce absorption of phenytoin

• Antipsychotics: avoid concomitant use of cytotoxics with ●clozapine (increased risk of agranulocytosis)

Cardiac Glycosides: cytotoxics reduce absorption of digoxin tablets

Muscle Relaxants: thiotepa enhances effects of suxamethonium

**Thioxanthenes** *see* Antipsychotics

**Thyroid Hormones**

Antacids: absorption of levothyroxine (thyroxine) possibly reduced by antacids

Anti-arrhythmics: for concomitant use of thyroid hormones and amiodarone see p. 83

Antibacterials: metabolism of levothyroxine (thyroxine) accelerated by rifampicin (may increase requirements for levothyroxine (thyroxine) in hypothyroidism)

• Anticoagulants: thyroid hormones enhance anticoagulant effect of ●coumarins and ●phenindione

Antidepressants: thyroid hormones enhance effects of amitriptyline and imipramine; thyroid hormones possibly enhance effects of tricyclics

Antiepileptics: metabolism of thyroid hormones accelerated by carbamazepine and primidone (may increase requirements for thyroid hormones in hypothyroidism); metabolism of thyroid hormones accelerated by phenytoin (may increase requirements in hypothyroidism), also plasma concentration of phenytoin possibly increased

Barbiturates: metabolism of thyroid hormones accelerated by barbiturates (may increase requirements for thyroid hormones in hypothyroidism)

Beta-blockers: levothyroxine (thyroxine) accelerates metabolism of propranolol

Calcium Salts: absorption of levothyroxine (thyroxine) reduced by calcium salts

Cytotoxics: plasma concentration of levothyroxine (thyroxine) possibly reduced by imatinib

Iron: absorption of levothyroxine (thyroxine) reduced by *oral* iron (give at least 2 hours apart)

**Thyroid Hormones** *(continued)*

Lipid-regulating Drugs: absorption of thyroid hormones reduced by colestipol and colestyramine

Oestrogens: requirements for thyroid hormones in hypothyroidism may be increased by oestrogens

Polystyrene Sulphonate Resins: absorption of levothyroxine (thyroxine) reduced by polystyrene sulphonate resins

Ulcer-healing Drugs: absorption of levothyroxine (thyroxine) reduced by cimetidine and sucralfate

**Tiagabine**

• Antidepressants: anticonvulsant effect of antiepileptics possibly antagonised by MAOIs and ●tricyclic-related antidepressants (convulsive threshold lowered); anticonvulsant effect of antiepileptics antagonised by ●SSRIs and ●tricyclics (convulsive threshold lowered); avoid concomitant use of antiepileptics with ●St John's wort

Antiepileptics: plasma concentration of tiagabine reduced by carbamazepine, phenytoin and primidone

• Antimalarials: possible increased risk of convulsions when antiepileptics given with chloroquine and hydroxychloroquine; anticonvulsant effect of antiepileptics antagonised by ●mefloquine

Barbiturates: plasma concentration of tiagabine reduced by phenobarbital

**Tiaprofenic Acid** *see* NSAIDs

**Tibolone**

Antibacterials: metabolism of tibolone accelerated by rifampicin (reduced plasma concentration)

Antiepileptics: metabolism of tibolone accelerated by carbamazepine and primidone (reduced plasma concentration); metabolism of tibolone accelerated by phenytoin

Barbiturates: metabolism of tibolone accelerated by barbiturates (reduced plasma concentration)

**Ticarcillin** *see* Penicillins

**Tigecycline**

Anticoagulants: tigecycline possibly enhances anticoagulant effect of coumarins

Oestrogens: antibacterials that do not induce liver enzymes possibly reduce contraceptive effect of oestrogens (risk probably small, see p. 445)

Vaccines: antibacterials inactivate oral typhoid vaccine–see p. 688

**Tiludronic Acid** *see* Bisphosphonates

**Timolol** *see* Beta-blockers

**Tinidazole**

Alcohol: possibility of disulfiram-like reaction when tinidazole given with alcohol

Oestrogens: antibacterials that do not induce liver enzymes possibly reduce contraceptive effect of oestrogens (risk probably small, see p. 445)

Vaccines: antibacterials inactivate oral typhoid vaccine–see p. 688

**Tinzaparin** *see* Heparins

**Tioguanine**

Antiepileptics: cytotoxics possibly reduce absorption of phenytoin

• Antipsychotics: avoid concomitant use of cytotoxics with ●clozapine (increased risk of agranulocytosis)

Cardiac Glycosides: cytotoxics reduce absorption of digoxin tablets

Cytotoxics: increased risk of hepatotoxicity when tioguanine given with busulfan

**Tiotropium** *see* Antimuscarinics

**Tipranavir**

Antacids: absorption of tipranavir reduced by antacids

• Antibacterials: tipranavir increases plasma concentration of ●clarithromycin (reduce dose of clarithromycin in renal impairment), also plasma concentration of tipranavir increased by clarithromycin; tipranavir increases plasma concentration of ●rifabutin (reduce dose of rifabutin); plasma concentration of tipranavir possibly reduced by ●rifampicin—avoid concomitant use; avoidance of concomitant tipranavir in severe renal and hepatic impairment advised by manufacturer of ●telithromycin

**Tipranavir** *(continued)*
  Anticoagulants: avoidance of tipranavir advised by manufacturer of rivaroxaban
- Antidepressants: plasma concentration of tipranavir possibly reduced by ●St John's wort—avoid concomitant use
  Antiepileptics: plasma concentration of tipranavir possibly reduced by carbamazepine
  Antifungals: plasma concentration of tipranavir increased by fluconazole
  Antimalarials: caution with tipranavir advised by manufacturer of artemether/lumefantrine
  Antimuscarinics: avoidance of tipranavir advised by manufacturer of darifenacin
- Antivirals: tipranavir reduces plasma concentration of ●abacavir, ●didanosine, ●fosamprenavir, ●lopinavir, ●saquinavir and ●zidovudine; plasma concentration of tipranavir increased by atazanavir (also plasma concentration of atazanavir reduced); tipranavir reduces plasma concentration of ●etravirine, also plasma concentration of tipranavir increased (avoid concomitant use)
- Beta-blockers: manufacturer of tipranavir advises avoid concomitant use with ●metoprolol for heart failure
- Lipid-regulating Drugs: possible increased risk of myopathy when tipranavir given with ●rosuvastatin—avoid concomitant use
- Ranolazine: tipranavir possibly increases plasma concentration of ●ranolazine—manufacturer of ranolazine advises avoid concomitant use
- Ulcer-healing Drugs: tipranavir reduces plasma concentration of ●esomeprazole and ●omeprazole
  Vitamins: increased risk of bleeding when tipranavir given with high doses of vitamin E

**Tirofiban**
  Iloprost: increased risk of bleeding when tirofiban given with iloprost

**Tizanidine** *see* Muscle Relaxants

**Tobacco**
  Cinacalcet: tobacco smoking increases cinacalcet metabolism (reduced plasma concentration)
  Cytotoxics: tobacco smoking reduces plasma concentration of erlotinib
  Theophylline: tobacco smoking increases theophylline metabolism (reduced plasma concentration)

**Tobramycin** *see* Aminoglycosides

**Tolazoline** *see* Alpha-blockers

**Tolbutamide** *see* Antidiabetics

**Tolcapone**
  Antidepressants: avoid concomitant use of tolcapone with MAOIs
  Memantine: effects of dopaminergics possibly enhanced by memantine
  Methyldopa: antiparkinsonian effect of dopaminergics antagonised by methyldopa

**Tolfenamic Acid** *see* NSAIDs

**Tolterodine** *see* Antimuscarinics

**Topiramate**
- Antidepressants: anticonvulsant effect of antiepileptics possibly antagonised by MAOIs and ●tricyclic-related antidepressants (convulsive threshold lowered); anticonvulsant effect of antiepileptics antagonised by ●SSRIs and ●tricyclics (convulsive threshold lowered); avoid concomitant use of antiepileptics with ●St John's wort
  Antidiabetics: topiramate possibly reduces plasma concentration of glibenclamide
- Antiepileptics: plasma concentration of topiramate often reduced by carbamazepine; topiramate increases plasma concentration of ●phenytoin (also plasma concentration of topiramate reduced)
- Antimalarials: possible increased risk of convulsions when antiepileptics given with chloroquine and hydroxychloroquine; anticonvulsant effect of antiepileptics antagonised by ●mefloquine
  Lithium: topiramate possibly affects plasma concentration of lithium

**Topiramate** *(continued)*
- Oestrogens: topiramate accelerates metabolism of ●oestrogens (reduced contraceptive effect—see p. 445)
- Progestogens: topiramate accelerates metabolism of ●progestogens (reduced contraceptive effect—see p. 445)

**Torasemide** *see* Diuretics

**Toremifene**
- Anticoagulants: toremifene possibly enhances anticoagulant effect of ●coumarins
  Antiepileptics: metabolism of toremifene possibly accelerated by carbamazepine (reduced plasma concentration); metabolism of toremifene possibly accelerated by phenytoin; metabolism of toremifene accelerated by primidone (reduced plasma concentration)
  Barbiturates: metabolism of toremifene possibly accelerated by barbiturates (reduced plasma concentration)
  Diuretics: increased risk of hypercalcaemia when toremifene given with thiazides and related diuretics
  Sugammadex: toremifene possibly reduces response to sugammadex

**Trabectedin**
  Antiepileptics: cytotoxics possibly reduce absorption of phenytoin
- Antipsychotics: avoid concomitant use of cytotoxics with ●clozapine (increased risk of agranulocytosis)
  Cardiac Glycosides: cytotoxics reduce absorption of digoxin tablets

**Tramadol** *see* Opioid Analgesics

**Trandolapril** *see* ACE Inhibitors

**Tranylcypromine** *see* MAOIs

**Trazodone** *see* Antidepressants, Tricyclic (related)

**Tretinoin** *see* Retinoids

**Triamcinolone** *see* Corticosteroids

**Triamterene** *see* Diuretics

**Triclofos** *see* Anxiolytics and Hypnotics

**Trientine**
  Iron: trientine reduces absorption of *oral* iron
  Zinc: trientine reduces absorption of zinc, also absorption of trientine reduced by zinc

**Trifluoperazine** *see* Antipsychotics

**Trihexyphenidyl (benzhexol)** *see* Antimuscarinics

**Trilostane**
  Diuretics: increased risk of hyperkalaemia when trilostane given with potassium-sparing diuretics and aldosterone antagonists

**Trimethoprim**
- Anti-arrhythmics: increased risk of ventricular arrhythmias when trimethoprim (as co-trimoxazole) given with ●amiodarone—avoid concomitant use of co-trimoxazole
  Antibacterials: plasma concentration of trimethoprim possibly reduced by rifampicin; plasma concentration of both drugs may increase when trimethoprim given with dapsone
  Anticoagulants: trimethoprim possibly enhances anticoagulant effect of coumarins
- Antidiabetics: trimethoprim possibly enhances hypoglycaemic effect of repaglinide—manufacturer advises avoid concomitant use; trimethoprim rarely enhances the effects of sulphonylureas
- Antiepileptics: trimethoprim increases plasma concentration of ●phenytoin (also increased antifolate effect)
- Antimalarials: increased antifolate effect when trimethoprim given with ●pyrimethamine
  Antivirals: trimethoprim (as co-trimoxazole) increases plasma concentration of lamivudine—avoid concomitant use of high-dose co-trimoxazole
- Azathioprine: increased risk of haematological toxicity when trimethoprim (also with co-trimoxazole) given with ●azathioprine
  Cardiac Glycosides: trimethoprim possibly increases plasma concentration of digoxin
- Ciclosporin: increased risk of nephrotoxicity when trimethoprim given with ●ciclosporin, also plasma

**Trimethoprim**
- Ciclosporin *(continued)*
  concentration of ciclosporin reduced by intravenous trimethoprim
- Cytotoxics: increased risk of haematological toxicity when trimethoprim (also with co-trimoxazole) given with ●mercaptopurine or ●methotrexate
  Diuretics: increased risk of hyperkalaemia when trimethoprim given with eplerenone
  Oestrogens: antibacterials that do not induce liver enzymes possibly reduce contraceptive effect of oestrogens (risk probably small, see p. 445)
  Vaccines: antibacterials inactivate oral typhoid vaccine–see p. 688

**Trimipramine** *see* Antidepressants, Tricyclic

**Tripotassium Dicitratobismuthate**
  Antibacterials: tripotassium dicitratobismuthate reduces absorption of tetracyclines

**Tropicamide** *see* Antimuscarinics

**Trospium** *see* Antimuscarinics

**Tryptophan**
- Antidepressants: possible increased serotonergic effects when tryptophan given with duloxetine; CNS excitation and confusion when tryptophan given with ●MAOIs (reduce dose of tryptophan); agitation and nausea may occur when tryptophan given with ●SSRIs
- Antimalarials: avoidance of antidepressants advised by manufacturer of ●artemether/lumefantrine
  Atomoxetine: possible increased risk of convulsions when antidepressants given with atomoxetine
- Sibutramine: increased risk of CNS toxicity when tryptophan given with ●sibutramine (manufacturer of sibutramine advises avoid concomitant use)

**Typhoid Vaccine (oral)** *see* Vaccines

**Typhoid Vaccine (parenteral)** *see* Vaccines

**Ubidecarenone**
  Anticoagulants: ubidecarenone may enhance or reduce anticoagulant effect of warfarin

**Ulcer-healing Drugs** *see* Histamine H₂-antagonists, Proton Pump Inhibitors, Sucralfate, and Tripotassium Dicitratobismuthate

**Ursodeoxycholic Acid**
  Antacids: absorption of bile acids possibly reduced by antacids
- Ciclosporin: ursodeoxycholic acid increases absorption of ●ciclosporin
  Lipid-regulating Drugs: absorption of bile acids possibly reduced by colestipol and colestyramine
  Oestrogens: elimination of cholesterol in bile increased when bile acids given with oestrogens

**Ustekinumab**
- Vaccines: avoid concomitant use of ustekinumab with live ●vaccines (see p. 669)

**Vaccines**
  Note  For a general warning on live vaccines and high doses of corticosteroids or other immunosuppressive drugs, see p. 669 ; for advice on live vaccines and immunoglobulins, see under Normal Immunoglobulin, p. 690
- Abatacept: avoid concomitant use of live vaccines with ●abatacept (see p. 669)
- Adalimumab: avoid concomitant use of live vaccines with ●adalimumab (see p. 669)
- Anakinra: avoid concomitant use of live vaccines with ●anakinra (see p. 669)
  Antibacterials: oral typhoid vaccine inactivated by antibacterials–see p. 688
  Anticoagulants: influenza vaccine possibly enhances anticoagulant effect of warfarin
  Antiepileptics: influenza vaccine enhances effects of phenytoin
  Antimalarials: oral typhoid vaccine inactivated by antimalarials–see p. 688
- Corticosteroids: immune response to vaccines impaired by high doses of ●corticosteroids, avoid concomitant use with live vaccines (see p. 669)
- Etanercept: avoid concomitant use of live vaccines with ●etanercept (see p. 669)

**Vaccines** *(continued)*
- Infliximab: avoid concomitant use of live vaccines with ●infliximab (see p. 669)
  Interferons: avoidance of vaccines advised by manufacturer of interferon gamma
- Leflunomide: avoid concomitant use of live vaccines with ●leflunomide (see p. 669)
  Theophylline: influenza vaccine possibly increases plasma concentration of theophylline
- Ustekinumab: avoid concomitant use of live vaccines with ●ustekinumab (see p. 669)

**Valaciclovir** *see* Aciclovir

**Valganciclovir** *see* Ganciclovir

**Valproate**
  Analgesics: effects of valproate enhanced by aspirin
  Antibacterials: plasma concentration of valproate possibly reduced by doripenem and ertapenem; plasma concentration of valproate reduced by imipenem with cilastatin and meropenem; metabolism of valproate possibly inhibited by erythromycin (increased plasma concentration)
  Anticoagulants: valproate possibly enhances anticoagulant effect of coumarins
- Antidepressants: anticonvulsant effect of antiepileptics possibly antagonised by MAOIs and ●tricyclic-related antidepressants (convulsive threshold lowered); anticonvulsant effect of antiepileptics antagonised by ●SSRIs and ●tricyclics (convulsive threshold lowered); avoid concomitant use of antiepileptics with ●St John's wort
- Antiepileptics: plasma concentration of valproate reduced by carbamazepine, also plasma concentration of active metabolite of carbamazepine increased; valproate possibly increases plasma concentration of ethosuximide; valproate increases plasma concentration of lamotrigine; valproate sometimes reduces plasma concentration of an active metabolite of oxcarbazepine; valproate increases or possibly decreases plasma concentration of phenytoin, also plasma concentration of valproate reduced; valproate possibly increases plasma concentration of ●primidone (plasma concentration of active metabolite of primidone increased), also plasma concentration of valproate reduced; valproate possibly increases plasma concentration of rufinamide (reduce dose of rufinamide)
- Antimalarials: possible increased risk of convulsions when antiepileptics given with chloroquine and hydroxychloroquine; anticonvulsant effect of antiepileptics antagonised by ●mefloquine
- Antipsychotics: anticonvulsant effect of valproate antagonised by ●antipsychotics (convulsive threshold lowered); increased risk of neutropenia when valproate given with ●olanzapine
  Antivirals: valproate possibly increases plasma concentration of zidovudine (increased risk of toxicity)
  Anxiolytics and Hypnotics: plasma concentration of valproate possibly increased by clobazam; increased risk of side-effects when valproate given with clonazepam; valproate possibly increases plasma concentration of diazepam and lorazepam
  Barbiturates: valproate increases plasma concentration of phenobarbital (also plasma concentration of valproate reduced)
  Bupropion: valproate inhibits the metabolism of bupropion
  Cytotoxics: valproate increases plasma concentration of temozolomide
  Lipid-regulating Drugs: absorption of valproate possibly reduced by colestyramine
  Sodium Benzoate: valproate possibly reduces effects of sodium benzoate
  Sodium Phenylbutyrate: valproate possibly reduces effects of sodium phenylbutyrate
- Ulcer-healing Drugs: metabolism of valproate inhibited by ●cimetidine (increased plasma concentration)

**Valsartan** *see* Angiotensin-II Receptor Antagonists

## Vancomycin

Anaesthetics, General: hypersensitivity-like reactions can occur when intravenous vancomycin given with general anaesthetics

Antibacterials: increased risk of nephrotoxicity and ototoxicity when vancomycin given with aminoglycosides, capreomycin or colistin; increased risk of nephrotoxicity when vancomycin given with polymyxins

Antifungals: possible increased risk of nephrotoxicity when vancomycin given with amphotericin

- Ciclosporin: increased risk of nephrotoxicity when vancomycin given with •ciclosporin

Cytotoxics: increased risk of nephrotoxicity and possibly of ototoxicity when vancomycin given with cisplatin

- Diuretics: increased risk of ototoxicity when vancomycin given with •loop diuretics

Lipid-regulating Drugs: effects of oral vancomycin antagonised by colestyramine

- Muscle Relaxants: vancomycin enhances effects of •suxamethonium

Oestrogens: antibacterials that do not induce liver enzymes possibly reduce contraceptive effect of oestrogens (risk probably small, see p. 445)

Tacrolimus: possible increased risk of nephrotoxicity when vancomycin given with tacrolimus

Vaccines: antibacterials inactivate oral typhoid vaccine–see p. 688

## Vardenafil

- Alpha-blockers: enhanced hypotensive effect when vardenafil given with •alpha-blockers (excludes tamsulosin)—separate doses by 6 hours—see also p. 463

Antibacterials: plasma concentration of vardenafil increased by erythromycin (reduce dose of vardenafil)

- Antifungals: plasma concentration of vardenafil increased by •ketoconazole—avoid concomitant use; plasma concentration of vardenafil possibly increased by •itraconazole—avoid concomitant use

- Antivirals: plasma concentration of vardenafil possibly increased by fosamprenavir; plasma concentration of vardenafil increased by •indinavir—avoid concomitant use; plasma concentration of vardenafil possibly increased by •ritonavir—avoid concomitant use; plasma concentration of vardenafil possibly increased by saquinavir—reduce initial dose of vardenafil

Calcium-channel Blockers: enhanced hypotensive effect when vardenafil given with nifedipine

- Grapefruit Juice: plasma concentration of vardenafil possibly increased by •grapefruit juice—avoid concomitant use

- Nicorandil: possible increased hypotensive effect when vardenafil given with •nicorandil—avoid concomitant use

- Nitrates: possible increased hypotensive effect when vardenafil given with •nitrates—avoid concomitant use

## Vasodilator Antihypertensives

ACE Inhibitors: enhanced hypotensive effect when hydralazine, minoxidil or sodium nitroprusside given with ACE inhibitors

Adrenergic Neurone Blockers: enhanced hypotensive effect when hydralazine, minoxidil or sodium nitroprusside given with adrenergic neurone blockers

Alcohol: enhanced hypotensive effect when hydralazine, minoxidil or sodium nitroprusside given with alcohol

Aldesleukin: enhanced hypotensive effect when hydralazine, minoxidil or sodium nitroprusside given with aldesleukin

Alpha-blockers: enhanced hypotensive effect when hydralazine, minoxidil or sodium nitroprusside given with alpha-blockers

Anaesthetics, General: enhanced hypotensive effect when hydralazine, minoxidil or sodium nitroprusside given with general anaesthetics

## Vasodilator Antihypertensives *(continued)*

Analgesics: hypotensive effect of hydralazine, minoxidil and sodium nitroprusside antagonised by NSAIDs

Angiotensin-II Receptor Antagonists: enhanced hypotensive effect when hydralazine, minoxidil or sodium nitroprusside given with angiotensin-II receptor antagonists

Antidepressants: enhanced hypotensive effect when hydralazine, minoxidil or sodium nitroprusside given with MAOIs; enhanced hypotensive effect when hydralazine or sodium nitroprusside given with tricyclic-related antidepressants

Antipsychotics: enhanced hypotensive effect when hydralazine, minoxidil or sodium nitroprusside given with phenothiazines

Anxiolytics and Hypnotics: enhanced hypotensive effect when hydralazine, minoxidil or sodium nitroprusside given with anxiolytics and hypnotics

Beta-blockers: enhanced hypotensive effect when hydralazine, minoxidil or sodium nitroprusside given with beta-blockers

Calcium-channel Blockers: enhanced hypotensive effect when hydralazine, minoxidil or sodium nitroprusside given with calcium-channel blockers

Clonidine: enhanced hypotensive effect when hydralazine, minoxidil or sodium nitroprusside given with clonidine

Corticosteroids: hypotensive effect of hydralazine, minoxidil and sodium nitroprusside antagonised by corticosteroids

Diazoxide: enhanced hypotensive effect when hydralazine, minoxidil or sodium nitroprusside given with diazoxide

Diuretics: enhanced hypotensive effect when hydralazine, minoxidil or sodium nitroprusside given with diuretics

Dopaminergics: enhanced hypotensive effect when hydralazine, minoxidil or sodium nitroprusside given with levodopa

Methyldopa: enhanced hypotensive effect when hydralazine, minoxidil or sodium nitroprusside given with methyldopa

Moxisylyte (thymoxamine): enhanced hypotensive effect when hydralazine, minoxidil or sodium nitroprusside given with moxisylyte

Moxonidine: enhanced hypotensive effect when hydralazine, minoxidil or sodium nitroprusside given with moxonidine

Muscle Relaxants: enhanced hypotensive effect when hydralazine, minoxidil or sodium nitroprusside given with baclofen; enhanced hypotensive effect when hydralazine, minoxidil or sodium nitroprusside given with tizanidine

Nicorandil: possible enhanced hypotensive effect when hydralazine, minoxidil or sodium nitroprusside given with nicorandil

Nitrates: enhanced hypotensive effect when hydralazine, minoxidil or sodium nitroprusside given with nitrates

Oestrogens: hypotensive effect of hydralazine, minoxidil and sodium nitroprusside antagonised by oestrogens

Prostaglandins: enhanced hypotensive effect when hydralazine, minoxidil or sodium nitroprusside given with alprostadil

Vasodilator Antihypertensives: enhanced hypotensive effect when hydralazine given with minoxidil or sodium nitroprusside; enhanced hypotensive effect when minoxidil given with sodium nitroprusside

**Vecuronium** *see* Muscle Relaxants

## Venlafaxine

- Analgesics: increased risk of bleeding when venlafaxine given with •NSAIDs or •aspirin

- Anticoagulants: venlafaxine possibly enhances anticoagulant effect of •warfarin

- Antidepressants: possible increased serotonergic effects when venlafaxine given with duloxetine or mirtazapine; enhanced CNS effects and toxicity when

Venlafaxine
- Antidepressants *(continued)*
venlafaxine given with ●MAOIs (venlafaxine
should not be started until 2 weeks after stopping
MAOIs, avoid MAOIs for 1 week after stopping
venlafaxine); after stopping SSRI-related antidepressants do not start ●moclobemide for at
least 1 week
- Antimalarials: avoidance of antidepressants advised by
manufacturer of ●artemether/lumefantrine
- Antipsychotics: venlafaxine increases plasma concentration of ●clozapine and haloperidol
Atomoxetine: possible increased risk of convulsions
when antidepressants given with atomoxetine
- Dopaminergics: caution with venlafaxine advised by
manufacturer of entacapone; increased risk of
hypertension and CNS excitation when venlafaxine
given with ●selegiline (selegiline should not be
started until 1 week after stopping venlafaxine, avoid
venlafaxine for 2 weeks after stopping selegiline)
Lithium: possible increased serotonergic effects when
venlafaxine given with lithium
- Sibutramine: increased risk of CNS toxicity when
SSRI-related antidepressants given with ●sibutramine
(manufacturer of sibutramine advises avoid concomitant use)

Verapamil *see* Calcium-channel Blockers

Vigabatrin
- Antidepressants: anticonvulsant effect of antiepileptics
possibly antagonised by MAOIs and ●tricyclic-related
antidepressants (convulsive threshold lowered); anticonvulsant effect of antiepileptics antagonised by
●SSRIs and ●tricyclics (convulsive threshold
lowered); avoid concomitant use of antiepileptics
with ●St John's wort
Antiepileptics: vigabatrin reduces plasma concentration of phenytoin; vigabatrin possibly reduces plasma
concentration of primidone
- Antimalarials: possible increased risk of convulsions
when antiepileptics given with chloroquine and
hydroxychloroquine; anticonvulsant effect of antiepileptics antagonised by ●mefloquine
Barbiturates: vigabatrin possibly reduces plasma concentration of phenobarbital

Vildagliptin *see* Antidiabetics

Vinblastine
- Antibacterials: toxicity of vinblastine increased by
●erythromycin—avoid concomitant use
Antiepileptics: cytotoxics possibly reduce absorption
of phenytoin
- Antifungals: metabolism of vinblastine possibly inhibited by ●posaconazole (increased risk of neurotoxicity)
- Antipsychotics: avoid concomitant use of cytotoxics
with ●clozapine (increased risk of agranulocytosis)
Cardiac Glycosides: cytotoxics reduce absorption of
digoxin tablets

Vincristine
Antiepileptics: cytotoxics possibly reduce absorption
of phenytoin
- Antifungals: metabolism of vincristine possibly inhibited by ●itraconazole and ●posaconazole (increased
risk of neurotoxicity)
- Antipsychotics: avoid concomitant use of cytotoxics
with ●clozapine (increased risk of agranulocytosis)
Calcium-channel Blockers: metabolism of vincristine
possibly inhibited by nifedipine
Cardiac Glycosides: cytotoxics reduce absorption of
digoxin tablets

Vinorelbine
Antiepileptics: cytotoxics possibly reduce absorption
of phenytoin
- Antipsychotics: avoid concomitant use of cytotoxics
with ●clozapine (increased risk of agranulocytosis)
Cardiac Glycosides: cytotoxics reduce absorption of
digoxin tablets

Vitamin A *see* Vitamins
Vitamin D *see* Vitamins

Vitamin E *see* Vitamins
Vitamin K (Phytomenadione) *see* Vitamins
Vitamins
Antibacterials: absorption of vitamin A possibly
reduced by neomycin
- Anticoagulants: vitamin K antagonises anticoagulant
effect of ●coumarins and ●phenindione
Antiepileptics: vitamin D requirements possibly
increased when given with carbamazepine,
phenytoin or primidone
Antifungals: plasma concentration of paricalcitol pos-
sibly increased by ketoconazole
Antivirals: increased risk of bleeding when high doses
of vitamin E given with tipranavir
Barbiturates: vitamin D requirements possibly
increased when given with barbiturates
Diuretics: increased risk of hypercalcaemia when
vitamin D given with thiazides and related diuretics
Dopaminergics: pyridoxine reduces effects of levodopa when given without dopa-decarboxylase inhibitor
Retinoids: risk of hypervitaminosis A when vitamin A
given with retinoids
Selenium: ascorbic acid possibly reduces absorption of
selenium (give at least 4 hours apart)

Voriconazole *see* Antifungals, Triazole
Warfarin *see* Coumarins
Xipamide *see* Diuretics
Xylometazoline *see* Sympathomimetics
Zafirlukast *see* Leukotriene Receptor Antagonists
Zaleplon *see* Anxiolytics and Hypnotics
Zidovudine
Note Increased risk of toxicity with nephrotoxic and mye-
losuppressive drugs—for further details consult product literature
Analgesics: increased risk of haematological toxicity
when zidovudine given with NSAIDs; plasma concentration of zidovudine possibly increased by
methadone
Antibacterials: absorption of zidovudine reduced by
clarithromycin tablets (give at least 2 hours apart);
manufacturer of zidovudine advises avoid concomitant use with rifampicin
Antiepileptics: zidovudine increases or decreases
plasma concentration of phenytoin; plasma concentration of zidovudine possibly increased by valproate
(increased risk of toxicity)
- Antifungals: plasma concentration of zidovudine
increased by ●fluconazole (increased risk of toxicity)
Antimalarials: increased antifolate effect when zidovudine given with pyrimethamine
- Antivirals: profound myelosuppression when zidovudine given with ●ganciclovir (if possible avoid
concomitant administration, particularly during initial
ganciclovir therapy); increased risk of anaemia when
zidovudine given with ●ribavirin—avoid concomitant
use; zidovudine possibly inhibits effects of ●stavudine
(manufacturers advise avoid concomitant use);
plasma concentration of zidovudine reduced by
●tipranavir
Atovaquone: metabolism of zidovudine possibly
inhibited by atovaquone (increased plasma concentration)
- Probenecid: excretion of zidovudine reduced by
●probenecid (increased plasma concentration and
risk of toxicity)
Zinc
Antibacterials: zinc reduces absorption of ciprofloxacin, levofloxacin, moxifloxacin, norfloxacin and
ofloxacin; zinc reduces absorption of tetracyclines,
also absorption of zinc reduced by tetracyclines
Calcium Salts: absorption of zinc reduced by calcium
salts
Iron: absorption of zinc reduced by *oral* iron, also
absorption of *oral* iron reduced by zinc
Penicillamine: absorption of zinc reduced by penicillamine, also absorption of penicillamine reduced by
zinc

**Zinc** *(continued)*

  Trientine: absorption of zinc reduced by trientine, also absorption of trientine reduced by zinc

**Zoledronic Acid** *see* Bisphosphonates

**Zolmitriptan** *see* 5HT₁ Agonists

**Zolpidem** *see* Anxiolytics and Hypnotics

**Zonisamide**

- Antidepressants: anticonvulsant effect of antiepileptics possibly antagonised by MAOIs and ●tricyclic-related antidepressants (convulsive threshold lowered); anticonvulsant effect of antiepileptics antagonised by ●SSRIs and ●tricyclics (convulsive threshold lowered); avoid concomitant use of antiepileptics with ●St John's wort

  Antiepileptics: plasma concentration of zonisamide reduced by carbamazepine and phenytoin

- Antimalarials: possible increased risk of convulsions when antiepileptics given with chloroquine and hydroxychloroquine; anticonvulsant effect of antiepileptics antagonised by ●mefloquine

  Barbiturates: plasma concentration of zonisamide reduced by phenobarbital

**Zopiclone** *see* Anxiolytics and Hypnotics

**Zotepine** *see* Antipsychotics

**Zuclopenthixol** *see* Antipsychotics

# A2 Liver disease

Liver disease may alter the response to drugs in several ways as indicated below, and drug prescribing should be kept to a minimum in all patients with severe liver disease. The main problems occur in patients with jaundice, ascites, or evidence of encephalopathy.

**Impaired drug metabolism** Metabolism by the liver is the main route of elimination for many drugs, but hepatic reserve is large and liver disease has to be severe before important changes in drug metabolism occur. Routine liver-function tests are a poor guide to the capacity of the liver to metabolise drugs, and in the individual patient it is not possible to predict the extent to which the metabolism of a particular drug may be impaired.

A few drugs, e.g. rifampicin and fusidic acid, are excreted in the bile unchanged and can accumulate in patients with intrahepatic or extrahepatic obstructive jaundice.

**Hypoproteinaemia** The hypoalbuminaemia in severe liver disease is associated with reduced protein binding and increased toxicity of some highly protein-bound drugs such as phenytoin and prednisolone.

**Reduced clotting** Reduced hepatic synthesis of blood-clotting factors, indicated by a prolonged prothrombin time, increases the sensitivity to oral anticoagulants such as warfarin and phenindione.

**Hepatic encephalopathy** In severe liver disease many drugs can further impair cerebral function and may precipitate hepatic encephalopathy. These include all sedative drugs, opioid analgesics, those diuretics that produce hypokalaemia, and drugs that cause constipation.

**Fluid overload** Oedema and ascites in chronic liver disease can be exacerbated by drugs that give rise to fluid retention, e.g. NSAIDs and corticosteroids.

**Hepatotoxic drugs** Hepatotoxicity is either dose-related or unpredictable (idiosyncratic). Drugs that cause dose-related toxicity may do so at lower doses in the presence of hepatic impairment than in individuals with normal liver function, and some drugs that produce reactions of the idiosyncratic kind do so more frequently in patients with liver disease. These drugs should be avoided or used very carefully in patients with liver disease.

## Table of drugs to be avoided or used with caution in liver disease

The list of drugs given below is not comprehensive and is based on current information concerning the use of prescribed drugs in therapeutic dosage. Products introduced or amended since publication of BNF No. 57 (March 2009) are underlined.

| Drug | Comment |
|---|---|
| Abacavir | Avoid in moderate hepatic impairment unless essential; avoid in severe hepatic impairment |
| Abciximab | Avoid in severe liver disease—increased risk of bleeding |
| Acamprosate | Avoid in severe liver disease |
| Acarbose | Avoid |
| ACE inhibitors | Use of prodrugs such as cilazapril, enalapril, fosinopril, imidapril, moexipril, perindopril, quinapril, ramipril, and trandolapril requires close monitoring in patients with impaired liver function |
| Aceclofenac | see NSAIDs |
| Acemetacin | see NSAIDs |
| Acenocoumarol (nicoumalone) | see Anticoagulants, Oral |
| Acitretin | Avoid—further impairment of liver function may occur |
| Agomelatine | Avoid |
| Alfentanil | see Opioid Analgesics |
| Alfuzosin | Reduce dose in mild to moderate liver disease; avoid if severe |
| Alimemazine (trimeprazine) | Avoid—may precipitate coma in severe liver disease; hepatotoxic |
| Alitretinoin | Manufacturer advises avoid—no information available |
| Allopurinol | Reduce dose |
| Almotriptan | Manufacturer advises caution in mild to moderate liver disease; avoid in severe liver disease |
| Alprazolam | see Anxiolytics and Hypnotics |
| Alteplase | see Fibrinolytics |
| Ambrisentan | Avoid in severe hepatic impairment |
| Amfebutamone | see Bupropion |
| Aminophylline | see Theophylline |
| Amitriptyline | see Antidepressants, Tricyclic (and related) |
| Amlodipine | Half-life prolonged—may need dose reduction |
| Amsacrine | Reduce dose |
| Anabolic steroids | Preferably avoid—dose-related toxicity |
| Anagrelide | Manufacturer advises caution in mild hepatic impairment; avoid in moderate to severe impairment |
| Analgesics | see Aspirin, NSAIDs, Opioid Analgesics and Paracetamol |
| Anastrozole | Avoid in moderate to severe liver disease |
| Androgens | Preferably avoid—dose-related toxicity with some, and produce fluid retention |

| Drug | Comment |
|------|---------|
| Antacids | In patients with fluid retention, avoid those containing large amounts of sodium |
| | Avoid those causing constipation—can precipitate coma |
| Anticoagulants, oral | Avoid in severe liver disease, especially if prothrombin time already prolonged; *see also* Rivaroxaban |
| Antidepressants, MAOI | May cause idiosyncratic hepatotoxicity; see also Moclobemide |
| Antidepressants, SSRI | Reduce dose or avoid; *see also* Escitalopram |
| Antidepressants, tricyclic (and related) | Tricyclics preferable to MAOIs but sedative effects increased (avoid in severe liver disease) |
| Antihistamines | *see* individual entries |
| Antipsychotics | All can precipitate coma; phenothiazines are hepatotoxic; *see also* Aripiprazole, Clozapine, Droperidol, Olanzapine, Paliperidone, Quetiapine, Risperidone, and Sertindole |
| Anxiolytics and hypnotics | All can precipitate coma; small dose of oxazepam or temazepam probably safest; reduce oral dose of clomethiazole; reduce dose of zaleplon to 5 mg (avoid if severe); reduce dose of zolpidem to 5 mg (avoid if severe); reduce dose of zopiclone (avoid if severe); *see also* Buspirone, Chloral Hydrate, Clonazepam, Melatonin, and Sodium Oxybate |
| Apomorphine | Manufacturer of *APO-go*® advises avoid |
| Aprepitant | *see* Neurokinin Receptor Antagonists |
| Aripiprazole | Manufacturer advises use with caution in severe impairment |
| Arsenic trioxide | Manufacturer advises caution—limited information available |
| Artemether [ingredient] | *see Riamet*® |
| Aspirin | Avoid in severe hepatic impairment—increased risk of gastro-intestinal bleeding |
| Atazanavir | Manufacturer advises caution in mild hepatic impairment; avoid in moderate to severe hepatic impairment |
| Atomoxetine | Halve dose in moderate liver disease; quarter dose in severe liver disease |
| Atorvastatin | *see* Statins |
| Atosiban | No information available |
| Atovaquone | Manufacturer advises caution—monitor more closely |
| Auranofin | Caution in mild to moderate liver disease; avoid in severe liver disease |
| Azacitidine | Caution in severe hepatic impairment |
| Azapropazone | *see* NSAIDs |
| Azathioprine | May need dose reduction |

| Drug | Comment |
|------|---------|
| Azithromycin | Manufacturer advises avoid in severe liver disease—no information available |
| Bambuterol | Avoid in severe liver disease |
| Beclometasone dipropionate | Manufacturer advises avoid tablets in severe hepatic impairment—no information available |
| Bemiparin | Manufacturer advises avoid in severe liver disease |
| Bendrofluazide | *see* Thiazides and Related Diuretics |
| Bendroflumethiazide (bendrofluazide) | *see* Thiazides and Related Diuretics |
| Benperidol | *see* Antipsychotics |
| Benzthiazide | *see* Thiazides and Related Diuretics |
| Betamethasone | *see* Corticosteroids |
| Bexarotene | Avoid |
| Bezafibrate | Avoid in severe liver disease |
| Bicalutamide | Increased accumulation possible in moderate to severe hepatic impairment |
| Bisoprolol | Max. 10 mg daily in severe liver impairment |
| Bortezomib | Manufacturer advises caution in mild to moderate hepatic impairment—consider dose reduction; avoid in severe hepatic impairment |
| Bosentan | Avoid in moderate and severe hepatic impairment |
| Bromocriptine | Dose reduction may be necessary |
| Buclizine | Sedation inappropriate in severe liver disease—avoid |
| Budesonide | Plasma-budesonide concentration may increase on oral administration |
| Bumetanide | *see* Loop Diuretics |
| Bupivacaine | Manufacturer advises caution in severe hepatic impairment |
| Buprenorphine | *see* Opioid Analgesics |
| Bupropion | Manufacturer recommends 150 mg daily; avoid in severe hepatic cirrhosis |
| Buspirone | Reduce dose in mild to moderate liver disease; avoid in severe liver disease |
| Busulfan | Manufacturer advises monitor liver function—no information available |
| Cabergoline | Reduce dose in severe hepatic impairment |
| Calcitriol | Manufacturer of topical calcitriol advises avoid—no information available |
| Candesartan | For hypertension, initially 2 mg once daily in mild or moderate hepatic impairment (no initial dose adjustment necessary in heart failure); avoid in severe hepatic impairment |
| Capecitabine | Manufacturer advises avoid in severe hepatic impairment |
| Carbamazepine | Metabolism impaired in advanced liver disease |
| Carbetocin | Manufacturer advises avoid |

| Drug | Comment |
|---|---|
| Carbimazole | Manufacturers advise caution in mild to moderate hepatic impairment; avoid in severe hepatic impairment |
| Carboprost | Manufacturer advises avoid |
| Carvedilol | Avoid |
| Caspofungin | 70 mg on first day then 35 mg once daily in moderate hepatic impairment; no information available for severe hepatic impairment |
| Ceftriaxone | Reduce dose and monitor plasma concentration if both hepatic and severe renal impairment |
| Celecoxib | see NSAIDs |
| Cetrorelix | Manufacturer advises avoid in moderate or severe liver impairment |
| Chloral hydrate | Reduce dose in mild to moderate hepatic impairment; avoid in severe impairment; see also Anxiolytics and Hypnotics |
| Chlorambucil | Manufacturer advises consider dose reduction in severe hepatic impairment—limited information available |
| Chloramphenicol | Avoid if possible—increased risk of bone-marrow depression; reduce dose and monitor plasma-chloramphenicol concentration |
| Chlordiazepoxide | see Anxiolytics and Hypnotics |
| Chloroquine | Use with caution in moderate to severe hepatic impairment |
| Chlorphenamine (chlorpheniramine) | Sedation inappropriate in severe liver disease—avoid |
| Chlorpheniramine | see Chlorphenamine |
| Chlorpromazine | see Antipsychotics |
| Chlorpropamide | see Sulphonylureas |
| Chlortalidone | see Thiazides and Related Diuretics |
| Ciclosporin | May need dose adjustment |
| Cilazapril | see ACE Inhibitors |
| Cilostazol | Avoid in moderate or severe liver disease |
| Cimetidine | Increased risk of confusion; reduce dose |
| Cinacalcet | Manufacturer advises caution in moderate to severe hepatic impairment—monitor closely especially when increasing dose |
| Cinnarizine | Sedation inappropriate in severe liver disease—avoid |
| Ciprofibrate | Avoid in severe liver disease |
| Citalopram | Use doses at lower end of range |
| Cladribine | Regular monitoring recommended |
| Clarithromycin | Hepatic dysfunction including jaundice reported |
| Clavulanic acid [ingredient] | see Co-amoxiclav, below and Timentin®, p. 814 |
| Clemastine | Sedation inappropriate in severe liver disease—avoid |
| Clobazam | see Anxiolytics and Hypnotics |

| Drug | Comment |
|---|---|
| Clofarabine | No information available—manufacturer advises caution in mild to moderate hepatic impairment; avoid in severe hepatic impairment |
| Clomethiazole | see Anxiolytics and Hypnotics |
| Clomifene | Avoid in severe liver disease |
| Clomipramine | see Antidepressants, Tricyclic (and related) |
| Clonazepam | Reduce dose in mild to moderate impairment; avoid in severe liver impairment; see also Anxiolytics and Hypnotics |
| Clopamide | see Thiazides and Related Diuretics |
| Clopidogrel | Manufacturer advises caution (risk of bleeding); avoid in severe hepatic impairment |
| Clozapine | Monitor hepatic function regularly; avoid in symptomatic or progressive liver disease or hepatic failure |
| Co-amoxiclav | Monitor liver function in liver disease. Cholestatic jaundice, see p. 300 |
| Codeine | see Opioid Analgesics |
| Colchicine | Caution |
| Colesevelam | Manufacturer advises caution |
| Contraceptives, oral | Avoid in active liver disease and if history of pruritus or cholestasis during pregnancy |
| Corticosteroids | For oral and parental administration, plasma-drug concentration may increase, use with caution and monitor closely; see also Beclometasone Dipropionate, Budesonide and Cortisone |
| Cortisone | Use with caution; hepatic conversion to active metabolite hydrocortisone may be affected |
| Co-trimoxazole | Manufacturer advises avoid in severe liver disease |
| Cyclizine | Sedation inappropriate in severe liver disease—avoid |
| Cyclopenthiazide | see Thiazides and Related Diuretics |
| Cyclophosphamide | Reduce dose |
| Cyclosporin | see Ciclosporin |
| Cyproheptadine | Sedation inappropriate in severe liver disease—avoid |
| Cyproterone acetate | Dose-related toxicity; see also side-effects, p. 509 |
| Cytarabine | Reduce dose |
| Dabigatran etexilate | see Anticoagulants, Oral |
| Dacarbazine | Dose reduction may be required in mild to moderate liver disease; avoid if severe |
| Dalfopristin [ingredient] | see Synercid® |
| Dalteparin | see Heparin |
| Danaparoid | Use with caution in moderate hepatic impairment (increased risk of bleeding); avoid in severe hepatic impairment unless patient has heparin-induced thrombocytopenia and no alternative |

| Drug | Comment |
|------|---------|
| Dantrolene | Avoid oral use—may cause severe liver damage; injection may be used in emergency for malignant hyperthermia |
| Daptomycin | Manufacturer advises caution in severe hepatic impairment—no information available |
| Darbepoetin | Manufacturer advises caution |
| Darifenacin | Max. 7.5 mg daily in moderate hepatic impairment; avoid in severe hepatic impairment |
| Darunavir | Manufacturer advises caution in mild to moderate hepatic impairment; avoid in severe hepatic impairment—no information available |
| Dasatinib | Manufacturer advises caution in moderate to severe hepatic impairment—no information available |
| Daunorubicin | Reduce dose |
| Deferasirox | Manufacturer advises caution—no information available; avoid in severe hepatic impairment |
| Deferiprone | Manufacturer advises monitor liver function—interrupt treatment if persistent elevation in serum alanine aminotransferase |
| Deflazacort | see Corticosteroids |
| Degarelix | Manufacturer advises caution in severe hepatic impairment—no information available |
| Demeclocycline | see Tetracyclines |
| Desogestrel | Avoid; see also Contraceptives, Oral |
| Dexamethasone | see Corticosteroids |
| Dexibuprofen | see NSAIDs |
| Dexketoprofen | see NSAIDs |
| Dexrazoxane | Monitor liver function in patients with liver disease |
| Dextromethorphan | see Opioid Analgesics |
| Diamorphine | see Opioid Analgesics |
| Diazepam | see Anxiolytics and Hypnotics |
| Diclofenac | see NSAIDs |
| Didanosine | Insufficient information but monitor for toxicity |
| Diethylstilbestrol | Avoid; see also Contraceptives, Oral |
| Dihydrocodeine | see Opioid Analgesics |
| Diltiazem | Reduce dose |
| Dinoprostone | Manufacturers advise avoid |
| Diphenoxylate | see Opioid Analgesics |
| Dipipanone | see Opioid Analgesics |
| Disodium pamidronate | Manufacturer advises caution in severe hepatic impairment—no information available |
| Disopyramide | Half-life prolonged—may need dose reduction |
| Docetaxel | Monitor liver function—reduce dose according to liver enzymes; avoid in severe hepatic impairment |
| Domperidone | Avoid |

| Drug | Comment |
|------|---------|
| Donepezil | Manufacturer advises caution in mild to moderate hepatic impairment |
| Dosulepin (dothiepin) | see Antidepressants, Tricyclic (and related) |
| Dothiepin | see Antidepressants, Tricyclic (and related) |
| Doxazosin | No information—manufacturer advises caution |
| Doxepin | see Antidepressants, Tricyclic (and related) |
| Doxorubicin | Reduce dose according to bilirubin concentration |
| Doxycycline | see Tetracyclines |
| Droperidol | In postoperative nausea and vomiting, max. 625 micrograms repeated every 6 hours as required; for nausea and vomiting caused by opioid analgesics in postoperative patient-controlled analgesia, reduce dose |
| Drotrecogin alfa (activated) | Avoid in chronic severe liver disease |
| Duloxetine | Manufacturer advises avoid |
| Dutasteride | Manufacturer advises avoid in severe liver impairment—no information available |
| Dydrogesterone | Avoid; see also Contraceptives, Oral |
| Efavirenz | In mild to moderate liver disease, monitor for dose related side-effects (e.g. CNS effects) and monitor liver function; avoid in severe hepatic impairment |
| Eletriptan | Manufacturer advises avoid in severe hepatic impairment |
| Enalapril | see ACE Inhibitors |
| Enfuvirtide | Manufacturer advises caution—no information available |
| Enoxaparin | see Heparin |
| Enoximone | Dose reduction may be required |
| Entacapone | Avoid |
| Epirubicin | Reduce dose according to bilirubin concentration |
| Eplerenone | Avoid in severe liver disease |
| Epoetin | Manufacturers advise caution in chronic hepatic failure |
| Eprosartan | Halve initial dose in mild or moderate liver disease; avoid if severe |
| Eptifibatide | Avoid in severe liver disease—increased risk of bleeding |
| Erdosteine | Manufacturer advises max. 300 mg daily in mild to moderate hepatic impairment; avoid in severe hepatic impairment |
| Ergometrine | Avoid in severe liver disease |
| Ergotamine | Avoid in severe liver disease—risk of toxicity increased |
| Erlotinib | Manufacturer advises caution in mild to moderate impairment; avoid in severe impairment |
| Erythromycin | May cause idiosyncratic hepatotoxicity |

Appendix 2: Liver disease

| Drug | Comment |
|------|---------|
| Escitalopram | Initial dose 5 mg daily in mild to moderate hepatic impairment (for 2 weeks), increased to 10 mg daily according to response; manufacturer advises caution in severe hepatic impairment |
| Esomeprazole | In severe liver disease dose should not exceed 20 mg daily |
| Estradiol | Avoid; *see also* Contraceptives, Oral |
| Estramustine | Manufacturer advises caution and regular liver function tests; avoid in severe liver disease |
| Estriol | Avoid; *see also* Contraceptives, Oral |
| Estrone | Avoid; *see also* Contraceptives, Oral |
| Estropipate | Avoid; *see also* Contraceptives, Oral |
| Ethinylestradiol | Avoid; *see also* Contraceptives, Oral |
| Etodolac | *see* NSAIDs |
| Etomidate | Reduce dose in liver cirrhosis |
| Etoposide | Avoid in severe hepatic impairment |
| Etoricoxib | Max. 60 mg daily in mild hepatic impairment; max. 60 mg on alternate days or 30 mg once daily in moderate hepatic impairment; avoid in severe hepatic impairment; *see also* NSAIDs |
| Etravirine | Manufacturer advises caution in moderate hepatic impairment; avoid in severe hepatic impairment—no information available |
| Etynodiol diacetate | Avoid; *see also* Contraceptives, Oral |
| Exemestane | Manufacturer advises caution |
| Ezetimibe | Avoid in moderate and severe hepatic impairment—may accumulate |
| Famciclovir | Usual dose in well compensated liver disease (information not available on decompensated) |
| Felodipine | Reduce dose |
| Fenbufen | *see* NSAIDs |
| Fenofibrate | Avoid in severe liver disease |
| Fenoprofen | *see* NSAIDs |
| Fentanyl | *see* Opioid Analgesics |
| Ferric carboxymaltose | Use with caution; avoid in conditions where iron overload increases risk of impairment |
| Fesoterodine | Manufacturer advises increase dose cautiously; max. 4 mg daily in moderate hepatic impairment; avoid in severe hepatic impairment; consult product literature before concomitant use of cytochrome P450 enzyme inhibitors |
| Fibrinolytics | Avoid in severe hepatic impairment—increased risk of bleeding |
| Flecainide | Avoid (or reduce dose) in severe liver disease |

| Drug | Comment |
|------|---------|
| Flucloxacillin | Caution in hepatic impairment (risk of cholestatic jaundice and hepatitis, *see* p. 297) |
| Fluconazole | Toxicity with related drugs |
| Fludrocortisone | *see* Corticosteroids |
| Flumazenil | Carefully titrate dose |
| Fluorouracil | Manufacturer advises caution |
| Fluoxetine | *see* Antidepressants, SSRI |
| Flupentixol | *see* Antipsychotics |
| Fluphenazine | *see* Antipsychotics |
| Flurazepam | *see* Anxiolytics and Hypnotics |
| Flurbiprofen | *see* NSAIDs |
| Flutamide | Use with caution (hepatotoxic) |
| Fluvastatin | *see* Statins |
| Fluvoxamine | *see* Antidepressants, SSRI |
| Fondaparinux sodium | Caution in severe hepatic impairment (increased risk of bleeding) |
| Formoterol (eformoterol) | Metabolism possibly reduced in severe cirrhosis |
| Fosamprenavir | Manufacturer advises caution in mild hepatic impairment; reduce dose to 450 mg twice daily in moderate hepatic impairment; reduce dose to 300 mg twice daily in severe hepatic impairment |
| Fosaprepitant | *see* Neurokinin Receptor Antagonists |
| Fosinopril | *see* ACE Inhibitors |
| Fosphenytoin | Consider 10–25% reduction in dose or infusion rate (except initial dose for status epilepticus) |
| Frovatriptan | Avoid in severe hepatic impairment |
| Frusemide | *see* Loop Diuretics |
| Fulvestrant | Manufacturer advises caution in mild to moderate hepatic impairment; avoid in severe hepatic impairment |
| Furosemide (frusemide) | *see* Loop Diuretics |
| Fusidic acid | *see* Sodium Fusidate |
| Galantamine | Reduce dose in moderate hepatic impairment; avoid in severe impairment |
| Ganirelix | Manufacturer advises avoid in moderate or severe hepatic impairment |
| Gemcitabine | Manufacturer advises caution |
| Gemfibrozil | Avoid in liver disease |
| Gestodene | Avoid; *see also* Contraceptives, Oral |
| Gestrinone | Avoid in severe liver disease |
| Glibenclamide | *see* Sulphonylureas |
| Gliclazide | *see* Sulphonylureas |
| Glimepiride | Manufacturer advises avoid in severe hepatic impairment |
| Glipizide | *see* Sulphonylureas |
| Glyceryl trinitrate | *see* Nitrates |
| Griseofulvin | Avoid in severe liver disease |
| Haloperidol | *see* Antipsychotics |
| Halothane | Avoid if history of unexplained pyrexia or jaundice following previous exposure to halothane |

| Drug | Comment |
|------|---------|
| Heparin | Reduce dose in severe liver disease |
| Hydralazine | Reduce dose |
| Hydrochlorothiazide | see Thiazides and Related Diuretics |
| Hydrocortisone | see Corticosteroids |
| Hydroflumethiazide | see Thiazides and Related Diuretics |
| Hydromorphone | see Opioid Analgesics |
| Hydroxycarbamide (hydroxyurea) | For sickle-cell disease, manufacturer advises caution in mild to moderate hepatic impairment; avoid in severe hepatic impairment |
| Hydroxychloroquine | Use with caution in moderate to severe hepatic impairment |
| Hydroxyzine | Sedation inappropriate in severe liver disease—avoid |
| Hyoscine hydro-bromide | Manufacturer advises caution |
| Hypnotics | see Anxiolytics and Hypnotics |
| Ibuprofen | see NSAIDs |
| Idarubicin | Reduce dose according to serum-bilirubin concentration; avoid in severe hepatic impairment |
| Ifosfamide | Avoid |
| Iloprost | Elimination reduced in hepatic impairment—initially 2.5 micrograms no more frequently than every 3 hours (max. 6 times daily), adjusted according to response (consult product literature) |
| Imatinib | Max. 400 mg daily; reduce dose further if not tolerated |
| Imidapril | see ACE Inhibitors |
| Imipramine | see Antidepressants, Tricyclic (and related) |
| Indapamide | see Thiazides and Related Diuretics |
| Indinavir | Increased risk of nephrolithiasis; reduce dose to 600 mg every 8 hours in mild to moderate hepatic impairment; not studied in severe impairment |
| Indometacin | see NSAIDs |
| Indoramin | Manufacturer advises caution |
| Interferon alfa | Close monitoring in mild to moderate hepatic impairment; avoid if severe |
| Interferon beta | Avoid in decompensated liver disease |
| Interferon gamma-1b | Manufacturer advises caution in severe liver disease |
| Irinotecan | Monitor closely for neutropenia if plasma-bilirubin concentration 1.5–3 times upper limit of normal range; avoid if plasma-bilirubin concentration greater than 3 times upper limit of normal range |
| Iron dextran | Avoid in severe hepatic impairment |
| Iron sucrose | Use with caution; avoid in conditions where iron overload increases risk of impairment |
| Isocarboxazid | see Antidepressants, MAOI |

| Drug | Comment |
|------|---------|
| Isometheptene [ingredient] | see Midrid® |
| Isoniazid | Use with caution; monitor liver function regularly and particularly frequently in first 2 months; see also p. 324 |
| Isosorbide dinitrate | see Nitrates |
| Isosorbide mono-nitrate | see Nitrates |
| Isotretinoin | Avoid—further impairment of liver function may occur |
| Isradipine | Reduce dose |
| Itraconazole | Use only if potential benefit outweighs risk of hepatotoxicity (see p. 336); dose reduction may be necessary |
| Ivabradine | Manufacturer advises caution in moderate hepatic impairment; avoid in severe hepatic impairment |
| Kaletra® | Avoid oral solution because of propylene glycol content; manufacturer advises avoid capsules and tablets in severe hepatic impairment |
| Ketoconazole | Avoid; see also p. 337 |
| Ketoprofen | see NSAIDs |
| Ketorolac | see NSAIDs |
| Ketotifen | Sedation inappropriate in severe liver disease—avoid |
| Labetalol | Avoid—severe hepatocellular injury reported |
| Lacidipine | Antihypertensive effect possibly increased |
| Lacosamide | Manufacturer advises caution in severe hepatic impairment — no information available |
| Lamotrigine | Halve dose in moderate hepatic impairment; quarter dose in severe hepatic impairment |
| Lansoprazole | In severe liver disease dose should not exceed 30 mg daily |
| Lapatinib | Manufacturer advises caution in moderate to severe hepatic impairment—metabolism reduced |
| Leflunomide | Avoid—active metabolite may accumulate |
| Lepirudin | No information—manufacturer advises that cirrhosis may affect renal excretion |
| Lercanidipine | Avoid in severe liver disease |
| Levetiracetam | Halve dose in severe hepatic impairment if eGFR less than 70 mL/minute/1.73m$^2$ |
| Levobupivacaine | Manufacturer advises caution in liver disease |
| Levomepromazine (methotrimeprazine) | see Antipsychotics |
| Levonorgestrel | Avoid (however levonorgestrel emergency contraception can be used); see also Contraceptives, Oral |
| Lidocaine (lignocaine) | Manufacturer advises caution—increased risk of side-effects |
| Lignocaine | see Lidocaine |

| Drug | Comment |
|------|---------|
| Linezolid | In severe hepatic impairment manufacturer advises use only if potential benefit outweighs risk |
| Lofepramine | see Antidepressants, Tricyclic (and related) |
| Loop diuretics | Hypokalaemia may precipitate coma (use potassium-sparing diuretic to prevent this); increased risk of hypomagnesaemia in alcoholic cirrhosis |
| Lopinavir [ingredient] | see Kaletra® |
| Loprazolam | see Anxiolytics and Hypnotics |
| Lorazepam | see Anxiolytics and Hypnotics |
| Lormetazepam | see Anxiolytics and Hypnotics |
| Losartan | Consider dose reduction in mild to moderate hepatic impairment; manufacturer advises avoid in severe impairment—no information available |
| Lumefantrine [ingredient] | see Riamet® |
| Lymecycline | see Tetracyclines |
| Magnesium salts | Avoid in hepatic coma if risk of renal failure |
| Maraviroc | Manufacturer advises caution |
| Medroxyprogesterone | Avoid; see also Contraceptives, Oral |
| Mefenamic acid | see NSAIDs |
| Mefloquine | Avoid for prophylaxis in severe liver disease |
| Megestrol | Avoid; see also Contraceptives, Oral |
| Melatonin | Manufacturer advises avoid |
| Meloxicam | see NSAIDs |
| Meprobamate | see Anxiolytics and Hypnotics |
| Meptazinol | see Opioid Analgesics |
| Mercaptopurine | May need dose reduction |
| Meropenem | Monitor transaminase and bilirubin concentrations |
| Mesalazine | Avoid in severe hepatic impairment |
| Mesterolone | see Androgens |
| Mestranol | Avoid; see also Contraceptives, Oral |
| Metformin | Withdraw if tissue hypoxia likely |
| Methadone | see Opioid Analgesics |
| Methenamine | Avoid |
| Methionine | May precipitate coma |
| Methocarbamol | Manufacturer advises caution; half-life may be prolonged |
| Methotrexate | Dose-related toxicity—avoid in non-malignant conditions (e.g. psoriasis); avoid for all indications in severe hepatic impairment |
| Methotrimeprazine | see Antipsychotics |
| Methoxy polyethylene glycol-epoetin beta | Manufacturer advises caution in severe liver disease—no information available |
| Methyldopa | Manufacturer advises caution in history of liver disease; avoid in active liver disease |
| Methylnaltrexone | Manufacturer advises avoid in severe hepatic impairment—no information available |
| Methylprednisolone | see Corticosteroids |

| Drug | Comment |
|------|---------|
| Methysergide | Avoid |
| Metoclopramide | Reduce dose |
| Metolazone | see Thiazides and Related Diuretics |
| Metoprolol | Reduce dose in severe hepatic impairment |
| Metronidazole | In severe liver disease reduce total daily dose to one-third, and give once daily |
| Mianserin | see Antidepressants, Tricyclic (and related) |
| Micafungin | Use with caution in mild to moderate hepatic impairment; avoid in severe hepatic impairment—no information available |
| Miconazole | Avoid |
| Midazolam | see Anxiolytics and Hypnotics |
| Midrid® | Avoid in severe liver disease; see also Paracetamol |
| Mifepristone | Manufacturer advises avoid |
| Miglustat | No information available—manufacturer advises caution |
| Minocycline | see Tetracyclines |
| Mirtazapine | Manufacturer advises caution |
| Mitotane | Manufacturer advises caution in mild to moderate hepatic impairment—monitoring of plasma-mitotane concentration recommended; avoid in severe impairment |
| Mitoxantrone | Manufacturer advises caution in severe hepatic impairment |
| Mivacurium | Reduce dose in severe liver impairment |
| Mizolastine | Manufacturer recommends avoid in significant hepatic impairment |
| Moclobemide | Reduce dose in severe liver disease |
| Modafinil | Halve dose in severe liver disease |
| Moexipril | see ACE Inhibitors |
| Morphine | see Opioid Analgesics |
| Moxifloxacin | Manufacturer advises avoid in severe hepatic impairment |
| Moxonidine | Avoid in severe liver disease |
| Nabilone | Avoid in severe liver disease |
| Nabumetone | see NSAIDs |
| Nadolol | Manufacturer advises caution |
| Nalidixic acid | Manufacturer advises caution in liver disease |
| Naltrexone | Manufacturer advises caution; avoid in acute hepatitis or hepatic failure |
| Nandrolone | see Anabolic Steroids |
| Naproxen | see NSAIDs |
| Naratriptan | Max. 2.5 mg in 24 hours in moderate hepatic impairment; avoid if severe |
| Nateglinide | Manufacturer advises caution in moderate hepatic impairment; avoid in severe impairment—no information available |
| Nebivolol | No information available—manufacturer advises avoid |
| Nelfinavir | Manufacturer advises caution |

| Drug | Comment |
|------|---------|
| Neomycin | Absorbed from gastro-intestinal tract in liver disease—increased risk of ototoxicity |
| Neurokinin receptor antagonists | Manufacturer advises caution in moderate to severe hepatic impairment |
| Nevirapine | Manufacturer advises caution in moderate hepatic impairment; avoid in severe hepatic impairment; see also p. 347 |
| Nicardipine | Half-life prolonged in severe hepatic impairment—may need dose reduction |
| Nicotine | Manufacturers advise caution in moderate to severe hepatic impairment |
| Nicotinic acid | Manufacturer advises monitor liver function in mild to moderate hepatic impairment and avoid in severe impairment; discontinue if severe abnormalities in liver function tests |
| Nicoumalone | see Anticoagulants, Oral |
| Nifedipine | Dose reduction may be required in severe liver disease |
| Nilotinib | Manufacturer advises caution—no information available |
| Nimodipine | Elimination reduced in cirrhosis—monitor blood pressure |
| Nitrates | Caution in severe hepatic impairment |
| Nitrazepam | see Anxiolytics and Hypnotics |
| Nitrofurantoin | Cholestatic jaundice and chronic active hepatitis reported |
| Nitroprusside | see Sodium Nitroprusside |
| Nizatidine | Manufacturer advises caution |
| Norethisterone | Avoid; see also Contraceptives, Oral |
| Norgestimate | Avoid; see also Contraceptives, Oral |
| Norgestrel | Avoid; see also Contraceptives, Oral |
| Nortriptyline | see Antidepressants, Tricyclic (and related) |
| NSAIDs | Increased risk of gastro-intestinal bleeding and can cause fluid retention; avoid in severe liver disease; aceclofenac, initially 100 mg daily; celecoxib, halve initial dose in moderate liver disease; dexketoprofen, reduce initial dose to max. 50 mg daily in mild to moderate hepatic impairment; parecoxib, halve dose in moderate hepatic impairment (max. 40 mg daily); tiaprofenic acid, reduce dose in mild or moderate hepatic impairment; see also Etoricoxib |
| Oestrogens | Avoid; see also Contraceptives, Oral |
| Ofloxacin | Elimination may be reduced in severe hepatic impairment |
| Olanzapine | Consider initial dose of 5 mg daily |

| Drug | Comment |
|------|---------|
| Olmesartan | Dose should not exceed 20 mg daily in moderate impairment; manufacturer advises avoid in severe impairment—no information available |
| Omalizumab | Manufacturer advises caution—no information available |
| Omega-3-acid ethyl esters | Monitor liver function |
| Omeprazole | In liver disease not more than 20 mg daily should be needed |
| Ondansetron | Max. 8 mg daily in moderate or severe hepatic impairment |
| Opioid analgesics | Avoid or reduce dose—may precipitate coma |
| Oral contraceptives | see Contraceptives, Oral |
| Oxazepam | see Anxiolytics and Hypnotics |
| Oxcarbazepine | Manufacturer advises caution in severe hepatic impairment—no information available |
| Oxprenolol | Reduce dose |
| Oxybutynin | Manufacturer advises caution |
| Oxycodone | see Opioid Analgesics |
| Oxytetracycline | see Tetracyclines |
| Paclitaxel | Avoid in severe liver disease |
| Paliperidone | Manufacturer advises caution in severe hepatic impairment—no information available |
| Pancuronium | Possibly slower onset, higher dose requirement and prolonged recovery time |
| Pantoprazole | Max. 20 mg daily in severe hepatic impairment and cirrhosis—monitor liver function (discontinue if deterioration) |
| Papaveretum | see Opioid Analgesics |
| Paracetamol | Dose-related toxicity—avoid large doses |
| Parathyroid hormone | Avoid |
| Parecoxib | see NSAIDs |
| Paroxetine | see Antidepressants, SSRI |
| Peginterferon alfa | Avoid in severe hepatic impairment |
| Pentazocine | see Opioid Analgesics |
| Pentostatin | Manufacturer advises caution—limited information available |
| Pericyazine | see Antipsychotics |
| Perindopril | see ACE Inhibitors |
| Perphenazine | see Antipsychotics |
| Pethidine | see Opioid Analgesics |
| Phenelzine | see Antidepressants, MAOI |
| Phenindione | see Anticoagulants, Oral |
| Phenobarbital | May precipitate coma; avoid in severe hepatic impairment |
| Phenothiazines | see Antipsychotics |
| Phenytoin | Reduce dose to avoid toxicity |
| Pholcodine | see Opioid Analgesics |
| Pilocarpine | Reduce initial oral dose in moderate or severe cirrhosis |
| Pimozide | see Antipsychotics |
| Pioglitazone | Avoid |
| Piperazine | Manufacturer advises avoid |
| Pipotiazine | see Antipsychotics |
| Piracetam | Avoid |
| Piroxicam | see NSAIDs |

Appendix 2: Liver disease

| Drug | Comment |
|------|---------|
| Posaconazole | Monitor liver function; use with caution in severe hepatic impairment |
| Prasugrel | Use with caution—increased risk of bleeding; avoid in severe hepatic impairment |
| Pravastatin | *see* Statins |
| Prazosin | Initially 500 micrograms daily; increased with caution |
| Prednisolone | *see* Corticosteroids |
| Prilocaine | Manufacturer advises caution |
| Primidone | Reduce dose; may precipitate coma |
| Procarbazine | Avoid in severe hepatic impairment |
| Prochlorperazine | *see* Antipsychotics |
| Progesterone | Avoid; *see also* Contraceptives, Oral |
| Progestogens | Avoid; *see also* Contraceptives, Oral |
| Promazine | *see* Antipsychotics |
| Promethazine | Avoid—may precipitate coma in severe liver disease; hepatotoxic |
| Propafenone | Reduce dose |
| Propantheline | Manufacturer advises caution |
| Propiverine | Avoid in moderate to severe hepatic impairment |
| Propofol | Use with caution |
| Propranolol | Reduce oral dose |
| Propylthiouracil | Reduce dose |
| Prothrombin Complex, Dried | Increased risk of thromboembolic events—manufacturer advises use with caution |
| Pyrazinamide | Monitor hepatic function—idiosyncratic hepatotoxicity more common; avoid in severe hepatic impairment; *see also* p. 324 |
| Pyrimethamine | Manufacturer advises caution |
| Quetiapine | For *immediate-release tablets*, initially 25 mg daily, increased daily in steps of 25–50 mg; for *modified-release tablets*, initially 50 mg daily, increased daily in steps of 50 mg |
| Quinagolide | Manufacturer advises avoid—no information available |
| Quinapril | *see* ACE Inhibitors |
| Quinine | For treatment of malaria in severe hepatic impairment, reduce parenteral maintenance dose to 5–7 mg/kg of salt |
| Quinupristin [ingredient] | *see* Synercid® |
| Rabeprazole | Manufacturer advises caution in severe hepatic dysfunction |
| Raloxifene | Manufacturer advises avoid |
| Raltegravir | Manufacturer advises caution in severe hepatic impairment—no information available |
| Raltitrexed | Caution in mild or moderate disease; avoid if severe |
| Ramipril | *see* ACE Inhibitors |
| Ranolazine | Use with caution in mild hepatic impairment; avoid in moderate and severe hepatic impairment |

| Drug | Comment |
|------|---------|
| Rasagiline | Manufacturer advises caution in mild hepatic impairment; avoid in moderate to severe impairment |
| Reboxetine | Initial dose 2 mg twice daily, increased according to tolerance |
| Remifentanil | *see* Opioid Analgesics |
| Repaglinide | Manufacturer advises avoid in severe liver disease |
| Reteplase | *see* Fibrinolytics |
| Riamet® | Manufacturer advises caution in severe hepatic impairment—monitor ECG and plasma-potassium concentration |
| Ribavirin | No dosage adjustment required; use oral ribavirin with caution in severe hepatic dysfunction or decompensated cirrhosis |
| Rifabutin | Reduce dose in severe hepatic impairment |
| Rifampicin | Impaired elimination; monitor liver function; avoid or do not exceed 8 mg/kg daily; *see also* p. 325 |
| Riluzole | Avoid |
| Rimonabant | Manufacturer advises caution in moderate hepatic impairment; avoid in severe impairment |
| Risperidone | Manufacturer advises initial and subsequent oral doses should be halved; if an oral dose of at least 2 mg daily tolerated, 25 mg as a depot injection can be given every 2 weeks |
| Ritonavir | Avoid in decompensated liver disease; in severe hepatic impairment without decompensation, use 'booster' doses with caution (avoid treatment doses) |
| Rivaroxaban | Manufacturer advises caution in cirrhotic patients with moderate hepatic impairment; avoid in liver disease with coagulopathy |
| Rivastigmine | No information available—manufacturer advises avoid in severe liver disease |
| Rizatriptan | Reduce dose to 5 mg in mild to moderate liver disease; avoid in severe liver disease |
| Rocuronium | Reduce dose |
| Ropinirole | Manufacturer advises caution in moderate hepatic impairment; avoid in severe hepatic impairment |
| Ropivacaine | Manufacturer advises caution in severe liver disease |
| Rosiglitazone | Avoid |
| Rosuvastatin | *see* Statins |
| Rotigotine | Manufacturer advises caution in severe hepatic impairment—no information available |

| Drug | Comment |
|------|---------|
| Rufinamide | Manufacturer advises caution and careful dose titration in mild to moderate hepatic impairment; avoid in severe impairment |
| Sapropterin | Manufacturer advises caution—no information available |
| Saquinavir | Manufacturer advises caution in moderate hepatic impairment; avoid in severe impairment |
| Sertindole | Slower titration and lower maintenance dose in mild to moderate hepatic impairment; avoid in severe hepatic impairment; see also Antipsychotics |
| Sertraline | see Antidepressants, SSRI |
| Sibutramine | Increased plasma-sibutramine concentration; manufacturer advises caution in mild to moderate hepatic impairment; avoid if severe impairment |
| Sildenafil | For erectile dysfunction, initial dose 25 mg; for pulmonary hypertension reduce to 20 mg twice daily if usual dose not tolerated; manufacturer advises avoid in severe hepatic impairment |
| Simvastatin | see Statins |
| Sirolimus | Decrease dose by 50%; monitor blood-sirolimus trough concentration every 5–7 days until 3 consecutive measurements have shown stable blood-sirolimus concentrations |
| Sitaxentan sodium | Avoid |
| Sodium aurothiomalate | Caution in mild to moderate liver disease; avoid in severe liver disease |
| Sodium bicarbonate | see Antacids |
| Sodium fusidate | Impaired biliary excretion; possibly increased risk of hepatotoxicity; avoid or reduce dose |
| Sodium nitroprusside | Avoid in severe liver disease |
| Sodium oxybate | Halve initial dose |
| Sodium phenylbutyrate | Manufacturer advises caution |
| Sodium valproate | see Valproate |
| Solifenacin | Max. 5 mg daily in moderate liver disease; avoid if severe |
| Sorafenib | Manufacturer advises caution in severe hepatic impairment—no information available |
| Statins | Avoid in active liver disease or unexplained persistent elevations in serum transaminases |
| Stilboestrol (diethylstilbestrol) | Avoid; see also Contraceptives, Oral |
| Streptokinase | see Fibrinolytics |
| Sulindac | see NSAIDs |
| Sulphonylureas | Increased risk of hypoglycaemia in severe liver disease; avoid or use small dose; can produce jaundice; see also Glimepiride |

| Drug | Comment |
|------|---------|
| Sulpiride | see Antipsychotics |
| Sumatriptan | Manufacturer advises 50 mg oral dose in hepatic impairment; avoid in severe hepatic impairment |
| Suxamethonium | Prolonged apnoea may occur in severe liver disease because of reduced hepatic synthesis of pseudocholinesterase |
| Synercid® | Consider reducing dose to 5 mg/kg every 8 hours in moderate hepatic impairment, adjusted according to clinical response; avoid in severe hepatic impairment or if plasma-bilirubin concentration greater than 3 times upper limit of reference range |
| Tacrolimus | Dose reduction may be necessary in severe hepatic impairment |
| Tadalafil | Max. dose 10 mg; manufacturer advises monitor patient in severe hepatic impairment |
| Tamsulosin | Avoid in severe hepatic impairment |
| Tegafur with uracil | see Uftoral® |
| Telithromycin | Manufacturer advises caution; see also p. 314 |
| Telmisartan | 20–40 mg once daily in mild or moderate impairment; avoid in severe hepatic impairment or biliary obstruction |
| Temazepam | see Anxiolytics and Hypnotics |
| Temsirolimus | Manufacturer advises caution in mild to moderate hepatic impairment; avoid in severe hepatic impairment—no information available |
| Tenecteplase | see Fibrinolytics |
| Tenoxicam | see NSAIDs |
| Terbinafine | Manufacturer advises avoid—elimination reduced |
| Testosterone and esters | see Androgens |
| Tetracosactide | See Corticosteroids |
| Tetracyclines | Avoid (or use with caution); tetracycline and demeclocycline max. 1 g daily in divided doses; see also Tigecycline |
| Thalidomide | Manufacturer advises caution in severe hepatic impairment—no information available |
| Theophylline | Reduce dose |
| Thiazides and related diuretics | Use with caution in mild to moderate impairment; avoid in severe liver disease; hypokalaemia may precipitate coma (potassium-sparing diuretic can prevent); increased risk of hypomagnesaemia in alcoholic cirrhosis |
| Thiopental | Reduce dose for induction in severe liver disease |
| Tiagabine | Maintenance dose 5–10 mg 1–2 times daily initially in mild to moderate hepatic impairment; avoid in severe impairment |

| Drug | Comment |
|---|---|
| Tiaprofenic acid | *see* NSAIDs |
| Tibolone | Avoid in severe liver disease |
| Ticarcillin [ingredient] | *see Timentin®* |
| Tigecycline | Initially 100 mg then 25 mg every 12 hours in severe hepatic impairment |
| *Timentin®* | Cholestatic jaundice, *see* under Co-amoxiclav p. 300 |
| Timolol | Dose reduction may be necessary |
| Tinzaparin | *see* Heparin |
| Tioguanine | Reduce dose in hepatic impairment |
| Tipranavir | Manufacturer advises caution in mild hepatic impairment; avoid in moderate or severe hepatic impairment—no information available |
| Tirofiban | Caution in mild to moderate liver disease; avoid in severe liver disease—increased risk of bleeding |
| Tizanidine | Avoid in severe liver disease |
| Tolbutamide | *see* Sulphonylureas |
| Tolcapone | Avoid |
| Tolfenamic acid | *see* NSAIDs |
| Tolterodine | Reduce dose to 1 mg twice daily |
| Topiramate | Use with caution in hepatic impairment—clearance may be decreased |
| Topotecan | Avoid in severe hepatic impairment |
| Torasemide | *see* Loop Diuretics |
| Toremifene | Elimination decreased in hepatic impairment—avoid if severe |
| Trabectedin | Manufacturer advises caution in liver impairment—consider dose reduction; avoid in patients with raised bilirubin |
| Tramadol | *see* Opioid Analgesics |
| Trandolapril | *see* ACE Inhibitors |
| Tranylcypromine | *see* Antidepressants, MAOI |
| Trazodone | *see* Antidepressants, Tricyclic (and related) |
| Tretinoin (oral) | Reduce dose |
| Triamcinolone | *see* Corticosteroids |
| Tribavirin | *see* Ribavirin |
| Triclofos | *see* Anxiolytics and Hypnotics |
| Trifluoperazine | *see* Antipsychotics |
| Trimeprazine | *see* Alimemazine |
| Trimipramine | *see* Antidepressants, Tricyclic (and related) |
| Trospium | Manufacturer advises avoid—no information available |
| *Uftoral®* | Manufacturer advises monitor liver function in mild to moderate hepatic impairment and avoid in severe impairment |
| Urokinase | *see* Fibrinolytics |
| Ursodeoxycholic acid | Avoid in chronic liver disease (but used in primary biliary cirrhosis) |
| Valaciclovir | Manufacturer advises caution with high doses used for preventing cytomegalovirus disease—no information available |

| Drug | Comment |
|---|---|
| Valproate | Avoid if possible—hepatotoxicity and hepatic failure may occasionally occur (usually in first 6 months); *see also* p. 262 |
| Valproic acid | *see* Valproate |
| Valsartan | Max. dose 80 mg daily in mild to moderate hepatic impairment; avoid if severe |
| Vardenafil | Initial dose 5 mg in mild to moderate hepatic impairment, increased subsequently according to response (max. 10 mg in moderate hepatic impairment); manufacturer advises avoid in severe hepatic impairment |
| Venlafaxine | Halve dose in moderate hepatic impairment; avoid if severe |
| Verapamil | Reduce oral dose |
| Verteporfin | Avoid in severe hepatic impairment |
| Vildagliptin | Manufacturer advises avoid |
| Vinblastine | Dose reduction may be necessary |
| Vincristine | Dose reduction may be necessary |
| Vindesine | Dose reduction may be necessary |
| Vinorelbine | Dose reduction may be required in significant hepatic impairment |
| Voriconazole | In mild to moderate hepatic cirrhosis use usual initial dose then halve subsequent doses; no information available for severe hepatic cirrhosis—manufacturer advises use only if potential benefit outweighs risk |
| Warfarin | *see* Anticoagulants, Oral |
| Xipamide | *see* Thiazides and Related Diuretics |
| Zafirlukast | Manufacturer advises avoid |
| Zaleplon | *see* Anxiolytics and Hypnotics |
| Zidovudine | Accumulation may occur |
| Zoledronic acid | Manufacturer advises caution in severe hepatic impairment—limited information available |
| Zolmitriptan | Max. 5 mg in 24 hours in moderate or severe hepatic impairment |
| Zolpidem | *see* Anxiolytics and Hypnotics |
| Zonisamide | Initially, increase dose at 2-week intervals if mild or moderate hepatic impairment; avoid in severe impairment |
| Zopiclone | *see* Anxiolytics and Hypnotics |
| Zotepine | Initial dose 25 mg twice daily, increased gradually according to response (max. 75 mg twice daily); monitor liver function at weekly intervals for first 3 months |
| Zuclopenthixol | *see* Antipsychotics |

# A3 Renal impairment

The use of drugs in patients with reduced renal function can give rise to problems for several reasons:

- reduced renal excretion of a drug or its metabolites may cause toxicity;

- sensitivity to some drugs is increased even if elimination is unimpaired;

- many side-effects are tolerated poorly by patients with renal impairment;

- some drugs are not effective when renal function is reduced.

Many of these problems can be avoided by reducing the dose or by using alternative drugs.

## Principles of dose adjustment in renal impairment

The level of renal function below which the dose of a drug must be reduced depends on the proportion of the drug eliminated by renal excretion and its toxicity.

For many drugs with only minor or no dose-related side-effects very precise modification of the dose regimen is unnecessary and a simple scheme for dose reduction is sufficient.

For more toxic drugs with a small safety margin or patients at extremes of weight, dose regimens based on creatinine clearance (see Use of Dosage Table for details) should be used. When both efficacy and toxicity are closely related to plasma-drug concentration, recommended regimens should be regarded only as a guide to initial treatment; subsequent doses must be adjusted according to clinical response and plasma-drug concentration.

Renal function declines with age; many elderly patients have renal impairment but, because of reduced muscle mass, this may not be indicated by a raised serum creatinine. It is wise to assume at least mild impairment of renal function when prescribing for the elderly.

The total daily maintenance dose of a drug can be reduced either by reducing the size of the individual doses or by increasing the interval between doses. For some drugs, although the size of the maintenance dose is reduced it is important to give a loading dose if an immediate effect is required. This is because it takes about five times the half-life of the drug to achieve steady-state plasma concentrations. Because the plasma half-life of drugs excreted by the kidney is prolonged in renal impairment it can take many doses for the reduced dosage to achieve a therapeutic plasma concentration. The loading dose should usually be the same size as the initial dose for a patient with normal renal function.

**Nephrotoxic drugs** should, if possible, be avoided in patients with renal disease because the consequences of nephrotoxicity are likely to be more serious when renal reserve is already reduced.

## Use of dosage table

Dose recommendations are based on the severity of renal impairment.

Renal function is measured either in terms of estimated **glomerular filtration rate** (eGFR) calculated from a formula derived from the Modification of Diet in Renal Disease study ('MDRD formula' that uses serum creatinine, age, sex, and race (for Afro-Caribbean patients)) or it can be expressed as **creatinine clearance** (best derived from a 24-hour urine collection but often calculated from the Cockcroft and Gault formula (CG).

| Cockcroft and Gault formula | |
|---|---|
| Estimated Creatinine Clearance in mL/minute | $= \dfrac{(140 - \text{Age}) \times \text{Weight} \times \text{Constant}}{\text{Serum creatinine}}$ |

Age in years
Weight in kilograms; use ideal body-weight
Serum creatinine in micromol/litre
Constant = 1.23 for men; 1.04 for women

The serum-creatinine concentration is sometimes used instead as a measure of renal function but it is only a **rough guide** to drug dosing.

### Important

Renal function in adults is increasingly being reported on the basis of estimated glomerular filtration rate (eGFR) normalised to a body surface area of $1.73\,m^2$ and derived from the Modification of Diet in Renal Disease (MDRD) formula. However, published information on the effects of renal impairment on drug elimination is usually stated in terms of creatinine clearance as a surrogate for glomerular filtration rate (GFR).

The information on dosage adjustment in the BNF is expressed in terms of eGFR, rather than creatinine clearance, for most drugs (see exceptions below: Toxic Drugs and Patients at Extremes of Weight). Although the two measures of renal function are not interchangeable, in practice, for most drugs and for most patients (over 18 years) of average build and height, eGFR (MDRD 'formula') can be used to determine dosage adjustments in place of creatinine clearance. An individual's absolute glomerular filtration rate can be calculated from the eGFR as follows: $GFR_{Absolute} = eGFR \times$ (individual's body surface area/1.73)

**Toxic drugs** For potentially toxic drugs with a small safety margin, creatinine clearance (calculated from the Cockcroft and Gault formula) should be used to adjust drug dosages in addition to plasma-drug concentration and clinical response.

**Patients at extremes of weight** In patients at both extremes of weight (BMI of less than $18.5\,kg/m^2$ or greater than $30\,kg/m^2$) the absolute glomerular filtration rate or creatinine clearance (calculated from the Cockcroft and Gault formula) should be used to adjust drug dosages.

In the BNF, values for eGFR, creatinine clearance (for toxic drugs), or another measure of renal function are included where possible. However, where such values are not available, the BNF reflects the terms used in the published information.

*Chronic kidney disease in adults: UK guidelines for identification, management and referral (March 2006)* define renal function as follows:

| Degree of impairment | eGFR mL/minute/1.73 m² |
|---|---|
| Normal - Stage 1 | More than 90 (with other evidence of kidney damage) |
| Mild - Stage 2 | 60–89 (with other evidence of kidney damage) |
| Moderate¹ - Stage 3 | 30–59 |
| Severe - Stage 4 | 15–29 |
| Established renal failure - Stage 5 | Less than 15 |

1. NICE clinical guideline 73 (September 2008)—Chronic kidney disease: Stage 3A eGFR 45–59, Stage 3B eGFR 30–44

### Dialysis
For prescribing in patients on continuous ambulatory peritoneal dialysis (CAPD) or haemodialysis, consult specialist literature.

The following table can be used as a guide to drugs which require a reduction in dose in renal impairment, and to those which are potentially harmful or are ineffective. Drug prescribing should be kept to the minimum in all patients with severe renal disease.

If even mild renal impairment is considered likely on clinical grounds, renal function should be checked before prescribing **any** drug which requires dose modification.

Absence of a drug from the table does not imply safety.

For adjusting drug doses in renal impairment, see Important on p. 815.

## Table of drugs to be avoided or used with caution in renal impairment
The list of drugs given below may not be comprehensive and is based on current information concerning the use of prescribed drugs in therapeutic dosage.

Products introduced or amended since publication of BNF No. 57 (March 2009) are underlined.

| Drug | Comment |
|---|---|
| Abacavir | Manufacturer advises avoid in end-stage renal disease; *see also Kivexa® and Trizivir®* |
| Abciximab | Use with caution in severe renal impairment—increased risk of bleeding |
| Acamprosate | Avoid if serum-creatinine greater than 120 micromol/litre |
| Acarbose | Avoid if eGFR less than 25 mL/minute/1.73 m² |
| ACE inhibitors | Use with caution and monitor response (*see also* p. 103); hyperkalaemia and other side-effects more common; *see also* individual drugs |

| Drug | Comment |
|---|---|
| Acebutolol | Halve dose if eGFR 25–50 mL/minute/1.73 m²; use quarter dose if eGFR less than 25 mL/minute/1.73 m²; do not administer more than once daily |
| Aceclofenac | *see* NSAIDs; avoid in moderate to severe renal impairment |
| Acemetacin | *see* NSAIDs |
| Acenocoumarol (nicoumalone) | *see* Anticoagulants, Oral |
| Acetazolamide | Avoid; metabolic acidosis |
| Aciclovir | Risk of neurological reactions increased; use normal *intravenous* dose every 12 hours if eGFR 25–50 mL/minute/1.73 m² (every 24 hours if eGFR 10–25 mL/minute/1.73 m²); consult product literature for intravenous dose if eGFR less than 10 mL/minute/1.73 m²; for *herpes zoster*, use normal oral dose every 8 hours if eGFR 10–25 mL/minute/1.73 m² (every 12 hours if eGFR less than 10 mL/minute/1.73 m²); for *herpes simplex*, use normal oral dose every 12 hours if eGFR less than 10 mL/minute/1.73 m² |
| Acipimox | Reduce dose if eGFR 30–60 mL/minute/1.73 m²; avoid if eGFR less than 30 mL/minute/1.73 m² |
| Acitretin | Avoid; increased risk of toxicity |
| Adefovir dipivoxil | 10 mg every 48 hours if eGFR 30–50 mL/minute/1.73 m²; 10 mg every 72 hours if eGFR 10–30 mL/minute/1.73 m²; no information available if eGFR less than 10 mL/minute/1.73 m² |
| Agomelatine | Manufacturer advises caution in moderate to severe renal impairment |
| Alendronic acid | Avoid if eGFR less than 35 mL/minute/1.73 m² |
| Alfentanil | *see* Opioid Analgesics |
| Alfuzosin | Start at 2.5 mg twice daily and adjust according to response |
| Alimemazine (trimeprazine) | Avoid |
| Aliskiren | Caution if eGFR less than 30 mL/minute/1.73 m²—no information available |
| Alitretinoin | Manufacturer advises avoid in severe renal impairment—no information available |
| Allopurinol | Max. 100 mg daily, increased only if response inadequate; in severe renal impairment, reduce daily dose below 100 mg, or increase dose interval; if facilities available, adjust dose to maintain plasma-oxipurinol concentration below 100 micromol/litre |
| Almotriptan | Max. 12.5 mg in 24 hours if eGFR less than 30 mL/minute/1.73 m² |

| Drug | Comment |
|------|---------|
| Alprazolam | *see* Anxiolytics and Hypnotics |
| Aluminium salts | Risk of accumulation and aluminium toxicity<br>**Note** Absorption of aluminium from aluminium salts is increased by citrates, which are contained in many effervescent preparations (such as effervescent analgesics) |
| Amantadine | Reduce dose; avoid if eGFR less than 15 mL/minute/1.73 m² |
| Ambrisentan | Use with caution if eGFR less than 30 mL/minute/1.73 m² |
| Amfebutamone | *see* Bupropion |
| Amikacin | *see* Aminoglycosides |
| Amiloride | *see* Potassium-sparing Diuretics |
| Aminoglycosides | Reduce dose; monitor serum concentrations; *see also* Neomycin and section 5.1.4 |
| Amisulpride | Halve dose if eGFR 30–60 mL/minute/1.73 m²; use one-third dose if eGFR 10–30 mL/minute/1.73 m²; no information available if eGFR less than 10 mL/minute/1.73 m² |
| Amoxicillin | Risk of crystalluria with high doses (particularly during parenteral therapy). Reduce dose in severe impairment; rashes more common |
| Amphotericin | Use only if no alternative; nephrotoxicity may be reduced with use of lipid formulations |
| Ampicillin | Reduce dose if eGFR less than 10 mL/minute/1.73 m²; rashes more common |
| Amsacrine | Reduce dose |
| Anagrelide | Avoid if eGFR less than 50 mL/minute/1.73 m² |
| Anakinra | Caution if eGFR 30–50 mL/minute/1.73 m²; avoid if eGFR less than 30 mL/minute/1.73 m² |
| Analgesics | *see* Opioid Analgesics, NSAIDs, Paracetamol, *Solpadol*®, and *Tylex*® |
| Anastrozole | Avoid if creatinine clearance less than 20 mL/minute |
| *Angeliq*® | Avoid if eGFR less than 30 mL/minute/1.73 m² |
| Anticoagulants, oral | Manufacturer advises avoid in severe renal impairment; *see also* Dabigatran Etexilate and Rivaroxaban |
| Antipsychotics | Start with small doses in severe impairment; increased cerebral sensitivity; *see also* Amisulpride, Clozapine, Droperidol, Flupentixol, Fluphenazine, Haloperidol, Olanzapine, Paliperidone, Pericyazine, Quetiapine, Risperidone, Sulpiride, and Zotepine |
| Anxiolytics and hypnotics | Start with small doses in severe impairment; increased cerebral sensitivity; *see also* Buspirone, Chloral Hydrate, Melatonin, and Sodium Oxybate |

| Drug | Comment |
|------|---------|
| Arsenic trioxide | Manufacturer advises caution—limited information available |
| Artemether [ingredient] | *see Riamet*® |
| Aspirin | Use with caution; avoid in severe renal impairment; sodium and water retention; deterioration in renal function; increased risk of gastro-intestinal bleeding |
| Atenolol | Max. 50 mg daily (10 mg on alternate days *intravenously*) if eGFR 15–35 mL/minute/1.73 m²; max. 25 mg daily or 50 mg on alternate days (10 mg every 4 days *intravenously*) if eGFR less than 15 mL/minute/1.73 m² |
| Atosiban | No information available |
| Atovaquone | Manufacturer advises caution—monitor more closely |
| *Atripla*® | Manufacturer advises avoid if eGFR less than 50 mL/minute/1.73 m² |
| Auranofin | *see* Sodium Aurothiomalate |
| Azacitidine | Delay next treatment cycle if serum-creatinine or blood urea nitrogen greater than twice baseline value and above the upper level of normal until values return to normal or baseline, and then reduce dose by 50% on the next treatment cycle. Reduce dose by 50% on the next treatment cycle if serum-bicarbonate concentration less than 20 mmol/L |
| Azapropazone | *see* NSAIDs; reduce dose (max. 600 mg daily) in rheumatoid arthritis and ankylosing spondylitis; avoid in severe impairment (avoid in gout if eGFR less than 60 mL/minute/1.73 m²) |
| Azathioprine | Reduce dose and monitor full blood count |
| Aztreonam | If eGFR 10–30 mL/minute/1.73 m², usual initial dose, then half normal dose; if eGFR less than 10 mL/minute/1.73 m² usual initial dose, then one-quarter normal dose |
| Baclofen | Use smaller doses (e.g. 5 mg daily by mouth); excreted by kidney |
| Balsalazide | Manufacturer advises avoid in moderate to severe renal impairment |
| Bambuterol | Reduce initial dose by half if eGFR less than 50 mL/minute/1.73 m² |
| Barbiturates | Reduce dose in severe renal impairment; *see also* Phenobarbital |
| Bemiparin | Risk of bleeding may be increased—use with caution; monitoring of anti-Factor Xa may be required; use of unfractionated heparin may be preferable |

| Drug | Comment |
|---|---|
| Bendrofluazide | see Thiazides and Related Diuretics |
| Bendroflumethiazide (bendrofluazide) | see Thiazides and Related Diuretics |
| Benperidol | see Antipsychotics |
| Benzodiazepines | Use with caution; reduce dose |
| Benzylpenicillin | Reduce dose—consult product literature; high doses may cause cerebral irritation, convulsions, or coma |
| Beta-blockers | see under individual drugs |
| Betamethasone | see Corticosteroids |
| Bezafibrate | Reduce dose to 400 mg daily if eGFR 40–60 mL/minute/ 1.73 m²; reduce dose to 200 mg every 1–2 days if eGFR 15– 40 mL/minute/1.73 m²; avoid if eGFR less than 15 mL/ minute/1.73 m²; avoid modified-release preparations if eGFR less than 60 mL/ minute/1.73 m² |

For adjusting drug doses in renal impairment, see Important on p. 815.

| Drug | Comment |
|---|---|
| Bisoprolol | Reduce dose if eGFR less than 20 mL/minute/1.73 m² (max. 10 mg daily) |
| Bivalirudin | For percutaneous coronary intervention, reduce rate of infusion to 1.4 mg/kg/hour if eGFR 30–60 mL/minute/ 1.73 m² and monitor blood clotting parameters; for acute coronary syndromes and percutaneous coronary intervention, avoid if eGFR less than 30 mL/minute/1.73 m² |
| Bleomycin | Reduce dose by half if serum-creatinine 177–354 micromol/ litre; reduce dose further if serum-creatinine greater than 354 micromol/litre |
| Bortezomib | No information available for creatinine clearance less than 20 mL/minute/1.73 m² |
| Brinzolamide | Avoid if eGFR less than 30 mL/minute/1.73 m² |
| Bupivacaine | Manufacturer advises caution |
| Buprenorphine | see Opioid Analgesics |
| Bupropion | Manufacturer recommends 150 mg daily |
| Buspirone | Reduce dose; avoid if eGFR less than 20 mL/minute/ 1.73 m² |
| Calcitriol | Manufacturer of topical calcitriol advises avoid—no information available |
| Candesartan | Initially 4 mg daily |
| Capecitabine | Reduce starting dose of 1250 mg/m² to 75% if creatinine clearance 30–50 mL/ minute; avoid if creatinine clearance less than 30 mL/ minute |
| Capreomycin | Reduce dose—consult product literature; nephrotoxic; ototoxic |

| Drug | Comment |
|---|---|
| Captopril | see ACE inhibitors; reduce dose; max. initial dose 25 mg daily (do not exceed 100 mg daily) if eGFR 20–40 mL/ minute/1.73 m²; max. initial dose 12.5 mg daily (do not exceed 75 mg daily) if eGFR 10–20 mL/minute/1.73 m²; max. initial dose 6.25 mg daily (do not exceed 37.5 mg daily) if eGFR less than 10 mL/ minute/1.73 m² |
| Carbamazepine | Manufacturer advises caution |
| Carbetocin | Manufacturer advises avoid |
| Carboplatin | Reduce dose and monitor haematological parameters and renal function; avoid if creatinine clearance less than 20 mL/minute |
| Carboprost | Manufacturer advises avoid |
| Carnitine | Use with caution—accumulation of metabolites may occur with chronic oral administration in severe renal impairment |
| Cefaclor | No dose adjustment required—manufacturer advises caution |
| Cefadroxil | 0.5–1 g every 24 hours if eGFR 11–26 mL/minute/1.73 m²; 0.5–1 g every 36 hours if eGFR less than 11 mL/minute/ 1.73 m² |
| Cefalexin | Max. 3 g daily if eGFR 40– 50 mL/minute/1.73 m²; max. 1.5 g daily if eGFR 10–40 mL/ minute/1.73 m²; max. 750 mg daily if eGFR less than 10 mL/ minute/1.73 m² |
| Cefixime | Reduce dose if eGFR less than 20 mL/minute/1.73 m² (max. 200 mg once daily) |
| Cefotaxime | If eGFR less than 5 mL/ minute/1.73 m², initial dose of 1 g then use half normal dose |
| Cefpodoxime | Increase dose interval to every 24 hours if eGFR 10–40 mL/ minute/1.73 m²; increase dose interval to every 48 hours if eGFR less than 10 mL/ minute/1.73 m² |
| Cefradine | Use half normal dose if eGFR 5–20 mL/minute/1.73 m²; use one-quarter normal dose if eGFR less than 5 mL/minute/ 1.73 m² |
| Ceftazidime | Reduce dose if eGFR less than 50 mL/minute/1.73 m²—consult product literature |
| Ceftriaxone | Reduce dose if creatinine clearance less than 10 mL/ minute (max. 2 g daily); monitor plasma concentration if both hepatic and severe renal impairment |
| Cefuroxime | Use parenteral dose of 750 mg twice daily if eGFR 10–20 mL/ minute/1.73 m²; use parenteral dose of 750 mg once daily if eGFR less than 10 mL/ minute/1.73 m² |

| Drug | Comment |
|------|---------|
| Celecoxib | *see* NSAIDs; avoid if eGFR less than 30 mL/minute/1.73 m² |
| Celiprolol | Reduce dose by half if eGFR 15–40 mL/minute/1.73 m²; avoid if eGFR less than 15 mL/minute/1.73 m² |
| Cetirizine | Use half normal dose if eGFR less than 30 mL/minute/1.73 m² |
| Cetrorelix | Manufacturer advises avoid in moderate or severe renal impairment |
| Chloral hydrate | Manufacturer advises avoid in severe impairment |
| Chloramphenicol | Avoid in severe renal impairment unless no alternative; dose-related depression of haematopoiesis |
| Chlordiazepoxide | *see* Anxiolytics and Hypnotics |
| Chloroquine | Manufacturer advises caution; reduce dose (but for malaria prophylaxis *see* p. 360) |
| Chlorpromazine | *see* Antipsychotics |
| Chlorpropamide | Avoid |
| Chlortalidone | *see* Thiazides and Related Diuretics |
| Ciclosporin | *see* p. 495 (*see also* p. 644 if used in atopic dermatitis or psoriasis and p. 574 if used in rheumatoid arthritis) |
| Cidofovir | Avoid if creatinine clearance less than 55 mL/minute; nephrotoxic |
| Cilastatin [ingredient] | *see* Primaxin® |
| Cilazapril | *see* ACE inhibitors; max. initial dose 500 micrograms once daily (do not exceed 2.5 mg once daily) if eGFR 10–40 mL/minute/1.73 m²; avoid if eGFR less than 10 mL/minute/1.73 m² |
| Cilostazol | Avoid if eGFR less than 25 mL/minute/1.73 m² |
| Cimetidine | Reduce dose; 200 mg 4 times daily if eGFR 30–50 mL/minute/1.73 m²; 200 mg 3 times daily if eGFR 15–30 mL/minute/1.73 m²; 200 mg twice daily if eGFR less than 15 ml/minute/1.73 m²; occasional risk of confusion |
| Ciprofibrate | Manufacturer advises reduce dose to 100 mg on alternate days in moderate renal impairment; avoid in severe renal impairment |
| Ciprofloxacin | *By mouth*, 250–500 mg every 12 hours if eGFR 30–60 mL/minute/1.73 m² (every 24 hours if eGFR less than 30 mL/minute/1.73 m²); *by intravenous infusion* (200 mg over 30 minutes), 200–400 mg every 12 hours if eGFR 30–60 mL/minute/1.73 m² (every 24 hours if eGFR less than 30 mL/minute/1.73 m²) |
| Cisplatin | Avoid if possible; nephrotoxic |
| Citalopram | No information available for eGFR less than 20 mL/minute/1.73 m² |

| Drug | Comment |
|------|---------|
| *CitraFleet*® | Avoid if eGFR less than 30 mL/minute/1.73 m²—risk of hypermagnesaemia |
| *Citramag*® | Avoid if eGFR less than 30 mL/minute/1.73 m²—risk of hypermagnesaemia |
| Citrates | Absorption of aluminium from aluminium salts is increased by citrates, which are contained in many effervescent preparations (such as effervescent analgesics) |
| Cladribine | Regular monitoring recommended |
| Clarithromycin | Use half normal dose if eGFR less than 30 mL/minute/1.73 m²; avoid *Klaricid XL*® if eGFR less than 30 mL/minute/1.73 m² |
| Clavulanic acid [ingredient] | *see* Co-amoxiclav and *Timentin*® |
| Clobazam | *see* Anxiolytics and Hypnotics |
| Clodronate sodium | *see* Sodium Clodronate |
| Clofarabine | Manufacturer advises caution in mild to moderate renal impairment; avoid in severe renal impairment |
| Clomethiazole | *see* Anxiolytics and Hypnotics |
| Clopamide | *see* Thiazides and Related Diuretics |
| Clopidogrel | Manufacturer advises caution |
| Clozapine | Manufacturer advises avoid in severe renal impairment |
| Co-amoxiclav | Risk of crystalluria with high doses (particularly during parenteral therapy); reduce dose if eGFR less than 30 mL/minute/1.73 m²—consult product literature |
| Codeine | *see* Opioid Analgesics |
| Colchicine | Reduce dose if eGFR less than 50 mL/minute/1.73 m²; avoid if eGFR less than 10 mL/minute/1.73 m² |
| Colistin | Reduce dose and monitor plasma-colistin concentration during parenteral or nebulised treatment—consult product literature |
| *Combivir*® | Avoid if eGFR less than 50 mL/minute/1.73 m²; consult product literature |
| Corticosteroids | Use oral and parenteral preparations with caution |
| Cortisone | *see* Corticosteroids |
| Co-trimoxazole | Use half normal dose if eGFR 15–30 mL/minute/1.73 m²; avoid if eGFR less than 15 mL/minute/1.73 m² and if plasma-sulfamethoxazole concentration cannot be monitored |
| Cyclopenthiazide | *see* Thiazides and Related Diuretics |
| Cyclophosphamide | Reduce dose |
| Cycloserine | Reduce dose (see also p. 323); avoid in severe renal impairment |
| Cyclosporin | *see* Ciclosporin |

| Drug | Comment |
|------|---------|
| Dabigatran etexilate | Reduce initial dose to 75 mg and subsequent doses to 150 mg once daily if eGFR 30–50 mL/minute/1.73 m$^2$; avoid if eGFR less than 30 mL/minute/1.73 m$^2$ |
| Dacarbazine | Dose reduction may be required in combined renal and hepatic impairment; avoid in severe renal impairment |
| Dalteparin | Risk of bleeding may be increased—dose reduction, and monitoring of anti-Factor Xa, may be required; use of unfractionated heparin may be preferable |
| Danaparoid | Caution in moderate renal impairment; increased risk of bleeding (monitor anti-Factor Xa activity); avoid in severe renal impairment unless patient has heparin-induced thrombocytopenia and no alternative available |

For adjusting drug doses in renal impairment, see Important on p. 815.

| Drug | Comment |
|------|---------|
| Daptomycin | Monitor renal function if eGFR less than 80 mL/minute/1.73 m$^2$; for complicated skin and soft-tissue infections without bacteraemia use 4 mg/kg every 48 hours if eGFR less than 30 mL/minute/1.73 m$^2$; for other indications, consult product literature if eGFR less than 50 mL/minute/1.73 m$^2$ |
| Daunorubicin | Reduce dose by 25% if serum creatinine 105–265 micromol/litre and by 50% if serum creatinine greater than 265 micromol/litre |
| Deferasirox | Reduce dose by 10 mg/kg if eGFR 60–90 mL/minute/1.73 m$^2$ and if serum creatinine increased by more than 33% of baseline measurement on 2 consecutive occasions—interrupt treatment if deterioration in renal function persists after dose reduction; avoid if eGFR less than 60 mL/minute/1.73 m$^2$ |
| Deferiprone | Manufacturer advises caution—no information available |
| Deflazacort | see Corticosteroids |
| Degarelix | Manufacturer advises caution in severe renal impairment—no information available |
| Demeclocycline | Avoid |
| Desloratadine | Manufacturer advises caution in severe renal insufficiency |
| Desmopressin | Antidiuretic effect may be reduced |
| Dexamethasone | see Corticosteroids |
| Dexamfetamine | Manufacturer advises caution |
| Dexibuprofen | see NSAIDs; reduce initial dose; avoid if eGFR less than 30 mL/minute/1.73 m$^2$ |

| Drug | Comment |
|------|---------|
| Dexketoprofen | see NSAIDs; reduce initial dose to 50 mg daily; avoid in moderate to severe renal impairment |
| Dexrazoxane | Manufacturer of Cardioxane® advises reduce dose by 50% if creatinine clearance less than 40 mL/minute |
| Dextromethorphan | see Opioid Analgesics |
| Diafalk® | Manufacturer advises caution |
| Diamorphine | see Opioid Analgesics |
| Diazepam | see Anxiolytics and Hypnotics |
| Diazoxide | Dose reduction may be required |
| Diclofenac | see NSAIDs; avoid in severe renal impairment; avoid intravenous injection if serum creatinine greater than 160 micromol/litre |
| Didanosine | Reduce dose if eGFR less than 60 mL/minute/1.73 m$^2$; consult product literature |
| Digoxin | Reduce dose; toxicity increased by electrolyte disturbances |
| Dihydrocodeine | see Opioid Analgesics |
| Diltiazem | Start with smaller dose |
| Dinoprostone | Manufacturers advise avoid |
| Diphenoxylate | see Opioid Analgesics |
| Dipipanone | see Opioid Analgesics |
| Disodium etidronate | Reduce dose in mild renal impairment; avoid in moderate to severe renal impairment |
| Disodium pamidronate | Max. infusion rate 20 mg/hour; avoid if eGFR less than 30 mL/minute/1.73 m$^2$, except in life-threatening hypercalcaemia if benefit of use outweighs risk; if renal function deteriorates in patients with bone metastases, withhold dose until serum creatinine returns to within 10% of baseline value |
| Disopyramide | Reduce dose by increasing dose interval; adjust according to response; avoid sustained release preparation |
| Diuretics, potassium-sparing | see Potassium-sparing Diuretics |
| Domperidone | Manufacturer advises reduce dose |
| Doripenem | 250 mg every 8 hours if eGFR 30–50 mL/minute/1.73 m$^2$; 250 mg every 12 hours if eGFR less than 30 mL/minute/1.73 m$^2$ |
| Dorzolamide | Avoid if eGFR less than 30 mL/minute/1.73 m$^2$ |
| Doxycycline | Use with caution (avoid excessive doses) |
| Droperidol | In postoperative nausea and vomiting, max. 625 micrograms repeated every 6 hours as required; for nausea and vomiting caused by opioid analgesics in postoperative patient-controlled analgesia, reduce dose |
| Drospirenone [ingredient] | see Angeliq®, Yasmin®, and Yaz® |

| Drug | Comment |
|------|---------|
| Duloxetine | Avoid if eGFR less than 30 mL/minute/1.73 m² |
| Efavirenz | Manufacturer advises caution in severe renal failure—no information available; see also Atripla® |
| Eletriptan | Reduce initial dose to 20 mg; max. 40 mg in 24 hours; avoid if eGFR less than 30 mL/minute/1.73 m² |
| Emtricitabine | Reduce dose if eGFR less than 50 mL/minute/1.73 m²; consult product literature; see also Atripla® and Truvada® |
| Enalapril | see ACE inhibitors; max. initial dose 2.5 mg daily if eGFR less than 30 mL/minute/1.73 m² |
| Enoxaparin | Risk of bleeding increased; reduce dose if eGFR less than 30 mL/minute/1.73 m²—consult product literature for details; monitoring of anti-factor Xa may be required; use of unfractionated heparin may be preferable |
| Enoximone | Consider dose reduction |
| Entecavir | Reduce dose if eGFR less than 50 mL/minute/1.73 m²; consult product literature |
| Ephedrine | Use with caution |
| Eplerenone | Increased risk of hyperkalaemia—close monitoring required; avoid if eGFR less than 50 mL/minute/1.73 m² |
| Eprosartan | Halve initial dose if eGFR less than 60 mL/minute/1.73 m² |
| Eptifibatide | Reduce infusion to 1 microgram/kg/minute if eGFR 30–50 mL/minute/1.73 m²; avoid if eGFR less than 30 mL/minute/1.73 m² |
| Erdosteine | Avoid if eGFR less than 25 mL/minute/1.73 m²—no information available |
| Ergometrine | Manufacturer advises caution in mild or moderate renal impairment and avoid in severe renal impairment |
| Ergotamine | Avoid; risk of renal vasoconstriction |
| Erlotinib | Manufacturer advises avoid in severe renal impairment |
| Ertapenem | Risk of seizures; max. 500 mg daily if eGFR less than 30 mL/minute/1.73 m² |
| Erythromycin | Max. 1.5 g daily in severe renal impairment (ototoxicity) |
| Escitalopram | Manufacturer advises caution if eGFR less than 30 mL/minute/1.73 m² |
| Esmolol | Manufacturer advises caution |
| Esomeprazole | Manufacturer advises caution in severe renal insufficiency |
| Estramustine | Manufacturer advises caution |
| Ethambutol | Reduce dose; if creatinine clearance less than 30 mL/minute monitor plasma-ethambutol concentration; optic nerve damage |
| Etidronate disodium | see Disodium Etidronate |

| Drug | Comment |
|------|---------|
| Etodolac | see NSAIDs |
| Etoposide | Consider dose reduction |
| Etoricoxib | Avoid if eGFR less than 30 mL/minute/1.73 m²; see also NSAIDs |
| Exemestane | Manufacturer advises caution |
| Exenatide | Caution if eGFR 30–50 mL/minute/1.73 m²; avoid if eGFR less than 30 mL/minute/1.73 m² |
| Famciclovir | Reduce dose; consult product literature |
| Famotidine | Use normal dose every 36–48 hours or use half normal dose if eGFR less than 50 mL/minute/1.73 m²; seizures reported very rarely |
| Fenbufen | see NSAIDs |
| Fenofibrate | Reduce dose to 134 mg daily if eGFR less than 60 mL/minute/1.73 m²; reduce dose to 67 mg daily if eGFR less than 20 mL/minute/1.73 m²; avoid if eGFR less than 15 mL/minute/1.73 m² |
| Fenoprofen | see NSAIDs |
| Fentanyl | see Opioid Analgesics |
| Fesoterodine | Increase dose cautiously if eGFR 30–80 mL/minute/1.73 m²; max. 4 mg daily if eGFR less than 30 mL/minute/1.73 m²; consult product literature before concomitant use of cytochrome P450 enzyme inhibitors |
| Flecainide | Reduce initial oral dose to max. 100 mg daily or reduce intravenous dose by 50%, if eGFR less than 35 mL/minute/1.73 m² |
| Fleet Phospho-soda® | Manufacturer advises avoid in significant renal impairment |
| Flucloxacillin | Reduce dose if eGFR less than 10 mL/minute/1.73 m² |
| Fluconazole | Usual initial dose then halve subsequent doses if eGFR less than 50 mL/minute/1.73 m² |
| Flucytosine | Reduce dose and monitor plasma-flucytosine concentration—consult product literature |
| Fludarabine | Reduce dose by up to 50% if creatinine clearance 30–70 mL/minute; avoid if creatinine clearance less than 30 mL/minute |
| Fludrocortisone | see Corticosteroids |
| Flupentixol | see Antipsychotics; manufacturer advises caution; avoid in renal failure |
| Fluphenazine | see Antipsychotics; manufacturer advises caution; avoid in renal failure |
| Flurazepam | see Anxiolytics and Hypnotics |
| Flurbiprofen | see NSAIDs; avoid in severe renal impairment |
| Fluvoxamine | Start with smaller dose |

| Drug | Comment |
|------|---------|
| Fondaparinux | Increased risk of bleeding; for treatment of acute coronary syndromes avoid if eGFR less than 20 mL/minute/1.73 m²; for treatment of venous thromboembolism use with caution if eGFR 30–50 mL/minute/1.73 m², avoid if eGFR less than 30 mL/minute/1.73 m²; for prophylaxis of venous thromboembolism reduce dose to 1.5 mg daily if eGFR 20–50 mL/minute/1.73 m², avoid if less than 20 mL/minute/1.73 m² |
| Foscarnet | Reduce dose; consult product literature |
| Fosinopril | see ACE inhibitors |
| Fosphenytoin | Consider 10–25% reduction in dose or infusion rate (except initial dose for status epilepticus) |

> For adjusting drug doses in renal impairment, see Important on p. 815.

| Drug | Comment |
|------|---------|
| Frusemide | see Furosemide |
| Furosemide (frusemide) | May need high doses; deafness may follow rapid i/v injection |
| Fybogel Mebeverine® | Contains 2.5 mmol potassium per sachet |
| Gabapentin | Reduce dose if eGFR less than 80 mL/minute/1.73 m²; consult product literature |
| Galantamine | Avoid if eGFR less than 9 mL/minute/1.73 m² |
| Ganciclovir | Reduce dose if eGFR less than 70 mL/minute/1.73 m²; consult product literature |
| Ganirelix | Manufacturer advises avoid in moderate to severe renal impairment |
| Gemcitabine | Manufacturer advises caution |
| Gemeprost | Manufacturer advises avoid |
| Gemfibrozil | Initially 900 mg daily if eGFR 30–80 mL/minute/1.73 m²; avoid if eGFR less than 30 mL/minute/1.73 m² |
| Gentamicin | see Aminoglycosides |
| Gestrinone | Monitor closely; manufacturer advises avoid in severe renal impairment |
| Glatiramer | No information available—manufacturer advises caution |
| Glibenclamide | Avoid in severe renal impairment |
| Gliclazide | Reduce initial dose and monitor closely; avoid in severe renal impairment |
| Glimepiride | Avoid in severe renal impairment |
| Glipizide | Increased risk of hypoglycaemia; avoid in severe renal impairment or if hepatic impairment also present |
| Glyceryl trinitrate | see Nitrates |
| Guanethidine | Reduce dose if eGFR 40–65 mL/minute/1.73 m²; avoid if eGFR less than 40 mL/minute/1.73 m² |

| Drug | Comment |
|------|---------|
| Haloperidol | see Antipsychotics; manufacturer advises caution in renal impairment |
| Heparin | Risk of bleeding increased in severe renal impairment—dose may need to be reduced |
| Hetastarch | Avoid in severe renal impairment; excreted by kidney |
| Hydralazine | Reduce dose if eGFR less than 30 mL/minute/1.73 m² |
| Hydrochlorothiazide | see Thiazides and Related Diuretics |
| Hydrocortisone | see Corticosteroids |
| Hydroflumethiazide | see Thiazides and Related Diuretics |
| Hydromorphone | see Opioid Analgesics |
| Hydroxycarbamide (hydroxyurea) | For sickle-cell disease, reduce initial dose by 50% if eGFR less than 60 mL/minute/1.73 m²; avoid if eGFR less than 30 mL/minute/1.73 m² |
| Hydroxychloroquine | Manufacturer advises caution and monitoring of plasma-hydroxychloroquine concentration in severe renal impairment |
| Hydroxyzine | Use half normal dose |
| Hyoscine hydrobromide | Manufacturer advises caution |
| Hypnotics | see Anxiolytics and Hypnotics |
| Ibandronic acid | For treatment of osteoporosis, avoid if eGFR less than 30 mL/minute/1.73 m²; for reduction of bone damage in bone metastases, if eGFR 30–50 mL/minute/1.73 m² infuse normal dose over 1 hour, if eGFR less than 30 mL/minute/1.73 m² reduce intravenous dose to 2 mg and infuse over 1 hour, reduce oral dose to 50 mg once weekly |
| Ibuprofen | see NSAIDs; avoid in severe renal impairment |
| Idarubicin | Reduce dose; avoid in severe renal impairment |
| Ifosfamide | Avoid if serum creatinine concentration greater than 120 micromol/litre |
| Imatinib | Max. starting dose 400 mg daily if creatinine clearance less than 60 mL/minute |
| Imidapril | see ACE inhibitors; initial dose 2.5 mg daily if eGFR 30–80 mL/minute/1.73 m²; avoid if eGFR less than 30 mL/minute/1.73 m² |
| Imipenem [ingredient] | see Primaxin® |
| Indapamide | see Thiazides and Related Diuretics |
| Indometacin | see NSAIDs; avoid in severe renal impairment |
| Indoramin | Manufacturer advises caution |
| Inosine pranobex | Manufacturer advises caution; metabolised to uric acid |
| Insulin | May need dose reduction; insulin requirements fall; compensatory response to hypoglycaemia is impaired |

| Drug | Comment |
|---|---|
| Interferon alfa | Close monitoring required; avoid in severe renal impairment |
| Interferon beta | Manufacturers advise caution and close monitoring in severe renal impairment |
| Interferon gamma-1b | Manufacturer advises caution in severe renal impairment—risk of accumulation |
| Irinotecan | Manufacturer advises avoid—no information available |
| Iron dextran | Avoid in acute renal failure |
| Isometheptene [ingredient] | see *Midrid*® |
| Isoniazid | Max. 200 mg daily if eGFR less than 10 mL/minute/1.73 m²; peripheral neuropathy |
| Isosorbide dinitrate | see Nitrates |
| Isosorbide mono-nitrate | see Nitrates |
| Isotretinoin | Reduce initial dose (e.g. 10 mg daily) and increase gradually up to 1 mg/kg daily as tolerated |
| Itraconazole | Risk of congestive heart failure; bioavailability of oral formulations possibly reduced; use intravenous infusion with caution if eGFR 30–80 mL/minute/1.73 m² (monitor renal function); avoid intravenous infusion if eGFR less than 30 mL/minute/1.73 m² |
| Ivabradine | Use with caution if eGFR less than 15 mL/minute/1.73 m² |
| *Kaletra*® | Avoid oral solution due to propylene glycol content; use tablets with caution in severe renal impairment |
| Ketoprofen | see NSAIDs; avoid in severe renal impairment |
| Ketorolac | see NSAIDs; use lowest effective dose (max. 60 mg daily when given by intramuscular or intravenous injection); avoid if serum creatinine more than 160 micromol/litre |
| *Kivexa*® | Avoid if eGFR less than 50 mL/minute/1.73 m² |
| Labetalol | Dose reduction may be required |
| Lacosamide | Manufacturer advises caution; max. 250 mg daily if eGFR less than 30 mL/minute/1.73 m² |
| Lamivudine | Reduce dose if eGFR less than 50 mL/minute/1.73 m²; consult product literature; see also *Combivir*®, *Kivexa*®, and *Trizivir*® |
| Lamotrigine | Manufacturer advises caution in renal failure; metabolite may accumulate |
| Lapatinib | Manufacturer advises caution in severe renal impairment—no information available |
| Leflunomide | Manufacturer advises avoid in moderate or severe impairment—no information available |

| Drug | Comment |
|---|---|
| Lenalidomide | Starting dose 10 mg once daily if creatinine clearance 30–50 mL/minute; starting dose 15 mg on alternate days if creatinine clearance less than 30 mL/minute |
| Lepirudin | Reduce initial intravenous injection dose to 200 micrograms/kg and reduce subsequent infusion dose by 50–85% if eGFR less than 60 mL/minute/1.73 m²; but avoid or stop infusion if eGFR less than 15 mL/minute/1.73 m² (consult product literature) |
| Lercanidipine | Avoid if eGFR less than 30 mL/minute/1.73 m² |
| Letrozole | Manufacturer advises caution if creatinine clearance less than 10 mL/minute |
| Levetiracetam | Max. 2 g daily if eGFR 50–80 mL/minute/1.73 m²; max. 1.5 g daily if eGFR 30–50 mL/minute/1.73 m²; max. 1 g daily if eGFR less than 30 mL/minute/1.73 m² |
| Levocetirizine | 5 mg on alternate days if eGFR 30–50 mL/minute/1.73 m²; 5 mg every 3 days if eGFR 10–30 mL/minute/1.73 m²; avoid if eGFR less than 10 mL/minute/1.73 m² |
| Levofloxacin | Usual initial dose then reduce subsequent doses (consult product literature) if eGFR less than 50 mL/minute/1.73 m² |
| Levomepromazine (methotrimeprazine) | see Antipsychotics |
| Lidocaine | Possible accumulation of lidocaine and active metabolite; manufacturers advise caution in severe renal impairment |
| Linezolid | Manufacturer advises metabolites may accumulate if eGFR less than 30 mL/minute/1.73 m² |
| Lisinopril | see ACE inhibitors; max. initial doses 5–10 mg daily if eGFR 30–80 mL/minute/1.73 m² (max. 40 mg daily); 2.5–5 mg daily if eGFR 10–30 mL/minute/1.73 m² (max. 40 mg daily); 2.5 mg daily if eGFR less than 10 mL/minute/1.73 m² |
| Lithium salts | Avoid if possible or reduce dose and monitor serum-lithium concentration carefully |
| Lofepramine | Manufacturer advises avoid in severe impairment |
| Lofexidine | Manufacturer advises caution in chronic renal impairment |
| Lopinavir [ingredient] | see *Kaletra*® |
| Loprazolam | see Anxiolytics and Hypnotics |
| Lorazepam | see Anxiolytics and Hypnotics |
| Lormetazepam | see Anxiolytics and Hypnotics |
| Lumefantrine [ingredient] | see *Riamet*® |
| Lymecycline | Avoid |

| Drug | Comment |
|------|---------|
| Magnesium salts | Avoid or reduce dose; increased risk of toxicity; magnesium carbonate mixture and magnesium trisilicate mixture also have high sodium content |
| *Malarone*® | Avoid for malaria prophylaxis (and if possible for malaria treatment) if eGFR less than 30 mL/minute/1.73 m² |
| Mannitol | Use with caution in severe renal impairment |
| Maraviroc | If eGFR less than 80 mL/minute/1.73 m², consult product literature |
| Mefenamic acid | *see* NSAIDs; avoid in severe renal impairment |

For adjusting drug doses in renal impairment, see Important on p. 815.

| Drug | Comment |
|------|---------|
| Melatonin | No information available—manufacturer advises caution |
| Meloxicam | *see* NSAIDs; avoid if eGFR less than 25 mL/minute/1.73 m² |
| Melphalan | Reduce dose initially (consult product literature) |
| Memantine | Reduce dose to 10 mg daily if eGFR 30–49 mL/minute/1.73 m², if well tolerated after at least 7 days dose can be increased in steps to 20 mg daily; reduce dose to 10 mg daily if eGFR 5–29 mL/minute/1.73 m²; avoid if eGFR less than 5 mL/minute/1.73 m² |
| Meprobamate | *see* Anxiolytics and Hypnotics |
| Meptazinol | *see* Opioid Analgesics |
| Mercaptopurine | Reduce dose |
| Meropenem | Use normal dose every 12 hours if eGFR 26–50 mL/minute/1.73 m²; use half normal dose every 12 hours if eGFR 10–25 mL/minute/1.73 m²; use half normal dose every 24 hours if eGFR less than 10 mL/minute/1.73 m² |
| Mesalazine | Use with caution; avoid if eGFR less than 20 mL/minute/1.73 m² |
| Metformin | *see* Metformin, p. 383 |
| Methadone | *see* Opioid Analgesics |
| Methenamine | Avoid if eGFR less than 10 mL/minute/1.73 m²—risk of hippurate crystalluria |
| Methocarbamol | Manufacturer advises caution |
| Methotrexate | Reduce dose; risk of nephrotoxicity at high doses; avoid in severe renal impairment |
| Methotrimeprazine | *see* Antipsychotics |
| Methyldopa | Start with small dose; increased sensitivity to hypotensive and sedative effect |

| Drug | Comment |
|------|---------|
| Methylnaltrexone | If eGFR less than 30 mL/minute/1.73 m², reduce dose as follows: body-weight under 62 kg, 75 micrograms/kg on alternate days; body-weight 62–114 kg, 8 mg on alternate days; body-weight over 114 kg, 75 micrograms/kg on alternate days |
| Methylprednisolone | *see* Corticosteroids |
| Methysergide | Avoid |
| Metoclopramide | Avoid or use small dose in severe renal impairment; increased risk of extrapyramidal reactions |
| Metolazone | *see* Thiazides and Related Diuretics |
| Micafungin | Use with caution; renal function may deteriorate |
| Midazolam | *see* Anxiolytics and Hypnotics |
| *Midrid*® | Manufacturer advises avoid in severe renal impairment |
| Mifepristone | Manufacturer advises avoid |
| Miglustat | For Gaucher's disease initially 100 mg twice daily if eGFR 50–70 mL/minute/1.73 m²; initially 100 mg once daily if eGFR 30–50 mL/minute/1.73 m²; for Niemann-Pick type C disease, initially 200 mg twice daily if eGFR 50–70 mL/minute/1.73 m²; initially 100 mg twice daily if eGFR 30–50 mL/minute/1.73 m²; child under 12 years—consult product literature; avoid if eGFR less than 30 mL/minute/1.73 m² |
| Milrinone | Reduce dose if eGFR less than 50 mL/minute/1.73 m²—consult product literature for details |
| Minocycline | Use with caution (avoid excessive doses) |
| Minoxidil | Use with caution in significant renal impairment |
| Mirtazapine | Clearance reduced by 30% if eGFR less than 40 mL/minute/1.73 m²; clearance reduced by 50% if eGFR less than 10 mL/minute/1.73 m² |
| Mitotane | Manufacturer advises caution in mild to moderate renal impairment—monitoring of plasma-mitotane concentration recommended; avoid in severe renal impairment |
| Mivacurium | Clinical effect prolonged in renal failure—reduce dose according to response |
| Modafinil | Manufacturer advises use half normal dose in severe renal impairment |
| Moexipril | *see* ACE inhibitors; initial dose 3.75 mg once daily if eGFR less than 40 mL/minute/1.73 m² |
| Morphine | *see* Opioid Analgesics |
| *Moviprep*® | Caution if eGFR less than 30 mL/minute/1.73 m² |

| Drug | Comment |
|------|---------|
| Moxonidine | Max. single dose 200 micrograms and max. daily dose 400 micrograms if eGFR 30–60 mL/minute/1.73 m²; avoid if eGFR less than 30 mL/minute/1.73 m² |
| Nabumetone | see NSAIDs; avoid in severe renal impairment |
| Nadolol | Increase dosage interval if eGFR less than 50 mL/minute/1.73 m² |
| Nalidixic acid | Use with caution; avoid if eGFR less than 20 mL/minute/1.73 m² |
| Naltrexone | Manufacturers advise caution |
| Naproxen | see NSAIDs; avoid if eGFR less than 30 mL/minute/1.73 m² |
| Naratriptan | Max. 2.5 mg in 24 hours; avoid if eGFR less than 15 mL/minute/1.73 m² |
| Narcotic analgesics | see Opioid Analgesics |
| Nebivolol | For hypertension, initially 2.5 mg once daily, increased to 5 mg once daily if required; for heart failure, manufacturer advises avoid if serum creatinine greater than 250 micromol/litre |
| Nelfinavir | Manufacturer advises caution |
| Neomycin | Avoid; ototoxic; nephrotoxic |
| Neostigmine | May need dose reduction |
| Nicardipine | Start with small dose |
| Nicotine | Manufacturers advise caution in severe renal impairment |
| Nicoumalone | see Acenocoumarol |
| Nimodipine | Manufacturer advises caution with intravenous administration |
| Nitrates | Manufacturer advises use with caution in severe renal impairment |
| Nitrazepam | see Anxiolytics and Hypnotics |
| Nitrofurantoin | Avoid if eGFR less than 60 mL/minute/1.73 m²; ineffective because of inadequate urine concentrations |
| Nitroprusside | see Sodium Nitroprusside |
| Nizatidine | Use half normal dose if eGFR 20–50 mL/minute/1.73 m²; use one-quarter normal dose if eGFR less than 20 mL/minute/1.73 m² |
| Norfloxacin | Use half normal dose if eGFR less than 30 mL/minute/1.73 m² |
| NSAIDs | Use lowest effective dose for the shortest possible duration and monitor renal function; sodium and water retention; deterioration in renal function possibly leading to renal failure; deterioration also reported after topical use; see also individual drugs |
| Ofloxacin | Usual initial dose, then use half normal dose if eGFR 20–50 mL/minute/1.73 m²; 100 mg every 24 hours if eGFR less than 20 mL/minute/1.73 m² |

| Drug | Comment |
|------|---------|
| Olanzapine | Consider lower initial dose of 5 mg daily |
| Olmesartan | Max. 20 mg daily if eGFR 20–60 mL/minute/1.73 m²; avoid if eGFR less than 20 mL/minute/1.73 m² |
| Olsalazine | Use with caution; manufacturer advises avoid in significant renal impairment |
| Omalizumab | Manufacturer advises caution—no information available |
| Opioid analgesics | Reduce doses or avoid; increased and prolonged effect; increased cerebral sensitivity |
| Oseltamivir | For treatment, use 75 mg once daily or 30 mg twice daily if eGFR 10–30 mL/minute/1.73 m²; for prevention, use 75 mg every 48 hours or 30 mg once daily if eGFR 10–30 mL/minute/1.73 m²; avoid for treatment and prevention if eGFR less than 10 mL/minute/1.73 m² |
| Oxaliplatin | Manufacturer advises avoid if creatinine clearance less than 30 mL/minute |
| Oxazepam | see Anxiolytics and Hypnotics |
| Oxcarbazepine | Use half initial dose if eGFR less than 30 mL/minute/1.73 m²; increase according to response at intervals of at least 1 week |
| Oxpentifylline | see Pentoxifylline |
| Oxybutynin | Manufacturer advises caution |
| Oxycodone | see Opioid Analgesics |
| Oxytetracycline | Avoid |
| Paliperidone | Initially 3 mg once daily if eGFR 50–80 mL/minute/1.73 m² (max. 6 mg once daily); initially 1.5 mg once daily if eGFR 10–50 mL/minute/1.73 m² (max. 3 mg once daily); avoid if eGFR less than 10 mL/minute/1.73 m² |
| Pamidronate disodium | see Disodium Pamidronate |
| Pancuronium | Manufacturer advises caution; prolonged duration of block |
| Pantoprazole | Max. oral dose 40 mg daily |
| Papaveretum | see Opioid Analgesics |
| Paracetamol | Increase infusion dose interval to every 6 hours if eGFR less than 30 mL/minute/1.73 m² |
| Parathyroid hormone | Avoid if eGFR less than 30 mL/minute/1.73 m² |
| Parecoxib | see NSAIDs |
| Paroxetine | Reduce dose if eGFR less than 30 mL/minute/1.73 m² |
| Peginterferon alfa | Close monitoring required—reduce dose in moderate to severe renal impairment; consult product literature |
| Pemetrexed | Manufacturer advises avoid if creatinine clearance less than 45 mL/minute |
| Penicillamine | Reduce dose and monitor renal function or avoid (consult product literature) |

| Drug | Comment |
| --- | --- |
| Pentamidine | Reduce dose for pneumocystis pneumonia if eGFR less than 10 mL/minute/1.73 m$^2$—consult product literature |
| Pentazocine | *see* Opioid Analgesics |
| Pentostatin | Avoid if creatinine clearance less than 60 mL/minute |
| Pentoxifylline (oxpentifylline) | Reduce dose by 30–50% if eGFR less than 30 mL/minute/1.73 m$^2$ |
| Pericyazine | Manufacturer advises avoid |
| Perindopril arginine | *see* ACE inhibitors; max. initial doses 2.5 mg once daily if eGFR 30–60 mL/minute/1.73 m$^2$; 2.5 mg once daily on alternate days if eGFR 15–30 mL/minute/1.73 m$^2$ |
| Perindopril erbumine | *see* ACE inhibitors; max. initial doses 2 mg once daily if eGFR 30–60 mL/minute/1.73 m$^2$; 2 mg once daily on alternate days if eGFR 15–30 mL/minute/1.73 m$^2$ |
| Perphenazine | *see* Antipsychotics |

For adjusting drug doses in renal impairment, see Important on p. 815.

| Drug | Comment |
| --- | --- |
| Pethidine | *see* Opioid Analgesics |
| Phenindione | *see* Anticoagulants, Oral |
| Phenobarbital | Use with caution |
| Phenothiazines | *see* Antipsychotics |
| Pholcodine | *see* Opioid Analgesics |
| *Picolax*® | Avoid if eGFR less than 30 mL/minute/1.73 m$^2$—risk of hypermagnesaemia |
| Pilocarpine | Manufacturer advises caution with tablets |
| Pimozide | *see* Antipsychotics |
| Pindolol | May adversely affect renal function in severe impairment—manufacturer advises avoid |
| Piperacillin with tazobactam | Max. 4.5 g every 8 hours if eGFR 20–80 mL/minute/1.73 m$^2$; max. 4.5 g every 12 hours if eGFR less than 20 mL/minute/1.73 m$^2$; child under 12 years: Consult product literature |
| Piperazine | Use with caution; avoid in severe renal impairment; risk of neurotoxicity |
| Pipotiazine | *see* Antipsychotics |
| Piracetam | Use two-thirds of normal dose if eGFR 50–80 mL/minute/1.73 m$^2$; use one-third of normal dose in 2 divided doses if eGFR 30–50 mL/minute/1.73 m$^2$; use one-sixth normal dose as a single dose if eGFR 20–30 mL/minute/1.73 m$^2$; avoid if eGFR less than 20 mL/minute/1.73 m$^2$ |
| Piroxicam | *see* NSAIDs |
| Potassium salts | Close monitoring required—high risk of hyperkalaemia; avoid in severe renal impairment |

| Drug | Comment |
| --- | --- |
| Potassium-sparing diuretics | Monitor plasma-potassium concentration (high risk of hyperkalaemia in renal impairment); manufacturers advise avoid in severe renal impairment; *see also* Eplerenone |
| Povidone–iodine | Avoid regular application to inflamed or broken mucosa |
| Pramipexole | In Parkinson's disease, initially 88 micrograms twice daily if eGFR 20–50 mL/minute/1.73 m$^2$ (88 micrograms once daily if eGFR less than 20 mL/minute/1.73 m$^2$); if renal function declines during treatment, reduce dose by the same percentage as the decline in eGFR; in restless legs syndrome, reduce dose if eGFR less than 20 mL/minute/1.73 m$^2$ |
| Prasugrel | Use with caution in renal impairment—increased risk of bleeding |
| Pravastatin | Manufacturer advises initial dose of 10 mg once daily in moderate to severe renal impairment |
| Prazosin | Initially 500 micrograms daily in moderate to severe renal impairment; increased with caution |
| Prednisolone | *see* Corticosteroids |
| Pregabalin | Initially 75 mg daily and max. 300 mg daily if eGFR 30–60 mL/minute/1.73 m$^2$; initially 25–50 mg daily and max. 150 mg daily in 1–2 divided doses if eGFR 15–30 mL/minute/1.73 m$^2$; initially 25 mg once daily and max. 75 mg once daily if eGFR less than 15 mL/minute/1.73 m$^2$ |
| Prilocaine | Manufacturer advises caution |
| *Primaxin*® | Reduce dose if eGFR less than 70 mL/minute/1.73 m$^2$—consult product literature |
| Primidone | *see* Phenobarbital |
| Probenecid | Avoid if eGFR less than 30 mL/minute/1.73 m$^2$ |
| Procarbazine | Use with caution; avoid in severe renal impairment |
| Prochlorperazine | *see* Antipsychotics |
| Proguanil | 100 mg once daily if eGFR 20–60 mL/minute/1.73 m$^2$; 50 mg on alternate days if eGFR 10–20 mL/minute/1.73 m$^2$; 50 mg once weekly if eGFR less than 10 mL/minute/1.73 m$^2$ (increased risk of haematological toxicity) |
| Promazine | *see* Antipsychotics |
| Propantheline | Manufacturer advises caution |
| Propiverine | Doses above 30 mg daily should be used with caution if eGFR less than 30 mL/minute/1.73 m$^2$ |
| Propofol | Use with caution |
| Propranolol | Manufacturer advises caution—dose reduction may be required |

| Drug | Comment |
|---|---|
| Propylthiouracil | Use three-quarters normal dose if eGFR 10–50 mL/minute/1.73 m² ; use half normal dose if eGFR less than 10 mL/minute/1.73 m² |
| Pseudoephedrine | Manufacturer advises caution in moderate to severe renal impairment |
| Pyridostigmine | Reduce dose; excreted by kidney |
| Pyrimethamine | Manufacturer advises caution |
| Quetiapine | For *immediate-release tablets*, initially 25 mg daily, increased daily in steps of 25–50 mg; for *modified-release tablets*, initially 50 mg daily, increased daily in steps of 50 mg |
| Quinagolide | Manufacturer advises avoid—no information available |
| Quinapril | *see* ACE inhibitors; max. initial dose 2.5 mg once daily if eGFR less than 40 mL/minute/1.73 m² |
| Quinine | For treatment of malaria in severe renal impairment, reduce parenteral maintenance dose to 5–7 mg/kg of salt |
| Raloxifene | Manufacturer advises caution in mild to moderate renal impairment; avoid in severe renal impairment |
| Raltitrexed | Reduce dose and increase dosing interval if creatinine clearance less than 65 mL/minute (consult product literature); avoid if creatinine clearance less than 25 mL/minute |
| Ramipril | *see* ACE inhibitors; max. initial dose 1.25 mg once daily (do not exceed 5 mg once daily) if eGFR 10–30 mL/minute/1.73 m² ; max. initial dose 1.25 mg once daily (do not exceed 2.5 mg once daily) if eGFR less than 10 mL/minute/1.73 m² |
| Ranitidine | Use half normal dose if eGFR less than 50 mL/minute/1.73 m² |
| Ranolazine | Use with caution if eGFR 30–80 mL/minute/1.73 m² ; avoid if eGFR less than 30 mL/minute/1.73 m² |
| Reboxetine | Initial dose 2 mg twice daily, increased according to tolerance |
| *Riamet*® | Manufacturer advises caution in severe renal impairment—monitor ECG and plasma potassium concentration |
| Ribavirin | Plasma-ribavirin concentration increased; avoid oral ribavirin unless essential if eGFR less than 50 mL/minute/1.73 m²—monitor haemoglobin concentration closely |
| Rifabutin | Use half normal dose if eGFR less than 30 mL/minute/1.73 m² |
| Riluzole | No information available—manufacturer advises avoid |

| Drug | Comment |
|---|---|
| Rimonabant | Manufacturer advises avoid in severe impairment—no information available |
| Risedronate sodium | Avoid if eGFR less than 30 mL/minute/1.73 m² |
| Risperidone | Manufacturer advises initial and subsequent oral doses should be halved |
| Ritonavir [ingredient] | *see Kaletra*® |
| Rivaroxaban | Use with caution if eGFR 15–29 mL/minute/1.73 m² or if eGFR 30–49 mL/minute/1.73 m² and concomitant use of drugs that increase plasma-rivaroxaban concentration (consult product literature); avoid if eGFR less than 15 mL/minute/1.73 m² |
| Rivastigmine | Manufacturer advises caution |
| Rizatriptan | Manufacturer advises reduce dose to 5 mg in mild to moderate renal impairment; avoid in severe renal impairment |
| Rocuronium | Reduce maintenance dose; prolonged paralysis |
| Ropinirole | Avoid if eGFR less than 30 mL/minute/1.73 m² |
| Ropivacaine | Manufacturer advises caution in chronic renal impairment |
| Rosiglitazone | Caution if eGFR less than 30 mL/minute/1.73 m² |
| Rosuvastatin | Initially 5 mg once daily (do not exceed 20 mg daily) if eGFR 30–60 mL/minute/1.73 m² ; avoid if eGFR less than 30 mL/minute/1.73 m² |
| Sapropterin | Manufacturer advises caution—no information available |
| Saquinavir | Dose adjustment possibly required if eGFR less than 30 mL/minute/1.73 m²—no information available |
| Sertraline | Manufacturer advises caution |
| Sevoflurane | Manufacturer advises caution |
| Sibutramine | Use with caution if eGFR 30–80 mL/minute/1.73 m² ; avoid if eGFR less than 30 mL/minute/1.73 m² |
| Sildenafil | For erectile dysfunction initial dose 25 mg if eGFR less than 30 mL/minute/1.73 m² ; for pulmonary hypertension reduce to 20 mg twice daily if usual dose not tolerated |
| Simvastatin | Doses above 10 mg daily should be used with caution if eGFR less than 30 mL/minute/1.73 m² |
| Sitagliptin | Avoid if eGFR less than 50 mL/minute/1.73 m² |
| Sodium aurothiomalate | Caution in mild to moderate renal impairment; avoid in severe renal impairment |
| Sodium bicarbonate | Avoid; specialised role in some forms of renal disease, *see* section 9.2.1.3 |
| Sodium citrate | Use with caution, *see also* Citrates |

Appendix 3: Renal impairment

| Drug | Comment |
|------|---------|
| Sodium clodronate | Use half normal dose if eGFR 10–30 mL/minute/1.73 m²; avoid if eGFR less than 10 mL/minute/1.73 m² |
| Sodium nitroprusside | Cyanide or thiocyanate metabolites may accumulate—avoid prolonged use |
| Sodium oxybate | Caution—*Xyrem*® oral solution contains 3.96 mmol Na⁺/mL |
| Sodium phenylbutyrate | Manufacturer advises caution |
| Sodium valproate | *see* Valproate |
| Solifenacin | Max. 5 mg daily if eGFR less than 30 mL/minute/1.73 m² |
| Solpadol® | Avoid effervescent tablets; contains 16.9 mmol sodium per tablet; *see also* Opioid Analgesics |

For adjusting drug doses in renal impairment, see Important on p. 815.

| Drug | Comment |
|------|---------|
| Sotalol | Use half normal dose if eGFR 30–60 mL/minute/1.73 m²; use one-quarter normal dose if eGFR 10–30 mL/minute/1.73 m²; avoid if eGFR less than 10 mL/minute/1.73 m² |
| Spironolactone | *see* Potassium-sparing Diuretics |
| Stavudine | Use half normal dose every 12 hours if eGFR 25–50 mL/minute/1.73 m²; use half normal dose every 24 hours if eGFR less than 25 mL/minute/1.73 m² |
| Streptomycin | *see* Aminoglycosides |
| Strontium ranelate | Avoid if eGFR less than 30 mL/minute/1.73 m² |
| Sucralfate | Use with caution; aluminium is absorbed and may accumulate |
| Sugammadex | Avoid if eGFR less than 30 mL/minute/1.73 m² |
| Sulfadiazine | Use with caution; avoid in severe renal impairment; high risk of crystalluria |
| Sulfasalazine | Risk of toxicity including crystalluria—ensure high fluid intake; avoid in severe renal impairment |
| Sulfinpyrazone | Reduce dose; avoid in severe renal impairment |
| Sulindac | *see* NSAIDs; avoid in severe renal impairment |
| Sulphonamides | Ensure high fluid intake; rashes and blood disorders; crystalluria a risk; *see also* individual drugs |
| Sulphonylureas | *see under* individual drugs |
| Sulpiride | Reduce dose; avoid in severe renal impairment |
| Sumatriptan | Manufacturer advises caution |
| Tacalcitol | Monitor serum calcium concentration |
| Tadalafil | Max. dose 10 mg if eGFR less than 30 mL/minute/1.73 m² (avoid regular once-daily dosing) |
| Tamsulosin | Use with caution if eGFR less than 10 mL/minute/1.73 m² |

| Drug | Comment |
|------|---------|
| Tazobactam [ingredient] | *see* Piperacillin with tazobactam |
| Teicoplanin | On day 4 use half normal dose if eGFR is 40–60 mL/minute/1.73 m² and use one-third normal dose if eGFR is less than 40 mL/minute/1.73 m² |
| Telbivudine | 600 mg every 48 hours if eGFR 30–49 mL/minute/1.73 m²; 600 mg every 72 hours if eGFR less than 30 mL/minute/1.73 m² |
| Telithromycin | Manufacturer advises avoid if possible if eGFR less than 30 mL/minute/1.73 m²—if no alternative, use alternating daily doses of 800 mg and 400 mg, starting with 800 mg dose |
| Telmisartan | Manufacturer advises initial dose of 20 mg once daily in severe renal impairment |
| Temazepam | *see* Anxiolytics and Hypnotics |
| Temocillin | Use normal dose every 24 hours if eGFR 10–30 mL/minute/1.73 m²; use normal dose every 48 hours if eGFR less than 10 mL/minute/1.73 m² |
| Temsirolimus | Manufacturer advises caution in severe renal impairment—no information available |
| Tenofovir | Monitor renal function—interrupt treatment if further deterioration; 245 mg every 2 days if eGFR 30–50 mL/minute/1.73 m²; 245 mg every 3–4 days if eGFR 10–30 mL/minute/1.73 m²; *see also* Atripla® and Truvada® |
| Tenoxicam | *see* NSAIDs; avoid in severe renal impairment |
| Terbinafine | Use half normal dose if eGFR less than 50 mL/minute/1.73 m² |
| Tetracosactide | *see* Corticosteroids |
| Tetracyclines | Avoid tetracyclines except doxycycline or minocycline which may be used cautiously (avoid excessive doses) |
| Thalidomide | Manufacturer advises caution in severe renal impairment—no information available |
| Thiazides and related diuretics | Avoid if eGFR less than 30 mL/minute/1.73 m²—ineffective (metolazone remains effective but risk of excessive diuresis) |
| Tiaprofenic acid | *see* NSAIDs; avoid in severe renal impairment |
| Ticarcillin [ingredient] | *see* Timentin® |
| Tiludronic acid | Use with caution and monitor renal function regularly if eGFR 30–90 mL/minute/1.73 m²; avoid if eGFR less than 30 mL/minute/1.73 m² |

| Drug | Comment |
|------|---------|
| *Timentin®* | Reduce dose to 3.2 g every eight hours if eGFR 30–60 mL/minute/1.73 m²; 1.6 g every eight hours if eGFR 10–30 mL/minute/1.73 m²; 1.6 g every twelve hours if eGFR less than 10 mL/minute/1.73 m² |
| Timolol | Manufacturer advises caution—dose reduction may be required |
| Tinzaparin | Risk of bleeding may be increased—dose reduction, and monitoring of anti-Factor Xa may be required; use with caution in elderly and avoid if age over 90 years; unfractionated heparin may be preferable |
| Tioguanine | Reduce dose |
| Tiotropium | Plasma-tiotropium concentration raised; use with caution if eGFR less than 50 mL/minute/1.73 m² |
| Tirofiban | Increased risk of bleeding; monitor carefully if eGFR less than 60 mL/minute/1.73 m²; use half normal dose if eGFR less than 30 mL/minute/1.73 m² |
| Tizanidine | Manufacturer advises caution |
| Tobramycin | *see* Aminoglycosides |
| Tolbutamide | Reduce initial dose and monitor closely; avoid in severe renal impairment |
| Tolcapone | Caution if eGFR less than 30 mL/minute/1.73 m² |
| Iolfenamic acid | *see* NSAIDs |
| Tolterodine | Reduce dose to 1 mg twice daily if eGFR less than 30 mL/minute/1.73 m²; avoid *Detrusitol®* XL if eGFR less than 30 mL/minute/1.73 m² |
| Topiramate | Longer time to steady-state plasma concentrations |
| Topotecan | Reduce dose; avoid infusion if creatinine clearance less than 20 mL/minute; avoid oral route if creatinine clearance less than 60 mL/minute |
| Torasemide | May need high doses |
| Trabectedin | Avoid if creatinine clearance less than 30 mL/minute |
| Tramadol | *see* Opioid Analgesics |
| Trandolapril | *see* ACE Inhibitors; max. 2 mg daily if eGFR less than 10 mL/minute/1.73 m² |
| Tranexamic acid | Reduce dose—consult product literature for details |
| Tretinoin (oral) | Reduce dose to 25 mg/m² |
| Triamcinolone | *see* Corticosteroids |
| Triamterene | *see* Potassium-sparing Diuretics |
| Tribavirin | *see* Ribavirin |
| Triclofos | *see* Anxiolytics and Hypnotics |
| Trifluoperazine | *see* Antipsychotics |
| Trimeprazine | *see* Alimemazine |

| Drug | Comment |
|------|---------|
| Trimethoprim | Use half normal dose after 3 days if eGFR 15–30 mL/minute/1.73 m²; use half normal dose if eGFR less than 15 mL/minute/1.73 m²(monitor plasma-trimethoprim concentration if eGFR less than 10 mL/minute/1.73 m²) |
| Tripotassium dicitratobismuthate | Avoid in severe renal impairment |
| *Trizivir®* | Manufacturer advises avoid if eGFR less than 50 mL/minute/1.73m² or in end-stage renal disease; consult product literature |
| Trospium | Use with caution; reduce dose to 20 mg once daily or 20 mg on alternate days if eGFR 10–30 mL/minute/1.73 m² |
| *Truvada®* | Monitor renal function; use normal dose every 48 hours if eGFR 30–50 mL/minute/1.73 m²; avoid if eGFR less than 30 mL/minute/1.73 m² |
| *Tylex®* | Manufacturer advises caution in severe impairment; effervescent tablets contain 13.6 mmol sodium per tablet; *see also* Opioid Analgesics |
| Valaciclovir | For *herpes zoster*, 1 g every 12 hours if eGFR 15–30 mL/minute/1.73 m² (every 24 hours if eGFR less than 15 mL/minute/1.73 m²); for *treatment of herpes simplex*, 500 mg every 24 hours if eGFR less than 15 mL/minute/1.73 m²; for *suppression of herpes simplex*, 250 mg (500 mg in immunocompromised) every 24 hours if eGFR less than 15 mL/minute/1.73 m²; for *reduction of genital herpes transmission*, 250 mg every 24 hours if eGFR less than 15 mL/minute/1.73 m²; reduce dose according to eGFR for *cytomegalovirus prophylaxis* following renal transplantation (consult product literature) |
| Valganciclovir | Reduce dose; consult product literature |
| Valproate | Reduce dose; adjust dosage according to free serum valproic acid concentration |
| Valproic acid | *see* Valproate |
| Valsartan | Use with caution if eGFR less than 10 mL/minute/1.73 m²—no information available |
| Vancomycin | Reduce dose—monitor plasma-vancomycin concentration and renal function regularly |
| Vardenafil | Initial dose 5 mg if eGFR less than 30 mL/minute/1.73 m² |
| Varenicline | If eGFR less than 30 mL/minute/1.73 m², initial dose 500 micrograms once daily, increased after 3 days to 1 mg once daily |

| Drug | Comment |
|------|---------|
| Venlafaxine | Use half normal dose (immediate-release tablets may be given once daily) if eGFR 10–30 mL/minute/1.73 m$^2$; avoid if eGFR less than 10 mL/minute/1.73 m$^2$ |
| Vigabatrin | Consider reduced dose or increased dose interval if eGFR less than 60 mL/minute/1.73 m$^2$ |
| Vildagliptin | Avoid if eGFR less than 50 mL/minute/1.73 m$^2$ |
| Voriconazole | Intravenous vehicle may accumulate if eGFR less than 50 mL/minute/1.73 m$^2$—use intravenous infusion only if potential benefit outweighs risk, and monitor renal function; alternatively, use tablets or oral suspension (no dose adjustment required) |
| Warfarin | *see* Anticoagulants, Oral |

For adjusting drug doses in renal impairment, see Important on p. 815.

| Drug | Comment |
|------|---------|
| Xipamide | *see* Thiazides and Related Diuretics |
| *Yasmin*® | Avoid if eGFR less than 30 mL/minute/1.73 m$^2$ |
| *Yaz*® | Manufacturer advises avoid if creatinine clearance less than 30 mL/minute |
| Zafirlukast | Manufacturer advises caution in moderate to severe impairment |
| Zidovudine | Reduce oral dose to 300–400 mg daily in divided doses or intravenous dose to 1 mg/kg 3–4 times daily if eGFR less than 10 mL/minute/1.73 m$^2$; *see also* Combivir® and Trizivir® |
| Zoledronic acid | Avoid if serum creatinine above 400 micromol/litre in tumour-induced hypercalcaemia; in advanced malignancies involving bone, if eGFR 50–60 mL/minute/1.73 m$^2$ reduce dose to 3.5 mg every 3–4 weeks, if eGFR 40–50 mL/minute/1.73 m$^2$ reduce dose to 3.3 mg every 3–4 weeks, if eGFR 30–40 mL/minute/1.73 m$^2$ reduce dose to 3 mg every 3–4 weeks, avoid if eGFR less than 30 mL/minute/1.73 m$^2$ (or if serum creatinine greater than 265 micromol/litre); if renal function deteriorates in patients with bone metastases, withhold dose until serum creatinine returns to within 10% of baseline value; avoid in Paget's disease, treatment of postmenopausal osteoporosis and osteoporosis in men if eGFR less than 35 mL/minute/1.73 m$^2$ |
| Zonisamide | Initially increase dose at 2-week intervals; discontinue if renal function deteriorates |

| Drug | Comment |
|------|---------|
| Zopiclone | *see* Anxiolytics and Hypnotics |
| Zotepine | Initial dose 25 mg twice daily, increased gradually according to response (max. 75 mg twice daily) |
| Zuclopenthixol | *see* Antipsychotics |

# A4 Pregnancy

Drugs can have harmful effects on the embryo or fetus at any time during pregnancy. It is important to bear this in mind when prescribing for a woman of *childbearing age* or for men *trying to father* a child.

During the *first trimester* drugs can produce congenital malformations (teratogenesis), and the period of greatest risk is from the third to the eleventh week of pregnancy.

During the *second* and *third trimesters* drugs can affect the growth or functional development of the fetus, or they can have toxic effects on fetal tissues.

Drugs given shortly before term or during labour can have adverse effects on labour or on the neonate after delivery.

Not all the damaging effects of intrauterine exposure to drugs are obvious at birth, some may only manifest later in life. Such late-onset effects include malignancy, e.g. adenocarcinoma of the vagina after puberty in females exposed to diethylstilbestrol in the womb, and adverse effects on intellectual, social, and functional development.

The following list includes drugs which:

- may have harmful effects in pregnancy and indicates the trimester of risk
- are not known to be harmful in pregnancy

The list is based on human data, but information from *animal* studies has been included for some drugs when its omission might be misleading.

> Drugs should be prescribed in pregnancy only if the expected benefit to the mother is thought to be greater than the risk to the fetus, and all drugs should be avoided if possible during the first trimester. Drugs which have been extensively used in pregnancy and appear to be usually safe should be prescribed in preference to new or untried drugs; and the smallest effective dose should be used.
> Few drugs have been shown conclusively to be teratogenic in man, but no drug is safe beyond all doubt in early pregnancy. Screening procedures are available when there is a known risk of certain defects.
> **Absence of a drug from the list does not imply safety.**
> It should be noted that the BNF provides independent advice and may not always agree with the product literature.
> Information on drugs and pregnancy is also available from the National Teratology Information Service Telephone: (0191) 232 1525
> (0191) 282 5944 (out of hours emergency only)
> www.nyrdtc.nhs.uk/Services/teratology/teratology.html

## Table of drugs to be avoided or used with caution in pregnancy

Products introduced or amended since publication of BNF No. 57 (March 2009) are underlined.

| Drug (trimester of risk) | Comment |
|---|---|
| Abacavir | Manufacturer advises avoid (toxicity in *animal* studies); *see also* p. 340 |
| Abatacept | Manufacturer advises avoid unless essential—no information available; effective contraception required during treatment and for 14 weeks after last dose |
| Abciximab | Manufacturer advises use only if potential benefit outweighs risk—no information available |
| Acamprosate | Manufacturer advises avoid |
| Acarbose | Manufacturer advises avoid |
| ACE inhibitors (1, 2, 3) | Avoid unless essential; may adversely affect fetal and neonatal blood pressure control and renal function; also possible skull defects and oligohydramnios |
| Acebutolol | *see* Beta-blockers |
| Aceclofenac | *see* NSAIDs |
| Acemetacin | *see* NSAIDs |
| Acenocoumarol (nicoumalone) | *see* Anticoagulants, Oral |
| Acetazolamide | *see* Diuretics |
| Aciclovir | Not known to be harmful—manufacturers advise use only when potential benefit outweighs risk; limited absorption from topical aciclovir preparations |
| Acipimox | Manufacturer advises avoid |
| Acitretin (1, 2, 3) | Teratogenic; effective contraception must be used for at least 1 month before treatment, during treatment, and for at least 3 years after stopping (oral progestogen-only contraceptives not considered effective) |
| Adalimumab | Avoid; manufacturer advises adequate contraception during and for at least 5 months after last dose |
| Adapalene | Manufacturer advises teratogenicity in *animal* studies and recommends effective contraception during treatment |

Appendix 4: Pregnancy

| Drug (trimester of risk) | Comment |
|---|---|
| Adefovir dipivoxil | Toxicity in *animal* studies—manufacturer advises use only if potential benefit outweighs risk; effective contraception required during treatment |
| Agalsidase | Use with caution |
| Agomelatine | Manufacturer advises caution—no information available |
| Alclometasone | *see* Corticosteroids |
| Alcohol (1, 2) | Regular daily drinking is teratogenic (fetal alcohol syndrome) and may cause growth restriction; occasional single drinks are probably safe |
| (3) | Withdrawal syndrome may occur in babies of alcoholic mothers |
| Alemtuzumab | Avoid; manufacturer advises effective contraception during and for 6 months after treatment in men or women |
| Alendronic acid | *see* Bisphosphonates |
| Alfacalcidol | *see* Vitamin D |
| Alfentanil | *see* Opioid Analgesics |
| Alglucosidase alfa | Manufacturer advises avoid unless essential—no information available |
| Alimemazine (trimeprazine) | *see* Antihistamines |
| Aliskiren | Manufacturer advises avoid—no information available; other drugs acting on the renin-angiotensin system have been associated with fetal malformations and neonatal death |
| Alitretinoin (1, 2, 3) | Teratogenic; effective contraception must be used for at least 1 month before treatment, during treatment, and for 1 month after stopping; see also Pregnancy Prevention, p. 638 |
| Allopurinol | Toxicity not reported; manufacturer advises use only if no safer alternative and disease carries risk for mother or child |
| Almotriptan | *see* 5HT$_1$ Agonists |
| Alpha-blockers, post-synaptic | No evidence of teratogenicity; manufacturers advise use only when potential benefit outweighs risk |
| Alprazolam | *see* Benzodiazepines |
| Alprostadil (urethral application only) | Manufacturer advises barrier contraception if partner pregnant |
| Alteplase | *see* Fibrinolytics |
| Amantadine | Avoid; toxicity in *animal* studies |
| Ambrisentan | Avoid (teratogenic in *animal* studies); exclude pregnancy before treatment and ensure effective contraception during treatment; monthly pregnancy tests advised |
| Amfebutamone | *see* Bupropion |
| Amikacin | *see* Aminoglycosides |

| Drug (trimester of risk) | Comment |
|---|---|
| Amiloride | *see* Diuretics |
| Aminoglycosides (2, 3) | Auditory or vestibular nerve damage; risk greatest with streptomycin; probably very small with gentamicin and tobramycin, but avoid unless essential (if given, serum-aminoglycoside concentration monitoring essential) |
| Aminophylline | *see* Theophylline |
| Amiodarone (2, 3) | Possible risk of neonatal goitre; use only if no alternative |
| Amisulpride | Manufacturer advises avoid |
| Amitriptyline | *see* Antidepressants, Tricyclic (and related) |
| Amlodipine | No information available—manufacturer advises avoid, but risk to fetus should be balanced against risk of uncontrolled maternal hypertension |
| Amobarbital | *see* Barbiturates |
| Amorolfine | Systemic absorption very low, but manufacturer advises avoid—no information available |
| Amoxicillin | *see* Penicillins |
| Amphotericin | Not known to be harmful but manufacturers advise avoid unless potential benefit outweighs risk |
| Ampicillin | *see* Penicillins |
| Amsacrine | Avoid (teratogenic and toxic in *animal* studies); may reduce fertility; *see also* section 8.1 |
| Anabolic steroids (1, 2, 3) | Masculinisation of female fetus |
| Anaesthetics, general (3) | Depress neonatal respiration; for maintenance of anaesthesia, doses of propofol should not exceed 6 mg/kg/hour; dose of thiopental should not exceed 250 mg |
| Anaesthetics, local (3) | With large doses, neonatal respiratory depression, hypotonia, and bradycardia after paracervical or epidural block; neonatal methaemoglobinaemia with prilocaine; use lower doses of bupivacaine for intrathecal use during late pregnancy; *see also* Levobupivacaine and Ropivacaine |
| Anagrelide | Manufacturer advises avoid (toxicity in *animal* studies) |
| Anakinra | Manufacturer advises avoid; effective contraception must be used during treatment |
| Analgesics | *see* Opioid Analgesics, Nefopam, NSAIDs, and Paracetamol |
| Androgens (1, 2, 3) | Masculinisation of female fetus |

| Drug (trimester of risk) | Comment |
|---|---|
| Anidulafungin | Manufacturer advises avoid—no information available |
| Anticoagulants, oral (1, 2, 3) | Congenital malformations; fetal and neonatal haemorrhage; see also section 2.8.2; see also Dabigatran Etexilate and Rivaroxaban |
| Antidepressants, MAOI (1, 2, 3) | No evidence of harm but manufacturers advise avoid unless compelling reasons |
| Antidepressants, SSRI | Manufacturers advise use only if potential benefit outweighs risk; risk of neonatal withdrawal, particularly with fluoxetine and paroxetine; toxicity in animal studies with escitalopram and paroxetine |
| Antidepressants, tri-cyclic (and related) (3) | Tachycardia, irritability, and muscle spasms in neonate reported with imipramine |
| Antiepileptics | Benefit of treatment outweighs risk to fetus; risk of teratogenicity greater if more than one drug used; important: see also Carbamazepine, Ethosuximide, Gabapentin, Lamotrigine, Levetiracetam, Oxcarbazepine, Phenobarbital, Phenytoin, Pregabalin, Primidone, Rufinamide, Topiramate, Valproate, Vigabatrin, Zonisamide, and p. 253 |
| Antihistamines | No evidence of teratogenicity; embryotoxicity in animal studies with high doses of hydroxyzine and loratadine; manufacturers of cetirizine, cinnarizine, desloratadine, dimenhydrinate, hydroxyzine, ketotifen, loratadine, and mizolastine advise avoid |
| Antimalarials (1, 3) | Benefit of prophylaxis and treatment in malaria outweighs risk; important: see also individual drugs and p. 358 and p. 360 |
| Antipsychotics (3) | Extrapyramidal effects in neonate occasionally reported |
| | See also Amisulpride, Clozapine, Flupentixol, Olanzapine, Paliperidone, Quetiapine, Risperidone, Sertindole, Sulpiride, Zotepine |
| Antithymocyte immunoglobulin | Manufacturer advises use only if potential benefit outweighs risk—no information available |
| Apomorphine | Caution |
| Aprepitant | see Neurokinin Receptor Antagonists |
| Aripiprazole (1, 2, 3) | Manufacturer advises use only if potential benefit outweighs risk—no information available |

| Drug (trimester of risk) | Comment |
|---|---|
| Arsenic trioxide | Avoid (teratogenic and embryotoxic in animal studies); manufacturer advises effective contraception during treatment in men or women; see also section 8.1 |
| Artemether [ingredient] | see Riamet® |
| Aspirin (3) | Impaired platelet function and risk of haemorrhage; delayed onset and increased duration of labour with increased blood loss; avoid analgesic doses if possible in last few weeks (low doses probably not harmful); with high doses, closure of fetal ductus arteriosus in utero and possibly persistent pulmonary hypertension of newborn; kernicterus in jaundiced neonates |
| Atazanavir | Manufacturer advises use only if potential benefit outweighs risk; theoretical risk of hyperbilirubinaemia in neonate if used at term |
| Atenolol | see Beta-blockers |
| Atomoxetine | Manufacturer advises avoid unless potential benefit outweighs risk—no information available |
| Atorvastatin | see Statins |
| Atosiban | For use in premature labour see section 7.1.3 |
| Atovaquone | Manufacturer advises avoid unless potential benefit outweighs risk—no information available |
| Atracurium | Does not cross placenta in significant amounts but manufacturer advises use only if potential benefit outweighs risk |
| Atropine | Not known to be harmful; manufacturer advises caution |
| Auranofin | Manufacturer advises avoid (effective contraception should be used during and for at least 6 months after treatment) but limited data suggests usually not necessary to withdraw if condition well controlled—consider reducing dose and frequency |
| Azacitidine | Avoid (toxicity in animal studies); manufacturer advises effective contraception during and for 3 months after treatment in men or women; see also section 8.1 |
| Azapropazone | see NSAIDs |
| Azathioprine | see p. 493 |
| Azelastine | see Antihistamines |
| Azithromycin | Manufacturer advises use only if adequate alternatives not available |
| Aztreonam | Manufacturer advises avoid—no information available |

| Drug (trimester of risk) | Comment |
|---|---|
| Baclofen | Manufacturer advises use only if potential benefit outweighs risk (toxicity in *animal* studies) |
| Balsalazide | Manufacturer advises avoid |
| Bambuterol | *see* section 3.1 |
| Barbiturates (1, 2, 3) | Fetal abnormalities reported |
| (3) | Withdrawal effects in neonate; respiratory depression in neonate if used during labour; *see also* Phenobarbital |
| Basiliximab | Avoid—no information available; adequate contraception must be used during treatment and for 16 weeks after last dose |
| Beclometasone | *see* Corticosteroids |
| Bemiparin | Manufacturer advises avoid unless essential—no information available |
| Bendrofluazide | *see* Diuretics |
| Bendroflumethiazide (bendrofluazide) | *see* Diuretics |
| Benperidol | *see* Antipsychotics |
| Benzodiazepines | Avoid regular use (risk of neonatal withdrawal symptoms); use only if clear indication such as seizure control (high doses during late pregnancy or labour may cause neonatal hypothermia, hypotonia and respiratory depression) |
| Benzylpenicillin | *see* Penicillins |
| Beta-blockers | May cause intra-uterine growth restriction, neonatal hypoglycaemia, and bradycardia; risk greater in severe hypertension; *see also* section 2.5 |
| Betaine | Manufacturer advises avoid unless essential—limited information available |
| Betamethasone | *see* Corticosteroids |
| Bethanechol | Manufacturer advises avoid—no information available |
| Bevacizumab | Manufacturer advises avoid—toxicity in *animal* studies; effective contraception required during and for at least 6 months after treatment in women (*see also* section 8.1) |
| Bexarotene | Avoid; manufacturer advises effective contraception during and for at least 1 month after treatment in men or women; *see also* section 8.1 |
| Bezafibrate | *see* Fibrates |
| Bimatoprost | Manufacturer advises use only if potential benefit outweighs risk |
| Bisoprolol | *see* Beta-blockers |
| Bisphosphonates | Manufacturers advise avoid |
| Bivalirudin | Manufacturer advises avoid unless potential benefit outweighs risk—no information available |

| Drug (trimester of risk) | Comment |
|---|---|
| Bleomycin | Avoid (teratogenic and carcinogenic in *animal* studies); *see also* section 8.1 |
| Bortezomib | Manufacturer advises effective contraception during and for 3 months after treatment in men or women—toxicity in *animal* studies; *see also* section 8.1 |
| Bosentan | Avoid (teratogenic in *animal* studies); effective contraception required during and for at least 3 months after administration (hormonal contraception not considered effective); monthly pregnancy tests advised |
| Botulinum toxin | Manufacturers advise avoid unless essential—toxicity in *animal* studies |
| Brinzolamide | Manufacturer advises avoid unless essential |
| Buclizine | *see* Antihistamines |
| Budesonide | *see* Corticosteroids |
| Bumetanide | *see* Diuretics |
| Bupivacaine | *see* Anaesthetics, Local |
| Buprenorphine | *see* Opioid Analgesics |
| Bupropion | Manufacturer advises avoid—no information available |
| Buserelin | Avoid |
| Buspirone | Manufacturer advises avoid |
| Busulfan | Avoid (teratogenic in *animals*); manufacturers advise effective contraception during and for 6 months after treatment in men or women; *see also* section 8.1 |
| C1-esterase inhibitor | Manufacturer advises avoid unless essential |
| Cabergoline | No evidence of harm; manufacturer advises discontinuation one month before intended conception and avoidance during pregnancy; *see also* section 6.7.1 |
| Calcipotriol | Manufacturer advises avoid if possible; *see also* Vitamin D |
| Calcitonin (salmon) (salcatonin) | Manufacturer advises avoid unless potential benefit outweighs risk (toxicity in *animal* studies) |
| Calcitriol | *see* Vitamin D |
| Calcium folinate | Manufacturer advises caution—no information available |
| Calcium levofolinate | *see* Calcium Folinate |
| Candesartan | *As for* ACE Inhibitors |
| Capecitabine | Avoid (teratogenic in animal studies); *see also* section 8.1 |
| Capreomycin | Manufacturer advises use only if potential benefit outweighs risk—teratogenic in *animal* studies |
| Captopril | *see* ACE Inhibitors |
| Carbamazepine | Risk of teratogenesis including increased risk of neural tube defects; *see also* Antiepileptics |

| Drug (trimester of risk) | Comment | Drug (trimester of risk) | Comment |
|---|---|---|---|
| Carbimazole | Neonatal goitre and hypothyroidism; has been associated with congenital defects including aplasia cutis of the neonate | Cidofovir | Avoid (toxicity in *animal* studies); effective contraception required during and for 1 month after treatment; also men should avoid fathering a child during and for 3 months after treatment |
| Carbocisteine (1) | Manufacturer advises avoid | | |
| Carboplatin | Avoid (teratogenic and embryotoxic in *animal* studies); *see also* section 8.1 | Cilastatin [ingredient] | *see Primaxin®* |
| | | Cilazapril | *see* ACE Inhibitors |
| Carglumic acid | Manufacturer advises avoid unless essential—no information available | Cilostazol | Avoid—toxicity in *animal* studies |
| Carmustine | Avoid (teratogenic and embryotoxic in *animals*); manufacturer advises effective contraception during treatment in men or women; *see also* section 8.1 | Cimetidine | Manufacturer advises avoid unless essential |
| | | Cinacalcet | Manufacturer advises use only if potential benefit outweighs risk—no information available |
| | | Cinnarizine | *see* Antihistamines |
| Carnitine | Appropriate to use; no evidence of teratogenicity in *animal* studies | Ciprofibrate | *see* Fibrates |
| | | Ciprofloxacin | *see* Quinolones |
| Carvedilol | *see* Beta-blockers | Cisatracurium | Manufacturer advises avoid—no information available |
| Caspofungin | Manufacturer advises avoid unless essential—toxicity in *animal* studies | Cisplatin | Avoid (teratogenic and toxic in *animal* studies); *see also* section 8.1 |
| Cefaclor | Not known to be harmful | Citalopram | *see* Antidepressants, SSRI |
| Cefadroxil | Not known to be harmful | Cladribine | Avoid (teratogenic in *animal* studies); manufacturer advises that men should not father children during and for 6 months after treatment; *see also* section 8.1 |
| Cefalexin | Not known to be harmful | | |
| Cefixime | Not known to be harmful | | |
| Cefotaxime | Not known to be harmful | | |
| Cefpodoxime | Not known to be harmful | | |
| Cefradine | Not known to be harmful | | |
| Ceftazidime | Not known to be harmful | Clarithromycin | Manufacturer advises avoid unless potential benefit outweighs risk |
| Ceftriaxone | Not known to be harmful | | |
| Cefuroxime | Not known to be harmful | Clavulanic acid [ingredient] | *see* Co-amoxiclav, *Timentin®* |
| Celecoxib | Manufacturer advises avoid (teratogenic in *animal* studies); *see also* NSAIDs | Clemastine | *see* Antihistamines |
| | | Clindamycin | Not known to be harmful |
| | | Clobazam | *see* Benzodiazepines |
| Celiprolol | *see* Beta-blockers | Clobetasol | *see* Corticosteroids |
| Cetirizine | *see* Antihistamines | Clobetasone | *see* Corticosteroids |
| Cetrorelix | Manufacturer advises avoid in confirmed pregnancy | Clodronate sodium | *see* Bisphosphonates |
| Cetuximab | Manufacturer advises use only if potential benefit outweighs risk—no information available | Clofarabine | Manufacturer advises avoid (teratogenic in *animal* studies); *see also* section 8.1 |
| | | Clomethiazole | Avoid if possible—especially during first and third trimesters |
| Chloral hydrate | Avoid | | |
| Chlorambucil | Avoid; manufacturer advises effective contraception during treatment in men or women; *see also* section 8.1 | Clomifene | Possible effects on fetal development |
| | | Clomipramine | *see* Antidepressants, Tricyclic (and related) |
| Chloramphenicol (3) | Neonatal 'grey' syndrome | Clonazepam | *see* Benzodiazepines |
| Chlordiazepoxide | *see* Benzodiazepines | Clonidine | May lower fetal heart rate, but risk should be balanced against risk of uncontrolled maternal hypertension; avoid intravenous injection |
| Chloroquine | *see* Antimalarials | | |
| Chlorphenamine (chlorpheniramine) | *see* Antihistamines | | |
| Chlorpheniramine | *see* Antihistamines | Clopidogrel | Manufacturer advises avoid—no information available |
| Chlorpromazine | *see* Antipsychotics | | |
| Chlorpropamide | *see* Sulphonylureas | Clotrimazole | Minimal absorption from skin and vagina; not known to be harmful; see also section 7.2.2 |
| Chlortalidone | *see* Diuretics | | |
| Ciclesonide | *see* Corticosteroids | Clozapine | Manufacturer advises caution |
| Ciclosporin | *see* p. 493 | Co-amoxiclav | *see* Penicillins |
| | | Co-beneldopa | *see* Levodopa |
| | | Co-careldopa | *see* Levodopa |

Appendix 4: Pregnancy

| Drug (trimester of risk) | Comment |
|---|---|
| Co-cyprindiol (1, 2, 3) | Feminisation of male fetus (due to cyproterone) |
| Co-danthramer | Manufacturer advises avoid—no information available |
| Co-danthrusate | Manufacturer advises avoid—no information available |
| Codeine | *see* Opioid Analgesics |
| Co-fluampicil | *see* Penicillins |
| Colchicine | Avoid—teratogenicity in animal studies |
| Colecalciferol | *see* Vitamin D |
| Colesevelam | Use with caution—drug not absorbed but may cause fat-soluble vitamin deficiency on prolonged use |
| Colestipol | Use with caution—drug not absorbed but may cause fat-soluble vitamin deficiency on prolonged use |
| Colestyramine | Use with caution—drug not absorbed but may cause fat-soluble vitamin deficiency on prolonged use |
| Colistin (2, 3) | Avoid—possible risk of fetal toxicity |
| Contraceptives, hormonal | Not known to be harmful |
| Corticosteroids | Benefit of treatment, e.g. in asthma, outweighs risk (*see also* CSM advice, section 6.3.2); risk of intra-uterine growth restriction on prolonged or repeated systemic treatment; corticosteroid cover required by mother during labour; monitor closely if fluid retention |
| Co-trimoxazole (1) | Teratogenic risk (trimethoprim a folate antagonist) |
| (3) | Neonatal haemolysis and methaemoglobinaemia; fear of increased risk of kernicterus in neonates appears to be unfounded |
| Crisantaspase | Avoid; *see also* section 8.1 |
| Cromoglicate | *see* Sodium Cromoglicate |
| Cyclizine | *see* Antihistamines |
| Cyclopenthiazide | *see* Diuretics |
| Cyclophosphamide | Avoid (manufacturer advises effective contraception during and for at least 3 months after treatment in men or women); *see also* section 8.1 |
| Cycloserine | Manufacturer advises use only if potential benefit outweighs risk—crosses the placenta |
| Cyclosporin | *see* p. 493 |
| Cyproheptadine | *see* Antihistamines |
| Cyproterone [ingredient] | *see* Co-cyprindiol |
| Cytarabine | Avoid (teratogenic in animal studies); *see also* section 8.1 |
| Dabigatran etexilate | Manufacturer advises avoid—toxicity in animal studies |

| Drug (trimester of risk) | Comment |
|---|---|
| Dacarbazine | Avoid (carcinogenic and teratogenic in animal studies); ensure effective contraception during and for at least 6 months after treatment in men or women; *see also* section 8.1 |
| Dactinomycin | Avoid (teratogenic in animal studies); *see also* section 8.1 |
| Dalfopristin [ingredient] | *see* Synercid® |
| Dalteparin | Not known to be harmful; multidose vial contains benzyl alcohol—manufacturer advises avoid |
| Danaparoid | Limited information available but not known to be harmful—manufacturer advises avoid |
| Danazol (1, 2, 3) | Avoid; has weak androgenic effects and virilisation of female fetus reported |
| Dantrolene | Use only for malignant hyperthermia if potential benefit outweighs risk; avoid use in chronic spasticity—embryotoxic in animal studies |
| Dantron (danthron) | *see* Co-danthramer, Co-danthrusate |
| Dapsone | Folic acid 5 mg daily should be given to mother throughout pregnancy |
| (3) | Neonatal haemolysis and methaemoglobinaemia reported |
| Daptomycin | Manufacturer advises use only if potential benefit outweighs risk—no information available |
| Darbepoetin | No evidence of harm in animal studies—manufacturer advises caution |
| Darifenacin | Manufacturer advises avoid—toxicity in animal studies |
| Darunavir | Manufacturer advises use only if potential benefit outweighs risk—no information available |
| Dasatinib | Manufacturer advises avoid unless potential benefit outweighs risk—toxicity in animal studies; effective contraception required during treatment |
| Daunorubicin | Avoid (teratogenic and carcinogenic in animal studies); *see also* section 8.1 |
| Deferasirox | Manufacturer advises avoid unless potential benefit outweighs risk—toxicity in animal studies |
| Deferiprone | Manufacturer advises avoid before intended conception and during pregnancy—teratogenic and embryotoxic in animal studies; contraception advised in women of child-bearing potential |
| Deflazacort | *see* Corticosteroids |
| Demeclocycline | *see* Tetracyclines |

| Drug (trimester of risk) | Comment |
|---|---|
| Desferrioxamine | Teratogenic in *animal* studies; manufacturer advises use only if potential benefit outweighs risk |
| Desflurane | *see* Anaesthetics, General |
| Desloratadine | *see* Antihistamines |
| Desmopressin (3) | Small oxytocic effect in third trimester; increased risk of pre-eclampsia |
| Desogestrel | *see* Contraceptives, hormonal |
| Dexamethasone | *see* Corticosteroids |
| Dexamfetamine | Manufacturer advises avoid (retrospective evidence of uncertain significance suggesting possible embryotoxicity) |
| Dexibuprofen | *see* NSAIDs |
| Dexketoprofen | *see* NSAIDs |
| Dexrazoxane | Manufacturer advises avoid unless essential; ensure effective contraception during and for 3 months after treatment in men and women |
| Dextran | Avoid—reports of anaphylaxis in mother causing fetal anoxia, neurological damage and death |
| Dextromethorphan | *see* Opioid Analgesics |
| Diamorphine | *see* Opioid Analgesics |
| Diazepam | *see* Benzodiazepines |
| Diazoxide (2, 3) | Prolonged use may produce alopecia and impaired glucose tolerance in neonate; inhibits uterine activity during labour |
| Diclofenac | *see* NSAIDs |
| Didanosine | Manufacturer advises use only if potential benefit outweighs risk |
| Diethylstilbestrol (1) | High doses associated with vaginal carcinoma, urogenital abnormalities, and reduced fertility in female offspring; increased risk of hypospadias in male offspring |
| Diflucortolone | *see* Corticosteroids |
| Digoxin | May need dosage adjustment |
| Dihydrocodeine | *see* Opioid Analgesics |
| Dihydrotachysterol | *see* Vitamin D |
| Diloxanide | Manufacturer advises avoid—no information available |
| Diltiazem | Avoid |
| Dimenhydrinate | *see* Antihistamines |
| Diphenoxylate | *see* Opioid Analgesics |
| Dipipanone | *see* Opioid Analgesics |
| Dipyridamole | Not known to be harmful |
| Disodium etidronate | *see* Bisphosphonates |
| Disodium pamidronate | *see* Bisphosphonates |
| Disopyramide (3) | May induce labour |
| Distigmine | Manufacturer advises avoid (may stimulate uterine contractions) |

| Drug (trimester of risk) | Comment |
|---|---|
| Disulfiram (1) | High concentrations of acetaldehyde which occur in presence of alcohol may be teratogenic |
| Diuretics | Not used to treat gestational hypertension; *see also* Thiazides and Related Diuretics Manufacturers advise avoid acetazolamide and torasemide (toxicity in *animal* studies) |
| Dobutamine | No information available |
| Docetaxel | Avoid (toxicity and reduced fertility in *animal* studies); manufacturer advises effective contraception during and for at least 3 months after treatment; *see also* section 8.1 |
| Docusate sodium | Not known to be harmful—manufacturer advises caution |
| Dolasetron | Not known to be harmful but manufacturer advises avoid unless potential benefit outweighs risk |
| Domperidone | Manufacturer advises avoid |
| Donepezil | Manufacturer advises use only if potential benefit outweighs risk |
| Dopamine | Manufacturer advises use only if potential benefit outweighs risk |
| Dopexamine | No information available—manufacturer advises avoid |
| Doripenem | Manufacturer advises avoid unless essential—no information available |
| Dornase alfa | No evidence of teratogenicity; manufacturer advises use only if potential benefit outweighs risk |
| Dosulepin (dothiepin) | *see* Antidepressants, Tricyclic (and related) |
| Dothiepin | *see* Antidepressants, Tricyclic (and related) |
| Doxazosin | *see* Alpha-blockers, Post-synaptic |
| Doxepin | *see* Antidepressants, Tricyclic (and related) |
| Doxorubicin | Avoid (teratogenic and toxic in *animal* studies); manufacturer of liposomal product advises effective contraception during and for at least 6 months after treatment in men or women; *see also* section 8.1 |
| Doxycycline | *see* Tetracyclines |
| Droperidol | *see* Antipsychotics |
| Drospirenone | *see* Contraceptives, hormonal |
| Drotrecogin alfa (activated) | Manufacturer advises avoid unless benefit outweighs risk—no information available |

Appendix 4: Pregnancy

| Drug (trimester of risk) | Comment |
| --- | --- |
| Duloxetine | Toxicity in *animal* studies—manufacturer advises avoid in patients with stress urinary incontinence and use only if potential benefit outweighs risk in depression; risk of neonatal withdrawal symptoms if used near term |
| Dutasteride (1, 2, 3) | Avoid unprotected intercourse (*see* section 6.4.2). May cause feminisation of male fetus |
| Dydrogesterone | Not known to be harmful |
| Econazole | Minimal absorption from skin and vagina; not known to be harmful; *see also* section 7.2.2 |
| Eculizumab | No information available—use only if potential benefit outweighs risk; human IgG antibodies known to cross placenta; manufacturer advises effective contraception during and for 5 months after treatment |
| Edrophonium | Manufacturer advises use only if potential benefit outweighs risk |
| Efavirenz | Manufacturer advises avoid (effective contraception required during treatment and for 12 weeks after treatment); use efavirenz only if no alternative available |
| Eflornithine | Toxicity in *animal* studies—manufacturer advises avoid |
| Eletriptan | *see* 5HT$_1$ Agonists |
| Emtricitabine | No information available—manufacturer advises use only if essential |
| Enalapril | *see* ACE Inhibitors |
| Enfuvirtide | Manufacturer advises use only if potential benefit outweighs risk |
| Enoxaparin | Not known to be harmful |
| Enoximone | Manufacturer advises use only if potential benefit outweighs risk |
| Entacapone | Manufacturer advises avoid—no information available |
| Entecavir | Toxicity in *animal* studies—manufacturer advises use only if potential benefit outweighs risk; effective contraception required during treatment |
| Ephedrine | Increased fetal heart rate reported with parenteral ephedrine |
| Epinastine | *see* Antihistamines |
| Epirubicin | Avoid (carcinogenic in *animal* studies); *see also* section 8.1 |
| Eplerenone | Manufacturer advises caution—no information available |
| Epoetin | No evidence of harm; benefits probably outweigh risk of anaemia and of transfusion in pregnancy |

| Drug (trimester of risk) | Comment |
| --- | --- |
| Epoprostenol | Manufacturer advises use with caution—no information available |
| Eprosartan | *As for* ACE Inhibitors |
| Eptifibatide | Manufacturer advises use only if potential benefit outweighs risk—no information available |
| Erdosteine | Manufacturer advises avoid—no information available |
| Ergocalciferol | *see* Vitamin D |
| Ergotamine (1, 2, 3) | Avoid; oxytocic effect on the uterus |
| Erlotinib | Manufacturer advises avoid—toxicity in *animal* studies; effective contraception required during and for at least 2 weeks after treatment; *see also* section 8.1 |
| Ertapenem | Manufacturer advises avoid unless potential benefit outweighs risk |
| Erythromycin | Not known to be harmful |
| Escitalopram | *see* Antidepressants, SSRI |
| Esmolol | *see* Beta-blockers |
| Esomeprazole | Manufacturer advises caution—no information available |
| Estradiol | *see* Contraceptives, hormonal |
| Etanercept | Manufacturer advises avoid—no information available |
| Ethambutol | Not known to be harmful; *see also* p. 322 |
| Ethinylestradiol | *see* Contraceptives, hormonal |
| Ethosuximide (1) | May possibly be teratogenic; *see also* Antiepileptics |
| Etidronate disodium | *see* Bisphosphonates |
| Etodolac | *see* NSAIDs |
| Etomidate | *see* Anaesthetics, General |
| Etonogestrel | *see* Contraceptives, hormonal |
| Etoposide | Avoid (teratogenic in *animal* studies); *see also* section 8.1 |
| Etoricoxib | *see* NSAIDs |
| Etravirine | Manufacturer advises use only if potential benefit outweighs risk |
| Etynodiol | *see* Contraceptives, hormonal |
| Exenatide | Manufacturer advises avoid—toxicity in *animal* studies |
| Ezetimibe | Manufacturer advises use only if potential benefit outweighs risk—no information available |
| Famciclovir | *see* Aciclovir |
| Famotidine | Manufacturer advises avoid unless potential benefit outweighs risk |
| Felodipine | Avoid; toxicity in *animal* studies; may inhibit labour |
| Fenbufen | *see* NSAIDs |
| Fenofibrate | *see* Fibrates |
| Fenoprofen | *see* NSAIDs |
| Fenoterol | *see* section 3.1 |
| Fentanyl | *see* Opioid Analgesics |

| Drug (trimester of risk) | Comment | Drug (trimester of risk) | Comment |
|---|---|---|---|
| Ferric carboxymaltose | Avoid in first trimester; crosses the placenta in *animal* studies; may influence skeletal development | Flupentixol | Manufacturer advises avoid unless potential benefit outweighs risk |
| Fesoterodine | Manufacturer advises avoid—toxicity in *animal* studies | Fluphenazine | *see* Antipsychotics |
| Fexofenadine | *see* Antihistamines | Flurandrenolone | *see* Corticosteroids |
| Fibrates | Embryotoxicity in *animal* studies—manufacturers advise avoid | Flurazepam | *see* Benzodiazepines |
| | | Flurbiprofen | *see* NSAIDs |
| | | Fluticasone | *see* Corticosteroids |
| Fibrinolytics (1, 2, 3) | Possibility of premature separation of placenta in first 18 weeks; risk of maternal haemorrhage throughout pregnancy and on postpartum; theoretical risk of fetal haemorrhage throughout pregnancy | Fluvastatin | *see* Statins |
| | | Fluvoxamine | *see* Antidepressants, SSRI |
| | | Follitropin alfa and beta | Avoid |
| | | Fondaparinux | Manufacturer advises avoid unless potential benefit outweighs possible risk—no information available |
| Filgrastim | Toxicity in *animal* studies; manufacturer advises use only if potential benefit outweighs risk | Formoterol (eformoterol) | Manufacturers advise use only if potential benefit outweighs risk; *see also* section 3.1 |
| Finasteride (1, 2, 3) | Avoid unprotected intercourse (*see* section 6.4.2). May cause feminisation of male fetus | Fosamprenavir | Toxicity in *animal* studies; manufacturer advises use only if potential benefit outweighs risk |
| Flavoxate | Manufacturer advises avoid unless no safer alternative | Fosaprepitant | *see* Neurokinin Receptor Antagonists |
| Flecainide | Used in pregnancy to treat maternal and fetal arrhythmias in specialist centres; toxicity reported in *animal* studies; infant hyperbilirubinaemia also reported | Foscarnet | Manufacturer advises avoid |
| | | Fosinopril | *see* ACE Inhibitors |
| | | Fosphenytoin | *see* Phenytoin |
| | | Framycetin | *see* Aminoglycosides |
| | | Frovatriptan | *see* 5HT$_1$ Agonists |
| | | Frusemide | *see* Diuretics |
| Flucloxacillin | *see* Penicillins | Fulvestrant | Manufacturer advises avoid—increased incidence of fetal abnormalities and death in *animal* studies |
| Fluconazole | Manufacturer advises avoid—multiple congenital abnormalities reported with long-term high doses | Furosemide (frusemide) | *see* Diuretics |
| | | Fusidic acid | *see* Sodium Fusidate |
| Flucytosine | Teratogenic in *animal* studies; manufacturer advises use only if potential benefit outweighs risk | Gabapentin | Toxicity in *animal* studies; *see also* Antiepileptics |
| | | Galantamine | Developmental delay in *animal* studies |
| Fludarabine | Avoid (embryotoxic and teratogenic in *animal* studies); manufacturer advises effective contraception during and for at least 6 months after treatment in men or women; *see also* section 8.1 | Galsulfase | Manufacturer advises avoid unless essential |
| | | Ganciclovir | Avoid—teratogenic risk; *see also* p. 352 |
| | | Ganirelix | Manufacturer advises avoid in confirmed pregnancy—toxicity in *animal* studies |
| Fludrocortisone | *see* Corticosteroids | Gelatin | Manufacturer of *Geloplasma*® advises avoid at the end of pregnancy |
| Fludroxycortide (flurandrenolone) | *see* Corticosteroids | Gemcitabine | Avoid (teratogenic in *animal* studies); manufacturer advises effective contraception during treatment; men must avoid fathering a child during and for 6 months after treatment; *see also* p. 467 |
| Flumazenil | May cross placenta in small amounts—manufacturer advises avoid unless potential benefit outweighs risk | | |
| Flunisolide | *see* Corticosteroids | | |
| Fluocinolone | *see* Corticosteroids | | |
| Fluocinonide | *see* Corticosteroids | Gemfibrozil | *see* Fibrates |
| Fluocortolone | *see* Corticosteroids | Gentamicin | *see* Aminoglycosides |
| Fluorometholone | *see* Corticosteroids | Gestodene | *see* Contraceptives, hormonal |
| Fluorouracil | Avoid (teratogenic); *see also* section 8.1 | Gestrinone (1, 2, 3) | Avoid |
| | | Glatiramer | Manufacturer advises avoid—no information available |
| Fluoxetine | *see* Antidepressants, SSRI | Glibenclamide | *see* Sulphonylureas |

| Drug (trimester of risk) | Comment |
|---|---|
| Gliclazide | *see* Sulphonylureas |
| Glimepiride | *see* Sulphonylureas |
| Glipizide | *see* Sulphonylureas |
| Glucosamine | Manufacturer advises avoid—no information available |
| Glyceryl trinitrate | Not known to be harmful but most manufacturers advise avoid unless potential benefit outweighs risk |
| Gonadorelin analogues | *see* individual entries |
| Goserelin | Manufacturer advises avoid in pregnancy—exclude pregnancy before treatment and use non-hormonal contraceptives during treatment |
| Granisetron | Manufacturer advises use only when compelling reasons—no information available |
| Griseofulvin | Avoid (fetotoxicity and teratogenicity in *animals*); effective contraception required during and for at least 1 month after administration (**important:** effectiveness of oral contraceptives reduced, see p. 445); also men should avoid fathering a child during and for at least 6 months after administration |
| Guanethidine (3) | Postural hypotension and reduced uteroplacental perfusion; should not be used to treat hypertension in pregnancy |
| Haem arginate | Manufacturer advises avoid unless essential |
| Haloperidol | *see* Antipsychotics |
| Halothane | *see* Anaesthetics, General |
| Heparin (1, 2, 3) | Does not cross the placenta; maternal osteoporosis reported after prolonged use; multidose vials may contain benzyl alcohol—some manufacturers advise avoid; *see also* Bemiparin, Dalteparin, Enoxaparin, and Tinzaparin |
| 5HT₁ agonists | Limited experience—manufacturers advise avoid unless potential benefit outweighs risk |
| Human menopausal gonadotrophins | Avoid |
| Hydralazine (1, 2) | Manufacturer advises avoid before third trimester; no reports of serious harm following use in third trimester |
| Hydrochlorothiazide | *see* Diuretics |
| Hydrocortisone | *see* Corticosteroids |
| Hydroflumethiazide | *see* Diuretics |
| Hydromorphone | *see* Opioid Analgesics |
| Hydroxycarbamide (hydroxyurea) | Avoid (teratogenic in *animal* studies); manufacturer advises effective contraception before and during treatment *see also* section 8.1 |

| Drug (trimester of risk) | Comment |
|---|---|
| Hydroxychloroquine | Manufacturer advises avoid but see p. 573 |
| Hydroxyurea | *see* Hydroxycarbamide |
| Hydroxyzine | *see* Antihistamines |
| Hyoscine butylbromide | Manufacturer advises use only if potential benefit outweighs risk |
| Hyoscine hydrobromide | Manufacturer advises use only if potential benefit outweighs risk; injection may depress neonatal respiration |
| Ibandronic acid | *see* Bisphosphonates |
| Ibuprofen | *see* NSAIDs |
| Icatibant | Manufacturer advises use only if potential benefit outweighs risk—toxicity in *animal* studies |
| Idarubicin | Avoid (teratogenic and toxic in *animal* studies); *see also* section 8.1 |
| Idoxuridine | Teratogenic in *animal* studies—manufacturer advises avoid |
| Idursulfase | Manufacturer advises avoid—no information available |
| Ifosfamide | Avoid (teratogenic and carcinogenic in *animals*); manufacturer advises adequate contraception during and for at least 6 months after treatment in men or women; *see also* section 8.1 |
| Iloprost | Manufacturer advises avoid (toxicity in *animal* studies); effective contraception must be used during treatment |
| Imatinib | Manufacturer advises avoid unless potential benefit outweighs risk; *see also* section 8.1 |
| Imidapril | *see* ACE Inhibitors |
| Imiglucerase | Manufacturer advises use with caution—limited information available |
| Imipenem [ingredient] | *see* Primaxin® |
| Imipramine | *see* Antidepressants, Tricyclic (and related) |
| Imiquimod | No evidence of teratogenicity or toxicity in *animal* studies; manufacturer advises caution |
| Indapamide | *see* Diuretics |
| Indinavir | Toxicity in *animal* studies; manufacturer advises use only if potential benefit outweighs risk; theoretical risk of hyperbilirubinaemia and renal stones in neonate if used at term |
| Indometacin | *see* NSAIDs |
| Infliximab | Avoid; manufacturer advises adequate contraception during and for at least 6 months after last dose |
| Influenza vaccine | Not known to be harmful |
| Inosine pranobex | Manufacturer advises avoid |
| Inositol nicotinate | No information available—manufacturer advises avoid unless potential benefit outweighs risk |

| Drug (trimester of risk) | Comment |
|---|---|
| Insulin | Insulin requirements should be assessed frequently by an experienced diabetes physician; safety of long-acting insulin analogues not established; short-acting insulin analogues, insulin aspart and insulin lispro, not known to be harmful; see also p. 374 |
| Interferon beta | Manufacturers advise avoid—increased risk of spontaneous abortion; effective contraception required during treatment |
| Interferons | Manufacturers recommend avoid unless compelling reasons; effective contraception to be used by men and women receiving treatment; see also Interferon Beta and Peginterferon Alfa |
| Iodine and iodides (2, 3) | Neonatal goitre and hypothyroidism; see also Iodine, Radioactive and Povidone–iodine |
| Iodine, radioactive (1, 2, 3) | Permanent hypothyroidism—avoid |
| Iodoform | see Povidone–iodine |
| Ipratropium | Not known to be harmful; see section 3.1 |
| Irbesartan | As for ACE Inhibitors |
| Irinotecan | Avoid (teratogenic and toxic in animal studies); manufacturer advises effective contraception during and for at least 3 months after treatment; see also section 8.1 |
| Iron (parenteral) | Avoid in first trimester; see also Ferric Carboxymaltose |
| Iron dextran | see Iron (parenteral) |
| Iron sucrose | see Iron (parenteral) |
| Isocarboxazid | see Antidepressants, MAOI |
| Isoflurane | see Anaesthetics, General |
| Isometheptene [ingredient] | see Midrid® |
| Isoniazid | Not known to be harmful; see also p. 322 |
| Isosorbide dinitrate | May cross placenta—manufacturers advise avoid unless potential benefit outweighs risk |
| Isosorbide mononitrate | Manufacturers advise avoid unless potential benefit outweighs risk |
| Isotretinoin (1, 2, 3) | Teratogenic; effective contraception must be used for at least 1 month before oral treatment, during treatment and for at least 1 month after stopping (oral progestogen-only contraceptives not considered effective); also avoid topical treatment; see also Pregnancy Prevention, p. 650 |

| Drug (trimester of risk) | Comment |
|---|---|
| Isradipine | May inhibit labour; risk to fetus should be balanced against risk of uncontrolled maternal hypertension |
| Itraconazole | Manufacturer advises use only in life-threatening situations (toxicity at high doses in animal studies); ensure effective contraception during treatment and until the next menstrual period following end of treatment |
| Ivabradine | Manufacturer advises avoid—toxicity in animal studies |
| Kaletra® | Avoid oral solution due to high propylene glycol content; manufacturer advises use capsules and tablets only if potential benefit outweighs risk (toxicity in animal studies) |
| Ketamine | see Anaesthetics, General |
| Ketoconazole | Manufacturer advises avoid unless potential benefit outweighs risk (teratogenicity in animal studies) |
| Ketoprofen | see NSAIDs |
| Ketorolac | see NSAIDs |
| Ketotifen | see Antihistamines |
| Labetalol | see Beta-blockers |
| Lacidipine | Manufacturer advises avoid; may inhibit labour |
| Lacosamide | Manufacturer advises avoid unless potential benefit outweighs risk |
| Lactulose | Not known to be harmful |
| Lamivudine (1) | Manufacturer advises avoid during first trimester; see also p. 340 |
| Lamotrigine | Risk of teratogenesis; see also Antiepileptics |
| Lanreotide | Manufacturer advises use only if potential benefit outweighs risk |
| Lansoprazole | Manufacturer advises avoid |
| Lanthanum | Manufacturer advises avoid—toxicity in animal studies |
| Lapatinib | Manufacturer advises avoid unless potential benefit outweighs risk—toxicity in animal studies; see also section 8.1 |
| Laronidase | Manufacturer advises avoid unless essential—no information available |
| Latanoprost | Manufacturer advises avoid |
| Leflunomide | Avoid—active metabolite teratogenic in animal studies; effective contraception essential during treatment and for at least 2 years after treatment in women and at least 3 months after treatment in men (see also Leflunomide section 10.1.3) |

Appendix 4: Pregnancy

| Drug (trimester of risk) | Comment |
|---|---|
| Lenalidomide | Teratogenic risk; effective contraception must be used for at least 1 month before, during, and for at least 1 month after treatment (oral combined hormonal contraceptives and copper-releasing intrauterine devices not recommended); men should use condoms during treatment and for at least 1 week after stopping |
| Lenograstim | Toxicity in *animal* studies; manufacturer advises use only if potential benefit outweighs risk |
| Lepirudin | Avoid |
| Lercanidipine | Manufacturer advises avoid—no information available |
| Letrozole | Avoid (toxicity in *animal* studies); manufacturer advises effective contraception required until postmenopausal status fully established |
| Leuprorelin | Avoid—teratogenic in *animal* studies |
| Levetiracetam | Toxicity in *animal* studies—manufacturer advises use only if potential benefit outweighs risk; *see also* Antiepileptics |
| Levobupivacaine (1) | Manufacturer advises avoid if possible—toxicity in *animal* studies; *see also* Anaesthetics, Local |
| Levocetirizine | *see* Antihistamines |
| Levodopa | Manufacturers advise toxicity in *animal* studies |
| Levofloxacin | *see* Quinolones |
| Levomepromazine (methotrimeprazine) | *see* Antipsychotics |
| Levonorgestrel | *see* Contraceptives, hormonal |
| Levothyroxine (thyroxine) | Monitor maternal serum-thyrotrophin concentration—levothyroxine may cross the placenta and excessive maternal concentration can be detrimental to fetus |
| Lidocaine (lignocaine) | *see* Anaesthetics, Local |
| Lignocaine | *see* Anaesthetics, Local |
| Linezolid | Manufacturer advises use only if potential benefit outweighs risk—no information available |
| Liothyronine | Does not cross the placenta in significant amounts; monitor maternal thyroid function tests—dosage adjustment may be necessary |
| Lisinopril | *see* ACE Inhibitors |
| Lithium salts (1) | Avoid if possible (risk of teratogenicity, including cardiac abnormalities) |
| (2, 3) | Dose requirements increased (but on delivery return to normal abruptly); close monitoring of serum-lithium concentration advised (risk of toxicity in neonate) |

| Drug (trimester of risk) | Comment |
|---|---|
| Lofepramine | *see* Antidepressants, Tricyclic (and related) |
| Lofexidine | Manufacturer advises use only if benefit outweighs risk—no information available |
| Lomustine | Avoid (manufacturer advises effective contraception during and for at least 6 months after treatment in men or women); *see also* section 8.1 |
| Loperamide | Manufacturers advise avoid—no information available |
| Lopinavir [ingredient] | *see* Kaletra® |
| Loprazolam | *see* Benzodiazepines |
| Loratadine | Embryotoxic in *animal* studies; *see also* Antihistamines |
| Lorazepam | *see* Benzodiazepines |
| Lormetazepam | *see* Benzodiazepines |
| Losartan | *As for* ACE Inhibitors |
| Lumefantrine [ingredient] | *see* Riamet® |
| Lymecycline | *see* Tetracyclines |
| Macrogols (oral) | Manufacturers advise use only if essential—no information available |
| Magnesium sulphate (3) | Not known to be harmful for short-term intravenous administration in eclampsia but excessive doses cause neonatal respiratory depression |
| Malarone® | Manufacturer advises avoid unless essential |
| Mannitol | Manufacturer advises avoid unless essential—no information available |
| Maraviroc | Manufacturer advises use only if potential benefit outweighs risk—toxicity in *animal* studies |
| Mebendazole | Manufacturer advises toxicity in *animal* studies |
| Mebeverine | Not known to be harmful; manufacturers advise caution |
| Mecasermin | Manufacturer advises avoid unless essential; contraception advised in women of child-bearing potential |
| Mecysteine | Manufacturer advises avoid |
| Medroxyprogesterone | Avoid—genital malformations and cardiac defects reported with high doses; *see also* Contraceptives, hormonal |
| Mefenamic acid | *see* NSAIDs |
| Mefloquine (1) | Manufacturer advises teratogenicity in *animal* studies, but *see* p. 360 |
| Melatonin | No information available—manufacturer advises avoid |
| Meloxicam | *see* NSAIDs |
| Melphalan | Avoid (manufacturer advises adequate contraception during treatment in men or women); *see also* section 8.1 |
| Memantine | Manufacturer advises avoid unless essential—intra-uterine growth restriction in *animal* studies |

| Drug (trimester of risk) | Comment |
|---|---|
| Menadiol (3) | Neonatal haemolytic anaemia, hyperbilirubinaemia and increased risk of kernicterus in jaundiced infants |
| Menotrophin | Avoid |
| Meprobamate | Manufacturer advises avoid if possible |
| Meptazinol | see Opioid Analgesics |
| Mercaptamine | Manufacturer advises avoid |
| Mercaptopurine | Avoid (teratogenic); see also section 8.1 |
| Meropenem | Manufacturer advises use only if potential benefit outweighs risk—no information available |
| Mesalazine | Negligible quantities cross placenta |
| Mesna | Not known to be harmful; see also section 8.1 |
| Mesterolone | see Androgens |
| Mestranol | see Contraceptives, hormonal |
| Metaraminol | May reduce placental perfusion—manufacturer advises use only if potential benefit outweighs risk |
| Metformin | Used in pregnancy for both pre-existing and gestational diabetes—see also p. 381; manufacturer advises avoid |
| Methadone | see Opioid Analgesics |
| Methocarbamol | Manufacturer advises avoid unless potential benefit outweighs risk |
| Methotrexate | Avoid (teratogenic; fertility may be reduced during therapy but this may be reversible); manufacturer advises effective contraception during and for at least 3 months after treatment in men or women; see also section 8.1 |
| Methotrimeprazine | see Antipsychotics |
| Methoxy polyethylene glycol-epoetin beta | No evidence of harm in animal studies—manufacturer advises caution |
| Methyldopa | Not known to be harmful |
| Methylnaltrexone | Toxicity at high doses in animal studies—manufacturer advises avoid unless essential |
| Methylphenidate | Limited experience—manufacturer advises avoid unless potential benefit outweighs risk; toxicity in animals |
| Methylprednisolone | see Corticosteroids |
| Methysergide | Manufacturer advises avoid |
| Metoclopramide | Not known to be harmful but manufacturer advises use only when compelling reasons |
| Metolazone | see Diuretics |
| Metoprolol | see Beta-blockers |
| Metronidazole | Manufacturer advises avoidance of high-dose regimens |
| Metyrapone | Avoid (may impair biosynthesis of fetal-placental steroids) |
| Mianserin | see Antidepressants, Tricyclic (and related) |

| Drug (trimester of risk) | Comment |
|---|---|
| Micafungin | Manufacturer advises avoid unless essential—toxicity in animal studies |
| Miconazole | Manufacturer advises avoid if possible—toxicity at high doses in animal studies; small amount absorbed from vagina—not known to be harmful (see also section 7.2.2) |
| Midazolam | see Benzodiazepines |
| Midrid® | Manufacturer advises avoid |
| Mifepristone | Manufacturer advises that if treatment fails, essential that pregnancy be terminated by another method |
| Miglustat | Manufacturer advises avoid (toxicity in animal studies)—effective contraception must be used during treatment; also men should avoid fathering a child during and for 3 months after treatment |
| Milrinone | Manufacturer advises use only if potential benefit outweighs risk |
| Minocycline | see Tetracyclines |
| Minoxidil (3) | Neonatal hirsutism reported |
| Mirtazapine | Manufacturers advise caution—toxicity in animal studies; monitor neonate for withdrawal effects |
| Misoprostol (1, 2, 3) | Avoid—potent uterine stimulant (has been used to induce abortion) and may be teratogenic |
| Mitomycin | Avoid (teratogenic in animal studies); see also section 8.1 |
| Mitotane | Manufacturer advises avoid—women of childbearing age should use effective contraception during and after treatment; see also section 8.1 |
| Mitoxantrone (mitozantrone) | Avoid; manufacturer advises effective contraception during and for at least 6 months after treatment in men or women; see also section 8.1 |
| Mitozantrone | see Mitoxantrone |
| Mivacurium | Manufacturer advises avoid—no information available |
| Mizolastine | Manufacturer advises avoid; see also Antihistamines |
| MMR vaccine, live | see Vaccines (live) |
| Moclobemide | see Antidepressants, MAOI |
| Modafinil | Manufacturer advises avoid |
| Moexipril | see ACE Inhibitors |
| Montelukast | Manufacturer advises avoid unless essential |
| Morphine | see Opioid Analgesics |
| Moxifloxacin | see Quinolones |
| Moxisylyte (thymoxamine) | Manufacturer advises avoid |
| Moxonidine | Manufacturer advises avoid—no information available |

| Drug (trimester of risk) | Comment | Drug (trimester of risk) | Comment |
|---|---|---|---|
| Mupirocin | Manufacturer advises avoid unless potential benefit outweighs risk—no information available | Nicotine | Use only if smoking cessation without nicotine replacement fails; intermittent therapy preferable but avoid liquorice-flavoured nicotine products |
| Mycophenolate mofetil | Manufacturer advises avoid—congenital malformations reported; effective contraception required before treatment, during treatment, and for 6 weeks after discontinuation of treatment | Nicotinic acid | No information available—manufacturer advises avoid unless potential benefit outweighs risk |
| Mycophenolic acid | *see* Mycophenolate mofetil | Nicoumalone | *see* Anticoagulants, Oral |
| Nabilone | Manufacturer advises avoid unless essential | Nifedipine | May inhibit labour; manufacturer advises avoid before week 20; risk to fetus should be balanced against risk of uncontrolled maternal hypertension; use only if other treatment options are not indicated or have failed |
| Nabumetone | *see* NSAIDs | | |
| Nadolol | *see* Beta-blockers | | |
| Nafarelin | Avoid | | |
| Nalidixic acid | *see* Quinolones | | |
| Naloxone | Manufacturer advises use only if potential benefit outweighs risk | | |
| Naltrexone | Manufacturers advise use only if potential benefit outweighs risk | Nilotinib | Manufacturer advises avoid unless potential benefit outweighs risk—toxicity in *animal* studies; effective contraception required during treatment; *see also* section 8.1 |
| Nandrolone | *see* Anabolic Steroids | | |
| Naproxen | *see* NSAIDs | | |
| Naratriptan | *see* 5HT₁ Agonists | Nimodipine | Manufacturer advises use only if potential benefit outweighs risk |
| Narcotic analgesics | *see* Opioid Analgesics | | |
| Natalizumab | Manufacturer advises avoid unless essential—toxicity in *animal* studies | Nitisinone | Manufacturer advises avoid unless potential benefit outweighs risk—toxicity in *animal* studies |
| Nateglinide | Manufacturer advises avoid—toxicity in *animal* studies | | |
| Nebivolol | *see* Beta-blockers | Nitrazepam | *see* Benzodiazepines |
| Nedocromil | *see* section 3.1 | Nitrofurantoin (3) | May produce neonatal haemolysis if used at term |
| Nefopam | No information available—manufacturer advises avoid unless no safer treatment | Nitroprusside | *see* Sodium Nitroprusside |
| | | Nitrous oxide | *see* Anaesthetics, General |
| Nelarabine | Avoid (toxicity in *animal* studies); manufacturer advises effective contraception during and for at least 3 months after treatment in men and women; see also Section 8.1 | Nizatidine | Manufacturer advises avoid unless essential |
| | | Noradrenaline (norepinephrine) (1, 2, 3) | Avoid—may reduce placental perfusion |
| Nelfinavir | No information available—manufacturer advises use only if potential benefit outweighs risk | Norelgestromin | *see* Contraceptives, hormonal |
| | | Norethisterone | Masculinisation of female fetuses and other defects reported; *see also* Contraceptives, hormonal |
| Neomycin | *see* Aminoglycosides | | |
| Neostigmine | Manufacturer advises use only if potential benefit outweighs risk | Norfloxacin | *see* Quinolones |
| | | Norgestimate | *see* Contraceptives, hormonal |
| Neurokinin receptor antagonists | Manufacturer advises avoid unless potential benefit outweighs risk—no information available | Norgestrel | *see* Contraceptives, hormonal |
| | | Nortriptyline | *see* Antidepressants, Tricyclic (and related) |
| Nevirapine | Although manufacturers advise avoid, may be appropriate to use if clearly indicated; *see also* p. 340 | NSAIDs | Most manufacturers advise avoid (or avoid unless potential benefit outweighs risk); ketorolac contra-indicated during pregnancy, labour and delivery; *see also* Celecoxib |
| Nicardipine | May inhibit labour; manufacturer advises avoid, but risk to fetus should be balanced against risk of uncontrolled maternal hypertension | (3) | With regular use closure of fetal ductus arteriosus *in utero* and possibly persistent pulmonary hypertension of the newborn. Delayed onset and increased duration of labour |
| Nicorandil | Manufacturer advises use only if potential benefit outweighs risk—no information available | Nystatin | No information available, but absorption from gastro-intestinal tract negligible |

| Drug (trimester of risk) | Comment |
|---|---|
| Octreotide (1, 2, 3) | Possible effect on fetal growth; manufacturer advises use only if potential benefit outweighs risk |
| Oestrogens | see Contraceptives, hormonal |
| Ofloxacin | see Quinolones |
| Olanzapine (3) | Manufacturer advises use only if potential benefit outweighs risk; neonatal lethargy, tremor, and hypertonia reported |
| Olmesartan | As for ACE inhibitors |
| Olsalazine | Manufacturer advises avoid unless potential benefit outweighs risk |
| Omalizumab | Manufacturer advises avoid unless essential; no evidence of teratogenicity in animal studies |
| Omega-3-acid ethyl esters | Manufacturer advises use only if potential benefit outweighs risk—no information available |
| Omeprazole | Not known to be harmful |
| Ondansetron | No information available; manufacturer advises avoid unless potential benefit outweighs risk |
| Opioid analgesics (3) | Depress neonatal respiration; withdrawal effects in neonates of dependent mothers; gastric stasis and risk of inhalation pneumonia in mother during labour; see also Tramadol |
| Oral contraceptives | see Contraceptives, hormonal |
| Orlistat | Manufacturer advises caution |
| Orphenadrine | Manufacturer advises caution |
| Oseltamivir | Use only if potential benefit outweighs risk (e.g. during a pandemic); see also p. 354 |
| Oxaliplatin | Manufacturer advises avoid—toxicity in animal studies; effective contraception required during and for 4 months after treatment in women and 6 months after treatment in men; see also section 8.1 |
| Oxazepam | see Benzodiazepines |
| Oxcarbazepine | Risk of teratogenesis including increased risk of neural tube defects; see also Antiepileptics |
| Oxprenolol | see Beta-blockers |
| Oxybutynin | Manufacturer advises avoid unless potential benefit outweighs risk—toxicity in animal studies |
| Oxycodone | see Opioid Analgesics |
| Oxytetracycline | see Tetracyclines |
| Paclitaxel | Avoid (toxicity in animal studies); ensure effective contraception during and for at least 6 months after treatment in men or women; see also section 8.1 |

| Drug (trimester of risk) | Comment |
|---|---|
| Palifermin | Manufacturer advises avoid unless potential benefit outweighs risk—toxicity in animal studies |
| Paliperidone | Manufacturer advises use only if potential benefit outweighs risk—toxicity in animal studies; if discontinuation during pregnancy is necessary, paliperidone should be withdrawn gradually |
| Palonosetron | Manufacturer advises avoid—no information available |
| Pamidronate disodium | see Bisphosphonates |
| Pancreatin | Not known to be harmful |
| Pancuronium | Manufacturer advises avoid unless potential benefit outweighs risk—no information available |
| Panitumumab | Avoid (toxicity in animal studies); manufacturer advises effective contraception during and for 6 months after treatment; see also section 8.1 |
| Pantoprazole | Manufacturer advises avoid unless potential benefit outweighs risk—fetotoxic in animals |
| Papaveretum | see Opioid Analgesics |
| Paracetamol | Not known to be harmful |
| Paraldehyde | Manufacturer advises avoid unless essential—crosses the placenta |
| Parecoxib | see NSAIDS |
| Paricalcitol | Toxicity in animal studies—manufacturer advises avoid unless potential benefit outweighs risk; see also Vitamin D |
| Paroxetine | see Antidepressants, SSRI |
| Pegaptinib | Manufacturer advises avoid unless potential benefit outweighs risk |
| Pegfilgrastim | Toxicity in animal studies; manufacturer advises use only if potential benefit outweighs risk |
| Peginterferon alfa | manufacturer advises avoid unless potential benefit outweighs risk (toxicity in animal studies); effective contraception required during treatment |
| Pemetrexed | Avoid (toxicity in animal studies); manufacturer advises effective contraception during treatment; men must avoid fathering a child during and for 6 months after treatment; see also section 8.1 |
| Penicillamine (1, 2, 3) | Fetal abnormalities reported rarely; avoid if possible |
| Penicillins | Not known to be harmful |
| Pentamidine isetionate | Manufacturer advises avoid unless essential |
| Pentazocine | see Opioid Analgesics |

Appendix 4: Pregnancy

| Drug (trimester of risk) | Comment |
|---|---|
| Pentostatin | Avoid (teratogenic in *animal* studies); manufacturer advises that men should not father children during and for 6 months after treatment; *see also* section 8.1 |
| Pergolide | Manufacturer advises use only if potential benefit outweighs risk |
| Pericyazine | *see* Antipsychotics |
| Perindopril | *see* ACE Inhibitors |
| Perphenazine | *see* Antipsychotics |
| Pethidine | *see* Opioid Analgesics |
| Phenelzine | *see* Antidepressants, MAOI |
| Phenindione | *see* Anticoagulants, Oral |
| Phenobarbital | Congenital malformations; *see also* Antiepileptics |
| Phenothiazines | *see* Antipsychotics |
| Phenoxybenzamine | Hypotension may occur in newborn |
| Phenoxymethylpenicillin | *see* Penicillins |
| Phentolamine | Use with caution—may cause marked decrease in maternal blood pressure with resulting fetal anoxia |
| Phenylephrine (1) | Malformations reported |
| (3) | Avoid if possible—fetal hypoxia and bradycardia reported in late pregnancy and labour |
| Phenytoin | Congenital malformations; caution in interpreting plasma concentrations—bound may be reduced but free (i.e. effective) unchanged; *see also* Antiepileptics |
| Pholcodine | *see* Opioid Analgesics |
| Phytomenadione | Manufacturer advises use only if potential benefit outweighs risk—no specific information available |
| Pilocarpine | Avoid—smooth muscle stimulant; toxicity in *animal* studies |
| Pimozide | *see* Antipsychotics |
| Pindolol | *see* Beta-blockers |
| Pioglitazone | Manufacturer advises avoid—toxicity in *animal* studies |
| Piperacillin with tazobactam | Manufacturers advise use only if potential benefit outweighs risk |
| Piperazine | Not known to be harmful but manufacturer advises avoid in first trimester |
| Pipotiazine | *see* Antipsychotics |
| Piracetam | Manufacturer advises avoid |
| Piroxicam | *see* NSAIDs |
| Pivmecillinam | *see* Penicillins |
| Pizotifen | Manufacturer advises avoid unless potential benefit outweighs risk |
| Podophyllotoxin | Manufacturers advise avoid |
| Podophyllum | Avoid—neonatal death and teratogenesis have been reported |

| Drug (trimester of risk) | Comment |
|---|---|
| Polystyrene sulphonate resins | Manufacturers advise use only if potential benefit outweighs risk—no information available |
| Porfimer | Manufacturer advises avoid unless essential |
| Posaconazole | Manufacturer advises avoid unless potential benefit outweighs risk and recommends effective contraception during treatment; toxicity in *animal* studies |
| Povidone–iodine (2, 3) | Sufficient iodine may be absorbed to affect the fetal thyroid |
| Pramipexole | Manufacturer advises use only if potential benefit outweighs risk—no information available |
| Prasugrel | Manufacturer advises use only if potential benefit outweighs risk |
| Pravastatin | *see* Statins |
| Prazosin | *see* Alpha-blockers, Post-synaptic |
| Prednisolone | *see* Corticosteroids |
| Pregabalin | Toxicity in *animal* studies—manufacturer advises use only if potential benefit outweighs risk; *see also* Antiepileptics |
| Prilocaine (3) | Neonatal methaemoglobinaemia reported after paracervical block or pudendal block; *see also* Anaesthetics, Local |
| Primaquine (3) | Neonatal haemolysis and methaemoglobinaemia; *see also* Antimalarials |
| *Primaxin®* | Manufacturer advises avoid unless potential benefit outweighs risk (toxicity in *animal* studies) |
| Primidone | *see* Phenobarbital |
| Procarbazine | Avoid (teratogenic in *animal* studies and isolated reports in humans); *see also* section 8.1 |
| Prochlorperazine | *see* Antipsychotics |
| Procyclidine | Manufacturers advise use only if potential benefit outweighs risk |
| Progesterone | Not known to be harmful |
| Proguanil | Adequate folate supplements should be given to mother; *see also* Antimalarials |
| Promazine | *see* Antipsychotics |
| Promethazine | *see* Antihistamines |
| Propafenone | Manufacturer advises avoid—no information available |
| Propantheline | Manufacturer advises avoid—no information available |
| Propiverine | Manufacturer advises avoid (restriction of skeletal development in *animals*) |
| Propofol | *see* Anaesthetics, General |
| Propranolol | *see* Beta-blockers |
| Propylthiouracil (2, 3) | Neonatal goitre and hypothyroidism |

| Drug (trimester of risk) | Comment |
|---|---|
| Protionamide (1) | May be teratogenic |
| Pseudoephedrine | Defective closure of the abdominal wall (gastroschisis) reported very rarely in newborns after first trimester exposure |
| Pyrazinamide | Manufacturer advises use only if potential benefit outweighs risk; *see also* p. 322 |
| Pyridostigmine | Manufacturer advises use only if potential benefit outweighs risk |
| Pyrimethamine (1) | Theoretical teratogenic risk (folate antagonist); adequate folate supplements should be given to mother; *see also* Antimalarials |
| Pyrimethamine with sulfadoxine (1) | Possible teratogenic risk (pyrimethamine a folate antagonist) |
| (3) | Neonatal haemolysis and methaemoglobinaemia; fear of increased risk of kernicterus in neonates appears to be unfounded |
| | *see also* Antimalarials |
| Quetiapine | Manufacturer advises use only if potential benefit outweighs risk |
| Quinagolide | Manufacturer advises discontinue when pregnancy confirmed unless medical reason for continuing |
| Quinapril | *see* ACE Inhibitors |
| Quinine (1) | High doses are teratogenic; but in malaria benefit of treatment outweighs risk |
| Quinolones (1, 2, 3) | Avoid—arthropathy in *animal* studies; safer alternatives available |
| Quinupristin [ingredient] | *see* Synercid® |
| Rabeprazole | Manufacturer advises avoid—no information available |
| Raltegravir | Manufacturer advises avoid—toxicity in *animal* studies |
| Raltitrexed | Pregnancy must be excluded before treatment; ensure effective contraception during and for at least 6 months after treatment in men or women; *see also* section 8.1 |
| Ramipril | *see* ACE Inhibitors |
| Ranibizumab | Manufacturer advises avoid unless potential benefit outweighs risk and recommends effective contraception during treatment |
| Ranitidine | Manufacturer advises avoid unless essential, but not known to be harmful |
| Ranolazine | Manufacturer advises avoid unless essential—no information available |

| Drug (trimester of risk) | Comment |
|---|---|
| Rasagiline | Manufacturer advises caution |
| Rasburicase | Manufacturer advises avoid—no information available |
| Reboxetine | Manufacturer advises use only if potential benefit outweighs risk—limited information available |
| Remifentanil | No information available; *see also* Opioid Analgesics |
| Repaglinide | Manufacturer advises avoid |
| Reteplase | *see* Fibrinolytics |
| *Riamet*® | Toxicity in *animal* studies with artemether; manufacturer advises use only if potential benefit outweighs risk |
| Ribavirin | Avoid; teratogenicity in *animal* studies; ensure effective contraception during oral administration and for 4 months after treatment in women and for 7 months after treatment in men; *see also* Ribavirin section 5.3.5 |
| Rifabutin | Manufacturer advises avoid—no information available |
| Rifampicin (1) | Manufacturers advise very high doses teratogenic in *animal* studies; *see also* p. 322 |
| (3) | Risk of neonatal bleeding may be increased |
| Riluzole | No information available; manufacturer advises avoid |
| Rimonabant | Manufacturer advises avoid |
| Risedronate sodium | *see* Bisphosphonates |
| Risperidone | Manufacturer advises use only if potential benefit outweighs risk. |
| (3) | Extrapyramidal effects reported in neonates |
| Ritodrine | For use in premature labour *see* section 7.1.3 |
| Ritonavir | Manufacturer advises use only if potential benefit outweighs risk—no information available |
| Rituximab | Avoid unless potential benefit to mother outweighs risk of B-lymphocyte depletion in fetus—effective contraception required during and for 12 months after treatment |
| Rivaroxaban | Manufacturer advises avoid—toxicity in *animal* studies |
| Rivastigmine | Manufacturer advises use only if potential benefit outweighs risk |
| Rizatriptan | *see* 5HT₁ Agonists |
| Rocuronium | Manufacturer advises caution |
| Ropinirole (1) | Manufacturer advises avoid unless potential benefit outweighs risk—toxicity in *animal* studies |
| Ropivacaine | Safety not established but not known to be harmful |
| Rosiglitazone | Manufacturer advises avoid—toxicity in *animal* studies |
| Rosuvastatin | *see* Statins |

| Drug (trimester of risk) | Comment |
|---|---|
| Rotigotine | Manufacturer advises avoid—no information available |
| Rufinamide | Manufacturer advises avoid unless potential benefit outweighs risk—fetotoxic in *animal* studies; effective contraception must be used during treatment; *see also* Antiepileptics |
| Salbutamol | For use in asthma *see* section 3.1 |
| (3) | For use in premature labour *see* section 7.1.3 |
| Salcatonin | *see* Calcitonin (salmon) |
| Salmeterol | *see* section 3.1 |
| Sapropterin | Manufacturer advises caution—consider only if dietary management inadequate |
| Saquinavir | Manufacturer advises use only if potential benefit outweighs risk |
| Selegiline | Manufacturer advises avoid—no information available |
| Sertindole | Manufacturer advises avoid |
| Sertraline | *see* Antidepressants, SSRI |
| Sevelamer | Manufacturer advises use only if potential benefit outweighs risk |
| Sevoflurane | *see* Anaesthetics, General |
| Sibutramine | Manufacturer advises avoid—toxicity in *animal* studies |
| Sildenafil | Manufacturer advises use only if potential benefit outweighs risk—toxicity in *animal* studies |
| Silver sulfadiazine | *see* Sulphonamides |
| Simvastatin | *see* Statins |
| Sirolimus | Manufacturer advises avoid (toxicity in *animal* studies); effective contraception must be used during treatment and for 12 weeks after stopping |
| Sitagliptin | Manufacturer advises avoid—toxicity in *animal* studies |
| Sitaxentan sodium | Avoid unless essential—toxicity in *animal* studies; manufacturer advises effective contraception during treatment |
| Sodium aurothiomalate | Manufacturer advises avoid but limited data suggests usually not necessary to withdraw if condition well controlled—consider reducing dose and frequency |
| Sodium clodronate | *see* Bisphosphonates |
| Sodium cromoglicate | Not known to be harmful; *see also* section 3.1 |
| Sodium fusidate | Not known to be harmful; manufacturer advises use only if potential benefit outweighs risk |
| Sodium nitroprusside | Potential for accumulation of cyanide in fetus—avoid prolonged use |
| Sodium oxybate | Manufacturer advises avoid |

| Drug (trimester of risk) | Comment |
|---|---|
| Sodium phenylbutyrate | Avoid (toxicity in *animal* studies); manufacturer advises adequate contraception during administration |
| Sodium stibogluconate | Manufacturer advises use only if potential benefit outweighs risk |
| Sodium valproate | *see* Valproate |
| Solifenacin | Manufacturer advises caution—no information available |
| Somatropin | Discontinue if pregnancy occurs—no information available but theoretical risk |
| Sorafenib | Manufacturer advises avoid unless essential—toxicity in *animal* studies; *see also* section 8.1 |
| Sotalol | *see* Beta-blockers |
| Spironolactone | Manufacturers advise toxicity in *animal* studies |
| Statins | Avoid—congenital anomalies reported; decreased synthesis of cholesterol possibly affects fetal development |
| Stavudine | Manufacturer advises use only if potential benefit outweighs risk |
| Streptokinase | *see* Fibrinolytics |
| Streptomycin | *see* Aminoglycosides |
| Strontium ranelate | Avoid—toxicity in *animal* studies |
| Sugammadex | Manufacturer advises caution—no information available |
| Sulfadiazine | *see* Sulphonamides |
| Sulfadoxine | *see* Sulphonamides |
| Sulfasalazine | |
| (3) | Theoretical risk of neonatal haemolysis; adequate folate supplements should be given to mother |
| Sulindac | *see* NSAIDs |
| Sulphonamides | |
| (3) | Neonatal haemolysis and methaemoglobinaemia; fear of increased risk of kernicterus in neonates appears to be unfounded |
| Sulphonylureas | Avoid; possible neonatal hypoglycaemia |
| Sulpiride | Limited experience but no evidence of harm in *animal* studies |
| Sumatriptan | *see* 5HT₁ Agonists |
| Sunitinib | Manufacturer advises avoid unless potential benefit outweighs risk—toxicity in *animal* studies; *see also* section 8.1 |
| Suxamethonium | Mildly prolonged maternal paralysis may occur |
| Synercid® | Manufacturer advises avoid unless potential benefit outweighs risk—no information available |
| Tacalcitol | Manufacturer advises avoid unless no safer alternative—no information available; *see also* Vitamin D |

| Drug (trimester of risk) | Comment |
|---|---|
| Tacrolimus | Avoid unless potential benefit outweighs risk—risk of premature delivery and hyperkalaemia; toxicity in *animal* studies following systemic administration |
| Tamoxifen | Avoid—possible effects on fetal development; effective contraception must be used during treatment and for 2 months after stopping |
| Tazarotene | Avoid; effective contraception required (oral progestogen-only contraceptives not considered effective) |
| Tazobactam [ingredient] | *see* Piperacillin with tazobactam |
| Tegafur with uracil | *see Uftoral*® |
| Teicoplanin | Manufacturer advises use only if potential benefit outweighs risk |
| Telbivudine | Manufacturer advises use only if potential benefit outweighs risk |
| Telithromycin | Toxicity in animal studies—manufacturer advises use only if potential benefit outweighs risk |
| Telmisartan | *As for* ACE Inhibitors |
| Temazepam | *see* Benzodiazepines |
| Temocillin | Temocillin *see* Penicillins |
| Temoporfin | Toxicity in *animal* studies—manufacturer advises avoid pregnancy for at least 3 months after treatment |
| Temozolomide | Avoid (teratogenic and embryotoxic in *animal* studies); manufacturer advises adequate contraception during treatment; *see also* section 8.1; also men should avoid fathering a child during and for at least 6 months after treatment |
| Temsirolimus | Manufacturer advises avoid (toxicity in *animal* studies); ensure effective contraception during treatment in men and women; *see also* section 8.1 |
| Tenecteplase | *see* Fibrinolytics |
| Tenofovir | No information available—manufacturer advises use only if potential benefit outweighs risk |
| Tenoxicam | *see* NSAIDs |
| Terazosin | *see* Alpha-blockers, Post-synaptic |
| Terbinafine | Manufacturer advises use only if potential benefit outweighs risk—no information available |
| Terbutaline | For use in asthma *see* section 3.1 |
| (3) | For use in premature labour *see* section 7.1.3 |
| Testosterone | *see* Androgens |
| Tetrabenazine | Inadequate information but no evidence of harm |

| Drug (trimester of risk) | Comment |
|---|---|
| Tetracosactide | Manufacturer advises avoid (but may be used diagnostically if essential) |
| Tetracyclines (1) | Effects on skeletal development in *animal* studies |
| (2, 3) | Dental discoloration; maternal hepatotoxicity with large parenteral doses |
| Thalidomide | Teratogenic risk; effective contraception must be used for at least 1 month before, during, and for at least 1 month after treatment (oral combined hormonal contraceptives and copper-releasing intrauterine devices not recommended); men should use condoms during treatment and for at least 1 week after stopping |
| Theophylline (3) | Neonatal irritability and apnoea have been reported |
| Thiazides and related diuretics | Not used to treat gestational hypertension; may cause neonatal thrombocytopenia, bone marrow suppression, jaundice, electrolyte disturbances, and hypoglycaemia; placental perfusion may also be reduced; stimulation of labour, uterine inertia, and meconium staining also reported |
| Thiopental | *see* Anaesthetics, General |
| Thiotepa | Avoid (teratogenic and embryotoxic in *animals*); *see also* section 8.1 |
| Thymoxamine | *see* Moxisylyte |
| Thyroxine | *see* Levothyroxine |
| Tiagabine | Manufacturer advises avoid unless potential benefit outweighs risk; *see also* Antiepileptics |
| Tiaprofenic acid | *see* NSAIDs |
| Ticarcillin [ingredient] | *see* Penicillins |
| Tigecycline | *see* Tetracyclines |
| Tiludronic acid | *see* Bisphosphonates |
| *Timentin*® | *see* Penicillins |
| Timolol | *see* Beta-blockers |
| Tinidazole | Manufacturer advises avoid in first trimester |
| Tinzaparin | Not known to be harmful; vials contain benzyl alcohol—manufacturer advises avoid |
| Tioconazole | Manufacturer advises avoid |
| Tioguanine | Avoid (teratogenicity reported when men receiving tioguanine have fathered children); ensure effective contraception during treatment in men or women; *see also* section 8.1 |
| Tiotropium | Toxicity in *animal* studies—manufacturer advises use only if potential benefit outweighs risk |
| Tipranavir | Manufacturer advises use only if potential benefit outweighs risk—toxicity in *animal* studies |

| Drug (trimester of risk) | Comment |
| --- | --- |
| Tirofiban | Manufacturer advises use only if potential benefit outweighs risk—no information available |
| Tizanidine | Manufacturer advises use only if potential benefit outweighs risk—no information available |
| Tobramycin | *see* Aminoglycosides |
| Tocopheryl acetate (1, 2, 3) | No evidence of safety of high doses |
| Tolbutamide | *see* Sulphonylureas |
| Tolcapone | Toxicity in *animal* studies—manufacturer advises use only if potential benefit outweighs risk |
| Tolfenamic acid | *see* NSAIDs |
| Tolterodine | Manufacturer advises avoid—toxicity in *animal* studies |
| Topiramate | Manufacturer advises avoid unless potential benefit outweighs risk—toxicity in *animal* studies; *see also* Antiepileptics |
| Topotecan | Avoid (teratogenicity and fetal loss in *animal* studies); *see also* section 8.1 |
| Torasemide | *see* Diuretics |
| Trabectedin | Effective contraception recommended during and for at least 3 months after treatment in women and at least 5 months after treatment in men; *see also* section 8.1 |
| Tramadol | Embryotoxic in animal studies—manufacturers advise avoid; *see also* Opioid Analgesics |
| Trandolapril | *see* ACE Inhibitors |
| Tranexamic acid | No evidence of teratogenicity in *animal* studies; manufacturer advises use only if potential benefit outweighs risk—crosses the placenta |
| Tranylcypromine | *see* Antidepressants, MAOI |
| Trastuzumab | Avoid unless potential benefit outweighs risk |
| Travoprost | Manufacturer advises use only if potential benefit outweighs risk |
| Trazodone | *see* Antidepressants, Tricyclic (and related) |
| Treosulfan | Avoid; *see also* section 8.1 |
| Tretinoin (1, 2, 3) | Teratogenic; effective contraception must be used for at least 1 month before oral treatment, during treatment and for at least 1 month after stopping (oral progestogen-only contraceptives not considered effective); also avoid topical treatment |
| Triamcinolone | *see* Corticosteroids |
| Triamterene | *see* Diuretics |
| Tribavirin | *see* Ribavirin |
| Triclofos | Avoid |

| Drug (trimester of risk) | Comment |
| --- | --- |
| Trientine | Manufacturer advises use only if potential benefit outweighs risk; monitor maternal and neonatal serum-copper concentration; teratogenic in *animal* studies |
| Trifluoperazine | *see* Antipsychotics |
| Trihexyphenidyl | Manufacturer advises use only if potential benefit outweighs risk |
| Trilostane (1, 2, 3) | Interferes with placental sex hormone production |
| Trimeprazine | *see* Antihistamines |
| Trimethoprim (1) | Teratogenic risk (folate antagonist); manufacturers advise avoid |
| Trimipramine | *see* Antidepressants, Tricyclic (and related) |
| Tripotassium dicitratobismuthate | Manufacturer advises avoid on theoretical grounds |
| Triptorelin | Manufacturers advise avoid |
| Trospium | Manufacturer advises caution—no information available |
| Tryptophan | No information available |
| *Uftoral*® | Avoid; manufacturer advises effective contraception during and for 3 months after treatment in men or women |
| Urokinase | *see* Fibrinolytics |
| Ursodeoxycholic acid | No evidence of harm but manufacturer advises avoid |
| Ustekinumab | Avoid; manufacturer advises effective contraception during treatment and for 15 weeks after stopping treatment |
| Vaccines (live) | Theoretical risk of fetal infection, but need for vaccination may outweigh possible risk to fetus (*see also* p. 670); avoid MMR vaccine, live and see, p. 683; avoid varicella–zoster vaccine, see p. 689; *see also* yellow fever vaccine (live), p. 690 |
| Valaciclovir | *see* Aciclovir |
| Valganciclovir | *see* Ganciclovir |
| Valproate (1, 3) | Increased risk of congenital malformations and developmental delay (counselling and screening advised—**important**: *see also* Antiepileptics and p. 253); neonatal bleeding (related to hypofibrinaemia) and neonatal hepatotoxicity also reported |
| Valproic acid | *see* Valproate |
| Valsartan | As for ACE Inhibitors |
| Vancomycin | Manufacturer advises use only if potential benefit outweighs risk—plasma-vancomycin concentration monitoring essential to reduce risk of fetal toxicity |
| Varenicline | Manufacturer advises avoid—toxicity in *animal* studies |

| Drug (trimester of risk) | Comment |
|---|---|
| Varicella-zoster vaccine | *see* Vaccines (live) |
| Vasopressin | Oxytocic effect in third trimester |
| Vecuronium | Manufacturer advises avoid unless potential benefit outweighs risk—no information available |
| Venlafaxine | Manufacturer advises avoid unless potential benefit outweighs risk; risk of withdrawal effects in neonate |
| Verapamil | May reduce uterine blood flow with fetal hypoxia; manufacturer advises avoid in first trimester unless absolutely necessary; may inhibit labour |
| Verteporfin | Manufacturer advises use only if potential benefit outweighs risk (teratogenic in *animal* studies) |
| Vigabatrin | Congenital anomalies reported—manufacturer advises avoid unless potential benefit outweighs risk; *see also* Antiepileptics |
| Vildagliptin | Manufacturer advises avoid—toxicity in *animal* studies |
| Vinblastine | Avoid (limited experience suggests fetal harm; teratogenic in *animal* studies); *see also* section 8.1 |
| Vincristine | Avoid (teratogenicity and fetal loss in *animal* studies); *see also* section 8.1 |
| Vindesine | Avoid (teratogenic in *animal* studies); *see also* section 8.1 |
| Vinorelbine | Avoid (teratogenicity and fetal loss in *animal* studies); *see also* section 8.1 |
| Vitamin A (1) | Excessive doses may be teratogenic; *see also* p. 547 |
| Vitamin D | High systemic doses teratogenic in *animals* but therapeutic doses unlikely to be harmful; avoid *topical* calcitriol—use in restricted amounts if clearly necessary (significant systemic absorption; monitor urine and plasma-calcium concentration); *see also* Calcipotriol, Paricalcitol, and Tacalcitol |
| Voriconazole | Toxicity in *animal* studies—manufacturer advises avoid unless potential benefit outweighs risk; effective contraception required during treatment |
| Warfarin | *see* Anticoagulants, Oral |
| Xipamide | *see* Diuretics |
| Yellow fever vaccine, live | *see* Vaccines (live) |
| Zafirlukast | Manufacturer advises use only if potential benefit outweighs risk |

| Drug (trimester of risk) | Comment |
|---|---|
| Zaleplon | Use only if necessary and restrict to occasional short-term use; risk of withdrawal symptoms in neonate if used in late pregnancy |
| Zanamivir | Use only if potential benefit outweighs risk (e.g. during a pandemic); *see also* p. 354 |
| Zidovudine | Limited information available; manufacturer advises use only if clearly indicated; *see also* p. 340 |
| Zinc acetate | Usual dose 25 mg 3 times daily adjusted according to plasma-copper concentration and urinary copper excretion |
| Zinc sulphate | Safety not established—crosses placenta |
| Zoledronic acid | Manufacturer advises avoid—toxicity in *animal* studies |
| Zolmitriptan | *see* 5HT₁ Agonists |
| Zolpidem | *see* Benzodiazepines |
| Zonisamide | Toxicity in *animal* studies; manufacturer advises use only if potential benefit outweighs risk—effective contraception required during and for 4 weeks after treatment; *see also* Antiepileptics |
| Zopiclone | *see* Benzodiazepines |
| Zotepine | Manufacturer advises avoid unless potential benefit outweighs risk |
| Zuclopenthixol | *see* Antipsychotics |

# A5 Breast-feeding

Appendix 5: Breast-feeding

Breast-feeding is beneficial; the immunological and nutritional value of breast milk to the infant is greater than that of formula feeds.

Although there is concern that drugs taken by the mother might affect the infant, there is very little information on this. In the absence of evidence of an effect, the potential for harm to the infant can be inferred from:

- the amount of drug or active metabolite of the drug delivered to the infant (dependent on the pharmacokinetic characteristics of the drug in the mother);

- the efficiency of absorption, distribution, and elimination of the drug by the infant (infant pharmacokinetics);

- the nature of the effect of the drug on the infant (pharmacodynamic properties of the drug in the infant).

The amount of drug transferred in breast milk is rarely sufficient to produce a discernible effect on the infant. This applies particularly to drugs that are poorly absorbed and need to be given parenterally. However, there is a theoretical possibility that a small amount of drug present in breast milk can induce a hypersensitivity reaction.

A clinical effect can occur in the infant if a pharmacologically significant quantity of the drug is present in milk. For some drugs (e.g. fluvastatin), the ratio between the concentration in milk and that in maternal plasma may be high enough to expose the infant to adverse effects. Some infants, such as those born prematurely or who have jaundice, are at a slightly higher risk of toxicity.

Some drugs inhibit the infant's sucking reflex (e.g. phenobarbital) while others can affect lactation (e.g. bromocriptine)

The following table identifies drugs:

- that should be used with caution or are contraindicated in breast-feeding;

- that can be given to the mother during breast-feeding because they are present in milk in amounts which are too small to be harmful to the infant;

- that might be present in milk in significant amount but are not known to be harmful.

> For many drugs insufficient evidence is available to provide guidance and it is advisable to use only essential drugs to a mother during breast-feeding. Because of the inadequacy of information on drugs in breast-feeding, absence from the table does not imply safety.

## Table of drugs present in breast milk

Products introduced or amended since publication of BNF No. 57 (March 2009) are underlined.

| Drug | Comment |
| --- | --- |
| Abacavir | Breast-feeding not advised in HIV infection |
| Abatacept | Present in milk in *animal* studies—manufacturer advises avoid breast-feeding during treatment and for 14 weeks after last dose |
| Abciximab | Manufacturer advises avoid—no information available |
| Acamprosate | Manufacturer advises avoid |
| Acarbose | Manufacturer advises avoid |
| Acebutolol | *see* Beta-blockers |
| Aceclofenac | Manufacturer advises avoid—no information available |
| Acemetacin | Manufacturer advises avoid |
| Acenocoumarol (nicoumalone) | *see* Anticoagulants, Oral |
| Acetazolamide | Amount too small to be harmful |
| Aciclovir | Significant amount in milk after systemic administration—not known to be harmful but manufacturer advises caution |
| Acipimox | Manufacturer advises avoid |
| Acitretin | Avoid |
| Adalimumab | Avoid; manufacturer advises avoid for at least 5 months after last dose |
| Adapalene | Manufacturer advises avoid (if used, avoid application to chest)—no information available |
| Adefovir dipivoxil | Manufacturer advises avoid—no information available |
| Agalsidase | Use with caution—no information available |
| Agomelatine | Manufacturer advises avoid—present in milk in *animal* studies |
| Alcohol | Large amounts may affect infant and reduce milk consumption |
| Alemtuzumab | Avoid; manufacturer advises avoid breast-feeding for at least 4 weeks after administration |
| Alendronic acid | No information available |
| Alfacalcidol | *see* Vitamin D |
| Alfentanil | Present in milk—manufacturer advises withhold breast-feeding for 24 hours |
| Alglucosidase alfa | Manufacturer advises avoid—no information available |
| Alimemazine (trimeprazine) | *see* Antihistamines |

| Drug | Comment |
|------|---------|
| Aliskiren | Present in milk in *animal* studies—manufacturer advises avoid |
| Alitretinoin | Manufacturer advises avoid |
| Allopurinol | Present in milk—not known to be harmful |
| Almotriptan | Present in milk in *animal* studies—withhold breast-feeding for 24 hours |
| Alprazolam | *see* Benzodiazepines |
| Alverine | Manufacturer advises avoid—little information available |
| Amantadine | Avoid; present in milk; toxicity in infant reported |
| Ambrisentan | Manufacturer advises avoid—no information available |
| Amfebutamone | *see* Bupropion |
| Amiloride | Manufacturer advises avoid—no information available |
| Aminophylline | *see* Theophylline |
| Amiodarone | Avoid; present in milk in significant amounts; theoretical risk from release of iodine; *see also* Iodine |
| Amisulpride | Manufacturer advises avoid—no information available |
| Amitriptyline | *see* Antidepressants, Tricyclic (and related) |
| Amlodipine | Manufacturer advises avoid—no information available |
| Amobarbital | *see* Barbiturates |
| Amorolfine | Manufacturer advises avoid—no information available |
| Amoxicillin | *see* Penicillins |
| Amphetamines | Significant amount in milk. Avoid |
| Amphotericin | No information available |
| Ampicillin | *see* Penicillins |
| Amsacrine | *see* Cytotoxic Drugs |
| Anagrelide | Manufacturer advises avoid—no information available |
| Anakinra | Manufacturer advises avoid—no information available |
| Analgesics | *see* Aspirin, NSAIDs, Opioid Analgesics and Paracetamol |
| Androgens | Avoid; may cause masculinisation in the female infant or precocious development in the male infant; high doses suppress lactation |
| Anidulafungin | Manufacturer advises avoid unless potential benefit outweighs risk—present in milk in *animal* studies |
| Anticoagulants, oral | Risk of haemorrhage; increased by vitamin-K deficiency; warfarin appears safe but phenindione should be avoided; manufacturer of acenocoumarol (nicoumalone) recommends prophylactic vitamin K for the infant (consult product literature); *see also* Dabigatran Etexilate and Rivaroxaban |
| Antidepressants, SSRI | *see* individual entries |

| Drug | Comment |
|------|---------|
| Antidepressants, tricyclic (and related) | Amount of tricyclic antidepressants (including related drugs such as mianserin and trazodone) too small to be harmful but most manufacturers advise avoid; accumulation of doxepin metabolite may cause sedation and respiratory depression |
| Antihistamines | Significant amount of some antihistamines present in milk; although not known to be harmful, manufacturers of alimemazine, cetirizine, cinnarizine, cyproheptadine, desloratadine, dimenhydrinate, fexofenadine, hydroxyzine, loratadine, and mizolastine advise avoid; manufacturer of ketotifen advises avoid; adverse effects in infant reported with clemastine |
| Antipsychotics | Although amount present in milk probably too small to be harmful, *animal* studies indicate possible adverse effects of these drugs on developing nervous system therefore avoid unless absolutely necessary; *see also* Amisulpride, Chlorpromazine, Clozapine, Droperidol, Olanzapine, Paliperidone, Quetiapine, Risperidone, Sertindole, Sulpiride, Zotepine |
| Antithymocyte immunoglobulin | Manufacturer advises avoid—no information available |
| Apomorphine | Manufacturer advises avoid—no information available |
| Aprepitant | *see* Neurokinin Receptor Antagonists |
| Aripiprazole | Manufacturer advises avoid—present in milk in *animal* studies |
| Arsenic trioxide | *see* Cytotoxic Drugs |
| Artemether [ingredient] | *see* Riamet® |
| Aspirin | Avoid—possible risk of Reye's syndrome; regular use of high doses could impair platelet function and produce hypoprothrombinaemia in infant if neonatal vitamin K stores low |
| Atazanavir | Breast-feeding not advised in HIV infection |
| Atenolol | *see* Beta-blockers |
| Atomoxetine | Manufacturer advises avoid—present in milk in *animal* studies |
| Atorvastatin | *see* Statins |
| Atosiban | Small amounts present in milk |
| Atovaquone | Manufacturer advises avoid; for malaria prophylaxis or treatment *see* Malarone® |
| Atracurium | Breast-feeding unlikely to be harmful following recovery from neuromuscular block; some manufacturers advise avoiding breast-feeding for 24 hours after administration |

| Drug | Comment |
| --- | --- |
| Atropine | Small amount present in milk—manufacturer advises caution |
| Auranofin | Present in milk; manufacturer advises avoid |
| Azacitidine | see Cytotoxic Drugs |
| Azapropazone | Small amount present in milk—manufacturer advises avoid |
| Azathioprine | Teratogenic metabolite present in milk in low concentration but no evidence of harm in small studies—consider if potential benefit outweighs risk |
| Azithromycin | Present in milk; use only if no suitable alternative |
| Aztreonam | Amount probably too small to be harmful—manufacturer advises avoid |
| Baclofen | Amount too small to be harmful |
| Balsalazide | Manufacturer advises avoid |
| Barbiturates | Avoid if possible (see also Phenobarbital); large doses may produce drowsiness |
| Basiliximab | Avoid |
| Beclometasone | see Corticosteroids |
| Bemiparin | Manufacturer advises avoid—no information available |
| Bendrofluazide | see Thiazides and Related Diuretics |
| Bendroflumethiazide (bendrofluazide) | see Thiazides and Related Diuretics |
| Benperidol | see Antipsychotics |
| Benzodiazepines | Present in milk—avoid if possible; see also Midazolam |
| Benzylpenicillin | see Penicillins |
| Beta-blockers | Monitor infant; possible toxicity due to beta-blockade but amount of most beta-blockers present in milk too small to affect infant; acebutolol, atenolol, nadolol, and sotalol are present in greater amounts than other beta-blockers; manufacturers advise avoid celiprolol and nebivolol |
| Betaine | Manufacturer advises caution—no information available |
| Betamethasone | see Corticosteroids |
| Bethanechol | Manufacturer advises avoid |
| Bevacizumab | Manufacturer advises avoid breast-feeding during and for at least 6 months after treatment |
| Bexarotene | see Cytotoxic Drugs |
| Bezafibrate | Manufacturer advises avoid—no information available |
| Bimatoprost | Manufacturer advises avoid |
| Bisoprolol | see Beta-blockers |
| Bivalirudin | Manufacturer advises caution—no information available |
| Bleomycin | see Cytotoxic Drugs |
| Bortezomib | see Cytotoxic Drugs |
| Bosentan | Manufacturer advises avoid—no information available |
| Botulinum toxin | Manufacturers advise avoid (or avoid unless essential)—no information available |

| Drug | Comment |
| --- | --- |
| Bromocriptine | Suppresses lactation |
| Buclizine | see Antihistamines |
| Budesonide | see Corticosteroids |
| Bumetanide | Manufacturer advises avoid if possible—no information available |
| Bupivacaine | Amount too small to be harmful |
| Buprenorphine | Avoid unless essential—may inhibit lactation; manufacturer advises contra-indicated in the treatment of opioid dependence |
| Bupropion | Present in milk—manufacturer advises avoid |
| Buserelin | Small amount present in milk—manufacturer advises avoid |
| Buspirone | Manufacturer advises avoid |
| Busulfan | see Cytotoxic Drugs |
| Butobarbital | see Barbiturates |
| C1-esterase inhibitor | Manufacturer advises use only if potential benefit outweighs risk—no information available |
| Cabergoline | Suppresses lactation |
| Caffeine | Regular intake of large amounts can affect infant |
| Calciferol | see Vitamin D |
| Calcipotriol | No information available; see also Vitamin D |
| Calcitonin (salmon) (salcatonin) | Avoid; inhibits lactation in animals |
| Calcitriol | see Vitamin D |
| Calcium folinate | Manufacturer advises caution—no information available |
| Calcium levofolinate | see Calcium Folinate |
| Candesartan | Avoid—no information available |
| Capecitabine | Discontinue breast-feeding |
| Capreomycin | Manufacturer advises caution—no information available |
| Captopril | Avoid in first few weeks after delivery—risk of profound neonatal hypotension; can be used when infant is older if essential but monitor infant's blood pressure |
| Carbamazepine | Amount probably too small to be harmful |
| Carbimazole | Amounts in milk may be sufficient to affect neonatal thyroid function therefore lowest effective dose should be used (see also section 6.2.2) |
| Carbocisteine | No information available |
| Carboplatin | see Cytotoxic Drugs |
| Carglumic acid | Manufacturer advises avoid—present in milk in animal studies |
| Carisoprodol | Concentrated in milk; no adverse effects reported but best avoided |
| Carmustine | see Cytotoxic Drugs |
| Carvedilol | see Beta-blockers |
| Caspofungin | Present in milk in animal studies—manufacturer advises avoid |
| Cefaclor | Present in milk in low concentration |

| Drug | Comment |
|------|---------|
| Cefadroxil | Present in milk in low concentration |
| Cefalexin | Present in milk in low concentration |
| Cefixime | Manufacturer advises avoid—no information available |
| Cefotaxime | Present in milk in low concentration |
| Cefpodoxime | Present in milk in low concentration |
| Cefradine | Present in milk in low concentration |
| Ceftazidime | Present in milk in low concentration |
| Ceftriaxone | Present in milk in low concentration |
| Cefuroxime | Present in milk in low concentration |
| Celecoxib | Manufacturer advises avoid—present in milk in *animal* studies |
| Celiprolol | *see* Beta-blockers |
| Cetirizine | *see* Antihistamines |
| Cetrorelix | Manufacturer advises avoid |
| Cetuximab | Manufacturer advises avoid breast-feeding during and for 2 months after treatment—no information available |
| Chloral hydrate | Sedation in infant—manufacturer advises avoid |
| Chlorambucil | *see* Cytotoxic Drugs |
| Chloramphenicol | Use another antibiotic; may cause bone-marrow toxicity in infant; concentration in milk usually insufficient to cause 'grey syndrome' |
| Chlordiazepoxide | *see* Benzodiazepines |
| Chloroquine | Amount probably too small to be harmful when used for malaria prophylaxis; inadequate for reliable protection against malaria, *see* section 5.4.1; avoid breast-feeding when used for rheumatic diseases |
| Chlorphenamine (chlorpheniramine) | *see* Antihistamines |
| Chlorpheniramine | *see* Antihistamines |
| Chlorpromazine | Drowsiness in infant reported; *see* Antipsychotics |
| Chlorpropamide | *see* Sulphonylureas |
| Chlortalidone | *see* Thiazides and Related Diuretics |
| Ciclesonide | *see* Corticosteroids |
| Ciclosporin | Present in milk—manufacturer advises avoid |
| Cidofovir | Manufacturer advises avoid |
| Cilastatin [ingredient] | *see* Primaxin® |
| Cilazapril | Avoid—no information available |
| Cilostazol | Present in milk in *animal* studies—manufacturer advises avoid |
| Cimetidine | Significant amount—not known to be harmful but manufacturer advises avoid |
| Cinacalcet | Manufacturer advises avoid—present in milk in *animal* studies |

| Drug | Comment |
|------|---------|
| Cinnarizine | *see* Antihistamines |
| Ciprofibrate | Manufacturer advises avoid—present in milk in *animal* studies |
| Ciprofloxacin | Amount probably too small to be harmful but manufacturer advises avoid |
| Cisatracurium | No information available |
| Cisplatin | *see* Cytotoxic Drugs |
| Citalopram | Present in milk—manufacturer advises avoid |
| Cladribine | *see* Cytotoxic Drugs |
| Clarithromycin | Manufacturer advises avoid unless potential benefit outweighs risk—present in milk |
| Clavulanic acid [ingredient] | see Co-amoxiclav, Timentin® |
| Clemastine | *see* Antihistamines |
| Clindamycin | Amount probably too small to be harmful but bloody diarrhoea reported in 1 infant |
| Clobazam | *see* Benzodiazepines |
| Clodronate sodium | *see* Sodium Clodronate |
| Clofarabine | *see* Cytotoxic Drugs |
| Clofazimine | May alter colour of milk; skin discoloration of infant |
| Clomethiazole | Amount too small to be harmful |
| Clomifene | May inhibit lactation |
| Clomipramine | *see* Antidepressants, Tricyclic (and related) |
| Clonazepam | *see* Benzodiazepines |
| Clonidine | Present in milk—manufacturer advises avoid |
| Clopidogrel | Manufacturer advises avoid |
| Clozapine | Manufacturer advises avoid |
| Co-amoxiclav | *see* Penicillins |
| Co-beneldopa | *see* Levodopa |
| Co-careldopa | *see* Levodopa |
| Co-danthramer | Manufacturer advises avoid—limited information available |
| Co-danthrusate | Manufacturer advises avoid—limited information available |
| Codeine | Amount usually too small to be harmful; however mothers vary considerably in their capacity to metabolise codeine—risk of morphine overdose in infant |
| Co-fluampicil | *see* Penicillins |
| Colchicine | Present in milk but no adverse effects reported; manufacturers advise avoid because of risk of cytotoxicity |
| Colecalciferol | *see* Vitamin D |
| Colesevelam | Use with caution—drug not absorbed but may cause fat-soluble vitamin deficiency on prolonged use |
| Colestipol | Use with caution—drug not absorbed but may cause fat-soluble vitamin deficiency on prolonged use |
| Colestyramine | Use with caution—drug not absorbed but may cause fat-soluble vitamin deficiency on prolonged use |

| Drug | Comment |
|------|---------|
| Colistin | Present in milk but poorly absorbed from gut; manufacturers advise avoid (or use only if potential benefit outweighs risk) |
| Contraceptives, hormonal | Avoid combined hormonal contraceptives until weaning or for 6 months after birth (adverse effects on lactation); progestogen-only contraceptives do not affect lactation (start 3 weeks after birth or later) |
| Corticosteroids | Systemic effects in infant unlikely with maternal dose of prednisolone up to 40 mg daily; monitor infant's adrenal function with higher doses—the amount of inhaled drugs in breast milk is probably too small to be harmful |
| Cortisone acetate | see Corticosteroids |
| Co-trimoxazole | Small risk of kernicterus in jaundiced infants and of haemolysis in G6PD-deficient infants (due to sulfamethoxazole) |
| Crisantaspase | see Cytotoxic Drugs |
| Cromoglicate | see Sodium Cromoglicate |
| Cyclopenthiazide | see Thiazides and Related Diuretics |
| Cyclophosphamide | Discontinue breast-feeding during and for 36 hours after stopping treatment |
| Cycloserine | Amount too small to be harmful |
| Cyclosporin | see Ciclosporin |
| Cyproheptadine | see Antihistamines |
| Cyproterone | Caution; possibility of anti-androgen effects in neonate |
| Cytarabine | see Cytotoxic Drugs |
| Cytotoxic drugs | Discontinue breast-feeding; see also Azathioprine, Natalizumab, Nilotinib, Panitumumab, Rituximab, and Trabectedin |
| Dabigatran etexilate | Manufacturer advises avoid—no information available |
| Dacarbazine | see Cytotoxic Drugs |
| Dactinomycin | see Cytotoxic Drugs |
| Dalfopristin [ingredient] | see Synercid® |
| Dalteparin | No information available |
| Danaparoid | Amount probably too small to be harmful but manufacturer advises avoid |
| Danazol | No data available but avoid because of possible androgenic effects in infant |
| Dantrolene | Present in milk—manufacturer advises avoid use in chronic spasticity; use only for malignant hyperthermia if potential benefit outweighs risk |
| Dantron (danthron) | see Co-danthramer, Co-danthrusate |
| Dapsone | Haemolytic anaemia; although significant amount in milk, risk to infant very small unless infant is G6PD deficient |

| Drug | Comment |
|------|---------|
| Daptomycin | Manufacturer advises avoid—no information available |
| Darbepoetin | Manufacturer advises avoid—no information available |
| Darifenacin | Present in milk in animal studies—manufacturer advises caution |
| Darunavir | Breast-feeding not advised in HIV infection |
| Dasatinib | see Cytotoxic Drugs |
| Daunorubicin | see Cytotoxic Drugs |
| Deferasirox | Manufacturer advises avoid—present in milk in animal studies |
| Deferiprone | Manufacturer advises avoid—no information available |
| Deflazacort | see Corticosteroids |
| Demeclocycline | see Tetracyclines |
| Desferrioxamine | Manufacturer advises use only if potential benefit outweighs risk—no information available |
| Desflurane | Manufacturer advises avoid—no information available |
| Desloratadine | see Antihistamines |
| Desmopressin | Not known to be harmful |
| Desogestrel | see Contraceptives, hormonal |
| Dexamethasone | see Corticosteroids |
| Dexamfetamine | see Amphetamines |
| Dexibuprofen | Present in milk—but risk to infant minimal |
| Dexketoprofen | Manufacturer advises avoid—no information available |
| Dexrazoxane | see Cytotoxic Drugs |
| Diamorphine | Therapeutic doses unlikely to affect infant; withdrawal symptoms in infants of dependent mothers; breast-feeding not best method of treating dependence in offspring |
| Diazepam | see Benzodiazepines |
| Diclofenac | Amount too small to be harmful |
| Dicycloverine | Avoid—present in milk; apnoea reported in infant |
| Didanosine | Breast-feeding not advised in HIV infection |
| Digoxin | Amount too small to be harmful |
| Dihydrocodeine | Manufacturer advises use only if potential benefit outweighs risk |
| Dihydrotachysterol | see Vitamin D |
| Diloxanide | Manufacturer advises avoid |
| Diltiazem | Significant amount present in milk—no evidence of harm but avoid unless no safer alternative |
| Dimenhydrinate | see Antihistamines |
| Dipyridamole | Small amount present in milk—manufacturer advises caution |
| Disodium etidronate | No information available |
| Disodium pamidronate | Manufacturer advises avoid |
| Disopyramide | Present in milk—use only if essential and monitor infant for antimuscarinic effects |
| Distigmine | Manufacturer advises avoid—no information available |

| Drug | Comment |
|---|---|
| Disulfiram | Manufacturer advises avoid—no information available |
| Docetaxel | *see* Cytotoxic Drugs |
| Docusate sodium | Present in milk following oral administration—manufacturer advises caution; rectal administration not known to be harmful |
| Dolasetron | Not known to be harmful but manufacturer advises avoid |
| Domperidone | Amount probably too small to be harmful |
| Donepezil | Manufacturer advises avoid—no information available |
| Doripenem | Manufacturer advises use only if potential benefit outweighs risk—present in milk in *animal* studies |
| Dornase alfa | Amount probably too small to be harmful—manufacturer advises caution |
| Dosulepin (dothiepin) | *see* Antidepressants, Tricyclic (and related) |
| Dothiepin | *see* Antidepressants, Tricyclic (and related) |
| Doxazosin | Accumulates in milk—manufacturer advises avoid |
| Doxepin | *see* Antidepressants, Tricyclic (and related) |
| Doxorubicin | *see* Cytotoxic Drugs |
| Doxycycline | *see* Tetracyclines |
| Droperidol | Limited information available—manufacturer advises avoid repeated administration |
| Drospirenone | *see* Contraceptives, hormonal |
| Drotrecogin alfa (activated) | Manufacturer advises avoid—no information available |
| Duloxetine | Present in milk—manufacturer advises avoid |
| Dydrogesterone | Present in milk—no adverse effects reported |
| Eculizumab | No information available—manufacturer advises avoid breast-feeding during and for 5 months after treatment |
| Edrophonium | Amount probably too small to be harmful |
| Efavirenz | Breast-feeding not advised in HIV infection |
| Eflornithine | Manufacturer advises avoid—no information available |
| Eletriptan | Present in milk—avoid breast-feeding for 24 hours |
| Emtricitabine | Breast-feeding not advised in HIV infection |
| Enalapril | Avoid in first few weeks after delivery—risk of profound neonatal hypotension; can be used when infant is older if essential but monitor infant's blood pressure |
| Enfuvirtide | Breast-feeding not advised in HIV infection |
| Enoxaparin | Manufacturer advises avoid—no information available |
| Enoximone | Manufacturer advises caution—no information available |
| Entacapone | Manufacturer advises avoid—present in milk in *animal* studies |

| Drug | Comment |
|---|---|
| Entecavir | Manufacturer advises avoid—present in milk in *animal* studies |
| Ephedrine | Irritability and disturbed sleep reported |
| Epinastine | Present in milk in *animal* studies—manufacturer advises caution |
| Epirubicin | *see* Cytotoxic Drugs |
| Eplerenone | Manufacturer advises use only if potential benefit outweighs risk |
| Epoetin | Unlikely to be present in milk; minimal effect on infant |
| Eprosartan | Avoid—no information available |
| Eptifibatide | No information available—manufacturer advises avoid |
| Erdosteine | Manufacturer advises avoid—no information available |
| Ergocalciferol | *see* Vitamin D |
| Ergotamine | Avoid; ergotism may occur in infant; repeated doses may inhibit lactation |
| Erlotinib | Manufacturer advises avoid—no information available |
| Ertapenem | Present in milk—manufacturer advises avoid |
| Erythromycin | Only small amounts in milk—not known to be harmful |
| Escitalopram | Present in milk; manufacturer advises avoid |
| Esmolol | *see* Beta-blockers |
| Esomeprazole | Manufacturer advises avoid—no information available |
| Estradiol | *see* Oestrogens |
| Etamsylate | Significant amount but not known to be harmful |
| Etanercept | Manufacturer advises avoid—present in milk in *animal* studies |
| Ethambutol | Amount too small to be harmful |
| Ethinylestradiol | *see* Oestrogens |
| Ethosuximide | Present in milk but unlikely to be harmful; manufacturer advises avoid |
| Etidronate disodium | *see* Disodium Etidronate |
| Etodolac | Manufacturer advises avoid—no information available |
| Etomidate | Avoid breast-feeding for 24 hours after administration |
| Etonogestrel | *see* Contraceptives, hormonal |
| Etoposide | *see* Cytotoxic Drugs |
| Etoricoxib | Manufacturer advises avoid—present in milk in *animal* studies |
| Etravirine | Breast-feeding not advised in HIV infection |
| Etynodiol | *see* Contraceptives, hormonal |
| Exenatide | Manufacturer advises avoid—no information available |
| Ezetimibe | Present in milk in *animal* studies—manufacturer advises avoid |
| Famciclovir | Manufacturer advises avoid unless potential benefit outweighs risk—present in milk in *animal* studies |

| Drug | Comment |
|---|---|
| Famotidine | Present in milk—not known to be harmful but manufacturer advises avoid |
| Felodipine | Present in milk |
| Fenbufen | Small amount present in milk—manufacturer advises avoid |
| Fenofibrate | Manufacturer advises avoid—no information available |
| Fenoprofen | Amount too small to be harmful |
| Fentanyl | Amount too small to be harmful |
| Fesoterodine | Manufacturer advises avoid—no information available |
| Fexofenadine | *see* Antihistamines |
| Filgrastim | No information available—manufacturer advises avoid |
| Flavoxate | Manufacturer advises caution—no information available |
| Flecainide | Significant amount present in milk but not known to be harmful |
| Flucloxacillin | *see* Penicillins |
| Fluconazole | Present in milk but amount probably too small to be harmful |
| Flucytosine | Manufacturer advises avoid |
| Fludarabine | *see* Cytotoxic Drugs |
| Fludrocortisone | see Corticosteroids |
| Fluorouracil | *see* Cytotoxic Drugs |
| Fluoxetine | Present in milk—manufacturer advises avoid |
| Flupentixol | see Antipsychotics |
| Fluphenazine | *see* Antipsychotics |
| Flurazepam | *see* Benzodiazepines |
| Flurbiprofen | Amount too small to be harmful |
| Fluticasone | *see* Corticosteroids |
| Fluvastatin | *see* Statins |
| Fluvoxamine | Present in milk—manufacturer advises avoid |
| Follitropin alfa and beta | Avoid |
| Fomepizole | Manufacturer advises caution—no information available |
| Fondaparinux | Present in milk in *animal* studies—manufacturer advises avoid |
| Formoterol (eformoterol) | Amount in milk probably too small to be harmful but manufacturers advise avoid |
| Fosamprenavir | Breast-feeding not advised in HIV infection |
| Fosaprepitant | *see* Neurokinin Receptor Antagonists |
| Foscarnet | Avoid—present in milk in *animal* studies |
| Fosinopril | Avoid—present in milk |
| Fosphenytoin | *see* Phenytoin |
| Frovatriptan | Present in milk in *animal* studies—withhold breast-feeding for 24 hours |
| Frusemide | *see* Furosemide |
| Fulvestrant | Manufacturer advises avoid—present in milk in *animal* studies |

| Drug | Comment |
|---|---|
| Furosemide (frusemide) | Amount too small to be harmful; may inhibit lactation |
| Fusidic acid | *see* Sodium Fusidate |
| Gabapentin | Present in milk—manufacturer advises use only if potential benefit outweighs risk |
| Galantamine | Manufacturer advises avoid—no information available |
| Galsulfase | Manufacturer advises avoid—no information available |
| Ganciclovir | Avoid—no information available |
| Ganirelix | Manufacturer advises avoid—no information available |
| Gemcitabine | *see* Cytotoxic Drugs |
| Gemfibrozil | Manufacturer advises avoid—no information available |
| Gestodene | *see* Contraceptives, hormonal |
| Gestrinone | Manufacturer advises avoid |
| Glatiramer | Manufacturer advises caution—no information available |
| Glibenclamide | *see* Sulphonylureas |
| Gliclazide | *see* Sulphonylureas |
| Glimepiride | *see* Sulphonylureas |
| Glipizide | *see* Sulphonylureas |
| Glucosamine | Manufacturer advises avoid—no information available |
| Glyceryl trinitrate | No information available—manufacturers advise use only if potential benefit outweighs risk |
| Goserelin | Manufacturer advises avoid |
| Granisetron | Not known to be harmful but manufacturer advises avoid |
| Griseofulvin | Avoid—no information available |
| Haem arginate | Manufacturer advises avoid unless essential—no information available |
| Haloperidol | *see* Antipsychotics |
| Halothane | Present in milk—withhold breast-feeding for 24 hours after termination of anaesthesia |
| Heparin | Not excreted into milk due to high molecular weight |
| Hepatitis A vaccine | No information available |
| Human menopausal gonadotrophins | Avoid |
| Hydralazine | Present in milk but not known to be harmful; monitor infant |
| Hydrochlorothiazide | *see* Thiazides and Related Diuretics |
| Hydrocortisone | *see* Corticosteroids |
| Hydroflumethiazide | *see* Thiazides and Related Diuretics |
| Hydromorphone | Manufacturer advises avoid—no information available |
| Hydroxocobalamin | Present in milk but not known to be harmful |
| Hydroxycarbamide (hydroxyurea) | *see* Cytotoxic Drugs |
| Hydroxychloroquine | Avoid—risk of toxicity in infant |
| Hydroxyurea | *see* Cytotoxic Drugs |
| Hydroxyzine | *see* Antihistamines |
| Hyoscine | Amount too small to be harmful |

| Drug | Comment |
|------|---------|
| Ibandronic acid | Manufacturer advises avoid—present in milk in *animal* studies |
| Ibuprofen | Amount too small to be harmful but some manufacturers advise avoid (including topical use) |
| Icatibant | Manufacturer advises avoid in breast-feeding for 12 hours after administration |
| Idarubicin | see Cytotoxic Drugs |
| Idoxuridine | May make milk taste unpleasant |
| Idursulfase | No information available |
| Ifosfamide | see Cytotoxic Drugs |
| Iloprost | Manufacturer advises avoid—no information available |
| Imatinib | see Cytotoxic Drugs |
| Imidapril | Avoid—no information available |
| Imiglucerase | No information available |
| Imipenem [ingredient] | see Primaxin® |
| Imipramine | see Antidepressants, Tricyclic (and related) |
| Imiquimod | Manufacturer advises no information available |
| Indapamide | Present in milk—manufacturer advises avoid |
| Indinavir | Breast-feeding not advised in HIV infection |
| Indometacin | Amount probably too small to be harmful but convulsions reported in one infant—manufacturers advise avoid |
| Infliximab | Amount probably too small to be harmful |
| Influenza vaccine | Not known to be harmful |
| Interferons | Manufacturers advise avoid—no information available |
| Iodine and iodides | Stop breast-feeding; danger of neonatal hypothyroidism or goitre; appears to be concentrated in milk; see also Povidone–iodine |
| Iodine, radioactive | Breast-feeding contra-indicated after therapeutic doses. With diagnostic doses withhold breast-feeding for at least 24 hours |
| Ipratropium | Amount probably too small to be harmful |
| Irbesartan | Avoid—no information available |
| Irinotecan | see Cytotoxic Drugs |
| Isoflurane | Manufacturer advises avoid—withhold breast-feeding for at least 12 hours after termination of anaesthesia |
| Isoniazid | Monitor infant for possible toxicity; theoretical risk of convulsions and neuropathy; prophylactic pyridoxine advisable in mother and infant |
| Isosorbide dinitrate | No information available—manufacturers advise use only if potential benefit outweighs risk |

| Drug | Comment |
|------|---------|
| Isosorbide mononitrate | No information available—manufacturers advise use only if potential benefit outweighs risk |
| Isotretinoin | Avoid |
| Isradipine | Manufacturer advises avoid—present in milk in *animal* studies |
| Itraconazole | Small amounts present in milk—may accumulate; manufacturer advises avoid |
| Ivabradine | Present in milk in *animal* studies—manufacturer advises avoid |
| Kaletra® | Breast-feeding not advised in HIV infection |
| Ketoconazole | Manufacturer advises avoid |
| Ketoprofen | Amount probably too small to be harmful but manufacturer advises avoid unless essential |
| Ketorolac | Amount too small to be harmful but manufacturer advises avoid |
| Ketotifen | see Antihistamines |
| Labetalol | see Beta-blockers |
| Lacidipine | Manufacturer advises avoid—no information available |
| Lacosamide | Manufacturer advises avoid—present in milk in *animal* studies |
| Lamivudine | Present in milk—manufacturer advises avoid; breast-feeding not advised in HIV infection |
| Lamotrigine | Present in milk but limited data suggest no harmful effects on infants |
| Lanreotide | Manufacturer advises avoid unless potential benefit outweighs risk—no information available |
| Lansoprazole | Manufacturer advises avoid unless essential—present in milk in *animal* studies |
| Lanthanum | Manufacturer advises caution—no information available |
| Lapatinib | see Cytotoxic Drugs |
| Laronidase | Manufacturer advises avoid—no information available |
| Latanoprost | May be present in milk—manufacturer advises avoid |
| Leflunomide | Present in milk in *animal* studies—manufacturer advises avoid |
| Lenalidomide | Manufacturer advises discontinue breast-feeding—no information available |
| Lenograstim | Manufacturer advises avoid—no information available |
| Lepirudin | Avoid |
| Lercanidipine | Manufacturer advises avoid |
| Letrozole | Manufacturer advises avoid |
| Leuprorelin | Manufacturer advises avoid |
| Levetiracetam | Present in milk—manufacturer advises avoid |
| Levobupivacaine | Likely to be present in milk but risk to infant minimal |
| Levocetirizine | see Antihistamines |

| Drug | Comment |
|------|---------|
| Levodopa | May suppress lactation; present in milk—manufacturers advise avoid |
| Levofloxacin | Manufacturer advises avoid |
| Levomepromazine (methotrimeprazine) | see Antipsychotics |
| Levonorgestrel | see Contraceptives, hormonal |
| Levothyroxine (thyroxine) | Amount too small to affect tests for neonatal hypothyroidism |
| Lidocaine (lignocaine) | Amount too small to be harmful |
| Lignocaine | see Lidocaine |
| Linezolid | Manufacturer advises avoid—present in milk in animal studies |
| Liothyronine | Amount too small to affect tests for neonatal hypothyroidism |
| Lisinopril | Avoid—no information available |
| Lithium salts | Present in milk and risk of toxicity in infant—manufacturers advise avoid |
| Lofepramine | see Antidepressants, Tricyclic (and related) |
| Lofexidine | Manufacturer advises use only if potential benefit outweighs risk—no information available |
| Loperamide | Amount probably too small to be harmful |
| Lopinavir [ingredient] | see Kaletra® |
| Loprazolam | see Benzodiazepines |
| Loratadine | see Antihistamines |
| Lorazepam | see Benzodiazepines |
| Lormetazepam | see Benzodiazepines |
| Losartan | Avoid—no information available |
| Lumefantrine [ingredient] | see Riamet® |
| Lymecycline | see Tetracyclines |
| Macrogols | Manufacturers advise use only if essential—no information available |
| Malarone® | Use only if no suitable alternative available; see also p. 360 |
| Mannitol | Manufacturer advises avoid unless essential—no information available |
| Maraviroc | Breast-feeding not advised in HIV infection |
| Mebendazole | Amount too small to be harmful but manufacturer advises avoid |
| Mecysteine | Manufacturer advises avoid |
| Medroxyprogesterone | Present in milk—no adverse effects reported; see also Contraceptives, hormonal |
| Mefenamic acid | Amount too small to be harmful but manufacturer advises avoid |
| Mefloquine | Present in milk but risk to infant minimal |
| Melatonin | Present in milk—manufacturer advises avoid |
| Meloxicam | No information available—manufacturer advises avoid |
| Melphalan | see Cytotoxic Drugs |

| Drug | Comment |
|------|---------|
| Memantine | Manufacturer advises avoid—no information available |
| Menotrophin | Avoid |
| Meprobamate | Avoid; concentration in milk may exceed maternal plasma concentrations fourfold and may cause drowsiness in infant |
| Meptazinol | Manufacturer advises use only if potential benefit outweighs risk |
| Mercaptamine | Manufacturer advises avoid |
| Mercaptopurine | see Cytotoxic Drugs |
| Meropenem | Unlikely to be absorbed (however, manufacturer advises avoid unless potential benefit justifies potential risk) |
| Mesalazine | Diarrhoea reported but manufacturers advise negligible amounts detected in breast milk |
| Mesterolone | see Androgens |
| Mestranol | see Oestrogens |
| Metaraminol | Manufacturer advises caution—no information available |
| Metformin | May be used during breast-feeding—see section 6.1.2; manufacturer advises avoid |
| Methadone | Withdrawal symptoms in infant; breast-feeding permissible during maintenance but dose should be as low as possible and infant monitored to avoid sedation |
| Methenamine | Amount too small to be harmful |
| Methocarbamol | Present in milk in animal studies—manufacturer advises caution |
| Methotrexate | see Cytotoxic Drugs |
| Methotrimeprazine | see Antipsychotics |
| Methoxy polyethylene glycol-epoetin beta | Manufacturer advises use only if potential benefit outweighs risk—present in milk in animal studies |
| Methyldopa | Amount too small to be harmful |
| Methylnaltrexone | Manufacturer advises use only if potential benefit outweighs risk—present in milk in animal studies |
| Methylphenidate | No information available—manufacturer advises avoid |
| Methylprednisolone | see Corticosteroids |
| Methysergide | Manufacturer advises avoid |
| Metoclopramide | Small amount present in milk; manufacturer advises avoid |
| Metolazone | see Thiazides and Related Diuretics |
| Metoprolol | see Beta-blockers |
| Metronidazole | Significant amount in milk; manufacturer advises avoid large single doses |
| Metyrapone | Manufacturer advises avoid—no information available |
| Mianserin | see Antidepressants, Tricyclic (and related) |
| Micafungin | Manufacturer advises use only if potential benefit outweighs risk—present in milk in animal studies |

| Drug | Comment |
|------|---------|
| Miconazole | Manufacturer advises caution—no information available |
| Midazolam | Present in milk—manufacturer advises avoid breast feeding for 24 hours after administration |
| Mifepristone | No information available—manufacturer advises avoid |
| Miglustat | Manufacturer advises avoid—no information available |
| Milrinone | Manufacturer advises caution—no information available |
| Minocycline | *see* Tetracyclines |
| Minoxidil | Present in milk but not known to be harmful |
| Mirtazapine | Small amount present in milk; manufacturer advises avoid |
| Misoprostol | No information available—manufacturer advises avoid |
| Mitomycin | *see* Cytotoxic Drugs |
| Mitotane | *see* Cytotoxic Drugs |
| Mitoxantrone (mitozantrone) | *see* Cytotoxic Drugs |
| Mitozantrone | *see* Cytotoxic Drugs |
| Mizolastine | *see* Antihistamines |
| Moclobemide | Amount too small to be harmful, but patient leaflet advises avoid |
| Modafinil | Manufacturer advises avoid—present in milk in *animal* studies |
| Moexipril | Avoid—no information available |
| Montelukast | Manufacturer advises avoid unless essential |
| Morphine | Therapeutic doses unlikely to affect infant; withdrawal symptoms in infants of dependent mothers; breast-feeding not best method of treating dependence in offspring |
| Moxifloxacin | Manufacturer advises avoid—present in milk in *animal* studies |
| Moxonidine | Present in milk—manufacturer advises avoid |
| Mupirocin | Manufacturer advises avoid unless potential benefit outweighs risk—no information available |
| Mycophenolate mofetil | Manufacturer advises avoid—present in milk in *animal* studies |
| Nabilone | Manufacturer advises avoid—no information available |
| Nabumetone | No information available—manufacturer advises avoid |
| Nadolol | *see* Beta-blockers |
| Nafarelin | Manufacturer advises avoid—no information available |
| Nalidixic acid | Risk to infant very small but one case of haemolytic anaemia reported |
| Naloxone | No information available |
| Naltrexone | Manufacturers advise avoid—present in milk in *animal* studies |

| Drug | Comment |
|------|---------|
| Naproxen | Amount too small to be harmful but manufacturer advises avoid |
| Naratriptan | Manufacturer advises caution—no information available |
| Natalizumab | Present in milk in *animal* studies—manufacturer advises avoid |
| Nateglinide | Manufacturer advises avoid—present in milk in *animal* studies |
| Nebivolol | *see* Beta-blockers |
| Nedocromil | Unlikely to be present in milk |
| Nelarabine | *see* Cytotoxic Drugs |
| Nelfinavir | Breast-feeding not advised in HIV infection |
| Neostigmine | Amount probably too small to be harmful; monitor infant |
| Neurokinin receptor antagonists | Manufacturer advises avoid—present in milk in *animal* studies |
| Nevirapine | Breast-feeding not advised in HIV infection |
| Nicardipine | Manufacturer advises avoid—no information available |
| Nicorandil | No information available—manufacturer advises avoid |
| Nicotine | Present in milk; intermittent therapy preferable |
| Nicotinic acid | Present in milk—avoid |
| Nicoumalone | *see* Anticoagulants, Oral |
| Nifedipine | Amount too small to be harmful but manufacturers advise avoid |
| Nilotinib | Manufacturer advises avoid—present in milk in *animal* studies |
| Nimodipine | No information available |
| Nitisinone | Manufacturer advises avoid—adverse effects in *animal* studies |
| Nitrazepam | *see* Benzodiazepines |
| Nitrofurantoin | Only small amounts in milk but could be enough to produce haemolysis in G6PD-deficient infants |
| Nitroprusside | *see* Sodium Nitroprusside |
| Nizatidine | Amount too small to be harmful |
| Nonoxinol 9 | Present in milk in *animal* studies |
| Norelgestromin | *see* Contraceptives, hormonal |
| Norethisterone | Higher doses may suppress lactation and alter milk composition—use lowest effective dose; *see also* Contraceptives, hormonal |
| Norfloxacin | No information available—manufacturer advises avoid |
| Norgestimate | *see* Contraceptives, hormonal |
| Norgestrel | *see* Contraceptives, hormonal |
| Nortriptyline | *see* Antidepressants, Tricyclic (and related) |
| NSAIDs | *see* individual entries |
| Nystatin | No information available, but absorption from gastro-intestinal tract negligible |

| Drug | Comment |
|------|---------|
| Octreotide | Manufacturer advises avoid unless essential—no information available |
| Oestrogens | Avoid; adverse effects on lactation; see also Contraceptives, hormonal |
| Ofloxacin | Amount probably too small to be harmful but manufacturer advises avoid |
| Olanzapine | Manufacturer advises avoid—present in milk |
| Olmesartan | Avoid—no information available |
| Olsalazine | Manufacturer advises use only if potential benefit outweighs risk; monitor infant for diarrhoea |
| Omalizumab | Manufacturer advises avoid—present in milk in animal studies |
| Omega-3-acid ethyl esters | Manufacturer advises avoid—no information available |
| Omeprazole | Present in milk but not known to be harmful |
| Ondansetron | Not known to be harmful but manufacturer advises avoid |
| Opioid analgesics | see individual entries |
| Oral contraceptives | see Contraceptives, hormonal |
| Orlistat | Manufacturer advises avoid—no information available |
| Orphenadrine | Manufacturers advise caution |
| Oseltamivir | Amount probably too small to be harmful; use only if potential benefit outweighs risk (e.g. during a pandemic); see also p. 354 |
| Oxaliplatin | see Cytotoxic Drugs |
| Oxazepam | see Benzodiazepines |
| Oxcarbazepine | Present in milk—manufacturer advises avoid |
| Oxprenolol | see Beta-blockers |
| Oxybutynin | Present in milk—manufacturers advise avoid |
| Oxycodone | Present in milk—manufacturer advises avoid |
| Oxytetracycline | see Tetracyclines |
| Paclitaxel | see Cytotoxic Drugs |
| Palifermin | Manufacturer advises avoid—no information available |
| Paliperidone | Manufacturer advises avoid—present in milk |
| Palonosetron | Manufacturer advises avoid—no information available |
| Pamidronate disodium | see Disodium Pamidronate |
| Pancuronium | Manufacturer advises avoid unless potential benefit outweighs possble risk—no information available |
| Panitumumab | Manufacturer advises avoid breast-feeding during and for 3 months after treatment |
| Pantoprazole | Manufacturer advises avoid unless potential benefit outweighs risk—small amount present in milk in animal studies |
| Papaveretum | see Morphine |
| Paracetamol | Amount too small to be harmful |
| Paraldehyde | Manufacturer advises avoid unless essential—present in milk |
| Parecoxib | Manufacturer advises avoid—present in milk in animal studies |
| Paricalcitol | Manufacturer advises caution—no information available; see also Vitamin D |
| Paroxetine | Present in milk but amount too small to be harmful |
| Pegaptinib | Manufacturer advises avoid—no information available |
| Pegfilgrastim | No information available—manufacturer advises avoid |
| Peginterferon alfa | see Interferons |
| Pemetrexed | see Cytotoxic Drugs |
| Penicillamine | Manufacturer advises avoid unless potential benefit outweighs risk—no information available |
| Penicillins | Trace amounts in milk |
| Pentamidine isetionate | Manufacturer advises avoid unless essential |
| Pentazocine | Small amount present in milk—manufacturer advises caution |
| Pentostatin | see Cytotoxic Drugs |
| Pergolide | May suppress lactation |
| Pericyazine | see Antipsychotics |
| Perindopril | Avoid—no information available |
| Perphenazine | see Antipsychotics |
| Pethidine | Present in milk but not known to be harmful |
| Phenindione | see Anticoagulants, Oral |
| Phenobarbital | Avoid when possible; drowsiness may occur but risk probably small; one report of methaemoglobinaemia with phenobarbital and phenytoin |
| Phenoxybenzamine | May be present in milk |
| Phenoxymethylpenicillin | see Penicillins |
| Phentolamine | Manufacturer advises avoid—no information available |
| Phenytoin | Small amount present in milk; manufacturer advises avoid—but see section 4.8.1 |
| Phytomenadione | Present in milk |
| Pilocarpine | Manufacturer advises avoid—present in milk in animal studies |
| Pimozide | see Antipsychotics |
| Pindolol | see Beta-blockers |
| Pioglitazone | Manufacturer advises avoid—present in milk in animal studies |
| Piperacillin with tazobactam | Present in milk—manufacturers advise use only if potential benefit outweighs risk |
| Piperazine | Present in milk—manufacturer advises avoid breast-feeding for 8 hours after dose (express and discard milk during this time) |
| Piracetam | Manufacturer advises avoid |

| Drug | Comment |
|------|---------|
| Piroxicam | Amount too small to be harmful |
| Pivmecillinam | see Penicillins |
| Pizotifen | Amount probably too small to be harmful, but manufacturer advises avoid |
| Podophyllotoxin | Manufacturers advise avoid |
| Podophyllum | Avoid |
| Porfimer | No information available—manufacturer advises avoid |
| Posaconazole | Manufacturer advises avoid—present in milk in *animal* studies |
| Povidone–iodine | Avoid; iodine absorbed from vaginal preparations is concentrated in milk |
| Pramipexole | May suppress lactation; manufacturer advises avoid—present in milk in *animal* studies |
| Prasugrel | Manufacturer advises avoid—no information available |
| Pravastatin | Small amount present in milk—manufacturer advises avoid |
| Prazosin | Amount probably too small to be harmful |
| Prednisolone | see Corticosteroids |
| Pregabalin | Present in milk in *animal* studies—manufacturer advises avoid |
| Prilocaine | Present in milk but not known to be harmful |
| *Primaxin*® | Present in milk but unlikely to be absorbed (however, manufacturer advises avoid) |
| Primidone | see Phenobarbital |
| Probenecid | No information available |
| Procarbazine | see Cytotoxic Drugs |
| Prochlorperazine | see Antipsychotics |
| Procyclidine | No information available |
| Progesterone | Manufacturers advise avoid—present in milk |
| Proguanil | Amount probably too small to be harmful when used for malaria prophylaxis; inadequate for reliable protection against malaria in breast-fed infant, *see* p. 360; for Proguanil with Atovaquone *see* *Malarone*® |
| Promazine | see Antipsychotics |
| Promethazine | see Antihistamines |
| Propafenone | Manufacturer advises avoid—no information available |
| Propantheline | May suppress lactation |
| Propiverine | Manufacturer advises avoid—present in milk in *animal* studies |
| Propofol | Present in milk but amount probably too small to be harmful |
| Propranolol | see Beta-blockers |
| Propylthiouracil | Monitor infant's thyroid status but amounts in milk probably too small to affect infant; high doses might affect neonatal thyroid function |
| Protirelin | Breast enlargement and leaking of milk reported |

| Drug | Comment |
|------|---------|
| Pseudoephedrine | Amount too small to be harmful |
| Pyrazinamide | Amount too small to be harmful |
| Pyridostigmine | Amount probably too small to be harmful |
| Pyrimethamine | Significant amount—avoid administration of other folate antagonists to infant; avoid breast-feeding during toxoplasmosis treatment |
| Pyrimethamine with sulfadoxine | Small risk of kernicterus in jaundiced infants and of haemolysis in G6PD-deficient infants (due to sulfadoxine) |
| Quetiapine | Manufacturer advises avoid—no information available |
| Quinagolide | Suppresses lactation |
| Quinapril | Avoid in first few weeks after delivery—risk of profound neonatal hypotension; can be used when infant is older if essential but monitor infant's blood pressure |
| Quinupristin [ingredient] | see Synercid® |
| Rabeprazole | Manufacturer advises avoid—no information available |
| Raltegravir | Breast-feeding not advised in HIV infection |
| Raltitrexed | see Cytotoxic Drugs |
| Ramipril | Avoid—no information available |
| Ranibizumab | Manufacturer advises avoid—no information available |
| Ranitidine | Significant amount but not known to be harmful |
| Ranolazine | Manufacturer advises avoid—no information available |
| Rasagiline | Manufacturer advises caution—may suppress lactation |
| Rasburicase | Manufacturer advises avoid—no information available |
| Reboxetine | Small amount present in milk—manufacturer advises use only if potential benefit outweighs risk |
| Remifentanil | Manufacturer advises caution—present in milk in *animal* studies |
| Repaglinide | Manufacturer advises avoid—present in milk in *animal* studies |
| Reteplase | Manufacturer advises avoid breast-feeding for 24 hours after dose (express and discard milk during this time) |
| *Riamet*® | Manufacturer advises avoid breast-feeding for at least 1 week after last dose; present in milk in *animal* studies |
| Ribavirin | Avoid—no information available |
| Rifabutin | Manufacturer advises avoid—no information available |
| Rifampicin | Amount too small to be harmful |
| Riluzole | Manufacturer advises avoid—no information available |

| Drug | Comment |
|------|---------|
| Rimonabant | Manufacturer advises avoid—present in milk in *animal* studies |
| Risedronate sodium | Manufacturer advises avoid |
| Risperidone | Manufacturer advises use only if potential benefit outweighs risk—small amount present in milk |
| Ritonavir | Breast-feeding not advised in HIV infection |
| Rituximab | Avoid breast-feeding during and for 12 months after treatment |
| Rivaroxaban | Manufacturer advises avoid—present in milk in *animal* studies |
| Rivastigmine | Present in milk in *animal* studies—manufacturer advises avoid |
| Rizatriptan | Present in milk in *animal* studies—withhold breast-feeding for 24 hours |
| Rocuronium | Manufacturer advises avoid unless potential benefit outweighs risk—present in milk in *animal* studies |
| Ropinirole | May suppress lactation—manufacturer advises avoid |
| Ropivacaine | Not known to be harmful |
| Rosiglitazone | Manufacturer advises avoid—present in milk in *animal* studies |
| Rosuvastatin | *see* Statins |
| Rotigotine | May suppress lactation; manufacturer advises avoid—present in milk in *animal* studies |
| Rufinamide | Manufacturer advises avoid—no information available |
| Salbutamol | Probably present in milk; manufacturer advises avoid unless potential benefit outweighs risk—the amount of inhaled drugs in breast milk is probably too small to be harmful |
| Salcatonin | *see* Calcitonin (salmon) |
| Sapropterin | Manufacturer advises avoid—no information available |
| Saquinavir | Breast-feeding not advised in HIV infection |
| Secobarbital | *see* Barbiturates |
| Selegiline | Manufacturer advises avoid—no information available |
| Senna | Not known to be harmful |
| Sertindole | Manufacturer advises avoid—no information available |
| Sertraline | Present in milk but not known to be harmful in short-term use |
| Sevelamer | Manufacturer advises use only if potential benefit outweighs risk |
| Sevoflurane | Manufacturer advises caution—no information available |
| Sibutramine | Manufacturer advises avoid—no information available |
| Sildenafil | Manufacturer advises avoid—no information available |
| Silver sulfadiazine | *see* Sulphonamides |
| Simvastatin | *see* Statins |

| Drug | Comment |
|------|---------|
| Sirolimus | Discontinue breast-feeding |
| Sitagliptin | Manufacturer advises avoid—present in milk in *animal* studies |
| Sitaxentan sodium | Manufacturer advises avoid—present in milk in *animal* studies |
| Sodium aurothiomalate | Caution—present in milk; theoretical possibility of rashes and idiosyncratic reactions |
| Sodium clodronate | No information available |
| Sodium cromoglicate | Unlikely to be present in milk |
| Sodium fusidate | Present in milk—manufacturer advises caution |
| Sodium nitroprusside | No information available; caution advised due to thiocyanate metabolite |
| Sodium oxybate | No information available |
| Sodium phenylbutyrate | Manufacturer advises avoid—no information available |
| Sodium picosulfate | Not known to be present in milk but manufacturer advises avoid unless potential benefit outweighs risk |
| Sodium stibogluconate | Amount probably too small to be harmful |
| Sodium valproate | *see* Valproate |
| Solifenacin | Manufacturer advises avoid—present in milk in *animal* studies |
| Somatropin | No information available |
| Sorafenib | *see* Cytotoxic Drugs |
| Sotalol | *see* Beta-blockers |
| Spironolactone | Amount probably too small to be harmful but manufacturer advises avoid |
| Statins | Manufacturers of atorvastatin, fluvastatin, rosuvastatin and simvastatin advise avoid—no information available; *see also* pravastatin |
| Stavudine | Breast-feeding not advised in HIV infection |
| Strontium ranelate | Avoid |
| Sulfadiazine | *see* Sulphonamides |
| Sulfasalazine | Small amounts in milk (1 report of bloody diarrhoea and rashes); theoretical risk of neonatal haemolysis especially in G6PD-deficient infants |
| Sulfinpyrazone | No information available |
| Sulindac | No information available |
| Sulphonamides | Small risk of kernicterus in jaundiced infants particularly with long-acting sulphonamides, and of haemolysis in G6PD-deficient infants |
| Sulphonylureas | Theoretical possibility of hypoglycaemia in infant; see section 6.1.2 |
| Sulpiride | Best avoided; present in milk; *see also* Antipsychotics |
| Sumatriptan | Present in milk—withhold breast-feeding for 12 hours |
| Sunitinib | *see* Cytotoxic Drugs |
| Suxamethonium | No information available |
| Synercid® | Manufacturer advises avoid—no information available |

| Drug | Comment |
|------|---------|
| Tacalcitol | Manufacturer advises avoid application to breast area—no information available; *see also* Vitamin D |
| Tacrolimus | Avoid—present in milk following systemic administration |
| Tamoxifen | Supresses lactation; manufacturer advises avoid unless potential benefit outweighs risk |
| Tazarotene | Manufacturer advises avoid—present in milk in *animal* studies |
| Tazobactam [ingredient] | *see* Piperacillin with tazobactam |
| Tegafur with uracil | *see* Cytotoxic Drugs |
| Teicoplanin | No information available |
| Telbivudine | Manufacturer advises avoid—present in milk in *animal* studies |
| Telithromycin | Manufacturer advises avoid—present in milk in *animal* studies |
| Telmisartan | Avoid—no information available |
| Temazepam | *see* Benzodiazepines |
| Temocillin | *see* Penicillins |
| Temoporfin | Manufacturer advises avoid breast-feeding for at least 1 month after treatment—no information available |
| Temozolomide | *see* Cytotoxic Drugs |
| Temsirolimus | *see* Cytotoxic Drugs |
| Tenecteplase | Manufacturer advises avoid breast-feeding for 24 hours after dose (express and discard milk during this time) |
| Tenofovir | Breast-feeding not advised in HIV infection |
| Tenoxicam | Present in milk in *animal* studies |
| Terazosin | No information available |
| Terbinafine | Avoid systemic use; absorption from gastro-intestinal tract negligible after topical application, but avoid topical application to the nipple |
| Terbutaline | Amount too small to be harmful |
| Terlipressin | Not known to be harmful |
| Testosterone | *see* Androgens |
| Tetrabenazine | Manufacturer advises avoid |
| Tetracosactide | Manufacturer advises avoid (but may be used diagnostically if essential) |
| Tetracyclines | Avoid (although absorption and therefore discoloration of teeth in infant probably usually prevented by chelation with calcium in milk); *see also* tigecycline |
| Thalidomide | Manufacturer advises avoid—present in milk in *animal* studies |
| Theophylline | Present in milk—irritability in infant reported; modified-release preparations preferable |
| Thiamine | Severely thiamine-deficient mothers should avoid breast-feeding as toxic methyl-glyoxal present in milk |

| Drug | Comment |
|------|---------|
| Thiazides and related diuretics | Amount too small to be harmful; large doses may suppress lactation |
| Thiopental | Present in milk—manufacturer advises avoid |
| Thiotepa | *see* Cytotoxic Drugs |
| Thyroxine | *see* Levothyroxine |
| Tiagabine | Manufacturer advises avoid unless potential benefit outweighs risk |
| Tiaprofenic acid | Amount too small to be harmful |
| Ticarcillin [ingredient] | *see* Penicillins |
| Tigecycline | Manufacturer advises caution—present in milk in *animal* studies |
| Tiludronic acid | Manufacturer advises avoid—no information available |
| Timentin® | *see* Penicillins |
| Timolol | *see* Beta-blockers |
| Tinidazole | Present in milk—manufacturer advises avoid breast-feeding during and for 3 days after stopping treatment |
| Tinzaparin | Manufacturer advises avoid—no information available |
| Tioguanine | *see* Cytotoxic Drugs |
| Tiotropium | Amount in milk probably too small to be harmful (present in milk in *animal* studies)—manufacturer advises use only if potential benefit outweighs risk |
| Tipranavir | Breast-feeding not advised in HIV infection |
| Tirofiban | Manufacturer advises avoid—no information available |
| Tizanidine | Manufacturer advises use only if potential benefit outweighs risk—no information available |
| Tolbutamide | *see* Sulphonylureas |
| Tolcapone | Manufacturer advises avoid—present in milk in *animal* studies |
| Tolfenamic acid | Amount too small to be harmful |
| Tolterodine | Manufacturer advises avoid—no information available |
| Topiramate | Manufacturer advises avoid—present in milk |
| Topotecan | *see* Cytotoxic Drugs |
| Torasemide | No information available |
| Trabectedin | Manufacturer advises avoid breast-feeding during and for 3 months after treatment |
| Tramadol | Amount probably too small to be harmful, but manufacturer advises avoid |
| Trandolapril | Avoid—no information available |
| Tranexamic acid | Small amount present in milk—antifibrinolytic effect in infant unlikely |
| Trastuzumab | Avoid breast-feeding during treatment and for six months after |
| Travoprost | Present in milk in animal studies; manufacturer advises avoid |

| Drug | Comment |
|------|---------|
| Trazodone | *see* Antidepressants, Tricyclic (and related) |
| Treosulfan | *see* Cytotoxic Drugs |
| Tretinoin | Avoid |
| Triamcinolone | *see* Corticosteroids |
| Triamterene | Present in milk—manufacturer advises avoid |
| Tribavirin | *see* Ribavirin |
| Triclofos | Avoid |
| Trifluoperazine | *see* Antipsychotics |
| Trihexyphenidyl | Manufacturer advises avoid |
| Trimeprazine | *see* Antihistamines |
| Trimethoprim | Present in milk—short-term use not known to be harmful |
| Trimipramine | *see* Antidepressants, Tricyclic (and related) |
| Triptorelin | Manufacturers advise avoid |
| Trospium | Manufacturer advises caution—no information available |
| Tryptophan | No information available |
| Urokinase | Manufacturer advises avoid—no information available |
| Ursodeoxycholic acid | Not known to be harmful but manufacturer advises avoid |
| Ustekinumab | Manufacturer advises avoid—present in milk in *animal* studies |
| Valaciclovir | No information available; *see also* Aciclovir |
| Valganciclovir | *see* Ganciclovir |
| Valproate | Amount too small to be harmful |
| Valproic acid | *see* Valproate |
| Valsartan | Avoid—no information available |
| Vancomycin | Present in milk—significant absorption following oral administration unlikely |
| Varenicline | Present in milk in *animal* studies |
| Vasopressin | Not known to be harmful |
| Vecuronium | No information available |
| Venlafaxine | Present in milk—manufacturer advises avoid |
| Verapamil | Amount too small to be harmful |
| Verteporfin | No information available—manufacturer advises avoid breast-feeding for 48 hours after administration |
| Vigabatrin | Present in milk—manufacturer advises avoid |
| Vildagliptin | Manufacturer advises avoid—present in milk in *animal* studies |
| Vinblastine | *see* Cytotoxic Drugs |
| Vincristine | *see* Cytotoxic Drugs |
| Vindesine | *see* Cytotoxic Drugs |
| Vinorelbine | *see* Cytotoxic Drugs |
| Vitamin A | Theoretical risk of toxicity in infants of mothers taking large doses |

| Drug | Comment |
|------|---------|
| Vitamin D | Caution with high systemic doses; may cause hypercalcaemia in infant—monitor serum-calcium concentration; manufacturer of *topical* calcitriol advises avoid; *see also* Calcipotriol, Paricalcitol, and Tacalcitol |
| Voriconazole | Manufacturer advises avoid—no information available |
| Warfarin | *see* Anticoagulants, Oral |
| Xipamide | No information available |
| Zafirlukast | Present in milk—manufacturer advises avoid |
| Zaleplon | Present in milk but amount probably too small to be harmful |
| Zanamivir | Amount probably too small to be harmful; use only if potential benefit outweighs risk (e.g. during a pandemic); *see also* p. 354 |
| Zidovudine | Breast-feeding not advised in HIV infection |
| Zoledronic acid | Manufacturer advises avoid—no information available |
| Zolmitriptan | Manufacturer advises caution—present in milk in *animal* studies |
| Zolpidem | Small amounts present in milk—manufacturer advises avoid |
| Zonisamide | Avoid; manufacturer advises avoid breast-feeding for 4 weeks after administration |
| Zopiclone | Present in milk—manufacturer advises avoid |
| Zotepine | Manufacturer advises avoid |
| Zuclopenthixol | *see* Antipsychotics |

# A6 Intravenous additives

**Intravenous additives policies** A local policy on the addition of drugs to intravenous fluids should be drawn up by a multi-disciplinary team in each Strategic Health Authority (or equivalent) and issued as a document to the members of staff concerned.

Centralised additive services are provided in a number of hospital pharmacy departments and should be used in preference to making additions on wards.

The information that follows should be read in conjunction with local policy documents.

## Guidelines

1. Drugs should only be added to infusion containers when constant plasma concentrations are needed or when the administration of a more concentrated solution would be harmful.

2. In general, only one drug should be added to any infusion container and the components should be compatible. Ready-prepared solutions should be used whenever possible. Drugs should not normally be added to blood products, mannitol, or sodium bicarbonate. Only specially formulated additives should be used with fat emulsions or amino-acid solutions (section 9.3).

3. Solutions should be thoroughly mixed by shaking and checked for absence of particulate matter before use.

4. Strict asepsis should be maintained throughout and in general the giving set should not be used for more than 24 hours (for drug admixtures).

5. The infusion container should be labelled with the patient's name, the name and quantity of additives, and the date and time of addition (and the new expiry date or time). Such additional labelling should not interfere with information on the manufacturer's label that is still valid. When possible, containers should be retained for a period after use in case they are needed for investigation.

6. It is good practice to examine intravenous infusions from time to time while they are running. If cloudiness, crystallisation, change of colour, or any other sign of interaction or contamination is observed the infusion should be discontinued.

## Problems

**Microbial contamination** The accidental entry and subsequent growth of micro-organisms converts the infusion fluid pathway into a potential vehicle for infection with micro-organisms, particularly species of Candida, Enterobacter, and Klebsiella. Ready-prepared infusions containing the additional drugs, or infusions prepared by an additive service (when available) should therefore be used in preference to making extemporaneous additions to infusion containers on wards etc.

However, when this is necessary strict aseptic procedure should be followed.

**Incompatibility** Physical and chemical incompatibilities may occur with loss of potency, increase in toxicity, or other adverse effect. The solutions may become opalescent or precipitation may occur, but in many instances there is no visual indication of incompatibility. Interaction may take place at any point in the infusion fluid pathway, and the potential for incompatibility is increased when more than one substance is added to the infusion fluid.

**Common incompatibilities** Precipitation reactions are numerous and varied and may occur as a result of pH, concentration changes, 'salting-out' effects, complexation or other chemical changes. Precipitation or other particle formation must be avoided since, apart from lack of control of dosage on administration, it may initiate or exacerbate adverse effects. This is particularly important in the case of drugs which have been implicated in either thrombophlebitis (e.g. diazepam) or in skin sloughing or necrosis caused by extravasation (e.g. sodium bicarbonate and certain cytotoxic drugs). It is also especially important to effect solution of colloidal drugs and to prevent their subsequent precipitation in order to avoid a pyrogenic reaction (e.g. amphotericin).

It is considered undesirable to mix beta-lactam antibiotics, such as semi-synthetic penicillins and cephalosporins, with proteinaceous materials on the grounds that immunogenic and allergenic conjugates could be formed.

A number of preparations undergo significant loss of potency when added singly or in combination to large volume infusions. Examples include ampicillin in infusions that contain glucose or lactates. The breakdown products of dacarbazine have been implicated in adverse effects.

**Blood** Because of the large number of incompatibilities, drugs should not normally be added to blood and blood products for infusion purposes. Examples of incompatibility with blood include hypertonic mannitol solutions (irreversible crenation of red cells), dextrans (rouleaux formation and interference with cross-matching), glucose (clumping of red cells), and oxytocin (inactivated).

If the giving set is not changed after the administration of blood, but used for other infusion fluids, a fibrin clot may form which, apart from blocking the set, increases the likelihood of microbial growth.

**Intravenous fat emulsions** These may break down with coalescence of fat globules and separation of phases when additions such as antibacterials or electrolytes are made, thus increasing the possibility of embolism. Only specially formulated products such as *Vitlipid N*® (section 9.3) may be added to appropriate intravenous fat emulsions.

**Other infusions** Infusions that frequently give rise to incompatibility include amino acids, mannitol, and sodium bicarbonate.

**Bactericides** Bactericides such as chlorocresol 0.1% or phenylmercuric nitrate 0.001% are present in some injection solutions. The total volume of such solutions added to a container for infusion on one occasion should not exceed 15 mL.

## Method

Ready-prepared infusions should be used whenever available. **Potassium chloride** is usually available in concentrations of 20, 27, and 40 mmol/litre in sodium chloride intravenous infusion (0.9%), glucose intravenous infusion (5%) or sodium chloride and glucose intravenous infusion. **Lidocaine hydrochloride** (lignocaine hydrochloride) is usually available in concentrations of 0.1 or 0.2% in glucose intravenous infusion (5%).

When addition is required to be made extemporaneously, any product reconstitution instructions such as those relating to concentration, vehicle, mixing, and handling precautions should be strictly followed using an aseptic technique throughout. Once the product has been reconstituted, addition to the infusion fluid should be made immediately in order to minimise microbial contamination and, with certain products, to prevent degradation or other formulation change which may occur; e.g. reconstituted ampicillin injection degrades rapidly on standing, and also may form polymers which could cause sensitivity reactions.

It is also important in certain instances that an infusion fluid of specific pH be used (e.g. **furosemide** (frusemide) injection requires dilution in infusions of pH greater than 5.5).

When drug additions are made it is important to mix thoroughly; additions should not be made to an infusion container that has been connected to a giving set, mixing is hampered. If the solutions are not thoroughly mixed a concentrated layer of the additive may form owing to differences in density. **Potassium chloride** is particularly prone to this 'layering' effect when added without adequate mixing to infusions packed in non-rigid infusion containers; if such a mixture is administered it may have a serious effect on the heart.

A time limit between addition and completion of administration must be imposed for certain admixtures to guarantee satisfactory drug potency and compatibility. For admixtures in which degradation occurs without the formation of toxic substances, an acceptable limit is the time taken for 10% decomposition of the drug. When toxic substances are produced stricter limits may be imposed. Because of the risk of microbial contamination a maximum time limit of 24 hours may be appropriate for additions made elsewhere than in hospital pharmacies offering central additive service.

Certain injections must be protected from light during continuous infusion to minimise oxidation, e.g. amphotericin, dacarbazine, and sodium nitroprusside.

Dilution with a small volume of an appropriate vehicle and administration using a motorised infusion pump is advocated for preparations such as heparin where strict control over administration is required. In this case the appropriate dose may be dissolved in a convenient volume (e.g. 24–48 mL) of sodium chloride intravenous infusion (0.9%).

## Use of table

The table lists preparations given by three methods:

- continuous infusion;
- intermittent infusion;
- addition via the drip tubing.

Drugs for **continuous infusion** must be diluted in a large volume infusion. Penicillins and cephalosporins are not usually given by continuous infusion because of stability problems and because adequate plasma and tissue concentrations are best obtained by intermittent infusion. Where it is necessary to administer them by continuous infusion, detailed literature should be consulted.

Drugs that are both compatible and clinically suitable may be given by **intermittent infusion** in a relatively small volume of infusion over a short period of time, e.g. 100 mL in 30 minutes. The method is used if the product is incompatible or unstable over the period necessary for continuous infusion; the limited stability of ampicillin or amoxicillin in large volume glucose or lactate infusions may be overcome in this way.

Intermittent infusion is also used if adequate plasma and tissue concentrations are not produced by continuous infusion as in the case of drugs such as dacarbazine, gentamicin, and ticarcillin.

An in-line burette may be used for intermittent infusion techniques in order to achieve strict control over the time and rate of administration, especially for infants and children and in intensive care units. Intermittent infusion may also make use of the 'piggy-back' technique provided that no additions are made to the primary infusion. In this method the drug is added to a small secondary container connected to a Y-type injection site on the primary infusion giving set; the secondary solution is usually infused within 30 minutes.

**Addition via the drip tubing** is indicated for a number of cytotoxic drugs in order to minimise extravasation. The preparation is added aseptically via the rubber septum of the injection site of a fast-running infusion. In general, drug preparations intended for a bolus effect should be given directly into a separate vein where possible. Failing this, administration may be made via the drip tubing provided that the preparation is compatible with the infusion fluid when given in this manner.

## Table of drugs given by intravenous infusion

Covers addition to *Glucose intravenous infusion* 5 and 10%, *Sodium chloride intravenous infusion* 0.9%, *Compound sodium chloride intravenous infusion* (Ringer's solution), and *Compound sodium lactate intravenous infusion* (Hartmann's solution). Compatibility with glucose 5% and with sodium chloride 0.9% indicates compatibility with *Sodium chloride and glucose intravenous infusion*. Infusion of a large volume of hypotonic solution should be avoided therefore care should be taken if water for injections is used. The information in the Table relates to the proprietary preparations indicated; for other preparations suitability should be checked with the manufacturer

**Abatacept**  (*Orencia*®)

Intermittent *in* Sodium chloride 0.9%

Reconstitute each vial with 10 mL water for injections using the silicone-free syringe provided; dilute requisite dose in infusion fluid to 100 mL (using the same silicone-free syringe); give over 30 minutes through a low protein-binding filter (pore size 0.2–1.2 micron)

**Abciximab**  (*ReoPro*®)

Continuous *in* Glucose 5% *or* Sodium chloride 0.9%

Dilute requisite dose in infusion fluid and give *via* infusion pump; filter upon dilution with infusion fluid through a non-pyrogenic low protein-binding 0.2, 0.22, or 5 micron filter *or* upon administration through an in-line non-pyrogenic low protein-binding 0.2 or 0.22 micron filter

**Acetylcysteine**  (*Parvolex*®)

Continuous *in* Glucose 5% *or* Sodium chloride 0.9%

Glucose 5% is preferable—see Emergency Treatment of Poisoning

**Aciclovir (as sodium salt)**  (*Zovirax IV*®; *Aciclovir IV*, Hospira; *Aciclovir IV*, Genus; *Aciclovir Sodium*, Zurich)

Intermittent *in* Sodium chloride 0.9% *or* Sodium chloride and glucose *or* Compound sodium lactate

For *Zovirax IV*®, *Aciclovir IV* (Genus) initially reconstitute to 25 mg/mL in water for injections or sodium chloride 0.9% then dilute to not more than 5 mg/mL with the infusion fluid; to be given over 1 hour; alternatively, may be administered in a concentration of 25 mg/mL using a suitable infusion pump and given over 1 hour; for *Aciclovir IV* (Hospira) dilute to not more than 5 mg/mL with infusion fluid; give over 1 hour

**Agalsidase alfa**  (*Replagal*®)

Intermittent *in* Sodium chloride 0.9%

Dilute requisite dose with 100 mL infusion fluid and give over 40 minutes using an in-line filter; use within 3 hours of dilution

**Agalsidase beta**  (*Fabrazyme*®)

Intermittent *in* Sodium chloride 0.9%

Reconstitute with water for injections (35 mg in 7.2 mL, 5 mg in 1.1 mL) to produce a solution containing 5 mg/mL; dilute with infusion fluid (for doses less than 35 mg dilute with at least 50 mL; doses 35–70 mg dilute with at least 100 mL; doses 70–100 mg dilute with at least 250 mL; doses greater than 100 mg dilute with 500 mL) and give through an in-line low protein-binding 0.2 micron filter at an initial rate of no more than 15 mg/hour; for subsequent infusions, infusion rate may be increased gradually once tolerance has been established

**Alemtuzumab**  (*MabCampath*®)

Intermittent in Glucose 5% *or* Sodium chloride 0.9%

Add requisite dose to 100 mL infusion fluid; infuse over 2 hours

**Alfentanil (as hydrochloride)**  (*Rapifen*®)

Continuous *or* intermittent *in* Glucose 5% *or* Sodium chloride 0.9% *or* Compound sodium lactate

**Alglucosidase alfa**  (*Myozyme*®)

Intermittent *in* Sodium chloride 0.9%

Reconstitute 50 mg with 10.3 mL water for injections to produce 5 mg/mL solution; gently rotate vial without shaking; dilute requisite dose with infusion fluid to give a final concentration of 0.5–4 mg/mL; give through a low protein-binding in-line filter (0.2 micron) at an initial rate of 1 mg/kg/hour increased by 2 mg/kg/hour every 30 minutes to max. 7 mg/kg/hour

**Alprostadil**  (*Prostin VR*®)

Continuous *in* Glucose 5% *or* Sodium chloride 0.9%

Dilute 150 micrograms/kg body-weight to a final volume of 50 mL with infusion fluid; an intravenous infusion rate of 0.1 mL/hour provides a dose of 5 nanograms/kg/minute. Undiluted solution must not come into contact with the barrel of the plastic syringe; add the required volume of alprostadil to a volume of infusion fluid, and then make up to final volume

**Alteplase**  (*Actilyse*®)

Continuous *or* intermittent *in* Sodium chloride 0.9%

Dissolve in water for injections to a concentration of 1 mg/mL or 2 mg/mL and infuse intravenously; alternatively dilute the solution further in the infusion fluid to a concentration of not less than 200 micrograms/mL; not to be infused in glucose solution

**Amikacin sulphate**  (*Amikin*®)

Intermittent *in* Glucose 5% *or* Sodium chloride 0.9% *or* Compound sodium lactate

To be given over 30 minutes

**Aminophylline**

Continuous *in* Glucose 5% *or* Sodium chloride 0.9% *or* Compound sodium lactate

**Amiodarone hydrochloride**  (*Cordarone X*®)

Continuous *or* intermittent *in* Glucose 5%

Suggested initial infusion volume 250 mL given over 20–120 minutes; for repeat infusions up to 1.2 g in max. 500 mL; infusion in extreme emergency see section 2.7.3; should not be diluted to less than 600 micrograms/mL; incompatible with sodium chloride infusion; avoid equipment containing the plasticizer di-2-ethyl-hexyphthalate (DEHP)

**Amoxicillin (as sodium salt)**  (*Amoxil*®)

Intermittent *in* Glucose 5% *or* Sodium chloride 0.9%

Reconstituted solutions diluted and given without delay; suggested volume 100 mL given over 30–60 minutes

*via* drip tubing *in* Glucose 5% *or* Sodium chloride 0.9%

Continuous infusion not usually recommended

**Amphotericin (colloidal)**  (*Amphocil*®)

Intermittent *in* Glucose 5%

Initially reconstitute with water for injections (50 mg in 10 mL, 100 mg in 20 mL), shaking gently to dissolve (fluid may be opalescent) then dilute to a concentration of 625 micrograms/mL (1 volume of reconstituted solution with 7 volumes of infusion fluid); give at a rate of 1–2 mg/kg/hour or slower if not tolerated (initial test dose 2 mg of a 100 microgram/mL solution over 10 minutes); incompatible with sodium chloride or other electrolyte solutions, flush existing intravenous line with glucose 5% or use separate line

**Amphotericin (lipid complex)**  (*Abelcet*®)

Intermittent *in* Glucose 5%

Allow suspension to reach room temperature, shake gently to ensure no yellow settlement, withdraw requisite dose (using 17–19 gauge needle) into one or more 20-mL syringes; replace needle on syringe with a 5-micron filter needle provided (fresh needle for each syringe) and dilute to a concentration of 1 mg/mL (2 mg/mL can be used in fluid restriction and in children); preferably give *via* an infusion pump at a rate of 2.5 mg/kg/hour (initial test dose of 1 mg given over 15 minutes); an in-line filter (pore size no less than 15 micron) may be used; do not use sodium chloride or other electrolyte solutions, flush existing intravenous line with glucose 5% or use separate line

**Amphotericin (liposomal)**  (*AmBisome*®)

Intermittent *in* Glucose 5%

Reconstitute each vial with 12 mL water for injections and shake vigorously to produce a preparation containing 4 mg/mL; withdraw requisite dose from vial and introduce into infusion fluid through the 5 micron filter provided to produce a final concentration of 0.2–2 mg/mL; infuse over 30–60 minutes (initial test dose 1 mg over 10 minutes); incompatible with sodium chloride solutions, flush existing intravenous line with glucose 5% or use separate line

### Amphotericin (as sodium deoxycholate complex)
(*Fungizone®*)

Intermittent *in* Glucose 5%

Reconstitute each vial with 10 mL water for injections and shake immediately to produce a 5 mg/mL colloidal solution; dilute further in infusion fluid to a concentration of 100 micrograms/mL; pH of the glucose must not be below 4.2 (check each container—consult product literature for details of buffer); infuse over 2–4 hours, or longer if not tolerated (initial test dose 1 mg over 20–30 minutes); begin infusion immediately after dilution and protect from light; incompatible with sodium chloride solutions, flush existing intravenous line with glucose 5% or use separate line; an in-line filter (pore size no less than 1 micron) may be used

### Ampicillin sodium  (*Penbritin®*)

Intermittent *in* Glucose 5% *or* Sodium chloride 0.9%

Reconstituted solutions diluted and given without delay; suggested volume 100 mL given over 30–60 minutes

*via* drip tubing *in* Glucose 5% *or* Sodium chloride 0.9% *or* Ringer's solution *or* Compound sodium lactate

Continuous infusion not usually recommended

### Amsacrine  (*Amsidine®*)

Intermittent *in* Glucose 5%

Reconstitute with diluent provided and dilute to suggested volume 500 mL; give over 60–90 minutes; use glass syringes; incompatible with sodium chloride infusion

### Anidulafungin  (*Ecalta®*)

Intermittent *in* Glucose 5% *or* Sodium chloride 0.9%

Reconstitute each 100 mg with solvent provided, allow up to 5 minutes for reconstitution; dilute dose in infusion fluid to a concentration of 360 micrograms/mL; give at a rate not exceeding 1.1 mg/minute

### Antithymocyte immunoglobulin  (*Thymoglobuline®*)

Continuous *in* Glucose 5% *or* Sodium chloride 0.9%

Reconstitute each vial with 5 mL water for injections to produce a solution of 5 mg/mL; gently rotate to dissolve. Dilute requisite dose with infusion fluid to a total volume of 50–500 mL (usually 50 mL/vial); begin infusion immediately after dilution; give through an in-line filter (pore size 0.22 micron); not to be given with heparin and hydrocortisone in glucose infusion as precipitation reported

### Arsenic trioxide  (*Trisenox®*)

Intermittent *in* Glucose 5% *or* Sodium chloride 0.9%

Dilute requisite dose with 100–250 mL infusion fluid; infuse over 1–2 hours (up to 4 hours if vasomotor reactions observed)

### Atenolol  (*Tenormin®*)

Intermittent *in* Glucose 5% *or* Sodium chloride 0.9%

Suggested infusion time 20 minutes

### Atosiban  (*Tractocile®* concentrate for intravenous infusion)

Continuous *in* Glucose 5% *or* Sodium chloride 0.9% *or* Compound sodium lactate

Withdraw 10 mL infusion fluid from 100-mL bag and replace with 10 mL atosiban concentrate (7.5 mg/mL) to produce a final concentration of 750 micrograms/mL

### Atracurium besilate  (*Tracrium®*; *Atracurium besilate injection*, Hospira; *Atracurium injection/infusion*, Genus)

Continuous *in* Glucose 5% *or* Sodium chloride 0.9% *or* Ringer's solution *or* Compound sodium lactate

Stability varies with diluent; dilute requisite dose with infusion fluid to a concentration of 0.5–5 mg/mL

### Azathioprine (as sodium salt)  (*Imuran®*)

Intermittent *in* Sodium chloride 0.9% *or* Sodium chloride and glucose

Reconstitute 50 mg with 5–15 mL water for injections; dilute with 20–200 mL infusion fluid

### Aztreonam  (*Azactam®*)

Intermittent *in* Glucose 5% *or* Sodium chloride 0.9% *or* Ringer's solution *or* Compound sodium lactate

Dissolve initially in water for injections (1 g per 3 mL) then dilute to a concentration of less than 20 mg/mL; to be given over 20–60 minutes

### Basiliximab  (*Simulect®*)

Intermittent in Glucose 5% *or* Sodium chloride 0.9%

Reconstitute 10 mg with 2.5 mL water for injections then dilute to at least 25 mL with infusion fluid; reconstitute 20 mg with 5 mL water for injections then dilute to at least 50 mL with infusion fluid; give over 20–30 minutes

### Benzylpenicillin sodium  (*Crystapen®*)

Intermittent *in* Glucose 5% *or* Sodium chloride 0.9%

Suggested volume 100 mL given over 30–60 minutes
Continuous infusion not usually recommended

### Betamethasone (as sodium phosphate)  (*Betnesol®*)

Continuous *or* intermittent *or via* drip tubing *in* Glucose 5% *or* Sodium chloride 0.9%

### Bevacizumab  (*Avastin®*)

Intermittent *in* Sodium chloride 0.9%

Dilute requisite dose in infusion fluid to 100 mL and give over 90 minutes; if initial dose well tolerated give second dose over 60 minutes; if second dose well tolerated give subsequent doses over 30 minutes; incompatible with glucose solutions

### Bivalirudin  (*Angiox®*)

Continuous *in* Glucose 5% *or* Sodium chloride 0.9%

Reconstitute each 250-mg vial with 5 mL water for injections then withdraw 5 mL and dilute to 50 mL with infusion fluid

### Bleomycin sulphate

Intermittent *in* Sodium chloride 0.9%

To be given slowly; suggested volume 200 mL

### Bumetanide

Intermittent *in* Glucose 5% *or* Sodium chloride 0.9%

Suggested volume 500 mL given over 30–60 minutes; concentrations above 25 mg/litre may cause precipitation

### Busulfan  (*Busilvex®*)

Intermittent *in* Glucose 5% *or* Sodium chloride 0.9%

Dilute to a concentration of 500 micrograms/mL; give through a central venous catheter over 2 hours

### Calcitonin (salmon)/Salcatonin  (*Miacalcic®*)

Intermittent *in* Sodium chloride 0.9%

Diluted solution given without delay; dilute in 500 mL and give over at least 6 hours; glass or hard plastic containers should not be used; some loss of potency on dilution and administration

### Calcium folinate  (*Refolinon®*; *Calcium folinate injection*, Hospira, Wockhardt)

Intermittent *in* Sodium chloride 0.9%

*Calcium folinate* (Hospira and Wockhardt) can also be infused in Glucose 5%
Protect from light

### Calcium gluconate

Continuous *in* Glucose 5% *or* Sodium chloride 0.9%

Avoid bicarbonates, phosphates, or sulphates

### Calcium levofolinate  (*Isovorin®*)

Intermittent *in* Glucose 5 and 10% *or* Sodium chloride 0.9% *or* Compound sodium lactate

Protect from light

### Carboplatin  (*Paraplatin®*)

Intermittent *in* Glucose 5% *or* Sodium chloride 0.9%

Final concentration as low as 500 micrograms/mL; give over 15–60 minutes

**Caspofungin** (*Cancidas®*)

Intermittent *in* Sodium chloride 0.9% *or* Compound sodium lactate

Allow vial to reach room temperature; initially reconstitute each vial with 10.5 mL water for injections, mixing gently to dissolve then dilute requisite dose in 250 mL infusion fluid (35- or 50-mg doses may be diluted in 100 mL infusion fluid if necessary); give over 60 minutes; incompatible with glucose solutions

**Cefotaxime (as sodium salt)**

Intermittent *in* Glucose 5% *or* Sodium chloride 0.9% *or* Compound sodium lactate *or* Water for injections

Suggested volume 40–100 mL given over 20–60 minutes; incompatible with alkaline solutions

**Cefradine** (*Velosef®*)

Continuous *or* intermittent *in* Glucose 5 and 10% *or* Sodium chloride 0.9% *or* Ringer's solution *or* Compound sodium lactate

Reconstitute 500 mg with 5 mL water for injections or glucose 5% or sodium chloride 0.9% then dilute with infusion fluid

**Ceftazidime (as pentahydrate)** (*Fortum®*, *Kefadim®*)

Intermittent *or via* drip tubing *in* Glucose 5 and 10% *or* Sodium chloride 0.9% *or* Compound sodium lactate

Dissolve 2 g initially in 10 mL (3 g in 15 mL) infusion fluid; for *Fortum®* dilute further to a concentration of 40 mg/mL; for *Kefadim®* dilute further to a concentration of 20 mg/mL; give over up to 30 minutes

**Ceftriaxone (as sodium salt)** (*Rocephin®*; *Ceftriaxone Injection*, Genus)

Intermittent *or via* drip tubing *in* Glucose 5 and 10% *or* Sodium chloride 0.9%

Reconstitute 2-g vial with 40 mL infusion fluid; give intermittent infusion over at least 30 minutes (60 minutes in neonates); not to be given with total parenteral nutrition or infusion fluids containing calcium, even by different infusion lines

**Cefuroxime (as sodium salt)** (*Zinacef®*)

Intermittent *or via* drip tubing *in* Glucose 5% *or* Sodium chloride 0.9% *or* Compound sodium lactate

Dissolve in water for injections 2 mL for each 250 mg, 15 mL for 1.5 g); suggested volume 50–100 mL given over 30 minutes

**Chloramphenicol (as sodium succinate)** (*Kemicetine®*)

Intermittent *or via* drip tubing *in* Glucose 5% *or* Sodium chloride 0.9%

**Ciclosporin** (*Sandimmun®*)

Intermittent *or* continuous *in* Glucose 5% *or* Sodium chloride 0.9%

Dilute to a concentration of 50 mg in 20–100 mL; give intermittent infusion over 2–6 hours; not to be used with PVC equipment

**Cidofovir** (*Vistide®*)

Intermittent *in* Sodium chloride 0.9%

Dilute requisite dose with 100 mL infusion fluid; infuse over 1 hour

**Cisatracurium** (*Nimbex®*, *Nimbex Forte®*)

Continuous *in* Glucose 5% *or* Sodium chloride 0.9%

Solutions of 2 mg/mL and 5 mg/mL may be infused undiluted; alternatively dilute with infusion fluid to a concentration of 0.1–2 mg/mL

**Cisplatin** (*Cisplatin powder*, Pharmacia; *Cisplatin injection solution*, Hospira, Wockhardt)

Intermittent *in* Sodium chloride 0.9%

Cisplatin *injection solution* (Wockhardt) and *powder* can also be infused in Sodium chloride and Glucose

Reconstitute powder initially with water for injections to produce 1 mg/mL solution.

Dilute in 2 litres infusion fluid; give over 6–8 hours; avoid equipment containing aluminium; protect from light

**Cladribine** (*Leustat®*)

Continuous *in* Sodium chloride 0.9%

Dilute with 100–500 mL; glucose solutions are unsuitable

**Clarithromycin** (*Klaricid® I.V.*)

Intermittent *in* Glucose 5% *or* Sodium chloride 0.9% *or* Ringer's solution *or* Compound sodium lactate

Dissolve initially in water for injections (500 mg in 10 mL) then dilute to a concentration of 2 mg/mL; give over 60 minutes

**Clindamycin (as phosphate)** (*Dalacin® C Phosphate*)

Continuous *or* intermittent *in* Glucose 5% *or* Sodium chloride 0.9%

Dilute to not more than 18 mg/mL and give over 10–60 minutes at a rate not exceeding 30 mg/minute (1.2 g over at least 60 minutes; higher doses by continuous infusion)

**Clofarabine** (*Evoltra®*)

Intermittent *in* Sodium chloride 0.9%

Filter requisite dose through a 0.2 micron filter and dilute with infusion fluid; give over 2 hours

**Clonazepam** (*Rivotril®*)

Intermittent *in* Glucose 5 and 10% *or* Sodium chloride 0.9%

Suggested volume 250 mL

**Co-amoxiclav** (*Augmentin®*; *Co-amoxiclav Injection*, Wockhardt)

Intermittent *in* Sodium chloride 0.9% *or* Water for injections; see also package leaflet

Suggested volume 50–100 mL given over 30–40 minutes and completed within 4 hours of reconstitution

*via* drip tubing *in* Glucose 5% *or* Sodium chloride 0.9%

**Co-fluampicil (as sodium salts)** (*Magnapen®*)

Intermittent *in* Glucose 5% *or* Sodium chloride 0.9%

Reconstituted solutions diluted and given without delay; suggested volume 100 mL given over 30–60 minutes

*via* drip tubing *in* Glucose 5% *or* Sodium chloride 0.9% *or* Ringer's solution *or* Compound sodium lactate

**Colistimethate sodium** (*Colomycin®*)

Intermittent *in* Sodium chloride 0.9% *or* Water for injections

Dilute with 50 mL infusion fluid and give over 30 minutes

**Co-trimoxazole** (*Septrin® for infusion*)

Intermittent *in* Glucose 5 and 10% *or* Sodium chloride 0.9% *or* Ringer's solution

Dilute contents of 1 ampoule (5 mL) to 125 mL, 2 ampoules (10 mL) to 250 mL or 3 ampoules (15 mL) to 500 mL; suggested duration of infusion 60–90 minutes (but may be adjusted according to fluid requirements); if fluid restriction necessary, 1 ampoule (5 mL) may be diluted with 75 mL glucose 5% and infused over max. 60 minutes

**Cyclophosphamide** (*Endoxana®*)

*via* drip tubing *in* Glucose 5% *or* Sodium chloride 0.9%

Reconstitute with sodium chloride 0.9%

**Cytarabine** (*Cytarabine injection solution*, Pharmacia, Hospira)

Continuous *or* intermittent *in* Glucose 5% *or* Sodium chloride 0.9%

For *Cytarabine injection solution* 100 mg/mL (Pharmacia) before use, vials should be warmed to 55°C for 30 minutes, with adequate shaking, and allowed to cool to room temperature

**Dacarbazine** (*Dacarbazine*, Medac)

Intermittent *in* Glucose 5% *or* Sodium chloride 0.9%

Reconstitute initially with water for injections then dilute in 200–300 mL infusion fluid; give over 15–30 minutes; protect infusion from light

**Dactinomycin** (*Cosmegen Lyovac®*)

Intermittent *or via* drip tubing *in* Glucose 5% *or* Sodium chloride 0.9%

Reconstitute with water for injections

**Danaparoid sodium** (*Orgaran®*)

Continuous *in* Glucose 5% *or* Sodium chloride 0.9%

**Daptomycin** (*Cubicin®*)

Intermittent *in* Sodium chloride 0.9%

Reconstitute with water for injections or sodium chloride 0.9% (350 mg in 7 mL, 500 mg in 10 mL); gently rotate vial without shaking; allow to stand for at least 10 minutes then rotate gently to dissolve; dilute requisite dose in 50 mL infusion fluid and give over 30 minutes

**Daunorubicin (as hydrochloride)** (*Daunorubicin*, Winthrop)

Intermittent *via* drip tubing *in* Sodium chloride 0.9%

Reconstitute vial with 4 mL water for injections to give 5 mg/mL solution; dilute requisite dose with infusion fluid to a concentration of 1 mg/mL; give over 20 minutes; protect from light

**Daunorubicin (liposomal)** (*DaunoXome®*)

Intermittent *in* Glucose 5%

Dilute to a concentration of 0.2–1 mg/mL; give over 30–60 minutes; incompatible with sodium chloride solutions; in-line filter not recommended (if used, pore size should be no less than 5 micron)

**Desferrioxamine mesilate** (*Desferal®*)

Continuous *or* intermittent *in* Glucose 5% *or* Sodium chloride 0.9%

Reconstitute with water for injections to a concentration of 100 mg/mL; dilute with infusion fluid

**Desmopressin** (*DDAVP®*, *Octim®*)

Intermittent *in* Sodium chloride 0.9%

Dilute with 50 mL and give over 20 minutes

**Dexamethasone sodium phosphate** (*Dexamethasone*, Hospira; *Dexamethasone*, Organon)

Continuous *or* intermittent *or via* drip tubing *in* Glucose 5% *or* Sodium chloride 0.9%

*Dexamethasone* (Organon) can also be infused in Ringer's solution *or* Compound sodium lactate

**Dexrazoxane** (*Savene®*)

Intermittent *in* Savene® diluent

Reconstitute 500 mg with 25 mL of Water for Injections then dilute in 500 mL Savene® diluent; give over 1–2 hours into a large vein in an area other than the one affected

**Diamorphine hydrochloride** (*Diamorphine Injection*, Wockhardt)

Continuous *in* Glucose 5% *or* Sodium chloride 0.9%

Glucose is preferred as infusion fluid

**Diazepam (solution)** (*Diazepam*, Wockhardt)

Continuous *in* Glucose 5% *or* Sodium chloride 0.9%

Dilute to a concentration of not more than 10 mg in 200 mL; adsorbed to some extent by the plastics of bags and infusion sets

**Diazepam (emulsion)** (*Diazemuls®*)

Continuous *in* Glucose 5 and 10%

May be diluted to a max. concentration of 200 mg in 500 mL; max. 6 hours between addition and completion of administration; adsorbed to some extent by the plastics of the infusion set

*via* drip tubing *in* Glucose 5 and 10% *or* Sodium chloride 0.9%

Adsorbed to some extent by the plastics of the infusion set

**Diclofenac sodium** (*Voltarol®*)

Continuous *or* intermittent *in* Glucose 5% *or* Sodium chloride 0.9%

Dilute 75 mg with 100–500 mL infusion fluid (previously buffered with 0.5 mL sodium bicarbonate 8.4% solution *or* with 1 mL sodium bicarbonate 4.2% solution); for intermittent infusion give 25–50 mg over 15–60 minutes or 75 mg over 30–120 minutes; for continuous infusion give at a rate of 5 mg/hour

**Digoxin** (*Lanoxin®*)

Intermittent *in* Glucose 5% *or* Sodium chloride 0.9%

Dilute to a concentration of not more than 62.5 micrograms/mL. To be given over at least 2 hours. Protect from light

**Digoxin-specific antibody fragments** (*Digibind®*)

Intermittent *in* Sodium chloride 0.9%

Dissolve initially in water for injections (4 mL/vial) then dilute with the sodium chloride 0.9% and give through a 0.22 micron sterile, disposable filter over 30 minutes

**Dinoprostone** (*Prostin E2®*)

Continuous *or* intermittent *in* Glucose 5% *or* Sodium chloride 0.9%

**Disodium folinate** (*Sodiofolin®*)

Intermittent *in* Sodium chloride 0.9%

Protect from light

Avoid bicarbonate containing infusions

**Disodium levofolinate** (*Levofolinic acid*, Medac)

Intermittent in Glucose 5% *or* Sodium chloride 0.9%

**Disodium pamidronate** (*Aredia®*; *Disodium pamidronate*, Forum, Hospira, Medac)

Intermittent *in* Glucose 5% *or* Sodium chloride 0.9%

For *Aredia®* and *Pamidronate disodium* (Britannia), reconstitute initially with water for injections (15 mg in 5 mL, 30 mg or 90 mg in 10 mL); for *Aredia®*, *Pamidronate disodium* (Britannia), *Disodium pamidronate* (Hospira), dilute with infusion fluid to a concentration of not more than 60 mg in 250 mL; for *Disodium pamidronate* (Medac) dilute with infusion fluid to a concentration of not more than 90 mg in 250 mL; give at a rate not exceeding 1 mg/minute; not to be given with infusion fluids containing calcium

**Disopyramide (as phosphate)** (*Rythmodan®*)

Continuous *or* intermittent *in* Glucose 5% *or* Sodium chloride 0.9% *or* Ringer's solution *or* Compound sodium lactate

Max. rate by continuous infusion 20–30 mg/hour (or 400 micrograms/kg/hour)

**Dobutamine (as hydrochloride)**

Continuous *in* Glucose 5% *or* Sodium chloride 0.9%

Dilute to a concentration of 0.5–1 mg/mL and give *via* a controlled infusion device; give higher concentration (max. 5 mg/mL) with infusion pump; incompatible with bicarbonate

**Docetaxel** (*Taxotere®*)

Intermittent *in* Glucose 5% *or* Sodium chloride 0.9%

Stand docetaxel vials and diluent at room temperature for 5 minutes; add diluent to produce a concentrate containing 10 mg/mL and allow to stand for a further 5 minutes; dilute the requisite dose with at least 250 mL infusion fluid to a final concentration not exceeding 740 micrograms/mL; infuse over 1 hour

**Dolasetron mesilate** (*Anzemet®*)

Intermittent *in* Glucose 5% *or* Sodium chloride 0.9% *or* Compound sodium lactate

Suggested volume 50 mL given over 30 seconds–15 minutes

**Dopamine hydrochloride**

Continuous *in* Glucose 5% *or* Sodium chloride 0.9% *or* Compound sodium lactate

Dilute to max concentration of 3.2 mg/mL; incompatible with bicarbonate

**Dopexamine hydrochloride** (*Dopacard®*)

Continuous *in* Glucose 5% *or* Sodium chloride 0.9%

Dilute to a concentration of 400 or 800 micrograms/mL; max. concentration *via* large peripheral vein 1 mg/mL, concentrations up to 4 mg/mL may be infused *via* central vein; give *via* infusion pump or other device which provides accurate control of rate; contact with metal should be minimised; incompatible with bicarbonate

**Doripenem** (*Doribax®*)

Intermittent *in* Glucose 5% *or* Sodium chloride 0.9%

Reconstitute 500 mg with 10 mL water for injections or sodium chloride 0.9% then dilute with 100 mL infusion fluid; give over 1 hour (for severe hospital-acquired pneumonia or hospital-acquired pneumonia caused by less sensitive organisms, may extend infusion time to 4 hours using sodium chloride 0.9% as the infusion fluid)

**Doxorubicin hydrochloride**

Continuous *or via* drip tubing *in* Glucose 5% *or* Sodium chloride 0.9%

Reconstitute with water for injections or sodium chloride 0.9% (10 mg in 5 mL, 50 mg in 25 mL); give over 3–5 minutes; for continuous infusion over 24 hours (*Doxorubicin*, Medac and *Doxorubicin*, Teva UK only), consult local protocol

**Doxorubicin hydrochloride (liposomal)** (*Caelyx®*)

*via* drip tubing *in* Glucose 5%

Dilute up to 90 mg in 250 mL infusion fluid and over 90 mg in 500 mL infusion fluid

**Eculizumab** (*Soliris®*)

Intermittent *in* Glucose 5% *or* Sodium chloride 0.9%

Dilute requisite dose to a concentration of 5 mg/mL and mix gently; give over 25–45 minutes (infusion time may be increased to 2 hours if infusion-related reactions occur)

**Enoximone** (*Perfan®*)

Continuous *or* intermittent *in* Sodium chloride 0.9% *or* Water for injections

Dilute to a concentration of 2.5 mg/mL; incompatible with glucose solutions; use only plastic containers or syringes

**Epirubicin hydrochloride** (*Pharmorubicin® Rapid Dissolution, Pharmorubicin® Solution*)

*via* drip tubing *in* Glucose 5% *or* Sodium chloride 0.9%

Reconstitute *Pharmorubicin® Rapid Dissolution* with sodium chloride 0.9% or with water for injections (10 mg in 5 mL, 20 mg in 10 mL, 50 mg in 25 mL); give over 3–5 minutes

**Epoprostenol** (*Flolan®*)

Continuous *in* Sodium chloride 0.9% (but see also below)

Reconstitute using the filter and solvent (glycine buffer diluent) provided to make a concentrate; may be diluted further (consult product literature); for *pulmonary hypertension* dilute further with glycine buffer diluent only, for *renal dialysis* may be diluted further with sodium chloride 0.9%

**Ertapenem** (*Invanz®*)

Intermittent *in* Sodium chloride 0.9%

Reconstitute 1 g with 10 mL water for injections or sodium chloride 0.9%; dilute requisite dose in infusion fluid to a final concentration not exceeding 20 mg/mL; give over 30 minutes; incompatible with glucose solutions

**Erythromycin (as lactobionate)**

Continuous *or* intermittent *in* Glucose 5% (neutralised with sodium bicarbonate) *or* Sodium chloride 0.9%

Dissolve initially in water for injections (1 g in 20 mL) then dilute to a concentration of 1 mg/mL for continuous infusion and 1–5 mg/mL for intermittent infusion; give intermittent infusion over 20–60 minutes

**Esomeprazole (as sodium salt)** (*Nexium®*)

Intermittent *in* Sodium chloride 0.9%

Reconstitute 40 mg with 5 mL sodium chloride 0.9% then dilute with up to 100 mL infusion fluid, give requisite dose over 10–30 minutes

**Ethanol**

Continuous *in* Glucose 5% *or* Sodium chloride 0.9% *or* Ringer's solution *or* Compound sodium lactate

Dilute to a concentration of 5–10%

**Etoposide** (*Eposin®*; *Etoposide*, TEVA UK and Hospira)

Intermittent *in* Sodium chloride 0.9%

For *Etoposide* (TEVA UK) dilute with either sodium chloride 0.9% or glucose 5% to a concentration of 200 micrograms/mL and give over 30–60 minutes; for *Etoposide* (Hospira) dilute with either sodium chloride 0.9% or glucose 5% to a concentration of not more than 250 micrograms/mL and give over not less than 30 minutes; for *Eposin®* dilute with either sodium chloride 0.9% or glucose 5% to a concentration of 200–400 micrograms/mL and give over at least 30 minutes; check container for haze or precipitate during infusion

**Etoposide (as phosphate)** (*Etopophos®*)

Intermittent *in* Glucose 5% *or* Sodium chloride 0.9%

Reconstitute with 5–10 mL of either water for injections or with infusion fluid then dilute further with infusion fluid to a concentration as low as 100 micrograms/mL and give over 5 minutes to 3.5 hours

**Fentanyl** (*Sublimaze®*)

Continuous *or* intermittent *in* Glucose 5% *or* Sodium chloride 0.9%

**Ferric carboxymaltose** (*Ferinject®*)

Intermittent *in* Sodium chloride 0.9%

Dilute 200–500 mg in up to 100 mL infusion fluid and give over at least 6 minutes; dilute 0.5–1 g in up to 250 mL infusion fluid and give over at least 15 minutes

**Filgrastim** (*Neupogen®*; *Ratiograstim®*)

Continuous *or* intermittent *in* Glucose 5%

For a filgrastim concentration of less than 1 500 000 units/mL (15 micrograms/mL) albumin solution (human serum albumin) is added to produce a final albumin concentration of 2 mg/mL; should not be diluted to a filgrastim concentration of less than 200 000 units/mL (2 micrograms/mL) and should not be diluted with sodium chloride solution

**Flecainide acetate** (*Tambocor®*)

Continuous *or* intermittent *in* Glucose 5% *or* Sodium chloride 0.9% *or* Compound sodium lactate

Minimum volume in infusion fluids containing chlorides 500 mL

**Flucloxacillin (as sodium salt)** (*Floxapen®*)

Intermittent *in* Glucose 5% *or* Sodium chloride 0.9%

Suggested volume 100 mL given over 30–60 minutes

*via* drip tubing *in* Glucose 5% *or* Sodium chloride 0.9% *or* Ringer's solution *or* Compound sodium lactate

Continuous infusion not usually recommended

**Fludarabine phosphate** (*Fludara®*)

Intermittent *in* Sodium chloride 0.9%

Reconstitute each 50 mg with 2 mL water for injections and dilute requisite dose in 100 mL; give over 30 minutes

**Flumazenil** (*Anexate®*)

Continuous *in* Glucose 5% *or* Sodium chloride 0.9%

**Fluorouracil (as sodium salt)**

Continuous *or* intermittent *or via* drip tubing *in* Glucose 5% *or* Sodium chloride 0.9%

Give intermittent infusion over 30–60 minutes or over 4 hours

**Fondaparinux** (*Arixtra®*)

Intermittent *in* Sodium chloride 0.9%

For ST-segment elevation myocardial infarction, add requisite dose to 25–50 mL infusion fluid and give over 1–2 minutes

**Fosaprepitant** (*Ivemend®*)

Intermittent *in* Sodium chloride 0.9%

Reconstitute each 115-mg vial with 5 mL sodium chloride 0.9% gently without shaking to avoid foaming, then dilute in 110 mL infusion fluid; give over 15 minutes

**Foscarnet sodium** (*Foscavir®*)

Intermittent *in* Glucose 5% *or* Sodium chloride 0.9%

Dilute to a concentration of 12 mg/mL for infusion into peripheral vein (undiluted solution *via* central venous line only); infuse over at least 1 hour (infuse doses greater than 60 mg/kg over 2 hours)

**Fosphenytoin Sodium** (*Pro-Epanutin®*)

Intermittent *in* Glucose 5% *or* Sodium chloride 0.9%

Dilute to a concentration of 1.5–25 mg (phenytoin sodium equivalent)/mL

**Furosemide/Frusemide (as sodium salt)** (*Lasix®*)

Continuous *in* Sodium chloride 0.9% *or* Ringer's solution

Infusion pH must be above 5.5 and rate should not exceed 4 mg/ minute; glucose solutions are unsuitable

**Fusidic acid (as sodium salt)**

Continuous *in* Glucose 5% (but see below) *or* Sodium chloride 0.9%

Reconstitute with the buffer solution provided and dilute to 500 mL; give through central venous line over 2 hours (or over 6 hours if superficial vein used); incompatible in solution of pH less than 7.4

**Galsulfase** (*Naglazyme®*)

Intermittent *in* Sodium chloride 0.9%

Dilute requisite dose with infusion fluid to final volume of 250 mL and mix gently; infuse through a 0.2 micron in-line filter; give approx. 2.5% of the total volume over 1 hour, then infuse remaining volume over next 3 hours; if body-weight under 20 kg and at risk of fluid overload, dilute requisite dose in 100 mL infusion fluid and give over at least 4 hours

**Ganciclovir (as sodium salt)** (*Cymevene®*)

Intermittent *in* Glucose 5% *or* Sodium chloride 0.9% *or* Ringer's solution *or* Compound sodium lactate

Reconstitute initially in water for injections (500 mg/10 mL) then dilute to not more than 10 mg/mL with infusion fluid (usually 100 mL); give over 1 hour

**Gemcitabine** (*Gemzar®*)

Intermittent *in* Sodium chloride 0.9%

Reconstitute initially with sodium chloride 0.9% (200 mg in at least 5 mL, 1 g in at least 25 mL); may be diluted further with infusion fluid; give over 30 minutes

**Gentamicin (as sulphate)** (*Cidomycin®*; *Gentamicin Paediatric Injection*, Beacon; *Gentamicin Injection*, Hospira)

Intermittent *or via* drip tubing *in* Glucose 5% *or* Sodium chloride 0.9%

Suggested volume for intermittent infusion 50–100 mL given over 20–30 minutes

**Glyceryl trinitrate** (*Nitrocine®*, *Nitronal®*)

Continuous *in* Glucose 5% *or* Sodium chloride 0.9%

For *Nitrocine®* suggested infusion concentration 100 micrograms/ mL; incompatible with polyvinyl chloride infusion containers such as *Viaflex®* or *Steriflex®*; use glass or polyethylene containers or give *via* a syringe pump

**Granisetron (as hydrochloride)** (*Kytril®*)

Intermittent *in* Glucose 5% *or* Sodium chloride 0.9% *or* Compound sodium lactate

Dilute 3 mL in 20–50 mL infusion fluid (up to 3 mL in 10–30 mL for children); give over 5 minutes

**Haem arginate** (*Normosang®*)

Intermittent *in* Sodium chloride 0.9%

Dilute requisite dose in 100 mL infusion fluid in glass bottle and give over at least 30 minutes *via* large antebrachial vein; administer within 1 hour after dilution

**Heparin sodium**

Continuous *in* Glucose 5% *or* Sodium chloride 0.9%

Administration with a motorised pump advisable

**Hydralazine hydrochloride** (*Apresoline®*)

Continuous *in* Sodium chloride 0.9% *or* Ringer's solution

Suggested infusion volume 500 mL

**Hydrocortisone (as sodium phosphate)** (*Efcortesol®*)

Continuous *or* intermittent *or via* drip tubing *in* Glucose 5% *or* Sodium chloride 0.9%

**Hydrocortisone (as sodium succinate)** (*SoluCortef®*)

Continuous *or* intermittent *or via* drip tubing *in* Glucose 5% *or* Sodium chloride 0.9%

**Ibandronic acid** (*Bondronat®*)

Intermittent *in* Glucose 5% *or* Sodium chloride 0.9%

Dilute requisite dose in 500 mL infusion fluid and give over 1–2 hours

**Idarubicin hydrochloride** (*Zavedos®*)

*via* drip tubing *in* Sodium chloride 0.9%

Reconstitute with water for injections to produce a 1 mg/mL solution; give over 5–10 minutes

**Idursulfase** (*Elaprase®*)

Intermittent *in* Sodium chloride 0.9%

Dilute requisite dose in 100 mL infusion fluid and mix gently (do not shake); give over 3 hours (gradually reduced to 1 hour if no infusion-related reactions)

**Ifosfamide** (*Mitoxana®*)

Continuous *or* intermittent *or via* drip tubing *in* Glucose 5% *or* Sodium chloride 0.9%

For continuous infusion, suggested volume 3 litres given over 24 hours; for intermittent infusion, give over 30–120 minutes

**Imiglucerase** (*Cerezyme®*)

Intermittent *in* Sodium chloride 0.9%

Initially reconstitute with water for injections (200 units in 5.1 mL, 400 units in 10.2 mL) to give 40 units/mL solution; dilute requisite dose with infusion fluid to a final volume of 100–200 mL and give over 1–2 hours *or* at a rate not exceeding 1 unit/kg/minute; administer within 3 hours after reconstitution

**Imipenem with cilastatin (as sodium salt)** (*Primaxin®*)

Intermittent *in* Sodium chloride 0.9% *or* Sodium chloride and Glucose

Dilute to a concentration of 5 mg (as imipenem)/mL; infuse 250–500 mg (as imipenem) over 20–30 minutes, 1 g over 40–60 minutes

Continuous infusion not usually recommended

**Infliximab** (*Remicade®*)

Intermittent *in* Sodium chloride 0.9%

Reconstitute each 100-mg vial with 10 mL water for injections using a 21-gauge or smaller needle; gently swirl vial without shaking to dissolve; allow to stand for 5 minutes; dilute requisite dose with infusion fluid to a final volume of 250 mL and give through a low protein-binding filter (1.2 micron or less) over at least 2 hours (patients being treated for rheumatoid arthritis who have tolerated 3 initial 2-hour infusions may be given subsequent infusions of up to 6 mg/kg over at least 1 hour); start infusion within 3 hours of reconstitution

**Insulin (soluble)**

Continuous *in* Sodium chloride 0.9%

Adsorbed to some extent by plastics of infusion set; see also section 6.1.3; ensure insulin is not injected into 'dead space' of injection port of the infusion bag

**Insulin aspart**

Continuous *in* Sodium chloride 0.9% *or* Glucose 5%

Dilute to 0.05–1 unit/mL with infusion fluid; adsorbed to some extent by plastics of infusion set

**Insulin lispro**

Continuous *in* Sodium chloride 0.9% *or* Glucose 5%

### Interferon alfa-2b (*IntronA*®)

Intermittent *in* Sodium chloride 0.9%

For *IntronA*® solution, dilute requisite dose in 50 mL infusion fluid and administer over 20 minutes; not to be diluted to less than 300 000 units/mL

For *IntronA*® powder, reconstitute with 1 mL water for injections; dilute requisite dose in 100 mL infusion fluid and administer over 20 minutes; not to be diluted to less than 100 000 units/mL

### Irinotecan hydrochloride (*Campto*®)

Intermittent *in* Glucose 5% *or* Sodium chloride 0.9%

Dilute requisite dose in 250 mL infusion fluid; give over 30–90 minutes

### Iron dextran (*Cosmofer*®)

Intermittent *in* Glucose 5% *or* Sodium chloride 0.9%

Dilute 100–200 mg in 100 mL infusion fluid; give 25 mg over 15 minutes as a test dose initially, then give at a rate not exceeding 6.67 mg/minute; *total dose infusion* diluted in 500 mL infusion fluid and given over 4–6 hours (initial test dose 25 mg over 15 minutes)

### Iron sucrose (*Venofer*®)

Intermittent *in* Sodium chloride 0.9%

Dilute 100 mg in up to 100 mL infusion fluid; give 25 mg over 15 minutes as a test dose initially, then give at a rate not exceeding 3.33 mg/minute

### Isosorbide dinitrate (*Isoket 0.05%*®, *Isoket 0.1%*®)

Continuous *in* Glucose 5% *or* Sodium chloride 0.9%

Adsorbed to some extent by polyvinyl chloride infusion containers, preferably use glass or polyethylene containers or give *via* a syringe pump; *Isoket 0.05%*® can alternatively be administered undiluted using a syringe pump with a glass or rigid plastic syringe

### Itraconazole (*Sporanox*®)

Intermittent *in* Sodium chloride 0.9%

Dilute 250 mg in 50 mL infusion fluid and infuse only **60 mL** through an in-line filter (0.2 micron) over 60 minutes

### Ketamine (as hydrochloride) (*Ketalar*®)

Continuous *in* Glucose 5% *or* Sodium chloride 0.9%

Dilute to 1 mg/mL; microdrip infusion for maintenance of anaesthesia

### Labetalol hydrochloride (*Trandate*®)

Intermittent *in* Glucose 5% *or* Sodium chloride and glucose

Dilute to a concentration of 1 mg/mL; suggested volume 200 mL; adjust rate with in-line burette

### Lacosamide (*Vimpat*®)

Intermittent *in* Glucose 5% *or* Sodium chloride 0.9% *or* Compound sodium lactate solution

May be administered undiluted

### Laronidase (*Aldurazyme*®)

Intermittent *in* Sodium chloride 0.9%

Body-weight under 20 kg, use 100 mL infusion fluid; body-weight over 20 kg use 250 mL infusion fluid; withdraw volume of infusion fluid equivalent to volume of laronidase concentrate being added; give through an in-line filter (0.22 micron) at an initial rate of 2 units/kg/hour then increasing gradually every 15 minutes to max. 43 units/kg/hour

### Lenograstim (*Granocyte*®)

Intermittent *in* Sodium chloride 0.9%

Initially reconstitute with 1 mL water for injection provided (do not shake vigorously) then dilute with up to 50 mL infusion fluid for each vial of *Granocyte-13* or up to 100 mL infusion fluid for *Granocyte-34*; give over 30 minutes

### Lepirudin (*Refludan*®)

Continuous *in* Glucose 5% *or* Sodium chloride 0.9%

Reconstitute initially with water for injections *or* sodium chloride 0.9% then dilute to a concentration of 2 mg/mL with infusion fluid

### Levetiracetam (*Keppra*®)

Intermittent *in* Glucose 5% *or* Sodium chloride 0.9% *or* Compound sodium lactate

Dilute requisite dose with at least 100 mL of infusion fluid; give over 15 minutes

### Magnesium sulphate

Continuous *in* Glucose 5% *or* Sodium chloride 0.9%

Suggested concentration up to 200 mg/mL; max. rate 150 mg/minute

### Melphalan (*Alkeran*®)

Intermittent *or via* drip tubing *in* Sodium chloride 0.9%

Reconstitute with the solvent provided then dilute with infusion fluid; max. 90 minutes between addition and completion of administration; incompatible with glucose infusion

### Meropenem (*Meronem*®)

Intermittent *in* Glucose 5 and 10% *or* Sodium chloride 0.9%

Dilute in 50–200 mL infusion fluid and give over 15–30 minutes

### Mesna (*Uromitexan*®)

Continuous *or via* drip tubing *in* Glucose 5% *or* Sodium chloride 0.9%

### Metaraminol (as tartrate) (*Aramine*®)

Continuous *or via* drip tubing *in* Glucose 5% *or* Sodium chloride 0.9%

Suggested volume 500 mL

### Methotrexate (as sodium salt) (*Methotrexate*, Lederle)

Continuous *or via* drip tubing *in* Glucose 5% *or* Sodium chloride 0.9% *or* Compound sodium lactate *or* Ringer's solution

Dilute in a large-volume infusion; max. 24 hours between addition and completion of administration

### Methylprednisolone (as sodium succinate) (*Solu-Medrone*®)

Continuous *or* intermittent *or via* drip tubing *in* Glucose 5% *or* Sodium chloride 0.9%

Reconstitute initially with water for injections; doses up to 250 mg should be given over at least 5 minutes, high doses over at least 30 minutes

### Metoclopramide hydrochloride (*Maxolon High Dose*®)

Continuous *or* intermittent *in* Glucose 5% *or* Sodium chloride 0.9% *or* Compound sodium lactate

Continuous infusion recommended; loading dose, dilute with 50–100 mL and give over 15–20 minutes; maintenance dose, dilute with 500 mL and give over 8–12 hours; for intermittent infusion dilute with at least 50 mL and give over at least 15 minutes

### Micafungin (*Mycamine*®)

Intermittent *in* Glucose 5% *or* Sodium chloride 0.9%

Reconstitute each vial with 5 mL infusion fluid; gently rotate vial, without shaking, to dissolve; dilute requisite dose with infusion fluid to 100 mL (final concentration 0.5–2 mg/mL); protect from light; give over 60 minutes

### Midazolam (*Hypnovel*®)

Continuous *in* Glucose 5% *or* Sodium chloride 0.9%

For neonates and children under 15 kg dilute to a max. concentration of 1 mg/mL

### Milrinone (*Primacor*®)

Continuous *in* Glucose 5% *or* Sodium chloride 0.9%

Dilute to a suggested concentration of 200 micrograms/mL

### Mitoxantrone/Mitozantrone (as hydrochloride)
(*Onkotrone®*)

Intermittent *or via* drip tubing *in* Glucose 5% *or* Sodium chloride 0.9%

For administration *via* drip tubing suggested volume at least 50 mL given over at least 3–5 minutes; for intermittent infusion, dilute with 50–100 mL and give over 15–30 minutes

### Mivacurium (as chloride) (*Mivacron®*)

Continuous *in* Glucose 5% *or* Sodium chloride 0.9%

Dilute to a concentration of 500 micrograms/mL; may also be given undiluted

### Mycophenolate mofetil (as hydrochloride)
(*CellCept®*)

Intermittent *in* Glucose 5%

Reconstitute each 500-mg vial with 14 mL glucose 5% and dilute the contents of 2 vials in 140 mL infusion fluid; give over 2 hours

### Naloxone (*Minijet® Naloxone Hydrochloride*)

Continuous *in* Glucose 5% *or* Sodium chloride 0.9%

Reversal of opioid-induced respiratory depression, dilute to a concentration of 4 micrograms/mL; opioid overdose only, dilute 10 mg in 50 mL glucose 5%, see Emergency Treatment of Poisoning

### Natalizumab (*Tysabri®*)

Intermittent *in* Sodium chloride 0.9%

Dilute 300 mg in 100 mL infusion fluid; gently invert to mix, do not shake. Use within 8 hours of dilution and give over 1 hour

### Nimodipine (*Nimotop®*)

*via* drip tubing *in* Glucose 5% *or* Sodium chloride 0.9% *or* Compound sodium lactate

Not to be added to infusion container; administer *via* an infusion pump through a Y-piece into a central catheter; incompatible with polyvinyl chloride giving sets or containers; protect infusion from light

### Nizatidine (*Axid®*)

Continuous *or* intermittent *in* Glucose 5% *or* Sodium chloride 0.9% *or* Compound sodium lactate

For continuous infusion, dilute 300 mg in 150 mL and give at a rate of 10 mg/hour; for intermittent infusion, dilute 100 mg in 50 mL and give over 15 minutes

### Noradrenaline acid tartrate/Norepinephrine bitartrate

Continuous *in* Glucose 5% *or* Sodium chloride and glucose

Give *via* controlled infusion device; for administration *via* syringe pump, dilute 4 mg noradrenaline acid tartrate (2 mL solution) with 48 mL; for administration *via* drip counter dilute 40 mg (20 mL solution) with 480 mL; give through a central venous catheter; incompatible with alkalis

### Omeprazole (as sodium salt) (*Losec®*)

Intermittent *or* continuous *in* Glucose 5% *or* Sodium chloride 0.9%

Reconstitute each 40 mg vial with infusion fluid and dilute to 100 mL; for intermittent infusion, give 40 mg over 20–30 minutes; stable for 3 hours in glucose 5% or 12 hours in sodium chloride 0.9%

### Ondansetron (as hydrochloride) (*Zofran®*)

Continuous *or* intermittent *in* Glucose 5% *or* Sodium chloride 0.9% *or* Ringer's solution

For intermittent infusion, dilute 32 mg in 50–100 mL and give over at least 15 minutes

### Oxaliplatin (*Eloxatin®*)

Continuous *in* Glucose 5%

Dilute requisite dose to a concentration of 200–700 micrograms/mL and give over 2–6 hours; incompatible with alkaline or chloride-containing fluids; avoid equipment containing aluminium

### Oxycodone hydrochloride (*OxyNorm®*)

Continuous *or* intermittent *in* Glucose 5% *or* Sodium chloride 0.9%

Dilute to a concentration of 1 mg/mL

### Oxytocin (*Syntocinon®*)

Continuous *in* Glucose 5% *or* Sodium chloride 0.9% *or* Compound sodium lactate *or* Ringer's solution

Preferably given *via* a variable-speed infusion pump in a concentration appropriate to the pump; if given by drip infusion for *induction or enhancement of labour*, dilute 5 units in 500 mL infusion fluid or for higher doses, 10 units in 500 mL; for *treatment of postpartum uterine haemorrhage* dilute 5–30 units in 500 mL; if high doses given for prolonged period (e.g. for inevitable or missed abortion or for postpartum haemorrhage), use low volume of an electrolyte-containing infusion fluid (not Glucose 5%) given at higher concentration than for induction or enhancement of labour; close attention to patient's fluid and electrolyte status essential

### Paclitaxel (*Abraxane®*)

Intermittent *in* Sodium chloride 0.9%

Reconstitute to a concentration of 5 mg/mL. Inject requisite dose volume into an empty, sterile, intravenous bag and give over 30 minutes; in-line filter not recommended

### Paclitaxel (*Taxol®*)

Continuous *in* Glucose 5% *or* Sodium chloride 0.9%

Dilute to a concentration of 0.3–1.2 mg/mL and give through an in-line filter (0.22 micron or less) over 3 hours; not to be used with PVC equipment (short PVC inlet or outlet on filter may be acceptable)

### Panitumumab (*Vectibix®*)

Intermittent *in* Sodium chloride 0.9%

Flush intravenous line with Sodium chloride 0.9% before and after infusion; dilute requisite dose with infusion fluid to 100 mL (final concentration not to exceed 10 mg/mL); gently invert to mix, do not shake; give *via* infusion pump through a low protein-binding in-line filter (0.2 or 0.22 micron) over 60 minutes; for doses higher than 1 g, dilute requisite dose with infusion fluid to 150 mL and give over 90 minutes

### Pantoprazole (as sodium sesquihydrate)
(*Protium®*)

Intermittent *in* Glucose 5% *or* Sodium chloride 0.9%

Reconstitute 40 mg with 10 mL sodium chloride 0.9% and dilute with 100 mL of infusion fluid; give 40 mg over 15 minutes

### Paracetamol (*Perfalgan®*)

Intermittent *in* Sodium chloride 0.9% *or* Glucose 5%

Dilute to a concentration of 1 mg/mL and use within 1 hour; may also be given undiluted

### Pemetrexed (*Alimta®*)

Intermittent *in* Sodium chloride 0.9%

Reconstitute 500-mg vial with 20 mL sodium chloride 0.9% to produce a 25 mg/mL solution; dilute requisite dose with infusion fluid to 100 mL; give over 10 minutes

### Pentamidine isetionate (*Pentacarinat®*)

Intermittent *in* Glucose 5% *or* Sodium chloride 0.9%

Dissolve initially in water for injections (300 mg in 3–5 mL) then dilute in 50–250 mL; give over at least 60 minutes

### Pentostatin (*Nipent®*)

Intermittent *in* Glucose 5% *or* Sodium chloride 0.9%

Reconstitute initially with 5 mL water for injections to produce a 2 mg/mL solution; dilute requisite dose in 25–50 mL infusion fluid (final concentration 180–330 micrograms/mL) and give over 20–30 minutes

### Phenoxybenzamine hydrochloride

Intermittent *in* Sodium chloride 0.9%

Dilute in 200–500 mL infusion; give over at least 2 hours; max. 4 hours between dilution and completion of administration

#### Phenylephrine hydrochloride

Intermittent *in* Glucose 5% *or* Sodium chloride 0.9%

Dilute 10 mg in 500 mL infusion fluid

#### Phenytoin sodium (*Epanutin®*)

Intermittent *in* Sodium chloride 0.9%

Flush intravenous line with Sodium chloride 0.9% before and after infusion; dilute in 50–100 mL infusion fluid (final concentration not to exceed 10 mg/mL) and give through an in-line filter (0.22–0.50 micron) at a rate not exceeding 50 mg/minute (neonates, give at a rate of 1–3 mg/kg/minute); complete administration within 1 hour of preparation

#### Phytomenadione (in mixed micelles vehicle)
(*Konakion® MM*)

Intermittent *in* Glucose 5%

Dilute with 55 mL; may be injected into lower part of infusion apparatus

#### Piperacillin with tazobactam (as sodium salts)

Intermittent *in* Glucose 5% *or* Sodium chloride 0.9% *or* Water for injections (*or* Compound sodium lactate for *Tazocin®* brand only)

Reconstitute initially with water for injections or sodium chloride 0.9% (2.25 g in 10 mL, 4.5 g in 20 mL), then dilute to 50–150 mL with infusion fluid (to max. 50 mL with water for injections); give over 20–30 minutes

#### Potassium chloride

Continuous *in* Glucose 5% *or* Sodium chloride 0.9%

Dilute in a large-volume infusion; mix thoroughly to avoid 'layering', especially in non-rigid infusion containers; use ready-prepared solutions when possible

#### Propofol (emulsion) (*Diprivan®*; Abbott; Baxter; *Propofol-Lipuro®*, *Propofen®*, Braun; Hospira; Fresenius Kabi)

**1% or 2% emulsion**

*via* drip tubing *in* Glucose 5% *or* Sodium chloride 0.9%

To be administered *via* a Y-piece close to injection site; microbiological filter not recommended

**1% emulsion only**

Continuous *in* Glucose 5% (*or* Sodium chloride 0.9% for *Propofol-Lipuro®*, *Propofen®*, Braun, and Fresenius Kabi brands only)

Dilute to a concentration not less than 2 mg/mL; microbiological filter not recommended; administer using suitable device to control infusion rate; use glass or PVC containers (if PVC bag used it should be full—withdraw volume of infusion fluid equal to that of propofol to be added); give within 6 hours of preparation; propofol may alternatively be infused undiluted using a suitable infusion pump

#### Quinine dihydrochloride

Continuous *in* Glucose 5% *or* Sodium chloride 0.9%

To be given over 4 hours; see also section 5.4.1

#### Quinupristin with dalfopristin (*Synercid®*)

Intermittent *in* Glucose 5%

Reconstitute 500 mg with 5 mL water for injections or glucose 5%; gently swirl vial without shaking to dissolve; allow to stand for at least 2 minutes until foam disappears; dilute requisite dose in 100 mL infusion fluid and give over 60 minutes *via* central venous catheter (in an emergency, first dose may be diluted in 250 mL infusion fluid and given over 60 minutes *via* peripheral line); flush line with glucose 5% before and after infusion; incompatible with sodium chloride solutions

#### Raltitrexed (*Tomudex®*)

Intermittent *in* Glucose 5% *or* Sodium chloride 0.9%

Reconstitute with water for injections; dilute requisite dose in 50–250 mL infusion fluid and give over 15 minutes

#### Ranitidine (as hydrochloride) (*Zantac®*)

Intermittent *in* Glucose 5% *or* Sodium chloride 0.9% *or* Compound sodium lactate

#### Rasburicase (*Fasturtec®*)

Intermittent *in* Sodium chloride 0.9%

Reconstitute with solvent provided; gently swirl vial without shaking to dissolve; dilute requisite dose to 50 mL with infusion fluid and give over 30 minutes

#### Remifentanil (*Ultiva®*)

Continuous *in* Glucose 5% *or* Sodium chloride 0.9% *or* Water for injections

Reconstitute with infusion fluid to a concentration of 1 mg/mL then dilute further to a concentration of 20–250 micrograms/mL (50 micrograms/mL recommended for general anaesthesia, 20–25 micrograms/mL recommended for children 1–12 years; 20–50 micrograms/mL recommended when used with target controlled infusion (TCI) device)

#### Rifampicin (*Rifadin®*)

Intermittent *in* Glucose 5 and 10% *or* Sodium chloride 0.9% *or* Ringer's solution

Reconstitute with solvent provided then dilute with 500 mL infusion fluid; give over 2–3 hours

#### Ritodrine hydrochloride (*Yutopar®*)

Continuous *in* Glucose 5%

Give *via* controlled infusion device, preferably a syringe pump; if syringe pump available dilute to a concentration of 3 mg/mL; if syringe pump not available dilute to a concentration of 300 micrograms/mL; close attention to patient's fluid and electrolyte status essential

#### Rituximab (*MabThera®*)

Intermittent *in* Glucose 5% *or* Sodium chloride 0.9%

Dilute to 1–4 mg/mL and gently invert bag to avoid foaming

#### Rocuronium bromide (*Esmeron®*)

Continuous *or via* drip tubing *in* Glucose 5% *or* Sodium chloride 0.9%

#### Salbutamol (as sulphate) (*Ventolin® For Intravenous Infusion*)

Continuous *in* Glucose 5%

For *bronchodilatation* dilute to a concentration of 200 micrograms/mL with glucose 5%, sodium chloride 0.9%, or water for injections; for *premature labour* dilute with glucose 5% to a concentration of 200 micrograms/mL for use in a syringe pump or for other infusion methods (preferably *via* controlled infusion device), dilute to a concentration of 20 micrograms/mL; close attention to patient's fluid and electrolyte status essential

#### Sodium calcium edetate (*Ledclair®*)

Continuous *in* Glucose 5% *or* Sodium chloride 0.9%

Dilute to a concentration of not more than 3%; suggested volume 250–500 mL given over at least 1 hour

#### Sodium clodronate (*Bonefos® Concentrate*)

Continuous *in* Glucose 5% *or* Sodium chloride 0.9%

Dilute 300 mg in 500 mL and give over at least 2 hours or 1.5 g in 500 mL and give over at least 4 hours

#### Sodium nitroprusside

Continuous *in* Glucose 5%

Infuse *via* infusion device to allow precise control; protect infusion from light. For further details consult product literature

#### Sodium valproate (*Epilim®*, *Episenta®*)

Continuous *or* intermittent *in* Glucose 5% *or* Sodium chloride 0.9%

Reconstitute *Epilim®* with solvent provided then dilute with infusion fluid

#### Sotalol hydrochloride (*Sotacor®*)

Continuous *or* intermittent *in* Glucose 5% *or* Sodium chloride 0.9%

Dilute to a concentration of between 0.01–2 mg/mL

**Streptokinase** (*Streptase®*)

Continuous *or* intermittent *in* Glucose 5% *or* Sodium chloride 0.9%

Reconstitute with sodium chloride 0.9%, then dilute further with infusion fluid

**Sulfadiazine sodium**

Continuous *in* Sodium chloride 0.9%

Suggested volume 500 mL; ampoule solution has a pH of over 10

**Suxamethonium chloride** (*Anectine®*)

Continuous *in* Glucose 5% *or* Sodium chloride 0.9%

**Tacrolimus** (*Prograf®*)

Continuous *in* Glucose 5% *or* Sodium chloride 0.9%

Dilute concentrate in infusion fluid to a final concentration of 4–100 micrograms/mL; give over 24 hours; incompatible with PVC

**Teicoplanin** (*Targocid®*)

Intermittent *in* Glucose 5% *or* Sodium chloride 0.9% *or* Compound sodium lactate

Reconstitute initially with water for injections provided; infuse over 30 minutes

Continuous infusion not usually recommended

**Temocillin** (*Negaban®*)

Intermittent *in* Glucose 5% or 10% *or* Sodium chloride 0.9% *or* Ringer's solution *or* Compound sodium lactate

Reconstitute 1 g with 20 mL water for injections then dilute with 50–150 mL infusion fluid; give over 30–40 minutes

**Temsirolimus** (*Torisel®*)

Intermittent *in* Sodium chloride 0.9%

Add 1.8 mL of the supplied diluent to the vial of concentrate to produce a concentration of 10 mg/mL; dilute requisite dose with 250 mL of sodium chloride 0.9%; give (preferably via infusion pump) through an in-line filter with a maximum pore size of 5 microns; avoid PVC equipment; protect from light and administer within 6 hours of dilution

**Terbutaline sulphate** (*Bricanyl®*)

Continuous *in* Glucose 5%

For *bronchodilatation* dilute 1.5–2.5 mg with 500 mL glucose 5% or sodium chloride 0.9% and give over 8–10 hours; for *premature labour* dilute in glucose 5% and give *via* controlled infusion device preferably a syringe pump; if syringe pump available dilute to a concentration of 100 micrograms/mL; if syringe pump not available dilute to a concentration of 10 micrograms/mL; close attention to patient's fluid and electrolyte status essential

**Ticarcillin sodium with clavulanic acid** (*Timentin®*)

Intermittent *in* Glucose 5% *or* Water for injections

Suggested volume (depending on dose) glucose 5% 100–150 mL or water for injections 50–100 mL; given over 30–40 minutes

**Tigecycline** (*Tygacil®*)

Intermittent *in* Glucose 5% *or* Sodium chloride 0.9%

Reconstitute each vial with 5.3 mL infusion fluid to produce a 10 mg/mL solution; dilute requisite dose in 100 mL infusion fluid; give over 30–60 minutes

**Tirofiban** (*Aggrastat®*)

Continuous *in* Glucose 5% *or* Sodium chloride 0.9%

Withdraw 50 mL infusion fluid from 250-mL bag and replace with 50 mL tirofiban concentrate (250 micrograms/mL) to give a final concentration of 50 micrograms/mL

**Tobramycin (as sulphate)** (*Nebcin®*)

Intermittent *or via* drip tubing *in* Glucose 5% *or* Sodium chloride 0.9%

For adult intermittent infusion suggested volume 50–100 mL (children proportionately smaller volume) given over 20–60 minutes

**Topotecan (as hydrochloride)** (*Hycamtin®*)

Intermittent *in* Glucose 5% *or* Sodium chloride 0.9%

Reconstitute 4 mg with 4 mL water for injections then dilute to a final concentration of 25–50 micrograms/mL; give over 30 minutes

**Tramadol hydrochloride** (*Zydol®*)

Continuous *or* intermittent *in* Glucose 5% *or* Sodium chloride 0.9% *or* Ringer's solution *or* Compound sodium lactate

**Tranexamic acid** (*Cyklokapron®*)

Continuous *in* Glucose 5% *or* Sodium chloride 0.9% *or* Ringer's solution

**Trastuzumab** (*Herceptin®*)

Intermittent *in* Sodium chloride 0.9%

Reconstitute each 150-mg vial with 7.2 mL water for injections to produce 21 mg/mL solution, swirl vial gently to avoid excessive foaming and allow to stand for approximately 5 minutes; dilute requisite dose in 250 mL infusion fluid

**Treosulfan** (*Treosulfan*) (Medac)

Intermittent *in* Water for injections

Infusion suggested for doses above 5 g; dilute to a concentration of 5 g in 100 mL

**Urokinase** (*Syner-KINASE®*)

Continuous *or* intermittent *in* Sodium chloride 0.9%

**Vancomycin (as hydrochloride)** (*Vancocin®*)

Intermittent *in* Glucose 5% *or* Sodium chloride 0.9%

Reconstitute each 500 mg with 10 mL water for injections and dilute with infusion fluid to a concentration of up to 5 mg/mL (10 mg/mL in fluid restriction but increased risk of infusion-related effects); give over at least 60 minutes (rate not to exceed 10 mg/minute for doses over 500 mg); use continuous infusion only if intermittent not feasible

**Vasopressin, synthetic** (*Pitressin®*)

Intermittent *in* Glucose 5%

Suggested concentration 20 units/100 mL given over 15 minutes

**Vecuronium bromide** (*Norcuron®*)

Continuous *or* via drip tubing *in* Glucose 5% *or* Sodium chloride 0.9% *or* Ringer's solution

Reconstitute each vial with 5 mL water for injections to give 2 mg/mL solution; *alternatively* reconstitute with up to 10 mL glucose 5% *or* sodium chloride 0.9% *or* water for injections—unsuitable for further dilution if not reconstituted with water for injections. For *continuous intravenous infusion*, dilute to a concentration up to 40 micrograms/mL

**Verteporfin** (*Visudyne®*)

Intermittent *in* Glucose 5%

Reconstitute each 15 mg with 7 mL water for injections to produce a 2 mg/mL solution then dilute requisite dose with infusion fluid to a final volume of 30 mL and give over 10 minutes; protect from light and administer within 4 hours of reconstitution. Incompatible with sodium chloride infusion

**Vinblastine sulphate** (*Velbe®*)

*via* drip tubing *in* Sodium chloride 0.9%

Reconstitute with sodium chloride 0.9%; give over approx. 1 minute

**Vincristine sulphate** (*Oncovin®*)

*via* drip tubing *in* Glucose 5% *or* Sodium chloride 0.9%

**Vindesine sulphate** (*Eldisine®*)

*via* drip tubing *in* Glucose 5% *or* Sodium chloride 0.9%

Reconstitute with sodium chloride 0.9%; give over 1–3 minutes

**Vinorelbine** (*Navelbine®*)

Intermittent *in* Glucose 5% *or* Sodium chloride 0.9%

Dilute in 125 mL infusion fluid; give over 20–30 minutes

**Vitamins B & C**  (*Pabrinex® I/V High potency*)

Intermittent *or via* drip tubing *in* Glucose 5% *or* Sodium chloride 0.9%

Ampoule contents should be mixed, diluted, and administered without delay; give over 30 minutes (see MHRA/CHM advice, section 9.6.2)

**Vitamins, multiple**

(*Cernevit®*)

Intermittent *in* Glucose 5% *or* Sodium chloride 0.9%

Dissolve initially in 5 mL water for injections (or infusion fluid)

(*Solivito N®*)

Intermittent *in* Glucose 5 and 10%

Suggested volume 500–1000 mL given over 2–3 hours; see also section 9.3

**Voriconazole**  (*Vfend®*)

Intermittent *in* Glucose 5% *or* Sodium chloride 0.9% *or* Compound sodium lactate

Reconstitute each 200 mg with 19 mL water for injections to produce a 10 mg/mL solution; dilute dose in infusion fluid to concentration of 0.5–5 mg/mL; give at a rate not exceeding 3 mg/kg/hour

**Zidovudine**  (*Retrovir®*)

Intermittent *in* Glucose 5%

Dilute to a concentration of 2 mg/mL or 4 mg/mL and give over 1 hour

**Zoledronic acid**  (*Zometa®*)

Intermittent *in* Glucose 5% *or* Sodium chloride 0.9%

Dilute requisite dose with 100 mL infusion fluid; infuse over at least 15 minutes; administer as a single intravenous solution in a separate infusion line; do not mix with calcium or other divalent cation-containing infusion solutions such as lactated Ringer's solution

# A7 Borderline substances

**A7.1 Enteral feeds (non-disease specific)** 881

A7.1.1 Enteral feeds (non-disease specific): less than 5 g protein/ 100 mL 881

A7.1.2 Enteral feeds (non-disease specific): 5 g (or more) protein/ 100 mL 883

A7.1.3 Enteral feeds (non-disease specific): Child under 12 years 887

**A7.2 Nutritional supplements (non-disease specific)** 887

A7.2.1 Nutritional supplements: less than 5 g protein/100 mL 887

A7.2.2 Nutritional supplements: 5 g (or more) protein/100 mL 888

**A7.3 Specialised formulas** 894

A7.3.1 Specialised formulas: Infant and child 894

A7.3.2 Specialised formulas for specific clinical conditions 894

**A7.4 Feed supplements** 898

A7.4.1 High-energy supplements 898

A7.4.2 Fibre, vitamin, and mineral supplements 902

**A7.5 Feed additives** 903

A7.5.1 Special foods for conditions of intolerance 903

A7.5.2 Feed thickeners and pre-thickened foods 903

A7.5.3 Flavouring preparations 903

**A7.6 Foods for special diets** 903

A7.6.1 Gluten-free foods 903

A7.6.2 Low-protein foods 905

**A7.7 Nutritional supplements for metabolic diseases** 905

*Appendix 7: Borderline substances*

In certain conditions some foods (and toilet preparations) have characteristics of drugs and the Advisory Committee on Borderline Substances advises as to the circumstances in which such substances may be regarded as drugs. Prescriptions issued in accordance with the Committee's advice and endorsed 'ACBS' will normally not be investigated.

General Practitioners are reminded that the ACBS recommends products on the basis that they may be regarded as drugs for the management of specified conditions. Doctors should satisfy themselves that the products can safely be prescribed, that patients are adequately monitored and that, where necessary, expert hospital supervision is available.

**Foods which may be prescribed on FP10, GP10 (Scotland), or WP10 (Wales)**
Note All the food products listed in this appendix have ACBS approval. The clinical condition for which the product has been approved is included with each entry.
Foods included in this appendix may contain cariogenic sugars and patients should be advised to take appropriate oral hygiene measures.

**Enteral feeds and supplements** For most enteral feeds and nutritional supplements, the main source of carbohydrate is either maltodextrin or glucose syrup; other carbohydrate sources are listed in the relevant table, below. Feeds containing residual lactose (less than 1 g lactose/100 mL formula) are described as 'clinically lactose-free' or 'lactose-free' by some manufacturers. The presence of lactose (including residual lactose) in feeds is indicated in the relevant table, below. The primary sources of protein or amino acids are included with each product entry. The fat or oil content is derived from a variety of sources such as vegetables, soya bean, corn, palm nuts, and seeds; where the fat content is derived from animal or fish sources, this information is included in the relevant table, below. The presence of medium chain triglycerides (MCT) is also noted where the quantity exceeds 30% of the fat content.

Enteral feeds and nutritional supplements can contain varying amounts of **vitamins**, **minerals**, and **trace elements**—the manufacturer's product literature should be consulted for more detailed information. For further information on enteral nutrition, see section 9.4.2. Feeds containing vitamin K may affect the INR in patients receiving warfarin; see **interactions**: Appendix 1 (vitamins).

The suitability of food products for patients requiring a vegan, kosher, halal, or other compliant diet should be confirmed with individual manufacturers.

For details of enteral feeds, nutritional supplements, and specialised formulas suitable for infants and children under 12 years see *BNF for Children* (Appendix 2)
Note Feeds containing more than 6 g/100 mL protein or 2 g/ 100 mL fibre should be avoided in children unless recommended by an appropriate specialist or dietician.

**Standard ACBS indications**
Disease-related malnutrition, intractable malabsorption, pre-operative preparation of malnourished patients, dysphagia, proven inflammatory bowel disease, following total gastrectomy, short-bowel syndrome, bowel fistula

## A7.1  Enteral feeds (non-disease specific)

### A7.1.1  Enteral feeds (non-disease specific): less than 5 g protein/100 mL

For further information on composition of feeds, see p. 880

### A7.1.1.1  Enteral feeds: 1 kcal/mL and less than 5 g protein/100 mL

Not suitable for use in child under 1 year; not recommended for child 1–6 years unless otherwise stated

| Product | Formulation | Energy | Protein | Carbohydrate | Fat | Fibre | Special Characteristics | ACBS Indications | Presentation & Flavour |
|---|---|---|---|---|---|---|---|---|---|
| Fresubin® Original (Fresenius Kabi) | Liquid (sip or tube feed) | 420 kJ (100 kcal) **per 100 mL** | 3.8 g cows' milk soya | 13.8 g (sugars 3.5 g[1]) | 3.4 g | Nil | Gluten-free Residual lactose Contains fish gelatin Feed in flexible pack contains fish fish and fish gelatin | Standard, p. 880 | Bottle: 200 mL = £1.74 Black currant, chocolate, mocha, nut, peach, vanilla Flexible pack: 500 mL = £3.36 1000 mL = £6.63 1500 mL = £9.97 |
| Fresubin® Original Fibre (Fresenius Kabi) | Liquid (tube feed) | 420 kJ (100 kcal) **per 100 mL** | 3.8 g cows' milk soya | 13.8 g (sugars 1 g) | 3.4 g | 2 g | Gluten-free Residual lactose Contains fish oil and fish gelatin | Standard, p. 880 except bowel fistula. Not suitable for child under 2 years | Flexible pack: 500 mL = £3.80 1000 mL = £7.59 1500 mL = £10.69 |
| Isosource® Fibre (Nestlé) | Liquid (tube feed) | 422 kJ (100 kcal) **per 100 mL** | 3.8 g cows' milk | 13.6 g | 3.4 g | 1.4 g | Gluten-free Residual lactose | Standard, p. 880 Not suitable for child under 2 years | Flexible pack: 500 mL = £3.39 1000 mL = £6.77 |
| Isosource® Standard (Nestlé) | Liquid (tube feed) | 420 kJ (100 kcal) **per 100 mL** | 4 g cows' milk | 13.6 g | 3.3 g | Nil | Gluten-free Residual lactose | Standard, p. 880 | Flexible pack: 500 mL = £2.98 1000 mL = £5.95 |
| Jevity® (Abbott) | Liquid (tube feed) | 441 kJ (106 kcal) **per 100 mL** | 4 g caseinates | 14.1 g (sugars 470 mg) | 3.47 g | 1.76 g | Gluten-free Residual lactose | Standard, p. 880 except bowel fistula. Not suitable for child under 2 years | Flexible pack: 500 mL = £4.04 1000 mL = £7.59 1500 mL = £11.40 |
| Novasource® GI Control (Nestlé) | Liquid (tube feed) | 444 kJ (106 kcal) **per 100 mL** | 4.1 g cows' milk | 14.4 g (sugars 500 mg) | 3.5 g (MCT 40 %) | 2.2 g | Gluten-free Residual lactose | Standard, p. 880 | Flexible pack: 500 mL = £4.52 |
| Nutrison® (Nutricia Clinical) Formerly *Nutrison® Standard* | Liquid (tube feed) | 420 kJ (100 kcal) **per 100 mL** | 4 g cows' milk | 12.3 g (sugars 1 g) | 3.9 g | Nil | Gluten-free Residual lactose | Standard, p. 880 | Bottle: 500 mL = £3.76 Flexible pack: 500 mL = £4.17 1000 mL = £7.32 1500 mL = £10.97 |

1. Sugar content varies with flavour

## Appendix 7: Borderline substances

### A7.1.1.1 Enteral feeds: 1 kcal/mL and less than 5 g protein/100 mL (product list continued)

Not suitable for use in child under 1 year; not recommended for child 1–6 years unless otherwise stated

| Product | Formulation | Energy | Protein | Carbohydrate | Fat | Fibre | Special Characteristics | ACBS Indications | Presentation & Flavour |
|---|---|---|---|---|---|---|---|---|---|
| Nutrison® Multi Fibre (Nutricia Clinical) | Liquid (tube feed) | 420 kJ (100 kcal) **per 100 mL** | 4 g cows' milk | 12.3 g (sugars 1 g) | 3.9 g | 1.5 g | Gluten-free Residual lactose | Standard, p. 880 except bowel fistula | Bottle: 500 mL = £4.09 Flexible pack: 500 mL = £4.51 1000 mL = £8.16 1500 mL = £12.25 |
| Osmolite® (Abbott) | Liquid (tube feed) | 424 kJ (100 kcal) **per 100 mL** | 4 g caseinates soy isolate | 13.6 g (sugars 630 mg) | 3.4 g | Nil | Gluten-free Residual lactose | Standard, p. 880 | Can: 250 mL = £1.83 Bottle: 500 mL = £3.47 1000 mL = £6.62 1500 mL = £9.93 |
| **■ Soya protein formula** | | | | | | | | | |
| Nutrison® Soya (Nutricia Clinical) | Liquid (tube feed) | 420 kJ (100 kcal) **per 100 mL** | 4 g soy isolate | 12.3 g (sugars 1 g) | 3.9 g | Nil | Gluten-free Residual lactose Milk protein-free | Standard, p. 880; *also* cows' milk and protein and lactose intolerance | Bottle: 500 mL = £4.24 Flexible pack: 1000 mL = £8.49 |
| Nutrison® Soya Multi Fibre (Nutricia Clinical) | Liquid (tube feed) | 420 kJ (100 kcal) **per 100 mL** | 4 g soy isolate | 12.3 g (sugars 700 mg) | 3.9 g | 1.5 g | Gluten-free Residual lactose Milk protein-free | Standard, p. 880 except bowel fistula; *also* cows' milk protein and lactose intolerance | Flexible pack: 1500 mL = £14.12 |
| **■ Peptide-based formula** | | | | | | | | | |
| Peptamen® (Nestlé) | Liquid (sip or tube feed) | 420 kJ (100 kcal) **per 100 mL** | 4 g whey peptides | 12.7 g (sugars 480 mg)[1] | 3.7 g (MCT 70 %) | Nil | Gluten-free Residual lactose | Short bowel syndrome, intractable malabsorption, proven inflammatory bowel disease, bowel fistula | Cup (vanilla flavour): 200 mL = £2.68 Can (unflavoured)[2]: 375 mL = £4.84 Flexible pack: 500 mL = £5.38 1000 mL = £10.10 |
| Peptisorb® (Nutricia Clinical) | Liquid (tube feed) | 425 kJ (100 kcal) **per 100 mL** | 4 g whey protein hydrolysate | 17.6 g (sugars 1.7 g) | 1.7 g (MCT 47 %) | Nil | Gluten-free Residual lactose | Short bowel syndrome, intractable malabsorption, proven inflammatory bowel disease, bowel fistula | Bottle: 500 mL = £5.76 Flexible pack: 500 mL = £6.31 1000 mL = £11.41 |
| Survimed® OPD (Fresenius Kabi) | Liquid (tube feed) | 420 kJ (100 kcal) **per 100 mL** | 4.5 g lactalbumin hydrolysate | 15 g (sugars 300 mg) | 2.4 g (MCT 54 %) | Nil | Gluten-free Residual lactose Contains fish oil and fish gelatin | Standard, p. 880; *also* growth failure | Flexible pack: 500 mL = £5.60 |

1. Sugar content varies with flavour
2. Flavouring: see *Flavour Mix*, p. 903

## A7.1.1.2 Enteral feeds: Less than 1 kcal/mL and less than 5 g protein/100 mL

Not suitable for use in child under 1 year; not recommended for child 1–6 years unless otherwise stated

### ◼ Amino acid formula (essential and non-essential amino acids)

| Product | Formulation | Energy | Protein | Carbohydrate | Fat | Fibre | Special Characteristics | ACBS Indications | Presentation & Flavour |
|---|---|---|---|---|---|---|---|---|---|
| Elemental 028® Extra (SHS) | Liquid (sip or tube feed) | 360 kJ (86 kcal) **per 100 mL** | 2.5 g (protein equivalent) | 11 g (sugars 4.7 g) | 3.5 g (MCT 35%) | Nil | | Short bowel syndrome, intractable malabsorption, proven inflammatory bowel disease, bowel fistula | Carton: 250 mL = £2.88 Grapefruit, orange-pineapple, summer fruits |
| | Standard dilution (20%) of powder (sip or tube feed) | 374 kJ [1] (89 kcal) **per 100 mL** | 2.5 g (protein equivalent) | 11.8 g (sugars 1.8 g) | 3.5 g (MCT 35%) | Nil | | | Sachet: 100 g = £5.60 Banana, citrus, orange, unflavoured[2] |

Powder provides protein equivalent 12.5 g, carbohydrate 59 g, fat 17.45 g, energy 1871 kJ (443 kcal)/100 g

1. Minor nutritional variations between flavours—consult product literature
2. Flavouring: see *Modjul® Flavour System*, p. 903

## A7.1.2 Enteral feeds (non-disease specific): 5 g (or more) protein/100 mL

For further information on composition of feeds, see p. 880

## A7.1.2.1 Enteral feeds: 1.5 kcal/mL and 5 g (or more) protein/100 mL

Not suitable for use in child under 1 year; not recommended for child 1–6 years unless otherwise stated

| Product | Formulation | Energy | Protein | Carbohydrate | Fat | Fibre | Special Characteristics | ACBS Indications | Presentation & Flavour |
|---|---|---|---|---|---|---|---|---|---|
| Clinutren® 1.5 (Nestlé) | Liquid (sip feed) | 630 kJ (150 kcal) **per 100 mL** | 5.6 g cows' milk | 21 g (sugars 5.2 g)[1] | 5 g | less than 500 mg | Gluten-free Residual lactose | Standard, p. 880 Not suitable for child under 3 years | Plastic cup: 4 × 200 mL = £6.59 Apricot, banana, chocolate, coffee, strawberry-raspberry, vanilla |
| Clinutren® 1.5 Fibre (Nestlé) | Liquid (sip feed) | 630 kJ (150 kcal) **per 100 mL** | 5.7 g cows' milk | 19 g (sugars 6.1 g) | 5.9 g | 2.6 g | Gluten-free Residual lactose | Standard, p. 880 except bowel fistula Not suitable for child under 3 years | Plastic cup: 4 × 200 mL = £6.59 Plum or vanilla |
| Fresubin® 2250 Complete (Fresenius Kabi) (Formerly *Fresubin® Energy Fibre*) | Liquid (tube feed) | 630 kJ (150 kcal) **per 100 mL** | 5.6 g cows' milk | 18.8 g (sugars 1.5 g) | 5.8 g | 2 g | Gluten-free Residual lactose Contains fish oil and fish gelatin | Standard, p. 880 | Flexible pack: 1500 mL = £11.94 |

1. Sugar content varies with flavour

**Appendix 7: Borderline substances**

## Appendix 7: Borderline substances

### A7.1.2.1 Enteral feeds: 1.5 kcal/mL and 5 g (or more) protein/100 mL (product list continued)

Not suitable for use in child under 1 year; not recommended for child 1–6 years unless otherwise stated

| Product | Formulation | Energy | Protein | Carbohydrate | Fat | Fibre | Special Characteristics | ACBS Indications | Presentation & Flavour |
|---|---|---|---|---|---|---|---|---|---|
| Fresubin® Energy (Fresenius Kabi) | Liquid (sip feed) | 630 kJ (150 kcal) per 100 mL | 5.6 g cows' milk | 18.8 g (sugars)[1] | 5.8 g | Nil | [2]Gluten-free Residual lactose Contains fish gelatin | Standard, p. 880 | Bottle: 200 mL = £1.74 Banana, black currant, cappuccino, chocolate, lemon, neutral, strawberry, tropical fruits, vanilla |
| | Liquid (tube feed) | 630 kJ (150 kcal) per 100 mL | 5.6 g cows' milk | 18.8 g (sugars 1.4 g) | 5.8 g | Nil | Gluten-free Residual lactose Contains fish oil and fish gelatin | Standard, p. 880 | Flexible pack: 500 mL = £4.10 1000 mL = £8.07 1500 mL = £10.82 |
| Fresubin® Energy Fibre (Fresenius Kabi) | Liquid (sip feed) | 630 kJ (150 kcal) per 100 mL | 5.6 g cows' milk | 18.8 g (sugars)[1] | 5.8 g | 2 g | Gluten-free Residual lactose Contains fish gelatin | Standard, p. 880 | Bottle: 200 mL = £1.82 Banana, caramel, cherry, chocolate, strawberry, vanilla |
| | Liquid (tube feed) | 630 kJ (150 kcal) per 100 mL | 5.6 g cows' milk | 18.8 g (sugars 1.5 g) | 5.8 g | 2 g | Gluten-free Residual lactose Contains fish oil and fish gelatin | Standard, p. 880 | Flexible pack: 500 mL = £4.51 1000 mL = £8.59 |
| Fresubin® HP Energy (Fresenius Kabi) | Liquid (tube feed) | 630 kJ (150 kcal) per 100 mL | 7.5 g cows' milk | 17 g (sugars 1 g) | 5.8 g (MCT 57%) | Nil | Gluten-free Residual lactose Contains fish oil and fish gelatin | Standard, p. 880; also CAPD and haemodialysis | Flexible pack: 500 mL = £4.18 1000 mL = £8.38 |
| Isosource® Energy Fibre (Nestlé) | Liquid (tube feed) | 630 kJ (150 kcal) per 100 mL | 4.9 g cows' milk | 20.2 g | 5.5 g | 1.5 g | Gluten-free Residual lactose | Standard, p. 880 except bowel fistula | Flexible pack: 500 mL = £3.96 1000 mL = £7.93 |
| Jevity® 1.5 kcal (Abbott) | Liquid (tube feed) | 640 kJ (152 kcal) per 100 mL | 6.38 g caseinates soy isolate | 20.1 g (sugars 1.47 g) | 4.9 g | 2.2 g | Gluten-free Residual lactose | Standard, p. 880. Not suitable for child under 2 years; not recommended for child 2–10 years | Flexible pack: 500 mL = £4.78 1000 mL = £9.14 1500 mL = £14.26 |
| Novasource® GI Forte (Nestlé) | Liquid (tube feed) | 631 kJ (150 kcal) per 100 mL | 6 g cows' milk | 18.3 g (sugars 1.8 g) | 5.9 g | 2.2 g | Gluten-free Residual lactose | Standard, p. 880 | Flexible pack: 500 mL = £4.49 1000 mL = £8.98 |

1. Sugar content varies with flavour
2. Strawberry flavour may contain traces of wheat starch and egg

| Product | Formulation | Energy | Protein | Carbohydrate | Fat | Fibre | Special Characteristics | ACBS Indications | Presentation & Flavour |
|---|---|---|---|---|---|---|---|---|---|
| Nutrison® Energy (Nutricia Clinical) | Liquid (tube feed) | 630 kJ (150 kcal) per 100 mL | 6 g cows' milk | 18.5 g (sugars 1.5 g) | 5.8 g | Nil | Gluten-free Residual lactose | Standard, p. 880 | Bottle: 500 mL = £4.38; Flexible pack: 500 mL = £4.86; 1000 mL = £8.81; 1500 mL = £13.18 |
| Nutrison® Energy Multi Fibre (Nutricia Clinical) | Liquid (tube feed) | 630 kJ (150 kcal) per 100 mL | 6 g cows' milk | 18.5 g (sugars 1.5 g) | 5.8 g | 1.5 g | Gluten-free Residual lactose | Standard, p. 880 | Bottle: 500 mL = £4.90; Flexible pack: 500 mL = £5.39; 1000 mL = £9.77; 1500 mL = £15.66 |
| Osmolite® 1.5 kcal (Abbott) | Liquid (tube feed) | 632 kJ (150 kcal) per 100 mL | 6.25 g cows' milk soya protein isolate | 20 g (sugars 4.9 g) | 5 g | Nil | Gluten-free Residual lactose | Standard, p. 880 | Flexible pack: 500 mL = £4.15; 1000 mL = £8.10; 1500 mL = £12.13 |

Formerly *Ensure® Plus* (Ready to Hang)

## A7.1.2.2 Enteral feeds: Less than 1.5 kcal/mL and 5 g (or more) protein/100 mL

Not suitable for use in child under 1 year; not recommended for child 1–6 years unless otherwise stated

| Product | Formulation | Energy | Protein | Carbohydrate | Fat | Fibre | Special Characteristics | ACBS Indications | Presentation & Flavour |
|---|---|---|---|---|---|---|---|---|---|
| Fresubin® 1000 Complete (Fresenius Kabi) | Liquid (tube feed) | 420 kJ (100 kcal) per 100 mL | 5.5 g cows' milk | 12.5 g (sugars 1.1 g) | 3.1 g | 2 g | Gluten-free Residual lactose Contains fish oil | Standard, p. 880 | Flexible pack: 1000 mL = £8.59 |
| Fresubin® 1200 Complete (Fresenius Kabi) | Liquid (tube feed) | 500 kJ (120 kcal) per 100 mL | 6 g cows' milk | 15 g (sugars 1.22 g) | 4.1 g | 2 g | Gluten-free Residual lactose Contains fish oil | Standard, p. 880 | Flexible pack: 1000 mL = £11.12 |
| Jevity® Plus (Abbott) | Liquid (tube feed) | 504 kJ (120 kcal) per 100 mL | 5.5 g caseinates soy isolates | 15.1 g (sugars 890 mg) | 3.93 g | 2.2 g | Gluten-free Residual lactose | Standard, p. 880 Not suitable for child under 2 years; not recommended for child 2–10 years | Flexible pack: 500 mL = £4.35; 1000 mL = £8.90; 1500 mL = £13.36 |
| Jevity® Promote (Abbott) | Liquid (tube feed) | 427 kJ (101 kcal) per 100 mL | 5.55 g caseinates soy isolates | 12 g (sugars 670 mg) | 3.32 g | 1.7 g | Gluten-free Residual lactose | Standard, p. 880 Not suitable for child under 2 years; not recommended for child 2–10 years | Flexible pack: 1000 mL = £8.70 |
| Nutrison® MCT (Nutricia Clinical) | Liquid (tube feed) | 420 kJ (100 kcal) per 100 mL | 5 g cows' milk | 12.6 g (sugars 1 g) | 3.3 g (MCT 61%) | Nil | Gluten-free Residual lactose | Standard, p. 880 | Flexible pack: 1000 mL = £7.96 |

Appendix 7: Borderline substances

## Appendix 7: Borderline substances

### A7.1.2.2 Enteral feeds: Less than 1.5 kcal/mL and 5 g (or more) protein/100 mL *(product list continued)*

Not suitable for use in child under 1 year; not recommended for child 1–6 years unless otherwise stated

| Product | Formulation | Energy | Protein | Carbohydrate | Fat | Fibre | Special Characteristics | ACBS Indications | Presentation & Flavour |
|---|---|---|---|---|---|---|---|---|---|
| Nutrison® Protein Plus (Nutricia Clinical) | Liquid (tube feed) | 525 kJ (125 kcal) **per 100 mL** | 6.3 g cows' milk | 14.2 g (sugars 1.1 g) | 4.9 g | Nil | Gluten-free Residual lactose | Standard, p. 880 | Flexible pack: 1000 mL = £8.19 |
| Nutrison® Protein Plus Multi Fibre (Nutricia Clinical) | Liquid (tube feed) | 525 kJ (125 kcal) **per 100 mL** | 6.3 g cow's milk | 14.1 g (sugars 1.1 g) | 4.9 g | 1.5 g | Gluten-free Residual lactose | Disease-related malnutrition | Flexible pack: 1000 mL = £9.12 |
| Nutrison® 1000 Complete Multi Fibre (Nutricia Clinical) | Liquid (tube feed) | 420 kJ (100 kcal) **per 100 mL** | 5.5 g cows' milk | 11.3 g (sugars 700 mg) | 3.7 g | 2 g | Gluten-free Residual lactose | Disease-related malnutrition in patients with low energy and/or low fluid requirements | Flexible pack: 1000 mL = £8.85 |
| Nutrison® 1200 Complete Multi Fibre (Nutricia Clinical) | Liquid (tube feed) | 505 kJ (120 kcal) **per 100 mL** | 5.5 g cows' milk | 15 g (sugars 1.2 g) | 4.3 g | 2 g | Gluten-free Residual lactose | Standard, p. 880 except bowel fistula | Bottle: 500 mL = £4.69 Flexible pack: 1000 mL = £9.37 1500 mL = £14.07 |
| Osmolite® Plus (Abbott) | Liquid (tube feed) | 508 kJ (121 kcal) **per 100 mL** | 5.55 g caseinates | 15.8 g (sugars 730 mg) | 3.93 g | Nil | Gluten-free Residual lactose | Standard, p. 880 Not recommended for child under 10 years | Flexible pack: 500 mL = £4.06 1000 mL = £7.83 1500 mL = £11.73 |
| Peptamen® HN (Nestlé) | Liquid (tube feed) | 556 kJ (133 kcal) **per 100 mL** | 6.6 g whey protein hydrolysates | 15.6 g (sugars 1.4 g) | 4.9 g (MCT 70%) | Nil | Gluten-free Residual lactose Hydrolysed with pork trypsin | Short bowel syndrome, intractable malabsorption, proven inflammatory bowel disease, bowel fistula Not suitable for child under 3 years | Flexible pack: 500 mL = £5.97 |
| Perative® (Abbott) | Liquid (sip or tube feed) | 552 kJ (131 kcal) **per 100 mL** | 6.7 g caseinate whey protein hydrolysates | 17.7 g (sugars 660 mg) | 3.7 g (MCT 42%) | Nil | Gluten-free Residual lactose | Standard, p. 880 Not suitable for child under 5 years | Flexible pack: 500 mL = £5.66 1000 mL = £11.32 |

## A7.1.2.3 Enteral feeds: More than 1.5 kcal/mL and 5 g (or more) protein/100 mL

Not suitable for use in child under 1 year; not recommended for child 1–6 years unless otherwise stated

| Product | Formulation | Energy | Protein | Carbohydrate | Fat | Fibre | Special Characteristics | ACBS Indications | Presentation & Flavour |
|---|---|---|---|---|---|---|---|---|---|
| Ensure® Twocal (Abbott) | Liquid (sip or tube feed) | 838 kJ (200 kcal) **per 100 mL** | 8.4 g cows' milk | 21 g (sugars 4.5 g) | 8.9 g | ¹ g | Gluten-free Residual lactose | Standard, p. 880; *also* haemodialysis, CAPD | Bottle: 200 mL = £2.08 Banana, neutral, strawberry, vanilla |
| Isosource® Energy (Nestlé) | Liquid (tube feed) | 670 kJ (160 kcal) **per 100 mL** | 5.7 g cows' milk | 20 g | 5.2 g | Nil | Gluten-free Residual lactose | Standard, p. 880 | Flexible pack: 500 mL = £3.66 1000 mL = £7.31 |

## A7.1.3 Enteral feeds (non-disease specific): Child under 12 years see *BNF for Children*

## A7.2 Nutritional supplements (non-disease specific)

### A7.2.1 Nutritional supplements: less than 5 g protein/100 mL

For further information on composition of feeds, see p. 880

### A7.2.1.1 Nutritional supplements: 1 kcal/mL and less than 5 g protein/100 mL

Not suitable for use in child under 1 year; use with caution in child 1–5 years unless otherwise stated

| Product | Formulation | Energy | Protein | Carbohydrate | Fat | Fibre | Special Characteristics | ACBS Indications | Presentation & Flavour |
|---|---|---|---|---|---|---|---|---|---|
| Ensure® (Abbott) | Liquid (sip or tube feed) | 423 kJ (100 kcal)¹ **per 100 mL** | 4 g caseinates soy isolate | 13.6 g (sugars 3.93 g) | 3.36 g | Nil | Gluten-free Residual lactose | Standard, p. 880 | Can: 250 mL = £2.01 Chocolate, vanilla |

1. Nutritional values vary with flavour—consult product literature

Appendix 7: Borderline substances

Appendix 7: Borderline substances

## A7.2.1.2 Nutritional supplements: More than 1 kcal/mL and less than 5 g protein/100 mL

Not suitable for use in child under 1 year; use with caution in child 1–5 years unless otherwise stated

| Product | Formulation | Energy | Protein | Carbohydrate | Fat | Fibre | Special Characteristics | ACBS Indications | Presentation & Flavour |
|---|---|---|---|---|---|---|---|---|---|
| Clinutren® Fruit (Nestlé) | Liquid (sip feed) | 520 kJ (125 kcal) **per 100 mL** | 4 g whey protein hydrolysate | 27 g (sugars 9.5 g[1]) | less than 200 mg | less than 200 mg[2] | Gluten-free Residual lactose Non-milk taste | Standard, p. 880 Not suitable for child under 3 years | Carton: 4 × 200 mL = £6.63 Apple, grapefruit, orange, pear-cherry, raspberry-black currant |
| Ensure® Plus Juce (Abbott) | Liquid (sip feed) | 638 kJ (150 kcal) **per 100 mL** | 4.8 g whey protein isolate | 32.7 g (sugars 9.4 g[1]) | Nil | Nil | Gluten-free Residual lactose Non-milk taste | Standard, p. 880 | Bottle: 220 mL = £1.75 Apple, fruit punch, grapefruit, lemon-lime, orange, peach, pineapple, strawberry |
| Fortijuce® (Nutricia Clinical) | Liquid (sip feed) | 640 kJ (150 kcal) **per 100 mL** | 4.0 g cows' milk | 33.5 g (sugars 13.1 g[1]) | Nil | Nil | Gluten-free Residual lactose Non-milk taste | Standard, p. 880 Not suitable for child under 3 years | Bottle: 200 mL = £1.85 Apple, black currant, forest fruits, lemon, orange, strawberry, tropical Starter pack (mixed): 4 × 200 mL = £7.40 |
| Provide® Xtra Juice Drink (Fresenius Kabi) | Liquid (sip feed) | 525 kJ (125 kcal) **per 100 mL** | 3.75 g pea and soya protein hydrolysates | 27.5 g[1] | Nil | Nil[2] | Gluten-free Lactose-free Sweet-flavoured products contain fish gelatin | Standard, p. 880 | Bottle: 200 mL = £1.71 Apple, black currant, carrot-apple, cherry, citrus-cola, lemon-lime, melon, orange-pineapple, tomato |
| Resource® Dessert Energy (Nestlé) | Semi-solid | 671 kJ (160 kcal) **per 100 g** | 4.8 g cows' milk | 21.2 g (sugars 9.9 g[1]) | 6.2 g | Nil | Gluten-free Contains lactose | Standard, p. 880; *also* CAPD, haemodialysis | Cup: 125 g = £1.35 Caramel, chocolate, vanilla |
| Resource® Fruit Flavour Drink (Nestlé) | Liquid (sip feed) | 638 kJ (150 kcal) **per 100 mL** | 4.0 g cows' milk | 33.5 g (sugars 8 g[1]) | Nil | Nil | Gluten-free Residual lactose Non-milk taste | Standard, p. 880 Not suitable for child under 3 years | Carton: 200 mL = £1.53 Apple, orange, pineapple |

1. Sugar content varies with flavour
2. Fibre content varies with flavour

## A7.2.2 Nutritional supplements: 5 g (or more) protein/100 mL

For further information on composition of feeds, see p. 880

### A7.2.2.1 Nutritional supplements: 1.5 kcal/mL and 5 g (or more) protein/100 mL

Not suitable for use in child under 1 year; use with caution in child 1–5 years unless otherwise stated

| Product | Formulation | Energy | Protein | Carbohydrate | Fat | Fibre | Special Characteristics | ACBS Indications | Presentation & Flavour |
|---|---|---|---|---|---|---|---|---|---|
| Ensure® Plus Fibre (Abbott) | Liquid (sip or tube feed) | 642 kJ (153 kcal)[1] **per 100 mL** | 6.25 g cows' milk soya protein isolate | 20.2 g (sugars 5.5 g) | 4.92 g | 2.5 g | Gluten-free Residual lactose | Standard, p. 880; *also* CAPD, haemodialysis | Bottle: 200 mL = £1.80 Banana, chocolate, fruits of the forest, raspberry, strawberry, vanilla |
| Ensure® Plus Milkshake style (Abbott) | Liquid (sip or tube feed) | 632 kJ (150 kcal)[1] **per 100 mL** | 6.25 g cows' milk soya protein isolate | 20.2 g (sugars 5.6 g) | 4.92 g | Nil | Gluten-free Residual lactose | Standard, p. 880; *also* CAPD, haemodialysis | Can: 250 mL = £2.28 (vanilla) 250 mL = £2.28 (chicken or mushroom) Bottle: 220 mL = £1.80 Banana, black currant, caramel, chocolate, coffee, fruits of the forest, orange, peach, raspberry, strawberry, vanilla, neutral |
| Ensure® Plus Yoghurt style (Abbott) | Liquid (sip feed) | 632 kJ (150 kcal)[1] **per 100 mL** | 6.25 g cows' milk | 20.2 g (sugars 11.7 g) | 4.92 g | Nil | Gluten-free Residual lactose | Standard, p. 880; *also* CAPD, haemodialysis | Bottle: 220 mL = £1.80 Orange, peach, p neapple, straw-berry |
| Ensure® Plus Commence (Abbott) | Starter pack (5–10 day's supply), contains: *Ensure® Plus Milkshake Style* (various flavours), 1 pack (10 × 220-mL) = £18.00. | | | | | | | | |
| Enmix® Plus Commence (Abbott) | Starter pack (5–10 day's supply), contains: *Ensure® Plus* (Milkshake, Yoghurt, & Juce style; various flavours), 1 pack (10 × 220-mL) = £18.00. | | | | | | | | |
| Fortisip® Bottle (Nutricia Clinical) | Liquid (sip feed) | 630 kJ (150 kcal) **per 100 mL** | 6 g cows' milk | 18.4 g[2] | 5.8 g | Nil | Gluten-free Residual lactose | Standard, p. 880 Not suitable for child under 3 years | Bottle: 200 mL = £1.85 Banana, chocolate, neutral, orange, strawberry, toffee, tropical fruits, vanilla |

1. Minor nutritional variations between flavours—consult product literature
2. Sugar content varies with flavour

**Appendix 7: Borderline substances**

## Appendix 7: Borderline substances

### A7.2.2.1 Nutritional supplements: 1.5 kcal/mL and 5 g (or more) protein/100 mL *(product list continued)*

Not suitable for use in child under 1 year; use with caution in child 1–5 years unless otherwise stated

| Product | Formulation | Energy | Protein | Carbohydrate | Fat | Fibre | Special Characteristics | ACBS Indications | Presentation & Flavour |
|---|---|---|---|---|---|---|---|---|---|
| Fortisip® Multi Fibre (Nutricia Clinical) | Liquid (sip feed) | 630 kJ (150 kcal) **per 100 mL** | 6 g cows' milk | 18.4 g (sugars 7.0 g) | 5.8 g | 2.3 g | Gluten-free Residual lactose | Standard, p. 880 Not suitable for child under 3 years | Bottle: 200 mL = £1.91 Banana, chocolate, orange, strawberry, tomato, vanilla |
| Fortisip® Yogurt Style (Nutricia Clinical) | Liquid (sip feed) | 630 kJ (150 kcal) **per 100 mL** | 6 g cows' milk | 18.7 g (sugars 10.8 g) | 5.8 g | 200 mg | Gluten-free Contains lactose | Standard, p. 880 Not suitable for child under 3 years | Bottle: 200 mL = £1.85 Peach-orange, raspberry, vanilla-lemon |
| Fortisip® Range (Nutricia Clinical) | Starter pack contains 4 × *Fortisip®* Bottle, 4 × *Fortijuce®*, 2 × *Fortisip®* Yogurt Style, 1 pack (10 × 200 mL) = £18.50. | | | | | | | | |
| Fresubin® Protein Energy Drink (Fresenius Kabi) | Liquid (sip feed) | 630 kJ (150 kcal) **per 100 mL** | 10 g cows' milk | 12.4 g (sugars 6.4 g[1]) | 6.7 g | Nil[2] | Gluten-free Residual lactose Contains fish gelatin | Standard, p. 880; *also* CAPD, haemodialysis | Bottle: 200 mL = £1.77 Cappuccino, chocolate, strawberry, tropical fruits, vanilla |

1. Sugar content varies with flavour
2. Fibre content varies with flavour

### A7.2.2.2 Nutritional supplements: Less than 1.5 kcal/mL and 5 g (or more) protein/100 mL

Not suitable for use in child under 1 year; use with caution in child 1–5 years unless otherwise stated

| Product | Formulation | Energy | Protein | Carbohydrate | Fat | Fibre | Special Characteristics | ACBS Indications | Presentation & Flavour |
|---|---|---|---|---|---|---|---|---|---|
| Clinutren® Dessert (Nestlé) | Semi-solid | 520 kJ (125 kcal) **per 100 g** | 9.5 g cows' milk | 15.5 g (sugars 14 g[1]) | 2.6 g | 500 mg[2] | Gluten-free Contains lactose | Standard, p. 880; *also* CAPD, haemodialysis Not suitable for child under 3 years | Pot: 4 × 125 g = £5.40 Caramel, chocolate, peach, vanilla |

1. Sugar content varies with flavour
2. Fibre content varies with flavour

| Product | Formulation | Energy | Protein | Carbohydrate | Fat | Fibre | Special Characteristics | ACBS Indications | Presentation & Flavour |
|---|---|---|---|---|---|---|---|---|---|
| Ensure® Plus Crème (Abbott) | Semi-solid | 574 kJ (137 kcal)[1] **per 100 g** | 5.68 g milk protein isolate soy protein isolate | 18.4 g (sugars 12.4 g) | 4.47 g | Nil | Gluten-free Residual lactose Contains soya | Standard, p. 880; *also* CAPD, haemodialysis Not suitable for child under 3 years | Pot: 125 g = £1.67 Banana, chocolate, neutral, vanilla |
| Fortimel® Regular (Abbott) (Formerly *Fortimel®*) | Liquid (sip feed) | 420 kJ (100 kcal) **per 100 mL** | 10 g cows' milk | 10.3 g (sugars 8.1 g[2]) | 2.1 g | Nil | Gluten-free Contains lactose | Standard, p. 880 Not suitable for child under 3 years | Bottle: 200 mL = £1.57 Chocolate, forest fruits, strawberry, vanilla |
| Fortisip® Fruit Dessert (Nutricia Clinical) | Semi-Solid | 560 kJ (133 kcal) **per 100 g** | 7 g whey isolate | 16.7 g (sugars 11.3 g[2]) | 4 g | 2.6 g | Residual lactose Gluten-free | Standard, p. 880 except bowel fistula; *also* CAPD, haemodialysis Not suitable for child under 3 years | Pot: 3 × 150 g = £6.49 Apple 3 × 150 g = £6.49 Strawberry |
| Resource® Protein (Nestlé) | Liquid (sip feed) | 530 kJ (125 kcal)[3] **per 100 mL** | 9.4 g cows' milk | 14 g (sugars 4.5 g) | 3.5 g | Nil | Gluten-free Contains lactose | Standard, p. 880 Not suitable for child under 3 years | Bottle: 200 mL = £1.33 Apricot, chocolate, forest fruits, strawberry, vanilla |

1. Minor nutritional variations between flavours—consult product literature
2. Sugar content varies with flavour
3. Nutritional values vary with flavour—consult product literature

## A7.2.2.3 Nutritional supplements: More than 1.5 kcal/mL and 5 g (or more) protein/100 mL

Not suitable for use in child under 1 year; use with caution in child 1–5 years unless otherwise stated

| Product | Formulation | Energy | Protein | Carbohydrate | Fat | Fibre | Special Characteristics | ACBS Indications | Presentation & Flavour |
|---|---|---|---|---|---|---|---|---|---|
| Complan® Shake (Complan Foods) | Powder | 1057 kJ (251 kcal)[1] **per 57 g** | 8.8 g cows' milk | 35.2 g (sugars 22.7 g) | 8.4 g | Trace | Gluten-free Contains lactose | Standard, p. 880 | Sachet: 4 × 57 g = £3.26 Banana, chocolate, milk, strawberry, vanilla |

Powder 57 g reconstituted with 200 mL whole milk provides: protein 15.6 g, carbohydrate 44.5 g, fat 16.4 g, energy 1621 kJ (387 kcal)
1. Nutritional values vary with flavour—consult product literature

**Appendix 7: Borderline substances**

## Appendix 7: Borderline substances

### A7.2.2.3 Nutritional supplements: More than 1.5 kcal/mL and 5 g (or more) protein/100 mL (product list continued)

Not suitable for use in child under 1 year; use with caution in child 1–5 years unless otherwise stated

| Product | Formulation | Energy | Protein | Carbohydrate | Fat | Fibre | Special Characteristics | ACBS Indications | Presentation & Flavour |
|---|---|---|---|---|---|---|---|---|---|
| Foodlink® Complete (Foodlink) | Powder | 1838 kJ[1] (437 kcal) **per 100 g** | 21.9 g cows' milk | 57.3 g | 13.3 g | Nil | Contains lactose | Standard, p. 880 | Carton: 450 g = £3.29 Banana, chocolate, neutral, strawberry |
| Recommended serving = 3 heaped tablespoonfuls in 250 mL water provides: protein 12.5 g, carbohydrate 32.7 g, fat 7.6 g, energy 1048 kJ (249 kcal) | | | | | | | | | |
| Foodlink® Complete with Fibre (Foodlink) | Powder | 1804 kJ (428 kcal)[1] **per 100 g** | 19.5 g cows' milk | 57.1 g (sugars 36.8 g) | 12.3 g | 8 g | Contains lactose | Standard, p. 880 | Sachet: 10 × 63 g = £6.67 Vanilla + fibre |
| Recommended serving = 4 heaped tablespoonfuls in 250 mL water provides: protein 12.3 g, carbohydrate 38 g, fat 7.5 g, fibre 5 g, energy 1137 kJ (270 kcal) | | | | | | | | | |
| Forticreme® Complete (Nutricia Clinical) | Semi-solid | 675 kJ (160 kcal) **per 100 g** | 9.5 g cows' milk | 19.2 g (sugars 10.6 g) | 5 g | 100 mg[2] | Gluten-free Residual lactose | Standard, p. 880; also CAPD, haemodialysis Not suitable for child under 3 years | Pot: 4 × 125 g = £7.20 Banana, chocolate, forest fruits, vanilla |
| Fortisip® Extra (Nutricia Clinical) | Liquid (sip feed) | 675 kJ (160 kcal) **per 100 mL** | 10 g cows' milk | 18.1 g (sugars 9 g) | 5.3 g | Nil[2] | Gluten-free Contains lactose | Standard, p. 880 Not suitable for child under 3 years | Bottle: 200 mL = £1.85 Chocolate, forest fruits, mocha, strawberry, vanilla Starter pack: 4 × 200 mL = £7.40 |
| Fresubin® 2kcal Drink (Fresenius Kabi) | Liquid (sip feed) | 840 kJ (200 kcal) **per 100 mL** | 10 g cows' milk | 22.5 g (sugars 5.8 g) | 7.8 g | Nil | Gluten-free Contains lactose | Standard, p. 880; also CAPD, haemodialysis | Bottle: 200 mL = £1.69 Apricot-peach, cappuccino, fruits of the forest, toffee, vanilla |
| Fresubin® 2kcal Fibre Drink (Fresenius Kabi) | Liquid (sip feed) | 840 kJ (200 kcal) **per 100 mL** | 10 g cows' milk | 22.5 g (sugars 5.8 g) | 7.8 g | 1.6 g | Gluten-free Contains lactose | Standard, p. 880; also CAPD, haemodialysis | Bottle: 200 mL = £1.69 Cappuccino, chocolate, lemon, vanilla |
| Fresubin® Crème (Fresenius Kabi) | Semi-solid | 756 kJ (180 kcal) **per 100 g** | 10 g cows' milk | 19 g (sugars 14.4 g) | 7.2 g | 2 g | Gluten-free Residual lactose | Standard, p. 880; also CAPD, haemodialysis Not suitable for child under 3 years | Pot: 4 × 125 g = £6.92 Cappuccino, strawberry, vanilla |

1. Nutritional values vary with flavour—consult product literature
2. Fibre content varies with flavour

| Product | Form | Energy | Protein | Carbohydrate | Fat | Special characteristics | | Presentation / Flavour |
|---|---|---|---|---|---|---|---|---|
| Renilon® 7.5 (Nutricia Clinical) | Liquid (sip feed) | 840 kJ (200 kcal) **per 100 mL** | 7.5 g cows' milk | 20 g (sugars 4.8 g) | 10 g | Nil | Gluten-free Residual lactose | Standard, p. 880 Not suitable for child under 3 years | Carton: 125 mL = £1.85 Apricot, caramel |
| Resource® 2.0 Fibre (Nestlé) | Liquid (sip feed) | 836 kJ (200 kcal)[1] **per 100 mL** | 9 g cows' milk | 21.4 g (sugars 5.5 g) | 8.7 g | 2.5 g | Gluten-free Residual lactose | Standard, p. 880 Not suitable for child under 6 years; caution in child 6–10 years | Carton: 200 mL = £1.65 Apricot, coffee, neutral, strawberry, summer fruits, vanilla |
| Resource® Dessert Fruit (Nestlé) | Semi-solid | 678 kJ (160 kcal)[1] **per 100 g** | 5 g cows' milk | 24 g (sugars 16.4 g) | 5 g | 1.4 g | Gluten-free Residual lactose | Standard, p. 880; also CAPD, haemodialysis | Cup: 3 × 125 g = £4.05 Apple, apple-peach, apple-strawberry[2] |
| Resource® Shake (Nestlé) | Liquid (sip feed) | 730 kJ (174 kcal)[1] **per 100 mL** | 5.1 g cows' milk | 22.6 g (sugars 6.4 g) | 7 g | Nil | Gluten-free Residual lactose | Standard, p. 880 | Carton: 175 mL = £1.50 Banana, chocolate, lemon, strawberry, summer fruits, toffee, vanilla |
| Vegenat®-med Balanced Protein (Vegenat) | Powder | 1924 kJ (458 kcal) **per 110 g serving** | 18 g cows' milk | 62 g | 15.35 g | 5.8 g | Gluten-free Residual lactose | Standard, p. 880 except bowel fistula Not suitable for child under 14 years | Sachet: 12 × 110 g = £35.58 Apple, chocolate, honey, orange |
| Vegenat®-med High Protein (Vegenat) | Powder | 1940 kJ (463 kcal) **per 110 g serving** | 23.3 g cows' milk | 57.2 g | 15.6 g | 6 g | Gluten-free Residual lactose | Standard, p. 880 except bowel fistula Not suitable for child under 14 years | Sachet: 12 × 110 g = £49.81 Chicken, chickpea, fish, fish-vegetable, ham, lentil, veal, vegetable, winter vegetable 12 × 110 g = £48.04 Curry chicken 12 × 110 g = £47.32 Lemon, rice with lemon 24 × 55 g = £45.63 Rice with apple |

1. Nutritional values vary with flavour—consult product literature
2. Flavour not suitable for child under 3 years

**Appendix 7: Borderline substances**

## Appendix 7: Borderline substances

### A7.3 Specialised formulas

### A7.3.1 Specialised formulas: Infant and child see BNF for Children

### A7.3.2 Specialised formulas for specific clinical conditions

For further information on composition of feeds, see p. 880

| Product | Formulation | Energy | Protein | Carbohydrate | Fat | Fibre | Special Characteristics | ACBS Indications | Presentation & Flavour |
|---|---|---|---|---|---|---|---|---|---|
| Alicalm® (SHS) | Standard dilution (30%) of powder | 567 kJ (135 kcal) **per 100 mL** | 4.5 g caseinate whey | 17.4 g (sugars 3.2 g) | 5.3 g | Nil | Residual lactose | Crohn's disease Not suitable for child under 1 year; use as nutritional supplement only in children 1–6 years. | Powder: 400 g = £16.85 Vanilla |
| | Powder provides: protein 15 g, carbohydrate 58 g, fat 17.5 g, energy 1889 kJ (450 kcal)/100 g | | | | | | | | |
| Casilan® 90 (Heinz) | Powder | 1572 kJ (370 kcal) **per 100 g** | 90 g cows' milk | 300 mg | 1 g | Nil | Gluten-free Electrolytes/100 g: Na⁺ 1.3 mmol K⁺ 8.7 mmol Ca²⁺ 35 mmol P⁺ 22.6 mmol | Nutritional supplement for use in biochemically proven hypoprotein-aemia | Can: 250 g = £5.90 |
| Forticare® (Nutricia Clinical) | Liquid (sip feed) | 675 kJ (160 kcal) **per 100 mL** | 9 g cows' milk | 19.1 g (sugars 13.6 g) | 5.3 g | 2.1 g | Gluten-free Residual lactose Contains fish oil | Nutritional supplement in patients with lung cancer undergoing chemotherapy, or with pancreatic cancer Not suitable in child under 3 years | Carton: 125 mL = £1.98 Cappuccino, orange-lemon, peach-ginger . |
| Generaid® (SHS) | Powder | 1586 kJ (374 kcal) **per 100 g** | 76 g protein equivalent (whey protein, plus branched chain amino acids) | 5 g (sugars 5 g) | 5.5 g | Nil | Electrolytes/100 g: Na⁺ 6.1 mmol K⁺ 10.8 mmol Ca²⁺ 6.5 mmol P⁺ 6.45 mmol | Nutritional supplement for use in chronic liver disease and/or porto-hepatic encephalopathy | Tub: 200 g = £23.97 Unflavoured[1] |

1. Flavouring: see Modjul® Flavour System, p. 903

| Product | Presentation | Energy | Protein | Carbohydrate | Fat | | Electrolytes / Special properties | Indications | Packaging |
|---|---|---|---|---|---|---|---|---|---|
| Generaid® Plus (SHS) | Standard dilution (22%) of powder | 428 kJ (102 kcal) per 100 mL | 2.4 g protein equivalent (whey protein, branched chain amino acids) | 13.6 g (sugars 1.4 g) | 4.2 g (MCT 32%) | Nil | Electrolytes/100 mL: Na⁺ 0.7 mmol K⁺ 2.7 mmol Ca²⁺ 1.72 mmol P⁺ 1.67 mmol | A sole source of nutrition or nutritional supplement in children over 1 year with hepatic disorders | Can: 400 g = £17.15 Unflavoured[1] (5-g measuring scoop provided) |
| *Powder provides: protein equivalent 11 g, carbohydrate 62 g, fat 19 g, energy 1944 kJ (463 kcal)/100 g* | | | | | | | | | |
| KetoCal® (SHS) | Standard dilution (20%) of powder | 602 kJ (146 kcal) per 100 mL | 3.1 g cows' milk with additional amino acids | 600 mg (sugars 120 mg) | 14.6 g (LCT 100%) | Nil | Electrolytes/100 mL: Na⁺ 4.3 mmol K⁺ 4.1 mmol Ca²⁺ 2.15 mmol P⁺ 2.77 mmol | Sole source of nutrition or nutritional supplement as part of ketogenic diet in management of epilepsy resistant to drug therapy, in children over 1 year, only on the advice of secondary care physician with experience of ketogenic diet | Can: 300 g = £23.87 Vanilla, Unflavoured |
| *Powder provides: protein 15.25 g, carbohydrate 3 g, fat 73 g, energy 3011 kJ (730 kcal)/100 g* | | | | | | | | | |
| Kindergen® (SHS) | Standard dilution (20%) of powder | 421 kJ (101 kcal) per 100 mL | 1.5 g whey protein | 11.8 g (sugars 1.2 g) | 5.3 g (LCT 93%) | Nil | Electrolytes/100 mL: Na⁺ 2 mmol K⁺ 0.6 mmol Ca²⁺ 2.8 mmol P⁺ 3 mmol Low Vitamin A | Sole source of nutrition or nutritional supplement for infants and children with chronic renal failure receiving peritoneal rapid overnight dialysis | Tub: 400 g = £22.77 (5-g measuring scoop provided) |
| *Powder provides: protein 7.5 g, carbohydrate 59 g, fat 26.3 g, energy 2104 kJ (504 kcal)/100 g* | | | | | | | | | |
| Medium-chain Triglyceride (MCT) Oil | Liquid | 3515 kJ (855 kcal) per 100 mL | Nil | Nil | MCT 100% | Nil | | Nutritional supplement for steatorrhoea associated with cystic fibrosis of the pancreas, intestinal lymphangiectasia, intestinal surgery, chronic liver disease and liver cirrhosis, other proven malabsorption syndromes, ketogenic diet in management of epilepsy, type 1 hyperlipoproteinaemia | Bottle: 500 mL = £11.50 |
| Modulen IBD® (Nestlé) | Standard dilution (20%) of powder (sip or tube feed) | 420 kJ (100 kcal) per 100 mL | 3.6 g casein | 11 g (sugars 3.98 g) | 4.7 g | Nil | Gluten-free Residual lactose | Crohn's disease active phase, and in remission if malnourished | Can: 400 g = £13.60 Unflavoured[2] (8.3-g measuring scoop provided) |
| *Powder provides: protein 18 g, carbohydrate 54 g, fat 23 g, energy 2070 kJ (500 kcal)/100 g* | | | | | | | | | |

1. Flavouring: see *Modjul® Flavour System*, p. 903
2. Flavouring: see *Flavour Mix*, p. 903

**Appendix 7: Borderline substances**

## Appendix 7: Borderline substances

### A7.3.2 Specialised formulas for specific clinical conditions (product list continued)

For further information on composition of feeds, see p. 880

| Product | Formulation | Energy | Protein | Carbohydrate | Fat | Fibre | Special Characteristics | ACBS Indications | Presentation & Flavour |
|---|---|---|---|---|---|---|---|---|---|
| Nepro® (Abbott) | Liquid (sip or tube feed) | 838 kJ (200 kcal)[1] **per 100 mL** | 7 g cows' milk | 20.6 g (sugars 3.26 g) | 9.6 g | 1.56 g | Gluten-free Residual lactose Electrolytes/100 mL: Na⁺ 3.67 mmol K⁺ 2.72 mmol Ca²⁺ 3.43 mmol P⁻ 2.23 mmol | Sole source of nutrition or nutritional supplement in patients with chronic renal failure who are on haemodialysis or CAPD, or with cirrhosis, or other conditions requiring a high energy, low fluid, low electrolyte diet. Not suitable for child under 1 year; use with caution in child 1–5 years | Carton: 200 mL = £2.34 Strawberry, vanilla Flexible pack: 500 mL = £5.07 Vanilla |
| ProSure® (Abbott) | Liquid (sip or tube feed) | 529 kJ (125 kcal)[1] **per 100 mL** | 6.65 g cows' milk | 18.3 g (sugars 2.95 g) | 2.56 g | 2.07 g | Gluten-free Residual lactose Contains fish oil | Nutritional supplement for patients with pancreatic cancer Not suitable for child under 1 year; use with caution in child 1–4 years | Carton: 240 mL = £2.77 Banana, vanilla |
| Protifar® (Nutricia Clinical) | Powder | 1580 kJ (373 kcal) **per 100 g** | 88.5 g cows' milk | less than 1.5 g | 1.6 g | Nil | Gluten-free Residual lactose Electrolytes/100 mL: Na⁺ 1.3 mmol K⁺ 1.28 mmol Ca²⁺ 33.75 mmol P⁻ 22.58 mmol | Nutritional supplement for use in biochemically proven hypoproteinaemia | Can: 225 g = £7.44 Unflavoured (2.5-g measuring scoop provided) |
| Renamil® (KoRa) Powder provides: protein 2.2 g per 2.5 g | Powder (sip or tube feed when reconstituted) | 2003 kJ (477 kcal) **per 100 g** | 4.6 g cows' milk | 70.8 g | 19.3 g | Nil | Contains lactose Gluten-free Electrolytes/100 g: Na⁺ 1.04 mmol K⁺ 0.13 mmol Ca²⁺ 10.22 mmol P⁻ 1.06 mmol Contains no vitamin A or vitamin D | Sole source of nutrition or nutritional supplement for adults and children over 1 year with chronic renal failure | Sachet: 10 × 100 g = £25.40 |

1. Minor nutritional variations between flavours—consult product literature

| Product | Form | Energy | Protein | Carbohydrate | Fat | Fibre | Special characteristics | Presentation/Indications | Presentation |
|---|---|---|---|---|---|---|---|---|---|
| Renapro® (KoRa) | Powder | 1580 kJ (372 kcal) **per 100 g** | 90 g whey protein | 800 mg | 1 g | Nil | Gluten-free Residual lactose Electrolytes/100 g: Na+ 23 mmol K+ 2 mmol Ca2+ 4.99 mmol P+ 4.84 mmol | Nutritional supplement for bio-chemically proven hypoprotein-aemia and patients undergoing dialysis. Not suitable for child under 1 year | Sachet: 30 × 20 g = £69.60 |

Powder provides: protein 18 g, energy 316 kJ (74 kcal)/20-g sachet

| Renastart® (Vitaflo) | Standard dilution (20%) of powder | 411 kJ (98 kcal) **per 100 mL** | 1.5 g cows' milk soya | 12.6 g (sugars 1.2 g) | 4.6 g | Nil | Contains lactose Electrolytes/100 mL: Na+ 2.1 mmol K+ 0.6 mmol Ca2+ 0.58 mmol P+ 0.58 mmol | Dietary management of renal failure in neonates and children 1 month–10 years | Powder: 10 × 100 g = £56.93 Unflavoured (7-g measuring scoop provided) |

Powder provides: protein 7.5 g, carbohydrate 63 g, fat 23.2 g, energy 2053 kJ (491 kcal)/100 g

| Respifor® (Nutricia Clinical) | Liquid (sip feed) | 633 kJ (150 kcal) **per 100 mL** | 7.5 g cows' milk | 22.5 g (sugars 6.4 g[1]) | 3.3 g | Nil[2] | Contains lactose | Nutritional supplement for dietary management of disease-related malnutrition in patients with chronic obstructive pulmonary disease and body-mass index less than 20. Not suitable for child under 3 years; caution in child 3–5 years | Bottle: 125 mL = £1.85 Chocolate, strawberry, vanilla |
| Suplena® (Abbott) | Liquid (sip or tube feed) | 840 kJ (200 kcal) **per 100 mL** | 3 g caseinates | 25.5 g (sugars 2.7 g) | 9.6 g | Nil | Gluten-free Residual lactose Electrolytes/100 mL: Na+ 3.39 mmol K+ 2.87 mmol Ca2+ 3.48 mmol P+ 2.39 mmol | A sole source of nutrition or nutritional supplement in patients with chronic or acute renal failure who are not undergoing dialysis, or with chronic or acute liver disease with fluid restriction; other conditions requiring high energy, low protein, low electrolyte, low volume enteral feed. Not suitable for child under 1 year; use with caution in child 1–5 years | Can: 237 mL = £2.40 Vanilla |

1. Sugar content varies with flavour
2. Fibre content varies with flavour

Appendix 7: Borderline substances

## A7.4 Feed supplements

### A7.4.1 High-energy supplements

For further information on composition of feeds, see p. 880

### A7.4.1.1 High-energy supplements: carbohydrate

Flavoured carbohydrate supplements are not suitable for child under 1 year; liquid supplements should be diluted before use in child under 5 years

**ACBS Indications:** disease-related malnutrition, malabsorption states, or other conditions requiring fortification with a high or readily available carbohydrate supplement

| Product | Formulation | Energy | Protein | Carbohydrate | Fat | Fibre | Special Characteristics | ACBS Indications | Presentation & Flavour |
|---|---|---|---|---|---|---|---|---|---|
| Caloreen® (Nestlé) | Powder | 1640 kJ (390 kcal) **per 100 g** | Nil | 96 g Maltodextrin | Nil | Nil | Gluten-free Lactose-free | See above Not suitable for child under 3 years | Powder: 500 g = £3.42 Unflavoured (10-g measuring scoop provided) |
| Maxijul® Super Soluble (SHS) | Powder | 1615 kJ (380 kcal) **per 100 g** | Nil | 95 g Glucose polymer (sugars 8.6 g) | Nil | Nil | Gluten-free Lactose-free | See above | Sachets: 4 × 132 g = £5.04 Can: 200 g = £1.96 2.5 kg = £17.94 25 kg = £121.85 Unflavoured |
| Maxijul® Liquid (SHS) | Liquid | 850 kJ (200 kcal) **per 100 mL** | Nil | 50 g Glucose polymer (sugars 4.5 g[1]) | Nil | Nil | Gluten-free Lactose-free | See above | Carton: 200 mL = £1.28 Orange, unflavoured |
| Polycal® (Nutricia Clinical) | Powder | 1630 kJ (384 kcal) **per 100 g** | Nil | 96 g Maltodextrin (sugars 6 g) | Nil | Nil | Gluten-free Lactose-free | See above | Can: 400 g = £3.66 Neutral (5-g measuring scoop provided) |
| | Liquid | 1050 kJ (247 kcal) **per 100 mL** | Nil | 61.9 g Maltodextrin (sugars 12.2 g) | Nil | Nil | | Liquid not suitable for child under 3 years | Bottle: 200 mL = £1.46 Neutral, orange |
| Vitajoule® (Vitaflo) | Powder | 1610 kJ (380 kcal) **per 100 g** | Nil | 96 g Dried glucose syrup | Nil | Nil | Gluten-free Lactose-free | See above | Can: 500 g = £3.58 2.5 kg = £17.65 25 kg = £105.03 (10-g measuring scoop provided) |

1. Sugar content varies with flavour

## A7.4.1.2 High-energy supplements: fat

Liquid supplements should be diluted before use in child under 5 years

**ACBS indications:** disease-related malnutrition, malabsorption states, or other conditions requiring fortification with a high fat (or fat and carbohydrate) supplement

| Product | Formulation | Energy | Protein | Carbohydrate | Fat | Fibre | Special Characteristics | ACBS Indications | Presentation & Flavour |
|---|---|---|---|---|---|---|---|---|---|
| Calogen® (Nutricia Clinical) | Liquid (emulsion) | 1850 kJ (450 kcal)[1] **per 100 mL** | Nil | 100 mg | 50 g (LCT 100%) | Nil | Gluten-free Lactose-free | See above | Bottle: 200 mL = £3.91 500 mL = £9.60 Banana[2], neutral, strawberry[2] |
| Liquigen® (SHS) | Liquid (emulsion) | 1850 kJ (450 kcal) **per 100 mL** | Nil | Nil | 50 g (MCT 97%) Fractio-nated coconut oil | Nil | Gluten-free Lactose-free | Steatorrhoea associated with cystic fibrosis of the pancreas, intestinal lymphangiectasia, intestinal surgery, chronic liver disease, liver cirrhosis, other proven malabsorption syndromes, ketogenic diet in epilepsy, and in type 1 lipoproteinaemia Not suitable for child under 1 year | Bottle: 250 mL = £7.26 |
| **■ Fat and Carbohydrate** | | | | | | | | | |
| Duobar® (SHS) | Bar | 1211 kJ (292 kcal) **per 45 g** | Less than 20 mg | 22.5 g (sucrose) | 22.5 g | Nil | Contains phenylalanine 180 micrograms/45-g bar Gluten-free Lactose-free | See above | Bar: 45 g = £1.54 Neutral, strawberry, toffee |
| Duocal® (SHS) | Liquid | 695 kJ (166 kcal) **per 100 mL** | Nil | 23.7 g (sugars 2.1 g) | 7.9 g (MCT 30%) | Nil | Contains vitamin E | See above | Bottle: 250 mL = £3.14 |
| Duocal® Super Soluble (SHS) | Powder | 2061 kJ (492 kcal) **per 100 g** | Nil | 72.7 g (sugars 6.5 g) | 22.3 g (MCT 35%) | Nil | Gluten-free Lactose-free | See above | Can: 400 g = £14.16 (5-g measuring scoop provided) |
| Energivit® (SHS) | Standard dilution (15%) of powder | 309 kJ (74 kcal) **per 100 mL** | Nil | 10 g (sugars 900 mg) | 3.75 g | Nil | Lactose-free With vitamins, minerals, and trace elements | For children requiring additional energy, vitamins, minerals, and trace elements following a protein-restricted diet | Can: 400 g = £17.23 (5-g measuring scoop provided) |

Powder provides: carbohydrate 66.7 g, fat 25 g, energy 2059 kJ (492 kcal)/100 g

1. Nutritional values vary with flavour—consult product literature
2. Flavour not suitable for child under 3 years

**Appendix 7: Borderline substances**

**Appendix 7: Borderline substances**

### A7.4.1.2 High-energy supplements: fat *(product list continued)*

Liquid supplements should be diluted before use in child under 5 years

**ACBS indications:** disease-related malnutrition, malabsorption states, or other conditions requiring fortification with a high fat (or fat and carbohydrate) supplement

| Product | Formulation | Energy | Protein | Carbohydrate | Fat | Fibre | Special Characteristics | ACBS Indications | Presentation & Flavour |
|---|---|---|---|---|---|---|---|---|---|
| MCT Duocal® (SHS) | Powder | 2082 kJ (497 kcal) **per 100 g** | Nil | 72 g (sugars 10.1 g) | 23.2 g (MCT 83%) | Nil | | See above | Can: 400 g = £16.84 |

### A7.4.1.3 High-energy supplements: protein

**ACBS indications:** disease-related malnutrition, malabsorption states, or other conditions requiring fortification with a high fat or carbohydrate (with protein) supplement

| Product | Formulation | Energy | Protein | Carbohydrate | Fat | Fibre | Special Characteristics | ACBS Indications | Presentation & Flavour |
|---|---|---|---|---|---|---|---|---|---|
| Vitapro® (Vitaflo) | Powder | 1506 kJ (360 kcal) **per 100 g** | 75 g whey protein isolate | 9 g | 6 g | Nil | Contains lactose | Biochemically proven hypoprotein-aemia | Tub: 250 g = £7.31 2 kg = £57.40 (5-g measuring scoop provided) |

**■ Protein and carbohydrate**

| Product | Formulation | Energy | Protein | Carbohydrate | Fat | Fibre | Special Characteristics | ACBS Indications | Presentation & Flavour |
|---|---|---|---|---|---|---|---|---|---|
| Dialamine® (SHS) | Standard dilution (20%) of powder | 264 kJ (62 kcal) **per 100 mL** | 4.3 g protein equivalent (essential and non-essential amino acids) | 11.2 g (sugars 10.2 g) | Nil | Nil | Contains vitamin C | Hypoproteinaemia, chronic renal failure, wound fistula leakage with excessive protein loss, conditions requiring a controlled nitrogen intake, and haemodialysis Not suitable for child under 6 months | Can: 400 g = £57.53 Orange |

Powder provides: protein equivalent 25 g, carbohydrate 65 g, vitamin C 125 mg, energy 1530 kJ (360 kcal)/100 g

**■ Protein, fat, and carbohydrate**

| Product | Formulation | Energy | Protein | Carbohydrate | Fat | Fibre | Special Characteristics | ACBS Indications | Presentation & Flavour |
|---|---|---|---|---|---|---|---|---|---|
| Calogen® Extra (Nutricia Clinical) | Liquid | 1650 kJ (400 kcal) **per 100 mL** | 5 g cows' milk | 4.5 g (sugars 3.5 g) | 40.3 g | Nil | Residual lactose With vitamins, minerals, and trace elements | See above Not suitable for child under 3 years; may require dilution for child 3–5 years | Bottle: 200 mL = £4.45 Neutral, strawberry |
| Calshake® (Fresenius Kabi) | Powder | 1841 kJ (439 kcal)[1] **per 87 g** | 4.1 g cows' milk | 56.4 g (sugars 20 g) | 22 g | Nil | Contains lactose Gluten-free | See above Not suitable for child under 1 year | Sachet: 87 g = £1.96 Banana, neutral, strawberry, vanilla 90 g = £1.96 Chocolate |

Powder, one sachet reconstituted with 240 mL whole milk provides approx. 2 kcal/mL and protein 12 g

1. Nutritional values vary with flavour—consult product literature

| Product | Form | Energy | Protein / source | Carbohydrate | Fat | Residual lactose / vitamins | Suitability | Presentation / price |
|---|---|---|---|---|---|---|---|---|
| Enshake® (Abbott) | Powder | 1893 kJ (450 kcal[1]) **per 100 g** | 8.4 g cows' milk, soy protein isolate | 69 g (sugars 14.5 g) | 15.6 g | Nil | With vitamins and minerals | See above. Not suitable for child under 1 year; use with caution in child 1–6 years | Sachet: 96.5 g = £1.92. Banana, chocolate, strawberry, vanilla |

**Powder: 96.5 g reconstituted with 240 mL whole milk provides approx. 2 kcal/mL and protein 16 g**

| Product | Form | Energy | Protein / source | Carbohydrate | Fat | Residual lactose | Suitability | Presentation / price |
|---|---|---|---|---|---|---|---|---|
| Pro-Cal® (Vitaflo) | Powder | 2788 kJ (667 kcal) **per 100 g** | 13.5 g cows' milk | 27 g | 56 g | Nil | Contains lactose | Not suitable for child under 1 year | Sachets: 25 × 15 g = £13.21; Tub: 510 g = £12.24; 1.5 kg = £24.94; 12.5 kg = £177.29; 25 kg = £273.21 (15-g measuring scoop provided) |

**Powder 15 g provides: protein 2 g, carbohydrate 4 g, fat 8.4 g, energy 418 kJ (100 kcal)**

| Product | Form | Energy | Protein / source | Carbohydrate | Fat | Residual lactose | Suitability | Presentation / price |
|---|---|---|---|---|---|---|---|---|
| Pro-Cal® Shot (Vitaflo) | Liquid | 1393 kJ (334 kcal) **per 100 mL** | 6.7 g cows' milk | 13.4 g | 28.2 g | Nil | Contains lactose | Not suitable for child under 1 year | Bottle: 6 × 250 mL = £26.22. Banana, neutral, strawberry[2] |
| QuickCal® (Vitaflo) | Powder | 3263 kJ (780 kcal) **per 100 g** | 4.6 g cows' milk | 17 g | 77 g | Nil | Contains lactose | Not suitable for child under 1 year | Sachets: 25 × 13 g = £11.89 |

**Powder 13 g provides: protein 600 mg, carbohydrate 2.2 g, fat 10 g, energy 418 kJ (100 kcal)**

| Product | Form | Energy | Protein / source | Carbohydrate | Fat | Residual lactose | Suitability | Presentation / price |
|---|---|---|---|---|---|---|---|---|
| Scandishake® Mix (Nutricia Clinical) | Powder | 2099 kJ (500 kcal)[1] **per 100 g** | 4.7 g cows' milk | 65 g (sugars 14.3 g) | 24.7 g | Nil | Gluten-free. Contains lactose | Not suitable for child under 3 years | Sachet: 85 g = £2.08. Banana, caramel, chocolate, strawberry, vanilla, unflavoured |

**Powder 85 g reconstituted with 240 mL whole milk provides: protein 11.7 g, carbohydrate 66.8 g, fat 30.4 g, energy 2457 kJ (588 kcal)**

| Product | Form | Energy | Protein / source | Carbohydrate | Fat | Residual lactose | Suitability | Presentation / price |
|---|---|---|---|---|---|---|---|---|
| Vitasavoury® (Vitaflo) | Powder | 2590 kJ (619 kcal)[1] **per 100 g** | 12.7 g cows' milk | 23.5 g (sugars 1.5 g) | 52.3 g | 6.2 g | Contains lactose | Not suitable for child under 3 years | Cup (200 kcal): 24 × 33 g = £26.53; Sachet (300 kcal) 10 × 50 g = £15.99. Chicken, leek and potato, mushroom, vegetable |

1. Nutritional values vary with flavour—consult product literature
2. Flavour not suitable for child under 3 years

**Appendix 7: Borderline substances**

# Appendix 7: Borderline substances

## A7.4.2 Fibre, vitamin, and mineral supplements

| Product | Formulation | Energy | Protein | Carbohydrate | Fat | Fibre | Special Characteristics | ACBS Indications | Presentation & Flavour |
|---|---|---|---|---|---|---|---|---|---|
| **High-fibre supplements** | | | | | | | | | |
| Resource® Benefiber® (Nestlé) | Powder | 323 kJ (76 kcal) **per 100 g** | Nil | 19 g guar gum, partially hydrolysed | Nil | 78 g | Gluten-free Lactose-free | Standard, p. 880 except dysphagia Not suitable for child under 5 years | Sachets 16 x 8 g = £5.72 Can: 250 g = £8.76 (5-g measuring scoop provided) |
| **Vitamin and Mineral supplements** | | | | | | | | | |
| Metabolic Mineral Mixture® (SHS) | Powder | 729 kJ (175 kcal) **per 100 g** | Nil | Nil | Nil | Nil | Contains trace elements Electrolytes/100 g: $Na^+$ 172 mmol $K^+$ 212 mmol $Ca^{2+}$ 205 mmol $P^+$ 192 mmol Energy source: Calcium lactate | Mineral supplement for synthetic diets Suitable for infants (but may require further dilution) | Tub: 100 g = £9.94 |
| Paediatric Seravit® (SHS) | Powder | 1275 kJ (300 kcal) **per 100 g** | Nil | 75 g (sugars 6.75 g)[1] | Nil | Nil | | Vitamin and mineral supplement in infants and children with restrictive therapeutic diets | Tub: 200 g = £14.03 Unflavoured[2] 200 g = £14.94 Pineapple[3] (5-g measuring scoop provided) |

1. Sugar content varies with flavour
2. Flavouring: see *Modjul® Flavour System*, p. 903
3. Flavour not suitable for child under 3 years

## A7.5 Feed additives

### A7.5.1 Special foods for conditions of intolerance

**Colief®** (Forum)

Liquid, lactase 50 000 units/g, Net price 7-mL dropper bottle = £7.00

For the relief of symptoms associated with lactose intolerance in infants, provided that lactose intolerance is confirmed by the presence of reducing substances and/or excessive acid in stools, a low concentration of the corresponding disaccharide enzyme on intestinal biopsy or by breath hydrogen test or lactose intolerance test. For dosage and administration details, consult product literature

**Fructose**
**(Laevulose)**

For proven glucose/galactose intolerance

**VSL#3®** (Ferring)

Powder, containing 8 strains of live, freeze-dried, lactic acid bacteria. Contains traces of soya, gluten, and lactose. Net price 30 × 4.4-g sachets = £32.98

Nutritional supplement for use under the supervision of a physician, for the maintenance of remission of ileoanal pouchitis induced by antibacterials in adults. For dosage and administration details, consult product literature

### A7.5.2 Feed thickeners and pre-thickened foods

For pre-thickened infant feeds see *BNF for Children* (Appendix 2)

**Carobel, Instant®** (Cow & Gate)

Powder, carob seed flour. Net price 135 g = £2.92
For thickening feeds in the treatment of vomiting

**Nutilis®** (Nutricia Clinical)

Powder, modified maize starch, gluten- and lactose-free, Net price 20 × 9-g sachets = £5.88; 225 g = £4.51.
For thickening of foods in dysphagia. Not suitable for children under 3 years

**Resource® Thickened Drink** (Nestlé)

Liquid, carbohydrate 22 g, energy: orange 382 kJ (90 kcal); apple 375 kJ (89 kcal)/100 mL. Syrup and custard consistencies. Gluten- and lactose-free, net price 12 × 114-mL cups = £7.08.
For dysphagia. Not suitable for children under 1 year

**Resource® ThickenUp®** (Nestlé)

Powder, modified maize starch. Gluten- and lactose-free, net price 227 g = £4.11; 75 × 4.5-g sachet = £15.75.
For thickening of foods in dysphagia. Not suitable for children under 1 year

**SLO Drinks®** (SLO Drinks)

Powder, carbohydrate content varies with flavour and chosen consistency (3 consistencies available), see product literature. Flavours: black currant, lemon, orange, or peach, net price 25 × 115 mL = £7.50.
Nutritional supplement for patient hydration in the dietary management of dysphagia. Not suitable for children under 3 years

**Thick and Easy®** (Fresenius Kabi)

Powder. Modified maize starch, net price 225-g can = £4.35; 100 × 9-g sachets = £26.35; 4.54 kg = £70.53.

Thickened Juices, liquid, modified food starch. Flavours: apple, orange, net price 118-mL pot = 57p; apple, black currant, cranberry, kiwi-strawberry, and orange, 1.42-litre bottle = £3.61.
For thickening of foods in dysphagia. Not suitable for children under 1 year except in cases of failure to thrive

**Thixo-D®** (Sutherland)

Powder, modified maize starch, gluten-free. Net price 375-g tub = £6.75.
For thickening of foods in dysphagia. Not suitable for children under 1 year except in cases of failure to thrive

**Vitaquick®** (Vitaflo)

Powder. Modified maize starch. Net price 300 g = £6.59; 2 kg = £33.57; 6 kg = £85.90.
For thickening of foods in dysphagia. Not suitable for children under 1 year except in cases of failure to thrive

### A7.5.3 Flavouring preparations

**Flavour Mix®** (Nestlé)

Powder. Flavours: banana, chocolate, coffee, lemon-lime, strawberry. Net price 60 g = £5.62

**FlavourPac®** (Vitaflo)

Powder, flavours: black currant, lemon, orange, tropical or raspberry, net price 30 × 4-g sachets = £11.29
For use with Vitaflo's range of unflavoured protein substitutes for metabolic diseases

**Modjul® Flavour System** (SHS)

Powder, flavours: black currant, orange, pineapple, 100 g = £9.54; cherry-vanilla, grapefruit, lemon-lime, 20 × 5-g sachets = £9.54.
For use with unflavoured SHS products based on peptides or amino acids; not suitable for child under 6 months

### A7.6 Foods for special diets

### A7.6.1 Gluten-free foods

> **ACBS indications:** gluten-sensitive enteropathies including steatorrhoea due to gluten sensitivity, coeliac disease, and dermatitis herpetiformis.

**Aproten®** (Ultrapharm)

Gluten-free. Flour. Net price 500 g = £4.99.

**Barkat®** (Gluten Free Foods Ltd)

Gluten-free. Baguettes (par-baked), net price 200 g = £3.36. Bread (white, sliced, par-baked), 300 g = £2.70; country loaf (par-baked, sliced), 250 g = £3.36; rolls (par-baked), 200 g = £2.48. Bread mix, 500 g = £5.74. Multi Grain Bread, 500 g = £4.44. Rice bread, brown or white, 500 g = £4.44. Crackers (matzo), 200 g = £2.52. Biscuits (coffee) 200 g = £1.68. Pasta, (animal shapes, macaroni, spaghetti, spirals, tagliatelle), 500 g = £4.95. buckwheat (penne or spirals), 250 g = £2.03. Rice pizza crust, brown or white, 150 g = £3.83. Flour mix, 750 g = £5.35.

**Bi-Aglut®** (Ultrapharm)

Gluten-free. Bread flour mix or plain flour, net price 500 g = £4.75. Bread rolls, 150 g = £1.77. Bread sticks, 150 g = £1.95.Biscuits, 180 g = £2.89. Crackers, 150 g = £2.36. Cracker toast, 240 g = £4.18. Pasta (fusilli, macaroni, penne, spaghetti), 500 g = £5.23.

**Dietary Specials** (Nutrition Point)

Gluten-free. Bread, loaf, sliced (white, brown or white multigrain) 400 g = £2.94; bread rolls, long (white) 3 = £1.84. Bread mix, 500 g = £5.20; cracker bread, 150 g = £1.89; cake mix (white), 750 g = £5.20; white mix, 500 g = £5.20. Tea biscuits, 220 g = £2.10. Pasta (spaghetti, penne, fusilli), 500 g = £3.36. Pizza base, 2 = £5.15

**Ener-G®** (General Dietary)

Gluten-free. Cookies (vanilla flavour), net price 435 g = £5.00. Rolls, dinner 6 × 280 g = £2.97, long, white 220 g = £2.39; round, white 200 g = £2.39. Rice bread (sliced), brown, 474 g = £4.39; white, 456 g = £4.39. Rice loaf (sliced) 612 g = £4.39. Seattle brown loaf, 600 g = £5.05. Tapioca bread (sliced), 480 g = £4.39. Rice pasta (macaroni, shells, small shells, and lasagne), 454 g = £4.08; spaghetti, 447 g = £3.98; tagliatelle, 400 g = £3.98; vermicelli, 300 g = £4.08; cannelloni, 335 g = £3.98. Brown rice pasta: lasagne, 454 g = £3.98; macaroni, 454 g = £3.98; spaghetti, 447 g = £3.98. Xanthan gum, 170 g = £6.93.

**Freebake®** (Freebake)

Gluten-free. Bread mix, net price 2.4 kg = £12.15, cake mix, 2.4 kg = £11.90, pizza base mix, 2.4 kg = £12.00. Flour (plain), 2.4 kg = £11.50.

**Gadsby's**

Gluten-free. White bread flour, net price 1 kg = £4.99. White bread (sliced or unsliced), 400 g = £2.50. White bread rolls, 4 × 75 g = £2.00

**Glutafin®** (Nutrition Point)

Gluten-free. Bread loaf, fibre or white (sliced or unsliced), 400 g = £3.41; rolls, fibre or white, 4 = £3.41. Biscuits, savoury, 125 g = £1.89; savoury shorts, 150 g = £2.59. Biscuits, digestive, sweet or tea, 150 g = £1.89. Biscuits, 200 g = £3.68. Biscuits, shortbread, 100 g = £1.56. Mixes, bread, fibre or white, 500 g = £5.91. Crackers, 200 g = £3.08. High fibre crackers, 200 g = £2.58. Pasta (penne, shells, spirals, spaghetti), 500 g = £5.97; (lasagne, tagliatelle), 250 g = £3.13. Pizza bases, 2 × 150 g = £5.83.

Select Gluten-free. Bread, fibre loaf (sliced), 400 g = £3.04; part-baked, 400 g = £3.41; fresh, white or brown, (sliced), 400 g = £3.17. Seeded loaf, 400 g = £3.31. White loaf (sliced), 400 g = £3.04; part-baked, 400 g = £3.41. Fibre rolls, 4 = £3.17. White rolls, 4 = £3.17, part-baked 4 = £3.41; long (part-baked), 2 = £3.41. Mixes (bread, cake, fibre, fibre bread, pastry, and white), 500 g = £5.91

**Heron Foods®** (Gluten Free Foods Ltd)

Gluten-free. Bread mix, organic (standard or fibre), net price 500 g = £4.12

**Il Pane di Anna®** (Gluten Free Foods Ltd)

Gluten-free. Bread mix, white, net price 500 g = £5.25, cake mix, white 500 g = £5.25, pizza base mix, 500 g = £5.25

**Juvela®** (Juvela)

Gluten-free. Harvest mix, fibre mix, and flour mix, net price 500 g = £6.33. Bread mix (whole or sliced), 400-g loaf = £3.05; part-baked loaf (with or without fibre), 400g = £3.27; fresh sliced loaf (white) 400 g = £3.17, (fibre) 400 g = £3.05. Fibre bread (sliced and unsliced), 400-g loaf = £3.05. Bread rolls (white), 5 × 85 g = £4.11, fibre bread rolls, 5 × 85 g = £4.11, part-baked rolls (with or without fibre), 5 × 75 g = £4.25. Crispbread, 210 g = £3.82. Pasta (fibre linguine, fibre penne, fusilli, macaroni, spaghetti), 500 g = £6.20; lasagne, 250 g = £3.16; tagliatelle, 250 g = £2.99. Pizza bases, 2 × 180 g = £7.56. Digestive biscuits, 150 g = £2.62. Savoury biscuits, 150 g = £3.29. Sweet biscuits, 150 g = £2.48. Tea biscuits, 150 g = £2.62.

**Lifestyle®** (Ultrapharm)

Gluten-free. Brown bread (sliced and unsliced), net price 400 g = £2.82. White bread (sliced and unsliced), 400 g = £2.82. High fibre bread (sliced and unsliced), 400 g = £2.82. Bread rolls, (brown, white, or high-fibre) 400 g = £2.82.

**Livwell®** (Livwell)

Gluten-free. Bread, sliced, (brown or white), 200 g = £2.25; baguette (white) 250 g = £2.50; rolls (white), 4 = £2.50; flat bread, 4 = £3.00

**Orgran®** (Community)

Gluten-free. Pasta: lasagne (corn, rice and maize), 150 g = £2.89; macaroni (rice and maize), 250 g = £2.35; shells (split pea and soya), 200 g = £2.25; spaghetti (corn, rice, rice and maize), 250 g = £2.25; spirals (buckwheat, corn, rice, rice and millet, rice and maize), 250 g = £2.35, spirals (organic brown rice), 250 g = £2.60. Crispbread (corn or rice), 200 g = £2.70. Pizza and pastry mix, 375 g = £3.52. Flour, self-raising, 500 g = £2.89. Bread mix, 450 g = £3.10

**Proceli** (Generpharm)

Gluten-free. Bread, (white, sliced), net price 165 g = £2.19; sandwich bread, 155 g = £2.06. Baguettes (part-baked), 2 × 125 g = £2.90. Bread buns, 4 × 50 g = £3.26. Dinner rolls (white, part-baked), 4 × 35 g = £4.04. Hotdog rolls (white, part-baked) 3 × 35 g = £1.96. Long rolls (white, part-baked), 3 × 83 g = £2.74. Lunch rolls (white), 6 × 45 g = £3.11. Flour (white), 1 kg = £5.14. Pasta (macaroni, small macaroni, puntini, short spaghetti, spirals), 250 g = £2.59. Pizza bases, 3 × 125 g = £5.18. Rice bread (sandwich loaf), 200 g = £2.32; rice bread (brown), 220 g = £2.19.

**Pure®** (Innovative)

Gluten-free. Blended flour, net price 1 kg = £3.56; potato starch flour 500 g = £1.42; rice flour (brown) 500 g = £1.33, (white) 500 g = £1.42; tapioca starch flour 500 g = £1.89; teff flour, (brown or white), 1 kg = £3.99; xanthan gum 100 g = £5.46

**Rite-Diet® Gluten-free** (Nutricia Dietary)

Gluten-free Flour mix (white or fibre), 500 g = £5.22.

**Rizopia®** (PGR Health Foods)

Gluten-free. Brown rice pasta (fusilli, penne, spaghetti) 500 g = £2.50, (lasagne) 375 g = £2.50

**Schar®** (Nutrition Point)

Gluten-free. Bread.(white, sliced), net price 2 x 200 g = £3.05. Baguette (french bread), 400 g = £3.20. Bread rolls, 150 g = £1.91. Lunch rolls, 150 g = £1.94. Bread mix, 1 kg = £4.99. Ertha brown bread, 2 x 250 g = £3.26. Cake mix, 500 g = £4.99. Flour mix, 1 kg = £4.99. Breadsticks (Grissini), 150 g = £2.05. Cracker toast, 150 g = £2.21. Crackers, 200 g = £2.68. Crispbread, 250 g = £3.68. Pasta (fusilli, penne), 500 g = £3.47; lasagne, 250 g = £3.47; macaroni pipette, 500 g = £3.47; spaghetti, 500 g = £3.47. Biscuits (frollini tea), 200 g = £2.36. Savoy biscuits, 200 g = £2.57.

**Sunnyvale®** (Everfresh)

Gluten-free. Mixed grain bread (sour dough), net price 400 g = £1.91.

**Tobia Teff** (Tobia Teff)

Gluten-free. Teff flour (brown or white), net price 1 kg = £2.95

**Tritamyl®** (Gluten Free Foods Ltd)

Gluten-free. Flour, net price 1 kg = £5.60. Bread mix (brown or white), 1 kg = £5.60.

**Ultra®** (Ultrapharm)

Gluten-free. Baguette, net price 400 g = £2.46. Bread, 400 g = £2.46. High-fibre bread, 500 g = £3.35. Bread rolls, 400 g = £2.46. Crackerbread, 100 g = £1.77. Sweet biscuits, 250 g = £2.93. Pasta (fusilli, penne, spaghetti, tagliatelle), 250 g = £2.95. Pizza base, 400 g = £2.65.

**Valpiform®** (Ultrapharm)

Gluten-free. Bread mix, 2 × 500 g = £6.73; country loaf (sliced), 400 g = £3.75. Crac'form toast, 2 × 125 g = £3.52. Crisp rolls, 220 g = £3.60; Baguettes, maxi, 2 × 200 g = £4.49, petites, 2 × 160 g = £2.99. Pastry mix, 2 × 500 g = £6.73.

**Wellfoods®** (Wellfoods)

Gluten-free. Bread, loaf (unsliced), net price 600 g = £4.85, (sliced) 600 g = £4.95; burger buns, 4 = £3.95; rolls, 4 = £3.65. Flour alternative 1 kg = £7.65. Pizza base, 2 = £8.95

### A7.6.1.1 Gluten- and wheat-free foods

**ACBS indications:** established gluten enteropathy (including steatorrhoea due to gluten sensitivity, coeliac disease, and dermatitis herpetiformis) with coexisting established wheat sensitivity only.

**Ener-G®** (General Dietary)

Gluten-free, wheat-free. Pizza bases, 372 g = £3.75. Six flour bread loaf, 576 g = £3.60. Seattle brown rolls (round or long), 4 × 119 g = £3.00

**Glutafin®** (Nutricia Dietary)

Gluten-free, wheat-free. Crisp bread, 2 × 125 g = £3.82. Mixes (fibre bread, bread), 500 g = £5.63; cake or pastry mix, 500 g = £5.63.

**Heron Foods®** (Gluten Free Foods Ltd)

Gluten-free, wheat-free. Bread mix, organic (fibre), net price 500 g = £4.12; bread and cake mix, organic, 500 g = £4.12

### A7.6.2 Low-protein foods

**ACBS indications:** inherited metabolic disorders, renal or liver failure, requiring a low-protein diet

**Aproten®** (Ultrapharm)

Low protein. Low Na$^+$ and K$^+$. Biscuits, net price 180 g (36) = £2.88; bread mix 250 g = £2.17; crispbread 260 g = £4.06; pasta (anellini, ditalini, rigatini, spaghetti) 500 g = £4.06; tagliatelle 250 g = £2.16.

**Ener-G®** (General Dietary)

Low protein. Egg replacer, net price 454 g = £4.05. Rice bread, 600 g − £4.39.

**Fate®** (Fate)

Low protein. All-purpose mix, net price 500 g = £6.39; Cake mix, 2 × 250 g = £6.39, chocolate-flavour, 2 × 250 g = £6.39.

**Harifen®** (Ultrapharm)

Low protein. Cracker toast, net price 200 g = £2.75. Cookies, white chip, 200 g = £2.25

**Juvela®** (SHS)

Low Protein. Mix, net price 500 g = £6.66. Bread (sliced), 400-g loaf = £3.12. Bread rolls, 5 × 70 g = £3.87. Biscuits, orange and cinnamon flavour, 125 g = £6.51; chocolate chip, 130 g = £6.51. Pizza base, 2 = £7.37

**Loprofin®** (SHS)

Low protein. Sweet biscuits, net price 150 g = £2.08; chocolate cream-filled biscuits, 125 g = £2.08; cookies (chocolate chip or cinnamon), 100 g = £5.51; crunch bar, 8 × 41 g = £11.09; wafers (orange, vanilla, or chocolate), 100 g = £2.02. Breakfast cereal, flakes (apple, chocolate, or strawberry), 375 g = £6.24, loops 375 g = £6.48. Egg replacer, 500 g = £12.14. Egg-white replacer, 100 g = £7.81. Bread (sliced), 400-g loaf = £3.12. Bread rolls (white) 4 = £2.91, (part-baked) 4 × 65 g = £3.28. Mix, 500 g = £6.61. Cake mix (chocolate or lemon), 500 g = £6.99. Dessert mix (chocolate, strawberry, vanilla), 150 g = £3.82. Crackers, 150 g = £2.84. Herb crackers, 150 g = £2.84. Pasta (fusilli, penne, spaghetti), 500 g = £6.91, (macaroni, puntoni, tagliatelle) 250 g = £3.32, (conchigle, gnocchetti sardi) 500 g = £6.66, (lasagne), 250 g = £3.36, (vermicelli), 250 g = £3.44, (animal shapes) 500 g = £6.64. Snack Pot (unflavoured, curry, or tomato and basil), 47 g = £3.67, Rice, 500 g = £6.71.

**Low protein drink** (Milupa)

Powder, whey protein 500 mg, carbohydrate 6 g, fat 3 g, energy 220 kJ (53 kcal)/10 g, with vitamins, minerals, and trace elements. Net price 400 g = £7.23.

For inherited disorders of amino acid metabolism in children over 1 year

Note Termed *Milupa® lpd* by manufacturer

**PK Foods®** (Gluten Free Foods Ltd)

Low-protein. Bread (white sliced) net price 550 g = £4.00. Crispbread, 75 g = £2.00. Pasta (spirals) 250 g = £2.00. *Aminex®* biscuits, 150 g = £4.25; cookies, 200 g = £4.25; rusks, 200 g = £4.25

For phenylketonuria and similar amino acid abnormalities

Cookies (chocolate chip, orange, or cinnamon), 150 g = £4.25. Egg replacer, 350 g = £4.25. Flour mix, 750 g = £9.60. Jelly (orange or cherry flavour), 4 × 80 g = £6.76.

For phenylketonuria only

**Promin®** (Firstplay Dietary)

Low protein. Burger mix, 2 × 62 g = £5.60, (lamb and mint), 4 × 72 g = £5.50. Sausage mix (apple and sage, tomato and basil, or original), 4 × 30 g = £6.30. Cous Cous, 500 g = £6.35. Pasta (alphabets, macaroni, shells, shortcut spaghetti, spirals) and pasta tricolour (alphabets, shells, spirals), 500 g = £6.35; Lasagne sheets, 200 g = £2.70. Pasta shells in tomato, pepper and herb sauce, 4 × 72-g sachets = £7.32; Pasta elbows in cheese and broccoli sauce, 4 × 66-g sachets = £7.32. Pasta spirals in Moroccan sauce, 4 × 72 g = £7.32. Pasta meal, 500 g = £6.35. Pasta imitation rice, 500 g = £6.35. Rice pudding imitation (apple, banana, strawberry, and original flavours), 4 × 69-g sachets = £5.60. Dessert (chocolate and banana, strawberry and vanilla, custard, or caramel) 6 × 36.5-g = £5.60. Hot breakfast (apple and cinnamon, banana, chocolate, original) 6 × 57-g = £7.14. Spread, chocolate and hazelnut, 230 g = £6.80

**Rite-Diet® Low-protein** (SHS)

Low protein. Baking mix, net price 500 g = £6.61

**Sno-Pro®** (SHS)

Low-protein. Drink, protein 220 mg (phenylalanine 12.5 mg), carbohydrate 8 g, fat 3.8 g, energy 280 kJ (67 kcal)/100 mL. Net price 200 mL = 98p.

For phenylketonuria, chronic renal failure, and other inborn errors of metabolism

**Taranis** (Firstplay Dietary)

Low protein. Cake bars (lemon), net price 6 × 40 g = £5.10

**Ultra®** (Ultrapharm)

Low protein. PKU bread, 400 g = £2.65. PKU flour, 500 g = £3.07. PKU biscuits, 200 g = £2.21. PKU pizza base, 400 g = £2.45. PKU savoy biscuits, 150 g = £2.06.

**Valpiform®** (Ultrapharm)

Low protein. Biscuits, shortbread, net price 120 g = £4.06

**Vita Bite®** (Vitaflo)

Low-protein. Bar, protein 30 mg (less than 2.5 mg phenylalanine), carbohydrate 15.35 g, fat 8.4 g, energy 572 kJ (137 kcal)/25 g. Chocolate flavoured, net price 25 g = 99p.

Not recommended for children under 1 year

### A7.7 Nutritional supplements for metabolic diseases

◀ **Glutaric aciduria (type 1)**

**GA Gel®** (Vitaflo)

Gel, protein equivalent (essential and non-essential amino acids except lysine, and low tryptophan) 8.4 g, carbohydrate 8.6 g, fat trace, energy 286 kJ (68 kcal)/20 g, with vitamins, minerals, and trace elements. Unflavoured (flavouring: see *FlavourPac®*, p. 903), net price 30 × 20-g sachets = £145.76

Nutritional supplement for dietary management of type 1 glutaric aciduria in children 1–10 years

**[1]XLYS, Low TRY, Analog** (SHS)

Powder, protein equivalent (essential and non-essential amino acids except lysine, and low tryptophan) 13 g, carbohydrate 54 g, fat 23 g, energy 1990 kJ (475 kcal)/100 g, with vitamins, minerals, and trace elements; *standard dilution* (15%) provides protein equivalent 1.95 g, carbohydrate 8.1 g, fat 3.5 g, energy 300 kJ (72 kcal)/100 mL. Unflavoured, net price 400 g = £28.22. (5-g measuring scoop provided)

Nutritional supplement for the dietary management of type 1 glutaric aciduria

**[2]XLYS, Low TRY, Maxamaid** (SHS)

Powder, protein equivalent (essential and non-essential amino acids except lysine, and low tryptophan) 25 g, carbohydrate 51 g, fat less than 500 mg, energy 1311 kJ (309 kcal)/100 g, with vitamins, minerals, and trace elements. Unflavoured, (flavouring: see *Modjul® Flavour System*, p. 903), net price 500 g = £76.94.

Nutritional supplement for the dietary management of type 1 glutaric aciduria

**XLYS, TRY Glutaridon** (SHS)

Powder, protein equivalent (essential and non-essential amino acids except lysine and tryptophan) 79 g, carbohydrate 4 g, energy 1411 kJ (332 kcal)/100 g. Unflavoured (flavouring: see *Modjul® Flavour System*, p. 903), net price 2 × 500 g = £291.46.

Nutritional supplement for the dietary management of type 1 glutaric aciduria in children and adults; requires additional source of vitamins, minerals, and trace elements

◢**Glucogen storage disease**

**Corn flour and corn starch**

> For hypoglycaemia associated with glycogen-storage disease

**Glucose**

**(Dextrose monohydrate)**

Net price 500 g = £1.14.

For glycogen storage disease and sucrose/isomaltose intolerance

**Glycosade®** (Vitaflo)

Powder, protein 200 mg, carbohydrate (maize starch) 47.6 g, fat 100 mg, fibre less than 600 mg, energy 803 kJ (192 kcal)/60 g, net price 30 × 60-g sachets = £90.00

Nutritional supplement for use in the dietary management of glycogen storage disease and other metabolic conditions where a constant supply of glucose is essential. Not suitable for children under 2 years

◢**Homocystinuria or hypermethioninaemia**

**HCU cooler®** (Vitaflo)

Liquid, protein (essential and non-essential amino acids except methionine) 15 g, carbohydrate 7.8 g, fat trace, energy 386 kJ (92 kcal)/130 mL, with vitamins, minerals and trace elements. Orange flavour, net price 30 × 130-mL pouch = £271.20

A methionine-free protein substitute for use as a nutritional supplement in patients over 3 years of age with homocystinuria

**HCU Express®** (Vitaflo)

Powder, protein (essential and non-essential amino acids except methionine) 15 g, carbohydrate 3.8 g, fat 30 mg, energy 315 kJ (75.3 kcal)/25 g with vitamins, minerals and trace elements. Unflavoured (flavouring: see *FlavourPac®*, p. 903), net price 30 × 25-g sachets = £265.90

A methionine-free protein substitute for use as a nutritional supplement in patients over 8 years of age with homocystinuria

**HCU gel®** (Vitaflo)

Powder, protein (essential and non-essential amino acids except methionine) 8.4 g, carbohydrate 8.6 g, fat 30 mg, energy 286 kJ (68 kcal)/20 g with vitamins, minerals and trace elements. Unflavoured (flavouring: see *FlavourPac®*, p. 903), net price 30 × 20-g sachets = £148.59

A methionine-free protein substitute for use as a nutritional supplement for the dietary management of children 1–10 years with homocystinuria

**HCU LV®** (SHS)

Powder, protein (essential and non-essential amino acids except methionine) 20 g, carbohydrate 2.5 g, fat 190 mg, energy 390 kJ (92 kcal)/27.8-g sachet, with vitamins, minerals and trace elements. Unflavoured (flavouring: see *Modjul® Flavour System*, p. 903) or tropical flavour (formulation varies slightly), net price 30 × 27.8-g sachets = £386.17

A nutritional supplement for the dietary management of hypermethioninaemia or vitamin B$_6$ non-responsive homocystinuria in patients over 8 years.

**[1]XMET Analog** (SHS)

Powder, protein equivalent (essential and non-essential amino acids except methionine) 13 g, carbohydrate 54 g, fat 23 g, energy 1990 kJ (475 kcal)/100 g, with vitamins, minerals, and trace elements; *standard dilution* (15%) provides protein equivalent 1.95 g, carbohydrate 8.1 g, fat 3.5 g, energy 300 kJ (72 kcal)/100 mL. Unflavoured, net price 400 g = £28.22 (5-g measuring scoop provided)

Nutritional supplement for the dietary management of hypermethioninaemia or homocystinuria

**XMET Homidon** (SHS)

Powder, protein equivalent (essential and non-essential amino acids except methionine) 77 g, carbohydrate 4.5 g, fat nil, energy 1386 kJ (326 kcal)/100 g, with vitamins, minerals, and trace elements. Unflavoured (flavouring: see *Modjul® Flavour system*, p. 903), net price 500 g = £145.76.

Nutritional supplement for the dietary management of hypermethioninaemia or homocystinuria in children and adults

**[2]XMET Maxamaid** (SHS)

Powder, protein equivalent (essential and non-essential amino acids except methionine) 25 g, carbohydrate 51 g, fat less than 500 mg, energy 1311 kJ (309 kcal)/100 g, with vitamins, minerals, and trace elements. Unflavoured (flavouring: see *Modjul® Flavour Sytem*, p. 903), net price 500 g = £76.94

Nutritional supplement for the dietary management of hypermethioninaemia or homocystinuria

**[3]XMET Maxamum®** (SHS)

Powder, protein equivalent (essential and non-essential amino acids except methionine) 39 g, carbohydrate 34 g, fat less than 500 mg, energy 1260 kJ (297 kcal)/100 g, with vitamins, minerals, and trace elements. Unflavoured (flavouring: see *Modjul® Flavour System*, p. 903), net price 500 g = £123.34.

Nutritional supplement for the dietary management of hypermethioninaemia or homocystinuria

◢**Hyperlysinamia**

**[1]XLYS Analog** (SHS)

Powder, protein equivalent (essential and non-essential amino acids except lysine) 13 g, carbohydrate 54 g, fat 23 g, energy 1990 kJ (475 kcal)/100 g, with vitamins, and trace elements; *standard dilution* (15%) provides protein equivalent 1.95 g carbohydrate 8.1 g, fat 3.5 g, energy 300 kJ (72 kcal)/100 mL. Unflavoured, net price 400 g = £28.22. (5-g measuring scoop provided)

Nutritional supplement for the dietary management of hyperlysinaemia

**[2]XLYS Maxamaid** (SHS)

Powder, protein equivalent (essential and non-essential amino acids except lysine) 25 g, carbohydrate 51 g, fat less than 500 mg, energy 1311 kJ (309 kcal)/100 g, with vitamins, minerals, and trace elements. Unflavoured (flavouring: see *Modjul® Flavour System*, p. 903), net price 500 g = £76.94.

Nutritional supplement for the dietary management of hyperlysinaemia

◢**Isovaleric acidaemia**

**[1]XLEU Analog** (SHS)

Powder, protein equivalent (essential and non-essential amino acids except leucine) 13 g, carbohydrate 54 g, fat 23 g, energy 1990 kJ (475 kcal)/100 g, with vitamins, minerals, and trace elements; *standard dilution* (15%) provides protein

---

1. Analog products are generally intended for use in children up to 1 year
2. Maxamaid products are generally intended for use in children 1–8 years

3. Maxamum products are generally intended for use in children over 8 years and adults

equivalent 1.95 g, carbohydrate 8.1 g, fat 3.5 g, energy 300 kJ (72 kcal)/100 mL. Unflavoured, net price 400 g = £28.22. (5-g measuring scoop provided)

Nutritional supplement for the dietary management of isovaleric acidaemia

**XLEU Faladon** (SHS)

Powder, protein equivalent (essential and non-essential amino acids except leucine) 77 g, carbohydrate 4.5 g, fat nil, energy 1386 kJ (326 kcal)/100 g, with vitamins, minerals, and trace elements. Unflavoured (flavouring: see *Modjul® Flavour System*, p. 903), net price 200 g = £58.29.

Nutritional supplement for the dietary management of isovaleric acidaemia

**¹XLEU Maxamaid** (SHS)

Powder, protein equivalent (essential and non-essential amino acids except leucine) 25 g, carbohydrate 51 g, fat less than 500 mg, energy 1311 kJ (309 kcal)/100 g, with vitamins, minerals, and trace elements. Unflavoured (flavouring: see *Modjul® Flavour System*, p. 903), net price 500 g = £76.94.

Nutritional supplement for the dietary management of isovaleric acidaemia

◢ **Maple syrup urine disease**

**Isoleucine Amino Acid Supplement** (Vitaflo)

Powder, isoleucine 50 mg, carbohydrate 4 g, fat nil, energy 64 kJ (15 kcal)/4 g, net price 30 × 4-g sachets = £43.50

Nutritional supplement for the dietary management of maple syrup urine disease and other inborn errors of amino acid metabolism in children over 1 year and adults

**Mapleflex®** (SHS)

Powder, protein equivalent (essential and non-essential amino acids except isoleucine, leucine, and valine) 8.4 g, carbohydrate 11 g, fat 3.9 g, energy 474 kJ (113 kcal)/29-g sachet, with vitamins, minerals, and trace elements. Unflavoured (flavouring: see *Modjul® Flavour System*, p. 903), net price 30 × 29-g sachets = £162.82.

Nutritional supplement for the dietary management of maple syrup urine disease in children 1–10 years

**MSUD Aid III®** (SHS)

Powder, protein equivalent (essential and non-essential amino acids except isoleucine, leucine, and valine) 77 g, carbohydrate 4.5 g, energy 1386 kJ (326 kcal)/100 g, with vitamins, minerals, and trace elements. Unflavoured, (flavouring: see *Modjul® Flavour System*, p. 903), net price 500 g = £145.76.

Nutritional supplement for the dietary management of maple syrup urine disease and related conditions in children and adults where it is necessary to limit the intake of branched chain amino acids

**²MSUD Analog** (SHS)

Powder, protein equivalent (essential and non-essential amino acids except isoleucine, leucine, and valine) 13 g, carbohydrate 54 g, fat 23 g, energy 1990 kJ (475 kcal)/100 g, with vitamins, minerals, and trace elements; *standard dilution* (15%) provides protein equivalent 1.95 g, carbohydrate 8.1 g, fat 3.5 g, energy 300 kJ (72 kcal)/100 mL. Unflavoured, net price 400 g = £28.22. (5-g measuring scoop provided)

Nutritional supplement for the dietary management of maple syrup urine disease

**MSUD express®** (Vitaflo)

Powder, protein equivalent (essential and non-essential amino acids except leucine, isoleucine, and valine) 15 g, carbohydrate 3.8 g, fat less than 100 mg, energy 315 kJ (75 kcal)/25 g with vitamins, minerals, and trace elements. Unflavoured (flavouring: see *FlavourPac®* sachets, p. 903), net price 30 × 25-g sachets = £265.90.

Nutritional supplement for the dietary management of maple syrup urine disease in children over 8 years and adults

**MSUD express cooler®** (Vitaflo)

Liquid, protein equivalent (essential and non-essential amino acids except leucine, isoleucine, and valine) 15 g, carbohydrate 7.8 g, fat trace, energy 386 kJ (92 kcal)/130-mL pouch, with vitamins, minerals, and trace elements. Orange flavour, net price 30 × 130-mL = £271.20.

Nutritional supplement for the dietary management of maple syrup urine disease in children over 3 years and adults

**MSUD Gel®** (Vitaflo)

Powder, protein equivalent (essential and non-essential amino acids except leucine, isoleucine, and valine) 8.4 g, carbohydrate 8.6 g, fat less than 100 mg, energy 286 kJ (68 kcal)/20 g with vitamins, minerals, and trace elements. Unflavoured (flavouring: see *FlavourPac®* sachets, p. 903), net price 30 × 20-g sachets = £148.59.

Nutritional supplement for the dietary management of maple syrup urine disease in children 1–10 years

**¹MSUD Maxamaid®** (SHS)

Powder, protein equivalent (essential and non-essential amino acids except isoleucine, leucine, and valine) 25 g, carbohydrate 51 g, fat less than 500 mg, energy 1311 kJ (309 kcal)/100 g, with vitamins, minerals, and trace elements. Unflavoured, (flavouring: see *Modjul® Flavour System*, p. 903), net price 500 g = £76.94.

Nutritional supplement for the dietary management of maple syrup urine disease

**³MSUD Maxamum®** (SHS)

Powder, protein equivalent (essential and non-essential amino acids except isoleucine, leucine, and valine) 39 g, carbohydrate 34 g, fat less than 500 mg, energy 1260 kJ (297 kcal)/100 g, with vitamins, minerals, and trace elements. Orange flavour or unflavoured (flavouring: see *Modjul® Flavour System*, p. 903), net price 500 g = £123.34.

Nutritional supplement for the dietary management of maple syrup urine disease

**Valine Amino Acid Supplement** (Vitaflo)

Powder, valine 50 mg, carbohydrate 4 g, fat nil, energy 64 kJ (15 kcal)/4 g, net price 30 × 4-g sachets = £43.50

Nutritional supplement for the dietary management of maple syrup urine disease and other inborn errors of amino acid metabolism in children over 1 year and adults

◢ **Methylmalonic or propionic acidaemia**

**²XMTVI Analog** (SHS)

Powder, protein equivalent (essential and non-essential amino acids except methionine, threonine, and valine, and low isoleucine) 13 g, carbohydrate 54 g, fat 23 g, energy 1990 kJ (475 kcal)/100 g, with vitamins, minerals, and trace elements; *standard dilution* (15%) provides protein equivalent 1.95 g, carbohydrate 8.1 g, fat 3.5 g, energy 300 kJ (72 kcal)/100 mL. Unflavoured, net price 400 g = £28.22 (5-g measuring scoop provided).

Nutritional supplement for the dietary management of methylmalonic acidaemia or propionic acidaemia

**XMTVI Asadon** (SHS)

Powder, protein equivalent (essential and non-essential amino acids except methionine, threonine, and valine, and low isoleucine) 77 g, carbohydrate 4.5 g, fat nil, energy 1386 kJ (326 kcal)/100 g, with vitamins, minerals, and trace elements. Unflavoured, (flavouring: see *Modjul® Flavour System*, p. 903), net price 200 g = £58.29.

Nutritional supplement for the dietary management of methylmalonic acidaemia or propionic acidaemia in children and adults

**¹XMTVI Maxamaid** (SHS)

Powder, protein equivalent (essential and non-essential amino acids except methionine, threonine, and valine, and low isoleucine) 25 g, carbohydrate 51 g, fat less than 500 mg, energy 1311 kJ (309 kcal)/100 g, with vitamins, minerals, and trace elements. Unflavoured, (flavouring: see *Modjul® Flavour System*, p. 903), net price 500 g = £76.94.

Nutritional supplement for the dietary management of methylmalonic acidaemia or propionic acidaemia

---

1. Maxamaid products are generally intended for use in children 1–8 years
2. Analog products are generally intended for use in children up to 1 year

3. Maxamum products are generally intended for use in children over 8 years and adults

[1]**XMTVI Maxamum®** (SHS)

Powder, protein equivalent (essential and non-essential amino acids except methionine, threonine, and valine, and low isoleucine) 39 g, carbohydrate 34 g, fat less than 500 mg, energy 1260 kJ (297 kcal)/100 g, with vitamins, minerals, and trace elements. Unflavoured (flavouring: see *Modjul® Flavour System*, p. 903), net price 500 g = £123.34.

Nutritional supplement for the dietary management of methyl-malonic acidaemia or propionic acidaemia

◢**Other inborn errors of metabolism**

**Cystine Amino Acid Supplement** (Vitaflo)

Powder, cystine 500 mg, carbohydrate 3.4 g, fat nil, energy 63 kJ (15 kcal)/4 g, net price 30 x 4-g sachets = £43.50

Nutritional supplement for the dietary management of inborn errors of amino acid metabolism in children over 1 year and adults

**EAA® Supplement** (Vitaflo)

Powder, protein equivalent (essential amino acids) 5 g, carbohydrate 4 g, fat nil, energy 151 kJ (36 kcal)/12.5 g, with vitamins, minerals, and trace elements. Tropical flavour, net price 50 x 12.5-g sachets = £170.64

Nutritional supplement for the dietary management of disorders of protein metabolism including urea cycle disorders. Not suitable for children under 3 years

**KeyOmega®** (Vitaflo)

Powder, protein (cows' milk, soya) 170 mg, carbohydrate 2.8 g, fat 800 mg (of which arachidonic acid 200 mg, doco-sahexaenoic acid 100 mg), energy 80 kJ (19 kcal)/4 g, net price 30 × 4-g sachet = £32.30

A nutritional supplement for the dietary management of inborn errors of metabolism

**Leucine Amino Acid Supplement** (Vitaflo)

Powder, leucine 0.1 g, carbohydrate 4 g, fat nil, energy 64 kJ (15 kcal)/4 g, net price 30 x 4-g sachets = £43.50

Nutritional supplement for the dietary management of inborn errors of amino acid metabolism in children over 1 year and adults

**Phenylalanine Amino Acid Supplement** (Vitaflo)

Powder, phenylalanine 50 mg, carbohydrate 3.8 g, energy 64 kJ (15 kcal)/4 g, net price 30 × 4-g sachets = £43.50

Nutritional supplement for use in the dietary management of inborn errors of metabolism only

◢**Phenylketonuria**

**Add-Ins®** (SHS)

Powder, protein equivalent (containing essential and non-essential amino acids except phenylalanine) 10 g, carbohy-drate nil, fat 5.1 g, energy 359 kJ (86 kcal)/18.2-g sachet, with vitamins, minerals, and trace elements. Unflavoured (flavouring: see *Modjul® Flavour System*, p. 903), net price 60 × 18.2-g sachets = £294.00.

Nutritional supplement for the dietary management of proven phenylketonuria. Not suitable for children under 4 years

**Easiphen®** (SHS)

Liquid, protein equivalent (containing essential and non-essential amino acids except phenylalanine) 6.7 g, carbohy-drate 5.1 g, fat 2 g, energy 275 kJ (65 kcal)/100 mL with vitamins, minerals, and trace elements. Forest berries, orange, or tropical flavour, net price 250-mL carton = £7.56.

Nutritional supplement for the dietary management of proven phenylketonuria. Not suitable for children under 8 years

**Lophlex®** (SHS)

Powder, protein equivalent (containing essential and non-essential amino acids except phenylalanine) 20 g, carbohy-drate 2.5 g, fat 60 mg, fibre 220 mg, energy[2] 385 kJ (91 kcal)/27.8-g sachet, with vitamins, minerals, and trace elements. Flavours: berry, orange or unflavoured, net price 30 × 27.8-g sachets = £226.87.

Nutritional supplement for the dietary management of proven phenylketonuria in children over 8 years and adults including pregnant women

1. Maxamum products are generally intended for use in children over 8 years and adults
2. Minor nutritional variations between flavours—consult product literature

**Lophlex® LQ** (SHS)

Liquid, protein equivalent (containing essential and non-essential amino acids except phenylalanine) 20 g, carbohy-drate 8.8 g, fibre 340 mg, energy 490 kJ (115 kcal)/125 mL, with vitamins, minerals, and trace elements. Flavours: berry, citrus, or orange, net price 3 × 125 mL = £24.27.

Nutritional supplement for the dietary management of phenyl-ketonuria in children over 8 years and adults including pregnant women

**Lophlex® LQ 10** (SHS)

Liquid, protein equivalent (containing essential and non-essential amino acids except phenylalanine) 10 g, carbohy-drate 4.4 g, fibre 170 mg, energy 245 kJ (58 kcal)/62.5 mL, with vitamins, minerals, and trace elements. Berry flavour, net price 60 × 62.5 mL = £243.00.

Nutritional supplement for dietary management of phenylketon-uria in children over 4 years and adults including pregnant women

**Loprofin® PKU Drink** (SHS)

Liquid, protein (cows' milk) 400 mg (phenylalanine 10 mg), lactose 9.4 g, fat 2 g, energy 165 kJ (40 kcal)/100 mL. Net price 200-mL carton = 60p.

Nutritional supplement for the dietary management of phenyl-ketonuria in children over 1 year and adults

**Milupa PKU 2-prima®** (Milupa)

Powder, protein equivalent (essential and non-essential amino acids except phenylalanine) 60 g, carbohydrate 10 g, fat nil, energy 1190 kJ (280 kcal)/100 g, with vitamins, minerals, and trace elements. Vanilla flavour, net price 500 g = £122.70

Nutritional supplement for the dietary management of phenyl-ketonuria in children 1–8 years

**Milupa PKU 2-secunda®** (Milupa)

Powder, protein equivalent (essential and non-essential amino acids except phenylalanine) 70 g, carbohydrate 6.8 g, fat nil, energy 1306 kJ (307 kcal)/100 g, with vitamins, minerals, and trace elements. Vanilla flavour, net price 500 g = £143.15

Nutritional supplement for the dietary management of phenyl-ketonuria in children 9–14 years

**Milupa PKU 3-advanta®** (Milupa)

Powder, protein equivalent (essential and non-essential amino acids except phenylalanine) 70 g, carbohydrate 4.7 g, fat nil, energy 1270 kJ (299 kcal)/100 g, with vitamins, minerals, and trace elements. Vanilla flavour, net price 500 g = £143.15

Nutritional supplement for the dietary management of phenyl-ketonuria in patients 15 years and over

**Minaphlex®** (SHS)

Liquid, protein equivalent (essential and non-essential amino acids except phenylalanine) 8.4 g, carbohydrate 9.9 g, fat 3.9 g, energy 455 (108 kcal)/29-g sachet, with vitamins, minerals, and trace elements. Chocolate, pineapple-vanilla. Unflavoured (carbohydrate 11 g, energy 474 kJ (113 kcal)/29-g sachet), net price 30 × 29-g sachets = £98.92.

Nutritional supplement for the dietary management of phenyl-ketonuria in children 1–10 years

**Phlexy-10® Exchange System** (SHS)

Bar, protein equivalent (essential and non-essential amino acids except phenylalanine) 8.33 g, carbohydrate 20.5 g, fat 3.7 g, fibre 1.7 g/42-g bar. Citrus fruit flavour. Net price per bar = £4.76

Capsules, protein equivalent (essential and non-essential amino acids except phenylalanine) 416.5 mg/capsule. Net price 200-cap pack = £33.33

Tablets, protein equivalent (essential and non-essential amino acids except phenylalanine), 833 mg/tablet. Net price 75-tab pack = £21.59

Drink Mix, powder, protein equivalent (essential and non-essential amino acids except phenylalanine) 8.33 g, carbo-hydrate 8.8 g/20-g sachet. Apple-black currant, citrus, or tropical flavour. Net price 30 × 20-g sachet = £100.51

Nutritional supplement for the dietary management of phenyl-ketonuria

**Phlexy-Vits®** (SHS)

Powder, vitamins, minerals, and trace elements, net price 30 × 7-g sachets = £56.08.

Tablets, vitamins, minerals, and trace elements, net price 180-tab pack = £68.69.

For use as a vitamin and mineral component of restricted therapeutic diets in children 11 years and over and adults with phenylketonuria and similar amino acid abnormalities

**PK Aid-4®** (SHS)

Powder, protein equivalent (essential and non-essential amino acids except phenylalanine) 79 g, carbohydrate 4.5 g, fat nil, energy 1420 kJ (334 kcal)/100 g. Unflavoured, (flavouring: see *Modjul® Flavour System*, p. 903), net price 500 g = £112.04 (5-g measuring scoop provided).

Nutritional supplement for the dietary management of phenylketonuria in children and adults

**PKU Anamix Junior LQ®** (SHS)

Liquid, protein equivalent (essential and non-essential amino acids except phenylalanine) 10 g, carbohydrate 8.8 g, fat 4.8 g, fibre 310 mg, energy 497 kJ (118 kcal)/125 mL, with vitamins, minerals, and trace elements. Lactose-free. Flavours: Berry or orange, net price 125-mL carton = £4.50

Nutritional supplement for the dietary management of phenylketonuria in children 1–10 years

**PKU cooler10®** (Vitaflo)

Liquid, protein equivalent (essential and non-essential amino acids except phenylalanine) 10 g, carbohydrate 5.1 g, energy 258 kJ (62 kcal)/87-mL pouch, with vitamins, minerals, and trace elements. Orange or purple option. Net price 30 × 87 mL = £110.40.

Nutritional supplement for the dietary management of phenylketonuria. Not recommended for children under 3 years

**PKU cooler15®** (Vitaflo)

Liquid, protein equivalent (essential and non-essential amino acids except phenylalanine) 15 g, carbohydrate 7.8 g, energy 386 kJ (92 kcal)/130-mL pouch, with vitamins, minerals, and trace elements. Orange or purple option, net price 30 x 130 mL = £164.40.

Nutritional supplement for the dietary management of phenylketonuria, not recommended for children under 3 years

**PKU cooler20®** (Vitaflo)

Liquid, protein equivalent (essential and non-essential amino acids except phenylalanine) 20 g, carbohydrate 10.2 g, energy 517 kJ (124 kcal)/174-mL pouch, with vitamins, minerals, and trace elements. Orange or purple option. Net price 30 × 174 mL = £220.50.

Nutritional supplement for the dietary management of phenylketonuria. Not recommended for children under 3 years

**PKU express®** (Vitaflo)

Powder, protein equivalent (essential and non-essential amino acids except phenylalanine) 15 g, carbohydrate 3.8 g, energy 315 kJ (76 kcal)/25-g sachet, with vitamins, minerals, and trace elements. Lemon, orange, tropical or unflavoured (flavouring: see *Flavour Pac®*, p. 903), net price 30 x 25-g sachets = £161.21.

Nutritional supplement for the dietary management of phenylketonuria. Not recommended for children under 8 years

**PKU gel®** (Vitaflo)

Powder, protein equivalent (essential and non-essential amino acids except phenylalanine) 8.4 g, carbohydrate 8.6 g, fat less than 100 mg, energy 286 kJ (68 kcal)/20-g sachet with vitamins, minerals, and trace elements. Orange, raspberry, or unflavoured (flavouring: see *Flavour Pac®*, p. 903), net price 30 × 20-g sachets = £92.94.

Nutritional supplement for use as part of the low-protein dietary management of phenylketonuria in children 1–10 years.

**PKU Start®** (Vitaflo)

Liquid, protein equivalent (essential and non-essential amino acids except phenylalanine) 2 g, carbohydrate 8.3 g, fat 2.9 g, energy 286 kJ (68 kcal)/100 mL with vitamins, minerals, and trace elements. Contains lactose and fish oil. Net price 500-mL bottle = £5.46

Nutritional supplement for the dietary management of phenylketonuria in children under 1 year

**L-Tyrosine** (SHS)

Powder, net price 100 g = £12.53.

For use as a supplement in maternal phenylketonurics who have low plasma tyrosine concentrations

**¹XP Analog** (SHS)

Powder, protein equivalent (essential and non-essential amino acids except phenylalanine) 13 g, carbohydrate 54 g, fat 23 g (of which LCT 95%), energy 1990 kJ (475 kcal)/100 g, with vitamins, minerals, and trace elements; *standard dilution* (15%) provides protein equivalent 1.95 g, carbohydrate 8.1 g, fat 3.5 g, energy 300 kJ (72 kcal)/100 mL, net price 400 g = £22.54 (5-g measuring scoop provided)

Nutritional supplement for the dietary management of phenylketonuria in children under 1 year

**XP Analog LCP** (SHS)

Powder, protein equivalent (essential and non-essential amino acids except phenylalanine) 13 g, carbohydrate 54 g, fat 23 g (of which LCT 98.7%), energy 1990 kJ (475 kcal)/100 g, with vitamins, minerals, and trace elements; *standard dilution* (15%) provides protein equivalent 1.95 g, carbohydrate 8.1 g, fat 3.5 g, energy 300 kJ (72 kcal)/100 mL, net price 400 g = £25.64 (5-g measuring scoop provided)

Nutritional supplement for the dietary management of phenylketonuria in children under 1 year

**²XP Maxamaid** (SHS)

Powder, protein equivalent (essential and non-essential amino acids except phenylalanine) 25 g, carbohydrate 51 g, fat less than 500 mg, energy 1311 kJ (309 kcal)/100 g, with vitamins, minerals, and trace elements. Orange flavour or unflavoured (flavouring: see *Modjul® Flavour System*, p. 903), net price 500 g = £45.52

Nutritional supplement for the dietary management of phenylketonuria in children 1–8 years

**³XP Maxamum®** (SHS)

Powder, protein equivalent (essential and non-essential amino acids except phenylalanine) 39 g, carbohydrate 34 g, fat less than 500 mg, energy 1260 kJ (297 kcal)/100 g, with vitamins, minerals, and trace elements. Flavours: orange, unflavoured (flavouring: see *Modjul® Flavour System*, p. 903). Net price 30 × 50-g sachets = £211.14, 500 g = £70.39.

Nutritional supplement for the dietary management of phenylketonuria in children over 8 years and adults

## ◢Tyrosinaemia

**TYR cooler®** (Vitaflo)

Liquid, protein equivalent (essential and non-essential amino acids except tyrosine and phenylalanine) 15 g, carbohydrate 7.8 g, fat nil, energy 386 kJ (92 kcal)/130 mL, with vitamins, minerals, and trace elements. Orange flavour, net price 30 x 130-mL pouch = £271.20.

Nutritional supplement for the dietary management of tyrosinaemia in children over 8 years and adults

**TYR express®** (Vitaflo)

Powder, protein equivalent (essential and non-essential amino acids except tyrosine and phenylalanine) 15 g, carbohydrate 3.8 g, fat less than 100 mg, energy 315 kJ (76 kcal)/25 g, with vitamins, minerals, and trace elements. Unflavoured (flavouring: see *FlavourPac®* sachets, p. 903), net price 30 × 25-g sachets = £265.90

Nutritional supplement for the dietary management of tyrosinaemia. Not recommended for children under 8 years

1. Analog products are generally intended for use in children up to 1 year
2. Maxamaid products are generally intended for use in children 1–8 years
3. Maxamum products are generally intended for use in children over 8 years and adults

Appendix 7: Borderline substances

**TYR Gel®** (Vitaflo)

Gel, protein equivalent (essential and non-essential amino acids except tyrosine and phenylalanine) 8.4 g, carbohydrate 8.6 g, fat less than 100 mg, energy 286 kJ (68 kcal)/20 g, with vitamins, minerals and trace elements. Unflavoured (flavouring: see *Flavourpac®* sachets, p. 903), net price 30 × 20-g sachets = £148.59

Nutritional supplement for the dietary management of tyrosinaemia in children 1–10 years

**Tyrosine Amino Acid Supplement** (Vitaflo)

Powder, tyrosine 1 g, carbohydrate 2.9 g, energy 62 kJ (15 kcal)/4-g sachet, net price 30 × 4-g sachets = £37.80.

Nutritional supplement for the dietary management of tyrosinaemia and other inborn errors of amino acid metabolism

**¹XPHEN TYR Analog** (SHS)

Powder, protein equivalent (essential and non-essential amino acids except phenylalanine and tyrosine) 13 g, carbohydrate 54 g, fat 23 g (of which LCT 95%), energy 1990 kJ (475 kcal)/100 g, with vitamins, minerals, and trace elements; *standard dilution* (15%) provides protein equivalent 1.95 g, carbohydrate 8.1 g, fat 3.5 g, energy 300 kJ (72 kcal)/100 mL. Unflavoured, net price 400 g = £28.22.

Nutritional supplement for the dietary management of tyrosinaemia in children under 1 year

**²XPHEN TYR Maxamaid** (SHS)

Powder, protein equivalent (essential and non-essential amino acids except phenylalanine and tyrosine) 25 g, carbohydrate 51 g, fat less than 500 mg, energy 1311 kJ (309 kcal)/100 g with vitamins, minerals, and trace elements. Unflavoured (flavouring: see *Modjul® Flavour System*, p. 903). Net price 500 g = £76.94.

Nutritional supplement for the dietary management of tyrosinaemia in children 1–8 years

**XPHEN TYR Tyrosidon** (SHS)

Powder, protein equivalent (essential and non-essential amino acids except phenylalanine and tyrosine) 77 g, carbohydrate 4.5 g, fat nil, energy 1386 kJ (326 kcal)/100 g, with vitamins, minerals, and trace elements. Unflavoured (flavouring: see *Modjul® Flavour System*, p. 903). Net price 500 g = £145.76

Nutritional supplement for the dietary management of tyrosinaemia in children and adults where plasma-methionine concentrations are normal

**¹XPTM Analog** (SHS)

Powder, protein equivalent (essential and non-essential amino acids except phenylalanine, tyrosine, and methionine) 13 g, carbohydrate 54 g, fat 23 g (of whick LCT 95%), energy 1990 kJ (475 kcal)/100 g, with vitamins, minerals, and trace elements; *standard dilution* (15%) provides protein equivalent 1.95 g, carbohydrate 8.1 g, fat 3.5 g, energy 300 kJ (72 kcal)/100 mL. Unflavoured Net price 400 g = £28.22.

Nutritional supplement for the dietary management of tyrosinaemia type 1 in children under 1 year

**XPTM Tyrosidon** (SHS)

Powder, protein equivalent (essential and non-essential amino acids except phenylalanine, tyrosine, and methionine) 77 g, carbohydrate 4.5 g, fat nil, energy 1386 kJ (326 kcal)/100 g, with vitamins, minerals, and trace elements. Unflavoured (flavouring: see *Modjul® Flavour System*, p. 903). Net price 500 g = £145.76.

Nutritional supplement for the dietary management of tyrosinaemia type 1 in children and adults where plasma-methionine concentrations are above normal

◀**Urea cycle disorders (other than arginase deficiency)**

**L-Arginine** (SHS)

Powder, net price 100 g = £10.64.

Nutritional supplement for the dietary management of urea cycle disorders other than arginase deficiency, such as hyperammonaemia types I and II, citrullaemia, arginosuccinic aciduria, and deficiency of N-acetyl glutamate synthetase

## Conditions for which ACBS products can be prescribed

**Birthmarks** See Disfiguring skin lesions, below

**Dermatitis** Aveeno Bath Oil; Aveeno Cream; Aveeno Colloidal; Aveeno Lotion; E45 Emollient Bath Oil; E45 Emollient Wash Cream; E45 Lotion

For details of preparations see section 13.2.1, p. 625

**Dermatitis herpetiformis** See also Gluten-free foods, p. 903

**Disfiguring skin lesions (birthmarks, mutilating lesions, scars, vitiligo)** Covermark classic foundation and finishing powder; Dermacolor Camouflage cream and fixing powder; Keromask masking cream and finishing powder; Veil Cover cream and Finishing Powder. (Cleansing Creams, Cleansing Milks, and Cleansing Lotions are excluded)

For details of preparations see section 13.8.2, p. 654

**Disinfectants (antiseptics)** May be prescribed on an FP10 only when ordered in such quantities and with such directions as are appropriate for the treatment of patients, but not for general hygenic purposes.

**Dry mouth (xerostomia)** For patients suffering from dry mouth as a result of having (or having undergone) radiotherapy, or sicca syndrome.

AS Saliva Orthana; Biotène Oralbalance; BioXtra; Glandosane; Saliveze; Salivix.

For details of preparations see section 12.3.5, p. 621

**Eczema** See Dermatitis, above

**Photodermatoses (skin protection in)** Delph Sun Lotion SPF 30; E45 Sun SPF 50; Spectraban Ultra; Sunsense Ultra; Uvistat Lipscreen SPF 50, Uvistat Suncream SPF 30 and 50.

For details of preparations see section 13.8.1, p. 653

**Pruritus** See Dermatitis, above

---

1. Analog products are generally intended for use in children up to 1 year
2. Maxamaid products are generally intended for use in children 1–8 years

# A8 Wound management products and elasticated garments

**A8.1 Basic wound contact dressings 912**
**A8.1.1** Low adherence dressings — 912
**A8.1.2** Absorbent dressings — 913

**A8.2 Advanced wound dressings 913**
**A8.2.1** Hydrogel dressings — 913
**A8.2.2** Vapour-permeable films and membranes — 914
**A8.2.3** Soft polymer dressings — 915
**A8.2.4** Hydrocolloid dressings — 916
**A8.2.5** Foam dressings — 917
**A8.2.6** Alginate dressings — 918
**A8.2.7** Capillary-action dressings — 919
**A8.2.8** Odour absorbent dressings — 919

**A8.3 Antimicrobial dressings 919**
**A8.3.1** Honey — 920
**A8.3.2** Iodine — 920
**A8.3.3** Silver — 921
**A8.3.4** Other antimicrobials — 922

**A8.4 Specialised dressings 922**
**A8.4.1** Protease-modulating matrix dressings — 922
**A8.4.2** Silicone keloid dressings — 922

**A8.5 Adjunct dressings and appliances 923**
**A8.5.1** Surgical absorbents — 923
**A8.5.2** Wound drainage pouches — 923

**A8.6 Complex adjunct therapies 924**
**A8.6.1** Topical negative pressure therapy — 924

**A8.7 Wound care accessories 924**
**A8.7.1** Dressing packs — 924
**A8.7.2** Woven and fabric swabs — 924
**A8.7.3** Surgical adhesive tapes — 925
**A8.7.4** Adhesive dressings — 925
**A8.7.5** Skin closure dressings — 926

**A8.8 Bandages 926**
**A8.8.1** Non-extensible bandages — 926
**A8.8.2** Light-weight conforming bandages — 926

**A8.8.3** Tubular bandages and garments — 926
**A8.8.4** Support bandages — 927
**A8.8.5** Adhesive bandages — 928
**A8.8.6** Cohesive bandages — 928
**A8.8.7** Compression bandages — 928
**A8.8.8** Multi-layer compression bandaging — 929
**A8.8.9** Medicated bandages — 930

**A8.9 Compression hosiery and garments 930**
**A8.9.1** Graduated compression hosiery — 930
**A8.9.2** Lymphoedema garments — 931

**Wound dressings** The correct dressing for wound management depends not only on the type of wound but also on the stage of the healing process.
The principal stages of healing are:

- cleansing, removal of debris;
- granulation, vascularisation;
- epithelialisation.

The ideal dressing for moist wound healing needs to ensure that the wound remains:

- moist with exudate, but not macerated;
- free of clinical infection and excessive slough;
- free of toxic chemicals, particles or fibres;
- at the optimum temperature for healing;
- undisturbed by the need for frequent changes;
- at the optimum pH value.

As wound healing passes through its different stages, different types of dressings may be required to satisfy better one or other of these requirements. Under normal circumstances, a moist environment is a necessary part of the wound healing process; exudate provides a moist environment and promotes healing, but excessive exudate can cause maceration of the wound and surrounding healthy tissue. The volume and viscosity of exudate changes as the wound heals. There are certain circumstances where moist wound healing is not appropriate (e.g. gangrenous toes associated with vascular disease).

**Advanced wound dressings**, (section A8.2) are designed to control the environment for wound healing, for example to donate fluid (**hydrogels**), maintain hydration (**hydrocolloids**), or to absorb wound exudate (**alginates, foams**).

Appendix 8: Wound management

Practices such as the use of irritant cleansers and desloughing agents may be harmful and are largely obsolete; removal of debris and dressing remnants should need minimal irrigation with physiological saline.

Hydrogel, hydrocolloid, and medical grade honey dressings can be used to deslough wounds by promoting autolytic debridement; there is insufficient evidence to support any particular method of debridement for difficult-to-heal surgical wounds. Sterile larvae (maggots) are also available for biosurgical removal of wound debris.

There have been few clinical trials able to establish a clear advantage for any particular product. The choice between different dressings depends not only on the type and stage of the wound, but also on patient preference or tolerance, site of the wound, and cost. For further information, see *Buyers' Guide: Advanced wound dressings* (October 2008); NHS Purchasing and Supply Agency, Centre for Evidence-based Purchasing.

The table below gives suggestions for choices of primary dressing depending on the type of wound (a secondary dressing may be needed in some cases).

## A8.1 Basic wound contact dressings

## A8.1.1 Low adherence dressings

Low adherence dressings are used as interface layers under secondary absorbent dressings. Placed directly on the wound bed, non-absorbent, low adherence dressings are suitable for clean, granulating, lightly exuding wounds without necrosis, and protect the wound bed from direct contact with secondary dressings. Care must be taken to avoid granulation tissue growing into the weave of these dressings

**Tulle dressings** are manufactured from cotton or viscose fibres which are impregnated with white or yellow soft paraffin to prevent the fibres from sticking, but this is only partly successful and it may be necessary to change the dressings frequently. The paraffin reduces

**Appendix 8: Wound management**

### Wound contact material for different types of wounds

| Wound PINK (Epithelialising) | | |
|---|---|---|
| **Low Exudate** | **Moderate Exudate** | |
| Low adherence A8.1.1<br>Vapour-permeable film A8.2.2<br>Soft polymer A.8.2.3<br>Hydrocolloid A8.2.4 | Soft polymer A8.2.3<br>Foam, low absorbent A8.2.5<br>Alginate A8.2.6 | |

| Wound RED (Granulating)<br>Symptoms or signs of infection, see **Wounds with signs of infection** | | |
|---|---|---|
| **Low Exudate** | **Moderate Exudate** | **Heavy Exudate** |
| Low adherence A8.1.1<br>Soft polymer A8.2.3<br>Hydrocolloid A8.2.4<br>Foam, low absorbent A8.2.5 | Hydrocolloid-fibrous A8.2.4<br>Foam A8.2.5<br>Alginate A8.2.6 | Foam with extra absorbency A8.2.5<br>Hydrocolloid-fibrous A8.2.4<br>Alginate A8.2.6 |

| Wound YELLOW (Sloughy)<br>Symptoms or signs of infection, see **Wounds with signs of infection** | | |
|---|---|---|
| **Low Exudate** | **Moderate Exudate** | **Heavy Exudate** |
| Hydrogel A8.2.1<br>Hydrocolloid A8.2.4 | Hydrocolloid-fibrous A8.2.4<br>Alginate A8.2.6 | Hydrocolloid-fibrous A8.2.4<br>Alginate A8.2.6<br>Capillary-action A8.2.7 |

| Wound BLACK (Necrotic/Eschar)<br>Consider mechanical debridement alongside autolytic debridement | | |
|---|---|---|
| **Low Exudate or Dry** | **Moderate Exudate** | **Heavy Exudate** |
| Hydrogel A8.2.1<br>Hydrocolloid A8.2.4 | Hydrocolloid A8.2.4<br>Hydrocolloid-fibrous A8.2.4<br>Foam A8.2.5 | Seek advice from wound care specialist |

| Wounds with signs of infection<br>**Consider systemic antibacterials if appropriate;** also consider odour-absorbent dressings (section A8.2.8)<br>For malodourous wounds with slough or necrotic tissue, consider mechanical or autolytic debridement | | |
|---|---|---|
| **Low Exudate** | **Moderate Exudate** | **Heavy Exudate** |
| Low adherence with honey A8.3.1<br>Low adherence with iodine A8.3.2<br>Low adherence with silver A8.3.3<br>Hydrocolloid with silver A8.3.3<br>Honey—topical A8.3.1 | Hydrocolloid-fibrous with silver A8.3.3<br>Foam with silver A8.3.3<br>Alginate with silver A8.3.3<br>Honey—topical A8.3.1<br>Cadexomer–iodine A8.3.2 | Hydrocolloid-fibrous with silver A8.3.3<br>Foam, extra absorbent, with silver<br>A8.3.3<br>Alginate with honey A8.3.1<br>Alginate with silver A8.3.3 |

**Note** In each section of this table the dressings are listed in order of increasing absorbency. Some wound contact (primary) dressings require a secondary dressing absorbency of the dressing. Dressings with a reduced content of soft paraffin are less liable to interfere with absorption; those containing the traditional amount (such as *Jelonet*®) have been considered more suitable for skin graft transfer.

**Knitted viscose primary dressing** is an alternative to tulle dressings for exuding wounds; it can be used as the initial layer of multi-layer compression bandaging in the treatment of venous leg ulcers.

### Knitted Viscose Primary Dressing, BP 1993

Warp knitted fabric manufactured from a bright viscose monofilament.

N-A Dressing®, 9.5 cm × 9.5 cm = 35p, 9.5 cm × 19 cm = 66p (Systagenix)

N-A Ultra® (silicone-coated), 9.5 cm × 9.5 cm = 33p, 9.5 cm × 19 cm = 62p (Systagenix)

Paratex®, 9.5 cm × 9.5 cm = 24p (Urgo)

Profore® wound contact layer, 14 cm × 20 cm = 29p (S&N Hlth.)

Tricotex®, 9.5 cm × 9.5 cm = 31p (S&N Hlth.)

### Paraffin Gauze Dressing, BP 1993

(Tulle Gras). Fabric of leno weave, weft and warp threads of cotton and/or viscose yarn, impregnated with white or yellow soft paraffin, 10 cm × 10 cm, (light loading) = 25p; (normal loading) = 37p (most suppliers including Synergy Healthcare—*Paranet*® (light loading ); BSN Medical—*Cuticell*® *Classic* (normal loading); S&N Hlth.—*Jelonet*® (normal loading); Neomedic—*Neotulle*® (normal loading); C D Medical—*Paragauze*® (normal loading))

**Atrauman**® (Hartmann)

Non-adherent knitted polyester primary dressing impregnated with neutral triglycerides, 5 cm × 5 cm = 24p, 7.5 cm × 10 cm = 25p, 10 cm × 20 cm = 57p, 20 cm × 30 cm = £1.57

## A8.1.2 Absorbent dressings

**Perforated film absorbent dressings** are suitable only for wounds with mild to moderate amounts of exudate; they are **not** appropriate for leg ulcers or for other lesions that produce large quantities of viscous exudate.

◢**For lightly exuding wounds**
**Absorbent Perforated Dressing with Adhesive Border**
Low adherence dressing consisting of viscose and rayon absorbent pad with adhesive border.

Cosmopor E®, 5 cm × 7.2 cm = 7p, 8 cm × 10 cm = 16p, 8 cm × 15 cm = 25p, 10 cm × 20 cm = 41p, 10 cm × 25 cm = 51p, 10 cm × 35 cm = 71p (Hartmann)

Leukomed®, 7.2 cm × 5 cm = 8p, 8 cm × 10 cm = 17p, 8 cm × 15 cm = 30p, 10 cm × 20 cm = 40p, 10 cm × 25 cm = 45p, 10 cm × 30 cm = 58p , 10 cm × 35 cm = 67p (BSN Medical)

Medipore® +Pad, 5 cm × 7.2 cm = 7p, 10 cm × 10 cm = 15p, 10 cm × 15 cm = 24p, 10 cm × 20 cm = 36p, 10 cm × 25 cm = 45p, 10 cm × 35 cm = 62p (3M)

Medisafe®, 6 cm × 8 cm = 8p, 8 cm × 10 cm = 13p, 8 cm × 12 cm = 23p, 9 cm × 15 cm = 29p, 9 cm × 20 cm = 34p, 9 cm × 25 cm = 36p (Neomedic)

Mepore®, 7 cm × 8 cm = 10p, 10 cm × 11 cm = 20p, 11 cm × 15 cm = 34p, 9 cm × 20 cm = 41p, 9 cm × 25 cm = 57p, 9 cm × 30 cm = 65p, 9 cm × 35 cm = 71p (Mölnlycke)

PremierPore®, 5 cm × 7 cm = 5p, 10 cm × 10 cm = 12p, 10 cm × 15 cm = 18p, 10 cm × 20 cm = 32p, 10 cm × 25 cm = 36p, 10 cm × 30 cm = 45p, 10 cm × 35 cm = 52p (Shermond)

Primapore®, 6 cm × 8.3 cm = 16p, 8 cm × 10 cm = 18p, 8 cm × 15 cm = 30p, 10 cm × 20 cm = 40p, 10 cm × 25 cm = 46p, 10 cm × 30 cm = 57p, 10 cm × 35 cm = 88p (S&N Hlth)

Softpore®, 6 cm × 7 cm = 6p, 10 cm × 10 cm = 13p, 10 cm × 15 cm = 20p, 10 cm × 20 cm = 35p, 10 cm × 25 cm = 40p, 10 cm × 30 cm = 49p, 10 cm × 35 cm = 58p (Richardson)

Sterifix®, 5 cm × 7 cm = 18p, 7 cm × 10 cm = 30p, 10 cm × 14 cm = 53p (Hartmann)

Telfa® Island, 5 cm × 10 cm = 8p, 10 cm × 12.5 cm = 27p, 10 cm × 20 cm = 35p, 10 cm × 25.5 cm = 44p, 10 cm × 35 cm = 61p (Covidien)

**Absorbent Perforated Plastic Film Faced Dressing**
Low-adherence dressing consisting of 3 layers. Where no size specified by the prescriber, the 5 cm size to be supplied

Askina® Pad, 5 cm × 5 cm = 13p, 10 cm × 10 cm = 20p, 10 cm × 20 cm = 40p (Braun)

Cutisorb® LA, 5 cm × 5 cm = 8p, 10 cm × 10 cm = 14p, 10 cm × 20 cm = 29p (BSN Medical)

Interpose®, 5 cm × 5 cm = 9p, 10 cm × 10 cm = 15p, 10 cm × 20 cm = 32p (Frontier)

Melolin®, 5 cm × 5 cm = 16p, 10 cm × 10 cm = 25p, 20 cm × 10 cm = 49p (S&N Hlth)

Release®, 5 cm × 5 cm = 14p, 10 cm × 10 cm = 23p, 20 cm × 10 cm = 43p (Systagenix)

Skintact®, 5 cm × 5 cm = 10p, 10 cm × 10 cm = 17p, 20 cm × 10 cm = 34p (Robinson)

Solvaline N®, 5 cm × 5 cm = 9p, 10 cm × 10 cm = 16p, 10 cm × 20 cm = 33p (Activa)

Telfa®, 5 cm × 7.5 cm = 12p, 10 cm × 7.5 cm = 15p, 15 cm × 7.5 cm = 17p, 20 cm × 7.5 cm = 29p (Covidien)

◢**For moderately to heavily exuding wounds**
**Absorbent Cellulose Dressing with Fluid Repellent Backing**

Eclypse®, 15 cm × 15 cm = 97p, 20 cm × 30 cm = £2.14, 60 cm × 40 cm = £8.15, 80 cm × 50 cm = £9.35 (Advancis)

Exu-Dry®, 10 cm × 15 cm = £1.03, 15 cm × 23 cm = £2.11, 23 cm × 38 cm = £4.90 (S&N Hlth.)

Mesorb®, cellulose wadding pad with gauze wound contact layer and non-woven repellent backing, 10 cm × 10 cm = 58p, 10 cm × 15 cm = 75p, 10 cm × 20 cm = 93p, 15 cm × 20 cm = £1.32, 20 cm × 25 cm = £2.08, 20 cm × 30 cm = £2.36 (Mölnlycke)

Telfa Max®, 22.8 cm × 38 cm = £4.62, 38 cm × 45.7 cm = £5.61, 38 cm × 60.9 cm = £8.16 (Covidien)

Zetuvit® E, *non-sterile*, 10 cm × 10 cm = 6p, 10 cm × 20 cm = 8p, 20 cm × 20 cm = 13p, 20 cm × 40 cm = 25p; *sterile*, 10 cm × 10 cm = 19p, 10 cm × 20 cm = 22p, 20 cm × 20 cm = 35p, 20 cm × 40 cm = 98p (Hartmann)

**KerraMax**® (Ark Therapeutics)
Super absorbent polyacrylate primary dressing, 10 cm × 22 cm = £1.02, 20 cm × 22 cm = £1.80

## A8.2 Advanced wound dressings

**Advanced wound dressings** can be used for both acute and chronic wounds. Categories for dressings in this section (A8.2) start with the least absorptive, moisture-donating hydrogel dressings, followed by increasingly more absorptive hydrogel dressings. These dressings are classified according to their primary component; some dressings are comprised of several components

## A8.2.1 Hydrogel dressings

Hydrogel dressings are most commonly supplied as an amorphous, cohesive topical application that can take up the shape of a wound. A secondary, non-absorbent

Appendix 8: Wound management

dressing is needed. These dressings are generally used to donate liquid to dry sloughy wounds and facilitate autolytic debridement of necrotic tissue; some also have the ability to absorb very small amounts of exudate. Hydrogel products that do not contain propylene glycol should be used if the wound is to be treated with larval therapy.

Hydrogel sheets have a fixed structure and limited fluid-handling capacity; hydrogel sheet dressings are best avoided in the presence of infection, and are unsuitable for heavily exuding wounds

◢Hydrogel sheet dressings

**ActiFormCool®** (Activa)

Hydrogel dressing, 5 cm × 6.5 cm = £1.65, 10 cm × 10 cm = £2.43, 20 cm × 20 cm = £7.45, 10 cm × 15 cm = £3.49

**Aquaflo®** (Covidien)

Hydrogel dressing, 7.5 cm diameter = £2.55, 12 cm diameter = £5.26

**Coolie®** (Zeroderma)

Hydrogel dressing with lint backing, 7 cm diameter = £1.96

**Gel FX®** (Synergy Healthcare)

Hydrogel dressing (without adhesive border) 10 cm × 10 cm = £1.60, 15 cm × 15 cm = £3.20

**Geliperm®** (Geistlich)

Hydrogel sheets, 10 cm × 10 cm = £2.27

**Hydrosorb®** (Hartmann)

Absorbent, transparent, hydrogel sheets containing polyurethane polymers covered with a semi-permeable film, 5 cm × 7.5 cm = £1.43; 10 cm × 10 cm = £2.04; 20 cm × 20 cm = £6.12

Hydrosorb® comfort (with adhesive border, waterproof), 4.5 cm × 6.5 cm = £1.69; 7.5 cm × 10 cm = £2.24; 12.5 cm × 12.5 cm = £3.26

**Intrasite Conformable®** (S&N Hlth.)

Soft non-woven dressing impregnated with *Intrasite®* gel, 10 cm × 10 cm = £1.66; 10 cm × 20 cm = £2.23; 10 cm × 40 cm = £3.99

**Novogel®** (Ford)

Glycerol-based hydrogel sheets, 10 cm × 10 cm = £3.07; 30 cm × 30 cm, standard = £13.00, thin = £12.27; 5 cm × 7.5 cm = £1.95; 15 cm × 20 cm = £5.86; 20 cm × 40 cm = £11.16; 7.5 cm diameter = £2.79

**Vacunet®** (Protex)

Non-adherent, hydrogel coated polyester net dressing, 10 cm × 10 cm = £1.93, 10 cm × 15 cm = £2.86

◢Hydrogel application (amorphous)

**ActivHeal® Hydrogel** (MedLogic)

Hydrogel containing guar gum and propylene glycol, 15 g = £1.36

**Aquaform®** (Unomedical)

Hydrogel containing modified starch copolymer, 8 g = £1.57, 15 g = £1.91

**Askina® Gel** (Braun)

Hydrogel containing modified starch and glycerol, 15 g = £1.89

**Cutimed®** (BSN Medical)

Hydrogel, 8 g = £1.56, 15 g = £1.90, 25 g = £2.80

**Flexigran®** (A1 Pharmaceuticals)

Hydrogel containing starch polymer and glycerol, 15 g = £1.90

**GranuGel®** (ConvaTec)

Hydrogel containing carboxymethylcellulose, pectin, and propylene glycol, 15 g = £2.13

**Intrasite® Gel** (S&N Hlth.)

Hydrogel containing modified carmellose polymer and propylene glycol, 8-g sachet = £1.66, 15-g sachet = £2.22, 25-g sachet = £3.29

**Nu-Gel®** (Systagenix)

Hydrogel containing alginate and propylene glycol, 15 g = £2.05

**Purilon® Gel** (Coloplast)

Hydrogel containing carboxymethylcellulose and calcium alginate, 8 g = £1.61, 15 g = £2.10

## A8.2.2 Vapour-permeable films and membranes

Vapour-permeable films and membranes allow the passage of water vapour and oxygen but are impermeable to water and micro-organisms, and are suitable for lightly exuding wounds. They are highly conformable, provide protection, and a moist healing environment; transparent film dressings permit constant observation of the wound. Water vapour loss can occur at a slower rate than exudate is generated, so that fluid accumulates under the dressing, which can lead to tissue maceration and to wrinkling at the adhesive contact site (with risk of bacterial entry). Newer versions of these dressings have increased moisture vapour permeability. Despite these advances, vapour-permeable films and membranes are unsuitable for infected, large heavily exuding wounds, and chronic leg ulcers.

Vapour-permeable films and membranes are suitable for partial-thickness wounds with minimal exudate, or wounds with eschar. Most commonly, they are used as a secondary dressing over alginates or hydrogels; film dressings can also be used to protect the fragile skin of patients at risk of developing minor skin damage caused by friction or pressure.

### Vapour-permeable Adhesive Film Dressing, BP 1993 (Semi-permeable Adhesive Dressing)

Extensible, waterproof, water vapour-permeable polyurethane film coated with synthetic adhesive mass; transparent. Supplied in single-use pieces.

**ActivHeal® Film**, 6 cm × 7 cm = 31p, 10 cm × 12.7 cm = 73p, 15 cm × 17.8 cm = £1.78 (MedLogic)

**Askina® Derm**, 6 cm × 7 cm = 35p, 10 cm × 12 cm = £1.02, 10 cm × 20 cm = £1.94, 15 cm × 20 cm = £2.35, 20 cm × 30 cm = £4.20 (Braun)

**Bioclusive®**, 10.2 cm × 12.7 cm = £1.51 (Systagenix)

**Blisterfilm®**, 5 cm × 7.5 cm = 41p, 9 cm × 10 cm = 71p, 10 cm × 12.5 cm = 92p, 14 cm × 15 cm = £1.25 (Covidien)

**C-View®**, 6 cm × 7 cm = 39p, 10 cm × 12 cm = £1.08, 12 cm × 12 cm = £1.25, 15 cm × 20 cm = £2.47 (Unomedical)

**Episil®**, 12 cm × 12 cm = £1.10, 12 cm × 35 cm = £2.75, 15 cm × 20 cm = £2.10 (Advancis)

**Hydrofilm®**, 6 cm × 7 cm = 21p, 6 cm × 9 cm = 51p, 10 cm × 12.5 cm = 39p, 10 cm × 15 cm = 49p, 10 cm × 25 cm = 76p, 12 cm × 25 cm = 80p, 15 cm × 20 cm = 90p, 20 cm × 30 cm = £1.49 (Hartmann)

**Hypafix®** Transparent, 10 cm × 2 m = £8.15 (BSN Medical)

**Leukomed T®**, 7.2 cm × 5 cm = 35p, 8 cm × 10 cm = 65p, 10 cm × 12.5 cm = 95p, 11 cm × 14 cm = £1.15, 15 cm × 20 cm = £2.20, 15 cm × 25 cm = £2.35 (BSN Medical)

**Mepore® Film**, 6 cm × 7 cm = 43p, 10 cm × 12 cm = £1.14, 10 cm × 25 cm = £2.23, 15 cm × 20 cm = £2.83 (Mölnlycke)

**OpSite® Flexifix**, (non-sterile) 5 cm × 1 m = £3.59, 10 cm × 1 m = £6.05, *OpSite® Flexigrid*, 6 cm × 7 cm = 36p, 12 cm × 12 cm = £1.04, 15 cm × 20 cm = £2.62, (S&N Hlth)

Polyskin® II, 4 cm × 4 cm = 36p, 5 cm × 7 cm = 39p, 10 cm × 12 cm = £1.01, 10 cm × 20 cm = £2.00, 15 cm × 20 cm = £2.31, 20 cm × 25 cm = £4.03 (Covidien)

ProtectFilm®, 6 cm × 7 cm = 11p, 10 cm × 12 cm = 20p, 15 cm × 20 cm = 40p (Wallace Cameron)

Suprasorb F®, 5 cm × 7 cm = 31p, 10 cm × 12 cm = 73p, 15 cm × 20 cm = £2.30, (Activa)

Tegaderm®, 6 cm × 7 cm = 38p, 12 cm × 12 cm = £1.23, 15 cm × 20 cm = £2.34 (3M)

Vacuskin®, 6 cm × 7 cm = 40p, 10 cm × 12 cm = £1.06, 10 cm × 25 cm = £2.06, 15 cm × 20 cm = £2.19 (Protex)

◢**With absorbent pad**
**Vapour-permeable Adhesive Film Dressing with absorbent pad**

Alldress®, with absorbent pad, 10 cm × 10 cm = 88p, 15 cm × 15 cm = £1.92, 15 cm × 20 cm = £2.37 (Mölnlycke)

Hydrofilm® Plus, with absorbent pad, 5 cm × 7.2 cm = 15p, 9 cm × 10 cm = 20p, 9 cm × 15 cm = 22p, 10 cm × 20 cm = 34p, 10 cm × 25 cm = 36p, 10 cm × 30 cm = 53p (Hartmann)

*Leukomed T*® Plus, with absorbent pad, 7.2 cm × 5 cm = 25p, 8 cm × 10 cm = 50p, 8 cm × 15 cm = 75p, 10 cm × 20 cm = £1.25, 10 cm × 25 cm = £1.40, 10 cm × 30 cm = £2.35, 10 cm × 35 cm = £2.85 (BSN Medical)

Mepore® Ultra, with absorbent pad, 6 cm × 7 cm = 28p, 7 cm × 8 cm = 38p, 9 cm × 10 cm = 61p, 9 cm × 15 cm = 92p, 9 cm × 20 cm = £1.39, 9 cm × 25 cm = £1.54, 9 cm × 30 cm = £2.54, 10 cm × 11 cm = 74p, 11 cm × 15 cm = £1.10 (Mölnlycke)

OpSite® Plus, with absorbent pad, 5 cm × 5 cm = 29p, 9.5 cm × 8.5 cm = 81p, 10 cm × 12 cm = £1.10, 10 cm × 20 cm = £1.85, 35 cm × 10 cm = £3.07 (S&N Hlth)

Pharmapore-PU®, with absorbent pad, 8.5 cm × 15.5 cm = 20p, 10 cm × 25 cm = 38p, 10 cm × 30 cm = 58p (Wallace Cameron)

PremierPore VP®, with absorbent pad, 5 cm × 7 cm = 13p, 6 cm × 7 cm = 21p, 10 cm × 10 cm = 16p, 10 cm × 15 cm = 24p, 10 cm × 20 cm = 36p, 10 cm × 25 cm = 38p, 10 cm × 30 cm = 57p, 10 cm × 35 cm = 69p (Shermond)

Tegaderm®, with absorbent pad, 5 cm × 7 cm = 25p, 9 cm × 10 cm = 62p, 9 cm × 15 cm = 92p, 9 cm × 20 cm = £1.34, 9 cm × 25 cm = £1.51, 9 cm × 35 cm = £2.50 (3M)

◢**For intravenous and subcutaneous catheter sites**
**Central Gard®** (Unomedical)

16 cm × 7 cm (central venous catheter) = 94p, 16 cm × 8.8 cm (central venous catheter) = £1.03

**Easi-V®** (ConvaTec)

7 cm × 7.5 cm (intravenous peripheral cannula) = 38p

**IV3000®** (S&N Hlth.)

5 cm × 6 cm (1-hand) = 39p, 6 cm × 7 cm (non-winged peripheral catheter) = 51p, 7 cm × 9 cm (ported peripheral catheter) = 67p, 9 cm × 12 cm (PICC line) = £1.34, 10 cm × 12 cm (central venous catheter) = £1.28

**Mepore® IV** (Mölnlycke)

5 cm × 5.5 cm = 29p, 8 cm × 9 cm = 37p, 10 cm × 11 cm = 97p

**Niko Fix®** (Unomedical)

7 cm × 8.5 cm (intravenous ported peripheral catheter) = 19p

**Pharmapore-PU® IV** (Wallace Cameron)

8.5 cm × 7 cm = 7p, 6 cm × 7 cm (ported peripheral cannula) = 8p, 7 cm × 9 cm (peripheral cannula, hand) = 17p

**Tegaderm® IV** (3M)

7 cm × 8.5 cm (peripheral catheter) = 57p, 8.5 cm × 10.5 cm (central venous catheter) = £1.11, 10 cm × 15.5 cm (peripherally inserted central venous catheter) = £1.60

## A8.2.3 Soft polymer dressings

Dressings with soft polymer, often a soft silicone polymer, in a non-adherent layer are suitable for use on lightly to moderately exuding wounds. For moderately to heavily exuding wounds, an absorbent secondary dressing can be added, or a soft polymer dressing with an absorbent pad can be used.

Wound contact dressings coated with soft silicone have gentle adhesive properties and can be used on fragile skin areas or where it is beneficial to reduce the frequency of primary dressing changes.

Soft polymer dressings should not be used on heavily bleeding wounds; blood clots can cause the dressing to adhere to the wound surface.

For *silicone keloid dressings* see section A8.4.2.

**Mepitel®** (Mölnlycke)

Soft silicone wound contact dressing. 5 cm × 7 cm = £1.52, 8 cm × 10 cm = £3.05, 12 cm × 15 cm = £6.17, 20 cm × 30 cm = £16.61

**Physiotulle®** (Coloplast)

Non-adherent soft polymer wound contact dressing, 10 cm × 10 cm = £2.09, 15 cm × 20 cm = £6.37

**Silon-TSR®** (Jobskin)

Soft silicone polymer wound contact dressing, 13 cm × 13 cm = £3.52, 13 cm × 25 cm = £5.47, 28 cm × 30 cm = £7.37

**Siltex®** (Advancis)

Soft silicone-coated polyester wound contact dressing, 5 cm × 7 cm = £1.25, 8 cm × 10 cm = £2.55, 12 cm × 15 cm = £5.15, 20 cm × 30 cm = £13.25

**Tegaderm® Contact** (3M)

Non-adherent soft polymer wound contact dressing, 7.5 cm × 10 cm = £2.14, 7.5 cm × 20 cm = £4.20, 20 cm × 25 cm = £10.23

**Urgotul®** (Urgo)

Non adherent soft polymer wound contact dressing, 11 cm × 11 cm = £3.00, 10 cm × 40 cm = £9.89, 16 cm × 21 cm = £8.49

Urgotul® Start, soft polymer wound contact dressing, 5 cm × 7 cm = £2.80, 11 cm × 11 cm = £3.98, 16 cm × 21 cm = £9.50

◢**With absorbent pad**
**Allevyn® Gentle** (S&N Hlth.)

Soft gel wound contact dressing, with polyurethane foam film backing, 5 cm × 5 cm = £1.23, 10 cm × 10 cm = £2.43, 10 cm × 20 cm = £3.91, 15 cm × 15 cm = £4.40, 20 cm × 20 cm = £6.52

Allevyn® Gentle Border, silicone gel wound contact dressing, with polyurethane foam film backing, 7.5 cm × 7.5 cm = £1.43, 10 cm × 10 cm = £2.44, 12.5 cm × 12.5 cm = £3.14, 17.5 cm × 17.5 cm = £6.11, 23 cm × 23.2 cm (heel) = £8.95

**Eclypse® Adherent** (Advancis)

Soft silicone wound contact layer with absorbent pad and film-backing, 10 cm × 10 cm = £2.99, 10 cm × 20 cm = £3.75, 15 cm × 15 cm = £4.99, 20 cm × 30 cm = £9.99

**Episil® Absorbent** (Advancis)

Soft silicone wound contact dressing, with polyurethane foam film backing, 7.5 cm × 7.5 cm = £1.19, 10 cm × 10 cm = £2.16, 10 cm × 20 cm = £2.90, 10 cm × 30 cm = £4.25, 15 cm × 15 cm = £3.15, 15 cm × 20 cm = £4.10

**Flivasorb®** (Activa)

Absorbent polymer dressing with non-adherent wound contact layer, 10 cm × 10 cm = £2.09, 20 cm × 20 cm = £6.58, 10 cm × 20 cm = £3.50

**Appendix 8: Wound management**

**Mepilex®** (Mölnlycke)

Absorbent soft silicone dressing with polyurethane foam film backing, 10 cm × 11 cm = £2.53, 11 cm × 20 cm = £4.18, 15 cm × 16 cm = £4.59, 20 cm × 21 cm = £6.93, 20 cm × 50 cm = £27.24

Mepilex® Border, absorbent soft silicone dressing with polyurethane foam and adhesive border, 7 cm × 7.5 cm = £1.31, 10 cm × 12.5 cm = £2.59, 10 cm × 20 cm = £3.47, 10 cm × 30 cm = £5.21, 15 cm × 17.5 cm = £4.46, 17 cm × 20 cm = £5.78

Mepilex® Border Lite, thin absorbent soft silicone dressing with polyurethane foam and adhesive border, 4 cm × 5 cm = 88p, 7.5 cm × 7.5 cm = £1.33, 5 cm × 12.5 cm = £1.92, 10 cm × 10 cm = £2.42, 15 cm × 15 cm = £3.95; 18 cm × 18 cm (sacrum) = £4.56, 23 cm × 23 cm (sacrum) = £7.44; 13 cm × 20 cm (heel) = £5.15

Mepilex® Lite, thin absorbent soft silicone dressing with polyurethane foam, 6 cm × 8.5 cm = £1.69, 10 cm × 10 cm = £2.02, 15 cm × 15 cm = £3.92, 20 cm × 50 cm = £24.77

Mepilex® Transfer, soft silicone exudate transfer dressing, 7.5 cm × 8.5 cm = £2.10, 10 cm × 12 cm = £3.30, 15 cm × 20 cm = £9.89, 20 cm × 50 cm = £25.27

**Proguide®** (S&N Hlth.)

Non-adherent polyurethane wound contact layer with absorbent pad, 10 cm × 10 cm = £2.00

**Sorbion® Sana** (H&R)

Non-adherent polyethylene wound contact dressing with absorbent core, 8.5 cm × 8.5 cm = £4.93, 12 cm × 12 cm = £6.68, 12 cm × 22 cm = £12.37, 22 cm × 22 cm = £19.84

**UrgoCell®** (Urgo)

Non-adherent soft polymer wound contact dressing with polyurethane foam film backing, 10 cm × 12 cm = £4.44, 15 cm × 20 cm = £9.00; with adhesive border 13 cm × 13 cm = £4.44, 15 cm × 20 cm = £9.00

UrgoCell Start®, soft polymer wound contact dressing with polyurethane foam backing, 6 cm × 6 cm = £4.30, 10 cm × 10 cm = £5.95, 15 cm × 20 cm = £10.70

**Urgotul® Duo** (Urgo)

Non-adherent, soft polymer wound contact dressing with absorbent pad, 5 cm × 10 cm = £2.29, 10 cm × 12 cm = £3.54, 15 cm × 20 cm = £8.22

Urgotul® Duo Border, soft polymer wound contact dressing with absorbent pad and adhesive polyurethane film backing, 8 cm × 8 cm = £2.24, 10 cm × 12 cm = £3.47, 15 cm × 20 cm = £8.05

◢**Bio-cellulose dressings**

**Suprasorb® X** (Activa)

Biosynthetic cellulose fibre dressing, 5 cm × 5 cm = £1.87, 9 cm × 9 cm = £3.89, 14 cm × 20 cm = £7.71; 2 cm × 21 cm (rope) = £5.99

## A8.2.4 Hydrocolloid dressings

Hydrocolloid dressings are usually presented as a hydrocolloid layer on a vapour-permeable film or foam pad. Semi-permeable to water vapour and oxygen, these dressings form a gel in the presence of exudate to facilitate rehydration in lightly to moderately exuding wounds and promote autolytic debridement of dry, sloughy, or necrotic wounds; they are also suitable for promoting granulation.

Hydrocolloid-fibrous dressings made from modified carmellose fibres resemble alginate dressings; hydrocolloid-fibrous dressings are more absorptive and suitable for moderately to heavily exuding wounds.

◢**Without adhesive border**

**ActivHeal® Hydrocolloid** (MedLogic)

Semi-permeable polyurethane film backing, hydrocolloid wound contact layer, 5 cm × 7.5 cm = 75p, 10 cm × 10 cm =

£1.52, 15 cm × 15 cm = £3.31, 15 cm × 18 cm (sacral) = £3.84; with polyurethane foam layer, 5 cm × 7.5 cm = 94p, 10 cm × 10 cm = £1.49, 15 cm × 15 cm = £2.81, 15 cm × 18 cm (sacral) = £3.24

**Alione®** (Coloplast)

Semi-permeable hydrocolloid dressing without adhesive border, 10 cm × 10 cm = £2.96, 12.5 cm × 12.5 cm = £4.07, 12 cm × 20 cm = £5.34, 15 cm × 15 cm = £5.14, 20 cm × 20 cm = £7.68

**Askina® Biofilm Transparent** (Braun)

Semi-permeable, polyurethane film dressing with hydrocolloid adhesive, 10 cm × 10 cm = £1.02, 15 cm × 15 cm = £2.31, 20 cm × 20 cm = £3.02

**Comfeel® Plus** (Coloplast)

Hydrocolloid dressings containing carmellose sodium and calcium alginate. contour, 6 cm × 8 cm = £2.04, 9 cm × 11 cm = £3.54; ulcer, 4 cm × 6 cm = 88p, 10 cm × 10 cm = £2.25, 15 cm × 15 cm = £4.82, 18 cm × 20 cm (triangular) = £5.25, 20 cm × 20 cm = £6.94; transparent, 5 cm × 7 cm = 61p, 5 cm × 15 cm = £1.46, 5 cm × 25 cm = £2.37, 9 cm × 14 cm = £2.24, 9 cm × 25 cm = £3.18, 10 cm × 10 cm = £1.17, 15 cm × 15 cm = £3.06, 15 cm × 20 cm = £3.11, 17 cm × 17 cm (sacral) = £3.44, 20 cm × 20 cm = £3.13; pressure relieving, 7 cm diameter = £3.18, 10 cm = £4.26, 15 cm = £6.42

**DuoDERM® Extra Thin** (ConvaTec)

Semi-permeable hydrocolloid dressing, 5 cm × 10 cm = 71p, 7.5 cm × 7.5 cm = 73p, 10 cm × 10 cm = £1.21, 9 cm × 15 cm = £1.63, 9 cm × 25 cm = £2.61, 9 cm × 35 cm = £3.65, 15 cm × 15 cm = £2.61

DuoDERM® Signal, hydrocolloid dressing with 'Time to change' indicator, 10 cm × 10 cm = £1.97, 14 cm × 14 cm = £3.45, 20 cm × 20 cm = £6.86, 11 cm × 19 cm (oval) = £2.99, 18.5 cm × 19.5 cm (heel) = £4.82, 22.5 cm × 20 cm (sacral) = £5.64

**Flexigran®** (A1 Pharmaceuticals)

Semi-permeable hydrocolloid dressing without adhesive border, 10 cm × 10 cm = £2.19; thin, 10 cm × 10 cm = £1.08

**Granuflex®** (ConvaTec)

Hydrocolloid wound contact layer bonded to plastic foam layer, with outer semi-permeable polyurethane film, 10 cm × 10 cm = £2.56, 15 cm × 15 cm = £4.87, 15 cm × 20 cm = £5.27, 20 cm × 20 cm = £7.32

**Hydrocoll® Basic** (Hartmann)

Hydrocolloid dressing with absorbent wound contact pad, 10 cm × 10 cm = £2.23; thin, 7.5 cm × 7.5 cm = 63p, 10 cm × 10 cm = £1.05, 15 cm × 15 cm = £2.36

**NU DERM®** (Systagenix)

Semi-permeable hydrocolloid dressing, 5 cm × 5 cm = 83p, 10 cm × 10 cm = £1.53, 15 cm × 15 cm = £3.12, 20 cm × 20 cm = £6.24, 8 cm × 12 cm (heel/elbow) = £3.12, 15 cm × 18 cm (sacral) = £4.37; thin, 10 cm × 10 cm = £1.04

**Suprasorb® H** (Activa)

Semi-permeable hydrocolloid dressing, without adhesive border 10 cm × 10 cm = £1.54, 15 cm × 15 cm = £3.37; thin, 5 cm × 10 cm = 66p, 10 cm × 10 cm = £1.01, 15 cm × 15 cm = £2.31

**Tegaderm® Hydrocolloid** (3M)

Hydrocolloid dressing without adhesive border, 10 cm × 10 cm = £2.30, 15 cm × 15 cm = £4.46; thin, semi-permeable, clear film dressing with hydrocolloid, 10 cm × 10 cm = £1.51

**Ultec Pro®** (Covidien)

Semi-permeable hydrocolloid dressing; without adhesive border 10 cm × 10 cm = £2.23, 15 cm × 15 cm = £4.36, 20 cm × 20 cm = £6.56

◢**With adhesive border**

**Alione®** (Coloplast)

Semi-permeable hydrocolloid dressing with adhesive border, 10 cm × 10 cm = £2.96, 12.5 cm × 12.5 cm = £4.07, 12 cm × 20 cm = £5.34, 15 cm × 15 cm = £5.14, 20 cm × 20 cm = £7.68

**Granuflex® Bordered** (ConvaTec)

Hydrocolloid wound contact layer bonded to plastic foam layer, with outer semi-permeable polyurethane film, 6 cm × 6 cm = £1.63, 10 cm × 10 cm = £3.06, 15 cm × 15 cm = £5.88, 10 cm × 13 cm (triangular) = £3.61, 15 cm × 18 cm (triangular) = £5.62

**Hydrocoll® Border** (Hartmann)

Hydrocolloid dressing with adhesive border and absorbent wound contact pad, 5 cm × 5 cm = 92p, 7.5 cm × 7.5 cm = £1.51, 10 cm × 10 cm = £2.20, 15 cm × 15 cm = £4.13; 8 cm × 12 cm (concave) = £1.93; 12 cm × 18 cm (sacral) = £3.29

**Suprasorb® H** (Activa)

Semi-permeable hydrocolloid dressing with adhesive border, 14 cm × 14 cm = £2.27

**Tegaderm® Hydrocolloid** (3M)

Hydrocolloid dressing with adhesive border, 10 cm × 12 cm (oval) = £2.26, 13 cm × 15 cm (oval) = £4.22; 17.1 cm × 16.1 cm (sacral) = £4.71; *thin*, semi-permeable, clear film dressing with hydrocolloid 10 cm × 12 cm (oval) = £1.50; 13 cm × 15 cm (oval) = £2.81

**Ultec Pro®** (Covidien)

Semi-permeable hydrocolloid dressing with adhesive border, 21 cm × 21 cm = £4.58, 15 cm × 18 cm (sacral) = £3.23, 19.5 cm × 23 cm (sacral) = £4.88

◢**Hydrocolloid-fibrous dressings**
**Aquacel®** (ConvaTec)

Soft non-woven pad containing hydrocolloid-fibres, 4 cm × 10 cm = £1.38, 4 cm × 20 cm = £2.04, 4 cm × 30 cm = £3.05, 5 cm × 5 cm = £1.07; 10 cm × 10 cm = £2.54; 15 cm × 15 cm = £4.78; 2 cm × 45 cm (ribbon) = £2.59

**Versiva® XC** (ConvaTec)

Hydrocolloid gelling foam dressing, without adhesive border, 7.5 cm × 7.5 cm = £1.35, 11 cm × 11 cm = £2.25, 15 cm × 15 cm = £4.15, 20 cm × 20 cm = £6.20; with adhesive border, 10 cm × 10 cm = £2.30, 14 cm × 14 cm = £3.10, 19 cm × 19 cm = £4.95, 22 cm × 22 cm = £5.50, 18.5 cm × 20.5 cm (heel) = £5.50, 21 cm × 25 cm (sacral) = £5.90

◢**Polyurethane matrix dressing**
**Cutinova® Hydro** (S&N Hlth.)

Polyurethane matrix with absorbent particles and waterproof polyurethane film, 5 cm × 6 cm = £1.16, 10 cm × 10 cm = £2.33, 15 cm × 20 cm = £4.94

## A8.2.5 Foam dressings

Dressings containing hydrophilic polyurethane foam (adhesive or non-adhesive), with or without plastic film-backing, are suitable for all types of exuding wounds, but not for dry wounds; some foam dressings have a moisture-sensitive film backing with variable permeability dependant on the level of exudate

Foam dressings vary in their ability to absorb exudate; some are suitable only for lightly to moderately exuding wounds, others have greater fluid-handing capacity and are suitable for heavily exuding wounds. Saturated foam dressings can cause maceration of healthy skin if left in contact with the wound.

Foam dressings can be used in combination with other primary wound contact dressings. If used under compression bandaging or compression garments, the fluid-handling capacity of the foam dressing may be reduced. Foam dressings can also be used to provide a protective cushion for fragile skin.

◢**For lightly exuding wounds**
**Polyurethane Foam Film Dressing with Adhesive Border**

PolyMem®, 5 cm × 5 cm = 48p (Unomedical)

Tielle® Lite, 11 cm × 11 cm = £2.24; 7 cm × 9 cm = £1.19; 8 cm × 15 cm = £2.76; 8 cm × 20 cm = £2.91 (Systagenix)

◢**For lightly to moderately exuding wounds**
**Polyurethane Foam Dressing, BP 1993**

Lyofoam®, 7.5 cm × 7.5 cm = £1.02, 10 cm × 10 cm = £1.17, 10 cm × 17.5 cm = £1.88, 15 cm × 20 cm = £2.54

Suprasorb® M, 10 cm × 10 cm = £1.75, 10 cm × 20 cm = £3.09, 20 cm × 20 cm = £5.15 (Activa)

**Polyurethane Foam Film Dressing with Adhesive Border**

Suprasorb® P, 7.5 cm × 7.5 cm = £1.18, 10 cm × 10 cm = £1.28, 15 cm × 15 cm = £2.28 (Activa)

Tielle®, 11 cm × 11 cm = £2.33; 15 cm × 15 cm = £3.81, 18 cm × 18 cm = £4.85; 7 cm × 9 cm = £1.25, 15 cm × 20 cm = £4.77, 18 cm × 18 cm (sacral) = £3.53 (Systagenix)

**Polyurethane Foam Film Dressing without Adhesive Border**

ActivHeal FlexiPore®, self-adhesive, 6 cm × 7 cm = 93p; 10 cm × 10 cm = £1.73, 15 cm × 20 cm = £3.70; 20 cm × 20 cm = £5.06; 10 cm × 30 cm = £3.60 (MedLogic)

Allevyn® Lite, 5 cm × 5 cm = £1.04; 10 cm × 10 cm = £1.88; 10 cm × 20 cm = £3.22; 15 cm × 20 cm = £4.02 (S&N Hlth.)

Allevyn® Thin, self-adhesive, 5 cm × 6 cm = 98p, 10 cm × 10 cm = £1.98, 15 cm × 15 cm = £3.26, 15 cm × 20 cm = £3.96 (S&N Hlth)

Suprasorb® P, 5 cm × 5 cm = 92p, 7.5 cm × 7.5 cm = 98p, 10 cm × 10 cm = £1.15, 15 cm × 15 cm = £3.07 (Activa)

Transorbent®, self-adhesive, 5 cm × 7 cm = £1.00; 10 cm × 10 cm = £1.89; 15 cm × 15 cm = £3.47; 20 cm × 20 cm = £5.55 (Unomedical)

◢**For moderately to heavily exuding wounds**
**Polyurethane Foam Dressing**

Copa®, 5 cm × 5 cm = 70p, 7.5 cm × 7.5 cm = £1.19, 10 cm × 10 cm = £1.04, 12.5 cm × 12.5 cm = £1.77, 15 cm × 15 cm = £2.55, 20 cm × 20 cm = £2.95, 10 cm × 20 cm = £2.01, 0.5 cm × 7.5 cm (fenestrated) = 89p (Covidien)

**Polyurethane Foam Film Dressing with Adhesive Border**

ActivHeal® Foam Island, 10 cm × 10 cm = £1.57, 12.5 cm × 12.5 cm = £1.50, 15 cm × 15 cm = £1.92, 20 cm × 20 cm = £4.34 (MedLogic)

Avazorb® Border, 6 cm × 10 cm = £1.10, 8 cm × 12 cm = £1.90 (Advancis)

Allevyn® Adhesive, 7.5 cm × 7.5 cm = £1.39, 10 cm × 10 cm = £2.00, 12.5 cm × 12.5 cm = £2.50, 17.5 cm × 17.5 cm = £4.93, 22.5 cm × 22.5 cm = £3.89, 22.5 cm × 22.5 cm = £7.18; (sacral) 17 cm x 17 cm = £3.70, 22 cm x 22 cm = £5.32 (S&N Hlth.)

Allevyn® Plus Adhesive, 12.5 cm × 12.5 cm = £3.08; 17.5 cm × 17.5 cm = £5.93; 12.5 cm × 22.5 cm = £5.45; (sacral) 17 cm × 17 cm = £4.48, 22 cm × 22 cm = £6.49 (S&N Hlth)

Biatain® Adhesive, 10 cm × 10 cm = £1.62; 12 cm × 12 cm = £2.38, 18 cm × 18 cm = £4.77, 18 cm × 28 cm = £7.06, 23 cm × 23 cm (sacral) = £4.08, 19 cm × 20 cm (heel) = £4.76; 17 cm diameter (contour) = £4.59 (Coloplast)

Copa® Island, 10 cm × 10 cm = £1.51, 15 cm × 15 cm = £2.84, 20 cm × 20 cm = £5.36 (Coviden)

Lyofoam® Extra Adhesive, 9 cm × 9 cm = £1.27; 15 cm × 15 cm = £2.39; 22 cm × 22 cm = £4.70; 15 cm × 13 cm (sacral) = £1.95 (Medlock)

PermaFoam®, 16.5 cm × 18 cm (concave) = £ 3.67; 18 cm × 18 cm (sacral) = £3.02; 22 cm × 22 cm (sacral) = £3.47; *PermaFoam Comfort®* 8 cm × 8 cm = £1.02, 10 cm × 20 cm = £3.06, 11 cm × 11 cm = £1.94, 15 cm × 15 cm = £3.16, 15 cm × 20 cm = £4.59 (Hartmann)

*Appendix 8: Wound management*

Appendix 8: Wound management

PolyMem®, 5 cm × 7.6 cm = £1.07, 8.8 cm × 12.7 cm = £1.90, 10 cm × 13 cm = £2.06, 15 cm × 15 cm = £2.77, 16.5 cm × 20.9 cm = £6.25, 18.4 cm × 20 cm (sacral) = £4.28 (Unomedical)

Tegaderm® Foam Adhesive, 10 cm × 11 cm = £2.30, 14 cm × 14 cm = £3.40, 14 cm × 15 cm = £4.08, 19 cm × 22.5 cm = £6.69, 14 cm × 14 cm (heel) = £4.09 (3M)

Tielle® Plus, 11 cm × 11 cm = £2.58; 15 cm × 15 cm = £4.21; 15 cm × 20 cm = £5.28; 15 cm × 15 cm (sacrum) = £3.07; 20 cm × 26.5 cm (heel) = £4.37 (Systagenix)

Trufoam®, 11 cm × 11 cm = £2.16, 15 cm × 15 cm = £3.62, 7 cm × 9 cm = £1.13, 15 cm × 20 cm = £4.53 (Unomedical)

**Polyurethane Foam Film Dressing without Adhesive Border**

ActivHeal® Foam Non-Adhesive, 5 cm × 5 cm = 72p, 10 cm × 10 cm £1.09, 10 cm × 17.8 cm = £2.26, 20 cm × 20 cm = £3.78 (MedLogic)

Advazorb® Plus, 5 cm × 7.5 cm = 70p, 10 cm × 10 cm = £1.08, 15 cm × 15 cm = £2.10, 20 cm × 20 cm = £3.75 (Advancis)

Allevyn®, 5 cm × 5 cm = £1.18, 10 cm × 10 cm = £2.33, 10 cm × 20 cm = £3.75, 20 cm × 20 cm = £6.27, 10.5 cm × 13.5 cm (heel) = £4.68 (S&N Hlth.)

Allevyn® Cavity, circular, 5 cm diameter = £3.86, 10 cm diameter = £9.21; tubular, 9 cm × 2.5 cm = £3.75, 12 cm × 4 cm = £6.60 (S&N Hlth.)

Allevyn® Compression, 5 cm × 6 cm = £1.15; 10 cm × 10 cm = £2.36; 15 cm × 15 cm = £4.01, 15 cm × 20 cm = £4.49 (S&N Hlth.)

Allevyn® Plus Cavity, 5 cm × 6 cm = £1.74, 10 cm × 10 cm = £2.89, 15 cm × 20 cm = £5.79 (S&N Hlth.)

Askina® Foam, 10 cm × 10 cm = £2.06, 10 cm × 20 cm = £3.25, 20 cm × 20 cm = £5.43, 12 cm × 20 cm (heel) = £4.40; cavity dressing, 2.4 cm × 40 cm = £2.30 (Braun)

Biatain® Non-Adhesive, 10 cm × 10 cm = £2.20, 10 cm × 20 cm = £3.63, 15 cm × 15 cm = £4.05, 20 cm × 20 cm = £6.01; 5 cm × 7 cm = £1.21, 5 cm diameter = £1.13, 8 cm diameter = £1.59; *Biatain® Soft-Hold*, 10 cm × 10 cm = £2.39, 15 cm × 15 cm = £3.97, 5 cm × 7 cm = £1.21, 10 cm × 20 cm = £3.63 (Coloplast)

Copa® Plus, 5 cm × 5 cm = 80p, 7.5 cm × 7.5 cm = £1.39, 10 cm × 10 cm = £1.44, 12.5 cm × 12.5 cm = £2.20, 15 cm × 15 cm = £3.32, 20 cm × 20 cm = £3.96, 10 cm × 20 cm = £2.64, 8.5 cm × 7.5 cm (fenestrated) = £1.22 (Covidien)

Kerraboot®, (clear or white), foot-shaped, extra small = £14.38, small = £14.66, large = £14.66, extra large = £14.38 (Ark)

Lyofoam® Extra, 10 cm × 10 cm = £2.02, 17.5 cm × 10 cm = £3.43, 20 cm × 15 cm = £4.44 (Medlock)

PermaFoam®, 10 cm × 10 cm = £1.94, 10 cm × 20 cm = £3.32, 15 cm × 15 cm = £3.67, 20 cm × 20 cm = £5.61; 6 cm diameter = £1.00, 8 cm × 8 cm (fenestrated) = £1.14; cavity dressing, 10 cm × 10 cm = £1.84 (Hartmann)

PolyMem®, 8 cm × 8 cm = £1.50, 10 cm × 10 cm = £2.34, 13 cm × 13 cm = £3.90, 17 cm × 19 cm = £5.75, 10 cm × 61 cm = £12.39; *PolyMem® Max* 11 cm × 11 cm = £2.81 (Unomedical)

Tegaderm® Foam, 8.8 cm × 8.8 cm (fenestrated) = £2.14, 10 cm × 10 cm = £2.10, 10 cm × 20 cm = £3.57, 20 cm × 20 cm = £5.69, 10 cm × 60 cm = £12.05 (3M)

Tielle® Plus Borderless, 11 cm × 11 cm = £3.04; 15 cm × 20 cm = £5.51 (Systagenix)

Tielle® Xtra, 11 cm × 11 cm = £2.20; 15 cm × 15 cm = £3.30, 15 cm × 20 cm = £5.40 (Systagenix)

Trufoam® NA, 5 cm × 5 cm = £1.08, 10 cm × 10 cm = £2.05, 15 cm × 15 cm = £3.78 (Unomedical)

**Cavi-Care®** (S&N Hlth.)

Soft, conforming cavity wound dressing prepared by mixing thoroughly for 15 seconds immediately before use and allowing to expand its volume within the cavity. 20 g = £18.12

## A8.2.6 Alginate dressings

Non-woven or fibrous, non-occlusive, alginate dressings, made from calcium alginate, or calcium sodium alginate, derived from brown seaweed, form a soft gel in contact with wound exudate.

Alginate dressings are highly absorbent and suitable for use on exuding wounds, and for the promotion of autolytic debridement of debris in very moist wounds. Alginate dressings also act as a haemostatic, but caution is needed because blood clots can cause the dressing to adhere to the wound surface. Alginate dressings should not be used if bleeding is heavy and extreme caution is needed if used for tumours with friable tissue.

Alginate sheets are suitable for use as a wound contact dressing for moderately to heavily exuding wounds and can be layered into deep wounds; alginate rope can be used in sinus and cavity wounds to improve absorption of exudate and prevent maceration. If the dressing does not have an adhesive border or integral adhesive plastic film backing, a secondary dressing will be required.

**ActivHeal®** (MedLogic)

Activheal® Alginate, calcium sodium alginate dressing, 5 cm × 5 cm = 57p, 10 cm × 10 cm = £1.11, 10 cm × 20 cm = £2.73; cavity dressing, 2 cm × 30 cm = £2.05

ActivHeal Aquafiber®, non-woven, calcium sodium alginate dressing, 5 cm × 5 cm = 73p, 10 cm × 10 cm = £1.74, 15 cm × 15 cm = £3.28; cavity dressing, 2 cm × 42 cm = £1.75

**Algisite® M** (S&N Hlth.)

Calcium alginate fibre, non-woven dressing, 5 cm × 5 cm = 85p, 10 cm × 10 cm = £1.75, 15 cm × 20 cm = £4.71; cavity dressing, 2 cm × 30 cm = £3.18

**Algosteril®** (S&N Hlth.)

Calcium alginate dressing. 5 cm × 5 cm = 84p, 10 cm × 10 cm = £1.92, 10 cm × 20 cm = £3.25; cavity dressing, 2 g, 30 cm = £3.47

**Curasorb®** (Covidien)

Calcium alginate dressing, 5 cm × 5 cm = 70p, 10 cm × 10 cm = £1.49, 10 cm × 14 cm = £2.41, 10 cm × 20 cm = £2.93, 15 cm × 25 cm = £5.15, 30 cm × 61 cm = £27.03; cavity dressing, 30 cm = £2.84, 61 cm = £4.98, 91 cm = £5.36

Curasorb® Plus, calcium alginate dressing, 10 cm × 10 cm = £2.04

Curasorb® Zn, calcium alginate and zinc dressing, 5 cm × 5 cm = 80p, 10 cm × 10 cm = £1.68, 10 cm × 20 cm = £3.30

**Kaltostat®** (ConvaTec)

Calcium alginate fibre, non-woven, 5 cm × 5 cm, = 87p, 7.5 cm × 12 cm = £1.91, 10 cm × 20 cm = £3.77, 15 cm × 25 cm = £6.48; cavity dressing, 2 g = £3.54

**Melgisorb®** (Mölnlycke)

Calcium sodium alginate fibre, highly absorbent, gelling dressing, non-woven, 5 cm × 5 cm = 84p, 10 cm × 10 cm = £1.74, 10 cm × 20 cm = £3.27; cavity dressing, 32 cm × 2.2 cm, (2 g) = £3.30

**SeaSorb®** (Coloplast)

SeaSorb® Soft, alginate containing hydrocolloid dressing, highly absorbent, gelling dressing, 5 cm × 5 cm = 90p, 10 cm × 10 cm = £2.14, 15 cm × 15 cm = £4.05

SeaSorb® Soft Filler, calcium sodium alginate fibre, highly absorbent, gelling filler, 44 cm = £2.52

**Sorbalgon®** (Hartmann)

Calcium alginate dressing, 5 cm × 5 cm = 74p, 10 cm × 10 cm = £1.55; cavity dressing, 2 g, 32 cm = £3.17

**Sorbsan®** (Unomedical)

Sorbsan® Flat, calcium alginate fibre, highly absorbent, flat non-woven pads, 5 cm × 5 cm = 78p, 10 cm × 10 cm = £1.64, 10 cm × 20 cm = £3.08

Sorbsan® Plus, alginate dressing bonded to a secondary absorbent viscose pad, 7.5 cm × 10 cm = £1.66, 10 cm × 15 cm = £2.93, 10 cm × 20 cm = £3.74, 15 cm × 20 cm = £5.20

Sorbsan® Plus SA, alginate dressing with adhesive border and absorbent backing, 11.5 cm × 14 cm = £2.89, 14 cm × 19 cm = £4.22, 14 cm × 24 cm = £5.10, 19 cm × 24 cm = £6.40

Sorbsan® Ribbon, 40 cm (with probe) = £1.99

Sorbsan® Surgical Packing, 30 cm (2 g, with probe) = £3.41

**Suprasorb® A** (Activa)

Calcium alginate dressing, 5 cm × 5 cm = 57p, 10 cm × 10 cm = £1.12; cavity dressing, 2 g × 30 cm = £2.08

**Tegaderm® Alginate** (3M)

5 cm × 5 cm = 77p, 10 cm × 10 cm = £1.62; cavity dressing, 2 cm × 30 cm = £2.70

**Tielle® Packing** (Systagenix)

Tielle® Packing, 9.5 cm × 9.5 cm = £2.08

**Urgosorb®** (Urgo)

Alginate and hydrocolloid dressing without adhesive border, 5 cm × 5 cm = 81p, 10 cm × 10 cm = £1.93, 10 cm × 20 cm = £3.55; cavity dressing, 30 cm = £2.58

## A8.2.7 Capillary-action dressings

Capillary-action dressings consist of an absorbent core of hydrophilic fibres sandwiched between two low-adherent wound-contact layers to ensure no fibres are shed on to the wound surface. Wound exudate is taken up by the dressing and retained within the highly absorbent central layer.

The dressing may be applied intact to relatively superficial areas, but for deeper wounds or cavities it may be cut to shape to ensure good contact with the wound base. Multiple layers may be applied to heavily exuding wounds to further increase the fluid-absorbing capacity of the dressing. A secondary adhesive dressing is necessary.

Capillary-action dressings are suitable for use on all types of exuding wounds, but particularly on sloughy wounds where removal of fluid from the wound aids debridement; capillary-action dressings are contra-indicated for heavily bleeding wounds or arterial bleeding.

**Advadraw®** (Advancis)

Non-adherent dressing consisting of a soft viscose and polyester absorbent pad with central wicking layer between two perforated permeable wound contact layers. 5 cm × 7.5 cm = 56p, 10 cm × 10 cm = 87p, 10 cm × 15 cm = £1.17, 15 cm × 20 cm = £1.54

Advadraw Spiral®, 0.5 cm × 40 cm = 81p

**Cerdak® Basic** (CliniMed)

Non-adhesive wound contact sachet containing ceramic spheres, 5 cm × 5 cm = 70p, 10 cm × 10 cm = £1.56, 10 cm × 15 cm = £2.08; cavity dressing, 10 cm × 10 cm = £2.10, 10 cm × 15 cm = £2.63

Cerdak® Aerocloth, non-adhesive wound contact sachet containing ceramic spheres, with non-woven fabric adhesive backing, 5 cm × 5 cm = £1.37, 5 cm × 10 cm = £1.94

Cerdak® Aerofilm, non-adhesive wound contact sachet containing ceramic spheres, with waterproof transparent adhesive film backing, 5 cm × 5 cm = £1.51, 5 cm × 10 cm = £2.07

**Sumar®** (Lantor)

Sumar® Lite, for light to moderately exuding wounds and cavities, 5 cm × 5 cm = 93p, 10 cm × 10 cm = £1.59, 10 cm × 15 cm = £2.12

Sumar® Max, for heavily exuding wounds, 5 cm × 5 cm = 95p, 10 cm × 10 cm = £1.61, 10 cm × 15 cm = £2.15

Sumar®Spiral, 0.5 cm × 40 cm = £1.57

**Vacutex®** (Protex)

Low-adherent dressing consisting of two external polyester wound contact layers with central wicking polyester/cotton mix absorbent layer. 5 cm × 5 cm = 94p, 10 cm × 10 cm = £1.66, 10 cm × 15 cm = £2.23, 10 cm × 20 cm = £2.68, 15 cm × 20 cm = £3.14, 20 cm × 20 cm = £4.28

## A8.2.8 Odour absorbent dressings

Dressings containing activated charcoal are used to absorb odour from wounds. The underlying cause of wound odour should be identified. Wound odour is most effectively reduced by debridement of slough, reduction in bacterial levels, and frequent dressing changes.

Fungating wounds and chronic infected wounds produce high volumes of exudate. Many odour absorbent dressings are intended for use in combination with other dressings; odour absorbent dressings with a suitable wound contact layer can be used as a primary dressing.

**Askina® Carbosorb** (Braun)

Activated charcoal and non-woven viscose rayon dressing, 10 cm × 10 cm = £2.72, 10 cm × 20 cm = £5.25

**CarboFLEX®** (ConvaTec)

Dressing in 5 layers: wound-facing absorbent layer containing alginate and hydrocolloid; water-resistant second layer; third layer containing activated charcoal; non-woven absorbent fourth layer; water-resistant backing layer. 10 cm × 10 cm = £2.95, 8 cm × 15 cm = £3.55, 15 cm × 20 cm = £6.72

**Carbopad® VC** (Synergy Healthcare)

Activated charcoal non-absorbent dressing, 10 cm × 10 cm = £1.59, 10 cm × 20 cm = £2.15

**CliniSorb® Odour Control Dressings** (CliniMed)

Activated charcoal cloth enclosed in viscose rayon with outer polyamide coating. 10 cm × 10 cm = £1.75, 10 cm × 20 cm = £2.33, 15 cm × 25 cm = £3.75

**Lyofoam® C** (Medlock)

Lyofoam sheet with layer of activated charcoal cloth and additional outer envelope of polyurethane foam. 10 cm × 10 cm = £2.85, 15 cm × 20 cm = £6.47

**Sorbsan® Plus Carbon** (Unomedical)

Alginate dressing with activated carbon, 7.5 cm × 10 cm = £2.42, 10 cm × 15 cm = £4.70, 10 cm × 20 cm = £5.62, 15 cm × 20 cm = £6.47

## A8.3 Antimicrobial dressings

Spreading infection at the wound site requires treatment with systemic antibacterials.

For local wound infection, a topical antimicrobial dressing can be used to reduce the level of bacteria at the wound surface but will not eliminate a spreading infection. Some dressings are designed to release the antimicrobial into the wound, others act upon the bacteria after absorption from the wound. The amount of exudate present and the level of infection should be taken into account when selecting an antimicrobial dressing.

Appendix 8: Wound management

Medical grade honey (section A8.3.1), has anti-microbial and anti-inflammatory properties. Dressings impregnated with **iodine** (section A8.3.2), can be used to treat clinically infected wounds. Dressings containing **silver** (section A8.3.3), should be used only when clinical signs or symptoms of infection are present.

Dressings containing other **antimicrobials** (section A8.3.4) such as polihexanide (polyhexamethylene biguanide) or dialkylcarbamoyl chloride are available for use on infected wounds. Although hypersensitivity is unlikely with chlorhexidine impregnated tulle dressing, the antibacterial efficacy of these dressings has not been established.

## A8.3.1 Honey

**Medical grade honey** has antimicrobial and anti-inflammatory properties and can be used for acute or chronic wounds. Medical grade honey has osmotic properties, producing an environment that promotes autolytic debridement; it can help control wound malodour. Honey dressings should not be used on patients with extreme sensitivity to honey, bee stings or bee products. Patients with diabetes should be monitored for changes in blood-glucose concentrations during treatment with topical honey or honey-impregnated dressings.

◢**Sheet dressing**

**Actilite®** (Advancis)

Knitted viscose impregnated with medical grade manuka honey and manuka oil, 10 cm × 10 cm = 95p, 10 cm × 20 cm = £1.85

**Activon Tulle®** (Advancis)

Knitted viscose impregnated with medical grade manuka honey, 5 cm × 5 cm = £1.78, 10 cm × 10 cm = £3.01
Where no size stated by the prescriber the 5 cm size to be supplied

**Algivon®** (Advancis)

Absorbent, non-adherent calcium alginate dressing impregnated with medical grade manuka honey, 5 cm × 5 cm = £2.09, 10 cm × 10 cm = £3.53

**Medihoney®** (Medihoney)

Antibacterial Honey Tulle, woven fabric impregnated with medical grade manuka honey, 10 cm × 10 cm = £2.98

Gel sheet, sodium alginate dressing impregnated with medical grade honey, 5 cm × 5 cm = £1.75, 10 cm × 10 cm = £4.20

**Mesitran®** (Unomedical)

Hydrogel, semi-permeable dressing impregnated with medical grade honey, 10 cm × 10 cm = £2.51, 10 cm × 17.5 cm = £4.52, 15 cm × 20 cm = £5.22; *with adhesive border,* 10 cm × 10 cm = £2.61, 15 cm × 13 cm (sacral) = £4.42, 15 cm × 15 cm = £4.62

Mesitran® Mesh, hydrogel, non-adherent wound contact layer, without adhesive border, 10 cm × 10 cm = £2.41

◢**Honey-based topical application**

Medical grade honey is applied directly to the wound and covered with a primary low adherence wound dressing; an additional secondary dressing may be required for exuding wounds.

**Activon®** (Advancis)

Manuka honey, (medical grade), 25-g tube = £1.99

**Medihoney®** (Medihoney)

Antibacterial Medical Honey, honey (medical grade, *Leptospermum* sp.), 20-g tube = £3.96, 50-g tube = £9.90

Antibacterial Wound Gel, honey (medical grade, *Leptospermum* sp.), 80% in natural waxes and oils, 10-g tube = £2.69, 20-g tube = £4.02
Note *Antibacterial Wound Gel* is not recommended for use in deep wounds or body cavities where removal of waxes may be difficult

**Melladerm®** (Danetre)

Honey (medical grade; S. African, Fynbos) 45% in basis containing polyethylene glycol, 50-g tube = £7.50

Melladerm® Plus, honey (medical grade; Bulgarian, mountain flower) 45% in basis containing polyethylene glycol, 20-g tube = £4.49, 50-g tube = £8.50

**Mesitran®** (Unomedical)

Ointment, honey (medical grade) 47%, 15-g tube = £3.47, 50-g tube = £9.55
Excipients include lanolin

Ointment S, honey (medical grade) 40%, 15-g tube = £3.46
Excipients include lanolin

## A8.3.2 Iodine

**Cadexomer–iodine**, like povidone–iodine, releases free iodine when exposed to wound exudate. The free iodine acts as an antiseptic on the wound surface, the cadexomer absorbs wound exudate and encourages desloughing.

Two-component hydrogel dressings containing glucose oxidase and iodide ions generate a low level of free iodine in the presence of moisture and oxygen.

**Povidone–iodine fabric dressing** is a knitted viscose dressing with povidone–iodine incorporated in a hydrophilic polyethylene glycol basis; this facilitates diffusion of the iodine into the wound and permits removal of the dressing by irrigation. The iodine has a wide spectrum of antimicrobial activity but it is rapidly deactivated by wound exudate.

Systemic absorption of iodine may occur, particularly from large wounds or with prolonged use.

**Iodoflex®** (S&N Hlth.)

Paste, iodine 0.9% as cadexomer–iodine in a paste basis with gauze backing, 5-g unit = £3.73; 10 g = £7.46; 17 g = £11.81
Uses  for treatment of chronic exuding wounds; max. single application 50 g, max. weekly application 150 g; max. duration up to 3 months in any single course of treatment
Cautions  iodine may be absorbed, particularly from large wounds or during prolonged use; severe renal impairment; history of thyroid disorder
Contra-indications  children; patients receiving lithium; thyroid disorders; pregnancy and breast-feeding

**Iodosorb®** (S&N Hlth.)

Ointment, iodine 0.9% as cadexomer–iodine in an ointment basis, 10 g = £4.04; 20 g = £8.24

Powder, iodine 0.9% as cadexomer–iodine microbeads, 3-g sachet = £1.76
Uses  for treatment of chronic exuding wounds; max. single application 50 g, max. weekly application 150 g; max. duration up to 3 months in any single course of treatment
Cautions  iodine may be absorbed, particularly from large wounds or during prolonged use; severe renal impairment; history of thyroid disorder
Contra-indications  children; patients receiving lithium; thyroid disorders; pregnancy and breast-feeding

**Iodozyme®** (Insense)

Hydrogel (two-component dressing containing glucose oxidase and iodide ions), 10 cm × 10 cm = £12.50
Uses  antimicrobial dressing for lightly to moderately exuding wounds
Cautions  children; pregnancy and breast-feeding
Contra-indications  thyroid disorders; patients receiving lithium

**Appendix 8: Wound management**

### Oxyzyme® (Insense)

Hydrogel (two-component dressing containing glucose oxidase and iodide ions), 6.5 cm × 5 cm = £6.00, 10 cm × 10 cm = £10.00

**Uses** non-infected, dry to moderately exuding wounds

**Cautions** children; pregnancy and breast-feeding

**Contra-indications** thyroid disorders; patients receiving lithium

### Povidone–iodine Fabric Dressing

(Drug Tariff specification 43). Knitted viscose primary dressing impregnated with povidone–iodine ointment 10%, 5 cm × 5 cm = 32p; 9.5 cm × 9.5 cm = 47p (Systagenix—*Inadine*®)

**Uses** wound contact layer for abrasions and superficial burns

**Cautions** iodine may be absorbed particularly if large wounds treated; children under 6 months; thyroid disease

**Contra-indications** severe renal impairment; pregnancy; breast-feeding

## A8.3.3 Silver

Antimicrobial dressings containing **silver** should be used only when infection is suspected as a result of clinical signs or symptoms (see also p. 919). Silver ions exert an antimicrobial effect in the presence of wound exudate; the volume of wound exudate as well as the presence of infection should be considered when selecting a silver-containing dressing.

Dressings impregnated with silver sulfadiazine have broad antimicrobial activity; if silver sulfadiazine is applied to large areas, or used for prolonged periods, there is a risk of blood disorders and skin discolouration (see section 13.10.1.1). The use of silver sulfadiazine-impregnated dressings is contra-indicated in neonates, in pregnancy, and in patients with significant renal or hepatic impairment.

### ◢ Low adherence dressings

**Acticoat®** (S&N Hlth.)

Three layer antimicrobial barrier dressing consisting of a polyester core between low adherent silver coated high density polyethylene mesh, 5 cm × 5 cm = £3.22, 10 cm × 10 cm = £7.85, 10 cm × 20 cm = £12.28, 20 cm × 40 cm = £42.01

Acticoat® 7 five layer antimicrobial barrier dressing consisting of a polyester core between low adherent silver coated high density polyethylene mesh, 5 cm × 5 cm = £5.59, 10 cm × 12.5 cm = £16.65, 15 cm × 15 cm = £29.93

**Atrauman® Ag** (Hartmann)

Non-adherent polyamide fabric impregnated with silver and neutral triglycerides, 5 cm × 5 cm = 47p, 10 cm × 10 cm = £1.14, 10 cm × 20 cm = £2.23

### ◢ With charcoal

**Actisorb® Silver 220** (Systagenix)

Knitted fabric of activated charcoal, with one-way stretch, with silver residues, within spun-bonded nylon sleeve. 6.5 cm × 9.5 cm = £1.61, 10.5 cm × 10.5 cm = £2.53, 10.5 cm × 19 cm = £4.60

### ◢ Soft polymer dressings

**Mepilex® Ag** (Mölnlycke)

Soft silicone wound contact dressing with polyurethane foam film backing, with silver, 10 cm × 10 cm = £5.80, 10 cm × 20 cm = £9.57, 15 cm × 15 cm = £10.77, 20 cm × 20 cm = £15.96

**UrgoCell® Silver** (Urgo)

Non-adherent soft polymer wound contact dressing with polyurethane foam film backing, with silver, 6 cm × 6 cm = £4.00, 10 cm × 10 cm = £5.50, 15 cm × 20 cm = £9.90

### Urgotul® Silver (Urgo)

Non-adherent soft polymer wound contact dressing, with silver, 10 cm × 12 cm = £3.32, 15 cm × 20 cm = £9.03

Urgotul® Duo Silver, non-adherent, soft polymer wound contact dressing, with silver, 5 cm × 7 cm = £1.94, 11 cm × 11 cm = £3.85, 15 cm × 20 cm = £9.28

### ◢ Hydrocolloid dressings

**Aquacel® Ag** (ConvaTec)

Soft non-woven pad containing hydrocolloid fibres, (silver impregnated), 4 cm × 10 cm = £2.65, 4 cm × 20 cm = £3.46, 4 cm × 30 cm = £5.17, 5 cm × 5 cm = £1.81, 10 cm × 10 cm = £4.32, 15 cm × 15 cm = £8.13, 20 cm × 30 cm = £20.17; 2 cm × 45 cm (ribbon) = £4.34

**Biatain® Ag Hydrocolloid** (Coloplast)

Semi-permeable, antimicrobial barrier dressing with ionic silver (silver sodium thiosulphate), 10 cm × 10 cm = £6.72, 15 cm × 15 cm = £13.44

**Physiotulle® Ag** (Coloplast)

Non-adherent polyester fabric with hydrocolloid and silver sulfadiazine, 10 cm × 10 cm = £2.10

**Urgotul® SSD** (Urgo)

Non-adherent, polyester fabric with hydrocolloid and silver sulfadiazine, 11 cm × 11 cm = £2.97, 16 cm × 21 cm = £8.42

**Contra-indications** pregnancy, renal, or hepatic impairment, neonates

### ◢ Foam dressings

**Acticoat® Moisture Control** (S&N Hlth.)

Three layer polyurethane dressing consisting of a silver coated layer, a foam layer, and a waterproof layer, 5 cm × 5 cm = £6.58, 10 cm × 10 cm = £15.39, 10 cm × 20 cm = £29.99

**Allevyn® Ag** (S&N Hlth.)

Silver sulfadiazine impregnated polyurethane foam film dressing *with adhesive border*, 7.5 cm × 7.5 cm = £3.21, 10 cm × 10 cm = £5.06, 12.5 cm × 12.5 cm = £6.65, 17.5 cm × 17.5 cm = £12.79, 17 cm × 17 cm (sacral) = £9.99, 22 cm × 22 cm (sacral) = £13.38; *without adhesive border*, 5 cm × 5 cm = £3.00, 10 cm × 10 cm = £5.65, 15 cm × 15 cm = £10.71, 20 cm × 20 cm = £15.69, 10.5 cm × 13.5 cm (heel) = £9.99

**Cautions** large open wounds; sensitivity to sulphonamides; G6PD deficiency; significant hepatic or renal impairment; **interactions**: Appendix 1 (sulphonamides)

**Avance®** (Medlock)

Silver impregnated polyurethane foam film dressing, *without adhesive border*, 10 cm × 10 cm = £2.75, 10 cm × 17.5 cm = £4.38, 15 cm × 20 cm = £6.05; *with adhesive border*, 9 cm × 9 cm = £2.31, 12 cm × 12 cm = £3.83, 15 cm × 15 cm = £4.69, 15 cm × 13 cm (sacral) = £3.45

**Biatain® Ag** (Coloplast)

Silver impregnated polyurethane foam film dressing *with adhesive border*, 12.5 cm × 12.5 cm = £8.55, 18 cm × 18 cm = £17.14, 19 cm × 20 cm (heel) = £16.91, 23 cm × 23 cm (sacral) = £17.97; *without adhesive border*, 10 cm × 10 cm = £7.47, 5 cm × 7 cm = £3.07, 10 cm × 20 cm = £13.73, 15 cm × 15 cm = £15.00, 20 cm × 20 cm = £21.15, 5 cm diameter = £3.13; cavity dressing 5 cm × 8 cm = £3.72

**PolyMem®** (Unomedical)

Silver impregnated polyurethane foam film dressing, *with adhesive border*, 5 cm × 7.6 cm (oval) = £2.15, 12.7 cm × 8.8 cm (oval) = £5.30; *without adhesive border*, 10.8 cm × 10.8 cm = £8.20, 17 cm × 19 cm = £16.93

### ◢ Alginate dressings

**Acticoat® Absorbent** (S&N Hlth.)

Calcium alginate dressing with a silver coated antimicrobial barrier, 5 cm × 5 cm = £4.91, 10 cm × 12.5 cm = £11.78; 2 cm × 30 cm (cavity) = £11.85

**Algisite® Ag** (S&N Hlth.)

Calcium alginate dressing, with silver, 5 cm × 5 cm = £1.53, 10 cm × 10 cm = £3.83, 10 cm × 20 cm = £7.04; 2 g, 30 cm (cavity) = £5.28

**Silvercel®** (Systagenix)

Alginate and hydrocollid dressing impregnated with silver, 2.5 cm × 30.5 cm = £4.37, 5 cm × 5 cm = £1.64, 10 cm × 20 cm = £7.53, 11 cm × 11 cm = £4.06

**Sorbsan®** (Unomedical)

Sorbsan® Silver Flat, calcium alginate fibre, highly absorbent, flat non-woven pads, with silver, 5 cm × 5 cm = £1.50, 10 cm × 10 cm = £3.80, 10 cm × 20 cm = £6.94

Sorbsan® Silver Plus, calcium alginate dressing with absorbent backing, with silver, 7.5 cm × 10 cm = £3.25, 10 cm × 15 cm = £5.41, 10 cm × 20 cm = £6.58, 15 cm × 20 cm = £8.82

Sorbsan® Silver Plus SA, calcium alginate dressing with absorbent backing and adhesive border, with silver, 11.5 cm × 14 cm = £5.28, 14 cm × 19 cm = £7.60, 14 cm × 24 cm = £8.36, 19 cm × 24 cm = £9.32

Sorbsan® Silver Ribbon, with silver, 40 cm (with probe) = £3.97

Sorbsan® Silver Surgical Packing, with silver, 30 cm (2 g, with probe) = £5.55

**Urgosorb®Silver** (Urgo)

Alginate and hydrocollid dressing, impregnated with silver, 5 cm × 5 cm = £1.42, 10 cm × 10 cm = £3.39, 10 cm × 20 cm = £6.39; cavity dressing, 2.5 cm × 30 cm = £3.41

## A8.3.4 Other antimicrobials

**Chlorhexidine Gauze Dressing, BP 1993**

Fabric of leno weave, weft and warp threads of cotton and/or viscose yarn, impregnated with ointment containing chlorhexidine acetate, 5 cm × 5 cm = 27p; 10 cm × 10 cm = 56p (S&N Hlth.—*Bactigras®*)

**Cutimed® Sorbact** (BSN Medical)

Low adherence acetate tissue impregnated with dialkylcarbamoyl chloride, (dressing pad) 7 cm × 9 cm = £3.20, 10 cm × 10 cm = £5.00, 10 cm × 20 cm = £7.80; (swabs) 4 cm × 6 cm = £1.50, 7 cm × 9 cm = £2.50, (round swabs) 3 cm, 5 pad pack = £3.00; (cavity dressing, cotton) 2 cm × 50 cm = £3.74, 5 cm × 2 m = £7.37

**Flaminal®** (Ark Therapeutics)

Forte gel, alginate with glucose oxidase and lactoperoxidase, for moderately to heavily exuding wounds, 15 g = £7.18, 50 g = £23.77

Hydro gel, alginate with glucose oxidase and lactoperoxidase, for lightly to moderately exuding wounds, 15 g = £7.18, 50 g = £23.77

**Prontosan® Wound Gel** (Braun)

Hydrogel containing betaine surfactant and polyhexanide, 30 mL = £5.97

**Suprasorb® X + PHMB** (Activa)

Biosynthetic cellulose fibre dressing with polihexanide, 5 cm × 5 cm = £2.34, 9 cm × 9 cm = £4.66, 14 cm × 20 cm = £10.60; 2 cm × 21 cm (rope) = £6.60

**Telfa® AMD** (Covidien)

Low adherence absorbent perforated plastic film faced dressing with polihexanide, 7.5 cm × 10 cm = 17p, 7.5 cm × 20 cm = 28p

Telfa® AMD Island Low adherence dressing with adhesive border and absorbent pad, with polihexanide, 10 cm × 12.5 cm = 58p, 10 cm × 20 cm = 85p, 10 cm × 25.5 cm = 96p, 10 cm × 35 cm = £1.19

## A8.4 Specialised dressings

## A8.4.1 Protease-modulating matrix dressings

Protease-modulating matrix dressings alter the activity of *proteolytic enzymes* in chronic wounds; the clinical significance of this approach is yet to be demonstrated.

**Cadesorb®** (S&N Hlth.)

Ointment, starch-based, 10 g = £4.96, 20 g = £8.46

**Promogran®** (Systagenix)

Collagen and oxidised regenerated cellulose matrix, applied directly to wound and covered with suitable dressing, 28 cm² (hexagonal) = £5.09, 123 cm² (hexagonal) = £15.32

**Promogran® Prisma® Matrix** (Systagenix)

Collagen, silver and oxidised regenerated cellulose matrix, applied directly to wound and covered with suitable dressing, 28 cm² (hexagonal) = £6.19, 123 cm² (hexagonal) = £17.63

**Sorbion® S** (H&R)

Absorbent polymers in cellulose matrix, hypoallergenic fleece envelope, 7.5 cm × 7.5 cm = £1.75, 10 cm × 10 cm = £2.22, 20 cm × 20 cm = £6.90, 20 cm × 10 cm = £3.68, 30 cm × 10 cm = £5.29, 30 cm × 20 cm = £9.92, 12 cm × 5 cm = £1.86

**Suprasorb® C** (Activa)

Collagen, 4 cm × 6 cm = £2.60, 6 cm × 8 cm = £3.98, 8 cm × 12 cm = £7.80

**Tegaderm® Matrix** (3M)

Cellulose acetate matrix, impregnated with polyhydrated ionogens ointment in polyethylene glycol basis, 5 cm × 6 cm = £4.75, 8 cm × 10 cm = £9.75

## A8.4.2 Silicone keloid dressings

Silicone gel and gel sheets are used to reduce or prevent hypertrophic and keloid scarring. They should not be used on open wounds. Application times should be increased gradually. Silicone sheets can be washed and reused.

**Advasil® Conform** (Advancis)

Self-adhesive silicone gel sheet with polyurethane film backing, 10 cm × 10 cm = £5.20, 10 cm × 15 cm = £9.17

**Cica-Care®** (S&N Hlth.)

Soft, self-adhesive, semi-occlusive silicone gel sheet with backing. 6 cm × 12 cm = £13.42; 15 cm × 12 cm = £26.16

**Ciltech®** (Su-Med)

Silicone gel sheet, 10 cm × 10 cm = £7.50, 15 cm × 15 cm = £14.00, 10 cm × 20 cm = £12.50

Silicone gel, 15 g = £17.50, 60 g = £50.00

**Dermatix®** (Valeant)

Self-adhesive silicone gel sheet (clear- or fabric-backed), 4 cm × 13 cm = £6.61, 13 cm × 13 cm = £15.17, 13 cm × 25 cm = £27.41, 20 cm × 30 cm = £49.92; Silicone gel, 15 g = £19.38, 60 g = £58.14

**Kelo-cote®** (ABT Healthcare)

Silicone gel, 15 g = £17.88, 60 g = £51.00

Silicone spray, 100 mL = £51.00

**Mepiform®** (Mölnlycke)

Self-adhesive silicone gel sheet with polyurethane film backing, 5 cm × 7 cm = £3.20, 9 cm × 18 cm = £12.53, 4 cm × 31 cm = £10.12

**Silgel®** (Nagor)

Silicone gel sheet, 10 cm × 10 cm = £13.50; 20 cm × 20 cm = £40.00; 40 cm × 40 cm = £144.00; 10 cm × 5 cm = £7.50; 15 cm x 10 cm = £19.50; 30 cm × 5 cm = £19.50; 10 cm × 30 cm = £31.50; 25 cm × 15 cm (submammary) = £21.12; 46 cm × 8.5 cm (abdominal) = £39.46; 5.5 cm diameter (circular) = £4.00

Silgel® STC-SE silicone gel, 20-mL tube = £19.00

## A8.5 Adjunct dressings and appliances

## A8.5.1 Surgical absorbents

Surgical absorbent dressings, applied directly to the wound, have many disadvantages, since they adhere to the wound, shed fibres into it, and dehydrate it; they also permit leakage of exudate ('strike through') with an associated risk of infection. Surgical absorbents may be used as secondary absorbent layers in the management of heavily exuding wounds.

◀Cotton

**Absorbent Cotton, BP**

Carded cotton fibres of not less than 10 mm average staple length, available in rolls and balls, 25 g = 69p; 100 g = £1.58; 500 g = £5.31 (most suppliers). 25-g pack to be supplied when weight not stated

Uses general purpose cleansing and swabbing, pre-operative skin preparation, application of medicaments; supplementary absorbent pad to absorb excess wound exudate

**Absorbent Cotton, Hospital Quality**

As for absorbent cotton but lower quality materials, shorter staple length etc. 100 g = £1.10; 500 g = £3.46 (most suppliers)

Drug Tariff specifies to be supplied only where specifically ordered

Uses suitable only as general purpose absorbent, for swabbing, and routine cleansing of incontinent patients; not for wound cleansing

◀Gauze and tissue

**Absorbent Cotton Gauze, BP 1988**

Cotton fabric of plain weave, in rolls and as swabs (see below), usually Type 13 light, sterile, 90 cm (all) × 1 m = £1.04; 3 m = £2.17; 5 m = £3.38; 10 m = £6.47 (most suppliers). 1-m packet supplied when no size stated

Uses pre-operative preparation, for cleansing and swabbing

Note Drug Tariff also includes unsterilised absorbent cotton gauze, 25 m roll = £14.82

**Absorbent Cotton Ribbon Gauze, BP 1993** ⒨

Cotton fabric of plain weave in ribbon form with fast selvedge edges

Uses post-surgery cavity packing for sinus, dental, throat cavities etc.

**Absorbent Cotton and Viscose Ribbon Gauze, BP 1993**

Woven fabric in ribbon form with fast selvedge edges, warp threads of cotton, weft threads of viscose or combined cotton and viscose yarn, sterile. 5 m (both) × 1.25 cm = 78p; 2.5 cm = 86p

Uses post-surgery cavity packing for sinus, dental, throat cavities etc.

**Gauze and Cotton Tissue, BP 1988**

Consists of absorbent cotton enclosed in absorbent cotton gauze type 12 or absorbent cotton and viscose gauze type 2. 500 g = £6.74 (most suppliers, including Robinsons—*Gamgee Tissue®* (blue label))

Uses absorbent and protective pad, as burns dressing on non-adherent layer

**Gauze and Cotton Tissue**

(Drug Tariff specification 14). Similar to above. 500 g = £4.92 (most suppliers, including Robinsons—*Gamgee Tissue®* (pink label))

Drug Tariff specifies to be supplied only where specifically ordered

Uses absorbent and protective pad, as burns dressing on non-adherent layer

◀Lint and muslin

**Absorbent Lint, BPC** ◢

Cotton cloth of plain weave with nap raised on one side from warp yarns. 25 g = 86p; 100 g = £2.63; 500 g = £11.07 (most suppliers). 25-g pack supplied where no quantity stated

Note Not recommended for wound management

**Absorbent Muslin, BP 1988** ⒨

Fabric of plain weave, warp threads of cotton, weft threads of cotton and/or viscose

Uses wet dressing, soaked in 0.9% sterile sodium chloride solution

◀Pads

**Absorbent Dressing Pads, Sterile**

Drisorb®, 10 cm × 20 cm = 17p (Synergy Healthcare)

Xupad®, 10 cm × 20 cm = 17p, 20 cm × 20 cm = 28p, 20 cm × 40 cm = 40p (Richardson)

¹**Surgipad®** (Systagenix) ⒨

Absorbent pad of absorbent cotton and viscose in sleeve of non-woven viscose fabric, pouch 12 cm × 10 cm = 18p, 20 cm × 10 cm = 25p, 20 cm × 20 cm = 30p, 40 cm × 20 cm = 41p; *non sterile* pouch 12 cm × 10 cm = 5p, 20 cm × 10 cm = 10p, 20 cm × 20 cm = 17p, 40 cm × 20 cm = 28p

1. ⒨ Except in Sterile Dressing Pack with Non-woven Pads

## A8.5.2 Wound drainage pouches

**Biotrol®** (Braun)

Draina S Fistula, wound drainage pouch, mini (cut to 20 mm), 150-mL capacity = £2.40; medium (cut to 50 mm), 350-mL capacity = £3.59; large (cut to 88 mm), 500-mL capacity = £4.41

Draina S Vision, wound drainage pouch, (cut to 50 mm), 150-mL capacity = £9.39; (cut to 88 mm), 250-mL capacity = £9.92; (cut to 100 mm), 300-mL capacity = £11.51

**Dermasure®** (ADI Medical)

Pouch, small (wound size up to 9 cm × 16 cm) = £15.60; medium (wound size up to 15 cm × 27 cm) = £20.80

**Eakin®** (Eakin)

Wound pouch, *fold and tuck closure*, small (wound size up to 45 mm × 30 mm) = £4.50; medium (wound size up to 110 mm × 75 mm) = £6.50; large (wound size up to 175 mm × 110 mm) = £8.50; extra large (horizontal wound up to 245 mm × 160 mm) = £15.00

Wound pouch, *bung closure*, small (wound size up to 45 mm × 30 mm) = £5.00; medium (wound size up to 110 mm × 75 mm) = £7.00; large (wound size up to 175 mm × 110 mm) = £9.50; extra large (horizontal or vertical wound up to 245 mm × 160 mm) = £17.00, (vertical incision wound up to 290 mm × 130 mm) = £17.00; (horizontal wound up to 245 mm × 160 mm), *with access window* = £19.00

Access window, for use with *Eakin®* pouches = £7.00

**Oakmed® Option** (Oakmed)

Wound Manager, extra small (wound size up to 90 mm × 180 mm) = £10.91; small (horizontal wound size up to 245 mm × 160 mm) = £12.13; medium (vertical wound size up to 90 mm × 260 mm) = £12.41; large (wound size up to 160 mm × 200 mm) = £12.95

Wound manager, with access port, extra small (wound size up to 90 mm × 180 mm) = £11.93; small (horizontal wound size up to 245 mm × 160 mm) = £12.68; medium (vertical wound size up to 90 mm × 260 mm) = £12.95; large (wound size up to 160 mm × 260 mm) = £15.81; square (vertical wound size up to 160 mm × 200 mm) = £13.49

Wound manager, cut-to-fit, small (10–30 mm) = £2.23, medium (10–50 mm) = £2.47, large (10–50 mm) = £2.59

**Welland®** (CliniMed)
Fistula bag, *wound manager*, cut-to-fit (wound size up ro 40 mm × 70 mm) = £2.54

## A8.6 Complex adjunct therapies

Topical negative pressure (or vacuum-assisted) therapy requires specific wound dressings for use with the vacuum-pump equipment.

Other complex adjunct therapies include sterile larvae (maggots), and growth factors such as becalpermin (see section 13.11.7)

### A8.6.1 Topical negative pressure therapy

◀**Vacuum assisted closure products**
**Exsu-Fast®** (Synergy Healthcare)
Dressing kit, Kit 1 (small wound, low exudate) = £28.04; Kit 2 (large wound, heavy exudate) = £35.83; Kit 3 (large wound, medium to low exudate) = £35.83; Kit 4 (small wound, heavy exudate) = £28.04

**V.A.C. GranuFoam®** (KCI Medical)
Dressing kit, polyurethane foam dressing (with adhesive drapes and pad connector), 10 cm × 7.5 cm × 3.3 cm (small) = £21.41, 18 cm × 12.5 cm × 3.3 cm (medium) = £25.49, 26 cm × 15 cm × 3.3 cm (large) = £29.57

**Venturi®** (Talley)
Wound sealing kit, flat drain, standard = £15.00, large = £17.50; channel drain = £15.00

**V1STA®** (S&N Hlth.)
Dressing kit, flat drain, small = £16.52, medium = £20.70, large = £26.28; round drain, small = £16.52, large = £26.28; channel drain, medium = £20.70

**WoundASSIST®** (Huntleigh)
Wound pack, small–medium = £20.50, medium–large = £23.50

◀**Wound drainage collection devices**
**V.A.C Freedom®** (KCI Medical)
Canister (with gel), 300 mL = £26.51

**Venturi®** (Talley)
Canister kit (with solidifier) = £12.50

**V1STA®** (S&N Hlth.)
Canister kit, 250 mL (with solidifier) = £18.63, 800 mL (with solidifier) = £20.70

**WoundASSIST®** (Huntleigh)
Canister, 500 mL = £20.00

## A8.7 Wound care acccessories

### A8.7.1 Dressing packs

The role of dressing packs is very limited. They are used to provide a clean or sterile working surface; some packs shown below include cotton wool balls, which are not recommended for use on wounds.

**Non-Drug Tariff Specification Sterile Dressing Pack**
Dressit® contains vitrex gloves, large apron, disposable bag, paper towel, softswabs, adsorbent pad, sterile field = 60p (Richardson)

Nurse It® contains powder-free vinyl gloves, sterile polythene sheet, non-woven swabs, paper towel, disposable bag, compartmention tray, plastic forceps = 52p (Medicare)

Polyfield® Nitrile Patient Pack contains powder-free nitrile gloves, laminate sheet, non-woven swabs, towel, polythene disposable bag, apron = 52p (Shermond)

Polyfield® Soft Vinyl Patient Pack contains powder-free sterile soft vinyl gloves, polythene sheet, non-woven swabs, towel, polythene disposable bag, apron = 52p (Shermond)

Propax® SDP contains paper towel, disposable bag, gauze swabs, dressing pad, sterile field = 45p (BSN Medical)

Woundcare® contains nitrile gloves, sterile field, compartmented tray, large apron, disposable bag, non-woven swabs, drape = 44p (Frontier)

**Sterile Dressing Pack**
(Drug Tariff specification 10). Contains gauze and cotton tissue pad, gauze swabs, absorbent cotton wool balls, absorbent paper towel, water repellent inner wrapper. 1 pack = 49p (Synergy Healthcare—*Vernaid®*)

**Sterile Dressing Pack with Non-woven Pads**
(Drug Tariff specification 35). Contains non-woven fabric covered dressing pad, non-woven fabric swabs, absorbent cotton wool balls, absorbent paper towel, water repellent inner wrapper. 1 pack = 48p (Synergy Healthcare—*Vernaid®*)

### A8.7.2 Woven and fabric swabs

**Gauze Swab, BP 1988**
Consists of absorbent cotton gauze type 13 light or absorbent cotton and viscose gauze type 1 folded into squares or rectangles of 8-ply with no cut edges exposed, sterile, 7.5 cm × 7.5 cm 5-pad packet = 38p; non-sterile, 10 cm × 10 cm, 100-pad packet = £1.31 (most suppliers)

**Filmated Gauze Swab, BP 1988**
As for Gauze Swab, but with thin layer of Absorbent Cotton enclosed within, non-sterile, 10 cm × 10 cm, 100-pad packet = £3.52 (Synergy Healthcare—*Cotfil®*)

**Non-woven Fabric Swab**
(Drug Tariff specification 28). Consists of non-woven fabric folded 4-ply; alternative to gauze swabs, type 13 light, sterile, 7.5 cm × 7.5 cm, 5-pad packet = 24p; non-sterile, 10 cm × 10 cm, 100-pad packet = 76p

**Filmated Non-woven Fabric Swab**
(Drug Tariff specification 29). Film of viscose fibres enclosed within non-woven viscose fabric folded 8-ply, non-sterile, 10 cm × 10 cm, 100-pad packet = £3.52 (Systagenix—*Regal®*)

# A8.7.3 Surgical adhesive tapes

Adhesive tapes are useful for retaining dressings on joints or awkward body parts. These tapes, particularly those containing rubber, can cause irritant and allergic reactions in susceptible patients; synthetic adhesives have been developed to overcome this problem, but they, too, may sometimes be associated with reactions. Synthetic adhesive, or silicon adhesive, tapes can be used for patients with skin reactions to plasters and strapping containing rubber, or undergoing prolonged treatment.

Adhesive tapes that are occlusive may cause skin maceration. Care is needed not to apply these tapes under tension, to avoid creating a tourniquet effect. If applied over joints they need to be orientated so that the area of maximum extensibility of the fabric is in the direction of movement of the limb.

◄Permeable adhesive tapes
**Elastic Adhesive Tape, BP 1988**

(Elastic Adhesive Plaster). Woven fabric, elastic in warp (crepe-twisted cotton threads), weft of cotton and/or viscose threads, spread with adhesive mass containing zinc oxide. 4.5 m stretched × 2.5 cm = £1.64 (Robinsons—*Flexoplast*®; S&N —*Elastoplast*®)

For 5 cm width, see Elastic Adhesive Bandage

**Permeable, Apertured Non-Woven Synthetic Adhesive Tape, BP 1988**

Non-woven fabric with a polyacrylate adhesive.

Hypafix®, 5 cm × 5 m = £1.34, 10 cm × 5 m = £2.25, 10 m (all): 2.5 cm = £1.56, 5 cm = £2.48, 10 cm = £4.33, 15 cm = £6.42, 20 cm = £8.51, 30 cm = £12.31 (BSN Medical)

Mefix®, 5 m (all): 2.5 cm = 95p, 5 cm = £1.68; 10 cm = £2.69, 15 cm = £3.66, 20 cm = £4.69, 30 cm = £6.72 (Mölnlycke)

Omnifix®, 10 m (all): 5 cm = £2.19, 10 cm = £3.69, 15 cm = £5.44 (Hartmann)

**Permeable Non-woven Synthetic Adhesive Tape, BP 1988**

Backing of paper-based or non-woven textile material spread with a polymeric adhesive mass:

Clinipore®, 5 m (all) 1.25 cm = 35p, 2.5 cm = 59p, 5 cm = 99p; 2.5 cm × 10 m = 73p (Clinisupplies)

Leukofix®, 5 m (all) 1.25 cm = 52p, 2.5 cm = 83p, 5 cm = £1.45 (BSN Medical)

Leukopor®, 5 m (all) 1.25 cm = 46p, 2.5 cm = 72p, 5 cm = £1.26 (BSN Medical)

Mediplast®, 5 m (all) 1.25 cm = 30p, 2.5 cm = 50p (Neomedic)

Micropore®, 5 m (all) 1.25 cm = 60p, 2.5 cm = 89p, 5 cm = £1.57 (3M)

Scanpor®, 5 m (all) 1.25 cm = 40p, 2.5 cm = 65p, 5 cm = £1.12; 10 m (all), 1.25 cm = 52p, 2.5 cm = 87p, 5 cm = £1.65, 7.5 cm = £2.42 (BioDiagnostics)

Where no brand stated by prescriber, net price of tape supplied not to exceed 35p (1.25 cm), 59p (2.5 cm), 99p (5 cm)

**Permeable Woven Synthetic Adhesive Tape, BP 1988**

Non-extensible closely woven fabric, spread with a polymeric adhesive. 5 m (all): 1.25 cm = 77p; 2.5 cm = £1.12; 5 cm = £1.95 (Beiersdorf—*Leukosilk*®)

**Silicone adhesive tape**

Soft silicone, water-resistant, knitted fabric, polyurethane film adhesive tape

Insil®, 2 cm × 3 m = £5.60, 4 cm × 1.5 m = £5.60 (Insight)

Mepitac®, 2 cm × 3 m = £6.39, 4 cm × 1.5 m = £6.39 (Mölnlycke)

Siltape®, 2 cm × 3 m = £5.60, 4 cm × 1.5 m = £5.60 (Advancis)

**Zinc Oxide Adhesive Tape, BP 1988**

(Zinc Oxide Plaster). Fabric, plain weave, warp and weft of cotton and/or viscose, spread with an adhesive containing zinc oxide. 5 m (all): 1.25 cm = 93p; 2.5 cm = £1.35; 5 cm = £2.28; 7.5 cm = £3.43 (most suppliers)

**Zinc Oxide Adhesive Tape**

Mediplast®, 5 m (all), 1.25 cm = 82p, 2.5 cm = £1.19, 5 cm = £1.99, 7.5 cm = £2.99 (Neomedic)

Strappal®, 5 m (all): 1.25 cm = 89p, 2.5 cm = £1.29, 5 cm = £2.17, 7.5 cm = £3.27 (BSN Medical)

◄Occlusive adhesive tapes
**Impermeable Plastic Adhesive Tape, BP 1988**

Extensible water-impermeable plastic film spread with an adhesive mass. 2.5 cm × 3 m = £1.30; 2.5 cm × 5 m = £1.95; 5 cm × 5 m = £2.47; 7.5 cm × 5 m = £3.59 (BSN Medical—*Sleek*®)

**Impermeable Plastic Synthetic Adhesive Tape, BP 1988**

Extensible water-impermeable plastic film spread with a polymeric adhesive mass. 5 m (both): 2.5 cm = £1.72; 5 cm = £3.27 (3M—*Blenderm*®)

# A8.7.4 Adhesive dressings

Adhesive dressings (also termed 'island dressings') have a limited role for minor wounds only. The inclusion of an antiseptic is not particularly useful and may cause skin irritation in susceptible subjects.

◄Permeable adhesive dressings
**Elastic Adhesive Dressing, BP 1993** ⒿⒽⓈ

Wound dressing or dressing strip, pad attached to piece of extension plaster, leaving suitable adhesive margin; both pad and margin covered with suitable protector; pad may be dyed yellow and may be impregnated with suitable antiseptic (see below); extension plaster may be perforated or ventilated

Note Permitted antiseptics are aminoacridine hydrochloride (aminacrine hydrochloride), chlorhexidine hydrochloride (both 0.07–0.13%), chlorhexidine gluconate (0.11–0.20%); domiphen bromide (0.05–0.25%)

**Permeable Plastic Wound Dressing, BP 1993** ⒿⒽⓈ

Consisting of an absorbent pad, which may be dyed and impregnated with a suitable antiseptic (see under Elastic Adhesive Dressing), attached to a piece of permeable plastic surgical adhesive tape, to leave a suitable adhesive margin; both pad and margin covered with suitable protector (most suppliers)

◄Vapour permeable adhesive dressings
**Vapour-permeable Waterproof Plastic Wound Dressing, BP 1993**

(former Drug Tariff title: Semipermeable Waterproof Plastic Wound Dressing). Consists of absorbent pad, may be dyed and impregnated with suitable antiseptic (see under Elastic Adhesive Dressing), attached to piece of semi-permeable waterproof surgical adhesive tape, to leave suitable adhesive margin; both pad and margin covered with suitable protector.(S&N Hlth—*Elastoplast Airstrip*®)

◄Occlusive adhesive tapes
**Impermeable Plastic Wound Dressing, BP 1993** ⒿⒽⓈ

Consists of absorbent pad, may be dyed and impregnated with suitable antiseptic (see under Elastic Adhesive Dressing), attached to piece of impermeable plastic surgical adhesive tape, to leave suitable adhesive margin; both pad and margin covered with suitable protector (most suppliers)

Appendix 8: Wound management

## A8.7.5 Skin closure dressings

Skin closure strips are used as an alternative to sutures for minor cuts and lacerations. Skin tissue adhesive (section 13.10.5) can be used for closure of minor skin wounds and for additional suture support.

**Skin closure strips, sterile**
Leukostrip®, 6.4 mm × 76 mm, 3 strips per envelope. 10 envelopes = £5.79 (S&N Hlth.)
Steri-strip®, 6 mm × 75 mm, 3 strips per envelope. 12 envelopes = £8.52 (3M)
Drug Tariff specifies that these are specifically for personal administration by the prescriber

## A8.8 Bandages

According to their structure and performance bandages are used for dressing retention, for support, and for compression.

## A8.8.1 Non-extensible bandages

Bandages made from non-extensible woven fabrics have generally been replaced by more conformable products, therefore their role is now extremely limited. Triangular calico bandage has a role as a sling.

**Domette Bandage, BP 1988** [NHS]
Fabric, plain weave, cotton warp and wool weft (hospital quality also available, all cotton). 5 m (all): 5 cm = 54p; 7.5 cm = 81p; 10 cm = £1.08; 15 cm = £1.61 (Steraid)

**Multiple Pack Dressing No. 1**
(Drug Tariff). Contains absorbent cotton, absorbent cotton gauze type 13 light (sterile), open-wove bandages (banded). 1 pack = £3.93

**Open-wove Bandage, BP 1988**
Cotton cloth, plain weave, warp of cotton, weft of cotton, viscose, or combination, one continuous length. Type 1, 5 m (all): 2.5 cm = 30p; 5 cm = 51p; 7.5 cm = 72p; 10 cm = 94p (most suppliers) 5 m × 5 cm supplied when size not stated

**Triangular Calico Bandage, BP 1980**
Unbleached calico right-angled triangle, 90 cm × 90 cm × 1.27 m = £1.13 (most suppliers)

## A8.8.2 Light-weight conforming bandages

Lightweight conforming bandages are used for dressing retention, with the aim of keeping the dressing close to the wound without inhibiting movement or restricting blood flow. The elasticity of **conforming-stretch bandages** (also termed contour bandages) is greater than that of **cotton conforming bandages**.

**Conforming Bandage (Synthetic)**
Fabric, plain weave, warp of polyamide, weft of viscose. 4 m stretched (all):
Hospiform® (formerly Peha Crepp® E), 6 cm = 12p, 8 cm = 15p, 10 cm = 17p, 12 cm = 21p (Hartmann)

**Cotton Conforming Bandage, BP 1988**
Cotton fabric, plain weave, treated to impart some elasticity to warp and weft. 3.5 m (all): type A, 5 cm = 63p, 7.5 cm = 77p, 10 cm = 96p, 15 cm = £1.30 (S&N Hlth— Easifix Crinx®)

**Knitted Polyamide and Cellulose Contour Bandage, BP 1988**
Fabric, knitted warp of polyamide filament, weft of cotton or viscose, fast edges, one continuous length. 4 m stretched (all):
K-Band®, 5 cm = 19p, 7 cm = 24p, 10 cm = 26p, 15 cm = 46p (Urgo)
Knit-Band®, 5 cm = 10p, 7 cm = 15p, 10 cm = 17p, 15 cm = 30p (CliniMed)
Knit Fix®, 5 cm = 12p, 7 cm = 17p, 10 cm = 17p, 15 cm = 33p (Steraid)

**Polyamide and Cellulose Contour Bandage, BP 1988 (formerly Nylon and Viscose Stretch Bandage)**
Fabric, plain weave, warp of polyamide filament, weft of cotton or viscose, fast edges, one continuous length, 4 m stretched (all):
Acti-Wrap®, cohesive, latex-free, 6 cm = 43p, 8 cm = 62p, 10 cm = 74p (Activa)
Easifix®, 5 cm = 33p, 7.5 cm = 40p, 10 cm = 47p, 15 cm = 80p (S&N Hlth)
Kontour®, cohesive, 5 cm = 28p, 7.5 cm = 35p, 10 cm = 40p, 15 cm = 66p (Easigrip)
Slinky®, 5 cm = 39p, 7.5 cm = 55p, 10 cm = 66p, 15 cm = 95p (Medlock)
Stayform®, 5 cm = 29p, 7.5 cm = 36p, 10 cm = 40p, 15 cm = 68p (Robinsons)

## A8.8.3 Tubular bandages and garments

**Tubular bandages** are available in different forms, according to the function required of them. Some are used under orthopaedic casts and some are suitable for protecting areas to which creams or ointments (other than those containing potent corticosteroids) have been applied. The conformability of the elasticated versions makes them particularly suitable for retaining dressings on difficult parts of the body or for soft tissue injury, but their use as the only means of applying pressure to an oedematous limb or to a varicose ulcer is not appropriate, since the pressure they exert is inadequate.

**Compression hosiery** (section A8.9.1) reduces the recurrence of venous leg ulcers and should be considered after wound healing.

**Silk clothing** is available as an alternative to elasticated viscose stockinette garments, for use in the management of severe eczema and allergic skin conditions (see below)

◀ **Elasticated**
**Elasticated Surgical Tubular Stockinette, Foam padded**
(Drug Tariff specification 25). Fabric as for Elasticated Tubular Bandage with polyurethane foam lining. Heel, elbow, knee, small = £2.68, medium = £2.83, large = £3.09; sacral,, medium, and large (all) = £13.82 (Medlock—Tubipad®)
Uses relief of pressure and elimination of friction in relevant area; porosity of foam lining allows normal water loss from skin surface

**Elasticated Tubular Bandage, BP 1993**
(formerly Elasticated Surgical Tubular Stockinette). Knitted fabric, elasticated threads of rubber-cored polyamide or polyester with cotton or cotton and viscose yarn, tubular. Lengths 50 cm and 1 m, widths 6.25 cm, 6.75 cm, 7.5 cm, 8.75 cm, 10 cm, 12 cm; Synergy—Comfigrip®; Easigrip—EasiGRIP®; Sallis—Eesiban®; Sigma—Sigma ETB®; Medlock—Tubigrip®. Where no size stated by prescriber the 50 cm length should be supplied and width endorsed

## Elasticated Viscose Stockinette

(Drug Tariff specification 46). Lightweight plain-knitted elasticated tubular bandage.

Acti-Fast®, 3.5 cm red line (small limb), length 1 m = 62p; 5 cm green line (medium limb), length 1 m = 65p, 3 m = £1.90, 5 m = £3.30; 7.5 cm blue line (large limb), length 1 m = 90p, 3 m = £2.50, 5 m = £4.40; 10.75 cm yellow line (child trunk), length 1 m = £1.45, 3 m = £4.10, 5 m = £7.10; 17.5 cm beige line (adult trunk), length 1 m = £2.15 (Activa)

CliniFast®, 3.5 cm red line (small limb), length 1 m = 56p; 5 cm green line (medium limb), length 1 m = 58p, 3 m = £1.62, 5 m = £2.81; 7.5 cm blue line (large limb), length 1 m = 77p, 3 m = £2.13, 5 m = £3.74; 10.75 cm yellow line (child trunk), length 1 m = £1.20, 3 m = £3.49, 5 m = £6.04; 17.5 cm beige line (adult trunk), length 1 m = £1.83; vest (long-sleeved), 6–24 months = £7.13, 2–5 years = £9.50, 5–8 years = £10.69, 8–11 years = £11.88, 11–14 years = £11.88, adult, small, = £12.75, medium = £14.54, large = £16.58; vest (short-sleeved), adult, small = £12.50, medium = £14.25, large = £16.25; tights (pair) 6–24 months = £7.13; leggings (pair) 2–5 years = £9.50, 5–8 years = £10.69, 8–11 years = £11.88, 11–14 years = £11.88, adult, small, = £12.75, medium = £14.54, large = £16.58; cycle shorts, adult, small = £12.50, medium = £14.25, large = £16.25; socks (pair) up to 8 years = £2.97, 8–14 years = £2.97; mittens (pair) up to 24 months = £2.97, 2–8 years = £2.97, 8–14 years = £2.97; clava 6 months–5 years = £5.85, 5–14 years = £6.75 (Clinisupplies)

Comfifast®, 3.5 cm red line (small limb), length 1 m = 59p; 5 cm green line (medium limb), length 1 m = 61p, 3 m = £1.67, 5 m = £2.86; 7.5 cm blue line (large limb), length 1 m = 81p, 3 m = £2.19, 5 m = £3.80; 10.75 cm yellow line (child trunk), length 1 m = £1.26, 3 m = £3.54, 5 m = £6.09; 17.5 cm beige line (adult trunk), length 1 m = £1.88 (Synergy)

Comfifast® Easy Wrap, vest (long-sleeved), 6–24 months = £8.08, 2–5 years = £10.77, 5–8 years = £12.12, 8–11 years = £13.46, 11–14 years = £13.46, adult, small = £15.30, medium = £17.44, large = 19.89; tights (pair) 6–24 months = £8.08; leggings (pair) 2–5 years = £10.77, 5–8 years = £12.12, 8–11 years = £13.46, 11–14 years = £13.46, adult, small = £15.30, medium = £17.44, large = £19.89; socks (pair) up to 8 years = £3.37, 8–14 = £3.37; mittens (pair) up to 24 months = £3.37, 2–8 years = £3.37, 8–14 years = £3.37; clava, 6 months–5 years = £6.63, 5–14 years = £7.65 (Synergy)

Coverflex®, 3.5 cm red line (small limb), length 1 m = 75p; 5 cm green line (medium limb), length 1 m = 78p, 3 m = £2.28, 5 m = £3.94; 7.5 cm blue line (large limb), length 1 m = £1.09, 3 m = £2.60, 5 m = £5.14; 10.75 cm yellow line (child trunk), length 1 m = £1.71, 3 m = £4.93, 5 m = £8.67; 17.5 cm beige line (adult trunk), length 1 m = £2.28 (Hartmann)

Easifast®, 3.5 cm red line (small limb), length 1 m = 65p; 5 cm green line (medium limb), length 1 m = 69p, 3 m = £1.95, 5 m = £3.40; 7.5 cm blue line (large limb), length 1 m = 94p, 3 m = £2.60, 5 m = £4.50; 10.75 cm yellow line (child trunk), length 1 m = £1.50, 3 m = £4.25, 5 m = £7.20; 17.5 cm beige line (adult trunk), length 1 m = £1.90 (Easigrip)

Skinnies®, clava 6 months–5 years = £6.62, 5–14 years = £7.60; vest (long-sleeved) 6–24 months = £10.30, 2–5 years = £13.50, 5–8 years = £15.25, 8–11 years or 11–14 years = £16.90, adult (small) = £20.90, (medium) = £22.80, (large) = £24.70; body-suit 0–3 months or 3–6 months = £15.90; leggings (pair) 6–24 months = £10.30, 2–5 years = £13.50, 5–8 years = £15.25, 8–11 years or 11–14 years = £16.90, adult (small) = £20.90, (medium) = £22.80, (large) = £24.70; socks (pair) 6 months–8 years or 8–14 years = £4.20; mittens 0–24 months, 2–8 years, or 8–14 years = £3.80; gloves child (small) = £5.20, (medium or large) = £5.25, adult (small) = £5.20, (medium or large) = £5.25. (Skinnies)

Tubifast®, 3.5 cm red line (small limb), length 1 m = 85p; 5 cm green line (medium limb), length 1 m = 92p, 3 m = £2.62, 5 m = £4.49; 7.5 cm blue line (large limb), length 1 m = £1.23, 3 m = £3.45, 5 m = £6.02; 10.75 cm yellow line (child trunk), length 1 m = £1.97, 3 m = £5.62, 5 m = £9.66; 20 cm purple line (large adult trunk), length 1 m = £3.18, 5 m = £15.57; vest (long-sleeved), 6–24 months = £10.68, 2–5 years = £14.23, 5–8 years = £16.01, 8–11 years = £17.79, 11–14 years = £17.79; tights (pair) 6–24 months = £10.68; leggings (pair) 2–5 years = £14.23, 5–8 years = £16.01, 8–11 years = £17.79, 11–14 years = £17.79; socks (pair) up to 8 years = £4.45; gloves (small, medium or large adult, medium or large child) = £5.46 (Medlock)

### ◀ Non-elasticated

#### Cotton Stockinette, Bleached, BP 1988

Knitted fabric, cotton yarn, tubular length, 1 m (all), 2.5 cm = 33p; 5 cm = 51p; 7.5 cm = 62p; 6 m × 10 cm = £4.23 (J&J, Medlock)

Uses 1 m lengths, basis (with wadding) for Plaster of Paris bandages etc.; 6 m length, compression bandage

#### Ribbed Cotton and Viscose Surgical Tubular Stockinette, BP 1988

Knitted fabric of 1:1 ribbed structure, singles yarn spun from blend of two-thirds cotton and one-third viscose fibres, tubular. Length 5 m (all):

type A (lightweight): arm/leg (child), arm (adult) 5 cm = £2.40; arm (OS adult), leg (adult) 7.5 cm = £3.15; leg (OS adult) 10 cm = £4.18; trunk (child) 15 cm = £6.02; trunk (adult) 20 cm = £6.95; trunk (OS adult) 25 cm = £8.31 (Mölnlycke)

type B (heavyweight): sizes as for type A, net price £2.30–£7.97 (Sallis—Eesiban®)

Drug Tariff specifies various combinations of sizes to provide sufficient material for part or full body coverage

Uses protective dressings with tar-based and other non-steroid ointments

### ◀ Silk Clothing

Knitted, medical grade silk clothing can be used as an adjunct to normal treatment for severe eczema and allergic skin conditions. When used in combination with medical creams and ointments, care should be taken to ensure that the medication is fully absorbed into the skin before the silk clothing is worn; silk garments are not suitable for use in direct contact with emollients used in 'wet wrapping techniques'.

#### DermaSilk® (Espere)

Knitted silk fabric, hypoallergenic, sericin-free, body suit, child up to 6 months (height 68 cm) = £35.65, 6–9 months (height 74 cm) = £36.67, 12–18 months (height 86 cm) = £36.69, 2–3 years (height 98 cm) = £38.71, 3–4 years (height 110 cm) = £39.73; Facial mask, child 6–12 months = £15.30, 1–6 years = £15.30; Gloves, adult (small, medium or large) = £19.33, child 3–4 years = £13.77, 5–9 years = £13.77; Leggings, child up to 6 months (height 68 cm) = £25.45, 6–9 months (height 74 cm) = £26.47, 12–18 months (height 80 cm) = £27.49, 2–3 years (height 90 cm) = £28.51, 3–4 years (height 110 cm) = £29.53; Pyjamas, child 3–4 years (height 110 cm) = £66.25, 5–6 years (height 120 cm) = £70.53, 7–8 years (height 135 cm) = £73.39, 10–12 years (height 150 cm) = £76.45; Sleeves (tubular) one size = £25.45; Undersocks, (heel-less), 2 pairs standard or longer length = £22.95; Undersocks, adult shoe-size 5½–6½, 7–8½, 9–10½, 11–13, child shoe-size 3–8, 9–1, 2–5, 2 pairs = £17.45

## A8.8.4 Support bandages

Light support bandages, which include the various forms of crepe bandage, are used in the prevention of oedema; they are also used to provide support for mild sprains and joints but their effectiveness has not been proven for this purpose. Since they have limited extensibility, they are able to provide light support without exerting undue pressure. For a warning against injudicious compression see section A8.8.7.

#### Crepe Bandage, BP 1988

Fabric, plain weave, warp of wool threads and crepe-twisted cotton threads, weft of cotton threads; stretch bandage. 4.5 m stretched (all): 5 cm = 90p; 7.5 cm = £1.26; 10 cm = £1.65; 15 cm = £2.39 (most suppliers)

#### Cotton Crepe Bandage

Light support bandage, 4.5 m stretched (all): 5 cm = 48p; 7.5 cm = 67p; 10 cm = 87p; 15 cm = £1.27 (Steraid—Hospicrepe® 239)

**Appendix 8: Wound management**

**Cotton Crepe Bandage, BP 1988**

Fabric, plain weave, warp of crepe-twisted cotton threads, weft of cotton and/or viscose threads; stretch bandage. 4.5 m stretched (both): 7.5 cm = £2.81; 10 cm = £3.62; other sizes ⟨MHS⟩ (most suppliers)

**Cotton, Polyamide and Elastane Bandage**

Fabric, cotton, polyamide, and elastane; light support bandage (Type 2), 4.5 m stretched (all): 5 cm = 54p, 7.5 cm = 73p, 10 cm = 91p, 15 cm = £1.12 (Neomedic—*Neosport*®); 5 cm = 64p, 7.5 cm = 91p, 10 cm = £1.16, 15 cm = £1.67 (BSN Medical—*Softcrepe*®); 10 cm = £1.10 (Mölnlycke—*Setocrepe*®); 10 cm = £1.24, latex-free = £1.31 (S&N Hlth.—*Profore*® #2)

**Cotton Stretch Bandage, BP 1988**

Fabric, plain weave, warp of crepe-twisted cotton threads, weft of cotton threads; stretch bandage, lighter than cotton crepe, 4.5 m stretched (all):

Hospicrepe® 233, 5 cm = 52p; 7.5 cm = 72p; 10 cm = 96p; 15 cm = £1.36 (Steraid)

PremierBand®, 5 cm = 45p, 7.5 cm = 63p, 10 cm = 79p, 15 cm = £1.18 (Shermond)

**Cotton Suspensory Bandage**

(Drug Tariff). Type 1: cotton net bag with draw tapes and webbing waistband; small, medium, and large (all) = £1.55, extra large = £1.65. Type 2: cotton net bag with elastic edge and webbing waistband; small = £1.72, medium = £1.77, large = £1.83, extra large = £1.91. Type 3: cotton net bag with elastic edge and webbing waistband with elastic insertion; small, medium, and large (all) = £1.86; extra large = £1.92. Type supplied to be endorsed

**Knitted Elastomer and Viscose Bandage**

Knitted fabric, viscose and elastomer yarn.

*Type 2 (light support bandage)*

CliniLite®, 4.5 m (all), 5 cm = 44p, 7.5 cm = 61p, 10 cm = 80p, 15 cm = £1.16 (Clinisupplies)

K-Lite®, 4.5 m stretched, 5 cm = 51p, 7 cm = 71p, 10 cm = 93p, 15 cm = £1.34; 5.2 m stretched, 10 cm = £1.06 (Urgo)

Knit-Firm®, 4.5 m stretched, 5 cm = 36p, 7 cm = 51p, 10 cm = 66p, 15 cm = 96p (Steraid)

*Type 3a (light compression bandage)*:

CliniPlus®, 8.7 m × 10 cm = £1.80 (Clinisupplies)

Elset®, 6 m stretched, 10 cm = £2.39, 15 cm = £2.59; 8 m stretched, 10 cm = £3.06; 12 m stretched, 15 cm = £5.13 (Mölnlycke)

K-Plus®, 8.7 m stretched, 10 cm = £2.08 (Urgo)

K-Plus® Long, 10.25 m stretched, 10 cm = £2.41 (Urgo)

Profore® #3, 8.7 m stretched, 10 cm = £3.60, latex-free = £3.91 (S&N Hlth.)

L3, 8.6 m stretched, 10 cm = £2.04 (S&N Hlth.)

## A8.8.5 Adhesive bandages

**Elastic adhesive bandages** are used to provide compression in the treatment of varicose veins and for the support of injured joints; they should no longer be used for the support of fractured ribs and clavicles. They have also been used with **zinc paste bandage** in the treatment of venous ulcers, but they can cause skin reactions in susceptible patients and may not produce sufficient pressures for healing (significantly lower than those provided by other compression bandages).

**Elastic Adhesive Bandage, BP 1993**

Woven fabric, elastic in warp (crepe-twisted cotton threads), weft of cotton and/or viscose threads spread with adhesive mass containing zinc oxide. 4.5 m stretched (all): 5 cm = £3.31; 7.5 cm = £4.80; 10 cm = £6.38 (Robinsons—

*Flexoplast*®; S&N Hlth—*Elastoplast*® Bandage). 7.5 cm width supplied when size not stated

## A8.8.6 Cohesive bandages

**Cohesive bandages** adhere to themselves, but not to the skin, and are useful for providing support for sports use where ordinary stretch bandages might become displaced and adhesive bandages are inappropriate. Care is needed in their application, however, since the loss of ability for movement between turns of the bandage to equalise local areas of high tension carries the potential for creating a tourniquet effect. They should not be used if arterial disease is suspected.

◢**Cohesive extensible bandages**

These elastic bandages adhere to themselves and not to skin; this prevents slipping during use.

*Uses:* support of sprained joints; outer layer of multi-layer compression bandaging

**Coban®** (3M)

6 m (stretched), 10 cm = £2.76; other sizes ⟨MHS⟩ 4.5 m stretched (all): 2.5 cm = £1.29; 5 cm = £1.81; 7.5 cm = £2.74; 10 cm = £3.61; 15 cm = £5.33

**K-Press®** (Urgo)

6.5 m × 10 cm (0, short) = £2.76, 7.5 m × 10 cm (18–25 cm ankle circumference) = £3.22, 10.5 m × 10 cm (25–32 cm ankle circumference) = £3.53

**Profore®** #4 (S&N Hlth.)

2.5 m (unstretched) = £2.97, latex-free = £3.23

**Ultra Fast®** (Robinsons)

6.3 m (stretched), 10 cm = £2.59

## A8.8.7 Compression bandages

High compression products are used to provide the high compression needed for the management of gross varices, post-thrombotic venous insufficiency, venous leg ulcers, and gross oedema in average-sized limbs. Their use calls for an expert knowledge of the elastic properties of the products and experience in the technique of providing careful graduated compression. Incorrect application can lead to uneven and inadequate pressures or to hazardous levels of pressure. In particular, injudicious use of compression in limbs with arterial disease has been reported to cause severe skin and tissue necrosis (in some instances calling for amputation). Doppler testing is required before treatment with compression. Oral pentoxifylline (section 2.6.4) can be used as adjunct therapy if a chronic venous leg ulcer does not respond to compression bandaging [unlicensed indication].

◢**High compression bandages**

**PEC High Compression Bandage**

Polyamide, elastane, and cotton compression (high) extensible bandage, 3.5 m unstretched (both): 7.5 cm = £2.51; 10 cm = £3.25 (Mölnlycke—*Setopress*®)

**VEC High Compression Bandage**

Viscose, elastane, and cotton compression (high) extensible bandage, 3 m unstretched (both): 7.5 cm = £2.53; 10 cm = £3.25 (S&N—*Tensopress*®)

**High Compression Bandage**

Cotton, viscose, nylon, and Lycra® extensible bandage, 3 m (unstretched), 10 cm = £3.33 (ConvaTec— *SurePress*®);

Appendix 8: Wound management

3 m (unstretched), 10 cm = £2.64 (Urgo—*K-ThreeC*®); 3.5 m (unstretched), 10 cm = £1.82 (Advancis—*Adva-Co*®)

**ProGuide® #2** (S&N Hlth.)

Woven, elastomer, cohesive, extensible, compression bandage, 3 m (unstretched), 10 cm (red) = £5.37, 10 cm (yellow) = £5.85, 10 cm (green) = £6.34

◀ **Short stretch compression bandage**

Short stretch bandages help to reduce oedema and promote healing of venous leg ulcers. They are also used to reduce swelling associated with lymphoedema. They are applied at full stretch over padding (*see* Sub-compression Wadding Bandage below) which protects areas of high pressure and sites at high risk of pressure damage.

**Actiban®** (Activa)

All 5 m, 8 cm = £3.08; 10 cm = £3.31; 12 cm = £4.02

**Actico®** (Activa)

Cohesive, all 6 m, 4 cm = £2.19, 6 cm = £2.57, 8 cm = £2.95, 10 cm = £3.07, 12 cm = £3.91

**Comprilan®** (BSN Medical)

All 5 m, 6 cm = £2.52; 8 cm = £2.96; 10 cm = £3.18; 12 cm = £3.87

**Rosidal K®** (Activa)

All 5 m, 4cm = £1.73, 6cm = £2.42, 8 cm = £2.89, 10 cm = £3.15, 12 cm = £3.83; 10m x 10cm = £5.49

**Silkolan®** (Urgo)

All 5 m, 8 cm = £3.00; 10 cm = £3.39

◀ **Sub-compression wadding bandage**

**Advasoft®** (Advancis)

3.5 m unstretched, 10 cm = 37p

**Cellona® Undercast Padding** (Activa)

2.75 m unstretched (all): 5 cm = 29p, 7.5 cm = 35p; 10 cm = 43p; 15 cm = 55p

**Flexi-Ban®** (Activa)

Padding, 3.5 m unstretched, 10cm = 46p

**K-Soft®** (Urgo)

3.5 m unstretched, 10 cm = 42p; 4.5 m unstretched, 10 cm = 52p

**K-Tech®** (Urgo)

5 m unstretched, 10 cm (0, short) = £3.73, 6 m unstretched, 10 cm (18–25 cm ankle circumference) = £4.48, 7.3 m unstretched, 10 cm (25–32 cm ankle circumference) = £4.89

**Ortho-Band Plus®** (Steraid)

10 cm × 3.5 cm unstretched = 37p

**Profore® #1** (S&N Hlth.)

Viscose fleece, 3.5 m unstretched, 10 cm = 64p, latex-free = 70p

**ProGuide® #1** (S&N Hlth.)

Polyester and viscose fleece, 4 m unstretched, 10 cm = £1.49

**Softexe®** (Mölnlycke)

3.5 m unstretched, 10 cm = 58p

**SurePress®** (ConvaTec)

Absorbent padding, 3 m unstretched, 10 cm = 56p

**Ultra Soft®** (Robinsons)

Soft absorbent bandage, 3.5 m unstretched, 10 cm = 39p

**Velband®** (BSN Medical)

Absorbent padding, 4.5 m unstretched, 10 cm = 67p

## A8.8.8 Multi-layer compression bandaging

Multi-layer compression bandaging systems are an alternative to High Compression Bandages (section A8.8.7) for the treatment of venous leg ulcers. Compression is achieved by the combined effects of two or three extensible bandages applied over a layer of orthopaedic wadding and a wound contact dressing.

◀ **Four layer systems**

**K-Four®** (Urgo)

*K-Four® Wound Dressing* (*Paratex*®—see Knitted Viscose Primary Dressing, p. 913); *K-Four® # 1* (*K-Soft*®—see Sub-compression Wadding Bandage, above); *K-Four® # 2* (*K-Lite*®—see Knitted Elastomer and Viscose Bandage, p. 928); *K-Four® # 3* (*K-Plus*®—see Knitted Elastomer and Viscose Bandage, p. 928); *K-Three C*®—see High compression bandages, p. 928); *K-Four® # 4* (*Ko-Flex*®), 6 m (stretched), 10 cm = £2.76; 7 m (stretched), 10 cm = £3.16

Multi-layer compression bandaging kit, four layer system, for ankle circumference up to 18 cm = £6.93, 18–25 cm = £6.51, 25–30 cm = £6.64, above 30 cm = £9.05; *reduced compression*, 18 cm+ = £4.43

**Profore®** (S&N Hlth.)

*Profore®* wound contact layer (see Knitted Viscose Primary Dressing, p. 913); *Profore® #1* (see Sub-compression Wadding Bandage, above); *Profore® #2* (see Cotton, Polyamide and Elastane Bandage, p. 928); *Profore® #3* (see Knitted Elastomer and Viscose Bandage, p. 928); *Profore® #4* (see Cohesive bandages, p. 928); *Profore® Plus* 3 m (unstretched), 10 cm = £3.37, latex-free = £3.60

Multi-layer compression bandaging kit, four layer system, for ankle circumference up to 18 cm = £9.32, 18–25 cm = £8.68, 25–30 cm = £7.21, above 30 cm = £10.79, latex-free, 18–25 cm = £9.28; *Profore Lite*® above 18 cm = £5.01, latex-free = £5.45

**System 4®** (Mölnlycke)

*System 4® #1* (*Softexe*®—see Sub-compression Wadding Bandage, above); *System 4® #2* (*Setocrepe*®—see Cotton, Polyamide and Elastane Bandage, p. 928); *System 4® #3* (*Elset*®—see Knitted Elastomer and Viscose Bandage, p. 928); *System 4® #4* (*Coban*®—see Cohesive Bandages, p. 928)

Multi-layer compression bandaging kit, four layer system, for ankle circumference 18–25 cm = £7.51

**Ultra Four®** (Robinsons)

*Ultra Four® #1* (*Ultra Soft*®—see Sub-compression Wadding Bandage, above); *Ultra Four® #2* (*Ultra Lite*®) 10 cm × 4.5 cm (stretched) = 85p; *Ultra Four® #3* (*Ultra Plus*®) 10 cm × 8.7 cm (stretched) = £1.89; *Ultra Four® #4* (*Ultra Fast*®—see Cohesive Bandages, p. 928)

Multi-layer compression bandaging kit, four layer system, for ankle circumference up to 18 cm = £6.41, 18–25 cm = £5.67; *Ultra Four® RC* (reduced compression) 18–25 cm = £4.14

◀ **Two layer systems**

**Coban®** (3M)

Multi-layer compression bandaging kit, two layer system (latex-free, foam bandage and cohesive compression bandage), one size = £8.08

**K-Two®** (Urgo)

*K-Tech*® (see Sub-compression Wadding Bandages, above); *K-Press*® (see Cohesive Bandages, p. 928)

Multi-layer compression bandaging kit, two layer system, ankle circumference 18–25 cm (short) = £6.50, ankle circumference 18–25 cm= £7.70, ankle circumference 25–32 cm = £8.41

*K-Two® Start, Urgotul® Start* (see Soft polymer dressings, p. 915); *K-Tech®* (see Sub-compression Wadding Bandages, p. 929); *K-Press®* (see Cohesive Bandages, p. 928)

Multi-layer compression bandaging kit, two-layer system, for ankle circumference 18–25cm = £9.68; 25–32cm = £10.33

**ProGuide®** (S&N Hlth.)

*ProGuide®* wound contact layer (see Soft polymer dressings, p. 916); *ProGuide®* #1 (see Sub-compression Wadding Bandage, p. 929); *ProGuide®* #2 (see High Compression Bandages, p. 929)

Multi-layer compression bandaging kit, two layer system, for ankle circumference 18–22 cm (red) = £8.98; 22–28 cm (yellow) = £9.48; 28–32 cm (green) = £9.96

## A8.8.9 Medicated bandages

**Zinc Paste Bandage** has been used with compression bandaging for the treatment of venous leg ulcers. However, paste bandages are associated with hypersensitivity reactions and should be used with caution.

Zinc paste bandages are also used with **coal tar** or **ichthammol** in chronic lichenified skin conditions such as chronic eczema (ichthammol often being preferred since its action is considered to be milder). They are also used with **calamine** in milder eczematous skin conditions.

**Zinc Paste Bandage, BP 1993**

Cotton fabric, plain weave, impregnated with suitable paste containing zinc oxide; requires additional bandaging, 6 m × 7.5 cm = £3.23 (S&N Hlth.—*Viscopaste PB7®* (10%), *excipients: include* cetostearyl alcohol, hydroxybenzoates)

**Zinc Paste and Calamine Bandage**

(Drug Tariff specification 5). Cotton fabric, plain weave, impregnated with suitable paste containing calamine and zinc oxide; requires additional bandaging. 6 m × 7.5 cm = £3.33 (Mölnlycke—*Calaband®*)

**Zinc Paste and Ichthammol Bandage, BP 1993**

Cotton fabric, plain weave, impregnated with suitable paste containing zinc oxide and ichthammol; requires additional bandaging, 6 m × 7.5 cm = £3.31 S&N Hlth.—*Ichthopaste®* (6/2%), *excipients: include* cetostearyl alcohol

Uses see section 13.5

**Steripaste®** (Mölnlycke)

Cotton fabric, selvedge weave impregnated with paste containing zinc oxide (requires additional bandaging), 6 m × 7.5 cm = £3.24

Excipients include polysorbate 80

◢ **Medicated stocking**

**Zipzoc®** (S&N Hlth.)

Sterile rayon stocking impregnated with ointment containing zinc oxide 20%. 4-pouch carton = £12.52; 10-pouch carton = £31.30

Note Can be used under appropriate compression bandages or hosiery in chronic venous insufficiency

## A8.9 Compression hosiery and garments

**Compression (elastic) hosiery** is used to treat conditions associated with chronic venous insufficiency, to prevent recurrence of thrombosis, or to reduce the risk of further venous ulceration after treatment with compression bandaging (section A8.8.7). Doppler testing to confirm arterial sufficiency is required before recommending the use of compression hosiery.

Before elastic hosiery can be dispensed, the quantity (single or pair), article (including accessories), and compression class must be specified by the prescriber. There are different compression values for graduated compression hosiery and lymphoedema garments (see table below). All dispensed elastic hosiery articles must state on the packaging that they conform with Drug Tariff technical specification No. 40, for further details see Drug Tariff.

Note Graduated compression tights are [NHS]

### Compression values for hosiery and lymphoedema garments

| Compression class | Compression hosiery (British standard) | Lymphoedema garments (European classification) |
| --- | --- | --- |
| Class 1 | 14–17 mmHg | 18–21 mmHg |
| Class 2 | 18–24 mmHg | 23–32 mmHg |
| Class 3 | 25–35 mmHg | 34–46 mmHg |
| Class 4 | Not available | 49–70 mmHg |
| Class 4 super | Not available | 60–90 mmHg |

## A8.9.1 Graduated compression hosiery

**Class 1 Light Support**

Hosiery, compression at ankle 14–17 mmHg, thigh length or below knee with knitted in heel. 1 pair, circular knit (standard), thigh length = £7.44, below knee = £6.80, (made-to-measure), thigh length = £36.95, below knee = £23.12; lightweight elastic net (made-to-measure), thigh length = £19.93, below knee = £15.55

Uses superficial or early varices, varicosis during pregnancy

**Class 2 Medium Support**

Hosiery, compression at ankle 18–24 mmHg, thigh length or below knee with knitted in heel. 1 pair, circular knit (standard), thigh length = £11.06, below knee = £9.94, (made-to-measure), thigh length = £36.95, below knee = £23.12; net (made-to-measure), thigh length = £19.93, below knee = £15.55; flat bed (made-to-measure, only with closed heel and open toe), thigh length = £36.95, below knee = £23.12

Uses varices of medium severity, ulcer treatment and prophylaxis, mild oedema, varicosis during pregnancy

**Class 3 Strong Support**

Hosiery, compression at ankle 25–35 mmHg, thigh length or below knee with open or knitted in heel. 1 pair, circular knit (standard), thigh length = £13.11, below knee = £11.27, (made-to-measure), thigh length = £36.95, below knee = £23.12; flat bed (made-to-measure, only with open heel and open toe), thigh length = £36.95, below knee = £23.12

Uses gross varices, post thrombotic venous insufficiency, gross oedema, ulcer treatment and prophylaxis

◢ **Accessories**

In addition to the product listed below, accessories such as application aids for hosiery are available, see Drug Tariff for details

**Suspender**

Suspender, for thigh stockings = 65p, belt (specification 13), = £4.96, fitted (additional price) = 62p

Appendix 8: Wound management

◀Anklets
**Class 2 Medium Support**
Anklets, compression 18–24 mmHg, circular knit (standard and made-to-measure), 1 pair = £6.51; flat bed (standard and made-to-measure) = £13.53; net (made-to-measure) = £12.80

**Class 3 Strong Support**
Anklets, compression 25–35 mmHg, circular knit (standard and made-to-measure), 1 pair = £9.09; flat bed (standard) = £9.09, (made-to-measure) = £13.53

◀Knee caps
**Class 2 Medium Support**
Kneecaps, compression 18–24 mmHg, circular knit (standard and made-to-measure), 1 pair = £6.51; flat bed (standard and made-to-measure) = £13.53; net (made-to-measure) = £10.63

**Class 3 Strong Support**
Kneecaps, compression 25–35 mmHg, circular knit (standard and made-to-measure), 1 pair = £8.68; flat bed (standard) = £8.68, (made-to-measure) = £13.53

## A8.9.2 Lymphoedema garments

**Lymphoedema compression garments** are used to maintain limb shape and prevent additional fluid retention.

In addition to the products listed below, made-to-measure garments up to compression 90 mmHg and accessories also available; see Drug Tariff for details. There are different compression values for lymphoedema garments and graduated compression hosiery, see table, p. 930

**Low Compression**
Armsleeves (with grip top), compression 12–16 mmHg, small, medium, and large sizes all available short or long, 1 pair = £16.70

**Class 1 Light support**
Hosiery and armsleeves, compression 18–21 mmHg, small, medium, large, and extra large (hosiery only) sizes all available standard length (some available petite), 1 pair below knee closed toe (no top band) = £25.50, thigh closed toe (with top band) = £49.00; 1 piece armsleeve (no top band) = £13.50, armsleeve (with top band) = £18.00, combined armsleeve (no top band) = £24.50, combined armsleeve (with top band) = £29.00
Armsleeves (with grip top), compression 18–22 mmHg, small, medium, and large sizes all available short or long, 1 pair = £16.70

**Class 2 Medium support**
Hosiery and armsleeves, compression 23–32 mmHg, small, medium, large, and extra large (hosiery only) sizes all available standard length (some available petite), 1 pair below knee closed or open toe (no top band) = £25.50, thigh closed or open toe (with top band) = £49.00; 1 piece armsleeve (no top band) = £14.50, armsleeve (with top band) = £19.00, combined armsleeve (no top band) = £25.50, combined armsleeve (with top band) = £30.00

**Class 3 Strong support**
Hosiery, compression 34–46 mmHg, small, medium, large, and extra large sizes all available standard length (some available petite), 1 pair below knee open toe (no top band) = £28.00, thigh open toe (with top band) = £51.00

Appendix 8: Wound management

# A9 Cautionary and advisory labels for dispensed medicines

Numbers following the preparation entries in the BNF correspond to the code numbers of the cautionary labels that pharmacists are recommended to add when dispensing. It is also expected that pharmacists will counsel patients when necessary.

Counselling needs to be related to the age, experience, background, and understanding of the individual patient. The pharmacist should ensure that the patient understands how to take or use the medicine and how to follow the correct dosage schedule. Any effects of the medicine on driving or work, any foods or medicines to be avoided, and what to do if a dose is missed should also be explained. Other matters, such as the possibility of staining of the clothes or skin by a medicine should also be mentioned.

For some preparations there is a special need for counselling, such as an unusual method or time of administration or a potential interaction with a common food or domestic remedy, and this is indicated where necessary.

**Original packs** Most preparations are now dispensed in unbroken original packs (see Patient Packs, p. x) that include further advice for the patient in the form of patient information leaflets. Label 10 may be of value where appropriate. More general leaflets advising on the administration of preparations such as eye drops, eye ointments, inhalers, and suppositories are also available.

**Scope of labels** In general no label recommendations have been made for injections on the assumption that they will be administered by a healthcare professional or a well-instructed patient. The labelling is not exhaustive and pharmacists are recommended to use their professional discretion in labelling new preparations and those for which no labels are shown.

Individual labelling advice is not given on the administration of the large variety of antacids. In the absence of instructions from the prescriber, and if on enquiry the patient has had no verbal instructions, the directions given under 'Dose' should be used on the label.

It is recognised that there may be occasions when pharmacists will use their knowledge and professional discretion and decide to omit one or more of the recommended labels for a particular patient. In this case counselling is of the utmost importance. There may also be an occasion when a prescriber does not wish additional cautionary labels to be used, in which case the prescription should be endorsed 'NCL' (no cautionary labels). The exact wording that is required instead should then be specified on the prescription.

Pharmacists label medicines with various wordings in addition to those directions specified on the prescription. Such labels include 'Shake the bottle', 'For external use only', and 'Store in a cool place', as well as 'Discard . . . . days after opening' and 'Do not use after . . . .', which apply particularly to antibiotic mixtures, diluted liquid and topical preparations, and to eye-drops. Although not listed in the BNF these labels should continue to be used when appropriate; indeed, 'For external use only' is a legal requirement on external liquid preparations, while 'Keep out of the reach of children' is a legal requirement on all dispensed medicines. Care should be taken not to obscure other relevant information with adhesive labelling.

It is the usual practice for patients to take standard tablets with water or other liquid and for this reason no separate label has been recommended.

The label wordings recommended by the BNF apply to medicines dispensed against a prescription. Patients should be aware that a dispensed medicine should never be taken by, or shared with, anyone other than for whom the prescriber intended it. Therefore, the BNF does not include warnings against the use of a dispensed medicine by persons other than for whom it was specifically prescribed.

The label or labels for each preparation are recommended after careful consideration of the information available. However, it is recognised that in some cases this information may be either incomplete or open to a different interpretation. The BNF will therefore be grateful to receive any constructive comments on the labelling suggested for any preparation.

## Recommended label wordings

Wordings which can be given as separate warnings are labels 1–19 and 29–33. Wordings which can be incorporated in an appropriate position in the directions for dosage or administration are labels 21–28. A label has been omitted for number 20.

If separate labels are used it is recommended that the wordings be used without modification. If changes are made to suit computer requirements, care should be taken to retain the sense of the original.

1   **Warning. May cause drowsiness**
    To be used on *preparations for children* containing antihistamines, or other preparations given to children where the warnings of label 2 on driving or alcohol would not be appropriate.

2   **Warning. May cause drowsiness. If affected do not drive or operate machinery. Avoid alcoholic drink**
    To be used on *preparations for adults that can cause drowsiness*, thereby affecting the ability to drive and operate hazardous machinery; label 1 is more appropriate for children. *It is an offence to drive while under the influence of drink or drugs.*

Some of these preparations only cause drowsiness in the first few days of treatment and some only cause drowsiness in higher doses.

In such cases the patient should be told that the advice applies until the effects have worn off. However many of these preparations can produce a slowing of reaction time and a loss of mental concentration that can have the same effects as drowsiness.

Avoidance of alcoholic drink is recommended because the effects of CNS depressants are enhanced by alcohol. Strict prohibition however could lead to some patients not taking the medicine. Pharmacists should therefore explain the risk and encourage compliance, particularly in patients who may think they already tolerate the effects of alcohol (see also label 3).

Queries from patients with epilepsy regarding fitness to drive should be referred back to the patient's doctor.

Side-effects unrelated to drowsiness that may affect a patient's ability to drive or operate machinery safely include *blurred vision, dizziness, or nausea*. In general, no label has been recommended to cover these cases, but the patient should be suitably counselled.

**3    Warning. May cause drowsiness. If affected do not drive or operate machinery**

To be used on *preparations containing monoamine-oxidase inhibitors*; the warning to avoid alcohol and dealcoholised (low alcohol) drink is covered by the patient information leaflet.

Also to be used as for label 2 but where alcohol is not an issue.

**4    Warning. Avoid alcoholic drink**

To be used on *preparations where a reaction such as flushing may occur if alcohol is taken* (e.g. metronidazole and chlorpropamide). Alcohol may also enhance the hypoglycaemia produced by some oral antidiabetic drugs but routine application of a warning label is not considered necessary.

**5    Do not take indigestion remedies at the same time of day as this medicine**

To be used with label 25 on *preparations coated to resist gastric acid* (e.g. enteric-coated tablets). This is to avoid the possibility of premature dissolution of the coating in the presence of an alkaline pH.

Label 5 also applies to drugs such as ketoconazole *where the absorption is significantly affected by antacids*; the usual period of avoidance recommended is 2 to 4 hours.

**6    Do not take indigestion remedies or medicines containing iron or zinc at the same time of day as this medicine**

To be used on *preparations containing ofloxacin and some other quinolones, doxycycline, lymecycline, minocycline, and penicillamine*. These drugs chelate calcium, iron and zinc and are less well absorbed when taken with calcium-containing antacids or preparations containing iron or zinc. These incompatible preparations should be taken 2–3 hours apart.

**7    Do not take milk, indigestion remedies, or medicines containing iron or zinc at the same time of day as this medicine**

To be used on *preparations containing ciprofloxacin, norfloxacin or tetracyclines that chelate calcium, iron, magnesium, and zinc* and are thus less available for absorption; these incompatible preparations should be taken 2–3 hours apart. Doxycycline, lymecycline and minocycline are less liable to form chelates and therefore only require label 6 (see above).

**8    Do not stop taking this medicine except on your doctor's advice**

To be used on *preparations that contain a drug which is required to be taken over long periods without the patient necessarily perceiving any benefit* (e.g. antituberculous drugs).

Also to be used on *preparations that contain a drug whose withdrawal is likely to be a particular hazard*

(e.g. clonidine for hypertension). Label 10 (see below) is more appropriate for corticosteroids.

**9    Take at regular intervals. Complete the prescribed course unless otherwise directed**

To be used on *preparations where a course of treatment should be completed* to reduce the incidence of relapse or failure of treatment.

The preparations are antimicrobial drugs given by mouth. Very occasionally, some may have severe side-effects (e.g. diarrhoea in patients receiving clindamycin) and in such cases the patient may need to be advised of reasons for stopping treatment quickly and returning to the doctor.

**10    Warning. Follow the printed instructions you have been given with this medicine**

To be used particularly on *preparations containing anticoagulants, lithium and oral corticosteroids*. The appropriate treatment card should be given to the patient and any necessary explanations given.

This label may also be used on other preparations to remind the patient of the instructions that have been given.

**11    Avoid exposure of skin to direct sunlight or sun lamps**

To be used on *preparations that may cause phototoxic or photoallergic reactions* if the patient is exposed to ultraviolet radiation. Many drugs other than those listed in Appendix 9 (e.g. phenothiazines and sulphonamides) may, on rare occasions, cause reactions in susceptible patients. Exposure to high intensity ultraviolet radiation from sunray lamps and sunbeds is particularly likely to cause reactions.

**12    Do not take anything containing aspirin while taking this medicine**

To be used on *preparations containing probenecid and sulfinpyrazone* whose activity is reduced by aspirin.

Label 12 should not be used for anticoagulants since label 10 is more appropriate.

**13    Dissolve or *mix with water* before taking**

To be used on *preparations that are intended to be dissolved in water* (e.g. soluble tablets) or *mixed with water* (e.g. powders, granules) before use. In a few cases other liquids such as fruit juice or milk may be used.

**14    This medicine may colour the urine**

To be used on *preparations that may cause the patient's urine to turn an unusual colour*. These include phenolphthalein (alkaline urine pink), triamterene (blue under some lights), levodopa (dark reddish), and rifampicin (red).

**15    Caution flammable: keep away from fire or flames**

To be used on *preparations containing sufficient flammable solvent to render them flammable if exposed to a naked flame.*

**16    Allow to dissolve under the tongue. Do not transfer from this container. Keep tightly closed. Discard eight weeks after opening**

To be used on *glyceryl trinitrate tablets* to remind the patient not to transfer the tablets to plastic or less suitable containers.

**17    Do not take more than . . . in 24 hours**

To be used on *preparations for the treatment of acute migraine* except those containing ergotamine, for which label 18 is used. The dose form should be specified, e.g. tablets or capsules.

It may also be used on preparations for which no dose has been specified by the prescriber.

**18    Do not take more than . . . in 24 hours or . . . in any one week**

To be used on preparations containing ergotamine. The dose form should be specified, e.g. tablets or suppositories.

**19** **Warning. Causes drowsiness which may continue the next day. If affected do not drive or operate machinery. Avoid alcoholic drink**

To be used on *preparations containing hypnotics (or some other drugs with sedative effects) prescribed to be taken at night.* On the rare occasions (e.g. nitrazepam in epilepsy) when hypnotics are prescribed for daytime administration this label would clearly not be appropriate. Also to be used as an *alternative to the label 2 wording* (the choice being at the discretion of the pharmacist) *for anxiolytics prescribed to be taken at night.*

It is hoped that this wording will convey adequately the problem of residual morning sedation after taking 'sleeping tablets'.

**21** **. . . with or after food**

To be used on *preparations that are liable to cause gastric irritation, or those that are better absorbed with food.*

Patients should be advised that a *small amount of food is sufficient.*

**22** **. . . half to one hour before food**

To be used on some preparations *whose absorption is thereby improved.*

Most oral antibacterials require label 23 instead (see below).

**23** **. . . an hour before food or on an empty stomach**

To be used on *oral preparations whose absorption may be reduced by the presence of food and acid in the stomach.*

**24** **. . . sucked or chewed**

To be used on *preparations that should be sucked or chewed.*

The pharmacist should use discretion as to which of these words is appropriate.

**25** **. . . swallowed whole, not chewed**

To be used on *preparations that are enteric-coated or designed for modified-release.*

Also to be used on *preparations that taste very unpleasant or may damage the mouth* if not swallowed whole.

**26** **. . . dissolved under the tongue**

To be used on *preparations designed for sublingual use.* Patients should be advised to hold under the tongue and avoid swallowing until dissolved. The buccal mucosa between the gum and cheek is occasionally specified by the prescriber.

**27** **. . . with plenty of water**

To be used on *preparations that should be well diluted* (e.g. chloral hydrate), *where a high fluid intake is required* (e.g. sulphonamides), or *where water is required to aid the action* (e.g. methylcellulose). The patient should be advised that 'plenty' means at least 150 mL (about a tumblerful). In most cases fruit juice, tea, or coffee may be used.

**28** **To be spread thinly . . .**

To be used on *external preparations* that should be applied sparingly (e.g. corticosteroids, dithranol).

**29** **Do not take more than 2 at any one time. Do not take more than 8 in 24 hours**

To be used on containers of dispensed *solid dose preparations containing paracetamol for adults when* the instruction on the label indicates that the dose can be taken on an *'as required' basis.* The dose form should be specified, e.g. tablets or capsules.

This label has been introduced because of the serious consequences of overdosage with paracetamol.

**30** **Do not take with any other paracetamol products**

To be used on all containers of dispensed *preparations containing paracetamol.*

**31** **Contains aspirin and paracetamol. Do not take with any other paracetamol products**

To be used on all containers of dispensed *preparations containing aspirin and paracetamol.*

**32** **Contains aspirin**

To be used on containers of dispensed *preparations containing aspirin when the name on the label does not include the word 'aspirin'.*

**33** **Contains an aspirin-like medicine**

To be used on containers of dispensed *preparations containing aspirin derivatives.*

# Products and their labels

Products introduced or amended since publication of BNF No. 57 (March 2009) are underlined.
Proprietary names are in *italic*.
C = counselling advised; see BNF = consult product entry in BNF

Abacavir, C, hypersensitivity reactions, see BNF

*Abilify*, 2

*Abilify orodispersible tabs*, 2, C, administration, see BNF

*Abstral*, 2, 26

Acamprosate, 21, 25

Acarbose, C, administration, see BNF

*Accolate*, 23

Acebutolol, 8

Aceclofenac, 21

Acemetacin, 21, C, driving

Acenocoumarol, 10, anticoagulant card

Acetazolamide, 3

Acetazolamide m/r, 3, 25

Aciclovir susp and tabs, 9

Acipimox, 21

Acitretin, 10, patient information leaflet, 21

*Acomplia*, C, depression, see BNF

*Actinac*, 28

*Actiq*, 2

*Actonel*, C, administration, food and calcium, see BNF

*Acupan*, 2, 14, (urine pink)

*Adalat LA*, 25

*Adalat Retard*, 25

Adalimumab, C, tuberculosis

*Adcal*, 24

*Adcal-D₃*, 24

*Adcal-D₃ Dissolve*, 13

*Adipine MR*, 21, 25

*Adipine XL*, 25

*Adizem preps*, 25

*Advagraf*, 23, 25, C, driving, see BNF

*Airomir*, C, dose, change to CFC-free inhaler, see BNF

Albendazole, 9

Alclometasone external preps, 28, C, application, see BNF

Aldactone, 21

*Aldara*, 10, patient information leaflet

*Aldomet*, 3, 8

Alendronic acid, C, administration, see BNF

Alfuzosin, 3, C, dose, see BNF

Alfuzosin m/r, 3, 21, 25, C, dose, see BNF

Alimemazine, 2

Aliskiren, 21

Alitretinoin, 10, patient information leaflet, 11, 21

*Allegron*, 2

Allopurinol, 8, 21, 27

*Almogran*, 3

Almotriptan, 3

*Alphosyl HC*, 28

*Alphaderm*, 28, C, application, see BNF

Alprazolam, 2
Altargo, 28
Alvedon, 30
Alvesco, 8, C, dose
Amantadine, C, driving
Aminophylline m/r, see preps
Amiodarone, 11
Amisulpride, 2
Amitriptyline, 2
Amobarbital sodium, 19
Amorolfine, 10, patient information leaflet
Amoxicillin, 9
Amoxicillin dispersible sachets, 9, 13
Amoxil, 9
Amoxil dispersible sachets, 9, 13
Amoxil paed susp, 9, C, use of pipette
Amphotericin loz, 9, 24, C, after food
Ampicillin, 9, 23
Anafranil, 2
Anafranil m/r, 2, 25
Anagrelide, C, driving
Anakinra, C, blood disorder symptoms
Androcur, 21
Andropatch, C, administration, see BNF
Angettes-75, 32
Angitil SR, 25
Angitil XL, 25
Anhydrol Forte, 15
Anquil, 2
Antabuse, 2, C, alcohol reaction, see BNF
Antacids, see BNF dose statements
Antepsin, 5
Anticoagulants, oral, 10, anticoagulant card
Antihistamines, (see individual preparations)
Anturan, 12, 21
Aptivus, 5, 21
Arava, 4
Aricept Evess, C, administration
Aripiprazole, 2
Aripiprazole orodispersible tabs, 2, C, administration, see BNF
Arlevert, 2
Aromasin, 21
Arpicolin, C, driving
Artemether with lumefantrine, 21, C, driving
Arythmol, 21, 25
Arthrotec, 21, 25
Asacol MR tabs, 5, 25, C, blood disorder symptoms, see BNF
Asacol enema and supps, C, blood disorder symptoms, see BNF
Asasantin Retard, 21, 25
Ascorbic acid tabs (500 mg), 24
Asmabec preps, 8, C, dose; with high doses, 10, steroid card
Asmanex, 8, 10, steroid card, C, dose

Asmasal, C, dose, see BNF
Aspav, 2, 13, 21, 32
Aspirin and papaveretum dispersible tabs, 2, 13, 21, also 32 (if 'aspirin' not on label)
Aspirin dispersible tabs, 13, 21, also 32 (if 'aspirin' not on label)
Aspirin e/c, 5, 25, also 32 (if 'aspirin' not on label)
Aspirin m/r, 25, also 32 (if 'aspirin' not on label)
Aspirin supps, 32, (if 'aspirin' not on label)
Aspirin tabs, 21, also 32 (if 'aspirin' not on label)
Atarax, 2
Atazanavir, 5, 21
Atenolol, 8
Atomoxetine, 3
Atorvastatin, C, muscle effects, see BNF
Atovaquone, 21
Atripla, 23, 25
Atrovent inhalations, C, dose, see BNF
Augmentin susp and tabs, 9
Augmentin Duo, 9
Augmentin dispersible tabs, 9, 13
Auranofin, 11, 21, C, blood disorder symptoms, see BNF
Aureocort, 28, C, application, see BNF
Avandamet, 21
Avelox, 6, 9, C, driving
Avloclor, 5, C, malaria prophylaxis, see BNF
Avodart, 25
Avomine, 2
Azathioprine, 21
Azithromycin caps, 5, 9, 23
Azithromycin susp and tabs, 5, 9

Baclofen, 2, 8
Balsalazide, 21, 25
Baraclude, C, administration
Baratol, 2
Baxan, 9
Beclazone, 8, C, dose; with high doses, 10, steroid card
Beclometasone inhalations, 8, C, dose; with high doses, 10, steroid card
Becodisks, 8, C, dose; with high doses, 10, steroid card
Benemid, 12, 21, 27
Benperidol, 2
Benzoin tincture, compound, 15
Beta-Adalat, 8, 25
Betacap, 15, 28, C, application, see BNF
Beta-Cardone, 8
Betahistine, 21
Betaloc-SA, 8, 25
Betamethasone inj, 10, steroid card

Betamethasone soluble tab, 10, steroid card, 13, 21, (when used as a mouthwash, Label: 10, 13, C, administration)
Betamethasone tab, 10, steroid card, 21
Betamethasone external preps, 28, C, application, see BNF
Betamethasone scalp application, 15, 28, C, application, see BNF
Bethanechol, 22
Betim, 8
Betnelan, 10, steroid card, 21
Betnesol injection, 10, steroid card
Betnesol tabs, 10, steroid card, 13, 21, (when used as a mouthwash, Label: 10, 13, C, administration)
Betnovate external preps, 28, C, application, see BNF
Betnovate scalp application, 15, 28, C, application, see BNF
Betnovate-RD, 28, C, application, see BNF
Bettamousse, 28, C, application, see BNF
Bezafibrate, 21
Bezafibrate m/r, 21, 25
Bezalip, 21
Bezalip-Mono, 21, 25
Biorphen, C, driving
Bisacodyl tabs, 5, 25
Bisoprolol, 8
Bolamyn SR, 21, 25
Bondronat tabs, C, administration, see BNF
Bonefos caps and tabs, C, food and calcium, see BNF
Bonviva tabs, C, administration, see BNF
Brexidol, 21
Bricanyl inhalations, C, dose, see BNF
Britlofex, 2
Broflex, C, driving, see BNF
Bromocriptine, 21, C, hypotensive reactions, see BNF
Brufen, 21
Brufen gran, 13, 21
Brufen Retard, 25, 27
Buccastem, 2, C, administration, see BNF
Budenofalk, 5, 10, steroid card, 22, 25
Budesonide inhalations, 8, C, dose; with high doses, 10, steroid card
Budesonide caps, 5, 10, steroid card, 22, 25
Budesonide m/r caps, 5, 10, steroid card, 25
Buprenorphine, 2, 26
Bupropion, 25, C, driving
Buserelin nasal spray, C, nasal decongestants, see BNF
Buspar, C, driving
Buspirone, C, driving

Butobarbital, 19
*BuTrans*, 2
*Byetta*, C, administration, see BNF

*Cabaser*, 21, C, driving, hypotensive reactions, see BNF
Cabergoline, 21, C, driving, hypotensive reactions, see BNF
*Cacit*, 13
*Cacit D3*, 13
*Cafergot*, 18, C, dosage
*Calceos*, 24
*Calcicard CR*, 25
*Calcichew preps*, 24
*Calcium-500*, 25
Calcium acetate tabs, 25, C, with meals
Calcium carbonate tabs, chewable, 24
Calcium carbonate tabs and gran effervescent, 13
Calcium gluconate tabs, 24
Calcium phosphate sachets, 13
*Calcium Resonium*, 13
Calcium and ergocalciferol tabs, C, administration, see BNF
*Calcort*, 5, 10, steroid card
*Calfovit D3*, 13, 21
*Calmurid HC*, 28, C, application, see BNF
*Calpol susp*, 30
*Camcolit 250 tabs*, 10, lithium card, C, fluid and salt intake, see BNF
*Camcolit 400 tabs*, 10, lithium card, 25, C, fluid and salt intake, see BNF
*Campral EC*, 21, 25
*Canesten HC*, 28, C, application, see BNF
*Canesten spray*, 15
Capecitabine, 21
*Caprin*, 5, 25, 32
*Carbaglu*, 13
Carbamazepine chewable, 3, 8, 21, 24, C, blood, hepatic or skin disorder symptoms (see BNF), driving (see BNF)
Carbamazepine liq, supps and tabs, 3, 8, C, blood, hepatic or skin disorder symptoms (see BNF), driving (see BNF)
Carbamazepine m/r, 3, 8, 25, C, blood, hepatic or skin disorder symptoms (see BNF), driving (see BNF)
Carbimazole, C, blood disorder symptoms, see BNF
*Cardene SR*, 25
*Cardura*, C, initial dose, driving
*Cardura XL*, 25, C, initial dose, driving
Carglumic acid, 13
*Carisoma*, 2
Carisoprodol, 2
Carvedilol, 8
*Catapres*, 3, 8

*Cefaclor*, 9
*Cefaclor m/r*, 9, 21, 25
Cefadroxil, 9
Cefalexin, 9
Cefixime, 9
Cefpodoxime, 5, 9, 21
Cefradine, 9
Cefuroxime susp, 9, 21
Cefuroxime tab, 9, 21, 25
*Celance*, C, driving, hypotensive reactions, see BNF
*Celectol*, 8, 22
*Celevac (constipation or diarrhoea)*, C, administration, see BNF
*Celevac tabs (anorectic)*, C, administration, see BNF
Celiprolol, 8, 22
*Centyl K*, 25, 27, C, posture, see BNF
*Ceporex*, 9
Cetirizine, C, driving, alcohol, see BNF
*Champix*, 3
*Chemydur 60XL*, 25
Chloral hydrate, 19, 27
Chloral paed elixir, 1, 27
Chloral mixt, 19, 27
Chlordiazepoxide, 2
Chloroquine, 5, C, malaria prophylaxis, see BNF
Chlorphenamine, 2
Chlorpromazine solution, supps and tabs, 2, 11
Chlorpropamide, 4
Cholera vaccine (oral), C, administration
*Cholestagel*, 21
Ciclesonide, 8, C, dose
Ciclosporin, C, administration, see BNF
*Cinacalcet*, 21
Cinnarizine, 2
*Cipralex drops*, C, driving, administration
*Cipralex tabs*, C, driving
*Cipramil drops*, C, driving, administration
*Cipramil tabs*, C, driving
Ciprofloxacin, 7, 9, 25, C, driving
*Ciproxin susp and tabs*, 7, 9, 25, C, driving
*Circadin*, 2, 21, 25
Citalopram drops, C, driving, administration
Citalopram tabs, C, driving
*CitraFleet*, 10, patient information leaflet, 13, C, administration
*Citramag*, 10, patient information leaflet, 13, C, administration
*Clarelux*, 15, 28, C, application, see BNF
Clarithromycin, 9
Clarithromycin m/r, 9, 21, 25
Clarithromycin sachets, 9, 13
*Clasteon*, C, food and calcium, see BNF

Clemastine, 2
*Clenil Modulite*, 8, C, dose; with high doses, 10, steroid card
Clindamycin, 9, 27, C, diarrhoea, see BNF
*Clipper*, 25
Clobazam, 2 or 19, 8, C, driving (see BNF)
Clobetasol external preps, 28, C, application, see BNF
Clobetasol scalp application, 15, 28, C, application, see BNF
Clobetasone butyrate, 28, C, application, see BNF
Clofazimine, 8, 14, (urine red), 21
Clomethiazole, 19
Clomipramine, 2
Clomipramine m/r, 2, 25
Clonazepam, 2, 8, C, driving (see BNF)
Clonidine, *see Catapres*
*Clopixol*, 2
*Clotam Rapid*, 21
Clotrimazole spray, 15
*Clozapine tabs*, 2, 10, patient information leaflet
*Clozapine susp*, 2, 10, patient information leaflet, C, administration
*Clozaril*, 2, 10, patient information leaflet
Coal tar paint, 15
Co-amoxiclav, 9
Co-amoxiclav dispersible tabs, 9, 13
Co-beneldopa, 14, (urine reddish), C, driving
Co-beneldopa dispersible tabs, 14, (urine reddish), C, administration, driving, see BNF
Co-beneldopa m/r, 14, (urine reddish), 25, C, driving
Co-careldopa, 14, (urine reddish), C, driving
Co-careldopa intestinal gel, 14, (urine reddish), C, driving
Co-careldopa m/r, 14, (urine reddish), 25, C, driving
Co-codamol, see preps
Co-codaprin dispersible tabs, 13, 21, 32
*Codalax*, 14, (urine red)
Co-danthramer, 14, (urine red)
Co-danthrusate, 14, (urine red)
Codeine phosphate syr and tabs, 2
*Codipar*, 2, 29, 30
Co-dydramol, 21, 29, 30
Co-fluampicil, 9, 22
*Colazide*, 21, 25
Colesevelam, 21
*Colestid*, 13, C, avoid other drugs at same time, see BNF
Colestipol preps, 13, C, avoid other drugs at same time, see BNF

Colestyramine, 13, C, avoid other drugs at same time, see BNF

Collodion, flexible, 15

Colofac, C, administration, see BNF

Colofac MR, 25, C, administration, see BNF

Colpermin, 5, 22, 25

Co-methiamol, 29, 30

Competact, 21

Comtess, 14, (urine reddish-brown), C, driving, avoid iron-containing preparations at the same time of day

Concerta XL, 25

Condyline, 15

Convulex, 8, 25, C, blood or hepatic disorder symptoms (see BNF), driving (see BNF)

Copegus, 21

Co-prenozide, 8, 25

Coracten preps, 25

Cordarone X, 11

Corgard, 8

Cortisone tab, 10, steroid card, 21

Co-tenidone, 8

Co-triamterzide, 14, (urine blue in some tablets), 21

Co-trimoxazole susp and tabs, 9

Coversyl, 22

Coversyl Arginine, 22

Coversyl Plus, 22

Coversyl Arginine Plus, 22

Creon preps, C, administration, see BNF

Crixivan, 27, C, administration, see BNF

Cuplex, 15

Cutivate, 28, C, application, see BNF

Cyclizine, 2

Cyclophosphamide, 23, 25, 27

Cycloserine caps, 2, 8

Cymbalta, 2

Cymevene, 21

Cyproheptadine, 2

Cyprostat, 21

Cyproterone, 21

Cystrin, 3

Cytotec, 21

Dabigatran, 25

Daktacort, 28, C, application, see BNF

Daktarin oral gel, 9, C, hold in mouth, after food

Dalacin C, 9, 27, C, diarrhoea, see BNF

Dalmane, 19

Dantrium, 2, C, driving, hepatotoxicity (see BNF)

Dantrolene, 2, C, driving, hepatotoxicity (see BNF)

Dapsone, 8

Darifenacin m/r, 3, 25

Darunavir, 21, C, missed dose, see BNF

Dasatinib, 25

DDAVP Melt, 26, C, fluid intake, see BNF

DDAVP tabs and intranasal, C, fluid intake, see BNF

Deferasirox, 13, 22

Deferiprone, 14, C, blood disorders

Deflazacort, 5, 10, steroid card

Deltacortril e/c, 5, 10, steroid card, 21

Deltastab inj, 10, steroid card

Demeclocycline, 7, 9, 11, 23

De-Noltab, C, administration, see BNF

Denzapine tabs, 2, 10, patient information leaflet

Denzapine susp, 2, 10, patient information leaflet, C, administration

Depakote, 25

Depixol, 2

Depo-Medrone (systemic), 10, steroid card

Dermovate cream and oint, 28, C, application, see BNF

Dermovate scalp application, 15, 28, C, application, see BNF

Deseril, 2, 21

DesmoMelt, 26, C, fluid intake, see BNF

Desmopressin sublingual tabs, 26, C, fluid intake, see BNF

Desmopressin tabs and intranasal, C, fluid intake, see BNF

Desmospray, C, fluid intake, see BNF

Desmotabs, C, fluid intake, see BNF

Destolit, 21

Detrunorm, 3

Detrunorm XL, 3, 25

Detrusitol, 3

Detrusitol XL, 3, 25

Dexamethasone inj, 10, steroid card

Dexamethasone tabs and solution, 10, steroid card, 21

Dexamfetamine, C, driving

Dexedrine, C, driving

Dexibuprofen, 21

Dexketoprofen, 22

DF118 Forte, 2, 21

DHC Continus, 2, 25

Diafalk, 10, patient information leaflet, C, administration

Diamicron MR, 25

Diamorphine preps, 2

Diamox tabs, 3

Diamox SR, 3, 25

Diazepam, 2 or 19

Diclofenac dispersible tabs, 13, 21

Diclofenac e/c, 5, 25

Diclofenac m/r, 21, 25

Dicloflex Retard, 21, 25

Diclomax 75 mg SR and Retard, 21, 25

Diconal, 2

Didanosine e/c caps, 25, C, administration

Didanosine tabs, 23, C, administration

Didronel, C, food and calcium, see BNF

Didronel PMO, 10, patient leaflet, C, food and calcium, see BNF

Diflucan 50 and 200 mg, 9

Diflucan susp, 9

Diflucortolone external preps, 28, C, application, see BNF

Digoxin elixir, C, use of pipette

Dihydrocodeine, 2, 21

Dihydrocodeine m/r, 2, 25

Dilcardia SR, 25

Diloxanide, 9

Diltiazem, 25

Dilzem preps, 25

Dioderm, 28, C, application, see BNF

Dipentum, 21, C, blood disorder symptoms, see BNF

Diprosalic, 28, C, application, see BNF

Diprosone, 28, C, application, see BNF

Dipyridamole, 22

Dipyridamole m/r, 21, 25

Disipal, C, driving

Disodium etidronate, C, food and calcium, see BNF

Disopyramide m/r, 25

Disprol, 30

Distaclor, 9

Distaclor MR, 9, 21, 25

Distamine, 6, 22, C, blood disorder symptoms, see BNF

Distigmine, 22

Disulfiram, 2, C, alcohol reaction, see BNF

Dithranol preps, 28

Dithrocream preps, 28

Dithrolan, 28

Ditropan, 3

Diumide-K Continus, 25, 27

Dolmatil, 2

Donepezil orodispersible tabs, C, administration

Doralese, 2

Dostinex, 21, C, hypotensive reactions, see BNF

Dosulepin, 2

Dovobet, 28

Doxazosin, C, initial dose, driving

Doxazosin m/r, 25, C, initial dose, driving

Doxepin, 2

Doxepin topical, 2, 10, patient information leaflet

Doxycycline caps, 6, 9, 11, 27, C, posture, see BNF

Doxycycline dispersible tabs, 6, 9, 11, 13

Doxycycline tabs, 6, 11, 27, C, posture, see BNF
*Dozic*, 2
*Driclor*, 15
*Dromadol SR*, 2, 25
*Dukoral*, C, administration
Duloxetine, 2
*Duodopa*, 14, (urine reddish), C, driving
*Duofilm*, 15
*Duovent inhalations*, C, dose
*Duraphat toothpaste*, C, administration
<u>*Durogesic DTrans*</u>, 2, C, administration
Dutasteride, 25
*Dyazide*, 14, (urine blue in some lights), 21
*Dytac*, 14, (urine blue in some lights), 21
*Dytide*, 14, (urine blue in some lights), 21

*Econacort*, 28, C, application, see BNF
Eculizumab, C, meningococcal infection, patient information card
*Edronax*, C, driving
Efavirenz caps and tabs, 23
*Efcortesol*, 10, steroid card
*Efexor*, 3, C, driving
*Efexor XL*, 3, 25, C, driving
<u>*Effentora*</u>, 2, C, administration, see BNF
*Elantan preps*, 25
*Elidel*, 4, 28
*Elleste Solo MX patches*, C, administration, see BNF
*Elocon*, 28, C, application, see BNF
*Emcor preps*, 8
*Emeside*, 8, C, blood disorder symptoms (see BNF), driving (see BNF)
*Emflex*, 21, C, driving
*Emselex*, 3, 25
*En-De-Kay mouthwash*, C, food and drink, see BNF
*Endoxana*, 23, 25, 27
Enfuvirtide, C, hypersensitivity reactions, see BNF
Entacapone, 14, (urine reddish-brown), C, driving, avoid iron-containing preparations at the same time of day
Entecavir, C, administration
*Entocort CR*, 5, 10, steroid card, 25
*Epanutin caps*, 8, C, administration, blood or skin disorder symptoms (see BNF), driving (see BNF)
*Epanutin Infatabs*, 8, 24, C, blood or skin disorder symptoms (see BNF), driving (see BNF)

*Epanutin susp*, 8, C, administration, blood or skin disorder symptoms (see BNF), driving (see BNF)
*Epilim Chrono*, 8, 25, C, blood or hepatic disorder symptoms (see BNF), driving (see BNF)
*Epilim Chronosphere*, 8, 25, C, administration, blood or hepatic disorder symptoms (see BNF), driving (see BNF)
*Epilim crushable tabs, liquid and syrup*, 8, C, blood or hepatic disorder symptoms (see BNF), driving (see BNF)
*Epilim e/c tabs*, 5, 8, 25, C, blood or hepatic disorder symptoms (see BNF), driving (see BNF)
*Episenta*, 8, 25, C, administration, blood or hepatic disorder symptoms (see BNF), driving (see BNF)
Eprosartan, 21
*Equasym XL*, 25
Ergotamine, 18, C, dosage
Erlotinib, 23
*Erymax*, 5, 9, 25
*Erythrocin*, 9
Erythromycin caps, 5, 9, 25
Erythromycin ethyl succinate, 9
Erythromycin stearate tabs, 9
Erythromycin tabs, 5, 9, 25
*Erythroped*, 9
*Erythroped A tabs*, 9
Escitalopram drops, C, driving, administration
Escitalopram tabs, C, driving
Esomeprazole, C, administration, see BNF
*Estracombi*, C, administration, see BNF
*Estracyt*, 23, C, dairy products, see BNF
*Estraderm MX*, C, administration, see BNF
*Estraderm TTS*, C, administration, see BNF
*Estradot*, C, administration, see BNF
Estramustine, 23, C, dairy products, see BNF
*Estring*, 10, patient information leaflet
Estriol, 25
Ethambutol, 8
*Ethibide XL*, 25
Ethosuximide, 8, C, blood disorder symptoms (see BNF), driving (see BNF)
Etidronate, C, food and calcium, see BNF
Etodolac m/r, 25
Etonogestrel implant, C, see patient information leaflet
Etoposide caps, 23
Etravirine, 21
*Etrivex*, 28, C, application, see BNF

*Eucardic*, 8
*Eucreas*, 21
*Eumovate external preps*, 28, C, application, see BNF
*Eurax-Hydrocortisone*, 28, C, application, see BNF
*Evorel preps*, C, administration, see BNF
*Exelon caps*, 21, 25
*Exelon solution*, 21
Exemestane, 21
Exenatide, C, administration, see BNF
*Exjade*, 13, 22, C, administration, see BNF

Famciclovir, 9
*Famvir*, 9
*Fasigyn*, 4, 9, 21, 25
*Faverin*, C, driving, see BNF
*Fefol*, 25
Felbinac foam, 15
*Feldene caps*, 21
*Feldene Melt*, 10, patient information leaflet, 21
Felodipine m/r, 25
*Fematrix*, C, administration, see BNF
*Femapak*, C, administration, see BNF
*FemSeven*, C, administration, see BNF
*Fenbid*, 25
Fenbufen, 21
Fenofibrate, 21
Fenoprofen, 21
*Fenopron*, 21
<u>Fentanyl buccal tablets</u>, 2, C, administration, see BNF
Fentanyl lozenges, 2
<u>Fentanyl patches</u>, 2, C, administration
Fentanyl sublingual tablets, 2, 26
*Fentazin*, 2
*Feospan*, 25
*Ferriprox*, 14, C, blood disorders
*Ferrograd*, 25
*Ferrograd C*, 25
*Ferrograd Folic*, 25
Ferrous salts m/r, see preps
Fesoterodine, 3, 25
Fexofenadine, 5, C, driving, see BNF
*Fibrelief*, 13, C, administration, see BNF
*Flagyl S*, 4, 9, 23
*Flagyl supps*, 4, 9
*Flagyl tabs*, 4, 9, 21, 25, 27
<u>*Flamasacard*</u>, 25, 32
Flavoxate, 3
Flecainide m/r, 25
*Fleet Phospho-soda*, 10, patient information leaflet, C, administration
*Flixotide*, 8, C, dose; with high doses, 10, steroid card

*Flixotide Evohaler*, 8, C, dose, change to CFC-free inhaler (see BNF); with high doses, 10, steroid card

*Flomaxtra XL*, 25

*Florinef*, 10, steroid card

*Floxapen*, 9, 23

*Fluanxol*, 2, C, administration, driving, see BNF

Flucloxacillin, 9, 23

Fluconazole 50 and 200 mg, 9

Fluconazole susp, 9

Fludrocortisone, 10, steroid card

Fludroxycortide external preps, 28, C, application, see BNF

Fluocinolone external preps, 28, C, application, see BNF

Fluocinonide external preps, 28, C, application, see BNF

Fluocortolone external preps, 28, C, application, see BNF

*Fluorigard mouthwash*, C, food and drink, see BNF

Fluoxetine, C, driving, see BNF

Flupentixol, see preps

Flurazepam, 19

Flurbiprofen, 21

Flurbiprofen m/r, 21, 25

Fluticasone external preps, 28, C, application, see BNF

Fluticasone inhalations, 8, C, dose; with high doses, 10, steroid card

Fluticasone inhalations (CFC-free), 8, C, dose, change to CFC-free inhaler (see BNF); with high doses, 10, steroid card

Fluvastatin, C, muscle effects, see BNF

Fluvastatin m/r, 25, C, muscle effects, see BNF

Fluvoxamine, C, driving, see BNF

*Foradil*, C, dose, see BNF

*Foraven XL*, 3, 25, C, driving

*Forceval caps*, 25

Formoterol fumarate, C, dose, see BNF

*Fortipine LA 40*, 21, 25

*Fortral caps and tabs*, 2, 21

*Fosamax*, C, administration, see BNF

Fosamprenavir susp, C, administration, see BNF

*Fosavance*, C, administration, see BNF

*Fosrenol*, 21, C, to be chewed

*Fostair*, 8, C, dose, 10, steroid card

*Frisium*, 2 or 19, 8, C, driving (see BNF)

*Froben*, 21

*Froben SR*, 21, 25

Frovatriptan, 3

*Frusene*, 14, (urine blue in some lights), 21

*Fucibet*, 28, C, application, see BNF

*Fucidin susp*, 9, 21

*Fucidin tabs*, 9

*Fucidin H*, 28, C, application, see BNF

*Full Marks lotion, mousse*, 15

*Fungilin loz*, 9, 24, C, after food

*Furadantin*, 9, 14, (urine yellow or brown), 21

*Fuzeon*, C, hypersensitivity reactions, see BNF

*Fybogel*, 13, C, administration, see BNF

*Fybogel Mebeverine*, 13, 22, C, administration, see BNF

Gabapentin, 3, 5, 8, C, driving (see BNF)

*Gabitril*, 21

Galantamine, 3, 21

Galantamine m/r, 3, 21, 25

Ganciclovir, 21

Gemfibrozil, 22

*Gliclazide m/r*, 25

*Glivec*, 21, 27

*Glucobay*, C, administration, see BNF

*Glucophage tabs*, 21

*Glucophage powder*, 13, 21, C, administration, see BNF

*Glucophage SR*, 21, 25

Glyceryl trinitrate patch, see preps

Glyceryl trinitrate m/r, 25

Glyceryl trinitrate tabs, 16

Griseofulvin spray, 15

Griseofulvin tabs, 9, 21, C, driving

*Grisol AF*, 15

*GTN 300 mcg*, 16

*Haelan*, 28, C, application, see BNF

*Haldol*, 2

*Half-Inderal LA*, 8, 25

*Half-Securon SR*, 25

*Half-Sinemet CR*, 14, (urine reddish), 25

Haloperidol, 2

*Heminevrin*, 19

*Hiprex*, 9

*Humira*, C, tuberculosis

*Hycamtin*, 25

Hydrocortisone inj, 10, steroid card

Hydrocortisone external preps, 28, C, application, see BNF

Hydrocortisone tabs, 10, steroid card, 21

Hydrocortisone butyrate external preps, 28, C, application, see BNF

Hydrocortisone butyrate scalp lotion, 15, 28, C, application, see BNF

*Hydrocortistab inj*, 10, steroid card

Hydromorphone caps, 2, C, administration, see BNF

Hydromorphone m/r, 2, C, administration, see BNF

Hydroxychloroquine, 5, 21

Hydroxyzine, 2

Hyoscine hydrobromide tabs, see preps

Hyoscine hydrobromide patches, 19, C, application, see BNF

*Hypolar Retard*, 25

*Hypovase*, C, initial dose, driving, see BNF

*Hytrin*, C, initial dose, driving

Ibandronic acid tabs, C, administration, see BNF

Ibuprofen, 21

Ibuprofen gran, 13, 21

Ibuprofen m/r, 25, 27

Idarubicin caps, 25

*Imatinib*, 21, 27

*Imdur*, 25

*Imigran*, 3, 10, patient information leaflet

*Imigran RADIS*, 3, 10, patient information leaflet

Imipramine, 2

Imiquimod, 10, patient information leaflet

*Imodium Plus*, 24

*Implanon*, C, see patient information leaflet

*Imunovir*, 9

*Imuran*, 21

*Increlex*, C, administration, see BNF

Indapamide m/r, 25

*Inderal-LA*, 8, 25

Indinavir, 27, C, administration, see BNF

*Indolar SR*, 21, 25, C, driving

Indometacin caps and mixt, 21, C, driving

Indometacin m/r, see preps

Indometacin supps, C, driving

Indoramin, 2

Industrial methylated spirit, 15

*Inegy*, C, muscle effects, see BNF

*Infacol*, C, use of dropper

Infliximab, 10, Alert card, C, tuberculosis and hypersensitivity reactions

Inosine pranobex, 9

*Inovelon*, 21, C, driving, see BNF

Insulin, C, see BNF

*Intal*, 8, C, change to CFC-free inhaler

*Intelence*, 21

*Invega*, 2, 25

*Invirase*, 21

Iodine Solution, Aqueous, 27

*Ipocol*, 5, 25, C, blood disorder symptoms, see BNF

Ipratropium inhalations, C, dose, see BNF

*Isentress*, 25

*Isib 60XL*, 25

*Ismo Retard*, 25

*Ismo tabs*, 25

Isocarboxazid, 3, 10, patient information leaflet

*Isodur XL*, 25
*Isogel*, 13, C, administration, see BNF
*Isoket Retard*, 25
Isoniazid elixir and tabs, 8, 22
Isosorbide dinitrate m/r, 25
Isosorbide mononitrate, 25
Isosorbide mononitrate m/r, 25
*Isotard XL*, 25
Isotretinoin, 10, patient information leaflet, 11, 21
Isotretinoin gel, 10, patient information leaflet
*Isotrex*, 10, patient information leaflet
*Isotrexin*, 10, patient information leaflet
*Ispagel*, 13, C, administration, see BNF
Ispaghula, 13, C, administration, see BNF
Itraconazole caps, 5, 9, 21, 25, C, hepatotoxicity
Itraconazole liq, 9, 23, C, hepatotoxicity

*Joy-Rides*, 2, 24

*Kaletra solution*, 21
*Kaletra tabs*, 25
*Kalspare*, 14, (urine blue in some lights), 21
*Kalten*, 8
*Kapake caps and tabs*, 2, 29, 30
*Kay-Cee-L*, 21
*Keflex*, 9
Kemadrin, C, driving
*Kenalog (systemic)*, 10, steroid card
*Kentera*, 3, C, administration, see BNF
*Keppra*, 8
*Keral*, 22
*Ketek*, 9, C, driving, hepatic disorders
Ketoconazole tabs, 5, 9, 21, C, hepatotoxicity
Ketoprofen caps, 21
Ketoprofen m/r caps, 21, 25
Ketotifen, 2, 21
Ketorolac tabs, 17, 21
*Ketovail*, 21, 25
*Kineret*, C, blood disorder symptoms
*Kivexa*, C, hypersensitivity reactions, see BNF
*Klaricid*, 9
*Klaricid sachets*, 9, 13
*Klaricid XL*, 9, 21, 25
*Klean-Prep*, 10, patient information leaflet, 13, C, administration
*Konakion tabs*, 24
*Kuvan*, 13, 21, C, administration, see BNF
*Kwells*, 2

Labetalol, 8, 21
Lacosamide tabs and syrup, 8, C, driving, see BNF
*Lamictal dispersible tabs*, 8, 13, C, driving (see BNF), skin reactions
*Lamictal tabs*, 8, C, driving (see BNF), skin reactions
*Lamisil*, 9
Lamotrigine dispersible tabs, 8, 13, C, driving (see BNF), skin reactions
Lamotrigine tabs, 8, C, driving (see BNF), skin reactions
*Lanoxin-PG elixir*, C, use of pipette
Lansoprazole caps, 5, 22, 25
Lansoprazole oro-dispersible tabs, 5, 22, C, administration, see BNF
Lanthanum, 21, C, to be chewed
Lapatinib, C, see BNF
*Larapam SR*, 2, 25
*Largactil*, 2, 11
*Lariam*, 21, 25, 27, C, driving, malaria prophylaxis, see BNF
*Laxido*, 13
*Lederfen*, 21
*Ledermycin*, 7, 9, 11, 23
Leflunomide, 4
Lenalidomide, 25, C, symptoms of thromboembolism, neutropenia, or thrombocytopenia, patient information leaflet
Lercanidipine, 22
*Lescol*, C, muscle effects, see BNF
*Lescol XL*, 25, C, muscle effects, see BNF
Levetiracetam, 8
Levocetirizine, C, driving
Levofloxacin, 6, 9, 25, C, driving
Levomepromazine, 2
*Librium*, 2
*Li-Liquid*, 10, lithium card, C, fluid and salt intake, see BNF
Linezolid susp and tabs, 9, 10, patient information leaflet
*Lioresal*, 2, 8
*Lipantil*, 21
*Lipitor*, C, muscle effects, see BNF
*Lipostat*, C, muscle effects, see BNF
Liquid paraffin, C, administration, see BNF
*Liskonum*, 10, lithium card, 25, C, fluid and salt intake, see BNF
Lithium carbonate, 10, lithium card, C, fluid and salt intake, see BNF
Lithium carbonate m/r, 10, lithium card, 25, C, fluid and salt intake, see BNF
Lithium citrate liq, 10, lithium card, C, fluid and salt intake, see BNF
*Lithonate*, 10, lithium card, 25, C, fluid and salt intake, see BNF

*Loceryl*, 10, patient information leaflet
*Locoid cream, oint, and topical emulsion*, 28, C, application, see BNF
*Locoid scalp lotion*, 15, 28, C, application, see BNF
Lofepramine, 2
Lofexidine, 2
*Lopid*, 22
Loprazolam, 19
*Lopresor*, 8
*Lopresor SR*, 8, 25
*Loramyc C*, 10, C, administration, see BNF
Loratadine, C, driving, alcohol, see BNF
Lorazepam, 2 or 19
Lormetazepam, 19
*Loron tabs*, 10, patient information leaflet, C, food and calcium, see BNF
*Losec*, C, administration, see BNF
*Lotriderm*, 28, C, application, see BNF
Lugol's solution, 27
*Lustral*, C, driving, see BNF
*Lyclear Dermal cream*, 10, patient information leaflet
Lymecycline, 6, 9
*Lyrica*, 3, 8, C, driving
*Lysodren*, 2, 10, 21, C, driving, adrenal suppression
*Lysovir*, C, driving

*Mabron*, 2, 25
*Macrobid*, 9, 14, (urine yellow or brown), 21, 25
*Macrodantin*, 9, 14, (urine yellow or brown), 21
Macrogols, 13
*Madopar*, 14, (urine reddish), C, driving
*Madopar dispersible tabs*, 14, (urine reddish), C, administration, driving, see BNF
*Madopar CR*, 5, 14, (urine reddish), 25, C, driving
*Magnapen*, 9, 22
Magnesium citrate effervescent pdr, 10, patient information leaflet, 13, C, administration
Magnesium sulphate, 13, 23
*Malarivon*, 5, C, malaria prophylaxis
*Malarone preps*, 21, C, malaria prophylaxis
*Manerix*, 10, patient information leaflet, 21
*Manevac*, 25, 27
*Marevan*, 10, anticoagulant card
*Maxalt*, 3
*Maxalt Melt*, 3, C, administration
*Maxepa*, 21
*Maxitram SR*, 2, 25
*Maxolon SR*, 25

*Maxtrex (methotrexate)*, C, NSAIDs (see BNF)

*Mebeverine*, C, administration, see BNF

*Mecasermin*, C, administration, see BNF

*Mecysteine*, 5, 22, 25

*Medikinet XL*, 25

*Medrone tabs*, 10, steroid card, 21

Mefenamic acid caps, paed susp, and tabs, 21

*Mefloquine*, 21, 25, 27, C, driving, malaria prophylaxis, see BNF

Melatonin, 2, 21, 25

Meloxicam tabs, 21

Mepacrine, 4, 9, 14, 21

Meprobamate, 2

Meptazinol, 2

*Meptid*, 2

Mesalazine e/c, see preps

Mesalazine m/r, see preps

Mesalazine enema and supps, C, blood disorder symptoms, see BNF

Mesalazine gran, see preps

*Mesren MR*, 5, 25, C, blood disorder symptoms, see BNF

Metformin m/r, 21, 25

<u>Metformin powder</u>, 13, 21, C, administration, see BNF

Metformin solution and tabs, 21

Methadone, 2

*Methadose*, 2

Methenamine, 9

Methocarbamol, 2

Methotrexate tabs, C, NSAIDs (see BNF)

Methylcellulose (constipation or diarrhoea), C, administration, see BNF

Methylcellulose tabs (anorectic), C, administration, see BNF

Methyldopa, 3, 8

Methylphenidate m/r, 25

Methylprednisolone inj, 10, steroid card

Methylprednisolone tabs, 10, steroid card, 21

Methysergide, 2, 21

Metirosine, 2

<u>Metoclopramide oral solution</u>, C, use of pipette

<u>Metoclopramide m/r</u>, 25

Metopirone, 21, C, driving

Metoprolol, 8

Metoprolol m/r, see preps

*Metosyn cream and oint*, 28, C, application, see BNF

*Metrolyl supps*, 4, 9

Metronidazole mixt, 4, 9, 23

Metronidazole supps, 4, 9

Metronidazole tabs, 4, 9, 21, 25, 27

Metyrapone, 21, C, driving

*Mezavant XL*, 21, 25, C, blood disorder symptoms, see BNF

Mianserin, 2, 25

*Micanol*, 28

Miconazole buccal tabs, 10, C, administration, see BNF

Miconazole oral gel, 9, C, hold in mouth, after food

*Midrid*, 30, C, dosage

*Mifegyne*, 10, patient information leaflet

Mifepristone, 10, patient information leaflet

*Migard*, 3

*Migraleve*, 2, (pink tablets), 17, 30

*Migril*, 2, 18, C, dosage

*Mildison*, 28, C, application, see BNF

*Mimpara*, 21

*Minocin MR*, 6, 25

Minocycline, 6, 9, C, posture, see BNF

Minocycline m/r, 6, 25

*Mintec*, 5, 22, 25

*Mirapexin*, C, hypotensive reactions, driving, see BNF

Mirtazapine oral solution, 2

Mirtazapine orodispersible tablets, 2, C, administration, see BNF

Mirtazapine tabs, 2, 25

Misoprostol, 21

Mitotane, 2, 10, 21, C, driving, adrenal suppression

Mizolastine, 25, C, driving

*Mizollen*, 25, C, driving

*Mobic tabs*, 21

*Mobiflex*, 21

Moclobemide, 10, patient information leaflet, 21

*Modisal LA*, 25

*Modisal XL*, 25

*Modrasone*, 28, C, application, see BNF

*Modrenal*, 21

*Molipaxin*, 2, 21

Mometasone external preps, 28, C, application, see BNF

Mometasone inhaler, 8, 10, steroid card, C, dose

*Monomax SR*, 25

*Monomax XL*, 25

*Monomil XL*, 25

*Monosorb XL*, 25

*Montelukast chewable tabs*, 23, 24

Morphine preps, 2

Morphine m/r susp, 2, 13

Morphine m/r caps and tabs, see preps

*Motifene*, 25

*Movicol preps*, 13

*Moviprep*, 10, patient information leaflet, 13, C, administration

Moxifloxacin, 6, 9, C, driving

Moxisylyte, 21

Moxonidine, 3

*MST Continus susp*, 2, 13

*MST Continus tabs*, 2, 25

*MXL*, 2, C, administration, see BNF

*Mycobutin*, 8, 14, (urine orange-red), C, soft lenses

Mycophenolic acid, 25

*Myfortic*, 25

*Myocrisin inj*, 11, C, blood disorder symptoms, see BNF

*Myotonine Chloride*, 22

*Mysoline*, 2, 8, C, driving (see BNF)

Nabilone, 2, C, behavioural effects, see BNF

Nabumetone, 21

Nabumetone susp, 21

Nadolol, 8

Nafarelin spray, 10, patient information leaflet, C, nasal decongestants, see BNF

Naftidrofuryl, 25, 27

*Nalcrom*, 22, C, administration, see BNF

Nalidixic acid, 9, 11

*Napratec*, 21

*Naprosyn EC*, 5, 25

*Naprosyn tabs*, 21

Naproxen e/c, 5, 25

Naproxen tabs, 21

*Naramig*, 3

Naratriptan, 3

*Nardil*, 3, 10, patient information leaflet

*Natecal D3*, 24

*Natrilix SR*, 25

*Navelbine caps*, 21, 25

*Nebilet*, 8

Nebivolol, 8

Nedocromil sodium inhalation, 8, C, change to CFC-free inhaler

Nefopam, 2, 14, (urine pink)

Nelfinavir tabs, 21

*Neo-Mercazole*, C, blood disorder symptoms, see BNF

*Neo-NaClex-K*, 25, 27, C, posture, see BNF

*Neoral*, C, administration, see BNF

*Neotigason*, 10, patient information leaflet, 21

*Nerisone*, 28, C, application, see BNF

*Nerisone Forte*, 28, application, see BNF

*Neulactil*, 2

*Neupro*, C, hypotensive reactions, driving

*Neurontin*, 3, 5, 8, C, driving (see BNF)

Nevirapine, C, hypersensitivity reactions, see BNF

*Nexavar*, 23

*Nexium*, C, administration, see BNF

*Niaspan*, 21, 25

Nicardipine m/r, 25

*Nicopass*, 24

*Nicotinell lozenges*, 24

Nicorette Microtab, 26
Nicotine (sublingual), 26
Nicotinic acid m/r, see preps
Nifedipine m/r, see preps
Nifedipress MR, 25
Niferex elixir, C, infants, use of dropper
Nilotinib, 23, 25, 27
NiQuitin lozenges, 24
Nitrazepam, 19, (infantile spasms 1, 8)
Nitrofurantoin, 9, 14, (urine yellow or brown), 21
Nitrofurantoin m/r, 9, 14, (urine yellow or brown), 21, 25
Nivaquine, 5, C, malaria prophylaxis, see BNF
Nizoral, 5, 9, 21, C, hepatotoxicity
Nootropil, 3
Norfloxacin, 7, 9, 23, C, driving
Normacol preps, 25, 27, C, administration, see BNF
Normax, 14, (urine red)
Norprolac, 21, C, hypotensive reactions, see BNF
Nortriptyline, 2
Norvir, 21, C, administration, see BNF
Novolizer, 8, C, dose; with high doses, 10, steroid card
Noxafil, 9, 21
Nozinan, 2
Nuelin SA preps, 21, 25
Nurofen for children, 21
Nu-Seals Aspirin, 5, 25, 32
Nystaform-HC, 28, C, application, see BNF
Nystan susp (g.i.), 9, C, use of pipette
Nystan susp (mouth), 9, C, use of pipette, hold in mouth, after food
Nystan tabs, 9
Nystatin susp (g.i.), 9, C, use of pipette
Nystatin susp (mouth), 9, C, use of pipette, hold in mouth, after food
Nystatin tabs, 9

Occlusal, 15
Octim, C, fluid intake, see BNF
Oestrogel, C, administration, see BNF
Ofloxacin, 6, 9, 11, C, driving
Olanzapine tabs, 2
Olanzapine orodispersible tabs, 2, C, administration, see BNF
Olbetam, 21
Olsalazine, 21, C, blood disorder symptoms, see BNF
Omacor, 21
Omega-3-acid ethyl esters, 21
Omeprazole caps, C, administration, see BNF
Omeprazole tabs, 25

Ondansetron oral lyophilisates, C, administration, see BNF
Opilon, 21
Optimax, 3
Oramorph preps, 2
Oramorph SR, 2, 25
Orap, 2
Orelox, 5, 9, 21
Orphenadrine, C, driving
Orudis caps, 21
Oruvail, 21, 25
Oseltamivir, 9
Ovestin, 25
Oxazepam, 2
Oxcarbazepine, 3, 8, C, see BNF
Oxerutins, 21
Oxis, C, dose, see BNF
Oxprenolol, 8
Oxprenolol m/r, 8, 25
Oxybutynin tabs and elixir, 3
Oxybutynin patch, 3, C, administration, see BNF
Oxycodone caps and liq, 2
Oxycodone m/r, 2, 25
OxyContin, 2, 25
OxyNorm, 2
Oxytetracycline, 7, 9, 23

Paliperidone, 2, 25
Palladone, 2, C, administration, see BNF
Palladone SR, 2, C, administration, see BNF
Paludrine, 21, C, malaria prophylaxis, see BNF
Panadeine, 29, 30
Panadeine effervescent, 13, 29, 30
Panadol tabs, 29, 30
Panadol Soluble, 13, 29, 30
Panadol susp, 30
Pancrease preps, C, administration, see BNF
Pancreatin, C, administration, see BNF
Pancrex gran, 25, C, dose, see BNF
Pancrex V Forte tabs, 5, 25, C, dose, see BNF
Pancrex V caps, 125 caps and pdr, C, administration, see BNF
Pancrex V tabs, 5, 25, C, dose, see BNF
Pantoprazole, 25
Paracetamol liq and supps, 30
Paracetamol tabs and caps, 29, 30
Paracetamol tabs, soluble, 13, 29, 30
Paracodol caps, 29, 30
Paracodol effervescent tabs, 13, 29, 30
Paradote, 29, 30
Paramax sachets, 13, 17, 30
Paramax tabs, 17, 30
Pariet, 25
Parlodel, 21, C, hypotensive reactions, see BNF

Paroven, 21
Paroxetine tabs, 21, C, driving
Paroxetine susp, 5, 21, C, driving
Penbritin, 9, 23
Penicillamine, 6, 22, C, blood disorder symptoms, see BNF
Pentasa tabs and gran, C, administration, blood disorder symptoms, see BNF
Pentasa enema and supps, C, blood disorder symptoms, see BNF
Pentazocine caps and tabs, 2, 21
Pentoxifylline m/r, 21, 25
Peppermint oil caps, 5, 22, 25
Percutol, C, administration, see BNF
Pergolide, C, driving, hypotensive reactions, see BNF
Periactin, 2
Pericyazine, 2
Perindopril, 22
Periostat, 6, 11, 27, C, posture, see BNF
Permethrin dermal cream, 10, patient information leaflet
Perphenazine, 2
Persantin, 22
Persantin Retard, 21, 25
Pethidine, 2
Phenelzine, 3, 10, patient information leaflet
Phenergan, 2
Phenindione, 10, anticoagulant card, 14, (urine pink or orange)
Phenobarbital elixir and tabs, 2, 8, C, driving (see BNF)
Phenothrin lotion, mousse, 15
Phenoxymethylpenicillin, 9, 23
Phenytoin caps and tabs, 8, C, administration, blood or skin disorder symptoms (see BNF), driving (see BNF)
Phenytoin chewable tabs, 8, 24, C, blood or skin disorder symptoms (see BNF), driving (see BNF)
Phenytoin susp, 8, C, administration, blood or skin disorder symptoms (see BNF), driving (see BNF)
Phosex, 25, C, with meals
Phosphate-Sandoz, 13
Phyllocontin Continus, 25
Physeptone, 2
Physiotens, 3
Phytomenadione, 24
Picolax, 10, patient information leaflet, 13, C, solution, see BNF
Pilocarpine tabs, 21, 27, C, driving
Pimecrolimus, 4, 28
Pimozide, 2
Pindolol, 8
Piperazine powder, 13
Piracetam, 3
Piriton, 2
Piroxicam caps and tabs, 21

Piroxicam dispersible tabs, 13, 21

Pivmecillinam, 9, 21, 27, C, posture, see BNF

Pizotifen, 2

*Plaquenil*, 5, 21

*Plendil*, 25

Podophyllin paint cpd, 15, C, application, see BNF

*Ponstan*, 21

Posaconazole, 9, 21

*Potaba caps and tabs*, 21

*Potaba Envules*, 13, 21

Potassium chloride m/r, see preps

Potassium citrate mixt, 27

Potassium effervescent tabs, 13, 21

*Pradaxa*, 25

Pramipexole, C, hypotensive reactions, driving, see BNF

Pravastatin, C, muscle effects, see BNF

*Praxilene*, 25, 27

Prazosin, C, initial dose, driving, see BNF

Prednisolone inj, 10, steroid card

Prednisolone tabs, 10, steroid card, 21

Prednisolone e/c, 5, 10, steroid card, 25

Pregabalin, 3, 8, C, driving

*Preservex*, 21

*Prestim*, 8

*Prezista*, 21, C, missed dose, see BNF

*Priadel liq*, 10, lithium card, C, fluid and salt intake, see BNF

*Priadel tabs*, 10, lithium card, 25, C, fluid and salt intake, see BNF

Primidone, 2, 8, C, driving (see BNF)

*Prioderm lotion*, 15

*Pripsen*, 13

*Pro-Banthine*, 23

Probenecid, 12, 21, 27

Procarbazine, 4

Prochlorperazine, 2

Prochlorperazine buccal tabs, 2, C, administration, see BNF

Procyclidine, C, driving

Progesterone (micronised), C, administration, see BNF

*Prograf*, 23, C, driving, see BNF

Proguanil, 21, C, malaria prophylaxis, see BNF

*Progynova TS preps*, C, administration, see BNF

Promazine, 2

Promethazine, 2

Propafenone, 21, 25

Propantheline, 23

Propiverine hydrochloride, 3

Propiverine hydrochloride m/r, 3, 25

Propranolol oral solution and tabs, 8

Propranolol m/r, 8, 25

*Protelos*, 5, 13, C, administration, see BNF

*Prothiaden*, 2

*Protium*, 25

*Protopic*, 4, 11, 28

*Prozac*, C, driving, see BNF

*Psorin*, 28

*Pulmicort*, 8, C, dose; with high doses, 10, steroid card

*Pulmicort Respules*, 8, 10, steroid card, C, dose

Pyrazinamide, 8

*Questran preps*, 13, C, avoid other drugs at same time, see BNF

Quetiapine, 2

Quetiapine m/r, 2, 23, 25

Quinagolide, 21, C, hypotensive reactions, see BNF

*Qvar preps*, 8, C, dose; with high doses, 10, steroid card

Rabeprazole, 25

Raltegravir, 25

*Ranexa*, 25, patient alert card

Ranitidine effervescent tabs, 13

*Ranolazine*, 25, patient alert card

*Rapamune*, C, administration

*Rasilez*, 21

*Rebetol*, 21

Reboxetine, C, driving

*Regulan*, 13, C, administration, see BNF

*Regurin*, 23

*Relifex*, 21

*Relifex susp*, 21

*Remedeine*, 2, 21, 29, 30

*Remicade*, 10, Alert card, C, tuberculosis and hypersensitivity reactions

*Reminyl*, 3, 21

*Reminyl XL*, 3, 21, 25

*Renagel*, 25, C, with meals

*Requip*, 21, C, driving, see BNF

*Requip XL*, 25, C, driving (see BNF)

*Resonium A*, 13

*Restandol*, 21, 25

Retapamulin, 28

*Retrovir oral solution*, C, use of oral syringe

*Revlimid*, 25, C, symptoms of thromboembolism, neutropenia, or thrombocytopenia, patient information leaflet

*Reyataz*, 5, 21

*Rhumalgan*, 5, 25

*Riamet*, 21, C, driving

Ribavirin caps, tabs, and solution, 21

*Ridaura*, 11, 21, C, blood disorder symptoms, see BNF

Rifabutin, 8, 14, (urine orange-red), C, soft lenses

*Rifadin*, 8, 14, (urine orange-red), 22, C, soft lenses

Rifampicin caps and syrup, 8, 14, (urine orange-red), 22, C, soft lenses

*Rifater*, 8, 14, (urine orange-red), 22, C, soft lenses

*Rifinah*, 8, 14, (urine orange-red), 22, C, soft lenses

*Rilutek*, C, blood disorders, driving

*Rimactane*, 8, 14, (urine orange-red), 22, C, soft lenses

Rimonabant, C, depression, see BNF

Risedronate sodium, C, administration, food and calcium, see BNF

Risperdal liquid, 2, C, use of dose syringe

*Risperdal orodispersible tabs*, 2, C, administration, see BNF

*Risperdal tabs*, 2

Risperidone liquid, 2, C, use of dose syringe

Risperidone orodispersible tabs, 2, C, administration, see BNF

Risperidone tabs, 2

Ritonavir, 21, C, administration, see BNF

Rivastigmine, 21, 25

*Rivotril*, 2, 8, C, driving (see BNF)

Rizatriptan tabs, 3

Rizatriptan wafers, 3, C, administration

*Roaccutane*, 10, patient information leaflet, 11, 21

*Robaxin*, 2

Ropinirole, 21, C, driving, see BNF

Ropinirole m/r, 25, C, driving (see BNF)

Rotigotine, C, hypotensive reactions, driving

*Rowachol*, 22

*Rowatinex caps*, 25

Rufinamide, 21, C, driving (see BNF)

*Rythmodan Retard*, 25

*Sabril sachets*, 3, 8, 13, C, driving (see BNF)

*Sabril tabs*, 3, 8, C, driving (see BNF)

*Salactol*, 15

*Salagen*, 21, 27, C, driving

*Salatac*, 15

*Salazopyrin*, 14, (urine orange-yellow), C, blood disorder symptoms and soft lenses, see BNF

*Salazopyrin EN-tabs*, 5, 14, (urine orange-yellow), 25, C, blood disorder symptoms and soft lenses, see BNF

*Salbulin Novolizer*, C, dose, see BNF

Salbutamol inhalations, C, dose, see BNF

Salbutamol inhalations (CFC-free), C, dose, change to CFC-free inhaler, see BNF

Salbutamol m/r, 25

Salicylic acid collodion, 15

Salmeterol, C, dose, see BNF

Salmeterol (CFC-free), C, dose, change to CFC-free inhaler, see BNF

Salofalk enema and supps, C, blood disorder symptoms, see BNF

Salofalk gran, 25, C, administration, blood disorder symptoms, see BNF

Salofalk tabs, 5, 25, C, blood disorder symptoms, see BNF

Sandrena, C, administration, see BNF

Sando-K, 13, 21

Sandocal, 13

Sandocal +D 600, 13

Sanomigran, 2

Sapropterin, 13, 21, C, administration, see BNF

Saquinavir, 21

Scopoderm TTS, 19, C, administration, see BNF

Sebivo, C, muscle effects

Sebomin MR, 6, 25

Secobarbital, 19

Seconal, 19

Sectral, 8

Securon SR, 25

Selegiline (freeze-dried tablets), C, administration, see BNF

Selexid, 9, 21, 27, C, posture, see BNF

Septrin susp and tabs, 9

Seractil, 21

Serc, 21

Serenace, 2

Seretide, 8, 10, steroid card (250- and 500-Accuhaler only), C, dose

Seretide Evohaler, 8, C, dose, change to CFC-free inhaler (see BNF), 10, steroid card (125- and 250-Evohaler only)

Serevent, C, dose, see BNF

Serevent (CFC-free), C, dose, change to CFC-free inhaler, see BNF

Seroquel, 2

Seroquel XL, 2, 23, 25

Seroxat tabs, 21, C, driving

Seroxat susp, 5, 21, C, driving

Sertraline, C, driving, see BNF

Sevelamer, 25, C, with meals

Sevredol, 2

Simeticone, see paediatric prep

Simvastatin, C, muscle effects, see BNF

Sinemet CR, 14, (urine reddish), 25, C, driving

Sinemet preps, 14, (urine reddish), C, driving

Sinepin, 2

Singulair chewable tabs, 23, 24

Sinthrome, 10, anticoagulant card

Sirolimus, C, administration

Skelid, C, food and calcium

Slo-Indo, 21, 25, C, driving

Slo-Phyllin, 25 or C, administration, see BNF

Sloprolol, 8, 25

Slow Sodium, 25

Slow-Fe, 25

Slow-Fe Folic, 25

Slow-K, 25, 27, C, posture, see BNF

Slow-Trasicor, 8, 25

Slozem, 25

Sodium Amytal, 19

Sodium aurothiomalate, 11, C, blood disorder symptoms, see BNF

Sodium chloride m/r, 25

Sodium chloride and glucose oral pdr, cpd, 13

Sodium clodronate, C, food and calcium, see BNF

Sodium cromoglicate (oral), 22, C, administration, see BNF

Sodium cromoglicate inhalation, 8, C, change to CFC-free inhaler

Sodium fusidate susp, 9, 21

Sodium fusidate tabs, 9

Sodium picosulfate pdr, 10, patient information leaflet, 13, C, see BNF

Sodium valproate e/c, 5, 8, 25, C, blood or hepatic disorder symptoms (see BNF), driving (see BNF)

Sodium valproate m/r and granules, 8, 25, C, blood or hepatic disorder symptoms (see BNF), driving (see BNF)

Sodium valproate crushable tabs, liquid and syrup, 8, C, blood or hepatic disorder symptoms (see BNF), driving (see BNF)

Solian, 2

Solifenacin, 3

Soliris, C, meningococcal infection, patient information card

Solpadol caps and caplets, 2, 29, 30

Solpadol Effervescent, 2, 13, 29, 30

Solu-Cortef, 10, steroid card

Solu-Medrone, 10, steroid card

Solvazinc, 13, 21

Somnite, 19

Sonata, 2

Soneryl, 19

Sorafenib, 23

Sotacor, 8

Sotalol, 8

Spironolactone, 21

Sporanox caps, 5, 9, 21, 25, C, hepatotoxicity

Sporanox liq, 9, 23, C, administration, hepatotoxicity

Sprycel, 25

Stalevo, 14, (urine reddish-brown), C, driving, avoid iron-containing preparations at the same time of day

Stavudine, 23

Stelara, 10, C, tuberculosis, see BNF

Stelazine syrup and tabs, 2

Stemetil, 2

Sterculia, C, administration, see BNF

Stilnoct, 19

Strattera, 3

Striant SR, C, administration, see BNF

Strontium, 5, 13, C, administration, see BNF

Stugeron, 2

Suboxone, 2, 26

Subutex, 2, 26

Sucralfate, 5

Sulfadiazine, 9, 27

Sulfasalazine, 14, (urine orange-yellow), C, blood disorder symptoms and soft lenses, see BNF

Sulfasalazine e/c, 5, 14, (urine orange-yellow), 25, C, blood disorder symptoms and soft lenses, see BNF

Sulfinpyrazone, 12, 21

Sulindac, 21

Sulpiride, 2

Sulpor, 2

Sumatriptan, 3, 10, patient information leaflet

Sunitinib, 14

Suprax, 9

Supralip, 21

Suprecur, C, nasal decongestants, see BNF

Suprefact nasal spray, C, nasal decongestants, see BNF

Surgam tabs, 21

Surgical spirit, 15

Surmontil, 2

Suscard Buccal, C, administration, see BNF

Sustiva caps and tabs, 23

Sutent, 14

Symbicort, 8, C, dose, 10, steroid card (200/6- and 400/12-Turbohaler only)

Symmetrel, C, driving

Synalar external preps, 28, C, application, see BNF

Synarel, 10, patient information leaflet, C, nasal decongestants, see BNF

Synflex, 21

Tacrolimus caps, 23, C, driving, see BNF

Tacrolimus topical, 4, 11, 28

Tambocor XL, 25

*Tamiflu*, 9
Tamsulosin m/r, 25
*Tarceva*, 23
*Tarivid*, 6, 9, 11, C, driving
*Tarka*, 25
*Tasigna*, 23, 25, 27
*Tasmar*, 14, 25
*Tavanic*, 6, 9, 25, C, driving
*Tavegil*, 2
*Tegretol Chewtabs*, 3, 8, 21, 24, C, blood, hepatic or skin disorder symptoms (see BNF), driving (see BNF)
*Tegretol liq, supps and tabs*, 3, 8, C, blood, hepatic or skin disorder symptoms (see BNF), driving (see BNF)
*Tegretol Retard*, 3, 8, 25, C, blood, hepatic or skin disorder symptoms (see BNF), driving (see BNF)
Telbivudine, C, muscle effects
*Telfast*, 5, C, driving, see BNF
Telithromycin, 9, C, driving, hepatic disorders
*Telzir susp*, C, administration, see BNF
Temazepam, 19
*Temgesic*, 2, 26
*Temodal*, 23, 25
Temozolomide, 23, 25
*Tenif*, 8, 25
Tenofovir, 21, C, administration, see BNF
*Tenoret 50*, 8
*Tenoretic*, 8
*Tenormin*, 8
Tenoxicam tabs, 21
*Tensipine MR*, 21, 25
Terazosin, C, initial dose, driving
Terbinafine, 9
Terbutaline inhalations, C, dose, see BNF
Terbutaline m/r, 25
*Testim*, C, administration, see BNF
*Testogel*, C, administration, see BNF
Testosterone buccal tablets, C, administration, see BNF
Testosterone gel, C, administration, see BNF
Testosterone patch, C, administration, see BNF
Testosterone undecanoate caps, 21, 25
Tetrabenazine, 2
Tetracycline, 7, 9, 23, C, posture
*Tetralysal preps*, 6, 9
*Teveten*, 21
Thalidomide, 2, C, symptoms of peripheral neuropathy and thromboembolism, see BNF
*Thalidomide Pharmion*, 2, C, symptoms of peripheral neuropathy and thromboembolism, see BNF
Theophylline m/r, see preps
Tiagabine, 21

Tiaprofenic acid tabs, 21
*Tifaxin XL*, 3, 25, C, driving
*Tilade*, 8, C, change to CFC-free inhaler
*Tildiem preps*, 25
Tiludronic acid, C, food and calcium
*Timodine*, 28, C, application, see BNF
Timolol, 8
Tinidazole tabs, 4, 9, 21, 25
Tipranavir, 5, 21
Tizanidine, 2
*Toctino*, 10, patient information leaflet, 11, 21
Tolcapone, 14, 25
Tolfenamic acid, 21
Tolterodine, 3
Tolterodine m/r, 3, 25
*Topamax Sprinkle*, 3, 8, C, administration, driving (see BNF)
*Topamax tabs*, 3, 8, C, driving (see BNF)
Topiramate Sprinkle caps, 3, 8, C, administration, driving (see BNF)
Topiramate tabs, 3, 8, C, driving (see BNF)
*Topotecan*, 25
*Toradol tabs*, 17, 21
*Tostran*, C, administration
*Toviaz*, 3, 25
*Tradorec XL*, 2, 25
*Tramacet*, 2, 25, 29, 30
Tramadol, 2
Tramadol m/r, 2, 25
Tramadol soluble, 2, 13
*Tramake*, 2
*Tramquel SR*, 2, C, administration, see BNF
*Trandate*, 8, 21
*Trasicor*, 8
*Trasidrex*, 8, 25
*Traxam foam*, 15
Trazodone, 2, 21
*Trental m/r*, 21, 25
Treosulfan, 25
Tretinoin caps, 21, 25
Triamcinolone inj, 10, steroid card
Triamterene, 14, (urine blue in some lights), 21
*Triapin preps*, 25
Triclofos sodium, 19
Trientine, 6, 22
Trifluoperazine, 2
Trihexyphenidyl syrup, C, driving, see BNF
Trihexyphenidyl tabs, C, with or after food, driving, see BNF
*Trileptal*, 3, 8, C, see BNF
Trilostane, 21
Trimethoprim susp and tabs, 9
Trimipramine, 2
*Trimopan*, 9
*Trimovate*, 28, C, application, see BNF

Tripotassium dicitratobismuthate, C, administration, see BNF
*Triptafen preps*, 2
*Trizivir*, C, hypersensitivity reactions, see BNF
*Tropium*, 2
Trospium chloride, 23
Truvada, 21, C, administration, see BNF
*Tryptophan*, 3
*Tuinal*, 19
*Tylex caps*, 2, 29, 30
*Tylex effervescent tabs*, 2, 13, 29, 30
Typhoid vaccine, oral, 23, 25, C, administration, see BNF
*Tyverb*, C, see BNF

*Ubretid*, 22
*Ucerax*, 2
*Ultralanum Plain*, 28, C, application, see BNF
*Uniphyllin Continus*, 25
*Univer*, 25
*Urdox*, 21
*Uriben*, 9, 11
*Urispas*, 3
Ursodeoxycholic acid, 21
*Ursogal*, 21
*Ursofalk*, 21
*Ustekinumab*, 10, C, tuberculosis, see BNF
*Utinor*, 7, 9, 23, C, driving
*Utrogestan*, C, administration, see BNF

Valaciclovir, 9
*Valcyte*, 21
Valganciclovir, 21
*Vallergan*, 2
*Valoid*, 2
*Valni XL*, 25
Valproic acid, see individual preparations
*Valtrex*, 9
Vancocin caps, 9
Vancomycin caps, 9
Varenicline, 3
*Velosef*, 9
*Venaxx XL*, 3, 25, C, driving
Venlafaxine, 3, C, driving
Venlafaxine m/r, 3, 25, C, driving
*Venlalic XL*, 3, 25, C, driving
*Ventmax SR*, 25
*Ventolin Evohaler*, C, dose, change to CFC-free inhaler, see BNF
*Ventolin inhalations*, C, dose, see BNF
*Vepesid caps*, 23
Verapamil m/r, 2, 25
*Verapress*, 25
*Vertab SR*, 25
*Vesanoid*, 21, 25
*Vesicare*, 3
*Vfend*, 9, 11, 23
*Viazem XL*, 25

*Vibramycin-D*, 6, 9, 11, 13
*Videx e/c caps*, 25, C, administration, see BNF
*Videx tabs*, 23, C, administration, see BNF
*Vigabatrin sachets*, 3, 8, 13, C, driving (see BNF)
*Vigabatrin tabs*, 3, 8, C, driving (see BNF)
*Vimpat tabs and syrup*, 8, C, driving, see BNF
*Vinorelbine caps*, 21, 25
*Vioform-Hydrocortisone*, 28, C, application, see BNF
*Viracept tabs*, 21
*Viramune*, C, hypersensitivity reactions, see BNF
*Viread*, 21, C, administration, see BNF
*Visclair*, 5, 22, 25
*Viskaldix*, 8
*Visken*, 8
*Vivotif*, 23, 25, C, administration, see BNF
*Voltarol dispersible tabs*, 13, 21
*Voltarol 75 mg SR and Retard*, 21, 25
*Voltarol tabs*, 5, 25
*Voriconazole*, 9, 11, 23

*Warfarin*, 10, anticoagulant card
*Warticon*, 15
*Welldorm*, 19, 27
*Wellvone*, 21
*Wilzin*, 23

*Xagrid*, C, driving
*Xamiol*, 28

*Xanax*, 2
*Xatral*, 3, C, dose, see BNF
*Xatral XL*, 3, 21, 25, C, dose, see BNF
*Xeloda*, 21
*Xepin*, 2, 10, patient information leaflet
*Xismox XL*, 25
*Xyzal*, C, driving

*Yentreve*, 2

*Zaditen*, 2, 21
*Zafirlukast*, 23
*Zaleplon*, 2
*Zamadol*, 2
*Zamadol 24hr*, 2, 25
*Zamadol SR*, 2, C, administration, see BNF
*Zanaflex*, 2
*Zanidip*, 22
*Zantac effervescent tabs*, 13
*Zaponex*, 2, 10, patient information leaflet
*Zarontin*, 8, C, blood disorder symptoms (see BNF), driving (see BNF)
*Zavedos caps*, 25
*Zelapar*, C, administration, see BNF
*Zemon XL*, 25
*Zemtard XL*, 25
*Zeridame SR*, 2, 25
*Zerit*, 23
*Ziagen*, C, hypersensitivity reactions, see BNF
*Zidovudine oral solution*, C, use of oral syringe

*Zimbacol XL*, 21, 25
*Zimovane*, 19
Zinc acetate, 23
Zinc sulphate, see preps
*Zinnat susp*, 9, 21
*Zinnat tabs*, 9, 21, 25
*Zispin SolTab*, 2
*Zithromax caps*, 5, 9, 23
*Zithromax susp*, 5, 9
*Zocor*, C, muscle effects, see BNF
*Zofran Melt*, C, administration, see BNF
Zolmitriptan orodispersible tabs, C, administration, see BNF
*Zolpidem*, 19
*Zomig Rapimelt*, C, administration, see BNF
*Zomorph*, 2, C, administration, see BNF
*Zonegran*, 3
Zonisamide, 3
Zopiclone, 19
Zotepine, 2
*Zoton FasTab*, 5, 22, C, administration, see BNF
*Zovirax susp and tabs*, 9
Zuclopenthixol, 2
*Zyban*, 25, C, driving
*Zydol*, 2
*Zydol soluble tabs*, 2, 13
*Zydol SR*, 2, 25
*Zydol XL*, 2, 25
*Zyloric*, 8, 21, 27
*Zyprexa tabs*, 2
*Zyprexa Velotab*, 2, C, administration, see BNF
*Zyvox susp and tabs*, 9, 10, patient information leaflet

# Dental Practitioners' Formulary

## List of Dental Preparations

The following list has been approved by the appropriate Secretaries of State, and the preparations therein may be prescribed by dental practitioners on form FP10D (GP14 in Scotland, WP10D in Wales).

**Sugar-free** versions, where available, are preferred.
Aciclovir Cream, BP
Aciclovir Oral Suspension, BP, 200 mg/5 mL
Aciclovir Tablets, BP, 200 mg
Aciclovir Tablets, BP, 800 mg
Amoxicillin Capsules, BP
Amoxicillin Oral Powder, DPF[1]
Amoxicillin Oral Suspension, BP
Amphotericin Lozenges, BP
Ampicillin Capsules, BP
Ampicillin Oral Suspension, BP
Artificial Saliva Liquid, DPF
Artificial Saliva Oral Spray, DPF[2]
Artificial Saliva Substitutes as listed below (to be prescribed only for indications approved by ACBS[3]):
  AS Saliva Orthana®
  Glandosane®
  Biotene Oralbalance®
  BioXtra®
  Saliveze®
  Salivix®
Aspirin Tablets, Dispersible, BP[4]
Azithromycin Oral Suspension, 200 mg/5 mL, DPF
Beclometasone Pressurised Inhalation, BP, 50 micrograms/metered inhalation, CFC-free, as:
  Clenil Modulite®
Benzydamine Mouthwash, BP 0.15%
Benzydamine Oromucosal Spray, BP 0.15%
Betamethasone Soluble Tablets, 500 micrograms, DPF
Carbamazepine Tablets, BP
Carmellose Gelatin Paste, DPF
Cefalexin Capsules, BP
Cefalexin Oral Suspension, BP
Cefalexin Tablets, BP
Cefradine Capsules, BP
Cefradine Oral Solution, DPF
Cetirizine Hydrochloride Tablets, 10 mg, DPF
Chlorhexidine Gluconate Gel, BP
Chlorhexidine Mouthwash, BP
Chlorhexidine Oral Spray, DPF
Chlorhexidine Oromucosal Solution, Alcohol-free, 0.2%, DPF
Chlorphenamine Oral Solution, BP
Chlorphenamine Tablets, BP
Choline Salicylate Dental Gel, BP

Co-amoxiclav Tablets, BP, 250/125 (amoxicillin 250 mg as trihydrate, clavulanic acid 125 mg as potassium salt)
Co-amoxiclav Oral Suspension, 125/31 (amoxicillin 125 mg as trihydrate, clavulanic acid 31.25 mg as potassium salt)/5 mL, DPF
Co-amoxiclav Oral Suspension, 250/62 (amoxicillin 250 mg as trihydrate, clavulanic acid 62.5 mg as potassium salt)/5 mL, DPF
Diazepam Oral Solution, BP, 2 mg/5 mL
Diazepam Tablets, BP
Diclofenac Sodium Tablets, BP
Dihydrocodeine Tablets, BP, 30 mg
Doxycycline Capsules, BP, 100 mg
Doxycycline Tablets, 20 mg, DPF
Ephedrine Nasal Drops, BP
Erythromycin Ethyl Succinate Oral Suspension, BP
Erythromycin Ethyl Succinate Tablets, BP
Erythromycin Stearate Tablets, BP
Erythromycin Tablets, BP
Fluconazole Capsules, 50 mg, DPF
Fluconazole Oral Suspension, 50 mg/5 mL, DPF
Hydrocortisone Cream, BP, 1%
Hydrocortisone Oromucosal Tablets, BP
Hydrogen Peroxide Mouthwash, BP
Ibuprofen Oral Suspension, BP, sugar-free
Ibuprofen Tablets, BP
Lansoprazole Capsules, DPF
Lidocaine 5% Ointment, DPF
Lidocaine Spray 10%, DPF
Loratadine Tablets, 10 mg, DPF
Menthol and Eucalyptus Inhalation, BP 1980[5]
Metronidazole Oral Suspension, BP
Metronidazole Tablets, BP
Miconazole Cream, BP
Miconazole Oromucosal Gel, BP
Miconazole and Hydrocortisone Cream, BP
Miconazole and Hydrocortisone Ointment, BP
Mouthwash Solution-tablets, DPF
Nitrazepam Tablets, BP
Nystatin Oral Suspension, BP
Gastro-resistant Omeprazole Capsules, BP
Oxytetracycline Tablets, BP
Paracetamol Oral Suspension, BP[6]
Paracetamol Tablets, BP
Paracetamol Tablets, Soluble, BP
Penciclovir Cream, DPF
Phenoxymethylpenicillin Oral Solution, BP
Phenoxymethylpenicillin Tablets, BP
Promethazine Hydrochloride Tablets, BP
Promethazine Oral Solution, BP
Saliva Stimulating Tablets, DPF
Sodium Chloride Mouthwash, Compound, BP

---

1. Amoxicillin Dispersible Tablets are no longer available
2. Supplies may be difficult to obtain
3. Indications approved by the ACBS are: patients suffering from dry mouth as a result of having (or having undergone) radiotherapy or sicca syndrome
4. The BP directs that when soluble aspirin tablets are prescribed, dispersible aspirin tablets should be dispensed

5. This preparation does not appear in subsequent editions of the BP
6. The BP directs that when Paediatric Paracetamol Oral Suspension or Paediatric Paracetamol Mixture is prescribed and no strength stated Paracetamol Oral Suspension 120 mg/5 mL should be dispensed

Dental Practitioners' Formulary

Sodium Fluoride Mouthwash, BP
Sodium Fluoride Oral Drops, BP
Sodium Fluoride Tablets, BP
Sodium Fluoride Toothpaste 0.619%, DPF
Sodium Fluoride Toothpaste 1.1%, DPF
Sodium Fusidate Ointment, BP
Temazepam Oral Solution, BP
Temazepam Tablets, BP
Tetracycline Tablets, BP
Triamcinolone Dental Paste, BP

> Preparations in this list which are not included in the
> BP or BPC are described under Details of DPF
> preparations, below

## Details of DPF preparations

Preparations on the List of Dental Preparations which
are specified as DPF are described as follows in the DPF.

Although brand names have sometimes been included
for identification purposes preparations on the list
should be prescribed by non-proprietary name.

**Amoxicillin Oral Powder** (PoM)

amoxicillin (as trihydrate) 3 g sachet

**Artificial Saliva Liquid**

(proprietary product: *Salinum*) consists of linseed
extract (containing polysaccharides) with dipotassium
phosphate buffer and preservatives, pH 6–7

**Artificial Saliva Oral Spray**

(proprietary product: *Luborant*) consists of sorbitol
1.8 g, carmellose sodium (sodium carboxymethylcellulose) 390 mg, dibasic potassium phosphate
48.23 mg, potassium chloride 37.5 mg, monobasic
potassium phosphate 21.97 mg, calcium chloride
9.972 mg, magnesium chloride 3.528 mg, sodium
fluoride 258 micrograms/60 mL, with preservatives
and colouring agents

**Azithromycin Oral Suspension 200 mg/5 mL** (PoM)

(proprietary product: *Zithromax*); azithromycin (as
dihydrate) 200 mg/5 mL when reconstituted with
water

**Betamethasone Soluble Tablets 500 micrograms**
(PoM)

(proprietary product: *Betnesol Soluble Tablets*), betamethasone (as sodium phosphate) 500 micrograms

**Carmellose Gelatin Paste**

(proprietary product: *Orabase Oral Paste*), gelatin,
pectin, carmellose sodium, 16.58% of each in a suitable basis

**Cefradine Oral Solution** (PoM)

(proprietary product: *Velosef Syrup*), cefradine
250 mg/5 mL when reconstituted with water

**Cetirizine Hydrochloride Tablets**

cetirizine hydrochloride 10 mg

**Chlorhexidine Oral Spray**

(proprietary product: *Corsodyl Oral Spray*), chlorhexidine gluconate 0.2%

**Chlorhexidine Oromucosal Solution, Alcohol-free,
0.2%**

(proprietary product: *Periogard Oromucosal Solution*),
chlorhexidine gluconate 0.2%

**Co-amoxiclav Oral Suspension 125/31** (PoM)

amoxicillin 125 mg as trihydrate, clavulanic acid
31.25 mg as potassium salt/5 mL when reconstituted
with water

**Co-amoxiclav Oral Suspension 250/62** (PoM)

amoxicillin 250 mg as trihydrate, clavulanic acid
62.5 mg as potassium salt/5 mL when reconstituted
with water

**Doxycycline Tablets 20 mg** (PoM)

(proprietary product: *Periostat*), doxycycline (as
hyclate) 20 mg

**Fluconazole Capsules 50 mg** (PoM)

fluconazole 50 mg

**Fluconazole Oral Suspension 50 mg/5 mL** (PoM)

(proprietary product: *Diflucan*), fluconazole 50 mg/
5 mL when reconstituted with water

**Lansoprazole Capsules** (PoM)

lansoprazole 15 mg and 30 mg capsules, enclosing
e/c granules

**Lidocaine 5% Ointment**

lidocaine 5% in a suitable basis

**Lidocaine Spray 10%**

(proprietary product: *Xylocaine Spray*), lidocaine 10%
supplying 10 mg lidocaine/spray

**Loratadine Tablets**

loratadine 10 mg

**Mouthwash Solution-tablets**

consist of tablets which may contain antimicrobial,
colouring and flavouring agents in a suitable soluble
effervescent basis to make a mouthwash suitable for
dental purposes

**Penciclovir Cream** (PoM)

(proprietary product: *Vectavir Cream*), penciclovir 1%

**Saliva Stimulating Tablets**

(proprietary product: *SST*), citric acid, malic acid and
other ingredients in a sorbitol base

**Sodium Fluoride Toothpaste 0.619%** (PoM)

(proprietary product: *Duraphat '2800 ppm' Toothpaste*),
sodium fluoride 0.619%

**Sodium Fluoride Toothpaste 1.1%** (PoM)

(proprietary product: *Duraphat '5000 ppm' Toothpaste*),
sodium fluoride 1.1%

## Changes to Dental Practitioners' Formulary since September 2008

### Additions

Artificial Saliva Liquid, DPF

Beclometasone Pressurised Inhalation, BP, 50 micr-
ograms/metered inhalation, CFC-free, as:
   *Clenil Modulite®*

Cetirizine Hydrochloride Tablets, 10 mg, DPF

Chlorhexidine Oromucosal Solution, Alcohol-free, 0.2%,
DPF

Chlorphenamine Oral Solution, BP

Co-amoxiclav Oral Suspension 125/31 (amoxicillin
125 mg as trihydrate, clavulanic acid 31.25 mg as potassium salt)/5 mL, DPF

Co-amoxiclav Oral Suspension 250/62 (amoxicillin
250 mg as trihydrate, clavulanic acid 62.5 mg as potassium salt)/5 mL, DPF

Co-amoxiclav Tablets, BP, 250/125 (amoxicillin 250 mg
as trihydrate, clavulanic acid 125 mg as potassium salt)

Lansoprazole Capsules, DPF

Loratadine Tablets, 10 mg, DPF

Gastro-resistant Omeprazole Capsules, BP

## Deletions

Ascorbic Acid Tablets, BP

Beclometasone Dipropionate Aerosol Inhalation
50 micrograms/metered dose, DPF

Nystatin Ointment, BP

Pethidine Tablets, BP

Vitamin B Tablets, Compound, Strong, BPC

## Changes of title

| Old | New |
|-----|-----|
| Artificial Saliva, DPF | Artificial Saliva Oral Spray, DPF |
| Chlorhexidine Gluconate 1% Gel, DPF | Chlorhexidine Gluconate Gel, BP |
| Metronidazole Oral Suspension, DPF | Metronidazole Oral Suspension, BP |

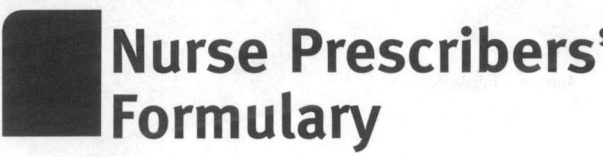

# Nurse Prescribers' Formulary

## Nurse Prescribers' Formulary for Community Practitioners

**Nurse Prescribers' Formulary Appendix** (Appendix NPF). List of preparations approved by the Secretary of State which may be prescribed on form FP10P (form HS21(N) in Northern Ireland, form GP10(N) in Scotland, forms WP10CN and WP10PN in Wales) by Nurses for National Health Service patients.

Community practitioners who have completed the necessary training may only prescribe items appearing in the nurse prescribers' list set out below. Community Practitioner Nurse Prescribers are recommended to prescribe generically, except where this would not be clinically appropriate or where there is no approved generic name.

## Medicinal Preparations

> Preparations on this list which are not included in the BP or BPC are described on p. 951

Almond Oil Ear Drops, BP
Arachis Oil Enema, NPF
[1]Aspirin Tablets, Dispersible, 300 mg, BP
Bisacodyl Suppositories, BP (includes 5-mg and 10-mg strengths)
Bisacodyl Tablets, BP
Catheter Maintenance Solution, Chlorhexidine, NPF
Catheter Maintenance Solution, Sodium Chloride, NPF
Catheter Maintenance Solution, 'Solution G', NPF
Catheter Maintenance Solution, 'Solution R', NPF
Chlorhexidine Gluconate Alcoholic Solutions containing at least 0.05%
Chlorhexidine Gluconate Aqueous Solutions containing at least 0.05%
Choline Salicylate Dental Gel, BP
Clotrimazole Cream 1%, BP
Co-danthramer Capsules, NPF
Co-danthramer Capsules, Strong, NPF
Co-danthramer Oral Suspension, NPF
Co-danthramer Oral Suspension, Strong, NPF
Co-danthrusate Capsules, BP
Co-danthrusate Oral Suspension, NPF
Crotamiton Cream, BP
Crotamiton Lotion, BP
Dimeticone barrier creams containing at least 10%
Dimeticone Lotion, NPF
Docusate Capsules, BP
Docusate Enema, NPF
Docusate Oral Solution, BP
Docusate Oral Solution, Paediatric, BP
Econazole Cream 1%, BP

Emollients as listed below:
 Aqueous Cream, BP
 Arachis Oil, BP
 Cetraben® Emollient Cream
 Dermamist®
 Diprobase® Cream
 Diprobase® Ointment
 Doublebase®
 E45® Cream
 Emulsifying Ointment, BP
 Hydromol® Cream
 Hydromol® Ointment
 Hydrous Ointment, BP
 Linola® Gamma Cream
 Lipobase®
 Liquid and White Soft Paraffin Ointment, NPF
 Neutrogena® Dermatological Cream
 Oilatum® Cream
 Oilatum® Junior Cream
 Paraffin, White Soft, BP
 Paraffin, Yellow Soft, BP
 QV® Cream
 QV® Lotion
 QV® Wash
 Ultrabase®
 Unguentum M®
 Zerobase® Cream
Emollient Bath Additives as listed below:
 Alpha Keri® Bath Oil
 [2]Balneum®
 Cetraben® Emollient Bath Additive
 Dermalo® Bath Emollient
 Diprobath®
 Doublebase® Emollient Bath Additive
 Doublebase® Emollient Shower Gel
 Doublebase® Emollient Wash Gel
 Hydromol® Emollient
 Imuderm® Bath Oil
 Oilatum® Emollient
 Oilatum® Junior Emollient Bath Additive
 Oilatum® Gel
 QV® Bath Oil
Folic Acid 400 micrograms/5 mL Oral Solution, NPF
Folic Acid Tablets 400 micrograms, BP
Glycerol Suppositories, BP
[3]Ibuprofen Oral Suspension, BP
[3]Ibuprofen Tablets, BP
Ispaghula Husk Granules, BP
Ispaghula Husk Granules, Effervescent, BP
Ispaghula Husk Oral Powder, BP
Lactulose Solution, BP
Lidocaine Ointment, BP
Lidocaine and Chlorhexidine Gel, BP
Macrogol Oral Powder, Compound, NPF

---

1. Max. 96 tablets; max. pack size 32 tablets

2. Except pack sizes that are not to be prescribed under the NHS (see Part XVIIIA of the Drug Tariff, Part XI of the Northern Ireland Drug Tariff)
3. Except for indications and doses that are [PoM]

Macrogol Oral Powder, Compound, Half-strength, NPF
Magnesium Hydroxide Mixture, BP
Magnesium Sulphate Paste, BP
Malathion aqueous lotions containing at least 0.5%
Mebendazole Oral Suspension, NPF
Mebendazole Tablets, NPF
Methylcellulose Tablets, BP
Miconazole Cream 2%, BP
Miconazole Oromucosal Gel, BP
Mouthwash Solution-tablets, NPF
Nicotine Inhalation Cartridge for Oromucosal Use, NPF
Nicotine Lozenge, NPF
Nicotine Medicated Chewing Gum, NPF
Nicotine Nasal Spray, NPF
Nicotine Sublingual Tablets, NPF
Nicotine Transdermal Patches, NPF
Nystatin Oral Suspension, BP
Olive Oil Ear Drops, BP
Paracetamol Oral Suspension, BP (includes 120 mg/
    5 mL and 250 mg/5 mL strengths—both of which are
    available as sugar-free formulations)
[1]Paracetamol Tablets, BP
[1]Paracetamol Tablets, Soluble, BP (includes 120-mg and
    500-mg tablets)
Permethrin Cream, NPF
Phenothrin Aqueous Lotion, NPF
Phosphate Suppositories, NPF
Phosphates Enema, BP
Piperazine and Senna Powder, NPF
Povidone–Iodine Solution, BP
Senna Oral Solution, NPF
Senna Tablets, BP
Senna and Ispaghula Granules, NPF
Sodium Chloride Solution, Sterile, BP
Sodium Citrate Compound Enema, NPF
Sodium Picosulfate Capsules, NPF
Sodium Picosulfate Elixir, NPF
Spermicidal contraceptives as listed below:
    Gygel® Contraceptive Jelly
Sterculia Granules, NPF
Sterculia and Frangula Granules, NPF
Titanium Ointment, BP
Water for Injections, BP
Zinc and Castor Oil Ointment, BP
Zinc Cream, BP
Zinc Ointment, BP
Zinc Oxide and Dimeticone Spray, NPF
Zinc Oxide Impregnated Medicated Bandage, NPF
Zinc Oxide Impregnated Medicated Stocking, NPF
Zinc Paste Bandage, BP 1993
Zinc Paste and Calamine Bandage
Zinc Paste and Ichthammol Bandage, BP 1993

### Appliances and Reagents (including Wound Management Products)

Community Practitioner Nurse Prescribers in England, Wales and Northern Ireland can prescribe any appliance or reagent in the relevant Drug Tariff. In the Scottish Drug Tariff, Appliances and Reagents which may **not** be prescribed by Nurses are annotated **Nx**.

The Drug Tariffs can be accessed online at:
National Health Service Drug Tariff for England and Wales: www.ppa.org.uk/ppa/edt_intro.htm
Health and Personal Social Services for Northern Ireland Drug Tariff: www.centralservicesagency.com/display/ni_drug_tariff

Scottish Drug Tariff: www.isdscotland.org/isd/2245.html

**Appliances** (including Contraceptive Devices[2]) as listed in Part IXA of the Drug Tariff (Part III of the Northern Ireland Drug Tariff, Part 3 (Appliances) and Part 2 (Dressings) of the Scottish Drug Tariff)

**Incontinence Appliances** as listed in Part IXB of the Drug Tariff (Part III of the Northern Ireland Drug Tariff, Part 5 of the Scottish Drug Tariff)

**Stoma Appliances and Associated Products** as listed in Part IXC of the Drug Tariff (Part III of the Northern Ireland Drug Tariff, Part 6 of the Scottish Drug Tariff)

**Chemical Reagents** as listed in Part IXR of the Drug Tariff (Part II of the Northern Ireland Drug Tariff, Part 9 of the Scottish Drug Tariff)

## Details of NPF preparations

Preparations on the Nurse Prescribers' Formulary which are not included in the BP or BPC are described as follows in the Nurse Prescribers' Formulary.

Although brand names have sometimes been included for identification purposes, it is recommended that non-proprietary names should be used for prescribing medicinal preparations in the NPF except where a non-proprietary name is not available.

**Arachis Oil Enema**
    arachis oil 100%

**Catheter Maintenance Solution, Chlorhexidine**
    (proprietary products: *Uro-Tainer Chlorhexidine; Uriflex C*), chlorhexidine 0.02%

**Catheter Maintenance Solution, Sodium Chloride**
    (proprietary products: *OptiFlo S; Uro-Tainer Sodium Chloride; Uriflex-S*), sodium chloride 0.9%

**Catheter Maintenance Solution, 'Solution G'**
    (proprietary products: *OptiFlo G; Uro-Tainer Suby G; Uriflex G*), citric acid 3.23%, magnesium oxide 0.38%, sodium bicarbonate 0.7%, disodium edetate 0.01%

**Catheter Maintenance Solution, 'Solution R'**
    (proprietary products: *OptiFlo R; Uro-Tainer Solution R; Uriflex R*), citric acid 6%, gluconolactone 0.6%, magnesium carbonate 2.8%, disodium edetate 0.01%

**Chlorhexidine gluconate alcoholic solutions**
    (proprietary products: *ChloraPrep; Hydrex Solution; Hydrex spray*), chlorhexidine gluconate in alcoholic solution

**Chlorhexidine gluconate aqueous solutions**
    (proprietary product: *Unisept*) chlorhexidine gluconate in aqueous solution

**Co-danthramer Capsules** [PoM]
    co-danthramer 25/200 (dantron 25 mg, poloxamer '188' 200 mg)

**Co-danthramer Capsules, Strong** [PoM]
    co-danthramer 37.5/500 (dantron 37.5 mg, poloxamer '188' 500 mg)

---

1. Max. 96 tablets; max. pack size 32 tablets

2. Nurse Prescribers in Family Planning Clinics—where it is not appropriate for nurse prescribers in family planning clinics to prescribe contraceptive devices using form FP10(P) (forms WP10CN and WP10PN in Wales), they may prescribe using the same system as doctors in the clinic

### Co-danthramer Oral Suspension [PoM]

(proprietary product: *Codalax*), co-danthramer 25/200 in 5 mL (dantron 25 mg, poloxamer '188' 200 mg/5 mL)

### Co-danthramer Oral Suspension, Strong [PoM]

(proprietary product: *Codalax Forte*), co-danthramer 75/1000 in 5 mL (dantron 75 mg, poloxamer '188' 1 g/5 mL)

### Co-danthrusate Oral Suspension [PoM]

(proprietary product: *Normax*), co-danthrusate 50/60 (dantron 50 mg, docusate sodium 60 mg/5 mL)

### Dimeticone barrier creams

(proprietary products: *Conotrane Cream*, dimeticone '350' 22%; *Siopel Barrier Cream*, dimeticone '1000' 10%; *Vasogen Barrier Cream*, dimeticone 20%), dimeticone 10–22%

### Dimeticone Lotion

(proprietary product: *Hedrin*), dimeticone 4%

### Docusate Enema

(proprietary product: *Norgalax Micro-enema*) docusate sodium 120 mg in 10 g

### Folic Acid Oral Solution 400 micrograms/5 mL

(proprietary product: *Folicare*), folic acid 400 micrograms/5 mL

### Liquid and White Soft Paraffin Ointment

liquid paraffin 50%, white soft paraffin 50%

### Macrogol Oral Powder, Compound

macrogol '3350' (polyethylene glycol '3350') 13.125 g, sodium bicarbonate 178.5 mg, sodium chloride 350.7 mg, potassium chloride 46.6 mg/sachet (proprietary products: *Movicol*; *Movicol Plain*; *Laxido* (orange or natural flavour)) *or* macrogol '3350' (polyethelyene glycol '3350') 13.125 g, sodium bicarbonate 178.5 mg, sodium chloride 350.7 mg, potassium chloride 31.7 mg/sachet (proprietary product: *Movicol Chocolate*)

### Macrogol Oral Powder, Compound, Half-strength

(proprietary product: *Movicol-Half*), macrogol '3350' (polyethylene glycol '3350') 6.563 g, sodium bicarbonate 89.3 mg, sodium chloride 175.4 mg, potassium chloride 23.3 mg/sachet

### Malathion aqueous lotions

(proprietary products: *Derbac-M Liquid*; *Quellada M Liquid*), malathion 0.5% in an aqueous basis

### Mebendazole Oral Suspension [PoM]

(proprietary product: *Vermox*), mebendazole 100 mg/5 mL

### [1]Mebendazole Tablets [PoM]

(proprietary products: *Ovex*, *Vermox*), mebendazole 100 mg

### Mouthwash Solution-tablets

consist of tablets which may contain antimicrobial, colouring and flavouring agents in a suitable soluble effervescent basis to make a mouthwash

### [2]Nicotine Inhalation Cartridge for Oromucosal Use

(proprietary products: *Nicorette Inhalator*), nicotine 10 mg

### Nicotine Lozenge

nicotine (as bitartrate) 1 mg or 2 mg (proprietary product: *Nicotinell Mint Lozenge*) or nicotine (as polacrilex) 2 mg or 4 mg (proprietary product: *NiQuitin Lozenges*), or nicotine (as resinate complex) 1.5 mg (proprietary product: *Nicopass Lozenge*)

### Nicotine Medicated Chewing Gum

(proprietary products: *Nicorette Gum*, *Nicotinell Gum*, *NiQuitin Gum*), nicotine 2 mg or 4 mg

### Nicotine Nasal Spray

(proprietary product: *Nicorette Nasal Spray*), nicotine 500 micrograms/metered spray

### [3]Nicotine Sublingual Tablets

(proprietary product: *Nicorette Microtab*), nicotine (as a cyclodextrin complex) 2 mg

### [4]Nicotine Transdermal Patches

releasing in each 16 hours, nicotine approx. 5 mg, 10 mg, or 15 mg (proprietary product: *Boots NicAssist Patch*, *Nicorette Patch*) or releasing in each 24 hours nicotine approx. 7 mg, 14 mg, or 21 mg (proprietary products: *Nicopatch*, *Nicotinell TTS*, *NiQuitin*)

### Permethrin Cream

(proprietary product: *Lyclear Dermal Cream*), permethrin 5%

### Phenothrin Aqueous Lotion

(proprietary product: *Full Marks Liquid*), phenothrin 0.5% in an aqueous basis

### Phosphate Suppositories

(proprietary product: *Carbalax*), sodium acid phosphate (anhydrous) 1.3 g, sodium bicarbonate 1.08 g

### Piperazine and Senna Powder

(proprietary product: *Pripsen Oral Powder*), piperazine phosphate 4 g, sennosides 15.3 mg/sachet

### Senna Oral Solution

(proprietary product: *Senokot Syrup*), sennosides 7.5 mg/5 mL

### Senna and Ispaghula Granules

(proprietary product: *Manevac Granules*), senna fruit 12.4%, ispaghula 54.2%

### Sodium Citrate Compound Enema

(proprietary products: *Micolette Micro-enema*; *Micralax Micro-enema*; *Relaxit Micro-enema*), sodium citrate 450 mg with glycerol, sorbitol and an anionic surfactant

### Sodium Picosulfate Capsules

(proprietary products: *Dulco-lax Perles*), sodium picosulfate 2.5 mg

### Sodium Picosulfate Elixir

(proprietary products: *Dulco-lax Liquid*, *Laxoberal* (NHS)), sodium picosulfate 5 mg/5 mL

### Sterculia Granules

(proprietary product: *Normacol Granules*), sterculia 62%

---

1. For [PoM] exemption, see p. 370
2. For use with inhalation mouthpiece; to be prescribed as either a starter pack (6 cartridges with inhalator device and holder) or refill pack (42 cartridges with inhalator device)
3. To be prescribed as either a starter pack (2 x 15-tablet discs with dispenser) or refill pack (7 x 15-tablet discs)
4. Prescriber should specify the brand to be dispensed

**Sterculia and Frangula Granules**

(proprietary product: *Normacol Plus Granules*), sterculia 62%, frangula (standardised) 8%

**Zinc Oxide and Dimeticone Spray**

(proprietary product: *Sprilon*), dimeticone 1.04%, zinc oxide 12.5% in a pressurised aerosol unit

**Zinc Oxide Impregnated Medicated Bandage**

(proprietary product: *Steripaste*), sterile cotton bandage impregnated with paste containing zinc oxide 15%

**Zinc Oxide Impregnated Medicated Stocking**

(proprietary product: *Zipzoc*), sterile rayon stocking impregnated with ointment containing zinc oxide 20%

## Nurse Independent Prescribing

Nurse Independent Prescribers (formerly known as Extended Formulary Nurse Prescribers) are able to prescribe any licensed medicine for any medical condition, including some Controlled Drugs (see below).

Nurse Independent Prescribers must work within their own level of professional competence and expertise. They are recommended to prescribe generically, except where this would not be clinically appropriate or where there is no approved non-proprietary name.

Nurse Independent Prescribers are also able to prescribe independently the Controlled Drugs in the table below, *solely for the medical conditions indicated*.

Up-to-date information and guidance on nurse independent prescribing is available on the Department of Health website at
www.dh.gov.uk/nonmedicalprescribing

## Controlled drugs prescribable by Nurse Independent Prescribers solely for the medical conditions Indicated

| Drug | Indication | Route of Administration |
|---|---|---|
| Buprenorphine | Transdermal use in palliative care | Transdermal |
| Chlordiazepoxide hydrochloride | Treatment of initial or acute withdrawal symptoms caused by the withdrawal of alcohol from persons habituated to it | Oral |
| Codeine phosphate | – | Oral |
| Co-phenotrope | – | Oral |
| Diamorphine hydrochloride | Use in palliative care, pain relief in respect of suspected myocardial infarction or for relief of acute or severe pain after trauma, including in either case postoperative pain relief | Oral, parenteral |
| Diazepam | Use in palliative care, treatment of initial or acute withdrawal symptoms caused by the withdrawal of alcohol from persons habituated to it, tonic-clonic seizures | Oral, parenteral, rectal |
| Dihydrocodeine tartrate | – | Oral |
| Fentanyl | Transdermal use in palliative care | Transdermal |
| Lorazepam | Use in palliative care, tonic-clonic seizures | Oral, parenteral |
| Midazolam | Use in palliative care, tonic-clonic seizures | Parenteral, buccal |
| Morphine hydrochloride | Use in palliative care, pain relief in respect of suspected myocardial infarction or for relief of acute or severe pain after trauma, including in either case postoperative pain relief | Rectal |
| Morphine sulphate | Use in palliative care, pain relief in respect of suspected myocardial infarction or for relief of acute or severe pain after trauma, including in either case postoperative pain relief | Oral, parenteral, rectal |
| Oxycodone hydrochloride | Use in palliative care | Oral, parenteral |

**Note** For the purposes of nurse independent prescribing, palliative care means the care of patients with advanced, progressive illness

Nurse Prescribers' Formulary

# Non-medical prescribing

A range of non-medical healthcare professionals can prescribe medicines for patients as either Independent or Supplementary Prescribers.

Independent prescribers are practitioners responsible and accountable for the assessment of patients with previously undiagnosed or diagnosed conditions and for decisions about the clinical management required, including prescribing. They are recommended to prescribe generically, except where this would not be clinically appropriate or where there is no approved non-proprietary name.

Supplementary prescribing is a partnership between an independent prescriber (a doctor or a dentist) and a supplementary prescriber to implement an agreed Clinical Management Plan for an individual patient with that patient's agreement.

Independent and Supplementary Prescribers are identified by an annotation next to their name in the relevant professional register.

Up-to-date information and guidance on non-medical prescribing is available on the Department of Health website at www.dh.gov.uk/nonmedicalprescribing.

For information on the supply and administration of medicines to groups of patients using Patient Group Directions, see p. 3.

## Nurses

For further information on Nurse Independent Prescribing, see Nurse Prescribers' Formulary, p. 953.

## Optometrists

Optometrist Independent Prescribers can prescribe any licensed medicine for ocular conditions affecting the eye and the tissues surrounding the eye, except Controlled Drugs or medicines for parenteral administration. Optometrist Independent Prescribers must work within their own level of professional competence and expertise.

## Pharmacists

Pharmacist Independent Prescribers can prescribe any licensed medicine, except Controlled Drugs, for any medical condition. Pharmacist Independent Prescribers must work within their own level of professional competence and expertise.

# Index of manufacturers

**3M**
3M Health Care Ltd
3M House
Morley St
Loughborough
Leics, LE11 1EP.
tel: (01509) 611611
fax: (01509) 237288

**A&H**
Allen & Hanburys Ltd
See GSK

**A1 Pharmaceuticals**
A1 Pharmaceuticals Plc
Units 20+21 Easter Park
Site 8A Beam Reach
Ferry Lane South, Rainham
Essex, RM13 9BP.
tel: (01708) 528 900
fax: (01708) 528 928
sales@a1plc.co.uk

**Abbey**
Abbey Pharmaceuticals Ltd
13 Islet Park Drive
Maidenhead
Berks, SL6 8LF.
tel: (01628) 771 036
fax: (01628) 771 524

**Abbott**
Abbott Laboratories Ltd
Abbott House
Norden Rd, Maidenhead
Berks, SL6 4XE.
tel: (01628) 773 355
fax: (01628) 644 185
ukmedinfo@abbott.com

**Abraxis**
Abraxis BioScience Ltd
IDIS House
Churchfield Road
Weybridge
Surrey, KT13 8DB.
tel: 0207 081 0850
abraxismedical@idispharma.com

**ABT Healthcare**
ABT Healthcare UK Ltd
Springwood Booths Hall
Booths Park
Chelford Rd
Knutsford, WA16 8QZ.
tel: (01565) 757783

**Acorus**
Acorus Therapeutics Ltd
Office Village
Chester Business Park
Chester, CH4 9QZ.
tel: (01244) 625 152
fax: (01244) 625 151
enquiries@acorus-therapeutics.com

**Actavis**
Actavis UK Ltd
Whiddon Valley
Barnstaple
Devon, EX32 8NS.
tel: (01271) 311 257
fax: (01271) 346 106
medinfo@actavis.co.uk

**Actelion**
Actelion Pharmaceuticals UK Ltd
BSi Building, 13th Floor
389 Chiswick High Rd, London, W4
4AL.
tel: (020) 8987 3333
fax: (020) 8987 3322

**Activa**
Activa Healthcare
1 Lancaster Park
Newborough Rd, Needwood
Burton-upon-Trent, Staffs, DE13 9PD.
tel: (0845) 060 6707
fax: (01283) 576 808
advice@activahealthcare.co.uk

**ADI Medical**
ADI Medical Ltd
Sunny Hollow
Handleton Common
Lane End
Bucks, HP14 3LA.
tel: 01494 882 666
fax: 01494 883 086
info@adimedical.co.uk

**Advancis**
Advancis Medical Ltd
Lowmoor Business Park
Kirkby-in-Ashfield, Nottingham, NG17
7JZ.
tel: (01623) 751 500
fax: (0871) 264 8238
info@advancis.co.uk

**Agepha**
Agepha GmbH
9 High St
Woburn Sands, MK17 8RF.
tel: (0203) 239 6241
uk@agepha.com

**Aguettant**
Aguettant Ltd
The Barn
41a Main Rd, Cleeve
Somerset, BS49 4NZ.
tel: (01934) 835 694
fax: (01934) 876 790
info@aguettant.co.uk

**Air Products**
Air Products plc
Medical Group
2 Millennium Gate
Westmere Drive, Crewe
Cheshire, CW1 6AP.
tel: (0800) 373 580
fax: (0800) 214 709

**Alan Pharmaceuticals**
Alan Pharmaceuticals
2 Kingsgate Ave
London, N3 3BH.
tel: (020) 8346 4311
fax: (020) 8346 5218

**Alcon**
Alcon Laboratories (UK) Ltd
Pentagon Park
Boundary Way
Hemel Hempstead, Herts, HP2 7UD.
tel: (01442) 341 234
fax: (01442) 341 200

**Alembic Products**
Alembic Products Ltd
River Lane
Saltney, Chester, Cheshire, CH4 8RQ.
tel: (01244) 680 147
fax: (01244) 680 155

**Alexion**
Alexion Pharma UK Ltd
Unit 14, Horizon Business Village
1 Brooklands Rd
Weybridge
Surrey, KT13 0TJ.
tel: (01932) 359 220
fax: (01932) 349 793
alexion.uk@alxn.com

**ALK-Abelló**
ALK-Abelló (UK) Ltd
1 Tealgate
Hungerford, Berks, RG17 0YT.
tel: (01488) 686 016
fax: (01488) 685 423
info@uk.alk-abello.com

**Allergan**
Allergan Ltd
1st Floor Marlow International
The Parkway
Marlow
Bucks, SL7 1YL.
tel: (01628) 494 026
fax: (01628) 494 449

**Allergy**
Allergy Therapeutics Ltd
Dominion Way
Worthing, West Sussex, BN14 8SA.
tel: (01903) 844 702
fax: (01903) 844 744
infoservices@allergytherapeutics.com

**Alliance**
Alliance Pharmaceuticals Ltd
Avonbridge House
2 Bath Rd
Chippenham, Wilts, SN15 2BB.
tel: (01249) 466 966
fax: (01249) 466 977
medinfo@alliancepharma.co.uk

**Almirall**
Almirall Ltd
4 The Square
Stockley Park
Uxbridge, UB11 1ET.
tel: (0800) 0087399
almirall@professionalinformation.co.uk

**Alpharma**
See Actavis

**Alphashow**
Alphashow Ltd
10 South Rd
Amersham
Bucks, HP6 5LX.
tel: (0870) 240 2775
fax: (01672) 515 614
info@alphashow.co.uk

**Altacor**
Altacor Ltd
St. John's Innovation Centre
Cowley Road
Cambridge, CB4 0WS.
tel: (01223) 421 411
fax: (01223) 420 844
info@altacor-pharma.com

**Amdipharm**
Amdipharm plc
Regency House
Miles Gray Rd
Basildon, Essex, SS14 3AF.
tel: (0870) 777 7675
fax: (0870) 777 7875
medinfo@amdipharm.com

**Amgen**
Amgen Ltd
240 Cambridge Science Park
Milton Rd, Cambridge, CB4 0WD.
tel: (01223) 420 305
fax: (01223) 426 314
infoline@uk.amgen.com

**Anglian**
Anglian Pharma Sales & Marketing
Units 3 & 4 Quidhampton Business
Units
Polhampton Lane
Overton
Hants, RG25 3ED.
tel: (01256) 772 742
mail@anglianpharma.com

**Anpharm**
See Goldshield

**Antigen**
See Goldshield

**Archimedes**
Archimedes Pharma UK Ltd
250 South Oak Way
Green Park
Reading
Berks, RG2 6UG.
tel: (0118) 931 5060
fax: (0118) 931 5065
medicalinformation@
archimedespharma.com

**Ardana**
Ardana Bioscience Ltd
58 Queen St
Edinburgh, EH2 3NS.
tel: (0131) 226 8550
fax: (0131) 226 8551
info@ardana.co.uk

**Ardern**
Ardern Healthcare Ltd
Pipers Brook Farm
Eastham
Tenbury Wells, Worcs, WR15 8NP.
tel: (01584) 781 777
fax: (01584) 781 788
info@ardernhealthcare.com

**Ark Therapeutics**
Ark Therapeutics Group Plc
79 New Cavendish St
London, W1W 6XB.
tel: (020) 7388 7722
fax: (020) 7388 7805
info@arktherapeutics.com

**AS Pharma**
AS Pharma Ltd
PO Box 181
Polegate, East Sussex, BN26 6WD.
tel: (08700) 664 117
fax: (08700) 664 118
info@aspharma.co.uk

**Astellas**
Astellas Pharma Ltd
Lovett House, Lovett Rd
Staines, TW18 3AZ.
tel: (01784) 419 615
fax: (01784) 419 401

**AstraZeneca**
AstraZeneca UK Ltd
Horizon Place
600 Capability Green
Luton, Beds, LU1 3LU.
tel: 0800 7830 033
fax: (01582) 838 003
medical.informationuk@astrazeneca.
com

**Auden Mckenzie**
Auden Mckenzie (Pharma Division) Ltd
30 Stadium Business Centre
North End Rd
Wembley, Middx, HA9 0AT.
tel: (020) 8900 2122
fax: (020) 8903 9620

**Aurum**
Aurum Pharmaceuticals Ltd
Hubert Rd
Brentwood
Essex, CM14 4LZ.
tel: (01277) 266600
fax: (01277) 848 976
info@martindalepharma.co.uk

**Aventis Pharma**
See Sanofi-Aventis

**Ayrton Saunders**
Ayrton Saunders Ltd
Ayrton House
Commerce Way
Parliament Business Park
Liverpool, Merseyside, L8 7BA.
tel: (0151) 709 2074
fax: (0151) 709 7336
info@ayrtons.com

**Bard**
Bard Ltd
Forest House
Brighton Rd
Crawley, West Sussex, RH11 9BP.
tel: (01293) 527 888
fax: (01293) 552 428

**Basilea**
Basilea Pharmaceuticals Ltd
14/16 Frederick Sanger Road
The Surrey Research Park
Guildford
Surrey, GU2 7YD.
tel: (01483) 790 023
fax: (01483) 505 345
ukmedinfo@basilea.com

**Bausch & Lomb**
Bausch & Lomb UK Ltd
106 London Rd
Kingston-upon-Thames
Surrey, KT2 6TN.
tel: (020) 8781 2900
fax: (020) 8781 2901

**Baxter**
Baxter Healthcare Ltd
Wallingford Rd
Compton
Newbury
Berks, RG20 7QW.
tel: (01635) 206 345
fax: (01635) 206 071
surecall@baxter.com

**Bayer**
Bayer plc
Bayer Schering Pharma
Bayer House, Strawberry Hill
Newbury, Berks, RG14 1JA.
tel: (01635) 563 000
fax: (01635) 563 393
medical.science@bayer.co.uk

**Bayer Consumer Care**
See Bayer

**Bayer Diabetes Care**
See Bayer

**Bayer Diagnostics**
See Bayer

**BBI Healthcare**
BBI Healthcare
Unit A
Kestrel Way
Garngoch Industrial Estate
Gorseinon, Swansea, SA4 9WN.
tel: (01792) 229 333
fax: (01792) 897 311
info@bbihealthcare.com

**Beacon**
Beacon Pharmaceuticals Ltd
85 High St
Tunbridge Wells, TN1 1YG.
tel: (01892) 600 930
fax: (01892) 600 937
info@beaconpharma.co.uk

**Beiersdorf**
Beiersdorf UK Ltd
2010 Solihull Parkway
Birmingham Business Park
Birmingham, B37 7YS.
tel: (0121) 329 8800
fax: (0121) 329 8801

**Bell and Croyden**
John Bell and Croyden
50-54 Wigmore St
London, W1U 2AU.
tel: (020) 7935 5555
fax: (020) 7935 9605
jbc@johnbellcroyden.co.uk

**BHR**
BHR Pharmaceuticals Ltd
41 Centenary Business Centre
Hammond Close
Attleborough Fields, Nuneaton
Warwickshire, CV11 6RY.
tel: (024) 7635 3742
fax: (024) 7632 7812
info@bhr.co.uk

**Bioenvision**
Bioenvision Ltd
10 Lockside Place
Edinburgh Park
Edinburgh, EH12 9RG.
tel: (0131) 248 3555
fax: (0131) 2483300
info@bioenvision.com

**Biogen**
Biogen Idec Ltd
Innovation House
70 Norden Rd
Maidenhead
Berks, SL6 4AY.
tel: (0800) 008 7401
fax: (01628) 501 010

**Biolitec**
Biolitec Pharma Ltd
Unit 2, Broomhill Business Park
Broomhill Rd
Tallaght
Dublin 24, Ireland.
tel: (00353) 14637415
fax: (00353) 14637411
medical.info@biolitec.com

**BioMarin**
BioMarin Europe Ltd
164 Shaftsbury Ave
London, WC2 8HL.
tel: (020) 7420 0800
fax: (020) 7420 0829

**Biotest UK**
Biotest (UK) Ltd
28 Monkspath Business Park
Highlands Road
Shirley
Solihull, B90 4NZ.
tel: (0121) 733 3393
fax: (0121) 733 3066
MedicinesInformation@biotestuk.com

**Blackwell**
Blackwell Supplies Ltd
Medcare House
Centurion Close
Gillingham Business Park, Gillingham
Kent, ME8 0SB.
tel: (01634) 877 620
fax: (01634) 877 621

**Blake**
Thomas Blake Cosmetic Creams Ltd
Quantum House
Hobson Industrial Estate
Burnopfield
Co. Durham, NE16 6EA.
tel: (01207) 279 432
fax: (01207) 272 078
sales@veilcover.com

**BOC**
BOC Medical
The Priestley Centre,
10 Priestley Rd
Surrey Research Park
Guildford, Surrey, GU2 7XY.
tel: 0800 111 333
fax: 0800 111 555

**Boehringer Ingelheim**
Boehringer Ingelheim Ltd
Ellesfield Ave
Bracknell
Berks, RG12 8YS.
tel: (01344) 424 600
fax: (01344) 741 444
medinfo@bra.boehringer-ingelheim.
com

**Boots**
Boots The Chemists
Medical Services
Thane Rd
D90 East S10
Nottingham, NG90 1BS.
tel: (0115) 959 5165
fax: (0115) 959 2565

**BPC 100**
The Bolton Pharmaceutical 100 Ltd
2 Chapel Drive
Ambrosden
Oxfordshire, OX25 2RS.
tel: (0845) 602 3907
fax: (0845) 602 3908
info@bpc100.com

**BPL**
Bio Products Laboratory
Dagger Lane
Elstree, Herts, WD6 3BX.
tel: (020) 8258 2200
fax: (020) 8258 2601

**Braun**
B Braun (Medical) Ltd
Brookdale Rd
Thorncliffe Park Estate
Chapeltown, Sheffield, S35 2PW.
tel: (0114) 225 9000
fax: (0114) 225 9111
info.bbmuk@bbraun.com

**Bray**
Bray Health & Leisure
1 Regal Way
Faringdon
Oxon, SN7 7BX.
tel: (01367) 240 736
fax: (01367) 242 625
Info@bray.co.uk

**Bristol-Myers Squibb**
Bristol-Myers Squibb Pharmaceuticals
Ltd
Uxbridge Business Park
Sanderson Rd
Uxbridge
Middx, UB8 1DH.
tel: (01895) 523 000
fax: (01895) 523 010
medical.information@bms.com

**BSN Medical**
BSN Medical Ltd
PO Box 258
Willerby
Hull, HU10 6WT.
tel: (0845) 1223 600
fax: (0845) 1223 666

**Cambridge**
Cambridge Laboratories
Deltic House, Kingfisher Way
Silverlink Business Park, Wallsend
Tyne & Wear, NE28 9NX.
tel: (0191) 296 9300
fax: (0191) 296 9368
customer.services@camb-labs.com

**Cardinal**
Cardinal Health Martindale Products
Hubert Rd
Brentwood
Essex, CM14 4JY.
tel: (01277) 266 600
fax: (01277) 848 976
info@martindalepharma.co.uk

**Castlemead**
See Sanofi-Aventis

**C D Medical**
C D Medical Ltd
Aston Grange
Oker, Matlock, DE4 2JJ.
tel: (01629) 733 860
fax: (01629) 733 414

**Celgene**
Celgene Ltd
Morgan House
Madeira Walk
Windsor
Berks, SL4 1EP.
tel: (08448) 010 045
fax: (08448) 010 046
medinfo.uk.ire@celgene.com

**Centrapharm**
See Derma UK

**Cephalon**
Cephalon Ltd
1 Albany Place
Hyde Way
Welwyn Garden City
Herts, AL7 3BT.
tel: 0800 783 4869
fax: (01483) 765 008
ukmedinfo@cephalon.com

**Chattem UK**
Chattem UK Ltd
Guerry House
Ringway Centre
Edison Rd
Basingstoke, RG24 6YH.
tel: (01256) 844 144
fax: (01256) 844 145

**Chauvin**
See Bausch & Lomb

**Chefaro UK**
Chefaro UK Ltd
Unit 1, Tower Close
St. Peter's Industrial Park
Huntingdon
Cambs, PE29 7DH.
tel: (01480) 421 000
fax: (01480) 434 861

**Chemical Search**
Chemical Search International Ltd
29th floor
1 Canada Square
Canary Wharf
London, E14 5DY.
tel: (020) 7712 1758
fax: (020) 7712 1759
info@chemicalsearch.co.uk

**Chemidex**
Chemidex Pharma Ltd
Chemidex House
Egham Business Village
Crabtree Rd, Egham
Surrey, TW20 8RB.
tel: (01784) 477 167
fax: (01784) 471 776
info@chemidex.co.uk

**Chiesi**
Chiesi Ltd
Cheadle Royal Business Park
Highfield
Cheadle, SK8 3GY.
tel: (0161) 488 5555
fax: (0161) 488 5565
medinfo@chiesi.uk.com

**Chiron**
See Novartis

**CHS**
Cambridge Healthcare Supplies Ltd
14D Wendover Rd
Rackheath Industrial Estate
Rackheath
Norwich, NR13 6LH.
tel: (01603) 735 200
fax: (01603) 735 217
customerservices@typharm.com

**Chugai**
Chugai Pharma UK Ltd
Mulliner House, Flanders Rd
Turnham Green
London, W4 1NN.
tel: (020) 8987 5680
fax: (020) 8987 5661

**Clement Clarke**
Clement Clarke International Ltd
Edinburgh Way
Harlow
Essex, CM20 2TT.
tel: (01279) 414 969
fax: (01279) 456 304
resp@clement-clarke.com

**CliniMed**
CliniMed Ltd
Cavell House, Knaves Beech Way
Loudwater
High Wycombe
Bucks, HP10 9QY.
tel: (01628) 535 250
fax: (01628) 850 331
enquires@clinimed.co.uk

**Clinisupplies**
Clinisupplies Ltd
9 Crystal Way
Elmgrove Rd
Harrow
Middx, HA1 2HP.
tel: (020) 8863 4168
fax: (020) 8426 0768
info@clinisupplies.co.uk

**Colgate-Palmolive**
Colgate-Palmolive Ltd
Guildford Business Park
Middleton Rd
Guildford
Surrey, GU2 5LZ.
tel: (01483) 302 222
fax: (01483) 303 003

**Coloplast**
Coloplast Ltd
Peterborough Business Park
Peterborough, PE2 6FX.
tel: (01733) 392 000
fax: (01733) 233 348
gbcareteam@coloplast.com

**Community**
Community Foods Ltd
Micross, Brent Terrace
London, NW2 1LT.
tel: (020) 8450 9411
fax: (020) 8208 1803
email@communityfoods.co.uk

**Complan Foods**
Complan Foods Ltd
Imperial House
15–19 Kingsway
London, WC2B 6UN.
tel: (020) 7395 7565
fax: (08704) 434 018

**Concord**
See Archimedes

**ConvaTec**
ConvaTec Ltd
Harrington House, Milton Rd
Ickenham
Uxbridge
Middx, UB10 8PU.
tel: (01895) 628 400
fax: (01895) 628 456

**Covidien**
Covidien UK Commercial Ltd
154 Fareham Rd
Gosport
Hants, PO13 0AS.
tel: (01329) 224 226
fax: (01329) 224 334
medicalcustomerservices@covidien.
com

**Cow & Gate**
See Nutricia Clinical

**CP**
See Wockhardt

**Crawford**
Crawford Pharmaceuticals
Cheshire House
164 Main Rd
Goostrey
Cheshire, CW4 8NP.
tel: (01477) 537 596
fax: (01477) 534 262

**Credenhill**
Credenhill Ltd
10 Cossall Industrial Estate
Ilkeston
Derbyshire, DE7 5UG.
tel: (0800) 195 0650
fax: (0800) 028 5206
sales@credenhill.co.uk

**Crookes**
See Reckitt Benckiser

**CSL Behring**
CSL Behring UK Ltd
Hayworth House
Market Place
Haywards Heath
West Sussex, RH16 1DB.
tel: (01444) 447 400
fax: (01444) 447 403
medinfo@cslbehring.com

**Daiichi Sankyo**
Daiichi Sankyo UK Ltd
Chiltern Place
Chalfont Park
Gerrards Cross, SL9 0BG.
tel: (01753) 482 771
fax: (01753) 893 894
medinfo@daiichi-sankyo.co.uk

**Dallas Burston Ashbourne**
Dallas Burston Ashbourne Ltd
The Rectory
Braybrooke Rd
Arthingworth
Market Harborough, Leics, LE16 8JT.
tel: (01858) 525 643
sharonjackson@dbashbourne.com

**Danetre**
Danetre Health Products Ltd
Office 4, Broad March
Long March Industrial Estate
Daventry
Northants, NN11 4HE.
tel: (01327) 310 909
fax: (01327) 310 311
enquiries@danetrehealthproducts.com

**DDD**
DDD Ltd
94 Rickmansworth Rd
Watford
Herts, WD18 7JJ.
tel: (01923) 229 251
fax: (01923) 220 728

**Dee**
Dee Pharmaceuticals Ltd
Office 3K6 Redwither Tower
Redwither Business Park
Wrexham, LL13 9XT.
tel: (01978) 661993
fax: (01978) 661993
enquiries@deepharmaceuticalsltd.co.
uk

**Dental Health**
Dental Health Products Ltd
60 Boughton Lane
Maidstone
Kent, ME15 9QS.
tel: (01622) 749 222
fax: (01622) 744 672

**Dentsply**
Dentsply Ltd
Hamm Moor Lane
Addlestone
Weybridge
Surrey, KT15 2SE.
tel: (01932) 837 279
fax: (01932) 858 970

**Dermal**
Dermal Laboratories Ltd
Tatmore Place
Gosmore
Hitchin
Herts, SG4 7QR.
tel: (01462) 458 866
fax: (01462) 420 565

**Derma UK**
Derma UK Ltd
ARC Progress
Mill Lane
Stotfold
Beds, SG5 4NY.
tel: (01462) 733 500
fax: (01462) 733 600
info@dermauk.co.uk

**De Vilbiss**
De Vilbiss Health Care UK Ltd
High Street
Wollaston
West Midlands, DY8 4PS.
tel: (01384) 446 688
fax: (01384) 446 699

**De Witt**
E C De Witt & Co Ltd
Aegon House
Daresbury Park
Daresbury
Warrington, Cheshire, WA4 4HS.
tel: (01928) 756 800
fax: (01928) 756 818
info@ecdewitt.com

**Dexcel**
Dexcel-Pharma Ltd
1 Cottesbrooke Park
Heartlands Business Park
Daventry
Northamptonshire, NN11 8YL.
tel: (01327) 312 266
fax: (01327) 312 262
office@dexcelpharma.co.uk

**DHP Healthcare**
DHP Healthcare Ltd
60 Boughton Lane
Maidstone
Kent, ME15 9QS.
tel: (01622) 749 222
fax: (01622) 743 816
sales@dhphealthcare.co.uk

**Diatos**
Diatos SA
Immeuble Paris BioPark - 2 etage
11 Rue Watt
75013
Paris, France
tel: (00800) 3286 6966

**Dimethaid**
Dimethaid International
c/o Benoliel Partners
Linden House, Ewelme
Oxfordshire, OX10 6HQ.
tel: (01491) 825 016
fax: (01491) 834 592
medinfo@dimethaid.com

**Dr Falk**
Dr Falk Pharma UK Ltd
Bourne End Business, Cores End Rd
Bourne End, Bucks, SL8 5AS.
tel: (01628) 536 600

**Durbin**
Durbin plc
180 Northolt Rd
South Harrow
Middx, HA2 0LT.
tel: (020) 8869 6500
fax: (020) 8869 6565
info@durbin.co.uk

**Eakin**
T G Eakin
15 Ballystockart Rd
Comber
Newtownards
County Down, N. Ireland, BT23 5QY.
tel: (028) 9187 1000
fax: (028) 9187 1111
mail@eakin.co.uk

**Easigrip**
Easigrip Ltd
Unit 13, Scar Bank
Millers Rd
Warwick
Warwickshire, CV34 5DB.
tel: (01926) 497 108
fax: (01926) 497 109
enquiry@easigrip.co.uk

**Ecolab**
Ecolab UK
Lotherton Way
Garforth
Leeds, LS25 2JY.
tel: (0113) 232 0066
fax: (0113) 287 1317
info.healthcare@ecolab.co.uk

**Egis**
Egis Pharmaceuticals UK Ltd
127 Shirland Rd
London, W9 2EP.
tel: (020) 7266 2669
fax: (020) 7266 2702
enquiries@medimpexuk.com

**Eisai**
Eisai Ltd
European Knowledge Centre
Mosquito Way
Hatfield
Herts, AL10 9SN.
tel: (020) 8600 1400
fax: (020) 8600 1401
lmedinfo@eisai.net

**Elida Fabergé**
Elida Fabergé Ltd
Coal Rd
Seacroft
Leeds, LS14 2AR.
tel: (0113) 222 5000
fax: (0113) 222 5362

**Encysive**
Encysive (UK) Ltd
Regus House
Highbridge, Oxford Rd
Uxbridge
Middlesex, UB8 1HR.
tel: (01895) 876 168
fax: (01895) 876 320
enquiries@encysive.co.uk

**Enturia**
Enturia Ltd
Reigate Place
43 London Road
Reigate
Surrey, RH2 9PW.
tel: (0800) 043 7546
fax: (01737) 237 950
enquiries@enturia.co.uk

**Espere**
Espere Healthcare Ltd
Suite F11, Bedford i-Lab
Priory Business Park
Bedford
Beds, MK44 3RZ.
tel: (01234) 834 614
fax: (01234) 834 615
info@esperehealth.co.uk

**Ethicon**
Ethicon Ltd
P.O. Box 1988
Simpson Parkway
Kirkton Campus
Livingston, EH54 0AB.
tel: (01506) 594 500
fax: (01506) 460 714

**Eumedica**
Eumedica S.A.
Winston Churchill Avenue 67
1180 Brussels
Belgium
tel: (0208) 444 3377
fax: (0208) 444 6866
enquiries@eumedica.com

**EUSA Pharma**
EUSA Pharma (Europe) Ltd
Building 3, Gateway 1000
Whittle Way
Stevenage
Herts, SG1 2FP.
tel: (01438) 740 720
fax: (01438) 735 740
medinfo-uk@eusapharma.com

**Everfresh**
Everfresh Natural Foods
Gatehouse Close
Aylesbury
Bucks, HP19 3DE.
tel: (01296) 425 333
fax: (01296) 422 545

**Exelgyn**
Exelgyn Laboratories
PO Box 4511
Henley-on-Thames
Oxon, RG9 5ZQ.
tel: (01491) 642 137
fax: (0800) 731 6120

**Fabre**
Pierre Fabre Ltd
Hyde Abbey House
23 Hyde St
Winchester
Hants, SO23 7DR.
tel: (01962) 874 435
fax: (01962) 874 413
medicalinformation@pierre-fabre.co.
uk

**Fate**
Fate Special Foods
Unit E2
Brook Street Business Centre
Brook St, Tipton
West Midlands, DY4 9DD.
tel: (01215) 224 433
fax: (01215) 224 433

**Fenton**
Fenton Pharmaceuticals Ltd
4J Portman Mansions
Chiltern St
London, W1U 6NS.
tel: (020) 7224 1388
fax: (020) 7486 7258
mail@Fent-Pharm.co.uk

**Ferndale**
Ferndale Pharmaceuticals Ltd
Unit 124, Thorp Arch Estate
Wetherby
West Yorks, LS23 7BJ.
tel: (01937) 541 122
fax: (01937) 849 682
info@ferndalepharma.co.uk

**Ferring**
Ferring Pharmaceuticals (UK)
The Courtyard
Waterside Drive
Langley
Berks, SL3 6EZ.
tel: (01753) 214 800
fax: (01753) 214 801

**Firstplay Dietary**
Firstplay Dietary Foods Ltd
338 Turncroft Lane
Offerton
Stockport
Cheshire, SK1 4BP.
tel: (0161) 474 7576
fax: (0161) 474 7576

**Flynn**
Flynn Pharma Ltd
2nd Floor, The Maltings
Bridge St
Hitchin
Herts, SG5 2DE.
tel: (01462) 458 974
fax: (01462) 450 755

**Foodlink**
Foodlink (UK) Ltd
2B Plymouth Rd
Plympton
Plymouth, PL7 4JR.
tel: (01752) 344 544
fax: (01752) 342 412
info@foodlinkltd.co.uk

**Ford**
Ford Medical Associates Ltd
8 Wyndham Way
Orchard Heights
Ashford
Kent, TN25 4PZ.
tel: (01233) 633 224
fax: (01223) 646 595
enquiries@fordmedical.co.uk

**Forest**
Forest Laboratories UK Ltd
Bourne Rd
Bexley
Kent, DA5 1NX.
tel: (01322) 550 550
fax: (01322) 555 469
medinfo@forest-labs.co.uk

**Forum**
Forum Health Products Ltd
41-51 Brighton Rd
Redhill
Surrey, RH1 6YS.
tel: (01737) 773711
fax: (01737) 779382
health@forumgroup.co.uk

**Fox**
C. H. Fox Ltd
22 Tavistock St
London, WC2E 7PY.
tel: (020) 7240 3111
fax: (020) 7379 3410

**FP**
Family Planning Sales Ltd
Maerdy Industrial Estate
Rhymney
Gwent, NP22 5PY.
tel: (0870) 4444 620
fax: (0870) 4444 621

**Freebake**
Freebake Ltd
Unit E3 Blackpole East
Worcs, WR3 8SG.
tel: (0845) 603 9230
info@freebake.co.uk

**Fresenius Kabi**
Fresenius Kabi Ltd
Cestrian Court
Eastgate Way
Manor Park, Runcorn
Cheshire, WA7 1UF.
tel: (01928) 533 575
fax: (01928) 533 534
med.info-uk@fresenius-kabi.com

**Frontier**
Frontier Multigate
Newbridge Rd Industrial Estate
Blackwood
South Wales, NP12 2YL.
tel: (01495) 233 050
fax: (01495) 233 055
multigate@frontier-group.co.uk

**Galderma**
Galderma (UK) Ltd
Meridien House
69-71 Clarendon Rd
Watford
Herts, WD17 1DS.
tel: (01923) 208 950
fax: (01923) 208 998

**Galen**
Galen Ltd
Seagoe Industrial Estate
Craigavon
Northern Ireland, BT63 5UA.
tel: (028) 3833 4974
fax: (028) 3835 0206
customer.services@galen.co.uk

**GE Healthcare**
GE Healthcare
The Grove Centre, White Lion Rd
Amersham, Bucks, HP7 9LL.
tel: (01494) 544 000

**Geistlich**
Geistlich Pharma
Newton Bank
Long Lane
Chester, CH2 2PF.
tel: (01244) 347 534
fax: (01244) 319 327

**General Dietary**
General Dietary Ltd
PO Box 38
Kingston upon Thames
Surrey, KT2 7YP.
tel: (020) 8336 2323
fax: (020) 8942 8274

**Generics**
Generics (UK) Ltd
Albany Gate
Darkes Lane
Potters Bar
Herts, EN6 1AG.
tel: (01707) 853 000
fax: (01707) 643 148

**Generpharm**
Generpharm Ltd
See Sigma

**Genus**
Genus Pharmaceuticals
Park View House
65 London Rd
Newbury
Berks, RG14 1JN.
tel: (01635) 568 400
fax: (01635) 568 401
enquiries@genuspharma.com

**Genzyme**
Genzyme Therapeutics
4620 Kingsgate
Cascade Way
Oxford Business Park South
Oxford, OX4 2SU.
tel: (01865) 405 200
fax: (01865) 774 172

**Gilead**
Gilead Sciences Ltd
The Flowers Building
Granta Park
Great Abington
Cambs, CB21 6GT.
tel: (01223) 897 555
fax: (01223) 897 291
ukmedinfo@gilead.com

**GlaxoSmithKline**
See GSK

**Glenwood**
Glenwood Laboratories Ltd
Jenkins Dale
Chatham
Kent, ME4 5RD.
tel: (01634) 830 535
fax: (01634) 831 345
g.wooduk@virgin.net

**Gluten Free Foods Ltd**
Gluten Free Foods Ltd
Unit 270 Centennial Park
Centennial Ave
Elstree, Borehamwood
Herts, WD6 3SS.
tel: (020) 8953 4444
fax: (020) 8953 8285
info@glutenfree-foods.co.uk

**Goldshield**
Goldshield Pharmaceuticals Ltd
NLA Tower
12-16 Addiscombe Rd
Croydon, CR0 0XT.
tel: (08700) 703 033
fax: (020) 8686 0807
medicalinformation@goldshieldplc.
com

**GP Pharma**
See Derma UK

**Grifols**
Grifols UK Ltd
Byron House
Cambridge Business Park
Cowley Road
Cambridge , CB4 0WZ.
tel: (01223) 395 700
fax: (01223) 395 766
reception.uk@grifols.com

**Grünenthal**
Grünenthal Ltd
2 Beacon Heights Business Park
Ibstone Rd
Stokenchurch
Bucks, HP14 3XR.
tel: (0870) 351 8960
fax: (01494) 486 298
medicalinformationuk@grunenthal.
com

**GSK**
GlaxoSmithKline
Stockley Park West
Uxbridge
Middx, UB11 1BT.
tel: 0800 221 441
fax: (020) 8990 4328
customercontactuk@gsk.com

**GSK Consumer Healthcare**
GlaxoSmithKline Consumer Healthcare
GSK House
980 Great West Rd
Brentford
Middx, TW8 9GS.
tel: (020) 8047 2500
fax: (020) 8047 6860
customer.relations@gsk.com

**H&R**
H&R Healthcare Ltd
Melton Court, Gibson Lane
Melton
East Yorkshire, HU14 3HH.
tel: (01482) 638 491
fax: (01482) 638 485

**Hampton**
Hampton Pharmaceuticals Ltd
Unit 9 Park House
15-19 Greenhill Crescent
Watford Business Park
Watford, WD18 8PH.
tel: (01923) 251 777
fax: (01923) 251 999

**Hartmann**
Paul Hartmann Ltd
Unit P2, Parklands
Heywood Distribution Park
Pilsworth Rd, Heywood
Lancs, OL10 2TT.
tel: (01706) 363 200
fax: (01706) 363 201
info@uk.hartmann.info

**Healthcare Logistics**
See Movianto

**Heinz**
H. J. Heinz Company Ltd
South Building
Hayes Park
Hayes, UB4 8AL.
tel: (020) 8573 7757
fax: (020) 8848 2325
Farleys_Heinz@Heinz.co.uk

**Henleys**
Henleys Medical Supplies Ltd
Brownfields
Welwyn Garden City
Herts, AL7 1AN.
tel: (01707) 333 164
fax: (01707) 334 795

**HK Pharma**
HK Pharma Ltd
PO Box 105
Hitchin
Herts, SG5 2GG.
tel: (01462) 433 993
fax: (01462) 450 755

**Hoechst Marion Roussel**
See Sanofi-Aventis

**Home Diagnostics**
Home Diagnostics (UK) Ltd
25 Barnes Wallis Road
Segensworth East
Fareham
Hants, PO15 5TT.
tel: (01489) 569 469
fax: (01489) 569 424
info@homediagnostics-uk.com

**Hospira**
Hospira UK Ltd
Queensway
Royal Leamington Spa
Warwickshire, CV31 3RW.
tel: (01926) 834 400
fax: (01926) 821 041
medinfouk@hospira.com

**HRA Pharma**
Laboratoire HRA Pharma
15 rue Beranger
75003
Paris
France
tel: (0033) 1 40 33 11 30
fax: (0033) 1 40 33 12 31
info@lysodren-europe.com

**Huntleigh**
Huntleigh Healthcare Ltd
310 - 312 Dallow Rd
Luton, LU1 1TD.
tel: (01582) 413 104

**Hypoguard**
Hypoguard Ltd
Dock Lane
Melton
Woodbridge
Suffolk, IP12 1PE.
tel: (01394) 387 333
fax: (01394) 380 152
enquiries@hypoguard.com

**IDIS**
IDIS World Medicines
IDIS House
Churchfield Rd
Weybridge
Surrey, KT13 8DB.
tel: (01932) 824 000
fax: (01932) 824 200
idis@idispharma.com

**INCA-Pharm**
INCA-Pharm UK
PO Box 122
Richmond, DL10 5HX.
tel: (01748) 828 812
fax: (01748) 828 801
info@inca-pharm.com

**Infai**
Infai UK Ltd
Innovation Centre
University of York Science Park
University Rd
Heslington, York, YO10 5DG.
tel: (01904) 435 228
fax: (01904) 435 229
paul@infai.co.uk

**Innovative**
Innovative Solutions UK Ltd
Unit 28
Transpennine Industrial Estate
Gorrels Way, Queensway
Rochdale, Lancs, OL11 2QR.
tel: (01706) 746713
enquiries@innovative-solutions.org.uk

**Insense**
Insense Ltd
Colworth Science Park
Sharnbrook
Bedford, MK44 1LQ.
tel: (01234) 782 870
fax: (01234) 783 444
enquiries@insense.co.uk

**Insight**
Insight Medical Products Ltd
Units 1-4 Silk Mill Studios
2 Charlton Rd
Tetbury
Glos, GL8 8DY.
tel: (01666) 500 055
fax: (01666) 500 115
info@insightmedical.net

**Intrapharm**
Intrapharm Laboratories Ltd
60 Boughton Lane
Maidstone
Kent, ME15 9QS.
tel: (01622) 749 222
fax: (01622) 744 672
sales@intraphamlabs.com

**Ipsen**
Ipsen Ltd
190 Bath Rd
Slough
Berks, SL1 3XE.
tel: (01753) 627 777
fax: (01753) 627 778
medical.information.uk@ipsen.com

**IS Pharmaceuticals**
IS Pharmaceuticals Ltd
Office Village
Chester Business Park
Chester, CH4 9QZ.
tel: (01244) 625 152
fax: (01244) 625 151
enquiries@ispharma.plc.uk

**IVAX**
See TEVA UK

**J&J**
Johnson & Johnson Ltd
Foundation Park
Roxborough Way
Maidenhead
Berks, SL6 3UG.
tel: (01628) 822 222
fax: (01628) 821 222

**J&J Medical**
Johnson & Johnson Medical
Coronation Rd
Ascot
Berks, SL5 9EY.
tel: (01344) 871 000
fax: (01344) 872 599

**Janssen-Cilag**
Janssen-Cilag Ltd
50-100 Holmers Farm Way
High Wycombe
Bucks, HP12 4EG.
tel: (01494) 567 444
fax: (01494) 567 568

**Javelin**
Javelin Pharmaceuticals UK Ltd
Compass House, Vision Park
Chivers Way
Histon
Cambs, CB4 9AD.
tel: (0800) 066 5446
fax: (01223) 527 800

**Jerini**
Jerini AG
Invalidenstrasse 130
10115 Berlin
Germany
tel: (00800) 7020 7020

**JLB**
B. Braun JLB Ltd
Unit 2A
St Columb Industrial Estate
St Columb Major
Cornwall, TR9 6SF.
tel: (01637) 880 065
fax: (01637) 881 549

**Jobskin**
Jobskin Ltd
Unit 13 Harrington Mill
Leopold St
Long Eaton
Nottingham, NG10 4QG.
tel: (0115) 973 4300
fax: (0115) 973 3902
dw@jobskin.co.uk

**Juvela**
Juvela (Hero UK) Ltd
19 De-Havilland Drive
Liverpool, L24 8RN.
tel: (0151) 432 5300
fax: (0151) 432 5335
info@juvela.co.uk

**K/L**
K/L Pharmaceuticals Ltd
21 Macadam Place
South Newmoor
Irvine
Ayrshire, KA11 4HP.
tel: (01294) 215 951
fax: (01294) 221 600

**KCI Medical**
KCI Medical Ltd
Langford Business Park
Langford Locks
Kidlington
Oxon, OX5 1GF.
tel: (01865) 840 600
fax: (01865) 840 626

**Kestrel**
Kestrel Ltd
Ashfield House
Resolution Rd
Ashby de la Zouch
Leics, LE65 1HW.
tel: (01530) 562 301
fax: (01530) 562 430
kestrel@ventiv.co.uk

**Kestrel Ophthalmics**
Kestrel Ophthalmics Ltd
Kestrel House
7 Moor Rd
Broadstone
Dorset, BH18 8AZ.
tel: (01202) 658 444
fax: (01202) 659 599
info@kestrelophthalmics.co.uk

**King**
King Pharmaceuticals Ltd
2nd Floor, The Maltings
Bridge St
Hitchin
Herts, SG5 2DE.
tel: (01462) 434 366
fax: (01462) 450 755

**KoGEN**
KoGEN Ltd
Seagoe Industrial Estate
Craigavon, BT63 5UA.
tel: (028) 383 33933
fax: (028) 383 33665
info@kogen.co.uk

**KoRa**
KoRa Healthcare Ltd
First Floor, Unit 2
Swords Business Park, Swords
Co. Dublin
Ireland
tel: (01142) 994 979
fax: (00353) 1890 3016
info@kora.ie

**Kyowa Hakko**
Kyowa Hakko UK Ltd
258 Bath Rd
Slough
Berks, SL1 4DX.
tel: (01753) 566 020
fax: (01753) 566 030

**Labopharm**
Labopharm Europe Ltd
Unit 5, The Seapoint Building
44-45 Clontarf Rd
Dublin 3
Ireland
tel: (0800) 678 3765 (UK only) or
(01908) 542 374
labopharm.uk@canreginc.com

**Lantor**
Lantor UK Ltd
73 St Helens Rd
Bolton
Lancs, BL3 3PR.
tel: (01204) 855 000
help@lantor.co.uk

**Lederle**
See Wyeth

**LEO**
LEO Pharma
Longwick Rd
Princes Risborough
Bucks, HP27 9RR.
tel: (01844) 347 333
fax: (01844) 342 278
medical-info.uk@leo-pharma.com

**LifeScan**
LifeScan
50-100 Holmers Farm Way
High Wycombe
Bucks, HP12 4DP.
tel: (01494) 658 750
fax: (01494) 658 751

**Lilly**
Eli Lilly & Co Ltd
Lilly House
Priestley Rd
Basingstoke
Hants, RG24 9NL.
tel: (01256) 315 999
ukmedinfo@lilly.com

**Lincoln Medical**
Lincoln Medical Ltd
13 Boathouse Meadow Business Park
Cherry Orchard Lane
Salisbury
Wilts, SP2 7LD.
tel: (01722) 410 443

**Linderma**
Linderma Ltd
Allenby Laboratories
Wigan Rd
West Houghton
Bolton, BL5 2AL.
tel: (01942) 816 184
fax: (01942) 813 937
linderma@virgin.net

**Link**
See Archimedes

**Lipomed**
Lipomed GmbH
Schonaugasse 11
D-79713
Bad Sackingen
tel: (0049) 776 155 9222
fax: (0049) 776 155 9223
lipomed@lipomed.com

**Livwell**
Livwell Ltd
PO Box 22
Hull, HU2 0YX.
tel: (0845) 120 0038
info@livwell.eu

**Lornamead**
Lornamead UK Ltd
Sabre House
377-399 London Road
Camberley
Surrey, GU15 3HL.
tel: (01276) 674000
fax: (01276) 674098
lornamead@dhl.com

**LPC**
LPC Pharmaceuticals Ltd
30 Chaul End Lane
Luton, Beds, LU4 8EZ.
tel: (01582) 560 393
fax: (01582) 560 395
info@lpcpharma.com

**Lundbeck**
Lundbeck Ltd
Lundbeck House
Caldecotte Lake Business Park
Caldecotte, Milton Keynes
Bucks, MK7 8LF.
tel: (01908) 649 966
fax: (01908) 647 888
ukmedicalinformation@lundbeck.com

**M & A Pharmachem**
M & A Pharmachem Ltd
Allenby Laboratories
Wigan Road
West Houghton
Bolton, BL5 2AL.
tel: (01942) 816184
fax: (01942) 813937
buy@mapharmachem.co.uk

**Manx**
Manx Healthcare
Taylor Group House
Wedgnock Lane
Warwick, CV34 5YA.
tel: (01926) 482 511
fax: (01926) 498 711
info@manxhealthcare.com

**Marlborough**
Marlborough Pharmaceuticals
PO Box 2957
Marlborough
Wilts, SN8 1WS.
tel: (01672) 514 187
fax: (01672) 515 614
info@marlborough-pharma.co.uk

**Martindale**
See Cardinal

**MASTA**
MASTA
Moorfield Rd
Yeadon
Leeds, LS19 7BN.
tel: (0113) 238 7500
fax: (0113) 238 7501
medical@masta.org

**McNeil**
McNeil Products Ltd
Foundation Park
Roxborough Way
Maidenhead
Berks, SL6 3UG.
tel: (01628) 822 222

**MDE**
Medical Diagnostics Europe Ltd
Surrey Technology Centre
40 Occam Rd
Guildford
Surrey, GU2 7YG.
tel: (08453) 708 077
info@mdediagnostic.co.uk

**Mead Johnson**
Mead Johnson Nutritionals
Uxbridge Business Park
Sanderson Rd
Uxbridge
Middx, UB8 1DH.
tel: (01895) 523 764
fax: (01895) 523 103

**Meadow**
Meadow Laboratories Ltd
18 Avenue Rd
Chadwell Heath
Romford
Essex, RM6 4JF.
tel: (020) 8597 1203
enquiries@meadowlabs.fsnet.co.uk

**Meda**
Meda Pharmaceuticals Ltd
Skyway House
Parsonage Rd
Takeley
Bishop's Stortford, CM22 6PU.
tel: (01748) 828 810
fax: (0845) 460 0002
meda@professionalinformation.co.uk

**Medac**
Medac (UK)
Scion House, Stirling University
Innovation Park
Stirling, FK9 4NF.
tel: (01786) 458 086
fax: (01786) 458 032
Info@medac-uk.co.uk

**Medical House**
The Medical House plc
199 Newhall Rd
Sheffield, S9 2QJ.
tel: (0114) 261 9011
fax: (0114) 243 1597
info@themedicalhouse.com

**Medicare**
Medicare Plus International Ltd
Chemilines House
Alperton Lane
Wembley
Middlesex, HA0 1DX.
tel: (020) 8799 7891
fax: (020) 8799 7882
info@medicare-plus.com

**Medihoney**
Medihoney (Europe) Ltd
200 Brook Drive
Green Park
Reading, RG2 6UB.
tel: (0800) 071 3912

**Medix**
See Clement Clarke

**Medlock**
Medlock Medical Ltd
Tubiton House
Medlock St.
Oldham, OL1 3HS.
tel: (0161) 621 2100
fax: (0161) 627 0932
medical.information@
medlockmedical.com

**MedLogic**
MedLogic Global Ltd
Western Wood Way
Langage Science Park
Plympton
Plymouth, Devon, PL7 5BG.
tel: (01752) 209 955
fax: (01752) 209 956
enquiries@mlgl.co.uk

**Menarini**
A. Menarini Pharma UK SRL
Menarini House
Mercury Park
Wycombe Lane, Wooburn Green
Bucks, HP10 0HH.
tel: (01628) 856 400
fax: (01628) 856 402

**Menarini Diagnostics**
A. Menarini Diagnostics
Wharfedale Rd
Winnersh
Wokingham
Berks, RG41 5RA.
tel: (0118) 944 4100
fax: (0118) 944 4111

**Merck**
See Merck Serono

**Merck Serono**
Merck Serono Ltd
Bedfont Cross
Stanwell Rd
Feltham
Middx, TW14 8NX.
tel: (020) 8818 7373
fax: (020) 8818 7274
medinfo.uk@merckserono.net

**Merck Sharp & Dohme**
See MSD

**Merz**
Merz Pharma UK Ltd
260 Centennial Park
Elstree Hill South
Herts, WD6 3SR.
tel: (020) 8236 0000
fax: (020) 8236 3501
info@merzpharma.co.uk

**Micro Medical**
Micro Medical Ltd
Quayside
Chatham Maritime
Chatham
Kent, ME4 4QY.
tel: (01634) 893 500
fax: (01634) 893 600
sales@micromedical.co.uk

**Milupa**
Milupa Aptamil
White Horse Business Park
Trowbridge
Wilts, BA14 0XQ.
tel: (0845) 762 3676
fax: (01225) 768 847
careline@aptamil4hcps.co.uk

**Mölnlycke**
Mölnlycke Health Care Ltd
The Arenson Centre
Arenson Way
Dunstable
Beds, LU5 5UL.
tel: (0161) 777 2628
fax: (0161) 777 2601
info.uk@molnlycke.net

**Morningside**
Morningside Healthcare Ltd
115 Narborough Rd
Leicester, LE3 OPA.
tel: (0116) 204 5950
fax: (0116) 247 0756

**Movianto**
Movianto UK
1 Progress Park
Bedford, MK42 9XE.
tel: (01234) 248 500
fax: (01234) 248 700
movianto.uk@movianto.com

**MSD**
Merck Sharp & Dohme Ltd
Hertford Rd
Hoddesdon
Herts, EN11 9BU.
tel: (01992) 467 272
fax: (01992) 451 066

**Nagor**
Nagor Ltd
PO Box 21, Global House
Isle of Man Business Park
Douglas
Isle of Man, IM99 1AX.
tel: (01624) 625 556
fax: (01624) 661 656
enquiries@nagor.com

**Napp**
Napp Pharmaceuticals Ltd
Cambridge Science Park
Milton Rd
Cambs, CB4 0GW.
tel: (01223) 424 444
fax: (01223) 424 441

**Neolab**
Neolab Ltd
57 High St
Odiham
Hants, RG29 1LF.
tel: (01256) 704 110
fax: (01256) 701 144
info@neolab.co.uk

**Neomedic**
Neomedic Ltd
2a Crofters Rd
Northwood
Middx, HA6 3ED.
tel: (01923) 836 379
fax: (01923) 840 160
marketing@neomedic.co.uk

**Nestlé**
Nestlé Nutrition
St George's House
Park Lane
Croydon
Surrey, CR9 1NR.
tel: (020) 8667 5130
fax: (020) 8667 5616
nutrition@uk.nestle.com

**Nordic**
Nordic Pharma UK Ltd
Abbey House
1650 Arlington Business Park
Theale
Reading, RG7 4SA.
tel: (0118) 929 8233
fax: (0118) 929 8234
info@nordicpharma.co.uk

**Norgine**
Norgine Pharmaceuticals Ltd
Chaplin House
Moorhall Rd
Harefield
Middx, UB9 6NS.
tel: (01895) 826 600
fax: (01895) 825 865

**Novartis**
Novartis Pharmaceuticals UK Ltd
Frimley Business Park
Frimley
Camberley
Surrey, GU16 7SR.
tel: (01276) 692 255
fax: (01276) 692 508

**Novartis Consumer Health**
Novartis Consumer Health
Wimblehurst Rd
Horsham
West Sussex, RH12 5AB.
tel: (01403) 210 211
fax: (01403) 323 939
medicalaffairs.uk@novartis.com

**Novartis Vaccines**
Novartis Vaccines Ltd
Gaskill Rd
Speke
Liverpool, L24 9GR.
tel: (08457) 451 500
fax: (0151) 7055 669
serviceuk@chiron.com

**Novo Nordisk**
Novo Nordisk Ltd
Broadfield Park
Brighton Rd
Crawley
West Sussex, RH11 9RT.
tel: (01293) 613 555
fax: (01293) 613 535
customercareuk@novonordisk.com

**nSPIRE Health**
nSPIRE Health Ltd
Unit 10, Harforde Court
John Tate Rd
Hertford
Herts, SG13 7NW.
tel: (01992) 526 300
fax: (01992) 526 320
info@nspirehealth.com

**Nutricia Clinical**
Nutricia Clinical Care
Nutricia Ltd
White Horse Business Park
Trowbridge
Wilts, BA14 0XQ.
tel: (01225) 711 688
fax: (01225) 711 798
cndirect@nutricia.co.uk

**Nutricia Dietary**
Nutricia Dietary Care
see Nutricia Clinical

**Nutrition Point**
Nutrition Point Ltd
13 Taurus Park
Westbrook
Warrington
Cheshire, WA5 7ZT.
tel: (07041) 544 044
fax: (07041) 544 055
info@nutritionpoint.co.uk

**Nycomed**
Nycomed UK Ltd
3 Globeside Business Park
Fieldhouse Lane
Marlow
Bucks, SL7 1HZ.
tel: (0800) 633 5797
fax: (01628) 646 401
medinfo@nycomed.com

**OakMed**
OakMed Ltd
54 Adams Ave
Northampton, NN1 4LJ.
tel: (0800) 592 786
fax: (01604) 629 713
orders@oakmed.co.uk

**Octapharma**
Octapharma Ltd
The Zenith Building
26 Spring Gardens
Manchester, M2 1AB.
tel: (0161) 837 3770
octapharma@octapharma.co.uk

**Omron**
Omron Healthcare (UK) Ltd
Opal Drive
Fox Milne
Milton Keynes, MK15 0DG.
tel: (0870) 750 2771
fax: (0870) 750 2772
info.omronhealthcare.uk@eu.omron.com

**Organon**
Organon Laboratories Ltd
Cambridge Science Park
Milton Rd
Cambs, CB4 0FL.
tel: (01223) 432 700
fax: (01223) 424 368
medrequest@organon.co.uk

**Orion**
Orion Pharma (UK) Ltd
Oaklea Court
22 Park St
Newbury
Berks, RG14 1EA.
tel: (01635) 520 300
fax: (01635) 520 319
medicalinformation@orionpharma.com

**Orphan Europe**
Orphan Europe (UK) Ltd
Isis House
43 Station Rd
Henley-on-Thames
Oxon, RG9 1AT.
tel: (01491) 414 333
fax: (01491) 414 443
info.uk@orphan-europe.com

**Otsuka**
Otsuka Pharmaceutical (UK) Ltd
BSi Tower
389 Chiswick High Rd, London, W4 4AJ.
tel: (020) 8742 4300
fax: (020) 8994 8548
medinfo@otsuka.co.uk

**Ovation**
Ovation Healthcare International Ltd
1 Setanta Place
Dublin 2
Ireland
tel: (00353) 161 39 707
fax: (00353) 161 39 708

**Owen Mumford**
Owen Mumford Ltd
Brook Hill
Woodstock
Oxford, OX20 1TU.
tel: (01993) 812 021
fax: (01993) 813 466
customerservices@owenmumford.co.uk

**Oxford Nutrition**
Oxford Nutrition Ltd
Unit 5 Western Units
Pottery Rd
Bovey Tracey, TQ13 9JJ.
tel: (01626) 832 067
fax: (01626) 836 841
info@nutrinox.com

**Paines & Byrne**
Paines & Byrne Ltd
Lovett House
Lovett Rd
Staines
Middx, TW18 3AZ.
tel: (01784) 419 620
fax: (01784) 419 401

**Pari**
PARI Medical Ltd
The Old Sorting Office
Rosemount Ave
West Byfleet
Surrey, KT14 6LB.
tel: (01932) 341 122
fax: (01932) 341 134
infouk@pari.de

**Parkside**
Parkside Healthcare
12 Parkside Ave
Salford, M7 4HB.
tel: (0161) 795 2792
fax: (0161) 795 4076

**Peckforton**
Peckforton Pharmaceuticals Ltd
Crewe Hall
Crewe
Cheshire, CW1 6UL.
tel: (01270) 582 255
fax: (01270) 582 299
info@peckforton.com

**Penn**
Penn Pharmaceuticals Services Ltd
Unit 23 & 24, Tafarnaubach Industrial Estate
Tredegar
Gwent, NP22 3AA.
tel: (01495) 711 222
fax: (01495) 711 225
penn@pennpharm.co.uk

**Pfizer**
Pfizer Ltd
Walton Oaks
Dorking Rd
Walton-on-the-Hill
Surrey, KT20 7NS.
tel: (01304) 616 161
fax: (01304) 656 221

**PGR Health Foods**
PGR Health Foods Ltd
PO Box 214
Hertford, SG14 2ZX.
tel: (01992) 581715
fax: (01992) 536594
info@pgrhealthfoods.co.uk

**Pharmacia**
See Pfizer

**Pharma-Global**
Pharma-Global Ltd
Hudson Rd
Sandycove
Co. Dublin
Ireland
tel: (00353) 1280 1104
fax: (00353) 1280 2419
eyecare@pharmaglobal.ie

**Pharma Mar**
See IDIS

**Pharma Nord**
Pharma Nord (UK) Ltd
Telford Court
Morpeth
Northumberland, NE61 2DB.
tel: (01670) 519989
fax: (01670) 534903
info@pharmanord.co.uk

**Pharmasure**
Pharmasure Ltd
28 Watford Metro Centre
Dwight Rd
Watford, WD18 9SB.
tel: (01923) 233 466
fax: (01923) 233 113
info@pharmasure.co.uk

**Pinewood**
Pinewood Healthcare
Ballymacabry
Clonmel, Co Tipperary, Eire
tel: (00353) 523 6253
fax: (00353) 523 6311
info@pinewood.ie

**Potters**
Potters Herbal Medicines
1 Botanic Court
Martland Park
Wigan, WN5 0JZ.
tel: (01942) 219 960
fax: (01942) 219 966
info@pottersherbals.co.uk

**Procter & Gamble**
Procter & Gamble UK
The Heights
Brooklands
Weybridge
Surrey, KT13 0XP.
tel: (01932) 896 000
fax: (01932) 896 200

**Procter & Gamble Pharm.**
Procter & Gamble Technical Centres
Medical Dept
Rusham Park
Whitehall Lane
Egham, Surrey, TW20 9NW.
tel: (01784) 474 900
fax: (01784) 474 705

**Profile**
Profile Pharma Ltd
Chichester Business Park
City Fields Way
Chichester
West Sussex, PO20 2FT.
tel: (0800) 1300 855
fax: (0800) 1300 856
info@profilepharma.com

**Profile Respiratory**
See Respironics

**ProStrakan**
ProStrakan Ltd
Galabank Business Park
Galashiels, TD1 1QH.
tel: (01896) 664 000
fax: (01896) 664 001
medinfo@prostrakan.com

**Protex**
Protex Healthcare (UK) Ltd
Unit 5, Molly Millars Lane
Wokingham
Berks, RG41 2Q2.
tel: (08700) 114 112
orders@protexhealthcare.co.uk

**Provalis**
See KoGEN

**R&C**
See Reckitt Benckiser

**Ranbaxy**
Ranbaxy UK Ltd
20 Balderton St
London, W1K 6TL.
tel: (020) 8280 1986
fax: (020) 8280 1996
medinfoeurope@ranbaxy.com

**Ransom**
Ransom Consumer Healthcare
Alexander House
40A Wilbury Way
Hitchin
Herts, SG5 1LY.
tel: (01462) 437 615
fax: (01462) 420 528
info@williamransom.com

**Ratiopharm UK**
Ratiopharm UK Ltd
5 Jackson Close
Grove Rd
Cosham
Portsmouth, Hants, PO6 1UP.
tel: (02392) 313 587
fax: (02392) 386 208
info@ratiopharmdirect.co.uk

**Reckitt Benckiser**
Reckitt Benckiser Healthcare
Dansom Lane
Hull, HU8 7DS.
tel: (01482) 326 151
fax: (01482) 582 526
info.MIU@reckittbenckiser.com

**Recordati**
Recordati Pharmaceuticals Ltd
Knyvett House
The Causeway
Staines
Middx, TW18 3BA.
tel: (01784) 898 300
fax: (01784) 895 103

**Regent Medical**
See Mölnlycke

**ReSource Medical**
ReSource Medical UK Ltd
2 Thorne Rd
Thornton Lodge
Huddersfield, HD1 3JJ.
tel: (01484) 531 489
fax: (01484) 531 584
info@resource-medical.co.uk

**Respironics**
Philips Respironics (UK) Ltd
Chichester Business Park
City Fields Way
Tangmere, Chichester
West Sussex, PO20 2FT.
tel: (0800) 1300 840
fax: (0800) 1300 841
rukmarketing@respironics.com

**Rhône-Poulenc Rorer**
See Sanofi-Aventis

**Richardson**
Richardson Healthcare Ltd
Devonshire House
Manor Way
Borehamwood
Herts, WD6 1QQ.
tel: (08700) 111 126
fax: (08700) 111 127
info@richardsonhealthcare.com

**Riemser**
Riemser Arzneimittel AG
An der Wiek 7
17493 Greifswald - Insel Riems
Germany
tel: (0049) 38351 76 679
fax: (0049) 38351 76 778
info@RIEMSER.de

**RIS Products**
RIS Products Ltd
10 Prospect Place
Welwyn
Herts, AL6 9EW.
tel: (01438) 840 135
fax: (01438) 716 067
info@risproducts.co.uk

**Robinsons**
Robinson Healthcare Ltd
Lawn Rd
Carlton-in-Lindrick Industrial Estate
Worksop
Notts, S81 9LB.
tel: (01909) 735 001
fax: (01909) 731 103
enquiries@robinsoncare.com

**Roche**
Roche Products Ltd
Hexagon Place
6 Falcon Way, Shire Park
Welwyn Garden City
Herts, AL7 1TW.
tel: (0800) 328 1629
fax: (01707) 384 555
medinfo.uk@roche.com

**Roche Consumer Health**
See Bayer

**Roche Diagnostics**
Roche Diagnostics Ltd
Charles Avenue
Burgess Hill
West Sussex, RH15 9RY.
tel: (01444) 256 000
fax: (01444) 256 239
burgesshill.accu-chek@roche.com

**Rosemont**
Rosemont Pharmaceuticals Ltd
Rosemont House
Yorkdale Industrial Park
Braithwaite St
Leeds, LS11 9XE.
tel: (0113) 244 1999
fax: (0113) 246 0738
infodesk@rosemontpharma.com

Index of manufacturers

**Rowa**
Rowa Pharmaceuticals Ltd
Bantry
Co Cork
Ireland
tel: (00 353 27) 50077
fax: (00 353 27) 50417
rowa@rowa-pharma.ie

**S&N Hlth.**
Smith & Nephew Healthcare Ltd
Healthcare House
Goulton St
Hull, HU3 4DJ.
tel: (01482) 222 200
fax: (01482) 222 211
advice@smith-nephew.com

**Sallis**
Sallis Healthcare Ltd
Vernon Works
Waterford St
Basford
Nottingham, NG6 0DH.
tel: (0115) 978 7841
fax: (0115) 942 2272

**Sandoz**
Sandoz Ltd
37 Woolmer Way
Bordon
Hants, GU35 9QE.
tel: (01420) 478 301
fax: (01420) 474 427
uk.drugsafety@sandoz.com

**Sankyo**
See Daiichi Sankyo

**Sanochemia**
Sanochemia Diagnostics UK Ltd
Argentum
510 Bristol Business Park
Coldharbour Lane
Bristol, BS16 1EJ.
tel: (0117) 906 3562
fax: (0117) 906 3709

**Sanofi-Aventis**
Sanofi-Aventis Ltd
1 Onslow St
Guildford
Surrey, GU1 4YS.
tel: (01483) 505 515
fax: (01483) 535 432
uk-medicalinformation@
sanofi-aventis.com

**Sanofi Pasteur**
Sanofi Pasteur MSD Ltd
Mallards Reach
Bridge Avenue
Maidenhead
Berks, SL6 1QP.
tel: (01628) 785 291
fax: (01628) 671 722

**Sanofi-Synthelabo**
See Sanofi-Aventis

**Schering Health**
See Bayer

**Schering-Plough**
Schering-Plough Ltd
Shire Park
Welwyn Garden City
Herts, AL7 1TW.
tel: (01707) 363 636
fax: (01707) 363 763
medical.info@spcorp.com

**Schuco**
Schuco International Ltd
Challenge House
1 Lyndhurst Ave
London, N12 0NE.
tel: (020) 8368 1642
fax: (020) 8361 3761
sales@schuco.co.uk

**Serono**
See Merck Serono

**Servier**
Servier Laboratories Ltd
Gallions
Wexham Springs
Framewood Rd
Wexham, SL3 6RJ.
tel: (01753) 666 409
fax: (01753) 666 204
medical.information@uk.netgrs.com

**Seven Seas**
Seven Seas Ltd
Hedon Rd
Marfleet
Hull, HU9 5NJ.
tel: (01482) 375 234
fax: (01482) 374 345

**Shermond**
Shermond
Castle House
Sea View Way
Woodingdean
Brighton, East Sussex, BN2 6NT.
tel: (0870) 242 7701
fax: (01273) 391 028
sales@shermond.com

**Shire**
Shire Pharmaceuticals Ltd
Hampshire International Business Park
Chineham
Basingstoke
Hants, RG24 8EP.
tel: (0800) 055 6614
fax: (01256) 894 708
medinfoglobal@shire.com

**SHS**
SHS International Ltd
100 Wavertree Boulevard
Wavertree Technology Park
Liverpool, L7 9PT.
tel: (0151) 228 8161
fax: (0151) 230 5365
nutrition@shsint.co.uk

**Sigma**
Sigma Pharmaceuticals plc
PO Box 233
Unit 1-7 Colonial Way
Watford
Herts, WD24 4YR.
tel: (01923) 444 999
fax: (01923) 444 998
info@sigpharm.co.uk

**Sigma-Tau**
Sigma-Tau Pharma Ltd (UK)
Abbey House
1650 Arlington Business Park
Reading
Berks, RG7 4SA.
tel: (0800) 043 1268
fax: (0118) 929 8076
medical.information@sigma-tau.co.uk

**Sinclair**
Sinclair Pharmaceuticals Ltd
4 Godalming Business Centre
Woolsack Way
Godalming
Surrey, GU7 1XW.
tel: (01483) 410 600
fax: (01483) 410 620
info@sinclairpharma.com

**Skin Camouflage Co.**
The Skin Camouflage Company Ltd
Moor Lane
Sotby
Market Rasen, LN8 5LR.
tel: (01507) 343 091
fax: (01507) 343 092
smjcovermark@aol.com

**Skinnies**
Skinnies UK
Manor House
Manor Lane
Halesowen
West Midlands, B62 8PU.
tel: (01562) 546 123
fax: (0121) 259 0292
info@skinniesuk.com

**SLO Drinks**
SLO Drinks Ltd
Unit 1
Torr Top St
New Mills
High Peak, SK22 4BS.
tel: (08452) 22 22 05
fax: (08452) 22 22 06
info@slodrinks.com

**SMA Nutrition**
See Wyeth

**SNBTS**
Scottish National Blood Transfusion
Service
Protein Fractionation Centre
Ellen's Glen Rd
Edinburgh, EH17 7QT.
tel: (0131) 536 5700
fax: (0131) 536 5781
Contact.pfc@snbts.csa.scot.nhs.uk

**Solvay**
Solvay Healthcare Ltd
Mansbridge Rd
West End
Southampton, SO18 3JD.
tel: (023) 8046 7000
fax: (023) 8046 5350
medinfo.shl@solvay.com

**Sovereign**
See Amdipharm

**Spectrum**
Spectrum Thea Pharmaceuticals
Fernbank House
Springwood Way
Macclesfield
Cheshire, SK10 2XA.
tel: (0845) 521 1290
fax: (01625) 619 959
philiplewiswilliams@spectrum-thea.co.
uk

**SpePharm**
SpePharm UK Ltd
2B Bankside
Hanborough Business Park
Long Hanborough
Witney, Oxon, OX29 8LJ.
tel: (0844) 800 7579
fax: (0844) 800 7336
medinfo.uk@spepharm.com

**Squibb**
See Bristol-Myers Squibb

**SSL**
SSL International plc
Venus, 1 Old Park Lane
Trafford Park
Urmston
Manchester, M41 7HA.
tel: (08701) 222 690
fax: (08701) 222 692
medical.information@ssl-international.
com

**STD Pharmaceutical**
STD Pharmaceutical Products Ltd
Plough Lane
Hereford, HR4 0EL.
tel: (01432) 373 555
fax: (01432) 373 556
enquiries@stdpharm.co.uk

**Steraid**
Steraid (Gainsborough) Ltd
Unit 42
Corringham Road Industrial Estate
Gainsborough , DN21 1QB.
tel: (01427) 677 659
fax: (01427) 677 654

**Stiefel**
Stiefel Laboratories (UK) Ltd
Eurasia Headquarters
Concorde Rd
Maidenhead
Berks, SL6 4BY.
tel: (01628) 612 000
fax: (01628) 810 021
general@stiefel.co.uk

**Stragen**
Stragen UK Ltd
Castle Court
41 London Rd
Reigate
Surrey, RH2 9RJ.
tel: (0870) 351 8744
fax: (0870) 351 8745
info@stragenuk.com

**Strakan**
See ProStrakan

**Su-Med**
Su-Med International UK Ltd
Integrity House
Units 1-2 Graphite Way
Hadfield
Glossop, Derbyshire, SK13 1QH.
tel: (01457) 890 980
fax: (01457) 890 990
sales@sumed.co.uk

**Sutherland**
Sutherland Health Ltd
Unit 1, Rivermead
Pipers Way
Thatcham
Berks, RG19 4EP.
tel: (01635) 874 488
fax: (01635) 877 622

**Swedish Orphan**
Swedish Orphan International Ltd
1 Fordham House Court
Fordham House Estate
Newmarket Rd
Fordham, Cambs, CB7 5LL.
tel: (01638) 722 380
fax: (01638) 723 167

**Synergy Healthcare**
Synergy Healthcare (UK) Ltd
Lion Mill
Fitton St
Royton
Oldham, OL2 5JX.
tel: (0161) 624 5641
fax: (0161) 627 0902
healthcaresolutions@synergyhealthplc.
com

**Syner-Med**
Syner-Med (Pharmaceutical Products)
Ltd
Beech House
840 Brighton Rd
Purley, CR8 2BH.
tel: (0845) 634 2100
fax: (0845) 634 2101
mail@syner-med.com

**Systagenix**
Systagenix Wound Management
Coronation Rd
Ascot
Berks, SL5 9EY.
tel: (01344) 871 000
fax: (01344) 621 247

**Takeda**
Takeda UK Ltd
Takeda House, Mercury Park
Wycombe Lane
Wooburn Green
High Wycombe, Bucks, HP10 0HH.
tel: (01628) 537 900
fax: (01628) 526 615

**Talley**
Talley Group Ltd
Abbey Park Industrial Estate
Premier Way
Romsey
Hants, SO51 9DQ.
tel: (01794) 503 500
fax: (01794) 503 555

**Taro**
Taro Pharmaceuticals (UK) Ltd
Lakeside
1 Furzeground Way
Stockley Park East
Uxbridge, Middx, UB11 1BD.
tel: (08707) 369 544
fax: (08707) 369 545
customerservice@taropharma.co.uk

**Teofarma**
Teofarma S.r.l.
c/o Professional Information Ltd
Olliver
Richmond
North Yorkshire, DL10 5HX.
tel: (01748) 828 857
teofarma@professionalinformation.co.
uk

**Teva**
Teva Pharmaceuticals Ltd
The Gate House
Gatehouse Way
Aylesbury
Bucks, HP19 8DB.
med.info@tevapharma.co.uk

**TEVA UK**
TEVA UK Ltd
Building V
The London Road Campus
London Rd
Harlow, Essex, CM17 9LP.
tel: (08705) 020 304
fax: (08705) 323 334
medinfo@tevauk.com

**The Medicines Company**
The Medicines Company
c/o Quintiles AG, Medical Information
Group
Hochstrasse 50
CH-4053 Basel
Switzerland
tel: (00) 800 8436 3326
fax: (00) 800 5283 5460
GCHS.MI@Quintiles.com

**Thornton & Ross**
Thornton & Ross Ltd
Linthwaite Laboratories
Huddersfield, HD7 5QH.
tel: (01484) 842 217
fax: (01484) 847 301
mail@thorntonross.com

**Tillomed**
Tillomed Laboratories Ltd
3 Howard Rd
Eaton Socon, St Neots
Cambs, PE19 3ET.
tel: (01480) 402 400
fax: (01480) 402 402
info@tillomed.co.uk

**Tobia Teff**
Tobia Teff UK Ltd
27 Carlton House
Canterbury Terrace
London, NW6 5DY.
tel: (0207) 328 2045
info@tobiateff.co.uk

**TOL**
Tree of Life
Coaldale Rd
Lymedale Business Park
Newcastle Under Lyme
Staff, ST5 9QX.
tel: (01782) 567 100
fax: (01782) 567 199
health@tol-europe.com

**TopoTarget**
TopoTarget A/S
Symbion Science Park
Fruebjergvej 3
DK-2100
Copenhagen, Denmark
tel: (00 45 39) 178 392
fax: (00 45 39) 179 492

**Torbet**
Torbet Laboratories Ltd
14D Wendover Rd
Rackheath Industrial Estate
Rackheath
Norwich, NR13 6LH.
tel: (01603) 735 200
fax: (01603) 735 217
torbet@typharm.com

**Transdermal**
Transdermal Ltd
35 Grimwade Ave
Croydon
Surrey, CR0 5DJ.
tel: (020) 8654 2251
fax: (020) 8654 2252
transdermal@transdermal.co.uk

**TRB Chemedica**
TRB Chemedica (UK) Ltd
MED IC3
Keele University Science Park
Keele
Staffordshire, ST5 5NP.
tel: (0845) 330 7556
fax: (0845) 330 7557
phunt@trbchemedica.co.uk

**Typharm**
Typharm Ltd
14D Wendover Rd
Rackheath Industrial Estate
Rackheath
Norwich, NR13 6LH.
tel: (01603) 735 200
fax: (01603) 735 217
customerservices@typharm.com

**UCB Pharma**
UCB Pharma Ltd
208 Bath Rd
Slough, SL1 3WE.
tel: (01753) 534 655
fax: (01753) 447 647
medicalinformationuk@ucb.com

**Ultrapharm**
Ultrapharm Ltd
Centenary Business Park
Henley-on-Thames
Oxon, RG9 1DS.
tel: (01491) 578 016
fax: (01491) 570 001
orders@glutenfree.co.uk

**Univar**
Univar Ltd
International House
Zenith, Paycocke Rd
Basildon
Essex, SS14 3DW.
tel: (01268) 594 400
fax: (01268) 594 481
trientine@univareurope.com

**Unomedical**
Unomedical Ltd
Thornhill Rd
Redditch, B98 7NL.
tel: (01527) 587 700
fax: (01527) 592 111

**Urgo**
Urgo Ltd
Sullington Rd
Shepshed
Loughborough
Leics, LE12 9JJ.
tel: (01509) 502 051
fax: (01509) 650 898
medical@parema.com

**Valeant**
Valeant Pharmaceuticals Ltd
Cedarwood
Chineham Business Park
Crockford Lane, Basingstoke
Hants, RG24 8WD.
tel: (01256) 707 744
fax: (01256) 707 334
valeantuk@valeant.com

**Vegenat**
c/o Archaelis Ltd
23 Pembridge Gardens
London, W2 4EB.
tel: (0870) 803 2484
info@vegenat.co.uk

**Viatris**
See Meda

**Viridian**
Viridian Pharma Ltd
Yew Tree House
Hendrew Lane
Llandevaud
Newport, Gwent, NP18 2AB.
tel: (01633) 400 335
info@viridianpharma.co.uk

**Vitaflo**
Vitaflo International Ltd
11-16 Century Buildings
Brunswick Business Park
Liverpool, L3 4BL.
tel: (0151) 709 9020
fax: (0151) 709 9727
vitaflo@vitaflo.co.uk

**Vitaline**
Vitaline Pharmaceuticals UK Ltd
Chiltern House, Unit P
Howland Rd
Thame
Oxon, OX9 3GQ.
tel: (01844) 269 007
fax: (01844) 269 005
vitalineinfo@aol.com

**Vitalograph**
Vitalograph Ltd
Maids Moreton
Buckingham, MK18 1SW.
tel: (01280) 827 110
fax: (01280) 823 302
sales@vitalograph.co.uk

**Wallace Cameron**
Wallace Cameron Ltd
26 Netherhall Rd
Netherton Industrial Estate
Wishaw, ML2 0JG.
tel: (01698) 354 600
fax: (01698) 354 700
sales@wallacecameron.com

**Wallace Mfg**
Wallace Manufacturing Chemists Ltd
Wallace House
New Abbey Court
51-53 Stert St, Abingdon
Oxon, OX14 3JF.
tel: (01235) 538 700
fax: (01235) 538 800
info@alinter.co.uk

**WaveSense**
WaveSense Europe Ltd
Harwell Innovation Centre
173 Curie Ave
Harwell Science & Innovation Campus
Didcot, Oxon, OX11 0QG.
tel: (01235) 838 639
fax: (01235) 838 648
enquiries@wavesense.co.uk

**Wellfoods**
Wellfoods Ltd
Towngate
Mapplewell
Barnsley
South Yorks, S75 6LP.
tel: (01226) 381 712
fax: (01226) 390 087
wellfoods@talk21.com

**Winthrop**
Winthrop Pharmaceuticals UK Ltd
PO Box 611
Guildford, Surrey, GU1 4YS.
tel: (01483) 554 101
fax: (01483) 554 810
winthropsales@sanofi-aventis.com

**Wockhardt**
Wockhardt UK Ltd
Ash Rd North
Wrexham Industrial Estate
Wrexham, LL13 9UF.
tel: (01978) 661 261
fax: (01978) 660 130

**Wyeth**
Wyeth Pharmaceuticals
Huntercombe Lane South
Taplow
Maidenhead
Berks, SL6 0PH.
tel: (01628) 604 377
fax: (01628) 666 368
ukmedinfo@wyeth.com

**Wynlit**
Wynlit Laboratories
153 Furzehill Rd
Borehamwood
Herts, WD6 2DR.
tel: (07903) 370 130
fax: (020) 8292 6117

**Wyvern**
Wyvern Medical Ltd
PO Box 17
Ledbury
Herefordshire, HR8 2ES.
tel: (01531) 631 105
fax: (01531) 634 844

**Zeal**
G. H. Zeal Ltd
Deer Park Rd
London, SW19 3UU.
tel: (020) 8542 2283
fax: (020) 8543 7840
scientific@zeal.co.uk

**Zeneus**
See Cephalon

**Zeroderma**
Zeroderma Ltd
The Rectory
Braybrooke Rd
Arthingworth
Market Harborough, LE16 8JT.
tel: (01858) 525 643
fax: (01858) 525 383
info@ixlpharma.com

**ZooBiotic**
ZooBiotic Ltd
Biosurgical Research Unit
Surgical Materials Testing Laboratory
Princess of Wales Hospital, Coity Rd
Brigend, Mid Glamorgan, South Wales,
CF31 1RQ.
tel: (0845) 230 1810
fax: (01656) 752 830
maggots@smtl.co.uk

# Special-order Manufacturers

Unlicensed medicines are available from 'special-order' manufacturers and specialist-importing companies; the MHRA maintains a register of these companies at www.mhra.gov.uk

Licensed **hospital manufacturing units** also manufacture 'special-order' products as unlicensed medicines, the principal NHS units are listed below. A database (*Pro-File*; www.pro-file.nhs.uk) provides information on medicines manufactured in the NHS; access is restricted to NHS pharmacy staff.

> The MHRA recommends that an unlicensed medicine should only be used when a patient has special requirements that cannot be met by use of a licensed medicine

## England

### London

Mr P. Forsey
Production Manager
Guy's and St. Thomas' NHS Foundation Trust
Pharmacy Department
St. Thomas' Hospital
Lambeth Palace Rd
London, SE1 7EH.
tel: (020) 7188 5003
fax: (020) 7188 5013
paul.forsey@gstt.nhs.uk

Mr A. Krol
Director of Commercial Services
Pharmaceutical Manufacturing Unit
Moorfields Eye Hospital NHS Trust
34 Nile St
London, N1 7LX.
tel: (020) 7684 8561
fax: 0800 328 8191
alan.krol@moorfields.nhs.uk

Mr M. Lillywhite
Director of Technical Services
Barts and the London NHS Trust
Pathology and Pharmacy Building
80 Newark St
Whitechapel
London, EC1A 7BE.
tel: (020) 3246 0273
fax: (020) 3246 0268
mike.lillywhite@bartsandthelondon.nhs.uk

Dr K. Middleton
Principal Pharmacist, Technical Services
Department of Pharmacy
Northwick Park and St Mark's Hospital
Watford Rd
Harrow
Middx, HA1 3UJ.
tel: (020) 8869 2204/2223
keith.middleton@nwlh.nhs.uk

Ms C. Trehane
Production Manager
Royal Free Hospital
Pond Street
London, NW3 2QG.
tel: (020) 7830 2282 / orders: 2424
christine.trehane@royalfree.nhs.uk

### Midlands and Eastern

Mr J. Harwood
Production Manager
Pharmacy Manufacturing Unit
The Ipswich Hospital NHS Trust
Heath Rd
Ipswich, IP4 5PD.
tel: (01473) 703 440
fax: (01473) 703 609
john.harwood@ipswichhospital.nhs.uk

Ms J. Kendall
Assistant Chief Pharmacist
Pharmacy Production Units
Nottingham University Hospitals NHS Trust
Queens Medical Centre Campus
Nottingham, NG7 2UH.
tel: (0115) 875 4521
fax: (0115) 970 9744
jeanette.kendall@nuh.nhs.uk

Mrs R. Newton
Head of Production
Pharmacy Manufacturing Unit
University Hospital of North Staffs
City General Site
Stoke-on-Trent, ST4 6QG.
tel: (01782) 552 290
fax: (01782) 552 916
ruth.newton@uhns.nhs.uk

Mr S. Parrish
Associate Director of Pharmacy
Technical Services
UHB Medicines (SFMU)
32–34 Melchett Rd, Kings Norton
Business Centre, Kings Norton
Birmingham, B30 3HS.
tel: (0121) 627 2326
fax: (0121) 627 2168
Steve.Parrish@uhb.nhs.uk

Dr R. Needle
Chief Pharmacist
Essex Rivers Healthcare NHS Trust
Colchester General Hospital
Turner Rd
Colchester, CO4 5JL.
tel: (01206) 742 433
fax: (01206) 742 319
richard.needle@essexrivers.nhs.uk

Mr P.G. Williams
Technical and Support Services Manager
Pharmacy Manufacturing Unit
Queens Hospital
Burton Hospitals NHS Trust
Belvedere Rd
Burton-on-Trent, DE13 0RB.
tel: (01283) 511 511 Extn 5138
fax: (01283) 593 036
paul.williams@burtonh-tr.wmids.nhs.uk

### North East

Ms S. Klein
Production Manager
Pharmacy Production Unit
Royal Victoria Infirmary
Queen Victoria Rd
Newcastle-upon-Tyne, NE1 4LP.
tel: (0191) 282 0377
fax: (0191) 282 0376
stephanie.klein@nuth.nhs.uk

### North West

Mr M.D. Booth
Principal Pharmacist
Production & Aseptic Services Manager
Stockport Pharmaceuticals
Stepping Hill Hospital
Stockport
Cheshire, SK2 7JE.
tel: (0161) 419 5657
fax: (0161) 419 5664
mike.booth@stockport.nhs.uk

Mr N. Fletcher
Deputy Director of Pharmacy, Technical Services
Preston Pharmaceuticals
Royal Preston Hospital
Fulwood
Preston, PR2 9HT.
tel: (01772) 522 505
fax: (01772) 522 602
neil.fletcher@lthtr.nhs.uk

## South East

Mr F. Brown
Head of Production
Pharmacy Department
St Peter's Hospital
Guildford Rd
Chertsey
Surrey, KT16 OPZ.
tel: (01932) 722 886
fax: (01932) 723 209
fraser.brown@asph.nhs.uk

Ms G. Middlehurst
Quality Assurance and Business Manager
Pharmacy Manufacturing Unit
Queen Alexandra Hospital
Southwick Hill Rd
Cosham
Portsmouth
Hants, PO6 3LY.
tel: (02392) 286 335
fax: (02392) 378 288
gillian.middlehurst@porthosp.nhs.uk

Mr M. Sherwood
Principal Pharmacist (Production)
Eastbourne DGH Pharmaceuticals
Eastbourne DGH Hospital
East Sussex Hospitals NHS Trust
Kings Drive, Eastbourne
East Sussex, BN21 2UD.
tel: (01323) 414 906
fax: (01323) 414 931
mike.sherwood@esht.nhs.uk

## South West

Mr P. S. Bendell
Pharmacy Manufacturing Services
Manager
Torbay PMU
South Devon Healthcare
Kemmings Close, Long Rd
Paignton
Devon, TQ4 7TW.
tel: (01803) 664 707
fax: (01803) 664 354
phil.bendell@nhs.net

## Yorkshire

Mr R.W. Brookes
Technical Services Manager
Pharmacy Department
Royal Hallamshire Hospital
Glossop Rd
Sheffield, S10 2JF.
tel: (0114) 271 3104
fax: (0114) 271 2783
roger.brookes@sth.nhs.uk

Dr S. Langford
Pharmacy Production Director
Pharmacy Manufacturing Unit
Calderdale and Huddersfield NHS
Foundation Trust
Gate 2 Acre Mills, School St
Lindley
Huddersfield
West Yorks, HD3 3ET.
tel: (01484) 355 388
fax: (01484) 355 377
john.harwood@cht.nhs.uk

## Northern Ireland

Ms C. McBride
Assistant Director of Pharmaceutical
Services
Manufacturing and Royal Group of
Hospitals Belfast
77 Boucher Crescent
Belfast, BT12 6HU.
tel: (028) 9063 3310 or (028) 9055 3407
fax: (028) 9055 3498
colette.mcbride@royalhospitals.n-i.
nhs.uk

## Scotland

Mr G. Conkie
Manager, Pharmacy Production Unit
Western Infirmary
Dumbarton Road
Glasgow, G11 6NT.
tel: (0141) 211 2882
fax: (0141) 211 1967
graham.conkie@northglasgow.scot.
nhs.uk

Mr B. W. Millar
General Manager
Tayside Pharmaceuticals
Ninewells Hospital
Dundee, DD1 9SY.
tel: (01382) 632 183
fax: (01382) 632 060
baxter.w.millar@tuht.scot.nhs.uk

## Wales

Mr P. Spark
Principal Pharmacist (Production)
Cardiff and Vale NHS Trust
University Hospital of Wales
Heath Park
Cardiff, CF14 4XW.
tel: (029) 2074 4828
fax: (029) 2074 3114
paul.spark@cardiffandvale.wales.nhs.
uk

# Index

Principal page references are printed in **bold** type. Proprietary (trade) names and names of organisms are printed in *italic* type; where the BNF does not include a full entry for a branded product, the non-proprietary name is shown in brackets

## A

Abacavir, 340, **341**
   lamivudine and zidovudine with, 341
   lamivudine with, 341
Abatacept, **578**
   infusion table, 869
Abbreviations,
   *inside back cover*
   prescription writing, 4
*Abcare*, 380
Abciximab, **134**, 135
   infusion table, 869
Abdominal surgery, antibacterial prophylaxis, 293
*Abelcet*, 333, 334
*Abidec*, 552
*Abilify* preparations, 201
*Able Spacer*, 162
Abortion
   habitual *see* Miscarriage, recurrent, 408
   haemorrhage, 435
   induction, 434
Abrasive agents, acne, 649
*Abraxane*, 491
Abscess, dental, 292
Absence seizures, 254
   atypical, 254
Absorbent cotton, bandages, dressings, gauze, 913, 923, 924
*Abstral*, 240
*AC 2000 HI FLO*, 164
*AC 4000*, 164
Acamprosate, **280**
Acanthamoeba keratitis, 591, 607
Acarbose, 384, **385**
Acaricides, 662
ACBS
   foods, 880
   toilet preparations, 910
*Accolate*, 171
*Accu-Chek* preparations, 390
*Accuhaler*
   *Flixotide*, 168
   *Seretide*, 169
   *Serevent*, 158
   *Ventolin*, 157
*Accupro*, 106
*Accuretic*, 107
ACE inhibitors, 102
   heart failure, 102
   myocardial infarction, 138
   renal function, 103
*Acea*, 658
Acebutolol, **89**
   *see also* Beta-adrenoceptor blocking drugs
Aceclofenac, 560, **562**

Acemetacin, 562
   postoperative pain, 706
Acenocoumarol, 130, **132**
*Acepril* (captopril), 104
Acetaminophen *see* Paracetamol
Acetazolamide, **600**, 601
   diuretic, 80
   epilepsy, 265
   eye, 601
   glaucoma, 598, 600
Acetic acid, otitis externa, 608
Acetylcholine, 605
Acetylcysteine
   eye, 603
   infusion table, 869
   paracetamol poisoning, 29, **30**, 31
Acetylsalicylic acid *see* Aspirin
*Acezide* (co-zidocapt), 104
Aciclovir, **349**, 350
   herpes simplex, 349
      buccal, 620
      eye, 349, **593**
      genital, 349, 661
      labialis, 661, **662**
      skin, **662**
   herpes zoster, 349
   infusion table, 869
Acid aspiration, 45
   surgery, 698
*Acidex*, 40
Acidosis, metabolic, 529, 532
Acipimox, **148**
Acitretin, 640, **643**
Acknowledgements, iv
*Aclasta*, 425
*Acnamino MR*, 310
Acne, **647**
Acne rosacea *see* Rosacea, 647
*Acnecide*, 647
*Acnisal*, 649
*Acnocin* (co-cyprindiol), 650
*Acomplia*, 224
Acrolein, 469
Acromegaly, 416, 426, 510
ACTH *see* Corticotropin, 413
*Actiban*, 929
*Actico*, 929
*Acticoat* products, 921
*Actidose-Aqua Advance*, 28
*Acti-Fast*, 927
*ActiFormCool*, 914
*Actilite*, 920
*Actilyse*, 139
*Actinac*, 649
Actinic keratosis, 654
Actinomycin D *see* Dactinomycin
*Actiq*, 241
*Actisorb Silver*, 921
Activated charcoal
   dressings, 919
   poisoning, use in, **28**
*Active*, 390
*ActivHeal* products
   alginate, 918
   film dressing, 914
   foam, 917, 918
   hydrocolloid, 916
   hydrogel, 914
*Activon* products, 920
*Acti-Wrap*, 926
*Actonel* preparations, 424
*Actos*, 386
*Actrapid* preparations, 376
*Acular*, 606
*Acupan*, 236

Acute coronary syndrome, 134
Acute lymphoblastic leukaemia, 487
*ACWY Vax*, 684
Acyclovir *see* Aciclovir
*Adalat* preparations, 118, 119
Adalimumab, 579
   Crohn's disease, 53, **58**
   psoriasis, **578**, 644, **646**
   rheumatic diseases, 576, **578**
Adapalene, **648**
*Adartrel*, 271
*Adcal*, 541
*Adcal-D₃* preparations, 550
*Adcortyl*
   in Orabase, 617
   *Intra-articular/Intradermal*, 570
Addicts, notification of, 9
*Add-Ins*, 908
*Addiphos*, 539
Addison's disease, 394
Additives *see* Excipients
*Additrace*, 539
Adefovir, **353**, 354
*Adenocor*, 83
*Adenoscan* (adenosine), 83
Adenosine, 82, **83**
ADH *see* Antidiuretic hormone
ADHD *see* Attention deficit hyperactivity disorder, 220
Adhesive
   dressings, 925
   films, 914
   skin tissue, 665
*Adipine* preparations, 119
*Adizem* preparations, 116
Adrenal
   function test, 413
   hyperplasia, 395
   insufficiency, 394
      dental practice, 21
   suppression
      metyrapone, 432
      systemic corticosteroids, 395
      topical corticosteroids, 630
Adrenaline
   anaphylaxis, 176, **177**
   cardiopulmonary resuscitation, 125
   croup, 154
   eye, 600
   local anaesthesia, 714, 717
Adrenergic neurone blocking drugs, 99
Adrenoceptor agonists, 154
*Adriamycin* (doxorubicin), 473
Adsorbents
   gastro-intestinal, 51
   poisoning, 28
Adult advanced life support algorithm, *inside back cover*
*Adva-Co*, 929
*Advadraw* products, 919
*Advagraf*, 497
Advanced hypereosinophilic syndrome, 487
*Advantage Plus*, 390
*Advasil*, 922
*Advasoft*, 929
*Advate* (factor VIII fraction), 141
*Advazorb* products, 917, 918
Adverse reactions, reporting, 11
Advisory Committee on Borderline Substances *see* ACBS
Advisory labels *see* Cautionary and advisory labels
*AeroChamber*, 162
*AErrane*, 702

Agalsidase
    alfa, **554**
    beta, **554**
    infusion tables, 869
Agammaglobulinaemia, congenital,
    replacement therapy, 690
Age-related macular degeneration,
    606
*Aggrastat*, 137
Agomelatine, **218**
*Agrippal*, 681
AIDS, 339
    vaccines and, 670
*Airomir* preparations, 157
*Airstrip*, 925
*Aknemin* (minocycline), 309
*Aknemycin Plus*, 649
*Alateris*, 583
Albendazole
    hookworm infections, 371
    hydatid disease, 370
    strongyloidiasis, 371
Albumin solution, 532, **533**
*Albustix*, 391
Albuterol *see* Salbutamol
Alclometasone dipropionate,
    634
Alcohol
    dependence, 279
    hypnotic, 190
    nutrition, 539
    poisoning by, 29
    skin antiseptic, 665
    withdrawal, 279
Alcoholism, 279
    vitamin B, 547
*Aldactide* preparations (co-flumacto-
    ne), 80
*Aldactone*, 79
*Aldara*, 653
Aldesleukin, 501
*Aldioxa*, 668
*Aldomet*, 99
Aldosterone antagonists, 78, 79
*Aldurazyme*, 555
Alemtuzumab, **498**, 499
    infusion table, 869
Alendronate sodium *see* Alendronic
    acid
Alendronic acid, 419, 422
    colecalciferol with, 423
Alfacalcidol, 549, **550**
Alfentanil, 237, **707**, 708
    infusion table, 869
Alfuzosin, **455**
Alginates
    antacids, 39, 40
    dressings, 918–21
*Algisite* products, 918, 921
*Algivon*, 920
Alglucosidase alfa, **556**
    infusion table, 869
*Algosteril* products, 918
*Alicalm*, 894
Alimemazine
    allergic disorders, 171, **173**
    premedication, 173
*Alimta*, 479
*Alione*, 916
Aliskiren, **110**
Alitretinoin, **638**, 639
Alkalinisation of urine, 460
*Alkeran*, 471
Alkylating drugs, 469
*Alldress*, 915
*Allegron*, 212
Allergen extract vaccines, 174

Allergy, 395
    anaphylaxis, 176
    angioedema, 178
    conjunctivitis, 595
    food, 58
    rhinitis, 612
*Allevyn* products, 915, 917, 918, 921
Allopurinol, **581**, 582
Almond oil, ear, 611
Almotriptan, **248**
*Alomide*, 596
Alopecia
    androgenetic, 656
    cytotoxic drugs, 467
*Aloxi*, 230
Alpha *Keri* Bath Oil, 628
Alpha tocopheryl acetate, 551
Alpha₂-adrenoceptor stimulants
    cardiovascular, 98
    eye, 600, 605
    migraine, 252
Alpha-adrenoceptor blocking drugs
    cardiovascular, 99
    urinary tract, 455
Alpha-blockers *see* Alpha-adreno-
    ceptor blocking drugs
*Alphaderm*, 633
*Alphagan*, 600
*Alphanate* (factor VIII fraction), 141
*AlphaNine* (factor IX fraction), 142
*Alphosyl 2 in 1*, 655
*Alphosyl HC*, 642
Alprazolam, 191, **192**
Alprostadil
    ductus arteriosus, 437
    erectile dysfunction, **462**, 463
    infusion table, 869
*Altacite* preparations (hydrotalcite),
    39, 40
*Altargo*, 658
Alteplase, 138, **139**
    infusion table, 869
Alternative medicine, 1
*Alu-Cap*
    antacid, 39
    hyperphosphataemia, 544
Aluminium acetate, ear, 608, **609**
Aluminium chloride, 668
Aluminium hydroxide
    antacid, **39**, 40
    hyperphosphataemia, **544**
Aluminium oxide, 649
*Alupent* preparations, 159
*Alvedon* (paracetamol), 235
Alverine, **42**
*Alvesco*, 168
Alzheimer's disease, 285
Amantadine
    parkinsonism, **276**
    viral infections, 354, **355**
*Amaryl*, 382
*Ambirix*, 677
*AmBisome*, 333, 334
Ambrisentan, **95**, 96
Amethocaine *see* Tetracaine
*Ametop*, 718
Amfebutamone *see* Bupropion, 280,
    **281**
Amfetamine *see* Amphetamines
*Amias*, 108
Amikacin, 311, **312**
    infusion table, 869
    tuberculosis, 323
*Amikin*, 312
*Amilamont* (amiloride), 78

*Amil-Co* (co-amilozide), 79
Amiloride, **78**
    bumetanide with, 79
    cyclopenthiazide with, 79
    furosemide with, 79
    hydrochlorothiazide with, 79
*Aminex*, 905
Amino acids
    ACBS, 906, 907, 910
    intravenous nutrition, 539
Aminobenzoic acid, 547, **549**
Aminoglycosides
    ear, 608, 611
    eye, 591
    skin, 657
    systemic, 310
Aminophylline, 160, **161**
    infusion table, 869
    *see also* Theophylline
*Aminoplasmal* preparations, 535
Aminosalicylates, 52, 54
*Aminoven* preparations, 535
Amiodarone, 83, **84**
    cardiopulmonary resuscitation,
    125
    infusion table, 869
Amisulpride, 199, **200**
Amitriptyline, **211**
    neuropathic pain, 246
    perphenazine with, 211
    postherpetic neuralgia, 247
*Amix* (amoxicillin), 299
Amlodipine, **115**
    olmesartan with, 109
    *see also* Calcium-channel block-
    ers
    valsartan with, 115
*Amlostin* (amlodipine), 115
*Ammonaps*, 556
Ammonia and ipecacuanha mixture,
    184
Ammonia, poisoning by, 35
Amobarbital, 193
    secobarbital with, 193
Amoebiasis, 366
Amoebic
    abscess, 366
    dysentery, 366
Amoebicides, 366
*Amoram* (amoxicillin), 299
Amorolfine, **659**
Amoxicillin, **298**, 299
    infusion table, 869
    urinary tract infection, 331
*Amoxident* (amoxicillin), 299
*Amoxil* preparations, 299
Amoxycillin *see* Amoxicillin
Amphetamines
    abuse, 8
    poisoning by, 33
*Amphocil*, 333, 334
Amphotericin, 332, 333, **334**
    bladder infections, 461
    eye, 603
    infusion, 334
        lipid formulation, 333, 334
        liposomal, 334
    infusion table, 869, 870
    leishmaniasis, 367
    mouth, 618, 619
Ampicillin, 298, **299**
    flucloxacillin with [co-fluampi-
    cil], 298, **301**
    infusion table, 870
Amsacrine, 480, **481**
    infusion table, 870
*Amsidine*, 481

Amylobarbitone see Amobarbital
Amyotrophic lateral sclerosis, 277
*Anabact*, 658
Anabolic steroids, 412
   anaemias, 517
Anaemias, 512
   aplastic, 517
   chronic renal failure, 517
   haemolytic, 517, 523
   hypoplastic, 517
   iron-deficiency, 512
   megaloblastic, 515
   pernicious, 515
   sideroblastic, 517
Anaesthesia
   analgesics, 706
   antimuscarinics, 703
   corticosteroids, 395, 697
   dental practice, 698
   driving, 698
   general
      inhalational, 701
      intravenous, 698
   local, 713
      dental practice, 714
      eye, 602
      mouth, 616
      rectal, 67
      skin, 630
   muscle relaxants, 708
   status epilepticus, 265
*Anafranil* preparations, 211
Anagrelide, **524**
Anakinra, 578, **579**
Anal fissure, 68
Analeptics, 178
Analgesic-induced headache see Medication-overuse headache, 247
Analgesics, 232
   compound, 233
   non-opioid, 232
   NSAIDs, 232, 560
      anaesthesia, 706
      dental pain, 561
      elderly, 20
      orofacial pain, 561
      poisoning by, 29
      rheumatic diseases,
         560
      topical, 588, 589
   opioid, 237
      anaesthesia, 707
      cough suppressants, 182
      dependence on, 8
      diabetic neuropathy, 389
      diarrhoea, 51
      equivalent doses, 15
      neuropathic pain, 246
      palliative care, 15, 18
      poisoning by, 31
*Analog* products, 906, 907, 909, 910
*Anapen*, 177
Anaphylaxis, 176
Anastrozole, 505, **506**
*Ancotil*, 336
Ancylostomiasis, 371
*Androcur*, 411
Androgens, 409
   malignant disease, 505
*Andropatch*, 410
*Anectine*, 711
*Anexate*, 713
*Angeliq*, 403
*Angettes 75* (aspirin), 135
*Angeze* (isosorbide mononitrate)
   preparations, 113, 114
*Angilol* (propranolol), 88

Angina
   aspirin, 111
   beta-blockers, 87, 111
   calcium-channel blockers, 115
   dental practice, 22, 24
   heparins, 111
   nitrates, 111
   potassium-channel activators,
      120
   stable, 110
   statins, 111
   unstable, 111
Angioedema, 178
   hereditary, 178
      danazol, 428
      tranexamic acid, 140
Angiotensin-converting enzyme inhibitors see ACE inhibitors
Angiotensin-II receptor antagonists,
   107
*Angiox*, 129
*Angitak*, 113
*Angitil* preparations, 116
Angular cheilitis, 619
   bacterial infection, 658
   fungal infection, 659
   inflammation, 631
*Anhydrol Forte*, 668
Anidulafungin, **334**, 335
   infusion table, 870
Anistreplase, 139
Ankylosing spondylitis, 576
Anogenital warts, 652
Anorectics, 223
*Anquil*, 196
*Antabuse*, 280
Antacids
   alginates and, 39
   aluminium, 38
   bismuth, 38
   calcium, 38
   magnesium, 38
   simeticone and, 39
   sodium content, 39
Antazoline, **595**
*Antepsin*, 47
Anterior uveitis, 596
Anthelmintics, 369
Anthracyclines, 472
Anthralin see Dithranol
Anthraquinones, 60
Anthrax
   antibacterial treatment, 328
   vaccine, **672**
Anti-androgens, 411
Anti-arrhythmic drugs, 81
Antibacterial policies, 289
Antibacterials, 289
   acne, 648, 649
   diarrhoea, 50
   ear, 608
   eczema, 638
   eye, 591
   oral infections, 289
   prophylaxis, 293
   skin, 656
   summary of therapy, 290
   vaginal, 441
Antibiotic policies see Antibacterial
   policies, 289
Antibiotic-associated colitis see Clostridium difficile
Antibiotics see Antibacterials
Anticholinergic drugs see Antimuscarinics
Anticholinergic syndrome, 703
Anticholinesterases, 583
   anaesthesia, 711

Anticoagulant treatment booklets, 131
Anticoagulants
   oral, 130
      dental practice, 25
      reversal, 131
      surgery, 132, 698
   parenteral, 125
Anticonvulsants see Antiepileptics
Anti-D ($Rh_0$) immunoglobulin, 693,
   **694**, 695
Antidepressants
   anxiety, 209
   choice, 208, 210
   obsessive-compulsive disorder,
      209
   panic disorder, 209
   poisoning by, 31
   post-traumatic stress disorder,
      209
   see also Monoamine-oxidase
      inhibitors
   serotonin re-uptake inhibitors,
      215
   social anxiety disorder, 209
   surgery, 698
   tricyclic, 209
      diabetic neuropathy, 389
      enuresis, 460
      irritable bowel syndrome,
         54
      MAOIs with, 213
      migraine, 251
      urinary incontinence, 457
      withdrawal, 209
Antidiabetic drugs, 372
   insulin, 373
   oral, 380
Antidiarrhoeal drugs see Diarrhoea,
   50, 528
Antidiuretic hormone, 417
   antagonist, 419
   inappropriate secretion, 419
Anti-emetics, 225
   cytotoxic therapy and, 466
   migraine, 251
Antiepileptics, 252
   surgery, 697
Antifibrinolytic drugs, 140
Antifungal drugs, 332
   anogenital, 441
   oropharyngeal, 618
   skin, 659
Antigiardial drugs, 367
Antihaemophilic fraction, human, 141
Antihepatitis B immunoglobulin, 692
Antihistamines, 171
   allergic emergencies, 176
   allergy, 171
      eye, 595
      nose, 612
      skin, 630
   cough preparations, 182
   eczema, 638
   nasal decongestants, 184
   nausea and vertigo, 225, **226**
Antihypertensives, 102
   ACE inhibitors, 102
   adrenergic neurone blockers, 99
   alpha-blockers, 99
   angiotensin-II receptor
      antagonists, 107
   beta-blockers, 87
   calcium-channel blockers, 115
   centrally-acting, 98
   renin inhibitors, 110
   vasodilator, 95

Anti-inflammatory analgesics see Analgesics, NSAIDs
Antileprotic drugs, 326
Antilymphocyte immunoglobulin, 517
Antimalarials, 357
  rheumatic diseases, 572
Antimanic drugs, 206
Antimetabolites, 474
Antimicrobial dressings, 919
Antimigraine drugs, 247
Antimotility drugs, 51
Antimuscarinics
  antipsychotics and, 195
  bronchodilator, 159
  diabetic neuropathy, 389
  eye, 596
  gastro-intestinal, 41
  parkinsonism, 276
  premedication, 703
  quaternary ammonium, 41
  urinary tract, 457
Antineoplastic drugs, 465
  see also Cytotoxic drugs
Anti-oestrogens, 412, 505
Antiperspirants, 668
Antiplatelet drugs, 133
Antiprotozoal drugs, 357
Antipruritics, topical, 630
Antipsychotics, 194
  depot injections, 204
  equivalent doses
    depot, 205
    oral, 196
  high doses, 193
  mania, 206
  withdrawal, 194
Antipyretics, 233
Antirabies immunoglobulin, 692, 693
Antiretrovirals, 339, 340, 348
Antiseptics, 665
  ACBS, 910
  lozenges, 620
  mouthwashes, 620
  sprays, oropharynx, 620
Antiserum, 672
Antispasmodics, 41
Antitetanus immunoglobulin, 693
Antithrombin alfa, 141
Antithrombin III concentrate, **141**
Antithymocyte immunoglobulin, **495**
  infusion table, 870
Antithyroid drugs, 392
Antituberculous drugs, 321
Antitussives, 182
Antivaricella-zoster immunoglobulin, 693
Antivenoms, 36
Antiviral drugs, 339
  eye, 593
  mouth, 620
  skin, 661
*Anturan*, 582
*Anugesic-HC*, 67
*Anusol* preparations, 67
Anxiety, 190
  antipsychotics, 194
  chronic, 209
Anxiolytics, 185, **190**
  anaesthesia, 704
  benzodiazepines, 191
  poisoning by, 32
  withdrawal, 185
*Anzemet*, 229
APD *see* Disodium pamidronate
Aphthous ulcers, 616
*Apidra*, 377

Aplastic anaemia, 517
*APO-go*, 269
Apomorphine, **269**
Appetite
  stimulants, 553
  suppressants, 223
Applications, definition, 624
Apraclonidine, 600, **605**
Aprepitant, 225, **231**, 467
*Apresoline*, 97
Aprinox (bendroflumethiazide), 75
*Aproten*
  gluten-free, 903
  low-protein, 905
*Aprovel*, 108
*Aptivus*, 346
*Aquacel* products, 917, 921
*Aquadrate*, 627
*Aquaflo*, 914
*Aquaform*, 914
*Aquasept—discontinued*
Aqueous cream, 626
*Aquilon*, 164
Arachis oil
  enema, 62, 63
  presence of, 2, 176
*Aranesp* preparations, 519
*Arava*, 575
*Arcoxia*, 564
*Aredia Dry Powder*, 424
Arginine supplement, 910
Argipressin *(Pitressin)*, 418
*Aricept*, 286
*Aricept Evess*, 286
*Arimidex*, 506
Aripiprazole, 199, **200**, 201
*Arixtra*, 130
*Arlevert*, 226
*Aromasin*, 506
Aromatase inhibitors, 506
*Arpicolin*, 277
Arrhythmias, 81
  beta-blockers, 87
  dental practice, 24
  poisoning and, 27
  supraventricular, 81
  ventricular, 82
Arsenic trioxide, **481**
  infusion table, 870
*Artelac* (hypromellose), 604
*Artelac SDU*, 604
Artemether
  lumefantrine with, **362**
Arterial occlusion, 130
Arteritis, giant cell (temporal), 569
Artesunate, 358
Arthritis
  juvenile idiopathic, 571
  psoriatic, 570
  rheumatoid, 559
  septic, 292
*Arthrofen* (ibuprofen), 565
*Arthrotec* preparations, 564
*Arthroxen* (naproxen), 567
Articaine, 714
Artificial saliva, 621
*Arythmol*, 86
*AS Saliva Orthana*, 621
5-ASA, 54
*Asacol* preparations, 54
*Asasantin Retard*, 136
*Ascabiol* (benzyl benzoate), 663
Ascaricides, 370
*Ascaris*, 370
*Ascensia* products, 380, 390

Ascorbic acid, **549**
  iron excretion, 522
*Asilone* preparations, 40
*Askina* products
  charcoal, 919
  film dressing, 913, 914
  foam, 918
  hydrocolloid, 916
  hydrogel, 914
*Asmabec* preparations, 167
*Asmanex*, 169
*Asmasal* preparations, 157
Asparaginase, 483
Aspartame, 540
  presence of, 2
*Aspav*, 234
Aspergillosis, 332
Aspirin
  analgesia, 233, **234**, 561
    codeine with, 234
    papaveretum with, 234
  angina, 111
  antiplatelet, 133, **135**
    dipyridamole with, 136
  migraine, 247
    metoclopramide with, 247
  myocardial infarction, 133, 137
  rheumatic diseases, 569
Asplenia
  *Haemophilus influenzae* type b vaccine, 676
  *Haemophilus influenzae* type b, prophylaxis, 293
  influenza vaccine, 680
  malaria, 360
  pneumococcal infection, 293
  pneumococcal vaccine, 685
  vaccines and, 670
Asthma, 150
  acute (table), 152
  beta$_2$ agonists, 154
  chronic (table), 151
  emergency treatment, 153
    dental practice, 22
  exercise-induced, 154
  nocturnal, 154, 155
  pregnancy, 150
  prophylaxis, 170
Astringents
  ear, 608
  skin, 665
*AT-10*, 551
*Atarax*, 174
Atazanavir, 340, **344**
*Atenix* (atenolol) preparations, 89
Atenolol, **89**
  chlortalidone with, 89
  co-amilozide with, 89
  infusion table, 870
  nifedipine with, 89
  *see also* Beta-adrenoceptor blocking drugs
Athlete's foot, 659
*Atimos Modulite*, 156
*Ativan* (lorazepam), 192
Atomoxetine, 220, **221**
Atonic seizures, 254
Atorvastatin, 143, **144**
Atosiban, **439**
  infusion table, 870
Atovaquone, **368**, 369
  malaria, 358, 364
  pneumocystis pneumonia, 368
  proguanil with, 365

Atracurium, **709**, 710
  infusion table, 870
*Atrauman* products, 913, 921
Atrial fibrillation, 72, **81**, 130
Atrial flutter, 72, 81
*Atriance*, 478
*Atripla*, 343
Atropine sulphate
  anaesthesia, **703**
    bradycardia, 703
  anticholinesterases and, 711
  antispasmodic, **41**
  beta-blocker poisoning, 32
  bradycardia, 82
  cardiopulmonary resuscitation,
    125
  eye, 596, 597
  myocardial infarction, 82
  organophosphorus poisoning,
    36
*Atrovent* preparations, 159
*ATryn* (antithrombin alfa), 141
Attention deficit hyperactivity
  disorder, 220
Atypical antipsychotics, 199
  poisoning by, 33
  prolactin elevation, 199
*Augmentin* preparations, 300
Auranofin, **571**
*Aureocort*, 637
Aurothiomalate, **571**
*Autopen*, 380
*Avamys*, 614
*Avance* products, 921
*Avandamet*, 387
*Avandia*, 386
*Avastin*, 481
*Avaxim*, 677
*Aveeno* preparations, 626, 628
*Avelox*, 330
*Aviva*, 390
*Avloclor*, 363
*Avoca*, 652
*Avodart*, 412
*Avomine*, 227
*Avonex*, 500
*Axid*, 46
*Axsain*, 589
Azacitidine, **476**
*Azactam*, 308
*Azamune* (azathioprine), 494
Azapropazone, 560, **562**
*Azarga*, 601
Azathioprine, 476, **493**, 494
  eczema, 644
  inflammatory bowel disease,
    53, **57**
  infusion table, 870
  myasthenia gravis, 585
  rheumatic disease, 574
  transplant rejection, 494
Azelaic acid, 647
Azelastine
  eye, **595**
  nose, **612**
Azidothymidine, 343
*Azilect*, 274
Azithromycin, 312, **313**, 314
  trachoma, 591
*Azopt*, 601
AZT, 343
Aztreonam, 307, **308**
  infusion table, 870

# B

*Babyhaler*, 162
Bacillus Calmette-Guérin
  bladder instillation, 501
  vaccines, **673**
Bacitracin
  eye, 593
  skin, polymyxin with,
    657
Back pain, 560
Baclofen, **585**
  palliative care, 17
Bacterial vaginosis, 291
*Bacteroides fragilis* infections
    antipseudomonal penicillins, in,
      301
    clindamycin, in, 315
    metronidazole, in, 327
*Bactigras*, 922
*Bactroban*, 657
*Bactroban Nasal*, 616
BAL, 34
Balanced Salt Solution, 604
Baldness
    androgenetic alopecia, 656
    cytotoxic drugs, 467
*Balneum* preparations, 627, 628
Balsalazide, 52, **54**
*Bambec*, 155
Bambuterol, **155**
Bandages, 926–30
*Baraclude*, 354
*Baratol*, 100
Barbiturates, **193**
    anaesthesia, 699
*Barkat*, 903
Barrier preparations, 629
Basal cell carcinoma, 652, 654
Basiliximab, **495**
    infusion table, 870
Bath additives
    antimicrobial with, 629
    coal tar, 642
    emollient, 628
*Baxan*, 303
*Bazetham MR* (tamsulosin), 456
BCG
    bladder instillation, 501
    vaccines, **673**
*BD Micro-Fine* products, 380
*BD Safe-clip*, 380
Becaplermin, **668**
*Beclazone* (beclometasone)
  preparations, 166
    Easi-Breathe—*discontinued*
Beclomethasone dipropionate
    asthma, 165–7
    formoterol with, 167
    nasal allergy, 613
    oral ulceration, 616
    ulcerative colitis, 52, **56**
Beclomethasone dipropionate *see*
  Beclometasone dipropionate
*Becodisks*, 167
*Beconase* preparations, 613
*Bedol*, 405
*Bedranol SR* (propranolol), 89
Bedsores, 629
Bee sting allergy preparations,
  175
*Begrivac*, 681
Belladonna, 41
Bemiparin, **127**
Bendrofluazide *see* Bendroflumethia-
zide

Bendroflumethiazide, **75**
    hypercalciuria, 542
    potassium with, 80
    timolol with, 93
*BeneFIX* (factor IX fraction), 142
*Benerva* (thiamine), 548
Benign fibrocystic breast disease,
  428
Benoxinate *see* Oxybuprocaine, **602**
Benperidol, **196**
*Benquil*, 196
Benzathine benzylpenicillin, 291, 295
Benzbromarone, 581
Benzhexol *see* Trihexyphenidyl
Benzalkonium, 655
    cetrimide with, 629
    chlorhexidine with, 627
    dimeticone with, 629
Benzocaine, 718
Benzodiazepines, 185
    anaesthesia, 704
    antagonist, 712
    anxiolytics, 191
    epilepsy, 264
    hypnotics, 186
    mania, 206
    muscle spasm, 585
    poisoning by, 32
    withdrawal, 185
Benzoic acid ointment, compound,
  659, 660
Benzoin tincture, compound, 182
Benzoyl peroxide, 647
    clindamycin with, 647
    hydroxyquinoline with,
      647
Benzthiazide, 75
    triamterene with, 79
Benzydamine, 616, **617**
Benzyl alcohol, presence of, 2
Benzyl benzoate, 662, **663**
Benzylpenicillin sodium, 295, **296**
    infusion table, 870
Beractant, **179**
*Berinert*, 178
*Beriplex P/N*, 141
*Besavar XL*, 455
Beta₂ agonists, 154
*Beta-Adalat*, 89
Beta-adrenoceptor blocking drugs,
  86
    angina, 87, 111
    anxiety, 191
    arrhythmias, 83, 87
    eye, 597, **598**
    heart failure, 88, 102
    hypertension, 87
    migraine, 251
    myocardial infarction, 87, 138
    poisoning by, 32
    thyrotoxicosis, 88, 393
    verapamil and, 119
Beta-adrenoceptor stimulants
    asthma, 154
    premature labour, 439
Beta-blockers *see* Beta-adrenoceptor
  blocking drugs
*Betacap*, 634
*Beta-Cardone*, 93
*Betadine* preparations, 667
*Betaferon*, 501
*Betagan*, 598
Betahistine, 226, **232**
Betaine, **557**
*Betaject Light* (interferon beta-1b), 501
Beta-lactamases, 295

*Betaloc* preparations, 91
Betamethasone, 394, 395, **398**
  mouth, 617
  skin, **634**
Betamethasone dipropionate
  skin, 634
    calcipotriol with, 641
    clotrimazole with, 635
    salicylic acid with, 634
Betamethasone sodium phosphate, 398
    ear, 609
    eye, 594
    infusion table, 870
    nose, 613, 615
    oral ulceration, 398
    rheumatic disease, 570
Betamethasone valerate
    skin, 634
      clioquinol with, 634
      fusidic acid with, 635
      neomycin with, 635
*Beta-Prograne*, 89
Betaxolol, **598**
Bethanechol
    laxative, 61
    urinary retention, **456**
*Betim*, 93
*Betnelan*, 398
*Betnesol*, 398
    ear, 609
    eye, 594
    mouth, 617
    nose, 613
    parenteral, 570
*Betnesol-N*
    ear, 609
    eye, 594
    nose, 615
*Betnovate* preparations, 634, 635
*Betoptic*, 598
*Bettamousse*, 634
Bevacizumab, **481**
    infusion table, 870
Bexarotene, **481, 482**
Bezafibrate, **147**
*Bezalip* preparations, 147
*Bi-Aglut*, 903
*Biatain* products, 917, 918
    silver with, 921
Bicalutamide, **508**
Bicarbonate
    intravenous, 532
    oral, 529
    see also Sodium bicarbonate
Biguanides, 382
Bile acid sequestrants, 145
Bilharziasis, 371
Biliary-tract infection, 290
Bimatoprost, **599**
    timolol with, 599
*Binocrit*, 519
*BiNovum*, 448
*Bioclusive*, 914
*Biorphen*, 276
Biosimilar medicines, 1
*Biotène Oralbalance*, 622
Biotin, 14, 547
*Biotrol* products, 923
*BioXtra*, 622
Biphosphonates *see* Bisphosphonates
Bipolar disorder, 207
Birthmarks, ACBS, 910
Bisacodyl, 60, 61
Bismuth chelate, 47
Bismuth subgallate, 67

Bisoprolol, **90**
    see also Beta-adrenoceptor
      blocking drugs
Bisphosphonates
    breast cancer, 506
    hypercalcaemia, 542
    osteoporosis, 419, 422
Bites
    animal, 293
    human, 293
    snake, 36
Bitters, 553
Bivalirudin, **129**
    infusion table, 870
Black triangle symbol, 11
Bladder
    blood clot dissolution, 461
    irrigations, 461
      cytotoxic, 461
*Blenderm*, 925
*Bleo-Kyowa* (bleomycin), 473
Bleomycin, **472**, 473
    infusion table, 870
Blepharitis, 591
Blepharospasm, 278
*Blisterfilm*, 914
Blood incompatibilities, 867
Blood products, 141, 142
*BM-Accutest*, 390
Body-surface, dosage and, 14
Body-weight, dosage and, 14
Boils, 665
*Bolamyn SR*, 383
*Bondronat*, 424
Bone metabolism, drugs affecting, 419
Bone tumours, analgesia, 233
*Bonefos*, 425
    concentrate—*discontinued*
Bone-marrow suppression, cytotoxic
    drugs, 467
*Bonjela* (choline salicylate), 618
*Bonviva* preparations, 424
Borderline substances *see* ACBS
Bortezomib, **482**
Bosentan, 95, **96**
*Botox*, 279
Botulinum
    antitoxin, 674
    hyperhidrosis, 668
    toxin type A, **278**, 279
    toxin type B, **279**
Botulism antitoxin, 674
Bowel
    cleansing preparations, 65
    irrigation, 28
    sterilisation, 311, 319
Bradycardia, 82
    anaesthesia, 703
*Bramitob*, 312
Bran, 60
Brand names, symbol, 1
*Brasivol*, 649
Breast
    cancer, **505**
      bone metastases, 422
      trastuzumab, 492
    pain, **431**
Breast-feeding, prescribing during, 852
*Breeze* products, 390
*Brevibloc*, 91
*Brevinor*, 448
*Brevoxyl*, 647
*Brexidol* (piroxicam), 568
*Bricanyl* preparations, 158

*Bridion*, 712
Brimonidine, **600**
    timolol with, 600
Brinzolamide , 600, **601**
    timolol with, 601
*BritLofex*, 284
*Broflex*, 277
*Brolene*, 593
Bromocriptine, 426, **427**
    acromegaly, 426
    galactorrhoea, 426
    hypogonadism, 427
    lactation suppression, 427
    neuroleptic malignant
      syndrome, 195
    parkinsonism, 268, **270**
    prolactinoma, 427
Bronchiectasis, 181
Bronchitis, 181, 290
    bronchodilators, 153
Bronchodilators
    adrenoceptor agonist, 154
    antimuscarinic, 159
    surgery, 697
    sympathomimetic, 154
    theophylline, 160
Bronchospasm, 154
Brucellosis, 308, 325
*Brufen* preparations, 566
*Brugia malayi*, 371
Bruxism, 233
BSA, 14
*Buccastem*, 228
Buclizine, 247
*Budenofalk*, 56
Budesonide, 167
    asthma, 165, **167**, 168
    Crohn's, 52, 56
    croup, 154
    formoterol with, 168
    inflammatory bowel disease,
      52, 56
    nasal
      allergy, 613
      polyps, 613
Bumetanide, 76, **77**
    amiloride with, 79
    infusion table, 870
Bupivacaine, **716**, 717
    adrenaline with, 717
Buprenorphine
    intra-operative analgesia, 238
    opioid dependence, 283, **284**
      naloxone with, 284
    pain, 237, **238**, 239
    palliative care, 16
    premedication, 238
Bupropion, 280, **281**
*Burinex*, 77
*Burinex A—discontinued*
Burns, infected, 657
*Buscopan* preparations (Hyoscine
    butylbromide), 42
Buserelin
    endometriosis, **430**
    IVF, **430**
    prostate cancer, **508**
*Busilvex*, 470
*Buspar*, 193
Buspirone, **192**, 193
Busulfan, 469, **470**
    infusion table, 870
Busulphan *see* Busulfan
Butobarbital, 193
Butobarbitone *see* Butobarbital, 193
*BuTrans*, 238

Index

Butyrophenones, 195
*Byetta*, 385

# C

C1-esterase inhibitor, **178**
*Cabaser—discontinued*
Cabergoline
   hyperprolactinaemia, 426, **428**
   parkinsonism, 268, **270**
*Cacit*, 423, 541
*Cacit D3*, 550
*Cadesorb*, 922
Cadexomer–iodine, 920
*Caelyx*, 473
*Cafergot*, 251
Caffeine
   analgesia, 234
   respiratory stimulant, 178
*Calaband*, 930
Calamine, 630
   coal tar with, 641
*Calceos*, 551
*Calchan MR* (nifedipine), 119
*Calcicard CR*, 116
*Calcichew*, 541
*Calcichew D3*, 551
*Calcichew D3 Forte*, 551
Calciferol, 549, 550
*Calcijex*, 550
Calcipotriol, 639, **640**
   betamethasone with, 641
Calcitonin, 420
   hypercalcaemia, **421**, 542
   infusion table, 870
   osteoporosis, **421**
Calcitriol, 549, **550**
   osteoporosis, 420
   psoriasis, 639, 640, **641**
Calcium
   colecalciferol with, 549, 550, 551
   ergocalciferol with, 549
Calcium acetate, 544
Calcium alginate dressings, 918, 920, 921
Calcium and vitamin D tablets, 549
Calcium balance, maintenance, 421
Calcium carbonate, 541, 542, 551
   antacid, 38
   disodium etidronate with, 423
   risedronate and colecalciferol with, 424
Calcium chloride, 541, 542
Calcium folinate, **468**, 516
   infusion table, 870
Calcium gluconate, 541, 542
   infusion table, 870
Calcium lactate tablets, 541
Calcium leucovorin *see* Calcium folinate
Calcium levofolinate, **468**
   infusion table, 870
Calcium phosphate, 551
Calcium polystyrene sulphonate, 528
*Calcium Resonium*, 528
Calcium salts, 541, 544
Calcium supplements, 541, 542
*Calcium-500*, 542
Calcium-channel blockers, 114
   angina, 115
   hypertension, 115
   poisoning by, 32
*Calcium-Sandoz*, 542
*Calcort*, 398
*Calfovit D3*, 551
Calluses, 651

*Calmurid*, 627
*Calmurid HC*, 633
*Calogen* preparations, 899, 900
*Caloreen*, 898
*Calpol* (paracetamol) preparations, 235
*Calprofen* (ibuprofen), 565
*Calshake*, 900
*Camcolit*, 208
Camouflaging preparations, 654
*Campral EC*, 280
*Campto*, 491
Campylobacter enteritis, 290, 312
*Cancidas*, 335
Candesartan, 107, 108
Candidiasis, 332
   intestinal, 333
   oropharyngeal, 332, 618
   perianal, 67
   skin, 659
   systemic, 332
   vaginal, **441**
   vulval, 441
Candidosis *see* Candidiasis
*Canesten*
   anogenital, 442
   ear, 610
   *HC*, 633
   *Internal Cream* (clotrimazole), 442
   skin, 660
Cannabis, regulations, 8
*Capasal*, 655
*Capastat*, 323
Capecitabine, 474, **476**, 477
Capillary-action dressings, 919
*Caplenal* (allopurinol), 582
*Capoten*, 104
*Capozide*, 104
Capreomycin, **323**
*Caprin* (aspirin)
   analgesia, 234
   antiplatelet, 135
Caps, contraceptive, 454
Capsaicin, 589
   diabetic neuropathy, 389, 589
   neuropathic pain, 246
   osteoarthritis, 559, 589
   postherpetic neuralgia, 247, 589
*Capto-co* (co-zidocapt), 104
Captopril, **103**, 104
   hydrochlorothiazide with, 104
   *see also* ACE inhibitors
*Carace* preparations, 105
*Caramet CR*, 273
*Carbagen SR*, 255
*Carbaglu*, 556
*Carbalax*, 64
Carbamazepine
   bipolar disorder, 206
   diabetes insipidus, 417
   diabetic neuropathy, 389
   epilepsy, **254**, 255
   poisoning, elimination, 28
   trigeminal neuralgia, 247
Carbapenems, 306
Carbetocin, 434, **435**
Carbimazole, 392, **393**
Carbocisteine, **181**
*Carbo-Dome*, 642
*CarboFLEX*, 919
Carbomers, 603
*Carbomix*, 28
Carbon monoxide poisoning, 35
Carbonic anhydrase inhibitors, 80
   glaucoma, 600

*Carbopad VC*, 919
Carboplatin, **485**
   infusion table, 870
Carboprost, 435
Carbuncle, 665
Carcinoid tumour, 499, 511
*Cardene* preparations, 118
Cardiac arrest
   *see* Cardiopulmonary resuscitation
Cardiac glycosides, 72
   arrhythmias, 82
Cardiac problems, dental practice, 22
Cardiac *see also* Heart
*Cardicor*, 90
*Cardioplen XL* (felodipine), 117
Cardiopulmonary resuscitation, 125
   chart, *inside back cover*
Cardiovascular disease
   angina, 110
   myocardial infarction, 137
   prediction charts, *inside back cover*
   prevention
      antiplatelet therapy, 133
      diabetes, 94
      dyslipidaemia, 143
      hypertension, 93
      non-drug treatment, 93, 142
      obesity, 93
   risk assessment, 143
*Cardioxane*, 467
*Cardura* preparations, 100
Carglumic acid, 556
*Carisoma—discontinued*
Carmellose
   eye, **603**
   mouth, 616, **617**
Carmustine, **470**
Carnitine, 554
*Carnitor*, 554
*Carobel, Instant*, 903
Carpal tunnel syndrome, 569
Carteolol, **598**
*Carticaine see* Articaine, 714
Carvedilol, 87, **90**
   *see also* Beta-adrenoceptor blocking drugs
Cascara, 61
*Casilan-90*, 894
*Casodex*, 508
Caspofungin, 332, 334, **335**
   infusion table, 871
Castor oil, 61
*Catapres*, 98
Catarrh, vernal, 595
Catechol-*O*-methyltransferase inhibitors, 275
Catheter maintenance, 461
Catheter patency solutions
   chlorhexidine, 461
   sodium chloride, 461
   solution G, 461
   solution R, 461
Cautionary and advisory labels, 932
   also, *inside back cover*
   counselling, 932
   list of products, 934
   NCL, 932
   original packs, 932
*Caverject* preparations, 463
*Cavi-Care*, 918
*CCNU* (lomustine), 471
*Ceanel Concentrate*, 655
*Cedocard Retard—discontinued*
Cefaclor, 302, **303**

Cefadroxil, 302, **303**
Cefalexin, 302, **303**, 304
Cefixime, 303, **304**
Cefotaxime, 302, **304**
   infusion table, 871
Cefpodoxime, 303, **304**
Cefradine, 302, **304**, 305
   infusion table, 871
Ceftazidime, 302, **305**
   eye, 603
   infusion table, 871
Ceftriaxone, 302, **305**, 306
   infusion table, 871
Cefuroxime, 302, **306**
   eye, 603
   infusion table, 871
Cefuroxime axetil, 302, 306
*Celance*, 270
*Celebrex*, 563
Celecoxib, 561, **562**, 563
*Celectol*, 90
*Celevac*, 60
Celiprolol, 87, **90**
   *see also* Beta-adrenoceptor
      blocking drugs
*CellCept*, 494
*Cellona*, 929
Cellulitis, 292
*Celluvisc*, 603
*Celsentri*, 348
*Central Gard*, 915
Central nervous system stimulants,
   220
*Centyl K*, 80
Ceph... *see also* Cef...
Cephalosporins, 302
*Ceporex*, 304
*Ceprotin* (protein C concentrate), 142
*Cepton*, 666
*Cerazette*, 450
*Cerdak* products, 919
Cerebral oedema, 395
*Cerezyme*, 554
*Cernevit*, 539
*Cerubidin* (daunorubicin), 473
*Cerumol*, 611
*Cervarix*, 680
Cetirizine, **171**, 172
*Cetraben*, 626, 628
Cetrimide, 629, 665, **667**
   benzalkonium with, 629
   chlorhexidine with, 666
   dimeticone with, 629
Cetrorelix, **428**, 429
*Cetrotide*, 429
Cetuximab, 482, **483**
CFCs, 155, 165
*Champix*, 283
Charcoal, activated
   dressings, 919, 921
   poisoning, use in, **28**
*Charcodote*, 28
Cheilitis, angular, 619
   bacterial infection, 658
   fungal infection, 659
   inflammation, 631
*Chemydur*, 114
Chickenpox, 349
   corticosteroids, caution in, 396
Chilblains, 668
Children
   adverse reactions, 14
   medicine storage, 3
   prescribing for, 13
Child-resistant containers, 3
*Chirocaine*, 717

*Chlamydia*
   eye, 591
   genital, 291
   macrolides, in, 312
   quinolones, in, 328
   tetracyclines, in, 308
*Chloractil* (chlorpromazine), 196
Chloral betaine *see* Cloral betaine,
   189
Chloral hydrate, **188**, 189
Chlorambucil, 469, **470**
Chloramphenicol, **315**, 316
   ear, 608, **610**
   eye, 591, **592**
   infusion table, 871
   skin, hydrocortisone with, 649
*Chloraprep*, 666
Chlordiazepoxide, 191, **192**
Chlorhexidine, 665, 666
   benzalkonium with, 627
   bladder infections, 461
   cetrimide with, 666
   dressing, gauze, 922
   hydrocortisone and nystatin
      with, 633
   mouth, 616, **620**, 621
   neomycin with, 616
   nose, 616
   skin disinfection, 666
      dusting powder, 666
Chlorine poisoning, 35
Chlormethiazole *see* Clomethiazole
Chlorofluorocarbon propellants, 155,
   165
*Chlorohex*, 620
*Chloromycetin*, 592
Chloroquine, 363
   malaria
      prophylaxis, 359–61, **362**
      treatment, 359, **362**
   proguanil with, 363
   rheumatic disease, 570, 573
Chloroxylenol, 668
Chlorphenamine, 171, **173**
Chlorpheniramine *see* Chlorphenamine, 171, **173**
Chlorpromazine, 195, **196**
   hiccup, 196
   nausea, **227**
   nausea and vertigo, 225
   psychosis, 195
Chlorpropamide, **381**, 382
   diabetes insipidus, 417
Chlortalidone, **75**, 76
   atenolol with, 89
   diabetes insipidus, 417
   triamterene with, 80
Chlorthalidone *see* Chlortalidone
Cholecalciferol *see* Colecalciferol
Cholera vaccine, **674**
   travel, 695
*Cholestagel*, 146
Cholestyramine *see* Colestyramine
Choline, 547
Choline salicylate
   dental gel, 617, **618**
Cholinergic crises, 583
Cholinesterase inhibitors, 583, 711
*Choragon*, 413
Choreas, 277
Choriocarcinoma, 474
Choriogonadotropin alfa, **413**, 414
Chorionic gonadotrophin, **413**
Chronic eosinophilic leukaemia,
   487
Chronic myeloid leukaemia, 487

Chronic obstructive pulmonary
   disease, 153, 178
   oxygen, 179, 180
*Cialis*, 464
*Cibral 60XL* (isosorbide mononitrate),
   114
*Cica-Care*, 922
*Cicafem*, 650
Ciclesonide, **168**
Ciclosporin
   aplastic anaemia, 517
   eczema, 644, **645**
   immunosuppression, **495**, 496
   infusion table, 871
   nephrotic syndrome, 495
   psoriasis, 644, **645**
   rheumatic disease, **574**
   ulcerative colitis, 52, **57**
Cidofovir, **351**
   infusion table, 871
*Cidomycin*, 311
Cigarette smoking, 280
Cilastatin, imipenem with, 306, 307
   infusion table, 874
Cilazapril, **104**
   *see also* ACE inhibitors
*Cilest*, 448
Cilostazol, 121, **122**
*Ciloxan*, 592
*Ciltech*, 922
Cimetidine, **45**
Cinacalcet, 421, 542, **543**
Cinchocaine [ingredient], 68
Cinnarizine, 226
   dimenhydrinate with, 226
   nausea and vertigo, 226
*Cipralex*, 216
*Cipramil*, 216
Ciprofibrate, **147**
Ciprofloxacin, 328, **329**
   Crohn's disease, 53
   ear, 611
   eye, 591, **592**
   travellers' diarrhoea, 50
*Ciproxin*, 329
*Circadin*, 190
Cisatracurium, 709, **710**
   infusion table, 871
Cisplatin, **485**, 486
   infusion table, 871
Citalopram, **215**, 216
*Citanest*, 717
   with Octapressin, 717
*CitraFleet*, 66
*Citramag*, 65
Cladribine, 475, **477**
   infusion table, 871
*Clairette*, 650
*Clarelux*, 635
Clarithromycin, 312, **314**
   infusion table, 871
*Clarosip—discontinued*
Classification changes, xii
*Clasteon*, 425
Clavulanic acid, 298
   amoxicillin with, 298, 299
      infusion table (co-amoxi-
         clav), 871
   ticarcillin with, 301, 302
      infusion table, 878
*Cleanlet Fine*, 380
Cleansers, skin, 665
Clemastine, **173**
*Clenil Modulite*, 167
*Clexane* preparations, 128
*Climagest*, 403

*Climanor*, 408
*Climaval*, 405
*Climesse*, 403
Clindamycin, **315**
  acne, 648
  benzoyl peroxide with, 647
  infusion table, 871
  malaria treatment, 358
  oral infections, 315
  pneumocystis pneumonia, 368
  vaginal infections, 443
*CliniFast*, 927
*CliniLite*, 928
*Clinimix* preparations, 535
*Clinipak* syringe, 380
*CliniPlus*, 928
*Clinipore*, 925
*Clinisorb*, 919
*Clinistix*, 391
*Clinitar*, 642
  shampoo, 655
*Clinitas*, 604
*Clinitek Microalbumin*, 391
*Clinitest*, 391
*ClinOleic*, 535
*Clinorette*, 403
*Clinutren* preparations
  enteral feed, 883
  nutritional supplement, 888, 890
Clioquinol
  ear, 608, 609, **610**
  skin
    betamethasone with, 634
    fluocinolone with, 636
*Clipper*, 56
CLL *see* Leukaemia, chronic lympho-
  cytic, 469, 474
Clobazam
  anxiety, 191, **265**
  epilepsy, 254, 264, **265**
Clobetasol propionate, 635
Clobetasone butyrate
  skin, 635
  tetracycline with, 635
Clodronate sodium *see* Sodium
  clodronate
Clofarabine, 475, **477**
  infusion table, 871
Clofazimine, **326**
Clomethiazole, **189**
  alcohol withdrawal, 280
*Clomid*, 413
Clomifene, **412**, 413
Clomiphene *see* Clomifene, **412**, 413
Clomipramine, 210, **211**
Clonazepam, 264, 265
  epilepsy, 254, **265**
    status epilepticus, 265, **266**
  infusion table, 871
Clonidine
  hypertension, **98**
  menopausal flushing, 252, 400
  migraine, 251, **252**
  Tourette syndrome, 277
Clopamide, 75
  pindolol with, 92
Clopidogrel, 134, **135**, 136
*Clopixol*, 199, 206
*Clopixol Acuphase*, 199
*Clopixol Conc.*, 206
Cloral betaine, 189
*Clostridium botulinum*, 674
*Clostridium difficile*, 53
  antibacterial therapy, 290
    metronidazole in, 327
    vancomycin in, 316

*Clotam Rapid*, 248
Clotrimazole
  anogenital, 442
  ear, 610
  skin, 659, **660**
    betamethasone with, 635
    hydrocortisone with, 633
Clozapine, 199, 200, **201**, 202
*Clozaril*, 201
Cluster headache, 252
CMV, 351
Coal tar, 638, 639, 641, 642
  calamine with, 641
  dithranol and salicylic acid with,
    643
  hydrocortisone with, 642
  salicylic acid with, 641
  scalp, 642, 655, 656
  zinc with, 642
Co-amilofruse, 79
Co-amilozide, 79
  atenolol with, 89
Co-amoxiclav, 298, **299**, 300
  infusion table, 871
  urinary tract infection, 331
*CoAprovel*, 108
*Cobalin-H* (hydroxocobalamin), 516
*Coban*, 928, 929
Co-beneldopa, **272**, 273
COC *see* Contraception, oral, com-
  bined, 443
Cocaine, 223
  local anaesthesia, 718
  poisoning by, 33
Co-careldopa, **273**, 274
  entacapone with, 274
Cockroft and Gault formula, 815
Co-codamol preparations, 235, 236
Co-codaprin preparations, 234
*Cocois*, 642
Co-cyprindiol, **650**
Cod liver oil
  zinc oxide with, 629
*Codalax* preparations, 61
Codeine
  aspirin with, 234
  buclizine with, 247
  cough suppressant, 182, **183**
  diabetic neuropathy, 389
  diarrhoea, 51
  pain, 237, **239**
  paracetamol with, 235, 236, 247
*Co-Diovan*, 110
*Codipar*, 235
Co-dydramol, 236
Coeliac disease, 540
  ACBS, 903
Co-fluampicil, 298, **301**
  infusion table, 871
Co-flumactone, 80
*Colazide*, 54
Colchicine, **581**
Cold sores, 661
Colds, 184, 549
  decongestants
    nasal, 614
    systemic, 184
Colecalciferol, 549, **550**, 551
  alendronic acid with, 423
  risedronate and calcium carb-
    onate with, 424
Colesevelam, 145, **146**
*Colestid*, 146
Colestipol, 145, **146**

Colestyramine, **146**
  diarrhoea, 51, **70**
  hypercholesterolaemia, 145
  hyperlipidaemias, 146
  pruritus, 70
*Colief*, 903
*Colifoam*, 57
Colistimethate sodium *see* Colistin
Colistin, **319**, 320
  eye, 603
  infusion table (Colistimethate
    sodium), 871
Colistin sulphomethate sodium *see*
  Colistin
Colitis
  *Clostridium difficile* infection, 53
  ulcerative, 52
Collodion
  definition, 624
  flexible, 665
Colloid dressings, 916, 921
Colloidal oatmeal, 626, 628
*Colofac* preparations (mebeverine), 42
*Colomycin*, 320
*Colpermin*, 43
Coma
  hyperglycaemic, 387
  hyperosmolar nonketotic, 387
  hypoglycaemic, 388
  hypothyroid, 392
  insulin, 387
  ketoacidotic, 387
Co-magaldrox, 39
*Combigan*, 600
Combined hormonal contraceptives,
  446
  *see also* Contraception
*Combivent*, 161
*Combivir*, 344
*Combur-3 Test*, 391
Co-methiamol, 236
*Comfeel* products, 916
*Comfifast* products, 927
*Comfigrip*, 926
*Compact*, 390
*Competact*, 386
*Complan Shake*, 891
Complementary medicine, 1
Compliance, 1
Compression bandages, 928
Compression hosiery, graduated, 930
*Comprilan*, 929
*Comtess*, 275
*Concerta XL*, 222
*Condyline*, 653
Condylomata acuminata, 652, 653
Congenital agammaglobulinaemia,
  replacement therapy, 690
Conjugated oestrogens
  HRT, 405
    levonorgestrel with, 403
    medroxyprogesterone with,
      403
  vaginal, 441
Conjunctivitis
  allergy, 595
  infection, 292, 591
Conn's syndrome, 78
*Conotrane*, 629
Constipation, 59
Contact lenses, 607
Containers, child-resistant, 3
Contents, iv
*Contiflo XL* (tamsulosin), 456
*Contigen*, 457
Continuous infusion devices, palliative
  care, 17

Contour products, 390
Contraception, 443
  devices, 452, 453, 454
    contraceptive caps, 454
    contraceptive diaphragms, 454
  implants, 451
  intra-uterine system, 451, 452
  oral, 443
    combined hormonal, 443
    emergency, 454
    missed pill, 444, 450
    progestogen-only, 449
    starting routines, 447, 449
    surgery, **445**, 449, 698
    travel, 444
  parenteral, 450, **451**
  perimenopausal, 402
  spermicidal, 452
  transdermal, 443, 449
    detached patch, 444
    starting routines, 447
Controlled drugs, 7
  see also preparations identified by [CD] throughout BNF
  travel abroad, 9
Conversion tables, inside back cover
Convulex, 263
Convulsions
  dental practice, 22
  febrile, 268
  poisoning and, 28
  see also Epilepsy
Coolie, 914
Copa products, 917, 918
Copaxone, 502
COPD see Chronic obstructive pulmonary disease
Copegus, 357
Co-phenotrope, 51
Co-prenozide, 92
Co-proxamol, 234
Coracten preparations, 119
Cordarone X, 84
Cordilox preparations, 120
Corgard, 92
Corlan, 617
Corn flour, 906
Corn starch, 906
Corneal ulcers, 591, 593
Coro-Nitro Pump Spray, 112
Corsodyl preparations, 620
Corticosteroids, 394, 397
  adrenal suppression, 395
  allergic emergencies, 176
  allergy, 395
    nasal, 612
  anaesthesia, 395, 697
  anaphylactic shock, 395
  aphthous ulcers, 616, **617**
  asthma, acute severe, 153
  blood disorders, 517
  breast-feeding, 397
  cancer, 494
  croup, 154
  ear, 608
  equivalent doses, 394
  eye, 591, 593
  gout, 581
  haemorrhoids, 67
  hypercalcaemia, 542
  immunosuppression, 494
  infections, caution in, 396
  inflammatory bowel disease, 52, 56
  myasthenia gravis, 583, 584

Corticosteroids (continued)—
  nasal
    allergy, 612
    polyps, 612
  neuropathic pain, 246
  osteoarthritis, 560
  pneumocystis pneumonia, 368
  pregnancy, 397
  proctitis, 57
  proctosigmoiditis, 57
  psychiatric reactions, 396
  replacement therapy, 394
  rheumatic disease, 569
  septic shock, 395
  side-effects, 397
  skin
    acne, 649
    eczema, 630, 637
    psoriasis, 631
    suitable quantities, 632
  surgery, 395
  thrombocytopenic purpura, 523
  ulcerative colitis, 56, 57
  withdrawal of, 396
Corticotrophin see Corticotropin, 413
Corticotropin, 413
Cortisol, 394
Cortisone acetate, 398
Co-simalcite [ingredient], 40
Cosmegen Lyovac, 473
CosmoFer, 515
Cosmopor E, 913
Cosopt, 601
Cosuric (allopurinol), 582
Co-tenidone, 89
Cotfil, 924
Co-triamterzide, 79
Co-trimoxazole, **320**, 321
  infusion table, 871
  pneumocystis pneumonia, 368
Cotton
  absorbent, 923
  gauze, 923
Cough suppressants, 182
Coumarins, 130
Counter-irritants, 588
Coverflex, 927
Covering creams, 654
Covermark preparations, 654
Coversyl preparations, 106
Cozaar preparations, 109
Co-zidocapt, 104
Crab lice, 663
Cradle cap, 655
Cramps, nocturnal, 587
Creams
  definition, 624
  suitable quantities, 625
Creatinine clearance, dosage and, 815
Creon preparations, 70, 71
Crestor, 145
Cretinism see Hypothyroidism, neonatal, 391
Crinone, 409
Crisantaspase, **483**
Crixivan, 345
Crohn's disease, 52
  fistulating, 53
Cromoglicate (or cromoglycate) see Sodium cromoglicate
Crotamiton, 630
  hydrocortisone with, 633
  scabies, 663

Croup, 154
Cryptococcosis, 333
Crystacide, 667
Crystapen, 296
CS gas see CS spray, 35
CS spray, 35
Cubicin, 318
Cuplex, 651
Curasorb products, 918
Curatoderm, 641
Curosurf, 179
Cushing's syndrome, 432
  corticosteroid-induced, 398
Cutaneous larva migrans, 371
Cuticell Classic, 913
Cutimed gel, 914
Cutimed Sorbact products, 922
Cutinova products, 917
Cutisorb LA, 913
Cutivate, 637
C-View, 914
CX Antiseptic Dusting Powder, 666
Cyanides, poisoning by, 34
Cyanocobalamin, 516
Cyanokit, 34
Cyclimorph, 243
Cyclizine, **226**
  ergotamine and caffeine with, 251
Cyclocaps
  beclometasone, 167
  budesonide, 167
  salbutamol, 157
Cyclogest, 409
Cyclohaler
  beclometasone, 167
  budesonide, 167
  salbutamol, 157
Cyclopenthiazide, 75, **76**
  amiloride with, 79
  oxprenolol with, 92
Cyclopentolate, **597**
Cyclophosphamide, 469, **470**
  infusion table, 871
  rheumatic disease, 574
Cycloplegics, 596
Cyclo-Progynova, 403
Cycloserine, **323**, 324
Cyclosporin see Ciclosporin
Cyklokapron, 141
Cymbalta, 218
Cymevene, 352
Cyproheptadine, **173**
  migraine, 251
Cyprostat, 509
Cyproterone acetate
  acne, 650
  male hypersexuality, **411**
  malignant disease, 508, **509**
Cystadane, 557
Cystagon, 556
Cysteamine see Mercaptamine, **555**, 556
Cystic fibrosis, 70
Cysticide, 371
Cystine amino acid supplement, 908
Cystinosis, nephropathic, 555
Cystinuria, 553
Cystitis, 460
  haemorrhagic, 469
  interstitial, 461
Cystrin, 458
Cytacon (cyanocobalamin), 516
Cytamen (cyanocobalamin), 516
Cytarabine, 474, **477**
  infusion table, 871

Cytokine modulators
  Crohn's disease, 58
  psoriasis, 644
  rheumatoid arthritis, 576
  ulcerative colitis, 58
Cytomegalovirus
  infections, 351, 593
*Cytotec*, 48
Cytotoxic drugs, 465
  alopecia, 467
  bladder instillation, 461
  bone-marrow suppression, 467
  dosage, 466
  extravasation, 466
  handling guidelines, 465
  hyperuricaemia, 466
  nausea and vomiting, 466
  pregnancy, 467
  regimens, 466
  thromboembolism, 467

# D

d4T *see* Stavudine, 340, **343**
Dabigatran, **132**
Dacarbazine, **483**
  infusion table, 871
Dactinomycin, 472, **473**
  infusion table, 872
*Daktacort*, 633
*Daktarin*
  oral gel, 619
  skin, 660
*Dalacin*, 315
  acne, 648
  bacterial vaginosis, 443
Dalfopristin, quinupristin with, **319**
  infusion table, 877
*Dalivit*, 552
*Dalmane*, 187
Dalteparin, **127**
Danaparoid, **128**, 129
  infusion table, 872
Danazol, 428, **429**
*Dandrazol* (ketoconazole), 655
Dandruff, 655
*Danlax*, 61
*Danol*, 429
Danthron *see* Dantron, 60, 61
*Dantrium*, 586
  *Intravenous*, 713
Dantrolene, **586**
  malignant hyperthermia, **713**
  muscle spasm, 585
  neuroleptic malignant
    syndrome, 195
Dantron, 60, 61
Dapsone, **326**
  dermatitis herpetiformis, 326
  leprosy, 326
  pneumocystis pneumonia, 368
  poisoning, elimination, 28
  pyrimethamine with, 361
Daptomycin, 317, **318**
  infusion table, 872
*Daraprim*, 365
Darbepoetin, 517, **518**, 519
Darier's disease, 640
Darifenacin, **457**
Darunavir, 340, **344**
Dasatinib, 486, **488**

Daunorubicin, 472, **473**
  infusion table, 872
*DaunoXome*, 473
*DDAVP* preparations, 419
DDI *see* Didanosine, 340, **341**, 342
De Vilbiss nebulisers, 164
*Deca-Durabolin*, 412
*Decan*, 539
*Decapeptyl SR*, 431, 510
Decongestants
  nasal, 615
  systemic, 184
Deep-vein thrombosis, 125, 130
DEET *see* Diethyltoluamide, 359
Defective medicines, 13
*Defenac* (diclofenac), 563, 564
Deferasirox, **522**
Deferiprone, **522**, 523
Deferoxamine *see* Desferrioxamine
Deflazacort, 394, **398**
Degarelix, **510**
*Delph*, 653
*Deltacortril Enteric* (prednisolone), 400
*Deltaprim*, 361
*Deltastab*, 570
Demeclocycline, **309**
  hyponatraemia, 419
Dementia, 285
Demulcent cough preparations, 184
Dendritic ulcer, 593
*De-Noltab*, 49
Dental Practitioners' Formulary, 947
Dental prescribing
  abscess, 292
  anaesthesia
    general, 698
    local, 714
    vasoconstrictors, 714
  angular cheilitis, 619
  anticoagulation, 25
  anxiety, 186, 704
  caries, prevention, 545
  chronic facial pain, 247
  denture stomatitis, 618
  dry mouth, 621
  endocarditis prophylaxis, 24
  fluoride, 545
  herpes labialis, 348, 661
  herpetic gingivostomatitis, 348
  hypnotic, 186, 704
  infections
    bacterial, 289, 292, 658
    fungal, 618, 659
    viral, 348, 620, 661
  medical emergencies, 21
  medical problems, 23
  neuropathic pain, 246
  oral hygiene, 620
  oral side-effects, 12
  oral ulceration, 616
  pain, 232, 233, 238, 561
    orofacial, 246, 561
    postoperative, 233
  panic attacks, 186, 704
  postherpetic neuralgia, 247
  premedication, 186, 704
  prophylaxis
    joint prostheses, 295
  sinusitis, 615
  temporomandibular
    dysfunction, 233
  trigeminal neuralgia, 247
  vitamin deficiency, 547
*Dentinox* colic drops, 40
*Dentomycin*, 618
Denture stomatitis, 618

*Denzapine*, 202
*Depakote*, 207
Dependence *see* Drug dependence
*Depixol* preparations, 197, 205
*DepoCyte*, 477
*Depodur*, 237
Depolarising muscle relaxants *see*
  Muscle relaxants
*Depo-Medrone*, 399, 570
  with *Lidocaine*, 570
*Deponit*, 112
*Depo-Provera*, 451
  contraception, 450, 451
Depression, 208
  antipsychotics, 194
  manic, 207
*Derbac-M*, 664
*Dermabond ProPen*, 665
*Dermacolor* preparations, 654
*Dermalo*, 628
*Dermamist*, 626
*DermaSilk*, 927
*Dermasure* products, 923
Dermatitis
  ACBS, 910
  herpetiformis, 326, 903
  *see also* Eczema
*Dermatix* products, 922
Dermatophyte infections, 333
*Dermax*, 655
*Dermol* preparations, 627, 629
*Dermovate* preparations, 635
*Deseril*, 252
*Desferal*, 523
Desferrioxamine, **523**
  eye, 603
  infusion table, 872
  iron overload, 522
  poisoning, use in, 32, 33
Desflurane, **701**
Desloratadine, 171, **172**
Desloughing agents, 667
*DesmoMelt*, 419
Desmopressin, 417, **418**, 419
  fibrinolytic response, 417
  haemophilia, 140
  infusion table, 872
  nocturnal enuresis, **418**, 460
  von Willebrand's disease, 417
*Desmospray*, 419
*Desmotabs*, 419
Desogestrel
  contraception, 450
    ethinylestradiol with, 447,
      448
*Destolit*, 69
*Detrunorm* preparations, 459
*Detrusitol* preparations, 459
Dexamethasone, 394, 395, **398**, 399
  croup, 154
  inflammation
    ear, 609
    eye, 594, 603
  infusion table, 872
  nausea and vertigo, 225, 226
  nausea and vomiting, 466
  palliative care, 16, 17
  rheumatic disease, 570
  suppression test, 395
Dexamethasone sodium phosphate,
  399
Dexamfetamine, 220, **221**
Dexamphetamine *see* Dexamfetamine,
  220, **221**
*Dexedrine*, 221
Dexfenfluramine, 224

Dexibuprofen, 560, **563**
Dexketoprofen, 560, **563**
*Dexomon* (diclofenac), 564
Dexrazoxane, **467**
  infusion table, 872
*Dexsol* (dexamethasone), 399
Dextran
  eye, 604
  intravenous infusion, 533
*Dextrogel*, 388
Dextromethorphan, 182
Dextropropoxyphene, poisoning by, 31
Dextrose monohydrate *see* Glucose
*DF118 Forte*, 240
*D-Gam*, 694
*DHC Continus*, 240
*diabact UBT*, 44
Diabetes insipidus, 417
  diagnosis, 417
Diabetes mellitus, 373
  diagnosis, 391
  monitoring, 374
    ketone, 390, 391
    meters, 390, 391
    test strips, 390
Diabetic
  ketoacidosis, **387**, 530, 531
  nephropathy, 389
  neuropathy, 389
    skin ulcers, 668
*Diabur Test-5000*, 391
*Diacomit*, 254
*Diafalk*, 66
*DIAGLYK* (gliclazide), 382
*Dialamine*, 900
*Dialar* (diazepam), 191
*Diamicron* preparations, 382
Diamorphine, 237, **239**
  infusion table, 872
  morphine equivalence, 15
  pain, 237
    chronic, 16, 237
*Diamox* preparations, 601
*Dianette*, 650
Diaphragms, contraceptive, 454
Diarrhoea, 50, 528
*Diastix*, 391
*Diazemuls* (diazepam), 191, 266
Diazepam, **191**
  anaesthesia, 704, **705**
  anxiety, 191
  febrile convulsions, 268
  hypnotic, 187
  infusion table, 872
  muscle spasm, 233, 585, 586
  palliative care, 17
  status epilepticus, 265, **266**
  temporomandibular dysfunction, 233
*Diazepam Rectubes*, 191, 266
Diazoxide
  hypertension, 95, **96**
  hypoglycaemia, **388**
*Dibenyline*, 101
Dibucaine *see* Cinchocaine, 68
Diclofenac, **563**, 564
  actinic keratosis, 654
  eye, 605
  gout, 581
  infusion table, 872
  misoprostol with, 564
  postoperative pain, 706
  rheumatic disease, 560, 563
  topical, 589
  ureteric colic, 460, 563

*Dicloflex* (diclofenac), 563, 564
*Diclomax* (diclofenac), 564
*Diclozip* (diclofenac), 563
Dicobalt edetate, **34**
Dicyclomine *see* Dicycloverine, **41**, 42
Dicycloverine, **41**, 42
*Dicynene*, 140
Didanosine, 340, **341**, 342
*Didronel* preparations, 423
Dienogest, estradiol with, 449
*Dietary Specialities*, 904
Diethylcarbamazine, 371
Diethylpropion, 224
Diethylstilbestrol, **504**, 508
Diethyltoluamide, 359
*Differin*, 648
*Difflam*, 617
*Diffundox XL* (tamsulosin), 456
*Diflucan* preparations, 335
Diflucortolone valerate, 635, 636
*Digibind*, 74
Digital ulcer disease, 95
Digitoxin, **73**
Digoxin, 72, **73**
  heart failure, 102
  infusion table, 872
Digoxin-specific antibody fragments, 73, **74**
  infusion table, 872
Dihydrocodeine, 237, **239**, 240
  paracetamol with, 236
Dihydropyridine calcium-channel blockers, 114
Dihydrotachysterol, 549, **551**
Dihydroxycholecalciferol, 549, 550, 641
*Dilcardia SR*, 116
Diloxanide furoate, **366**
Diltiazem, **115**, 116, 117
  anal fissure, 68
  poisoning by, 32
  *see also* Calcium-channel blockers
*Dilzem* preparations, 116
Dimenhydrinate, cinnarizine with, 226
Dimercaprol, **34**, 35
Dimethicone, activated *see* Simeticone, 39, 40
Dimethyl sulfoxide
  idoxuridine with, 662
  interstitial cystitis, 461
Dimethyl sulphoxide *see* Dimethyl sulfoxide
Dimeticone, **663**
  benzalkonium with, 629
  cetrimide with, 629
  zinc oxide with, 629
  zinc with, 630
Dimeticone, activated *see* Simeticone, 39, 40
*Dimetriose*, 429
Dinoprostone, 434, 435, 436
  infusion table, 872
*Dioctyl*, 62
Dioctyl sodium sulphosuccinate *see* Docusate sodium
*Dioderm*, 633
*Dioralyte* preparations, 529
*Diovan*, 110
*Dip/Ser*, 676
*Dipentum*, 55
*Dipeptiven*, 539
Diphenoxylate, 51, 237
  *see also* Analgesics, opioid
Diphenylbutylpiperidines, 195
Diphosphonates *see* Bisphosphonates

Diphtheria
  antibacterial
    prophylaxis, 293
    treatment, 295
  antitoxin, 676
  immunisation
    travel, 675
    vaccines, 674
    vaccines, combined, **675**
Dipipanone, 237, **240**
  cyclizine with, 240
Dipivefrine, **600**
*Diprivan*, 700
*Diprobase*, 626
*Diprobath*, 628
*Diprosalic*, 634
*Diprosone*, 634
Dipyridamole, 134, **136**
  aspirin with, 136
Discontinued preparations, xii
Disease-modifying antirheumatic drugs *see* DMARDs
Disfiguring skin lesions, ACBS, 910
Disinfectants, 665
  ACBS, 910
*Disipal*, 276
*Diskhaler*
  *Becodisks*, 167
  *Flixotide*, 169
  *Relenza*, 356
  *Serevent*, 158
Disodium clodronate *see* Sodium clodronate
Disodium cromoglicate *see* Sodium cromoglicate
Disodium etidronate, 419, 423
  calcium carbonate with, 423
Disodium folinate, **468**
  infusion table, 872
Disodium levofolinate, **468**, 469
  infusion table, 872
Disodium pamidronate, 423, 424
  infusion table, 872
Disopyramide, **84**, 85
  infusion table, 872
*Disprol* (paracetamol) preparations, 235
*Distaclor* preparations, 303
*Distamine*, 572
Distigmine
  laxative, 61
  myasthenia gravis, 583, 584
  urinary retention, 456, **457**
Disulfiram, 279, **280**
Dithranol, 639, **642**, 643
  coal tar and salicylic acid with, 643
  salicylic acid and zinc with, 642
*Dithrocream*, 642
*Ditropan*, 459
*Diumide-K Continus*, 80
Diuretics
  carbonic anhydrase inhibitors, 80
  heart failure, 102
  loop, 76
  mercurial, 80
  osmotic, 80
  potassium with, 80, 527
  potassium-sparing, 78
    with other diuretics, 79
  *see also* Thiazides
*Diurexan*, 76
*Diva*, 650
Diverticular disease, 41, **53**
*Dixarit*, 252

DMARDs (disease-modifying anti-
  rheumatic drugs), 559, 570
DMPS see Unithiol, 34
DMSA see Succimer, 34
Dobutamine, **123**
  infusion table, 872
Docetaxel, **490**
  infusion table, 872
Docusate sodium
  ear, 611
  laxative, **61**, 62
Docusol, 62
Dolasetron, 225, **229**
  infusion table, 872
Dolmatil, 199
Domette bandage, 926
Domperidone, 228
  diabetic neuropathy, 389
  gastro-intestinal, 43
  migraine, 251
  nausea and vomiting, 225
    cytotoxic drugs, 466
    palliative care, 16
Donepezil, 285, **286**
Dopacard, 124
Dopamine, **123**
  infusion table, 872
Dopamine receptor agonists
  parkinsonism, 268
Dopaminergic drugs
  endocrine, 426
  parkinsonism, 268
Dopexamine, **123**, 124
  infusion table, 873
Dopram, 179
Doralese, 456
Doribax, 306
Doripenem, **306**
  infusion table, 873
Dornase alfa, 182
Dorzolamide, 600, **601**
  with timolol, 601
Dose changes, xi
Doses, 2
  children, 14
  elderly, 20
  liver disease, 804
  renal impairment, 815
Dostinex, 428
Dosulepin, 210, **211**, 212
DOT, 322
Dothiepin see Dosulepin, 210, **211**,
  212
Doublebase preparations, 626, 628
Dovobet, 641
Dovonex preparations, 640
Doxadura (doxazosin) preparations,
  100
Doxapram, **178**, 179
  respiratory depression, 178
Doxazosin
  cardiovascular, **99**, 100
  urinary tract, **455**
Doxepin, 210, **212**
  topical, 630
Doxorubicin, 472, **473**
  bladder, 461
  infusion table, 873
Doxycycline, **309**
  acne, 649
  aphthous ulcers, **617**
  Lyme disease, 298
  malaria
    prophylaxis, 359, 360, 361,
      362, **366**
    treatment, 358

malaria (continued)—
  mouth, 617
  oral infections, 308
  periodontitis, 617
  rosacea, 647
Doxylar (doxycycline), 309
Dozic, 197
Drapolene, 629
Dressing packs, 924, 926
Dressings
  absorbent, 911
  advanced, 911
  low adherence, 911
Dressit, 924
Driclor, 668
Dried prothrombin complex, 131, **141**
Drisorb, 923
Driver and Vehicle Licensing Agency,
  inside front cover
Driving and drugs, 3
Drogenil—discontinued
Dromadol preparations, 245
Droperidol, 225, **227**
Drospirenone
  contraception
    ethinylestradiol with, 449
  HRT, estradiol with, 403
Drotrecogin alfa (activated), **141**
Drug
  allergy, 171
  dependence, 7
    management, 279
  interactions, 720
  misusers, notification of, 9
Dry mouth, 621
  ACBS, 910
Duac, 647
Dual block, 711
Ductus arteriosus
  closure, 437
  patency, 437
Dukoral, 674
Dulcolax (bisacodyl), 61
Dulcolax (sodium picosulfate), 61, 62
Duloxetine
  depression, **218**
  diabetic neuropathy, **218**, 389
  generalised anxiety disorder,
    **218**
  urinary incontinence, 457, **458**
Duobar, 899
Duocal preparations, 899, 900
DuoDERM products, 916
Duodopa, 273
Duofilm, 651
DuoTrav, 600
Duovent preparations, 161
Duphalac (lactulose), 63
Duraphat preparations, 546
Durogesic DTrans, 241
Durolane, 560
Dusting powders, 625
Dutasteride, **411**, 412
Dyazide, 79
Dydrogesterone
  HRT, estradiol with, 404
  menstrual disorders, 407
Dyloject, 563
Dynastat, 707
Dysentery
  amoebic, 366
  bacillary see Shigellosis, 290
Dysmenorrhoea, 233
Dyspepsia, 37, 38
Dysport, 279
Dysthymia, 208

Dystonias, drug-induced, 276
Dytac, 78
Dytide, 79

# E

E numbers, inside back cover
E45 preparations, 626, 628
  Itch Relief, 627
  Sun, 653
EAA supplement, 908
Eakin products, 923
Ear
  infections, 608
  wax, removal, 611
EarCalm, 608
Easi-Breathe
  Qvar, 167
  Salamol, 157
Easifast, 927
Easifix products, 926
EasiGRIP, 926
Easiphen, 908
EasI-V, 915
Easyhaler
  beclometasone, 166
  budesonide, 167
  formoterol, 156
  salbutamol, 157
Ebixa preparations, 287
Ebufac (ibuprofen), 565
Ecalta, 335
Eccoxolac (etodolac), 564
Echinocandin antifungal drugs, 334
Echinococcosis, 370
Eclampsia, 543
Eclypse products, 913, 915
Econac (diclofenac), 563
Econacort, 633
Econazole
  anogenital, 442
  skin, 659, **660**
    hydrocortisone with, 633
  vaginal, 442
Econeb, 164
Ecopace (captopril), 104
Ecostatin
  anogenital, 442
  skin, 660
Ecstasy
  controlled drug, 7
  liquid (sodium oxybate), 33
  poisoning by, 33
ECT see Electroconvulsive therapy,
  208, 209
Ectopic beats, 81
Eculizumab, **523**
  infusion table, 873
Eczema, 637
  ACBS, 910
  ear, 609
Ednyt (enalapril), 104
Edronax, 219
Edrophonium
  anaesthesia, 711, **712**
  myasthenia gravis, 583, **584**
Eesiban, 926, 927
Efalizumab, 644
Efavirenz, 340, **346**, 347
  emtricitabine and tenofovir
    with, 343
Efcortesol, 399
Efexor preparations, 220
Effentora, 240
Effico, xii

*Efient*, 137
Eflornithine, **656**
Eformoterol *see* Formoterol
*Efudix*, 654
*Elantan* preparations, 113, 114
*Elaprase*, 555
Elastic adhesive
    dressing, 925
    plaster, 925
Elastic hosiery *see* Hosiery, elastic
*Elastoplast* products, 925, 928
*Eldepryl*, 275
Elderly
    diuretics and, 20
    hypertension in, 94
    prescribing for, 19
*Eldisine*, 480
Electroconvulsive therapy, 208, 209
*Electrolade*, 529
Electrolyte and water replacement
    intravenous, 530
    oral, 527
Electrolyte concentrations, 526
*Elemental-028* preparations, 883
Eletriptan, **248**
*Elidel*, 645
*Elleste Duet* preparations, 403
*Elleste Solo* preparations, 405
Elocon, 637
*Eloxatin*, 486
*Elset* products, 928
*Eltroxin* (levothyroxine), 392
*Eludril* preparations, 621
*Elyzol*, 618
*Emadine*, 596
*Emcor*, 90
Emedastine, **595**, 596
*Emend*, 231
Emergencies, dental practice, 21
Emergencies in the community, med-
    ical, *inside back cover*
Emergency
    contraception, 454
    supply of medicines, 6
*Emeside*, 256
Emesis, in poisoning, 28
*Emflex*, 562
*Emla*, 715
Emollients, 625
    eczema, 637
    psoriasis, 639
*Emollin*, 627
Emphysema, 153
*Emselex*, 457
Emtricitabine, 340, **342**
    efavirenz and tenofovir with,
    343
    tenofovir with, 343
*Emtriva*, 342
*Emulsiderm*, 629
Emulsifying ointment, 626, 627
Enalapril, **104**
    hydrochlorothiazide with, 105
    *see also* ACE inhibitors
*Enbrel* preparations, 579
Enbucrilate, 665
Encephalopathy, hepatic, 63
    drug usage, in, 804
*En-De-Kay* preparations, 545, 546
Endocarditis, 290, 311
    prophylaxis, 294
        dental practice, 24
Endometrial cancer, 504
Endometriosis, 407, 428
Endophthalmitis, 591
*Endoxana—discontinued*

*Ener-G*
    gluten- and wheat-free, 905
    gluten-free, 904
    low-protein, 905
*Energivit*, 899
Energy, intravenous nutrition, 539
Enfuvirtide, 340, **348**
*Engerix B*, 678
*Enmix Plus Commence*, 889
Enoxaparin, 127, **128**
Enoximone, **74**
    infusion table, 873
*Enshake*, 901
*Ensure Plus* preparations, 885, 888,
    889, 891
*Ensure* preparations, 887
Entacapone, **275**
*Entamoeba histolytica*, 366
Entecavir, 353, **354**
Enteral nutrition, 880
Enteric infections, 290
Enterobiasis, 369
*Entocort* preparations, 56
*Entonox*, 702
Enuresis, nocturnal, 460
*Enzira*, 681
Enzyme induction, 720
Enzymes, fibrinolytic, 138
*Epaderm*, 627
*Epanutin* preparations, 260
    *Ready Mixed Parenteral*, 268
*Epaxal*, 677
Ephedrine
    anaesthesia, **124**
    bronchospasm, **158**
    diabetic neuropathy, 389
    nasal congestion, 614, **615**
Epiglottitis, 290, 316
*Epiglu*, 665
Epilepsy, 254
    dental practice, 22
    driving, 253
    pregnancy, 253
    status epilepticus, 265
        non-convulsive, 266
    syndromes, 254
*Epilim* preparations, 263
*Epimaz* (carbamazepine), 255
Epinastine, 595, **596**
Epinephrine *see* Adrenaline
*EpiPen*, 177
Epirubicin, 472, **473**
    bladder, 461
    infusion table, 873
*Episenta* preparations, 263
*Episil* products, 914, 915
*Epistatus* (midazolam), 267
*Epivir*, 342
Eplerenone, **78**
Epoetin, 517
    alfa, **519**, 520
    beta, **519**, 520
    zeta, **519**, 520
Epoprostenol, 95, **130**
    infusion table, 873
*Eposin*, 480
*Eprex*, 520
Eprosartan, 107, **108**
Epsom salts *see* Magnesium sulphate
Eptacog alfa (activated), 141
*Eptadone* (methadone), 285
Eptifibatide, 111, 134, **136**
*Equanox*, 702
*Equasym* preparations, 222
*Erbitux*, 483
Erdosteine, **181**

Erdotin, 181
Erectile dysfunction, 409, 462
Ergocalciferol, **549**, 550
Ergometrine, 435, **436**
    oxytocin with, 436
Ergot alkaloids, 250
Ergotamine, 250
    caffeine with, 251
    cluster headache, 252
    cyclizine and caffeine with, 251
Erlotinib, 487, **488**
Ertapenem, 306, **307**
    infusion table, 873
*Erwinase*, 483
*Erymax*, 313
Erysipelas, 292
*Erythrocin*, 313
Erythromycin, 312, **313**
    acne, 648, 650
        isotretinoin with, 649
        tretinoin with, 649
    infusion table, 873
    rosacea, 647
*Erythroped* preparations, 313
Erythropoietins, 517
Escitalopram, 215, **216**
*Esmeron*, 710
Esmolol, 88, **90**, 91
    *see also* Beta-adrenoceptor
        blocking drugs
Esomeprazole, **48**
    infusion table, 873
Essential amino acids supplement,
    908
*Estracombi—discontinued*
*Estracyt*, 471
*Estraderm MX*, 405
*Estraderm TTS*, 405
Estradiol
    contraception
        dienogest with, 449
    HRT, 405, 406
        drospirenone with, 403
        dydrogesterone with, 404
        estriol and estrone with,
        406
        levonorgestrel with, 403,
        404
        medroxyprogesterone with,
        404, 405
        norethisterone with, 403,
        404, 405
    implants, 405
    vaginal, 441
*Estradot*, 405
Estramustine, 470, **471**
*Estring*, 441
Estriol
    HRT, 406
        estradiol and estrone with,
        406
    vaginal, 441
Estrone, estradiol and estriol with, 406
Estropipate, 406
Etamsylate, **140**
Etanercept
    psoriasis, 644, **646**
    rheumatic diseases, 576, **579**
Ethambutol, 321, 322, 323, **324**
Ethamsylate *see* Etamsylate, **140**
Ethanol, 539
    infusion table, 873
    poisoning, use in, 34
    *see also* Alcohol
Ethanolamine oleate, **149**
*Ethibide XL*, 76

Ethinylestradiol, 407
  acne *see* Co-cyprindiol, **650**
  contraception, 443
    desogestrel with, 447, 448
    drospirenone with, 449
    etonogestrel with, 447
    gestodene with, 447, 449
    levonorgestrel with, 448
    norelgestromin with, 449
    norethisterone with, 447,
      448
    norgestimate with, 448
  female hypogonadism, **407**
  HRT, **407**
  menstrual disorders, **407**
  prostate cancer, 504
Ethinyloestradiol *see* Ethinylestradiol
Ethosuximide, 254, **256**
Ethyl-2-cyanoacrylate, 665
Ethylene glycol, poisoning by, 34
Ethynodiol *see* Etynodiol, 450
Etidronate disodium *see* Disodium
  etidronate
Etodolac, 560, **564**
Etomidate, **699**
*Etomidate-Lipuro*, 699
Etonogestrel
  implant, 451
  vaginal ring, ethinylestradiol
    with, 447
*Etopan XL*, 564
*Etopophos*, 480
Etoposide, **479**, 480
  infusion table, 873
Etoricoxib, 561, **564**
  gout, 581
Etravirine, 340, **347**
Etretinate, 640
*Etrivex*, 635
Etynodiol, 450
*Eucardic*, 90
*Eucerin Intensive*, 627
*Eucreas*, 387
*Eudemine*
  hypertension, 96
  hypoglycaemia, 388
*Euflexxa*, 560
*Euglucon—discontinued*
*Eumovate*, 635
*Eurax*, 630
  *Hydrocortisone*, 633
European viper venom antiserum, 36
Evening primrose oil, 627
*Evista*, 407
*Evohaler*
  *Flixotide*, 169
  *Seretide*, 169
  *Ventolin*, 157
*Evoltra*, 477
*Evorel* preparations, 403, 405
*Evotrox*, 392
*Evra*, 449
Excipients
  details provided, 2
  skin preparations and, 625
  vaccines and, 669
*Exelderm*, 661
*Exelon* preparations, 287
Exemestane, 505, **506**
Exenatide, 384, **385**
Exfoliative dermatitis, 394
*Exforge*, 115
*Exjade*, 522
*Exocin*, 593
*Exorex*, 642
Expectorants, 184

*Exsu-Fast* products, 924
*Extavia*, 501
Extemporaneous preparation, 2
*Exterol*, 611
Extrapyramidal symptoms
  antipsychotics and, 194
  treatment, 276
Extravasation, 587
*Exu-Dry*, 913
Eye
  anaesthetics, local, 602
  antibacterials, 591
  antifungals, 593
  antivirals, 593
  contact lenses, 607
  cycloplegics, 596
  drops, 590
  glaucoma, 597
  inflammation, 593, 595
  lotions, 590
  microbial contamination, 591
  miotics, 601
  mydriatics, 596
  ointments, 590
  prostaglandins, 599
Ezetimibe, 146, **147**
  simvastatin with, 145
*Ezetrol*, 147

# F

*F16 Wave*, 164
*Fabrazyme*, 554
Fabry's disease, 554
Factor VIIa (recombinant), 141
Factor VIII fraction, 141
Factor VIII inhibitor bypassing
  fraction, 142
Factor IX fraction, 142
Factor XIII fraction, 142
Faecal softeners, 62
Fainting, dental practice, 23
Famciclovir, 349, **350**
Familial Mediterranean fever, 581
Famotidine, **46**
*Famvir*, 350
*Fanhdi* (factor VIII fraction), 141
*Fansidar*, 365
*Fareston*, 507
*Fasigyn*, 328
*Faslodex*, 506
*Fasturtec*, 582
Fat emulsions, intravenous, 539, 867
*Fate*, 905
*Faverin*, 217
Favism, 524
Febrile convulsions, 268
*Fectrim* (co-trimoxazole), 321
*Fefol*, 513
*FEIBA* (factor VIII inhibitor bypassing
  fraction), 142
Felbinac, 589
*Feldene* preparations, 568
    injection—*discontinued*, 588
    topical, 588
Felodipine, 115, **117**
    ramipril with, 107
    *see also* Calcium-channel block-
      ers
*Felogen XL* (felodipine), 117
*Felotens XL* (felodipine), 117

Felypressin, 714, 717
*Femapak*, 404
*Femara*, 507
*Fematrix*, 406
*FemCap* contraceptive cap, 454
*Femidom*, 443
*Femodene* preparations, 449
*Femodette*, 447
*Femoston* preparations, 404
*FemSeven* preparations, 404, 406
*Femulen*, 450
*Fenactol* (diclofenac), 563, 564
*Fenbid*
    *Forte Gel*, 588
    *Spansules*, 566
Fenbufen, 560, **565**
*Fendrix*, 679
Fenfluramine, 224
Fenofibrate, **147**, 148
Fenoprofen, 560
    pain, **565**
    rheumatic disease, **565**
*Fenopron* preparations, 565
Fenoterol, 154, **155**
    ipratropium with, 161
*Fenpaed* (ibuprofen), 565
*Fentalis* (fentanyl), 241
Fentanyl
    analgesia, 237, **240**, 241
      infusion table, 873
      palliative care, **16**
      perioperative, 707, **708**
*Fentazin*, 198
*Feospan*, 513
*Feprapax* (lofepramine), 212
*Ferinject*, 515
*Fermathron*, 560
Ferric carboxymaltose, 514, **515**
    infusion table, 873
*Ferriprox* preparations, 523
*Ferrograd* preparations, 513
Ferrous fumarate, 514
    folic acid with, 514
    vitamins with, 514
Ferrous gluconate, 514
Ferrous salts, 512
Ferrous sulphate, **513**
    ascorbic acid with, 513
    folic acid with, 513
*Fersaday*, 514
*Fersamal*, 514
Fertility
    female, 412, 413, 417
    male, 413
Fesoterodine, 457, **458**
*Feverfen* (ibuprofen), 565
Fexofenadine, 171, **172**
Fibrates, 147
*Fibrazate XL* (bezafibrate), 147
*Fibrelief*, 60
Fibrinolytic drugs, 138
*Fibrogammin P* (factor XIII fraction),
  142
*Fibro-Vein*, 149
Filaricides, 371
Filgrastim, xiii, **525**, 526
    infusion table, 873
*Finacea*, 647
Finasteride
    androgenetic alopecia,
      **656**
    benign prostatic hyperplasia,
      411, **412**
*Finepoint*, 380
Fingertip unit, 632
*Firazyr*, 178

*Firmagon*, 510
Fits *see* Epilepsy
*Flagyl* preparations, 327, 328
  intravenous infusion—*discontinued*
*Flamasacard*, 135
*Flamatak* (diclofenac), 564
*Flamazine*, 658
*Flaminal*, 922
*Flamrase* (diclofenac), 563, 564
*Flavour Mix*, 903
Flavouring preparations, 903
*FlavourPac*, 903
Flavoxate, 457, 458
*Flebogamma*, 692
Flecainide, 84, **85**
  infusion table, 873
*Fleet*
    *Phospho-soda*, 66
    *Ready-to-use enema*, 64
*Flexbumin* (albumin) preparations,
  533
*Flexi-Ban*, 929
Flexible collodion, 665
*Flexigran* products, 914, 916
*Flexi-T 300*, 453
*Flexi-T+ 380*, 453
*Flexoplast*, 925, 928
*Flexotard MR* (diclofenac), 564
*Flivasorb*, 915
*Flixonase* preparations, 613, 614
*Flixotide* preparations, 168
*Flolan*, 130
*Flomaxtra XL*, 456
*Florinef*, 394
*Flowfusor*, 666
*Floxapen* (flucloxacillin), 297, 298
*Flu-Amp* (co-fluampicil), 301
*Fluanxol*, 218
*Fluarix*, 681
*Fluclomix* (flucloxacillin), 297
Flucloxacillin, 296, **297**, 298
  ampicillin with [co-fluampicil],
  298, **301**
  ear infection, 609
  infusion table, 873
Fluconazole, 332, 333, **335**
  mouth, 618
Flucytosine, 333, 334, **335**, 336
*Fludara*, 477
Fludarabine, 474, **477**
  infusion table, 873
Fludrocortisone, **394**
  diabetic neuropathy, 389
Fludroxycortide, **636**
Fluid and electrolyte replacement,
  526
Fluid overload, liver disease, 804
Flumazenil, **712**, 713
  benzodiazepine poisoning, 32
  infusion table, 873
Flumetasone, **609**
Flumethasone *see* Flumetasone, **609**
Flunisolide, **613**
Fluocinolone acetonide, 636
  clioquinol with, 636
  neomycin with, 636
Fluocinonide, 636
Fluocortolone, **636**, 637
  [ingredient], 68
*Fluor-a-day*, 545
Fluorescein, 602, 604, **605**
  lidocaine with, 602
Fluoride, 545, 546
*FluoriGard* preparations, 545, 546
Fluorometholone, 594

Fluorouracil
  actinic keratosis, 654
  infusion table, 873
  malignant disease, 475, **477**, 478
  skin cancer, **654**
Fluoxetine, 215, **216**
Flupenthixol *see* Flupentixol
Flupentixol, **205**
  depot injections, **205**
  depression, **218**
  psychoses, 195, **197**, 205
Flupentixol decanoate, 205
Fluphenazine, 195
  depot injections, **205**
Flurandrenolone *see* Fludroxycortide,
  **636**
Flurazepam, 186, **187**
Flurbiprofen
  diabetic neuropathy, 389
  eye, 605
  pain, **565**
    postoperative, 706
  rheumatic disease, 560, **565**
  sore throat, 617, 618
Flutamide, 508, **509**
Fluticasone furoate, 614
Fluticasone propionate
  asthma, 165, **168**
  nasal allergy, 613, 614
  nasal polyps, 614
  salmeterol with, 169
  skin, 637
Fluvastatin, 143, **144**
*Fluvirin*, 681
Fluvoxamine, 215, **217**
*FML*, 594
Foam dressings, 917
Folate
  deficiency, 516
  rescue, 468
Folic acid, 516, **517**
  iron and, 513
  pregnancy, 513, 516
*Folicare* (folic acid), 517
Folinic acid
  rescue, 468
  *see* Calcium folinate
  *see also* Disodium folinate
Follicle-stimulating hormone, 413
Follitropin, **414**
  alfa, 414
    lutropin alfa with, 414
  beta, 414
Fomepizole, 34
Fondaparinux, **130**
  infusion table, 873
*Foodlink Complete* preparations, 892
Foods
  enteral, 880
  gluten-free, 903
  low-protein, 905
Foods for special diets, 540
  ACBS, 880
  vitamin supplements, 552, 553
*Foradil*, 156
*Foraven XL*, 220
*Forceval*, 552
Formaldehyde, 651, 652
Formoterol, 154, **155**, 156
  beclometasone dipropionate
  with, 167
  budesonide with, 168
Formulary
  Dental, 947
  Nurse, 950
*Forsteo*, 422

*Forticare*, 894
*Forticreme*, 892
*Fortijuce*, 888
*Fortimel*, 891
*Fortipine LA 40*, 119
*Fortisip* preparations, 889, 890, 891,
  892
*Fortral* (pentazocine), 245
*Fortum*, 305
*Fosamax* preparations, 422
Fosamprenavir, 340, **345**
Fosaprepitant, 225, **231**
  infusion table, 873
*Fosavance*, 423
*Foscan*, 486
Foscarnet, 351, **352**
  infusion table, 874
*Foscavir*, 352
Fosinopril, **105**
  *see also* ACE inhibitors
Fosphenytoin, **266**, 267
  infusion table, 874
  status epilepticus, 265
*Fosrenol*, 545
*Fostair*, 167
*Fostimon*, 414
*Fragmin*, 127
Framycetin
  ear, 609
  eye, 594
Frangula, 60
*Freebake* products, 904
*Freedom* products, 924
*FreeStyle* products, 380, 390
*Freeway Freedom*, 164
Fresh frozen plasma, 142
*Fresubin* preparations
  enteral feed, 881, 883, 884, 885
  nutritional supplement, 890, 892
Friars' Balsam, 182
*Frisium* (clobazam), 265
*Froben* preparations, 565
*Froop* (furosemide), 77
Frovatriptan, 248, **249**
Fructose, 539, 903
  presence of, 2
*Frumil* (co-amilofruse), 79
Frusemide *see* Furosemide
*Frusene*, 80
*Frusol* (furosemide), 77
FSH *see* Follicle-stimulating hormone,
  413
FTU *see* Fingertip unit, 632
*Fucibet*, 635
*Fucidin*, 316
  skin, 658
*Fucidin H*, 633
*Fucithalmic*, 592
*Full Marks*, 664
  lotion and mousse—*discontinued*
Fulvestrant, 505, **506**
Fungal infections, 332
  anogenital, 441
  eye, 593
  oral, 332, 618
  skin, 659
*Fungilin*, 619
*Fungizone*, 334
*Furadantin*, 332
Furosemide, 76, **77**
  amiloride with, 79
  infusion table, 874
  potassium with, 80
  spironolactone with, 80
  triamterene with, 80

Fusidic acid, 316
    angular cheilitis, 619
    eye, 591, **592**
    infusion gel, 874
    skin, 657, **658**
        betamethasone with, 635
        hydrocortisone with, 633
*Fuzeon*, 348
*Fybogel*, 60
*Fybogel Mebeverine*, 42

# G

G6PD deficiency, 524
    drugs to be avoided in, 524
*GA Gel*, 905
Gabapentin
    diabetic neuropathy, 389
    epilepsy, 254, **256**, 257
    neuropathic pain, 246, **256**
    postherpetic neuralgia, 247
    trigeminal neuralgia, 247
*Gabitril*, 261
*Gadsby's*, 904
Galactorrhoea, 427
Galantamine, 285, **286**
*Galcodine* preparations, 183
*Galenamox* (amoxicillin), 299
*Galenphol*, 183
*Galfer*, 514
*Galfer FA*, 514
Gallstones, 69
*Galpseud*, 184
Galsulfase, **555**
    infusion table, 874
*Galvus*, 387
*Gamgee Tissue*, 923
*Gammagard S/D*, 692
Gamma-hydroxybutyrate (sodium
    oxybate), 8, 33
Ganciclovir, **351**, 352
    eye infection, **593**
    infusion table, 874
*Ganfort*, 599
Canirelix, *128*, **429**
*Gardasil*, 680
*Gardnerella vaginalis*, 327
Gargles, 620
Gas cylinders, 698
Gas-gangrene
    prophylaxis, 293
    treatment, 295
Gastrectomy
    iron therapy, 512
    vitamin B₁₂, 515
Gastric emptying, poisoning and, 28
*Gastrocote*, 40
Gastro-enteritis, 50, 290
Gastro-intestinal procedures
    antibacterial prophylaxis, 293
Gastro-intestinal secretions
    electrolyte content, 526
Gastro-intestinal stromal tumour, 487
Gastro-oesophageal reflux disease, **38**
Gaucher's disease, 554
Gauze
    cotton ribbon, absorbent, 923
    swabs, 924
    viscose ribbon, absorbent cot-
        ton and, 923
*Gaviscon* preparations, 40
G-CSF, 525, 526
*Gel FX*, 914
Gelatin
    infusion, **533**, 534
    succinylated, 533, 534

*Geliperm*, 914
*Gelofusine*, 533
*Geloplasma*, 533
Gels, definition, 625
*GelTears*, 603
Gemcitabine, 475, **478**
    infusion table, 874
Gemeprost, 434, **436**, 438
Gemfibrozil, 147, **148**
*Gemzar*, 478
*Generaid* preparations, 894, 895
Generalised anxiety disorder, 209
Generic prescribing, 1
Genital warts, 652
*Genotropin* preparations, 415
Gentamicin, **311**
    ear, 610
    eye, 591, **592**, 603
    infusion table, 874
Gentian mixture, alkaline, xii
*Genticin*
    ear, 610
    eye, 592
    parenteral, 311
*Gentisone HC*, 610
German measles *see* Rubella
Gestodene, ethinylestradiol with, 447,
    449
*Gestone*, 409
Gestrinone, 428, **429**
GHB (sodium oxybate), 8, 33
Giant cell arteritis, 569
*Giardia lamblia*, 367
Giardiasis, 367
Gilles de la Tourette syndrome *see*
    Tourette syndrome, 277
Gingivitis, 620
    acute necrotising ulcerative
        antibacterial treatment,
            292, 327
    mouthwashes, 620
*Civitol*, 514
*Glamin*, 535
*Glandosane*, 622
Glatiramer, 501, **502**
Glaucoma, 597
    steroid, 594
*Gliadel*, 470
Glibenclamide, 381, **382**
*Glibenese*, 382
Gliclazide, 381, **382**
Glimepiride, **382**
Glipizide, 382
*Glivec*, 489
Glomerular filtration rate, dosage and,
    815
Glossopharyngeal neuralgia, 247
*GlucaGen HypoKit*, 388
Glucagon, **388**
    beta-blocker poisoning, 32
*Glucobay*, 385
Glucocorticoids
    equivalent doses, 394
    replacement therapy, 394
*GlucoGel*, 388
*GlucoMen* products, 380, 390, 391
*Glucophage*, 383
Glucosamine, **583**
Glucose, 531
    hypoglycaemia, 388
    infusion, 531
        potassium and, 531
        sodium and, 530
    intravenous nutrition, 539
    oral rehydration, 528
    presence of, 2

Glucose (*continued*)—
    special diets, 906
    tests
        blood, 389
        tolerance, 391
        urine, 391
Glucose 6-phosphate dehydrogenase
    deficiency, 524
    drugs to be avoided in, 524
Glucose syrup, hydrogenated, pre-
    sence of, 2
Glue ear, 611
*Glutafin*
    gluten- and wheat-free, 905
    gluten-free, 904
Glutaraldehyde, 651, 652
Glutaric aciduria, 905, 906
*Glutarol*, 652
Gluten, presence of, 2
Gluten-sensitive enteropathies, 903
Glycerol
    constipation, 61, 62
    glaucoma, 600
Glyceryl trinitrate
    anal fissure, **68**
    angina, 111, **112**, 113
    infusion table, 874
Glycine irrigation solution, **461**
Glycogen storage disease, dietary
    supplement, 906
Glycopeptide antibiotics, 316
*Glycophos*, 539
Glycoprotein IIb/IIIa inhibitors, 134
Glycopyrrolate *see* Glycopyrronium
    bromide
Glycopyrronium bromide
    hyperhidrosis, 668
    neostigmine with, 712
    palliative care, 18
    premedication, 703
*Glycosade*, 906
Glycylcycline antibiotic, 310
*Glypressin*, 419
*Glytrin Spray*, 112
GnRH *see* Gonadorelin, **417**
Goitre, 391
Gold, 570, 571
*Golden Eye Drops* (propamidine), 593
*Golden Eye Ointment* (dibromopropa-
    midine), 593
Golfer's elbow, 569
Gonadorelin, **417**
Gonadorelin analogues, 429
    malignant disease, 508
Gonadotrophin-releasing hormone *see*
    Gonadorelin, **417**
Gonadotrophins, 413
*Gonal-F*, 414
*Gonapeptyl Depot*, 431, 510
Gonorrhoea
    antibacterial treatment, 291
*Gopten*, 107
GORD *see* Gastro-oesophageal reflux
    disease, **38**
Goserelin
    endometriosis, 430
    IVF, 430
    malignant disease, 506, 508, **509**
Gout, 581
Gramicidin
    ear, 609
    eye, 592, 609
Granisetron, 225, **229**, 230
    infusion table, 874
*Granocyte*, 526
*Granuflex* products, 916

*GranuFoam see* Vacuum assisted closure products, 924
*GranuGel*, 914
*Granuflex* products, 917
Granulocyte-colony stimulating factor, 525, 526
Grass pollen allergy preparations, 175
*Grazax*, 175
Griseofulvin, 333, 334, **336**
  topical, 659, **660**
*Grisol AF*, 660
Ground-nut oil *see* Arachis oil
Growth factor, platelet derived, 668
Growth hormone, 415
  receptor antagonists, 416
*GTN 300-mcg*, 112
Guanethidine, **99**
Guillain-Barré syndrome, 690
*Gygel*, 452
*Gyne T*, 452
GyneFix, 453
*Gyno-Daktarin* preparations, 442
*Gyno-Pevaryl* preparations, 442

# H

*Haelan* preparations, 636
Haem arginate, **557**
  infusion table, 874
*Haemate P* (factor VIII fraction), 141
*Haemoctin* (factor VIII fraction), 141
Haemodialysis, 28
Haemolytic anaemia, 517
  G6PD deficiency, 524
Haemolytic disease of newborn, prevention, 693
Haemophilia
  blood products, 141, 142
  desmopressin, in, 417
*Haemophilus influenzae* type b (Hib), 676
  immunisation, **676**
    vaccines, 676
    vaccines, combined, 675
  prophylaxis, 293
Haemorrhage, 140
  abortion, 435
  gastro-intestinal, 45
  postpartum, 435
Haemorrhoids, 67
Haemostatics, 140
*HAES-steril*, 534
*Haldol*, 197
  depot injection, 205
*Haleraid*, 162
*Half-Beta-Prograne* (propranolol), 89
*Half-Inderal LA*, 89
*Half-Securon SR*, 120
*Half-Sinemet CR*, 274
Halibut-liver oil capsules, 547
Haloperidol, **197**
  hiccup, 196
  movement disorders, **277**
  nausea and vertigo, 225
  palliative care, 17, 18
  psychoses, 195, **197**, **205**
    depot injection, 205
Haloperidol decanoate, 205
Halothane, 701, **702**
*Halycitrol—discontinued*
Hansen's disease, 326
*Harifen* products, 905
*Harmogen*, 406

Hartmann's solution *see* Sodium lactate, intravenous infusion, compound
*Havrix* preparations, 677
Hay fever treatment
  systemic, 171
  topical, 612
*Hay-Crom* preparations (sodium cromoglicate), 596
*HBvaxPRO*, 679
HCG *see* Chorionic gonadotrophin, **413**
*HCU* products, 906
HCU products, 906
Head lice, 663
Headache, 233
  cluster, 252
  migraine, 247
Heaf test, 673
*Healthy Start* vitamins, 547
Heart failure, 101
  ACE inhibitors, 102
  beta-blockers, 88
  vasodilators, 102
Heart *see also* Cardiac
*Hedrin*, 663
Height-weight charts, 14
*Helicobacter pylori*
  eradication, **43**
  tests, 44
*Helixate NexGen* (factor VIII fraction), 141
Helminth infections, 369
*Hemabate*, 435
*Heminevrin*, 189
*Hemohes*, 534
Heparin, 125, **126**
  flushes, 129
  infusion table, 874
  low molecular weight, 127
  myocardial infarction, 137
Heparin calcium, 127
Heparin sodium, 126
Heparinoids
  thrombosis prophylaxis, 128
  topical, 668
Hepatic encephalopathy, 63, 311, 804
Hepatic *see also* Liver
Hepatitis A
  immunisation
    immunoglobulin, normal, 691
    travel, 695
    vaccine, 676, **677**
    vaccine, hepatitis B with, 677
    vaccine, typhoid with, 677, 678
Hepatitis B
  autoimmune
    corticosteroids, 395
    penicillamine, 553
  chronic, 353
  immunisation
    immunoglobulin, 692
    travel, 695
    vaccine, **678**, 679
Hepatitis C, chronic, 353
Hepatolenticular degeneration *see* Wilson's disease, 553
Hepatotoxicity, 804
*Hepatyrix*, 677
*Hepsera*, 354
Herbal medicines, 1
*Herceptin*, 492
Hereditary angioedema *see* Angioedema, hereditary
Heroin *see* Diamorphine

*Heron* products
  gluten- and wheat-free, 905
  gluten-free, 904
Herpes infections, 348
  eye, 593
  genital, 349
  immunoglobulin, 693
  mouth, 620
  skin, 661
*Herpid*, 662
Hetastarch, 533, **534**
*Hewletts*, 627
Hexamine *see* Methenamine, 331, **332**
Hexetidine, 621
*Hexopal*, 122
HFAs, 155, 165
HGH *see* Somatropin, 415, 416
Hib *see Haemophilus influenzae* type b vaccine
*Hibiscrub*, 666
*Hibisol—discontinued*
*Hibitane* preparations, 666
Hiccup, 196, 277
*Hiprex*, 332
Hirsutism, 650, 656
Hirudins, 129
*Hirudoid*, 668
Histamine H$_1$-antagonists, 171
Histamine H$_2$-antagonists, 45
*Histoacryl*, 665
Histoplasmosis, 333
Histrelin, xiii
HIV infection, 339
HNIG *see* Immunoglobulins, normal, 690, **691**, 692
Hodgkin's disease, 469, 483, 494
Homatropine, 597
Homocystinuria, 557
Honey, medical grade, 920
  impregnated dressings, 920
Hookworm infections, 371
Hormone antagonists
  hypersexuality, 411
  malignant disease, 505
Hormone replacement
  androgens, 409
  oestrogens, 400, **402**
    vaginal, 440
  progestogens, 400, 408
  surgery, 402
*Hormonin*, 406
Hosiery, elastic, 930
  accessories, 930
  anklets, 931
  compression values, 930
  knee caps, 931
*Hospicrepe* products, 927, 928
*Hospiform*, 926
HPV *see* Human papilloma virus, 679, **680**
*HRF*, 417
HRT, 400, 419
5HT$_1$ agonists, 247, **248**
5HT$_3$ antagonists, 225, 229, 230, 467
HTIG *see* Immunoglobulins, tetanus, 693
*Humalog* preparations, 377, 379
Human antihaemophilic fraction, 141
Human chorionic gonadotrophin *see* Chorionic gonadotrophin, **413**
Human factor VIII fraction, 141
Human factor IX fraction, 142
Human factor XIII fraction, 142
Human luteinising hormone *see* Lutropin alfa

Human menopausal gonadotrophins, 414

Human papilloma virus, vaccine, 679, **680**

Human prothrombin complex *see* Dried prothrombin complex, 131, **141**

*HumaPen* products, 380

*Humatrope*, 416

*Humira*, 579

*Humulin I*, 378

*Humulin M3*, 379

*Humulin S*, 376

Huntington's chorea, 277

*Hyalase*, 588

*Hyalgan*, 560

Hyaline membrane disease, 179

Hyaluronic acid, 560

Hyaluronidase, **588**

*Hycamtin*, 491

Hycanthone, 371

*Hycosan—discontinued*

Hydatid disease, 370

Hydralazine, 95, **96**, 97
  infusion table, 874

*Hydrea*, 484

*Hydrex*, 666

Hydrochlorothiazide, 75
  amiloride with, 79
  captopril with, 104
  enalapril with, 105
  irbesartan with, 108
  lisinopril with, 105, 106
  losartan with, 109
  olmesartan with, 109
  quinapril with, 107
  telmisartan with, 109
  triamterene with, 79
  valsartan with, 110

*Hydrocoll*, 916, 917

Hydrocolloid dressings, 916, 917, 922

Hydrocortisone, 395, **399**
  colitis, 57
  ear, 610
  eye, 594
  haemorrhoids, 67, 68
  mouth, 616, 617
  oral, 399
  parenteral, 399, 570
    infusion tables, 874
  pneumocystis pneumonia, 368
  replacement therapy, 394
  rheumatic disease, 570
  skin, 632, 633, 634
    chloramphenicol with, 649
    chlorhexidine and nystatin with, 633
    clotrimazole with, 633
    coal tar with, 642
    crotamiton with, 633
    econazole with, 633
    fusidic acid with, 633
    miconazole with, 633
    nystatin with, 633
    urea with, 633

*Hydrocortistab*, 570

*Hydrofilm* products, 914, 915

Hydroflumethiazide, 75
  spironolactone with, 80

Hydrofluoroalkane propellants, 155, 165

Hydrogel dressings, 913, 914, 917, 920, 921, 922

Hydrogen peroxide
  cream, 667
  mouthwash, 620, **621**
  solution, **667**

*Hydromol* preparations, 627, 628

Hydromorphone, 15, **241**
  morphine equivalence, 15

*Hydrosorb* products, 914

Hydrotalcite, 38, **39**

Hydrous ointment, 626

Hydroxocobalamin, **516**
  cyanide poisoning, 34

Hydroxycarbamide
  malignant disease, **484**
  psoriasis, 644
  sickle-cell disease, **521**, 522

Hydroxychloroquine, 570, **573**, 574

Hydroxycholecalciferol, 549, 550

Hydroxyethyl starch *see* Starch, etherified, 533, 534

Hydroxyethylcellulose, 603

Hydroxyquinoline
  benzoyl peroxide with, 647

Hydroxyurea *see* Hydroxycarbamide

Hydroxyzine, **173**, 174

*Hygroton*, 76

Hyoscine butylbromide, 41, **42**

Hyoscine hydrobromide, 232, 704
  nausea and vertigo, 226, **231**
  palliative care, 18
  premedication, 703, **704**

*Hypafix*
  adhesive tape, 925
  film dressing, 914

Hyperactive children, 220

Hyperaldosteronism, 432

*Hyperamine*, 535

Hypercalcaemia, 421, 422, 542

Hypercalciuria, 542

Hypercholesterolaemia, 142, 143, 145, 146, 147

Hyperemesis gravidarum, 226

Hyperglycaemia, 373
  coma, 387

*HyperHAES*, 534

Hyperhidrosis, 668

*Hypericum perforatum*, 209

Hyperkalaemia, 528

Hyperlipidaemia, 142

Hyperosmolar hyperglycaemic nonketotic coma *see* Hyperosmolar hyperglycaemic state

Hyperosmolar hyperglycaemic state, 387

Hyperparathyroidism, 542

Hyperphosphataemia, 544

Hypersensitivity *see* Allergy

Hypersexuality, 411

Hypertension, **93**
  ACE inhibitors, 102
  beta-blockers, 87
  calcium-channel blockers, 115
  crisis, 95
  diabetes, 94
  diuretics, 75
  elderly, 94
  malignant, 95
  poisoning and, 27
  pregnancy, 95
  pulmonary, 95, 130
  renal disease, 95
  systolic, 94

Hyperthermia
  malignant, 713
  poisoning and, 28

Hyperthyroidism *see* Thyrotoxicosis

Hypertonic sodium chloride, 182

Hyperuricaemia, 466, 581, 582

Hyperventilation, dental practice, 23

*Hypnomidate*, 699

Hypnotics, 186
  poisoning by, 32
  withdrawal, 185

*Hypnovel*, 706

Hypocalcaemia, 541

Hypodermic equipment, insulin, 379

Hypodermoclysis, 530, 588

Hypogammaglobulinaemia, 690

Hypoglycaemia, 375, 388
  acute, 388
  chronic, 388
  dental practice, 23

Hypogonadism, 409

*Hypoguard* products, 380, 390, 391

Hypokalaemia
  diuretics and, 75
  oral treatment, 527
  parenteral treatment, 531

*Hypolar Retard 20*, 119

*Hypoloc* (nebivolol), 92

Hypomagnesaemia, 543

Hyponatraemia, 530

Hypoparathyroidism, 549

Hypopituitarism, 394, 409, 413

Hypoproteinaemia, liver disease, 804

Hyposensitisation, 174

*Hypostop Gel*, 388

Hypotension
  poisoning and, 27
  sympathomimetics, 124

Hypothalamic hormones, 417

Hypothermia
  antipsychotics and, 195
  poisoning and, 27

Hypothyroidism, 391
  neonatal, 391

*Hypovase*, 100

Hypovolaemia, 532

Hypoxaemia, 179

Hypromellose, 603, 604

*Hypurin Isophane*, 378
  biphasic, 379

*Hypurin Lente*, 378

*Hypurin Neutral*, 376

*Hypurin Protamine Zinc*, 378

*Hytrin* preparations
  cardiovascular, 101
  urinary tract, 456

# I

Ibandronic acid, **424**
  infusion table, 874

*Ibugel*, 588

Ibuprofen
  pain, 560, 561, **565**, 566
    postoperative, 706
    topical, 588
  post-immunisation pyrexia, 670
  rheumatic disease, 560, **565**

Icatibant, **178**

*Ichthammol*, 637, **638**
  zinc with, 638

*Ichthopaste*, 930

Ichthyosis, 625

Idarubicin, 472, **473**, 474
  infusion table, 874

Idoxuridine, 349
  dimethyl sulfoxide with, 661, **662**

Idursulfase, **555**
  infusion table, 874

Ifosfamide, 469, **471**
   infusion table, 874
*Ikorel*, 121
*Il Pane di Anna* products, 904
Iloprost, 95, **97**
*Ilube*, 603
Imatinib, 487, **488**, 489
*Imdur*, 114
Imidapril, **105**
   *see also* ACE inhibitors
Imidazole antifungal drugs, 333
Imiglucerase, **554**
   infusion table, 874
*Imigran* preparations, 250
Imipenem, cilastatin with, 306, **307**
   infusion table, 874
Imipramine, 210, **212**, 457
Imiquimod, 652, 653
   actinic keratosis, **652**, 654
   genital warts, **652**
   malignant skin disease, **652**, 654
*ImmuCyst*, 501
*Immukin*, 501
Immune interferon *see* Interferon,
   gamma, 501
Immunisation, 669
   international travel, 695
   schedule, 671
Immunity
   active, 669
   passive, 672
Immunodeficiency, 690
   syndrome, acquired, 339
Immunoglobulins, **690**
   anti-D (Rh₀), 693, 694, 695
   antithymocyte, 495
   aplastic anaemia, 517
   hepatitis B, **692**
   myasthenia gravis, 583
   normal, 690, **691**, 692
   passive immunity, 672
   rabies, 692, **693**
   tetanus, 693
   thrombocytopenic purpura,
     idiopathic, 523
   varicella–zoster, 693
Immunostimulants, 498
Immunosuppressants
   malignant disease, 494
   myasthenia gravis, 584
   rheumatic disease, 570, 574
   skin disease, 643
   transplant rejection, 493
*Imodium* preparations, 52
Impetigo
   systemic treatment, 292
   topical treatment, 657
*Implanon*, 451
Impotence *see* Erectile dysfunction,
   409, 462
*Imuderm*, 628
*Imunovir*, 350
*Imuran*, 494
*Imuvac*, 681
*Inadine*, 921
Incontinence, urinary, 457
*Increlex*, 433
Indapamide, 75, **76**
   perindopril with, 106
Independent prescribing, 954
*Inderal* preparations, 88, 89
Indian hemp *see* Cannabis, 8
Indinavir, 340, **345**
*Indivina* preparations, 404
*Indocid PDA*, 438
*Indolar SR* (indometacin), 566

Indometacin
   ductus closure, **437**, 438
   gout, 581
   premature labour, 439
   rheumatic disease, 560, **566**
Indomethacin *see* Indometacin
Indoramin
   cardiovascular, 99, **100**
   urinary tract, 455, **456**
Industrial methylated spirit, 665
*Inegy*, 145
*Infacol*, 40
*Infanrix-IPV*, 675
*Infanrix-IPV+Hib*, 675
Infections
   amoebic, 366
   antisera, 672
   bladder, 331
     mycotic, 461
   ear, 608
   eye, 591
   fungal, 332
   helminth, 369
   immunoglobulins, 690
   nail, fungal, 333, 659
   notifiable diseases, 288
   oropharyngeal, 618
     bacterial, 289, 292
   protozoal, 357
   skin, 656
   trichomonal, 367
   vaccines, 669
   vaginal, 441
   viral, 339
   vulval, 441
Infertility
   female, 412, 413, 417
   male, 413
Inflammation, oral, 616
Inflammatory bowel disease, 52
Infliximab
   Crohn's disease, 52, 53, **58**
   infusion table, 874
   psoriasis, 644, **646**
   rheumatic diseases, 576, **579**,
     580
   ulcerative colitis, 52, **58**
Influenza
   prophylaxis, 354
   treatment, 354
   vaccines, **680**, 681
*Influvac Sub-unit*, 681
Information services
   poisons, 27
Inhalations
   aromatic, 182
   steam, 182, 614
Inhaler devices, 162
*Innohep*, 128
*Innovace*, 104
*Innovative* products *see* Pure products,
   904
*Innozide*, 105
Inosine acedoben dimepranol *see*
   Inosine pranobex
Inosine pranobex, 349, **350**
   anogenital warts, 652
Inositol, 547
Inositol nicotinate, 121, **122**
Inotropic drugs, positive, 72, 123
*Inovelon*, 261
Insect stings, 36, 171
Insecticides, poisoning by, 35
*Insil*, 925
Insomnia, 186
*Inspra*, 78

*Instillagel*, 715
*Insulatard* preparations, 378
Insulin, 373
   analogues, 376
   aspart, **376**
     biphasic, 377, **378**, 379
   detemir, **377**
   glargine, **377**
   glulisine, **376**, 377
   human, 373
   hypodermic equipment, 379
   infusion table, 874
   injection devices, 379, 380
   isophane, 377, **378**
     biphasic, 377, **379**
   lispro, 376, **377**
     biphasic, 377, **379**
   protamine zinc, 377, **378**
   soluble, **376**
   subcutaneous infusion, 374
   zinc suspension, 377, **378**
     mixed, 378
Insulin-like growth factor, 432
*Insuman Basal*, 378
*Insuman Comb* preparations, 379
*Insuman Rapid*, 376
*Insupak*, 380
*Intal*, 170
*Intanza*, 681
*Integrilin*, 136
*Intelence*, 347
Interactions, 720
Interferon
   alfa, **499**
     chronic hepatitis B, 353
     chronic hepatitis C, 353
     infusion table, 875
   beta, **500**, 501
   gamma, 501
   peginterferon alfa, **499**
     chronic hepatitis C, 353
Interferon gamma release assay, 674
Interleukin-2 *see* Aldesleukin, 501
Intermittent claudication, 121
International travel, immunisation for,
   695
*Interpose*, 913
Intracranial pressure, raised
   corticosteroids, 395
   palliative care, 17
   thiopental, 700
*Intralipid* preparations, 535
*Intrasite* products, 914
*Intratect*, 692
Intra-uterine devices, 452
   copper-bearing, 452, 453, 454
   progestogen-releasing, 451, 452
Intravenous infusions, 530
   addition to, 867
Intravenous nutrition, 534
*Intrinsa*, 410
*IntronA*, 499
*Invanz*, 307
*Invega*, 202
*Invirase*, 346
*Iocare*, 604
Iodine, **393**
   dressings, with, 920, 921
   oral solution, 393
   radioactive, 393
   topical, 667
*Iodoflex*, 920
*Iodosorb* products, 920
*Iodozyme*, 920
*IONSYS—discontinued*
*Iopidine*, 605

Ipecacuanha, poisoning in, 28
*Ipocol*, 55
Ipratropium, **159**
  asthma, 159
  fenoterol with, 161
  rhinorrhoea, **615**
  salbutamol with, 161
  *Steri-Neb*, 159
Irbesartan, 107, 108
  hydrochlorothiazide with, 108
Irinotecan, **491**
  infusion table, 875
Iron
  deficiency, 512
  folic acid and, 513
  overload, 522
  poisoning by, 32
  therapy
    oral, 512, 513, 514
    parenteral, 514, 515
Iron dextran, 514, **515**
  infusion table, 875
Iron sucrose, 514, **515**
  infusion table, 875
*Ironorm*, 513
*Irriclens*, 666
*Irripod*, 666
Irritable bowel syndrome, 41, **53**
*Isentress*, 348
*Isib 60XL*, 114
Island dressings, 925
*Ismelin*, 99
*Ismo* preparations, 113, 114
Isocarboxazid, 213, **214**
*Isodur* preparations, 114
Isoflurane, 701, **702**
*Isogel*, 60
*Isoket* preparations, 113
Isoleucine amino acid supplement,
  907
Isometheptene, 236
  paracetamol with, 236
Isoniazid, 321, 322, 323, **324**
Isophane protamine insulin *see* Insulin,
  isophane
*Isoplex*, 534
Isoprenaline, 123
*Isopto*
  Alkaline, 604
  Plain, 604
Isosorbide dinitrate, 111, **113**
  infusion table, 875
Isosorbide mononitrate, 111, **113**,
  114
*Isosource* preparations, 881, 884, 887
*Isotard* preparations, 114
Isotretinoin
  acne
    oral, 647, **650**, 651
    topical, 648, 649
  erythromycin with, 649
  rosacea, 647
*Isotrex*, 649
*Isotrexin*, 649
*Isovorin*, 468
*Ispagel Orange*, 60
Ispaghula
  constipation, **60**
  diarrhoea, 51
  mebeverine with, 42
Isradipine, 115, **117**
  *see also* Calcium-channel block-
    ers
*Istin*, 115
Itraconazole, 332, 333, **336**, 337
  infusion table, 875

IUDs *see* Intra-uterine devices
*IV3000*, 915
Ivabradine, **120**, 121
*Ivemend*, 231
Ivermectin
  larva migrans, 371
  onchocerciasis, 371
  scabies, 662
  strongyloidiasis, 371
*Ixiaro*, 681
IZS *see* Insulin, zinc suspension

**J**

*Januvia*, 387
Japanese encephalitis
  immunisation, 681
  vaccine, **681**
*Jelonet*, 913
Jet nebulisers, 163
*Jevity* preparations, 881, 884, 885
Joint prostheses
  endocarditis prophylaxis,
    295
*Joy Rides*, 232
*Juvela*
  gluten-free, 904
  low-protein, 905

**K**

*Kabiven* preparations, 535
Kala-azar, 367
*Kaletra*, 345
*Kalspare*, 80
*Kalten*, 89
*Kaltostat* products, 918
Kaolin, 51
  mixture, 51
  morphine with, 52
  poultices, 509
*Kapake*, 236
  effervescent tablets—*disconti-
    nued*
*Kaplon* (captopril), 104
*Karvol* preparations, 182
*Katya 30/75*, 449
Kawasaki syndrome, 690
*Kay-Cee-L*, 527
*K-Band*, 926
*Kefadim*, 305
*Keflex*, 304
*Keftid* (cefaclor), 303
*Keloc SR* (felodipine), 117
*Kelo-cote*, 922
Keloid dressings, 922, 923
*Kemadrin* preparations, 277
*Kemicetine*, 316
*Kenalog*, 400, 570
*Kentera*, 459
*Kentipine MR* (nifedipine), 119
*Kepivance*, 469
*Keppra*, 259
*Keral*, 563
Keratitis, 591
Keratolytics, warts and calluses, 651
Keratosis follicularis, 640
*Keromask* preparations, 654
*Kerraboot* products, 918
*KerraMax*, 913
*Ketalar*, 700
Ketamine, **699**, 700
  abuse, 8
  infusion table, 875
  neuropathic pain, 246

*Ketek*, 315
Ketoacidosis, diabetic, 387
*KetoCal*, 895
*Ketocid*, 566
Ketoconazole, 333, **337**
  anogenital, 442
  Cushing's syndrome, 432
  scalp, 655
  skin, 659, 660
*Ketodiastix*, 391
Ketolides, 313
Ketoprofen
  gout, 581
  pain, **566**
    postoperative, 706
    topical, 588, 589
  rheumatic disease, 560, **566**
Ketorolac
  eye, 605, 606
  postoperative, **706**, 707
*Ketostix*, 391
Ketotifen, 174
  eye, 595, **596**
*Ketovail*, 566
*Ketovite*, 553
*Ketur Test*, 391
*KeyOmega*, 908
*K-Four* products, 929
Kidney *see* Renal
*Kindergen*, 895
*Kineret*, 579
*Kivexa*, 341
*Klaricid* preparations, 314
*Klean-Prep*, 65
*Kliofem*, 404
*Kliovance*, 404
*K-Lite*, 928, 929
Knit Fix, 926
*Knit-Band*, 926
*Knit-Firm*, 928
Knitted viscose dressing, primary,
  913
*Ko-Flex*, 929
*Kogenate Bayer* (factor VIII fraction),
  141
*Kolanticon*, 42
*Konakion* preparations, 552
*Kontour*, 926
Korsakoff's psychosis, 547
*K-Plus*, 928, 929
*K-Press*, 928
*K-Soft*, 929
*K-Tech*, 929
*K-ThreeC*, 929
*K-Two* products, 929, 930
*Kuvan*, 540
*Kwells*, 232
*Kytril*, 230

**L**

*L3* bandage, 928
Labelling, cautionary and advisory *see*
  Cautionary and advisory labels
Labetalol, 87, **91**
  infusion table, 875
  *see also* Beta-adrenoceptor
    blocking drugs
Labour
  analgesia, 238
  induction, 434
  premature, 439
Labyrinthine disorders, 226
Lacidipine, 115, **117**
  *see also* Calcium-channel block-
    ers

Lacosamide, **257**
  infusion table, 875
*Lacri-Lube*, 604
Lactase, 903
Lactation, suppression
  dopaminergic drugs,
    427
  oestrogens, 400
Lactic acid
  hydrocortisone with, 633
  salicylic acid with, 651, 652
*Lactugal* (lactulose), 63
Lactulose, **63**
*Ladropen* (flucloxacillin), 297
Laevulose *see* Fructose
*Lamictal*, 258
*Lamisil*, 338
  cream, 661
Lamivudine, **342**
  chronic hepatitis B, **342**, 353
  HIV infection, 340, **342**
    abacavir and zidovudine
      with, 341
    abacavir with, 341
    zidovudine with, 344
Lamotrigine
  epilepsy, 254, **258**
    syndromes, 254
  trigeminal neuralgia, 247
Lancets, 380
Lanolin *see* Wool fat, hydrous,
  626
*Lanoxin* preparations, 73
Lanreotide, 510, **511**
Lansoprazole, **49**
Lanthanum, **544**, 545
*Lantus* preparations, 377
*Lanvis*, 479
Lapatinib, 487, **489**
*Larapam SR*, 246
*Largactil*, 196
*Lariam*, 364
Laronidase, **555**
  infusion table, 875
*LarvE*, 667
*Laryngojet*, 715
*Lasilactone*, 80
*Lasix*, 77
Lassar's paste, 643
Latanoprost, **599**
  timolol with, 599
Latin abbreviations, *inside back cover*
Laxatives
  bulk-forming, 59
  faecal softeners, 62
  osmotic, 63
  stimulant, 60
*Laxido*, 63
*Ledclair*, 35
*Lederfen* preparations, 565
*Ledermycin*, 309
Leflunomide, **575**
  rheumatic disease, 574
Left ventricular failure *see* Heart failure
Legionnaires' disease, 312
Leishmaniacides, 367
Leishmaniasis, 367
Lenalidomide, **502**
Lennox-Gastaut syndrome, 254
Lenograstim, 525, **526**
  infusion table, 875
Lepirudin, **129**
  infusion table, 875
Lepra reactions, 326
Leprosy, 326
Leptospirosis, 295, 308

Lercanidipine, 115, **117**, 118
  *see also* Calcium-channel block-
    ers
*Lescol* preparations, 144
Letrozole, 505, **506**, 507
Leucine amino acid supplement, 908
Leucovorin *see* Calcium folinate
Leukaemia
  acute, 472, 475
    lymphoblastic, 474, 483,
      494
  chronic lymphocytic, 469, 474
  chronic myeloid, 469, 484, 499
  CNS, prophylaxis, 474
  hairy cell, 499
  lymphoid, 517
*Leukeran*, 470
*Leukofix*, 925
*Leukomed* products, 913, 914, 915
*Leukopor*, 925
*Leukosilk*, 925
*Leukostrip*, 926
Leukotriene receptor antagonists, 170
Leuprorelin
  endometriosis, 431
  prostate cancer, 508, **509**, 510
  uterine fibroids, 430
*Leustat*, 477
Levamisole, 370
*Levemir* preparations, 377
Levetiracetam
  epilepsy, 254, **259**
  infusion table, 875
*Levitra*, 464
Levobunolol, **598**
Levobupivacaine, **717**
Levocetirizine, 171, **172**
Levodopa, 272
  benserazide with, **272**, 273
  carbidopa with, 272, **273**, 274
    and entacapone with,
      274
Levofloxacin, 328, **329**, 330
  eye, 591, **592**
Levofolinic acid
  *see* Calcium levofolinate
  *see also* Disodium levofolinate
Levomenthol, 182
Levomepromazine, **197**
  nausea and vertigo, 225
  palliative care, 17, 18
  psychosis, 197
*Levonelle 1500*, 455
*Levonelle One Step*, 454
Levonorgestrel, 451, **454**
  contraception, 450
    emergency, 454, 455
    ethinylestradiol with,
      448
  intra-uterine, 452
HRT
  conjugated oestrogens
    with, 403
  estradiol with, 403, 404
Levothyroxine, 391, 392
*Lexpec* (folic acid), 517
LH *see* Luteinising hormone, 413
LH-RH *see* Gonadorelin, **417**
*Liberty* nebuliser, 164
*Librium* (chlordiazepoxide), 192
Lice, 663
Lidocaine
  arrhythmias, **86**
  dental, 714
  fluorescein with, 602
  haemorrhoids, 67, 68

Lidocaine (*continued*)—
  local anaesthesia, **714**, 715, 716
    dental, 715
    eye, **602**
    mouth, 618
    postherpetic neuralgia, 247,
      716
    rectal, 67
    urethral, 715
    urethral pain, 460
  neuropathic pain, 246
  phenylephrine with, 716
  prilocaine with, 715
  tetracaine with, 716
*Lifestyle* preparations, 904
Lignocaine *see* Lidocaine
*Lignospan Special* , 715
*Li-Liquid*, 208
Linezolid, **318**, 319
*Linola Gamma*, 627
Lint, absorbent, 923
*Lioresal*, 585
Liothyronine, **392**
*Lipantil* preparations, 148
*Lipidem* preparations, 535
Lipid-regulating drugs, 142
*Lipitor*, 144
*Lipobase*, 627
Lipodystrophy syndrome, 340
*Lipofundin* preparations, 536
Lipopeptide antibiotic, 317
*Liposic*, 603
*Lipostat*, 145
*LiquiBand*, 665
Liquid and White Soft Paraffin
  Ointment, 626
Liquid paraffin
  constipation, 62, **63**
    emulsion, 63
    magnesium hydroxide and,
      64
  eye, lubricant, 604
*Liquifilm Tears*, 604
*Liquigen*, 899
*Liquivisc*, 603
*Lisicostad* preparations, 106
Lisinopril, **105**
  hydrochlorothiazide with, 105,
    106
  *see also* ACE inhibitors
*Liskonum*, 208
*Litak*, 477
Lithium
  cluster headache, 252
  mania, 207
  poisoning by, 33
  recurrent depression, 207
  surgery, 698
Lithium carbonate, **207**, 208
Lithium citrate, **208**
*Lithonate* (lithium carbonate), 208
Liver disease, prescribing in, 804
*Livial*, 407
*Livwell* products, 904
*LMX 4*, 715
*Loa loa*, 371
*Load 375*, 453
Local anaesthetics *see* Anaesthesia,
  local
*Loceryl*, 659
*Locoid* preparations, 633, 634
*Locorten-Vioform*, 609
*Lodine*, 564
Lodoxamide, 595, **596**
*Loestrin-20*, 447
*Loestrin-30*, 448

Lofepramine, 210, **212**
Lofexidine, 283, **284**
*Logynon* preparations, 448
*Lomont* (lofepramine), 212
*Lomotil*, 51
Lomustine, 469, **471**
*Loniten*, 97
Loop diuretics *see* Diuretics, loop, 76
Loperamide, 51, 52
    palliative care, 16
*Lophlex* preparations, 908
*Lopid*, 148
Lopinavir, 340, **345**
    ritonavir with, 345
Loprazolam, **187**
*Lopresor* preparations, 91
*Loprofin*
    low-protein, 905
    PKU drink, 908
*Loramyc*, 619
Loratadine, 171, **172**
Lorazepam
    anaesthesia, 704, **705**
    anxiety, 191, **192**
    nausea and vomiting, 466
    status epilepticus, 265, **267**
Lormetazepam, **187**
*Loron*, 425
Losartan, 107, **108**, 109
    hydrochlorothiazide with, 109
*Losec*, 49
*Lotemax*, 595
Loteprednol, **595**
Lotions
    definition, 625
    eye, 590
    suitable quantities, 625
*Lotriderm*, 635
*Low protein drink*, 905
Low sodium content (antacids), 38
Low-protein foods, 905
LSD *see* Lysergide, 8
*Luborant*, 622
*Lubri-Tears*, 604
Lucanthone, 371
*Lucentis*, 607
Lugol's solution, 393
Lumefantrine, 358, **362**
    artemether with, 362
*Lumigan*, 599
Lupus erythematosus
    discoid, 571
    systemic, 395, 569, 571, 574
*Lustral*, 217
Luteinising hormone, 413
Lutropin alfa, **414**
    follitropin alfa with, 414
*Luveris*, 414
*Lyclear*, 664
*Lyflex* (baclofen), 585
Lyme disease, 298
Lymecycline, **309**
    acne, 649
Lymphoedema garments, 931
    compression values, 930
Lymphogranuloma venereum, 308
*Lyofoam* products, 917, 918, 919
*Lyrica*, 257
*Lyrinel XL*, 459
Lysergic acid diethylamide *see* Lyser-
    gide, 8
Lysergide, regulations, 8
*Lysodren*, 484
Lysosomal storage disorder, 554, 555
*Lysovir*, 355

# M

*Maalox* preparations, 39, 40
*MabCampath*, 499
*Mabron*, 246
*MabThera*, 499
*Macrobid*, 332
*Macrodantin*, 332
Macrogol Oral Powder, Compound,
    NPF, 950, 952
Macrogols, 63
    bowel cleansing, **65**
    constipation, **63**, 64
    faecal impaction, **63**, 64
Macrolides, 312
*Macugen*, 606
Macular degeneration, age-related,
    606
*Madopar* preparations, 272, 273
*Magnapen*, 301
Magnesium carbonate, 38, **39**
Magnesium citrate, **65**
    sodium picosulfate with, **66**
Magnesium glycerophosphate, 543
Magnesium hydroxide, 38, 40, **64**
    liquid paraffin with, 64
Magnesium sulphate, **543**
    arrhythmias, 543
    asthma, 153
    eclampsia, 543
    infusion table, 875
    injection, 544
    laxative, 64
    myocardial infarction, 543
    paste, 665
    torsade de pointes, 543
Magnesium trisilicate, 38, **39**
Malabsorption syndromes, 54
    electrolytes, 527
    vitamin K, 551
Malaria
    prophylaxis, 359, 360, 361
    treatment, 357, 359
*Malarivon*, 363
*Malarone*
    malaria prophylaxis, 359, 360,
        361, 362, 364, **365**
    malaria treatment, 358, 364, **365**
*Malarone Paediatric*, 365
Malathion, 662, 663, **664**
Malignant disease, 465
    bladder, 461
    gonadorelin analogues, 508
    hormone antagonists, 505
    pain, 237
        bone, 233
    sex hormones, 504
Malignant effusions, 470
Malignant hyperthermia, 713
    antagonists, 713
*Manerix*, 215
*Manevac*, 62
Mania, 194, 206
Manic depression *see* Bipolar disorder,
    207
Mannitol, 80
    diuresis, **80**
    glaucoma, 598
    presence of, 2
Mantoux test, 673
Manufacturers, special order, 969
Manuka honey *see* Honey, medical
    grade
MAOIs *see* Monoamine-oxidase inhi-
    bitors
*Mapleflex*, 907

Maraviroc, 340, **348**
*Marcain* preparations, 716
*Marevan* (warfarin), 132
Marine stings, 36
Marketing authorisation, 1
*Marvelon*, 448
*Mastaflu*, 681
Mastalgia, **431**
*Matrifen* (fentanyl), 241
*Maxalt*, 249
*Maxamaid* preparations, 907
*Maxamaid* products, 906, 907, 909,
    910
*Maxamum* preparations, 907
*Maxamum* products, 906, 908, 909
*Maxepa*, 149
*Maxidex*, 594
*Maxijul* preparations, 898
*Maxitram SR*, 246
*Maxitrol*, 594
*Maxolon* preparations, 229
    liquid and syrup—*discontinued*
*Maxtrex* (methotrexate), 576
MCT Oil, 895
MDMA *see* Methylenedioxymetham-
    fetamine
Measles
    corticosteroids, caution in, 396
    immunisation, 681
        immunoglobulin, 691
        vaccines, combined, 681,
            **682**, 683
Mebendazole, **370**
    hookworm infections, 371
    roundworm infections, 370
    threadworm infections, 369
    whipworm infections, 370
Mebeverine, **42**
    ispaghula with, 42
Mecasermin, 432, **433**
Mecillinam, 302
Mecysteine, 182
*Medicaid*, 629
Medical emergencies in the commu-
    nity, *inside back cover*
Medical grade honey, 920
Medication-overuse headache, 247
Medicines information services, *inside
    front cover*
*Medihoney* products, 920
*Medikinet* preparations, 222
*Medinol* (paracetamol) preparations,
    235
*Mediplast*, 925
*Medipore+Pad*, 913
*Medisafe*, 913
*MediSense* products, 380, 390
Mediterranean fever, familial, 581
*Medi-Test* products, 391
Medium-chain triglyceride oil, 895
*Medix* nebulisers, 163
*Medocodene* (co-codamol 30/500),
    236
*Medrone*, 399
Medroxyprogesterone
    contraception, 450, 451
    HRT, 408
        conjugated oestrogens
            with, 403
        estradiol with, 404, 405
    malignant disease, **504**
    menstrual disorders, 407, **408**
Mefenamic acid
    menorrhagia, 566
    pain, 560, **566**, 567
    rheumatic disease, 560, **566**
*Mefix*, 925

Mefloquine, **363**, 364
  malaria
        prophylaxis, 359, 360, 361,
            362
        treatment, 358
*Megace*, 504
Megestrol, **504**
Melanoma, 483, 499
Melatonin, **190**
*Melgisorb* products, 918
*Melladerm* products, 920
*Melolin*, 913
Meloxicam, 560, **567**
Melphalan, 469, **471**
  infusion table, 875
Memantine, 285, **286**, 287
Menadiol sodium phosphate, **552**
Mendelson's syndrome, 45, 698
Meniere's disease, 226
Meningeal carcinoma, 474
*Meningitec*, 683
Meningitis
    cryptococcal, 335
    haemophilus, 291, 316
    immunisation, 683
        Hib with, 676
        vaccine, **683**, 684
    initial therapy, 291
    listerial, 291
    meningococcal, 291
        prophylaxis, 293
        travel, 683, 695
    pneumococcal, 291
Meningococcal *see* Meningitis
*Menitorix*, 676
*Menjugate*, 684
Menopausal symptoms, 252, 400
*Menopur*, 414
Menorrhagia, 408, 451, 452
    antifibrinolytics, 140
    NSAIDS, 566
Menotrophin, 414
Menthol and eucalyptus inhalation,
    182
Mepacrine
    discoid lupus erythematosus,
        573
    giardiasis, **367**
*Mepiform*, 922
*Mepilex* products, 916, 921
*Mepitac*, 925
*Mepitel*, 915, 916
Mepivacaine, 714
*Mepore* products, 913, 914, 915
*Mepradec* (omeprazole), 49
Meprobamate, **193**
    muscle spasm, 586
Meptazinol, 237, **241**
*Meptid*, 241
*Merbentyl* preparations, 41
Mercaptamine (cysteamine), **555**, 556
Mercaptopurine, 476, **478**
    inflammatory bowel disease,
        52, 53, **58**
*Mercilon*, 447
*Merional*, 414
*Meronem*, 307
Meropenem, 306, **307**
    infusion table, 875
Mesalazine, 52, **54**, 55
*Mesitran* products, 920
Mesna, **469**
    infusion fluid, 875
*Mesorb*, 913
*Mesren MR*, 55
Mesterolone, **411**

*Mestinon*, 584
Mestranol, norethisterone with, 449
Metabolic acidosis, 532
Metabolic Mineral Mixture, 902
Metals, poisoning by, 34, 35
*Metalyse*, 140
*Metanium*, 629
Metaraminol, **124**
    infusion table, 875
*Metastron* (strontium), 15
*Metatone*, xii
*Meted*, 655
*Metenix-5*, 76
Metformin, 382, **383**
    pioglitazone with, 386
    rosiglitazone with, 387
    vildagliptin with, 387
Methadone, **241**, 242
    cough, 183
    linctus, 183
    opioid dependence, 283, **284**
    oral solutions, 285
    pain, 237, 241
    palliative care, 15
    parenteral, 285
    poisoning by, 31
*Methadose*, 285
Methaemoglobinaemia, 717
Methanol, poisoning by, 34
*Metharose* (methadone), 285
Methenamine, 331, **332**
Methicillin-resistant *Staphylococcus
    aureus see* MRSA
Methionine, 29, **31**
    paracetamol with, 236
Methocarbamol, **586**, 587
Methotrexate
    Crohn's disease, 52, **58**
    infusion table, 875
    malignant disease, 474, **478**
    psoriasis, 644, **645**
    rheumatic disease, 571, 574,
        **575**, 576
Methotrimeprazine *see* Levomepro-
    mazine
Methoxy polyethylene glycol-epoetin
    beta, 517, **521**
Methyl alcohol *see* Methanol, 34
Methyl cysteine *see* Mecysteine, 182
Methyl salicylate, 665
    dithranol and salicylic acid with,
        643
Methyl-5-aminolevulinate, 654
Methylated spirit, industrial, 665
Methylcellulose, 223
    constipation, 60
    diarrhoea, 51
    obesity, 60, 223
Methylcysteine *see* Mecysteine, 182
Methyldopa, **98**, 99
Methylene blue *see* Methylthioninium
    chloride, 717
Methylenedioxymethamphetamine
    controlled drug, 7
    poisoning by, 33
Methylnaltrexone, **66**, 67
Methylphenidate, 220, **222**
Methylprednisolone, **399**
    lidocaine with, 570
    rheumatic disease, 570
Methylprednisolone acetate, 399
Methylprednisolone sodium
    succinate, 399
    infusion table, 875
Methylthioninium chloride, 717
Methysergide, 251, **252**
    cluster headache, 252

Meticillin-resistant *Staphylococcus aur-
    eus see* MRSA
Metipranolol, **598**
Metirosine, 101
Metoclopramide
    aspirin with, 247
    diabetic neuropathy, 389
    gastro-intestinal, 43
    infusion table, 875
    migraine, 251
    nausea and vomiting, 225, **228**,
        229
        cytotoxic drugs, 466
        postoperative, 226
        pregnancy, 225
    palliative care, 17
    paracetamol with, 248
*Metoject*, 576
Metolazone, 75, **76**
*Metopirone*, 432
Metoprolol, **91**
    migraine, 251
    *see also* Beta-adrenoceptor
        blocking drugs
*Metosyn*, 636
*Metrogel*, 658
*Metrolyl*, 328
Metronidazole, **327**, 328
    amoebiasis, 366
    Crohn's disease, 53
    giardiasis, 367
    protozoal infections, 366
    skin, 658, 659
    trichomoniasis, 367
    ulcerative gingivitis, 327, 618
    vaginal infections, 443
*Metrosa*, 658
*Metrotop*, 658
*Metsol* (metformin), 383
*Metvix*, 654
Metyrapone, **432**
Mexiletine, 84, 86
*Mezavant XL*, 55
*Mezolar* (fentanyl), 241
*Miacalcic*, 421
Mianserin, 210, **213**
Micafungin, 334, **337**, 338
    infusion table, 875
*Micanol*, 643
*Micardis* preparations, 109
*Micolette Micro-enema*, 65
Miconazole
    mouth, 618, **619**
    skin, 659, **660**
        hydrocortisone and, 633
    vaginal, 442
*Micralax Micro-enema*, 65
*Micral-Test II*, 391
*Microalbustix*, 391
*Microbumintest*, 391
*Microgynon* preparations, 448
*Microlance*, 380
*Micronor*, 450
*MicroPeak*, 161
*Micropirin* (aspirin), 135
*Micropore*, 925
Midazolam
    anaesthesia, **705**, 706
    infusion table, 875
    palliative care, 18
    status epilepticus, 265, **267**
*Midrid*, 236
*Mifegyne*, 439
Mifepristone, 434, **438**, 439
*Migard*, 249
Miglustat, 554, **557**

Index

Migraine, 247
    acute attack, 247
    prophylaxis, 251
*Migraleve*, 247
*MigraMax*, 247
*Migril*, 251
*Mildison*, 633
*Milex Arcing Style* diaphragm,
    454
*Milex Omniflex* diaphragm, 454
Milk, drugs in, 852
Milk-alkali syndrome, 38
*Milpar* (liquid paraffin emulsion and
    magnesium hydroxide), 64
Milrinone, **74**
    infusion table, 875
*Milupa*
    Low Protein Drink, 905
    PKU preparations, 908
*Milward Steri-Let*, 380
*Mimpara*, 543
*Minaphlex*, 908
Mineralocorticoids, replacement
    therapy, 394
*Mini TT 380 Slimline*, 453
*Minijet*
    *Adrenaline*, 125, 177
    *Aminophylline*, 161
    *Atropine sulphate*, 703
    *Calcium Chloride*, 542
    *Furosemide*, 77
    *Glucose*, 531
    *Lignocaine*, 86
    *Magnesium Sulphate*, 544
    *Morphine Sulphate*, 243
    *Naloxone*, 31
    *Sodium Bicarbonate*, 532
*Minims*
    Amethocaine, 602
    Artificial Tears, 603
    Atropine Sulphate, 597
    Chloramphenicol, 592
    Cyclopentolate, 597
    Dexamethasone, 594
    Fluorescein Sodium, 605
    Lignocaine and Fluorescein,
        602
    Metipranolol, 598
    Oxybuprocaine, 602
    Phenylephrine, 597
    Pilocarpine Nitrate, 602
    Prednisolone, 595
    Proxymetacaine, 602
    Proxymetacaine and Fluores-
        cein, 602
    Saline, 604
    Tropicamide, 597
*MiniQuick*, 416
*Minitran*, 113
*Miniversol*, 666
*Mini-Wright*, 161, 162
*Minocin* preparations, 310
Minocycline, 308, **309**
    acne, 649
    preparations, 309, 310
*Minodiab*, 382
Minoxidil
    androgenetic alopecia, 656
    hypertension, 95, **97**
    scalp, 656
*Mintec*, 43
*Miochol-E*, 605
*Mirapexin*, 271
*Mircera*, 521
*Mirena*, 451, 452
Mirtazapine, **218**, 219
Miscarriage, recurrent, 408

Misoprostol, 47, 48
    diclofenac with, 564
    naproxen with, 568
    obstetrics, 434
Misuse of drugs
    Act, 7
    Regulations 2001, 7
Mitobronitol, 470
Mitomycin, 472, **474**
    bladder, 461
*Mitomycin C Kyowa*, 474
Mitotane, **484**
*Mitoxana—discontinued*
Mitoxantrone, 472, **474**
    infusion table, 876
Mitozantrone *see* Mitoxantrone
*Mivacron*, 710
Mivacurium, 709, **710**
    infusion table, 876
*Mixtard* preparations, 379
Mizolastine, 171, **172**
*Mizollen*, 172
MMR vaccine, 681, 683
*MMRvaxPro*, 683
*Mobic*, 567
*Mobiflex*, 568
Moclobemide, **214**, 215
Modafinil, 220, **222**, 223
*Modalim*, 147
*Modecate* preparations, 205
Modification of Diet in Renal Disease
    study ('MDRD formula'), 815
*Modisal* preparations, 114
*Modjul Flavour System*, 903
*Modrasone*, 634
*Modrenal*, 432
*Modulen IBD*, 895
*Moduret-25* (co-amilozide), 79
*Moduretic* (co-amilozide), 79
Moexipril, **106**
    *see also* ACE inhibitors
*Mogadon* (nitrazepam), 187
*Molcer*, 611
*Molipaxin*, 213
Mometasone
    asthma, 165, **169**
    nasal allergy, 614
    skin, 637
*Monigen XL* (isosorbide mononitrate),
    114
Monoamine-oxidase inhibitors, 213
    reversible, 214
    surgery, 698
    type A, 214
    type B, 274
        parkinsonism, 274
Monoethanolamine oleate *see* Etha-
    nolamine oleate, **149**
Monofluorophosphate, 545
*Monoject*, 380
*Monoject Ultra*, 380
*Monolet*, 380
*Monomax* preparations, 114
*Monomil XL*, 114
*Mononine* (factor IX fraction), 142
*Monosorb XL*, 114
Montelukast, **170**
Moracizine, 86
*Morhulin*, 629
Moroctocog alfa, 141
*Morphgesic SR*, 243
Morphine, 238
    analgesia, 237, **242**, 243
    cyclizine with, 243
    palliative care, 15
    cough, 183
    kaolin with, 52

*Motens*, 117
*Motifene* (diclofenac), 564
*Motilium*, 228
    suspension—*discontinued*
Motion sickness, 226
Motor neurone disease, amyotrophic
    lateral sclerosis, 277
Mountain sickness, 80
Mouth ulceration, 616
Mouthwash solution-tablets, 621
Mouthwashes, 620
Movement disorders, 277
*Movicol* preparations, 63, 64
*Moviprep*, 65
Moxifloxacin, 328, **330**
*Moxisylyte*, **122**
Moxonidine, 98, **99**
*MPD Ultra Thin*, 380
MRSA, 297
    nasal, 616
*MST Continus*, 243
MSUD preparations, 907
*MucoClear*, 182
*Mucodyne*, 181
*Mucogel*, 39
Mucolytics, 181
    eye, 603
Mucopolysaccharidosis, 555
Mucosa, oral, side-effects on, 12
Mucositis, oral, 466
*Multiclix*, 380
*Multiload* IUDs, 453
Multiple myeloma, 482, 499, 517
Multiple sclerosis
    glatiramer, 502
    interferon beta, 500
    natalizumab, 503
    skeletal muscle relaxants, 585
        baclofen, 585
        tizanidine, 586
Multivitamin preparations, 552
Mumps, vaccines, combined, 681, 683
Mupirocin
    nose, 616
    skin, **657**
Muscle relaxants
    anaesthesia, 708
        depolarising, 711
        non-depolarising, 709
    skeletal, 585
Muscle spasm, 585
    temporomandibular
        dysfunction, 233
Musculoskeletal disorders, rheumatic,
    559
*MUSE*, 463
Muslin, absorbent, 923
*MXL*, 243
Myasthenia gravis, 583
    corticosteroids, 584
    diagnosis, 583
    immunosuppressants, 584
*Mycamine*, 338
*Mycobacterium avium* complex
    infections, 322, 325
*Mycobutin*, 325
Mycophenolate mofetil, 493, **494**
    eczema, 644
    infusion table, 876
Mycophenolic acid, 494
Mycoplasma infections, 308
*Mycota*, 661
*Mydriacyl*, 597
Mydriatics, 596
*Mydrilate*, 597
Myeloma, multiple *see* Multiple myel-
    oma, 482, 499, 517

*Myfortic*, 494
*Myleran*, 470
Myocardial infarction, 137
  analgesia, 242
  arrhythmias, 82
  beta-blockers, 87
  dental practice, 22, 24
  magnesium sulphate, 543
  secondary prevention, 149
  thrombolytics, 138
*Myocet*, 473
Myoclonic seizures, 254
*Myocrisin*, 572
Myometrial relaxants, 439
*Myotonine*, 456
*Myozyme*, 556
*Mysoline*, 260
Myxoedema, 391

# N

*N-A* products, 913
Nabilone, 225, **231**
Nabumetone, 560, **567**
Nadolol, **91**, 92
  cardiovascular, 91
  migraine, 251
  *see also* Beta-adrenoceptor
    blocking drugs
  thyrotoxicosis, 393
Nafarelin, 431
Naftidrofuryl, 121, **122**
*Naglazyme*, 555
*Nalcrom*, 59
Nalidixic acid, 328, **330**, 331
*Nalorex*, 285
Naloxone
  anaesthesia, 712, **713**
  buprenorphine with, 284
  infusion table, 876
  oxycodone with, 244
  poisoning, 31
Naltrexone, 283, **285**
Name changes, xiv
Nandrolone decanoate, 412
Nappy rash, 629
*Napratec*, 568
*Naprosyn* preparations, 567
Naproxen
  gout, 581
  misoprostol with, 568
  pain, 560
  rheumatic disease, 560, **567**
*Naramig*, 249
Naratriptan, 248, **249**
Narcolepsy, 222
Narcotic analgesics *see* Analgesics,
  opioid
Narcotic antagonists *see* Opioid
  antagonists
*Nardil*, 214
*Naropin*, 718
*Nasacort*, 614
Nasal
  allergy, 612
  congestion, 612, 614
  decongestants
    systemic, 171, 184
    topical, 614
  infection, 616
  polyps, 612
*Naseptin*, 616
*Nasobec* preparations, 613
*Nasofan*, 614

*Nasonex*, 614
Natalizumab, **503**
  infusion table, 870
*Natecal D3*, 551
Nateglinide, 384, **385**, 386
National Institute for Health and
  Clinical Excellence, 3
*Natrilix* preparations, 76
Nausea, 226
  cytotoxic drugs, 466
  motion sickness, 226
  palliative care, 17
  postoperative, 226
  pregnancy, 225
*Navelbine*, 480
*Navidrex*, 76
*Navispare*, 79
*Nebido*, 410
*Nebilet*, 92
Nebivolol, 87, **92**
  *see also* Beta-adrenoceptor
    blocking drugs
*Nebuchamber*, 162
Nebulisers, 163
Necatoriasis, 371
Nedocromil
  asthma, 170
  eye, 595, **596**
Needles, insulin, 380
  clipping device, 380
Nefopam, 233, **236**
*Negaban*, 298
*NeisVac-C*, 684
Nelarabine, 475, **478**
Nelfinavir, 340, **345**
*Neoclarityn*, 172
*Neo-Cortef—discontinued*
*Neo-Cytamen* (hydroxocobalamin),
  516
*Neofel XL* (felodipine), 117
*Neo-Mercazole*, 393
Neomycin, 311, **312**
  chlorhexidine with, 616
  ear, 608, 609, **610**
    betamethasone with, 609
    prednisolone with, 610
  eye, 591, **592**, 594
    betamethasone with, 594
  nose, 616
    betamethasone with, 615
  skin, **657**
    betamethasone with, 635
    fluocinolone with, 636
*Neo-NaClex* preparations, 75, 80
*Neoral*, 496
*NeoRecormon*, 520
*Neosporin*, 592
*Neosport*, 928
Neostigmine
  anaesthesia, 711, **712**
  glycopyrronium bromide with,
    712
  laxative, 61
  myasthenia gravis, 583, **584**
*Neotigason*, 643
*Neotulle*, 913
Nepafenac, 605, **606**
Nephropathic cystinosis, 555
Nephrotic syndrome, 395
*Nepro*, 896
*Nerisone* preparations, 635, 636
Nerve agent, poisoning by, 35
*Neulactil*, 198
*Neulasta*, 526
*Neupogen*, 525
*Neupro*, 272

Neural tube defects, prevention, 516
Neuralgia, 209, 246
  glossopharyngeal, 247
*NeuroBloc*, 279
Neuroleptic malignant syndrome, 195
Neuroleptics *see* Antipsychotics
Neuromuscular blocking drugs, 708
Neuromuscular disorders, 583
*Neurontin*, 257
Neuropathic pain, 246
Neuropathy, compression, 569
Neutral insulin *see* Insulin, soluble,
  **376**
Neutropenias, 517, 525
*Nevanac*, 606
Nevirapine, 340, **347**
New preparations, xiii
*Nexavar*, 489
*Nexium*, 48
NHS Direct, *inside front cover*
*Niaspan*, 149
*Nicam*, 649
Nicardipine, 115, **118**
  *see also* Calcium-channel block-
    ers
NICE *see* National Institute for Health
  and Clinical Excellence
*Nicef* (cefradine), 305
Niclosamide, 370
*Nicopass*, 281
*Nicopatch*, 281
Nicorandil, 120, **121**
*Nicorette* preparations, 281
Nicotinamide
  oral, 547, 548
  topical, 649
Nicotine
  replacement therapy, 280
  smoking cessation products,
    281, 282
*Nicotinell* preparations, 282
Nicotinic acid, 149
  hyperlipidaemia, **148**
*Nicoumalone see* Acenocoumarol,
  130, **132**
Niemann-Pick type C disease, 557
Nifedipine, 115, **118**, 119, 121, 439
  atenolol with, 89
  palliative care, 17
  *see also* Calcium-channel block-
    ers
*Nifedipress MR*, 119
*Niferex* preparations, 514
*Niko Fix IV*, 915
Nilotinib, 487, **489**
*Nimbex*, 710
Nimodipine, 115, **119**
  infusion table, 876
*Nimotop*, 119
*Nipent*, 485
*Niquitin* preparations, 282
Niridazole, 371
Nitisinone, **556**
Nitrates
  angina, 111
  heart failure, 111
  myocardial infarction, 138
  tolerance to, 111
Nitrazepam, 186, **187**
*Nitrocine*, 112
*Nitro-Dur*, 113
Nitrofurantoin, **331**, 332
*Nitrolingual Pumpspray*, 112
*Nitromin*, 112
*Nitronal*, 112
Nitroprusside *see* Sodium nitro-
  prusside

Nitrous oxide, **702**
Nitrous oxide-oxygen, 702
*Nivaquine*, 363
*Nivemycin* (neomycin), 312
Nizatidine, **46**
   infusion table, 876
*Nizoral*, 337
   anogenital, 442
   scalp, 655
   skin, 660
Nocturnal enuresis, 460
*Nolvadex* preparations, 507
Nonacog alfa, 142
Non-depolarising muscle relaxants *see*
   Muscle relaxants
Non-medical prescribing, 954
Non-nucleoside reverse transcriptase
   inhibitors, 339, 340
Nonoxinol, 452
*Nootropil*, 278
Noradrenaline, **124**
   infusion table, 876
*Norcuron*, 711
*Norditropin*, 416
Norelgestromin, ethinylestradiol with,
   449
Norepinephrine *see* Noradrenaline
Norethisterone
   contraception, 450
      ethinylestradiol with, 447,
      448
         mestranol with, 449
         parenteral, 451
   HRT, estradiol with, 403, 404,
   405
   malignant disease, 504
   menstrual disorders, **408**, 409
Norethisterone enantate, 451
Norfloxacin, 328, **330**
*Norgalax Micro-enema*, 62
Norgestimate, ethinylestradiol with,
   448
*Norgeston*, 450
Norgestrel
   *see* Levonorgestrel
*Noriday*, 450
*Norimin*, 448
*Norimode* (loperamide), 52
*Norinyl-1*, 449
*Noristerat*, 451
*Normacol* preparations, 60
Normal immunoglobulin *see* Immuno-
   globulins, normal, 690, **691**, 692
Normal saline *see* Sodium chloride
*Normasol*, 666
*Normax*, 61
*Normosang*, 557
*Norphyllin SR* (aminophylline), 161
*Norprolac*, 428
Nortriptyline, 210, **212**
   neuropathic pain, 246
*Norvir*, 346
*Norzol* (metronidazole), 327
Nose *see* Nasal
Notifiable diseases, 288
*Novasource* preparations, 881, 884
*Nova-T*, 453
*Novofem*, 404
*NovoFine*, 380
*Novogel*, 914
*Novolizer*, 168
*NovoMix 30*, 379
*NovoNorm see Prandin*, 386
*NovoPen* products, 380
*NovoRapid*, 376
*NovoSeven* (factor VIIa fraction), 141

*Noxafil*, 338
*Nozinan*, 197
NPH *see* Insulin, isophane
NSAIDs (non-steroidal anti-inflamm-
   atory drugs) *see* Analgesics
NTBC *see* Nitisinone, **556**
*NU DERM*, 916
Nucleoside analogues *see* Nucleoside
   reverse transcriptase inhibitors
Nucleoside reverse transcriptase
   inhibitors, 339, 340, 341
*Nuelin SA*, 160
*Nu-Gel*, 914
*Nurofen* (ibuprofen) preparations, 565
Nurse independent prescribing, 953
*Nurse It*, 924
Nurse Prescribers' Extended
   Formulary, 953
Nurse Prescribers' Formulary, 950
*Nu-Seals Aspirin*, 135
   analgesia, 234
*Nutilis*, 903
*Nutraplus*, 627
*NuTRIflex Lipid* preparations, 536, 537
*Nutriflex* preparations, 536
*Nutrison* preparations, 881, 882, 885,
   886
Nutrition, 534
   ACBS, 880
   enteral, 540, 880
   intravenous, 534
   oral, 540
   total parenteral, 534
*Nutrizym* preparations, 71
*NutropinAq*, 416
*NuvaRing*, 447
*Nuvelle* preparations, 404
*Nyogel*, 599
*Nystaform*, 660
*Nystaform-HC*, 633
*Nystan* tablets—*discontinued*
*Nystan* suspension
   intestinal, 338
   mouth, 619
Nystatin, 333, **338**
   mouth, 618, 619
   perianal, 67
   skin, 659, **660**
      chlorhexidine and hydro-
      cortisone with, 633
      hydrocortisone with, 633
      tolnaftate with, 661

# O

*Oakmed* products, 923, 924
Obesity, 223
Obsessive-compulsive disorder, 209
Obstetric and gynaecological surgery,
   antibacterial prophylaxis, 294
Obstructive pulmonary disease *see*
   Chronic obstructive pulmonary dis-
   ease
*Occlusal*, 651
*Octagam*, 692
*Octalbin* (albumin) preparations, 533
*Octanate* (factor VIII fraction), 141
*Octaplas* (fresh frozen plasma), 142
*Octim*, 419
Octocog alfa, 141
Octreotide, 510, **511**
   palliative care, 18
Octyl 2-cyanoacrylate, 665
*Ocufen*, 605
*Oculotect*, 604
*Ocusan*, 604

Oedema
   cerebral, 80
   pulmonary, 76
Oesophageal varices, 417
Oesophagitis *see* Gastro-oesophageal
   reflux disease, 38
Oestradiol *see* Estradiol
Oestriol *see* Estriol
*Oestrogel*, 406
Oestrogens
   HRT, 400, **402**
      conjugated, 405
      levonorgestrel with, 403
         medroxyprogesterone with,
         403
   malignant disease, 504
   oral contraceptives, 443
   vaginal, 440
Oestrone *see* Estrone, 406
Ofloxacin, 328, **330**, 331
   ear, 611
   eye, **592**, 593
*Oftaquix*, 592
*Oilatum*
   cream, 627
   *Emollient*, 628
   *Fragrance Free*, 628
   *Plus*, 629
   shower emollient, 627
Oily cream, 626
Ointments
   definition, 625
   eye, 590
   suitable quantities, 625
Olanzapine, 199, **202**
*Olbetam*, 148
*OliClinomel* preparations, 537
Olive oil
   cradle cap, 655
   ear, 611
Olmesartan, 107, **109**
   amlodipine with, 109
   hydrochlorothiazide with, 109
*Olmetec* preparations, 109
Olopatadine, 595, **596**
Olsalazine, 52, 54, **55**
*Omacor*, 149
Omalizumab, **175**
Omega-3 fatty acid compounds, 149
Omega-3-acid ethyl esters, **149**
Omega-3-marine triglycerides, **149**
*Omegaven* preparations, 537
Omeprazole, **49**
   infusion table, 876
*Omnic MR* (tamsulosin), 456
*Omnifix*, 925
*Omnikan*, 380
*Omnitrope*, 416
*Omnopon* (papaveretum), 244
*Omron* nebulisers, 164
Onchocerciasis, 371
*OncoTice*, 501
*Oncovin*, 480
Ondansetron, 225, **230**
   infusion table, 876
*Ondemet* (ondansetron), 230
*One Touch* products, 380, 390, 391
*One-Alpha*, 550
*Onkotrone*, 474
Onychomycosis *see* Fungal infections
*Opatanol*, 596
*Opilon*, 122
Opioid analgesics *see* Analgesics,
   opioid
Opioid antagonists, 712
   peripheral, 66, 67
   poisoning in, 31

Index

Opizone, 285
OpSite products, 914, 915
Optichamber, 162
OptiClik, 380
Opticrom preparations, 596
OptiFlo preparations, 461
Optil (diltiazem), 116
Optilast, 595
Optimax, 219
OptiPen Pro, 380
Optium products, 390, 391
Optivate (factor VIII and von Willebrand factor concentrate), 141
Optive, 603
Optometrist independent prescribing, 954
OPV see Poliomyelitis, immunisation
Orabase, 617
Orahesive, 617
Oral balance see Biotène Oralbalance
Oral contraceptives see Contraception, oral
Oral glucose tolerance test, 391
Oral hypoglycaemic drugs see Antidiabetic drugs, oral, 380
Oral rehydration, 528
Oral rehydration salts, 528, 529
    WHO formula, 529
Oral syringes, 2
Oraldene, 621
Oramorph preparations, 242
Orap, 198
Orbifen (ibuprofen), 565
Orciprenaline, 159
Orelox, 304
Orencia, 578
Orfadin, 556
Orgalutran, 429
Organophosphorus insecticides, poisoning by, 35
Orgaran, 129
Orgran, 904
Orlept (sodium valproate), 263
Orlistat, 223, 224
Oropharynx, 616
    anti-infective drugs, 618
Orphenadrine, 276
ORS, 529
ORT, 528
Ortho-Band Plus, 929
Ortho-Gynest, 441
Orthopaedic surgery
    antibacterial prophylaxis, 294
Orthovisc, 560
Orudis, 566
Oruvail preparations, 566
    topical, 588
Oseltamivir, 354, 355
Osmanil (fentanyl), 241
Osmolite preparations, 882, 885, 886
Ostenil, 560
Osteoarthritis, 559, 560
Osteomyelitis, 292, 315, 316
Osteonecrosis
    jaw, 422, 423, 424, 425
Osteoporosis, 419
    anabolic steroids, 412
    bisphosphonates, 420, 422
    calcitonin, 420
    calcitriol, 420, 549
    calcium, 419, 541
    corticosteroid-induced, 420
    HRT, 419
    parathyroid hormone, 420
    postmenopausal, 419
    raloxifene, 420
    strontium ranelate, 420
    teriparatide, 420

Otex, 611
Otitis externa, 608
    systemic treatment, 292
    topical treatment, 608
Otitis media, 611
    systemic treatment, 292
    with effusion, 611
Otomize, 609
Otosporin, 610
Otradrops (xylometazoline), 615
Otraspray (xylometazoline), 615
Otrivine (xylometazoline), 615
Otrivine-Antistin, 595
Ovestin
    cream, 441
    tablets, 406
Ovitrelle, 414
Ovranette, 448
Ovysmen, 448
Oxactin (fluoxetine), 216
Oxaliplatin, 485, 486
    infusion table, 876
Oxamniquine, 371
Oxazepam, 191, 192
Oxazolidinone antibacterials, 318
Oxcarbazepine
    epilepsy, 254, 255, 256
    trigeminal neuralgia, 247
Oxerutins, 122, 123
Oxidising agents see Hydrogen peroxide
Oxis, 156
Oxpentifylline see Pentoxifylline, 122, 928
Oxprenolol, 92
    cyclopenthiazide with, 92
    see also Beta-adrenoceptor blocking drugs
Oxyal, 604
Oxybuprocaine, 602
Oxybutynin, 457, 458, 459
Oxycodone, 15, 237, 243, 244
    infusion table, 876
    morphine equivalence, 15
    naloxone with, 244
OxyContin, 244
Oxygen
    acute asthma, 179
    alert card, 153
    anaphylaxis, 176
    chronic obstructive pulmonary disease, 179, 180
    cluster headache, 252
    equipment, 180
    myocardial infarction, 137
    nitrous oxide with, 702
    supply arrangements, 181
Oxymetazoline, 614
Oxymetholone, 517
Oxymycin (oxytetracycline), 310
OxyNorm, 244
Oxytetracycline, 310
    acne, 649
    clobetasone butyrate with, 635
    oral infections, 308
    rosacea, 647
Oxytocin, 435, 436, 437
    ergometrine with, 436
    infusion table, 876
Oxyzyme, 921

# P

Pabal, 435
Pabrinex, 548
Pacemakers
    dental practice, 24

Paclitaxel, 490, 491
    infusion table, 876
PACT, x
Paediatric doses, 14
Paediatric Seravit, 902
Paget's disease, 421
Pain, 232
    bone, 233
    dental, 232, 233, 238, 561
    dressings, 702
    musculoskeletal, 233, 588
    neuropathic, 246
    obstetric, 702
    orofacial, 232, 233, 238, 246, 561
        chronic, 247
    palliative care, 15, 18, 237
    perioperative, 238, 706
    rheumatic, 559
    sickle-cell disease, 232
    trigeminal neuralgia, 247
    urethral, 460
    visceral, 237
Paldesic (paracetamol) preparations, 235
Palifermin, 468, 469
Paliperidone, 199, 202
Palivizumab, 356
Palladone preparations, 241
Palliative care
    prescribing, 15
    subcutaneous infusion, 17
Palonosetron, 225, 230
Paludrine, 364
Paludrine/Avloclor, 363
Pamergan-P100, 245
Pamidronate disodium see Disodium pamidronate
Panadeine (co-codamol 8/500), 235
Panadol (paracetamol) preparations, 235
Pancrease HL, 71
Pancreatin, 70, 71
Pancreatitis, chronic, 70
Pancrex preparations, 71
Pancuronium, 709, 710
Panic disorder, 209
Panitumumab, 484
    infusion table, 876
Panoxyl preparations, 647
Panthenol, 547
Pantoprazole, 50
    infusion table, 876
Pantothenic acid, 547
Papaveretum, 244
    anaesthesia, 244
    aspirin with, 234
    hyoscine with, 244
Papaverine, impotence, 464
Paracetamol, 233, 234, 235
    buclizine with, 247
    codeine with, 235, 236, 247
    dihydrocodeine with, 236
    febrile convulsions, 268
    infusion table, 876
    isometheptene with, 236
    methionine with, 236
    metoclopramide with, 248
    migraine, 247
    poisoning by, 29
    post-immunisation pyrexia, 670
    postoperative pain, 706
    tramadol with, 246
Paracodol (co-codamol 8/500), 235
Paradote, 236

Index

Paraffin
    eye, 604
    gauze dressing, 913
    liquid and white soft, 626
    oral emulsion, 63
    white soft, 626
    yellow soft, 604, 626
*Paragauze*, 913
Paraldehyde
    injection—*discontinued*
    status epilepticus, 266, **267**
Paramax, 248
*Paramol* (co-dydramol), 236
*Paranet*, 913
*Paraplatin—discontinued*
Paraproteinaemias, 517
Parasiticidal preparations, 662
    suitable quantities, 662
Parasympathomimetics
    anaesthesia, 711
    eye, 601
    laxatives, 61
    myasthenia gravis, 583
    urinary retention, 456
*Paratex*, 913
Parathyroid hormone, 420, **421**
*Pardelprin* (indometacin), 566
Paromomycin, 367
*Paroven*, 123
Paroxetine, 215, **217**
Paroxysmal nocturnal
    haemoglobinuria, 523
Partial seizures, 254
*Partobulin SDF*, 694
*Parvolex*, 31
Pastes, definition, 625
Patents, 3
Patient group direction, 3
Patient packs, x
*Pavacol-D* (pholcodine), 183
Peak flow meters, 161, 162
Peanut oil *see* Arachis oil
PEC high compression bandage,
    928
*Pediacel*, 675
Pediculosis, 663
*Peditrace*, 540
Pegaptanib, **606**
*Pegasys*, 500
Pegfilgrastim, 525, **526**
Peginterferon alfa, 353, **499**, 500
Pegvisomant, **416**
Pegzerepoetin alfa *see* Methoxy poly-
    ethylene glycol-epoetin beta, 517,
    **521**
*Peha Crepp E*, 926
Pelvic inflammatory disease, 291
Pemetrexed, 475, **478**, 479
    infusion table, 876
Pemphigus, 394
*Penbritin*, 299
Penciclovir, 349, **662**
*Penfine*, 380

Penicillamine, 572
    autoimmune hepatitis, **553**
    cystinuria, **553**
    rheumatic disease, 570, 571,
        **572**
    Wilson's disease, **553**
Penicillin G *see* Benzylpenicillin sod-
    ium
Penicillin V *see* Phenoxymethylpeni-
    cillin, 295, **296**
Penicillin VK *see* Phenoxymethylpeni-
    cillin, 295, **296**
Penicillinases, 296
Penicillins, 295
    antipseudomonal, 301
    broad spectrum, 298
    penicillinase-resistant, 296
    penicillinase-sensitive, 295
*Pennsaid*, 589
*Pentacarinat*, 369
Pentamidine isetionate, **369**
    infusion table, 876
    leishmaniasis, 367
    pneumocystis pneumonia, 368
*Pentasa*, 55
Pentastarch, 533, **534**
Pentazocine, 238, **244**, 245
*Pentostam*, 367
Pentostatin, 484, **485**
    infusion table, 876
Pentoxifylline, **122**, 928
*Pentrax*, 655
*Pepcid* (famotidine) preparations, 46
Peppermint oil, 42, **43**
*Peptac*, 40
*Peptamen* preparations, 882, 886
*Peptisorb*, 882
*Perative*, 886
*Percutol*, 113
*Perdix*, 106
*Perfalgan*, 235
*Perfan*, 74
Pergolide, 268, **270**
*Pergoveris*, 414
*Periactin*, 173
Pericoronitis, 292
Pericyazine, **197**, 198
*Perinal*, 67
Perindopril, **106**
    indapamide with, 106
    *see also* ACE inhibitors
Periodontitis, 617
    antibacterial treatment, 292
*Periogard*, 621
*Periostat*, 617
Peripheral vascular disease, 121
Peritonitis, 290
*PermaFoam* products, 917, 918
Permethrin, 662, **664**
Permitabs, 667
*Peroxyl*, 621
Perphenazine
    depression
        amitriptyline with, 211
    nausea, 225, **227**
    psychoses, **198**
*Persantin* preparations, 136
*Personal Best*, 161
Pertussis
    immunisation, **684**
        vaccines, combined, 675,
            684
    prophylaxis, 293
Pethidine, **245**
    analgesia, 238
        postoperative, 238
        promethazine with, 245

Petroleum jelly, 626
Petroleum products, poisoning by,
    28
*Pevaryl*, 660
Peyronie's disease, 549
PGD *see* Patient group direction, 3
Phaeochromocytoma, 87, **101**
Pharmacist independent prescribing,
    954
*Pharma-Ject Morphine Sulphate*, 238
*Pharmalgen*, 175
*Pharmapore-PU* products, 915
*Pharmorubicin* preparations, 473
Pharyngitis *see* Throat infections
Pharynx *see* Oropharynx
Phenelzine, 213, **214**
*Phenergan* preparations, 174
Phenindione, 130, **132**
Phenobarbital, 259
    epilepsy, **259**
        status epilepticus, **267**
    poisoning, elimination, 28
Phenobarbital sodium, 267
Phenobarbitone *see* Phenobarbital
Phenol, 68
    haemorrhoids, 68
    injection, oily, 68
Phenothiazines, 195
    classification, 195
    nausea and vertigo, 225, 226
    poisoning by, 33
    psychoses, 195
*Phenothrin*, **664**
Phenoxybenzamine, **101**
    infusion table, 876
Phenoxymethylpenicillin, 295, **296**
Phentermine, 224
Phentolamine
    impotence, 464
    phaeochromocytoma, **101**
Phenylalanine amino acid
    supplement, 908
Phenylephrine, 597
    eye, **597**
    hypotension, 124
    infusion table, 877
    injection, 125
    lidocaine with, 716
Phenylketonuria, 540
Phenytoin
    diabetic neuropathy, 389
    epilepsy, **260**
        status epilepticus, 265, **267**,
            268
    infusion table, 877
    trigeminal neuralgia, 247
*Phlexy-10*, 908
*Phlexy-Vits* preparations, 909
Phobia, 213
Pholcodine, 182, **183**
*Phosex*, 544
Phosgene, poisoning by, 35
Phosphate supplements, 544
Phosphate-binding agents, 544
Phosphates
    enemas, 63
    intravenous, 544
    oral, **66**
    rectal, 64
*Phosphate-Sandoz*, 544
Phosphodiesterase inhibitors
    erectile dysfunction, 463
    heart failure, 74
    pulmonary hypertension, 97
Phosphorus, 544
Photodamage, skin, 654

Photodermatoses, 653
  ACBS, 910
Photodynamic therapy, 486
*Photofrin*, 486
Phototherapy, psoriasis, 640
*Phyllocontin Continus*, 161
*Physeptone* (methadone), 242, 285
Physiological saline *see* Sodium chloride
*Physiotens*, 99
*Physiotulle* products, 915, 921
*Phytex*, 661
Phytomenadione, 552
  infusion table, 877
Phytosterolaemia, 146
*Picolax*, 66
Piggy-back technique, 868
*Piko-1*, 161
Pilocarpine
  dry eyes, 621, **622**, 623
  dry mouth, 621, **622**, 623
  eye, **602**
*Pilogel*, 602
Pimecrolimus, 643, **645**
Pimozide, 195, **198**
  Tourette syndrome, 277
Pindolol, **92**
  clopamide with, 92
  *see also* Beta-adrenoceptor
    blocking drugs
*Pinetarsol*, 642
Pinworm infections, 369
Pioglitazone, 384, **386**
  with metformin, 386
Piperacillin
  tazobactam with, **301**
    infusion table, 877
Piperazine, **370**
  roundworm infections, 370
  threadworm infections, 369
Piperazine oestrone sulphate *see*
  Estropipate, 406
*Piportil Depot*, 206
Pipothiazine *see* Pipotiazine, **206**
Pipotiazine, **206**
Piracetam, 265, 277, **278**
Pirenzepine, 47
*Piriton*, 173
Piroxicam, **568**
  rheumatic disease, 560, 568
  topical, 588
*Pitressin*, 418
Pituitary
  function test, 432
  hormones
    anterior, 413
    posterior, 417
Pityriasis versicolor, 333, 659
Pivmecillinam, **302**
Pizotifen, **251**
*PK Aid 4*, 909
*PK Foods*, 905
*PKU* preparations, 908, 909
Plaque, 620
*Plaquenil*, 574
Plasma concentrations, electrolytes,
  526
Plasma substitutes, 532
Plasma, fresh frozen, 142
*Plasma-Lyte* preparations, 537
Plasmapheresis, myasthenia gravis,
  583
Plasters, 925
Plastic wound dressing
  impermeable, 925
  permeable, 925
*Plastipak*, 380

*Plavix*, 136
*Plendil*, 117
*Pletal*, 122
Pneumococcal infection
  antibacterial prophylaxis, 293
  immunisation
    vaccines, 684, **685**
Pneumocystis pneumonia, 368
Pneumonia, 179, 290, 291
  pneumococcal, 685
*Pneumovax II*, 685
*Pocket Chamber*, 162
*Pocketpeak*, 161, 162
*PocketScan* products, 390
Podagra, 581
Podophyllin, 651
Podophyllotoxin, 652, **653**
Podophyllum resin, 651
  *see also* Podophyllotoxin
Poisoning, 27
  active elimination, 28
  adsorbents, 28
  hospital admission, 27
Poisons information services, *inside
  front cover*
Polihexanide, 607
Poliomyelitis
  immunisation, 686
    travel, 686, 695
    vaccines, 685, **686**
    vaccines, combined, 675
*Pollinex*, 175
Polyacrylic acid *see* Carbomers, 603
Polyarteritis nodosa, 395, 569
*Polycal*, 898
  oral glucose tolerance test, 391
Polycystic ovary syndrome, 383
Polyene antifungal drugs, 333
Polyethoxylated castor oil *see* Polyoxyl
  castor oil, 2
Polyethylene glycols, 63
  [ingredient], 65
*Polyfax*
  eye, 593
  skin, 657
*Polyfield Nitrile Patient Pack*, 924
*Polyfield Soft Vinyl Patient Pack*, 924
Polyhexamethylene biguanide *see*
  Polihexanide, 607
Polyhexanide *see* Polihexanide, 607
*PolyMem* products, 917, 918, 921
Polymethylmethacrylate, 665
Polymyalgia rheumatica, 569
Polymyositis, 569, 574
Polymyxins, 319
  ear, 610, 611
  eye, 591, 592, 593, 594
  skin, 657
Polyoxyl castor oil, presence of, 2
Polyps, nasal, 612
Polysaccharide–iron complex, 514
Polyserositis, 581
*Polyskin* products, 915
Polystyrene sulphonate resins, 528
*Polytar*
  *AF*, 655
  *Emollient*, 642
  *Liquid*, 655
  *Plus*, 656
Polyurethane foam dressing, 917, 918,
  921
Polyvinyl alcohol, 604
Pompe disease, 556
*Ponstan* preparations, 567
POP *see* Progestogens, contraceptives,
  oral, 443, 449, **450**
Poractant alfa, **179**

Porfimer sodium, 486
Porphyrias, acute, 557
  drugs to be avoided in, 557, 558
Portal hypertension, 88
*Porta-Neb*, 164
Posaconazole, 333, **338**
*Posalfilin*, 652
Postherpetic neuralgia, 247, 349
Post-traumatic stress disorder, 209
*Potaba*, 549
Potable water, 3
Potassium aminobenzoate, 549
Potassium bicarbonate, **529**
  tablets, effervescent, 529
Potassium chloride, 527, 531
  concentrate, sterile, 532
  infusion
    glucose and, 531
    sodium chloride and, 532
    sodium chloride, glucose
      and, 532
  table, 877
  oral preparations, 527, 528
Potassium citrate, 460
Potassium permanganate, 638, 665,
  **667**
Potassium supplements, 527
  diuretic with, 80
Potassium tablets, effervescent, 529
Potassium-channel activators, 120
  angina, 111
Povidone, eye, 604
Povidone-iodine
  skin, 665, **667**
    dressing, 921
*Powergel*, 589
*Pradaxa*, 132
Prader-Willi syndrome, 415
Pralidoxime chloride, 35, **36**
Pramipexole, 268, **270**, 271
Pramocaine [ingredient], 67, 68
Pramoxine *see* Pramocaine, 67, 68
*Prandin*, 386
Prasugrel, 134, **136**, 137
Pravastatin, 143, **144**, 145
*Praxilene*, 122
Praziquantel, 370, 371
Prazosin, **100**
  cardiovascular, 99, 100
  preparations, 100
  urinary tract, 455, **456**
Precocious puberty, 430
*Pred Forte*, 595
*Predenema*, 57
*Predfoam*, 57
Prednisolone, 394, **399**, 400
  asthma, acute severe, 153
  Crohn's disease, 57
  ear, 610
    neomycin with, 610
  eye, 595
  haemorrhoids, 68
  injection, 570
  lepra reactions, 326
  malignant disease, 494
  myasthenia gravis, 584
  palliative care, 16
  pneumocystis pneumonia, 368
  rectal, 57
  rheumatic disease, 569, 570
  ulcerative colitis, 57
  withdrawal of, 396
*Predsol*
  ear, 610
  eye, 595
  rectal, 57

Index

*Predsol-N*
  ear, 610
  eye, 595
Pre-eclampsia, 95, 543
Preface, ii
Pregabalin
  epilepsy, 254, 256, **257**
  generalised anxiety disorder,
    **257**
  neuropathic pain, 246, **257**
*Pregaday*, 514
Pregnancy
  anticoagulants, 131
  asthma, 150
  epilepsy and, 253
  folate supplements, 513, 516
  hypertension in, 95
  iron, 512
    folic acid and, 513
  nausea and vomiting, 225
  prescribing in, 831
  termination, 434
*Pregnyl*, 413
*Premarin*
  oral, 405
  vaginal, 441
Premedication, 703
  children, 704
  dental procedures, 186, 704
Premenstrual syndrome, 408, 547
*PremierBand*, 928
*PremierPore* products, 913, 915
*Premique* preparations, 403
*Prempak-C*, 403
*Preotact*, 421
*Prescal*, 117
Prescribing, x
  ACBS, 880
  addicts, 9
  analyses and cost, x
  breast-feeding, 852
  children, 13
  computer-generated, 5
  controlled drugs, 8
  dental practice, 4
  drug misusers, 9
  elderly, 19
  generic, 1
  independent, 954
  instalments, 8
  liver disease, 804
  non-proprietary, 1
  palliative care, 15
  patient packs, x
  pregnancy, 831
  renal impairment, 815
  supplementary, 954
Prescription forms
  controlled drugs, 7
  dental, 4
  nurses, 950
  security, 3
Prescription only medicines *see* preparations identified by [PoM] throughout BNF
Prescription writing, 4
*Preservex*, 562
*Presinex* (desmopressin), 419
Pressure sores, 629
*Prestige* products, 390, 391
*Prestim*, 93
*Prevenar*, 685
*Prezista*, 344
*Priadel*, 208
*Prialt*, 233
Priapism, 462

Prices, x
Prilocaine, **717**
  felypressin with, 714, 717
  lidocaine with, 715
*Primacine* (erythromycin), 313
*Primacor*, 74
*Primapore*, 913
Primaquine, 359, **364**
  pneumocystis pneumonia, 368
*Primaxin*, 307
  infusion table, 874
*Primene*, 537
Primidone, 259, **260**
*Primolut N*, 409
*Prioderm*, 664
  lotion—*discontinued*
*Priorix*, 683
*Pripsen*, 370
*Privigen*, 692
*Pro-Banthine*, 42
Probenecid, 581, **582**
Procainamide, 83, 84, 86
Procaine—*discontinued*
*Pro-Cal* preparations, 901
Procarbazine, **486**
*Proceli* products, 904
Prochlorperazine
  nausea and vertigo, 225, **228**
  psychoses, **198**
*Procoralan*, 121
*Proctofoam HC*, 68
*Proctosedyl*, 68
Procyclidine, 276, **277**
*Prodose*, 97
Product licence, 1
*Pro-Epanutin*, 267
Proflavine cream, 665
*Profore* products, 913, 928, 929
Progesterone, 407, **409**
Progestogen-only pill *see* Progesto-
  gens, contraceptives, oral, 443, 449,
    **450**
Progestogens, 505
  contraceptives
    emergency, 454
    intra-uterine, 451, **452**
    oral, 443, 449, **450**
    parenteral, 450, **451**
  HRT, 408
  malignant disease, 504
  menstrual disorders, 407
*Prograf*, 497
Proguanil, 359–363
  atovaquone with, 358, 364, 365
*ProGuide* products, 916, 929, 930
*Progynova* preparations, 406
*Proleukin*, 501
Promazine, 196, **198**
Promethazine
  allergic disorders, 171, **174**
  analgesia, pethidine with, 245
  hypnotic, 189, **190**
  nausea and vertigo, 225, 226, **227**
  premedication, 174
Promethazine teoclate, 227
*Promin*, 905
*Promixin*, 320
*Promogran* products, 922
*Prontosan*, 922
Propafenone, 84, **85**, 86
Propamidine isetionate, 591, **593**
Propantheline, 42
  gastro-intestinal, 41, 42
  urinary tract, 457, 459
*Propax SDP*, 924
*Propecia*, 656

*Propess*, 436
Prophylaxis, antibacterial, 293
*Propine*, 600
*Propionibacterium acnes*, 648
Propiverine, 457, 459
Propofol, 699, **700**
  infusion table, 877
*Propofol-Lipuro*, 700
*Propoven*, 700
Propranolol, **88**, 89
  cardiovascular, 88
  migraine, 251
  *see also* Beta-adrenoceptor
    blocking drugs
  thyrotoxicosis, 393
  tremor, 277
Proprietary names, symbol, 1
Propylene glycol, presence of,
  2
Propylthiouracil, **393**
*Proscar*, 412
Prostacyclin *see* Epoprostenol
Prostaglandins
  anticoagulant, 130
  ductus arteriosus, 437
  eye, 597, 599
  gastro-intestinal, 47
  obstetrics, 434, 435, 436, 437
*Prostap* preparations, 510
Prostate cancer, 470, **508**, 510
Prostatic hyperplasia, benign, 411,
  412, 455
Prostatitis, 291, 331
*Prostin E2* preparations, 436
*Prostin VR*, 437
*ProSure*, 896
*Prosulf*—*discontinued*
Protamine sulphate, 126, **133**
Protease inhibitors, 339, 340, 344
Protease modulating matrix, 922
Proteasome inhibitors, 482
*ProtectFilm*, 915
Protein C concentrate, 142
Protein kinase inhibitors, 486
Protein, intravenous nutrition,
  539
*Protelos*, 426
*Prothiaden*, 212
Prothionamide *see* Protionamide, 323
Prothrombin complex, dried, 131, **141**
*Protifar*, 896
Protionamide, 323
Protirelin, **417**
*Protium*, 50
Proton pump inhibitors, 48
*Protopam*, 36
*Protopic*, 646
Protozoal infections, 357
*Provera*
  gynaecology, 408
  malignant disease, 504
*Provide*, 888
*Provigil*, 223
*Pro-Viron*, 411
Proxymetacaine, **602**
*Prozac*, 216
*Prozep* (fluoxetine), 216
Pruritus, 171, 630
  ACBS, 910
  ani, 67
Pseudoephedrine, **184**
Pseudomembranous colitis
  antibacterial therapy
    metronidazole, in, 327
    vancomycin, in, 316
  clindamycin, in, 315

Index

*Pseudomonas aeruginosa* infections, 306, 307, 310, 319
    antipseudomonal penicillins, in, 301
    cephalosporins, in, 302
    eye, 591
Psittacosis, 308
Psoriasis, 639
    corticosteroids, 631
Psoriatic arthropathy, 574
*Psoriderm* preparations, 642
    scalp, 655
*Psorin* preparations, 643
Psychoses, 193
Puberty
    delayed, 409, 413
    precocious, 430, 431
Pubic lice, 663
*Pulmicort* preparations, 168
Pulmonary
    embolism, 125, 138, 179
    fibrosis, 179
    hypertension, 95, 130, 180
    oedema, 76
    surfactants, 179
*Pulmozyme*, 182
*Pulvinal Beclometasone Dipropionate*, 166
*Pulvinal Salbutamol*, 157
*Pure* products, 904
*Puregon*, 414
*Purilon*, 914
*Puri-Nethol*, 478
Purpura, thrombocytopenic, 523
Pyelonephritis, 291, 331
*Pylobactell*, 44
*Pyralvex*, 618
Pyrazinamide, 321, 322, 323, **324**
Pyrexia, 233
    post immunisation, 670
Pyridostigmine, 583, **584**
    laxative, 61
Pyridoxine, 547, **548**
    anaemias, 517
    status epilepticus, 265
Pyrimethamine
    malaria, **365**
        sulfadoxine with, 358, **365**
    toxoplasmosis, 368
Pyrithione zinc shampoos, 655

# Q

Q-fever, 308
*Qlaira*, 449
*QuanitFERON TB Gold*, 674
Quaternary ammonium compounds, 41
*Quellada M*, 664
*Questran* preparations, 146
Quetiapine, 199, **203**
*QuickCal*, 901
Quinagolide, 426, **428**
Quinapril, **106**
    hydrochlorothiazide with, 107
    *see also* ACE inhibitors
*Quinil* (quinapril), 106
Quinine, **365**, 366
    infusion table, 877
    malaria, 358, 359, 365
    nocturnal cramps, 587
    poisoning
        elimination, 28
*Quinoderm*, 647

Quinolones, 328
    eye, 591
Quinupristin, dalfopristin with, **319**
    infusion table, 877
*QV* preparations, 627, 628
*Qvar* preparations, 167

# R

Rabeprazole, **50**
Rabies
    immunisation, 686
        travel, 695
    immunoglobulin, 692, 693
    vaccine, **686**, 687
*Rabipur*, 687
Raloxifene, **407**, 420
Raltegravir, 340, **348**
Raltitrexed, 476, **477**
    infusion table, 877
Ramipril, **107**
    felodipine with, 107
    *see also* ACE inhibitors
*Ranexa*, 121
Ranibizumab, **606**, 607
*Ranitic* (ranitidine), 46
Ranitidine, **46**, 47
    infusion table, 877
Ranolazine, 120, **121**
*Rapamune*, 497
*Rapifen*, 708
*Rapilysin*, 139
*Rapitil*, 596
*Rapolyte—discontinued*
*Raptiva—discontinued*
*Rapydan*, 716
Rasagiline, **274**
Rasburicase, 466, **582**
    infusion table, 877
Rashes, urticarial, 171
*Rasilez*, 110
*Ratiograstim*, 526
Raynaud's syndrome, 100, 118, 121
*Rebetol*, 357
*Rebif*, 500
Reboxetine, 218, **219**
Recombinant activated protein C, **141**
*Rectogesic*, 68
Red eye, 591, 594
*Redoxon* (ascorbic acid), 549
*Reductil*, 225
*ReFacto AF* (factor VIII fraction), 141
*Reflexions* diaphragm, 454
*Refludan*, 129
Reflux oesophagitis *see* Gastro-oeso-phageal reflux disease, **38**
*Refolinon* (calcium folinate), 468
*Regaine*, 656
*Regal*, 924
*Regranex*, 668
*Regulan*, 60
*Regulose* (lactulose), 63
*Regurin*, 460
Rehydration
    oral, 528
    parenteral, 530
*Relaxit*, 65
*Release*, 913
*Relenza*, 356
*Relestat*, 596
*Relifex*, 567
*Relistor*, 67
*Relpax*, 248
*Remedeine*, 236
*Remicade*, 580

Remifentanil, 237, 707, **708**
    infusion table, 877
*Reminyl* preparations, 206
*Remnos* (nitrazepam), 187
*Renagel*, 545
Renal colic *see* Ureteric colic, 460
Renal excretion, interactions affecting, 720
Renal impairment, prescribing in, 815
*Renamil*, 896
*Renapro*, 897
*Renastart*, 897
*Renilon 7.5*, 893
Renin inhibitors, 110
*Rennie Duo*, 40
*ReoPro*, 135
Repaglinide, 384, **386**
*Repevax*, 675
*Replagal*, 554
*Replenine-VF* (factor IX fraction), 142
*Replens*, 441
*Requip* preparations, 271
*RescueFlow*, 533
*Resonium A*, 528
*Resource* preparations
    fibre supplement, 902
    nutritional supplement, 888, 891, 893
    thickened, 903
*Respifor*, 897
Respiratory
    depression
        poisoning, 27
        postoperative, 712
    distress syndrome, 179
    failure, 178
    stimulants, 178
    syncytial virus infections , 356
*Respontin*, 159
*Resprin*, 234
*Restandol*, 410
Restless legs syndrome
    pramipexole, 270
    ropinirole, 271
Resuscitation
    cardiopulmonary, 125
    dental practice, 698
*Retacrit*, 520
Retapamulin, **657**, 658
Reteplase, 138, **139**
*Retin-A*, 649
Retinoids
    acne
        oral, 650
        topical, 648
    eczema, **638**
    leukaemia, 492
    psoriasis, 640, **643**
Retinol *see* Vitamin A
*Retrovir*, 344
*Revatio*, 97, 464
*Revaxis*, 675
*Revlimid*, 502
*Rexocaine*, 715
*Reyataz*, 344
Reye's syndrome, aspirin and, 234
Rhesus incompatibility, 693
*Rheumatac Retard* (diclofenac), 564
Rheumatic diseases, 559, 569
    corticosteroid injections, 569
    rubefacients, 588
Rheumatic fever
    prophylaxis, 293
Rheumatism, palindromic, 571
Rheumatoid arthritis, 395, 559
*Rheumox*, 562

Rhinitis
  allergic, 171, 612
  medicamentosa, 614
  vasomotor, 171, 614
*Rhinocort Aqua*, 613
*Rhinolast* preparations, 612
*Rhophylac*, 694
*Rhumalgan* (diclofenac), 564
*Riamet*, 358, 362
Ribavirin, **356**, 357
  chronic hepatitis C, 353, 356
  respiratory syncytial virus,
    356
Riboflavin, 547, 548
Rickets, hypophosphataemic, 544
Rickettsia, 308
*Ridaura*, 571
Rifabutin, 323, **324**, 325
*Rifadin*, 325
Rifampicin, **325**
  compound preparations, 325
  infusion table, 877
  leprosy, 326
  tuberculosis, 321, 322, 323
Rifamycins, 321–5
*Rifater*, 322, 325
*Rifinah*, 322, 325
*Rilutek*, 278
Riluzole, 277, **278**
RIMA, 214
*Rimacid* (indometacin), 566
*Rimacillin* (ampicillin), 299
*Rimactane*, 325
*Rimafen* (ibuprofen), 565
*Rimapam* (diazepam), 191
*Rimapurinol* (allopurinol), 582
Rimexolone, **595**
Rimonabant, 223, **224**
*Rimoxallin* (amoxicillin), 299
*Rimso-50*, 461
*Rinatec*, 615
Ringer's solution, 531
Ringer-Lactate solution, 531
Ringworm infection *see* Dermatophyte
  infection, 333
Risedronate sodium, 419, **424**
  calcium carbonate and colecal-
    ciferol with, 424
*Risperdal* preparations, 203, 206
Risperidone
  depot injection, **206**
  psychosis, 199, **203**
*Ritalin*, 222
*Rite-Diet*
  gluten-free, 904
  low protein, 905
Ritodrine, 439, **440**
  infusion table, 877
Ritonavir, 340, **346**
  lopinavir with, 345
  *see also* Kaletra
Rituximab
  infusion table, 877
  malignant diseases, 498, **499**
  rheumatic diseases, 577, 580
Rivaroxaban, 132, **133**
Rivastigmine, 285, **287**
*Rivotril*, 265, 266
Rizatriptan, 248, **249**
*Rizopia* products, 904
*Roaccutane*, 651
*Robaxin*, 587
*Robinul*, 668, 703
*Robinul-Neostigmine*, 712
*Rocaltrol*, 550
*Rocephin*, 306

Rocuronium, 709, **710**
  infusion table, 877
*Roferon-A*, 499
*Rogitine*, 101
Ropinirole, 268, **271**
Ropivacaine, **718**
Rosacea, 647
*Rosiced*, 658
Rosiglitazone, 384, **386**
  metformin with, 387
Rosuvastatin, 143, **145**
*Rotarix*, 687
Rotavirus vaccine, **687**
Rotigotine, 268, **271**, 272
Roundworm infections, 370
*Rowachol*, 70
*Rowatinex*, 461
*Rozex*, 659
rt-PA *see* Alteplase
Rubefacients, 588
Rubella
  immunisation, 687
    immunoglobulin, 691
    vaccines, combined, 681,
      683
Rufinamide, 254, **261**
*Rusyde* (furosemide), 77
Rutosides, 122
*Rynacrom*, 614
*Rythmodan* preparations, 85

## S

*Sabril*, 264
St John's Wort, 209
*Saizen*, 416
*Salactol*, 652
*Salagen*, 623
*Salamol* (salbutamol) preparations,
  157
*Salapin* (salbutamol), 156
Salatac, 652
*Salazopyrin*, 56, 581
*Salbulin Novolizer*, 157
Salbutamol, **156**, 157
  asthma, 154
  infusion table, 877
  ipratropium with, 161
  premature labour, 440
Salcatonin *see* Calcitonin
Salicylates
  aphthous ulcers, 618
  rheumatic disease
    topical, 588
Salicylic acid, 643
  acne, 649
  fungal infections, 661
  hyperkeratoses, 651
  psoriasis, 640
    betamethasone with, 634
    coal tar and dithranol with,
      643
    coal tar with, 641, 655
    dithranol and zinc with, 642
    sulphur with, 655
    zinc with, 643
  scalp, 655
  warts and calluses, 651, 652
    podophyllum with, 652
Saline *see* Sodium chloride
*Salinum*, 622
Saliva, artificial, 621

*Saliveze*, 622
*Salivix*, 622
Salmeterol, 154, **157**, 158
  fluticasone with, 169
Salmonellosis, 290
*Salofalk* preparations, 55
Salpingitis, 308
Salt substitutes, 527
*Sandimmun*, 496
*Sandocal* preparations, 542
  colecalciferol with, 551
*Sando-K*, 527
*Sandostatin*, 511
*Sandostatin LAR*, 511
*Sandrena*, 406
*Sanomigran*, 251
Sapropterin, **540**
Saquinavir, 340, **346**
*Savene*, 467
*Savlon Dry* powder, 667
Scabies, 662
*Scandishake*, 901
*Scandonest*, 714
*Scanpor*, 925
*Schar*, 904
*Scheriproct*, 68
Schistosoma, 371
Schistosomicides, 371
Schizophrenia, 194
Scleroderma, 549
Sclerosants, 149
*Scopoderm* preparations, 232
Scopolamine *see* Hyoscine, 41, **42**
Scottish Medicines Consortium, 3
Scottish Prescribing Analysis, x
Scurvy, 549
*SeaSorb* products, 918
*Sebco*, 642
*Sebivo*, 354
*Sebomin*, 310
Seborrhoeic dermatitis, 638
Seborrhoeic eczema, 638
Secobarbital
  amobarbital with, 193
*Seconal Sodium—discontinued*
*Sectral*, 89
*Securon* preparations, 120
Sedation, anaesthesia, 704
Sedatives, 185
  *see also* Anxiolytics
*Select-A-Jet Dopamine*, 123
Selegiline, **274**, 275
*Selenase*, 546
Selenium, **546**
Selenium sulphide, 655, 659
*Selexid*, 302
*Selsun*, 655
Semi-permeable adhesive film, 914
Semisodium valproate *see* Valproic
  acid
Senna, **62**
*Senokot*, 62
*Septanest*, 714
Septic arthritis, 292
Septicaemia
  catheter-related, 292
  community-acquired, 292
  hospital-acquired, 292
  meningococcal, 292
*Septrin*, 321
*Seractil*, 563
*Seravit, Paediatric*, 902
*Serc*, 232
*Serdolect*, 204
*Serenace*, 197
*Seretide*, 169

Index

*Serevent*, 158
*Seroquel* preparations, 203
Serotonin rc-uptakc inhibitor anti-
    depressants *see* Antidepressants
*Seroxat*, 217
Sertindole, 200, 204
Sertraline, 215, **217**
Sesame oil, presence of, 2
*Setocrepe*, 928
*Setopress*, 928
Sevelamer, 544, **545**
*Sevikar*, 109
Sevoflurane, 701, **702**
*Sevredol*, 242
Sex hormones
    androgens, 409
        antagonists, 411
    malignant disease, 504
    oestrogens, 400
        antagonists, 412
    progestogens, 407
Sexual deviation, 196, 411
Shampoos, 655
Shared care, 4
*Sharpsguard*, 380
Shigellosis, 290
Shingles, 349
Shock, 123
    anaphylactic, 176
        dental practice, 21
    cardiogenic, 123
    metabolic acidosis, 532
    plasma substitutes, 533
    septic, 123
        corticosteroids in, 395
Sibutramine, 223, **224**, 225
Sicca syndrome, 621
Sickle-cell disease, 521
    pain management, 232
*Sidestream Durable*, 164
*Sigma ETB*, 926
Significant changes, xi
*Siklos*, 522
Sildenafil, 464
    erectile dysfunction, 463, **464**
    pulmonary hypertension, 95, **97**
*Silgel*, 923
Silicone
    dressings, soft, 915
    gel dressings, 922, 923
    keloid spray, 922
Silk clothing, 927
*Silkis*, 641
*Silkolan*, 929
*Silon-TSR*, 915
*Siltape*, 925
*Siltex*, 915
Silver nitrate, 651, **652**
Silver sulfadiazine, 657, **658**
Silver sulphadiazine *see* Silver sulfa-
    diazine, 657, **658**
*Silvercel*, 922
Silver-containing dressings, 921, 922
Simeticone, 39, 40
Simple eye ointment, 604
Simple linctus, 184
    paediatric, 184
*SimpleXx*, 416
*Simulect*, 495
*Simvador* (simvastatin), 145
Simvastatin, 143, **145**
    ezetimibe with, 145
*Sinemet* preparations, 273, 274
*Sinepin*, 212
*Singulair*, 170
*Sinthrome*, 132

Sinusitis, 615
    antibacterial treatment, 292
    inhalation, 102
*Siopel*, 629
Sirolimus, 495, **496**, 497
Sitagliptin, 384, **387**
Sitaxentan, 95, **97**, 98
Sitosterolaemia, 146
*Skelid*, 425
Skin preparations
    anaesthetic, 630
    antibacterials, 656
    antipruritic, 630
    antiviral, 661
    barrier, 629
    cleansing, 665
    closure dressings, 926
    corticosteroids, 630
    emollient, 625
    excipients, 625
    tissue adhesive, 665
    ulcers, 667
*Skinnies*, 927
*Skinoren*, 647
*Skintact*, 913
*Sleek*, 925
*Slinky*, 926
*SLO Drinks*, 903
*Slocinx XL* (doxazosin), 100
*Slofenac* (diclofenac), 564
*Slo-Phyllin*, 160
*Slo-Pro* (propranolol), 89
*Slow-K*, 528
*Slow-Sodium*, 528
*Slow-Trasicor*, 92
*Slozem*, 116
Smallpox vaccine, 687
SMC *see* Scottish Medicines Consor-
    tium, 3
*SMOFlipid* preparations, 538
Smoking cessation, 280
Snake bites, 36
    antivenom, 36
*Sno Tears*, 604
*Sno-Pro*, 905
Social anxiety disorder, 209
Social phobia *see* social anxiety disor-
    der
*Sodiofolin*, 468
Sodium acid phosphate, 544
Sodium alendronate *see* Alendronic
    acid
*Sodium Amytal*, 193
Sodium aurothiomalate, **571**, 572
Sodium benzoate, 14
Sodium bicarbonate
    antacid, 38
    ear wax removal, 611
    intravenous, 532
    oral, 529
    urine alkalinisation, 460
Sodium calcium edetate, **35**
    infusion table, 877
Sodium calciumedetate *see* Sodium
    calcium edetate
Sodium carboxymethylcellulose *see*
    Carmellose
Sodium chloride
    bladder irrigation, 461, 666
    eye irrigation, 590, **604**
    infusion, 530
        glucose and, 530
        hypercalcaemia, 542
        potassium chloride and,
            532
        potassium chloride, glucose
            and, 532

Sodium chloride (*continued*)—
    mouthwash, compound, 620,
        **621**
    nasal solution, 614
    nebuliser solution, 164
        hypertonic, 182
    oral, 528
    skin cleansing, **665**, 666
Sodium citrate
    acid aspiration prophylaxis, 698
    bladder irrigation, **461**
    rectal, 65
    urine alkalinisation, 460
Sodium clodronate, 425
    infusion table, 877
Sodium content, antacids, 39
Sodium cromoglicate
    asthma, **170**
    eye, 595, **596**
    food allergy, 58, 59
    nose, 612, **614**
Sodium cromoglycate *see* Sodium
    cromoglicate
Sodium docusate *see* Docusate sodium
Sodium feredetate, 514
Sodium fluoride, **545**, 546
Sodium fusidate, **316**
    angular cheilitis, 619
    skin, 658
Sodium hyaluronate
    intra-articular, 560
    intra-ocular, 605
    tear deficiency, 603, **604**
Sodium ironedetate *see* Sodium fere-
    detate, 514
Sodium lactate, 532
    intravenous infusion, 532
        compound, 530, 531
Sodium nitrite, **34**
Sodium nitroprusside, 95, **98**
    infusion table, 877
Sodium oxybate, 33, **190**
Sodium phenylbutyrate, 556
Sodium picosulfate, **62**
    magnesium citrate with, **66**
Sodium picosulphate *see* Sodium
    picosulfate
Sodium pidolate, 627
Sodium polystyrene sulphonate, 528
Sodium risedronate *see* Risedronate
    sodium
Sodium stibocaptate, 371
Sodium stibogluconate, **367**
Sodium tetradecyl sulphate, **149**
Sodium thiosulphate, **34**
Sodium valproate *see* Valproate
*Soffcrepe*, 928
*Sofradex*
    ear, 609
    eye, 594
Soft polymer dressings, 915
Soft tissue disorders, 559
*Softclix* products, 380
*Softexe*, 929
*Softpore*, 913
*Solaraze*, 654
*Solian*, 200
Solifenacin, 457, **459**
*Soliris*, 523
*Solivito N*, 540
*Solpadol*, 236
*Soltamox* (tamoxifen), 507
*Solu-Cortef*, 399
*Solu-Medrone*, 399
*Solvaline N*, 913
*Solvazinc*, 546
Solvents, ear wax removal, 611

Somatomedins, 432
Somatostatin analogues, 510
Somatotrophin *see* Somatropin, 415, 416
Somatropin, 415, 416
*Somatuline* preparations, 511
*Somavert*, 416
*Somnite* (nitrazepam), 187
*Sonata*, 188
*Soneryl*, 193
Sorafenib, 487, **489**
*Sorbalgon* products, 918
*Sorbion* products, 916, 922
Sorbitol, 539
    presence of, 2
*Sorbsan* products, 918, 919, 922
*Sotacor*, 93
Sotalol, **92**, 93
    cardiovascular, 88
    infusion table, 877
    *see also* Beta-adrenoceptor blocking drugs
Soya oil, 628
SPA, x
Spacer devices, 162
*Spasmonal* preparations, 42
Spasticity, 585
*SpectraBan*, 653
Spermicides, 452
SPF, 653
Spiramycin, 312, 368
Spirit
    industrial methylated, 665
    surgical, 665
*Spiriva* preparations, 160
Spironolactone, 78, **79**
    furosemide with, 80
    heart failure, 102
    hydroflumethiazide with, 80
Splenectomy *see* Asplenia
*Sporanox* preparations, 337
Sports card, 26
*Sprilon*, 629
*Sprycel*, 488
SQ-PEN, 380
SSRIs *see* Antidepressants, serotonin re-uptake inhibitor, 215
*SST*, 622
*Stalevo*, 274
*Stamaril*, 690
Stannous fluoride, 546
Starch, etherified, 533, 534
*Staril*, 105
*Starlix*, 386
Statins, 143
    angina, 111
Status epilepticus, 265
    non-convulsive, 266
Stavudine, 340, **343**
*Stayform*, 926
*STD injection* see *Fibro-Vein*
Steam inhalations, 614
*Stelara*, 646
*Stelazine*, 199
*Stemetil*, 228
Sterculia, 60
    constipation, 60
    diarrhoea, 51
*Stericlens*, 666
*Sterifix*, 913
Sterile larvae, 667
*Steri-Neb*
    ipratropium, 159
    *Salamol*, 157
    sodium chloride, 164
*Steripaste*, 930

*Steripod* (sodium chloride), 666
*Steripoule* (sodium chloride), 164
*Steri-strip*, 926
Steroid cards, 397
*Ster-Zac—discontinued*
*Stesolid* (diazepam), 191, 266
Stibocaptate *see* Sodium stibocaptate, 371
*Stiemycin*, 648
Stilboestrol *see* Diethylstilbestrol, **504**, 508
Still's disease *see* Arthritis, juvenile idiopathic, 571
*Stilnoct*, 188
Stimulants
    central nervous system, 220
    respiratory, 178
Stings, 36
Stiripentol, 254
Stockinettes, 926, 927
Stoma, drugs and, 68
Stomatitis
    denture, 618
    herpetic, 620
*Strappal*, 925
*Strattera*, 221
*Strefen*, 618
*Streptase*, 140
Streptococcal infection
    antibacterial prophylaxis, 293
Streptogramin antibiotics, 319
Streptokinase, 138, **139**, 140
    infusion table, 878
Streptomycin, 321, 323, **325**, 326
*Striant SR*, 410
*Stronazon MR* (tamsulosin), 456
Strongyloidiasis, 371
Strontium ranelate, 420, **426**
*StructoKabiven* preparations, 538
Structolipid, 538
*Stugeron*, 226
*Subcuvia*, 691
*Subgam*, 691
*Sublimaze*, 708
*Suboxone*, 284
*Subutex*, 284
Succimer, 34
Succinylcholine *see* Suxamethonium
Sucralfate, **47**
Sucrose, presence of, 2
*Sudafed*, 184
*Sudocrem*, 630
Sugammadex, **712**
Sugar-free liquid medicines *see* preparations identified by 'sugar-free' throughout BNF
Sugar-free, definition, 2
*Sulazine EC* (sulfasalazine), 56, 581
Sulconazole, 659, **661**
Sulfa... *see also* Sulpha...
Sulfadiazine, **321**
    infusion table, 878
    toxoplasmosis, 368
Sulfadiazine, silver, 658
Sulfadoxine, pyrimethamine with, 358, 365
Sulfamethoxazole, trimethoprim with, *see* Co-trimoxazole
Sulfasalazine, 52
    Crohn's disease, 56
    inflammatory bowel disease, 54, **56**
    rheumatic disease, 570, 571, 580, 581
    ulcerative colitis, 54, **56**
Sulfinpyrazone, 581, **582**

Sulindac, 560, **568**
    gout, 581
Sulpha... *see also* Sulfa...
Sulphadiazine *see* Sulfadiazine
Sulphasalazine *see* Sulfasalazine
Sulphinpyrazone *see* Sulfinpyrazone, 581, **582**
Sulphites, presence of, 2
Sulphonamides, 320
Sulphonylureas, 381
Sulphur, 640, 649
    salicylic acid with, 655
Sulphur dioxide, poisoning, 35
Sulpiride, 195, **199**
    Tourette syndrome, 277
*Sulpor*, 199
*Sumar* products, 919
Sumatriptan, 248, **249**, 250
    cluster headache, 252
    migraine, 248
Sun protection factor, 653
Sunitinib, 487, **489**
*Sunnyvale*, 904
Sunscreens, 653
    ACBS, 910
*Sunsense Ultra*, 654
*Sunya 20/75*, 447
Superinfection, 290
*Suplasyn*, 560
*Suplena*, 897
Supplementary preparations, 539
Supplementary prescribing, 954
*Supralip*, 148
*Suprane*, 701
*Suprasorb* products, 922
    alginate, 919
    antimicrobial, 922
    bio-cellulose, 916
    film dressing, 915
    foam dressings, 917
    hydrocolloid, 916, 917
*Suprax*, 304
*Suprecur*, 430
*Suprefact*, 509
Suramin, 371
*SurePress*, 928, 929
Surfactants, pulmonary, 179
*Surgam* preparations, 569
Surgery
    antibacterial prophylaxis, 293, 294
    diabetes and, 375
    long-term medication and, 697
    tetanus vaccine, 687
Surgical
    absorbent dressings, 923
    adhesive tapes, 925
    spirit, 665
*Surgipad*, 923
*Surmontil*, 212
*Survanta*, 179
*Survimed* OPD, 882
*Suscard*, 112
*Sustanon* preparations, 410
*Sustiva*, 347
*Sutent*, 489
Suxamethonium, **711**
    infusion table, 878
Swabs, 924
*Sylk*, 441
*Symbicort*, 168
Symbols, *inside back cover*
*Symmetrel*, 276

Sympathomimetics
    asthma, 154
    decongestants, 614
    eye, 597, 600
    inotropic, 123
    premature labour, 439
    vasoconstrictor, 124
Synacthen preparations, 413
Synagis, 356
Synalar preparations, 636
Synarel, 431
Synastone (methadone), 242, 285
Syncope, dental practice, 23
Synercid, 319
Syner-KINASE, 140
Synflex, 567
Synocrom, 560
Synphase, 448
Syntaris, 613
Synthamin preparations, 538
Syntocinon, 435, 437
Syntometrine, 435, 436
Synvisc, 560
Syphilis, 291
Syprol (propranolol), 88
Syringe drivers, palliative care, 17
Syringes
    insulin, 380
        blind patients, 380
    oral, 2
System 4 products, 929
System 22 nebulisers, 164
Systemic sclerosis, 95
Sytron, 514


T

Tabphyn MR (tamsulosin), 456
Tacalcitol, 639, 640, 641
Tachycardias see Arrhythmias
Tacrolimus
    eczema, 643, 645, 646
    immunosuppression, 495, 497
        infusion table, 878
Tadalafil, 463, 464
Taenicides, 370
Tagamet preparations, 45
Tambocor preparations, 85
Tamiflu, 355
Tamoxifen, 505, 507
    breast pain, 432
    infertility, 412
Tamsulosin, 455, 456
Tanatril, 105
Tapes, surgical adhesive, 925
Tapeworm infections, 370
Tar, 642
    see also Coal tar
Taranis products, 905
Tarceva, 488
Tardive dyskinesia, 195
Targinact, 244
Targocid, 317
Targretin, 482
Tarivid, 331
Tarka, 107
Tartrazine, presence of, 2
Tasigna, 489
Tasmar, 275
Tavanic, 330
Tavegil, 173
Taxanes, 490
Taxol, 491

Taxotere, 490
Tazarotene, 639, 641
Tazobactam
    piperacillin with, 301
        infusion table, 877
Tazocin, 301
3TC see Lamivudine
Tear deficiency, 603
Tear gas, 35
Tears Naturale, 604
Tears, artificial, 603
Tegaderm products, 915, 916, 917, 918, 919, 922
Tegafur, 476, 479
    uracil with, 479
Tegretol preparations, 255
Teicoplanin, 316, 317
    infusion table, 878
Telangiectasia, hereditary haemorrhagic, 407
Telbivudine, 353, 354
Telfa products, 913, 922
Telfast, 172
Telithromycin, 313, 314, 315
Telmisartan, 107, 109
    hydrochlorothiazide with, 109
Telzir, 345
Temazepam, 187
    anaesthesia, 704, 706
Temgesic, 238
Temocillin, 296, 298
    infusion table, 878
Temodal, 483
Temoporfin, 486
Temozolomide, 483
Temporomandibular dysfunction, 233
Temsirolimus, 487, 489, 490
    infusion table, 878
Tendinitis, 569
Tenecteplase, 138, 140
Tenif, 89
Tennis elbow, 569
Tenofovir
    chronic hepatitis B, 343, 353
    HIV infection, 340, 343
        efavirenz and emtricitabine with, 343
        emtricitabine with, 343
Tenoret-50, 89
Tenoretic, 89
Tenormin, 89
Tenoxicam, 561, 568
TENS, 16
Tensipine MR, 119
Tensium (diazepam), 191
Tensopress, 928
Tensopril (captopril), 104
Teoptic, 598
Teratogenesis, 831
Teratology information service, inside front cover
Terazosin
    cardiovascular, 99, 100, 101
    urinary tract, 455, 456
Terbinafine, 333, 334, 338
    topical, 659, 661
Terbutaline
    asthma, 154, 158
    infusion table, 878
    premature labour, 440
Teriparatide, 420, 421, 422
Terlipressin, 419
Terminal care see Palliative care
Terpenes, gall bladder, 70
Testim, 410
Testogel, 410

Testosterone
    esters, 409
        enantate, 409, 410
        propionate, 409, 410
        undecanoate, 409, 410
    malignant disease, 505
    replacement therapy, 410, 411
Tetanus
    antibacterial treatment, 327
    immunisation, 687
        immunoglobulin, 693
        vaccines, combined, 675, 687
    muscle spasm, 586
    travel, 695
    wounds, 687
Tetany, hypocalcaemic, 541
Tetrabenazine, 277, 278
Tetracaine
    eye, 602
    local anaesthetic, 718
        lidocaine with, 716
    rectal, 67
Tetracosactide, 413
Tetracosactrin see Tetracosactide, 413
Tetracycline, 308, 309
    acne, 649
    diabetic neuropathy, 389
    oral infections, 308
    rosacea, 647
Tetracyclines see Tetracycline
Tetralysal-300, 309
Tetraspan preparations, 534
Tetrastarch, 533, 534
Teveten, 108
T-Gel, 655
Thalassaemia, 522
Thalidomide, 502, 503
    lepra reactions, 326
Thalidomide Pharmion, 503
Thelin, 98
Theophylline, 160
    poisoning, 33
        elimination, 28
    see also Aminophylline
Thiamine, 547, 548
    status epilepticus, 265
Thiazides, 75
    diabetes insipidus, 417
    see also Diuretics
Thiazolidinediones, 384
Thick and Easy, 903
Thioguanine see Tioguanine, 476, 479
Thiopental, 699, 700, 701
Thiopentone see Thiopental, 699, 700, 701
Thiopurine methyltransferase, 493
Thiotepa, 461, 470, 471
Thioxanthenes, 195
Thixo-D, 903
Threadworm infections, 369
Throat infections, 292
    gonorrhoea, 291
Thrombocythaemia, 524
Thrombocytopenia, 517
Thrombocytopenic purpura, 523
    immunoglobulin, 690
Thromboembolism, 130
    pulmonary, 125, 138, 179
Thrombolytics, 138
Thrombosis
    antiplatelet drugs, 133
    deep-vein, 125, 130
    prophylaxis, 126
    venous, 138
Thrush see Candidiasis

Index

*Thymoglobuline*, 495
Thymol, 621
Thymoxamine *see* Moxisylyte, **122**
*Thyrogen*, 417
Thyroid
    antagonists, 392
    carcinoma, 391
    function test, 417
    hormones, 391
    stimulating hormone, 416
    storm, 393
Thyroidectomy, 392
Thyrotoxic crisis, 393
Thyrotoxicosis, 392
    beta-blockers, 88, 393
Thyrotrophin-releasing hormone *see*
    Protirelin, **417**
Thyrotropin alfa, **416**, 417
Thyroxine *see* Levothyroxine, 391,
    392
Tiagabine, 254, **261**
Tiaprofenic acid, 560, **569**
Tibolone, 400, **406**, 407
Ticarcillin, **301**
    clavulanic acid with, 301, 302
        infusion table, 878
Tick-borne encephalitis, 695
    immunisation, vaccine, **688**
*TicoVac*, 688
Tics, 277
*Tielle* products, 917, 918, 919
*Tifaxin XL*, 220
Tigecycline, **310**
    infusion table, 878
*Tilade CFC-free Inhaler*, 170
*Tildiem* preparations, 116
*Tilofyl* (fentanyl), 241
*Tiloket CR*, 566
*Tiloryth* (erythromycin), 313
Tiludronic acid, 425
*Timentin*, 302
    infusion table, 878
*Timodine*, 633
Timolol
    cardiovascular, **93**
        bendroflumethiazide with,
        93
    eye, **598**, 599
        bimatoprost with, 599
        brimonidine with, 600
        brinzolamide with, 601
        dorzolamide with, 601
        latanoprost with, 599
        travoprost with, 600
    migraine, 251
    *see also* Beta-adrenoceptor
        blocking drugs
*Timoptol*, 599
*Timoptol LA*, 599
*Tinaderm-M*, 661
Tinea infections, 333, 659
Tinidazole, 327, **328**
    amoebiasis, 366
    giardiasis, 367
    protozoal infections, 366
    trichomoniasis, 367
Tinzaparin, 127, **128**
Tioconazole, 659, **661**
Tioguanine, 476, **479**
Tiotropium, **159**, 160
Tipranavir, 340, **346**
Tirofiban, 111, 134, **137**
    infusion table, 878
*Tisept*, 666
Tissue adhesive, 665
Titanium dioxide, 629

*Tixycolds* preparations, 615
Tizanidine, 585, **586**
*Tobi*, 312
*Tobia Teff* products, 904
*Tobradex*, 594
Tobramycin, 311, **312**
    eye, 594
    infusion table, 878
Tocopherols, 551
Tocopheryl, 551
*Toctino*, 639
Toilet preparations, ACBS, 910
Tolbutamide, 381, **382**
Tolcapone, **275**
Tolfenamic acid, **248**, 561
Tolnaftate, 659, 661
Tolterodine, 457, **459**
*Tomudex*, 479
Tonic seizures, 254
Tonic-clonic seizures, 254
Tonics, 553
Tonsillitis *see* Throat infections
*Topal*, 41
*Topamax*, 262
Topiramate
    epilepsy, 254, **261**, 262
    migraine, 251, **261**
Topotecan, **491**
    infusion table, 878
*Toradol*, 707
Torasemide, **77**
*Torem*, 77
Toremifene, 505, **507**
*Torisel*, 490
Torsade de pointes, **82**, 543
    magnesium sulphate, 543
Torsion dystonias, 278
*Tostran*, 411
Total parenteral nutrition, 534
*Tourer*, 164
Tourette syndrome, 277
*Toviaz*, 458
TOXBASE, 27
Toxoplasma choroidoretinitis, 368
Toxoplasmosis, 368
TPA *see* Alteplase
TPN, 534
Trabectedin, **492**
Trachoma, 308, 591
*Tracleer*, 96
*Tracrium*, 710
Trade marks, symbol, 1
*Tradorec XL*, 246
Tramadol, 238, **245**, 246
    infusion table, 878
    paracetamol with, 246
*Tramake* preparations, 245
*Tramquel SR*, 246
*Trandate*, 91
Trandolapril, **107**
    *see also* ACE inhibitors
    verapamil with, 107
Tranexamic acid, **140**, 141
    infusion table, 878
*Trangina XL* (isosorbide mononitrate),
    114
Tranquillisers, 185
Transcutaneous electrical nerve
    stimulation, 16
Transfusion reactions, 517
*Transiderm-Nitro*, 113
Transient ischaemic attacks, 130
*Transorbent*, 917
Transplant rejection, 493, 495

*Transtec*, 239
Tranylcypromine, 213, **214**
*Trasicor*, 92
*Trasidrex*, 92
Trastuzumab, **492**
    infusion table, 878
*Travasept-100*, 666
*Travatan*, 600
Travel, vaccination for, 695
Travellers' diarrhoea, 695
Travoprost, **599**, 600
    with timolol, 600
*Traxam* preparations, 589
Trazodone, 210, **213**
Treatment cards, anticoagulant, 131
Tree pollen allergy preparations, 175
Tremors, 277
*Trental*, 122
Treosulfan, 470, **471**
    infusion table, 878
Tretinoin
    acne, 648, 649
        erythromycin with, 649
    leukaemia, 492, 493
TRH *see* Protirelin, **417**
*Tri-Adcortyl Otic*—discontinued
*Triadene*, 449
Triamcinolone
    mouth, 617
    nose, 614
    parenteral
        allergic conditions, **400**
        rheumatic diseases, 570
    skin, 637
*Triam-Co* (co-triamterzide), 79
Triamterene, **78**
    benzthiazide with, 79
    chlortalidone with, 80
    furosemide with, 80
    hydrochlorothiazide with, 79
*Triapin* preparations, 107
Triazole antifungal drugs, 333
Tribavirin *see* Ribavirin
Trichomonacides, 367
Trichomonal infections, 367
Triclofos, 188, **189**
*Tricotex*, 913
Tricyclic antidepressants *see* Anti-
    depressants, tricyclic
*Tridestra*, 405
Trientine, **553**
Trifluoperazine
    nausea and vertigo, 225, **228**
    psychoses, 195, **199**
Trigeminal neuralgia, 247
Trihexyphenidyl, 276, **277**
    movement disorders, 277
Tri-iodothyronine, 392
*Trileptal*, 256
Trilostane, **432**
    malignant disease, 506
Trimeprazine *see* Alimemazine
Trimethoprim, 320, **321**, 331
    acne, 650
    pneumocystis pneumonia,
        368
    sulfamethoxazole with, *see* Co-
        trimoxazole
Trimipramine, 210, **212**
*Trimopan* (trimethoprim), 321
*Trimovate*, 635
*TriNovum*, 448
*Trintek*, 113
Tripotassium dicitratobismuthate, **47**
*Triptafen* preparations, 211
Triptans *see* 5HT$_1$ agonists, 247, **248**

Triptorelin
  endometriosis, **431**
  prostate cancer, 508, **510**
  uterine fibroids, 430, **431**
*Trisenox*, 481
*Trisequens* preparations, 405
*Tritace*, 107
*Tritamyl*, 904
*Trizivir*, 341
Tropical diseases, advice, 357
Tropicamide, 596, **597**
*Tropium* (chlordiazepoxide), 192
Trospium, 457, **459**, 460
*Trosyl*, 661
*TRUEone*, 390
*TRUETrack* products, 390, 391
*Trufoam* products, 918
*Trusopt*, 601
*Truvada*, 343
Trypanocides, 367
Trypanosomiasis, 367
Tryptophan, 218, **219**
*T-Safe CU 380 A*, 453
*T-SPOT.TB*, 674
*TT 380 Slimline*, 454
Tuberculin, 673, 674
Tuberculosis, 321
  diagnosis, 673
  immunisation
    travel, 695
    vaccines, 673
  prophylaxis, 293
*Tubifast*, 927
*Tubipad*, 926
*Tuinal*, 193
Tulle dressings, 913
Tumour lysis syndrome, 466
*Turbohaler*
  *Bricanyl*, 158
  *Oxis*, 156
  *Pulmicort*, 168
  *Symbicort*, 168
*Turboneb*, 164
Turner's syndrome, 415
*Twinrix* preparations, 677
*Tygacil*, 310
*Tylex*, 236
*Typherix*, 689
*Typhim Vi*, 689
Typhoid
  antibacterial treatment,
    290
  immunisation
    travel, 695
    vaccines, 688, **689**
*TYR* products, 909, 910
Tyrosine kinase inhibitors, 486
Tyrosine supplement, 909, 910
*Tysabri*, 503
*Tyverb*, 489

# U

*Ubretid*, 457
*Ucerax*, 174
*Uftoral*, 479
Ulcerative colitis, 52
Ulcerative gingivitis
  antibacterial treatment, 292, 327
  mouthwashes, 620
Ulcer-healing drugs, 43

Ulcers
  aphthous, 616
  corneal, 591, 593
  duodenal, 43, 45
  gastric, 43, 45
  Hunner's, 461
  mouth, 616
  NSAID-associated, 44
  skin, 667, 668
*Ultec Pro*, 916, 917
*Ultima*, 164
*Ultiva*, 708
*Ultra* bandages, 928, 929
*Ultra* foods
  gluten-free, 904
  low-protein, 905
*Ultra Neb-2000*, 164
*Ultrabase*, 627
*Ultralanum Plain*, 637
*Ultraproct*, 68
Ultrasonic nebulisers, 164
Ultraviolet radiation, 653
Undecenoates, **661**
*Unguentum M*, 627
*Unifine* products, 380
*Unilet* products, 380
*Uniphyllin Continus*, 160
*Uniroid-HC*, 68
*Unisept*, 666
*Unistik* products, 380
Unithiol, 34
*Univer*, 120
*Universal*, 380
Unresectable dermatofibrosarcoma
  protuberans, 487
Uracil, tegafur with, 479
*Urdox*, 69
Urea, 626, 627
  hydrocortisone with, 633
Urea cycle disorders, 556
  essential amino acids
    supplement, 908
Ureteric colic, 460
Urethritis, non-gonococcal, 291, 308
*UrgoCell* products, 916, 921
*Urgosorb* products, 919, 922
*Urgotul* products, 915, 916, 921
*Uriben*, 330
Uricosuric drugs, 581
*Uriflex* preparations, 461
Urinary
  frequency, 457
  incontinence, 457
  infections, 291, 331
  pH adjustment, 460
  retention, 455
Urine tests, 391
*Urispas-200*, 458
*Uristix*, 391
Urofollitrophin *see* Urofollitropin, 413,
  414
Urofollitropin, 413, 414
Urokinase, 138, **140**
  infusion table, 878
Urological procedures
  antibacterial prophylaxis,
    294
*Uro-Tainer* preparations, 461
Urothelial toxicity, 469
Ursodeoxycholic acid, **69**, 70
*Ursofalk*, 70
*Ursogal*, 70
Urticaria, 171
Ustekinumab, 644, **646**
*UT 380 Short*, 454
*UT 380 Standard*, 454

Uterine
  bleeding, 435
  relaxants, 439
  stimulants, 434
*Utinor*, 330
*Utovlan*, 409
*Utrogestan*, 409
UVB, psoriasis, 640
*Uvistat* preparations, 654

# V

*V.A.C.* products, 924
*VISTA* products, 924
Vaccination
  HIV-positive subjects, 670
  schedule, 671
  travel, 695
Vaccines
  active immunity, 669
    breast-feeding, 670
    pregnancy, 670
  allergen extract, 174
  cautions, 669
  contra-indication, 669
  post-immunisation pyrexia, 670
  side-effects, 670
  storage and use, 672
*Vacunet*, 914
*Vacuskin*, 915
*Vacutex*, 919
Vacuum assisted closure products,
  924
*Vagifem*, 441
Vaginitis
  candidal, 441
  herpes simplex, 443
  menopausal, 400, 440
  non-specific *see* Vaginosis, bac-
    terial, 291
  trichomonal, 442
Vaginosis, bacterial, 291
*Vaginyl* (metronidazole), 327
Valaciclovir, 349, **350**, 351
*Valclair* (diazepam), 191
*Valcyte*, 352
*Valdoxan*, 218
Valganciclovir, 351, 352
Valine amino acid supplement, 907
*Vallergan*, 173
*Valni XL*, 119
*Valoid*, 226
*Valpiform* products, 904, 905
Valproate
  epilepsy, 254, **262**, 263
  infusion table, 877
  migraine, 251
Valproic acid
  bipolar disorder, **206**, 207
  epilepsy, 263
Valsartan, 107, **110**
  amlodipine with, 115
  hydrochlorothiazide with, 110
*Valtrex*, 351
*Vamin* preparations, 538
*Vaminolact*, 538
*Vancocin*, 317
Vancomycin, **316**, 317
  eye, 603
  infusion table, 878

Index

Vancomycin-resistant enterococci, 310, 318
*Vaniqa*, 656
*Vantas*, xiii
Vapour-permeable adhesive film, 914
*Vaqta*, 677
Vardenafil, 463, **464**
Varenicline, 280, **283**
Variceal bleeding, 417, 510
Varicella-zoster, 349
    corticosteroids, caution in, 396
    immunisation
        vaccine, **689**, 693
        immunoglobulin, **693**
Varicose veins, 149, 668
*Varilrix*, 689
*Varivax*, 689
*Vascace*, 104
*Vascalpha* (felodipine), 117
Vascular surgery
    antibacterial prophylaxis,
    294
Vasoconstrictors
    local anaesthesia, 714
        dental practice, 714
    sympathomimetic, 124
Vasodilators
    antihypertensive, 95
    peripheral, 121
*Vasogen*, 630
Vasopressin, **417**
    diabetes insipidus, 417
    variceal bleeding, 417
    infusion table, 878
VEC high compression bandage,
    928
*Vectavir*, 662
*Vectibix*, 484
Vecuronium, 709, **711**
    infusion table, 878
*Vegenat-med* preparations, 893
*Veil* preparations, 654
*Velband*, 929
*Velbe*, 480
*Velcade*, 482
*Velosef*, 305
*Venaxx XL*, 220
Venlafaxine, 218, **219**, 220
*Venlalic XL*, 220
*Venofer*, 515
*Venofundin*, 534
*Venta-Neb*, 97
*Ventavis*, 97
Ventilatory failure, 178
*Ventmax SR* (salbutamol), 156
*Ventolin* preparations, 156, 157
*Ventstream*, 164
*Venturi* products, 924
*Vepesid*, 480
*Veracur*, 652
Verapamil, **119**, 120
    angina, 115
    arrhythmias, 82
    beta-blockers and, 119
    cluster headache, 252
    hypertension, 115
    poisoning by, 32
    *see also* Calcium-channel block-
        ers
    trandolapril with, 107
*Verapress MR*, 120
*Vermox*, 370
*Vernaid*, 924
Verrucas, 651
*Verrugon*, 652
*Versatis*, 716

*Versiva* products, 917
*Vertab SR 240*, 120
Verteporfin, 606, **607**
    infusion table, 878
*Vesanoid*, 493
*Vesicare*, 459
Vestibular disorders, 226
*Vexol*, 595
*Vfend*, 339
*Viagra*, 464
*ViATIM*, 678
*Viazem XL*, 117
*Vibramycin* preparations, 309
    capsules—*discontinued*
*Victanyl* (fentanyl), 241
*Vidaza*, 476
*Videne*, 667
*Videx* preparations, 342
Vigabatrin, 263, **264**
*Vigam*, 692
*Vigranon B*, 548
Vildagliptin, 384, **387**
    metformin with, 387
*Vimpat*, 257
Vinblastine, 479, **480**
    infusion table, 878
Vinca alkaloids, 479
Vincent's infection
    antibacterial treatment, 292, 327
    mouthwashes, 620
Vincristine, 479, **480**
    infusion table, 878
Vindesine, 479, **480**
    infusion table, 878
Vinorelbine, 479, **480**
    infusion table, 878
*Vioform-Hydrocortisone—discontinued*
*Viracept*, 345
*ViraferonPeg*, 500
*Viramune*, 347
*Virazole*, 357
*Viread*, 343
*Virgan*, 593
*Viridal Duo*, 463
*Viroflu*, 681
*Virormone* injection, 410
*Virovir* (aciclovir), 350
Virus infections, 339
*Visclair*, 182
*Viscopaste PB7*, 930
*Viscotears*, 603
*Viskaldix*, 92
*Visken*, 92
*Vismed*preparations, 604
*Vistabel*, 279
*Vistamethasone*
    ear, 609
    eye, 594
    nose, 613
*Vistamethasone N*
    ear, 609
    eye, 594
    nose, 615
*Vistide*, 351
*Visudyne*, 607
*Vita Bite*, 905
*Vitajoule*, 898
Vitalograph peak flow meters,
    161
Vitamin A, **547**
    vitamin D and, 547
Vitamin B group, 547, 548
    B and C injection, 548
        infusion table, 879
Vitamin B$_{12}$, 515, 516
Vitamin C *see* Ascorbic acid

Vitamin D, 549
    psoriasis, 639
Vitamin deficiency, 547
Vitamin E, 551
Vitamin K, 551, 552
Vitamins, 547
    children's drops, 547
    multivitamin preparations, 552,
        553
        infusion table, 879
    parenteral nutrition, 539
*Vitapro*, 900
*Vitaquick*, 903
*Vitasavoury*, 901
Vitiligo, 654
    ACBS, 910
*Vitlipid N*, 540
*Vitrex* products, 380
*Vivaglobin*, 692
*Vividrin* (sodium cromoglicate)
    eye, 596
    nose, 614
*Vivotif*, 689
*Volibris*, 96
*Volplex*, 534
*Volsaid* (diclofenac), 564
*Voltarol* preparations, 563, 564
    *Emulgel*, 589
    Gel patch, 589
    *Ophtha*, 605
    *Rapid*, 564
*Volulyte*, 534
*Volumatic*, 162
Volume expansion, 532
*Voluven*, 534
Vomiting, 225
    cytotoxic drugs, 466
    palliative care, 17
    postoperative, 226
    pregnancy, 225
von Willebrand's disease, 418
Voriconazole, 332, 334, **339**
    infusion table, 879
*VSL#3*, 903
Vulvitis, candidal, 441
VZIG *see* Immunoglobulins, varicella–
    zoster, 693

# W

Waldenstrom's macroglobulinaemia,
    469
Warfarin, 130, **131**, 132
*Warticon* preparations, 653
Warts, 651
Wasp sting allergy preparations, 175
Water
    for injections, 532
    potable, 3
*WaveSense* products, 380, 390, 391
*Waxsol*, 611
*Welland* products, 924
*Welldorm*, 189
*Wellfoods* products, 904
*Wellvone*, 369
Wernicke's encephalopathy, 547
West's syndrome, 264
Whooping cough *see* Pertussis
Wilson's disease, 553
*Wilzin*, 554
*WinRho SDF*, 695

Index

Withdrawal
  alcohol, 279
  anxiolytics, 185
  corticosteroids, 396
  hypnotics, 185
  nicotine, 280
  opioids, 283
Wolff-Parkinson-White syndrome, 83
Wool fat, hydrous, 626
*World Traveller HI FLO*, 164
Worm infestation, 369
Wound
  drainage collection devices, 924
  drainage pouches, 923, 924
  dressings, 911
    absorbent, 913
    advanced, 913
    low adherence, 912
*WoundASSIST* products, 924
*Woundcare*, 924
*Wuchereria bancrofti*, 371

## X

*Xagrid*, 524
*Xalacom*, 599
*Xalatan*, 599
*Xamiol*, 641
*Xanax* (alprazolam), 192
Xanthine bronchodilators *see* Theophylline
Xanthine-oxidase inhibitor, 581
*Xarelto*, 133
*Xatral* preparations, 455
*Xeloda*, 477
*Xenazine*, 278
*Xenical*, 224
*Xeomin*, 279
*Xepin*, 630
Xerostomia, 621
  ACBS, 910
*Xerotin*, 622
*Xigris* (drotrecogin alfa (activated)), 141
Xipamide, 75, **76**
*Xismox 60XL* (isosorbide mononitrate), 114
*XLEU* products, 906, 907
*XLYS Low TRY* products, 906
*XLYS* products, 906
*XLYS TRY* products, 906
*XMET* products, 906
*XMTVI* products, 907, 908
*Xolair*, 175
*Xomolix*, 227
*XP LCP* products, 909
*XP* products, 909
*XPHEN TYR* products, 910
*XPTM* products, 910
*Xupad*, 923
Xylitol, presence of, 2
*Xylocaine*, 618, 715, 716

Xylometazoline
  eye, 595
  nose, 614, **615**
*Xyloproct*, 68
*Xyrem*, 190
*Xyzal*, 172

## Y

*8Y* (factor VIII fraction), 141
*Yasmin*, 449
Yeasts, 333
Yellow Card Scheme, 11
  cards, *inside back cover*
Yellow fever
  immunisation
    travel, 695
    vaccine, 689, **690**
*Yentreve*, 458
*Yondelis*, 492
*Yutopar*, 440

## Z

*Zacin*, 589
*Zaditen*, 174, 596
Zafirlukast, 170, **171**
Zaleplon, 187, **188**
*Zamadol* preparations, 245, 246
*Zanaflex*, 586
Zanamivir, 354, **355**, 356
*Zanidip*, 118
*Zantac*, 47
*Zapain* (co-codamol 30/500), 236
*Zaponex*, 202
*Zarontin*, 256
*Zarzio*, xiii
*Zavedos*, 474
*Zavesca*, 557
*ZeaSORB*, 668
*Zeffix*, 342
*Zelapar*, 275
*Zemon* preparations, 114
*Zemplar*, 551
*Zemtard* preparations, 117
*Zenalb* (albumin) preparations, 533
*Zeridame SR*, 246
*Zerit*, 343
*Zerobase*, 627
*Zestoretic* preparations, 106
*Zestril*, 105
*Zetuvit E*, 913
*Ziagen*, 341
*Zibor*, 127
Ziconotide, 233
*Zidoval*, 443
Zidovudine, **343**, 344
  abacavir and lamivudine with, 341
  infusion table, 879
  lamivudine with, 344
*Zimbacol XL* (bezafibrate), 147
*Zimovane*, 188
*Zinacef*, 306

Zinc
  bandages, 930
    calamine and, 930
    ichthammol and, 637, 638, 930
    stocking, 930
  deficiency, **546**
  eye, 603, 604
  skin
    benzyl benzoate with, 630
    castor oil and, 629
    coal tar with, 642
    cod liver oil with, 629
    cream, 629
    dimeticone with, 629, 630
    ichthammol with, 638
    ointment, 629
    salicylic acid with, 643
    tape, adhesive, 925
  Wilson's disease (zinc acetate), **553**, 554
*Zindaclin*, 648
*Zineryt*, 648
*Zinnat*, 306
*Zipzoc*, 930
*Zispin* preparations, 219
*Zithromax*, 314
*Zocor* preparations, 145
*Zofran*, 230
*Zoladex* preparations, 509
  endometriosis, 430
  IVF, 430
Zoledronic acid, **425**, 426
  infusion table, 879
*Zoleptil*, 204
Zollinger-Ellison syndrome, 48
Zolmitriptan, 248, **250**
Zolpidem, 187, **188**
*Zolvera* (verapamil), 120
*Zomacton*, 416
*Zometa*, 426
*Zomig* preparations, 250
*Zomorph*, 243
*Zonegran*, 264
Zonisamide, 254, **264**
Zopiclone, 187, **188**
*Zorac*, 641
Zoster *see* Herpes infections
*Zotepine*, 199, **204**
*Zoton*, 49
*Zovirax* preparations
  cream, 662
  eye ointment, 593
  injection, 350
  tablets, 350
Zuclopenthixol, 195, 206
  depot injections, 205, 206
  injection, 199
  tablets, 199
Zuclopenthixol acetate, **199**
Zuclopenthixol decanoate, **206**
Zuclopenthixol dihydrochloride, **199**
*Zumenon*, 406
*Zuvogen*, 662
*Zyban*, 281
*Zydol* preparations, 245, 246
*Zyloric*, 582
*Zyomet*, 659
*Zyprexa*, 202
*Zyvox*, 319

# Yellowcard

## COMMISSION ON HUMAN MEDICINES

In Confidence

MHRA

## SUSPECTED ADVERSE DRUG REACTIONS

If you suspect that an adverse reaction may be related to a drug, or a combination of drugs, you should complete this Yellow Card or complete a report on the website at www.yellowcard.gov.uk. For *intensively monitored medicines* (identified by ▼) report **all** suspected reactions (including any considered not to be serious). For *established drugs* and *herbal remedies* report **all serious** adverse reactions in adults; report **all serious and minor** adverse reactions in **children** (under 18 years). You do not have to be certain about causality: if in doubt, please report. Do not be put off reporting just because some details are not known. See BNF (page 11) or the MHRA website (www.yellowcard.gov.uk) for additional advice.

| PATIENT DETAILS | Patient Initials: _____ | Sex: M / F | Weight if known (kg): _____ |
|---|---|---|---|
| Age (at time of reaction): _____ | Identification (Your Practice / Hospital Ref.)*: _____ | | |

**SUSPECTED DRUG(S)**

| Give brand name of drug and batch number if known | Route | Dosage | Date started | Date stopped | Prescribed for |
|---|---|---|---|---|---|
| _____ | ___ | ___ | ___ | ___ | |
| _____ | ___ | ___ | ___ | ___ | |

**SUSPECTED REACTION(S)**

**Please describe the reaction(s) and any treatment given:**

Outcome

Recovered ☐
Recovering ☐
Continuing ☐
Other ☐

Date reaction(s) started: _____     Date reaction(s) stopped: _____

Do you consider the reaction to be serious?   Yes / No

If *yes*, please indicate why the reaction is considered to be serious (please tick all that apply):

Patient died due to reaction ☐   Involved or prolonged inpatient hospitalisation ☐
Life threatening ☐   Involved persistent or significant disability or incapacity ☐
Congenital abnormality ☐   Medically significant; please give details: ☐

* This is to enable you to identify the patient in any future correspondence concerning this report

*Please attach additional pages if necessary*

**Please list other drugs taken in the last 3 months prior to the reaction (including self-medication & herbal remedies)**

Was the patient on any other medication?    Yes / No    If yes, please give the following information if known:

| Drug (Brand, if known) | Route | Dosage | Date started | Date stopped | Prescribed for |
|---|---|---|---|---|---|
| | | | | | |
| | | | | | |
| | | | | | |
| | | | | | |
| | | | | | |
| | | | | | / |

**Additional relevant information** e.g. medical history, test results, known allergies, rechallenge (if performed), suspected drug interactions. For congenital abnormalities please state all other drugs taken during pregnancy and the date of the last menstrual period.

**REPORTER DETAILS**
Name and Professional Address:

**CLINICIAN (if not the reporter)**
Name and Professional Address:

Post code: _____    Tel No: _____

Tel No: _____    Post code: _____

Speciality: _____    Speciality: _____

Signature: _____    Date: _____

If you would like information about other adverse reactions associated with the suspected drug, please tick this box ☐

If you report from an area served by a Yellow Card Centre (YCC), MHRA may ask the Centre to communicate with you, on its behalf, about your report. See BNF (page 11) for further details on YCCs. If you want only MHRA to contact you, please tick this box. ☐

Send to **Medicines and Healthcare products Regulatory Agency, CHM FREEPOST, LONDON SW8 5BR**

# Yellowcard®

## COMMISSION ON HUMAN MEDICINES

In Confidence

**MHRA**

## SUSPECTED ADVERSE DRUG REACTIONS

If you suspect that an adverse reaction may be related to a drug, or a combination of drugs, you should complete this Yellow Card or complete a report on the website at www.yellowcard.gov.uk. For *intensively monitored medicines* (identified by ▼) report **all** suspected reactions (including any considered not to be serious). For *established drugs* and *herbal remedies* report **all serious** adverse reactions in adults; report **all serious and minor** adverse reactions in **children** (under 18 years). You do not have to be certain about causality: if in doubt, please report. Do not be put off reporting just because some details are not known. See BNF (page 11) or the MHRA website (www.yellowcard.gov.uk) for additional advice.

---

**PATIENT DETAILS**    Patient Initials: _____    Sex: M / F    Weight if known (kg): _____

Age (at time of reaction): _____    Identification (Your Practice / Hospital Ref.)*: _____

---

**SUSPECTED DRUG(S)**

| Give brand name of drug and batch number if known | Route | Dosage | Date started | Date stopped | Prescribed for |
|---|---|---|---|---|---|
| | | | | | |
| | | | | | |

---

**SUSPECTED REACTION(S)**

**Please describe the reaction(s) and any treatment given:**

| | Outcome | |
|---|---|---|
| | Recovered | ☐ |
| | Recovering | ☐ |
| | Continuing | ☐ |
| | Other | ☐ |

Date reaction(s) started: _____    Date reaction(s) stopped: _____

Do you consider the reaction to be serious?    Yes / No

If *yes*, please indicate why the reaction is considered to be serious (please tick all that apply):

| | |
|---|---|
| Patient died due to reaction ☐ | Involved or prolonged inpatient hospitalisation ☐ |
| Life threatening ☐ | Involved persistent or significant disability or incapacity ☐ |
| Congenital abnormality ☐ | Medically significant; please give details: |

---

\* This is to enable you to identify the patient in any future correspondence concerning this report

*Please attach additional pages if necessary*

**Please list other drugs taken in the last 3 months prior to the reaction (including self-medication & herbal remedies)**

Was the patient on any other medication?   Yes / No   If yes, please give the following information if known:

| Drug (Brand, if known) | Route | Dosage | Date started | Date stopped | Prescribed for |
|---|---|---|---|---|---|
| | | | | | |
| | | | | | |
| | | | | | |
| | | | | | |

**Additional relevant information** e.g. medical history, test results, known allergies, rechallenge (if performed), suspected drug interactions. For congenital abnormalities please state all other drugs taken during pregnancy and the date of the last menstrual period.

**REPORTER DETAILS**
Name and Professional Address: _____

Post code: _____ Tel No: _____
Speciality: _____
Signature: _____   Date: _____

**CLINICIAN (if not the reporter)**
Name and Professional Address: _____

Post code: _____
Tel No: _____   Speciality: _____

If you would like information about other adverse reactions associated with the suspected drug, please tick this box ☐

If you report from an area served by a Yellow Card Centre (YCC), MHRA may ask the Centre to communicate with you, on its behalf, about your report. See BNF (page 11) for further details on YCCs. If you want only MHRA to contact you, please tick this box ☐

Send to **Medicines and Healthcare products Regulatory Agency, CHM FREEPOST, LONDON SW8 5BR**

# Yellowcard

## COMMISSION ON HUMAN MEDICINES

**MHRA**

In Confidence

## SUSPECTED ADVERSE DRUG REACTIONS

If you suspect that an adverse reaction may be related to a drug, or a combination of drugs, you should complete this Yellow Card or complete a report on the website at www.yellowcard.gov.uk. For *intensively monitored medicines* (identified by ▼) report **all** suspected reactions (including any considered not to be serious). For *established drugs* and *herbal remedies* report **all serious** adverse reactions in adults; report **all serious and minor** adverse reactions in **children** (under 18 years). You do not have to be certain about causality: if in doubt, please report. Do not be put off reporting just because some details are not known. See BNF (page 11) or the MHRA website (www.yellowcard.gov.uk) for additional advice.

| PATIENT DETAILS | Patient Initials: _____ | Sex: M / F | Weight if known (kg): _____ |
|---|---|---|---|
| Age (at time of reaction): _____ | Identification (Your Practice / Hospital Ref.)*: _____ | | |

### SUSPECTED DRUG(S)
Give brand name of drug
and batch number if known

| | Route | Dosage | Date started | Date stopped | Prescribed for |
|---|---|---|---|---|---|

### SUSPECTED REACTION(S)
**Please describe the reaction(s) and any treatment given:**

Outcome

Recovered ☐
Recovering ☐
Continuing ☐
Other ☐

Date reaction(s) started: _____        Date reaction(s) stopped: _____

Do you consider the reaction to be serious?    Yes / No

If *yes*, please indicate why the reaction is considered to be serious (please tick all that apply):

Patient died due to reaction ☐          Involved or prolonged inpatient hospitalisation ☐

Life threatening ☐          Involved persistent or significant disability or incapacity ☐

Congenital abnormality ☐          Medically significant; please give details:

\* This is to enable you to identify the patient in any future correspondence concerning this report

*Please attach additional pages if necessary*

**Please list other drugs taken in the last 3 months prior to the reaction (including self-medication & herbal remedies)**

Was the patient on any other medication?    Yes / No    If yes, please give the following information if known:

| Drug (Brand, if known) | Route | Dosage | Date started | Date stopped | Prescribed for |
|---|---|---|---|---|---|
| | | | | | |
| | | | | | |
| | | | | | |
| | | | | | |

**Additional relevant information** e.g. medical history, test results, known allergies, rechallenge (if performed), suspected drug interactions. For congenital abnormalities please state all other drugs taken during pregnancy and the date of the last menstrual period.

**REPORTER DETAILS**
Name and Professional Address:

Post code: _____ Tel No: _____
Speciality: _____
Signature: _____ Date: _____

**CLINICIAN (if not the reporter)**
Name and Professional Address:

Post code: _____
Tel No: _____ Speciality: _____

If you would like information about other adverse reactions associated with the suspected drug, please tick this box ☐

If you report from an area served by a Yellow Card Centre (YCC), MHRA may ask the Centre to communicate with you, on its behalf, about your report. See BNF (page 11) for further details on YCCs. If you want only MHRA to contact you, please tick this box. ☐

Send to **Medicines and Healthcare products Regulatory Agency, CHM FREEPOST, LONDON SW8 5BR**

# Yellowcard

**COMMISSION ON HUMAN MEDICINES**

In Confidence

**SUSPECTED ADVERSE DRUG REACTIONS**

MHRA

If you suspect that an adverse reaction may be related to a drug, or a combination of drugs, you should complete this Yellow Card or complete a report on the website at www.yellowcard.gov.uk. For *intensively monitored medicines* (identified by ▼) report **all** suspected reactions (including any considered not to be serious). For *established drugs* and *herbal remedies* report **all serious** adverse reactions in adults; report **all serious and minor** adverse reactions in **children** (under 18 years). You do not have to be certain about causality: if in doubt, please report. Do not be put off reporting just because some details are not known. See BNF (page 11) or the MHRA website (www.yellowcard.gov.uk) for additional advice.

| PATIENT DETAILS | Patient Initials: | Sex: M / F | Weight if known (kg): |
|---|---|---|---|
| Age (at time of reaction): | Identification (Your Practice / Hospital Ref.)*: | | |

**SUSPECTED DRUG(S)**

| Give brand name of drug and batch number if known | Route | Dosage | Date started | Date stopped | Prescribed for |
|---|---|---|---|---|---|

**SUSPECTED REACTION(S)**

**Please describe the reaction(s) and any treatment given:**

| | Outcome | |
|---|---|---|
| | Recovered | ☐ |
| | Recovering | ☐ |
| | Continuing | ☐ |
| | Other | ☐ |

Date reaction(s) started: Date reaction(s) stopped:

Do you consider the reaction to be serious? Yes / No

If *yes*, please indicate why the reaction is considered to be serious (please tick all that apply):

| | |
|---|---|
| Patient died due to reaction ☐ | Involved or prolonged inpatient hospitalisation ☐ |
| Life threatening ☐ | Involved persistent or significant disability or incapacity ☐ |
| Congenital abnormality ☐ | Medically significant; please give details: |

\* This is to enable you to identify the patient in any future correspondence concerning this report

*Please attach additional pages if necessary*

**Please list other drugs taken in the last 3 months prior to the reaction (including self-medication & herbal remedies)**

Was the patient on any other medication?  Yes / No   If yes, please give the following information if known:

| Drug (Brand, if known) | Route | Dosage | Date started | Date stopped | Prescribed for |
|---|---|---|---|---|---|
| —— | —— | —— | —— | —— | —— |
| —— | —— | —— | —— | —— | —— |
| —— | —— | —— | —— | —— | —— |
| —— | —— | —— | —— | —— | —— |

**Additional relevant information** e.g. medical history, test results, known allergies, rechallenge (if performed), suspected drug interactions. For congenital abnormalities please state all other drugs taken during pregnancy and the date of the last menstrual period.

**REPORTER DETAILS**
Name and Professional Address:

————————————

Post code: ————  Tel No: ————
Speciality: ————
Signature: ————  Date: ————

**CLINICIAN (if not the reporter)**
Name and Professional Address:

————————————

Post code: ————
Tel No: ————  Speciality: ————

If you would like information about other adverse reactions associated with the suspected drug, please tick this box ☐

If you report from an area served by a Yellow Card Centre (YCC), MHRA may ask the Centre to communicate with you, on its behalf, about your report. See BNF (page 11) for further details on YCCs. If you want only MHRA to contact you, please tick this box. ☐

Send to **Medicines and Healthcare products Regulatory Agency, CHM FREEPOST, LONDON SW8 5BR**

# Cardiovascular Risk Prediction Charts

Heart 2005; **91**(Suppl V): v1–v52

## How to use the Cardiovascular Risk Prediction Charts for Primary Prevention

These charts are for estimating cardiovascular disease (CVD) risk (non-fatal myocardial infarction and stroke, coronary and stroke death and new angina pectoris) for individuals who have **not** already developed coronary heart disease (CHD) or other major atherosclerotic disease. They are an aid to making clinical decisions about how intensively to intervene on lifestyle and whether to use antihypertensive, lipid lowering and anti-platelet medication, but should **not replace clinical judgment**.

- The use of these charts is **not appropriate** for patients who have existing diseases which already put them at high risk such as:

  - coronary heart disease or other major atherosclerotic disease;

  - familial hypercholesterolaemia or other inherited dyslipidaemias;

  - renal dysfunction including diabetic nephropathy;

  - type 1 and 2 diabetes mellitus.

- The charts should **not** be used to decide whether to introduce antihypertensive medication when blood pressure is persistently at or above 160/100 mmHg or when target organ damage due to hypertension is present. In both cases antihypertensive medication is recommended regardless of CVD risk. Similarly the charts should **not** be used to decide whether to introduce lipid-lowering medication when the ratio of serum total to HDL cholesterol exceeds 6. Such medication is generally then indicated regardless of estimated CVD risk.

- To estimate an individual's absolute 10-year risk of developing CVD choose the chart for his or her sex, lifetime smoking status and age. Within this square identify the level of risk according to the point where the coordinates for systolic blood pressure and the ratio of total cholesterol to high density lipoprotein (HDL) cholesterol meet. If no HDL cholesterol result is available, then assume this is 1.0 mmol/litre and the lipid scale can be used for total cholesterol alone.

- Higher risk individuals (red areas) are defined as those whose 10-year CVD risk exceeds 20%, which is approximately equivalent to the coronary heart disease risk of > 15% over the same period.

- The chart also assists in identifying individuals whose 10-year CVD risk is moderately increased in the range 10–20% (orange areas) and those in whom risk is lower than 10% over 10 years (green areas).

- Smoking status should reflect lifetime exposure to tobacco and not simply tobacco use at the time of assessment. For example, those who have given up smoking within 5 years should be regarded as current smokers for the purposes of the charts.

- The initial blood pressure and the first random (non-fasting) total cholesterol and HDL cholesterol can be used to estimate an individual's risk. However, the decision on using drug therapy should generally be based on repeat risk factor measurements over a period of time.

(Continued over)

- Men and women do not reach the level of risk predicted by the charts for the three age bands until they reach the ages 49, 59, and 69 years respectively. The charts will overestimate current risk most in the under 40s. Clinical judgement must be exercised in deciding on treatment in younger patients. However, it should be recognised that blood pressure and cholesterol tend to rise most and HDL cholesterol to decline most in younger people already with adverse levels. Left untreated, their risk at the age 49 years is likely to be higher than the projected risk shown on the age-under-50-years chart. From age 70 years the CVD risk, especially for men, is usually ≥ 20% over 10 years and the charts will underestimate true total CVD risk.

- These charts (and all other currently available methods of CVD risk prediction) are based on groups of people with **untreated** levels of blood pressure, total cholesterol and HDL cholesterol. In patients already receiving antihypertensive therapy in whom the decision is to be made about whether to introduce lipid-lowering medication, or vice versa, the charts can only act as a guide. Unless recent pre-treatment risk factor values are available it is generally safest to assume that CVD risk is higher than that predicted by current levels of blood pressure or lipids on treatment.

- CVD risk is also higher than indicated in the charts for:
  - those with a family history of premature CVD (male first-degree relatives aged < 55 years and female first-degree relatives aged < 65 years) which increases the risk by a factor of approximately 1.5;
  - men with HDL cholesterol < 1 mmol/litre or women with HDL cholesterol < 1.2 mmol/litre;
  - those with raised triglyceride levels (> 1.7 mmol/litre);
  - those with BMI ≥ 30 kg/m²;
  - women with premature menopause;
  - those who are not yet diabetic, but have impaired fasting glycaemia (6.1–6.9 mmol/litre) or impaired glucose tolerance (2 hour glucose ≥ 7.8 mmol/litre but < 11.1 mmol/litre in an oral glucose tolerance test).

- The charts have not been validated in ethnic minorities and in some may underestimate CVD risk. For example, in people originating from the Indian subcontinent it is safest to assume that the CVD risk is higher than predicted from the charts (1.4 times).

- An individual can be shown on the chart the direction in which his or her risk of CVD can be reduced by changing smoking status, blood pressure, or cholesterol, but it should be borne in mind that the estimate of risk is for a group of people with similar risk factors and that within that group there will be considerable variation in risk. It should also be pointed out in younger people that the estimated risk will generally not be reached before the age of 50, if their current blood pressure and lipid levels remain unchanged. The charts are primarily to assist in directing intervention to those who typically stand to benefit most.

---

The estimation of CVD risk in NICE clinical guideline 67 (May 2008): *Lipid modification–Cardiovascular risk assessment and the modification of blood lipids for the primary and secondary prevention of cardiovascular disease* (available at www.nice.org.uk) differs from that shown here as follows:
- estimated CVD risk increases by a factor of 1.5 in those with a family history of premature CHD (male first-degree relatives aged < 55 years and female first-degree relatives aged < 65 years)
- estimated CVD risk increases by a factor of 1.5–2 if more than one first-degree relative has a history of premature CHD
- estimated CVD risk for South Asian <u>men</u> is increased by a factor of 1.4
- CVD risk is higher than estimated in those with BMI > 40 kg/m²

The NICE guideline does not include the recommendation to treat all patients with a serum total to HDL cholesterol ratio of greater than 6 with lipid-lowering drugs.

The NICE guideline advises that the following factor is also taken into account when calculating CVD risk:
- presence of left ventricular hypertrophy

In addition, NICE advises that all patients over the age of 75 years should be considered at increased risk of CVD, and are likely to benefit from treatment.

(Continued over)

# Nondiabetic Men

## Non-smoker  Smoker

### Age under 50 years

### Age 50–59 years

### Age 60 years and over

SBP = systolic blood pressure mmHg

TC : HDL = serum total cholesterol to HDL cholesterol ratio

CVD risk <10% over next 10 years

CVD risk 10-20% over next 10 years

CVD risk >20% over next 10 years

CVD risk over next 10 years

30%

10% 20%

(Continued over)

# Nondiabetic Women

## Non-smoker  Smoker

### Age under 50 years

### Age 50–59 years

### Age 60 years and over

CVD risk <10% over next 10 years
CVD risk 10-20% over next 10 years
CVD risk >20% over next 10 years

CVD risk over
next 10 years
30%
10%  20%

SBP = systolic blood pressure mmHg
TC : HDL = serum total cholesterol to
HDL cholesterol ratio

© Central Manchester and Manchester
Children's University Hospitals NHS Trust

# ADULT ADVANCED LIFE SUPPORT ALGORITHM

**Unresponsive?**

**Open airway. Look for signs of life**

→ **Call Resuscitation Team**

**CPR 30:2**
Until defibrillator/monitor attached

**Assess rhythm**

| **Shockable**<br>(VF/pulseless VT) | ↔ | **Non-shockable**<br>(PEA/Asystole) |

**1 Shock**
150-360 J biphasic
or 360 J monophasic

**Immediately resume CPR 30:2 for 2 min**

### During CPR

- Correct reversible causes*
- Check electrode position and contact
- Attempt/verify: IV access, airway, and oxygen
- Give uninterrupted compressions when airway secure
- Give adrenaline every 3-5 min
- Consider: amiodarone, atropine, magnesium

**Immediately resume CPR 30:2 for 2 min**

---

**\*Reversible causes**

| | |
|---|---|
| Hypoxia | Tension pneumothorax |
| Hypovolaemia | Tamponade, cardiac |
| Hypo/hyperkalaemia/metabolic | Toxins |
| Hypothermia | Thrombosis (coronary or pulmonary) |

European Resuscitation Council

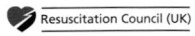

Resuscitation Council (UK)

Reprinted from *Resuscitation*, **67**(Suppl. 1): S45, © 2005, with permission from the European Resuscitation Council and Elsevier Ireland Ltd

# Medical emergencies in the community

**Drug treatment outlined below is intended for use by community healthcare professionals.** Only drugs that are used for immediate relief are shown; advice on supporting care is not given. Where the patient's condition requires investigation and further treatment, the patient should be transferred to hospital promptly.

## Anaphylaxis
(section 3.4.3)

**Adrenaline** injection 1 mg/mL (1 in 1000)

- By intramuscular injection
  CHILD UNDER 6 YEARS 150 micrograms (0.15 mL), repeated every 5 minutes if necessary
  CHILD 6–12 YEARS 300 micrograms (0.3 mL), repeated every 5 minutes if necessary
  CHILD 12–18 YEARS 500 micrograms (0.5 mL), repeated every 5 minutes if necessary; 300 micrograms (0.3 mL) if CHILD is small or prepubertal
  ADULT 500 micrograms (0.5 mL), repeated every 5 minutes if necessary

**Chlorphenamine** injection 10 mg/mL

- By intravenous injection over 1 minute or by intramuscular injection
  CHILD UNDER 6 MONTHS 250 micrograms/kg (max. 2.5 mg), repeated if required up to 4 times in 24 hours
  CHILD 6 MONTHS–6 YEARS 2.5 mg, repeated if required up to 4 times in 24 hours
  CHILD 6–12 YEARS 5 mg, repeated if required up to 4 times in 24 hours
  CHILD 12–18 YEARS 10 mg, repeated if required up to 4 times in 24 hours
  ADULT 10 mg, repeated if required up to 4 times in 24 hours

High-flow **oxygen** (section 3.6) and **intravenous fluids** should be given if required.

**Hydrocortisone** (preferably as sodium succinate) by intravenous injection (section 6.3.2) has delayed action but should be given to severely affected patients to prevent further deterioration.

## Angina: unstable
(section 2.6)

**Aspirin** dispersible tablets 75 mg, 300 mg

- By mouth (dispersed in water or chewed)
  ADULT 300 mg

*Plus*

*either* **Glyceryl trinitrate** aerosol spray 400 micrograms/metered dose

- Sublingually
  ADULT 1–2 sprays, repeated as required

*or* **Glyceryl trinitrate** tablets 300 micrograms, 500 micrograms, 600 micrograms

- Sublingually
  ADULT 0.3–1 mg, repeated as required

## Asthma: acute
(section 3.1)

Regard each emergency consultation as being for **severe acute asthma** until shown otherwise; failure to respond adequately **at any time** requires immediate transfer to hospital

*Either* **salbutamol** aerosol inhaler 100 micrograms metered inhalation

- By aerosol inhalation via large-volume spacer (and a close-fitting face mask if child under 3 years)
  ADULT and CHILD 4–10 puffs each inhaled separately repeated every 10–20 minutes or as necessary

*or* **salbutamol** nebuliser solution 1 mg/mL, 2 mg/mL

- By inhalation of nebulised solution (via oxygen-driven nebuliser if available)
  CHILD UNDER 5 YEARS 2.5 mg every 10–20 minutes or as necessary
  CHILD 5–12 YEARS 2.5–5 mg every 10–20 minutes or as necessary
  ADULT 2.5–5 mg every 10–20 minutes or as necessary

*or* **terbutaline** nebuliser solution 2.5 mg /mL

- By inhalation of nebulised solution (via oxygen-driven nebuliser if available)
  CHILD UNDER 5 YEARS 5 mg every 10–20 minutes or as necessary
  CHILD 5–12 YEARS 5–10 mg every 10–20 minutes or as necessary
  ADULT 10 mg every 10–20 minutes or as necessary

*Plus* (in all cases)

*either* **prednisolone** soluble tablets 5 mg

- By mouth
  CHILD UNDER 12 YEARS 1–2 mg/kg (max. 40 mg) once daily for 3–5 days; if child has been taking an oral corticosteroid for more than a few days, give prednisolone 2 mg/kg (CHILD UNDER 2 YEARS max. 40 mg, OVER 2 YEARS max. 50 mg) once daily
  ADULT 40–50 mg once daily for 5 days

*or* **hydrocortisone** (preferably as sodium succinate)

- By intravenous injection
  CHILD UNDER 12 YEARS 4 mg/kg every 6 hours until conversion to oral prednisolone is possible; CHILD UNDER 2 YEARS max. 25 mg, 2–5 YEARS max. 50 mg, 5–12 YEARS max. 100 mg
  ADULT 100 mg every 6 hours until conversion to oral prednisolone is possible

High-flow **oxygen** (section 3.6) if available (via face mask in children)

Monitor response 15 to 30 minutes after nebulisation; if any signs of acute asthma persist, arrange hospital admission. While awaiting ambulance, repeat **nebulised beta₂ agonist** (as above) and give with

**ipratropium** nebuliser solution 250 micrograms/mL

- By inhalation of nebulised solution (via oxygen-driven nebuliser if available)
  CHILD UNDER 12 YEARS 250 micrograms, repeated as necessary
  ADULT 500 micrograms, repeated as necessary

roup
ection 3.1)

**examethasone** oral solution 2 mg/5 mL

By mouth
CHILD 1 MONTH–2 YEARS 150 micrograms/kg as a single dose

## onvulsions
**section 4.8.2)**

*ither* **diazepam** rectal solution 2 mg/mL, 4 mg/mL

By rectum, repeated once after 10–15 minutes if necessary
NEONATE 1.25–2.5 mg
CHILD 1 MONTH–2 YEARS 5 mg
CHILD 2–12 YEARS 5–10 mg
CHILD 12–18 YEARS 10 mg
ADULT 10–20 mg (max. 30 mg), (ELDERLY 10 mg, max. 15 mg)

*r* **midazolam** buccal liquid 10 mg/mL or injection olution given by buccal route

By buccal administration, repeated once if necessary
NEONATE 300 micrograms/kg
CHILD 1–6 MONTHS 300 micrograms/kg (max. 2.5 mg)
CHILD 6 MONTHS–1 YEAR 2.5 mg
CHILD 1–5 YEARS 5 mg
CHILD 5–10 YEARS 7.5 mg
CHILD 10–18 YEARS 10 mg
ADULT 10 mg

## iabetic hypoglycaemia
**section 6.1.4)**

**lucose** or **sucrose**

By mouth
CHILD 2–18 YEARS approx. 10–20 g (2–4 teaspoonfuls of sugar *or* 3–6 sugar lumps *or*
55–110 mL *Lucozade*® *Energy Original or* 100–200 mL *Coca-Cola*®—both non-diet versions *or* *GlucoGel*® one or two 25-g tubes (containing glucose 10 g/25-g tube) *or Dextrogel*® one or two 25-g tubes (containing glucose 10-g/25-g tube)) repeated after 10–15 minutes if necessary
ADULT approx. 10–20 g (2–4 teaspoonfuls of sugar *or* 3–6 sugar lumps *or*
55–110 mL *Lucozade*® *Energy Original or* 100–200 mL *Coca-Cola*®—both non-diet versions *or* *GlucoGel*® one or two 25-g tubes (containing glucose 10 g/25-g tube) *or Dextrogel*® one or two 25-g tubes (containing glucose 10-g/25-g tube)) repeated after 10–15 minutes if necessary

*r* if hypoglycaemia unresponsive *or* if oral route cannot be used

**Glucagon** injection 1 mg/mL

By subcutaneous, intramuscular, or intravenous injection
CHILD BODY-WEIGHT UNDER 25 KG 500 micrograms (0.5 mL)
CHILD BODY-WEIGHT OVER 25 KG 1 mg (1 mL)
ADULT 1 mg (1 mL)

*or* if hypoglycaemia prolonged *or* unresponsive to glucagon after 10 minutes

**Glucose** intravenous infusion 10%

- By intravenous injection into large vein
CHILD 1 MONTH–18 YEARS 5 mL/kg (glucose 500 mg/kg)

**Glucose** intravenous infusion 20%

- By intravenous injection into large vein
ADULT 50 mL

## Febrile convulsions lasting longer than 15 minutes
(section 4.8.3)

**Diazepam** rectal solution 2 mg/mL, 4 mg/mL

- By rectum, repeated once after 10–15 minutes if necessary
NEONATE 1.25–2.5 mg
CHILD 1 MONTH–2 YEARS 5 mg
CHILD 2–12 YEARS 5–10 mg
CHILD 12–18 YEARS 10 mg

## Meningococcal disease
(Table 1, section 5.1)

**Benzylpenicillin sodium** injection 600 mg, 1.2 g

- By intravenous injection (or by intramuscular injection if venous access not available)
NEONATE 300 mg
CHILD 1 MONTH–1 YEAR 300 mg
CHILD 1–10 YEARS 600 mg
CHILD 10–18 YEARS 1.2 g
ADULT 1.2 g
Note Give single dose and transfer urgently to hospital

*or* if history of allergy to penicillin

**Cefotaxime** injection 1 g

- By intravenous injection (or by intramuscular injection if venous access not available)
NEONATE 50 mg/kg
CHILD 1 MONTH–12 YEARS 50 mg/kg (max. 1 g)
CHILD 12–18 YEARS 1 g
ADULT 1 g
Note Give single dose and transfer urgently to hospital

*or* if history of immediate hypersensitivity reaction (including anaphylaxis, angioedema, or urticarial reaction) to penicillin or to cephalosporins

**Chloramphenicol** injection 1 g

- By intravenous injection
CHILD 1 MONTH–18 YEARS 12.5–25 mg/kg
ADULT 12.5–25 mg/kg
Note Give single dose and transfer urgently to hospital

## Myocardial infarction
(section 2.10.1)

**Aspirin** dispersible tablets 75 mg, 300 mg

- By mouth (dispersed in water or chewed)
  ADULT 300 mg

**Glyceryl trinitrate** aerosol spray 400 micrograms/metered dose

- Sublingually
  ADULT 1–2 sprays, repeated as required

*or* **Glyceryl trinitrate** tablets 300 micrograms, 500 micrograms, 600 micrograms

- Sublingually
  ADULT 0.3–1 mg, repeated as required

**Metoclopramide** injection 5 mg/mL

- By intravenous injection
  ADULT (UNDER 60 KG) 18–19 YEARS 5 mg
  ADULT (OVER 60 KG) 18–19 YEARS 10 mg
  ADULT OVER 19 YEARS 10 mg

**Diamorphine** injection (5 mg powder for reconstitution)

- By slow intravenous injection (1–2 mg/minute)
  ADULT 5 mg followed by a further 2.5–5 mg if necessary; ELDERLY or FRAIL patients, reduce dose by half

**Oxygen**, if appropriate


## Pneumonia: uncomplicated
(Table 1, section 5.1)

**Amoxicillin** oral suspension 125 mg/5 mL, 250 mg/5 mL; capsules 250 mg

- By mouth
  CHILD 6 MONTHS–1 YEAR 125 mg 3 times daily
  CHILD 1–5 YEARS 250 mg 3 times daily
  CHILD 5–18 YEARS 500 mg 3 times daily
  ADULT 0.5–1 g 3 times daily

*or* if allergic to penicillin *or* atypical organism suspected

**Erythromycin** oral suspension 125 mg/5 mL, 250 mg/5 mL; tablets 250 mg

- By mouth
  CHILD 6 MONTHS–2 YEARS 125 mg 4 times daily
  CHILD 2–8 YEARS 250 mg 4 times daily
  CHILD 8–18 YEARS 250–500 mg 4 times daily
  ADULT 500 mg 4 times daily

## Approximate conversions and units

| lb | kg | stones | kg | mL | fl oz |
|----|------|--------|-------|------|-------|
| 1 | 0.45 | 1 | 6.35 | 50 | 1.8 |
| 2 | 0.91 | 2 | 12.70 | 100 | 3.5 |
| 3 | 1.36 | 3 | 19.05 | 150 | 5.3 |
| 4 | 1.81 | 4 | 25.40 | 200 | 7.0 |
| 5 | 2.27 | 5 | 31.75 | 500 | 17.6 |
| 6 | 2.72 | 6 | 38.10 | 1000 | 35.2 |
| 7 | 3.18 | 7 | 44.45 | | |
| 8 | 3.63 | 8 | 50.80 | | |
| 9 | 4.08 | 9 | 57.15 | | |
| 10 | 4.54 | 10 | 63.50 | | |
| 11 | 4.99 | 11 | 69.85 | | |
| 12 | 5.44 | 12 | 76.20 | | |
| 13 | 5.90 | 13 | 82.55 | | |
| 14 | 6.35 | 14 | 88.90 | | |
| | | 15 | 95.25 | | |

## Length

| | | |
|---|---|---|
| 1 metre (m) | | = 1000 millimetres (mm) |
| 1 centimetre (cm) | | = 10 mm |
| 1 inch (in) | | = 25.4 mm |
| 1 foot (ft) | =12 inches | = 304.8 mm |

## Mass

| | |
|---|---|
| 1 kilogram (kg) | = 1000 grams (g) |
| 1 gram (g) | = 1000 milligrams (mg) |
| 1 milligram (mg) | = 1000 micrograms |
| 1 microgram | = 1000 nanograms |
| 1 nanogram | = 1000 picograms |

## Volume

| | |
|---|---|
| 1 litre | − 1000 millilitres (mL) |
| 1 millilitre (1 mL) | = 1000 microlitres |
| 1 pint | ≈ 568 mL |

## Other units

| | |
|---|---|
| 1 kilocalorie (kcal) | = 4186.8 joules (J) |
| 1000 kilocalories (kcal) | = 4.1868 megajoules (MJ) |
| 1 megajoule (MJ) | = 238.8 kilocalories (kcal) |
| 1 millimetre of mercury (mmHg) | = 133.3 pascals (Pa) |
| 1 kilopascal (kPa) | = 7.5 mmHg (pressure) |

**Plasma-drug concentrations** in the BNF are expressed in mass units per litre (e.g. mg/litre). The approximate equivalent in terms of amount of substance units (e.g. micromol/litre) is given in brackets.

## Prescribing for children

### Weight, height, and gender

The table below shows the **mean values** for weight, height, and gender by age; these values have been derived from the UK-WHO growth charts 2009 and UK1990 standard centile charts, by extrapolating the 50th centile, and may be used to calculate doses in the absence of measurements. However, an individual's weight and height might vary considerably from the values in the table and it is important to ensure that the value chosen is appropriate. In most cases the actual measurement should be obtained as soon as possible and the dose re-calculated.

| Age | Weight | Height |
|-----|--------|--------|
| | kg | cm |
| Full-term neonate | 3.5 | 51 |
| 1 month | 4.3 | 55 |
| 2 months | 5.4 | 58 |
| 3 months | 6.1 | 61 |
| 4 months | 6.7 | 63 |
| 6 months | 7.6 | 67 |
| 1 year | 9 | 75 |
| 3 years | 14 | 96 |
| 5 years | 18 | 109 |
| 7 years | 23 | 122 |
| 10 years | 32 | 138 |
| 12 years | 39 | 149 |
| 14 year-old boy | 49 | 163 |
| 14 year-old girl | 50 | 159 |
| Adult male | 68 | 176 |
| Adult female | 58 | 164 |

## Recommended wording of cautionary and advisory labels

For details see Appendix 9

1 Warning. May cause drowsiness

2 Warning. May cause drowsiness. If affected do not drive or operate machinery. Avoid alcoholic drink

3 Warning. May cause drowsiness. If affected do not drive or operate machinery

4 Warning. Avoid alcoholic drink

5 Do not take indigestion remedies at the same time of day as this medicine

6 Do not take indigestion remedies or medicines containing iron or zinc at the same time of day as this medicine

7 Do not take milk, indigestion remedies, or medicines containing iron or zinc at the same time of day as this medicine

8 Do not stop taking this medicine except on your doctor's advice

9 Take at regular intervals. Complete the prescribed course unless otherwise directed

10 Warning. Follow the printed instructions you have been given with this medicine

11 Avoid exposure of skin to direct sunlight or sun lamps

12 Do not take anything containing aspirin while taking this medicine

13 Dissolve or mix with water before taking

14 This medicine may colour the urine

15 Caution flammable: keep away from fire or flames

16 Allow to dissolve under the tongue. Do not transfer from this container. Keep tightly closed. Discard 8 weeks after opening

17 Do not take more than ... in 24 hours

18 Do not take more than ... in 24 hours or ... in any one week

19 Warning. Causes drowsiness which may continue the next day. If affected do not drive or operate machinery. Avoid alcoholic drink

21 ... with or after food

22 ... half to one hour before food

23 ... an hour before food or on an empty stomach

24 ... sucked or chewed

25 ... swallowed whole, not chewed

26 ... dissolved under the tongue

27 ... with plenty of water

28 To be spread thinly ...

29 Do not take more than 2 at any one time. Do not take more than 8 in 24 hours

30 Do not take with any other paracetamol products

31 Contains aspirin and paracetamol. Do not take with any other paracetamol products

Contains aspirin

Contains an aspirin-like medicine